Newman and Carranza's
Clinical
Periodontology

Newman and Carranza's
Clinical Periodontology

THIRTEENTH EDITION

MICHAEL G. NEWMAN, DDS, FACD
Professor Emeritus
Section of Periodontics
School of Dentistry
University of California, Los Angeles
Los Angeles, California

HENRY H. TAKEI, DDS, MS, FACD
Distinguished Clinical Professor
Sections of Periodontics
School of Dentistry
University of California, Los Angeles
Los Angeles, California

PERRY R. KLOKKEVOLD, DDS, MS, FACD
Associate Professor
Program Director, Periodontics Residency
Section of Periodontics
School of Dentistry
University of California, Los Angeles
Los Angeles, California

Editor Emeritus
FERMIN A. CARRANZA, DR ODONT, FACD
Professor Emeritus
Section of Periodontics
School of Dentistry
University of California, Los Angeles
Los Angeles, California

ELSEVIER

ELSEVIER

1600 John F. Kennedy Blvd.
Ste 1800
Philadelphia, PA 19103-2899

NEWMAN AND CARRANZA'S CLINICAL PERIODONTOLOGY   ISBN: 978-0-323-52300-4
THIRTEENTH EDITION

Previous editions copyrighted 2015, 2012, 2006 by Saunders, an imprint of Elsevier Inc.

Library of Congress Control Number: 2018944001

Content Strategist: Alexandra Mortimer
Senior Content Development Manager: Lucia Gunzel
Publishing Services Manager: Catherine Albright Jackson
Senior Project Manager: Doug Turner
Designer: Brian Salisbury

Printed in India

Last digit is the print number: 9 8 7 6 5 4 3

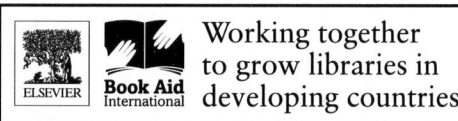

EDITORS

Associate and Section Editors

Fermin A. Carranza, DR ODONT, FACD
Professor Emeritus
Section of Periodontics
School of Dentistry
University of California, Los Angeles
Los Angeles, California

Satheesh Elangovan, BDS, DSc, DMSc
Professor
Department of Periodontics
University of Iowa College of Dentistry and Dental Clinics
Iowa City, Iowa

Marcelo Freire, DDS, PhD, DMSc
Associate Professor
Department of Genomic Medicine and Infectious Disease
J. Craig Venter Institute
La Jolla, California

Søren Jepsen, DDS, MD, MS, PhD
Professor and Chairman
Department of Periodontology
Operative and Preventative Dentistry
University of Bonn, Germany

Perry R. Klokkevold, DDS, MS, FACD
Associate Professor
Program Director, Periodontics Residency
Section of Periodontics
School of Dentistry
University of California, Los Angeles
Los Angeles, California

Michael G. Newman, DDS, FACD
Professor Emeritus
Section of Periodontics
School of Dentistry
University of California, Los Angeles
Los Angeles, California

Philip Preshaw, BDS, FDS RCSEd, FDS (Rest Dent) RCSEd, PhD
Professor of Periodontology
Institute of Cellular Medicine
School of Dental Sciences
Newcastle University
Newcastle upon Tyne, United Kingdom

Henry H. Takei, DDS, MS, FACD
Distinguished Clinical Professor
Section of Periodontics
School of Dentistry
University of California, Los Angeles
Los Angeles, California

Wim Teughels, DDS, PhD
Professor
Periodontology Section
University Hospitals Leuven
Department of Oral Health Services
KU Leuven
Leuven, Belgium

Online Editors

Satheesh Elangovan, BDS, DSc, DMSc
Professor
Department of Periodontics
University of Iowa College of Dentistry and Dental Clinics
Iowa City, Iowa

Michael G. Newman, DDS, FACD
Professor Emeritus
Section of Periodontics
School of Dentistry
University of California, Los Angeles
Los Angeles, California

v

CONTRIBUTORS

Alfredo Aguirre, DDS, MS
Professor
Department of Oral Diagnostic Sciences
School of Dental Medicine
University at Buffalo
The State University of New York
Buffalo, New York

Edward P. Allen, DD, PhD
Private Practice
Dallas, Texas

Robert R. Azzi, DDS
Department of Periodontology
University of Paris, VII
Paris, France

Janet G. Bauer, DDS
Advanced Education Services
Center for Dental Research
Loma Linda University School of Dentistry
Loma Linda, California
Professor Emerita
School of Dentistry
University of California, Los Angeles
Los Angeles, California

Mitchell J. Bloom, DMD
Clinical Associate Professor
Ashman Department of Periodontology and Implant Dentistry
New York University College of Dentistry
Private Practice
Periodontology and Implant Dentistry
New York, New York

Jaime Bulkacz, DR ODONT, PhD
Lecturer
Section of Periodontics
School of Dentistry
University of California, Los Angeles
Los Angeles, California

Bobby Butler, BS, DDS
Affiliate Faculty, Periodontics
School of Dentistry
University of Washington
Seattle, Washington

Paulo M. Camargo, DDS, MS, MBA, FACD
Professor and Tarrson Family Endowed Chair in Periodontics
Section of Periodontics
School of Dentistry
University of California, Los Angeles
Los Angeles, California

Fermin A. Carranza, DR ODONT, FACD
Professor Emeritus
Section of Periodontics
School of Dentistry
University of California, Los Angeles
Los Angeles, California

Ana B. Castro, DDS, MSc
Periodontology Section
University Hospitals Leuven
Department of Oral Health Services
KU Leuven
Leuven, Belgium

Frank Celenza, DDS
Associate Clinical Professor
Postgraduate Orthodontics
Rutgers School of Dental Medicine
Newark, New Jersey

Leandro Chambrone, DDS, MSc, PhD
Associate Professor
Unit of Basic Oral Investigation
School of Dentistry
El Bosque University
Bogota, Colombia
Professor
Master of Science Dentistry Program
Ibirapuera University
São Paulo, Brazil

Ting-Ling Chang, DDS
Clinical Professor
Chair of the Section of Prosthodontics
School of Dentistry
University of California, Los Angeles
Los Angeles, California

Yu-Cheng Chang, DDS, MS
Instructor
Department of Periodontics
The Robert Schattner Center
School of Dental Medicine
University of Pennsylvania
Philadelphia, Pennsylvania

Sang Choon Cho, DDS
Clinical Assistant Professor
Periodontology and Implant Dentistry
New York University College of Dentistry
New York, New York

Chih-Hung Chou, PhD
Manager
Molecular Biology Department
WuXi AppTec
Philadelphia, Pennsylvania

Evelyn Chung, DDS
Clinical Professor
Residency Program Director, GPR
Section of Hospital Dentistry
School of Dentistry
University of California, Los Angeles
Los Angeles, California

Sebastian G. Ciancio, DDS
Distinguished Service Professor and Chair
Department of Periodontics and Endodontics
University at Buffalo
The State University of New York
Buffalo, New York

David L. Cochran, DDS, MS, PhD, MMSci
Chair and Professor
Department of Periodontics
School of Dentistry
UT Health San Antonio
San Antonio, Texas

Joseph P. Cooney, BDS, MS
Clinical Professor Emeritus
Restorative Dentistry
University of California, Los Angeles
Los Angeles, California

Simone Cortellini, DDS, MSc
Periodontology Section
University Hospitals Leuven
Department of Oral Health Services
KU Leuven
Leuven, Belgium

J. David Cross, DDS
Private Practice
Springfield, Illinois

Sophie De Geest, DDS, MSc
Clinical Consultant
Periodontology Section
University Hospitals Leuven
Department of Oral Health Services
KU Leuven
Leuven, Belgium

Charlotte De Hous, DDS, MSc
Clinical Resident in Dentistry
Periodontology Section
University Hospitals Leuven
Department of Oral Health Services
KU Leuven
Leuven, Belgium

Christel Dekeyser, DDS
Head of Periodontology Section
Periodontology Section
University Hospitals Leuven
Department of Oral Health Services
KU Leuven
Leuven, Belgium

Raymond R. Derycke, DDS
CEO, Haptitude

Scott R. Diehl, BS, PhD
Professor
Department of Oral Biology
Rutgers School of Dental Medicine
Professor
Department of Health Informatics
Rutgers School of Health Professions
Newark, New Jersey

Jonathan H. Do, DDS
Assistant Clinical Professor
Section of Periodontics
School of Dentistry
University of California, Los Angeles
Los Angeles, California
Private Practice Limited to Periodontics and Implant Surgery
Poway, California

Henrik Dommisch, DDS, PhD
Professor
Periodontology and Synoptic Dentistry
Charité—Universitätsmedizin Berlin
Berlin, Germany
Associate Professor
Oral Health Sciences
University of Washington
Seattle, Washington

Donald F. Duperon, DDS, MSc
Professor Emeritus
Section of Pediatric Dentistry
School of Dentistry
University of California, Los Angeles
Los Angeles, California

Satheesh Elangovan, BDS, DSc, DMSc
Professor
Department of Periodontics
University of Iowa College of Dentistry and Dental Clinics
Iowa City, Iowa

Daniel H. Etienne, DDS, MS
Honorary Associate Professor in Periodontology
Pitié-Salpêtrière Hospital
Denis Diderot University
Paris, France

Richard D. Finkelman, DDS, PhD
Senior Clinical Pharmacology Medical Director
Clinical Pharmacology and Pharmacokinetics
Shire
Lexington, Massachusetts

Joseph P. Fiorellini, DMD, DMSc
Professor
Department of Periodontics
The Robert Schattner Center
School of Dental Medicine
University of Pennsylvania
Philadelphia, Pennsylvania

Jane L. Forrest, BSDH, MS, EdD
Professor of Clinical Dentistry
Dental Public Health and Pediatric Dentistry
Herman Ostrow School of Dentistry
University of Southern California
Los Angeles, California

Marcelo Freire, DDS, PhD, DMSc
Associate Professor
Department of Genomic Medicine and Infectious Disease
J. Craig Venter Institute
La Jolla, California

Scott H. Froum, DDS
Clinical Assistant Professor
Department of Peiodontology
School of Dental Medicine
Stony Brook University
Stony Brook, New York
Private Practice
New York, New York

Stuart J. Froum, DDS
Clinical Professor and Director of Clinical Research
Periodontology and Implant Dentistry
New York University College of Dentistry
New York, New York

Ying Gu, DDS, PhD
Associate Professor
General Dentistry
School of Dental Medicine
Stony Brook University
Stony Brook, New York

Thomas J. Han, DDS, MS
Clinical Professor
Department of Periodontics
Herman Ostrow School of Dentistry
University of Southern California
Los Angeles, California

M. Cenk Haytac, DDS, PhD
Professor
Department of Periodontology
Faculty of Dentistry
Cukurova University
Adana, Turkey

James E. Hinrichs, DDS, MS
Professor
Department of Developmental and Surgical Sciences
Division of Periodontology
School of Dentistry
University of Minnesota
Minneapolis, Minnesota

Eva L. Hogan, MD, DDS, MS
Lecturer
Section of Periodontics
School of Dentistry
University of California, Los Angeles
Los Angeles, California

Richard Holliday, BDS (Hons), MFDS RCSEd, MFDS an eundem RCSEng, MClinRes, MPerio RCSEd
NIHR Doctoral Research Fellow/Specialty Registrar in Restorative Dentistry
Newcastle Dental Hospital
Newcastle upon Tyne, United Kingdom

Ching-Yu Huang, PhD
Assistant Professor
Department of Computer Science
Kean University
Union, New Jersey

Philippe P. Hujoel, DDS, MS, MSD, PhD
Professor, Oral Health Sciences
Adjunct Professor, Epidemiology
School of Dentistry
University of Washington
Seattle, Washington

Carol A. Jahn, RDH, MS
Director Professional Relations and Education
Water Pik, Inc.
Fort Collins, Colorado

Nicholas Jakubovics, BSc, PhD
Senior Lecturer in Oral Microbiology
Centre for Oral Health Research, School of Dental Sciences
Newcastle University
Newcastle upon Tyne, United Kingdom

Mo K. Kang, DDS, PhD
Professor and Chairman
Jack A. Weichman Endowed Chair
Section of Endodontics
Division of Constitutive and Regenerative Sciences
School of Dentistry
University of California, Los Angeles
Los Angeles, California

Alpdogan Kantarci, DDS, PhD
Associate Staff Member
Applied Oral Sciences
Forsyth Institute
Cambridge, Massachusetts
Associate Professor
Cellular and Molecular Biology
Henry M. Goldman School of Dental Medicine
Boston University
Lecturer
Harvard School of Dental Medicine
Boston, Massachusetts

Richard T. Kao, DDS, PhD
Private Practice
Cupertino, California
Clinical Professor
Division of Periodontology
School of Dentistry
University of California, San Francisco
Adjunct Clinical Professor
Department of Periodontology
Arthur A. Dugoni School of Dentistry
University of the Pacific
San Francisco, California

Moritz Kebschull, DMD
Associate Professor
Department of Periodontology, Restorative and Preventive
University Hospital Bonn
Bonn, Germany
Adjunct Associate Professor of Dental Medicine
Division of Periodontics
Section of Oral, Diagnostic, and Rehabilitation Sciences
Columbia University College of Dental Medicine
New York, New York

David M. Kim, DDS, DMSc
Associate Professor
Department of Oral Medicine, Infection, and Immunity
Harvard School of Dental Medicine
Boston, Massachusetts

Keith L. Kirkwood, DDS, PhD
Professor and Chair
Craniofacial Biology
Medical University of South Carolina
Charleston, South Carolina

Perry R. Klokkevold, DDS, MS, FACD
Associate Professor
Program Director, Periodontics Residency
Section of Periodontics
School of Dentistry
University of California, Los Angeles
Los Angeles, California

†Vincent G. Kokich, DDS, MSD
Department of Orthodontics
School of Dentistry
University of Washington
Seattle, Washington

Olga A. Korczeniewska, PhD
Research Associate I
Department of Diagnostic Sciences
Rutgers School of Dental Medicine
Newark, New Jersey

Georgios A. Kotsakis, DDS, MS
Assistant Professor
Department of Periodontics
School of Dentistry
University of Washington
Seattle, Washington

Fengshen Kuo, PhD, MS
Bioinformatics Engineer III
Memorial Sloan Kettering Cancer Center
New York, New York

Isabelle Laleman, DDS, MSc
Periodontologist
Periodontology Section
University Hospitals Leuven
Department of Oral Health Services
KU Leuven
Leuven, Belgium

Clarice S. Law, DMD, MS
Associate Clinical Professor
Pediatric Dentistry and Orthodontics
Section of Pediatric Dentistry
School of Dentistry
University of California, Los Angeles
Los Angeles, California

Yasmin Mair, DDS, MS
Visiting Assistant Professor
Department of Oral Diagnostic Sciences
School of Dental Medicine
University at Buffalo
The State University of New York
Buffalo, New York
Assistant Professor
Oral Diagnostic Sciences
King Abdulaziz University
Jeddah, Saudi Arabia

Sanjay M. Mallya, BDS, MDS, PhD
Associate Professor, Program Director, and Chair
Section of Oral and Maxillofacial Radiology
School of Dentistry
University of California, Los Angeles
Los Angeles, California

Angelo J. Mariotti, DDS, PhD
Chair and Professor
Division of Periodontology
College of Dentistry
The Ohio State University
Columbus, Ohio

†Deceased.

Michael J. McDevitt, DDS
Visiting Faculty
Periodontics
College of Dental Medicine
Augusta, Georgia
Private Practice of Periodontics
Atlanta, Georgia

Adriana McGregor, DDS
Private Practice
Westlake Village, California

Brian L. Mealey, DDS, MS
Professor and Graduate Program Director
Department of Periodontics
University of Texas Health Science Center at San Antonio
San Antonio, Texas

Shebli Mehrazarin, DDS, PhD
Resident
Division of Periodontics
Section of Oral, Diagnostic, and Rehabilitation Sciences
Columbia University College of Dental Medicine
New York, New York

Philip R. Melnick, DMD
Lecturer
Section of Periodontics
School of Dentistry
University of California, Los Angeles
Los Angeles, California

Robert L. Merin, DDS, MS
Private Practice
Woodland Hills, California

Greg W. Miller, DDS
Private Practice
Deer Park, Washington

Syrene A. Miller, BA
Project Manager
National Center for Dental Hygiene Research and Practice
Culver City, California

Ian Needleman, BDS, MSc, PhD
Professor of Restorative Dentistry and Evidence-Based Healthcare
Department of Periodontology
UCL Eastman Dental Institute
London, United Kingdom

Michael G. Newman, DDS, FACD
Professor Emeritus
Section of Periodontics
School of Dentistry
University of California, Los Angeles
Los Angeles, California

Karen F. Novak, DDS, MS, PhD
Clinical Professor
Department of Periodontics and Dental Hygiene
Special Assistant to the Dean
School of Dentistry
Health Science Center at Houston
University of Texas
Houston, Texas

M. John Novak, BDS, LDS, MS, PhD
Professor of Periodontics, Retired
Director, Delta Dental of Kentucky Clinical Research Center
University of Kentucky College of Dentistry
Lexington, Kentucky

Chad M. Novince, DDS, MSD, PhD
Assistant Professor
Oral Health Sciences
Medical University of South Carolina
Charleston, South Carolina

Joan Otomo-Corgel, DDS, MPH
Associate Clinical Professor
Section of Periodontics
School of Dentistry
University of California, Los Angeles
Los Angeles, California

Kwang-Bum Park, DDS
Director
MINEC Institute of Clinical Periodontics and Implantology
Lecturer in Oral Anatomy and Histology
Kyung-Pook National University
Taegu, South Korea

Anna M. Pattison, BS, MS
Co-Director
Pattison Institute
Los Angeles, California

Gordon L. Pattison, DDS
Private Practice
Co-Director
Pattison Institute
Los Angeles, California

Dorothy A. Perry, RDH, PhD, MS
Professor Emeritus
School of Dentistry
University of California, San Francisco
San Francisco, California

Nelson R. Pinto, DDS
Periodontology and Implant Dentistry
University of Los Andes
Las Condes
Santiago, Chile

Flavia Q. Pirih, DDS, PhD
Associate Professor
Section of Periodontics
School of Dentistry
University of California, Los Angeles
Los Angeles, California

Alan M. Polson, DDS
Professor
Department of Periodontics
The Robert Schattner Center
School of Dental Medicine
University of Pennsylvania
Philadelphia, Pennsylvania

Philip M. Preshaw, BDS, FDS RCSEd, FDS (Rest Dent) RCSEd, PhD
Professor of Periodontology
School of Dental Sciences
Institute of Cellular Medicine
Newcastle University
Newcastle upon Tyne, United Kingdom

Marc Quirynen, DDS, PhD
Professor
Periodontology Section
University Hospitals Leuven
Department of Oral Health Services
KU Leuven
Leuven, Belgium

Terry D. Rees, DDS, MSD
Professor
Department of Periodontics
Baylor College of Dentistry
Texas A&M University
Dallas, Texas

Carlos Rossa, Jr., DDS, MSc, PhD
Associate Professor
Diagnosis and Surgery
School of Dentistry at Araraquara-Univ Estadual Paulista
Sao Paulo, Brazil

Maria Emanuel Ryan, DDS, PhD
Vice President and Chief Dental Officer
Colgate Palmolive Company
Piscataway, New Jersey

Hector L. Sarmiento, DMD, MSc
Assistant Clinical Professor
Department of Periodontics
The Robert Schattner Center
School of Dental Medicine
University of Pennsylvania
Philadelphia, Pennsylvania

E. Todd Scheyer, DDS, MS
Private Practice
Houston, Texas

Titus Schleyer, DMD, PhD
Professor of Biomedical Informatics
Indiana University School of Medicine
Research Scientist
Center for Biomedical Informatics
Regenstrief Institute
Indianapolis, Indiana

Todd R. Schoenbaum, DDS, FACD
Associate Clinical Professor
Director of Continuing Dental Education
School of Dentistry
University of California, Los Angeles
Los Angeles, California

Dennis A. Shanelec, DDS
Private Practice
Santa Barbara, California

Kitetsu Shin, DDS, PhD
Professor of Periodontology
Meikai University School of Dentistry
Sakado, Saitama, Japan

†Gerald Shklar, DDS
Department of Oral Medicine and Diagnostic Sciences
Harvard School of Dental Medicine
Boston, Massachusetts

Daniela R. Silva, DDS, MS
Chair and Residency Program Director
Associate Clinical Professor
Section of Pediatric Dentistry
School of Dentistry
University of California, Los Angeles
Los Angeles, California

Thomas N. Sims, BS, DDS
Senior Lecturer
Section of Periodontics
School of Dentistry
University of California, Los Angeles
Los Angeles, California

Sue S. Spackman, DDS
Division of General Dentistry
Center for Dental Research
Loma Linda University School of Dentistry
Loma Linda, California

Frank M. Spear, DDS, MSD
Founder and Director
Spear Education
Scottsdale, Arizona

Panagiota G. Stathopoulou, DDS
Assistant Professor
Department of Periodontics
The Robert Schattner Center
School of Dental Medicine
University of Pennsylvania
Philadelphia, Pennsylvania

Corey Stein, DMD, MS
College of Dental Medicine
Western University of Health Sciences
Pomona, California

†Deceased.

Henry H. Takei, DDS, MS, FACD
Distinguished Clinical Professor
Section of Periodontics
School of Dentistry
University of California, Los Angeles
Los Angeles, California

Dennis P. Tarnow, DDS
Clinical Professor
Director of Implant Education
Columbia University College of Dental Medicine
New York, New York

Andy Temmerman, DDS, MSc, PhD
Assistant Professor
Periodontology Section
University Hospitals Leuven
Department of Oral Health Services
KU Leuven
Leuven, Belgium

Sotirios Tetradis, DDS, PhD
Professor and Senior Associate Dean
Section of Oral and Maxillofacial Radiology
School of Dentistry
University of California, Los Angeles
Los Angeles, California

Wim Teughels, DDS, PhD
Professor
Periodontology Section
University Hospitals Leuven
Department of Oral Health Services
KU Leuven
Leuven, Belgium

Vivek Thumbigere-Math, BDS, PhD
Guest Researcher
National Institutes of Health
Bethesda, Maryland

Thankam P. Thyvalikakath, DMD, MDS, PhD
Associate Professor and Director of Dental Informatics Core
Department of Cariology, Operative Dentistry, and Dental
    Public Health
Indiana University School of Dentistry
Research Scientist
Center for Biomedical Informatics
Regenstrief Institute
Indianapolis, Indiana

Leonard S. Tibbetts, DDS, MSD
Private Practice
Arlington, Texas

Kenneth C. Trabert, DDS, MEd
Clinical Professor Emeritus
Section of Endodontics
Division of Constitutive and Regenerative Sciences
School of Dentistry
University of California, Los Angeles
Los Angeles, California

Onur Ucak Turer, DDS, PhD
Associate Professor
Department of Periodontology
Faculty of Dentistry
Cukurova University
Adana, Turkey

Istvan A. Urban, DMD, MD, PhD
Assistant Professor
Graduate Implant Dentistry
Loma Linda University
Loma Linda, California
Associate Professor
Periodontology
University of Szeged
Szeged, Hungary
Private Practice
Budapest, Hungary

Jose Luis Tapia Vazquez, DDS, MS
Assistant Professor
Department of Oral Diagnostic Sciences
School of Dental Medicine
University of Buffalo
The State University of New York
Buffalo, New York

Giuseppe Vercellotti, PhD
Adjunct Assistant Professor
School of Health and Rehabilitation Sciences
Division of Health Sciences
The Ohio State University
Columbus, Ohio

Tomas Vercellotti, DDS, MS
Honorary Professor and Faculty Member
University College of London
London, United Kingdom
Private Practice
Genoa, Italy

Keisuke Wada, DDS, PhD, DMSc, DMD
Associate Professor and Program Director
Kornberg School of Dentistry
Temple University
Philadelphia, Pennsylvania

Michael Whang, DDS
Lecturer
Section of Periodontics
School of Dentistry
University of California, Los Angeles
Los Angeles, California

Adrian K. Zacher, MBA
Founder and Managing Director
Snorer.com
Oxford, United Kingdom

ABOUT THE BOOK

Newman and Carranza's Clinical Periodontology, thirteenth edition, is the definitive global reference text in periodontics. Edited by Drs. Michael G. Newman, Henry H. Takei, Perry R. Klokkevold, editor emeritus Fermin A. Carranza, and associate editor Satheesh Elangovan, this book provides the highest quality information for students, residents, and practitioners.

The thirteenth edition is truly transformational. It fully engages modern information technology while maintaining and refining its decades of educational excellence. This edition improves on the previous one by more accurately reflecting the essential core information of periodontology and state-of-the-art methods in both the science and clinical knowledge base. Experts from more countries than ever have contributed to reflect a unifying view of the basic information related to the science and technology of modern periodontics.

The content on Expert Consult site is much improved in every aspect, including better speed, quality, functionality, access, and linking. There are more animations, videos, and case reports and one of the most comprehensive image libraries on periodontal pathology ever assembled. New case scenarios offer readers the opportunity to challenge their knowledge of integrated information in much more "real-life" patient encounters.

The print book is a complete and thorough presentation of periodontology essentials while retaining the style and quality that makes *Newman and Carranza's Clinical Periodontology* the number one periodontal textbook in the world. Advances in printing and digital technology make this edition more "readable" than ever before.

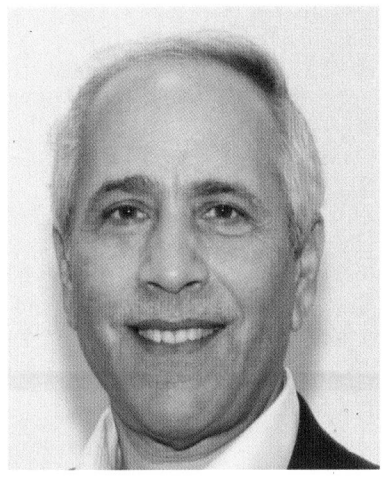

Michael G. Newman, DDS, FACD

Dr. Michael G. Newman graduated from the University of California, Los Angeles (UCLA), College of Letters and Sciences with a degree in psychology. He completed his dental training at the UCLA School of Dentistry in 1972. Dr. Newman received a Certificate in Periodontics and Oral Medicine at the Harvard School of Dental Medicine and a Certificate in Oral Microbiology from the Forsyth Dental Institute under the mentorship of Dr. Sigmund Socransky. He is a Diplomate of the American Board of Periodontology and is Professor Emeritus of Periodontics at the UCLA School of Dentistry. Dr. Newman is a fellow and past president of the American Academy of Periodontology. In 1975, he won the Balint Orban Memorial Prize from the American Academy of Periodontology. He has been in private practice of periodontics for more than 25 years. In 2007, Dr. Newman received the Gold Medal, the highest honor bestowed by the American Academy of Periodontology.

Dr. Newman has published more than 260 abstracts, journal articles, and book chapters and has co-edited nine textbooks. He has served as an ad-hoc reviewer for the National Institute of Dental and Craniofacial Research, was a consultant to the Council on Scientific Affairs of the American Dental Association, and is a reviewer for numerous scientific and professional journals and governmental research organizations.

Professor Newman has lectured throughout the world on microbiology, antimicrobials, evidence-based methodology, risk factors, and diagnostic strategies for periodontal disease. He has a strong interest in applied science and the transfer of new technology for practical use. Dr. Newman is a consultant to major dental and pharmaceutical companies throughout the world. He is the founding editor-in-chief of the *Journal of Evidence-Based Dental Practice (JEBDP)* and *The JEBDP Annual Report Series* and was the associate editor of the *International Journal of Oral and Maxillofacial Implants*.

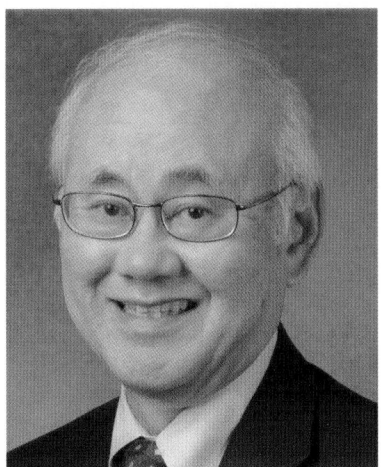

Henry H. Takei, DDS, MS, FACD

Dr. Henry H. Takei graduated in 1965 from the Marquette University School of Dentistry in Milwaukee, Wisconsin. He completed his Periodontics Certificate and Master of Science degree in 1967 at Marquette University and the Veterans Administration Hospital in Wood, Wisconsin.

Presently, Dr. Takei is a Distinguished Clinical Professor of Periodontics and Consultant in Periodontics at the University of California, Los Angeles (UCLA), School of Dentistry and a consultant in periodontics at the Veterans Administration Hospital in Los Angeles. In addition to his educational activities, he maintains a private practice limited to periodontics and implant surgery.

Dr. Takei has published numerous clinical and scientific articles on periodontal surgery and has contributed chapters to five textbooks. He has been actively involved in continuing education and has lectured throughout the world on clinical periodontology and implant surgery.

Dr. Takei has been honored nationally and internationally with awards from numerous periodontal organizations, universities, and study clubs for his contributions to education. He is also a Fellow of both the American College of Dentists and the International College of Dentists and has been elected into Omicron Kappa Upsilon.

He received the Distinguished Alumnus Award from Marquette University in 2001 and the Honorary Distinguished Alumnus Award from UCLA in 1998. The American Academy of Periodontology has honored Dr. Takei with the prestigious Master Clinician Award in 2006. This award is the highest clinical recognition from this national periodontal organization. In 2016, two universities in Japan, Meikai University and Asahi University, presented Dr. Takei with the Honorary Doctorate Degree for many years of academic and clinical collaboration.

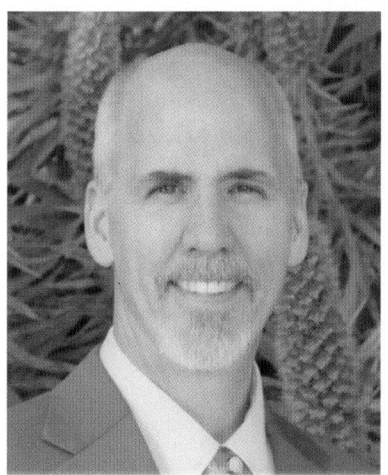

Perry R. Klokkevold, DDS, MS, FACD

Dr. Perry R. Klokkevold graduated from the University of California, San Francisco, School of Dentistry in 1986. His postdoctoral clinical training includes a General Practice Residency in Hospital Dentistry completed in 1987, a Postgraduate Periodontal Residency completed in 1994, and a Surgical Implant Fellowship completed in 1995. All of his postgraduate training was completed at the University of California, Los Angeles (UCLA), School of Dentistry. He earned a Master of Science degree in Oral Biology at UCLA in 1995.

Dr. Klokkevold is a Diplomate of the American Board of Periodontology and a Fellow of the American College of Dentists. He is an Associate Professor in the Division of Constitutive and Regenerative Sciences, Section of Periodontics, at the UCLA School of Dentistry and Program Director of the UCLA Postgraduate Periodontics Residency program. Dr. Klokkevold served as Clinical Director and Program Director of the General Practice Residency program in Hospital Dentistry at the UCLA School of Dentistry from 1987 to 1992. He has maintained a faculty practice limited to the specialty of periodontics and dental implant surgery at UCLA since 1995.

Dr. Klokkevold has published more than 60 articles for international peer-reviewed journals and has written more than 100 book chapters for 13 books, including five editions of *Clinical Periodontology*, on topics including periodontal medicine, influence of systemic disease and risk factors on periodontitis to bone regeneration, and dental implants. He has served as a reviewer for several journals, among them the *Journal of Periodontology* and the *International Journal of Oral and Maxillofacial Implants*. Dr. Klokkevold lectures nationally and internationally on many periodontal and implant-related topics. He has been invited to serve as an expert consultant/reviewer for five international conferences organized by the American Academy of Periodontology and the Academy of Osseointegration on topics that include implant therapy, bone augmentation and implant site development, periodontal regeneration, and lasers in periodontal therapy.

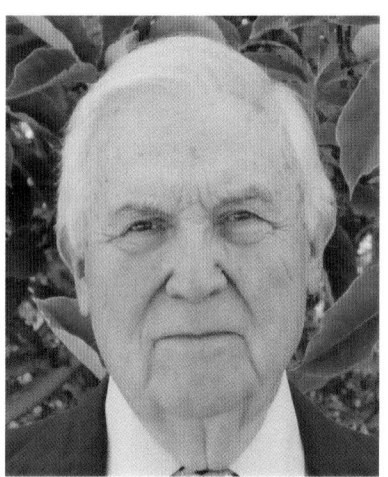

Fermin A. Carranza, DR ODONT, FACD

Dr. Fermin A. Carranza graduated from the University of Buenos Aires School of Dentistry in Argentina in 1948 and completed his postdoctoral training in periodontics at Tufts University School of Dental Medicine in 1952 under the mentorship of Dr. Irving Glickman.

Dr. Carranza is Professor Emeritus of Periodontology at the University of California, Los Angeles (UCLA), School of Dentistry. He was head of the Department of Periodontics at the University of Buenos Aires from 1966 to 1974 and at UCLA from 1974 until his retirement in 1994.

Dr. Carranza has published more than 218 scientific papers and abstracts on basic and applied aspects of periodontics and 18 books, including the past five editions of *Clinical Periodontology*. He has received numerous awards and recognition for his work, including the IADR Science Award in Periodontal Disease and the Gies Award of the American Academy of Periodontology.

Dr. Carranza has lectured throughout the world on clinical periodontology, pathology, and therapy.

PREFACE

With the help of Elsevier's advanced technology and high standards of quality, an international team of editors and contributors have developed the most comprehensive periodontal resource available, *Newman and Carranza's Clinical Periodontology*, thirteenth edition. The book's companion website is rich with images, animations, videos, question sets, case reports, PowerPoint slides, audio slides, virtual microscope, multidisciplinary case scenarios, and more. No other resource offers such a comprehensive approach to providing high quality content.

Since publication of the first edition of this book in 1953, periodontology has made tremendous advancements. Scientific analysis of periodontal tissues and the elucidation of mechanisms and causes of disease have extended far beyond histology and physiology into the realm of cellular and molecular biologic understanding.

Implant dentistry has become a major component of periodontology, and this book offers a wide coverage of important treatment modalities.

New therapeutic goals and clinical techniques, based on an improved understanding of disease and healing, have facilitated better outcomes and brought us closer to achieving the ultimate goal of optimal periodontal health and function. Today, reconstruction and regeneration of lost periodontal structures, replacement of compromised teeth with implants, and creation of aesthetic results are integral parts of clinical practice.

The multifaceted, complex task of producing the thirteenth edition required the collaboration of numerous experts from various fields, and their contributions are invaluable. We know that this new edition will continue to be a useful resource for to dentists, dental hygienists, periodontists, students, educators, and researchers.

Having this resource available will contribute to the continuous progress of our profession.

Michael G. Newman
Henry H. Takei
Perry R. Klokkevold
Fermin A. Carranza

ACKNOWLEDGMENTS

Clinical Periodontology has been a trusted and valuable periodontics resource for students, residents, academicians, scientists, and clinicians since the early 1950s. Dr. Irving Glickman was the originator and author of *Clinical Periodontology* for the first four editions, which were published in 1953, 1958, 1964, and 1972. Dr. Glickman was professor and chairman of the Department of Periodontology at Tufts University School of Dental Medicine, in Boston, Massachusetts.

Dr. Fermin A. Carranza, once a student of and collaborator with Dr. Glickman, assumed responsibility to author and continue the book after Dr. Glickman's death in 1972 at age 58. Dr. Carranza was professor and chairman of periodontics at the University of California, Los Angeles (UCLA), School of Dentistry. The subsequent four editions were published in 1979, 1984, 1990, and 1996 under the leadership and guidance of Dr. Carranza.

Dr. Michael G. Newman joined Dr. Carranza in 1996 as co-editor of the eighth edition. Dr. Newman was adjunct professor of periodontics at the UCLA School of Dentistry. Dr. Carranza retired to become professor emeritus at UCLA, and the responsibility of maintaining the book's tradition of almost half a century changed hands once again, this time to Dr. Newman. The subsequent four editions were published in 2002, 2006, 2012, and 2015 under the direction of Dr. Newman. The title of the ninth edition was changed from *Clinical Periodontology* to *Carranza's Clinical Periodontology* to acknowledge and honor Dr. Carranza for his leadership and dedication to this renowned resource.

Dr. Henry H. Takei joined Dr. Newman and Dr. Carranza in 2002 as co-editor of the ninth edition. Dr. Takei was clinical professor of periodontics at the UCLA School of Dentistry. Dr. Takei currently holds the title of Distinguished Clinical Professor of Periodontics at UCLA School of Dentistry.

Dr. Perry R. Klokkevold joined Drs. Newman, Takei, and Carranza in 2006 as co-editor of the tenth edition. Dr. Klokkevold is an associate professor and the program director of Postgraduate Periodontics at the UCLA School of Dentistry. Dr. Carranza became editor emeritus for the tenth and subsequent editions.

The title of the thirteenth edition has been changed to *Newman and Carranza's Clinical Periodontology* to acknowledge and recognize Dr. Newman's leadership in maintaining the book's reputation as a high-quality and forward-looking resource for those who practice periodontology and implant dentistry.

The level of understanding and the practice of clinical periodontics have evolved tremendously since the mid-20th century. Advances in basic science and clinical techniques have increased the knowledge base so dramatically that it is virtually impossible for individuals to master and retain all the information.

It is also certain that the task of researching, preparing, and assembling the enormous amount periodontology-related content necessary for this book had to be borne by many experts who shared their experience and knowledge. We express our deep gratitude to all the contributors whose expertise, ideas, and efforts built this valuable resource over the years. Many scientists and clinicians have shared their wisdom and expertise in previous editions of *Carranza's Clinical Periodontology,* as associate editors, section editors, and contributors, though some of their names no longer appear.

Our appreciation is given to Elsevier and particularly to Jennifer Flynn-Briggs and Lucia Gunzel. Their expertise and detailed attention to every word and every concept contributed greatly to producing a quality book and a truly useful website.

We also express appreciation to Dr. Satheesh Elangovan who joined the team for the thirteenth edition as associate editor. The online version of the book continues to assume greater importance to our readers. Elsevier's electronic capabilities provide a rich, useful, and complete resource and are directed by Dr. Elangovan.

We express gratitude to our parents, colleagues, friends, and mentors who have always been so tolerant, encouraging, and understanding and who guided our first steps in our profession and helped us develop our ideas in the field.

Dr. Newman: My family, Susan, Andrea, Kara, Callahan and Natalie, Scott, Zoey and Eleanor; my parents, Paul, Rose, John, and Inez. Sigmund S. Socransky, Fermin A. Carranza, Jr., and Henry H. Takei. My gratitude to my co-editors and contributors whose expertise and willingness to participate in this work have made this book an excellent educational standard.

Dr. Takei: My wife, June; my children, Scott and Akemi; their spouses, Kozue and David; my grandchildren, Hana, Markus, Carter, and Arden. My gratitude to my mentors Dr. Fermin A. Carranza, Jr., Dr. Donald Van Scotter, Dr. Delbert Nachazel, and Dr. John Pfeiffer. Thank you to my three co-editors and friends Michael G. Newman, Fermin A. Carranza, Jr., and Perry R. Klokkevold. Special gratitude to Laura Miyabe for her professional support. I would like to acknowledge and thank all of my periodontal postdoctoral students at UCLA for their help and support throughout the preparation of this classic textbook. Another note of thank you to Dr. Sasan Garakani for the many hours of collaboration and help that he provided in the review of literature and organizing the references for numerous chapters.

Dr. Klokkevold: My wife, Angie; my daughters, Ashley and Brianna; my parents Carl and Loretta; my gratitude and appreciation to my mentors Dr. Henry H. Takei, Dr. John Beumer III, Dr. Bradley G. Seto, Dr. Charles N. Bertolami, and Dr. Thomas Han. I am grateful to the many talented residents who matriculated through UCLA Postgraduate Periodontics for the passion and inspiration they bring to me as an educator and clinician. Finally, I give special thanks to my co-editors, Dr. Michael G. Newman, Dr. Henry H. Takei, and Dr. Fermin A. Carranza, Jr., for their friendship, support, and encouragement.

Dr. Carranza: My wife, Rita; my children, Fermin, Patricia, and Laura; and my grandchildren, Irving Glickman, Fermin Carranza, Sr., and Romulo L. Cabrini. My gratitude also to my co-editors, who will continue the tradition of this book.

Michael G. Newman
Henry H. Takei
Perry R. Klokkevold
Fermin A. Carranza

CONTENTS

†Deceased.

[†]Deceased.

VIDEO CONTENTS

CHAPTER **1**

Evidence-Based Decision Making

*Jane L. Forrest | Syrene A. Miller | Greg W. Miller | Satheesh Elangovan |
Michael G. Newman*

CHAPTER OUTLINE

Background and Definition
Principles of Evidence-Based Decision Making
Evidence-Based Decision-Making Process and Skills
Conclusion

Each day, dental care professionals make decisions about clinical care. It is important that these decisions incorporate the best available scientific evidence to maximize the potential for successful patient care outcomes. It is also important for readers of this book to have the background and skills necessary to evaluate information they read and hear about. These evaluative skills are as important as learning facts and clinical procedures. *The ability to find, discriminate, evaluate, and use information is the most important skill that can be learned as a professional and lifelong learner.* Becoming excellent at this skill will provide a rewarding and fulfilling professional career.

Background and Definition

Using evidence from the medical literature to answer questions, direct clinical action, and guide practice was pioneered at McMaster University, Ontario, Canada, in the 1980s. As clinical research and the publication of findings increased, so did the need to use the medical literature to guide practice. The traditional clinical problem-solving model based on individual experience or the use of information gained by consulting authorities (colleagues or textbooks) gave way to a new methodology for practice and restructured the way in which more effective clinical problem solving should be conducted. This new methodology was termed *evidence-based medicine* (EBM).[12]

KEY DEFINITIONS

Evidence: Evidence is considered the synthesis of all valid research that answers a specific question and that, in most cases, distinguishes it from a single research study.[2]

Evidence-based medicine: The integration of the best research evidence with our clinical expertise and our patient's unique values and circumstances.[31]

Evidence-based dentistry: An approach to oral health care that requires the judicious integration of systematic assessments of clinically relevant scientific evidence, relating to the patient's oral and medical condition and history, with the dentist's clinical expertise and the patient's treatment needs and preferences.[4]

The use of evidence to help guide clinical decisions is not new. However, the following aspects of EBM are new:
- The methods of generating high-quality evidence, such as randomized controlled trials (RCTs) and other well-designed methods
- The statistical tools for synthesizing and analyzing the evidence (systematic reviews [SRs] and meta-analysis [MA])
- The ways for accessing the evidence (electronic databases) and applying it (evidence-based decision making [EBDM] and practice guidelines)[9,10]

These changes have evolved along with the understanding of what constitutes the evidence and how to minimize sources of bias, quantify the magnitude of benefits and risks, and incorporate patient values.[13] "In other words, evidence-based practice is not just a new term for an old concept and as a result of advances, practitioners need (1) more efficient and effective online searching skills to find relevant evidence and (2) critical appraisal skills to rapidly evaluate and sort out what is valid and useful and what is not."[28]

EBDM is the formalized process and structure for learning and using the skills for identifying, searching for, and interpreting the results of the best scientific evidence, which is considered in conjunction with the clinician's experience and judgment, the patient's preferences and values, and the clinical and patient circumstances when making patient care decisions. Translating the EBDM process into action is based on the abilities and skills identified in Box 1.1.[31]

Principles of Evidence-Based Decision Making

The use of current best evidence does not replace clinical expertise or input from the patient, but rather provides another dimension to the decision-making process,[11,16,19] which is also placed in context with the patient's clinical circumstances (Fig. 1.1). It is this decision-making process that we refer to as "evidence-based decision making" and is not unique to medicine or any specific health discipline; it represents a concise way of referring to the application of evidence to clinical decision making.

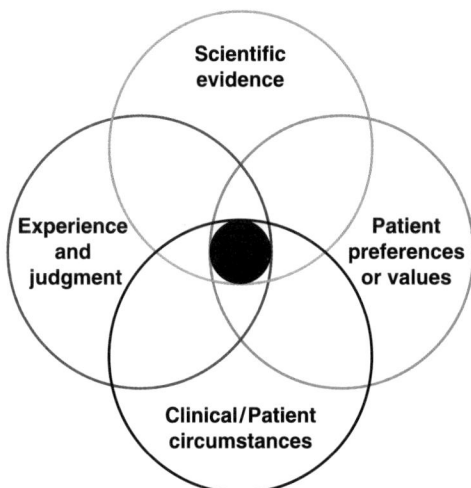

Fig. 1.1 Evidence-based decision making. *(Copyright Jane L. Forrest, reprinted with permission.)*

EBDM focuses on solving clinical problems and involves two fundamental principles, as follows[13]:
1. Evidence alone is never sufficient to make a clinical decision.
2. Hierarchies of quality and applicability of evidence exist to guide clinical decision making.

EBDM is a structured process that incorporates a formal set of rules for interpreting the results of clinical research and places a lower value on authority or custom. In contrast to EBDM, traditional decision making relies more on intuition, unsystematic clinical experience, and pathophysiologic rationale.[13]

Evidence-Based Dentistry

Since the 1990s, the evidence-based movement has continued to advance and is widely accepted among the health care professions, with some refining the definition to make it more specific to their area of health care. The American Dental Association (ADA) has defined evidence-based dentistry (EBD) as "an approach to oral health care that requires the judicious integration of systematic assessments of clinically relevant scientific evidence, relating to the patient's oral and medical condition and history, with the dentist's clinical expertise and the patient's treatment needs and preferences."[4] They also have established the ADA Center for Evidence-Based Dentistry (ebd.ada.org) to facilitate the integration of EBD into clinical practice.

The ADA's definition is now incorporated in the Accreditation Standards for Dental Education Programs.[3] Dental schools are expected to develop specific core competencies that focus on the need for graduates to become critical thinkers, problem solvers, and consumers

of current research findings to enable them to become lifelong learners. The accreditation standards require learning EBDM skills so that graduates are competent in being able to find, evaluate, and incorporate current evidence into their decision making.[3]

 KEY FACT

PICO
The first step in evidence-based decision making is asking the right question. The key is to frame a question that is simple and at the same time highly specific to the clinical scenario. Dissecting the question you want to ask into its components—problem or population (P), intervention (I), comparison group (C) and outcomes (O)—and then combining them will facilitate a thorough and precise evidence search.[31]

Evidence-Based Decision-Making Process and Skills

The growth of evidence-based practice has been made possible through the development of online scientific databases such as MEDLINE (PubMed) and Internet-based software, along with the use of computers and mobile devices, for example, smart phones, that enable users to quickly access relevant clinical evidence from almost anywhere. This combination of *technology* and *good evidence* allows health care professionals to apply the benefits from clinical research to patient care.[29] EBDM recognizes that clinicians can never be completely current with all conditions, medications, materials, or available products, and it provides a mechanism for assimilating current research findings into everyday practice to answer questions and to stay current with innovations in dentistry. Translating the EBDM process into action is based on the abilities and skills identified in Box 1.1.[31] This is illustrated clearly in a real patient case scenario (management of a patient with trauma-related avulsion and luxation of teeth) that is introduced in Case Scenario 1.1 (Figs. 1.2 and 1.3) and used throughout the chapter.

Asking Good Questions: The PICO Process

Converting information needs and problems into clinical questions is a difficult skill to learn, but it is fundamental to evidence-based practice. The EBDM process almost always begins with a patient question or problem. A "well-built" question should include four parts that identify the patient problem or population *(P)*, intervention *(I)*, comparison *(C)*, and outcome(s) *(O)*, referred to as PICO.[31] Once these four components are clearly and succinctly identified, the following format can be used to structure the question:

"For a patient with _____ (P), will _____ (I) as compared with _____ (C) increase/decrease/provide better/in doing _____ (O)?"

The formality of using PICO to frame the question serves two key purposes, as follows:
1. PICO forces the clinician to focus on what he or she and the patient believe to be the most important single issue and outcome.
2. PICO facilitates the next step in the process, the computerized search, by identifying key terms that will be used in the search.[31]

The conversion of information needs into a clinical question is demonstrated using Case Scenario 1.1 Two separate PICO questions were written as follows:
1. For a patient with replanted avulsed and luxated teeth (P), will early pulp extirpation (10 to 14 days) (I) as compared with late pulp extirpation (past 14 days) (C) increase the likelihood of successful tooth integration and functional periodontal healing and decrease the likelihood of resorption and ankylosis (O)?

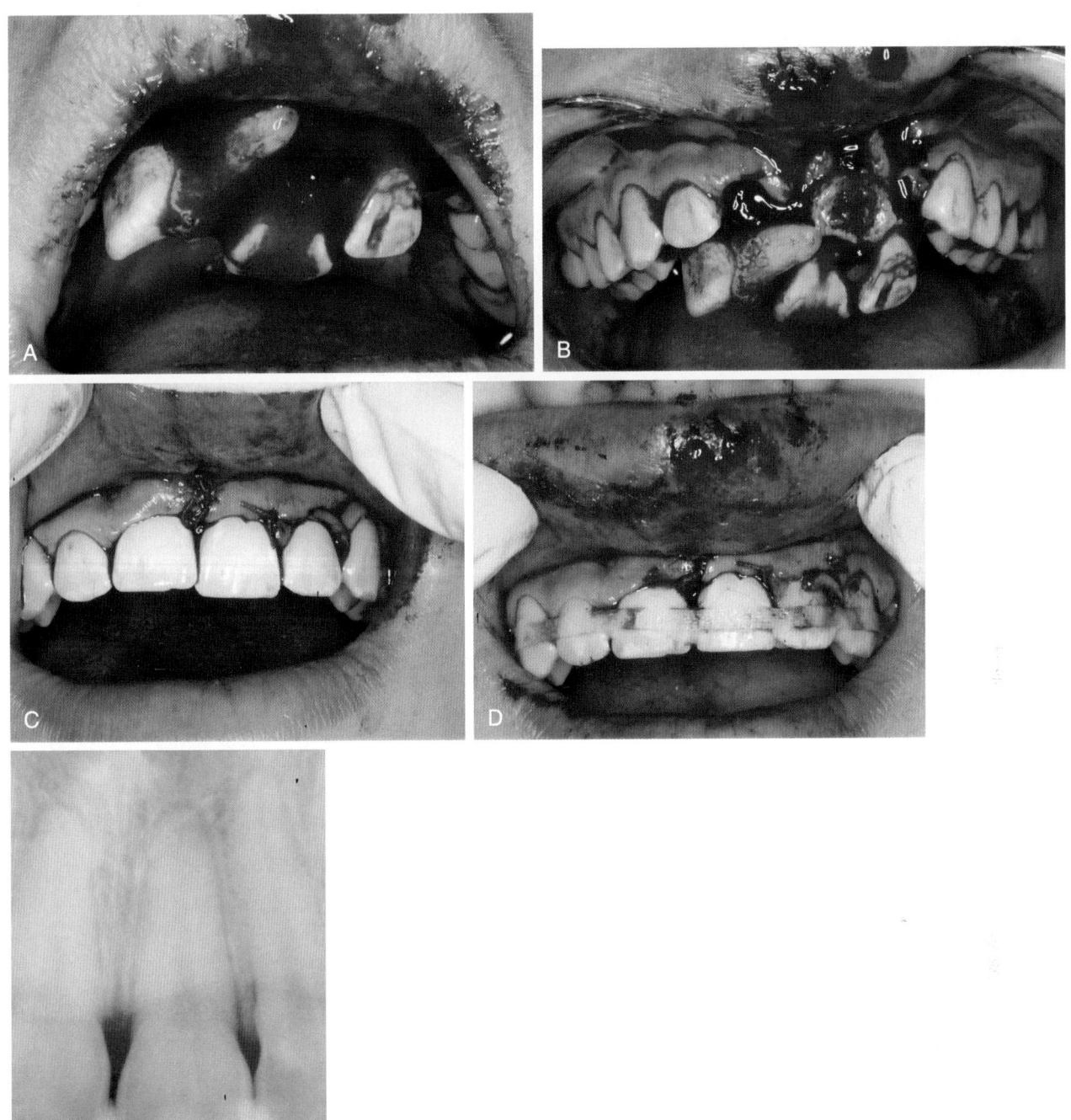

Fig. 1.2 (A) Initial examination of the patient. (B) Trauma site following irrigation. (C) Replantation of avulsed and luxated teeth. (D) Replanted and splinted teeth. (E) Radiograph after placement of the splint *(Copyright Greg W. Miller, DDS, reprinted with permission.)*

2. For a patient with replanted avulsed and luxated teeth (P), will short-term splinting (7 to 14 days) (I) as compared with long-term splinting (2 to 4 weeks) (C) increase the likelihood of successful tooth integration and functional periodontal healing and decrease the development of resorption and ankylosis (O)?

PICO directs the clinician to identify clearly the problem, the results, and the outcomes related to the specific care provided to that patient. This, in turn, helps identify the search terms that should be used to conduct an efficient search. It also allows identification of the type of evidence and information required to solve the problem, as well as considerations for measuring the effectiveness of the intervention and the application of the EBDM process. Thus EBDM

supports continuous quality improvements through measuring outcomes of care and self-reflection.

Before conducting a computerized search, it is important to have an understanding of the types of research study methodologies and the appropriate methodology that relates to different types of clinical questions. The methodology, in turn, relates to the levels of evidence. Table 1.1 shows these relationships.

Becoming a Competent Consumer of the Evidence

Evidence typically comes from studies related to questions about treatment and prevention, diagnosis, etiology and harm, and prognosis of disease, as well as from questions about the quality and economics

CASE SCENARIO 1.1

CLINICAL APPLICATION OF EVIDENCE-BASED DECISION MAKING

The clinician received a call from the parents of a 13-year-old female patient who had been struck in the face with a softball. She was being examined by paramedics in a town 30 minutes north of the dental office. The paramedics cleared the patient of any head or neck injury and other medical issues and informed the dentist that dental trauma was her primary injury. The dentist and his assistant met the parents and the patient at the office 45 minutes following the dental trauma. The patient's teeth remained in her mouth following the incident. Fig. 1.2A shows the initial examination of the patient. The preference of the patient and her parents was to "do anything to keep the teeth." After the site was cleaned and irrigated, it was apparent that there was complete avulsion of the maxillary right central incisor from the socket and lateral luxation of the maxillary left central and lateral incisors. In addition, there was alveolar bone fracture partially encasing the roots of the maxillary left central and lateral incisors (Fig. 1.2B.) The clinician replanted the teeth and reapproximated the gingival tissue with sutures (Fig. 1.2C). A stable and accurate ribbond and flowable composite splint were placed (Fig. 1.2D), and a radiograph was taken (Fig. 1.2E).

RADIOGRAPHIC EXAMINATION

The radiograph shows reimplantation of maxillary central incisors and left lateral incisor in correct socket location and confirmed proper reapproximation of the alveolar bone that was fractured with maxillary left central and lateral incisors. The stent also is apparent in this radiograph showing the splinting of the displaced teeth.

Due to the difficulty of splint placement and not wanting to risk displacing the teeth or breaking the splint prematurely, the clinician was hesitant to proceed with endodontic treatment until he had access to dependable information. The dentist had two questions regarding the treatment of the patient. He needed to determine the optimal timing of the pulp extirpation and splinting that would result in the best outcome and prognosis for healing. Fig. 1.3 diagrams the decision-making pathway from telephone call to resolution.[24]

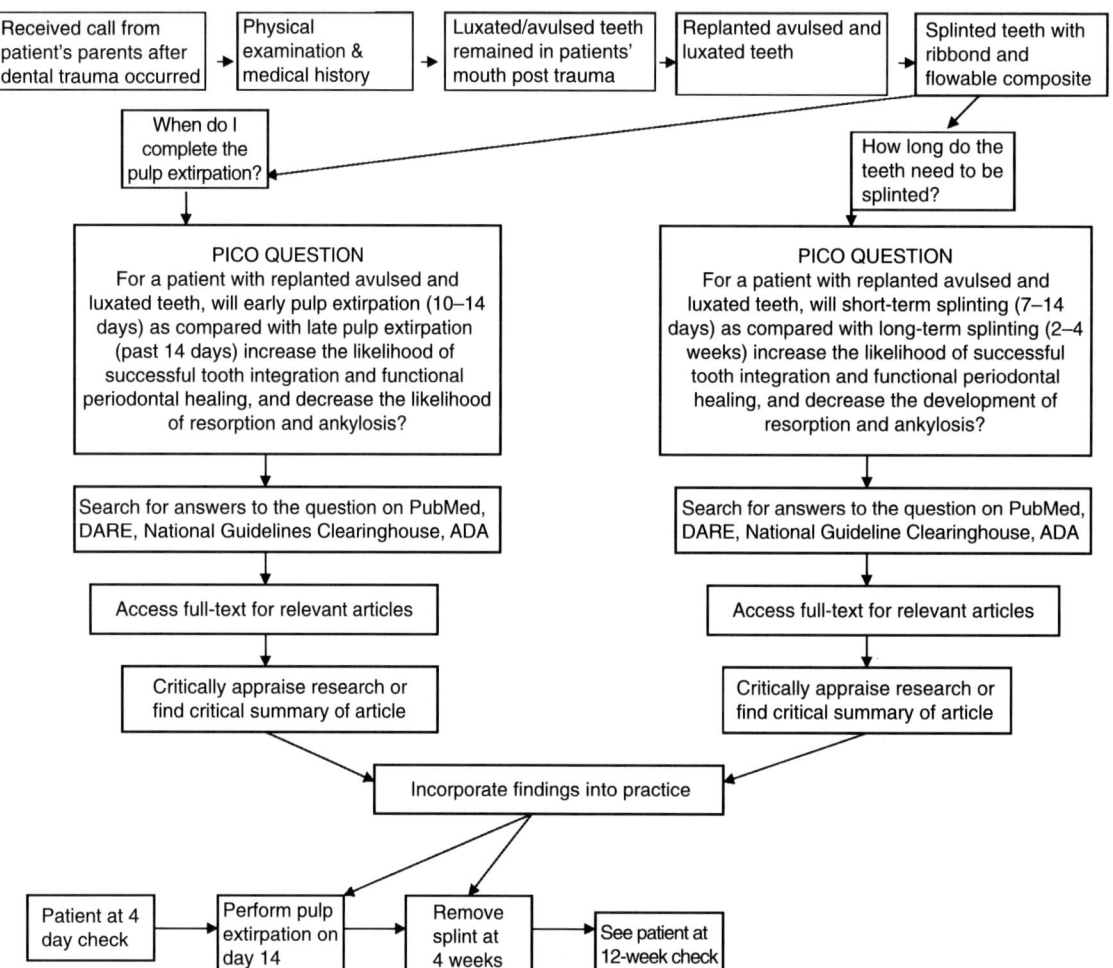

Fig. 1.3 Decision-making pathway from telephone call to resolution. *ADA,* American Dental Association; *DARE,* Database of Abstracts of Review of Effectiveness; *PICO,* patient problem or population, intervention, comparison, and outcome(s). *(Copyright Greg W. Miller, DDS, reprinted with permission.)*

TABLE 1.1   Type of Question Related to Type of Methodology and Levels of Evidence

Type of Question	Methodology of Choice[27]	Question Focus[22]
Therapy, prevention	MA or SR of randomized controlled trials SR of cohort studies	Study effect of therapy or test on real patients; allows for comparison between intervention and control groups; largest volume of evidence-based literature
Diagnosis	MA or SR of controlled trials (prospective cohort study) *Controlled trial* (Prospective: compare tests with a reference or "gold standard" test)	Measures reliability of a particular diagnostic measure for a disease against the "gold standard" diagnostic measure for the same disease
Etiology, causation, harm	MA or SR of cohort studies *Cohort study* (Prospective data collection with formal control group)	Compares a group exposed to a particular agent with an unexposed group; important for understanding prevention and control of disease
Prognosis	MA or SR of inception cohort studies *Inception cohort study* (All have disease but free of the outcome of interest) *Retrospective cohort*	Follows progression of a group with a particular disease and compares with a group without the disease

MA, Meta-analysis; *SR,* systematic review.

of care. Evidence is considered the synthesis of all valid research that answers a specific question and that, in most cases, distinguishes it from a single research study.[15] Once synthesized, evidence can help inform decisions about whether a method of diagnosis or a treatment is effective relative to other methods of diagnoses or to other treatments and under what circumstances. The challenge in using EBDM arises when only one research study is available on a particular topic. In these cases, individuals should be cautious in relying on the study because it can be contradicted by another study and it may test only efficacy and not effectiveness. This underscores the importance of staying current with the scientific literature because the body of evidence evolves over time as more research is conducted. Another challenge in using EBDM occurs when the limited research available is weak in quality or poorly conducted. In these cases, one may rely more heavily on clinical experience and patients' preferences and values than the scientific evidence (see Fig. 1.1).

Sources of Evidence

The two types of evidence-based sources are primary and secondary, as follows:

- *Primary sources* are original research studies and publications that have not been filtered or synthesized, such as an RCT or a cohort study.
- *Secondary sources* are synthesized studies and publications of the already conducted primary research. These include clinical practice guidelines (CPGs), SRs, MAs, and evidence-based article reviews and protocols. This terminology is often confusing to individuals new to the EBDM approach because, although SRs are *secondary* sources of evidence, they are considered a higher level of evidence than a *primary* source, such as an individual RCT.

Both primary and secondary sources can be found by conducting a search using such biomedical databases as MEDLINE (accessed through PubMed), EMBASE, and Database of Abstracts of Review of Effectiveness (DARE). Other sources of secondary evidence, such as CPGs, clinical recommendations, parameters of care, position papers, academy statements, and critical summaries related to dental practice can be found on the websites of professional organizations and journals as listed in Table 1.2.

TABLE 1.2   Sources of Secondary Evidence

Sources	Websites
American Academy of Pediatric Dentistry (AAPD): 2017–2018 definitions, oral health policies, and clinical practice guidelines	http://www.aapd.org/policies
American Academy of Periodontology (AAP): Clinical and scientific papers[1]	https://www.perio.org/resources-products/clinical-scientific-papers.html
American Dental Association (ADA), Center for Evidence-Based Dentistry	http://ebd.ada.org
American Heart Association (AHA): Prevention of bacterial endocarditis, recommendations	http://circ.ahajournals.org/content/116/15/1736.full.pdf+html?sid=ada268bd-1f10-4496-bae4-b91806aaf341
Centers for Disease Control and Prevention (CDC): Guidelines and recommendations	http://www.cdc.gov/OralHealth/guidelines.htm
Cochrane Collaboration: A nonprofit organization dedicated to producing systematic reviews as a reliable and relevant source of evidence about the effects of health care for making informed decisions.[7]	http://www.cochrane.org Cochrane Oral Health Group: http://ohg.cochrane.org
Journal: *Evidence-Based Dentistry*	http://www.nature.com/ebd/index.html
Journal: *Journal of Evidence-Based Dental Practice*	http://www.jebdp.com

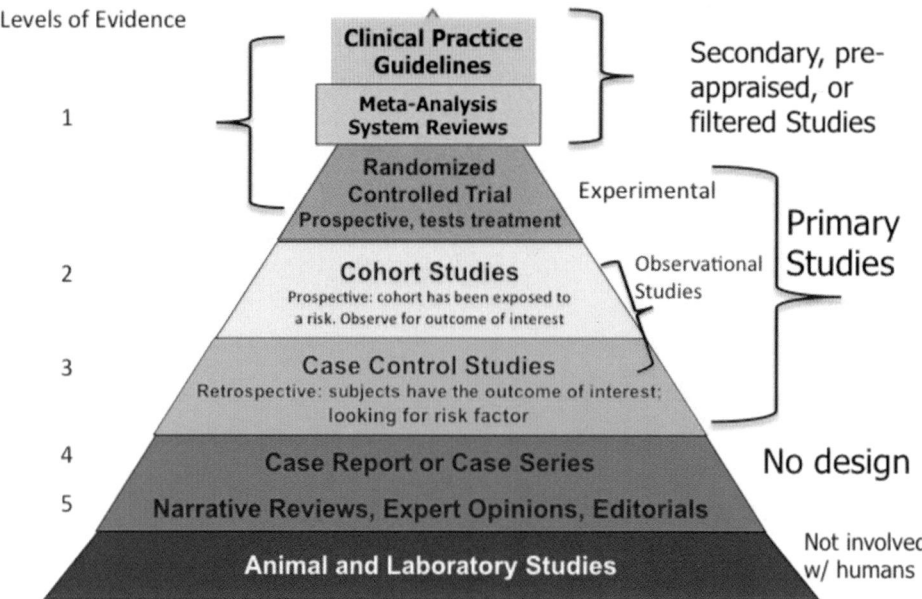

Levels of Evidence

Clinical Practice
Guidelines

1

Meta-Analysis
System Reviews

Secondary, pre-
appraised, or
filtered Studies

Randomized
Controlled Trial
Prospective, tests treatment

Experimental

Primary
Studies

2

Cohort Studies
Prospective: cohort has been exposed to
a risk. Observe for outcome of interest

Observational
Studies

3

Case Control Studies
Retrospective: subjects have the outcome of interest;
looking for risk factor

4

Case Report or Case Series

No design

5

Narrative Reviews, Expert Opinions, Editorials

Animal and Laboratory Studies

Not involved
w/ humans

Fig. 1.4 Hierarchy of research and levels of clinical evidence. *(Image Copyright 2012 JL Forrest, SA Miller: National Center for Dental Hygiene Research & Practice.)*

Levels of Evidence

As previously mentioned, one principle of EBDM is that hierarchies of evidence exist to guide decision making. At the top of the hierarchy for therapy are CPGs (Fig. 1.4). These are systematically developed statements to assist clinicians and patients about appropriate health care for specific clinical circumstances.[8] CPGs should be based on the best available scientific evidence typically from MAs and SRs, which put together all that is known about a topic in an objective manner. The level and quality of the evidence are then analyzed by a panel of experts who formulate the CPGs. Thus, guidelines are intended to translate the research into practical application.

Guidelines also will change over time as the evidence evolves, thereby underscoring the importance of keeping current with the scientific literature. One example of this is the change in the American Heart Association guidelines for the prevention of infective endocarditis related to the need for premedication before dental and dental hygiene procedures.[5] Before the 2007 guidelines, the last update was in 1997, and before then, eight updates were added to the primary regimens for dental procedures since the original guideline was first published in 1955. In the 2007 update, the rationale for revising the 1997 document was provided, notably that the prior guidelines were largely based on expert opinion and a few case-controlled studies. With more research conducted, the ability now existed to synthesize those findings to provide a more objective body of evidence on which to base recommendations.[5]

If a CPG does not exist, other sources of preappraised evidence (critical summaries, critically appraised topics [CATs], SRs, MAs, or reviews of individual research studies) are available to help stay current. MAs and SRs have strict protocols to reduce bias and the synthesis of research from more than one study. These reviews provide a summary of multiple research studies that have investigated the same specific question. SRs use explicit criteria for retrieval, assessment, and synthesis of evidence from individual RCTs and other well-controlled methods. SRs facilitate decision making by providing a clear summary of the current state of the existing evidence on a specific topic. SRs provide a way of managing large quantities of information,[25] thus making it easier to keep current with new research.

MA is a statistical process used when the data from the individual studies in the SR can be combined into one analysis. When data from these studies are pooled, the sample size and power usually increase. As a result, the combined effect can increase the precision of estimates of treatment effects and exposure risks.[25]

SRs and MAs are followed respectively by individual RCT studies, cohort studies, case–control studies, and then studies not involving human subjects.[27] In the absence of scientific evidence, the consensus opinion of experts in appropriate fields of research and clinical practice is used (see Fig. 1.4). This hierarchy of evidence is based on the concept of causation and the need to control bias.[21,22] Although each level may contribute to the total body of knowledge, "not all levels are equally useful for making patient care decisions."[22] In progressing up the pyramid, the number of studies and, correspondingly, the amount of available literature decrease, while at the same time their relevance to answering clinical questions increases.

Evidence is judged on its rigor of methodology, and the level of evidence is directly related to the type of question asked, such as those derived from issues of therapy or prevention, diagnosis, etiology, and prognosis (see Table 1.1). For example, the highest level of evidence associated with questions about therapy or prevention is from CPGs based on MAs and/or SRs of RCT studies. However, the highest level of evidence associated with questions about prognosis is from CPGs based on MAs and/or SRs of inception cohort studies.[27] Because the two case scenario questions are related to prognosis, the highest level of evidence for them is a CPG based on MAs and/or SRs of inception cohort studies. If no CPG is found, then the next highest level would be a critical summary of an MA or SR of cohort studies. In the event that a critical summary is not found, MAs or SRs of cohort studies followed by individual cohort studies provide the next highest levels of evidence.

Knowing what constitutes the highest levels of evidence and knowing how to apply evidence-based filters are necessary skills to search the literature with maximum efficiency.[22] By using filters, one can refine the search to limit the citations to publication types such as practice guidelines, MAs, SRs, RCTs, and clinical trials, the highest levels of evidence.

TABLE 1.3 Search Terms for Each PICO Question

PICO Question 1 Search Terms			PICO Question 2 Search Terms
Tooth avulsion (MeSH)[23] OR Tooth replantation (MeSH)[23]	**P**		Tooth avulsion (MeSH)[23] OR Tooth replantation (MeSH)[23]
Pulp extirpation OR Root canal therapy (MeSH)[23]	**I**		Splints (MeSH)[23]
(Same intervention as above, however, timing is the real comparison so that is the factor in the final article selection.)	**C**		(Same intervention as above, however, timing is the real comparison so that is the factor in the final article selection)
Tooth integration OR Functional periodontal healing OR Root resorption (MeSH)[23] OR Tooth ankylosis (MeSH)[23]	**O**	These terms were used as inclusion criteria and were not used when searching PubMed because only a few number of systematic reviews and guidelines were found just using the P, I, and C terms	Tooth integration OR Functional periodontal healing OR Root resorption (MeSH)[23] OR Tooth ankylosis (MeSH)[23]

MeSH, Medical Subject Heading (database); *PICO,* patient problem or population, intervention, comparison, and outcome(s).

Searching for and Acquiring the Evidence

PubMed is designed to provide access to both primary and secondary research from the biomedical literature. PubMed provides free access to MEDLINE, the National Library of Medicine's premier bibliographic database covering the fields of medicine, nursing, dentistry, veterinary medicine, the health care system, and the preclinical sciences. MEDLINE contains bibliographic citations and author abstracts from more than 5200 biomedical journals published in the United States and 80 other countries. The database contains more than 22 million citations dating back to 1966, and it adds more than 520,000 new citations each year.[26]

It is often helpful to identify the appropriate terminology when searching PubMed. This is done by using the Medical Subject Heading (MeSH) database. It provides the definition of terms and illustrates how the terms are indexed in MEDLINE. The PICO terms from the question can be typed into the MeSH database to maximize searching efficiency. For example, by typing "avulsed tooth" into the MeSH database, a term from the case scenario, it is learned that the MeSH term is "tooth avulsion." It is defined as partial or complete displacement of a tooth from its alveolar support. It is commonly the result of trauma. It also is learned that "tooth luxation" links to the MeSH term "tooth avulsion." This informs the searcher that "tooth avulsion" is the best term to use for the search because it encompasses both avulsed and luxated teeth.[23]

Using PubMed's Clinical Queries feature, one can quickly pinpoint a set of citations that will potentially provide an answer to the question being posed. Although online databases provide quicker access to the literature, knowing how databases filter information and having an understanding of how to use search terms and database features allow a more efficient search to be conducted.

Because two focused clinical (PICO) questions were generated from the clinical case, two separate searches were conducted, one for each PICO question. In addition to PubMed, several other databases were used to find high levels of evidence. These included the Database of Abstracts of Reviews of Effects (https://www.crd.york.ac.uk/CRDWeb/), the National Guideline Clearinghouse (http://www.guideline.gov), the ADA Center for Evidence-Based Dentistry website (http://ebd.ada.org), the American Academy of Pediatric Dentistry website (www.aapd.org), and the American Association of Endodontists (www.aae.org), resulting in several relevant references.

When searching for evidence, the PICO question guides the search[4,6] (Table 1.3). By using key terms identified in the PICO question and combining them using the Boolean operators "OR" and "AND," relevant articles can be narrowed to a manageable number.

The first search used the terms "(tooth avulsion OR tooth replantation) AND (pulp extirpation OR root canal therapy)." This resulted in 590 papers. Studies were limited to practice guidelines, MAs, and SRs by using each of these three filters separately so that each of these types of studies could be identified. The findings included four practice guidelines including those of the American Association of Endodontists and the International Association of Dental Traumatology, one critical summary of an SR, and one SR. The second search used the terms "(tooth avulsion OR tooth replantation) AND splints." This resulted in 340 papers. Again, studies were limited to practice guidelines, MAs, and SRs by using the filter for each publication type separately. Relevant results included four practice guidelines from the International Association of Dental Traumatology and Pediatric Dentistry, one MA, and one SR. Fig. 1.3 provides a detailed review of the decision-making steps in this case and the outcomes.[24]

The articles that were selected as relevant research included each aspect of the PICO question. Inclusion criteria included the following: The patient population studied had to have replanted avulsed or luxated teeth; the research studied the intervention for each of the two PICO questions, pulp extirpation and splint duration, respectively; and the research measured at least one of the outcomes of tooth integration, functional periodontal healing, or the levels of resorption or ankylosis. To reduce the requirement of critical appraisal, the search also looked for critical summaries of the SRs that were found.

Appraising the Evidence

After identifying the evidence gathered to answer a question, it is important to have the skills to understand the evidence found. In all cases, it is necessary to review the evidence, whether it is a CPG, MA, SR, or an original study, to determine whether the methods were conducted rigorously and appropriately. International evidence-based groups have made this easier by developing appraisal forms and checklists that guide the user through a structured series of "YES/NO" questions to determine the validity of the individual study or SR. Table 1.4 provides the names and websites of three different guides that can be used for critical analysis.

TABLE 1.4   Examples of Critical Analysis Guides

Guide	Purpose
CONSORT (Consolidated Standards of Reporting Trials) statement[3] http://www.consort-statement.org	To improve the reporting and review of RCTs
PRISMA (Preferred Reporting Items for Systematic Reviews and Meta-analyses) http://www.prisma-statement.org	To improve the reporting and review of SRs
CASP (Critical Appraisal Skills Program)[9] http://www.casp-uk.net	To review RCTs, SRs, and several other types of studies

RCTs, Randomized controlled trials; *SRs*, systematic reviews.

Common Ways Used to Report Results

Once the results are determined to be valid, the next step is to determine whether the results and potential benefits (or harms) are important. Straus and colleagues[31] identified the clinically useful measures for each type of study. For example, in determining the magnitude of therapy results, we would expect articles to report the control event rate (CER), the experimental event rate (EER), the absolute and relative risk reduction (ARR or RRR), and number needed to treat (NNT). The NNT provides the number of patients (e.g., surfaces, periodontal pockets) who would need to be treated with the experimental treatment or intervention to achieve one additional patient (surfaces, periodontal pockets) who has a favorable response. Another way of assessing evidence is presented in Chapter 2, which introduces 12 tools that may be useful in assessing causality in clinical sciences.

In appraising the evidence found for the case scenario, the first research study retrieved that answered the first PICO question was a well-conducted SR published in *Dental Traumatology* in 2009.[17] Results indicated an association between pulp extirpations performed after 14 days following replantation and the development of inflammatory resorption. A corresponding critical summary also was found.[30] This evidence was consistent with the 2007 clinical guidelines from the International Association of Dental Traumatology for pulp extirpation within 10 to 14 days of replantation.[14]

The Practice Guideline on the Management of Acute Dental Trauma from the American Academy of Pediatric Dentistry answered the second PICO question. It recommended a "flexible splint for 1 week" for avulsed teeth. However, for lateral luxation, an additional 2 to 4 weeks may be needed when there is breakdown of marginal bone.[2] In addition, a well-conducted SR about splinting duration reported inconclusive evidence of an association between short-term splinting and an increased likelihood of functional periodontal healing, acceptable healing, or decreased development of replacement resorption.[18] The study found no evidence to contraindicate the current guidelines and suggested that the likelihood of successful periodontal healing after replantation was unaffected by splinting duration. Although this SR excluded studies of luxated teeth, this SR is still applicable to the patient. It concluded that dentists should continue to use the currently recommended splinting periods when replanting avulsed permanent teeth, pending future research to the contrary.[18] Consistent with previous reviews, another SR on splinting luxated, avulsed, and root-fractured teeth reported that "the types of splint and the fixation period are generally not significant variables when related to healing outcomes."[20] These two SRs were appraised using the Critical Appraisal Skills Program (CASP) form for appraising reviews (see Table 1.4).

Applying the Evidence: Evidence-Based Dentistry in Action

Throughout this chapter, the EBDM process has illustrated the application of evidence in clinical decision making. The clinician used the EBDM process to answer two clinical questions. Several relevant resources were incorporated into the decision-making process and the treatment of the patient. The clinician performed pulp extirpations on the avulsed and luxated teeth within the recommended time period of 10 to 14 days (Fig. 1.5A). Healing at 2 weeks post trauma is seen in Fig. 1.5B. The clinician also removed the splint within the recommended time frame for luxated teeth of 2 to 4 weeks. The evidence, in combination with clinical experience, helped provide care for this patient that resulted in the best possible prognosis given the extent of the patient's dental trauma. It also allowed the patient to keep her own teeth, which incorporated the patient preferences aspect of the EBDM process. Fig. 1.5C shows the patient at 4 weeks post trauma; Fig. 1.5D shows the patient at 12 weeks; and Fig. 1.5E shows the patient 2 years post trauma.

Evaluating the Outcomes

The final steps in the EBDM process are to evaluate the effectiveness of the intervention and clinical outcomes and to determine how effectively the EBDM process was applied. For example, one question to ask in evaluating the effectiveness of the intervention is, "Did the selected intervention or treatment achieve the desired result?" In this specific case, the answer is yes.

EBDM is a valuable tool that guides practice decisions to achieve optimal results. In the case of tooth avulsion, the key PICO questions were established to identify research that studied the outcomes of reducing the risk of root resorption and tooth ankylosis and increasing periodontal healing. In using the EBDM process, providers can be confident that they have the most current and relevant evidence available on which to base treatment decisions to provide the best treatment to improve the possibility of a successful outcome.

Using an EBDM approach requires understanding new concepts and developing new skills. In addition to evaluating patient care outcomes, another aspect of evaluation is in using the EBDM process. Questions that parallel each step in the EBDM process can be asked in evaluating self-performance. For example, "How well was the search conducted to find appropriate and relevant evidence to answer the question?" As with most learning, time and practice are essential to mastering new techniques.

CHAPTER HIGHLIGHTS

- Evidence-based decision making (EBDM) provides clinicians the skills to find, efficiently filter, interpret, and apply research findings so that what is known is reflected in the care provided.
- EBDM takes time and practice to learn to use.
- When mastered, EBDM is an efficient way for clinicians to stay current, and it maximizes the potential for successful patient care outcomes

Conclusion

An EBDM approach closes the gap between clinical research and the realities of practice by providing dental practitioners with the skills to find, efficiently filter, interpret, and apply research findings so that what is known is reflected in the care provided. This approach assists clinicians in keeping current with conditions that a patient

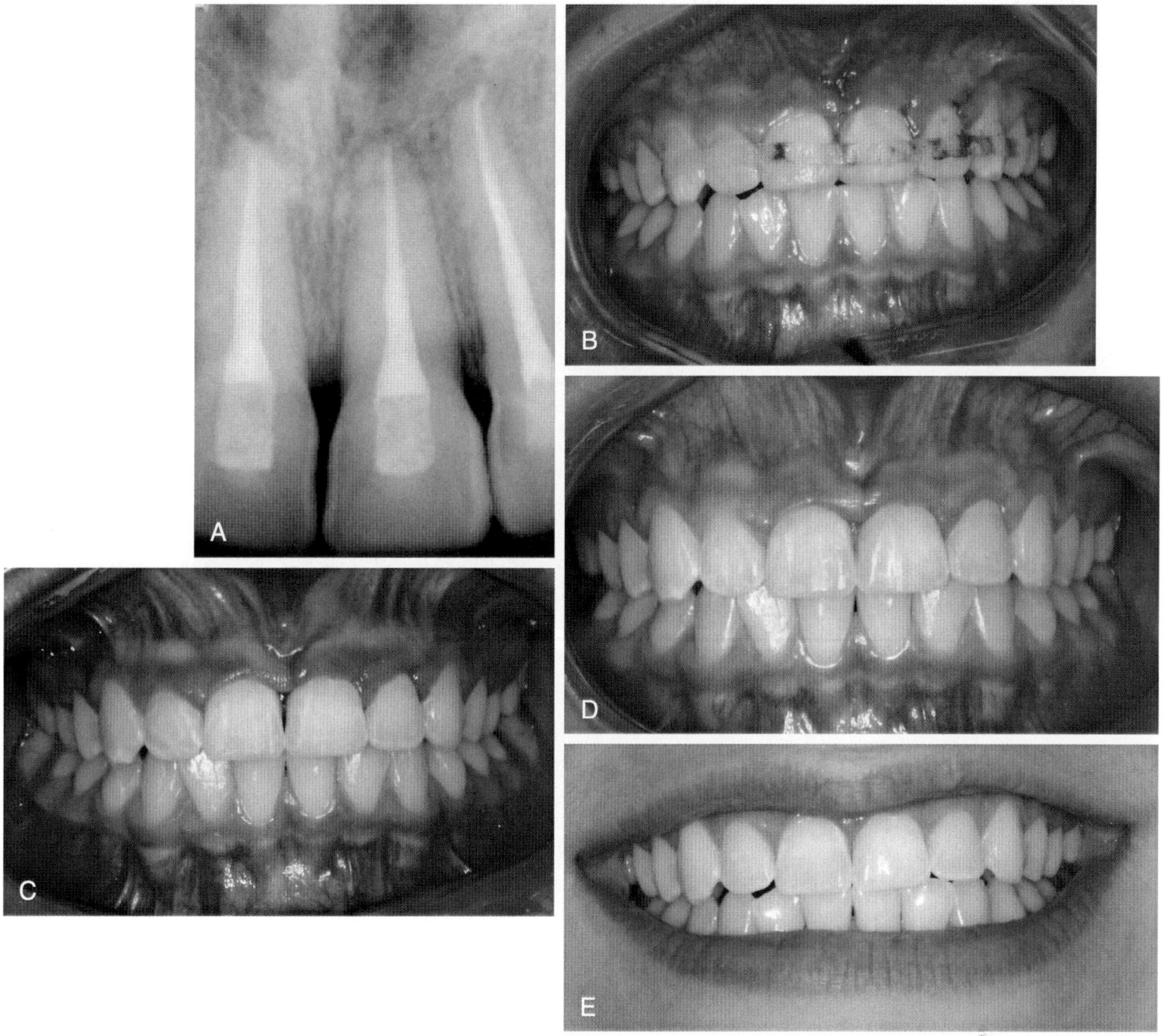

Fig. 1.5 (A) Periapical radiograph following pulp extirpations. (B) Healing at 2 weeks post trauma. (C) Healing at 4 weeks post trauma. (D) Healing at 12 weeks post trauma. (E) Patient 2 years post trauma *(Copyright Greg W. Miller, DDS, reprinted with permission.)*

may have by providing a mechanism for addressing gaps in knowledge to provide the best care possible.

As EBDM becomes standard practice, individuals must be knowledgeable about what constitutes the evidence and how it is reported. Understanding evidence-based methodology and distinctions among different types of articles allows the clinician to judge better the validity and relevance of reported findings. To assist practitioners with this endeavor, SRs and MAs are being conducted to answer specific clinical questions and to support the development of CPGs. Journals devoted to evidence-based practice are being published to alert readers about important advances in a concise and user-friendly manner. By integrating good science with clinical judgment and patient preferences, clinicians enhance their decision-making ability and maximize the potential for successful patient care outcomes.

References

 References for this chapter are found on the companion website www.expertconsult.com.

CHAPTER 2

Critical Thinking: Assessing Evidence

Philippe P. Hujoel

CHAPTER OUTLINE

Twelve Tools for Assessing Evidence
Conclusion

Between 1950 and 2016, 2290 scientific articles were published that have the terms "periodontal diseases" and "antibacterial agents" as Medical Subject Headings. Which of these articles provide information that is clinically relevant? Are those articles that are clinically relevant selected and accurately summarized in educational courses, textbooks, or systematic reviews? Relying completely on authority to ensure that this happens can be dangerous.

Einstein purportedly said that "his own major scientific talent was his ability to look at an enormous number of experiments and journal articles, select the very few that were both correct and important, ignore the rest, and build a theory on the right ones."[6] Most evidence-based clinicians aspire to the same goal when evaluating clinical evidence. In this search for good evidence, a "baloney detection kit"[71] can be helpful to separate salesmanship from science and suggestive hints from unequivocal evidence. This chapter introduces 12 tools that may be useful in assessing causality in clinical sciences.

Twelve Tools for Assessing Evidence

Be Skeptical

Of all machines ours is the most complicated and inexplicable.

—**Thomas Jefferson**

By 1990, it was concluded that "available data thus strongly support the hypothesis that dietary carotenoids reduce the risk of lung cancer."[85] Beta-carotene (β-carotene) was hypothesized to interfere passively with oxidative damage to deoxyribonucleic acid (DNA) and lipoproteins,[38] and these beliefs in part translated into $210 million sales of β-carotene in 1997 in the United States. Was this convincing evidence, or should it be evaluated skeptically? Two large randomized controlled trials (RCTs) were initiated, and both were stopped prematurely because β-carotene increased lung cancer risk, cardiovascular disease risk, and overall mortality risk.[60,79] In 2005, the primary investigator of one of the trials reported that "beta-carotene should be regulated as a human carcinogen."[59] In 2015, mechanistic studies started to demonstrate how antioxidants such as β-carotene accelerate the growth and invasiveness of tumors.[43,62] Similar dramatic turnarounds are in the process on the topic of the "heart-healthy" effects of vegetable oils,[66] dietary salt restriction,[2] or high-carbohydrate diets.[77]

Evidence on how to cure, manage, or prevent chronic diseases is notoriously contradictory, inconsistent, and unreliable. Mark Twain reminded people to be careful when reading health books because one may die of a misprint.[70] Powerful forces conspire to deliver a preponderance of misleading results:

1. Identifying a successful treatment for chronic diseases can be challenging. It has been estimated that less than 0.1% of all investigated treatments are effective. Because the odds of identifying successful interventions for chronic diseases are so small, most so-called effective treatments identified in small clinical trials turn out to be noneffective or harmful when they are evaluated in rigorously conducted pivotal trials.

2. Chronic diseases can be complex and include both environmental and genetic causes. The "obvious" causes of disease, such as tobacco and sugars for periodontitis, are often ignored.[47] As a result of such biased epidemiologic research, incomplete and mistaken understandings of chronic disease etiology can lead to a cascade of wrong turns in the exploration of possible diagnosis, prognosis, and treatment.

3. Poor scientific methodology is a common problem permeating most of the evidence that surrounds us. Popular press headlines tell it all: "Lies, Damned Lies And Medical Statistics,"[69] "Undermined by an Error of Significance: A Widespread Misconception Among Scientists Casts Doubt on the Reliability of a Huge Amount of Research,"[53] "Sloppy Stats Shame Science,"[72] or "How Science Goes Wrong."[27]

4. Finally, the possibility needs to be considered that no magic bullets exist against certain noxious aspects of civilized lifestyles. It was a popular idea in the 20th century that the harmful effects of smoking could be prevented by prescription (e.g., vitamin A), and not proscription (e.g., quit smoking). The experiences so far with finding prescriptions as protection against harmful lifestyles have been largely disastrous.

These factors may all be at play in periodontics, thus suggesting that skepticism is required in the evaluation of scientific evidence. First, the large number of "effective" periodontal treatments may be a telltale sign of a challenging chronic disease. Before 1917, hundreds of pneumonia treatments were available, none of which worked. Before the advent of antibiotics in the 1940s, the wealth of available tuberculosis treatments was misleading in the sense that none really worked. The current "therapeutic wealth" for periodontal diseases may well mean poverty—an indication of the absence of truly effective treatments—and a suggestion that we are dealing with a challenging chronic disease. Second, many no longer regard periodontal diseases as the simple, plaque-related diseases they were thought to be in the mid-20th century, but rather as complex diseases.

Complex diseases are challenging to diagnose, treat, and investigate. Third, the scientific quality of periodontal studies has been rated as low.[4] Major landmark trials were analyzed using wrong statistics,[34,46] most randomized studies were not properly randomized,[55] and the primary drivers of the periodontitis epidemic may have been misunderstood because of the definition of periodontal diseases as an infectious disease without properly controlled epidemiologic studies.[29,30,47] The chance that periodontal research somehow managed to escape the scientific challenges and hurdles that were present in research in medicine appears slim. The opposite appears more likely.

Do Not Trust Biologic Plausibility

Born but to die, and reasoning but to err.

—**Alexander Pope**

If an irregular heartbeat increases mortality risk and if encainide can turn an irregular heartbeat into a normal heartbeat, then encainide should improve survival.[64] If high serum lipid levels increase myocardial infarction risk and if clofibrate can successfully decrease lipid levels, clofibrate should improve survival.[67] If *Streptococcus mutans* causes dental decay and if chlorhexidine can eradicate *S. mutans*, then chlorhexidine can wipe out dental decay. Such "causal chain thinking" (A causes B, B causes C, therefore A causes C) is common and dangerous. These examples of treatment rationales, although seemingly reasonable and biologically plausible, turned out not to help but to harm patients. Causal chain thinking is sometimes referred to as "deductive inference," "deductive reasoning," or a "logical system."

In mathematics, "once the Greeks had developed the deductive method, they were correct in what they did, correct for all time."[5] In medicine or dentistry, decisions based on deductive reasoning have not been "correct for all time" and are certainly not universal. Because of an incomplete understanding of biology, the use of deductive reasoning for clinical decisions may be dangerous. For thousands of years, deductive reasoning largely failed to lead to medical breakthroughs. In evidence-based medicine, evidence that is based on deductive inference is classified as level 5, which is the lowest level of evidence available.

CLINICAL CORRELATION

The Dietary Guidelines for Americans dropped their recommendation to floss because of the lack of scientific evidence. Dental floss has been recommended by oral hygiene companies and the dental profession based on the following biologic plausibility argument: dental plaque causes dental caries; floss removes dental plaque. Therefore, flossing will lower the risk of dental caries. Such reasoning is no longer accepted as evidence for effectiveness in the 21st century.

Unfortunately, much of our knowledge on how to prevent, manage, and treat chronic periodontitis depends largely on deductive reasoning. Small, short-term changes in pocket depth or attachment levels have been assumed to translate into tangible, long-term benefits to patients, but minimal evidence to support this deductive inference leap is available. In one small study without statistical hypothesis testing, dental plaque was related to the transition from an unnatural, inflammation-free condition referred to as "Aarhus superhealthy gingiva" to experimental gingivitis (which is different from clinical gingivitis).[48] Such studies do not offer proof that dental plaque bacteria cause destructive periodontal disease. It is even unclear whether experimental gingivitis and plaque are correlated at a site-specific level above and beyond what would be expected by chance alone.

One subsequent study at the same university, using a similar population, and using a similar experimental design, failed to identify an association between plaque and gingivitis.[48] Evidence that personal plaque control affects the most common forms of periodontal diseases is still weak and largely based on "biologic plausibility" arguments.[31] A move toward a higher level of evidence (higher than biologic plausibility) is needed to put periodontics on a firmer scientific footing.

KEY FACT

Biologic plausibility will increasingly become an unacceptable rationale to recommend dental treatments.

What Level of Controlled Evidence Is Available?

Development of Western science is based on two great achievements: the invention of a formal logical system (in Euclidean geometry) by the Greek philosophers, and the discovery of the possibility to find out causal relationships by systematic experiment (during the Renaissance).

—**Albert Einstein**

Rational thought requires reliance on either deductive reasoning (biologic plausibility) or systematic experiments (sometimes referred to as inductive reasoning). Galileo is typically credited with the start of systematic experimentation in physics. Puzzlingly, it took until the latter half of the 20th century before systematic experiments became part of clinical research. Three systematic experiments are now routine in clinical research: the case-control study, the cohort study, and the RCT. In the following brief descriptions of these three systematic experimental designs, the term *exposure* refers to a suspected etiologic factor or an intervention, such as a treatment or a diagnostic test, and the term *endpoint* refers to the outcome of disease, quality-of-life measures, or any type of condition that may be of interest in clinical studies.

1. *RCT.* Individuals or clusters of individuals are randomly assigned to different exposures and monitored longitudinally for the endpoint of interest. An association between the exposure and the endpoint is present when frequency of the endpoint occurrence differs among the exposure groups. The RCT is the "gold standard" design in clinical research. In evidence-based medicine, RCTs, when properly executed, are referred to as level 1 evidence and the highest (best) level of evidence available.
2. *Cohort study.* Exposed individuals are compared with nonexposed individuals and monitored longitudinally for the occurrence of the primary endpoint of interest. An association between the exposure and endpoint is present when the frequency of endpoint occurrences differs between exposed and nonexposed individuals. A cohort study is often considered the optimal study design in nonexperimental clinical research (i.e., for those study designs where randomization may not be feasible). In evidence-based medicine, cohort studies, when properly executed, are referred to as level 2 evidence.
3. *Case-control study.* Cases (individuals with the endpoint of interest) are compared with controls (individuals without the endpoint of interest) with respect to the prevalence of the exposure. If the prevalence of exposure differs between cases and controls, an association between the exposure and the endpoint is present. In a case-control study, it is challenging to select cases and controls in an unbiased manner and to obtain reliable information on possible causes of disease that occurred in the past. The case-control study is the most challenging study design to use for

obtaining reliable evidence. As a result, in evidence-based medicine, case-control studies, when properly executed, are considered the lowest level of evidence.

All three study designs permit us to study the association between the exposure and the endpoint. This association can be represented schematically as follows:

Exposure → Endpoint

An important challenge in the assessment of controlled evidence is determining whether the association identified (→) is causal. Criteria used to assess causality include factors such as the assessment of temporality, the presence of a pretrial hypothesis, and the size or strength of the reported association. Unlike deductive reasoning, in which associations are either true or false, such absolute truths cannot be achieved with systematic experiments. Conclusions based on controlled study designs are always surrounded by a degree of uncertainty, a frustrating limitation to real-world clinicians who have to make yes/no decisions.

Did the Cause Precede the Effect?

You can't change the laws of physics, Captain.
— **"Scotty" in Star Trek**

In 2001, a study published in the *British Medical Journal* suggested that retroactive prayer shortened hospital stays in patients with bloodstream infection.[45] The only problem was that patients were already dismissed from the hospital when the nonspecified prayer to the nonspecified deity was made. To most scientists, findings in which the effect (shorter hospital stay) precedes the cause (the prayer) are impossible, and this provides an unequivocal example of a violation of correct temporality; the effect preceded the hypothesized cause. In chronic disease research, it is often challenging to disentangle temporality, and fundamental questions regarding temporality often remain disputed. For example, in Alzheimer disease research the amyloid in the senile plaques in the brain is often considered to be the cause of Alzheimer disease, but some researchers suggested that amyloid may be the result rather than the cause of Alzheimer disease and that the amyloid may be protective.[44] Or, it is widely believed that obesity is caused by overeating and insufficient physical activity. Yet, increasing evidence points to the opposite—that obesity is a disease induced by carbohydrates that leads to internal starvation and consequent overeating and physical inactivity.[76] Vigorous investigation of temporality is a key aspect in scientific investigation.

Temporality is the only criterion that needs to be satisfied for claiming causality; the cause needs to precede the effect. In periodontal research, almost all studies relating plaque or specific infections to periodontal diseases suffer from unclear temporality.[47] Are observed microbial profiles the result or the cause of periodontitis? No cohort studies in adults have established that an infectious cause precedes the onset of chronic periodontitis.[47] Unequivocal establishment of temporality is an essential element of causality and can be surprisingly difficult to establish for chronic diseases, including periodontal diseases.

No Betting on the Horse After the Race Is Over

Predictions are difficult, especially about the future.
— **Niels Bohr**

One of the most pervasive cancers in clinical research is the inability of researchers to stick to a hypothesis. Science is about formulating a specific hypothesis, testing it in a clinical experiment, and accepting the findings for what they are. Not only does this rarely happen, but also powerful forces sometimes actively try to prevent regulations that would enforce such scientific behavior.

An acquired immunodeficiency syndrome (AIDS) researcher at an international AIDS conference was jeered when she claimed that AIDS therapy provided a significant benefit for a subgroup of trial participants.[58] A study published in the *New England Journal of Medicine*[49] was taken as a textbook example of poor science[19] when it claimed that coffee drinking was responsible for more than 50% of the pancreatic cancers in the United States. Results of a large collaborative study demonstrating that aspirin use after myocardial infarction increased mortality risk in patients born under Gemini or Libra provided a comical example of an important scientific principle: data-generated ideas are unreliable.

An essential characteristic of science is that hypotheses or ideas predict observations, not that hypotheses or ideas can be fitted to observations. This essential characteristic of scientific enterprise—prediction—is often lost in medical and dental research when poorly defined prestudy hypotheses result in convoluted data-generated ideas or hypotheses that fit the observed data. It has been reported that even for well-organized studies with carefully written protocols, investigators often do not remember which hypotheses were defined in advance, which hypotheses were data derived, which hypotheses were "a priori" considered plausible, and which were unlikely.[87] A wealth of data-generated ideas can be created by exploring patient subgroups, exposures, and endpoints, as shown by the following:

1. Modifying study sample definition. A commonly observed posttrial modification of a hypothesis is to evaluate improper or proper subgroups of the original study sample. Improper subgroups are based on patients' characteristics that may have been influenced by the exposure. For example, one may evaluate tumor size only in those patients who survived or pocket depths only in those teeth that were not lost during maintenance. Results of improper subgroup analyses are almost always meaningless when establishing causality. Proper subgroups are based on patients' characteristics that cannot be influenced by the exposure, such as sex, race, or age. A review of trials in the area of cardiovascular disease suggested that even the results of proper subgroup analyses turn out to be misleading in a majority of cases.[87] In the human immunodeficiency virus (HIV) area, one proper subgroup analysis (based on racial characteristics) drew an investor lawsuit on the basis that company officials "deceived" investors with a "fraudulent scheme."[15]

2. Modifying exposure definition. After or during the conduct of a study, the exposure definition can be changed, or the number of exposures under study can be modified. In a controversial trial on the use of antibiotics for middle ear infections, the placebo treatment was replaced with a boutique antibiotic, thus causing a potentially misleading perception of the antibiotics' effectiveness.[16,17,50] In another example of "betting on the horse after the race was over," a negative finding for cigarette smoking (the primary exposure) as a cause of pancreatic cancer reportedly led to the data-generated hypothesis that coffee drinking increased pancreatic cancer risk.[49] When this study was repeated in the same hospital, using the same protocol, but now with the pretrial hypothesis to evaluate coffee drinking, the results of the prior study could not be duplicated.

3. Modifying endpoint definition. Almost all pivotal trials specify one primary endpoint in the pretrial hypothesis. In periodontal research the absence of a specific pretrial defined endpoint is common and permits effortless changing of the endpoint definition. The typical periodontal trial has six endpoints and does not specify

which endpoint is primary, and it is not always clear what is a good or a bad outcome.[19] Similarly, the definition of adverse pregnancy outcomes is flexible and susceptible to post hoc manipulations to squeeze out statistical significance. Statistical trickery to reach desired conclusions under such circumstances may be child's play. These problems have remained rampant in clinical research despite all efforts at preventing them. Two surveys of RCTs published in 2015 reported that 18% to 31% of the trials still changed primary endpoints, and 64% of the trials still changed secondary endpoints.[21,39]

Deviating from the pretrial hypothesis is often compared to data torturing.[54] Detecting the presence of data torturing in a published article is often challenging; just as the talented torturer leaves no scars on the victim's body, the talented data torturer leaves no marks on the published study. Long-term efforts at registering all trials (e.g., see www.alltrials.net) have still not solved this problem.[11] Opportunistic data torturing refers to exploring data without the goal of "proving" a particular point of view. Opportunistic data torturing is an essential aspect of scientific activity and hypothesis generation. Procrustean data torturing refers to exploring data with the goal of proving a particular point of view. Just as the Greek mortal Procrustes fitted guests perfectly to his guest bed either through bodily stretching or through chopping of the legs to ensure correspondence between body height and bed length, so can data be fitted to the pretrial hypothesis by Procrustean means.

What Is a Clinically Relevant Pretrial Hypothesis?

Clinically relevant questions are designed to have an impact on improving patients' outcomes. Usually, clinically relevant questions share four important characteristics of the pretrial hypothesis: (1) a clinically relevant endpoint (referred to as the Outcome in the PICO question), (2) relevant exposure comparisons (referred to as the Intervention and the Control in the PICO question, (3) a study sample representative of real-world clinical patients (should be representative of the Patient defined in the PICO question), and (4) small error rates.

Clinically Relevant Endpoint

An endpoint is a measurement related to a disease process or a condition and is used to assess the exposure effect. Two different types of endpoints are recognized. True endpoints are tangible outcomes that directly measure how a patient feels, functions, or survives[78]; examples include tooth loss, death, and pain. Surrogate endpoints are intangible outcomes used as a substitute for true endpoints[22]; examples include blood pressure and probing depths of periodontal pockets. Treatment effects on surrogates do not necessarily translate into real clinical benefit (Table 2.1). Reliance on surrogate endpoints in clinical trials has led to widespread use of deadly medications, and such disasters have prompted minor changes in the drug approval process.[65] Most major causes of human disease (e.g., cigarette smoking) were identified through studies using true endpoints. A first requirement for a clinically relevant study is the pretrial specification of a true endpoint.

Common and Relevant Comparisons

The more prevalent a studied exposure is, the more relevant is the clinical question. A clinically relevant comparison implies the absence of comparator bias, which is defined as the presence of contrived or unethical control groups.[51] Providing the control subjects with less than the standard dose of the standard treatment and providing a control therapy that avoids the real clinical questions are examples of clinically irrelevant research. Similarly, the presence of a placebo treatment instead of "no" treatment in clinical trials can be critical given the large therapeutic effects that can be obtained by proper attention and care in medical settings. For instance, the absence of placebo controls in fluoride varnish trials for primary teeth raises serious doubts whether fluoride varnish has an effect above and beyond what would be observed with just a placebo. In case-control or cohort studies, the measurement and characterization of exposures (e.g., mercury, fluoride, chewing tobacco) can be difficult and imprecise, thus making answers to the questions almost unavoidably imprecise.

Representative Study Sample

The larger the discrepancy between the typical subjects enrolled in clinical studies and the patient you seek to treat, the more questionable the applicability of the study's conclusions becomes. When cholesterol-lowering drugs provided a small benefit in middle-aged men with abnormally high cholesterol levels, it was concluded that those benefits "could and should be extended" to other age groups and women with "more modest elevations" of cholesterol levels.[80] Findings on blood lipids and heart disease that were derived mostly from Polish immigrants in the Framingham Study were generalized to a much more diverse population. An antidepressant that was approved for use in adults was widely prescribed for children, with unexpected, serious consequences.[1]

Ideally, clinical trials should use simple entry criteria in which the enrolled patients reflect the real-world clinical practice situation as closely as possible. Legislation has been enacted to reach this goal. In 1993, US policy ensured the recruitment of women and minority groups in clinical trials.[10] A US policy for the inclusion of children in clinical studies was then set into law in 1998. Experiments with long lists of inclusion and exclusion criteria can be expensive recipes for failure because they can lead to study subjects who are unrepresentative of most real-world clinical patients.

Small Type I and Type II Error Rates

The type I error rate is the likelihood of concluding that an effect exists when in truth no effect exists. The type I error rate is set by the investigator, and common values are 1% or 5%. The type II error rate is the likelihood of concluding that no effect exists when in truth an effect does exist. The type II error rate is typically set by the investigator at 10% or 20%. The complement of the type II error rate (i.e., 1 − type II error rate) is referred to as the power of the study. The likelihood of a false-positive or false-negative result depends, in addition to the type I and II error rates, on the likelihood that the treatment under investigation is truly effective. This last component is obviously not under the investigator's control, and yet it determines the likelihood of making correct conclusions. For chronic diseases, in which the likelihood of identifying effective treatments or true causes is low, the false-positive rate can be high even when the type I error rate is low. Clinically relevant studies require small type I and type II error rates to minimize false-positive and false-negative conclusions.[36]

Size Does Matter

Chronic hepatitis B infection increased the chances for liver cancer by more than 23,000%.[7] Proximity to electromagnetic radiation increased the chance for leukemia in children by 49%.[84] Periodontitis in populations with smokers increased the chance for coronary heart disease by 12%.[32] No one doubts the causality of the association between chronic hepatitis B infection and liver cancer, but the role of periodontitis in coronary heart disease or electromagnetic radiation in childhood leukemia remain controversial. Why? To a large extent, the size of the association drives the interpretation of causality.

TABLE 2.1 Examples of Potentially Misleading Surrogates[a]

Disease or Condition	Experimental Treatment	Control Treatment	Effect on Surrogate Endpoint	Effect on True Endpoint	Misleading Conclusion	Reference
AIDS	Immediate zidovudine	Delayed zidovudine	Significant increase of 30–35 CD4 cells/mm^3	No change in incidence of AIDS, AIDS-related complex, or survival	False-positive	80
Osteoporosis	Fluoride	Placebo	Significant increase of 16% in bone mineral density of lumbar spine	Nonvertebral fracture rates increased by 85%	False-positive	
Lung cancer	ZD1839 (Iressa)	Placebo	Dramatic tumor shrinkage in 10% of patients	No effect	False-positive	82
Aphthous ulcers	Thalidomide	Placebo	Although thalidomide expected to decrease TNF-α production, significant increase of 4.4 pg/mL in TNF-α production occurred, suggesting harm	Pain diminished and ability to eat improved	False-negative	32
Edentulism	Implant-supported dentures	Conventional dentures	No impact on chewing cycles	Improved oral health–related quality of life	False-negative	5
Prostate cancer	Radical prostatectomy	Watchful waiting	Substantial elimination of tumor mass	No effect on overall mortality risk	False-positive	78
Advanced colorectal cancer	5-FU + LV	5-FU	23% of patients had 50% or greater reduction in tumor volume	No effect on overall survival	False-positive	40
Periodontitis	Surgery	Scaling	Mean pocket depth reduced by 0.5 mm	Effect on tooth loss or quality of life unknown	?	30a

[a]For some examples, the experimental treatment led to improvements in surrogate endpoints, whereas the true endpoint was either unaffected or worsened (a false-positive conclusion). For other examples, the experimental treatment had no impact or worsened the surrogate endpoint, whereas the true endpoint improved (a false-negative conclusion).
AIDS, Acquired immunodeficiency syndrome; *5-FU,* 5-fluorouracil; *LV,* leucovorin; *TNF-α,* tumor necrosis factor-alpha.

The larger an association, the less likely it is to be caused by bias, and the more likely it is causal. One simple way to calculate the size of the association is to calculate an odds ratio. The odds of an event represent the probability that an event happens divided by the probability that an event does not happen. An odds ratio is a ratio of odds. To calculate an odds ratio, a two-by-two (2 × 2) table is constructed in which the outcome is cross-tabulated with the exposure (Table 2.2). Odds ratios can be calculated for data from RCTs, cohort studies, and case-control studies.

The odds ratio is the ratio of the cross-products (ad/bc). The odds ratio associated with penciclovir use for oral lesion healing is (376 × 757) / (526 × 878) = 0.62 (Table 2.3). The odds ratio associated with chronic periodontitis for a fatal myocardial infarction is (2 × 1241) / (8 × 257) = 1.21 (Table 2.4). The 95% confidence interval can be approximated by exp[ln(odds ratio) ± 1.96 $\sqrt{(1/a + 1/b + 1/c + 1/d)}$]. The 95% confidence intervals of the odds ratio for lesion healing and fatal myocardial infarction are, respectively, exp(−0.48 ± 1.96 $\sqrt{0.007}$), or 0.52 to 0.73, and exp(0.18 ± 1.96 $\sqrt{0.63}$), or 0.25 to 5.72.

The size of the odds ratio ranges between 0 and infinity. An odds ratio of 1 indicates the absence of an association, and if the two-by-two table is set up with the reference cell (poor outcome exposure of interest) in the left-hand side of the top data row, an odds ratio larger

TABLE 2.2 Two-by-Two Table Cross-Classifying Exposure and Endpoint[a]

		ENDPOINT	
		Failure	Success
Exposure	Experimental	A	B
	Control	C	D

[a]Note that the top left cell, by convention, tallies the number of failures for the experimental group.

TABLE 2.3 Two-by-Two Table on Association Between Penciclovir and Oral Lesion Healing

		ENDPOINT	
		No Lesion Healing by Day 6	Lesion Healing by Day 6
Exposure	1% Penciclovir	376	878
	Placebo	526	757

TABLE 2.4 Two-by-Two Table on Association Between Chronic Periodontitis and Fatal Myocardial Infarction

		ENDPOINT	
		Fatal MI	No Fatal MI
Exposure	CP	2	257
	No gingivitis or CP	8	1241

CP, Chronic periodontitis; *MI*, myocardial infarction.

than 1 means a harmful effect (e.g., periodontitis increases the odds of a fatal myocardial infarction by 20%), and an odds ratio smaller than 1 means a protective effect (e.g., penciclovir decreases the odds of failed lesion healing by day 6 by 38%).

The confidence interval is the range of numbers between the upper confidence limit and the lower confidence limit. The confidence interval contains the true odds ratio with a certain predetermined probability (e.g., 95%). In a properly executed randomized trial, a conclusion of causality is typically made if the 95% confidence interval does not include the possibility of "no association" (e.g., odds ratio = 1). For example, because the 95% confidence interval for the odds ratio associated with penciclovir use is 0.52 to 0.73 and does not include 1, the effect can be referred to as "statistically significant." For the chronic periodontitis–myocardial infarction example, the 95% confidence interval ranges from 0.25 to 5.72, includes 1, and is therefore referred to as "statistically insignificant."

In epidemiology, where no randomization of individuals to exposures occurs, the interpretation of a confidence interval is challenging because no probabilistic basis (in the form of randomization) exists for making causal inference. A pessimist will claim that because no randomization was present, no statistical interpretations are allowed.[24] The emphasis should be on visual display of the identified associations and on sensitivity analyses where the results are interpreted under "what if" assumptions. An optimist will argue that the absence of randomization does not preclude the making of statistical inferences, and that one always starts from the assumption that "assignments were random" (even when they were not).[88]

When individuals are randomly assigned to exposures, very small associations (i.e., associations very close to 1, such as 1.1) can reliably be identified. When individuals are not randomly assigned to exposures, as is the case in cohort studies and case-control studies, the size of the reported association (e.g., the odds ratio) becomes key in the interpretation of the findings. Because of the inherent biases in epidemiologic research, small odds ratios cannot be reliably identified. But what is small? Leading epidemiologists provide some guidelines on how to interpret the size of an association with respect to possible causality. Richard Doll, one of the founders of epidemiology, said, "No single epidemiological study is persuasive by itself unless the lower limit of its 95% confidence level falls above a threefold (200%) increased risk." Dimitrios Trichopoulos, past chairperson of the Department of Epidemiology at Harvard University, opted "for a fourfold (300%) increase at the lower limit (of the 95% confidence interval)." Marcia Angell, former editor of the *New England Journal of Medicine,* reported: "As a general rule of thumb we are looking for an odds ratio of 3 or more (≥200% increased odds) [before accepting a paper for publication]." Robert Temple, Director of the Food and Drug Administration, stated: "My basic rule is if the odds ratio isn't at least 3 or 4 (a 200% or 300% increased risk), forget it."[75] Textbooks on evidence-based medicine report an odds ratio of 3 for cohort studies and 4 for case-control studies as a reflection of a reliable result.[74] These opinions provide some guidelines on what size of odds ratio to look for when determining causality.

Periodontitis during pregnancy was reported to increase the risk for preterm low birth weight eightfold.[20]

Is a Better Alternative Explanation Available?

No amount of experimentation can ever prove me right; a single experiment can prove me wrong.

—**Albert Einstein**

When you have eliminated the impossible, whatever remains, however improbable, must be the truth.

—**Sir Arthur Conan Doyle**

Dozens of epidemiologic studies appeared to support the hypothesis that β-carotene intake lowered lung cancer risk. However, RCTs provided unequivocal evidence to the contrary. What went wrong? Different explanations that worked as well or better may have been inadequately explored. Possibly, smoking was not adequately considered as an alternative explanation and led to a misunderstanding of the health effects of β-carotene.[20,73] Similarly, a systematic review of epidemiologic studies appeared to support the hypothesis that chronic periodontitis caused low birth weight.[86] In contrast, however, a systematic review of RCTs suggested that the periodontitis–low birth weight theory may be dead.[83] Why was epidemiology misleading? Again, different explanations may have been inadequately explored. More efforts may have been expended toward proving associations by ignoring common causal factors rather than disproving associations. The highest goal of a scientist is the attempt to refute, disprove, and vigorously explore factors and alternative hypotheses that may "explain away" the observed association.[12] The efforts at refuting smoking and nutrition as potential confounders in periodontics have been minimal and may have led to a significant waste of clinical research resources.

Epidemiologic studies are by nature unreliable. It has been estimated that 80% of the epidemiologic studies report false-positive findings. Two large pivotal trials on periodontal treatments and adverse pregnancy outcomes funded by the National Institutes of Health,[20,73] as well as subsequent epidemiologic studies,[86] failed to confirm the dramatic claims of previously published epidemiologic studies.

For a factor (i.e., a potential confounder) to explain away an observed association, two criteria need to be fulfilled. First, the factor must be related to the exposure, but not necessarily in causal way. Second, the factor must be causally related to the outcome and must not be in the causal pathway. If both criteria are satisfied, the factor is referred to as a confounder, and confounding is said to be present. For example, smoking satisfied the criteria for a confounder in the β-carotene–lung cancer association because (1) cigarette smokers consumed less β-carotene than nonsmokers and (2) smoking caused lung cancer. Confounding is often represented schematically (Fig. 2.1).

In randomized studies, confounding is typically not an issue because randomization balances known and unknown confounders across the compared groups with a high degree of certainty. In epidemiologic studies, in which no randomization is present, three

Fig. 2.1 Schematic representation of the two necessary criteria for a variable to induce spurious associations (i.e., to be a confounding variable). The confounding variable has to be associated with the exposure and causally linked to the outcome. When both criteria are satisfied, confounding is said to be present.

questions related to confounding need to be considered in the assessment of the causality, as addressed next.

First, were all important confounders identified? Complex diseases have multiple risk factors, which may act as confounders in the reported association. The multiple confounders need to be included in the statistical analyses. An association unadjusted for any potential confounders is sometimes referred to as the *crude association*. When this crude association is adjusted for potential confounders, it is referred to as an *adjusted association*. Typically, crude and adjusted odds ratios are both presented so readers can evaluate the direction of the bias.

KEY FACT

Single epidemiologic studies reporting large odds ratios are unreliable.

Second, how accurately were confounders measured? Some potential confounders, such as age, sex, and race, can be measured relatively accurately. Other potential confounders, such as smoking or lifestyle factors such as nutrition, are notoriously more difficult to measure. A discrepancy between what is measured and what is the truth will result in the incomplete removal of bias and lead to spurious associations. The remaining bias is sometimes referred to as *residual confounding*. Residual confounding is common in epidemiology and is one of the reasons that case-control and cohort studies are less effective research tools than randomized trials in identifying small effects. For instance, an accurate summary of smoking history over a person's lifetime may be impossible.

Third, was the statistical modeling of the confounders appropriate? Any mis-specification of the functional relationships causes bias. For example, assuming a linear relationship between a confounder and an endpoint, whereas in truth the relationship is quadratic, causes bias.

Evaluating the impact of confounding can be a challenge. The goal of an epidemiologist is to come up with the best possible defense why an identified association is spurious. All possible efforts should be spent identifying known confounders, obtaining accurate measurements of the confounders, and exploring different analytic approaches to refute the observed association. Smoking, a potential confounder in many studies, has been found to be such a strong confounder that several leading epidemiologists have suggested that restriction to never-smokers is required to eliminate the potential for residual confounding by smoking. Control for confounding is the major methodologic challenge in epidemiology, and randomization is the only tool available to eliminate confounding reliably.

CLINICAL CORRELATION

Epidemiologic evidence has suggested that periodontal patients who comply with periodontal maintenance procedures lose fewer teeth.[33]

Was the Study Properly Randomized?

It is often taken for granted that randomization is properly performed in RCTs. This is unfortunately not the case. Attempts by physicians to circumvent randomization are not isolated events; they used to be part of an endemic problem stemming from ignorance.[58]

Randomization can be a counterintuitive process because it (1) creates heterogeneity, (2) takes control over treatment assignment away from the physician, and (3) leads to apparently illogical situations in which patients randomly assigned to a treatment but refusing compliance still are analyzed as if they received the treatment. Although randomization was a radical innovation introduced for agriculture, some have suggested that it is doubtful whether it would have ever been widely introduced into medicine (and subsequently dentistry) if not for a confluence of factors surrounding the end of World War II in Great Britain. Because of the revolutionary nature of randomization, fundamental misunderstandings of this process remained prevalent until recently. In 1994, about one-third of the clinical trials published in elite medical journals apparently did not ensure that patients are assigned to different treatments by chance.[58] The majority of reported periodontal trials failed to convince reviewers that (1) the studies were properly randomized, (2) randomization was concealed, or (3) randomized patients were accounted for.[55] Tampering with the delicate process of randomization can quickly, according to Ronald Fisher, a statistician and geneticist, turn an experiment into an experience.

KEY FACT

Patients who comply with medical or dental recommendations are typically healthier. As a result, interventions that increase mortality risk in randomized trials will spuriously appear to decrease mortality in epidemiologic studies. The reason for this discrepancy is healthy user bias. A Canadian study[17a] demonstrated that patients compliant with taking statins are less likely to have accidents (e.g., burns), more likely to undergo medical screening (e.g., eye examination), less likely to have dental problems, and less likely to have other serious medical problems such as deep vein thrombosis. Such effects are typically interpreted as examples of healthy user bias. The effectiveness of periodontal treatments in providing tangible patient benefits cannot reliably be estimated in epidemiologic studies due to the healthy user bias.

Several studies have shown how an inadequate randomization process will bias study findings. In one review study, the ability to reject patients from the study after random treatment assignment tripled the likelihood of finding significant results and doubled the likelihood that confounders were unequally distributed among the compared groups.[13] Trials where clinicians can break the randomization code reported treatment effects that averaged 30% larger than effects in trials where the randomization could not be broken.[13] The common desire to eliminate noncompliant patients can similarly lead to biases, as shown by the following two examples. First, in one cardiovascular disease trial, patients compliant with a placebo pill had a 10% reduction in mortality risk compared with patients who were noncompliant with the placebo.[67] Second, in a caries trial, adolescents compliant with a placebo varnish had on average 2.2 fewer new caries lesions than adolescents noncompliant with a placebo varnish.[23]

Such findings suggest that factors related to compliance and unrelated to the treatments under investigation have a powerful influence on the outcome measured. Deleting such noncompliant patients may lead to biases.

Proper randomization ideally includes the following elements. First, subjects are enrolled into a study before randomization: important baseline disease characteristics are recorded and provided to an independent person or organization. This step ensures that baseline information is available for every patient who will be randomized. Without this step, randomized patients can be "lost," thus leading to biases. Subsequently, an independent person or organization randomly assigns subjects to treatments and informs the clinician regarding the treatment assignment. This randomization process needs to be auditable, a requirement that makes pseudorandom processes such as coin tosses unacceptable. The concealment of the randomization process ensures that clinicians cannot crack the code and that they will enroll only those patients they think are suited for the treatment that will be assigned. Finally, the outcome in the subject is evaluated regardless of follow-up time or compliance and according to the treatment assigned, not the treatment received. Imputation is used in sensitivity analyses to determine the extent that subjects with missing information can bias the conclusions. The whole process of randomization is complex and often deviated from, thereby leading to unreliable results.

When to Rely on Nonrandomized Evidence

Randomize the first patient.
                                      —**Thomas Chalmers**

To tell the truth, all of the discussion today about the patient's informed consent still strikes me as absolute rubbish.
                              —**Sir Austin Bradford Hill**

Scores of epidemiologic studies reported evidence that hormone replacement therapy provided benefits to postmenopausal women. Despite this "strong" evidence from "leading" researchers, and despite the opposition on ethical grounds to begin a placebo-controlled trial, the Women's Health Initiative trial was initiated. The "miracle" of hormone replacement therapy was shown to lead to increased breast cancer risk, dementia, myocardial infarction, and stroke. This example illustrates the need for randomized studies and for questioning well-established and widely accepted beliefs based on numerous epidemiologic studies. Nonetheless, the initiation of randomized trials can become difficult because of ethical considerations and expensively large sample sizes.

Ethical principles dictate that proposed interventions do more good than harm, that the populations in whom the study will be conducted will benefit from the findings, that informed consent is obtained from enrolled subjects, and that a genuine uncertainty exists with respect to treatment efficacy. The interpretation of these ethical principles is largely determined by culture and era. Ethical principles also play an important role in determining which clinical questions are sufficiently important to warrant the conduct of an RCT.

Sample size requirements represent another consideration that may prevent the conduct of RCTs. The smaller the rate at which endpoints occur in an RCT, the larger the required sample size will be. For rare events, such as bacterial endocarditis subsequent to a dental procedure or HIV conversion after exposure to an HIV-contaminated dental needle, RCTs may never be possible because the required sample sizes are in the 100,000s or millions of subjects.

In addition to both ethical and practical reasons, powerful political issues can surround the decision to initiate clinical trials. It has been pointed out that specialists are unlikely to support clinical trials that evaluate their main source of income.[63] This observation for medical specialties may also hold for periodontics. Although dental professional organizations commonly claim that periodontal disease is a major cause of tooth loss, evidence indicates that standard periodontal therapy is not effective at reducing tooth loss. Hopefully, well-designed and well-conducted studies in the future will allow us to compare different treatments effectively. Unequivocal evidence requires the conduct of rigorously designed and executed RCTs. The absence of RCT evidence for important and answerable clinical questions can be frustrating to those who seek reliable, evidence-based practice guidelines.

Did the Investigators Take Into Account the Placebo or Nocebo Effects?

I never knew any advantage from electricity in (the treatment of) palsies that was permanent. And how far the apparent temporary advantage might arise from the exercise in the patient's journey, and coming daily to my house, or from the spirits given by the hope of success, enabling them to exert more strength in moving their limbs, I will not pretend to say.
                              —**Benjamin Franklin**[82]

Sham or mock surgical procedures have been used to evaluate whether implanting human fetal tissue in the brain decreases symptoms of Parkinson disease, whether surgical lavage and debridement decrease pain in arthritic knee joints,[56] whether mammary artery ligation improves heart disease outcomes,[14] and whether alveolar trephination relieves the pain of acute apical periodontitis.[26,57]

What motivates clinical investigators to subject patients to surgical risks and yet knowingly provide no hypothesized benefits to these patients? A partial answer to this question lies in a phenomenon known as placebo or nocebo effects: the beneficial or harmful effects patients may experience by participating in a study, by patient–physician interaction, by the patient's anticipation for improvement, or by the patient's desire to please the physician. One group of researchers suspects that the placebo or nocebo effect may be related to the balance of the parasympathetic and sympathetic nervous system, which could explain both placebo and nocebo effects.[41] Without mock surgical procedures it would be impossible to tell whether the improvements observed in clinical trials are caused by the placebo effects associated with the surgical procedures or by the hypothesized active ingredient of the surgery itself.

Two studies have quantified the placebo effect. In the first study, the magnitude of the placebo effect was estimated by evaluating patients' responses to ineffective treatments.[68] Five treatments were identified as ineffective (all these treatments had been abandoned by the medical profession and in at least one controlled study confirmed its ineffectiveness). With these ineffective treatments, good to excellent treatment responses were observed in 45% to 90% of the patients, a powerful placebo effect indeed. In the second study, placebo interventions (pharmacologic placebo, physical, or psychological interventions) were compared with true "no-treatment" interventions.[28] A significant placebo effect was observed for pain, the condition that was evaluated in the largest number of trials and that had the largest number of evaluated participants.

Placebo effects can reliably be estimated only when clinical trials randomly assign patients to a placebo treatment and no treatment. Such studies are rare. Some systematic reviews may provide a hint at the magnitude of placebo effects. One systematic review of 133 studies reported that the fluoride effect on caries was significantly larger when a no-treatment control group was used versus a placebo control group.[52] One possible interpretation for these differences is a placebo effect: the placebo lowered caries rates possible through re-equilibrating of parasympathetic and sympathetic nervous activity, which may influence factors such as improved saliva flow. Other explanations, such as the scientific quality of the studies, may, of course, also be responsible for such observed differences, especially for pain. Overall, sufficient evidence is available to suggest that placebo effects can be real and measurable, and that the magnitude of the placebo effect may depend on the treatment under study and the type of outcome evaluated.

Was Protection in Place Against Conflict of Interest?

In evidence-based medicine, the data from clinical research remain largely esoteric and of no real-world significance if the evidence fails to be translated into clinical practice. Spinal fusion, vertebroplasty, and arthroscopic surgery for knee pain have all shown noneffectiveness in clinical trials, yet these trials had no impact on clinical practice. In some instance, the use of surgical procedures actually increased after a demonstration of noneffectiveness.[37,42] Such discrepancies between clinical practice and science have been in part attributed to "perverse financial incentives."[37]

Can one trust clinical recommendations regarding a novel, noninvasive cardiac bypass operation by a physician who has a $100 million stake in the procedure he or she is recommending? Is it possible that financial stakes are preventing physicians from disclosing a 10-fold increased mortality risk? Can one trust guidelines establishing sharply lowered lipid levels while knowing that eight of the nine panel experts have financial connections to the manufacturers of lipid-lowering drugs? Is it possible that panelists are picked for ideology?[8] Can one trust clinical guidelines published by professional dental organizations? The answers to these questions are not straightforward and in general are discussed under the heading of "conflicts of interest."

Conflict of interest has been defined as "a set of conditions in which professional judgment concerning a primary interest (such as patient's welfare or validity of research) tends to be unduly influenced by a secondary interest."[3] A common secondary interest is financial but can include others, such as religious or scientific beliefs, ideologic or political beliefs, or academic interests (e.g., promotion). Some examples of how conflicts of interests can bias evidence are now given:

1. Evidence can be suppressed by lawsuits. For example, a company initiated a multimillion-dollar legal action[15] against the investigator who reported that the company's HIV vaccine was ineffective.[40] Companies can attempt to suppress submitted scientific articles that they perceive as incorrect.

2. Negative evidence can disappear into a "black hole."[25] One can expect that 2 of 40 trials of an ineffective treatment will provide positive results by chance if the experiments are run with a type I error rate of 5%. If the 38 negative trial reports go into a file drawer, and if the 2 positive reports lead to drug approval and are published in leading journals, a misleading perception of the drug's effectiveness will be given to the practicing community. Although a Food and Drug Administration official indicated that such situations have never happened,[18] reports on nondisclosed negative trials of an antidepressant drug suggests the contrary.[81] Although registries of clinical trials should succeed at eliminating the problem of disappearing trial results, and although many leading journals request a priori trial registration as a prerequisite for publishing, the problem of disappearing trial results remains with us today.

3. Conflicts of interest can lead to distortion of study designs and analyses to provide the desired results. Such distortions can range from data fabrication and data falsification to design and analysis "tweaks" such as contrived control groups, unplanned subgroup analyses, and only showing that time point in the analysis where the differences favor the investigated drug.

4. Conflicts of interests related to loss of patents or orphan drugs can shunt available research resources to the conduct of clinical trials that are not necessarily in the best interest of public health. The potential for conflict of interest appears to be ever increasing. The prevalence of industry-funded trials is increasing, and more and more universities hold stock in start-up companies that support clinical trials within those institutions. Such connections can be viewed with a skeptical eye. It has been confirmed over and over again that industry-sponsored studies are more likely to have proindustry conclusions than are non–industry-sponsored studies.[9]

Protection against potential conflict of interest is an important aspect of clinical research. Mandatory registration of clinical trials helps. The appointment of independent data and safety monitoring boards for trial monitoring provides protection against biases. Policy regulations established by journals, academic institutions, and governments can further decrease the impact of perceived conflicts of interests. For instance, all the work that has been done toward establishing registries of RCTs helps in decreasing biases.

Conflict of interest issues may be just as prevalent in dental research as in other medical areas dealing with chronic disease. In 2002, an article published in a leading dental journal ended up on the cover of the *New York Times*.[61] In part, the reason was a perceived conflict of interest; the article did not disclose that funding for the study came from an advertising company. Disclosure of conflict of interest is often poorly enforced, and some dental journals do not have regulations in place to reveal potential conflicts of interest of authors. Such situations (1) make it challenging for clinicians to recognize the potential for conflicts of interest, (2) may reduce trust in dental journals, and (3) may affect the scientific integrity of dental research.

Conclusion

Lessons learned from other chronic disease areas do apply to the evaluation of evidence in the periodontal disease research arena. Randomization and confounding are as important in periodontal research as they are in cancer research. Work remains to be done to integrate evidence-based thinking into clinical practice. One challenging task is to lessen the excessive reliance on biologic plausibility in determining both research priorities and patient management and to transition to clinical thinking that is based on controlled clinical observations. Maybe, however, the most challenging task for the dental profession to eliminate this bias will be to comply with the Institute of Medicine guideline largely to exclude experts from writing clinical guidelines.[35] Although the 12 discussed tools for assessing evidence do not cover all necessary tools, or maybe even the most important tools, it is hoped that they provide a useful starting point for the further exploration of the issues and principles involved in the conduct of systematic experiments in periodontal disease research.

References

 References for this chapter are found on the companion website www.expertconsult.com.

CHAPTER 3

Anatomy, Structure, and Function of the Periodontium

Joseph P. Fiorellini | David Kim | Yu-Cheng Chang

CHAPTER OUTLINE

Oral Mucosa
Gingiva
Periodontal Ligament
Cementum
Alveolar Process

Development of the Attachment
  Apparatus
External Forces and the
  Periodontium

Vascularization of the Supporting
  Structures

 For online-only content on the gingival epithelium, the alveolar process, and the attachment apparatus, please visit the companion website at www.expertconsult.com.

The normal periodontium provides the support necessary to maintain teeth in function. It consists of four principal components: gingiva, periodontal ligament, cementum, and alveolar bone. Each of these periodontal components is distinct in its location, tissue architecture, biochemical composition, and chemical composition, but all of these components function together as a single unit. Research has revealed that the extracellular matrix components of one periodontal compartment can influence the cellular activities of adjacent structures. Therefore the pathologic changes that occur in one periodontal component may have significant ramifications for the maintenance, repair, or regeneration of other components of the periodontium.[18]

This chapter first discusses the structural components of the normal periodontium; it then describes their development, vascularization, innervation, and functions.

Oral Mucosa

The *oral mucosa* consists of the following three zones:

1. The gingiva and the covering of the hard palate, termed the *masticatory mucosa* (the *gingiva* is the part of the oral mucosa that covers the alveolar processes of the jaws and surrounds the necks of the teeth)
2. The dorsum of the tongue, covered by *specialized mucosa*
3. The oral mucous membrane lining the remainder of the oral cavity

Gingiva

Clinical Features

In an adult, normal gingiva covers the alveolar bone and tooth root to a level just coronal to the cementoenamel junction. The gingiva is divided anatomically into *marginal, attached,* and *interdental areas.* Although each type of gingiva exhibits considerable variation in

differentiation, histology, and thickness according to its functional demands, all types are specifically structured to function appropriately against mechanical and microbial damage.[7] In other words, the specific structure of different types of gingiva reflects each one's effectiveness as a barrier to the penetration by microbes and noxious agents into the deeper tissue.

Marginal Gingiva

The marginal or unattached gingiva is the terminal edge or border of the gingiva that surrounds the teeth in collar-like fashion (Figs. 3.1 and 3.2).[6] In about 50% of cases, it is demarcated from the adjacent attached gingiva by a shallow linear depression called the *free gingival groove.*[6] The marginal gingiva is usually about 1 mm wide, and it forms the soft-tissue wall of the gingival sulcus. It may be separated from the tooth surface with a periodontal probe. The most apical point of the marginal gingival scallop is called the *gingival zenith.* Its apicocoronal and mesiodistal dimensions vary between 0.06 and 0.96 mm.[171]

Gingival Sulcus

The gingival sulcus is the shallow crevice or space around the tooth bounded by the surface of the tooth on one side and the epithelium lining the free margin of the gingiva on the other side. It is V-shaped and barely permits the entrance of a periodontal probe. The clinical determination of the depth of the gingival sulcus is an important diagnostic parameter. Under absolutely normal or ideal conditions, the depth of the gingival sulcus is 0 mm or close to 0 mm.[105] These strict conditions of normalcy can be produced experimentally only in germ-free animals or after intense and prolonged plaque control.[13,49]

In clinically healthy human gingiva, a sulcus of some depth can be found. The depth of this sulcus, as determined in histologic sections, has been reported as 1.8 mm, with variations from 0 to 6 mm[195]; other studies have reported 1.5 mm[289] and 0.69 mm.[93] The clinical

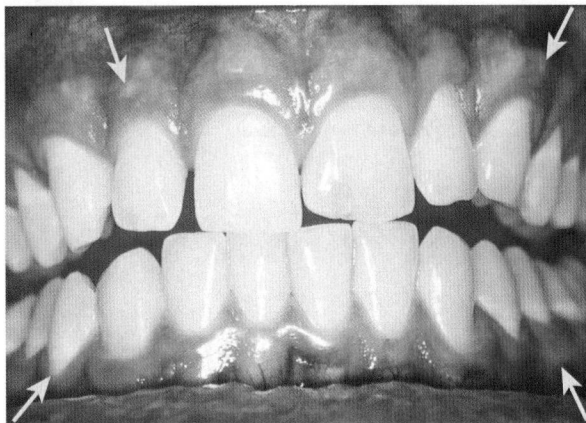

Fig. 3.1 Normal gingiva in a young adult. Note the demarcation (mucogingival line) *(arrows)* between the attached gingiva and the darker alveolar mucosa.

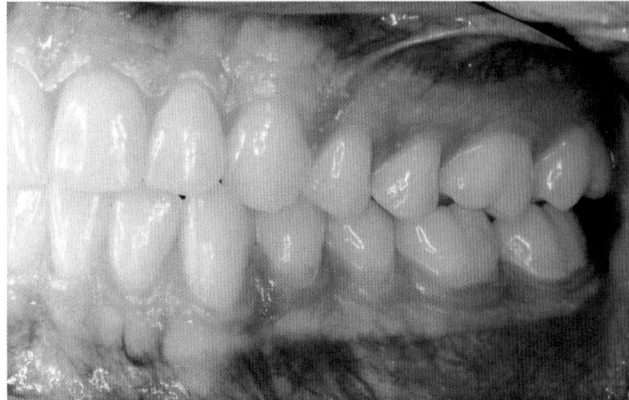

Fig. 3.3 Mean width of the attached gingiva in the human permanent dentition.

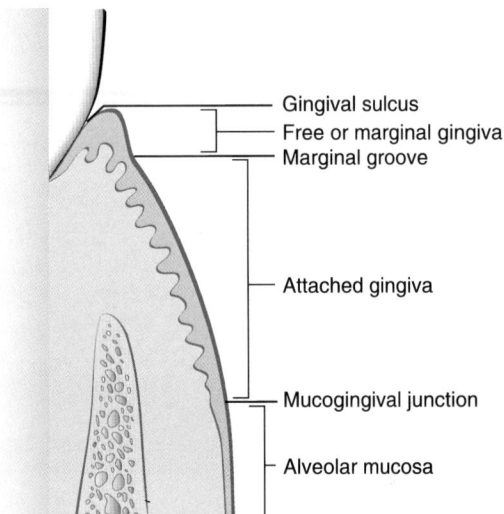

- Gingival sulcus
- Free or marginal gingiva
- Marginal groove
- Attached gingiva
- Mucogingival junction
- Alveolar mucosa

Fig. 3.2 Diagram showing the anatomic landmarks of the gingiva.

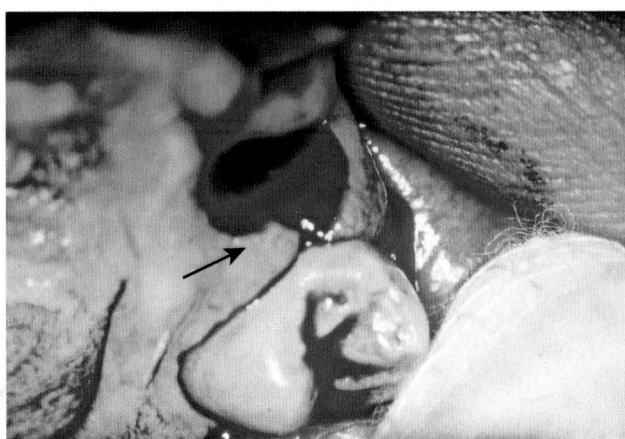

Fig. 3.4 Site of extraction showing the facial and palatal interdental papillae and the intervening col *(arrow).*

evaluation used to determine the depth of the sulcus involves the introduction of a metallic instrument (i.e., the periodontal probe) and the estimation of the distance it penetrates (i.e., the probing depth). The histologic depth of a sulcus does not need to be exactly equal to the depth of penetration of the probe. The penetration of the probe depends on several factors, such as probe diameter, probing force, and level of inflammation.[91] Consequently, the probing depth is not necessarily exactly equal to the histologic depth of the sulcus. The so-called probing depth of a clinically normal gingival sulcus in humans is 2 to 3 mm (see Chapter 32).

Attached Gingiva

The attached gingiva is continuous with the marginal gingiva. It is firm, resilient, and tightly bound to the underlying periosteum of alveolar bone. The facial aspect of the attached gingiva extends to the relatively loose and movable alveolar mucosa; it is demarcated by the *mucogingival junction* (see Fig. 3.2).

The *width of the attached gingiva* is another important clinical parameter.[7] It is the distance between the mucogingival junction and the projection on the external surface of the bottom of the gingival sulcus or the periodontal pocket. It should not be confused with the *width of the keratinized gingiva,* although this also includes the marginal gingiva (see Fig. 3.2).

The width of the attached gingiva on the facial aspect differs in different areas of the mouth.[40] It is generally greatest in the incisor region (i.e., 3.5 to 4.5 mm in the maxilla, 3.3 to 3.9 mm in the mandible) and narrower in the posterior segments (i.e., 1.9 mm in the maxillary first premolars and 1.8 mm in the mandibular first premolars)[6] (Fig. 3.3).

Because the mucogingival junction remains stationary throughout adult life,[4] changes in the width of the attached gingiva are caused by modifications in the position of its coronal portion. The width of the attached gingiva increases by the age of 4 years and in supraerupted teeth.[5] On the lingual aspect of the mandible, the attached gingiva terminates at the junction of the lingual alveolar mucosa, which is continuous with the mucous membrane that lines the floor of the mouth. The palatal surface of the attached gingiva in the maxilla blends imperceptibly with the equally firm and resilient palatal mucosa.

Interdental Gingiva

The interdental gingiva occupies the gingival embrasure, which is the interproximal space beneath the area of tooth contact. The interdental gingiva can be pyramidal, or it can have a "col" shape. In the former, the tip of one papilla is located immediately beneath the contact point; the latter presents a valley-like depression that connects a facial and lingual papilla and that conforms to the shape of the interproximal contact[62] (Figs. 3.4 and 3.5). The shape of the gingiva in a given interdental space depends on the presence or absence of a contact point between the adjacent teeth, the distance between the contact point and the osseous crest,[260] and the presence or absence of some degree of recession. Fig. 3.6 depicts the variations in normal interdental gingiva.

The facial and lingual surfaces are tapered toward the interproximal contact area, whereas the mesial and distal surfaces are slightly concave. The lateral borders and tips of the interdental papillae are formed by the marginal gingiva of the adjoining teeth. The intervening portion consists of attached gingiva (Fig. 3.7). If a diastema is present, the gingiva is firmly bound over the interdental bone to form a smooth, rounded surface without interdental papillae (Fig. 3.8).

Microscopic Features

Microscopic examination reveals that gingiva is composed of the overlying stratified squamous epithelium and the underlying central core of connective tissue. Although the epithelium is predominantly cellular in nature, the connective tissue is less cellular and composed primarily of collagen fibers and ground substance. These two tissues are considered separately. (A detailed description of gingival histology can be found in Schroeder HE: *The periodontium,* New York, 1986, Springer-Verlag; and in Biological structure of the normal and diseased periodontium, *Periodontol 2000* 13:1, 1997.)

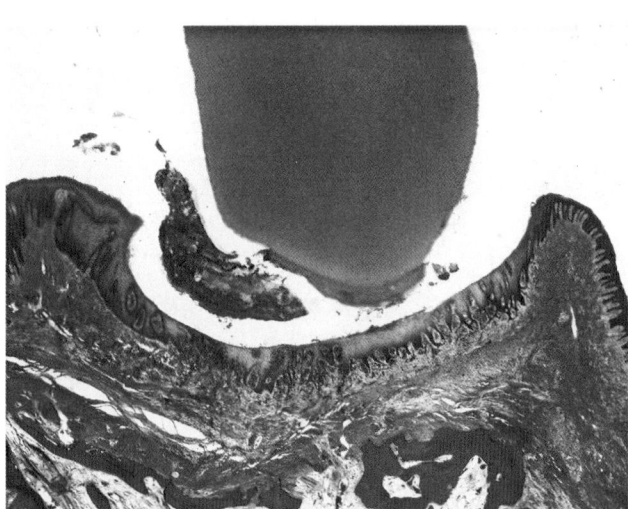

Fig. 3.5 Faciolingual section of a monkey showing the col between the facial and lingual interdental papillae. The col is covered with nonkeratinized stratified squamous epithelium.

Gingival Epithelium

General Aspects of Gingival Epithelium Biology

Historically, the epithelial compartment was thought to provide only a physical barrier to infection and the underlying gingival attachment. However, we now believe that epithelial cells play an active role in innate host defense by responding to bacteria in an interactive manner,[67] which means that the epithelium participates actively in responding to infection, in signaling further host reactions, and in

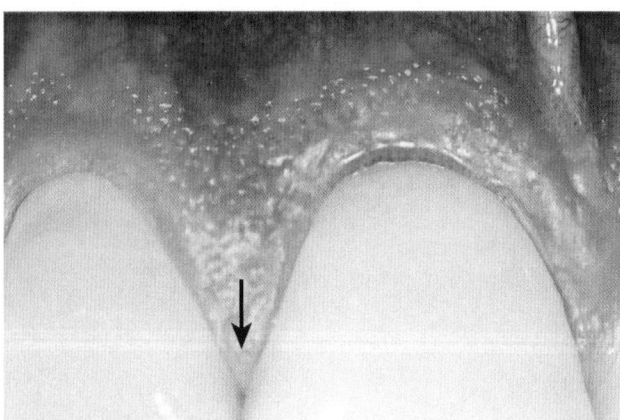

Fig. 3.7 Interdental papillae *(arrow)* with a central portion formed by the attached gingiva. The shape of the papillae varies according to the dimension of the gingival embrasure. *(Courtesy Dr. Osvaldo Costa.)*

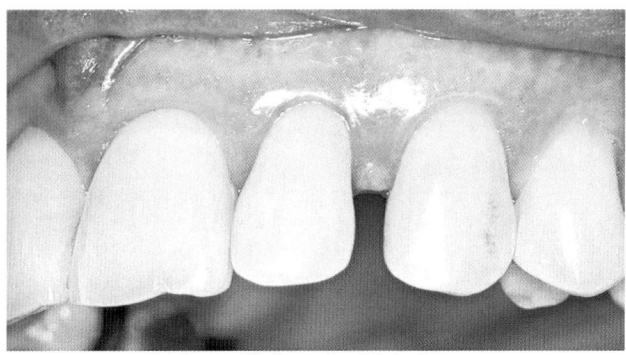

Fig. 3.8 An absence of interdental papillae and col where the proximal tooth contact is missing. *(Courtesy Dr. Osvaldo Costa.)*

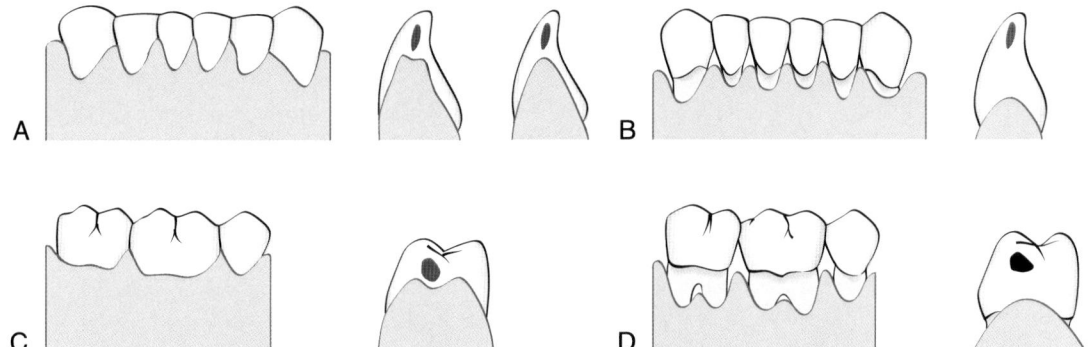

Fig. 3.6 A diagram that compares anatomic variations of the interdental col in the normal gingiva *(left side)* and after gingival recession *(right side).* (A–B) Mandibular anterior segment, facial and buccolingual views, respectively. (C–D) Mandibular posterior region, facial and buccolingual views, respectively. Tooth contact points are shown with black marks in the lower individual teeth.

integrating innate and acquired immune responses. For example, epithelial cells may respond to bacteria by increased proliferation, the alteration of cell-signaling events, changes in differentiation and cell death, and, ultimately, the alteration of tissue homeostasis.[67] To understand this new perspective of the epithelial innate defense responses and the role of epithelium in gingival health and disease, it is important to understand its basic structure and function (Box 3.1).

The gingival epithelium consists of a continuous lining of stratified squamous epithelium. There are three different areas that can be defined from the morphologic and functional points of view: the oral or outer epithelium, the sulcular epithelium, and the junctional epithelium.

The principal cell type of the gingival epithelium—as well as of other stratified squamous epithelia—is the *keratinocyte*. Other cells found in the epithelium are the clear cells or nonkeratinocytes, which include the Langerhans cells, the Merkel cells, and the melanocytes.

The main function of the gingival epithelium is to protect the deep structures while allowing for a selective interchange with the oral environment. This is achieved via the proliferation and differentiation of the keratinocytes. The *proliferation* of keratinocytes takes place by mitosis in the basal layer and less frequently in the suprabasal layers, in which a small proportion of cells remain as a proliferative compartment while a larger number begin to migrate to the surface.

Differentiation involves the process of keratinization, which consists of progressions of biochemical and morphologic events that occur in the cell as they migrate from the basal layer (Fig. 3.9). The main morphologic changes include the following: (1) the progressive flattening of the cell with an increasing prevalence of tonofilaments; (2) the couple of intercellular junctions with the production of keratohyalin granules; and (3) the disappearance of the nucleus. (See Schroeder[230] for further details.)

A complete keratinization process leads to the production of an *orthokeratinized* superficial horny layer similar to that of the skin, with no nuclei in the stratum corneum and a well-defined stratum granulosum (Fig. 3.10). Only some areas of the outer gingival epithelium are orthokeratinized; the other gingival areas are covered by parakeratinized or nonkeratinized epithelium[45] and are considered to be at intermediate stages of keratinization. These areas can progress to maturity or dedifferentiate under different physiologic or pathologic conditions.

In *parakeratinized epithelia,* the stratum corneum retains pyknotic nuclei, and the keratohyalin granules are dispersed rather than giving rise to a stratum granulosum. The *nonkeratinized epithelium* (although cytokeratins are the major component, as in all epithelia) has neither granulosum nor corneum strata, whereas superficial cells have viable nuclei.

BOX 3.1 Functions and Features of Gingival Epithelium

Functions
Mechanical, chemical, water, and microbial barrier
Signaling functions

Architectural Integrity
Cell–cell attachments
Basal lamina
Keratin cytoskeleton

Major Cell Type
Keratinocyte

Other Cell Types
Langerhans cells
Melanocytes
Merkel cells

Constant Renewal
Replacement of damaged cells

Cell–Cell Attachments
Desmosomes
Adherens junctions
Tight junctions
Gap junctions

Cell–Basal Lamina
Synthesis of basal lamina components
Hemidesmosome

Modified from Dale BA: Periodontal epithelium: a newly recognized role in health and disease. *Periodontol 2000* 30:71, 2002.

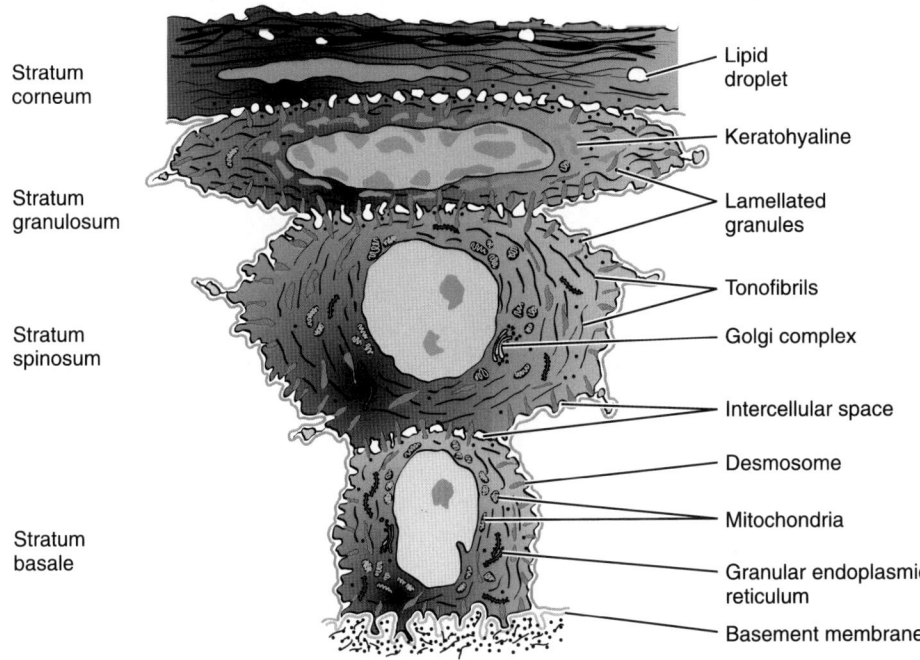

Stratum corneum
Stratum granulosum
Stratum spinosum
Stratum basale

Lipid droplet
Keratohyaline
Lamellated granules
Tonofibrils
Golgi complex
Intercellular space
Desmosome
Mitochondria
Granular endoplasmic reticulum
Basement membrane

Fig. 3.9 Diagram showing representative cells from the various layers of stratified squamous epithelium as seen by electron microscopy. *(Modified from Weinstock A: In Ham AW: Histology, ed 7, Philadelphia, 1974, Lippincott.)*

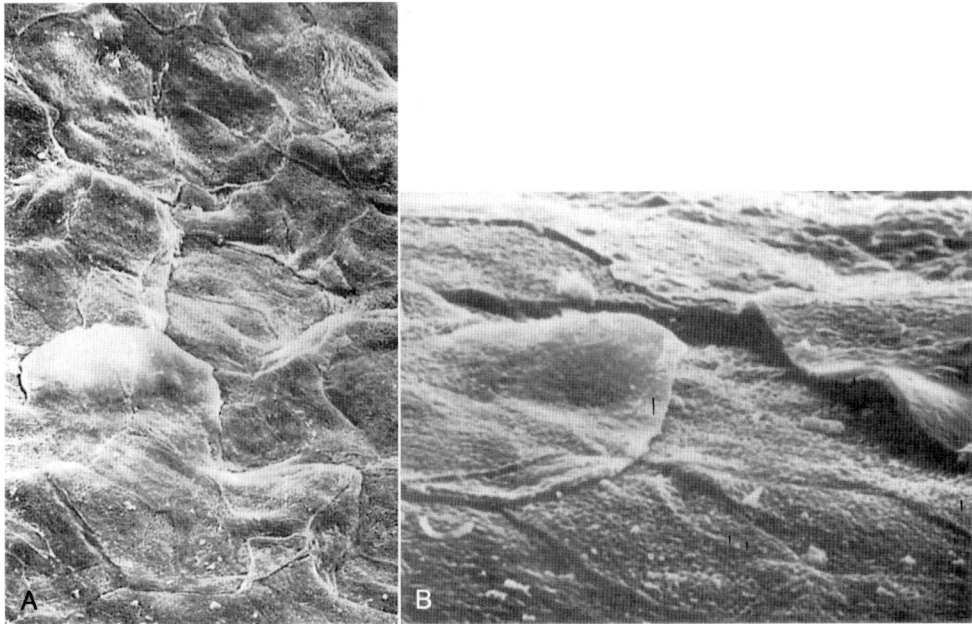

Fig. 3.10 (A) Scanning electron micrograph of keratinized gingiva showing the flattened keratinocytes and their boundaries on the surface of the gingiva (×1000). (B) Scanning electron micrograph of the gingival margin at the edge of the gingival sulcus showing several keratinocytes about to be exfoliated (×3000). *(From Kaplan GB, Pameijer CH, Ruben MP: J Periodontol 48:446, 1977.)*

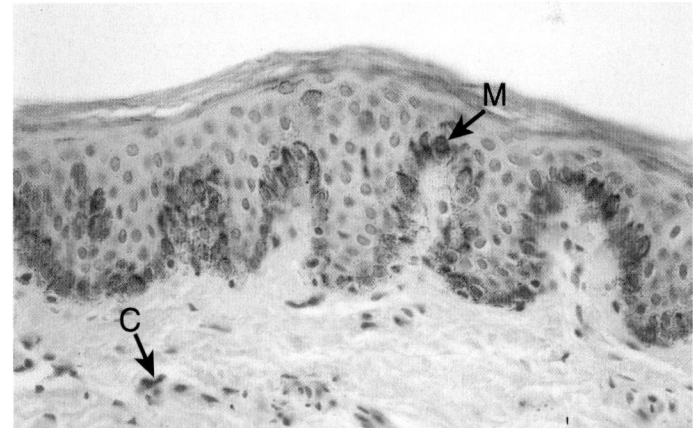

Fig. 3.11 Pigmented gingiva of dog showing melanocytes *(M)* in the basal epithelial layer and melanophores *(C)* in the connective tissue (Glucksman technique).

Nonkeratinocyte cells are present in gingival epithelium as in other malpighian epithelia. *Melanocytes* are dendritic cells located in the basal and spinous layers of the gingival epithelium. They synthesize melanin in organelles called *premelanosomes* or *melanosomes*[61,228,252] (Fig. 3.11).

Langerhans cells are dendritic cells located among keratinocytes at all suprabasal levels (Fig. 3.12). They belong to the mononuclear phagocyte system (reticuloendothelial system) as modified monocytes derived from the bone marrow. They contain elongated granules, and they are considered macrophages with possible antigenic properties.[72] Langerhans cells have an important role in the immune reaction as antigen-presenting cells for lymphocytes. They contain g-specific granules (Birbeck granules), and they have marked adenosine triphosphatase activity. They are found in the oral epithelium of normal gingiva and in smaller amounts in the sulcular epithelium; they are probably absent from the junctional epithelium of normal gingiva.

Merkel cells are located in the deeper layers of the epithelium; they harbor nerve endings, and they are connected to

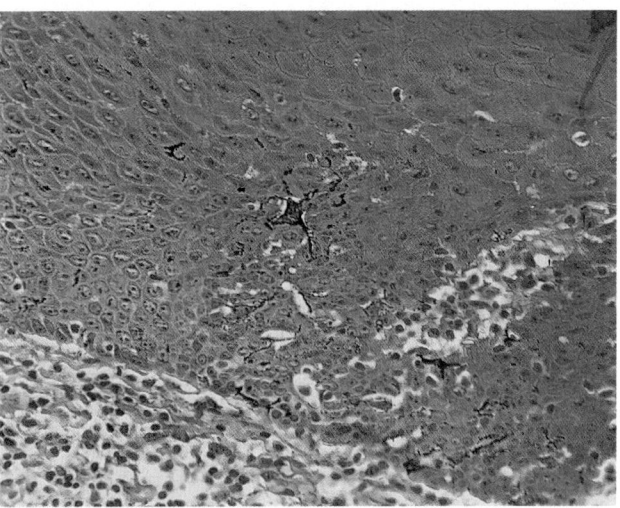

Fig. 3.12 Human gingival epithelium, oral aspect. Immunoperoxidase technique showing Langerhans cells.

adjacent cells by desmosomes. They have been identified as tactile perceptors.[188]

The epithelium is joined to the underlying connective tissue by a *basal lamina* 300 to 400 Å thick and lying approximately 400 Å beneath the epithelial basal layer.[147,235,254] The basal lamina consists of lamina lucida and lamina densa. Hemidesmosomes of the basal epithelial cells abut the lamina lucida, which is mainly composed of the glycoprotein laminin. The lamina densa is composed of type IV collagen.

The basal lamina, which is clearly distinguishable at the ultrastructural level, is connected to a reticular condensation of the underlying connective tissue fibrils (mainly collagen type IV) by the anchoring fibrils.[183,213,257] Anchoring fibrils have been measured at 750 nm in length from their epithelial end to their connective tissue end, where they appear to form loops around collagen fibers. The complex of basal lamina and fibrils is the periodic acid–Schiff–positive and argyrophilic line observed at the optical level[237,258] (Fig. 3.13). The basal lamina is permeable to fluids, but it acts as a barrier to particulate matter.

Structural and Metabolic Characteristics of Different Areas of Gingival Epithelium

The epithelial component of the gingiva shows regional morphologic variations that reflect tissue adaptation to the tooth and alveolar bone.[231] These variations include the oral epithelium, the sulcular epithelium, and the junctional epithelium. Whereas the oral epithelium and the sulcular epithelium are largely protective in function, the junctional epithelium serves many more roles and is of considerable importance in the regulation of tissue health.[18] It is now recognized that epithelial cells are not passive bystanders in the gingival tissues; rather, they are metabolically active and capable of reacting to external stimuli by synthesizing a number of cytokines, adhesion molecules, growth factors, and enzymes.[18]

The degree of gingival keratinization diminishes with age and the onset of menopause,[199] but it is not necessarily related to the different phases of the menstrual cycle.[131] Keratinization of the oral mucosa varies in different areas in the following order: palate (most

keratinized), gingiva, ventral aspect of the tongue, and cheek (least keratinized).[181]

Oral (Outer) Epithelium

The oral or outer epithelium covers the crest and outer surface of the marginal gingiva and the surface of the attached gingiva. On average, the oral epithelium is 0.2 to 0.3 mm in thickness. It is keratinized or parakeratinized, or it may present various combinations of these conditions (Fig. 3.14). The prevalent surface, however, is parakeratinized.[32,45,285] The oral epithelium is composed of four layers: stratum basale (basal layer), stratum spinosum (prickle cell layer), stratum granulosum (granular layer), and stratum corneum (cornified layer).

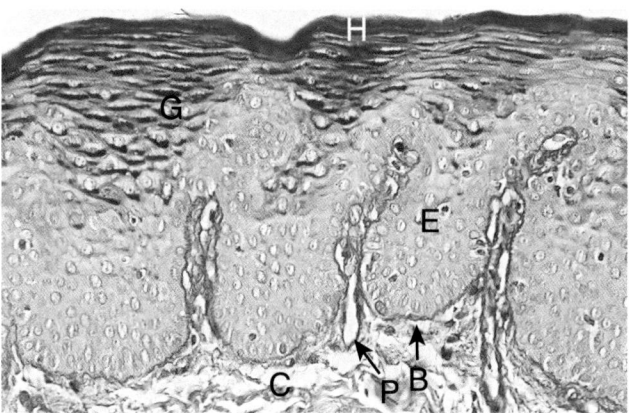

Fig. 3.13 Normal human gingiva stained with the periodic acid–Schiff histochemical method. The basement membrane *(B)* is seen between the epithelium *(E)* and the underlying connective tissue *(C)*. In the epithelium, glycoprotein material occurs in cells and cell membranes of the superficial hornified *(H)* and underlying granular layers *(G)*. The connective tissue presents a diffuse, amorphous ground substance and collagen fibers. The blood vessel walls stand out clearly in the papillary projections of the connective tissue *(P)*.

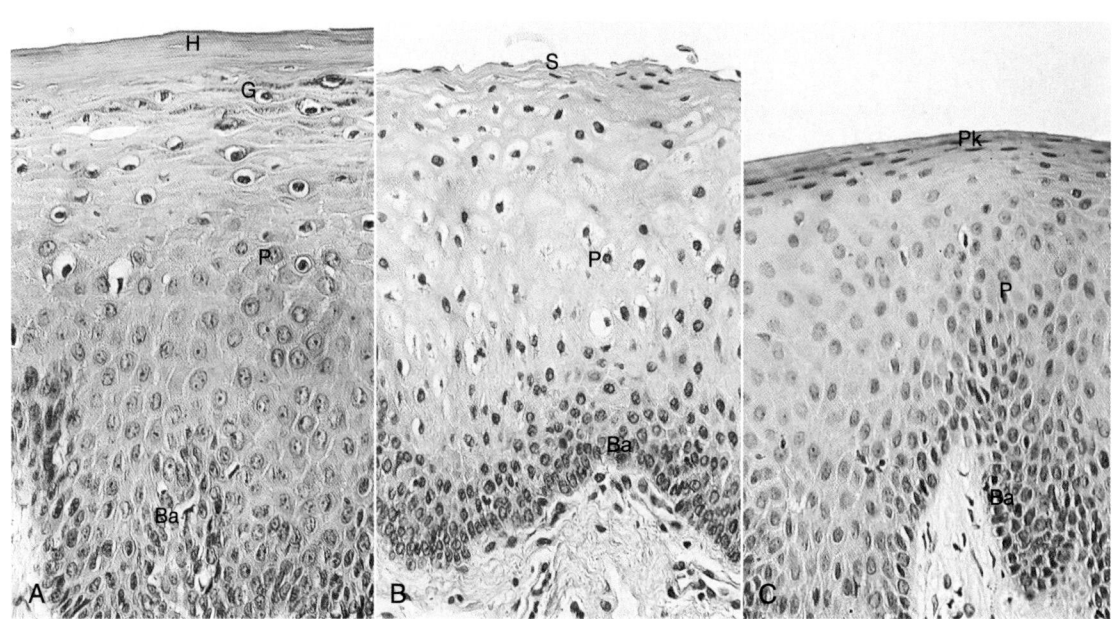

Fig. 3.14 Variations in the gingival epithelium. (A) Keratinized. (B) Nonkeratinized. (C) Parakeratinized. Horny layer *(H)*, granular layer *(G)*, prickle cell layer *(P)*, basal cell layer *(Ba)*, flattened surface cells *(S)*, and parakeratotic layer *(Pk)*.

Sulcular Epithelium

The sulcular epithelium lines the gingival sulcus (Fig. 3.15). It is a thin, nonkeratinized stratified squamous epithelium without rete pegs, and it extends from the coronal limit of the junctional epithelium to the crest of the gingival margin (Fig. 3.16). It usually shows many cells with hydropic degeneration.[32]

Despite these morphologic and chemical characteristics, the sulcular epithelium has the potential to keratinize if it is reflected and exposed to the oral cavity[44,48] or if the bacterial flora of the sulcus is totally eliminated.[50] Conversely, the outer epithelium loses its keratinization when it is placed in contact with the tooth.[50] These findings suggest that the local irritation of the sulcus prevents sulcular keratinization.

The sulcular epithelium is extremely important; it may act as a semipermeable membrane through which injurious bacterial products pass into the gingiva and through which tissue fluid from the gingiva seeps into the sulcus.[267] Unlike the junctional epithelium, however, the sulcular epithelium is not heavily infiltrated by polymorphonuclear neutrophil leukocytes, and it appears to be less permeable.[18]

Junctional Epithelium

The junctional epithelium consists of a collar-like band of stratified squamous nonkeratinizing epithelium. It is 3 to 4 layers thick in early life, but that number increases with age to 10 or even 20 layers. In addition, the junctional epithelium tapers from its coronal end, which may be 10 to 29 cells wide to 1 or 2 cells wide at its apical termination, which is located at the cementoenamel junction in healthy tissue. These cells can be grouped in two strata: the basal layer that faces the connective tissue and the suprabasal layer that extends to the tooth surface. The length of the junctional epithelium ranges from 0.25 to 1.35 mm (Fig. 3.17).

The junctional epithelium is formed by the confluence of the oral epithelium and the reduced enamel epithelium during tooth eruption. However, the reduced enamel epithelium is not essential for its formation; in fact, the junctional epithelium is completely restored after pocket instrumentation or surgery, and it forms around an implant.[151]

The junctional epithelium is attached to the tooth surface (epithelial attachment) by means of an internal basal lamina. It is attached to the gingival connective tissue by an external basal lamina that has the same structure as other epithelial–connective tissue attachments elsewhere in the body.[155,161]

The internal basal lamina consists of a lamina densa (adjacent to the enamel) and a lamina lucida to which hemidesmosomes are attached. Hemidesmosomes have a decisive role in the firm attachment of the cells to the internal basal lamina on the tooth surface.

Data suggest that the hemidesmosomes may also act as specific sites of signal transduction and thus may participate in the regulation of gene expression, cell proliferation, and cell differentiation.[134] Organic strands from the enamel appear to extend into the lamina densa.[256] The junctional epithelium attaches to afibrillar cementum that is present on the crown (usually restricted to an area within 1 mm of the cementoenamel junction)[233] and root cementum in a similar manner.

Histochemical evidence for the presence of neutral polysaccharides in the zone of the epithelial attachment has been reported.[272] Data also have shown that the basal lamina of the junctional epithelium resembles that of endothelial and epithelial cells in its laminin content but differs in its internal basal lamina, which has no type IV collagen.[142,223] These findings indicate that the cells of the junctional epithelium are involved in the production of laminin and play a key role in the adhesion mechanism.

The attachment of the junctional epithelium to the tooth is reinforced by the gingival fibers, which brace the marginal gingiva against the tooth surface. For this reason, the junctional epithelium and the gingival fibers are considered together as a functional unit referred to as the *dentogingival unit.*[158]

In conclusion, it is usually accepted that the junctional epithelium exhibits several unique structural and functional features that contribute to preventing pathogenic bacterial flora from colonizing the subgingival tooth surface.[205] First, junctional epithelium is firmly attached

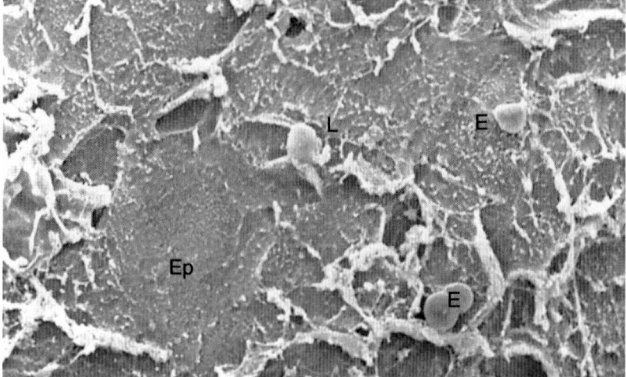

Fig. 3.15 Scanning electron microscopic view of the epithelial surface facing the tooth in a normal human gingival sulcus. The epithelium *(Ep)* shows desquamating cells, some scattered erythrocytes *(E)*, and a few emerging leukocytes *(L)*. (×1000.)

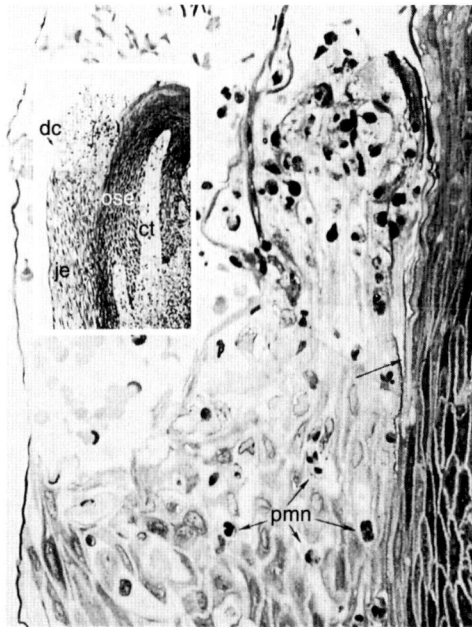

Fig. 3.16 Epon-embedded human biopsy specimen showing a relatively normal gingival sulcus. The soft-tissue wall of the gingival sulcus is made up of the oral sulcular epithelium *(ose)* and its underlying connective tissue *(ct)*, whereas the base of the gingival sulcus is formed by the sloughing surface of the junctional epithelium *(je)*. The enamel space is delineated by a dense cuticular structure *(dc)*. A relatively sharp line of demarcation exists between the junctional epithelium and the oral sulcular epithelium *(arrow)*, and several polymorphonuclear leukocytes *(pmn)* can be seen traversing the junctional epithelium. The sulcus contains red blood cells that resulted from the hemorrhage that occurred at the time of biopsy. (×391; inset ×55.) *(From Schluger S, Youdelis R, Page RC: Periodontal disease, ed 2, Philadelphia, 1990, Lea & Febiger.)*

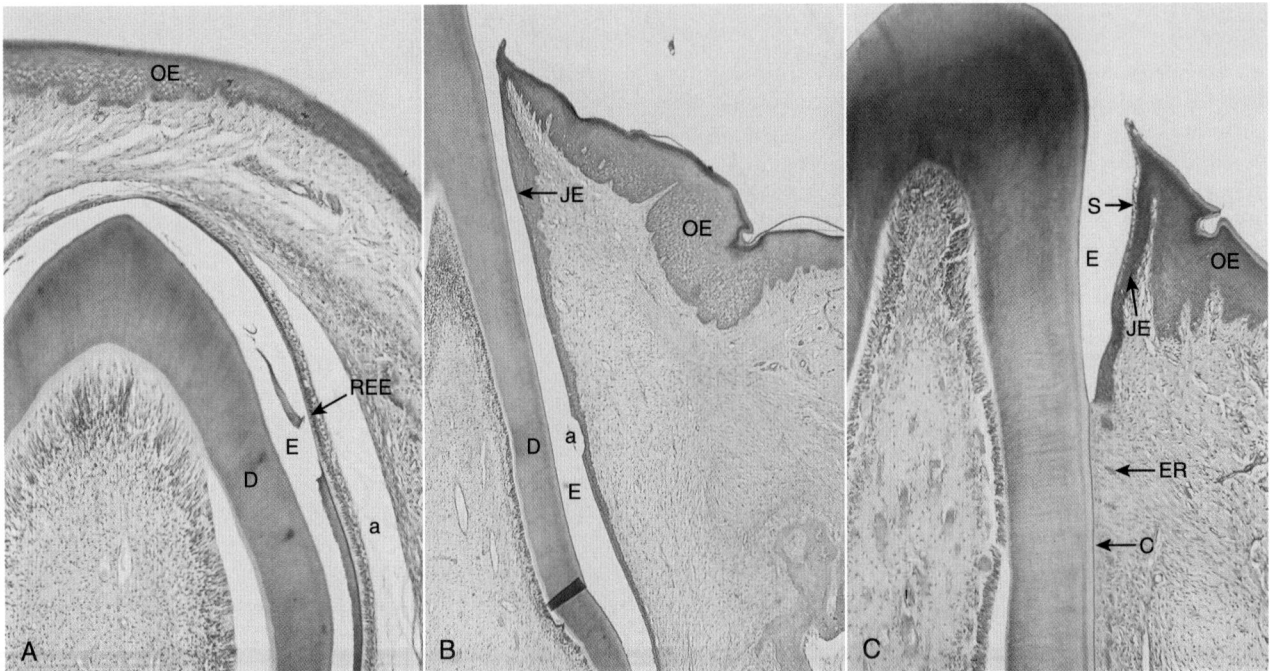

Fig. 3.17 Eruption process in cat's tooth. (A) Unerupted tooth. Dentin *(D)*, remnants of enamel matrix *(E)*, reduced enamel epithelium *(REE)*, oral epithelium *(OE)*, and artifact *(a)*. (B) Erupting tooth forming junctional epithelium *(JE)*. (C) Completely erupted tooth. Sulcus with epithelial debris *(S)*, cementum *(C)*, and epithelial rests *(ER)*.

to the tooth surface, thereby forming an epithelial barrier against plaque bacteria. Second, it allows access of gingival fluid, inflammatory cells, and components of the immunologic host defense to the gingival margin. Third, junctional epithelial cells exhibit rapid turnover, which contributes to the host–parasite equilibrium and the rapid repair of damaged tissue. Some investigators have also indicated that the cells of the junctional epithelium have an endocytic capacity equal to that of macrophages and neutrophils and that this activity may be protective in nature.[57]

Development of Gingival Sulcus

After enamel formation is complete, the enamel is covered with *reduced enamel epithelium* (REE), which is attached to the tooth by a basal lamina and hemidesmosomes.[156,255] When the tooth penetrates the oral mucosa, the REE unites with the oral epithelium and transforms into the junctional epithelium. As the tooth erupts, this united epithelium condenses along the crown, and the ameloblasts, which form the inner layer of the REE (see Fig. 3.17), gradually become squamous epithelial cells. The transformation of the REE into a junctional epithelium proceeds in an apical direction without interrupting the attachment to the tooth. According to Schroeder and Listgarten,[233] this process takes between 1 and 2 years.

The junctional epithelium is a continually self-renewing structure, with mitotic activity occurring in all cell layers.[156,255] The regenerating epithelial cells move toward the tooth surface and along it in a coronal direction to the gingival sulcus, where they are shed[22] (Fig. 3.18). The migrating daughter cells provide a continuous attachment to the tooth surface. The strength of the epithelial attachment to the tooth has not been measured.

The gingival sulcus is formed when the tooth erupts into the oral cavity. At that time, the junctional epithelium and the REE form a broad band that is attached to the tooth surface from near the tip of the crown to the cementoenamel junction. The gingival sulcus is the shallow, V-shaped space or groove between the tooth and the gingiva that encircles the newly erupted tip of the crown. In the fully erupted

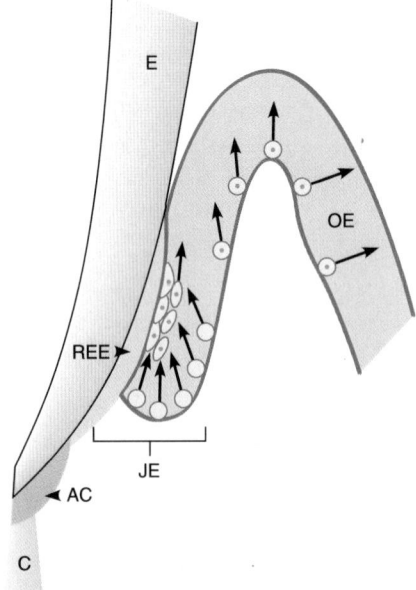

Fig. 3.18 Junctional epithelium on an erupting tooth. The junctional epithelium *(JE)* is formed by the joining of the oral epithelium *(OE)* and the reduced enamel epithelium *(REE)*. Afibrillar cementum *(AC)* is sometimes formed on enamel after the degeneration of the REE. The arrows indicate the coronal movement of the regenerating epithelial cells, which multiply more rapidly in the JE than in the OE. *E,* Enamel; *C,* root cementum. A similar cell turnover pattern exists in the fully erupted tooth. *(Modified from Listgarten MA: J Can Dent Assoc 36:70, 1970.)*

tooth, only the junctional epithelium persists. *The sulcus consists of the shallow space that is coronal to the attachment of the junctional epithelium and bounded by the tooth on one side and the sulcular epithelium on the other. The coronal extent of the gingival sulcus is the gingival margin.*

Renewal of Gingival Epithelium

The oral epithelium undergoes continuous renewal. Its thickness is maintained by a balance between new cell formation in the basal and spinous layers and the shedding of old cells at the surface. The mitotic activity exhibits a 24-hour periodicity, with the highest and lowest rates occurring in the morning and evening, respectively.[256] The mitotic rate is higher in nonkeratinized areas and increased in gingivitis, without significant gender differences. Opinions differ with regard to whether the mitotic rate is increased[160,161,179] or decreased[15] with age.

With regard to junctional epithelium, it was previously thought that only epithelial cells facing the external basal lamina were rapidly dividing. However, evidence indicates that a significant number of the cells (e.g., the basal cells along the connective tissue) are capable of synthesizing deoxyribonucleic acid (DNA), thereby demonstrating their mitotic activity.[221,222] The rapid shedding of cells effectively removes bacteria that adhere to the epithelial cells and therefore is an important part of the antimicrobial defense mechanisms at the dentogingival junction.[205]

Cuticular Structures on the Tooth

The term *cuticle* describes a thin acellular structure with a homogeneous matrix that is sometimes enclosed within clearly demarcated linear borders.

Listgarten[159] has classified cuticular structures into coatings of developmental origin and acquired coatings. *Acquired coatings* include those of exogenous origin such as saliva, bacteria, calculus, and surface stains (see Chapters 7 and 13). *Coatings of developmental origin* are those that are normally formed as part of tooth development. They include the REE, the coronal cementum, and the dental cuticle.

After enamel formation is completed, the ameloblastic epithelium is reduced to one or two layers of cells that remain attached to the enamel surface by hemidesmosomes and a basal lamina. This REE consists of postsecretory ameloblasts and cells from the stratum intermedium of the enamel organ. In some animal species, the REE disappears entirely and rapidly, thereby placing the enamel surface in contact with the connective tissue. Connective tissue cells then deposit a thin layer of cementum known as *coronal cementum* on the enamel. In humans, thin patches of afibrillar cementum sometimes may be seen in the cervical half of the crown.

Electron microscopy has demonstrated a dental cuticle that consists of a layer of homogeneous organic material of variable thickness (approximately 0.25 μm) overlying the enamel surface. It is nonmineralized, and it is not always present. In some cases, near the cementoenamel junction, it is deposited over a layer of afibrillar cementum, which in turn overlies enamel. The cuticle may be present between the junctional epithelium and the tooth. Ultrastructural histochemical studies have shown that the dental cuticle is proteinaceous,[143] and it may be an accumulation of tissue fluid components.[87,232]

Gingival Fluid (Sulcular Fluid)

The value of the gingival fluid is that it can be represented as either a transudate or an exudate. The gingival fluid contains a vast array of biochemical factors, thereby offering its potential use as a diagnostic or prognostic biomarker of the biologic state of the periodontium in health and disease[81] (see Chapter 16). It also contains components of connective tissue, epithelium, inflammatory cells, serum, and microbial flora that inhabit the gingival margin or the sulcus (pocket).[79]

In the healthy sulcus, the amount of gingival fluid is very small. During inflammation, however, the gingival fluid flow increases, and its composition starts to resemble that of an inflammatory exudate.[59] The main route of the gingival fluid diffusion is through the basement membrane, through the relatively wide intercellular spaces of the junctional epithelium, and then into the sulcus.[205] The gingival fluid is believed to do the following: (1) cleanse material from the sulcus; (2) contain plasma proteins that may improve adhesion of the epithelium to the tooth; (3) possess antimicrobial properties; and (4) exert antibody activity to defend the gingiva.

Gingival Connective Tissue

The major components of the gingival connective tissue are collagen fibers (about 60% by volume), fibroblasts (5%), vessels, nerves, and matrix (about 35%). The connective tissue of the gingiva is known as the *lamina propria*, and it consists of two layers: (1) a *papillary layer* subjacent to the epithelium that consists of papillary projections between the epithelial rete pegs and (2) a *reticular layer* that is contiguous with the periosteum of the alveolar bone.

Connective tissue has a cellular compartment and an extracellular compartment composed of fibers and ground substance. Thus the gingival connective tissue is largely a fibrous connective tissue that has elements that originate directly from the oral mucosal connective tissue as well as some fibers (dentogingival) that originate from the developing dental follicle.[18]

The *ground substance* fills the space between fibers and cells; it is amorphous, and it has a high water content. It is composed of proteoglycans (mainly hyaluronic acid and chondroitin sulfate) and glycoproteins (mainly fibronectin). Glycoproteins account for the faint periodic acid–Schiff–positive reaction of the ground substance.[82] Fibronectin binds fibroblasts to the fibers and many other components of the intercellular matrix, thereby helping to mediate cell adhesion and migration. Laminin, which is another glycoprotein found in the basal lamina, serves to attach it to epithelial cells.

The three types of connective tissue fibers are collagen, reticular, and elastic. Collagen type I forms the bulk of the lamina propria and provides the tensile strength to the gingival tissue. Type IV collagen (argyrophilic reticulum fiber) branches between the collagen type I bundles, and it is continuous with fibers of the basement membrane and the blood vessel walls.[161]

The elastic fiber system is composed of oxytalan, elaunin, and elastin fibers distributed among collagen fibers.[56] Therefore densely packed collagen bundles that are anchored into the acellular extrinsic fiber cementum just below the terminal point of the junctional epithelium form the connective tissue attachment. The stability of this attachment is a key factor in the limitation of the migration of junctional epithelium.[57]

Gingival Fibers

The connective tissue of the marginal gingiva is densely collagenous, and it contains a prominent system of collagen fiber bundles called the *gingival fibers*. These fibers consist of type I collagen.[213] The gingival fibers have the following functions:

1. To brace the marginal gingiva firmly against the tooth
2. To provide the rigidity necessary to withstand the forces of mastication without being deflected away from the tooth surface
3. To unite the free marginal gingiva with the cementum of the root and the adjacent attached gingiva

The gingival fibers are arranged in three groups: gingivodental, circular, and transseptal.[146]

The *gingivodental fibers* are those on the facial, lingual, and interproximal surfaces. They are embedded in the cementum just beneath the epithelium at the base of the gingival sulcus. On the

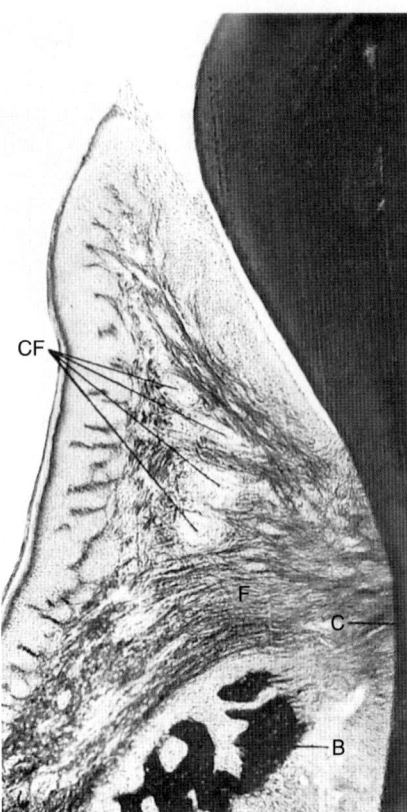

Fig. 3.19 Faciolingual section of marginal gingiva showing gingival fibers *(F)* that extend from the cementum *(C)* to the crest of the gingiva, to the outer gingival surface, and external to the periosteum of the bone *(B)*. Circular fibers *(CF)* are shown in cross-section between the other groups. *(Courtesy Sol Bernick.)*

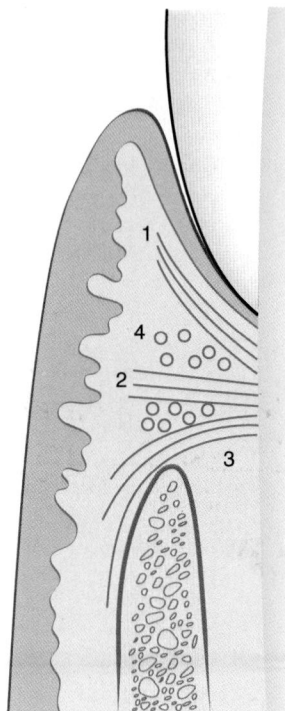

Fig. 3.20 Diagram of the gingivodental fibers that extend from the cementum *(1)* to the crest of the gingiva, *(2)* to the outer surface, and *(3)* external to the periosteum of the labial plate. Circular fibers *(4)* are shown in cross-section.

facial and lingual surfaces, they project from the cementum in a fanlike conformation toward the crest and outer surface of the marginal gingiva, where they terminate short of the epithelium (Figs. 3.19 and 3.20). They also extend externally to the periosteum of the facial and lingual alveolar bones, terminating in the attached gingiva or blending with the periosteum of the bone. Interproximally, the gingivodental fibers extend toward the crest of the interdental gingiva.

The *circular fibers* course through the connective tissue of the marginal and interdental gingivae and encircle the tooth in ringlike fashion.

The *transseptal fibers,* which are located interproximally, form horizontal bundles that extend between the cementum of the approximating teeth into which they are embedded. They lie in the area between the epithelium at the base of the gingival sulcus and the crest of the interdental bone, and they are sometimes classified with the principal fibers of the periodontal ligament.

Page and colleagues[198] described a group of *semicircular fibers* that attach at the proximal surface of a tooth immediately below the cementoenamel junction, go around the facial or lingual marginal gingiva of the tooth, and attach on the other proximal surface of the same tooth; they also discussed a group of *transgingival fibers* that attach in the proximal surface of one tooth, traverse the interdental space diagonally, go around the facial or lingual surface of the adjacent tooth, again traverse the interdental space diagonally, and then attach in the proximal surface of the next tooth.

Tractional forces in the extracellular matrix produced by fibroblasts are believed to be responsible for generating tension in the collagen. This keeps the teeth tightly bound to each other and to the alveolar bone.

Cellular Elements

The preponderant cellular element in the gingival connective tissue is the *fibroblast.* Numerous fibroblasts are found between the fiber bundles. Fibroblasts are of mesenchymal origin and play a major role in the development, maintenance, and repair of gingival connective tissue. As with connective tissue elsewhere in the body, fibroblasts synthesize collagen and elastic fibers as well as the glycoproteins and glycosaminoglycans of the amorphous intercellular substance. Fibroblasts also regulate collagen degradation through phagocytosis and the secretion of collagenases.

Fibroblast heterogeneity is now a well-established feature of fibroblasts in the periodontium.[226] Although the biologic and clinical significance of such heterogeneity is not yet clear, it seems that this is necessary for the normal functioning of tissues in health, disease, and repair.[18]

Mast cells, which are distributed throughout the body, are numerous in the connective tissue of the oral mucosa and the gingiva.[52,244,245,288] *Fixed macrophages* and *histiocytes* are present in the gingival connective tissue as components of the mononuclear phagocyte system (reticuloendothelial system) and are derived from blood monocytes. *Adipose cells* and *eosinophils,* although scarce, are also present in the lamina propria.

In clinically normal gingiva, small foci of plasma cells and lymphocytes are found in the connective tissue near the base of the sulcus (Fig. 3.21). Neutrophils can be seen in relatively high numbers in both the gingival connective tissue and the sulcus. These inflammatory cells are usually present in small amounts in clinically normal gingiva.

Repair of Gingival Connective Tissue

Because of the high turnover rate, the connective tissue of the gingiva has remarkably good healing and regenerative capacity. Indeed, it

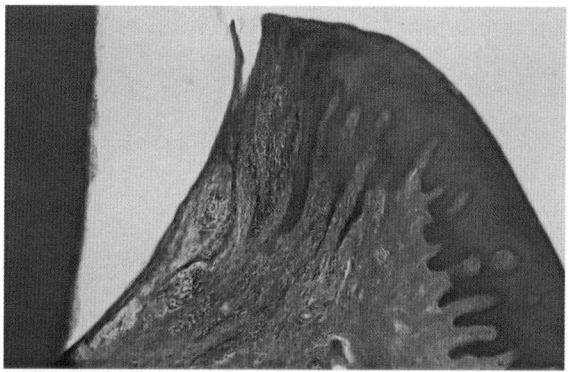

Fig. 3.21 Section of clinically normal gingiva showing some degree of inflammation, which is almost always present near the base of the sulcus.

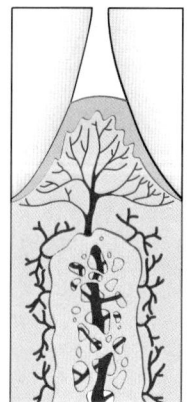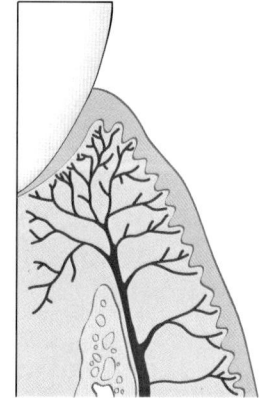

Fig. 3.22 Diagram of an arteriole penetrating the interdental alveolar bone to supply the interdental tissues *(left)* and a supraperiosteal arteriole overlying the facial alveolar bone, sending branches to the surrounding tissue *(right).*

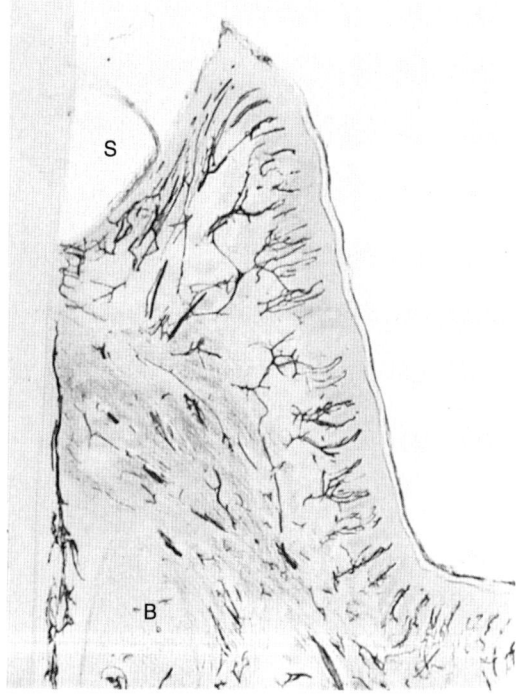

Fig. 3.23 Blood supply and peripheral circulation of the gingiva. Tissues perfused with India ink. Note the capillary plexus parallel to the sulcus *(S)* and the capillary loops in the outer papillary layer. Note also the supraperiosteal vessels external to the bone *(B),* which supply the gingiva, and a periodontal ligament vessel anastomosing with the sulcus plexus. *(Courtesy Sol Bernick.)*

may be one of the best healing tissues in the body, and it generally shows little evidence of scarring after surgical procedures. This is likely caused by the rapid reconstruction of the fibrous architecture of the tissues.[178] However, the reparative capacity of gingival connective tissue is not as great as that of the periodontal ligament or the epithelial tissue.

Blood Supply, Lymphatics, and Nerves

Microcirculatory tracts, blood vessels, and lymphatic vessels play an important role in the drainage of tissue fluid and in the spread of inflammation. In individuals with gingivitis and periodontitis, the microcirculation and vascular formation change greatly in the vascular network directly under the gingival sulcular epithelium and the junctional epithelium.[170]

Three sources of blood supply to the gingiva are as follows (Figs. 3.22 and 3.23):

1. *Supraperiosteal arterioles* along the facial and lingual surfaces of the alveolar bone from which capillaries extend along the sulcular epithelium and between the rete pegs of the external gingival surface[8,76,113]: Occasional branches of the arterioles pass through the alveolar bone to the periodontal ligament or run over the crest of the alveolar bone.
2. *Vessels of the periodontal ligament,* which extend into the gingiva, and anastomose with capillaries in the sulcus area.
3. *Arterioles,* which emerge from the crest of the interdental septa[84] and extend parallel to the crest of the bone to anastomose with

vessels of the periodontal ligament, with capillaries in the gingival crevicular areas and vessels that run over the alveolar crest.

Beneath the epithelium on the outer gingival surface, capillaries extend into the papillary connective tissue between the epithelial rete pegs in the form of terminal hairpin loops with efferent and afferent branches, spirals, and varices[54,113] (Fig. 3.24; also see Fig. 3.23). The loops are sometimes linked by cross-communications,[86] and flattened capillaries serve as reserve vessels when the circulation is increased in response to irritation.[99]

Along the sulcular epithelium, capillaries are arranged in a flat, anastomosing plexus that extends parallel to the enamel from the base of the sulcus to the gingival margin.[54] In the col area, a mixed pattern of anastomosing capillaries and loops occurs.

As mentioned previously, anatomic and histologic changes have been shown to occur in the gingival microcirculation of individuals with gingivitis. Prospective studies of the gingival vasculature in animals have demonstrated that, in the absence of inflammation, the vascular network is arranged in a regular, repetitive, and layered pattern.[54,216] By contrast, the inflamed gingival vasculature exhibits an irregular vascular plexus pattern, with the microvessels exhibiting a looped, dilated, and convoluted appearance.[216]

The role of the lymphatic system in removing excess fluids, cellular and protein debris, microorganisms, and other elements is important for controlling diffusion and the resolution of inflammatory processes.[168] The *lymphatic drainage of the gingiva* brings in the lymphatics of the connective tissue papillae.[238] It progresses into the collecting network external to the periosteum of the alveolar process and then moves to the regional lymph nodes, particularly the submaxillary group. In addition, lymphatics just beneath the junctional epithelium extend into the periodontal ligament and accompany the blood vessels.

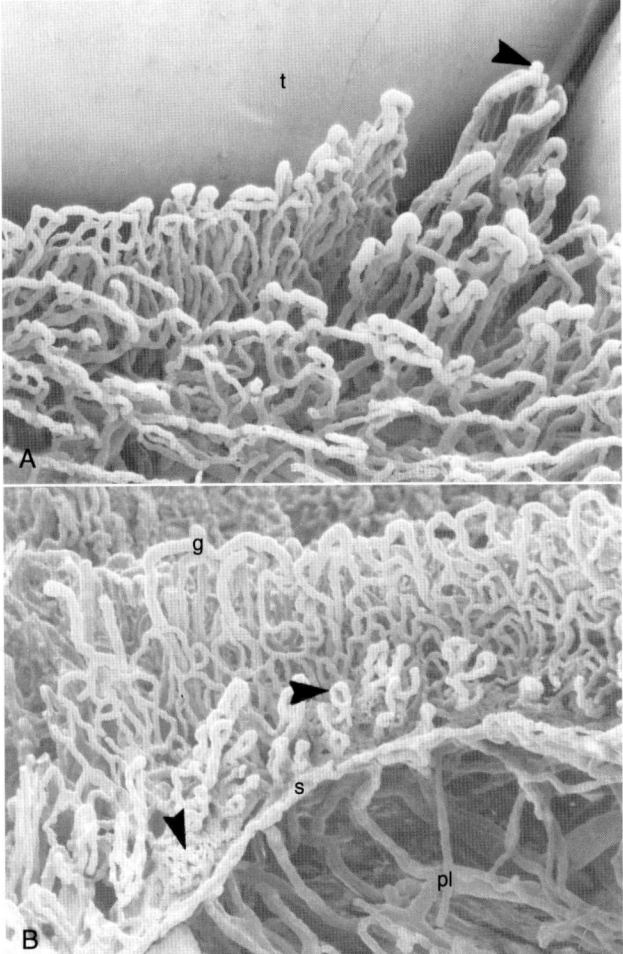

Fig. 3.24 Scanning electron microscopic view of the gingival tissues of rat molar palatal gingiva after the vascular perfusion of plastic and the corrosion of soft tissue. (A) Oral view of gingival capillaries: *t,* tooth; interdental papilla *(arrowhead)* (×180). (B) View from the tooth side. Note the vessels of the plexus next to the sulcular and junctional epithelium. The arrowheads point to vessels in the sulcus area with mild inflammatory changes. *g,* Crest of the marginal gingiva; *s,* bottom of the gingival sulcus; *pl,* periodontal ligament vessels. (×150.) *(Courtesy NJ Selliseth and K Selvig, University of Bergen, Norway.)*

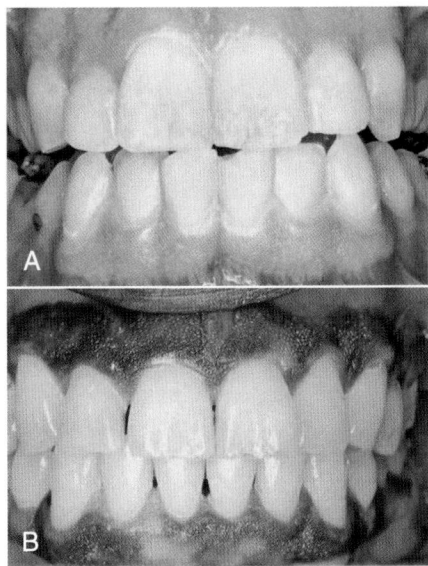

Fig. 3.25 (A) Clinically normal gingiva in a young adult. (B) Heavily pigmented (melanotic) gingiva in a middle-aged adult. (*From Glickman I, Smulow JB:* Periodontal disease: clinical, radiographic, and histopathologic features, *Philadelphia, 1974, Saunders.)*

Neural elements are extensively distributed throughout the gingival tissues. Within the gingival connective tissues, most nerve fibers are myelinated and closely associated with the blood vessels.[162] *Gingival innervation* is derived from fibers that arise from nerves in the periodontal ligament and from the labial, buccal, and palatal nerves.[30] The following nerve structures are present in the connective tissue: a meshwork of terminal argyrophilic fibers, some of which extend into the epithelium; Meissner-type tactile corpuscles; Krause-type end bulbs, which are temperature receptors; and encapsulated spindles.[14]

Correlation of Clinical and Microscopic Features

An understanding of the normal clinical features of the gingiva requires the ability to interpret them in terms of the microscopic structures that they represent.

Color

The color of the attached and marginal gingiva is generally described as "coral pink"; it is produced by the vascular supply, the thickness and degree of keratinization of the epithelium, and the presence of pigment-containing cells. The color varies among different persons and appears to be correlated with the cutaneous pigmentation. It is lighter in blond individuals with fair complexions than in swarthy, dark-haired individuals (Fig. 3.25).

The attached gingiva is demarcated from the adjacent alveolar mucosa on the buccal aspect by a clearly defined mucogingival line. The alveolar mucosa is red, smooth, and shiny rather than pink and stippled. A comparison of the microscopic structure of the attached gingiva with that of the alveolar mucosa provides an explanation for the difference in appearance. The epithelium of the alveolar mucosa is thinner and nonkeratinized, and it contains no rete pegs (Fig. 3.26). The connective tissue of the alveolar mucosa is loosely arranged, and the blood vessels are more numerous.

Physiologic Pigmentation (Melanin)

Melanin is a non–hemoglobin-derived brown pigment with the following characteristics:

- Melanin is responsible for the normal pigmentation of the skin, the gingiva, and the remainder of the oral mucous membrane.
- Melanin is present in all normal individuals (often not in sufficient quantities to be detected clinically), but it is absent or severely diminished in albinos.
- Melanin pigmentation in the oral cavity is prominent in black individuals (see Fig. 3.25).
- Ascorbic acid directly down-regulates melanin pigmentation in gingival tissues.[246]

According to Dummett,[73] the distribution of oral pigmentation in black individuals is as follows: gingiva, 60%; hard palate, 61%; mucous membrane, 22%; and tongue, 15%. Gingival pigmentation occurs as a diffuse, deep-purplish discoloration or as irregularly shaped brown and light-brown patches. It may appear in the gingiva as early as 3 hours after birth, and it is often the only evidence of pigmentation.[73]

Oral repigmentation refers to the clinical reappearance of melanin pigment after a period of clinical depigmentation of the oral mucosa as a result of chemical, thermal, surgical, pharmacologic, or idiopathic factors.[74] Information about the repigmentation of oral tissues after

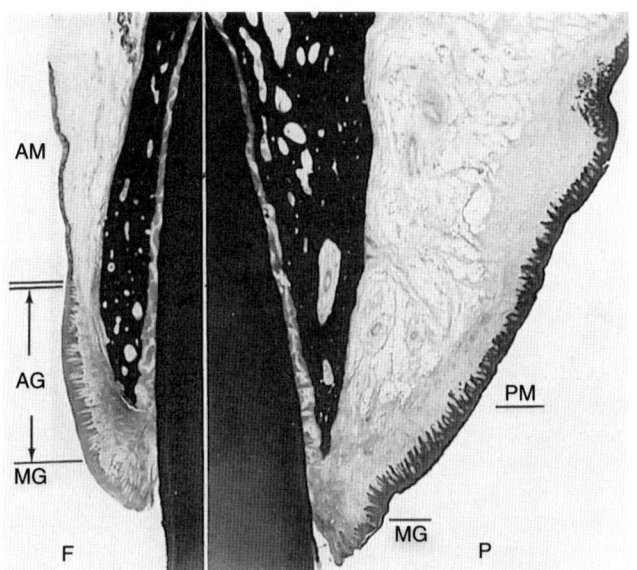

Fig. 3.26 Oral mucosa, facial and palatal surfaces. The facial surface *(F)* shows the marginal gingiva *(MG)*, the attached gingiva *(AG)*, and the alveolar mucosa *(AM)*. The double line marks the mucogingival junction. Note the differences in the epithelium and the connective tissue in the attached gingiva and the alveolar mucosa. The palatal surface *(P)* shows the marginal gingiva *(MG)* and the thick, keratinized palatal mucosa *(PM)*.

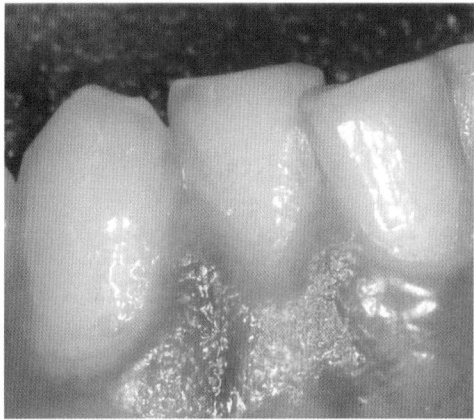

Fig. 3.27 A thickened, shelflike contour of gingiva on a tooth in lingual version aggravated by local irritation caused by plaque accumulation.

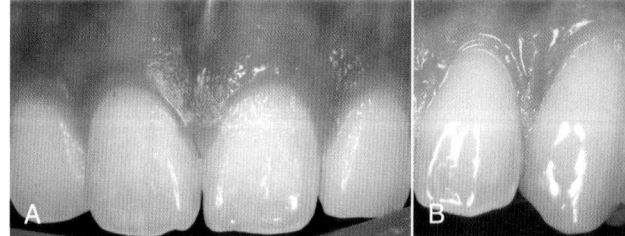

Fig. 3.28 Shape of the interdental gingival papillae correlated with the shape of the teeth and the embrasures. (A) Broad interdental papillae. (B) Narrow interdental papillae.

surgical procedures is extremely limited, and no definitive treatment is offered at this time.

Size

The size of the gingiva corresponds with the sum total of the bulk of cellular and intercellular elements and their vascular supply. Alteration in size is a common feature of gingival disease.

Contour

The contour or shape of the gingiva varies considerably and depends on the shape of the teeth and their alignment in the arch, the location and size of the area of proximal contact, and the dimensions of the facial and lingual gingival embrasures.

The marginal gingiva envelops the teeth in collar-like fashion and follows a scalloped outline on the facial and lingual surfaces. It forms a straight line along teeth with relatively flat surfaces. On teeth with pronounced mesiodistal convexity (e.g., maxillary canines) or teeth in labial version, the normal arcuate contour is accentuated, and the gingiva is located farther apically. On teeth in lingual version, the gingiva is horizontal and thickened (Fig. 3.27). In addition, the gingival tissue biotype varies significantly. A thin and clear gingiva is found in one-third of the population and primarily in females with slender teeth with a narrow zone of keratinized tissue, whereas a clear, thick gingiva with a broad zone of keratinized tissue is present in two-thirds of the population and primarily in males.[70]

Shape

The shape of the interdental gingiva is governed by the contour of the proximal tooth surfaces and the location and shape of the gingival embrasures.

When the proximal surfaces of the crowns are relatively flat faciolingually, the roots are close together, the interdental bone is thin mesiodistally, and the gingival embrasures and interdental gingiva are narrow mesiodistally. Conversely, with proximal surfaces that flare away from the area of contact, the mesiodistal diameter of the interdental gingiva is broad (Fig. 3.28). The height of the interdental gingiva varies with the location of the proximal contact. Thus in the anterior region of the dentition, the interdental papilla is pyramidal in form, whereas the papilla is more flattened in a buccolingual direction in the molar region.

Consistency

The gingiva is firm and resilient and, with the exception of the movable free margin, tightly bound to the underlying bone. The collagenous nature of the lamina propria and its contiguity with the mucoperiosteum of the alveolar bone determine the firmness of the attached gingiva. The gingival fibers contribute to the firmness of the gingival margin.

Surface Texture

The gingiva presents a textured surface similar to that of an orange peel and is referred to as *stippled* (see Fig. 3.25). Stippling is best viewed by drying the gingiva. *The attached gingiva is stippled; the marginal gingiva is not.* The central portion of the interdental papillae is usually stippled, but the marginal borders are smooth. The pattern and extent of stippling vary among individuals and among different areas of the same mouth.[108,216] Stippling is less prominent on lingual than facial surfaces and may be absent in some persons.

Stippling varies with age. It is absent during infancy, it appears in some children at about 5 years of age, it increases until adulthood, and it frequently begins to disappear during old age.

Microscopically, stippling is produced by alternate rounded protuberances and depressions in the gingival surface. The papillary layer of the connective tissue projects into the elevations, and the elevated and depressed areas are covered by stratified squamous epithelium (Fig. 3.29). The degree of keratinization and the prominence of stippling appear to be related.

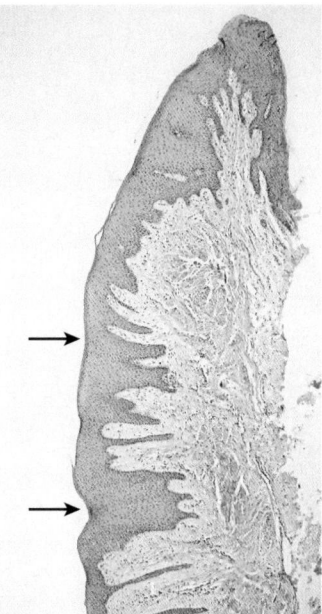

Fig. 3.29 Gingival biopsy of the patient shown in Fig. 3.7 demonstrating alternate elevations and depressions *(arrows)* in the attached gingiva that are responsible for the stippled appearance.

Scanning electron microscopy has shown considerable variation in shape but a relatively constant depth of stippling. At low magnification, a rippled surface is seen, and this is interrupted by irregular depressions that are 50 μm in diameter. At higher magnification, cell micropits are seen.[61]

Stippling is a form of adaptive specialization or reinforcement for function. It is a feature of healthy gingiva, and the reduction or loss of stippling is a common sign of gingival disease. When the gingiva is restored to health after treatment, the stippled appearance returns.

The surface texture of the gingiva is also related to the presence and degree of epithelial keratinization. Keratinization is considered a protective adaptation to function. It increases when the gingiva is stimulated by toothbrushing. However, research on free gingival grafts (see Chapter 65) has shown that when connective tissue is transplanted from a keratinized area to a nonkeratinized area, it becomes covered by a keratinized epithelium.[140] This finding suggests a connective-tissue–based genetic determination of the type of epithelial surface.

Position

The *position* of the gingiva is the level at which the gingival margin is attached to the tooth. When the tooth erupts into the oral cavity, the margin and sulcus are at the tip of the crown; as eruption progresses, they are seen closer to the root. During this eruption process, as described previously, the junctional epithelium, the oral epithelium, and the reduced enamel epithelium undergo extensive alterations and remodeling while maintaining the shallow physiologic depth of the sulcus. Without this remodeling of the epithelia, an abnormal anatomic relationship between the gingiva and the tooth would result.

Continuous Tooth Eruption

According to the concept of continuous eruption,[105] eruption does not cease when the teeth meet their functional antagonists; rather, it continues throughout life. Eruption consists of an active phase and a passive phase. *Active eruption* is the movement of the teeth in the direction of the occlusal plane, whereas *passive eruption* is the exposure of the teeth via apical migration of the gingiva.

This concept distinguishes between the anatomic crown (i.e., the portion of the tooth covered by enamel) and the anatomic root (i.e., the portion of the tooth covered by cementum) and between the clinical crown (i.e., the part of the tooth that has been denuded of its gingiva and projects into the oral cavity) and the clinical root (i.e., the portion of the tooth covered by periodontal tissues). When the teeth reach their functional antagonists, the gingival sulcus and the junctional epithelium are still on the enamel, and the clinical crown is approximately two-thirds of the anatomic crown.

Gottlieb and Orban[105] believed that active and passive eruption proceed together. Active eruption is coordinated with attrition; the teeth erupt to compensate for tooth substance that has been worn away by attrition. Attrition reduces the clinical crown and prevents it from becoming disproportionately long in relation to the clinical root, thus avoiding excessive leverage on the periodontal tissues. Ideally, the rate of active eruption keeps pace with tooth wear, thereby preserving the vertical dimension of the dentition.

As teeth erupt, cementum is deposited at the apices and furcations of the roots, and bone is formed along the fundus of the alveolus and at the crest of the alveolar bone. In this way, part of the tooth substance lost by attrition is replaced by the lengthening of the root, and the socket depth is maintained to support the root.

Although originally thought to be a normal physiologic process, passive eruption is now considered a pathologic process. Passive eruption is divided into the following four stages (Fig. 3.30):

Stage 1: The teeth reach the line of occlusion. The junctional epithelium and the base of the gingival sulcus are on the enamel.

Stage 2: The junctional epithelium proliferates so that part is on the cementum and part is on the enamel. The base of the sulcus is still on the enamel.

Stage 3: The entire junctional epithelium is on the cementum, and the base of the sulcus is at the cementoenamel junction. As the junctional epithelium proliferates from the crown onto the root, it does not remain at the cementoenamel junction any longer than at any other area of the tooth.

Stage 4: The junctional epithelium has proliferated farther on the cementum. The base of the sulcus is on the cementum, a portion of which is exposed. Proliferation of the junctional epithelium onto the root is accompanied by degeneration of the gingival and periodontal ligament fibers and their detachment from the tooth. The cause of this degeneration is not understood. At present, it is believed to be the result of chronic inflammation and therefore a pathologic process.

As noted, apposition of bone accompanies active eruption. The distance between the apical end of the junctional epithelium and the crest of the alveolus remains constant throughout continuous tooth eruption (i.e., 1.07 mm).[93]

Exposure of the tooth via the apical migration of the gingiva is called *gingival recession* or *atrophy*. According to the concept of continuous eruption, the gingival sulcus may be located on the crown, the cementoenamel junction, or the root, depending on the age of the patient and the stage of eruption. Therefore some root exposure with age would be considered normal and referred to as *physiologic recession*. Again, this concept is not accepted at present. Excessive exposure is termed *pathologic recession* (see Chapter 23).

Periodontal Ligament

The periodontal ligament is composed of a complex vascular and highly cellular connective tissue that surrounds the tooth root and connects it to the inner wall of the alveolar bone.[175] It is continuous

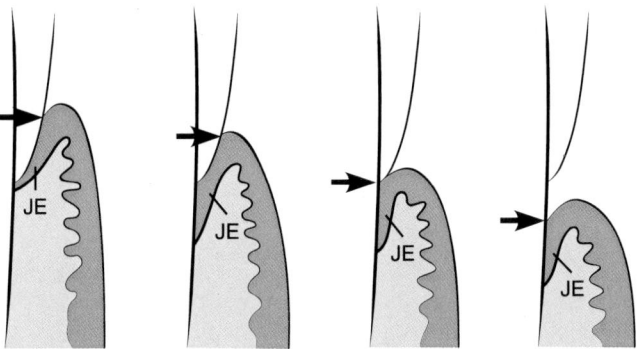

Fig. 3.30 Diagrammatic representation of the four steps of passive eruption according to Gottlieb and Orban.[105] **1,** The base of the gingival sulcus *(arrow)* and the junctional epithelium *(JE)* are on the enamel. **2,** The base of the gingival sulcus *(arrow)* is on the enamel, and part of the junctional epithelium is on the root. **3,** The base of the gingival sulcus *(arrow)* is at the cementoenamel line, and the entire junctional epithelium is on the root. **4,** The base of the gingival sulcus *(arrow)* and the junctional epithelium are on the root.

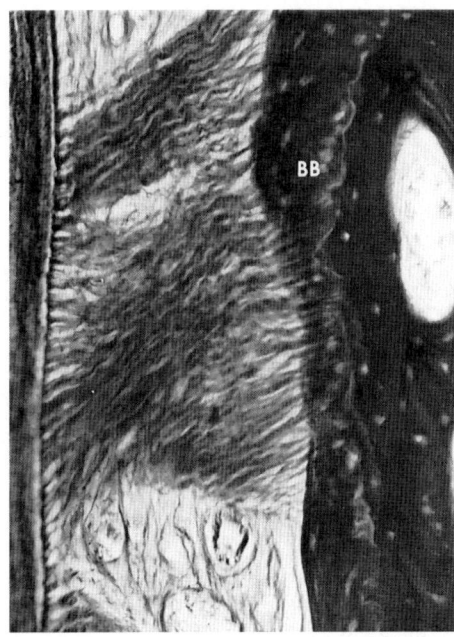

Fig. 3.32 Collagen fibers embedded in the cementum *(left)* and the bone *(right)* (silver stain). Note the Sharpey fibers within the bundle bone *(BB)* overlying the lamellar bone.

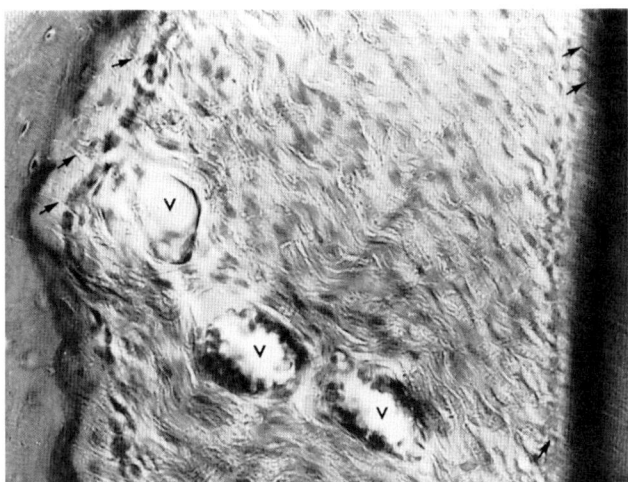

Fig. 3.31 Principal fibers of the periodontal ligament follow a wavy course when sectioned longitudinally. The formative function of the periodontal ligament is illustrated by the newly formed osteoid and osteoblasts along a previously resorbed bone surface *(left)* and the cementoid and cementoblasts *(right).* Note the fibers embedded in the forming calcified tissues *(arrows).* V, Vascular channels.

with the connective tissue of the gingiva, and it communicates with the marrow spaces through vascular channels in the bone. Although the average width of the periodontal ligament space is documented to be about 0.2 mm, considerable variation exists. The periodontal space is diminished around teeth that are not in function and in unerupted teeth, but it is increased in teeth that have been subjected to hyperfunction.

Periodontal Fibers

The most important elements of the periodontal ligament are the *principal fibers,* which are collagenous and arranged in bundles and which follow a wavy course when viewed in longitudinal section (Fig. 3.31). The terminal portions of the principal fibers that are inserted into cementum and bone are termed *Sharpey fibers* (Fig. 3.32). The principal fiber bundles consist of individual fibers that form a continuous anastomosing network between tooth and bone.[25,58] Once embedded in the wall of the alveolus or in the tooth, Sharpey

fibers calcify to a significant degree. They are associated with abundant noncollagenous proteins that are typically found in bone, and they have also been identified in tooth cementum.[33,132,175] Notable among these proteins are osteopontin and bone sialoprotein. These proteins are thought to contribute to the regulation of mineralization and to tissue cohesion at sites of increased biomechanical strain.[175]

Collagen is a protein that is composed of different amino acids, the most important of which are glycine, proline, hydroxylysine, and hydroxyproline.[51] The amount of collagen in a tissue can be determined by its hydroxyproline content. Collagen is responsible for the maintenance of the framework and the tone of tissue, and it exhibits a wide range of diversity.[80] There are at least 19 recognized collagen species encoded by at least 25 separate genes dispersed among 12 chromosomes.[80]

Collagen biosynthesis occurs inside the fibroblasts to form tropocollagen molecules. These aggregate into microfibrils that are packed together to form fibrils. Collagen fibrils have a transverse striation with a characteristic periodicity of 64 μm; this striation is caused by the overlapping arrangement of the tropocollagen molecules. In collagen types I and III, these fibrils associate to form fibers; in collagen type I, the fibers associate to form bundles (Fig. 3.33).

Collagen is synthesized by fibroblasts, chondroblasts, osteoblasts, odontoblasts, and other cells. The several types of collagen are all distinguishable by their chemical composition, distribution, function, and morphology.[138] The principal fibers are composed mainly of collagen type I,[211] whereas reticular fibers are composed of collagen type III. Collagen type IV is found in the basal lamina.[212,214] The expression of type XII collagen during tooth development is timed with the alignment and organization of periodontal fibers and is limited in tooth development to cells within the periodontal ligament.[164] Type VI collagen has also been immunolocalized in the periodontal ligament and the gingiva.[83]

The molecular configuration of collagen fibers provides them with a tensile strength that is greater than that of steel. Consequently, collagen imparts a unique combination of flexibility and strength to the tissues.[138]

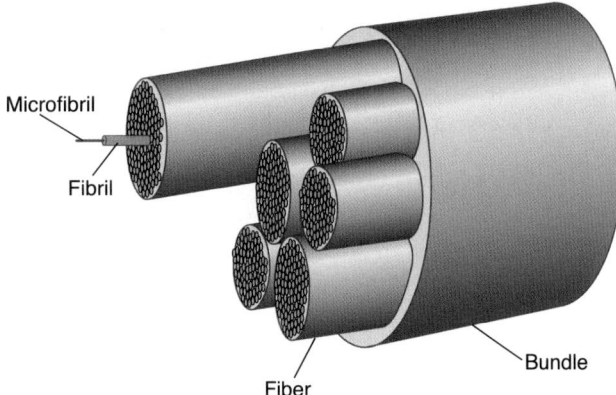

Fig. 3.33 Collagen microfibrils, fibrils, fibers, and bundles.

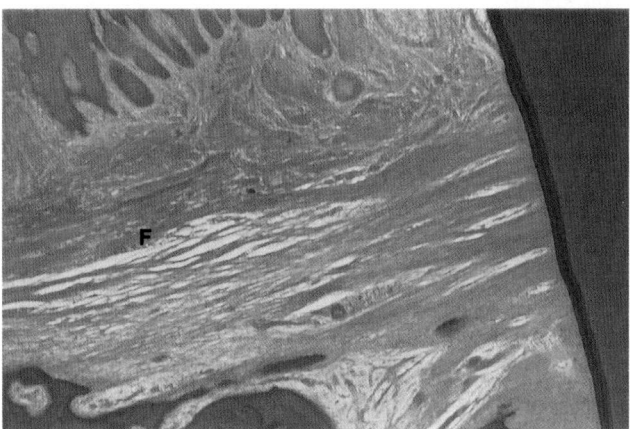

Fig. 3.35 Transseptal fibers *(F)* at the crest of the interdental bone.

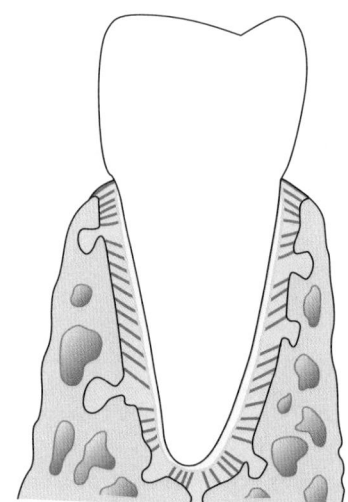

Fig. 3.34 Diagram of the principal fiber groups.

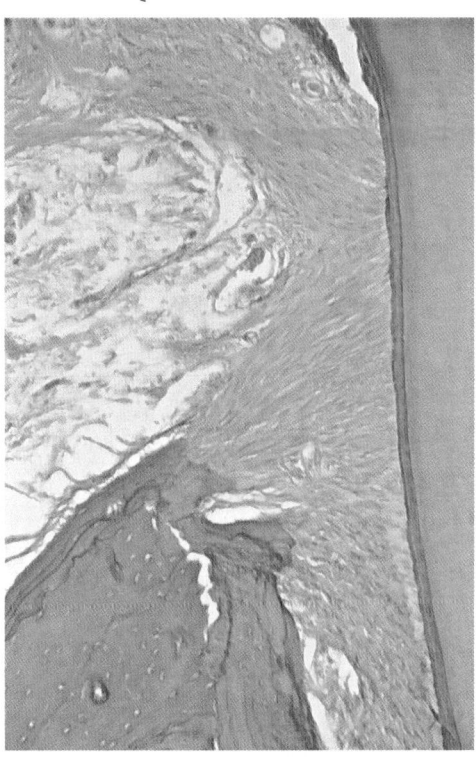

Fig. 3.36 Rat molar section showing alveolar crest fibers radiating coronally.

The principal fibers of the periodontal ligament are arranged in six groups that develop sequentially in the developing root: the transseptal, alveolar crest, horizontal, oblique, apical, and interradicular fibers (Fig. 3.34).

Transseptal fibers extend interproximally over the alveolar bone crest and are embedded in the cementum of adjacent teeth (Fig. 3.35). They are reconstructed even after destruction of the alveolar bone that results from periodontal disease. These fibers may be considered as belonging to the gingiva, because they do not have osseous attachment.

Alveolar crest fibers extend obliquely from the cementum just beneath the junctional epithelium to the alveolar crest (Fig. 3.36). Fibers also run from the cementum over the alveolar crest and to the fibrous layer of the periosteum that covers the alveolar bone. The alveolar crest fibers prevent the extrusion of the tooth[53] and resist lateral tooth movements. The incision of these fibers during periodontal surgery does not increase tooth mobility unless significant attachment loss has occurred.[97]

Horizontal fibers extend at right angles to the long axis of the tooth from the cementum to the alveolar bone.

Oblique fibers, which constitute the largest group in the periodontal ligament, extend from the cementum in a coronal direction obliquely to the bone (see Fig. 3.34). They bear the brunt of vertical masticatory stresses and transform such stresses into tension on the alveolar bone.

The *apical fibers* radiate in a rather irregular manner from the cementum to the bone at the apical region of the socket. They do not occur on incompletely formed roots.

The *interradicular fibers* fan out from the cementum to the tooth in the furcation areas of multirooted teeth.

Other well-formed fiber bundles interdigitate at right angles or splay around and between regularly arranged fiber bundles. Less regularly arranged collagen fibers are found in the interstitial connective tissue between the principal fiber groups; this tissue contains the blood vessels, lymphatics, and nerves.

Although the periodontal ligament does not contain mature elastin, two immature forms are found: oxytalan and elaunin. The so-called oxytalan fibers[89,103] run parallel to the root surface in a vertical direction and bend to attach to the cementum[89] in the cervical third of the root. They are thought to regulate vascular flow.[88] An elastic meshwork has been described in the periodontal ligament[133] as being composed of many elastin lamellae with peripheral oxytalan fibers and elaunin fibers. Oxytalan fibers have been shown to develop de novo in the regenerated periodontal ligament.[219]

The principal fibers are remodeled by the periodontal ligament cells to adapt to physiologic needs[265,295] and in response to different stimuli.[277] In addition to these fiber types, small collagen fibers associated with the larger principal collagen fibers have been described. These fibers run in all directions and form a plexus called the *indifferent fiber plexus*.[243]

Cellular Elements

Four types of cells have been identified in the periodontal ligament: connective tissue cells, epithelial rest cells, immune system cells, and cells associated with neurovascular elements.[26,27]

Connective tissue cells include fibroblasts, cementoblasts, and osteoblasts. Fibroblasts are the most common cells in the periodontal ligament; they appear as ovoid or elongated cells oriented along the principal fibers, and they exhibit pseudopodia-like processes.[210] These cells synthesize collagen and possess the capacity to phagocytose "old" collagen fibers and degrade them[265] via enzyme hydrolysis. Thus collagen turnover appears to be regulated by fibroblasts in a process of intracellular degradation of collagen that does not involve the action of collagenase.[24]

Phenotypically distinct and functionally different subpopulations of fibroblasts exist in the adult periodontal ligament. They appear to be identical at both the light and electron microscopic levels,[115] but they may have different functions, such as the secretion of different collagen types and the production of collagenase.

Osteoblasts, cementoblasts, osteoclasts, and odontoclasts are also seen in the cemental and osseous surfaces of the periodontal ligament.

The *epithelial rests of Malassez* form a latticework in the periodontal ligament and appear as either isolated clusters of cells or interlacing strands (Fig. 3.37), depending on the plane in which the microscopic section is cut. Continuity with the junctional epithelium has been suggested in experimental animals.[106] The epithelial rests are considered remnants of the Hertwig root sheath, which disintegrates during root development (Fig. 3.37A).

Epithelial rests are distributed close to the cementum throughout the periodontal ligament of most teeth; they are most numerous in the apical area[207] and the cervical area.[279,280] They diminish in number with age[248] by degenerating and disappearing or by undergoing calcification to become cementicles. The cells are surrounded by a distinct basal lamina, they are interconnected by hemidesmosomes, and they contain tonofilaments.[24]

Although their functional properties are still considered to be unclear,[259] the epithelial rests are reported to contain keratinocyte growth factors, and they have been shown to be positive for tyrosine kinase A neurotrophin receptor.[92,281,291] In addition, epithelial rests proliferate when stimulated,[261,266,275] and they participate in the formation of periapical cysts and lateral root cysts.

The *defense cells* in the periodontal ligament include neutrophils, lymphocytes, macrophages, mast cells, and eosinophils. These cells, as well as those associated with neurovascular elements, are similar to the cells found in other connective tissues.

Ground Substance

The periodontal ligament also contains a large proportion of ground substance that fills the spaces between fibers and cells. This substance consists of two main components: *glycosaminoglycans,* such as hyaluronic acid and proteoglycans, and *glycoproteins,* such as fibronectin and laminin. It also has a high water content (i.e., 70%).

The cell surface proteoglycans participate in several biologic functions, including cell adhesion, cell–cell and cell–matrix interactions, binding to various growth factors as coreceptors, and cell repair.[292] For example, fibromodulin (a small proteoglycan rich in keratan sulfate and leucine) has been identified in bovine periodontal ligament.[283] The most comprehensive study of the proteoglycans in periodontal ligament was performed with the use of fibroblast cultures of human ligament.[149]

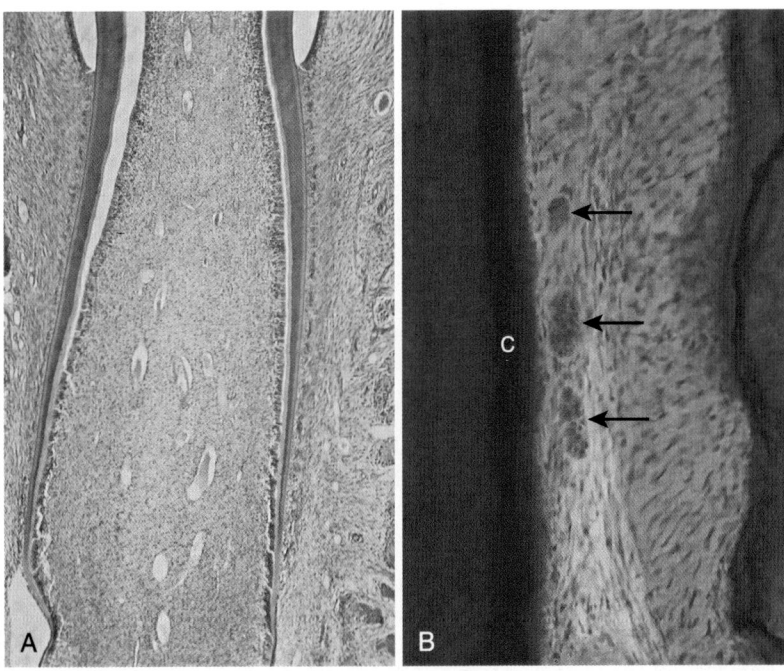

Fig. 3.37 Epithelial rests of Malassez. (A) Erupting tooth in a cat. Note the fragmentation of the Hertwig epithelial root sheath giving rise to epithelial rests located along and close to the root surface. (B) Human periodontal ligament with rosette-shaped epithelial rests *(arrows)* lying close to the cementum *(C)*.

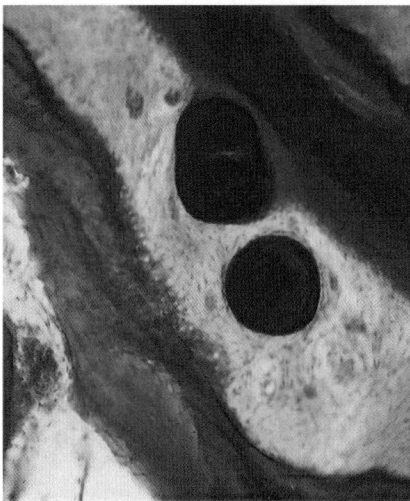

Fig. 3.38 Cementicles in the periodontal ligament. One is lying free and the other is adherent to the tooth surface.

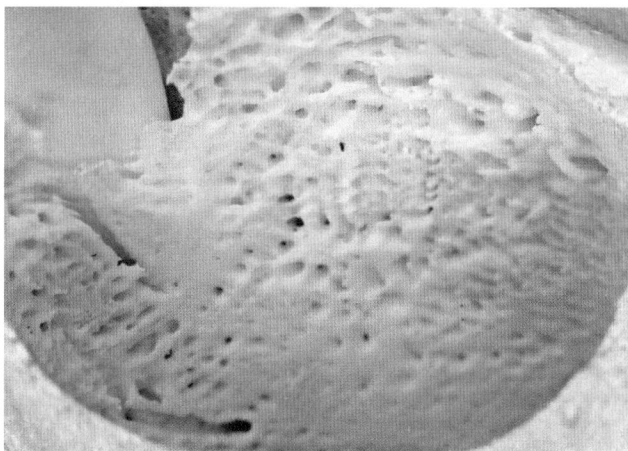

Fig. 3.39 Foramina perforating the lamina dura of a dog jaw.

The periodontal ligament may also contain calcified masses called *cementicles,* which are adherent to or detached from the root surfaces (Fig. 3.38).

Cementicles may develop from calcified epithelial rests; around small spicules of cementum or alveolar bone traumatically displaced into the periodontal ligament; from calcified Sharpey fibers; and from calcified, thrombosed vessels within the periodontal ligament.[180]

Functions of Periodontal Ligament

The functions of the periodontal ligament are categorized as physical, formative and remodeling, nutritional, and sensory.

Physical Functions

The physical functions of the periodontal ligament entail the following:

1. Provision of a soft-tissue "casing" to protect the vessels and nerves from injury by mechanical forces
2. Transmission of occlusal forces to the bone
3. Attachment of the teeth to the bone
4. Maintenance of the gingival tissues in their proper relationship to the teeth
5. Resistance to the impact of occlusal forces (i.e., shock absorption)

Resistance to Impact of Occlusal Forces (Shock Absorption)

Two theories pertaining to the mechanism of tooth support have been considered: the tensional theory and the viscoelastic system theory.

The tensional theory of tooth support states that the principal fibers of the periodontal ligament are the major factor in supporting the tooth and transmitting forces to the bone. When a force is applied to the crown, the principal fibers first unfold and straighten, and they then transmit forces to the alveolar bone, thereby causing an elastic deformation of the bony socket. Finally, when the alveolar bone has reached its limit, the load is transmitted to the basal bone. Many investigators find this theory insufficient to explain available experimental evidence.

The viscoelastic system theory states that the displacement of the tooth is largely controlled by fluid movements, with fibers having only a secondary role.[31,43] When forces are transmitted to the tooth,

the extracellular fluid passes from the periodontal ligament into the marrow spaces of the bone through the foramina in the cribriform plate. These perforations of the cribriform plate link the periodontal ligament with the cancellous portion of the alveolar bone; they are more abundant in the cervical third than in the middle and apical thirds (Fig. 3.39).

After the depletion of tissue fluids, the fiber bundles absorb the slack and tighten. This leads to a blood vessel stenosis. Arterial back pressure causes ballooning of the vessels and passage of the blood ultrafiltrates into the tissues, thereby replenishing the tissue fluids.[31]

Transmission of Occlusal Forces to Bone

The arrangement of the principal fibers is similar to that of a suspension bridge or a hammock. When an axial force is applied to a tooth, a tendency toward displacement of the root into the alveolus occurs. The oblique fibers alter their wavy, untensed pattern, assume their full length, and sustain the major part of the axial force. When a horizontal or tipping force is applied, two phases of tooth movement occur. The first is within the confines of the periodontal ligament, and the second produces a displacement of the facial and lingual bony plates.[69] The tooth rotates about an axis that may change as the force is increased.

The apical portion of the root moves in a direction that is opposite to the coronal portion. In areas of tension, the principal fiber bundles are taut rather than wavy. In areas of pressure, the fibers are compressed, the tooth is displaced, and a corresponding distortion of bone exists in the direction of root movement.[203]

In single-rooted teeth, the axis of rotation is located in the area between the apical third and the middle third of the root (Fig. 3.40). The root apex[184] and the coronal half of the clinical root have been suggested as other locations of the axis of rotation. The periodontal ligament, which has an hourglass shape, is narrowest in the region of the axis of rotation[65,145] (Table 3.1). In multirooted teeth, the axis of rotation is located in the bone between the roots (Fig. 3.41). In compliance with the physiologic mesial migration of the teeth, the periodontal ligament is thinner on the mesial root surface than on the distal surface.

Formative and Remodeling Function

Periodontal ligament and alveolar bone cells are exposed to physical forces in response to mastication, parafunction, speech, and orthodontic tooth movement.[173] Cells of the periodontal ligament participate in the formation and resorption of cementum and bone, which occur during physiologic tooth movement, during the accommodation of

TABLE 3.1 Thickness of the Periodontal Ligaments of 172 Teeth From 15 Human Subjects

	Average of Alveolar Crest (mm)	Average of Midroot (mm)	Average of Apex (mm)	Average of Tooth (mm)
Ages 11 through 16 years 83 teeth from 4 jaws	0.23	0.17	0.24	0.21
Ages 32 through 50 years 36 teeth from 5 jaws	0.20	0.14	0.19	0.18
Ages 51 through 67 years 35 teeth from 5 jaws	0.17	0.12	0.16	0.15
Age 24 years (1 case) 18 teeth from 1 jaw	0.16	0.09	0.15	0.13

Modified from Coolidge ED: The thickness of the human periodontal membrane. *J Am Dent Assoc* 24:1260, 1937.

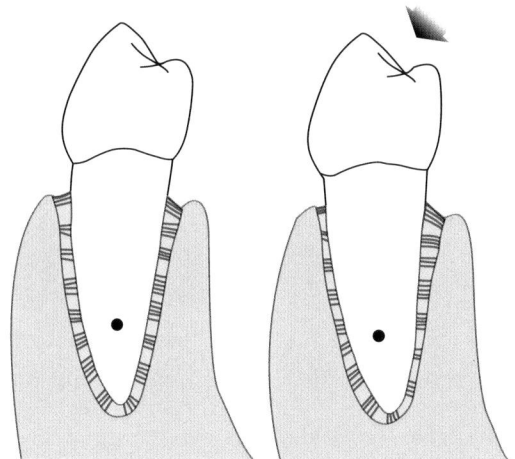

Fig. 3.40 *Left,* Diagram of a mandibular premolar in a resting state. *Right,* When a force is exerted on the tooth—in this case, in faciolingual direction *(arrow)*—the tooth rotates around the fulcrum or axis of rotation *(black circle on root)*. The periodontal ligament is compressed in areas of pressure and distended in areas of tension.

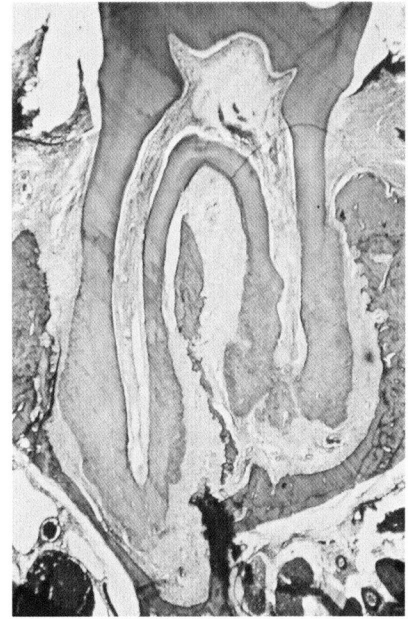

Fig. 3.41 Microscopic view of a rat molar subjected to occlusohorizontal forces. Note the alternating widened and narrowed areas of the periodontal ligament as the tooth rotates around its axis of rotation. The axis of rotation is in the interradicular space.

the periodontium to occlusal forces, and during the repair of injuries.

Variations in cellular enzyme activity are correlated with the remodeling process.[94-96] Although applied loads may induce vascular and inflammatory reactive changes in periodontal ligament cells, current evidence suggests that these cells have a mechanism to respond directly to mechanical forces via the activation of various mechanosensory signaling systems, including adenylate cyclase, stretch-activated ion channels, and via changes in cytoskeletal organization.[173]

Cartilage formation in the periodontal ligament, although unusual, may represent a metaplastic phenomenon in the repair of this ligament after injury.[20]

The periodontal ligament is constantly undergoing remodeling. Old cells and fibers are broken down and replaced by new ones, and mitotic activity can be observed in the fibroblasts and the endothelial cells.[185] Fibroblasts form the collagen fibers, and the residual mesenchymal cells develop into osteoblasts and cementoblasts. Therefore the rate of formation and the differentiation of osteoblasts, cementoblasts, and fibroblasts affect the rate of formation of collagen, cementum, and bone.

Radioautographic studies with radioactive thymidine, proline, and glycine indicate a high turnover rate of collagen in the periodontal ligament. The rate of collagen synthesis is twice as fast as that in the gingiva and four times as fast as that in the skin, as established in the rat molar.[250] A rapid turnover of sulfated glycosaminoglycans in the cells and amorphous ground substance of the periodontal ligament also occurs.[21] It should be noted that most of these studies have been performed in rodents and that information about primates and humans is scarce.[232]

Nutritional and Sensory Functions

The periodontal ligament supplies nutrients to the cementum, bone, and gingiva by way of the blood vessels, and it also provides lymphatic drainage as discussed later in this chapter. In relation to other ligaments and tendons, the periodontal ligament is highly vascularized tissue; almost 10% of its volume in the rodent molar is blood vessels.[35,174] This relatively high blood vessel content may provide hydrodynamic damping to applied forces as well as high perfusion rates to the periodontal ligament.[173]

The periodontal ligament is abundantly supplied with sensory nerve fibers that are capable of transmitting tactile, pressure, and pain sensations via the trigeminal pathways.[14,30] Nerve bundles pass into the periodontal ligament from the periapical area and through channels from the alveolar bone that follow the course of the blood vessels. The bundles divide into single myelinated fibers, which ultimately lose their myelin sheaths and end in one of four types of neural termination: (1) free endings, which have a treelike configuration and carry pain sensation; (2) Ruffini-like mechanoreceptors, which are located primarily in the apical area; (3) coiled Meissner corpuscles and mechanoreceptors, which are found mainly in the midroot region; and (4) spindle-like pressure and vibration endings, which are surrounded by a fibrous capsule and located mainly in the apex.[88,166]

Regulation of Periodontal Ligament Width

Some of the most interesting features of the periodontal ligament in animals are its adaptability to rapidly changing applied force and its capacity to maintain its width at constant dimensions throughout its lifetime.[174] These are important measures of periodontal ligament homeostasis that provide insight into the function of the biologic mechanisms that tightly regulate the metabolism and spatial locations of the cell populations involved in the formation of bone, cementum, and periodontal ligament fibers. In addition, the ability of periodontal ligament cells to synthesize and secrete a wide range of regulatory molecules is an essential component of tissue remodeling and periodontal ligament homeostasis.[173]

Cementum

Cementum is the calcified, avascular mesenchymal tissue that forms the outer covering of the anatomic root. The two main types of cementum are acellular *(primary)* and cellular *(secondary)* cementum.[104] Both consist of a calcified interfibrillar matrix and collagen fibrils.

The two main sources of collagen fibers in cementum are Sharpey fibers *(extrinsic)*, which are the embedded portion of the principal fibers of the periodontal ligament[214] and which are formed by the fibroblasts, and fibers that belong to the cementum matrix *(intrinsic)*, which are produced by the cementoblasts.[240] Cementoblasts also form the noncollagenous components of the interfibrillar ground substance, such as proteoglycans, glycoproteins, and phosphoproteins. Proteoglycans are most likely to play a role in regulating cell–cell and cell–matrix interactions, both during normal development and during the regeneration of the cementum.[17] In addition, immunohistochemical studies have shown that the distribution of proteoglycans is closely associated with the cementoblasts and the cementocytes.[1,2]

The major proportion of the organic matrix of cementum is composed of type I (90%) and type III (about 5%) collagens. Sharpey fibers, which constitute a considerable proportion of the bulk of cementum, are composed of mainly type I collagen.[206] Type III collagen appears to coat the type I collagen of the Sharpey fibers.[16]

Acellular cementum is the first cementum formed; it covers approximately the cervical third or half of the root, and it does not contain cells (Fig. 3.42). This cementum is formed before the tooth reaches the occlusal plane, and its thickness ranges from 30 to 230 μm.[248] Sharpey fibers make up most of the structure of acellular cementum, which has a principal role in supporting the tooth. Most fibers are inserted at approximately right angles into the root surface and penetrate deep into the cementum, but others enter from several different directions. Their size, number, and distribution increase with function.[123] Sharpey fibers are completely calcified, with the mineral crystals oriented parallel to the fibrils as in dentin and bone,

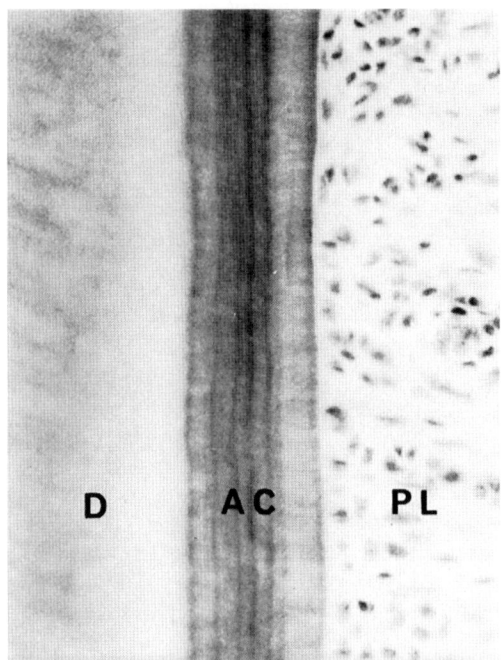

Fig. 3.42 Acellular cementum *(AC)* showing incremental lines running parallel to the long axis of the tooth. These lines represent the appositional growth of cementum. Note the thin, light lines running into the cementum perpendicular to the surface; these represent the Sharpey fibers of the periodontal ligament *(PL)*. D, Dentin. (×300.)

except in a 10- to 50-μm–wide zone near the cementodentinal junction, where they are only partially calcified. The peripheral portions of Sharpey fibers in actively mineralizing cementum tend to be more calcified than the interior regions, according to evidence obtained by scanning electron microscopy.[137] Acellular cementum also contains intrinsic collagen fibrils that are calcified and irregularly arranged or parallel to the surface.[232]

Cellular cementum, which is formed after the tooth reaches the occlusal plane, is more irregular and contains cells (cementocytes) in individual spaces (lacunae) that communicate with each other through a system of anastomosing canaliculi (Fig. 3.43). Cellular cementum is less calcified than the acellular type.[124] Sharpey fibers occupy a smaller portion of cellular cementum and are separated by other fibers that are arranged either parallel to the root surface or at random. Sharpey fibers may be completely or partially calcified, or they may have a central, uncalcified core surrounded by a calcified border.[135,240]

Both acellular cementum and cellular cementum are arranged in lamellae separated by incremental lines parallel to the long axis of the root (see Figs. 3.42 and 3.43). These lines represent "rest periods" in cementum formation, and they are more mineralized than the adjacent cementum.[215] In addition, the loss of the cervical part of the reduced enamel epithelium at the time of tooth eruption may place portions of mature enamel in contact with the connective tissue, which then will deposit an acellular and afibrillar type of cementum over the enamel.[157]

On the basis of these findings, Schroeder[133,134] has classified cementum as follows:

- Acellular afibrillar cementum contains neither cells nor extrinsic or intrinsic collagen fibers, except for a mineralized ground substance. Acellular afibrillar cementum is a product of cementoblasts and found as coronal cementum in humans, with a thickness of 1 to 15 μm.

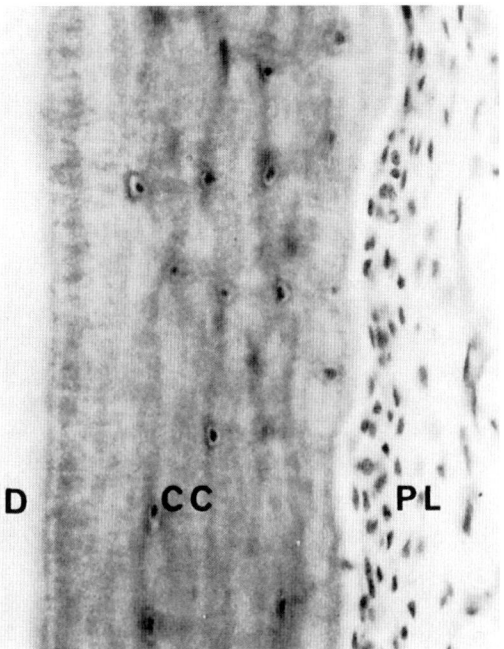

Fig. 3.43 Cellular cementum *(CC)* showing cementocytes lying within the lacunae. Cellular cementum is thicker than acellular cementum. The evidence of incremental lines also exists, but they are less distinct than in the acellular cementum. The cells adjacent to the surface of the cementum in the periodontal ligament *(PL)* space are cementoblasts. *D,* Dentin. (×300.)

- Acellular extrinsic fiber cementum is composed almost entirely of densely packed bundles of Sharpey fibers and lacks cells. Acellular extrinsic fiber cementum is a product of fibroblasts and cementoblasts. It is found in the cervical third of roots in humans, but it may extend farther apically. Its thickness is between 30 and 230 μm.
- Cellular mixed stratified cementum is composed of extrinsic (Sharpey) and intrinsic fibers, and it may contain cells. Cellular mixed stratified cementum is a co-product of fibroblasts and cementoblasts. In humans, it appears primarily in the apical third of the roots and apices and in furcation areas. Its thickness ranges from 100 to 1000 μm.
- Cellular intrinsic fiber cementum contains cells but no extrinsic collagen fibers. Cellular intrinsic fiber cementum is formed by cementoblasts, and, in humans, it fills the resorption lacunae.

Intermediate cementum is a poorly defined zone near the cementodentinal junction of certain teeth that appears to contain cellular remnants of the Hertwig sheath embedded in a calcified ground substance.[77,153]

Inorganic content of cementum (hydroxyapatite; $Ca_{10}[PO_4]_6[OH]_2$) is 45% to 50%, which is less than that of bone (65%), enamel (97%), or dentin (70%).[299] Opinions differ with regard to whether the microhardness increases[189] or decreases with age,[282] and no relationship has been established between aging and the mineral content of cementum.

Permeability of Cementum

In very young animals, acellular cementum and cellular cementum are very permeable and permit the diffusion of dyes from the pulp and the external root surface. In cellular cementum, the canaliculi in some areas are contiguous with the dentinal tubules. The permeability of cementum diminishes with age.[36]

Cementoenamel Junction

The cementum at and immediately subjacent to the *cementoenamel junction* is of particular clinical importance in root-scaling procedures. Three types of relationships involving the cementum may exist at the cementoenamel junction.[190] In about 60% to 65% of cases, cementum overlaps the enamel (Fig. 3.44); in about 30%, an edge-to-edge butt joint exists; and in 5% to 10%, the cementum and enamel fail to meet. In the last case, gingival recession may result in accentuated sensitivity as a result of exposed dentin.

Cementodentinal Junction

The terminal apical area of the cementum where it joins the internal root canal dentin is known as the *cementodentinal junction.* When root canal treatment is performed, the obturating material should be at the cementodentinal junction. There appears to be no increase or decrease in the width of the cementodentinal junction with age; its width appears to remain relatively stable.[253] Scanning electron microscopy of the human teeth reveals that the cementodentinal junction is 2 to 3 μm wide. The fibril-poor layer contains a significant amount of proteoglycans, and fibrils intermingle between the cementum and the dentin.[293,294]

Thickness of Cementum

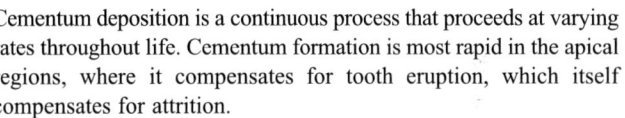

Cementum deposition is a continuous process that proceeds at varying rates throughout life. Cementum formation is most rapid in the apical regions, where it compensates for tooth eruption, which itself compensates for attrition.

The thickness of cementum on the coronal half of the root varies from 16 to 60 μm, which is about the thickness of a hair. It attains its greatest thickness (≤150 to 200 μm) in the apical third and in the furcation areas. It is thicker in distal surfaces than in mesial surfaces, probably because of functional stimulation from mesial drift over time.[68] Between the ages of 11 and 70 years, the average thickness of the cementum increases threefold, with the greatest increase seen in the apical region. Average thicknesses of 95 μm at the age of 20 years and of 215 μm at the age of 60 years have been reported.[298]

Abnormalities in the thickness of cementum may range from an absence or paucity of cellular cementum (i.e., cemental aplasia or hypoplasia) to an excessive deposition of cementum (i.e., cemental hyperplasia or hypercementosis).[152]

The term *hypercementosis* refers to a prominent thickening of the cementum. It is largely an age-related phenomenon, and it may be localized to one tooth or affect the entire dentition. As a result of considerable physiologic variation in the thickness of cementum among different teeth in the same person and also among different persons, distinguishing between hypercementosis and the physiologic thickening of cementum is sometimes difficult. Nevertheless, the excessive proliferation of cementum may occur with a broad spectrum of neoplastic and nonneoplastic conditions, including benign cementoblastoma, cementifying fibroma, periapical cemental dysplasia, florid cemento-osseous dysplasia, and other benign fibro-osseous lesions.[152]

Hypercementosis itself does not require treatment. It could pose a problem if an affected tooth requires extraction. In a multirooted tooth, sectioning of the tooth may be required before extraction.[19]

Cementum Resorption and Repair

Permanent teeth do not undergo physiologic resorption as primary teeth do. However, the cementum of erupted (as well as unerupted) teeth is subject to resorptive changes that may be of microscopic proportion or sufficiently extensive to present a radiographically detectable alteration in the root contour.

Microscopic cementum resorption is extremely common; in one study, it occurred in 236 of 261 teeth (90.5%).[118] The average number of resorption areas per tooth was 3.5. Of the 922 areas of resorption, 708 (76.8%) were located in the apical third of the root, 177 (19.2%) in the middle third, and 37 (4.0%) in the gingival third. Approximately 70% of all resorption areas were confined to the cementum without involving the dentin.

Cementum resorption may be caused by local or systemic factors, or it may occur without apparent etiology (i.e., idiopathic). Local conditions that cause cementum resorption include trauma from occlusion[194] (Fig. 3.45); orthodontic movement[117,193,217]; pressure from malaligned erupting teeth, cysts, and tumors[144]; teeth without functional antagonists; embedded teeth; replanted and transplanted teeth[3,135]; periapical disease; and periodontal disease. Systemic conditions that are cited as predisposing an individual to or inducing cemental resorption include calcium deficiency,[136] hypothyroidism,[23] hereditary fibrous osteodystrophy,[269] and Paget disease.[218]

Cementum resorption appears microscopically as baylike concavities in the root surface. (Fig. 3.46) Multinucleated giant cells and large mononuclear macrophages are generally found adjacent to

cementum that is undergoing active resorption (Fig. 3.47). Several sites of resorption may coalesce to form a large area of destruction. The resorptive process may extend into the underlying dentin and even into the pulp, but it is usually painless. Cementum resorption is not necessarily continuous and may alternate with periods of repair and the deposition of new cementum. The newly formed cementum is demarcated from the root by a deeply staining irregular line termed a *reversal line,* which delineates the border of the previous resorption. One study showed that the reversal lines of human teeth contain a few collagen fibrils and highly accumulated proteoglycans with mucopolysaccharides (glycosaminoglycans) and that fibril intermingling occurs only in some places between reparative cementum and resorbed dentin or cementum.[293,294] Embedded fibers of the periodontal ligament reestablish a functional relationship in the new cementum.

Cementum repair requires the presence of viable connective tissue. If epithelium proliferates into an area of resorption, repair will not

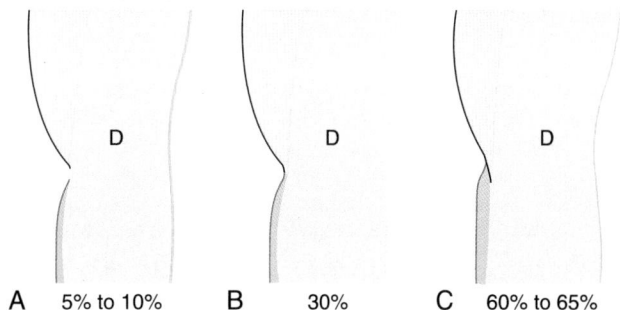

| A 5% to 10% | B 30% | C 60% to 65% |

Fig. 3.44 Normal variations in tooth morphology at the cementoenamel junction. (A) Space between the enamel and the cementum with the dentin *(D)* exposed. (B) End-to-end relationship of enamel and cementum. (C) Cementum overlapping the enamel.

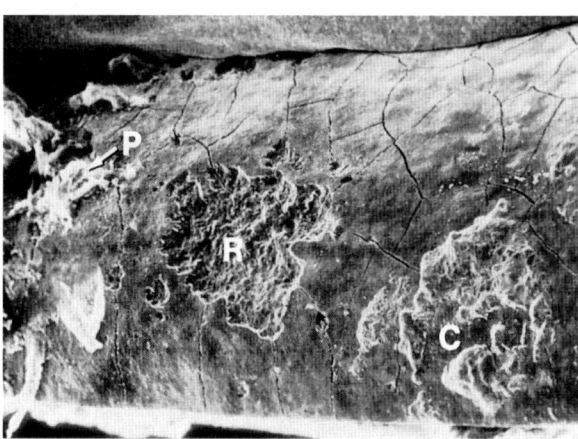

Fig. 3.46 Scanning electron micrograph of a root exposed by periodontal disease showing a large resorption bay *(R).* Remnants of the periodontal ligament *(P)* and calculus *(C)* are visible. Cracking of the tooth surface occurs as a result of the preparation technique. (×160.) *(Courtesy Dr. John Sottosanti, La Jolla, California.)*

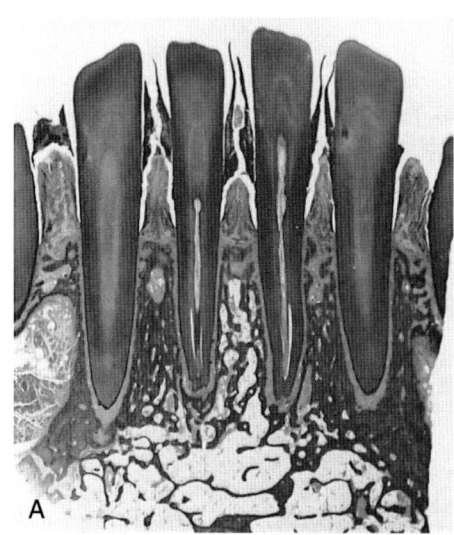
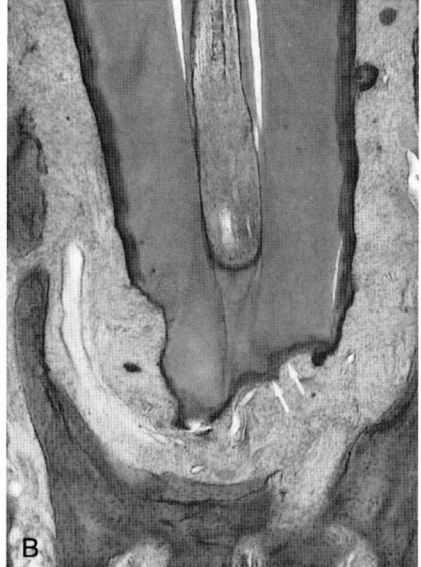

Fig. 3.45 Cemental resorption associated with excessive occlusal forces. (A) Low-power histologic section of the mandibular anterior teeth. (B) High-power micrograph of the apex of the left central incisor shortened by the resorption of cementum and dentin. Note the partial repair of the eroded areas *(arrows)* and the cementicle at the upper right.

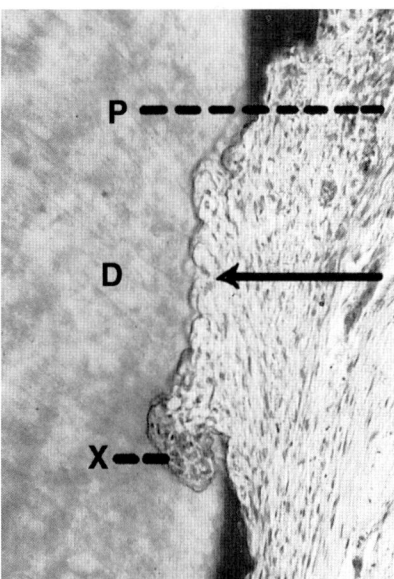

Fig. 3.47 Resorption of cementum and dentin. A multinuclear osteoclast in seen *(X)*. The direction of resorption is indicated by the arrow. Note the scalloped resorption front in the dentin *(D)*. The cementum is the darkly stained band at the upper and lower right. *P,* Periodontal ligament.

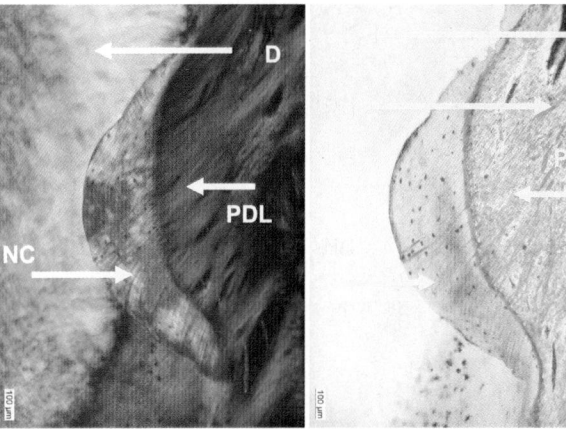

Fig. 3.48 A clinical human histology shows that new cementum and new periodontal ligament fiber formed at a previous periodontal defect treated with recombinant human platelet-derived growth factor-BB with β-tricalcium phosphate. *(Courtesy Dr. Daniel WK Kao, Philadelphia, Pennsylvania.)*

take place. Cementum repair can occur in devitalized as well as vital teeth.

Histologic evidence demonstrates that cementum formation is critical for the appropriate maturation of the periodontium, both during development and during the regeneration of lost periodontal tissues.[225] In other words, a variety of macromolecules present in the extracellular matrix of the periodontium are likely to play a regulatory role in cementogenesis.[169]

The regeneration of cementum requires cementoblasts, but the origin of the cementoblasts and the molecular factors that regulate their recruitment and differentiation are not fully understood. However, research provides a better understanding; for example, the epithelial cell rests of Malassez are the only odontogenic epithelial cells that remain in the periodontium after the eruption of teeth, and they may have some function in cementum repair and regeneration under specific conditions.[114] The rests of Malassez may be related to cementum repair by activating their potential to secrete matrix proteins that have been expressed in tooth development, such as amelogenins, enamelins, and sheath proteins. Several growth factors have been shown to be effective in cementum regeneration, including members of the transforming growth factor superfamily (i.e., bone morphogenetic proteins), platelet-derived growth factor, insulin-like growth factor, and enamel matrix derivatives[139,225] (Fig. 3.48).

Ankylosis

Fusion of the cementum and the alveolar bone with obliteration of the periodontal ligament is termed *ankylosis*. Ankylosis occurs in teeth with cemental resorption, which suggests that it may represent a form of abnormal repair. Ankylosis may also develop after chronic periapical inflammation, tooth replantation, and occlusal trauma and around embedded teeth. This condition is relatively uncommon, and it occurs most frequently in the primary dentition.[176]

Exposure of Cementum to the Oral Environment

Cementum becomes exposed to the oral environment in cases of gingival recession and as a result of the loss of attachment in pocket formation. The cementum is sufficiently permeable to be penetrated

in these cases by organic substances, inorganic ions, and bacteria. Bacterial invasion of the cementum occurs frequently in individuals with periodontal disease, and cementum caries can develop (see Chapter 23).

Alveolar Process

The alveolar process is the portion of the maxilla and mandible that forms and supports the tooth sockets (alveoli). It forms when the tooth erupts to provide the osseous attachment to the forming periodontal ligament; it disappears gradually after the tooth is lost.

Because the alveolar processes develop and undergo remodeling with tooth formation and eruption, they are tooth-dependent bony structures.[227] Therefore the size, shape, location, and function of the teeth determine their morphology. Interestingly, although the growth and development of the bones of the jaw determine the position of the teeth, a certain degree of repositioning of the teeth can be accomplished through occlusal forces and in response to orthodontic procedures that rely on the adaptability of the alveolar bone and the associated periodontal tissues.[251]

The alveolar process consists of the following:

1. An external plate of cortical bone is formed by haversian bone and compacted bone lamellae.
2. The inner socket wall of thin, compact bone called the *alveolar bone proper* is seen as the lamina dura in radiographs. Histologically, it contains a series of openings (i.e., the *cribriform plate*) through which neurovascular bundles link the periodontal ligament with the central component of the alveolar bone: the cancellous bone.
3. Cancellous trabeculae between these two compact layers act as supporting alveolar bone. The *interdental septum* consists of cancellous supporting bone enclosed within a compact border (Fig. 3.49).

In addition, the bones of the jaw include the basal bone, which is the portion of the jaw located apically but unrelated to the teeth (Fig. 3.50).

The alveolar process is divisible into separate areas on an anatomic basis, but it functions as a unit, with all parts interrelated in the support of the teeth. Figs. 3.51 and 3.52 show the relative proportions of cancellous bone and compact bone that form the alveolar process. Most of the facial and lingual portions of the sockets are formed by compact bone alone; cancellous bone surrounds the lamina dura in apical, apicolingual, and interradicular areas.

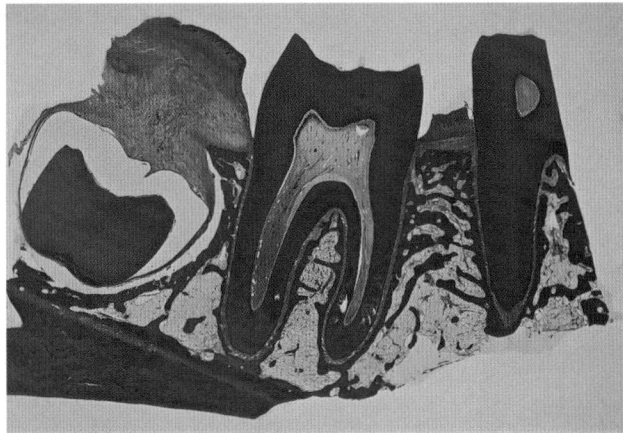

Fig. 3.49 Mesiodistal section through the mandibular molars of a 17-year-old girl obtained at autopsy. Note the interdental bony septa between the first and second molars. The dense cortical bony plates represent the alveolar bone proper (i.e., the cribriform plates) and are supported by cancellous bony trabeculae. The third molar is still in the early stages of root formation and eruption.

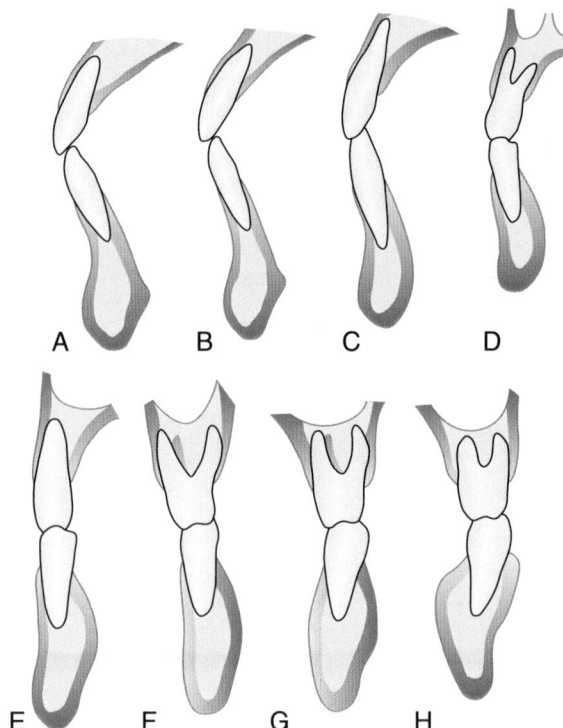

Fig. 3.51 Relative proportions of cancellous bone and compact bone in a longitudinal faciolingual section of (A) mandibular molars, (B) lateral incisors, (C) canines, (D) first premolars, (E) second premolars, (F) first molars, (G) second molars, and (H) third molars.

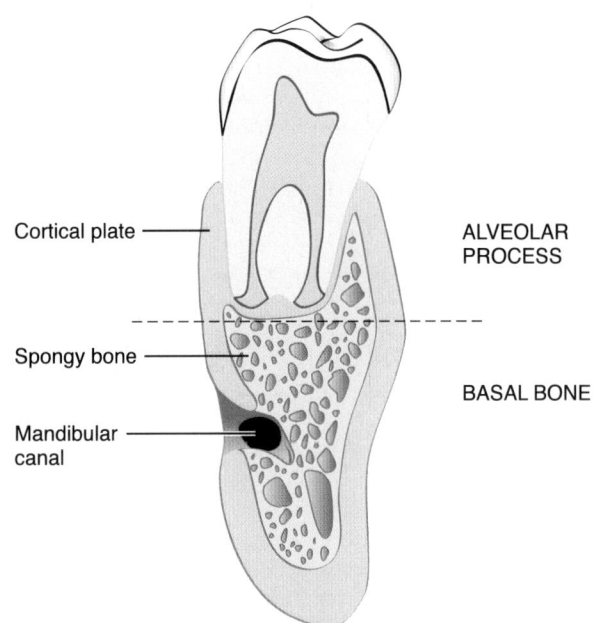

Cortical plate

ALVEOLAR PROCESS

Spongy bone

Mandibular canal

BASAL BONE

Fig. 3.50 Section through a human jaw with a tooth in situ. The dotted line indicates the separation between the basal bone and the alveolar bone. *(Redrawn from Ten Cate AR: Oral histology: development, structure, and function, ed 4, St Louis, 1994, Mosby.)*

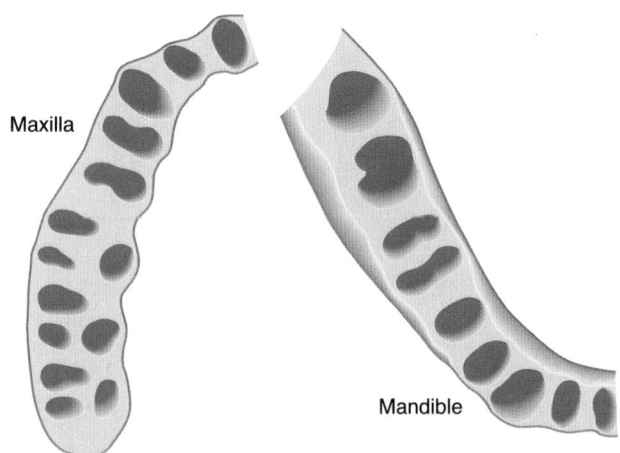

Maxilla

Mandible

Fig. 3.52 The shape of the roots and the surrounding bone distribution in a transverse section of maxilla and mandible at the midroot level.

Bone consists of two-thirds inorganic matter and one-third organic matrix. The inorganic matter is composed principally of the minerals calcium and phosphate, along with hydroxyl, carbonate, citrate, and trace amounts of other ions[101,102] such as sodium, magnesium, and fluorine. The mineral salts are in the form of hydroxyapatite crystals of ultramicroscopic size and constitute approximately two-thirds of the bone structure.

The organic matrix[75] consists mainly of collagen type I (90%),[185] with small amounts of noncollagenous proteins such as osteocalcin, osteonectin, bone morphogenetic protein, phosphoproteins, and proteoglycans.[209] Osteopontin and bone sialoprotein are cell-adhesion proteins that appear to be important for the adhesion of both osteoclasts and osteoblasts.[163] In addition, paracrine factors, including cytokines, chemokines, and growth factors, have been implicated in the local control of mesenchymal condensations that occur at the onset of organogenesis. These factors probably play a prominent role in the development of the alveolar processes.[251]

Although the alveolar bone tissue is constantly changing its internal organization, it retains approximately the same form from childhood through adult life. Bone deposition by osteoblasts is balanced by resorption by osteoclasts during tissue remodeling and renewal. It is well known that the number of osteoblasts decreases with aging; however, no remarkable change in the number of osteoclasts has ever been reported.[191]

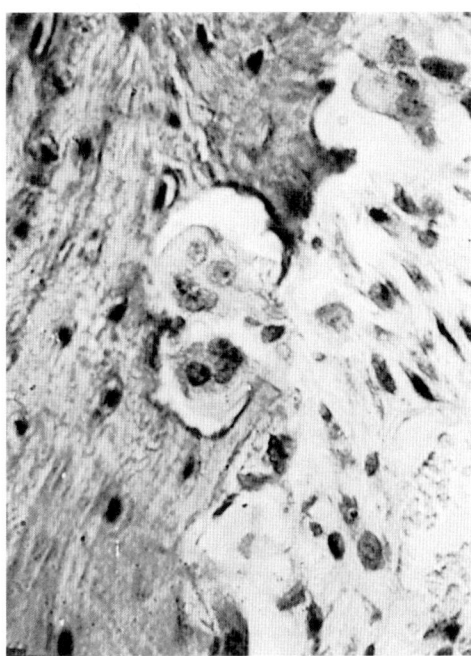

Fig. 3.53 Rat alveolar bone. This histologic view show two multinucleated osteoclasts in the Howship lacuna.

Remodeling is the major pathway of bony changes in shape, resistance to forces, repair of wounds, and calcium and phosphate homeostasis in the body. Indeed, the coupling of bone resorption with bone formation constitutes one of the fundamental principles by which bone is necessarily remodeled throughout its life. Bone remodeling involves the coordination of activities of cells from two distinct lineages, the osteoblasts and the osteoclasts, which form and resorb the mineralized connective tissues of bone.[251]

The bone matrix that is laid down by osteoblasts is nonmineralized osteoid. While new osteoid is being deposited, the older osteoid located below the surface becomes mineralized as the mineralization front advances.

Bone resorption is a complex process that is morphologically related to the appearance of eroded bone surfaces (i.e., Howship lacunae) and large, multinucleated cells (osteoclasts) (Fig. 3.53). Osteoclasts originate from hematopoietic tissue[55,110,197] and are formed by the fusion of mononuclear cells of asynchronous populations.[141,201,264] When osteoclasts are active rather than resting, they possess an elaborately developed ruffled border from which hydrolytic enzymes are thought to be secreted.[278] These enzymes digest the organic portion of bone. The activity of osteoclasts and the morphology of the ruffled border can be modified and regulated by hormones such as parathyroid hormone (indirectly) and calcitonin, which has receptors on the osteoclast membrane.

Another mechanism of bone resorption involves the creation of an acidic environment on the bone surface, thereby leading to the dissolution of the mineral component of bone. This event can be produced by different conditions, including a proton pump through the cell membrane of the osteoclast,[34] bone tumors, and local pressure[197] translated through the secretory activity of the osteoclast.

Ten Cate[264] described the sequence of events in the resorptive process as follows:

1. Attachment of osteoclasts to the mineralized surface of bone
2. Creation of a sealed acidic environment through the action of the proton pump, which demineralizes bone and exposes the organic matrix

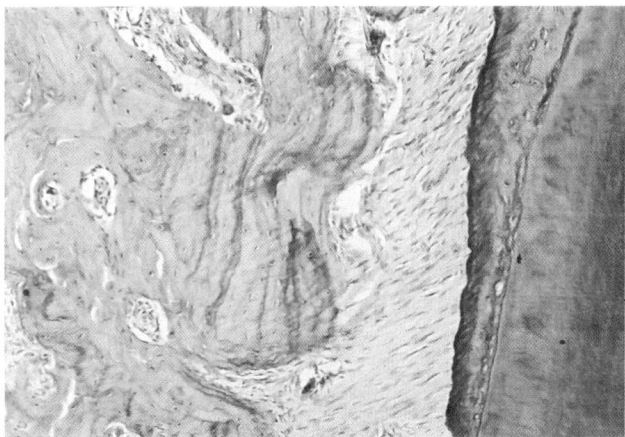

Fig. 3.54 Deep penetration of Sharpey fibers into bundle bone of a rat molar.

3. Degradation of the exposed organic matrix to its constituent amino acids via the action of released enzymes (e.g., acid phosphatase, cathepsin)
4. Sequestering of mineral ions and amino acids within the osteoclast

Notably, the cellular and molecular events involved in bone remodeling have a strong similarity to many aspects of inflammation and repair. The relationships among matrix molecules (e.g., osteopontin, bone sialoprotein, SPARC [secreted protein, acidic, rich in cysteine], osteocalcin), blood clotting, and wound healing are clearly evident.[251]

Cells and Intercellular Matrix

Osteoblasts, which are the cells that produce the organic matrix of bone, are differentiated from pluripotent follicle cells. Alveolar bone is formed during fetal growth by intramembranous ossification, and it consists of a calcified matrix with osteocytes enclosed within spaces called *lacunae.* The osteocytes extend processes into *canaliculi* that radiate from the lacunae. The canaliculi form an anastomosing system through the intercellular matrix of the bone, which brings oxygen and nutrients to the osteocytes through the blood and removes metabolic waste products. Blood vessels branch extensively and travel through the periosteum. The endosteum lies adjacent to the marrow vasculature. Bone growth occurs via the apposition of an organic matrix that is deposited by osteoblasts. Haversian systems (i.e., *osteons*) are the internal mechanisms that bring a vascular supply to bones that are too thick to be supplied only by surface vessels. These are found primarily in the outer cortical plates and the alveolar bone proper.

Socket Wall

The socket wall consists of dense, lamellated bone, some of which is arranged in haversian systems and bundle bone. *Bundle bone* is the term given to bone adjacent to the periodontal ligament that contains a great number of Sharpey fibers[286] (Fig. 3.54). It is characterized by thin lamellae arranged in layers parallel to the root, with intervening appositional lines (Fig. 3.55). Bundle bone is localized within the alveolar bone proper. Some Sharpey fibers are completely calcified, but most contain an uncalcified central core within a calcified outer layer.[240] Bundle bone is not unique to the jaws; it occurs throughout the skeletal system wherever ligaments and muscles are attached.

The cancellous portion of the alveolar bone consists of trabeculae that enclose irregularly shaped marrow spaces lined with a layer of thin, flattened endosteal cells. Wide variation occurs in the trabecular

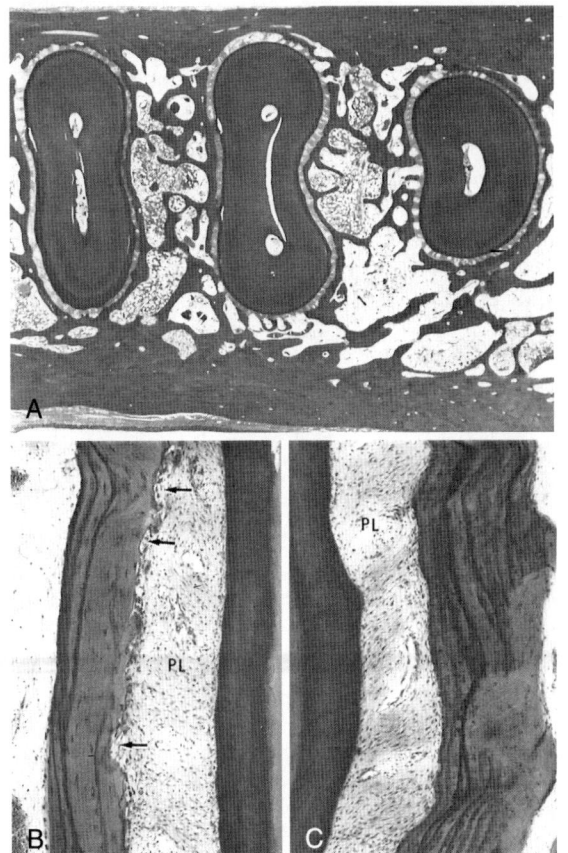

Fig. 3.55 Bundle bone associated with the physiologic mesial migration of the teeth. (A) Horizontal section through the molar roots during the process of mesial migration (*left*, mesial; *right*, distal). (B) Mesial root surface showing osteoclasis of bone *(arrows)*. (C) Distal root surface showing bundle bone that has been partially replaced with dense bone on the marrow side. *PL*, Periodontal ligament.

pattern of cancellous bone,[200] which is affected by occlusal forces. The matrix of the cancellous trabeculae consists of irregularly arranged lamellae separated by deeply staining incremental and resorption lines indicative of previous bone activity, with an occasional haversian system.

Cancellous bone is found predominantly in the interradicular and interdental spaces and in limited amounts facially or lingually, except in the palate. In the adult human, more cancellous bone exists in the maxilla than in the mandible.

Bone Marrow

In the embryo and the newborn, the cavities of all bones are occupied by red hematopoietic marrow. The red marrow gradually undergoes a physiologic change to the fatty or yellow inactive type of marrow. In the adult, the marrow of the jaw is normally of the latter type, and red marrow is found only in the ribs, sternum, vertebrae, skull, and humerus. However, foci of the red bone marrow are occasionally seen in the jaws, often accompanied by the resorption of bony trabeculae.[41] Common locations are the maxillary tuberosity, the maxillary and mandibular molar and premolar areas, and the mandibular symphysis and ramus angle, which may be visible radiographically as zones of radiolucency.

Periosteum and Endosteum

Layers of differentiated osteogenic connective tissue cover all of the bone surfaces. The tissue that covers the outer surface of bone

is termed *periosteum,* whereas the tissue that lines the internal bone cavities is called *endosteum.*

The periosteum consists of an *inner layer* composed of osteoblasts surrounded by osteoprogenitor cells, which have the potential to differentiate into osteoblasts, and an *outer layer* rich in blood vessels and nerves and composed of collagen fibers and fibroblasts. Bundles of periosteal collagen fibers penetrate the bone, thereby binding the periosteum to the bone. The endosteum is composed of a single layer of osteoblasts and sometimes a small amount of connective tissue. The inner layer is the osteogenic layer, and the outer layer is the fibrous layer.

Cellular events at the periosteum modulate bone size throughout an individual's life span, and a change in bone size is probably the result of the balance between periosteal osteoblastic and osteoclastic activities. Little is currently known about the control of periosteal osteoblastic activity or the clinical importance of variations in periosteal bone formation.[196] Moreover, the nature and impact of periosteal bone resorption are virtually unexplored.

Interdental Septum

The interdental septum consists of cancellous bone that is bordered by the socket wall cribriform plates (i.e., lamina dura or alveolar bone proper) of approximating teeth and the facial and lingual cortical plates (Fig. 3.56). If the interdental space is narrow, the septum may consist of only the cribriform plate. In one study, for example, the space between the mandibular second premolars and first molars consisted of cribriform plate and cancellous bone in 85% of the cases and of only cribriform plate in the remaining 15%.[116] If the roots are too close together, an irregular "window" can appear in the bone between adjacent roots (Fig. 3.57). Between maxillary molars, the septum consisted of cribriform plate and cancellous bone in 66.6% of cases; it was composed of only cribriform plate in 20.8%, and it had a fenestration in 12.5%.[116]

Determining root proximity radiographically is important (see Chapters 33 and 35). The mesiodistal angulation of the crest of the interdental septum usually parallels a line drawn between the cementoenamel junctions of the approximating teeth.[209] The distance between the crest of the alveolar bone and the cementoenamel junction in young adults varies between 0.75 and 1.49 mm (average, 1.08 mm). This distance increases with age to an average of 2.81 mm.[93] However, this phenomenon may not be as much a function of age as of periodontal disease.

The mesiodistal and faciolingual dimensions and shape of the interdental septum are governed by the size and convexity of the crowns of the two approximating teeth as well as by the position of the teeth in the jaw and their degree of eruption.[209]

Osseous Topography

The bone contour normally conforms to the prominence of the roots, with intervening vertical depressions that taper toward the margin (Fig. 3.58). Alveolar bone anatomy varies among patients and has important clinical implications. The height and thickness of the facial and lingual bony plates are affected by the alignment of the teeth, the angulation of the root to the bone, and occlusal forces.

On teeth in labial version, the margin of the labial bone is located farther apically than it is on teeth that are in proper alignment. The bone margin is thinned to a knife edge, and it presents an accentuated arc in the direction of the apex. On teeth in lingual version, the facial bony plate is thicker than normal. The margin is blunt, rounded, and horizontal rather than arcuate. The effect of the root-to-bone angulation on the height of alveolar bone is most noticeable on the palatal roots of the maxillary molars. The bone margin is located farther apically

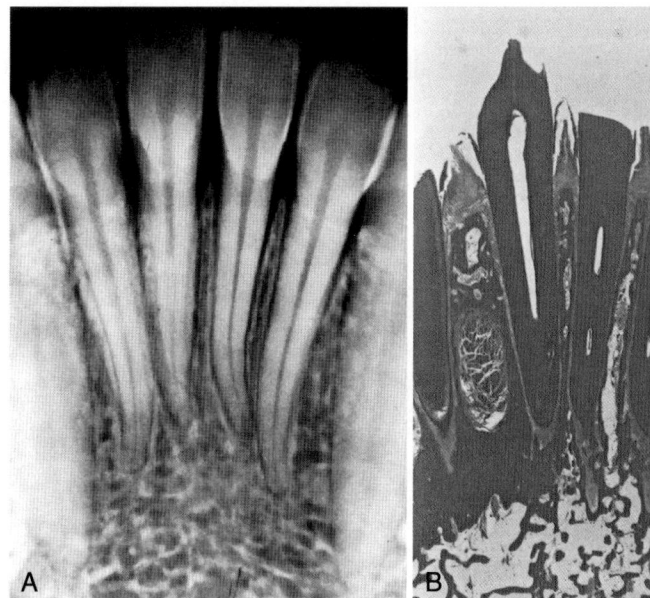

Fig. 3.56 Interdental septa. (A) Radiograph of the mandibular incisor area. Note the prominent lamina dura. (B) Interdental septa between the mandibular anterior teeth shown in A. There is a slight reduction in bone height with widening of the periodontal ligament in the coronal areas. The central cancellous portion is bordered by the dense bony cribriform plates of the socket, which form the lamina dura around the teeth in the radiograph. Attachments for the mentalis muscle are seen between the canine and lateral incisors. *(From Glickman I, Smulow J: Periodontal disease: clinical, radiographic, and histopathologic features, Philadelphia, 1974, Saunders.)*

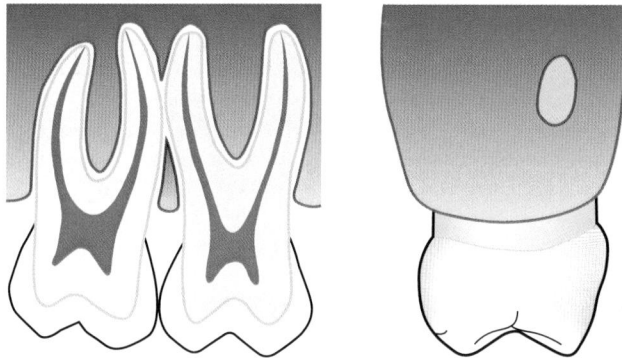

Fig. 3.57 Boneless "window" between adjoining close roots of molars.

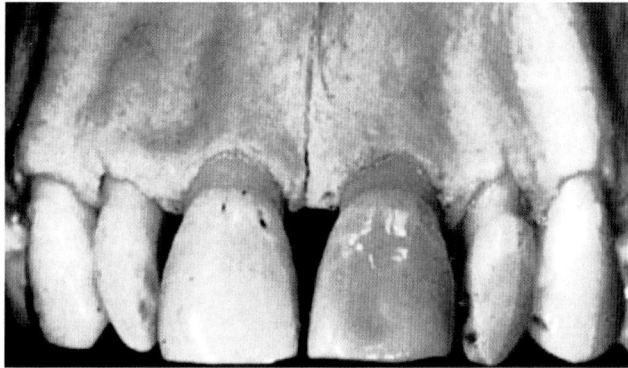

Fig. 3.58 Normal that the bone contour conforms to the prominence of the roots.

on the roots, and it forms relatively acute angles with the palatal bone.[120] The cervical portion of the alveolar plate is sometimes considerably thickened on the facial surface, apparently as reinforcement against occlusal forces (Fig. 3.59).

Fenestration and Dehiscence

Isolated areas in which the root is denuded of bone and the root surface is covered only by periosteum and overlying gingiva are termed *fenestrations*. In these areas, the marginal bone is intact. When the denuded areas extend through the marginal bone, the defect is called a *dehiscence* (Fig. 3.60).

Such defects occur on approximately 20% of the teeth; they occur more often on the facial bone than on the lingual bone, they are more common on anterior teeth than on posterior teeth, and they are frequently bilateral. Microscopic evidence of lacunar resorption may be present at the margins. The cause of these defects is not clear. Prominent root contours, malposition, and labial protrusion of the root in combination with a thin bony plate are predisposing factors.[78] Fenestration and dehiscence are important because they may complicate the outcome of periodontal surgery.

Remodeling of Alveolar Bone

In contrast with its apparent rigidity, alveolar bone is the least stable of the periodontal tissues, because its structure is in a constant state of flux. A considerable amount of internal remodeling takes place by means of resorption and formation, and this is regulated by local and systemic influences. Local influences include functional requirements on the tooth and age-related changes in bone cells. Systemic influences are probably hormonal (e.g., parathyroid hormone, calcitonin, vitamin D_3).

The remodeling of the alveolar bone affects its height, contour, and density and is manifested in the following three areas: adjacent to the periodontal ligament, in relation to the periosteum of the facial

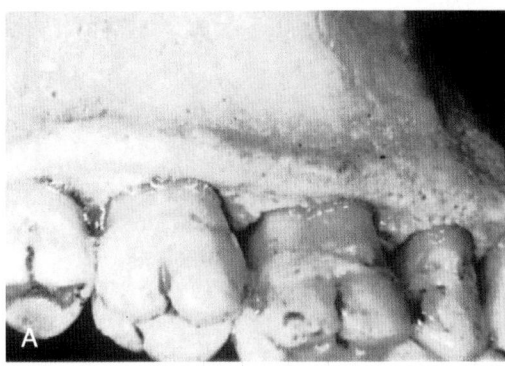
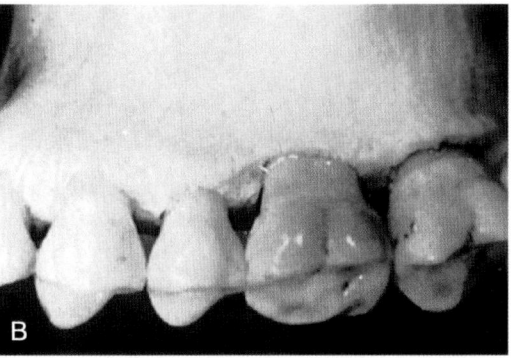

Fig. 3.59 Variations in the cervical portion of the buccal alveolar plate. (A) Shelflike conformation. (B) Comparatively thin buccal plate.

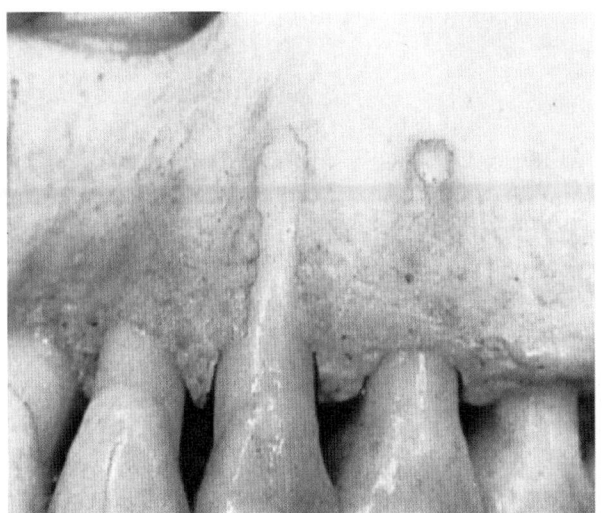

Fig. 3.60 Dehiscence on the canine and fenestration of the first premolar.

and lingual plates, and along the endosteal surface of the marrow spaces.

Development of the Attachment Apparatus

After the crown has formed, the stratum intermedium and the stellate reticulum of the enamel organ disappear. The outer and inner epithelia of the enamel organ remain and form REE. The apical portion of this constitutes the Hertwig epithelial root sheath, which will continue to grow apically and which determines the shape of the root. Before the beginning of root formation, the root sheath bends horizontally at the future cementoenamel junction, thereby narrowing the cervical opening and forming the epithelial diaphragm. The epithelial diaphragm separates the dental follicle from the dental papilla.

After root dentin formation begins, the Hertwig root sheath breaks up and partially disappears; the remaining cells form the epithelial clusters or strands known as the *epithelial rests of Malassez* (see Fig. 3.37A). In multirooted teeth, the epithelial diaphragm grows in such a way that tonguelike extensions develop horizontally, thereby leaving spaces for each of the future roots to form.

The role of the Hertwig epithelial root sheath in root development, especially as it relates to the initiation of cementogenesis, has become a focus of research.[271] On the basis of various studies, it is now generally accepted that there is a transient period of the secretion of proteins (e.g., bone sialoprotein, osteopontin, amelin) by the cells of the Hertwig epithelial root sheath.[38,85] In addition, research shows that growth and differentiation factors may play roles in the development of the attachment apparatus of periodontal tissues. Pluripotent dental follicle cells have been shown to differentiate into osteoblasts, cementoblasts, and periodontal fibroblasts.[241]

Cementum

The rupture of the Hertwig root sheath allows the mesenchymal cells of the dental follicle to contact the dentin, where they start forming a continuous layer of cementoblasts. On the basis of immunochemical and ultrastructural studies, Thomas[270] and others[35,165] have speculated that cementoblasts can be of epithelial origin (i.e., the Hertwig root sheath), having undergone an epithelial mesenchymal transformation.

Cementum formation begins with the deposition of a meshwork of irregularly arranged collagen fibrils sparsely distributed in a ground substance or matrix called *precementum* or *cementoid*. This is followed by a phase of matrix maturation, which subsequently mineralizes to form cementum. Cementoblasts, which are initially separated from the cementum by uncalcified cementoid, sometimes become enclosed within the matrix and are trapped. After they are enclosed, they are referred to as *cementocytes,* and they will remain viable in a manner similar to that of osteocytes.

A layer of connective tissue known as the *dental sac* surrounds the enamel organ and includes the epithelial root sheath as it develops. The zone that is immediately in contact with the dental organ and continuous with the ectomesenchyme of the dental papilla is called the *dental follicle,*[262,263,266] and it consists of undifferentiated fibroblasts.

Periodontal Ligament

As the crown approaches the oral mucosa during tooth eruption, these fibroblasts become active and start producing collagen fibrils. They initially lack orientation, but they soon acquire an orientation that is oblique to the tooth. The first collagen bundles then appear in the region immediately apical to the cementoenamel junction and give rise to the gingivodental fiber groups. As tooth eruption progresses, additional oblique fibers appear and become attached to the newly formed cementum and bone. The transseptal and alveolar crest fibers develop when the tooth merges into the oral cavity. Alveolar bone deposition occurs simultaneously with periodontal ligament organization.[250]

The developing periodontal ligament and the mature periodontal ligament contain undifferentiated stem cells that retain the potential to differentiate into osteoblasts, cementoblasts, and fibroblasts.[172]

Alveolar Bone

Just before mineralization, osteoblasts start producing matrix vesicles. These vesicles contain enzymes (e.g., alkaline phosphatase) that help to jump-start the nucleation of hydroxyapatite crystals. As these crystals grow and develop, they form coalescing bone nodules, which, with fast-growing nonoriented collagen fibers, are the substructure of woven bone and the first bone formed in the alveolus. Later, through bone deposition, remodeling, and the secretion of oriented collagen fibers in sheets, mature lamellar bone is formed.[28,29]

The hydroxyapatite crystals are generally aligned with their long axes parallel to the collagen fibers, and they appear to be deposited on and within the collagen fibers in mature lamellar bone. In this way, bone matrix is able to withstand the heavy mechanical stresses applied to it during function.

The alveolar bone develops around each tooth follicle during odontogenesis. When a deciduous tooth is shed, its alveolar bone is resorbed. The succedaneous permanent tooth moves into place and develops its own alveolar bone from its own dental follicle. As the tooth root forms and the surrounding tissues develop and mature, alveolar bone merges with the separately developing basal bone, and the two become one continuous structure. Although alveolar bone and basal bone have different intermediate origins, both are ultimately derived from neural crest ectomesenchyme.

Mandibular basal bone begins mineralization at the exit of the mental nerve from the mental foramen, whereas the maxillary basal bone begins at the exit of the infraorbital nerve from the infraorbital foramen.

Physiologic Migration of the Teeth

Tooth movement does not end when active eruption is completed and the tooth is in functional occlusion. With time and wear, the proximal contact areas of the teeth are flattened, and the teeth tend to move mesially. This is referred to as *physiologic mesial migration*. By the age of 40 years, this process results in a reduction of about 0.5 cm in the length of the dental arch from the midline to the third molars. Alveolar bone is reconstructed in compliance with the physiologic mesial migration of the teeth. Bone resorption is increased in areas of pressure along the mesial surfaces of the teeth, and new layers of bundle bone are formed in areas of tension on the distal surfaces (see Fig. 3.55).

External Forces and the Periodontium

The periodontium exists for the purpose of supporting teeth during function, and it depends on the stimulation that it receives from function for the preservation of its structure. Therefore a constant and sensitive balance is present between external forces and the periodontal structures.

Alveolar bone undergoes constant physiologic remodeling in response to external forces, particularly occlusal forces. Bone is removed from areas where it is no longer needed and added to areas where it is presently needed.

The socket wall reflects the responsiveness of alveolar bone to external forces. Osteoblasts and newly formed osteoid line the socket in areas of tension; osteoclasts and bone resorption occur in areas of pressure. Forces exerted on the tooth also influence the number, density, and alignment of cancellous trabeculae. The bony trabeculae are aligned in the path of the tensile and compressive stresses to provide maximal resistance to the occlusal force with a minimum of bone substance[100,247] (Fig. 3.61). When forces are increased, the cancellous bony trabeculae increase in number and thickness, and

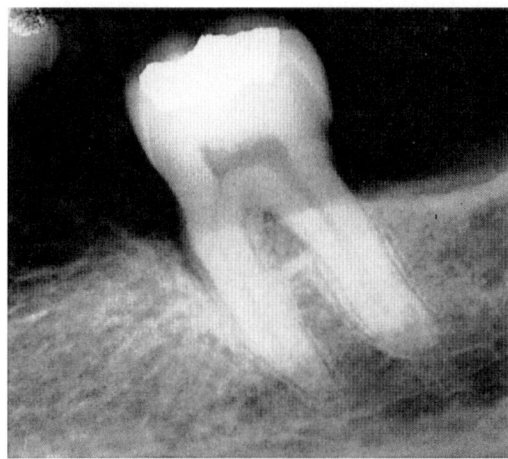

Fig. 3.61 Bony trabeculae realigned perpendicular to the mesial root of a tilted molar.

TABLE 3.2 Comparison of Periodontal Width of Functioning and Functionless Teeth in a 38-Year-Old Man

	AVERAGE WIDTH OF PERIODONTAL SPACE		
	Entrance of Alveolus (mm)	Middle of Alveolus (mm)	Fundus of Alveolus (mm)
Heavy Function Left upper second bicuspid	0.35	0.28	0.30
Light Function Left lower first bicuspid	0.14	0.10	0.12
Functionless Left upper third molar	0.10	0.06	0.06

Modified from Kronfeld R: Histologic study of the influence of function on the human periodontal membrane. *J Am Dent Assoc* 18:1242, 1931.

bone may be added to the external surface of the labial and lingual plates.

A study has shown that the presence of antagonists of occlusal force and the severity of periodontal disease increase the extension of periodontal tissue resorption.[66]

The periodontal ligament also depends on the stimulation provided by function to preserve its structure. Within physiologic limits, the periodontal ligament can accommodate increased function with an increase in width (Table 3.2), a thickening of its fiber bundles, and an increase in the diameter and number of Sharpey fibers. Forces that exceed the adaptive capacity of the periodontium produce injury called *trauma from occlusion*. Because trauma from occlusion can only be confirmed histologically, the clinician is challenged to use clinical and radiographic surrogate indicators in an attempt to facilitate and assist with its diagnosis[111] (see Chapter 26).

When occlusal forces are reduced, the number and thickness of the trabeculae are reduced.[64] The periodontal ligament also atrophies and appears thinned; the fibers are reduced in number and density, disoriented,[11,208] and ultimately arranged parallel to the root surface (Fig. 3.62). This phenomenon is termed *disuse atrophy* or *afunctional atrophy*. With this condition, the cementum is either unaffected[64] or thickened, and the distance from the cementoenamel junction to the alveolar crest is increased.[204]

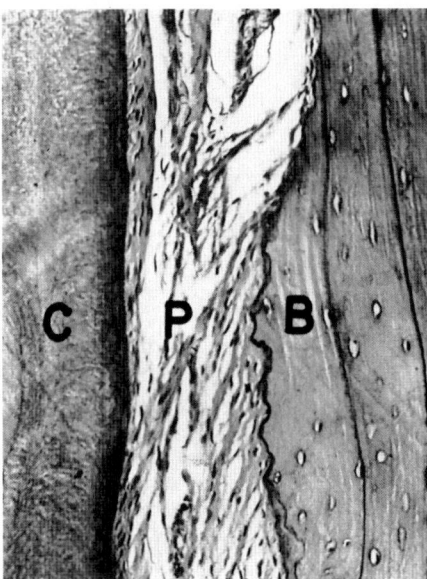

Fig. 3.62 Atrophic periodontal ligament *(P)* of a tooth devoid of function. Note the scalloped edge of the alveolar bone *(B)*, which indicates that resorption has occurred. *C,* Cementum.

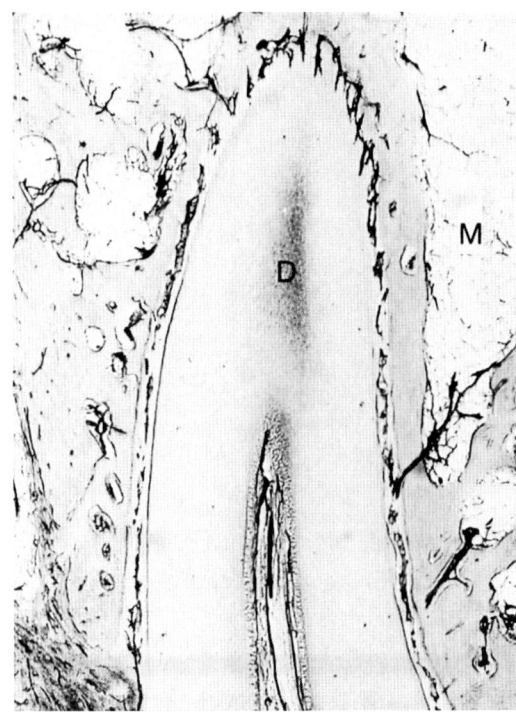

Fig. 3.63 Vascular supply of a monkey periodontium perfused with India ink. Note the longitudinal vessels in the periodontal ligament and the alveolar arteries passing through channels between the bone marrow *(M)* and the periodontal ligament. *D,* Dentin. *(Courtesy Dr. Sol Bernick, Los Angeles, California.)*

Decreased occlusal function causes changes in the periodontal microvasculature, such as the occlusion of blood vessels and a decrease in the number of blood vessels.[121] For example, Murrell and colleagues[187] reported that the application and removal of orthodontic force produced significant changes in blood vessel number and density; however, no evidence-based explanation exists for why the force stimulated such changes in the number of blood vessels.

Orthodontic tooth movement is thought to result from site-specific bone remodeling in the absence of inflammation. It is well recognized that tensional forces will stimulate the formation and activity of osteoblastic cells, whereas compressive forces promote osteoclastic activity.[251]

Vascularization of the Supporting Structures

The blood supply to the supporting structures of the tooth is derived from the inferior and superior alveolar arteries to the mandible and maxilla, and it reaches the periodontal ligament from three sources: apical vessels, penetrating vessels from the alveolar bone, and anastomosing vessels from the gingiva.[63]

The branches of the apical vessels supply the apical region of the periodontal ligament before the vessels enter the dental pulp. The transalveolar vessels are branches of the intraseptal vessels that perforate the lamina dura and enter the ligament. The intraseptal vessels continue to vascularize the gingiva; these gingival vessels in turn anastomose with the periodontal ligament vessels of the cervical region.[84]

The vessels within the periodontal ligament are contained in the interstitial spaces of loose connective tissue between the principal fibers, and they are connected in a netlike plexus that runs longitudinally and closer to the bone than the cementum[54] (Figs. 3.63 and 3.64). The blood supply increases from the incisors to the molars; it is greatest in the gingival third of single-rooted teeth, less in the apical third, and least in the middle; it is equal in the apical and middle thirds of multirooted teeth; it is slightly greater on the mesial and distal surfaces than on the facial and lingual surfaces; and it is greater on the mesial surfaces of the mandibular molars than on the distal surfaces.[33]

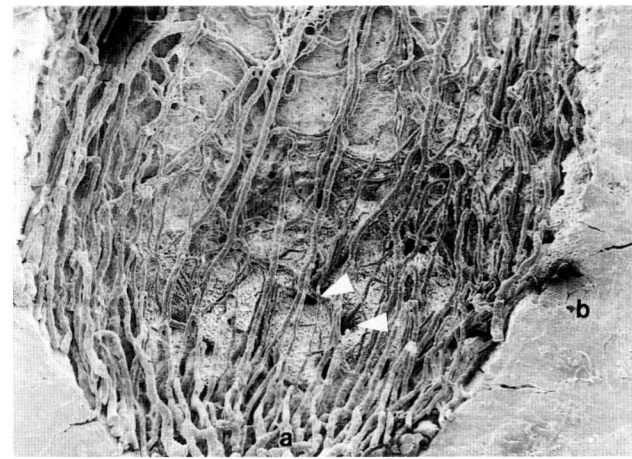

Fig. 3.64 Vascular supply to the periodontal ligament in a rat molar as viewed by scanning electron microscopy after perfusion with plastic and tissue corrosion. Middle and apical areas of the periodontal ligament are shown with longitudinal blood vessels from the apex *(below)* to the gingiva *(above)*, perforating vessels entering the bone *(b)*, and many transverse connections *(arrowheads)*. Apical vessels *(a)* form a cap that connects with the pulpal vessels. *(Courtesy NJ Selliseth and K Selvig, University of Bergen, Norway.)*

The vascular supply to the bone enters the interdental septa through nutrient canals together with veins, nerves, and lymphatics. Dental arterioles, which also branch off the alveolar arteries, send tributaries through the periodontal ligament, and some small branches enter the marrow spaces of the bone through the perforations in the cribriform plate. Small vessels that emanate from the facial and lingual compact bone also enter the marrow and spongy bone.

The *venous drainage* of the periodontal ligament accompanies the arterial supply. Venules receive the blood through the abundant capillary network. In addition, arteriovenous anastomoses bypass the capillaries and are seen more frequently in apical and interradicular regions; their significance is unknown.

Lymphatics supplement the venous drainage system. Lymphatic channels that drain the region just beneath the junctional epithelium pass into the periodontal ligament and accompany the blood vessels into the periapical region.[42] From there, they pass through the alveolar bone to the inferior dental canal in the mandible or the infraorbital canal in the maxilla and then go on to the submaxillary lymph nodes.

References

 References for this chapter are found on the companion website www.expertconsult.com.

CHAPTER 4

Aging and the Periodontium

Ian Needleman

CHAPTER OUTLINE

Effects of Aging on the Periodontium
Effects of Aging on the Progression of Periodontal Diseases
Aging and the Response to Treatment of the Periodontium

Increased health awareness and improvements in preventive dentistry have led to decreasing tooth loss for all age groups. The effects of this shift in tooth retention need to be considered carefully. In particular, increased life expectancy and greater health expectations may lead to changes in demand from older individuals for periodontal treatment and potentially a substantial increase in supportive periodontal therapy. Therefore, an understanding of the impact of aging on the periodontium is critical. This chapter first reviews the literature concerning the fundamental aspects of aging on the periodontal tissues; broader aspects of aging are then examined and their possible effects on treatment outcomes discussed. The chapter has been updated following a detailed search of new research published since 2012.

The evidence base is not without problems, many of which make it difficult to draw conclusions about the effects of aging. Some of these problems include inconsistency with regard to the definition of a true "older" group, the inadequate exclusion of adults with systemic diseases that can modify study findings, and attempts to extrapolate results from animal research. For the purposes of this chapter, the effects of aging are limited to a narrow review of possible biologic and microbiologic changes. (For further information on the effects of aging on the dental and periodontal patient, the reader should consult Holm-Pedersen P, Walls AW, Ship JA: *Textbook of geriatric dentistry,* ed 3, Oxford, UK, 2015, Wiley-Blackwell.[23]) The reader should be fully aware that this narrower scope excludes many important age-associated phenomena, including reductions in an individual's cognitive or motor function skills, which may have a direct impact on periodontal management. These issues are discussed more fully in Chapter 42. Several studies have reported associations between periodontitis and cognitive impairment and aging,[16,51] although whether these findings reflect causation or simply association remains unclear. These links are difficult to entangle because *"chronic inflammation is a prominent feature of aging and of age-related diseases."*[48]

CLINICAL CORRELATION

For a full understanding of aging and managing periodontal health, in addition to this chapter on biology readers should understand aging more broadly, including cognitive and motor function effects that could affect oral hygiene, for instance.

Since first writing this chapter in 1999, the volume of new research into aging and the periodontium has not increased substantially. Highly sensitive molecular and genomic techniques have been employed in related laboratory research, and these are starting to provide insight into age-associated effects. These approaches will likely prove fruitful in the future. Despite the limited data directly related to the periodontium, much effort and many resources have been used to research questions at least partially related to this topic. These include the effect of periodontal infection on general health (see Chapter 15) and the impact of osteoporosis on periodontal status (see Chapter 14).

Effects of Aging on the Periodontium
Gingival Epithelium

Thinning and decreased keratinization of the gingival epithelium have been reported with age.[52] The significance of these findings could mean an increase in epithelial permeability to bacterial antigens, a decreased resistance to functional trauma, or both. If so, such changes may influence long-term periodontal outcomes. However, other studies have found no age-related differences in the gingival epithelium of humans or dogs.[8,25] Other reported changes with aging include the flattening of rete pegs and altered cell density. Conflicting data regarding the surgical regeneration times for gingival epithelium have been ascribed to problems with research methodology.[57]

The effect of aging on the location of the junctional epithelium has been the subject of much speculation. Some reports show migration of the junctional epithelium from its position in healthy individuals (i.e., on the enamel) to a more apical position on the root surface, with accompanying gingival recession.[8] However, in other animal studies, no apical migration has been noted.[27] With continuing gingival recession, the width of the attached gingiva would be expected to decrease with age, but the opposite appears to be true.[2,3] Alternatively, the migration of the junctional epithelium to the root surface could be caused by the tooth erupting through the gingiva in an attempt to maintain occlusal contact with its opposing tooth (i.e., passive eruption) as a result of tooth surface loss from attrition (Fig. 4.1). The consensus is that gingival recession is not an inevitable physiologic process of aging, but rather that it can be explained by the cumulative effects of inflammation or trauma on the periodontium[6,8] (Fig. 4.2); this is discussed in more detail later in this chapter. Changes in the apoptotic gene expression of gingival tissue with age have

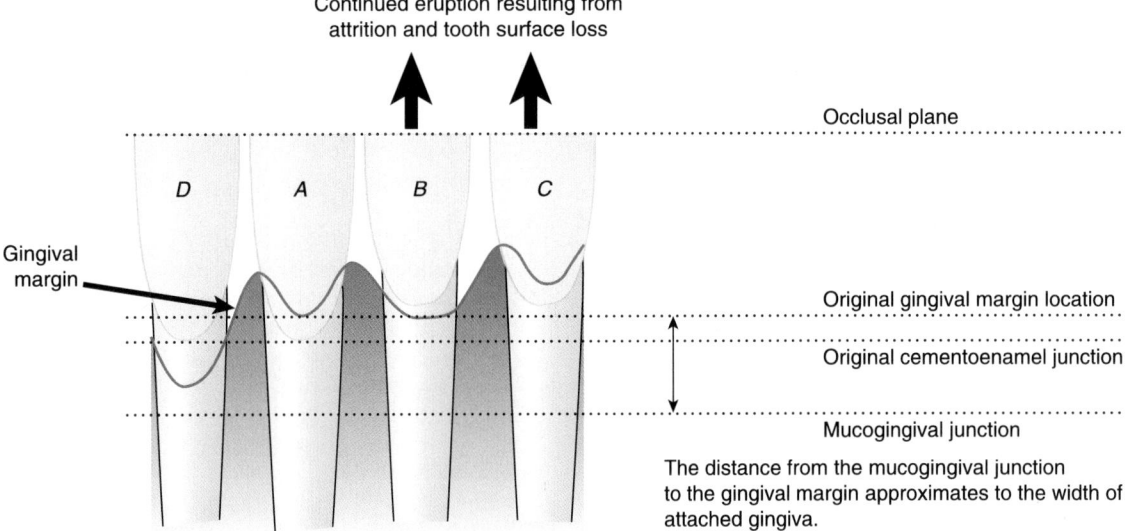

Fig. 4.1 Diagram showing the relationship of the gingival margin with the crown and root surface. *A,* Normal relationship with the gingival margin 1 to 2 mm above the cementoenamel junction. *B,* Wear of the incisal edge and continued tooth eruption. The gingival margin remains in the same position as shown in *A.* Therefore, the root surface is exposed, and clinical recession is evident. The width of the attached gingiva has not changed. *C,* Wear of the incisal edge and continued tooth eruption. The gingival margin has moved with the tooth; therefore, the entire dentogingival complex has moved coronally, with a resulting increase in the width of the attached gingiva. *D,* No wear of incisal edge is evident. The gingiva has moved apically, and clinical recession is evident. The width of attached gingiva is reduced.

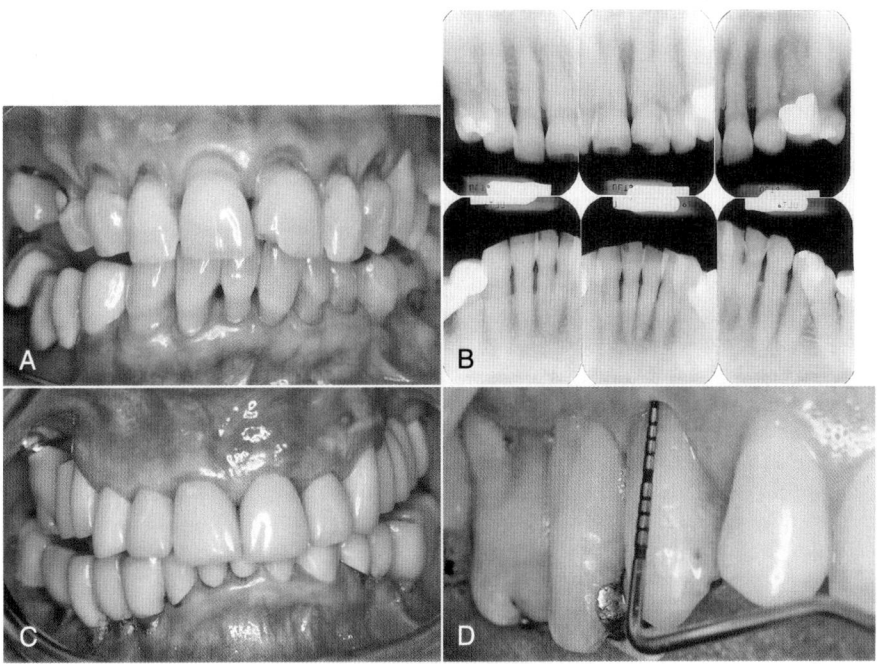

Fig. 4.2 Three scenarios illustrating the variation of the position of the gingival margin with age. (A) Overeruption with recession in an older individual (i.e., a 68-year-old woman) with generalized recession and a history of previously treated periodontitis. Note some overeruption of the lower anterior teeth and wear of teeth related to oral hygiene measures. (B) Radiographs of the patient shown in A. (C) Overeruption without recession in an older individual (i.e., a 72-year-old woman) with no periodontitis but marked lower incisor tooth wear and overeruption. Note how the gingival margin has migrated coronally with the erupting teeth. (D) Extensive recession in a younger individual (i.e., a 32-year-old man) with marked recession and no history of periodontitis. The recession has resulted from a combination of anatomically thin tissues and toothbrush-related trauma.

been reported in nonhuman primates.[19] This finding requires further research to understand its potential impact on gingival homeostasis and the pathogenesis of periodontal diseases.

KEY FACT

Gingival recession is not an inevitable consequence of aging but is the cumulative result of trauma or periodontitis.

Gingival Connective Tissue

Increasing age results in coarser and denser gingival connective tissues.[59] Qualitative and quantitative changes in collagen have been reported. These changes include an increased rate of conversion of soluble to insoluble collagen, increased mechanical strength, and increased denaturing temperature. These results indicate increased collagen stabilization caused by changes in the macromolecular conformation.[49] Not surprisingly, an increased collagen content has been found in the gingivae of older animals, despite a lower rate of collagen synthesis decreasing with age.[8,57]

Periodontal Ligament

Changes in the periodontal ligament that have been reported with aging include decreased numbers of fibroblasts and a more irregular structure, thus paralleling the changes seen in the gingival connective tissues.[8,49,57] Other findings include decreased organic matrix production, decreased epithelial cell rests, and increased amounts of elastic fiber.[57] Conflicting results have been reported for changes in the width of the periodontal ligament in human and animal models. Although true variation may exist, this finding probably reflects the functional status of the teeth in the studies: the width of the space will decrease if the tooth is unopposed (i.e., hypofunction) or increase with excessive occlusal loading.[57] Both scenarios can be anticipated as a result of tooth loss in this population. These effects may also explain the variability in studies that have reported qualitative changes within the periodontal ligament.

Recognition that the periodontal ligament has an important role in alveolar bone metabolism has led to an increased interest in investigating this role in relation to the maintenance of periodontal health and the pathogenesis of periodontitis. One approach to investigating this role is to examine mediators of bone homeostasis, such as receptor activator of nuclear factor-κB ligand (RANKL) and osteoprotegerin (OPG). RANKL is widely recognized for its role in activating osteoclasts, whereas OPG antagonizes RANKL binding, thus helping to maintain balance. The interplay of cytokines—and, in particular, the interleukin family—has also been extensively researched in periodontal pathogenesis. Some of the interleukins are potent mediators of inflammation (e.g., IL-1), whereas others have been shown to down-regulate this process (e.g., IL-4, IL-10). Therefore, evaluating the balance between these homeostatic processes would seem to be of great merit when assessing possible negative changes in the periodontium. Such a strategy appears to be predictive of hard tissue destruction among individuals with rheumatoid arthritis.[15] Findings comparing periodontal ligament cells in older individuals (i.e., >60 years old) with those of younger individuals (i.e., 15 to 20 years old) have suggested greater gene expression for proinflammatory cytokines.[7] This finding has been reported more widely as an age-associated change, although it is unclear whether it is a cause or an effect.[41] However, in addition to increased IL-1 and IL-6 expression, OPG was also increased, which suggests that increased OPG may be a homeostatic response to the up-regulation of inflammation.[7] If this homeostatic mechanism was effective, it may explain why an increase in inflammation did not result in greater

tissue damage with age. Periodontal ligament cell proliferation was decreased with age, thereby suggesting an impairment of repair potential, although such an impact does not appear to be manifested clinically.[58] Further research investigating periodontal ligament cells from individuals diagnosed with periodontitis will be important to understand the potentially important relationship between aging and periodontal ligament cells.

Cementum

Some consensus regarding the effect of aging on cementum exists. An increase in cemental width is a common finding; this increase may be 5 to 10 times wider than in those of younger age.[8] This finding is not surprising because deposition continues after tooth eruption. The increase in width is greater apically and lingually.[57] Although cementum has limited capacity for remodeling, an accumulation of resorption bays explains the finding of increasing surface irregularity.[20]

Alveolar Bone

Reports of morphologic changes in alveolar bone mirror age-related changes in other bony sites. Specific to the periodontium are findings of a more irregular periodontal surface of bone and the less-regular insertion of collagen fibers.[57] Although age is a risk factor for the bone mass reductions in individuals with osteoporosis, it is not causative and therefore should be distinguished from physiologic aging processes.[24] Overriding the diverse observations of bony changes with age is the important finding that the healing rate of bone in extraction sockets appears to be unaffected by increasing age.[4] Indeed, the success of osseointegrated dental implants, which relies on intact bone healing responses, does not appear to be age related.[9] However, balancing this view is the observation that bone graft preparations (i.e., decalcified freeze-dried bone) from donors who were more than 50 years old possessed significantly less osteogenic potential than graft material from younger donors.[50] The possible significance of this phenomenon for normal healing responses needs to be investigated.

Bacterial Plaque

Dentogingival plaque accumulation has been suggested to increase with age.[22] This may be explained by the increase in hard tissue surface area as a result of gingival recession and the surface characteristics of the exposed root surface as a substrate for plaque formation as compared with enamel. Other studies have shown no difference in plaque quantity with age. This contradiction may reflect the different age ranges of experimental groups as variable degrees of gingival recession and root surface exposure. For supragingival plaque, no real qualitative differences have been shown for plaque composition.[22] With regard to subgingival plaque, one study showed subgingival flora to be similar to normal flora, whereas another study reported increased numbers of enteric rods and pseudomonads in older adults.[37,55] Mombelli[35] suggested caution when interpreting this finding because of the increased oral carriage of these species among older adults. It has been speculated that a shift occurs in the importance of certain periodontal pathogens with age, specifically including an increased role for *Porphyromonas gingivalis* and a decreased role for *Aggregatibacter actinomycetemcomitans*. However, differentiating true age-related effects from the changes in ecologic determinants for periodontal bacteria will be difficult.

Another approach to investigating microbiology consists of conducting intervention studies and examining the impact on the microflora. Among individuals who were 60 to 75 years old, the prevalence of *P. gingivalis, Treponema forsythia, Treponema denticola, A. actinomycetemcomitans,* and *Prevotella intermedia* was high and was not clearly related to probing depth.[45] The finding of high levels of the organisms could have been related to the sample of individuals: the participants were mostly those with low incomes and with no recent dental care. Long-term use (i.e., 5 years) of a 0.12% chlorhexidine mouthrinse did not promote reductions in the proportions of the organisms in individuals experiencing alveolar bone loss as compared with the placebo mouthrinse, possibly because the mouthrinse routine may have been less frequent than daily.[45]

Immune and Inflammatory Responses

Advances in the study of the effects of aging on the immune response (i.e., immunosenescence) have altered the understanding of this phenomenon. In particular, more recent studies have set tighter controls on excluding individuals with systemic conditions known to affect the immune response. As a result, age has been recognized as having much less effect on the alteration of the host response than previously thought.[31] Differences between younger and older individuals can be demonstrated for T and B cells, cytokines, and natural killer cells, with increased inflammatory-type (M1) macrophage subset gene expression (in a nonhuman primate model),[18] but not for polymorphonuclear cells. McArthur[31] concluded the following: "Measurement of indicators of immune and inflammatory competency suggested that, within the parameters tested, there was no evidence for age-related changes in host defenses correlating with periodontitis in an elderly (65 to 75 years) group of individuals, with and without disease." Laboratory studies have shown age-related changes in the expression of proinflammatory mediators,[11] innate immunity[21] and major histocompatibility complex II (MHC II) pathway gene expression,[17] with the potential to alter the pathology of periodontal diseases or antimicrobial function. However, the relevance of these findings to the clinical situation has not been demonstrated. Age-related differences in the inflammatory response among individuals with gingivitis have been clearly demonstrated and are discussed later in this textbook.

In relation to systematic inflammatory responses, C-reactive protein (CRP) is an acute phase protein that is widely regarded as a marker of inflammatory burden and response to bacterial infection.[53] In an investigation of serum CRP levels among individuals who were 60 to 75 years old and comparing individuals with progressive periodontitis with those with stable disease, CRP levels were increased in people with progressive periodontitis and no other systemic conditions.[56] This finding may indicate that inflammatory burden can be investigated with the use of CRP, although growing evidence indicates that CRP alone may not be as reliable a marker in older people.[46]

A further modulator of the immune and inflammatory responses is nutrition. Interest in this field is increasing rapidly as part of both medicine and periodontology.[10] Nutrition has been studied extensively in geriatric medicine as a result of the nutritional intake changes that occur with age. The impact of nutrition as a potential risk factor for periodontal diseases and their progression is therefore of interest. Emerging data suggest a negative association of serum folate with periodontitis. After controlling for major known confounders, lower serum folate levels in dentate adults who are more than 60 years old are associated with greater levels of periodontitis.[61] These cross-sectional data cannot demonstrate causality alone, but the recognized relationship between folate protection and chronic inflammatory diseases (e.g., cardiovascular disease[33]) offers biologic plausibility to a potential relationship that merits further investigation with prospective studies.

Although many contradictions exist, a survey of the literature demonstrates that some age-related changes are evident in the periodontium and the host response. Whether these changes are significant in the alteration of the progression of periodontal diseases or the response of an older adult to periodontal treatment will be examined next.

Effects of Aging on the Progression of Periodontal Diseases

In a classic experimental gingivitis study, subjects were rendered free of plaque and inflammation through frequent professional cleaning. After this was achieved, the subjects abstained from oral hygiene measures for periods of 3 weeks to allow gingivitis to develop.[30] In this experimental model, a comparison of developing gingivitis between younger and older individuals demonstrated a greater inflammatory response in older subjects, both in humans and in dogs.[8,12,13,22] In the older age group (i.e., 65 to 80 years), the findings included a greater amount of infiltrated connective tissue, increased gingival crevicular fluid flow, and an increased gingival index.[12,13] Other studies have not demonstrated differences between subjects; this finding may be related to smaller differences between the ages of the younger and older experimental groups.[60] Intriguingly, even at the baseline level of excellent gingival health before the commencement of plaque accumulation, differences may exist between groups, with older individuals demonstrating more inflammation.[12,13]

The phrase "getting long in the tooth" expresses a widespread belief that age is inevitably associated with an increased loss of connective tissue attachment. However, this observation may equally reflect cumulative exposure to a number of potentially destructive processes. These exposures may include plaque-associated periodontitis, long-term mechanical trauma from toothbrushing, and iatrogenic damage from unfavorable restorative dentistry or repeated scaling and root planing. The effects of these exposures act in one direction only (i.e., an increased loss of attachment).

In an attempt to differentiate the effects of age from these other processes, several studies have been designed to eliminate confounding issues and to address more clearly the question of age as a risk factor for periodontitis. A *risk factor* is defined as "any characteristic, behavior, or exposure with an association to a particular disease. The relationship is not necessarily causal in nature. ... Some risk factors, if causal, can be modified to reduce one's risk of initiation or progression of disease, such as smoking or improved oral hygiene ... while other factors cannot be modified, such as genetic factors."[14] The conclusions from these studies are strikingly consistent and show that the effect of age is either nonexistent or provides a small and clinically insignificant increased risk of loss of periodontal support.[29,34,38,42,43] Indeed, in comparison with the odds ratio of 20.52 for poor oral hygiene status and periodontitis, the odds ratio for age was only 1.24,[1] and smoking was much more influential than age.[38] Therefore, age has been suggested to be not a true risk factor but rather a background or associated factor for periodontitis.[42] In addition, the clarification of a genetic basis for susceptibility to severe forms of periodontitis underlines the overriding importance of plaque, smoking, and susceptibility in explaining most of the variations in periodontal disease severity among individuals.[26] Nevertheless, a longitudinal study of essentially untreated periodontitis in an older adult (≥70 years old) Japanese population indicated that 296 of 394 individuals (75%) had a least 1 site with 3 mm or more loss of attachment over a 2-year period.[39] Smoking and a baseline attachment level of 6 mm or more were significantly associated with disease progression. A more recent study modeling the transition of periodontal health states over a 2-year period estimated that the risk of transitioning from health to gingivitis was overall reduced by 3% with age.[32] Each year of age increase was associated with a 2% decreased risk of such a transition. Furthermore, increased age was not statistically associated with an increased risk of transitioning from health or gingivitis to periodontitis.

Aging and the Response to Treatment of the Periodontium

The successful treatment of periodontitis requires both meticulous home plaque control by the patient and meticulous supragingival and subgingival debridement by the therapist.[36] Unfortunately, only a few studies have directly compared such an approach among patients of different age groups. The few studies that have done so clearly demonstrate that, despite the histologic changes in the periodontium with aging, no differences in response to nonsurgical or surgical treatment have been shown for periodontitis.[5,28,58] However, if plaque control is not ideal, the continued loss of attachment is inevitable. Furthermore, without effective periodontal therapy, the progression of disease may be faster with increasing age.[44] Attempts to increase plaque control by chemical means have also been reported.[54]

A purely biologic or physiologic review indicates that aging has some impact on the structure and function of the periodontium, as well as on the immune response and the nature of either supragingival or subgingival plaque. However, these changes have a negligible impact on an individual's responsiveness to treatment. Aging may affect other aspects of the management of periodontal health (e.g., the risk of root caries[47]; see Chapter 42), and the resulting difficulties should not be underestimated. One study identified greater compliance with supportive maintenance among older individuals as compared with younger patients.[40]

KEY FACT

The biologic effects of aging have either no impact or a minimal impact on an individual's response to periodontal treatment. However, other factors may have a profound impact, including cognitive and motor skills as well as medical history.

 A Case Scenario is found on the companion website www.expertconsult.com.

References

 References for this chapter are found on the companion website www.expertconsult.com.

Classification of Diseases and Conditions Affecting the Periodontium

James E. Hinrichs | Georgios A. Kotsakis

CHAPTER OUTLINE

Our understanding of the causes and pathogenesis of oral diseases and conditions changes continually with increased scientific knowledge. In light of this fact, a classification can be most consistently defined by the differences in the clinical manifestations of diseases and conditions: they are clinically consistent and require little (if any) clarification by laboratory testing. The current classification of periodontal diseases is based on their extent (generalized versus localized), severity (slight, moderate, or severe), rate of progression (aggressive versus chronic), and localization (i.e., contained within the gingiva, as in gingivitis, or further involving periodontal bone loss, as in periodontitis). The existing definitions encompass the best available way to universally define a spectrum of diseases affecting the periodontal tissues and to guide therapeutic approaches. Nonetheless, the disease state is dynamic, and the appropriate diagnosis for an individual can change over time. For instance, a patient diagnosed with existing periodontitis who undergoes successful periodontal therapy may be classified as having a healthy but reduced periodontium (with slight, moderate, or severe attachment loss) at the reevaluation. Subsequently, if the same individual presents with gingival inflammation without signs of further attachment loss at a future appointment, the appropriate diagnosis would be "gingivitis on a reduced periodontium." Depending on their future compliance with home care and maintenance visits, patients may progress to periodontitis or maintain a healthy but reduced periodontium. The case example highlights the importance of conceptualizing the dynamic nature of inflammatory diseases that affect the periodontium, while appreciating the importance of commonly accepted definitions for periodontal diseases. If a case of gingivitis on a reduced periodontium relapses into periodontitis, the prognosis of the affected teeth will depend on the preexisting attachment loss.

The classification presented in this chapter is based on the most recent internationally accepted consensus on the diseases and conditions that affect the tissues of the periodontium. Box 5.1 presents the overall classification system that was proposed at the 1999 International Workshop for a Classification of Periodontal Diseases and Conditions. More recent views on the Classification of Periodontal Diseases and Conditions are also discussed. Each disease or condition

is explored where clarification is needed. In each case, the reader is referred to pertinent reviews on the subject and specific chapters within this book that discuss the topics in more detail.

 An updated classification system, which is currently being developed jointly by the American Academy of Periodontology (AAP) and the European Federation of Periodontology (EFP), is scheduled to publish around the time of the release of this book. The goal of this effort is to address some of the shortcomings that exist with the current classification system (discussed in this chapter), including diagnostic inaccuracy and significant overlap of disease entities. Several working groups were created to focus on specific disease entities using the currently available scientific evidence, resulting in the most substantial update to the classification system since 1999.

To view the **updated AAP/EFP 2018 classification system,** visit the companion website www.expertconsult.com.

Gingival Diseases

Dental Plaque–Induced Gingival Diseases

Gingivitis that is associated with retained dental plaque is the most common form of gingival disease (Fig. 5.1). Box 5.2 outlines the classifications of gingival diseases. These diseases may occur on a periodontium with no attachment loss or on a periodontium with attachment loss that is stable and not progressing (i.e., reduced periodontium). The epidemiology of periodontal diseases is reviewed in Chapter 6, and its causes are detailed in Chapters 7 through 15 in this textbook.[15,23,26,39,40] What separates gingivitis from periodontitis is the containment of the inflammatory lesion within the gingiva in the former. As such, gingivitis is not associated with progressive attachment loss. This is not to say that gingivitis is solely associated with teeth showing no attachment loss (Fig. 5.2). Gingivitis can also be diagnosed in the gingiva of periodontitis-affected teeth that have previously lost attachment but that have been successfully treated

---

BOX 5.1   Classification of Periodontal Diseases and Conditions

Gingival Diseases
Plaque-induced gingival diseases[a]
Non–plaque-induced gingival lesions

Chronic Periodontitis[b]
Localized
Generalized

Aggressive Periodontitis
Localized
Generalized

Periodontitis as a Manifestation of Systemic Diseases
Necrotizing Periodontal Diseases
Necrotizing ulcerative gingivitis (NUG)
Necrotizing ulcerative periodontitis (NUP)

Abscesses of the Periodontium
Gingival abscess
Periodontal abscess
Pericoronal abscess

Periodontitis Associated With Endodontic Lesions
Endodontic–periodontal lesion
Periodontal–endodontic lesion
Combined lesion

Developmental or Acquired Deformities and Conditions
Localized tooth-related factors that predispose to plaque-induced
    gingival diseases or periodontitis
Mucogingival deformities and conditions around teeth
Mucogingival deformities and conditions on edentulous ridges
Occlusal trauma

---

[a]These diseases may occur on a periodontium with no attachment loss or on a periodontium with attachment loss that is stable and not progressing.
[b]Chronic periodontitis can be further classified based on extent and severity. As a general guide, extent can be characterized as localized (<30% of teeth involved) or generalized (>30% of teeth involved). Severity can be characterized based on the amount of clinical attachment loss (CAL) as follows: *slight* = 1 or 2 mm CAL, *moderate* = 3 or 4 mm CAL, and *severe* ≥5 mm CAL.
Data from Armitage GC: Development of a classification system for periodontal diseases and conditions. *Ann Periodontol* 4:1, 1999.

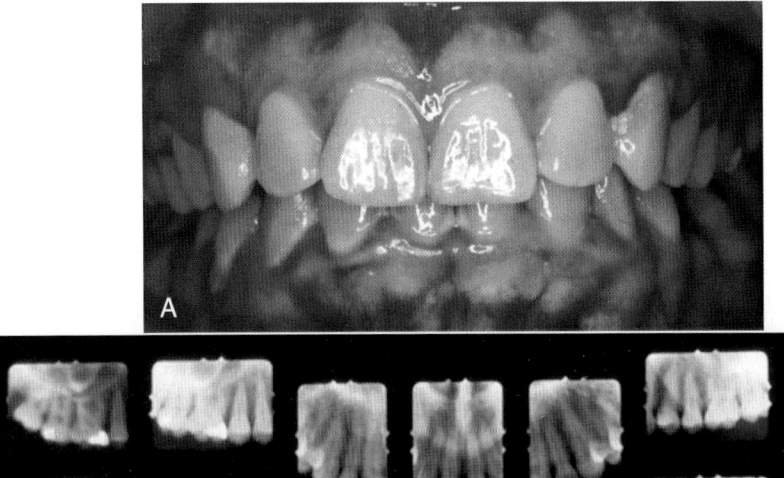

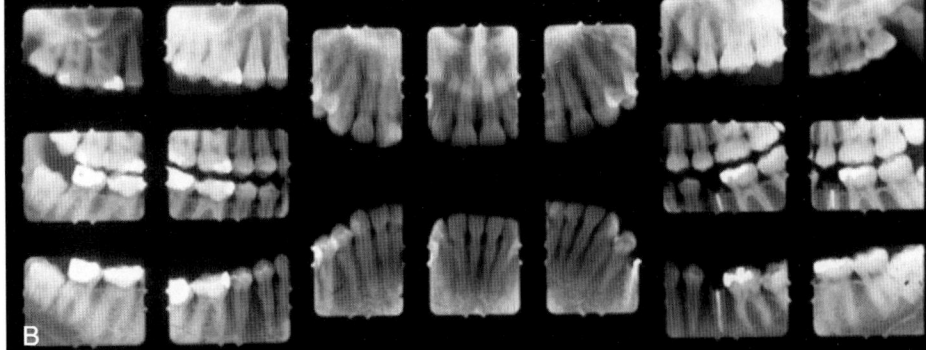

Fig. 5.1 (A) Plaque-related gingivitis depicts marginal and papillary inflammation, with 1- to 4-mm probing depths and generalized zero clinical attachment loss, except recession in tooth #28. (B) Radiographic images of the patient.

---

with periodontal therapy to prevent any further attachment loss. In these treated cases, where gingival inflammation recurs around teeth with existing attachment loss due to a history of treated periodontitis, the appropriate diagnosis would be gingivitis on a reduced periodontium. This implies that gingivitis may be the diagnosis for inflamed gingival tissues associated with a tooth with no previous attachment loss or with a tooth that has previously undergone attachment and bone loss (i.e., with reduced periodontal support) and is not currently losing attachment or bone, even though gingival inflammation is present. Clinical attachment levels and radiographic records are needed to establish this diagnosis.

KEY FACT

Gingivitis may be the diagnosis for inflamed gingival tissues associated with a tooth without previous attachment loss or with a tooth that has previously undergone attachment and bone loss (i.e., with reduced periodontal support) but is not currently losing attachment, even though gingival inflammation is present. In the latter case the appropriate definition would be "gingivitis on a reduced periodontium."

BOX 5.2 Gingival Diseases

Dental Plaque–Induced Gingival Diseases

These diseases may occur on a periodontium with no attachment loss or with attachment loss that is stable and not progressing.

I. Gingivitis associated with dental plaque only
    A. Without local contributing factors
    B. With local contributing factors (see Box 5.4)

II. Gingival diseases modified by systemic factors
    A. Associated with endocrine system
        1. Puberty-associated gingivitis
        2. Menstrual cycle–associated gingivitis
        3. Pregnancy associated
            a. Gingivitis
            b. Pyogenic granuloma
        4. Diabetes mellitus–associated gingivitis
    B. Associated with blood dyscrasias
        1. Leukemia-associated gingivitis
        2. Other

III. Gingival diseases modified by medications
    A. Drug-influenced gingival diseases
        1. Drug-influenced gingival enlargements
        2. Drug-influenced gingivitis
            a. Oral contraceptive–associated gingivitis
            b. Other

IV. Gingival diseases modified by malnutrition
    A. Ascorbic acid deficiency gingivitis
    B. Other

Non–Plaque-Induced Gingival Lesions

I. Gingival diseases of specific bacterial origin
    A. *Neisseria gonorrhoeae*
    B. *Treponema pallidum*
    C. *Streptococcus* species
    D. Other

II. Gingival diseases of viral origin
    A. Herpesvirus infections
        1. Primary herpetic gingivostomatitis
        2. Recurrent oral herpes
        3. Varicella zoster
    B. Other

III. Gingival diseases of fungal origin
    A. *Candida* species infections: generalized gingival candidiasis
    B. Linear gingival erythema
    C. Histoplasmosis
    D. Other

IV. Gingival lesions of genetic origin
    A. Hereditary gingival fibromatosis
    B. Other

V. Gingival manifestations of systemic conditions
    A. Mucocutaneous lesions
        1. Lichen planus
        2. Pemphigoid
        3. Pemphigus vulgaris
        4. Erythema multiforme
        5. Lupus erythematosus
        6. Drug induced
        7. Other
    B. Allergic reactions
        1. Dental restorative materials
            a. Mercury
            b. Nickel
            c. Acrylic
            d. Other
        2. Reactions attributable to the following:
            a. Toothpastes or dentifrices
            b. Mouth rinses or mouthwashes
            c. Chewing gum additives
            d. Foods and additives
        3. Other

VI. Traumatic lesions (factitious, iatrogenic, or accidental)
    A. Chemical injury
    B. Physical injury
    C. Thermal injury

VII. Foreign body reactions

VIII. Not otherwise specified

Data from Holmstrup P: Non–plaque-induced gingival lesions. *Ann Periodontol* 4:20, 1999; and Mariotti A: Dental plaque-induced gingival diseases. *Ann Periodontol* 4:7, 1999.

Gingivitis Associated With Dental Plaque Only

Plaque-induced gingival disease is the result of an interaction between the microorganisms found in the dental plaque biofilm and the inflammatory host response. A cause-and-effect relationship between microbial plaque and gingivitis has been elegantly demonstrated by a classic experiment demonstrating that the cessation of oral hygiene consistently leads to the manifestation of gingivitis within 2 to 3 weeks in healthy adults.[25] Clinical gingivitis is histologically characterized by a dense infiltrate of lymphocytes and other mononuclear cells, fibroblast alterations, increased vascular permeability, and continuing loss of collagen in response to the microbial challenge. However, the alveolar bone is not affected. Microbial plaque is thus considered to be the primary etiologic factor for gingivitis. The severity and duration of the inflammatory response interaction can be altered by the modifying local (see Chapter 13) or systemic modifying factors (see Chapters 14 and 15). Gingivitis is fully reversible in otherwise healthy persons within weeks following the removal of local factors and reduction of the microbial load around the teeth. As noted earlier, gingivitis is rapidly established in cases

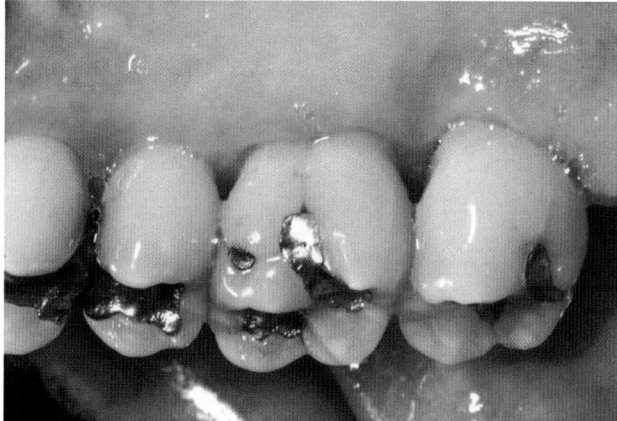

Fig. 5.2 Maxillary second molar exhibits mild inflammation at mesial-palatal surface. However, the clinical attachment loss has been stable for 15 years after apical positioned flap and periodontal maintenance, which is consistent with remission. The appropriate diagnosis is gingivitis on a reduced periodontium.

of generalized or localized inefficient plaque removal. Therefore it is crucial that patients are instructed in oral hygiene to maintain long-term gingival health.

Gingival Diseases Modified by Systemic Factors

Systemic factors that contribute to gingivitis—such as the endocrine changes associated with puberty (Fig. 5.3), the menstrual cycle, pregnancy (Fig. 5.4A), and diabetes—may exacerbate the gingival inflammatory response to plaque.[23,39] This altered response appears to result from the effects of systemic conditions on the host's cellular and immunologic functions, but the primary etiologic factor is still considered to be microbial plaque. One example of altered host response due to systemic factors is apparent during pregnancy when the incidence and severity of gingival

inflammation may increase even in the presence of low levels of plaque.

In blood dyscrasias (e.g., leukemia), the reduced number of immunocompetent lymphocytes in the periodontal tissues is associated with increased edema, erythema, and bleeding of the gingiva as well as gingival enlargement that may be associated with the swollen, spongy gingival tissues caused by the excessive infiltration of malignant blood cells (Fig. 5.5).

Gingival Diseases Modified by Medications

Gingival diseases that are modified by medications include gingival overgrowth due to anticonvulsant drugs such as phenytoin, immunosuppressive drugs such as cyclosporine (Fig. 5.6), and calcium channel blockers such as nifedipine (Fig. 5.7), verapamil, diltiazem,

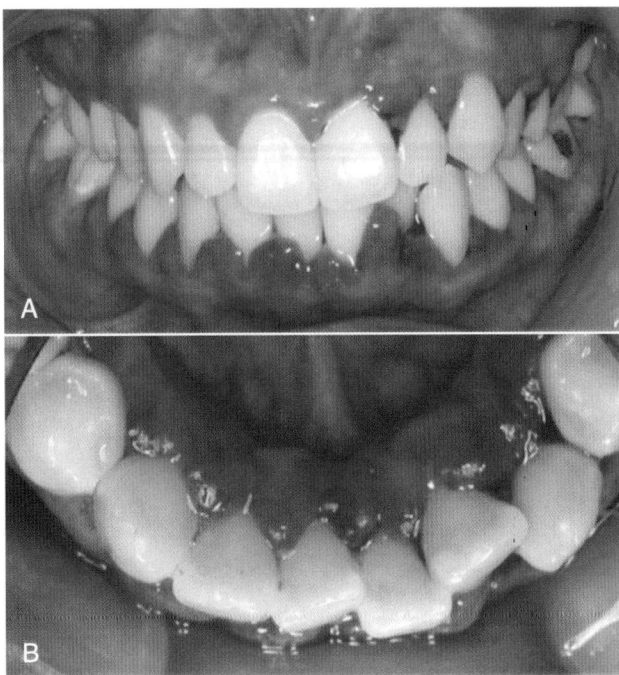

Fig. 5.3 A 13-year-old female with hormone-exaggerated marginal and papillary inflammation, with 1- to 4-mm probing depths yet minimal clinical attachment loss. (A) Facial view. (B) Lingual view.

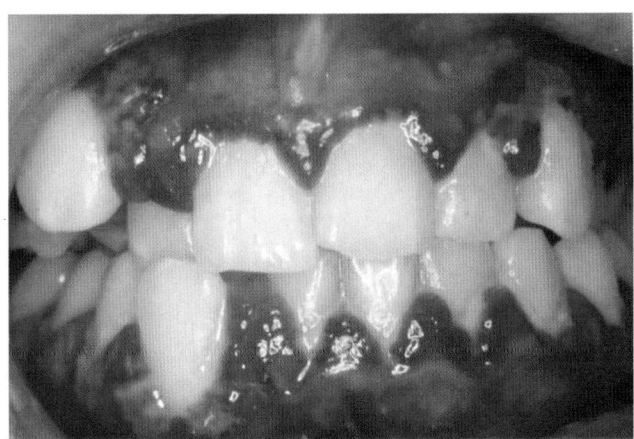

Fig. 5.5 A 12-year-old female with a primary medical diagnosis of leukemia that exhibits swollen/spongy gingiva.

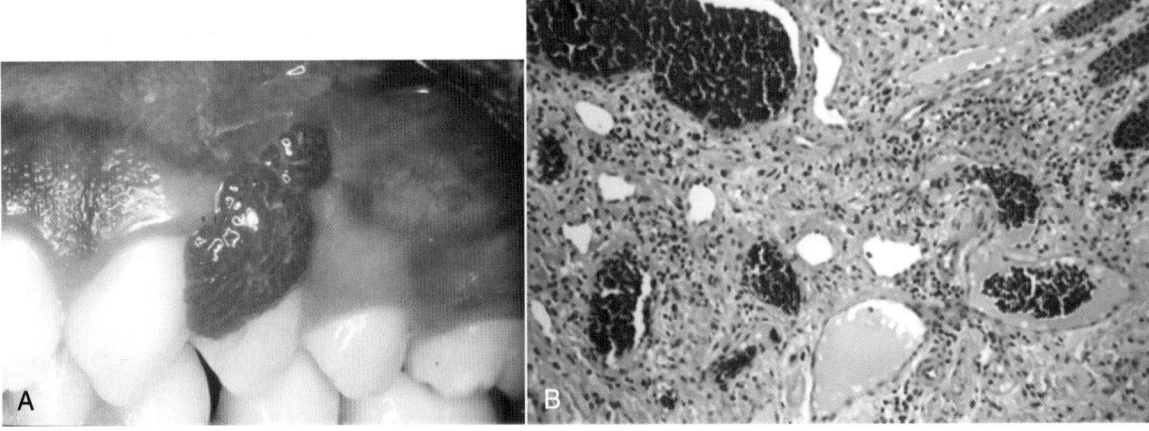

Fig. 5.4 (A) Clinical image of pyogenic granuloma in a 27-year-old pregnant female. (B) Histologic image depicts dense inflammatory infiltrate and prominent vessels.

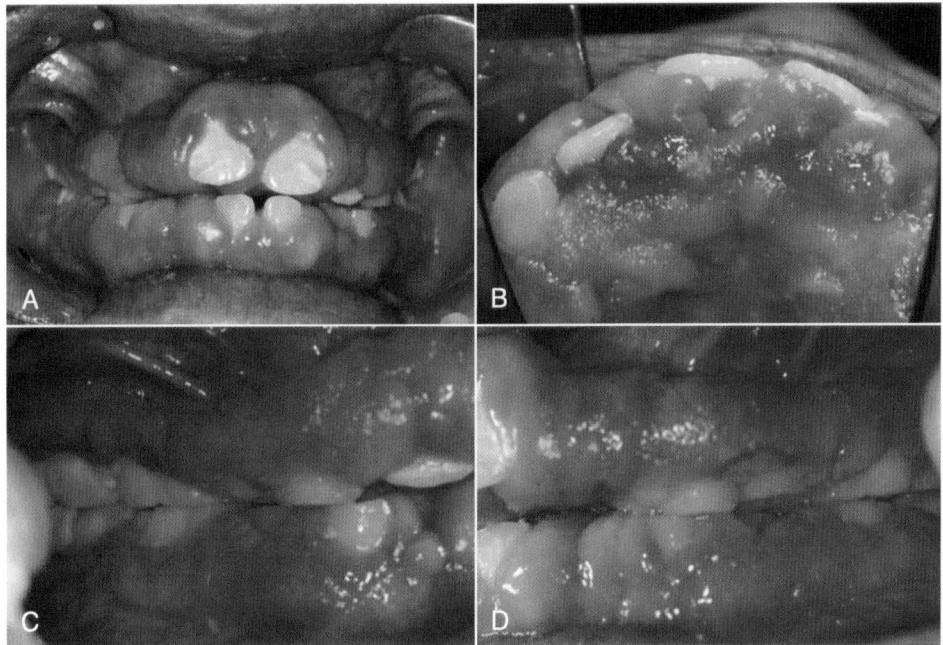

Fig. 5.6 Clinical images of a 9-year-old male with severe gingival overgrowth secondary to heart transplant and cyclosporine therapy.

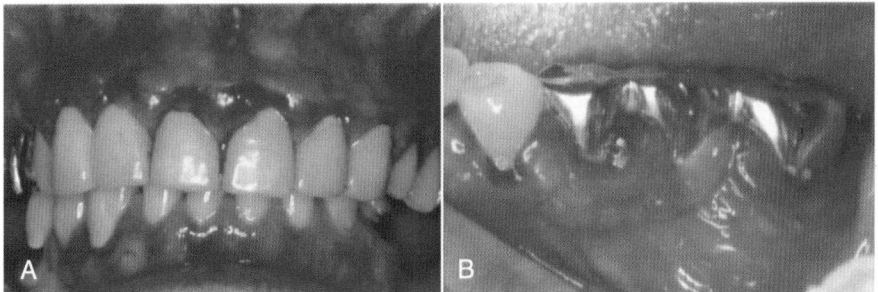

Fig. 5.7 Clinical images of gingival overgrowth following use a of calcium channel blocker to control hypertension.

and sodium valproate.[15,26,39] The development and severity of gingival enlargement in response to medications is patient specific and may be influenced by uncontrolled plaque accumulation as well as by elevated hormonal levels. The increased use of oral contraceptives by premenopausal women has also been previously associated with a higher incidence of gingival inflammation and gingival enlargement. Although this fact stood true for earlier contraceptive formulations, existing contraceptives that include more modest doses of active ingredients are not commonly associated with gingival inflammation.

Gingival Diseases Modified by Malnutrition

Gingival diseases modified by malnutrition have received attention because of clinical descriptions of bright red, swollen, and bleeding gingiva associated with severe ascorbic acid (vitamin C) deficiency or scurvy.[26] Various nutrients, such as long chain omega-3 fatty acids, have been found to have immunomodulatory properties, whereas others act to ameliorate the destructive effects of reactive oxygen species (ROS) functioning as ROS scavengers. Nonetheless, the available evidence to support a clinically impactful role for mild nutritional deficiencies in the development or severity of gingival inflammation in humans is limited. Data have shed light on the implication of increased dietary carbohydrate intake on gingivitis, in addition to its known causal role on the occurrence of dental caries.[19]

Non–Plaque-Induced Gingival Lesions

Oral manifestations of systemic conditions that produce lesions in the tissues of the periodontium are less common than plaque-induced gingivitis. This category mainly encompasses lesions of autoimmune or idiopathic etiology that can manifest in the gingiva. Benign mucous membrane pemphigoid is an example of a non–plaque-induced lesion associated with sloughing gingival tissues, which leave painful ulcerations of the gingiva (Fig. 5.8). In pemphigoid, autoimmune antibodies are targeted at the basement membrane, and histologically the destruction resembles a subepithelial blister (Fig. 5.8C–D). Case Scenario 5.2 depicts gingival recession accompanied by a mucosal lesion located on the gingiva manifesting with a white lacy pattern with characteristic striations.

Gingival Diseases of Specific Bacterial Origin

Gingival diseases of this category are attributed to specific bacteria that cause characteristic lesions in the gingiva. *Neisseria gonorrhoeae* and *Treponema pallidum* that can be transferred as a result of sexually transmitted diseases such as gonorrhea and syphilis, respectively, cause characteristic lesions in the gingiva.[41,46] Refer to the online references for further description. Streptococcal gingivitis or gingivostomatitis is a rare entity that may present as an acute condition with fever, malaise, and pain associated with acutely inflamed, diffuse,

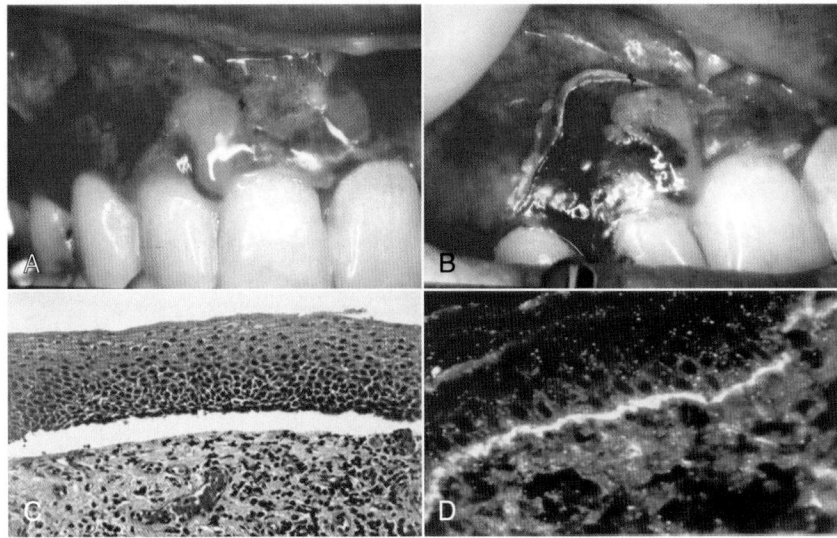

Fig. 5.8 A 62-year-old female with benign mucous membrane pemphigoid. (A–B) Clinical image with sloughing epithelial surface. (C) Hematoxylin and eosin (H&E) stain depicting separation of epithelium from connective tissue. (D) Immunofluorescent-labeled antibodies to basement membrane.

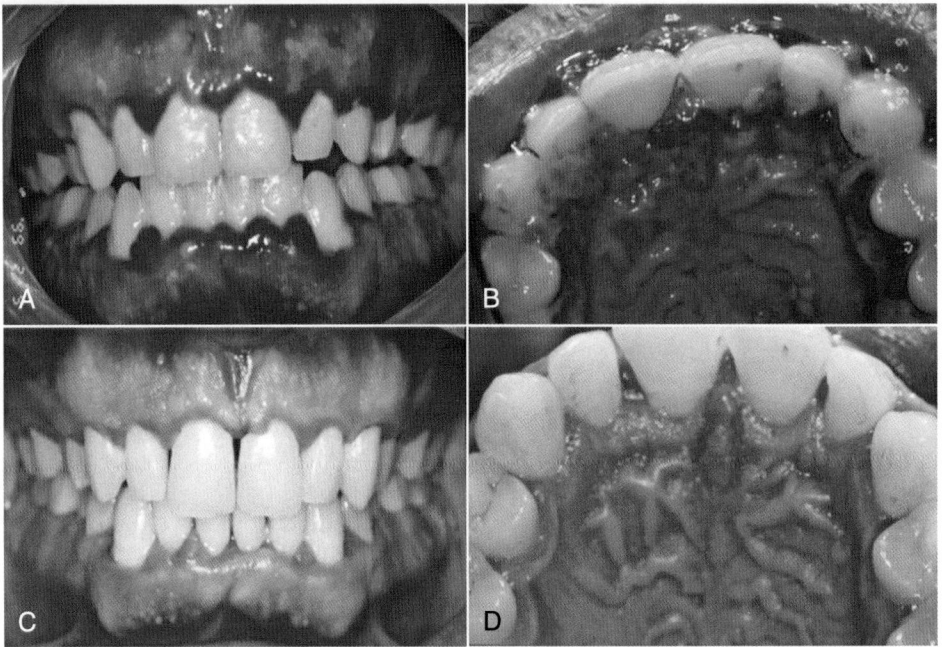

Fig. 5.9 (A–B) A 29-year-old male with primary herpetic infection and severe gingival inflammation. (C–D) Six weeks post systemic acyclovir.

red, and swollen gingiva with increased bleeding and occasional gingival abscess formation. The gingival infections are usually preceded by tonsillitis.

Gingival Diseases of Viral Origin

Gingival diseases of viral origin may be caused by a variety of deoxyribonucleic acid and ribonucleic acid viruses, with the most common being the herpesviruses. A case example of herpetic stomatitis is demonstrated in Fig. 5.9A–B. Herpetic lesions are not uncommon and develop as intraoral blisters, usually grouped together, that quickly burst, leaving minuscule ulcerations. Lesions are frequently related to the reactivation of latent viruses, especially as a result of reduced immune function. The oral manifestations of viral infection have been comprehensively reviewed.[20,45] Viral gingival diseases are treated with topical or systemic antiviral drugs (Fig. 5.9C–D).

Unlike other herpetic recurrences, varicella zoster virus (VZV) usually manifests with a prodrome of tingling, itching, burning, or a unilateral numbness at the affected dermatome. These symptoms are followed by moderate to severe pain shortly after initiation and are very important for differential diagnosis.

Gingival Diseases of Fungal Origin

Gingival diseases of fungal origin are relatively uncommon in immunocompetent individuals, but they occur more frequently in immunocompromised individuals and in those with disturbed microbiota by the long-term use of broad-spectrum antibiotics.[20,46,47] The most common oral fungal infection is candidiasis (*Candida albicans* is often implicated). Candidiasis can also be seen under prosthetic devices, in individuals using topical steroids, and in individuals with decreased salivary flow, increased salivary glucose, or decreased salivary pH. A generalized candidal infection may manifest as white patches on the gingiva, tongue, or oral mucous membrane that can potentially be removed with gauze and leave a red, bleeding surface. In human immunodeficiency virus (HIV) seropositive persons, candidal infection may present as continuous erythematous stripe of the attached gingiva; this has been referred to as *linear gingival erythema* or *HIV-associated gingivitis* (see Chapter 30). The diagnosis of candidal infection can be made by culture, smear, or biopsy. Less common fungal infections have also been described.[46,47]

Gingival Diseases of Genetic Origin

Gingival diseases of genetic origin may involve the tissues of the periodontium and have been described in detail.[2] One of the most clinically evident conditions is *hereditary gingival fibromatosis,* which exhibits autosomal-dominant or (rarely) autosomal-recessive modes of inheritance. The gingival enlargement may completely cover the teeth, delay eruption, and present as an isolated finding; alternatively, it may be associated with several more generalized syndromes.

Gingival Manifestations of Systemic Conditions

Gingival manifestations of systemic conditions may appear as desquamative lesions, ulcerations of the gingiva, or both.[20,38,46] Allergic reactions that manifest with gingival changes are uncommon but have been observed in association with several restorative materials (Fig. 5.10A), toothpastes, mouthwashes, chewing gums (Fig. 5.11), and foods (see Box 5.2). The diagnosis of these conditions may prove difficult and may require an extensive history and the selective elimination of potential causes. Conjoint assessment with an allergologist is indicated, and percutaneous tests are often recommended. Histologic traits of biopsies from gingival allergic reactions include a dense infiltrate of eosinophilic cells (Fig. 5.10B–C).

Traumatic Lesions

Traumatic lesions may be self-inflicted and *factitious* in origin, which means that they are intentionally or unintentionally produced by artificial means (Fig. 5.12). Other examples of traumatic lesions include toothbrush trauma that results in gingival ulceration, recession, or both.

> **CLINICAL CORRELATION**
>
> Individuals who perform aggressive horizontal brushing are often found to have gingival recession or cervical abrasion on the teeth quadrants contralateral to their dominant hand.

Iatrogenic trauma (i.e., induced by the dentist or health professional) to the gingiva may also lead to a gingival lesion. Such trauma may be caused directly (i.e., via use of dental instruments) or by the induction of cement or preventive or restorative materials (Fig. 5.13A). Peripheral ossifying fibroma may develop in response to the embedment of a foreign body (Fig. 5.13B–C). Self-inflicted *accidental damage* to the gingiva may also occur as a result of minor burns from hot foods and drinks.[20]

Foreign-Body Reactions

Foreign-body reactions lead to localized inflammatory conditions of the gingiva and are caused by the introduction of foreign material into the gingival connective tissues through breaks in the epithelium.[20] Common examples are the introduction of amalgam into the gingiva during the placement of a restoration, the extraction of a tooth, or an endodontic apicoectomy with retrofill leaving an amalgam tattoo (Fig. 5.14A), with resultant metal fragments observed during biopsies (Fig. 5.14B); abrasives may also be introduced during polishing procedures.

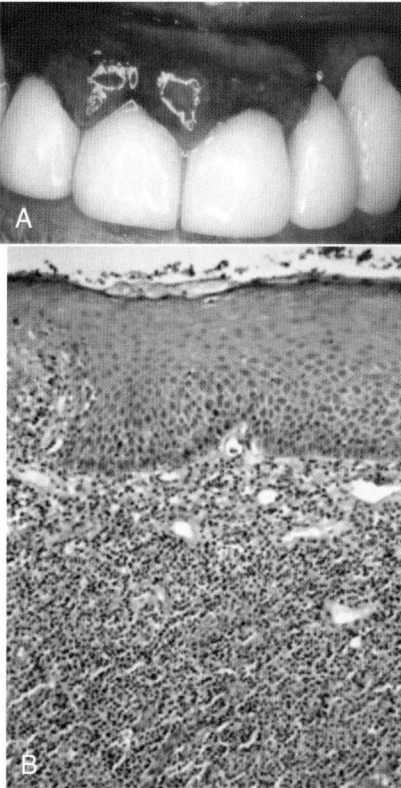
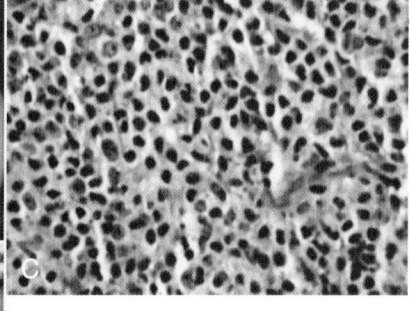

Fig. 5.10 (A) Localized pronounced gingival inflammation secondary to nickel allergy. (B–C) Biopsy depicts dense infiltrate of plasma cells.

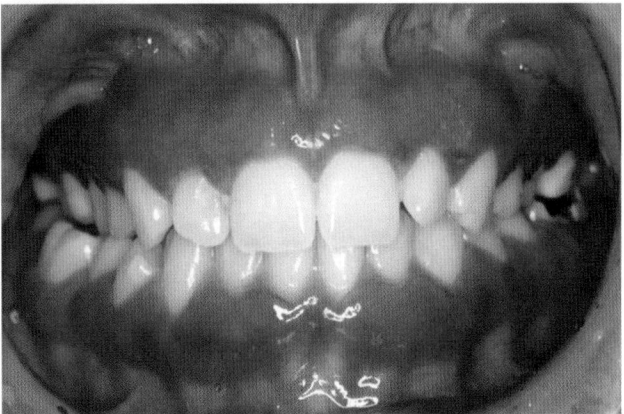

Fig. 5.11 Generalized severe allergic response of gingiva as a result of additive in chewing gum.

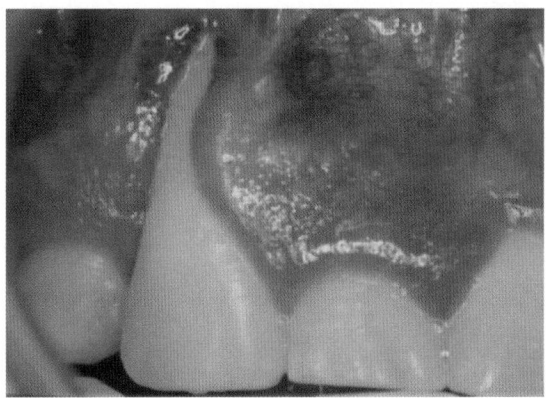

Fig. 5.12 Self-inflicted gingival dehiscence induced via patient's fingernail.

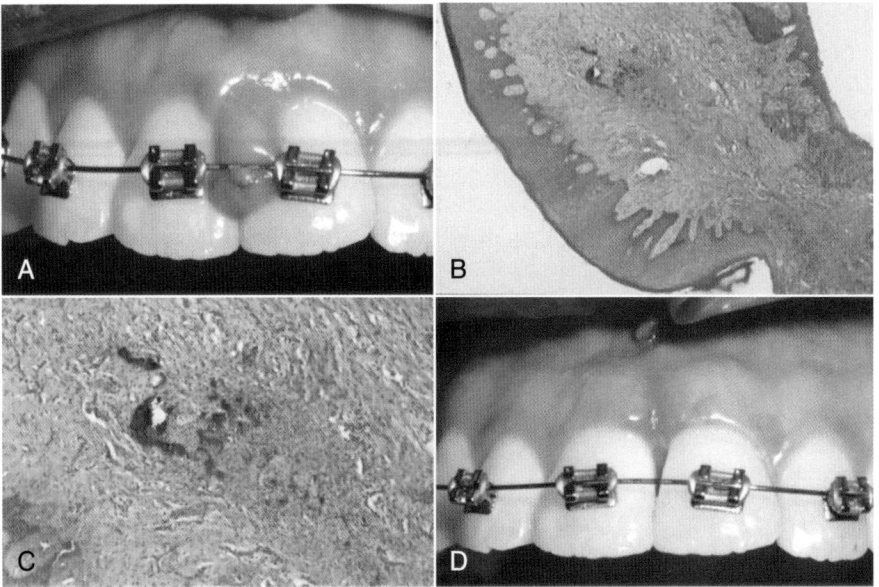

Fig. 5.13 (A) Proliferative gingival overgrowth secondary to impaction of foreign body. (B) Histology of peripheral ossifying fibroma. (C) Higher magnification of image in part B. (D) Four weeks post excisional biopsy.

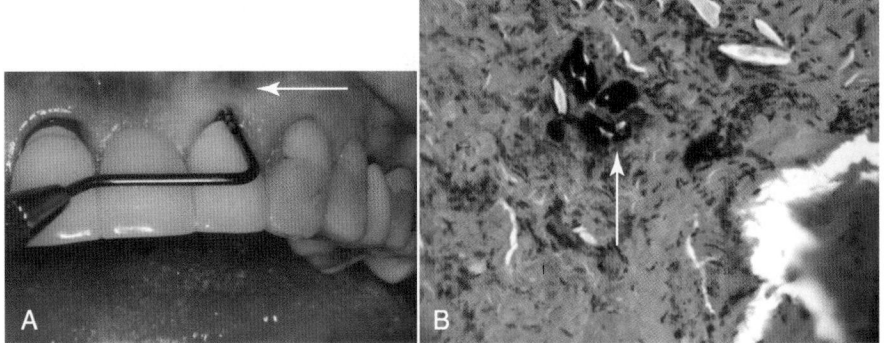

Fig. 5.14 (A) Gingival pigmentation associated with previous apicoectomy and amalgam retro-fill. (B) Biopsy depicts metal fragments.

Periodontitis

Periodontitis is defined as "an inflammatory disease of the supporting tissues of the teeth caused by specific microorganisms or groups of specific microorganisms, resulting in progressive destruction of the periodontal ligament and alveolar bone with increased probing depth formation, recession, or both."[51] The clinical feature that distinguishes periodontitis from gingivitis is the presence of clinically detectable attachment loss as a result of inflammatory destruction of the periodontal ligament and alveolar bone. This loss is often accompanied by periodontal pocket formation and changes in the density and height of the subjacent alveolar bone. In some cases, recession of the marginal gingiva may accompany attachment loss, thereby masking ongoing disease progression if only probing depth measurements are taken without measurements of clinical attachment levels.

KEY FACT

Probing depth measurement alone is inadequate for an assessment of periodontitis. Clinical attachment loss is usually assessed by adding the extent of gingival recession to the probing depth measurement to estimate the total extent of tissue loss from the cementoenamel junction (CEJ) of the tooth. However, when recession is not visible, it is essential that height of the marginal gingiva coronal to the CEJ be determined and that measurement subtracted from the probing depth to establish the extent of clinical attachment loss. The measurement of clinical attachment around a tooth provides insights on the history and extent of periodontal destruction around the tooth. One common pitfall of clinical periodontal examination is the direct translation of probing depths as clinical attachment levels when the gingival margin lies above the cementoenamel junction, leading to an overestimation of attachment levels.

Clinical signs of inflammation—such as changes in color, contour, and consistency as well as bleeding with probing—may not always be positive indicators of ongoing attachment loss. However, the presence of continued bleeding with probing during sequential visits has proved to be a reliable indicator of the presence of inflammation and an increased risk for subsequent attachment loss at the bleeding site. The attachment loss associated with periodontitis may occur in a cyclic fashion, with attachment loss progressing either continuously or in episodic bursts of disease activity. However, the available clinical instruments for detecting disease are not sensitive enough to capture the cycles of attachment loss and repair that occur during disease activity and remission, respectively (i.e., the periodontal probe is graded in 1-mm increments).

KEY FACT

In the AAP/EFP 2018 classification of periodontal diseases, a multidimensional staging and grading system will be introduced to subclassify periodontitis disease entities. The severity of periodontal disease at the time of presentation and the complexity of disease management will dictate the staging, while grading offers additional information, including the rate of past progression of the disease and the risk for future progression.

Although many classifications of the different clinical manifestations of periodontitis have been presented since the late 1990s, consensus workshops in North America in 1989[8] and in Europe in 1993[6] identified that periodontitis may present in early-onset, adult-onset, and necrotizing forms (Table 5.1). In addition, the AAP consensus concluded that periodontitis may be associated with systemic conditions (e.g., diabetes, HIV) and that some forms of periodontitis may be refractory to conventional therapy. Early-onset disease was distinguished from adult-onset disease by the age of onset (< 35 years of age was set as an arbitrary separation of diseases), the rate of disease progression, and the presence of alterations in host defenses. The early-onset diseases were more aggressive, occurred in individuals younger than 35 years old, and were associated with defects in host defenses. Adult forms of disease were slowly progressive, became clinically more evident during the fourth decade of life, and were not associated with defects in host defenses. In addition, early-onset periodontitis was subclassified into prepubertal, juvenile,

TABLE 5.1   Classification of the Various Forms of Periodontitis

Classification	Forms of Periodontitis	Disease Characteristics
AAP World Workshop in Clinical Periodontics, 1989[5]	Adult periodontitis	Age of onset >35 years Slow rate of disease progression No defects in host defenses
	Early-onset periodontitis (may be prepubertal, juvenile, or rapidly progressive)	Age of onset <35 years Rapid rate of disease progression Defects in host defenses Associated with specific microflora
	Periodontitis associated with systemic disease	Systemic diseases that predispose to rapid rates of periodontitis Diseases: diabetes, Down syndrome, HIV infection, Papillon–Lefèvre syndrome
	Necrotizing ulcerative periodontitis	Similar to acute necrotizing ulcerative gingivitis but with associated clinical attachment loss
	Refractory periodontitis	Recurrent periodontitis that does not respond to treatment
European Workshop in Periodontology, 1993[3]	Adult periodontitis	Age of onset: fourth decade of life Slow rate of disease progression No defects in host response
	Early-onset periodontitis	Age of onset: before fourth decade of life Rapid rate of disease progression Defects in host defense
	Necrotizing periodontitis	Tissue necrosis with attachment and bone loss
AAP International Workshop for Classification of Periodontal Diseases, 1999[2]	Chronic periodontitis Aggressive periodontitis Periodontitis as a manifestation of systemic diseases	See Box 5.3

AAP, American Academy of Periodontology; *HIV,* human immunodeficiency virus.

and rapidly progressive forms with localized or generalized disease distributions.

Extensive clinical and basic scientific research involving these disease entities has been performed in many countries, and emerging information has provided support for the unification of many of the preexisting disease categories.[13,23,49] In particular, supporting evidence was lacking for the distinct classifications of adult periodontitis, refractory periodontitis, and the various different forms of early-onset periodontitis as outlined by the AAP Workshop for the International Classification of Periodontal Diseases in 1999[5] (see Table 5.1). It has been observed that chronic periodontal destruction caused by the accumulation of local factors (e.g., plaque, calculus) can occur before the age of 35 years and that the aggressive disease seen in young patients may be independent of age and instead have a familial (genetic) association. With respect to refractory periodontitis, little

evidence supports the theory that this condition is indeed a distinct clinical entity. The causes of continued loss of clinical attachment and alveolar bone after periodontal therapy are currently poorly defined and apply to many disease entities. In addition, clinical data from the medical community emerged to support the belief that forms of periodontitis that were collectively referred to as prepubertal periodontitis were in fact representing periodontitis as a manifestation of distinct systemic diseases, such as in leukocyte adhesion deficiency syndromes. As a result, the AAP held an International Workshop for the Classification of Periodontal Diseases in 1999 to further refine the classification system with the use of current clinical and scientific data.[5] The resulting classification of the different forms of periodontitis was simplified to describe three general disease forms: chronic periodontitis, aggressive periodontitis, and periodontitis as a manifestation of systemic disease (Table 5.1 and Box 5.3).

BOX 5.3 Periodontitis

The disease periodontitis can be subclassified into the following three major types based on clinical, radiographic, historical, and laboratory characteristics.

Chronic Periodontitis
The following characteristics are common to patients with chronic periodontitis:
- Prevalent in adults but can occur in children
- Amount of destruction consistent with local factors
- Associated with a variable microbial pattern
- Subgingival calculus frequently found
- Slow-to-moderate rate of progression with possible periods of rapid progression
- Possibly modified by or associated with the following:
  - Systemic diseases such as diabetes mellitus and human immunodeficiency virus (HIV) infection
  - Local factors predisposing to periodontitis
  - Environmental factors such as cigarette smoking and emotional stress

Chronic periodontitis may be further subclassified into localized and generalized forms and characterized as mild, moderate, or severe based on the common features described previously and the following specific features:
- Localized form: <30% of teeth involved
- Generalized form: >30% of teeth involved
- Mild: 1 to 2 mm clinical attachment loss (CAL)
- Moderate: 3 to 4 mm CAL
- Severe: ≥5 mm CAL

Aggressive Periodontitis
The following characteristics are common to patients with aggressive periodontitis:
- Otherwise clinically healthy patient (note the distinction with periodontitis as a manifestation of systemic disease)
- Rapid attachment loss and bone destruction
- Familial aggregation of diseased individuals
  The following characteristics are common but not universal:
- Amount of microbial deposits inconsistent with disease severity
- Increased levels of *Actinobacillus actinomycetemcomitans*
- Abnormalities in phagocyte function
- Hyper-responsive macrophages, producing increased prostaglandin E$_2$ (PGE$_2$) and interleukin-1β (IL-1β)
- In some cases, self-arresting disease progression

Aggressive periodontitis may be further classified into localized and generalized forms based on the common features described here and the following specific features.

Localized Form
- Circumpubertal onset of disease
- Localized first molar or incisor disease with proximal attachment loss on at least two permanent teeth, one of which is a first molar
- Robust serum antibody response to infecting agents

Generalized Form
- Usually affecting persons under 30 years of age (however, may be older)
- Generalized proximal attachment loss affecting at least three teeth other than first molars and incisors
- Pronounced episodic nature of periodontal destruction
- Poor serum antibody response to infecting agents

Periodontitis as a Manifestation of Systemic Diseases
Periodontitis may be observed as a manifestation of the following systemic diseases:
1. Hematologic disorders
   a. Acquired neutropenia
   b. Leukemias
   c. Other
2. Genetic disorders
   a. Familial and cyclic neutropenia
   b. Down syndrome
   c. Leukocyte adhesion deficiency syndromes
   d. Papillon–Lefèvre syndrome
   e. Chédiak–Higashi syndrome
   f. Histiocytosis syndromes
   g. Glycogen storage disease
   h. Infantile genetic agranulocytosis
   i. Cohen syndrome
   j. Ehlers-Danlos syndrome (types IV and VIII autosomal dominant [AD])
   k. Hypophosphatasia
   l. Other
3. Not otherwise specified

Data from Flemmig TF: Periodontitis. *Ann Periodontol* 4:32, 1999; Kinane DF: Periodontitis modified by systemic factors. *Ann Periodontol* 4:54, 1999; and Tonetti MS, Mombelli A: Early-onset periodontitis. *Ann Periodontol* 4:39, 1999.

Since the establishment of the currently accepted 1999 classification, a taskforce commissioned by the AAP proposed an update to the existing classification scheme in 2015.[3] The update focused on suggestions to address the challenges in clinical documentation of attachment level changes and the distinction between chronic and aggressive periodontitis. In particular, the AAP task force recommended the consideration of probing depth levels, in addition to attachment levels, in determining the severity of periodontitis to avoid overestimation. The classification of diseases and conditions of the periodontium discussed in this chapter will focus on the currently accepted 1999 classification with references to the AAP update when appropriate.

Chronic Periodontitis

Chronic periodontitis is the most common form of periodontitis[13]; Box 5.3 includes the characteristics of this form of periodontitis. Chronic periodontitis is most prevalent in adults, but it can also be observed in children. Different classification schemes have confirmed or discarded the age range of more than 35 years to separate chronic versus aggressive periodontitis. According to the existing definition, persons younger than 35 years may exhibit a rate of progression of disease consistent with the definition of chronic periodontitis. Nonetheless, epidemiologic evidence supports the suggestion that persons younger than 25 years at disease onset are likely to exhibit aggressive periodontitis. Intraoral radiographs along with periodontal charting records are of paramount importance to the documentation of disease onset and rate of progression.

Chronic periodontitis is associated with the accumulation of plaque and calculus. It generally has a slow to moderate rate of disease progression, but periods of more rapid destruction may also be observed. Increases in the rate of disease progression may be caused by the impact of local, systemic, or environmental factors that may influence the normal host–bacteria interaction. Local factors may influence plaque accumulation (Box 5.4), whereas systemic diseases (e.g., diabetes mellitus, HIV) may influence the host's defenses, and environmental factors (e.g., cigarette smoking, stress) may influence the response of the host to plaque accumulation. Chronic periodontitis may occur as a localized disease in which less than 30% of evaluated teeth demonstrate attachment and bone loss, or it may occur as generalized when more than 30% of teeth are affected.

> ### KEY FACT
>
> Chronic periodontitis is classified by extent and severity of disease, such as generalized (extent), moderate (severity) chronic periodontitis.

Chronic periodontitis can be further classified on the basis of its extent and severity. The severity of disease has been traditionally determined as either slight/mild (1 to 2 mm of loss; Fig. 5.15), moderate (3 to 4 mm of loss; Fig. 5.16), or severe (≥5 mm of loss; Fig. 5.17) on the basis of the amount of clinical attachment loss (see Box 5.3). Clinical attachment levels provide important benefits over probing depth alone to monitor disease progression using the CEJ as a fixed reference point. In fact, probing depth levels only have poor to moderate sensitivity for predicting attachment level changes overtime. Nonetheless, clinical experience has revealed that oftentimes measurement of clinical attachment levels in practice may prove to be erroneous. The most common error occurs in the case of sites without gingival recession, whereby the location of the gingival margin is coronal to the CEJ. If the clinician in such a case only records the probing depth without charting the location of the CEJ (often charted as "positive recession" in electronic periodontal charts),

---

BOX 5.4 Developmental or Acquired Deformities and Conditions

Localized Tooth-Related Factors That Modify or Predispose to Plaque-Induced Gingival Diseases or Periodontitis
1. Tooth anatomic factors
2. Dental restorations or appliances
3. Root fractures
4. Cervical root resorption and cemental tears

Mucogingival Deformities and Conditions Around Teeth
1. Gingival or soft tissue recession
   a. Facial or lingual surfaces
   b. Interproximal (papillary)
2. Lack of keratinized gingiva
3. Decreased vestibular depth
4. Aberrant frenum or muscle position
5. Gingival excess
   a. Pseudopocket
   b. Inconsistent gingival margin
   c. Excessive gingival display
   d. Gingival enlargement (see Box 5.2)
   e. Abnormal color

Mucogingival Deformities and Conditions on Edentulous Edges
1. Vertical and/or horizontal ridge deficiency
2. Lack of gingiva or keratinized tissue
3. Gingival or soft tissue enlargements
4. Aberrant frenum or muscle position
5. Decreased vestibular depth
6. Abnormal color

Occlusal Trauma
1. Primary occlusal trauma
2. Secondary occlusal trauma

Data from Blieden TM: Tooth-related issues. *Ann Periodontol* 4:91, 1999; Halmon WW: Occlusal trauma: effect and impact on the periodontium. *Ann Periodontol* 4:102, 1999; and Pini Prato GP: Mucogingival deformities. *Ann Periodontol* 4:98, 1999.

---

the resulting attachment levels will be erroneously recorded as being equal to the probing depth. To prevent such an overestimate of disease, it has been suggested that clinicians consider that mild periodontitis be associated with probing depths of <4 mm, moderate periodontitis with probing depths of 5 to 6 mm, and severe periodontitis with probing depths of ≥7 mm. However, probing depths alone should not be used to classify periodontitis without simultaneous consideration of clinical attachment levels and radiographic bone loss.

>
>
> ### KEY FACT
>
> In the AAP/EFP 2018 classification of periodontal diseases, one of the major changes that will be implemented is avoidance of a separate category of "aggressive periodontitis." Both chronic and aggressive periodontitis disease entities will be grouped together and will be simply called *periodontitis*.

Aggressive Periodontitis

Aggressive periodontitis differs from the chronic form primarily by the rapid rate of disease progression seen in an otherwise healthy individual (Figs. 5.18 and 5.19). The absence of large accumulations

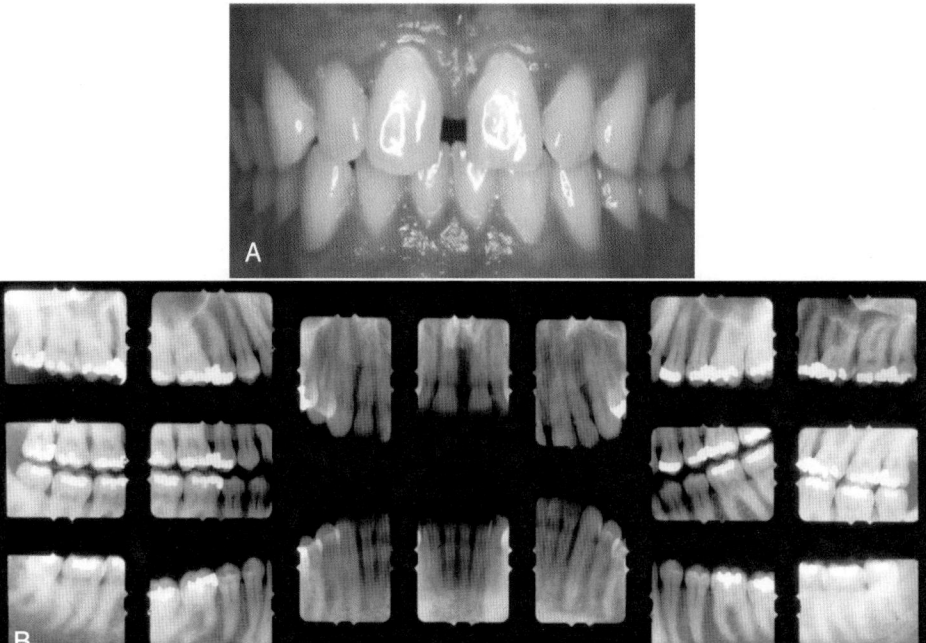

Fig. 5.15 (A) Clinical image of plaque-related slight/early chronic periodontitis with 1- to 2-mm clinical attachment loss in 40-year-old female. (B) Radiographic images of the patient.

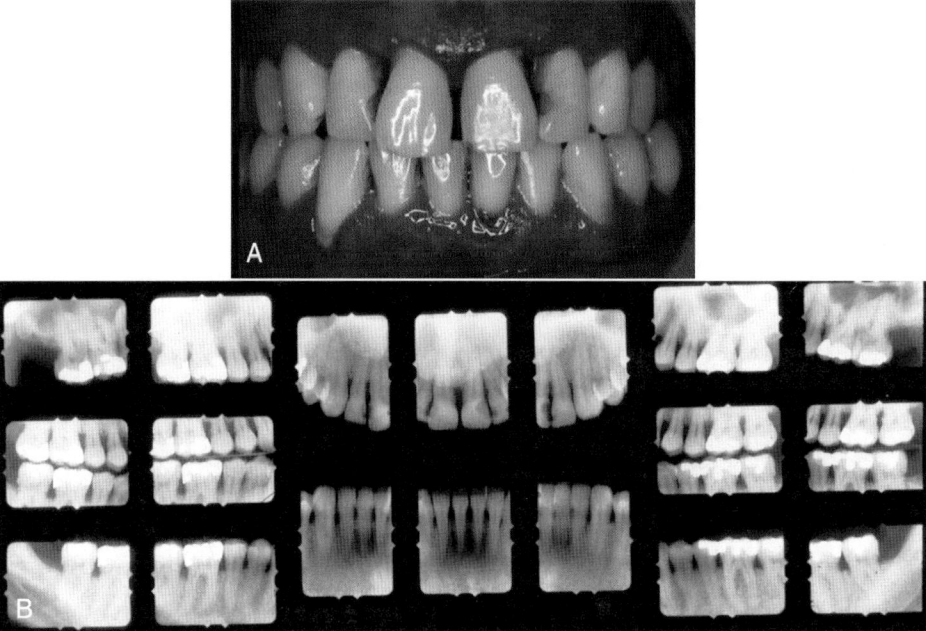

Fig. 5.16 (A) Clinical image of plaque-related moderate chronic periodontitis with 3- to 4-mm clinical attachment loss in a 53-year-old male smoker. (B) Radiographic images of the patient.

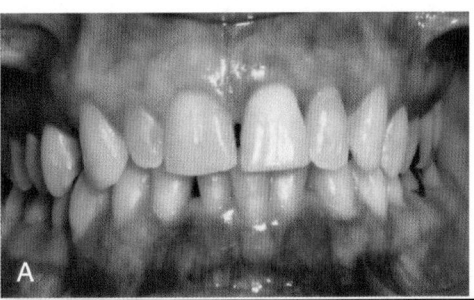

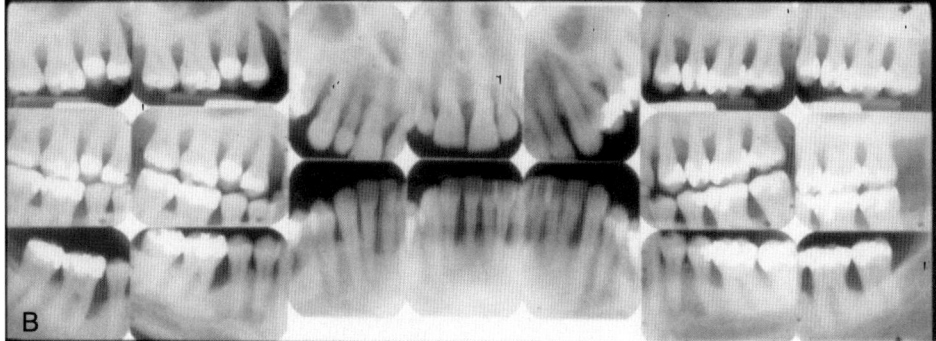

Fig. 5.17 (A) Clinical image of plaque-related severe/advanced chronic periodontitis with >5 mm clinical attachment loss in a 47-year-old female. (B) Radiographic images of the patient.

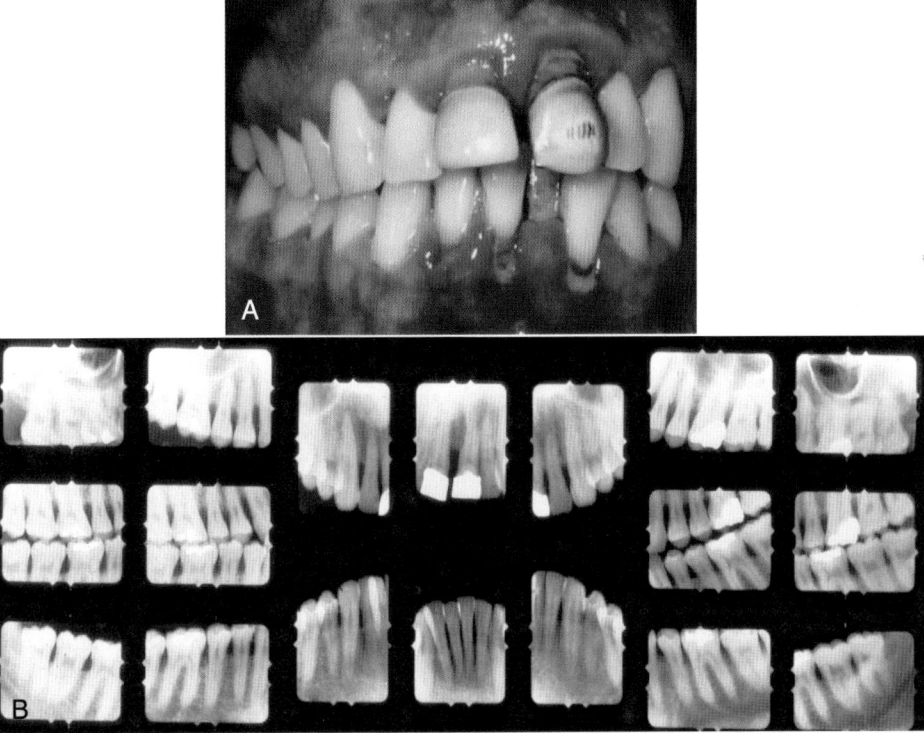

Fig. 5.18 (A) Clinical image of plaque-related aggressive moderate periodontitis with 1- to 7-mm PD and 3- to 4-mm clinical attachment loss in a 31-year-old male. (B) Radiographic images of the patient.

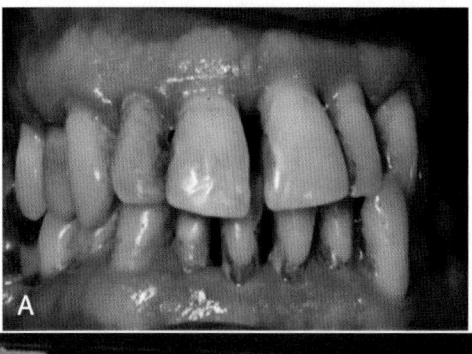

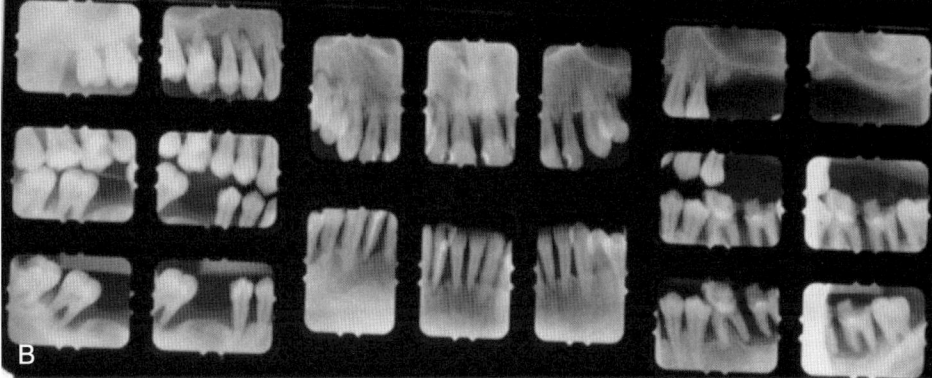

Fig. 5.19 (A) Clinical image of plaque-related aggressive severe periodontitis with 3- to 13-mm PD and 7- to 15-mm clinical attachment loss in a 32-year-old male. (B) Radiographic images of the patient.

of plaque and calculus, with a positive family history of aggressive disease, is suggestive of a genetic trait[34,49] (see Box 5.3). This form of periodontitis was previously classified as early-onset periodontitis (see Table 5.1) and therefore still includes many of the characteristics previously identified with the localized and generalized forms of early-onset periodontitis. Although the clinical presentation of aggressive disease appears to be universal, the causative factors involved are not always consistent. Box 5.3 outlines additional clinical, microbiologic, and immunologic characteristics of aggressive disease that may be present. As was previously described for early-onset disease, aggressive forms of periodontitis usually affect young individuals during or shortly after puberty and may be observed during the second and third decades of life (i.e., 10 to 30 years of age). The disease may be localized, as previously described for localized juvenile periodontitis, or generalized, as previously described for generalized juvenile periodontitis and rapidly progressive periodontitis (see Table 5.1). Box 5.3 describes the common features of the localized and generalized forms of aggressive periodontitis.

 FLASH BACK

Recall that chronic periodontitis is also categorized by the extent of *localized* or *generalized* disease according to the percentage of teeth involved with 30% of teeth being the cutoff between the two categories. Importantly, there is a distinct difference in the use of these definitions in the context of aggressive periodontitis. For aggressive periodontitis, the localized form is recognized to have a specific clinical phenotype, which is typically limited to incisor and first molar teeth.

Periodontitis as a Manifestation of Systemic Disease

Several hematologic and genetic disorders have been associated with the development of periodontitis in affected individuals[22,23] (see Box

5.3). The majority of existing publications are case reports, whereas only a few research studies have been performed to investigate the exact nature of the effect of the specific condition on the tissues of the periodontium primarily because of the rare occurrence of many of these diseases. It is speculated that the major effect of these disorders is through alterations in immune response, such as in the case of interleukin-17 overexpression in leukocyte adhesion deficiency[30] or due to tissue metabolic disorders such as in some forms of Ehlers–Danlos syndrome.[2] The clinical manifestation of many of these disorders appears at an early age and may be confused with aggressive forms of periodontitis depicting rapid attachment loss and the potential for early tooth loss. This was one of the drivers for the transition from the term *early-onset periodontitis,* which characterized a heterogeneous group of diseases, to the definitions of aggressive periodontitis and periodontitis as a manifestation of systemic diseases. With the introduction of this form of periodontitis (see Table 5.1), the potential exists for overlap and confusion between periodontitis as a manifestation of systemic disease in both the aggressive and the chronic forms of disease when a systemic component is suspected. At present, *periodontitis as a manifestation of systemic disease* is the diagnosis to be used when the systemic condition is the major predisposing factor and when local factors (e.g., large quantities of plaque and calculus) are not clearly evident or their presence alone does not justify the severity or progression of disease. This definition is reserved for a specific group of diseases and syndromes that have been documented to have a profound destructive effect on the periodontium. The removal of local factors as part of conventional periodontal therapy in such cases is often inadequate to arrest the periodontal destruction due to the systemic effect. When periodontal destruction is clearly the result of local factors but has been exacerbated by the onset of conditions such as diabetes mellitus (Figs. 5.20 and 5.21) or HIV infection, the diagnosis should be *chronic periodontitis modified by the systemic condition.*

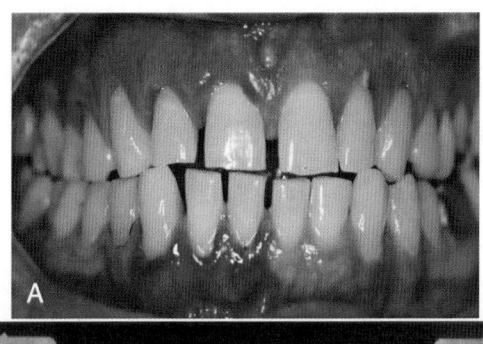

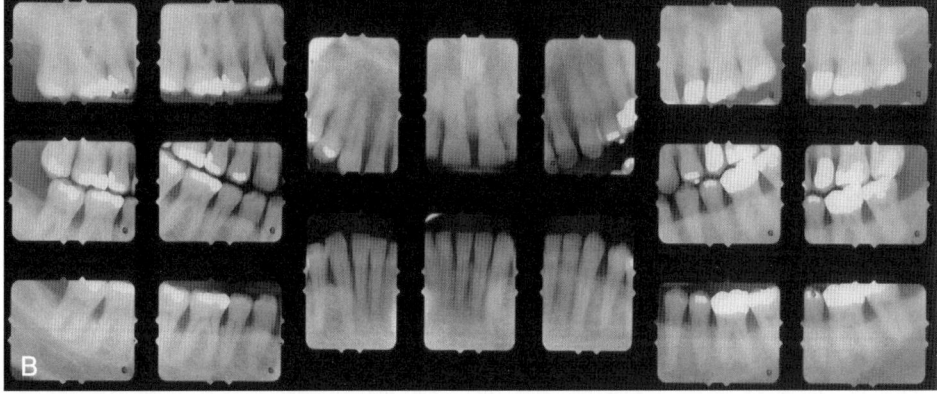

Fig. 5.20 (A) Clinical image of plaque-related severe aggressive periodontitis in a 53-year-old male, smoker with diabetes and hemoglobin A_{1c} (HbA_{1c}) = 10.7. (B) Radiographic images of the patient.

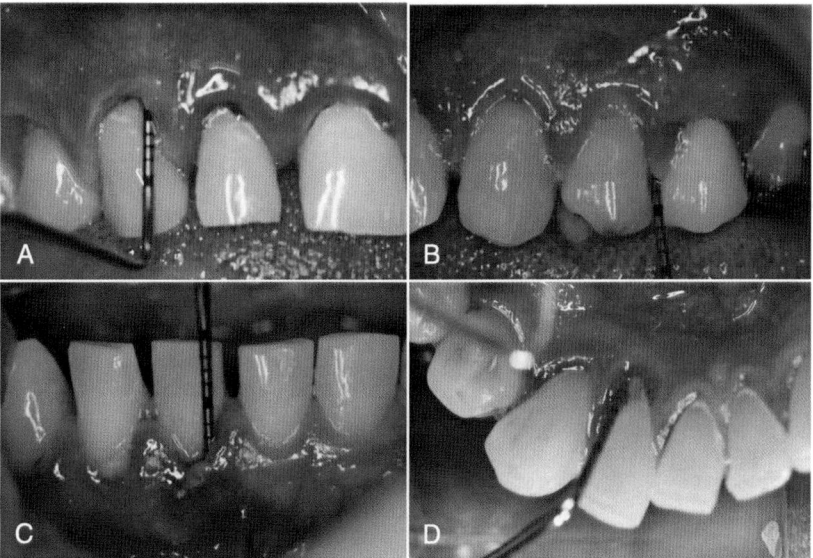

Fig. 5.21 Selective probing depths of the same 53-year-old diabetic patient shown in Fig. 5.20 with severe aggressive periodontitis.

Papillon–Lefèvre syndrome (PLS) is one example of a condition that causes severe periodontitis as one of its manifestations. PLS is an autosomal-recessive disorder caused by mutations in the cathepsin C gene located on chromosome 11q14.[17] The clinical manifestations of the syndrome include severe aggressive periodontitis and diffuse keratoderma on the palms, the soles, the knees, or all three[16] (Figs. 5.22 and 5.23). The consanguinity of the parents is a common finding in approximately one-third of the cases.[31]

 CLINICAL CORRELATION

When monogenic diseases are encountered, consanguinity can be a common finding particularly in certain ethnic cultures where it is socially acceptable. Appropriate genetic counseling is advisable. In addition, when the diagnosis for the proband (the first offspring for whom disease is noted) is established, it is crucial that the siblings are carefully examined for prompt diagnosis of additional cases.

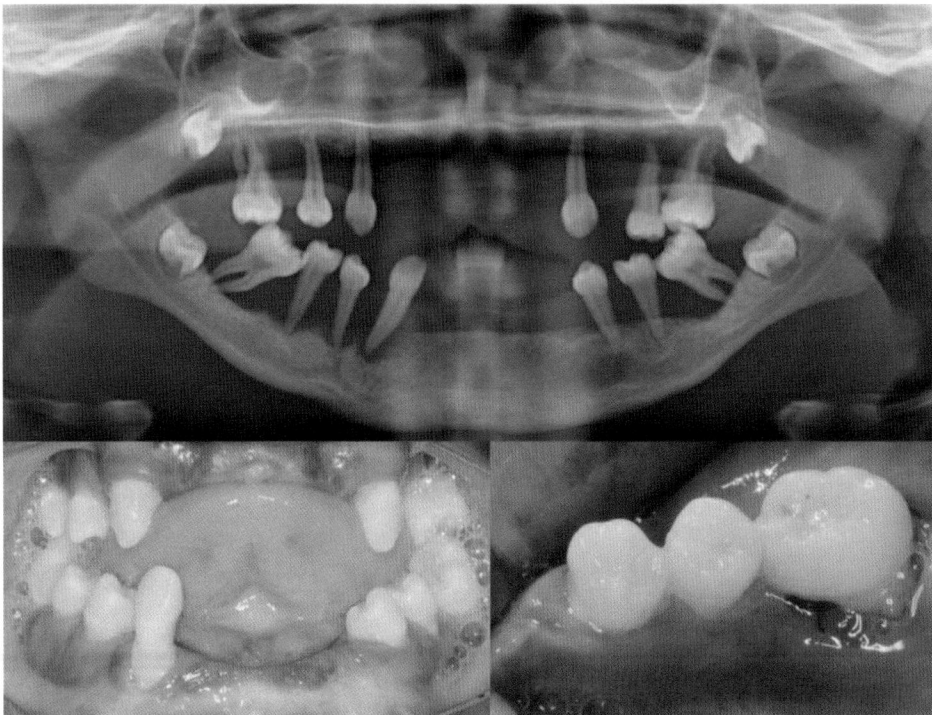

Fig. 5.22 Panoramic radiograph and clinical photos of a 13-year-old female with Papillon–Lefèvre syndrome (PLS). PLS is an autosomal recessive disorder caused by mutations in the cathepsin C gene located on chromosome 11q14. The clinical manifestations of the syndrome are severe aggressive periodontitis as well as diffuse keratoderma on the palms, soles, or knees. In PLS patients by the age of 4 to 5 years, the primary teeth have typically exfoliated or been extracted due to severe periodontal destruction. Subsequently, an edentulous phase occurs during which a reduction in the oral microbial load is noted and gingival health is restored. Following eruption of the permanent dentition, a similar cycle of severe periodontal inflammation is repeated that generally does not respond to conventional periodontal therapy. An increase in tooth mobility and periodontal abscesses is frequently observed shortly after the eruption of permanent teeth. *(Courtesy Dr. Georgios Kotsakis, Seattle, Washington.)*

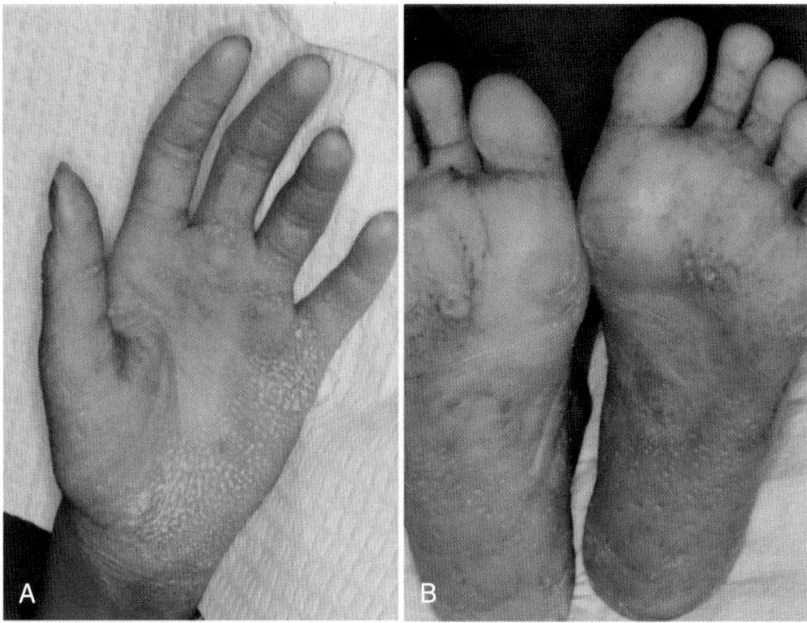

Fig. 5.23 Patient with Papillon-Lefèvre (PLS) syndrome exhibiting hyperkeratosis on palms of the hand and soles of the feet. PLS clinically affects both the primary and permanent dentition. Signs of palmoplantar keratoderma usually appear simultaneously with the eruption of the first primary teeth (5–6 months), but may appear as early as 1 month of age. *(Courtesy Dr. Georgios Kotsakis, Seattle, Washington.)*

Impaired neutrophil function is considered to be the primary cause of PLS and to eventually result in the deregulation of the polymorphonuclear leukocyte response to microbial infection.[11] Although the subgingival microbiota associated with PLS is diverse, opportunistic periodontal pathogens such as *Aggregatibacter actinomycetemcomitans* (Aa), *Porphyromonas gingivalis, Tannerella forsythia, Fusobacterium nucleatum,* and *Prevotella intermedia* are frequently identified among plaque samples from PLS patients.[1,50] Serum immunoglobulin G titers against Aa are typically elevated in individuals with PLS, thereby implicating Aa as a significant causative factor.[50] Individuals with PLS are often initially screened by a dermatologist or a pediatrician, and the phenotype of the syndrome may be mistaken for atopic dermatitis (eczema) or palmoplantar keratoderma.[35] The case presented in Figs. 5.22 and 5.23 was treated for several years by a dermatologist as atopic dermatitis with occasional cauterization of misdiagnosed "plantar warts." The diagnosis of PLS was established in a periodontal office. A multidisciplinary treatment approach for these patients including referral to a periodontist cannot be overemphasized. After a diagnosis of PLS has been established, it is important to collect a complete family history and to construct a pedigree to help identify undiagnosed or misdiagnosed siblings (Fig. 5.24). In 1979 Haneke proposed palmoplantar hyperkeratosis, the loss of primary and permanent teeth, and an autosomal-recessive pattern of inheritance as being essential criteria to verify a diagnosis of PLS.[16] Secondary manifestations of PLS may include ectopic intracranial calcifications and increased susceptibility to infections, including pyogenic liver abscesses that can be fatal.[9]

PLS clinically affects both the primary and permanent dentition. Signs of palmoplantar keratoderma usually appear simultaneously with the eruption of the first primary teeth (i.e., 5 to 6 months of age), but they may appear as early as the age of 1 month. By the age of 4 to 5 years, the primary teeth have typically exfoliated or been extracted as a result of severe periodontal destruction. Subsequently, an edentulous phase occurs during which a reduction in the oral microbial load is noted and gingival health is restored. After the eruption of the permanent dentition, a similar cycle of severe periodontal inflammation is repeated that generally does not respond to conventional periodontal therapy.[11] An increase in tooth mobility

and periodontal abscesses is frequently observed shortly after the eruption of the permanent teeth.

The periodontal prognosis for patients with PLS has significantly improved in response to an increase in the prompt and accurate diagnosis of the syndrome, the better understanding of its pathogenesis, and more efficient professional supervision. There appears to be a consensus among clinicians that the successful treatment of periodontitis among individuals with PLS requires the eradication of Aa.[10,12,43] Treatment of the primary dentition includes frequent prophylaxis appointments to ensure that the patient maintains adequate masticatory function and nutrition during early childhood. To create a healthy environment for the permanent teeth to erupt into, it has been advocated that a course of antibiotics effective against Aa be systemically administered along with the extraction of all primary teeth 6 to 12 months before the eruption of the first permanent tooth. However, culture and sensitivity testing of the subgingival plaque may enhance the selection of the most effective antibiotic regimen. De Vree and colleagues described two patients with PLS.[10] Aa was eradicated from one individual, who was able to retain most of his teeth over a 15-year period; the second individual's Aa was found to be resistant to the antibiotics combination, and he lost all of his teeth despite intensive treatment. The combination of trimethoprim and sulfamethoxazole (i.e., cotrimoxazole) has also been shown to be effective against Aa and to lead to a significant improvement in neutrophilic function against Aa.[24] A stringent periodontal maintenance schedule is of utmost importance to efficaciously monitor the patient's oral hygiene and to be able to intercede promptly if signs of inflammation reoccur.[32] Retinoids, which are synthetic analogues of vitamin A, a treatment modality against PLS skin manifestations, have also been considered as immunomodulatory adjuncts for the treatment of PLS-associated periodontitis.[12,24]

Sarcoidosis is a chronic disease that is expressed as a cell-mediated, delayed-type hypersensitivity that primarily affects the lungs, lymph nodes, skin, eyes, liver, spleen, and small bones of the hands and feet.[36] Sarcoidosis rarely affects the oral cavity, with incidence of occurrence in descending order noted in the lymph nodes, lips, soft palate, buccal mucosa, gingiva, tongue, and bone.[36] Fig. 5.25 depicts the pretreatment pattern of bone loss and recession associated with sarcoidosis, with pulmonary parenchymal fibrous infiltrate noted in the lungs as depicted by a white lacy pattern on a chest radiograph (Fig. 5.25C). Histologic features of sarcoidosis include the presence of an intense chronic inflammatory infiltrate with focal areas of noncaseating granulomas and a positive Kveim test (Fig. 5.26C). The remineralization of alveolar bone is noted on radiographs obtained 1 year after the systemic administration of steroids (e.g., prednisone) (Fig. 5.26A).

Medication-Related Osteonecrosis of the Jaw

Medication-related osteonecrosis of the jaw (MRONJ) is an updated term that has replaced the phrase bisphosphonate-related osteonecrosis of the jaw (BRONJ). Bisphosphonates (BPs) are pyrophosphate analogues with a high affinity for hydroxyapatite crystals. They inhibit osteoclast-mediated bone resorption and play a key role in the management of osteolytic bone disorders, including osteoporosis, Paget disease, bone metastasis, and multiple myeloma.[44] However, their prolonged use is associated with MRONJ.[18]

The American Association of Oral and Maxillofacial Surgeons defined MRONJ as "exposed bone in the maxillofacial area occurring in the absence of head and neck irradiation and showing no evidence of healing for at least 8 weeks after identification in patients treated with BP therapy"[4] (Figs. 5.27 and 5.28). To date, the true incidence

Pedigree chart

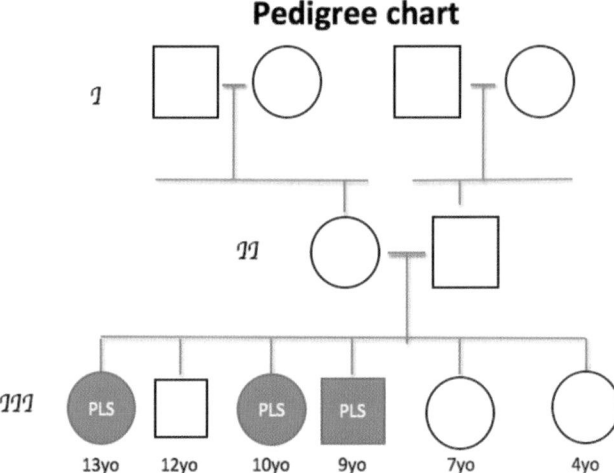

Fig. 5.24 No history of consanguinity was reported in this case. However, approximately one-third of the diagnosed Papillon-Lefèvre (PLS) cases descend from same ancestor. Offsprings III1, III3, and III4 display a PLS phenotype. All siblings should be thoroughly examined by a periodontist once a case of PLS has been diagnosed.

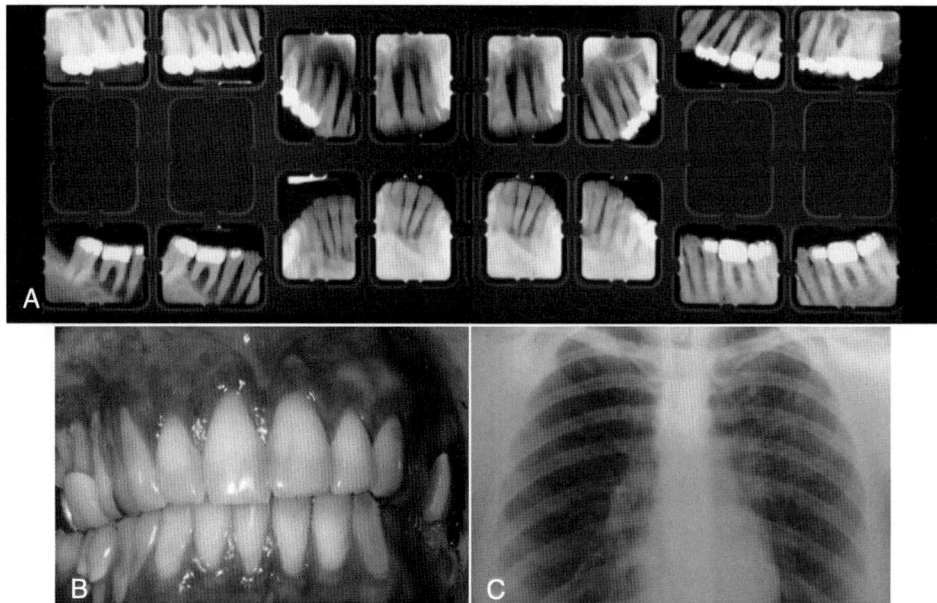

Fig. 5.25 Sarcoidosis pretreatment. (A) Intraoral x-rays depict more extensive bone loss for anterior teeth than clinical attachment loss. (B) Extensive recession plus clinical attachment loss. (C) Pulmonary parenchymal fibrous infiltrate.

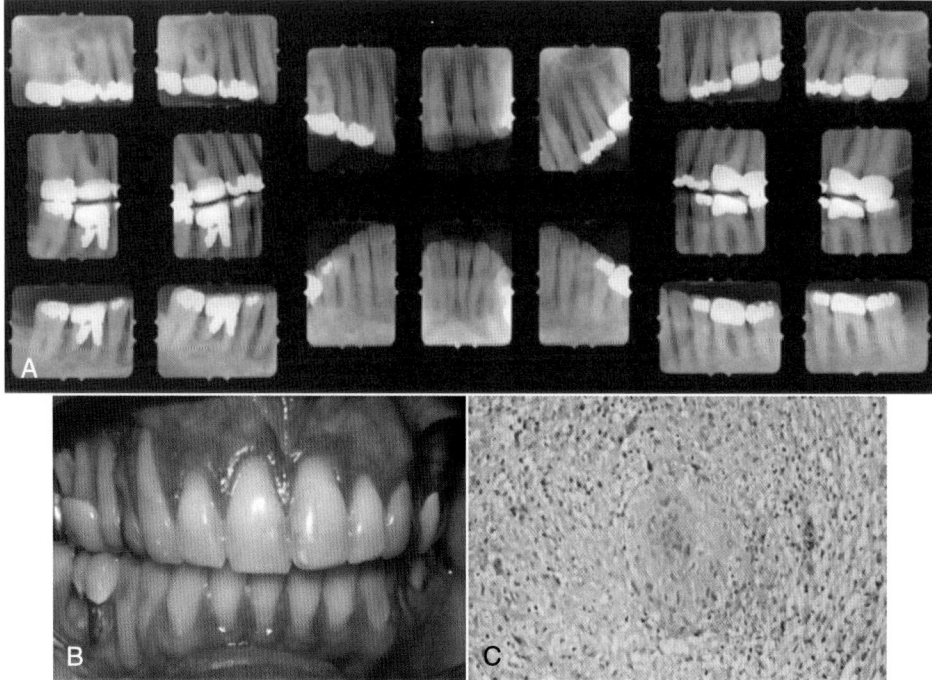

Fig. 5.26 Sarcoidosis after treatment with prednisone. (A) Intraoral x-rays depict remineralization of bone. (B) Reduction in gingival inflammation while extensive recession and clinical attachment loss persist. (C) Pretreatment biopsy.

of, causes of, and risk factors for the development of MRONJ are largely unknown. An overwhelming proportion (i.e., 97%) of the reported cases are related to the high-dose intravenous BP given to patients with cancer. However, a small fraction (i.e., 3%) has been reported in patients with osteoporosis and patients with Paget disease who are receiving oral BP.[18] The estimated incidence of MRONJ in patients with osteoporosis who are receiving oral BP is around 0.7 per 100,000 persons/years of exposure.[4] The incidence of MRONJ

among patients with cancer who are receiving intravenous BP ranges from 0.72% to 7.4%.[18]

MRONJ lesions may be asymptomatic, or they may present with pain, purulent discharge, swelling, tooth mobility, and paresthesia, culminating in a reduced ability to eat and speak. MRONJ occurs most frequently in the mandible (65%), followed by the maxilla (26%) and both jaws (95%).[52] The frequency of MRONJ is higher in the posterior region of the jaw. Among patients who develop

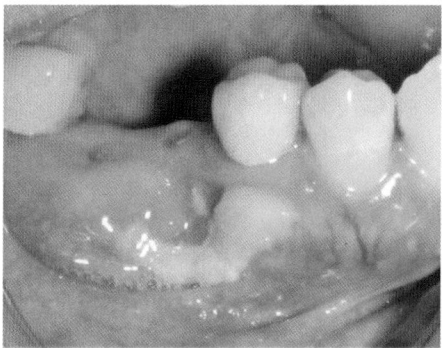

Fig. 5.27 Exposed bone on buccal lower premolar and molar in medication-related osteonecrosis of the jaw (MRONJ) patient following extraction of the first molar. *(Courtesy Dr. Vivek Thumbigere Math, Minneapolis.)*

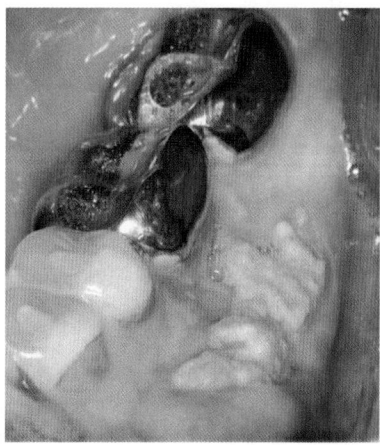

Fig. 5.28 Medication-related osteonecrosis of the jaw (MRONJ) patient with exposed bone on lingual aspect of lower premolar and molar following root canal treatment. *(Courtesy Dr. Vivek Thumbigere Math, Minneapolis.)*

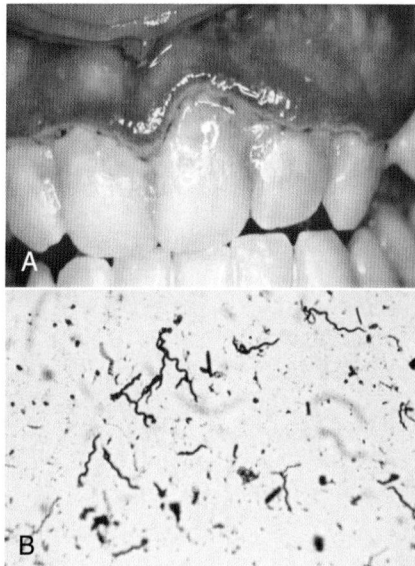

Fig. 5.29 (A) Ulcerative gingivitis illustrating sloughing of marginal gingiva. (B) Phase-contrast microscopy reveals spirochetes in subgingival plaque sample.

MRONJ, approximately 60% of cases occur after an invasive dental procedure (e.g., tooth extraction), whereas 40% develop spontaneously.[48] Radiographic evaluation is usually inconclusive for early lesions. In advanced cases, a poorly defined moth-eaten radiolucency is noted with radiopaque sequestra.

Currently, there is no effective treatment for MRONJ. The discontinuance of BP is not helpful because BPs tend to reside in the bone for very long periods of time. Radical surgical intervention often exacerbates the condition, and the merit of hyperbaric oxygen treatment for the management of MRONJ is not conclusive. Patients are typically treated via minimally invasive conservative debridement, antibiotics, and chlorhexidine mouth rinses to limit the extent of the damage and to facilitate wound healing.[48] The American Dental Association suggests that an oral health program that consists of sound hygiene practices and regular dental care is a valuable approach to lowering the risk of developing MRONJ.[18] Practitioners are encouraged to use atraumatic surgical techniques and to minimize the extent of dentoalveolar manipulation. Communication with the patient's physician and proper risk assessment are fundamental to the successful management of patients who are receiving BP therapy.

The use of the term *MRONJ* was introduced to capture the rising number of osteonecrosis cases of the jaw that are associated with new types of medication, such as other antiresorptive (denosumab) and antiangiogenic therapies, by the American Association of Oral and Maxillofacial Surgeons (AAOMS) in their 2014 update. Readers are referred to the position paper by the AAOMS for additional information on MRONJ.[4]

Necrotizing Periodontal Diseases

The clinical characteristics of necrotizing periodontal diseases may include (but are not limited to) ulcerated and necrotic papillary and marginal gingiva that is covered by a yellowish white or grayish slough or pseudomembrane, blunting and cratering of the papillae, bleeding on provocation or spontaneous bleeding, pain, and fetid breath. These diseases may be accompanied by fever, malaise, and lymphadenopathy, although these characteristics are not consistent. Two forms of necrotizing periodontal disease have been described: *necrotizing ulcerative gingivitis (NUG)* (Fig. 5.29) and *necrotizing ulcerative periodontitis (NUP)* (Fig. 5.30). NUG was previously classified as "gingival disease" or "gingivitis," because clinical attachment loss is not a consistent feature. NUP has been classified as a form of "periodontitis," because attachment loss is present. Nonetheless, NUP cases are almost exclusively reported in immunocompromised persons. Both NUG and NUP have been determined to constitute a separate group of diseases that have *tissue necrosis* as a primary clinical feature (see Box 5.1).

Necrotizing Ulcerative Gingivitis

The clinical and causative characteristics of NUG[42] are described in detail in Chapter 20. The defining characteristics of NUG are its bacterial cause, necrotic lesion, and predisposing factors, such as psychologic stress, smoking, and immunosuppression. In addition, malnutrition may be a contributing factor in developing countries. NUG is usually seen as an acute lesion that responds well to antimicrobial therapy in combination with professional plaque and calculus removal as well as improved oral hygiene.

Necrotizing Ulcerative Periodontitis

NUP differs from NUG in that the loss of clinical attachment and alveolar bone is a consistent feature originating from the proximal region.[33] The characteristics of NUP are described in detail in Chapter 29. NUP may be observed among HIV seropositive individuals with low CD4 counts. Clinical manifestations include local ulceration and the necrosis of gingival tissue with the exposure and rapid destruction of underlying bone as well as spontaneous bleeding and severe pain. HIV+ persons with NUP are 20.8 times more likely to have CD4+ cell counts of less than 200 cells/mm³ of peripheral blood as compared with those without NUP, which suggests that immunosuppression is a major contributing factor. NUP has also been associated with severe malnutrition in developing countries. More aggressive cases of necrotizing stomatitis exhibit tissue necrosis beyond the confines of the periodontium to include other oral tissues, such as the hard palate.

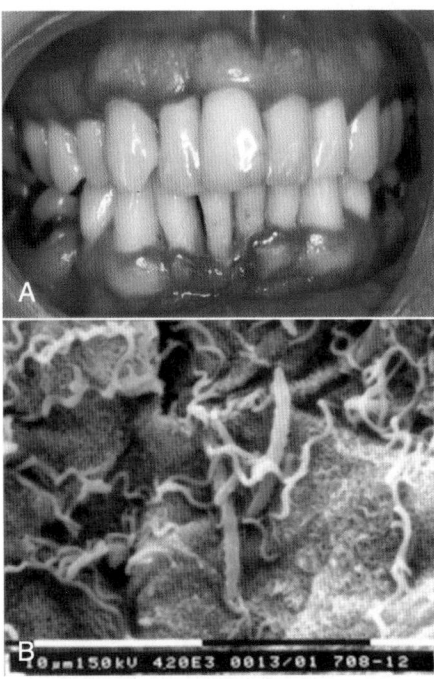

Fig. 5.30 (A) Necrotizing ulcerative periodontitis with severe clinical attachment loss in a 28-year-old male infected with human immunodeficiency virus (HIV). (B) Spirochetes noted on surface of sloughed epithelial cells.

 KEY FACT

Necrotizing stomatitis is a serious inflammatory condition that develops in systemically compromised individuals and is characterized by soft tissue necrosis that extends beyond the gingiva, with potential bony sequestrum formation. This disease entity is now included in the AAP/EFP 2018 classification of periodontal disease.

Abscesses of the Periodontium

A periodontal abscess is a localized purulent infection of periodontal tissues, and it is classified by its tissue of origin as gingival, periodontal, or pericoronal abscesses.[28] The clinical, microbiologic, immunologic, and predisposing characteristics are discussed in Chapters 8, 9, and 13.

Periodontitis Associated With Endodontic Lesions

The classification of lesions that affect the periodontium and the pulp is based on the sequence of the disease process.

Endodontic–Periodontal Lesions

Pulpal necrosis precedes periodontal changes in endodontic–periodontal lesions. A periapical lesion that originates with pulpal infection and necrosis may drain to the oral cavity through the periodontal ligament, resulting in the destruction of the periodontal ligament and the adjacent alveolar bone. This may present clinically as a localized, deep, periodontal probing depth that extends to the apex of the tooth (Fig. 5.31A). If the endodontic infection is left untreated in such cases, an extensive alveolar ridge defect may occur (Fig. 5.31B–C), thereby necessitating reconstructive surgery (Fig. 5.31D) before the placement of implants and prostheses (Fig. 5.32) to reestablish a functional and aesthetic outcome. Pulpal infection may also drain through accessory canals, especially in the area of the furcation, which may lead to furcal involvement through the loss of clinical attachment and alveolar bone.

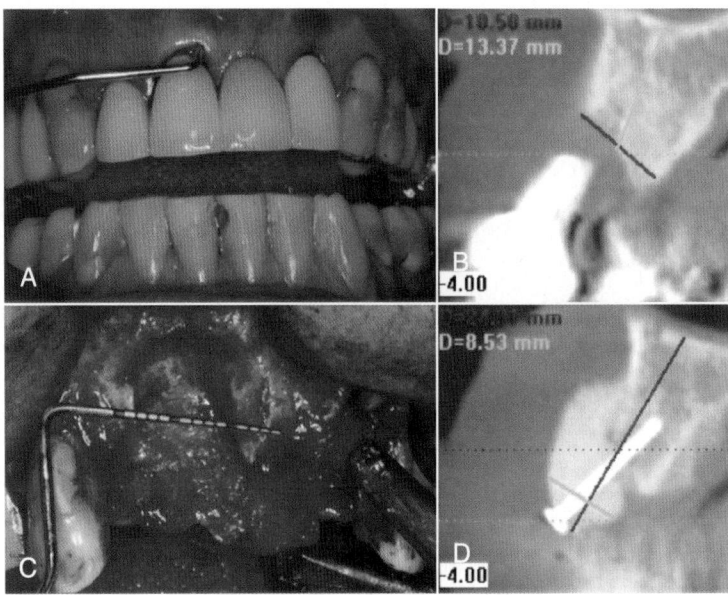

Fig. 5.31 (A and C) Clinical images of extensive loss of alveolar ridge secondary to periapical endodontic lesion. (B) CT scan depicts alveolar bone loss. (D) CT image of regenerated ridge via allogenic bone graft, tenting screw, and membrane.

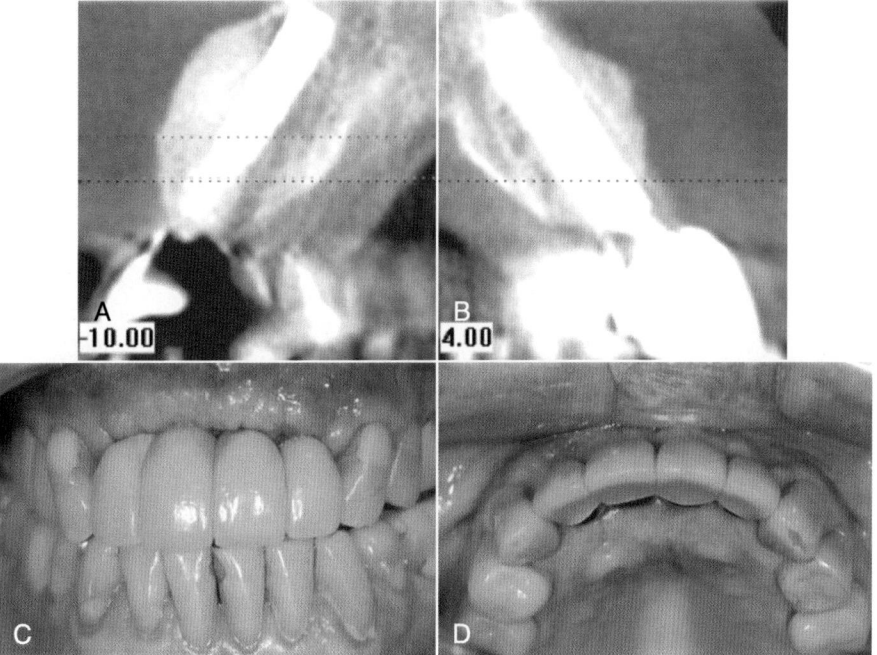

Fig. 5.32 Same patient depicted in Fig. 5.31. (A–B) CT scans of regenerated ridge with implants placed in areas 7, 9, and 10. (C–D) Clinical images of implant-supported bridge.

! CLINICAL CORRELATION

In early stages of primary endodontic lesions, root canal therapy may be the only treatment necessary to restore the periodontal apparatus.

Periodontal–Endodontic Lesions

It is more uncommon for periodontal disease to lead to endodontic disease than vice versa. In a periodontal–endodontic lesion, the bacterial infection from a periodontal pocket leads to loss of attachment, and root exposure then spreads to the pulp, resulting in pulpal necrosis. In the case of advanced periodontal disease, the infection may reach the pulp through the apical foramen. Nonetheless, existing studies have shown that although scaling and root planing remove cementum and underlying dentin, they may lead to dentine hypersensitivity but not to irreversible pulpitis.

Combined Lesions

Combined lesions occur when pulpal necrosis and a periapical lesion occur on a tooth that is also periodontally involved. An intrabony defect that communicates with a periapical lesion of pulpal origin results in a combined periodontal–endodontic lesion.

In all cases of periodontitis associated with endodontic lesions, the endodontic infection should be controlled before the definitive management of the periodontal lesion begins, especially when regenerative or bone-grafting techniques are planned.[29] Tooth prognosis in combined lesions highly depends on the outcome of the periodontal treatment.

Developmental or Acquired Deformities and Conditions

Localized Tooth-Related Factors That Modify or Predispose Individuals to Plaque-Induced Gingival Diseases or Periodontitis

In general, localized tooth-related factors contribute to the initiation and progression of periodontal disease through the enhancement of plaque accumulation or the prevention of effective plaque removal via normal oral hygiene measures.[7] These factors fall into the four subgroups outlined in Box 5.4.

Tooth Anatomic Factors

Tooth anatomic factors are associated with malformations of tooth development or tooth location. Anatomic factors (e.g., cervical enamel projections, palatal grooves, enamel pearls) have been associated with clinical attachment loss, especially in furcation areas. Cervical enamel projections are found on 15% to 24% of mandibular molars and on 9% to 25% of maxillary molars, and strong associations have been observed with furcation involvement.[27] Palatogingival grooves, which are found primarily on maxillary incisors, are observed in 8.5% of the population and are associated with increased plaque accumulation and clinical attachment as well as bone loss. Proximal root grooves on incisors and maxillary premolars also predispose individuals to plaque accumulation, inflammation, and the loss of clinical attachment and bone.

Tooth location is considered important for the initiation and development of disease. Misaligned teeth predispose individuals to plaque accumulation with resultant inflammation in children, and they may predispose adults to clinical attachment loss, especially when they are associated with poor oral hygiene habits. Open interproximal contacts that contribute to food impaction have been associated with an increased loss of attachment.[21]

Dental Restorations and Appliances

Dental restorations or appliances are frequently associated with the development of gingival inflammation. Restorations placed deep in the sulcus or within the junctional epithelium may impinge on the biologic width resulting in inflammation and the loss of clinical attachment and bone. Contour of a complete crown restoration can affect plaque retention with flat surfaces being more hygienic as compared to convex restorations exhibiting increased bulk of material at the cervical region.

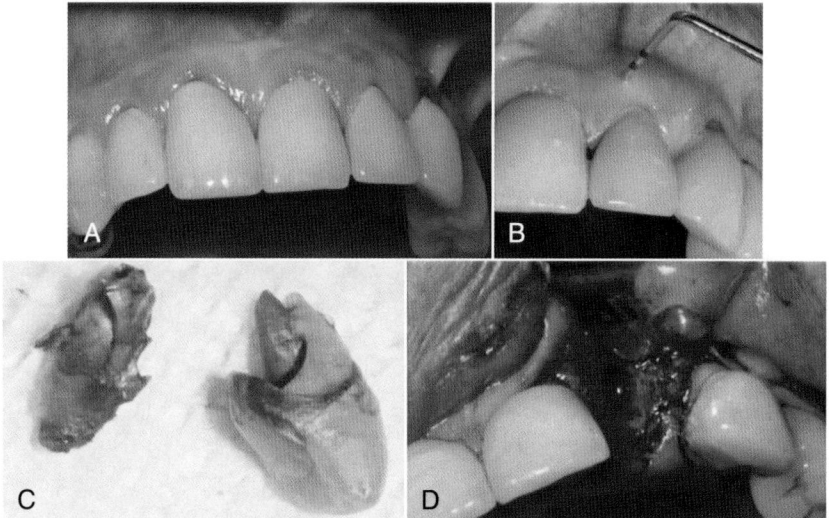

Fig. 5.33 (A–B) Clinical images of fistula tract. (C) Root fracture. (D) Resultant alveolar ridge defect.

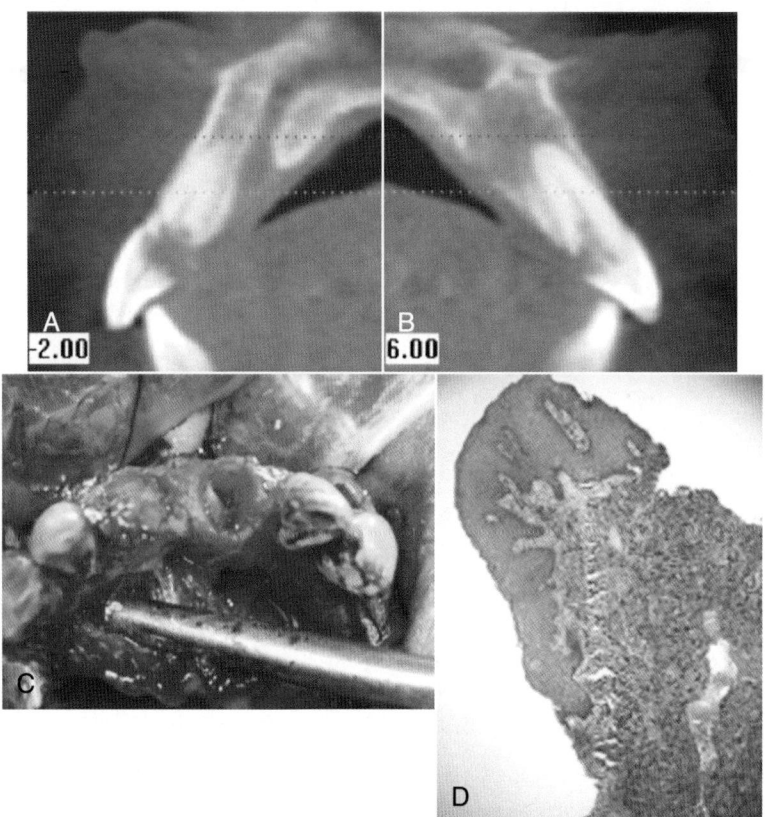

Fig. 5.34 (A–B) CT scans reveal severe cervical root resorption of maxillary central incisors and periapical abscess. (C) Crowns fractured because of resorption. (D) Biopsy of soft tissue from resorption.

Root Fractures

Root fractures may be associated with endodontic or restorative procedures as well as traumatic forces (Fig. 5.33A–C) and may lead to periodontal involvement through the apical migration of plaque along the fracture line (Fig. 5.33D).

 FLASH BACK

Vertical root fractures involving both the pulp and PDL are true combined endodontic–periodontal lesions.

Cervical Root Resorption and Cemental Tears

Invasive cervical root resorption (ICR) (as noted on the cone beam computed tomography scans shown in Fig. 5.34A–B) and cemental tears may lead to periodontal destruction when the lesion communicates with the oral cavity and allows bacteria to migrate subgingivally. The atraumatic removal of teeth with progressed cervical resorption lesions and the reconstruction of resultant ridge defects with bone grafts, dental implants, and prostheses are viable solutions for such defects (Fig. 5.35). Avulsed teeth that are reimplanted frequently develop ankylosis and cervical root resorption many years after reimplantation. If the patient is still in the phase of skeletal

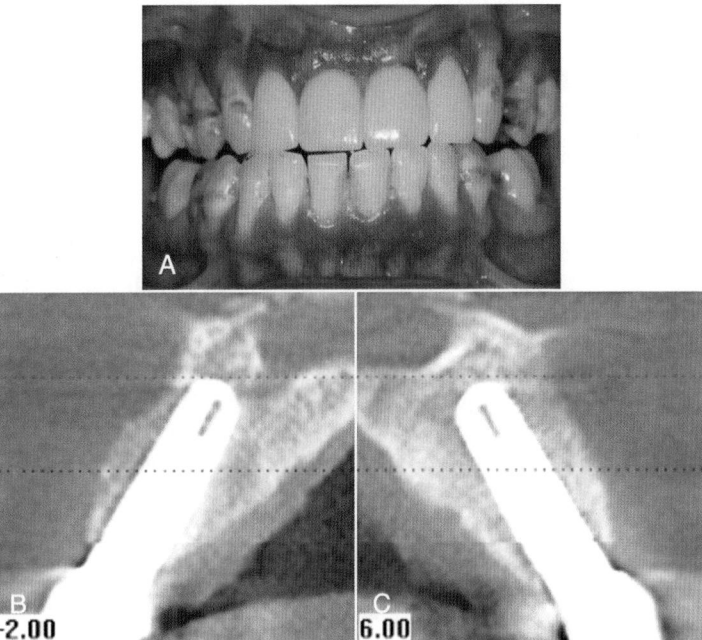

Fig. 5.35 (A) Posttreatment clinical image of same patient depicted in Fig. 5.34 with implant-supported crowns and veneers on laterals. (B–C) CT scans of bone grafts and implants replacing central incisors lost as the result of severe cervical root resorption.

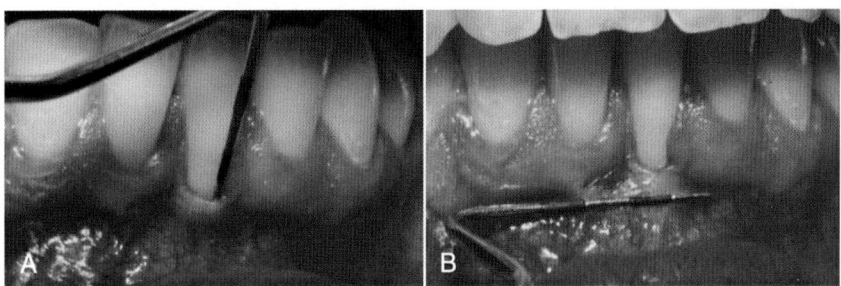

Fig. 5.36 (A) Mucogingival defect depicted by recession. (B) Defects extend into alveolar mucosa and lack keratinized gingiva.

growth, decoronation may be the treatment of choice for ridge preservation. In adults with completed skeletal growth, atraumatic removal of such ankylosed teeth, followed by ridge reconstruction and placement of implants and prosthesis, is a viable treatment option in adults (see Fig. 5.35).

Mucogingival Deformities and Conditions Around the Teeth

Mucogingival deformity is a generic term used to describe the mucogingival junction and its relationship to the gingiva (Fig. 5.36), the alveolar mucosa, and frenula muscle attachments. A mucogingival deformity is a significant departure from the normal shape of the gingiva and the alveolar mucosa, and it may involve the underlying alveolar bone. Mucogingival surgery and periodontal plastic and aesthetic surgery correct defects in the morphology, position, or amount of gingiva. This subject is described in detail in Chapter 65. The surgical correction of mucogingival deformities may be performed for aesthetic reasons, to enhance function, or to facilitate oral hygiene.[37]

Mucogingival Deformities and Conditions of the Edentulous Ridges

Mucogingival deformities, such as a lack of stable keratinized gingiva between the vestibular fornices and the floor of the mouth (Fig. 5.37A), may require soft-tissue grafting and vestibular deepening before prosthodontic reconstruction (Fig. 5.37B–D). Alveolar bone defects in edentulous ridges (Fig. 5.38A–B) usually require corrective surgery (Fig. 5.38C–D) to restore form and function before the placement of implants and prostheses to replace missing teeth (Fig. 5.39).[37]

Occlusal Trauma

The causes of trauma from occlusion and the effect of this trauma on the periodontium[14] are discussed in detail in Chapters 26 and 55.

 To view the **updated AAP/EFP 2018 classification system,** visit the the companion website www. expertconsult.com.

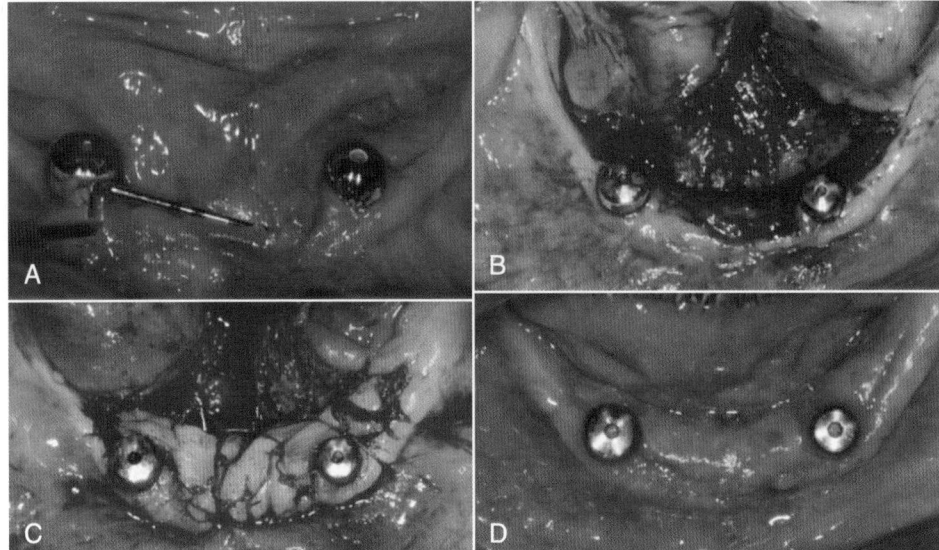

Fig. 5.37 (A) Mucogingival ridge defect from floor of mouth to vestibular fornix. (B) Partial thickness flap with vestibular deepening. (C) Placement of free gingival graft. (D) Reestablishment of vestibular depth and keratinized attached gingiva.

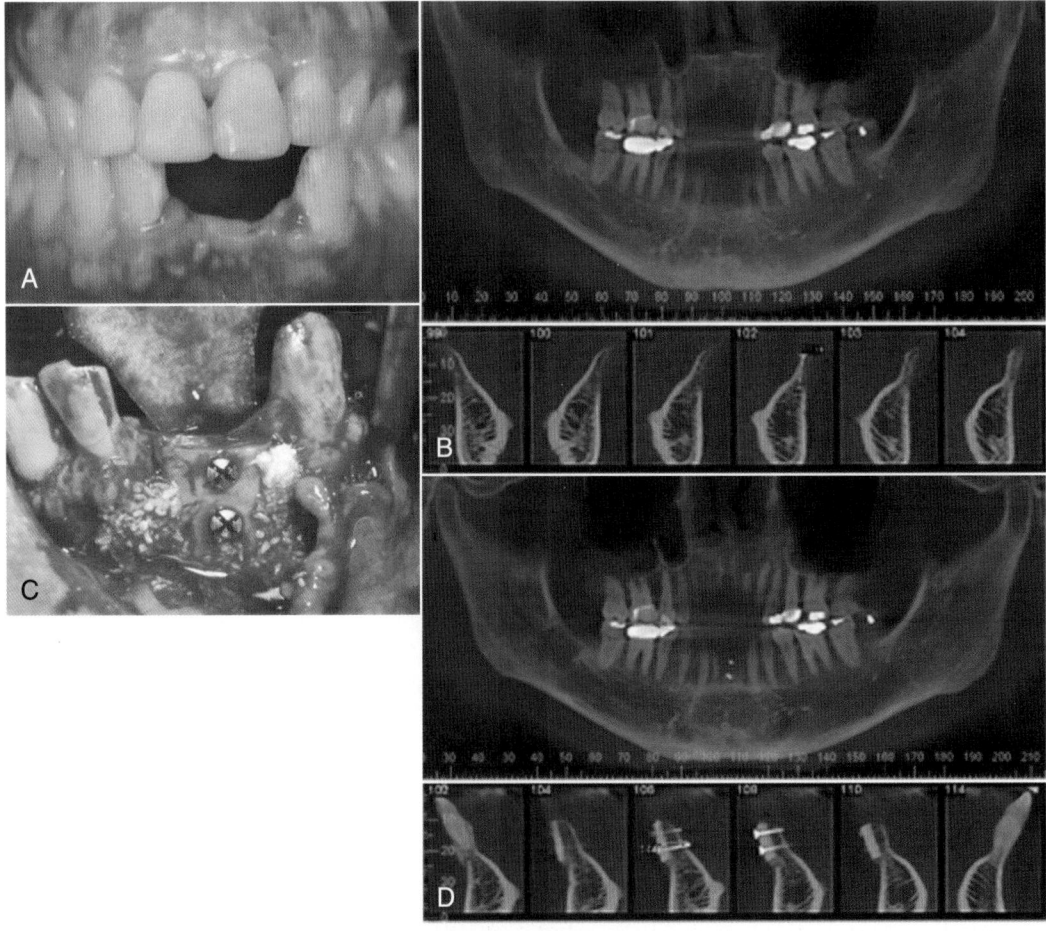

Fig. 5.38 (A) Clinical image of edentulous ridge defect. (B) Pretreatment CT image of defect. (C) Reconstructed ridge using ramus block graft. (D) CT scan of grafted site.

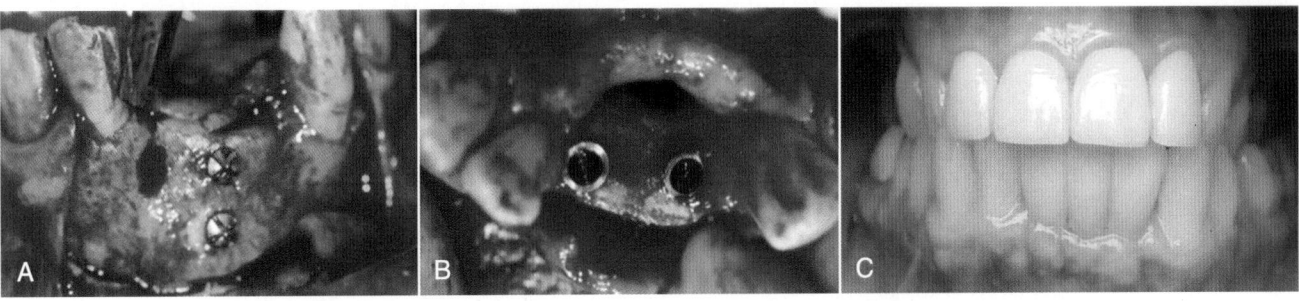

Fig. 5.39 (A) Clinical image of ridge 6 months after grafting. (B) Placement of implants in area of teeth #23 and #25. (C) Porcelain fused to metal (PFM) crowns for maxillary incisors and implant-supported bridge from teeth #23 to #25.

 Case Scenarios are found on the companion website www.expertconsult.com.

References

 References for this chapter are found on the companion website www.expertconsult.com.

CHAPTER 6

Fundamentals in the Methods of Periodontal Disease Epidemiology

Philippe P. Hujoel | Georgios A. Kotsakis

CHAPTER OUTLINE

The Need for Epidemiology
Epidemiologic Study Designs
Causes
Diagnosis

The Need for Epidemiology

The World Health Organization (WHO) defines epidemiology as "the study of the distribution and determinants of health-related states or events (including disease), and the application of this study to the control of diseases and other health problems." Distinct study designs are employed to examine the distribution of periodontal diseases in populations and to determine its etiology and its association with other diseases; the ultimate goal is to determine evidence-driven preventive and therapeutic strategies. "Periodontal [gum] diseases, including gingivitis and destructive periodontal disease, are serious infections."[72] This 2009 statement from a professional dental organization reflected the dominating belief accepted since the 1960s that bacteria cause periodontal conditions.[19] This bacterial dogma had several consequences. Clinical management and research became largely focused on vaccines, microbial diagnosis, antimicrobials, antibiotics, dental plaque, and immunology. Clinical diagnoses that did not fit the infection paradigm (e.g., periodontal atrophy) were eliminated from some periodontal disease classifications, and it was hypothesized that periodontal infections caused systemic diseases.

But are periodontal diseases really infectious diseases? A reliable answer to this question requires epidemiologic evidence. This chapter focuses on the role of epidemiology in the study of human diseases. *Case–control studies* and *cohort studies* are two epidemiologic study designs that identify common causes of chronic disease, such as smoking, ionizing radiation, hepatitis B, and high blood pressure. *Randomized controlled trials* are study designs that assess the diagnosis, management, and prognosis of chronic diseases and that either confirm or refute the suspected causes of disease identified in case–control or cohort studies. Prostate surface antigen screening, polio vaccination, and hormone replacement therapy are examples of diagnoses and treatments for chronic diseases that were evaluated by means of randomized controlled trials.

Study Designs

Epidemiologic study designs fall within two broad categories: observational and interventional studies. As the terms imply, assigning a study to one of these categories depends on if the investigators assess the efficacy of an intervention (interventional) or if the intervention is not under control of the investigators (observational). Examples of interventional studies in oral health research are randomized clinical trials and nonrandomized clinical trials. Examples of observational studies are cross-sectional studies, cohort studies, and case-control studies.

Some of the essential characteristics of epidemiologic studies are that they are conducted in humans, there is a control or a comparison group, and clinically relevant endpoints are evaluated. Such studies are available to support the direct effects that oral bacteria have on reversible gingival inflammation.[73] However, studies that are commonly cited in support of the periodontal infection hypothesis often lack these elements. For instance, is a "burst" of bone loss[21] subsequent to the implantation of *Bacteroides gingivalis* (now *Porphyromonas gingivalis*) in an animal model proof that "this microorganism [is] of great importance to the control of destructive periodontal disease"? Opponents of this hypothesis could argue that in similar animal models nicotine injections alone have a direct effect on periodontal bone loss, thus satisfying the biologic plausibility criterion for causality.[54] Nevertheless, in contemporary practice the strength of scientific evidence is formally ranked based on the study design. One widely used level of evidence classification by the Oxford Center for Evidence-Based Medicine (http://www.cebm.net/wp-content/uploads/2014/06/CEBM-Levels-of-Evidence-2.1.pdf) generally considers animal studies (i.e., mechanism-based reasoning) as having the lowest level of evidence to impact clinical thinking, whereas systematic reviews of randomized controlled trials are generally considered as having the highest available level of evidence.

Systematic Review versus Expert Opinion

A systematic review is considered a form of secondary research that aims to screen the entire breadth of information on a selected topic, identify relevant research studies, and summarize their findings. The key difference between an expert opinion review and a systematic review is that the latter is more objective in the sense that it intends to summarize the available body of literature inclusively and not based on the author's opinion on which studies are noteworthy or impactful. It goes without saying that systematic reviews are considered to be high level and are often used to guide clinical decision-making, but the clinicians should be aware that their conclusions suffer from the shortcomings of the included studies.

Epidemiologic studies, which are at a higher level than case reports and animal studies, have had a powerful impact on reducing the incidence of some chronic diseases by reliably identifying their primary causes. Reliable evidence on what causes disease allows laboratory research to focus on elucidating the causal pathways of disease, which can then lead to clinical trials. "Medical science continually passes the baton of discovery from [epidemiologic] observation to laboratory studies to human clinical trials."[42] For example, epidemiologic observations identified hepatitis B as the main cause of liver carcinoma, which is one of the most common cancers in the world.[3] Subsequently, the baton of discovery was passed to basic science, with which a recombinant engineered vaccine for hepatitis B was developed. Then, the baton of discovery was passed to clinical trialists, who assessed the effectiveness of vaccinations and documented dramatic declines in mortality rates from liver cancer.[41] Similar success stories in the management of chronic diseases in which epidemiology played a critical role include coronary heart disease and blood pressure medication, dental caries and fluoride, and lung cancer and smoking intervention programs.

 FLASH BACK

Recall that well-designed interventional studies generally are higher level than observational studies.

The emerging epidemiologic evidence regarding the cause of periodontal diseases suggests that factors such as cigarette smoking, sugar, cereals, and chronic diseases such as diabetes could be primary causes of periodontal disease.[5,22,64] Notably, the 2004 US Surgeon General report concluded that the evidence was sufficient to infer a causal relationship between smoking and periodontitis.[74] Organizations such as the WHO suggest that periodontal disease prevention be made an integral part of programs that focus on tobacco control, diet, and physical activity, which are also shared risk factors with other prevalent chronic diseases such as cardiovascular diseases.[56] Regardless of your current beliefs about the causes of periodontal disease, becoming familiar with the epidemiologic methodology may be important in order to judge this emerging evidence independently and critically.

Measuring the Occurrence of Conditions or Diseases

The fundamental tools of epidemiology are simple sums and divisions that reflect how many individuals or sites either have or develop a particular condition or disease.

The *prevalence* is the sum of all examined individuals or sites that exhibit the condition or disease of interest divided by the sum of the number of individuals or sites examined. The prevalence can range from 0% (no one has the condition or disease of interest) to 100% (everyone has the condition or disease of interest).

As an example of prevalence, the Centers for Disease Control and Prevention reported about the prevalence of individuals with at least one periodontal pocket depth of 4 mm or deeper. It was reported that, from 1988 to 1994, a little more than 1 in 5 Americans had such a condition, for a prevalence of a little more than 20%; from 1999 to 2004, only 1 in 10 Americans fell into this category,[15] for a prevalence of around 10%. These findings suggest a more than 50% decline in the prevalence of pocket depths greater than or equal to 4 mm for adults between the ages of 20 and 64 years, which occurred over approximately a decade. These epidemiologic data confirm another report of declining destructive periodontal disease prevalence in the United States.[7] Such information about prevalence measures of periodontal conditions may have implications for human resource needs in the United States and may provide clues with respect to the causative factors that drive such changes. Many countries do not have prevalence surveillance systems,[56] which makes it difficult to determine whether these trends observed in the United States are isolated events or part of a more general trend.

The *risk* is the probability that an individual or a site will develop a particular condition or disease during follow-up. The risk for a condition or a disease is a number that ranges between 0% and 100%. The simplest way to estimate risk is to have a fixed number of persons or sites at risk at some defining moment (i.e., time zero [t_0]). Individuals or sites within individuals are followed up over time after this defining moment. After a follow-up period (i.e., from t_0 to t_n), the risk can be calculated as the proportion of persons or sites in which the clinical outcome of interest develops during the follow-up period. Because the risk is estimated as a proportion, it is without dimension, and it ranges between 0 and 1. When a risk is reported, it should be accompanied by a specific time period to which it is applied. A 5% risk for death may be considered small when it refers to a 20-year period but large when it refers to a 3-month period.

As an example, consider concerns about occupational human immunodeficiency virus (HIV) infection among dentists. It has been reported that the risk for developing an HIV infection within the year subsequent to an accidental needle stick with HIV-contaminated blood is 0.3%. Such a statistic has an intuitive appeal and can be related to patients or colleagues. A risk of 0.003 (0.3%) indicates that for every 1000 individuals who have an accidental HIV-contaminated needle stick, 3 are expected to develop an HIV infection within a year of the event.

The *odds* for an event is the probability that an event occurred divided by the probability that an event did not occur. Whereas probability is a value that has to range between 0 and 1, odds values range from 0 to infinity. If the probability for observing an event is small, then the odds and the probability are almost identical. For example, if the probability for a vertical root fracture after an endodontic procedure is 0.001, then the odds are 0.001/0.999 or 0.001001. Odds are commonly reported in studies because they are often easier to estimate with statistical models than probabilities. For example, the odds for developing an HIV infection after an accidental needle stick with HIV-contaminated blood are 0.003 (0.003/0.997).

Incidence rates are an alternative measure to describe disease occurrence. One example of an incidence rate is the speedometer in a car that displays at any given time the number of kilometers being traveled per hour. In clinical trials or epidemiology, the rate reflects the number of disease occurrences per person-time or site-time. The disease rate is a ratio in which the numerator is the number of subjects or sites diagnosed with the disease of interest and the denominator is the sum of the time at risk over all subjects or sites in the population.

Incidence versus Prevalence

Recall that prevalence is the proportion of a population found to have a condition at a given point in time (e.g., 9% of the US population had severe periodontitis in the 2009-2010 NHANES survey), while incidence is the probability that a disease will occur in a previously healthy population over a period of time (e.g., the incidence of peri-implantitis for patients with mandibular over-dentures is 17% after 5 years).

Incidence rates—as opposed to the previously introduced measures of disease occurrence—imply an element of time. The denominator in the incidence rate has time as the dimension. Thus the dimension of incidence rate is 1/time. This dimension is often referred to as "person-time" or "site-time" to distinguish the time summation from ordinary clock-time. The magnitude of the incidence rate can vary between 0 and infinity. When there are no new disease onsets during the study period, the incidence rate is 0. When every person observed dies instantaneously at the start of the study (and thus the sum of the time periods is 0), then the incidence rate is infinity.

An example of the application of rates is provided in Fig. 6.1, in which the number of teeth lost per 1000 tooth-years is plotted as a function of the maximum probing depth at the start of follow-up. The plot suggests a nonlinear relationship between maximum pocket depth and tooth loss, with a substantial increase in tooth loss rate for teeth that have periodontal pockets of 7 mm or deeper.

For the study of risk, the population studied is usually limited to those individuals at risk for the outcome of interest. Thus if the outcome of interest is a disease, the following subjects are excluded from the cohort: persons who already have the disease, persons who have immunity to the disease, and persons who are biologically incapable of developing the disease.

Periodontal Measures Typically Recorded Clinically

A periodontal examination can measure various characteristics of the periodontium. Dental records of periodontal patients typically contain information about the teeth that are present, missing, or

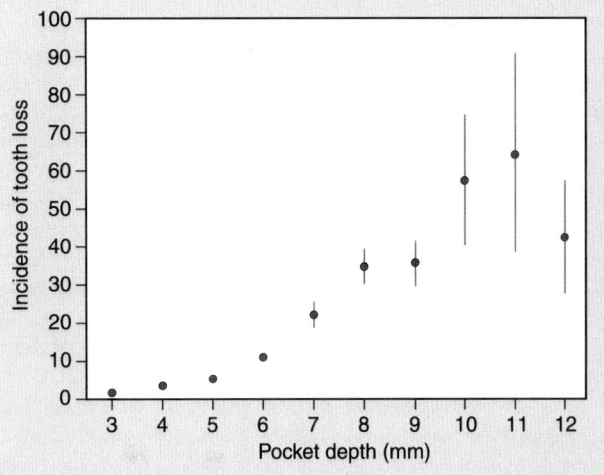

Fig. 6.1 Rate of tooth loss per 1000 tooth-years as a function of maximum probing depth per tooth in a cohort of 1021 patients between the ages of 40 and 65 years under periodontal specialist care for destructive periodontal disease. *(Data from Hujoel PP, Cunha-Cruz J, Selipsky H, et al: Abnormal pocket depth and gingival recession as distinct phenotypes. Periodontol 2000 39:22–29, 2005.)*

impacted as well as measurable information about the periodontal status of those teeth. Information such as clinical probing depth, bleeding on probing, gingival recession, mobility of teeth, and the presence of furcation involvements can be charted. In addition, some clinicians may collect information about the presence of gingivitis by evaluating the color and form of the gingival tissues. These measures can be complemented with radiographic examinations that may provide information about marginal bone levels.

In research settings or in some selected private practices, additional periodontal measures may be collected, such as clinical attachment levels, microbiologic measures, gingival crevicular fluid volume, biomarkers in the crevicular fluid, and indices that measure the amount of gingival inflammation or dental plaque or debris accumulation.

Two common measures of gingival inflammation are the Gingival Index (GI) and bleeding on probing.[25] The GI was proposed in 1963 as a method for assessing the severity and quantity of gingival inflammation.[46,47] With this particular index, only gingival tissues are assessed. Each of the four gingival areas of the tooth (i.e., facial, mesial, distal, and lingual) are assessed for inflammation and rated as normal gingiva (a score of 0) to severely inflamed gingiva with a tendency to spontaneously bleed (a score of 3). Gingiva that is mildly inflamed but without bleeding on probing is given a score of 1, whereas moderately inflamed gingiva with bleeding is given a score of 2. The scores can be averaged for each patient to provide patient means. Alternatively, site-specific analyses can relate local and patient-specific factors to the GI that is measured at individual sites.[13]

Bleeding on Probing versus Gingival Index

In clinical settings the term *gingival index* is often misused in lieu of bleeding on probing (BOP). According to the existing nomenclature, gingival index is a categorical index that assesses the severity of gingival inflammation on a scale from 0 to 3. On the other hand, BOP is a binary index (Yes/No) that determines whether a site is bleeding on probing or not. The two should not be confused.

Bleeding on probing is another measure of periodontal inflammation. The specific approach to obtain a bleeding measure can vary from one study to the next as well as from one clinician to another. For example, in the third National Health and Nutrition Examination Survey (NHANES III),[52] bleeding measures were obtained as follows. First, the facial and mesiofacial sites of teeth in two randomly selected quadrants—one maxillary and one mandibular—were selected. A special probe known as the *National Institute of Dental Research probe* was used in these assessments. This color-coded probe is marked at 2, 4, 6, 8, 10, and 12 mm. To begin the assessment, the examiner dried a quadrant of teeth with air. Then, starting with the most posterior tooth in the quadrant (excluding the third molar), the examiner placed a periodontal probe 2 mm into the gingival sulcus at the facial site and carefully swept the probe from the mesiofacial to the mesial interproximal area. After probing the sites in the quadrant, the examiner assesses the presence or absence of bleeding at each probed site. The same procedure was repeated for the remaining quadrant.

Commonly used measures of periodontal tissue destruction include mean probing depth, mean attachment loss, and mean recession level.[32] The clinical protocols regarding how such mean values are collected and calculated can vary considerably. One example of how such values can be ascertained clinically is described in the National Institute of Dental and Craniofacial Research "periodontal destruction" examination.[52] This examination includes an assessment of periodontal attachment loss[60] as the distance in millimeters from the cemento-enamel junction to the bottom of the gingival sulcus. This distance was measured at the facial and mesiofacial sites of teeth in a randomly selected maxillary and mandibular quadrant with the use of the indirect measurement method developed by Ramfjord.[60]

Sensitivity versus Specificity

Sensitivity is defined as the number of diseased patients who are correctly identified as having disease—that is, the diagnostic marker leads to a minimum number of false negative diagnoses. Specificity is defined as the number of healthy persons who are correctly determined to not have the disease—that is, the diagnostic marker leads to a minimum number of false positive diagnoses.

Translating Periodontal Measures Into Traditional Epidemiologic Measures of Disease Occurrence

The application of the traditional epidemiologic methods of risk, prevalence, and rate was challenging, because medical epidemiologists typically deal with patients. Dental epidemiologists deal with as many as 188 sites per patient. These periodontal sites within patients are correlated with many host-related factors. For example, gingival bleeding is suppressed in smokers.[6] Therefore bleeding on probing in periodontal sites in smokers tends to be more alike than bleeding on probing in periodontal sites among nonsmokers. Sites within patients are not statistically independent. The statistical methodology that is used to deal with correlated observations can be complex, and for most of the 20th century it was challenging to calculate the confidence intervals for site-specific risks or prevalence.[34] As a result, clinicians could not obtain reliable information about whether a periodontal site colonized with a particular microbiologic species was at an increased risk for periodontal attachment loss. These challenges may have hampered progress in the building of causal models of periodontal disease.

A common approach to dealing with this challenge of correlated observations was to summarize site-specific periodontal data at the patient level. These summaries could be calculated in a variety of ways. The information about the presence of bleeding in up to 188 periodontal sites in a patient could be summarized as the presence of at least 1 bleeding site, the presence of at least 5 bleeding sites, or a patient mean value.

The advent of modern statistical techniques to deal with the problem of correlated data made it possible to avoid summarizing site-specific information at a patient level.[13,14,28,33,34] These methods allow for the exploration of the role of patient- and site-specific factors in local site-specific events. For example, this can be used to determine whether the 3-mm loss of attachment at a site is related to site-specific factors (e.g., microflora present at that site), host factors (e.g., serum cotinine levels), or an interaction between a site-specific factor and a host factor.

True and Surrogate Measures of the Periodontal Condition

The epidemiology of true and surrogate endpoints of periodontal disease do not necessarily coincide. *True endpoints* are tangible outcomes that directly measure how a patient feels, functions, or survives.[17] True endpoints include oral health–related quality-of-life measurements[40,48,68] and self-reported problems, such as a positive answer to the following question: "When you brush or floss your teeth, do you notice bleeding that is both regular and that involves spitting blood-stained saliva?" *Surrogate endpoints* are intangible to the patient.[71] Surrogate endpoints in periodontal research include

anatomic measures (e.g., probing depth), measures of inflammation (e.g., bleeding), microbiologic measures, and immunologic measures.[13] Surrogate endpoints are often objective, because they can be measured by the clinician (rather than relying on self-report by patients) or by laboratory methods.

Surrogate endpoints can be misleading when the goal is to provide reliable information about clinical decisions related to diagnosis, etiology, treatment, or prognosis. An overview of situations in clinical research in which surrogate endpoints have led to misleading conclusions is provided in Table 2.1 on the Expert Consult website. One periodontal example is the use of systemic antibiotics that may have a beneficial impact on attachment gain[19] but a potential increased risk for tooth loss.[11]

Periodontal Endpoints: Examples

True endpoints: Tooth loss, patient's quality of life, and oral function
Surrogate endpoints: Probing depths, bleeding on probing, microbial measures

---

Challenges of Obtaining Epidemiologic Measures of Periodontal Conditions and Diseases

Among the challenges that periodontal epidemiologists face are the continuous changes in the type of surrogate data collected, the paucity of information about whether surrogate information provides reliable information regarding outcomes of tangible patient benefit (i.e., outcomes that the patient cares about), and the lack of diagnostic codes for the reasons for tooth loss. In fact, accruing evidence points in the direction of commonly used surrogate measures being poor predictors of periodontal status.[51]

The diversity of measures used to assess periodontal condition or disease is staggering. One survey of periodontal clinical trials conducted over a mere 4-year period indicated that 153 distinct surrogate endpoints were defined and that more than 80% of these endpoints were used in fewer than 5 of the 82 trials.[25] Another survey similarly identified the diversity of methodologies and definitions as a challenging issue when systematically reviewing evidence.[65] This continuous creation of "new and improved" surrogate outcomes in periodontal research is likely an important driver of false-positive conclusions.[27]

The types of periodontal measures that are favored also depend on the era. Russell developed the Periodontal Index,[63] which scored the supporting tissues for each tooth in the mouth according to a progressive scale that gives little weight to gingival inflammation and relatively great weight to advanced periodontal disease. Although the Periodontal Index was used in the first National Health and Nutrition Examination Survey (NHANES), thereby gaining national prominence in the United States, it was never used again in any of the subsequent NHANES versions. Since then, most periodontal surveys in the United States have employed different examination protocols. The survey methodology has been changed yet again, leading to large variations in disease estimates.[16] Studies of decreases in the use of scaling and root planing procedures in the state of Washington and at a national level,[8,61] long-term trends in decreasing edentulism, and decreasing periodontitis prevalence estimates in national surveys with consistent methodology[15] suggest that periodontitis prevalence in the United States is dropping rapidly (Tables 6.1 and 6.2).

A second challenge when interpreting periodontal statistics is the common lack of information about measures that matter to patients, such as tooth loss or quality-of-life issues related to oral health. This situation creates challenges when interpreting evidence. It is similar

TABLE 6.1 Periodontal Status of the US Population Among Adults Between the Ages of 20 and 64 Years

Status	1988 to 1994	1999 to 2004
Number of teeth present	24	25
Edentulism	6%	4%
Periodontal disease (i.e., one site with ≥3-mm attachment loss and ≥4-mm pocket depth)	15%	9%
Periodontal disease among the poor	28%	14%
Dental visits	66%	6%
Mean pocket depth	1.47 mm	1.02 mm
Mean loss of attachment	1.07 mm	0.72 mm
≥2-mm recession in at least one site	32%	21%
≥4-mm pocket depth in at least one site	23%	10%
≥4-mm attachment loss in at least one site	25%	17%

TABLE 6.2 Periodontal Status of the US Population Among Seniors 65 Years Old and Older

Status	1988 to 1994	1999 to 2004
Number of teeth present	18	19
Edentulism	34%	27%
Periodontal disease (one site with ≥3-mm attachment loss and ≥4-mm pocket depth)	19.5%	10.5%
Periodontal disease among the poor	26.3%	16.6%
Dental visits	54%	55%
Mean pocket depth	1.47 mm	1.07 mm
Mean loss of attachment	2.04 mm	1.55 mm
≥2-mm recession in at least one site	73%	48%
≥4-mm pocket depth in at least one site	22%	12%
≥4-mm attachment loss in at least one site	59%	50%

TABLE 6.3 Examples of Periodontal Randomized Controlled Trials

Periodontal Treatment	Outcome	Sample Size
Scaling and root planing for pregnant women[50]	Infants with low birth weights	823
Biphasic calcium phosphate ceramic[53]	Clinical attachment level	137

evaluated the effect of periodontal therapies on those teeth that survived the treatment. The more teeth that are lost, the more meaningless such data become. The imputation of data can provide an understanding of the extent to which such biases may alter the conclusions of studies.

In summary, the fundamental tool of periodontal epidemiology is a measure of the occurrence of periodontal conditions. These measures include epidemiologic statistics, such as prevalence, risk, and rate, and they focus on either patient-specific or site-specific markers, such as oral health–related quality of life, tooth loss, anatomic measures, and measures of gingival inflammation. This wealth of possibilities when defining periodontal conditions in combination with statistical challenges when handling correlated data has made it difficult to answer even a simple question such as whether a hidden periodontal disease epidemic occurred during the 20th century.[29]

Epidemiologic Study Designs

The essence of epidemiology and clinical epidemiology is to relate measures of disease occurrence to suspected causes or interventions. Can the dramatic drop in destructive periodontal disease prevalence in the United States be attributed to a change in smoking prevalence? Can the presence of particular microbiologic species around a tooth be related to the risk of future tooth loss? Can the rate of tooth loss in a sample of elderly patients be related to the use of an antimicrobial rinse? With an evidence-based approach, these questions can be most reliably answered by three epidemiologic study designs. As mentioned earlier in this chapter and as briefly introduced in Chapter 2, these study designs (in order of decreasing reliability) are the randomized controlled trial, the cohort study, and the case–control study.

Randomized Controlled Trials

Randomized controlled trials in periodontics typically assign patients or some teeth within a patient randomly to a treatment. Patients are then monitored, and subsequent outcomes are assessed. Table 6.3 provides two examples of randomized controlled trials.

The randomized controlled trial is the only study design that can provide a probabilistic basis for the making of a causal inference between an intervention and an outcome. Reliable inference regarding the causality of associations can be obtained if the delicate machinery of clinical trial design and analysis is strictly respected. For example, there needs to be a pretrial hypothesis that specifies the endpoint, the treatments to be compared, the patient population, and the degree of required precision. Other factors that are important for obtaining reliable answers include a secure randomization process, the masking of patients and clinicians, the presence of an independent data and safety monitoring board, and strict adherence to the pretrial hypothesis, which must include an intent-to-treat analysis. Trials with exquisite attention to detail are referred to as *definitive trials,* and they are rare in any field, including periodontal research. Definitive trials

to tracking prostate cancer by measuring inflammation or swelling of the prostate gland without knowing how this information relates to prostate cancer mortality. This challenge is further compounded by the absence of diagnostic codes for tooth loss, which has largely prevented the obtaining of reliable information about how many teeth are lost as a result of periodontal disease as opposed to dental caries.

Finally, the attempt to track a disease by only collecting a surrogate outcome measure such as probing depth from the teeth that are present leads to a type of bias that is typically referred to as *survival bias.* Most periodontal clinical trials performed during the 20th century

TABLE 6.4   Examples of Periodontal Cohort Studies

Periodontal Exposure	Outcome	Sample Size
Periodontal disease and tooth loss[35]	Coronary heart disease	51,529
Gingivitis[9]	Tooth loss	>500

TABLE 6.5   Examples of Periodontal Case–Control Studies

Case–Control Criteria	Investigated Risk Factors	Sample Size
Destructive periodontal disease[47a]	Smoking	177
Acute myocardial infarction[59a]	Dental health	202

are required to provide reliable answers about treatment efficacy. Most of the trials published in the literature are in the category of exploratory trials. These trials typically do not report a pretrial hypothesis, and they conclude that the intervention was successful when compared to the control.[26] These are almost always false-positive conclusions.[27]

Cohort Studies

Cohort studies can also be referred to as *exposure-based study designs.* Subjects who are free of the disease of interest are classified with respect to an exposure (e.g., cigarette smoking, diabetes) and followed longitudinally for the assessment of periodontal outcomes. Table 6.4 provides two examples of cohort studies.

Cohorts can be defined by a geographic area, records, exposure status, or a combination of different criteria. In one study of the causal factors of edentulism, the population of interest was defined as the inhabitants of the town of Tecumseh, Michigan. Persons within this community were examined in 1959 as part of a community-wide health study. Twenty-eight years later, a subset of these patients was reexamined to study the risk factors for edentulism.[52] Some natural disease history studies of destructive periodontal disease have been conducted on the basis of geographic location. Examples include the Norwegian Longitudinal Study,[1] the Veterans Administration Longitudinal Study,[39] and the Sri Lanka study.[2] A cohort can be defined by records (e.g., schools, health insurance plans, unions, industries, professional organizations). Many cohort studies of periodontal disease outcomes are performed in patients who belong to a particular dental insurance company[12] or to a professional group.[36] Finally, cohorts can be defined on the basis of a specific exposure. For example, different levels of fluoride concentrations in the water supply have been used for the definition of cohorts.

Case–Control Studies

Case–control studies are typically referred to as *outcome-based study designs.* Persons with a condition or outcome of interest (i.e., cases) are compared with persons without a condition of interest (i.e., controls) with respect to the history of the suspected causal factors. Many people intuitively think along the lines of a case–control study when evaluating disease causes. For example, if an individual suffers from food poisoning after a party, he or she is likely to compare past food intake with those individuals who did *not* experience food poisoning. Similarly, if one is diagnosed with a serious illness, a common reaction is to ask, "Why me?" This is usually followed by a comparison of one's history of exposures with those of other individuals who did *not* develop the serious illness. The primary goal of a case–control study is to find out what *past* exposures or factors are different between patients with a disease versus those without the disease. Table 6.5 provides two examples of case–control studies.

The case–control study is a challenging type of study to conduct. Trying to minimize the role of bias in case–control studies requires careful planning, conduct, and analysis. Even when everything is done perfectly, one can come to the wrong conclusions in case–control studies. A review of the quality of periodontal case–control studies

suggested that they are frequently inadequately conducted and reported.[45]

Two important elements of the case–control study design are the definitions of the terms *case* and *control.* A *case* is a person in the population or study group who has been identified as having a particular disease, health disorder, or condition.[10] The case definition should be rigorous to minimize bias and misclassification; it can be based on symptoms, signs, or the results of diagnostic tests. For example, the case definition for a myocardial infarction in a case–control study of the relationship between dental health and acute myocardial infarction was as follows[2]:

1. Symptoms start within 36 hours before the admission
2. No prior myocardial infarction
3. Residing in Helsinki or an immediate neighborhood
4. Age <60 years for men and <65 years for women
5. Blood samples available at admission and at 4 weeks

In a case–control study, the *controls* should be at risk for developing the investigated disease and come from the same population that generated the cases. For example, if the investigated disease is root caries, the controls should be at risk for developing root caries (i.e., have exposed root surfaces) and originate from the same population that generated the cases that have root caries.

Causes

Human chronic diseases such as cancer, diabetes, and destructive periodontal disease have complex causes. The terms *necessary cause, component cause,* and *sufficient cause* help to define the challenges of determining the cause of a disease and of verbalizing the complexity of chronic disease causes.[62]

The set of causes that initiate a chronic disease is referred to as a *sufficient cause.* Each sufficient cause consists of multiple component causes. Consider the hypothetical example in which four sufficient causes exist for noniatrogenic destructive periodontal disease (Fig. 6.2). The first sufficient cause in this example includes the following component causes: smoking, delayed neutrophil apoptosis, an interleukin-1 gene defect, dental plaque, a tooth, and an unspecified gene defect. These different elements of a sufficient cause are referred to as *component causes.* All component causes of a sufficient cause need to be present for the disease process to be initiated. Multiple sufficient causes may be responsible for a given disease. For example, two sufficient causes exist for destructive periodontal diseases that do not include smoking.

A component cause, which is an element of all the sufficient causes for a given disease, is referred to as a *necessary cause.* For example, fermentable carbohydrates are a necessary cause for dental caries. However, there are very few examples of necessary causes: smoking is not a necessary cause of lung cancer or destructive periodontal disease, hepatitis B infection is not a necessary cause of liver cancer, and *Streptococcus viridans* is not a necessary cause of bacterial endocarditis. The search for necessary causes of disease is important, because the elimination of such causes could eradicate a disease.

The proportion of disease that results from different component causes does not add up to 100%. The component cause "smoking"

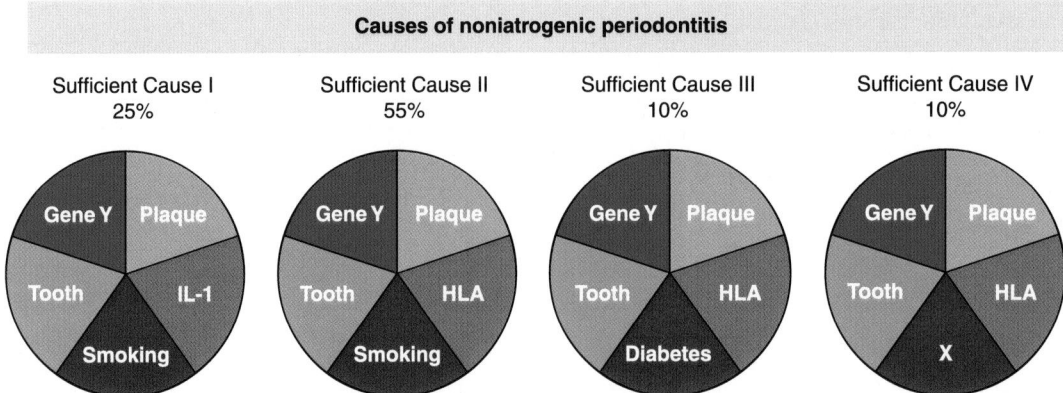

Fig. 6.2 Causes of noniatrogenic periodontitis. *(Data from Rothman KJ: Causes. 1976.* Am J Epidemiol *141:90–95, 1995.)*

is responsible for 80% of destructive periodontal disease cases; plaque is responsible for 100%, and diabetes is responsible for 10%.

The complex causal web that leads to the initiation and progression of chronic disease makes the reliable identification of causal components difficult. Since the 1960s, epidemiology has succeeded in reliably identifying some of the causes of human chronic diseases. Now that those component causes responsible for a large proportion of cases for particular diseases (e.g., smoking for lung cancer) have been identified, the search for new causes is becoming significantly more challenging. For example, the hope existed that the Human Genome Project would lead to quick advances, but these hopes have not yet been fulfilled. Chronic diseases are typically caused not by one gene but rather by a set of many different genes, with each one responsible for only a small proportion of cases and acting in a variety of synergistic mechanisms for disease initiation.

Suspected Modifiable Causative Factors for Periodontal Disease

Tobacco Smoking

Tobacco smoking is recognized by several organizations as one of the primary drivers of periodontal disease epidemiology.[3] Many criteria for causality have been satisfied,[18] and smoking cessation has been shown to slow the progression of periodontal disease.[38,39,57] The strong impact of tobacco smoking on periodontal disease has the potential to induce spurious causal associations in other suspected risk factors for periodontal disease. For example, smoking is a risk factor for both type 2 diabetes[75] and periodontal disease, thereby making associations between type 2 diabetes and periodontal disease susceptible to biases. To obtain reliable inferences about causal factors other than smoking, studies of periodontal disease epidemiology may need to be restricted to those who have never smoked.

Nutrition

Several studies have demonstrated relationships between periodontal disease and a variety of medical conditions that center on carbohydrate metabolism, including intake of dietary carbohydrates, exercise, obesity, prediabetes, and diabetes. A systematic review of randomized controlled trials involving carbohydrates suggested that the increased intake of fermentable carbohydrates may cause an increase in gingivitis.[26] Two systematic reviews suggested that diabetes was a risk factor for destructive periodontal disease.[64,67]

Dental Plaque

Several systematic reviews have provided evidence that chemotherapeutic and mechanical plaque control will reduce gingival inflammation. Essential oils[4] and cetylpyridinium-chloride–containing mouth rinses[20] may reduce gingival inflammation. Interdental brushes may reduce dental plaque, bleeding, and probing pocket depth.[69] Power-driven toothbrushes may be more effective than manual toothbrushes for removing plaque and reducing inflammation.[66] Self-performed dental flossing may not be effective for reducing plaque and gingival inflammation.[4] Although these systematic reviews provide evidence about the role of dental plaque in gingival inflammation, they do not necessarily suggest that dental plaque is the primary cause of gingival inflammation.[24] Stomach acids may cause heartburn, and antacids may be effective at eliminating heartburn symptoms. However, this evidence does not make stomach acids a primary cause of heartburn. The primary cause of heartburn may, for instance, be a gluten allergy, and thus the cure of the heartburn requires the elimination of gluten from the diet. Antacids can be considered a palliative that is needed as long as the primary cause has not been identified.

Neither is there reliable evidence that gingival inflammation precedes destructive periodontal disease. There is no reliable randomized controlled trial evidence that oral hygiene has a beneficial impact on the prevention of periodontal destruction.[27,30]

The Cause of Periodontal Disease for the Patient Sitting in Your Chair

In clinical epidemiology, in a court of a law, and in modern-day clinical practice, uncertainty regarding the "cause" is an important consideration when discussing causality. The term *attributable risk percentage* is used to express the probability that a disease is caused by a suspected causative agent. For example, in a smoker with lung cancer, there may be a 20% probability that the lung cancer was caused by a factor other than smoking (e.g., radon). In an obese person with diabetes, there may be a 10% chance that obesity played no role in the onset of diabetes. For a worker with leukemia in the nuclear industry, there may be an 80% chance that the leukemia was not caused by the low-level protracted radiation exposures. One can almost never determine with certainty what caused a particular condition or disease to appear in a patient; all one can do is assign probabilities to the likelihood that a particular causal factor was responsible for the disease diagnosed in the patient. Destructive periodontal disease and periodontal inflammation are no exception to this general rule of uncertainty for determining a disease's cause. As a result, diagnostic names (e.g., plaque-induced gingival disease, non–plaque-induced inflammatory gingival lesions[43]) can be considered misnomers, because such names imply diagnostic certainty that lead to circular reasoning.[2] The principle of diagnostic uncertainty is also important when it comes to the diagnosis of periodontal conditions.

Diagnosis

Periodontal Conditions Versus Periodontal Diseases

Disease is defined as an attribute or a characteristic of a person, and *diagnosis* is the clinician's belief that the person has the attribute.[70] The World Health Organization defined disease as those adverse health consequences that include physical or psychological impairment, activity restrictions, and role limitations.[70] Certain periodontal conditions have been associated with such adverse consequences, and thus certain periodontal conditions qualify as diseases according to the WHO's definition. In one study, about 1 in 5 patients who presented to a periodontal specialist reported that their teeth, gums, or dentures had an impact fairly often or very often on either eating; relaxing; avoiding going out; or feeling self-conscious, pain, or discomfort. In this same study, 4 out of 10 patients rated their oral health as fair or poor.[11] Other studies have shown that gingival conditions (e.g., necrotizing ulcerative gingivitis, attachment loss in high school students) are similarly related to oral health–related quality of life.[44]

An important thing to consider during periodontal diagnosis is to determine which periodontal conditions can be diagnosed as "diseased." Can a patient with a couple of sites with 1 or 2 mm of attachment loss be classified in this way? What about a patient with such subtle gingival inflammation that the majority of clinicians would not notice the inflammation and that even highly trained clinical examiners agree poorly about the presence of gingivitis? Disagreement regarding such questions is one of the reasons that the prevalence of gingivitis and destructive periodontal disease can range widely, depending on which reference levels are considered to be the cutoff for normal as compared with diseased.

Diagnostic Tests Available to Assess Periodontal Conditions

Diagnostic tests for periodontal disease can include anatomic measures of tissue destruction, such as probing pocket depth and clinical attachment loss; measures of gingival inflammation, such as redness, suppuration, bleeding, bleeding on probing, elevated gingival temperature, and gingival crevicular fluid markers; radiographic measures of bone destruction and tooth mobility; and microbiologic measures. These test results—in combination with factors such as age, dental history, and systemic conditions—can be translated into a distinct set of periodontal diagnoses.

Translating Periodontal Diagnostic Test Results Into Periodontal Disease Diagnosis

Three different methods can be distinguished to translate clinical conditions into diseases: (1) normative or arbitrary values, (2) risk-based reference values, and (3) treatment-based reference values.[32]

Normative or Arbitrary Values to Diagnose Periodontal Disease

Diseases can be defined on the basis of normative or arbitrary reference values. If the normal periodontium is assumed to have no pockets deeper than 3 mm, then one could define destructive periodontal disease as being present in a patient with any pocket equal to or deeper than 4 mm, or a patient with three pockets equal to or deeper than 5 mm could be classified as having destructive periodontal disease. Alternatively, normative values could be based on parametric or nonparametric percentage cutoff values as derived from national surveys. For instance, the 97.5th percentile of the age-specific number of pockets deeper than 5 mm could be used to define destructive periodontal disease. On the basis of the NHANES III data, a 28-year-old individual with two pockets deeper than 5 mm could be diagnosed as having destructive periodontal disease, whereas five periodontal pockets deeper than 5 mm would be required in a 58-year-old individual.[31]

Diagnoses that are based on normative or arbitrary cutoffs result in normative or arbitrary disease prevalence levels, regardless of the distribution of underlying risk factors. Whether 5% or 95% of the population smoked two packs a day for 40 years, the prevalence of destructive periodontal disease would remain equal to the selected cutoff value. If all human chronic diseases were defined on the basis of an arbitrary 10th percentile cutoff value, the prevalence of all chronic disease would be equal to 5% (e.g., 5% of the population would have blood pressure that is too high, 5% would have a blood glucose level that is too high).

Risk-Based Reference Values to Diagnose Periodontal Disease

The diagnosis of disease can be set at the point on the diagnostic marker at which a steep increased risk for adverse health outcomes is present. The cutoff is still somewhat arbitrary, but it is connected to clinical realities in terms of the risk of adverse health outcomes. There is a tradeoff between the dangers of missed diagnoses when the cutoff is made too high (i.e., more specific) and the dangers of false-positive diagnoses when the cutoff is too low (i.e., more sensitive).

A risk-based diagnosis of destructive periodontal disease requires the conducting of longitudinal studies in which pocket depth at baseline is related to the risk of subsequent adverse outcomes (e.g., tooth loss). Fig. 6.1 represents such a plot and suggests that a pocket depth of 6 mm could be a diagnostic marker for destructive periodontal disease, because a distinctive increased risk for tooth loss is associated with pocket depth values of 6 mm or deeper.

The risk-based diagnosis of chronic diseases, much like the use of normative or arbitrary values, can do more harm than good. A diagnosis of obesity that is based on a body mass index of 28 may do more harm than good if weight loss treatments increase mortality risk.[37] A diagnosis of high blood pressure[59] or diabetes[49] may cause more harm than good if the prescribed treatment further increases the mortality risk. Similarly, a diagnosis of destructive periodontal disease that is based on the presence of periodontal pockets 6 mm or deeper may cause more harm than good if the suggested periodontal treatments increase periodontal morbidity.

Therapeutic Reference Values to Diagnose Periodontal Disease

A more attractive definition of disease is the therapeutic or treatment-based diagnosis. With this definition, a person is defined as diseased only if the diagnosis of disease leads to tangible benefits. Most commonly, it is best to avoid diagnosing disease unless it can be shown that the diagnosis and the subsequent treatment actually provide tangible patient outcomes. With such an approach to diagnoses, periodontal disease should only be diagnosed if it leads to less morbidity.

Periodontal Disease Diagnoses

The Medical Subject Heading (MeSH) term headings for periodontal disease, the classification systems for periodontal diseases developed by professional organizations, and a sampling of English-language periodontal textbooks indicate that periodontal disease diagnoses come and go at a fast rate. On PubMed, seven different entry terms are currently listed under the MeSH heading of *Periodontitis,* which reflects some of the distinct periodontal diagnoses that have been used in the literature since 1965. However, a conference consensus[35] concluded that five of the seven terms listed were obsolete. The American Academy of Periodontology reported 10 different classification systems in 20 years.[2] Periodontal textbooks have similarly reported different sets of periodontal diagnoses every decade.

Periodontal dystrophies provide one example on the apparent arbitrariness by which periodontal diagnoses come and go. Periodontal dystrophies were commonly reported from the 18th century until the 1960s. However, this diagnosis was subsequently decided to be obsolete,[58] because it did not appear to fit the infection paradigm. Periodontal textbooks no longer referred to the diagnosis of "periodontosis." However, an argument was made that this diagnosis should be resurrected.[55]

This example illustrates how profoundly the belief that periodontal disease is infectious has influenced all aspects of clinical periodontics, including the system for classifying periodontal conditions. Periodontal diagnoses in some circles are based on the premise that periodontal diseases "follow an infection/host paradigm in which it is held that noxious materials from dental plaque bacteria induce an inflammatory response in the adjacent periodontal tissue. … Central to this paradigm is the notion that the destruction of periodontal tissues is accompanied by an inflammatory response."[1]

There are two reasons why the diagnostic classification of periodontal diseases should not be based on the infection paradigm or on any other assumed cause. First, high-level evidence from epidemiologic studies is required to determine that periodontal disease is indeed an infection. Such evidence remains largely missing.[23] Smoking and diabetes appear to be associated with destructive periodontal disease independent of microbial colonization. Second, for chronic diseases with multiple causes, it is not possible to determine the cause of the disease; therefore it is of little clinical value to name the disease after a suspected cause. For example, periodontal disease in a diabetic patient cannot be referred to as "diabetic periodontitis." The clinician can only say that there is a certain probability that the periodontal disease in a diabetic patient is attributable to the diabetic condition.

From a clinical perspective, the ever-changing diagnostic classification systems that result from consensus conferences may be irrelevant, because no reliable evidence exists that the clinical use of such diagnostic systems improves patient outcomes. Simple diagnostic systems of periodontal disease can have several advantages for patient care, because they provide useful information about both the severity of the disease and its prognosis. The readers are referred to Chapter 5 for an in-depth discussion of periodontitis classification systems.

References

 References for this chapter are found on the companion website www.expertconsult.com.

Periodontal Disease Pathogenesis

Philip M. Preshaw

CHAPTER OUTLINE

Histopathology of Periodontal
Disease
Inflammatory Responses in the
Periodontium

Linking Pathogenesis to Clinical
Signs of Disease
Resolution of Inflammation

Immune Responses in Periodontal
Pathogenesis
Concept of Host Susceptibility

Understanding periodontal pathogenesis is key to improving management strategies for this common, complex disease. The first challenge is to understand exactly what is meant by the term *pathogenesis.* According to *Merriam Webster's Collegiate Dictionary,* the word *pathogenesis* is defined as "the origination and development of a disease." Essentially, this refers to the step-by-step processes that lead to the development of a disease and that result in a series of changes in the structure and function of, in this case, the periodontium. In broad terms, the pathogenesis of a disease is the mechanism by which a causative factor (or factors) causes the disease. The word itself is derived from the Greek roots *pathos* (meaning "suffering") and *genesis* (meaning "generation or creation").

Our knowledge of periodontal pathogenesis has evolved over the years. It is important to be aware of this because treatment philosophies have changed in parallel with our improving understanding of the disease processes and will likely continue to change as our knowledge improves. During the late 1800s, Willoughby D. Miller[117] (an eminent dental researcher who established the important causal role of oral bacteria for dental caries) asserted that "during the last few years the conviction has grown continually stronger, among physicians as well as dentists, that the human mouth, as a gathering-place and incubator of diverse pathogenic germs, performs a significant role in the production of varied disorders of the body, and that if many diseases whose origin is enveloped in mystery could be traced to their source, they would be found to have originated in the oral cavity." This statement marked the beginning of an era of dental treatment strategies that aimed to treat systemic diseases by eliminating the so-called "foci of infection" in the mouth. As a result, many patients underwent unnecessary dental clearances to manage their systemic diseases.

By the 1930s, such approaches were beginning to be questioned. In an analysis of 200 patients with rheumatoid arthritis, of whom 92 had their tonsils removed as treatment for the arthritis (even though only about 15% gave any history of tonsillitis or sore throat) and of whom 52 had some or all of their teeth removed, no improvements in the rheumatoid arthritis symptoms were noted in any of the patients.[27] These authors wrote that "focal infection is a splendid example of a plausible medical theory which is in danger of being converted by its too enthusiastic supporters into the status of an accepted fact."[27] The end of the focal infection era was signaled by an editorial in the *Journal of the American Medical Association* in 1952, which stated that "many patients with diseases presumably caused by foci of infection have not been relieved of their symptoms by removal of the foci, many patients with these same systemic diseases have no evident focus of infection, foci of infection are as common in apparently healthy persons as in those with disease."[165]

In more recent times, advances in the management of periodontitis have been driven by improved knowledge of the epidemiology, causation, and pathogenesis of the disease.[192] During the 1970s, the role of plaque as the sole causative factor for periodontitis was unquestioned. In those days, nonsurgical treatment was in its infancy, and most treatment options involved surgery (e.g., gingivectomy for the treatment of shallower pockets, access flap surgery for the treatment of deeper sites). When looking back, it becomes clear that the treatment strategies used during a given time period entirely depend on the prevailing understanding of pathogenesis at that particular point in time. It is therefore very likely that the management options that we take for granted now will change again in the future. This is to be welcomed because a progressive clinical discipline such as periodontology that is well founded in science and with benefit to the patient as its primary value should strive to improve therapeutic strategies in parallel with continued discovery.

CLINICIAN'S CORNER

Why is studying periodontal pathogenesis important?
Pathogenesis refers to the processes that cause disease. In periodontitis, bacteria in the biofilm stimulate an immune–inflammatory response that causes the tissue damage that we recognize clinically as periodontitis. Understanding the disease processes is important because it may lead to the development of improved treatment strategies.

Periodontal disease results from a complex interplay between the subgingival biofilm and the host immune–inflammatory events that develop in the gingival and periodontal tissues in response to the challenge presented by the bacteria. The tissue damage that results from the immune–inflammatory response is recognized clinically as periodontitis. Gingivitis precedes periodontitis, but it is clear that not all cases of gingivitis progress to periodontitis. In gingivitis, the inflammatory lesion is confined to the gingiva; however, with periodontitis, the inflammatory processes extend to additionally affect the periodontal ligament and the alveolar bone. The net result of these inflammatory changes is the breakdown of the fibers of the periodontal ligament, resulting in clinical loss of attachment together with resorption of the alveolar bone.

During the 1970s and 1980s, bacterial plaque was generally considered to be preeminent as the cause of periodontitis. It was clear (as it is now) that poor oral hygiene results in increased plaque accumulation, and it was accepted that this, in turn, resulted in periodontal disease. However, this model failed to take into account observations such as the finding that there are many individuals with poor oral hygiene who do not develop advanced periodontal disease, and conversely, some individuals, despite good oral hygiene and compliance with periodontal treatment protocols, present with advanced and progressing periodontitis. These findings were confirmed by the work of Löe and colleagues,[108] who studied Sri Lankan tea laborers who had no access to dental care and who could be divided into three main categories: (1) individuals (≈8% of the population studied) who had rapid progression of periodontal disease, (2) those (≈81%) who had moderate progression of such disease, and (3) those (≈11%) who demonstrated no progression of periodontal disease beyond gingivitis. All patients in this population displayed abundant plaque and calculus deposits, so clearly susceptibility to disease is influenced by more than just presence of dental plaque. The causative role of bacteria in the biofilm is clear in that the bacteria initiate and perpetuate the inflammatory responses that develop in the gingival tissues. However, the main determinant of susceptibility to disease is the nature of the immune–inflammatory responses themselves. It is paradoxical that these defensive processes, which are protective by intent (i.e., to prevent the ingress of the bacteria and their products into the tissues), result in the majority of tissue damage that leads to the clinical manifestations of disease.

Periodontal disease is therefore a unique clinical entity. It is not an infection in the classic sense of the word. With many infections, a single infective organism causes the disease (e.g., human immuno-deficiency virus, syphilis, tuberculosis), and the identification of that organism can provide the basis for the diagnosis. With periodontal disease, many species are identifiable in the periodontal pocket, and it is impossible to conclude that a single species or even a group of species causes periodontal disease. Many of the species that are considered important in periodontal pathogenesis may predominate in deep pockets because the pocket is a favorable environment in which they can survive (i.e., it is warm, moist, and anaerobic, with a ready supply of nutrients). Many of the unique features of periodontitis are derived from the anatomy of the periodontium, in which a hard, nonshedding surface (the tooth) is partly embedded within the body (within connective tissue), crosses an epithelial surface, and is partly exposed to the outside world (within the confines of the mouth). The bacteria that colonize this surface are effectively outside of the body (although they are in the gingival crevice or pocket), yet the inflammatory response that develops is located within the body (i.e., within the tissues). These factors add complexity to our understanding of the role of the biofilm and the immune–inflammatory responses that are part of periodontal tissue breakdown.

Histopathology of Periodontal Disease

To understand periodontal pathogenesis better, it is important to have an appreciation of the histology of clinically healthy tissues, as well as of inflamed gingival and periodontal tissues. Even gingival tissues that clinically would be considered to be noninflamed and healthy always have evidence of inflammatory responses occurring at the microscopic level. This is normal given the chronic low-grade challenge presented by the subgingival biofilm. The low-grade inflammatory response that results is not detectable macroscopically at the clinical level, but it is an essential protective mechanism for combating the microbial challenge and for preventing bacteria and their products from infiltrating tissues and causing tissue damage. Our current understanding of susceptibility to periodontitis suggests that individuals who are susceptible to the disease mount an excessive or dysregulated immune–inflammatory response for a given bacterial challenge that leads to increased tissue breakdown as compared with those individuals who have a more normal inflammatory response.

Clinically Healthy Gingival Tissues

Clinically healthy gingival tissues appear pink, are not swollen or inflamed, and are firmly attached to the underlying tooth and bone, with minimal bleeding on probing. The dentogingival junction is a unique anatomic feature that functions to attach the gingiva to the tooth. It has an epithelial portion and a connective tissue portion, both of which are of fundamental importance for periodontal pathogenesis. The epithelial portion can be divided into three distinct epithelial structures: the gingival epithelium, the sulcular epithelium, and the junctional epithelium (Fig. 7.1). These epithelial structures are in continuity with each other, but they have distinct structures and functions, as indicated in Box 7.1.

The junctional epithelium is a unique epithelial structure because the surface cells are specialized for the purpose of attachment to the

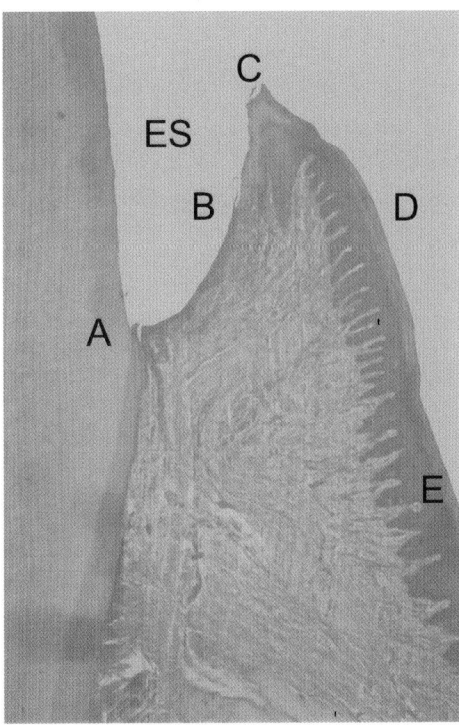

Fig. 7.1 Histologic appearance of healthy gingiva. A photomicrograph of a demineralized tooth with the gingival tissues in situ (hematoxylin and eosin staining, low magnification). Cementoenamel junction *(A)*. Enamel space *(ES)*. Gingival health is characterized by the organization of the epithelium into distinct zones; junctional epithelium *(A-B)*, sulcular epithelium *(B-C)*, free gingiva *(C-D)*, and attached gingiva *(D-E)*. The gingival connective tissue is composed of densely packed, organized, and interlacing collagen bundles. A few scattered inflammatory cells are present but no significant inflammatory cell infiltrate.

tooth.[12] Therefore, unlike other epithelial tissues elsewhere in the body, no opportunity exists for the sloughing of cells from the surface. Instead, cells at the basal layer continually divide and move to within two or three cell layers of the tooth surface and then migrate coronally and parallel to the tooth surface to reach the floor of the sulcus eventually and then be sloughed off into the gingival crevice. The spaces between cells of the junctional epithelium are also greater than those seen with other epithelial tissues, with the intercellular spaces comprising approximately 18% of the volume of the epithelium. This configuration is a result of a lower density of desmosomes in the junctional epithelium as compared with the gingival epithelium; the junctional epithelium is therefore intrinsically "leaky." This situation has great relevance for periodontal pathogenesis because the widened intercellular spaces in the junctional epithelium permit the migration of neutrophils (polymorphonuclear leukocytes); they also allow macrophages from the gingival connective tissues to enter the sulcus to phagocytose bacteria, and the ingress of bacterial products and antigens occurs as well.

The connective tissue component of the dentogingival unit contains densely packed collagen fiber bundles (a mixture of type I and III collagen fibers) that are arranged in distinct patterns that maintain the functional integrity of the tissues and the tight adaptation of the soft tissues to the teeth (see Chapter 3).

Even in clinically healthy gingiva, the gingival connective tissue contains at least some inflammatory cells, particularly neutrophils. Neutrophils continually migrate through the connective tissues and pass through the junctional epithelium to enter the sulcus or pocket.

These findings were reported in the classic investigations of the histology of periodontal disease reported by Page and Schroeder in 1976.[135] This low-grade inflammation occurs in response to the continued presence of bacteria and their products in the gingival crevice. There is a continuous exudate of fluid from the gingival tissues that enters the crevice and flows out as gingival crevicular fluid (GCF). In addition to the continuous migration of neutrophils through the gingival tissues, lymphocytes and macrophages also accumulate. The presence of leukocytes in the connective tissues results from the chemotactic stimulus created by the subgingival biofilm and bacterial products, as well as from the chemoattractant factors produced by the host.

In clinically healthy tissues, this steady-state equilibrium between low-grade inflammation in the tissues and the continual presence of the bacterial biofilm may persist for many years or indeed for the lifetime of the individual. Overt clinical signs of gingivitis (i.e., redness, swelling, and bleeding on probing) do not develop because of several innate and structural defense mechanisms, including the following:
- The maintenance of an intact epithelial barrier (the junctional and sulcular epithelium)
- The outflow of GCF from the sulcus (dilution effect and flushing action)
- The sloughing of surface epithelial cells of the junctional and sulcular epithelium
- The presence of neutrophils and macrophages in the sulcus that phagocytose bacteria
- The presence of antibodies in the GCF

However, if plaque accumulation increases, then inflammation and the classic clinical signs of gingivitis may develop. Although the development of gingivitis in response to the accumulation of plaque is fairly predictable, research has identified that a spectrum of responses may be observed, with some individuals developing more pronounced gingival inflammation for a given plaque challenge and others developing minimal gingival inflammation.[181] These observations underscore the importance of variations in host responses among individuals in terms of gingival inflammatory responses. Furthermore, many individuals may never develop periodontitis, despite having widespread gingivitis. The host's immune–inflammatory response is fundamental for determining which individuals may progress to developing periodontitis, and it is likely that inflammatory responses are different in those individuals who develop periodontitis as compared with those who never progress beyond gingivitis. The challenge that this presents clinically is that we do not yet know enough about susceptibility to periodontitis to identify these individuals before they actually develop signs of disease.

Histopathology of Gingivitis and Periodontitis

The development of gingivitis can be clearly observed from a clinical perspective. In addition, the changes that occur within the tissues are very obvious when examined under a microscope. In broad terms, infiltration of the connective tissues by numerous defense cells, particularly neutrophils, macrophages, plasma cells, and lymphocytes is noted. As a result of the accumulation of these defense cells and the extracellular release of their destructive enzymes, disruption of the normal anatomy of the connective tissues occurs and causes collagen depletion and subsequent proliferation of the junctional epithelium. Vasodilation and increased vascular permeability lead to increased leakage of fluid out of the vessels and facilitate the passage of defense cells from the vasculature into the tissues, thus resulting in enlargement of the tissues, which appear erythematous and edematous (i.e., the clinical appearance of gingivitis). These changes are all reversible if the bacterial challenge is substantially reduced by improved oral hygiene.

BOX 7.2   Key Features of the Histologic Stages of Gingivitis and Periodontitis

Initial Lesion (Corresponds With Clinically Healthy Gingival Tissues)
- Slightly elevated vascular permeability and vasodilation
- Gingival crevicular fluid flows out of the sulcus
- Migration of leukocytes, primarily neutrophils, in relatively small numbers through the gingival connective tissue, across the junctional epithelium, and into the sulcus

Early Lesion (Corresponds With Early Gingivitis That Is Evident Clinically)
- Increased vascular permeability, vasodilation, and gingival crevicular fluid flow
- Large numbers of infiltrating leukocytes (mainly neutrophils and lymphocytes)
- Degeneration of fibroblasts
- Collagen destruction that results in collagen-depleted areas of the connective tissue
- Proliferation of the junctional and sulcular epithelium into collagen-depleted areas

Established Lesion (Corresponds With Established Chronic Gingivitis)
- Dense inflammatory cell infiltrate (i.e., plasma cells, lymphocytes, and neutrophils)
- Accumulation of inflammatory cells in the connective tissues
- Elevated release of matrix metalloproteinases and lysosomal contents from neutrophils
- Significant collagen depletion and proliferation of epithelium
- Formation of pocket epithelium that contains large numbers of neutrophils

Advanced Lesion (Marks the Transition From Gingivitis to Periodontitis)
- Predominance of neutrophils in the pocket epithelium and in the pocket
- Dense inflammatory cell infiltrate in the connective tissues (primarily plasma cells)
- Apical migration of junctional epithelium to preserve an intact epithelial barrier
- Continued collagen breakdown that results in large areas of collagen-depleted connective tissue
- Osteoclastic resorption of alveolar bone

Adapted from Page RC, Schroeder HE: Pathogenesis of inflammatory periodontal disease: a summary of current work. *Lab Invest* 33:235–249, 1976.

Note: These classic descriptions are primarily based on findings in experimental animals, and the correlation with the clinical situation in humans is approximate.

The landmark studies of Page and Schroeder[135] described the histologic changes that occur in the gingival tissues as the *initial, early, established,* and *advanced* gingival lesions (Box 7.2). In broad terms, the initial lesion corresponds with clinically healthy tissues (but nonetheless with transmigrating defense cells such as neutrophils if examined histologically), the early lesion corresponds with the early stages of (clinically evident) gingivitis, the established lesion corresponds with chronic gingivitis, and the advanced lesion marks the transition to periodontitis, with attachment loss and bone resorption. These are *histologic descriptions only,* and they should not form part of a clinical diagnosis. Moreover, these classic descriptions are primarily based on findings in experimental animals. The histologic appearances of gingivitis and periodontitis are shown in Figs. 7.2 and 7.3, respectively.

The Initial Lesion

The initial lesion was reported to develop within 2 to 4 days of the accumulation of plaque at a site that was otherwise free of plaque and at which no inflammation was evident microscopically. However, this situation is probably never encountered in reality, and the gingival tissues always have characteristics of a low-grade chronic inflammatory response as a result of the continual presence of the subgingival biofilm. In other words, the initial lesion corresponds to the histologic picture that is evident in clinically healthy gingival tissues. This low-grade inflammation is characterized by dilation of the vascular network and increased vascular permeability, thus permitting the neutrophils and monocytes from the gingival vasculature to migrate through the connective tissues toward the source of the chemotactic stimulus: the bacterial products in the gingival sulcus. The up-regulation of adhesion molecules such as intercellular adhesion molecule-1 (ICAM-1) and E-selectin in the gingival vasculature facilitates the migration of neutrophils from the capillaries into the connective tissues. The increased leakage of fluid from the vessels increases the hydrostatic pressure in the local microcirculation, and, as a result, GCF flow increases. Increased GCF flow has the effect of diluting bacterial products, and it also potentially has a flushing action to remove bacteria and their products from the crevice. However, given the nature of the bacterial biofilm, it is likely that mainly only planktonic (free-floating) bacteria are removed in this way.

The Early Lesion

The early lesion was said to develop after about 1 week of continued plaque accumulation and corresponds to the early clinical signs of gingivitis. The gingiva are erythematous in appearance as a result of the proliferation of capillaries, the opening up of microvascular beds, and continued vasodilation.[105] Increasing vascular permeability leads to increased GCF flow, and transmigrating neutrophils increase significantly in number. The predominant infiltrating cell types are neutrophils and lymphocytes (primarily thymic lymphocytes [T cells]),[137] and the neutrophils migrate through the tissues to the sulcus and phagocytose bacteria. Fibroblasts degenerate, primarily by apoptosis (programmed cell death), which increases the space available for infiltrating leukocytes. Collagen destruction occurs, which results in collagen depletion in the areas apical and lateral to the junctional and sulcular epithelium. The basal cells of these epithelial structures begin to proliferate to maintain an intact barrier against the bacteria and their products, and the epithelium can then be seen proliferating into the collagen-depleted areas of the connective tissues (see Fig. 7.2).[153] As a result of edema of the gingival tissues, the gingiva may appear slightly swollen, and, accordingly, the gingival sulcus becomes slightly deeper. The subgingival biofilm exploits this ecologic niche and proliferates apically (thereby rendering effective plaque control more difficult). The early gingival lesion may persist indefinitely, or it may progress further.

The Established Lesion

The established lesion roughly corresponds to what clinicians would refer to as "chronic gingivitis." The progression from the early lesion to the established lesion depends on many factors, including the plaque challenge (the composition and quantity of the biofilm), host susceptibility factors, and risk factors (both local and systemic). In the initial work by Page and Schroeder,[135] the established lesion was defined as being dominated by plasma cells, and a significant inflammatory cell infiltrate in established gingivitis occupies a considerable volume of the inflamed connective tissues. Large numbers of infiltrating cells can be identified adjacent and lateral to the junctional and

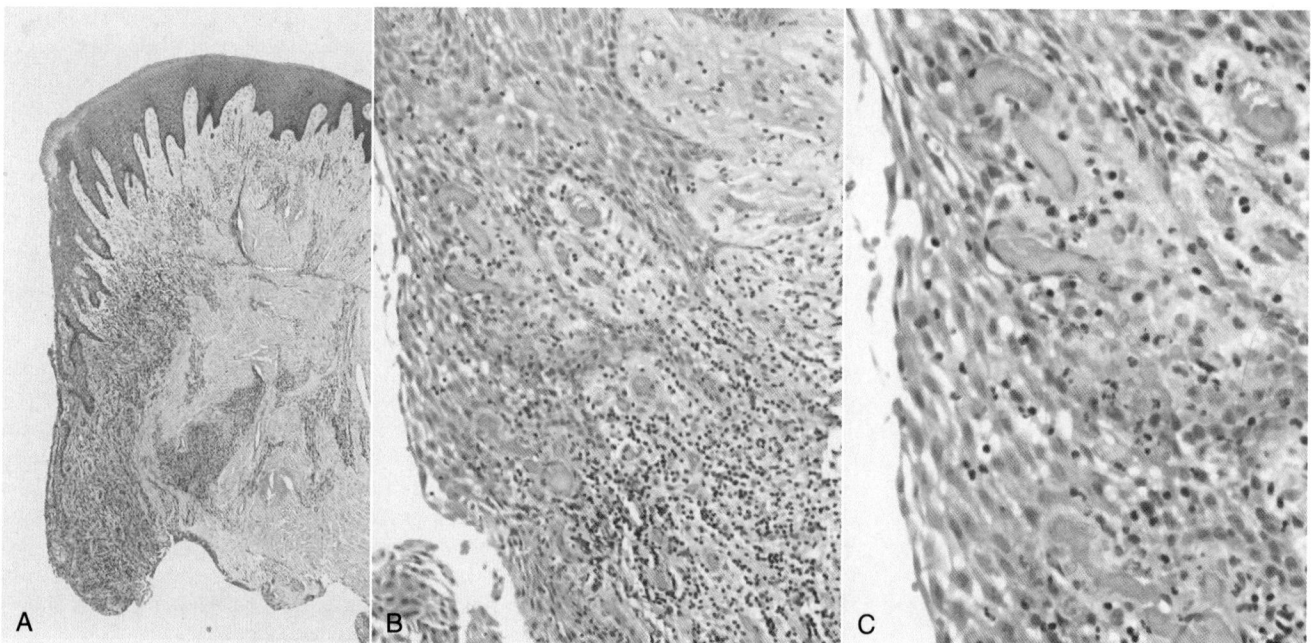

Fig. 7.2   A series of photomicrographs illustrating the histologic appearance of gingivitis (hematoxylin and eosin staining). In all cases, the tooth is to the left side of the image. (A) Low magnification of the gingiva demonstrates hyperplastic junctional and sulcular epithelium with a dense inflammatory cell infiltrate in the adjacent connective tissue. (B) Medium magnification of the epithelial–connective tissue interface shows numerous intraepithelial inflammatory cells along with intercellular edema. The connective tissue contains dilated capillaries (hyperemia), and a dense inflammatory cell infiltrate is noted. (C) High magnification shows neutrophils and small lymphocytes transiting the sulcular epithelium.

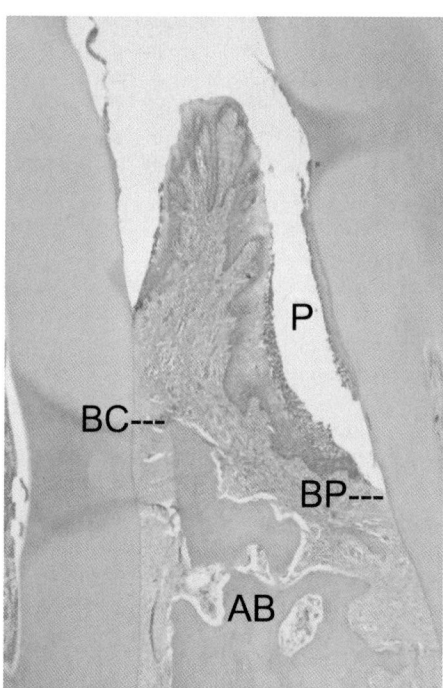

Fig. 7.3   Histologic appearance of periodontitis. A photomicrograph of adjacent demineralized teeth with the interproximal gingiva and periodontium in situ (hematoxylin and eosin staining, low magnification). The root of the tooth on the *right* is coated with a layer of dental biofilm or calculus, and attachment loss is noted with the formation of a periodontal pocket *(P)*. The periodontium is densely inflamed, and alveolar bone *(AB)* loss produces a triangular defect in addition to vertical bone loss. The base of the pocket *(BP)* is apical to the alveolar bone crest *(BC)*; this is called an *infrabony periodontal pocket*. (*From Soames JV, Southam JC:* Oral pathology, *ed 4, Oxford, UK, 2005, Oxford University Press.*)

sulcular epithelium, around blood vessels, and between collagen fiber bundles.[22] Collagen depletion continues, with further proliferation of the epithelium into the connective tissue spaces. Neutrophils accumulate in the tissues and release their lysosomal contents extracellularly (in an attempt to kill bacteria that are not phagocytosed), thereby resulting in further tissue destruction. Neutrophils are also a major source of matrix metalloproteinase-8 (MMP-8; neutrophil collagenase) and MMP-9 (gelatinase B), and these enzymes are produced in large quantities in the inflamed gingival tissues as the neutrophils migrate through the densely packed collagen fiber bundles to enter the sulcus. The junctional epithelium and sulcular epithelium form a pocket epithelium that is not firmly attached to the tooth surface, that contains large numbers of neutrophils, and that is more permeable to the passage of substances into or out of the underlying connective tissue. The pocket epithelium may be ulcerated and less able to resist the passage of the periodontal probe, so bleeding on probing is a common feature of chronic gingivitis. These inflammatory changes are still completely reversible if effective plaque control is reinstituted.

The Advanced Lesion

The advanced lesion, as described by Page and Schroeder,[135] marks the transition from gingivitis to periodontitis. This transition is determined by many factors, the relative importance of which is currently unknown but which includes the bacterial challenge (both the composition and the quantity of the biofilm), the host inflammatory response, and susceptibility factors, including environmental and genetic risk factors. Histologic examination reveals continued evidence of collagen destruction that extends into the periodontal ligament and the alveolar bone. Neutrophils predominate in the pocket epithelium and the periodontal pocket, and plasma cells dominate in the connective tissues. The junctional epithelium migrates apically along the root surface into the collagen-depleted areas to maintain an intact epithelial barrier. Osteoclastic bone resorption commences, and the bone retreats from the advancing inflammatory front as a defense mechanism to the prevent spread of bacteria into the bone (see Fig. 7.3). As the pocket deepens, plaque bacteria proliferate apically into a niche, which is very favorable for many of the species that are regarded as periodontal pathogens. The pocket presents a protected, warm, moist, and anaerobic environment with a ready nutrient supply, and because the bacteria are effectively outside of the body (even though they are in the periodontal pocket), they are not significantly eliminated by the inflammatory response. Thus a cycle develops in which chronic inflammation and associated tissue damage continue. The tissue damage is mainly caused by the inflammatory response, yet the initiating factor—the biofilm—is not eliminated. The destruction of collagen fibers in the periodontal ligament continues, bone resorption progresses, the junctional epithelium migrates apically to maintain an intact barrier, and as a result, the pocket deepens fractionally. This makes it even more difficult to remove the bacteria and to disrupt the biofilm through oral hygiene techniques, and thus the cycle is perpetuated.

Inflammatory Responses in the Periodontium

The molecules that play a role in the pathogenesis of periodontitis can be broadly divided into two main groups: those derived from the subgingival microbiota (i.e., microbial virulence factors) and those derived from the host immune–inflammatory response. In terms of the relative importance of each, it is now clear that most of the tissue breakdown results from the host's inflammatory processes.

Microbial Virulence Factors

The subgingival biofilm initiates and perpetuates inflammatory responses in the gingival and periodontal tissues. The subgingival bacteria also contribute directly to tissue damage by the release of noxious substances, but their primary importance in periodontal pathogenesis is that of activating immune–inflammatory responses that, in turn, result in tissue damage, which may well be beneficial to the bacteria located within the periodontal pocket by providing nutrient sources.

Lipopolysaccharide

Lipopolysaccharides (LPSs) are large molecules composed of a lipid component (lipid A) and a polysaccharide component. They are found in the outer membrane of gram-negative bacteria, they act as endotoxins (LPS is frequently referred to as *endotoxin*), and they elicit strong immune responses in animals. LPSs are highly conserved in gram-negative bacterial species, a finding that reflects their importance in maintaining the structural integrity of the bacterial cells. Immune systems in animals have evolved to recognize LPS through Toll-like receptors (TLRs), a family of cell surface molecules that are highly conserved in animal species ranging from *Drosophila* (a genus of fruit flies) to humans, thereby reflecting their importance in innate immune responses.[28] TLRs are cell surface receptors that recognize *microbe-associated molecular patterns* (MAMPs), which are conserved molecular structures located on pathogens. TLR-4 recognizes LPS from gram-negative bacteria and functions as part of a complex of cell surface molecules, including CD14 and MD-2 (also known as *lymphocyte antigen 96*). The interaction of this CD14/TLR-4/MD-2 complex with LPS triggers a series of intracellular events, the net results of which are the increased production of inflammatory mediators (most notably cytokines) and the differentiation of immune cells (e.g., dendritic cells) for the development of effective immune responses against the pathogens. LPS is of key importance

for initiating and sustaining inflammatory responses in the gingival and periodontal tissues. *Porphyromonas gingivalis* has an atypical form of LPS that is recognized by both TLR-2 and TLR-4.[38,45]

Biologic Properties of Lipopolysaccharide
- Located in the outer membrane of gram-negative bacteria
- Fundamental for maintaining structural integrity of the bacteria
- Elicits a strong response from animal immune systems
- Interacts with the CD14/TLR-4/MD-2 receptor complex on immune cells such as macrophages, monocytes, dendritic cells, and B cells, with resulting release of proinflammatory mediators such as cytokines from these cells

---

A component of gram-positive cell walls, lipoteichoic acid, also stimulates immune responses, although less potently than LPS. Lipoteichoic acid signals through TLR-2. Both LPS and lipoteichoic acid are released from the bacteria present in the biofilm and stimulate inflammatory responses in the tissues, thereby resulting in increased vasodilation and vascular permeability, the recruitment of inflammatory cells by chemotaxis, and the release of proinflammatory mediators by the leukocytes that are recruited to the area.

Bacterial Enzymes and Noxious Products

Plaque bacteria produce several metabolic waste products that contribute directly to tissue damage. These include noxious agents such as ammonia (NH_3) and hydrogen sulfide (H_2S), as well as short-chain carboxylic acids such as butyric acid and propionic acid. These acids are detectable in GCF and are found in increasing concentrations as the severity of periodontal disease increases. These substances have profound effects on host cells (e.g., butyric acid induces apoptosis in T cells, B cells, fibroblasts, and gingival epithelial cells).[95,96,166] The short-chain fatty acids may aid *P. gingivalis* infection through tissue destruction, and they may also create a nutrient supply for the organism by increasing bleeding into the periodontal pocket. The short-chain fatty acids also influence cytokine secretion by immune cells, and they may potentiate inflammatory responses after exposure to proinflammatory stimuli such as LPS, interleukin-1β (IL-1β), and tumor necrosis factor alpha (TNF-α).[125]

Plaque bacteria produce proteases, which are capable of breaking down structural proteins of the periodontium such as collagen, elastin, and fibronectin. Bacteria produce these proteases to digest proteins and thereby provide peptides for bacterial nutrition. Bacterial proteases disrupt host responses, compromise tissue integrity, and facilitate the microbial invasion of the tissues. *P. gingivalis* produces two classes of cysteine proteases that have been implicated in periodontal pathogenesis. These are known as *gingipains,* and they include the lysine-specific gingipain Kgp and the arginine-specific gingipains RgpA and RgpB. The gingipains can modulate the immune system and disrupt immune–inflammatory responses, thus potentially leading to increased tissue breakdown.[138] Gingipains can reduce the concentrations of cytokines in cell culture systems,[6] and they digest and inactivate TNF-α.[25] The gingipains can also stimulate cytokine secretion through the activation of protease-activated receptors (PARs). For example, RgpB activates two different PARs (PAR-1 and PAR-2), thereby stimulating cytokine secretion,[107] and both Rgp and Kgp gingipains stimulate IL-6 and IL-8 secretion by monocytes by the activation of PAR-1, PAR-2, and PAR-3.[182]

Microbial Invasion

Microbial invasion of the periodontal tissues has long been a contentious topic.[11] In histologic specimens, bacteria (including cocci, filaments, and rods) have been identified in the intercellular spaces of

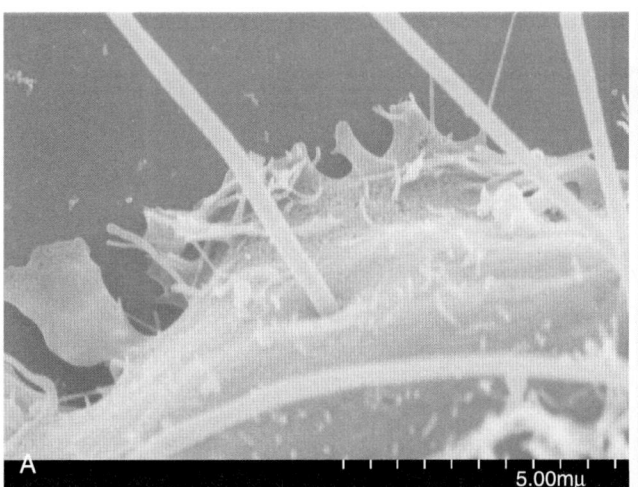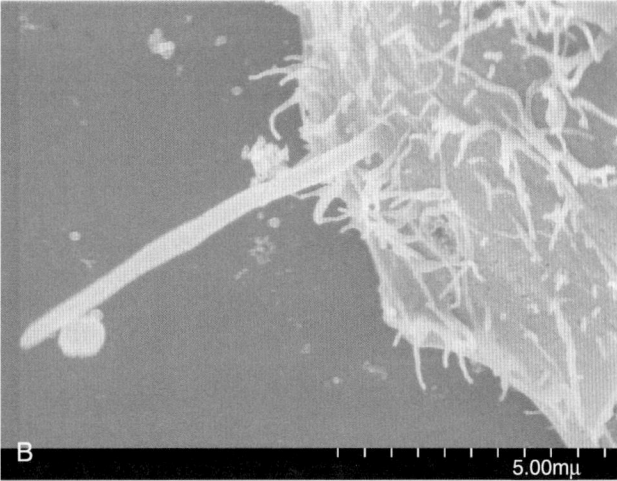

Fig. 7.4 Invasion of epithelial cells by *Fusobacterium nucleatum*. In both images, a single epithelial cell is shown being penetrated by invading *F. nucleatum* bacteria; three or four bacteria are evident in (A), and one bacterium is evident in (B). (A) The ruffled surface of the epithelial cells (multiple small fingerlike projections that are much smaller than the *F. nucleatum* bacteria) is likely to be an artifact. (B) *F. nucleatum* may facilitate the colonization of epithelial cells by bacteria that are unable to adhere or invade directly as evidenced by the single coccoid bacterium *(Streptococcus cristatus)* that has coaggregated with the *F. nucleatum* bacterium as it penetrates the epithelial cell. *(A and B, Courtesy Dr. A.E. Edwards, Imperial College, London, UK; Dr. J.D. Rudney, Bath University, Bath, UK; and Dr. T.J. Grossman, the University of Minnesota, Minneapolis, Minn.)*

the epithelium.[50] Periodontal pathogens such as *P. gingivalis* and *Aggregatibacter actinomycetemcomitans* have been reported to invade the gingival tissues,[30,73,148] including the connective tissues.[149] *Fusobacterium nucleatum* can invade oral epithelial cells, and bacteria that routinely invade host cells may facilitate the entry of noninvasive bacteria by coaggregating with them (Fig. 7.4).[47] It has also been shown that *A. actinomycetemcomitans* can invade epithelial cells and persist intracellularly.[49] The clinical relevance of these various findings is unclear, however, and more recent studies have reported that although species such as *P. gingivalis* can be found located within the tissues, they are mainly within the epithelium, and it is unusual for the bacteria to reach the connective tissue until extensive tissue destruction has occurred, and even then it is as a result of inflammation rather than "invading" bacteria.[11]

CLINICAL CORRELATION

Is bacterial invasion of the tissues a valid concept, and does it have implications for therapy?

Good evidence indicates that certain species of subgingival bacteria are able to invade epithelial cells, thereby providing a shelter from the host defenses (and also highlighting the important role of epithelium in host defenses by release of cytokines to activate inflammatory responses). However, invasion of the deeper connective tissues by live bacteria such as *Porphyromonas gingivalis* seems to occur (if it occurs!) at a much later stage in advanced disease, probably as a result of inflammation and resultant tissue destruction. Reports of bacteria present in the tissues (described as a "reservoir of infection") have sometimes been used to justify the use of antibiotics for treatment of periodontitis as a means to try to eliminate those organisms that are located in the tissues and that are therefore "protected" from mechanical disruption by root surface debridement. However, until the clinical relevance of the presence of bacteria in the tissues is better defined, it is inappropriate to make clinical treatment decisions (e.g., whether to use adjunctive systemic antibiotics) on this premise alone.

Fimbriae

The fimbriae of certain bacterial species, particularly *P. gingivalis*, may also play a role in periodontal pathogenesis. *P. gingivalis* fimbriae stimulate immune responses, such as IL-6 secretion,[97,129] and the major fimbrial structural component of *P. gingivalis*, FimA, has been shown to stimulate nuclear factor (NF)-κB and IL-8 in a gingival epithelial cell line through TLR-2.[5] Monocytes are also stimulated by *P. gingivalis* FimA, secreting IL-6, IL-8, and TNF-α.[48] *P. gingivalis* fimbriae also interact with complement receptor-3 (CR-3) to activate intracellular signaling pathways that inhibit IL-12 production mediated by TLR-2 signaling.[65] This may be of clinical relevance because IL-12 is important in the activation of natural killer (NK) cells and CD8+ cytotoxic T cells, which themselves may be important in killing *P. gingivalis*–infected host cells, such as epithelial cells. Indeed, the blockade of the CR-3 receptor promotes IL-12–mediated clearance of *P. gingivalis* and negates its virulence.[65] Bacterial fimbriae are therefore important for modifying and stimulating immune responses in the periodontium.

Bacterial Deoxyribonucleic Acid and Extracellular Deoxyribonucleic Acid

Bacterial deoxyribonucleic acid (DNA) stimulates immune cells through TLR-9, which recognizes hypomethylated CpG regions of the DNA.[93] (CpG sites are regions of DNA at which a cytosine nucleotide is found next to a guanine nucleotide, separated by a phosphate molecule, which links the C and G nucleotides together, hence "CpG".) Extracellular DNA (eDNA) is a ubiquitous constituent of all biofilms and of particular interest in biofilms associated with chronic diseases such as periodontitis.[79] eDNA is derived from the chromosomal DNA of bacteria in biofilms, and the majority of eDNA is released after bacterial cell lysis.[2,176] However, evidence also indicates that eDNA secretion may occur from bacterial cells by mechanisms that are independent of cell lysis.[66,143] The significance of this finding is not yet clear, but such "donated" DNA may be used by bacterial species as a means of increasing genetic diversity (if taken up by other bacteria), thereby contributing to antigenic variation and the spread of antibiotic resistance, and they may also modulate the host immune response. Thus eDNA may function as a source of genetic information for naturally transformable bacteria in the biofilm[189] or as a stimulus for host immunity. Perhaps more important, it is becoming increasingly clear that eDNA plays a number of important roles in biofilm integrity and formation on hard and soft tissues in the oral cavity. These include roles in adhesion and biofilm formation, protection against antimicrobial agents, and nutrient storage, as well as genetic exchange, and it is possible that eDNA may ultimately prove to be an important target for biofilm control.[79]

Host-Derived Inflammatory Mediators

The inflammatory and immune processes that develop in the periodontal tissues in response to the long-term presence of the subgingival biofilm are protective by intent but can result in considerable tissue damage, thereby leading to the clinical signs and symptoms of periodontal disease. It is paradoxical that the host response causes most of the tissue damage, although this is not unique to periodontal disease. For example, the tissue damage that occurs in the joints in patients with rheumatoid arthritis results from prolonged and excessive inflammatory responses, and it is characterized by the increased production of many of the cytokines that are also known to be important in periodontal pathogenesis. In the case of rheumatoid arthritis, the initiating factor is an autoimmune response to structural components of the joint; in periodontitis, the initiating factor is the subgingival biofilm. In both cases, the destructive inflammatory events are remarkably similar, although the pathogenesis varies as a result of the different anatomy. Key types of mediators that orchestrate the host responses in periodontitis are summarized in the following subsections.

Cytokines

Cytokines play a fundamental role in inflammation, and they are key inflammatory mediators in periodontal disease.[141] They are soluble proteins, and they act as messengers to transmit signals from one cell to another. Cytokines bind to specific receptors on target cells and initiate intracellular signaling cascades that result in phenotypic changes in the cell by altered gene regulation.[17,174] Cytokines are effective in very low concentrations, they are produced transiently in the tissues, and they primarily act locally in the tissues in which they are produced. Cytokines are able to induce their own expression in either an autocrine or paracrine fashion, and they have pleiotropic effects (i.e., multiple biologic activities) on a large number of cell types. (Autocrine signaling means that the autocrine agent [in this case cytokines] binds to receptors on the cell that secreted the agent, whereas paracrine signaling affects other nearby cells.) Simply put, cytokines bind to cell surface receptors and trigger a sequence of intracellular events that lead ultimately to the production of protein by the target cell that alters that cell's behavior and could result in, for example, the increased secretion of more cytokines in a positive feedback loop.

Cytokines are produced by a large number of cell types, including infiltrating inflammatory cells (e.g., neutrophils, macrophages, lymphocytes), as well as resident cells in the periodontium (e.g., fibroblasts, epithelial cells). Cytokines signal, broadcast, and amplify immune responses, and they are fundamentally important for regulating immune–inflammatory responses and for combating infections. They have profound biologic effects that also lead to tissue damage with chronic inflammation; the prolonged and excessive production of cytokines and other inflammatory mediators in the periodontium leads to the tissue damage that characterizes the clinical signs of the disease. For example, cytokines mediate connective tissue and alveolar bone destruction through the induction of fibroblasts and osteoclasts to produce proteolytic enzymes (i.e., MMPs) that break down structural components of these connective tissues.[10]

Significant overlap and redundancy exist in the functions of individual cytokines. Cytokines do not act in isolation; rather, they function in flexible and complex networks that involve both proinflammatory and antiinflammatory effects and that bring together aspects of both innate and acquired immunity.[7] Cytokines play a key role at all stages of the immune response in periodontal diseases.[141]

Prostaglandins

The prostaglandins (PGs) are a group of lipid compounds derived from arachidonic acid, a polyunsaturated fatty acid found in the plasma membrane of most cells. Arachidonic acid is metabolized by cyclooxygenase-1 and 2 (COX-1 and COX-2) to generate a series of related compounds called the *prostanoids,* which include the PGs, the thromboxanes, and the prostacyclins. PGs are important mediators of inflammation, particularly prostaglandin E_2 (PGE_2), which results in vasodilation and induces cytokine production by a variety of cell types. COX-2 is up-regulated by IL-1β, TNF-α, and bacterial LPS, thus resulting in increased production of PGE_2 in inflamed tissues. PGE_2 is produced by various types of cells and most significantly in the periodontium by macrophages and fibroblasts. PGE_2 results in the induction of MMPs and osteoclastic bone resorption, and it has a major role in contributing to the tissue damage that characterizes periodontitis.

Matrix Metalloproteinases

MMPs are a family of proteolytic enzymes that degrade extracellular matrix molecules such as collagen, gelatin, and elastin. They are produced by a variety of cell types, including neutrophils, macrophages, fibroblasts, epithelial cells, osteoblasts, and osteoclasts. The names and functions of key MMPs are shown in Table 7.1. The nomenclature of MMPs has been based on the perception that each enzyme has its own specific substrate; for example, MMP-8 and MMP-1 are both collagenases (i.e., they break down collagen). However, it is now appreciated that MMPs usually degrade multiple substrates, with significant substrate overlap among individual MMPs.[68] The substrate-based classification is still used, however, and MMPs can be divided into collagenases, gelatinases/type IV collagenases, stromelysins, matrilysins, membrane-type metalloproteinases, and others.

MMPs are secreted in a latent form (inactive) and are activated by the proteolytic cleavage of a portion of the latent enzyme. This is achieved by proteases, such as cathepsin G, produced by neutrophils. MMPs are inhibited by proteinase inhibitors, which have antiinflammatory properties. Key inhibitors of MMPs found in the serum include the glycoprotein $α_1$-antitrypsin and $α_2$-macroglobulin, a large plasma protein produced by the liver that is capable of inactivating a wide variety of proteinases. Inhibitors of MMPs that are found in the tissues include the tissue inhibitors of metalloproteinases (TIMPs), which are produced by many cell types; the most important in periodontal disease is TIMP-1.[18]

MMPs are also inhibited by the tetracycline class of antibiotics, which has led to the development of a subantimicrobial formulation of doxycycline as an adjunctive systemic drug treatment for periodontitis. Doxycycline, like all the tetracyclines, possesses the ability to down-regulate MMPs, and this was recognized as representing a potential novel treatment strategy for periodontitis. The subantimicrobial formulation has been shown to inhibit collagenase activity in the gingival tissues and GCF of patients with chronic periodontitis,[59] and some clinical trials have investigated the clinical effect of using this formulation of doxycycline as an adjunct to periodontal therapy.[139]

TABLE 7.1   Classification of Matrix Metalloproteinases

Group	Enzyme	Name
Collagenases	MMP-1	Collagenase 1, fibroblast collagenase
	MMP-8	Collagenase 2, neutrophil collagenase
	MMP-13	Collagenase 3
Gelatinases	MMP-2	Gelatinase A
	MMP-9	Gelatinase B
Stromelysins	MMP-3	Stromelysin 1
	MMP-10	Stromelysin 2
	MMP-11	Stromelysin 3
Matrilysins	MMP-7	Matrilysin 1, pump-1
	MMP-26	Matrilysin 2
Membrane-type MMPs	MMP-14	MT1-MMP
	MMP-15	MT2-MMP
	MMP-16	MT3-MMP
	MMP-17	MT4-MMP
	MMP-24	MT5-MMP
	MMP-25	MT6-MMP
Others	MMP-12	Macrophage elastase
	MMP-19	—
	MMP-20	Enamelysin

MMPs, Matrix metalloproteinases; *MT,* membrane type.
Adapted from Hannas AR, Pereira JC, Granjeiro JM, et al: The role of matrix metalloproteinases in the oral environment. *Acta Odontol Scand* 65:1–13, 2007.

Properties of Key Types of Inflammatory Mediators in Periodontitis

Cytokines	Proteins that transmit signals from one cell to another Bind to cell surface receptors to trigger production of protein by the cell There are proinflammatory and antiinflammatory cytokines. A key proinflammatory cytokine is interleukin-1β, which up-regulates inflammatory responses and is produced by multiple cell types in the periodontium.
Prostaglandins	Lipid compounds derived from arachidonic acid Prostaglandin E_2 (PGE_2) is a key inflammatory mediator, stimulating production of other inflammatory mediators and cytokine production. PGE_2 also stimulates bone resorption and plays a key role in periodontitis progression.
Matrix metalloproteinases (MMPs)	A group of enzymes that break down structural proteins of the body MMPs include collagenases, which break down collagen. Key MMPs in periodontitis include MMP-8 and MMP-9, which are produced by neutrophils as they migrate through the periodontal tissues, thus contributing to periodontal tissue breakdown.

Role of Specific Inflammatory Mediators in Periodontal Disease

Interleukin-1 Family Cytokines

The IL-1 family of cytokines comprises at least 11 members, including IL-1α, IL-1β, IL-1 receptor antagonist (IL-1Ra), IL-18, and IL-33.[141]

IL-1β plays a key role in inflammation and immunity; it is closely linked to the innate immune response, and it induces the synthesis and secretion of other mediators that contribute to inflammatory changes and tissue damage. For example, IL-1β stimulates the synthesis of PGE_2, platelet-activating factor, and nitrous oxide, thereby resulting in vascular changes associated with inflammation and increasing blood flow to the site of infection or tissue injury. IL-1β is mainly produced by monocytes, macrophages, and neutrophils and also by other cell types such as fibroblasts, keratinocytes, epithelial cells, B cells, and osteocytes.[40] IL-1β increases the expression of ICAM-1 on endothelial cells and stimulates the secretion of the chemokine CXCL8 (IL-8), thereby stimulating and facilitating the infiltration of neutrophils into the affected tissues. IL-1β also synergizes with other proinflammatory cytokines and PGE_2 to induce bone resorption. IL-1β has a role in adaptive immunity; it regulates the development of antigen-presenting cells (APCs) (e.g., dendritic cells), stimulates IL-6 secretion by macrophages (which, in turn, activates B cells), and has been shown to enhance the antigen-mediated stimulation of T cells.[13] GCF concentrations of IL-1β are increased at sites affected by gingivitis[70] and periodontitis,[99] and tissue levels of IL-1β correlate with clinical periodontal disease severity.[167] Studies in experimental animals have shown that IL-1β exacerbates inflammation and alveolar bone resorption.[88] It is clear from the multiplicity of studies that have investigated this cytokine that IL-1β plays a fundamental role in the pathogenesis of periodontal disease.[92]

IL-1α is primarily an intracellular protein that is not normally secreted and that therefore is not usually found in the extracellular environment or in the circulation.[43] Unlike IL-1β, biologically active IL-1α is constitutively expressed and likely mediates inflammation only when it is released from necrotic cells, thus acting as an "alarmin" to signal the immune system during cell and tissue damage.[16] The precise role of IL-1α in periodontal pathogenesis is not well defined, although studies have reported elevated IL-1α levels in GCF and gingival tissues in patients with periodontitis.[142] IL-1α is a potent bone-resorbing factor involved in the bone loss that is associated with inflammation.[172] It is possible that the measured level of IL-1α in gingival tissues represents intracellular IL-1α that has been released from damaged or necrotic cells, and it is probable that IL-1α plays a role in periodontal pathogenesis, possibly as a signaling cytokine (signaling tissue damage) and contributing to bone resorptive activity.

IL-1Ra has structural homology to IL-1β, and it binds to the IL-1 receptor (IL-1R1). However, the binding of IL-1Ra does not result in signal transduction; therefore, IL-1Ra antagonizes the action of IL-1β.[42] IL-1Ra is important for the regulation of inflammatory responses, and it can be considered an antiinflammatory cytokine. IL-1Ra levels have been reported to be elevated in the GCF and tissues of patients with periodontal disease, thereby suggesting that it has a role in immunoregulation in cases of periodontitis.[145]

IL-18 interacts with IL-1β and shares many of the proinflammatory effects of IL-1β.[141] It is mainly produced by stimulated monocytes and macrophages.[61] Increasing evidence suggests that IL-18 plays a significant role in inflammation and immunity. IL-18 results in proinflammatory responses, including the activation of neutrophils.[102] It is a chemoattractant for T cells,[89] and it interacts with IL-12 and IL-15 to induce interferon gamma (IFN-γ), thereby inducing T-helper (Th1) cells, which activate cell-mediated immunity.[197] Very limited

TABLE 7.2   Nomenclature of Interleukin-1 Family Cytokines

Cytokine	Systematic Name	Function
IL-1α	IL-1F1	Intracellular protein, proinflammatory, contributes to bone resorption, functions as an intracellular transcriptional regulator
IL-1β	IL-1F2	Key role in inflammation and innate immunity, synergizes with other proinflammatory mediators, major role in adaptive immunity (i.e., regulation of T cells and myeloid cells), stimulates connective tissue breakdown and bone resorption
IL-1Ra	IL-1F3	Inhibits the action of IL-1α and IL-1β
IL-18	IL-1F4	Similar proinflammatory profile to IL-1β, activates neutrophils, synergizes with IL-12 to activate T-helper 1 cells
IL-1F5	IL-1F5	Antiinflammatory effects via IL-4 induction, antagonizes IL-1F6 action
IL-1F6	IL-1F6	Proinflammatory but restricted expression (e.g., localized to skin)
IL-1F7	IL-1F7	Antiinflammatory, acts as an intracellular regulator, reduces production of lipopolysaccharide-stimulated proinflammatory cytokines
IL-1F8	IL-1F8	Proinflammatory but restricted expression (e.g., localized to skin and synovial tissues)
IL-1F9	IL-1F9	Proinflammatory but restricted expression (e.g., localized to skin, placenta, and esophagus)
IL-1F10	IL-1F10	Putative antagonist with antiinflammatory action
IL-33	IL-1F11	Activation of T-helper 2 cells and mast cells, functions as an intracellular transcriptional regulator but restricted expression (e.g., endothelial cells, smooth muscle cells, and fibroblasts)

IL, Interleukin; *IL-1F,* interleukin-1 family.

direct evidence exists for a role of IL-18 in periodontal pathogenesis. Oral epithelial cells secrete IL-18 in response to stimulation with LPS,[146] and a correlation between GCF IL-18 levels and sulcus depth has been reported.[81] IL-18 levels have been reported to be higher than those of IL-1β in patients with periodontitis, thereby suggesting that IL-18—along with IL-1β—is predominant in periodontitis lesions.[131] Because IL-18 has the ability to induce either Th1 or Th2 differentiation, it is likely to play an important role in periodontal disease pathogenesis.[132]

Other Interleukin-1 Family Cytokines

Six new members of the IL-1 family (IL-1F) of cytokines have been identified on the basis of their sequence homology, structure, gene location, and receptor binding.[4,9] Several of these cytokines were identified by different research groups, who gave them a variety of names, and proposals were suggested for renaming all the IL-1F cytokines in a more consistent manner, as indicated in Table 7.2. Our knowledge of the role of these cytokines in inflammation and immunity is very limited at present, and some of these cytokines may be evolutionarily redundant. IL-1F6, IL-1F8, and IL-1F9 are potential agonists (stimulating proinflammatory responses),[19,180] whereas IL-1F5 and IL-1F10 are potential antagonists.[19,33,103] IL-1F7 appears to have antiinflammatory action.[44] It has five splice variants and one isoform, IL-1F7b, which is highly expressed by monocytes and up-regulated by LPS.[23] An intracellular mode of action has been suggested for IL-1F7b; it translocates to the nucleus of macrophages, and it may act as a transcriptional modulator by reducing the production of LPS-stimulated proinflammatory cytokines, thus supporting an antiinflammatory role for this cytokine.[163]

The novel IL-1F cytokines have limited tissue expression. For example, the agonists IL-1F6, IL-1F8, and IL-1F9 are mainly expressed in skin.[180] Therefore, although the primary cellular sources of IL-1β and IL-18 are hematopoietic cells (e.g., neutrophils, macrophages, monocytes, lymphocytes), IL-1F5 through IL-1F10 are mainly expressed outside of these lineages. At present, no clear data support a role for IL-1F5 through IL-1F10 in periodontal pathogenesis. However, given that they are expressed mainly by epithelial cells, it will be interesting to learn whether they may play a role in inflammatory responses in the gingiva. This is relevant given the continual exposure of gingival epithelial cells to bacterial challenge, and these cytokines also have properties similar to the primary cytokines (e.g., IL-1β). For example, LPS results in the up-regulation of IL-1F6, IL-1F8, and IL-1F9, and these cytokines also stimulate the secretion of IL-6 and IL-8.[180] *P. gingivalis* LPS up-regulates IL-1F9 mRNA expression in monocytes, although it does not have an effect on IL-1F6, IL-1F7, IL-1F8, or IL-1F10.[9]

IL-33, which is also known as IL-1F11, is of interest because, uniquely among the IL-1 cytokines, it stimulates the production of Th2 cytokines (e.g., IL-5, IL-13), it activates Th2 cells, and it plays a role in mast cell development and function.[1,74,90,118,152] IL-33 is mainly found in nonimmune cells such as bronchial and arterial smooth muscle cells and epithelial cells from the bronchus.[152] It is constitutively expressed in the endothelial cells of small and large blood vessels, in the fibroblastic reticular cells of lymphoid tissues, and in epithelial cells.[26,119] Our knowledge of the expression of IL-33 in myeloid immune cells and of any role in periodontitis pathogenesis is very limited. However, it has been reported that IL-33 activates Th2 cells[152] and is chemoattractant for these cells.[90] Given that Th2 cells are likely to play a role in the destructive phases of periodontal disease and that the balance of T-cell subsets is an important factor in determining disease progression,[56] IL-33 may yet prove to play a role in periodontal pathogenesis.

Tumor Necrosis Factor Alpha

TNF-α is a key inflammatory mediator in periodontal disease, and it shares many of the cellular actions of IL-1β.[62] It plays a fundamental role in immune responses, it increases neutrophil activity, and it mediates cell and tissue turnover by inducing MMP secretion. TNF-α stimulates the development of osteoclasts and limits tissue repair by the induction of apoptosis in fibroblasts. TNF-α is secreted by activated macrophages, as well as by other cell types, particularly in response to bacterial LPS. The proinflammatory effects of TNF-α include the stimulation of endothelial cells to express selectins that facilitate leukocyte recruitment, the activation of macrophage IL-1β production, and the induction of PGE$_2$ by macrophages and gingival fibroblasts.[133] TNF-α—although possessing similar activity to IL-1β—has a less potent effect on osteoclasts, and it is present at lower levels in inflamed gingival tissues than IL-1β.[168] GCF levels of TNF-α increase as gingival inflammation develops, and higher levels are found in individuals with periodontitis.[62,70]

Interleukin-6 and Related Cytokines

The cytokines in this group—which include IL-6, IL-11, leukemia-inhibitory factor (LIF), and oncostatin M—share common signaling pathways through signal transducers glycoprotein (gp) 130.[71] IL-6 is the most extensively studied of this group, and it has pleiotropic proinflammatory properties.[86] IL-6 secretion is stimulated by cytokines such as IL-1β and TNF-α, and it is produced by a range of immune cells (e.g., T cells, B cells, macrophages, dendritic cells), as well as resident cells (e.g., keratinocytes, endothelial cells, fibroblasts).[186] IL-6 is also secreted by osteoblasts, and it stimulates bone resorption and the development of osteoclasts.[78,94] IL-6 is elevated in the cells, tissues, and GCF of patients with periodontal disease.[55,104] IL-6 may have an influence on monocyte differentiation into osteoclasts and a role in bone resorption in patients with periodontal disease.[130] IL-6 also has a key role in regulating the proliferation and differentiation of B cells and T cells, particularly the Th17 subset.[86] IL-6 therefore has an important role in periodontal pathogenesis, although less than that of IL-1β or TNF-α.

IL-6 also has many activities outside of the immune system, such as in the cardiovascular and nervous systems. It has an important role in hematopoiesis and in signaling the production of C-reactive protein (CRP) in the liver. Furthermore, IL-6 stimulates T-cell differentiation and function, and it is important in the regulation of the balance of T-cell subsets, particularly the activation of Th17 cells (a subset of T cells that produce IL-17) and the balance with regulatory T cells (T$_{reg}$ cells).[14]

Prostaglandin E$_2$

The cells primarily responsible for PGE$_2$ production in the periodontium are macrophages and fibroblasts. PGE$_2$ levels are increased in the tissues and in GCF at sites undergoing periodontal attachment loss. PGE$_2$ induces the secretion of MMPs, as well as osteoclastic bone resorption, and it contributes significantly to the alveolar bone loss seen with periodontitis. PGE$_2$ release from monocytes from patients with severe or aggressive periodontitis is greater than that from monocytes from patients who are periodontally healthy.[54,128] A large body of evidence has demonstrated the importance of PGE$_2$ in periodontal pathogenesis, and given that prostaglandins are inhibited by nonsteroidal antiinflammatory drugs (NSAIDs), researchers have investigated the use of NSAIDs as potential host–response modulators in the management of periodontal disease.[193,194] However, daily administration for extended periods is necessary for the periodontal benefits to become apparent, and NSAIDs are associated with significant unwanted side effects, including gastrointestinal problems, hemorrhage (from impaired platelet aggregation resulting from inhibition of thromboxane formation), and renal and hepatic impairment. NSAIDs are therefore not indicated as adjunctive treatments for the management of periodontitis (see Chapter 54).

The prostaglandins, including PGE$_2$, are derived from the COX pathway of arachidonic acid metabolism. The two main isoforms of the COX enzyme are COX-1 and COX-2. COX-1 is constitutively expressed and has antithrombogenic and cytoprotective functions. COX-2 is induced after stimulation with various cytokines, growth factors, and LPS. The inhibition of COX-1 by nonselective NSAIDs

results in the majority of the unwanted side effects associated with NSAID usage, such as gastrointestinal ulceration and impaired hemostasis. The induction of COX-2 results in the production of elevated quantities of prostaglandins (e.g., PGE$_2$); therefore, the inhibition of COX-2 by NSAIDs that selectively inhibit COX-2 results in a reduction of inflammation without the unwanted effects commonly seen after long-term NSAID use. Preliminary studies in animal models have shown that selective COX-2 inhibitors slowed alveolar bone loss,[15,75] and human studies confirmed that prostaglandin production in the periodontal tissues was modified.[187] However, in a dramatic and unfortunate development, the selective COX-2 inhibitors were later identified to be associated with significant and life-threatening adverse events, thereby resulting in several of these drugs being withdrawn from the market.[46] The selective COX-2 inhibitors therefore cannot be considered as adjunctive treatments for periodontal disease.

Matrix Metalloproteinases

MMPs are a family of zinc-dependent enzymes that are capable of degrading extracellular matrix molecules, including collagens.[18,147] MMPs play a key role in periodontal tissue destruction and are secreted by the majority of cell types in the periodontium, including fibroblasts, keratinocytes, endothelial cells, osteoclasts, neutrophils, and macrophages. In healthy tissues, MMPs are mainly produced by fibroblasts, which produce MMP-1 (also known as *collagenase-1*), and these have a role in the maintenance of the periodontal connective tissues. The transcription of genes coding for MMPs is up-regulated by cytokines such as IL-1β and TNF-α.[109] MMP activity is regulated by specific endogenous TIMPs and serum glycoproteins such as α-macroglobulins, which form complexes with active MMPs and their latent precursors.[144] TIMPs are produced by fibroblasts, macrophages, keratinocytes, and endothelial cells; they are specific inhibitors that bind to MMPs in a 1:1 stoichiometry.[68] MMPs are also produced by some periodontal pathogens, such as *A. actinomycetemcomitans* and *P. gingivalis,* but the relative contribution of these bacterially derived MMPs to periodontal pathogenesis is small. Most MMP activity in the periodontal tissues is derived from infiltrating inflammatory cells.

In healthy periodontal tissues, collagen homeostasis is a controlled process that is mediated extracellularly by MMP-1 (expressed by resident cells, primarily fibroblasts) and intracellularly by a variety of lysosomal-acid–dependent enzymes. In inflamed periodontal tissues, excessive quantities of MMPs are secreted by resident cells and by the large numbers of infiltrating inflammatory cells (particularly neutrophils) as they migrate through the tissues. As a result, the balance between MMPs and their inhibitors is disrupted, resulting in breakdown of the connective tissue matrix[18,175] and leading to the development of collagen-depleted areas within the connective tissues, as described previously. Neutrophils are key infiltrating cells in periodontitis that accumulate in large numbers in inflamed periodontal tissues (see Fig. 7.2). Neutrophils have evolved to respond rapidly and aggressively to external stimuli, such as bacterial LPS, and they release large quantities of destructive enzymes very rapidly.[124] The predominant MMPs in periodontitis, MMP-8 and MMP-9, are secreted by neutrophils,[60] and they are very effective at degrading type 1 collagen, which is the most abundant collagen type in the periodontal ligament.[111] MMP-8 and MMP-9 levels increase with increasing severity of periodontal disease and decrease after treatment.[59,60,84] The prolonged and excessive release of large quantities of MMPs in the periodontium leads to the significant breakdown of structural components of the connective tissues, thereby contributing to the clinical signs of disease.

MMPs play a fundamental role in connective tissue homeostasis, as well as disease pathogenesis, and they possess a wide range of

TABLE 7.3   Biologic Activities of Selected Matrix Metalloproteinases Relevant to Periodontal Disease

MMP Type	Enzyme	Biologic Activity
Collagenases	All	Degrade interstitial collagens (types I, II, and III)
		Digest ECM and non-ECM molecules
	MMP-1	Keratinocyte migration and re-epithelialization
		Platelet aggregation
	MMP-13	Osteoclast activation
Gelatinases	All	Degrade denatured collagens and gelatin
	MMP-2	Differentiation of mesenchymal cells with inflammatory phenotype
		Epithelial cell migration
		Increased bioavailability of MMP-9
Stromelysins	All	Digest ECM molecules
	MMP-3	Activate pro-MMPs
		Disrupted cell aggregation
		Increased cell invasion
Matrilysins	MMP-7	Disrupted cell aggregation
		Increased cell invasion
Membrane-type MMPs	All	Digest ECM molecules
		Activate pro-MMP-2 (except MT4-MMP)
	MT1-MMP	Epithelial cell migration
		Degrade collagen types I, II, and III

ECM, Extracellular matrix; *MMPs,* matrix metalloproteinases; *MT,* membrane type.
Adapted from Hannas AR, Pereira JC, Granjeiro JM, et al: The role of matrix metalloproteinases in the oral environment. *Acta Odontol Scand* 65:1–13, 2007.

biologic effects that are relevant in periodontitis (Table 7.3). MMPs are important in alveolar bone destruction. They are expressed by osteoclasts, which also express cathepsin K. Cathepsin K is a lysosomal cysteine protease that is mainly expressed in osteoclasts and that plays a key role in bone resorption and remodeling. This enzyme can catabolize collagen, gelatin, and elastin and can therefore contribute to the breakdown of bone and cartilage.

MMPs are critical for osteoclast access to the resorption site, particularly for MMP-9 and MMP-14. MMP-14 is located in the ruffled border of osteoclasts, and osteoblasts and osteocytes (but not osteoclasts) express MMP-13, which is present in resorption lacunae and functions to remove collagen remnants left over by osteoclasts.[68] MMPs also contribute to osteoclast recruitment and activity by releasing cytokines and receptor activator of nuclear factor-κB ligand (RANKL; see later). MMPs are also important in osteoblastic bone formation, including MMP-2, MMP-9, MMP-13, and MMP-14. MMP-14 also contributes to normal bone homeostasis, and MMP-14–activated transforming growth factor beta (TGF-β) inhibits osteoblast apoptosis.

Chemokines

Chemokines are cytokine-like molecules that are characterized by their chemotactic activity.[28] This activity gave rise to the term *chemokine* (i.e., they are chemotactic cytokines). Chemokines orchestrate leukocyte recruitment in physiologic and pathologic conditions,[20] so they are important for periodontal pathogenesis, which results in the chemotactic migration of neutrophils through the periodontal tissues toward the site of the bacterial challenge in the periodontal pocket.[164] Chemokines play a key role in neutrophil recruitment and the recruitment of other adaptive and innate immune cells to the site of immune and inflammatory responses. The chemokines are divided into two subfamilies according to structural similarity: the CC subfamily and the CXC subfamily.[162] The chemokine CXCL8, which is more familiarly known as IL-8, has been demonstrated to be localized in the gingival tissues in areas of plaque accumulation and in the presence of neutrophilic infiltration,[178] and it has also been found in GCF.[112] Interaction between bacteria and keratinocytes results in the up-regulation of IL-8 and ICAM-1 expression in the gingival epithelium and the development of a chemotactic gradient of these molecules in the gingiva, thereby stimulating neutrophil migration into the tissues and the gingival sulcus.[177,179] Similar chemotactic gradients are also present in the gingiva of periodontally healthy individuals; this suggests a role for this process in the maintenance of periodontal health and supports the findings of infiltrating neutrophils being present even in clinically healthy tissues.[179]

It is becoming clear that chemokines play an important role in leukocyte migration in periodontal disease. CCL2 and CCL5 (also known as *regulated on activation, normal T-cell expressed and secreted* [RANTES]) play a role in macrophage migration, and CCL3 (also known as *macrophage inflammatory protein-1α* [MIP-1α]) and CXCL10 play a role in T-cell migration in inflamed periodontal tissues.[164] Chemokines play important roles in immune responses, repair, and inflammation, and they regulate osteoclast activity by influencing myeloid cell differentiation into osteoclasts, which may be of particular importance in the context of periodontitis.

Antiinflammatory Cytokines

The balance between proinflammatory and antiinflammatory events is crucial for determining disease progression, and it is now clear that individual cytokines do not act in isolation but rather as part of complex networks of mediators that have different functional activities. Antiinflammatory cytokines include IL-10, TGF-β, IL-1Ra, IL-1F5, and possibly IL-1F10.

The IL-10 family of cytokines has multiple pleiotropic effects and possesses immunosuppressive properties.[32,34] IL-10 is produced by T$_{reg}$ cells, monocytes, and B cells, and it suppresses cytokine secretion by Th1 cells, Th2 cells, monocytes, and macrophages. The role of IL-10 in periodontal disease has been minimally studied, but animal models support that IL-10 down-regulates inflammatory responses. For example, IL-10 knockout mice are more susceptible to alveolar bone loss than wild-type mice.[150] IL-10 is also present in GCF and periodontal tissues.[76]

TGF-β is a growth factor that functions as a cytokine and has immunoregulatory roles, such as the regulation of T-cell subsets and the action of T$_{reg}$ cells, and it also plays a role in repair and regeneration.[195] It has multifunctional roles in various cellular functions, including angiogenesis, the synthesis of the extracellular matrix, apoptosis, and the inhibition of cell growth. TGF-β levels are higher in the GCF and periodontal tissues of patients with periodontitis and gingivitis than in patients who are periodontally healthy.[67]

Linking Pathogenesis to Clinical Signs of Disease

Advanced forms of periodontal disease are characterized by the symptoms of tooth mobility, tooth loss, and tooth migration. These result from the loss of attachment between the tooth and its supporting tissues after the breakdown of the inserting fibers of the periodontal ligament and the resorption of alveolar bone. Having reviewed the histopathology and the inflammatory processes that develop in the periodontal tissues as a result of prolonged accumulation of dental biofilm, it is now necessary to link these changes to the structural damage that occurs in the periodontium, thereby leading to the well-defined signs of disease.

Even clinically healthy tissues demonstrate signs of inflammation when histologic sections are examined. For example, transmigrating neutrophils are evident in clinically healthy gingival tissues moving toward the sulcus for the purpose of eliminating bacteria. If the inflammation becomes more extensive, then vasodilation and increased vascular permeability lead to edema of the tissues, as well as erythema, thereby causing gingival swelling and a slight deepening of the sulcus and further compromising plaque removal. The increased infiltration of inflammatory cells (particularly neutrophils) and the breakdown of collagen result in the development of collagen-depleted areas below the epithelium; as a result, the epithelium proliferates to maintain tissue integrity.

The epithelium provides a physical barrier to impede the ingress of bacteria and their products; therefore, the disruption of the epithelial barrier can lead to further bacterial invasion and inflammation. Antimicrobial peptides, which are also called *defensins,* are expressed by epithelial cells, and gingival epithelial cells express two human β-defensins (hBD-1 and hBD-2). Furthermore, a cathelicidin class antimicrobial peptide, LL-37, which is found in the lysosomes of neutrophils, is also expressed in gingiva. These antimicrobial peptides are important for determining the outcomes of the host–pathogen interactions at the epithelial barrier.[190] The epithelium is therefore more than simply a passive barrier: it also has an active role in innate immunity.[37] Epithelial cells in the junctional and sulcular epithelium are in constant contact with bacterial products and respond to these products by secreting chemokines (e.g., IL-8, CXCL8) to attract neutrophils, which migrate up the chemotactic gradient toward the pocket. Epithelial cells are therefore active in responding to infection and signaling further host responses.

If the bacterial challenge persists, the cellular and fluid infiltrate continues to develop, and neutrophils and other inflammatory cells soon occupy a significant volume of the inflamed gingival tissues. Neutrophils are key components of the innate immune system, and they play a fundamental role in maintaining periodontal health, despite the constant challenge presented by the plaque biofilm.[124] Neutrophils are protective leukocytes that phagocytose and kill bacteria, and deficiencies in neutrophil functioning result in increased susceptibility to infections in general, as well as periodontal disease.[100] Neutrophils also release large quantities of destructive enzymes (e.g., MMPs) as they migrate through the tissues (particularly MMP-8 and MMP-9), a process that results in the breakdown of structural components of the periodontium and the development of collagen-depleted areas. Neutrophils also release their potent lysosomal enzymes, cytokines, and reactive oxygen species (ROS) extracellularly, thereby causing further tissue damage.[82] Neutrophil hyperactivity in periodontitis has also been suggested, which leads to the overproduction of damaging ROS and other mediators.[52] Patients with periodontitis have been reported to have neutrophils that demonstrate enhanced enzymatic activity and that produce increased levels of ROS.[113,114] However, it is not yet clear whether the enhanced responsiveness of neutrophils is the result of the innate properties of the neutrophils in certain individuals, of priming by cytokines or bacteria, or of a combination of these factors. It is certainly clear, however, that the extracellular release of lysosomal enzymes contributes to continued tissue damage and collagen depletion in the periodontal tissues. The degeneration of fibroblasts limits opportunities for repair, and the epithelium continues to proliferate apically, thus deepening the pocket

further; the pocket is then rapidly colonized by the subgingival bacteria.

The very first steps in the development of the pocket result from a combination of factors, including the detachment of cells at the coronal aspect of the junctional epithelium, whereas cells at the apical aspect migrate apically into the collagen-depleted areas; intraepithelial cleavage occurs within the junctional epithelium.[106,155,171] Epithelial tissues do not have their own blood supply and must rely on the diffusion of nutrients from the underlying connective tissues. Thus, as the epithelium proliferates and thickens, necrosis of epithelial cells that are more distant from the connective tissues can lead to intraepithelial clefts and splits, which also contribute to the early stages of pocket formation.

CLINICIAN'S CORNER

How does a pocket develop?

The bacterial biofilm causes inflammation in the gingival tissues that causes swelling, and therefore the sulcus deepens slightly. The inflammatory response may subsequently spread to the deeper tissues and is characterized by infiltration by defense cells and breakdown of collagen in the connective tissues. The junctional epithelium migrates apically to maintain an intact epithelial barrier, and thus the sulcus becomes deeper again and is now referred to as a pocket. Bacteria in the biofilm proliferate apically, exploiting and perpetuating this environmental niche. The bacteria are never completely eradicated by the host response, and thus they continue to provoke an immune–inflammatory response, leading to progressing tissue breakdown, continued apical migration of the junctional epithelium, resorption of alveolar bone, and gradual deepening of the pocket.

A cycle of chronic inflammation is therefore established in which the presence of subgingival bacteria drives inflammatory responses in the periodontal tissues; this is characterized by infiltration by leukocytes, the release of inflammatory mediators and destructive enzymes, connective tissue breakdown, and the breakdown and proliferation of the epithelium in an apical direction. The junctional and pocket epithelia become thin and ulcerated and bleed more readily, a condition that results in bleeding on probing. The bacteria in the pocket are never fully eliminated because they are effectively outside the body, but their continued presence drives the destructive inflammatory response in the periodontal tissues. Attempts at effective oral hygiene are rendered more difficult by the deepening of the pocket, and the cycle continues.

Alveolar Bone Resorption

As the advancing inflammatory front approaches the alveolar bone, osteoclastic bone resorption commences.[31] This is a protective mechanism to prevent bacterial invasion of the bone, but it ultimately leads to tooth mobility and even tooth loss. The resorption of alveolar bone occurs simultaneously with the breakdown of the periodontal ligament in the inflamed periodontal tissues. Two critical factors determine whether bone loss occurs: (1) the concentration of inflammatory mediators in the gingival tissues must be sufficient to activate the pathways that lead to bone resorption; and (2) the inflammatory mediators must penetrate to within a critical distance of the alveolar bone.[62]

Histologic studies have confirmed that the bone resorbs so that a width of noninfiltrated connective tissue of about 0.5 to 1.0 mm overlying the bone is always present.[188] It has also been demonstrated that bone resorption ceases when at least a 2.5-mm distance is present between the site of bacteria in the pocket and the bone.[136] Osteoclasts are stimulated by proinflammatory cytokines and other mediators of inflammation to resorb the bone, and the alveolar bone "retreats" from the advancing inflammatory front. Osteoclasts are multinucleated cells that are formed from osteoclast progenitor cells and macrophages, and osteoclastic bone resorption is activated by a variety of mediators (e.g., IL-1β, TNF-α, IL-6, PGE$_2$).[122] Other mediators that also stimulate bone resorption include LIF, oncostatin M, bradykinin, thrombin, and various chemokines.[101]

Receptor Activator of Nuclear Factor-κB Ligand and Osteoprotegerin

A key system for controlling bone turnover is the receptor activator of nuclear factor-κB (RANK)/RANK ligand (RANKL)/osteoprotegerin (OPG) system. RANK is a cell surface receptor expressed by osteoclast progenitor cells, as well as by mature osteoclasts. RANKL is a ligand that binds to RANK and is produced as either a membrane-bound or secreted protein by a range of cells, including fibroblasts, osteoblasts, mesenchymal cells, and T- and B-lymphocytes. OPG is the inhibitor of RANKL and functions as a decoy receptor—that is, it binds to RANKL and prevents it from interacting with RANK. OPG is secreted primarily by osteoblasts, fibroblasts, and bone marrow stromal cells. The binding of RANKL to RANK results in osteoclast differentiation and activation, and thus bone resorption. The balance between RANKL and OPG activity (often referred to as the *RANKL:OPG ratio*) can therefore determine bone resorption or bone formation.

IL-1β and TNF-α regulate the expression of RANKL and OPG, and T cells express RANKL, which binds directly to RANK on the surfaces of osteoclast progenitors and osteoclasts, thereby resulting in cell activation and differentiation to form mature osteoclasts. In individuals with periodontitis, elevated levels of proinflammatory cytokines (e.g., IL-1β, TNF-α) and increasing numbers of infiltrating T cells result in the activation of osteoclasts by RANK, which results in alveolar bone loss. It has been reported that levels of RANKL are higher and that levels of OPG are lower in sites with active periodontal breakdown as compared with sites with healthy gingiva.[35] In addition, GCF RANKL/OPG ratios are higher in periodontitis than in healthy tissue.[21] It is clear that alterations in the relative levels of these key regulators of osteoclasts play a key role in the bone loss that characterizes periodontal disease.

RANK/RANKL/OPG System	
RANK (receptor activator of nuclear factor-κB)	Cell surface receptor on osteoclast progenitor cells
RANKL (RANK ligand)	Cytokine-like molecule that is the ligand for RANK (i.e., binds to RANK) and causes maturation into fully differentiated osteoclasts
OPG (osteoprotegerin)	Cytokine-like molecule that binds to RANKL and inhibits the interaction between RANKL and RANK

The RANK/RANKL/OPG signaling pathway plays a key role in regulating bone resorption. RANKL binds to RANK and stimulates osteoclast differentiation and activation. OPG antagonizes this action by binding to RANKL and preventing it from binding to RANK. The ratio of RANKL to OPG is important, with studies reporting higher levels of RANKL and lower levels of OPG in patients with advanced periodontitis compared with healthy controls.

Resolution of Inflammation

Inflammation is an important defense mechanism to combat the threat of bacterial infection, but inflammation also results in tissue damage associated with the development and progression of most chronic diseases associated with aging, including periodontal disease.[183,185] It is becoming evident that the resolution of inflammation (i.e., "turning off" inflammation) is an active process that is regulated by specific mechanisms that restore homeostasis (see Chapter 10). It is possible that controlling or augmenting these mechanisms may lead to the development of new treatment strategies for managing chronic diseases such as periodontitis.[83] The resolution of inflammation is an active process that results in a return to homeostasis, and it is mediated by specific molecules, including a class of endogenous, proresolving lipid mediators that includes the lipoxins, resolvins, and protectins.[158] These molecules are actively synthesized during the resolution phases of acute inflammation; they are antiinflammatory, and they inhibit neutrophil infiltration. They are also chemoattractants, but they do not cause inflammation. For example, lipoxins stimulate infiltration by monocytes but without stimulating the release of inflammatory cytokines.

Lipoxins

The lipoxins include lipoxin A$_4$ (LXA$_4$) and lipoxin B$_4$ (LXB$_4$), and the appearance of these molecules signals the resolution of inflammation.[157] Lipoxins are lipoxygenase (LO)–derived eicosanoids that are generated from arachidonic acid. They are highly potent, they possess biologic activity at very low concentrations, and they inhibit neutrophil recruitment, chemotaxis, and adhesion.[170] Lipoxins also signal macrophages to phagocytose the remnants of apoptotic cells at sites of inflammation without generating an inflammatory response. Proinflammatory cytokines (e.g., IL-1β) released during acute inflammation can induce the expression of lipoxins, which promote the resolution of the inflammatory response.[115]

Resolvins and Protectins

Resolvins (i.e., resolution phase interaction products) are derived from the omega-3 fatty acids eicosapentaenoic acid and docosahexaenoic acid; they are classified as E series resolvins (RvE) and D series resolvins (RvD).[159] Resolvins inhibit neutrophil infiltration and transmigration, as well as the production of proinflammatory mediators, and they have potent antiinflammatory and immunoregulatory effects.[156] Resolvins are highly potent and have been shown to reduce neutrophil transmigration by around 50% at concentrations of as low as 10 nM.[169] Protectins are also derived from docosahexaenoic acid. They are produced by glial cells, and they reduce cytokine expression.[77] They also inhibit neutrophil infiltration, and they have been reported to reduce retinal injury[120] and stroke damage.[110]

The release of endogenous proresolving molecules (e.g., lipoxins, resolvins, protectins) that "switch off" inflammation indicates that the control of inflammation is an active process rather than simply being a passive dwindling of proinflammatory signals. These molecules could potentially offer benefit for the management of chronic diseases such as periodontitis. This concept has been tested in animal models of periodontitis.[184] In a rabbit model of *P. gingivalis* and ligature-induced experimental periodontitis, periodontal inflammation was clearly evident after 6 weeks; this was characterized by collagen breakdown and the resorption of alveolar bone. As the experiment progressed beyond 6 weeks, 4 μg/tooth of topical resolvin E1 (RvE1) was applied three times per week for an additional 6 weeks, whereas the control group continued to receive applications of topical *P. gingivalis*. In the control group, inflammation continued and led to further alveolar bone loss, with large increases in the numbers of osteoclasts and infiltrating neutrophils, as well as significant collagen breakdown. However, in the animals that received the topical RvE1, the progression of periodontitis was prevented, the resolution of inflammation occurred, and the bone loss that had occurred during the first 6 weeks of the study was reversed, with evidence of bone gain in the RvE1-treated animals.[69] These experiments suggest that the endogenous lipid mediators that resolve inflammation could offer potential for the development of new adjunctive treatments for the management of periodontitis.

Immune Responses in Periodontal Pathogenesis

The immune system is essential for the maintenance of periodontal health, and it is central to the host response to periodontal pathogens. However, if the immune response is dysregulated, inappropriate, persistent, or excessive in some way, then damaging chronic inflammatory responses such as those observed in periodontal disease can ensue. The immune response to plaque bacteria involves the integration at the molecular, cellular, and organ level of elements that are often categorized as being part of the innate immune system or the adaptive immune system. Furthermore, host responses in periodontal disease (and other major human diseases) were until recently represented as a linear progression from the host's recognition of microbial pathogens, to innate immune responses dominated by the action of phagocytic neutrophils, and culminating in the establishment of adaptive immune responses led by antigen-specific effector functions (e.g., cytotoxic T cells, antibodies). It is now widely appreciated that immune responses are complex biologic networks in which pathogen recognition, innate immunity, and adaptive immunity are integrated and mutually dependent.[51] This complex network is flexible and dynamic, with aspects of positive and negative regulation, as well as feedback control; signals are amplified and broadcast, which leads to diverse effector functions. Furthermore, the immune system is integrated with other systems and processes, including the nervous system, hematopoiesis, and hemostasis, as well as elements of tissue repair and regeneration.[123]

Observational studies of periodontal tissues and investigations of animal models and cell and tissue systems have allowed us to identify aspects of the immune response that are relevant to periodontitis.[92,135] Immune responses, which underpin periodontal disease, have unique facets that must be considered before we can truly rationalize the detailed information that we have about individual immune cell functions and their responses to specific periodontal pathogens. Thus we need to understand how the polymicrobial biofilm (as opposed to individual species of periodontal pathogens) interacts with host immune defenses. We also need to appreciate specific immunologic properties that relate to the unique anatomy of the periodontium, to understand how immune responses contribute to the dynamic aspects of periodontal disease and its various clinical courses, and to gain a comprehension of how elements of host immunity contribute to tissue destruction, resolution, repair, and regeneration.

Innate Immunity

Defenses against infection include a wide range of mechanical, chemical, and microbiologic barriers that prevent pathogens from invading the cells and tissues of the body. Saliva, GCF, and the epithelial keratinocytes of the oral mucosa all protect the underlying tissues of the oral cavity and the periodontium. The commensal microbiota (e.g., in dental biofilm) may also be important for providing protection against infection by pathogenic microorganisms through

effective competition for resources and ecologic niches and also by stimulating protective immune responses. The complex microanatomy of the periodontium, including the diversity of specialized epithelial tissues, presents many interesting challenges for the study of the immunopathogenesis of periodontal disease.

If bacterial products enter the tissues, then the cellular and molecular elements of the innate immune response are activated. The term *innate immunity* refers to the elements of the immune response that are determined by inherited factors (and therefore "innate"), that have limited specificity, and that are "fixed" in that they do not change or improve during an immune response or as a result of previous exposure to a pathogen. The recognition of pathogenic microorganisms and the recruitment of effector cells (e.g., neutrophils) and molecules (e.g., the complement system) are central to effective innate immunity. Innate immune responses are orchestrated by a broad range of cytokines, chemokines, and cell surface receptors, and the stimulation of innate immunity leads to a state of inflammation. If innate immune responses fail to eliminate infection, then the effector cells of adaptive immune responses (lymphocytes) are activated. It is increasingly appreciated that the immune response functions as a network of interacting molecular and cellular elements in which innate immunity and adaptive (antigen-specific) immunity work together toward a common purpose. Aspects of innate immunity that are relevant to periodontal disease are now considered.

Innate Immunity	Adaptive Immunity
Refers to nonspecific defense mechanisms that act as barriers to infection. Components include: • Barriers to infection such as skin, mucosa, acid pH in the stomach • Antimicrobial molecules such as lysozyme, antimicrobial peptides • Immune system cells such as neutrophils and macrophages that kill infecting organisms • Receptors (e.g., Toll-like receptors) that recognize pathogen-derived molecules and activate immune–inflammatory responses • Antigen presentation to activate adaptive immune responses	Refers to antigen-specific immune responses. Components include: • Recognition of specific molecules on infecting organisms at the species and strain level • Cellular immune responses focused on defense from intracellular pathogens (e.g., viruses), involving cytokines from T helper cells, macrophages, and natural killer cells • Humoral immune responses focused on defense from extracellular pathogens (e.g., bacteria), involving B cells that differentiate into antibody-producing plasma cells

Innate and adaptive immunity do not function in isolation; close integration exists between the innate and adaptive arms of the immune response.

Saliva

Saliva that is secreted from the three major salivary glands (i.e., parotid, submandibular, and sublingual), as well as from the numerous minor salivary glands, has an important role in the maintenance of oral and dental health. The action of shear forces associated with

TABLE 7.4   Constituents of Saliva That Contribute to Innate Immunity

Saliva Constituent	Host Defense Function
Antibodies (e.g., immunoglobulin A)	Inhibit bacterial adherence, promote agglutination
Histatins	Neutralize lipopolysaccharides, inhibit destructive enzymes
Cystatins	Inhibit bacterial growth
Lactoferrin	Inhibits bacterial growth
Lysozyme	Lyses bacterial cell walls
Mucins	Inhibits bacterial adherence, promotes agglutination
Peroxidase	Neutralizes bacterial hydrogen peroxide

saliva flow is important for preventing the attachment of bacteria to the dentition and oral mucosal surfaces. Human saliva also contains numerous molecular components that contribute to host defenses against bacterial colonization and periodontal disease (Table 7.4). These components include molecules that non-specifically inhibit the formation of the plaque biofilm by inhibiting adherence to oral surfaces and promoting agglutination (e.g., mucins), those that inhibit specific virulence factors (e.g., histatins that neutralize LPS), and those that inhibit bacterial cell growth (e.g., lactoferrin) and that may induce cell death.[58,98] Saliva also contains specific immunoglobulin A (IgA) antibodies to periodontal pathogens that target specific antigens and that inhibit bacterial adherence.

Epithelial Tissues

The epithelial tissues play a key role in host defense because they are the main site of the initial interactions between plaque bacteria and the host, and they are also the site of the invasion of microbial pathogens. The keratinized epithelium of the sulcular and gingival epithelial tissues provides protection for the underlying periodontal tissue in addition to acting as a barrier against bacteria and their products.[12,154] By contrast, the junctional epithelium has significant intercellular spaces, it is not keratinized, and it exhibits a higher cellular turnover rate. These properties render the junctional epithelium permeable, thereby allowing for the inward movement of microbes and their products and the outward movement of GCF and the cells and molecules of innate immunity. Furthermore, the spaces between the cells of the junctional epithelium widen with inflammation, which results in increased GCF flow.[154]

Some species of periodontal bacteria invade host epithelial tissues; at the molecular level, the processes of adhesion and invasion are coupled. Studies of the invasion of gingival epithelial cells by *P. gingivalis* have served as a paradigm for the study of this process; the infection of host cells by *P. gingivalis* involves the action of proteases and cell surface fimbriae.[3,97] Invasion by *P. gingivalis* is initiated through signaling by interaction of bacterial components with surface integrins PAR-1 and PAR-2, as well as TLRs.[64,97,196] This, in turn, activates intracellular signaling pathways (e.g., mitogen-activated protein kinase) and results in the reorganization of actin filaments and microtubules and a modulation of calcium cation (Ca^{2+}) influx. It is thought that the inhibition of host cell apoptosis may facilitate the survival of intracellular bacteria and that bacteria inside of the cell are protected from the host immune response. The invasion of host cells could therefore be relevant to the spread and persistence of certain periodontal bacteria. In addition, in vivo analysis

and the studies of a three-dimensional–engineered human oral mucosa model demonstrated that *P. gingivalis* can migrate through the basement membrane of epithelial layers and invade connective tissue.[3] Histologic analysis reveals that, in the presence of periodontitis, epithelial cells become more rounded and tend to detach from the underlying connective tissue.[154] Proteases break down cell-to-cell junctions in epithelial tissues by digesting transmembrane proteins and adhesion molecules (e.g., E-cadherin). Microanatomic changes associated with the onset of periodontitis, such as the widening of the spaces between the cells of the junctional epithelium and the development of the pocket epithelium, further facilitate bacterial invasion. Bacterial spread through the basement membrane and into the underlying connective tissues is facilitated by bacterially derived proteases and host proteases derived from infiltrating neutrophils (e.g., MMPs).

At the cellular and molecular levels, most in vitro studies of epithelial cell responses to periodontal bacteria have been carried out in primary gingival epithelial cells or various immortalized cell lines derived from oral epithelial tissue; these studies have provided insight into host cell responses to periodontal bacteria.[3,64,67,196] Epithelial cells also constitutively express antimicrobial peptides (e.g., hBDs, LL-37), and the synthesis and secretion of these molecules is up-regulated in response to periodontal bacteria. Neutrophils are also a source of antimicrobial peptides (i.e., α-defensins). Antimicrobial peptides are small, polycationic peptides that disrupt bacterial cell membranes and thereby directly kill bacteria with broad specificity.

The different categories of antimicrobial peptides are defined on the basis of structural homology. The α-defensins (e.g., human neutrophil peptides 1 through 4) are expressed by neutrophils and as such are commonly found in GCF. The hBDs (e.g., hBDs 1 through 3) are expressed in the gingival epithelial cells, the salivary glands, and the tongue, as well as in immune cells (e.g., macrophages, dendritic cells); some hBDs are constitutively expressed, and others are expressed only in response to cytokines and bacterial products (e.g., gingipains of *P. gingivalis*).[3,37] A third class of antimicrobial peptides are the cathelicidins, of which LL-37 is expressed in high levels in the junctional epithelium. Like the hBDs, LL-37 has a widespread expression pattern in the mouth; it is found in the salivary glands, the tongue, and the leukocytes as well as in the connective tissue. Antimicrobial peptides have more recently assumed greater importance because it has been recognized that they have a wider role in regulating innate and adaptive immune responses to infection.[41] Thus these molecules have chemokine-like activity in that they stimulate the chemotaxis of a range of leukocytes involved in innate and acquired immunity. Antimicrobial peptides also stimulate mast cell degranulation and cytokine production, and they likely have a role in wound healing through their effect on keratinocyte differentiation. Furthermore, some interest has been expressed in their possible role in therapy for oral inflammatory diseases.[41]

Epithelial cells that are directly stimulated with bacterial components and cytokines can produce MMPs, which contribute to a loss of connective tissue. Epithelial cells also secrete a range of cytokines in response to periodontal bacteria (e.g., *P. gingivalis, A. actinomycetemcomitans, F. nucleatum, Prevotella intermedia*), which signal immune responses. These include the proinflammatory cytokines IL-1β, TNF-α, and IL-6, as well as the chemokine IL-8 (CXCL8) and the monocyte chemoattractant protein-1 (MCP-1), which serve to signal neutrophil and monocyte migration from the vasculature into the periodontal tissue. In some (but not all) experimental systems, *P. gingivalis* has been shown to inhibit IL-8; it has been suggested that this may result in a temporary local immune suppression in the periodontium and facilitate the accumulation and invasion of pathogenic periodontal bacteria and the initiation of periodontitis.[39,64] *P. gingivalis* is an example of one periodontal pathogen with a range

TABLE 7.5 Virulence Factors of *Porphyromonas gingivalis* That Interact With the Immune System

Virulence Factor	Effect on Immune System
Proteases (gingipains)	Degradation of signaling molecules (CD14) and cytokines (e.g., interleukin-1β, interleukin-6)
Cell invasion capabilities	Inhibition of interleukin-8 secretion
Lipopolysaccharides	Antagonism of the stimulatory effects of lipopolysaccharides from other species; no up-regulation of E-selectin
Fimbriae	Inhibition of interleukin-12 secretion in macrophages
Cell surface polysaccharides	Resistance to complement
Short-chain fatty acids	Induction of apoptosis in host cells

of virulence factors that affect host immune defenses,[64,97] as indicated in Table 7.5.

Gingival Crevicular Fluid

GCF originates from the postcapillary venules of the gingival plexus. It has a flushing action in the gingival crevice, but it also likely functions to bring the blood components (e.g., neutrophils, antibodies, complement components) of the host defenses into the sulcus.[63] The flow of GCF increases in inflammation, and neutrophils are an especially important component of GCF in periodontal health and disease.[92]

Pathogen Recognition and Activation of Cellular Innate Responses

If plaque bacteria and their products penetrate the periodontal tissues, specialized "sentinel cells" of the immune system recognize their presence and signal protective immune responses. These cells include macrophages and dendritic cells, which express a range of pattern recognition receptors (PRRs) that interact with microbe-associated molecular patterns (MAMPs). The activation of PRRs activates innate immune responses to provide immediate protection, and adaptive immunity is also activated with the aim of establishing a sustained antigen-specific defense. Excessive and inappropriate or dysregulated immune responses lead to chronic inflammation and the concomitant tissue destruction associated with periodontal disease.

 A glossary of terms relevant to periodontal immunobiology is presented in eTable 7.1, which can be accessed on the companion website www.expertconsult.com.

The best studied of the signaling systems involved in the recognition of plaque bacteria is the interaction of bacterial LPS with TLRs: *P. gingivalis*, *A. actinomycetemcomitans*, and *F. nucleatum* all possess LPS molecules that interact with TLR-4 to activate myeloid immune cells. However, individual species of plaque bacteria have a wide variety of MAMPs, which may interact with PRRs. For example, *P. gingivalis* LPS signals via TLRs (predominantly TLR-2), and fimbriae, proteases, and DNA from *P. gingivalis* are all recognized by host cells through interaction with specific PRRs. Certain nonimmune cells in the periodontium (e.g., epithelial cells, fibroblasts) also express PRRs and may recognize and respond to MAMPs from plaque bacteria.

Although the signaling pathways activated by PRRs may be diverse, in general terms, they converge to elicit similar host cell responses in the form of the up-regulation of cytokine secretion and, in the case of APCs such as dendritic cells, cell differentiation that leads to enhanced signaling of the adaptive immune response.

The signaling of cytokine responses by PRRs influences innate immunity (e.g., neutrophil activity), adaptive immunity (e.g., T-cell effector phenotype), and the development of destructive inflammation (e.g., the activation of fibroblasts and osteoclasts). Some cytokines are particularly important to innate immune signaling, and good evidence indicates that they have a role in immune responses in the periodontium. The archetypal proinflammatory cytokine is IL-1β, which exerts its action directly by activating other cells that express the IL-1R1 receptor (e.g., endothelial cells) or by stimulating the synthesis and secretion of other, secondary mediators such as PGE$_2$. The effect of IL-1β is amplified by a synergistic action with other cytokines such as TNF-α. The up-regulation of ICAM-1 and E-selectin on endothelial cells is central to the migration of neutrophils into the periodontium, and this is stimulated by IL-1β and TNF-α. IL-1β also stimulates the secretion of the chemokine IL-8, which stimulates neutrophil chemotaxis. IL-1β and TNF-α also activate MMP secretion from fibroblasts and osteoclasts; this facilitates the movement of neutrophils through the connective tissues (and thus protective innate responses), but it also contributes to the tissue destruction associated with periodontal disease, along with MMPs from neutrophils.

Other cytokines that are up-regulated as a result of the activation of PRRs include IL-6, which influences the development of a number of immune cells (e.g., B cells, dendritic cells) and stimulates osteoclast differentiation and thus bone turnover. Other cytokines provide specific signals that contribute to the development of specific CD4$^+$ T-helper cell subsets (e.g., IL-4, IL-12, IL-18). In addition to cytokines that activate immune responses, other cytokines are up-regulated that have a role in immune regulation by suppressing cytokine activity; these include IL-1Ra, IL-10, and TGF-β. Cytokines from T-cell subsets feed back to and modify innate immune responses; for example, IFN-γ from Th1 cells activates macrophages, IL-17 from Th17 cells synergizes with IL-1β and TNF-α to reinforce inflammatory reactions, and IL-10 and TGF-β suppress immune responses. The action of many cytokines produced in the periodontium is not limited to one aspect of the host immune response; in other words, cytokines are pleiotropic (i.e., they have multiple effects).

Neutrophil Function

Neutrophils are the "professional" phagocytes that are critical to the clearance of bacteria that invade host tissues.[124] Neutrophils are present in clinically healthy gingival tissues, and they migrate through the intercellular spaces of the junctional epithelium into the sulcus.[90,154] This is part of a "low-grade defense" against plaque bacteria, and it is necessary to prevent infection and periodontal tissue damage.[154] The importance of neutrophils to the maintenance of periodontal health is demonstrated clinically by the observations of severe periodontitis in patients with neutrophil defects.[124]

A small proportion (1% to 2%) of the intercellular spaces in healthy junctional epithelium is occupied by neutrophils (and other leukocytes at various stages of differentiation), but this can increase to 30% with even modest inflammation. In the inflammatory state, changes to the local vasculature occur in the gingiva: high endothelial venules develop from the postcapillary venules of the gingival plexus, which facilitates leukocyte emigration and increases the flow of GCF into the pocket.[154]

Neutrophils migrate from the gingival plexus to the extravascular connective tissue and then into the junctional epithelium through the basement membrane. The presence of a layer of neutrophils in the junctional epithelium forms a host defense barrier between subgingival biofilm and the gingival tissue. At the molecular level, the interaction of adhesion molecules (e.g., ICAM-1) on endothelial and epithelial cells with β2 integrins on neutrophils facilitates neutrophil migration. Indeed, evidence from immunohistochemistry studies indicate the existence of gradients of IL-8 (a "chemotactic gradient"), as well as gradients of ICAM-1, which direct the neutrophils from the vasculature into the tissues and toward the junctional epithelium.[179] The migration of neutrophils contributes to the disruption of the junctional epithelium by the degradation of the basement membrane through protease release and the action of ROS. An aspect of neutrophil-mediated immunity is the formation of neutrophil extracellular traps (NETs).[191] NETs constitute a highly conserved antimicrobial strategy in which decondensed nuclear DNA and associated histones are extruded from the neutrophil, thus forming weblike strands of DNA in the extracellular environment. These strands, in conjunction with antimicrobial peptides (AMPs), facilitate the extracellular killing of microorganisms that become trapped within the NETs. NETs can be released by viable neutrophils and also following a form of programmed cell death called NETosis. NETs are produced in response to a wide range of infecting pathogens and likely constitute an important defense strategy, but due to the concomitant release of cytotoxic molecules they can also contribute to host tissue damage. The potential role of NETs in periodontal pathogenesis is an area of ongoing research.

Adaptive Immunity

Adaptive immunity has evolved to provide a focused and intense defense against infections that overwhelm innate immune responses. Adaptive immunity is particularly important as ecologic, social, and demographic changes—which alter susceptibility to existing and emerging infective microorganisms—outpace the natural evolution of biologic systems. Furthermore, the development of effective vaccination is, along with the identification of antibiotics, perhaps one of the greatest triumphs of medical science; this success is based on knowledge of the elements and principles of adaptive immunity.

Adaptive immunity contrasts with innate immunity with regard to the dynamic of the underlying cellular and molecular responses: adaptive immunity is slower and reliant on complex interactions between APCs and T and B lymphocytes. A key element is the antigen specificity of the responses that facilitates the specific targeting of a diverse range of effector elements, including cytotoxic T cells and antibodies. Another facet is the ability of adaptive immune responses to improve during exposure to antigen and on subsequent reinfection events.[24] Our current understanding suggests that the cellular and molecular elements of adaptive immunity are more diverse than those of innate immunity, and although a role for many of these factors in periodontal disease has been identified, our knowledge is far from complete. The importance of adaptive immune responses in periodontal pathogenesis is endorsed by histologic studies of established lesions in periodontal disease.[92,135] The population of leukocytes in the periodontium in gingivitis (i.e., the early stages of responses to the plaque biofilm) and in stable periodontal lesions (i.e., those in which tissue destruction is apparently not progressing) has been reported to be dominated by T cells, and these cells are clustered mainly around blood vessels. Cell surface marker studies suggest that these cells are activated but not proliferating.[57] In addition, a predominance of the helper T-cell subset (i.e., CD4-expressing T cells) over the cytotoxic T-cell subset (i.e., CD8-expressing T cells) is observed. These T cells are considered to be proactively maintaining tissue homeostasis in the presence of the microbial challenge of the plaque biofilm.[57] By contrast, in active (progressing) periodontitis,

B cells and plasma cells predominate and are associated with pocket formation and the progression of disease.

Antigen-Presenting Cells

Central elements of the activation and function of T cells and B cells are the presentation of antigen by specialized APCs to T cells and the development of a specific cytokine milieu that influences the development of T cells with particular effector functions. APCs detect and take up microorganisms and their antigens, after which they may migrate to lymph nodes and interact with T cells to present antigen. The periodontium contains a number of APCs, including B cells, macrophages, and at least two types of dendritic cells (i.e., dermal dendritic cells and Langerhans cells).[36] It is increasingly recognized that the engagement of PRRs (and in particular TLRs) by MAMPs from pathogenic microorganisms is not only central to signaling innate immunity in the form of cytokine up-regulation but also a critical element of the activation of APCs and the elaboration of T-cell effector function. Thus TLR activation increases the expression of costimulatory molecules on APCs, which are critical to the interaction of these cells with T cells. In addition, TLR activation enhances antigen uptake and processing. Different APCs process and present antigens by different pathways and mechanisms, and this variation is one of the factors—along with the presence of specific combinations of cytokines—that influences the phenotype of T-cell effector function produced during specific immune responses.[57]

T Cells

Several different subsets of thymic lymphocytes (i.e., T cells) develop in the bone marrow and thymus and migrate to the peripheral tissues to participate in adaptive immune responses. The expression of the cell surface molecules (CD4 or CD8) or particular T-cell antigen receptors (αβ or γδ) broadly defines functional T-cell subsets that emerge from the thymus. The role of T cells in periodontal disease has been established through immunohistologic studies of diseased tissues.[161] CD4+ helper T cells are the predominant phenotype in the stable periodontal lesion, and it is thought that alterations in the balance of effector T-cell subsets within the CD4+ population may lead to progression toward a destructive, B-cell–dominated lesion.[57] CD4+ T-cell subsets are defined on the basis of their phenotypic characteristics and effector functions. The nature of the APCs, which present antigen to cognate T-cell receptors on T cells, and the presence of specific combinations of cytokines and chemokines locally influence the nature of the CD4+ T-cell effector subset that develops from naive T cells (Fig. 7.5). CD4+ T-cell subsets are defined by the expression of specific transcription factors, and their functional characteristics are associated with their cytokine secretion profile.

The best-defined functional subsets of CD4+ T cells are the Th1 and Th2 cells, and a dynamic interaction between Th1 and Th2 cells may provide, in part, an explanation for fluctuations in disease activity and the progression of periodontal disease (Box 7.3). Th1 cells secrete IFN-γ, which activates cell-mediated immunity (i.e., macrophages, NK cells, and CD8+ cytotoxic T cells) against pathogenic microorganisms. The activation of macrophages promotes phagocytosis and killing of microbial pathogens, whereas NK cells and CD8+ T cells are cytotoxic T cells that kill infected host cells. Conversely, Th2 cells regulate humoral (antibody-mediated) immunity and mast cell activity through the secretion of the cytokines IL-4, IL-5, and IL-13. Thus the predominance of Th2 cells leads to a B-cell response. The B-cell response may be protective, for example, as a result of the production of specific antibodies that would serve to clear tissue infections through interaction with the complement system and by enhancing neutrophil phagocytosis. However, B cells are also a source of proinflammatory cytokines that contribute to tissue destruction.

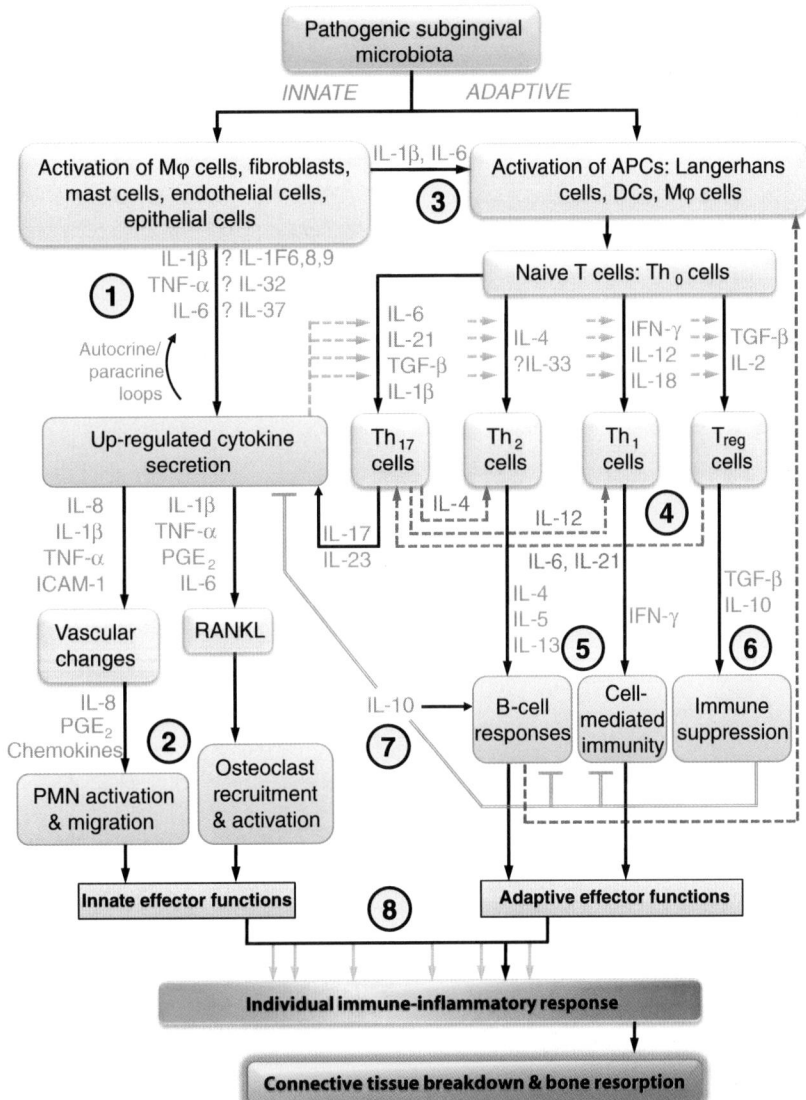

Fig. 7.5 Cytokine networks in periodontal diseases. Schematic to illustrate the multiple interactions between cytokines and cellular functions in periodontal diseases. *(1)* Resident and infiltrating cells in the periodontium respond to microbe-associated molecular patterns *(MAMPs)* signaling through pattern-recognition receptors *(PRRs)* by the production of cytokines as an early step in innate immune responses. Cytokine up-regulation is sustained by autocrine and paracrine feedback loops. (Note: *Question marks* indicate more speculative suggestions about the role of specific cytokines in periodontal pathogenesis than are known at present.) *(2)* Up-regulated cytokine activity leads to vascular changes, polymorphonuclear leukocyte *(PMN)* activation and migration, and, ultimately, osteoclastogenesis and osteoclast activation. *(3)* Cytokines produced in innate responses contribute to the activation of antigen-presenting cells *(APCs)*. These present specific antigens to naive CD4$^+$ T cells *(Th$_0$ cells)*, which differentiate into CD4$^+$ effector T cells (e.g., T-helper cells *[Th$_1$, Th$_2$, Th$_{17}$]*, and T-regulatory *[T$_{reg}$] cells*) according to the local cytokine milieu (as indicated by the groups of *four parallel horizontal gray dashed arrows*). For example, Th$_0$ cells differentiate into Th$_{17}$ cells under the influence of interleukin-6 *(IL-6)*, IL-21, transforming growth factor beta *(TGF-β)*, and IL-1β. (APCs are also activated by B cells, which are themselves activated at a later stage in the cytokine network [indicated by the *brown dashed arrow at the right edge of the figure*]; this is an example of the complexities of sequential feedback loops that develop). *(4)* Th$_1$ and Th$_2$ cells have a relatively stable phenotype, but other T-cell subsets can exhibit functional plasticity under the influence of different cytokine environments (indicated by *purple dashed arrows*). For example, Th$_{17}$ cells can develop into Th$_1$ cells under the influence of IL-12 and into Th$_2$ cells under the influence of IL-4. *(5)* Different T-cell subsets are associated with various cytokine secretion profiles that regulate different aspects of immune responses and that contribute to up-regulated cytokine activity. For example, Th$_1$ cells secrete interferon gamma *(IFN-γ)* (which activates cell-mediated immunity), and Th$_2$ cells regulate antibody-mediated (humoral) immunity through the secretion of cytokines IL-4, IL-5, and IL-13. Cytokines produced by different T-cell subsets increase their further secretion in positive feedback loops and also inhibit the development of other T-cell subsets (e.g., IL-4 from Th$_2$ cells inhibits Th$_1$ development, and IFN-γ from Th$_1$ cells inhibits Th$_2$ T-cell subsets). *(6)* T$_{reg}$ cells secrete TGF-β and IL-10, which have immunosuppressive functions. For example, IL-10 suppresses Th$_1$ and Th$_2$ responses, as well as cells of monocyte/macrophage lineage *(Mφ)* and dendritic cell *(DC)* function, and it also down-regulates cytokine production in various cells (i.e., Th$_1$ cells, Th$_2$ cells, PMNs, and natural killer *[NK]* cells). (Suppressive effects are indicated by *flat-ended green lines*.) *(7)* IL-10 functions as a regulatory mediator, but it can also exhibit other activities (e.g., the activation of B cells). The different aspects of IL-10 biology (i.e., immunosuppressive vs. immunostimulatory) likely depend on the local cytokine environment. These dual roles of IL-10 are indicated by the *green (inhibitory) line* and the *black (stimulatory) arrow*. *(8)* The sum total of innate and adaptive effector functions results in an immune–inflammatory response, the precise nature of which will vary from person to person (as indicated by the *multiple gray arrows*, with some patients being more susceptible to disease than others), as well as over time within an individual. In this case, the *black arrow* indicates an individual who has a proinflammatory response that leads to connective tissue breakdown and bone resorption. *ICAM-1*, intercellular adhesion molecule-1; *PGE$_2$*, prostaglandin E$_2$; *RANKL*, receptor activator of nuclear factor-κB ligand; *TNF-α*, tumor necrosis factor alpha. *(Reproduced with permission from Kinane DF, Preshaw PM, Loos BG: Host-response: understanding the cellular and molecular mechanisms of host-microbial interactions—consensus of the Seventh European Workshop on Periodontology. J Clin Periodontol 38[Suppl 11]:44–48, 2011.)*

BOX 7.3   The T-Helper 1/T-Helper 2 Concept of Periodontal Disease Progression

A dynamic interaction between T-helper 1 (Th1) and T-helper 2 (Th2) cells represents a possible explanation for aspects of the fluctuations in disease activity and clinical progression seen with periodontal disease. It has been hypothesized that a strong innate response results in interleukin-12 synthesis (e.g., by tissue macrophages) that leads to a Th1 response that provides protective cell-mediated immunity that would be manifested as a "stable" periodontal lesion. Conversely, a poor innate response would lead to reduced interleukin-12, which would permit the development of Th2 responses and lead to the activation of B cells; this, in turn, would mediate a destructive lesion, possibly through enhanced B-cell–derived interleukin-1β.[57,160] However, definitive evidence to support associations of Th1 and Th2 cells with different clinical presentations of periodontal disease has been difficult to obtain. Investigators have suggested that this is a result of variations among experimental studies, which have differed with respect to the material that has been used, the definitions of disease stages, the experimental designs, and analytic methods used.[53,57,160] In addition, in general terms, the Th1/Th2 dichotomy does not explain all aspects of the regulation of adaptive immune responses. More recently, other T-cell subsets have been identified and defined. For example, regulatory T cells secrete interleukin-10 and transforming growth factor beta and thereby suppress immune responses. Th17 cells have a proinflammatory action through the secretion of interleukin-17, a cytokine that synergizes with interleukin-1β and tumor necrosis factor alpha. Therefore, although it is widely accepted that Th1 and Th2 cells are likely to be important in the immunopathogenesis of periodontal disease, it is increasingly recognized that the Th1/Th2 model alone is probably inadequate to explain the role of T cells in this process.

T_{reg} cells have an immunosuppressive action that is mediated by the secretion of TGF-β and that is important to the prevention of autoimmune disease. These cells are increased in periodontitis lesions and may therefore have a role in disease pathogenesis.[121] Certain lines of evidence suggest that the pathogenesis of periodontal disease may involve some elements of autoimmunity.[57] For example, immunologic cross-reactivity occurs between HSP60 expressed on human cells and the GroEL molecule of *P. gingivalis*, and specific serum antibodies and antigen-specific T cells to these molecules have been detected in periodontal disease. Similarly, autoantibodies and specific T cells against other host (i.e., self) molecules, such as type I collagen, have been identified in periodontal disease.

Th17 cells comprise another subset of T cells, and they have a proinflammatory action that is important in immune responses against extracellular infections mediated by the cytokine IL-17. Infections with a diverse range of pathogens have been shown to activate strong Th17 cell responses, and Th17 cells are thought to provide a substantial inflammatory response to clear microorganisms that Th1/Th2 cells have failed to eradicate. IL-17 has a number of activities in common with IL-1β and TNF-α, and it has a synergistic activity with these cytokines, particularly TNF-α. IL-17 induces proinflammatory cytokine expression (including IL-1β and TNF-α) in macrophages, stimulates chemokine expression, and thereby activates neutrophil infiltration. Increasing evidence indicates a role of IL-17 and Th17 cells in periodontal disease.[53] IL-17 has been detected in periodontal tissues at sites of advanced disease. IL-17 induces IL-6 and IL-8 secretion by gingival fibroblasts and also up-regulates MMP-1 and MMP-3 in these cells. IL-17 also induces IL-1β and TNF-α secretion from macrophages and gingival epithelial cells. In a mouse model of periodontitis induced by *P. gingivalis*, IL-17 receptor deficiency (IL-17RA knockouts) resulted in increased susceptibility to alveolar bone loss, thereby suggesting a protective role of IL-17 in bone homeostasis, possibly by an effect on neutrophil function.

Several other effector CD4+ T-cell subsets have been defined on the basis of their cytokine secretion profile: these include Th9 cells and Th22 cells. In addition, T-cell subsets have been defined on the basis of their specific anatomic location. For example, Th22 cells home to the skin, in which they likely stimulate antimicrobial peptide (AMP) production and the differentiation of keratinocytes. In addition, T follicular helper cells are located in germinal centers in lymph nodes in which they provide B-cell help and stimulate Ig class switching. The homing of particular T-cell subsets to specific anatomic locations is defined by the expression of chemokine receptors that confer responsiveness to specific chemotactic signals that are produced in those locations. However, thus far, the majority of the work on these novel T-cell subsets has been carried out in mouse models and in vitro systems; their relevance to human biology in vivo and in disease remains to be fully elucidated.

Cytokines produced by differentiated T-cell subsets feed back to stimulate differentiation and to sustain the activity of the cells from which they are derived (i.e., in a positive feedback loop). Simultaneously, they inhibit the development of other competing subsets. For example, IL-4 from Th2 cells inhibits the development of Th1 cells, and IFN-γ from Th1 cells inhibits Th2 cells.

It is increasingly appreciated that individual CD4+ T-cell clones—after they have encountered antigen and differentiated in response under the influence of a specific cytokine environment (i.e., a milieu)—may not be terminally differentiated cells. Rather, functional flexibility appears to exist between T-cell subsets and in particular within the memory T-cell population (see Fig. 7.5). For example, Th17 and T_{reg} cells can interconvert, depending on the local concentrations of cytokines such as IL-6, IL-23, and TGF-β.[173] It is thought that the plethora of functional subsets of T cells, their anatomic location, and their ability to switch phenotype are reflections of the requirement for effective responses against diverse pathogens.

The complexities of the interactions between cellular and molecular aspects of innate and adaptive immune functioning are presented in Fig. 7.5. It is clear that multiple proinflammatory and antiinflammatory pathways, positive and negative feedback loops, and agonists and antagonists all play a role in determining the nature of the immune–inflammatory response to the bacterial challenge and the degree of tissue damage that is experienced. Furthermore, the nature of the inflammatory response varies among individuals; this could explain why certain people appear to be more susceptible to periodontitis than others.

CLINICIAN'S CORNER

What makes a person susceptible to periodontitis?

We have all seen patients with good oral hygiene yet advanced periodontitis and, conversely, patients with poor oral hygiene who may have gingivitis or mild periodontitis, but who do not develop advanced periodontitis. It is clear that immune functioning and inflammatory responses are highly complex processes that vary from person to person. Our understanding is that the sum total of all the immune–inflammatory events in the periodontal tissues (which are also influenced by environmental factors such as smoking or diabetes) is the main determinant of how much tissue damage occurs in response to the challenge presented by the bacterial biofilm. This tissue damage is what we recognize clinically as disease. Our challenge for the future is to learn how to identify susceptible patients at a much earlier stage in the disease process, before tissue damage occurs.

Antibodies

Specific antibodies are produced in response to the bacterial challenge in periodontal disease and are the endpoint of B-cell activation. Commensurate with the appearance of antibodies against bacterial antigens is the appearance of differentiated plasma cells. High levels of antibodies appear in GCF (in addition to those in the circulation), and these are produced locally by plasma cells in periodontal tissues.[8] Antibodies to periodontal pathogens are primarily IgG, with few IgM or IgA types produced.

Many species of oral bacteria elicit a polyclonal B-cell response (with the consequent production of specific antibodies against those bacteria). However, these responses augment responses against nonoral bacteria and may lead to the production of autoantibodies (e.g., antibodies against collagen and connective tissue proteins), which may contribute to tissue destruction in periodontal disease.[8,57] The incidence and levels of specific serum and GCF IgG antibodies are raised in chronic periodontitis, a finding suggesting that local and peripheral generation of antibodies may be important in the immune response to periodontal pathogens. Antibodies (i.e., IgA) to periodontal pathogens are also found in saliva. Variations in the levels of specific antibodies to different species in different clinical presentations suggest differences in pathogenesis. For example, antibodies to *A. actinomycetemcomitans* of the IgG_2 subclass predominate in aggressive periodontitis.[151]

Other *P. gingivalis* molecules (i.e., fimbriae and hemagglutinin) also act as antigens. Specific antibodies are also generated by serotype-specific carbohydrate antigens (e.g., capsular polysaccharide of *P. gingivalis,* carbohydrate of *A. actinomycetemcomitans* LPS). The subclass distribution of antibodies is influenced by cytokines that are derived from monocytes.[151] For example, IgG_2 production is regulated by IL-1α, IL-1β, and PGE_2 from monocytes as well as by platelet-activating factor from neutrophils. PGE_2 and platelet-activating factor indirectly induce Th1 responses and therefore IFN-γ, which stimulates IgG_2 production. Individuals with aggressive periodontitis have monocytes that are hyperresponsive to LPS and that produce elevated quantities of PGE_2.[8] *A. actinomycetemcomitans* is commonly associated with aggressive periodontitis, which induces IL-12 production that regulates NK cells and Th1 cells. These cells are a source of IFN-γ, which, in turn, regulates IgG_2.

Some studies have reported an effect of treatment on levels of specific antibodies to periodontal pathogens. For example, plaque removal reduces the titers of antibodies to *P. gingivalis* and *A. actinomycetemcomitans* in serum, GCF, and saliva.[8] Some studies have observed a transient increase in antibody titers after treatment, which may be due to the release of antigens into the tissue and circulation.

The significance of antibodies in periodontitis is not clear. It is not known whether these antibodies have a protective function or whether they participate in disease pathogenesis. Although some evidence indicates a correlation between clinical parameters of disease and titers of specific antibodies to periodontal pathogens, other studies report an inverse correlation of antibody levels and avidity with periodontal destruction. In addition, specific antibodies to periodontal pathogens are found in healthy individuals, as well as in persons with periodontal disease.

Concept of Host Susceptibility

The immune and inflammatory processes that result from the challenge presented by the subgingival biofilm are complex and are mediated by a large number of proinflammatory and antiinflammatory cytokines and enzymes that function as a network of mediators with overlapping roles and activity (see Fig. 7.5). Immune responses to the bacterial challenge do not occur in isolation, but rather take place in the context of other host and environmental factors that influence these responses and thereby determine the progression of disease. Certain risk factors increase susceptibility to periodontal disease, particularly smoking[126] and diabetes[140]; these are considered elsewhere in this book.

A feature of human development and evolution has been that quantitative and qualitative differences exist in immune responses among individuals.[72] Indeed, infectious agents (e.g., bacteria) exert evolutionary selection pressures on the species that they infect. This may be relevant in periodontal disease, and some studies have confirmed that immune cells from patients with periodontal disease secrete higher quantities of proinflammatory cytokines than do cells from persons who are periodontally healthy.[174] Cytokine profiles are also different in those individuals with immune-mediated diseases as compared with healthy control subjects.

These observations have led to the concept of the "hyperinflammatory" or "hyperresponsive" trait in which certain individuals possess a hyperinflammatory phenotype that accounts for their increased susceptibility to chronic inflammatory conditions such as periodontitis.[29] Such a trait may also underpin shared susceptibility between conditions such as periodontitis and cardiovascular disease or diabetes. However, at present, it is not possible to identify with certainty those patients who are hyperresponders. The hyperresponder concept was originally proposed in the context of the responsiveness of monocytes to LPS challenge; this suggests that patients with disease possess an individual hyperresponsive monocytic trait that is characterized by elevated levels of inflammatory mediators released from monocytes in response to bacterial challenge.[128] It is likely that many reasons contribute to disease variations among individuals, such as variations in immune responses, pathogenesis, and the plaque biofilm; this situation results in an uneven disease experience in the population.

Fig. 7.6 is a schematic illustration of how increasing bacterial challenge can result in differing levels of inflammatory response according to the response profile of an individual patient.[128] Most individuals would be considered normal, and for a given bacterial challenge, they would produce a certain level of inflammatory mediators in the periodontal tissues. For those who are hyperresponders, the same bacterial challenge results in a greater inflammatory response, which over time would result in increased tissue breakdown, earlier presentation of the clinical signs of disease, and a clinical interpretation of having increased susceptibility to periodontitis. Those individuals who are hyporesponsive produce lower levels of inflammatory mediators and are therefore somewhat resistant to the development of periodontitis, even though plaque may be present and they may have widespread gingivitis and/or mild periodontitis. The nature of the immune–inflammatory response is governed by genetic factors and environmental factors, and it may vary over time within the same individual (e.g., if environmental factors such as smoking status, stress, or systemic disease should change).[87]

A similar dose–response curve can also be expressed in the context of stable or progressing disease, and, as shown in Fig. 7.7, a certain level of bacterial challenge results in a moderate release of inflammatory cytokines, mediators, and enzymes. These mediators, together with the infiltrating defense cells, have a protective role to eliminate bacteria in the sulcus and do not trigger periodontal disease breakdown. Such a steady-state scenario may persist indefinitely. However, if something changes (e.g., the quantity or quality of the biofilm alters, or the host defenses alter as a result of a change in an environmental exposure), then the secretion of cytokines, prostanoids, MMPs, and

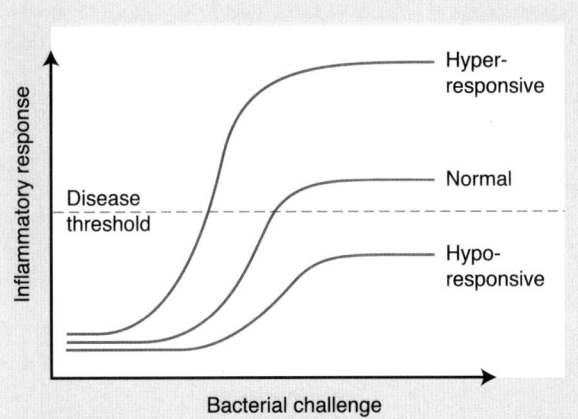

Fig. 7.6 Inflammatory response characteristics in relation to bacterial challenge. A given bacterial challenge results in differing levels of inflammatory response according to the response profile of an individual. Most people are close to normal and produce a certain level of inflammatory mediators for a given challenge. Those who are hyperresponders generate an excessive inflammatory response for the same bacterial challenge and cross the threshold into active disease at an earlier stage. Those who are hyporesponsive produce lower levels of inflammatory mediators and, despite a significant bacterial challenge, may never develop advanced periodontitis. *(Modified from Champagne CM, Buchanan W, Reddy MS, et al: Potential for gingival crevice fluid measures as predictors of risk for periodontal diseases.* Periodontol 2000 *31:167–180, 2003.)*

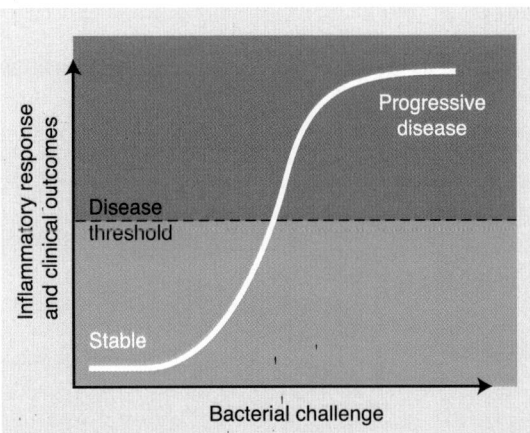

Fig. 7.7 Inflammatory response characteristics in relation to an individual's threshold for periodontitis. A certain level of bacterial challenge results in a moderate inflammatory response, which is protective by intent and may not be sufficient to transition to periodontal disease. This stable condition may persist for many years or even throughout the individual's lifetime. Changes in the bacterial burden (i.e., qualitative, quantitative, or both) or changes in the host response (e.g., as a result of a change in an environmental exposure) could result in an up-regulated inflammatory response characterized by marked cellular infiltrate and the increased secretion of inflammatory mediators leading to tissue damage and a transition from the stable situation to periodontitis. The location of the threshold between stable and active disease varies from person to person. In addition, the dose–response curve for any individual can shift to the left or the right in accordance with environmental changes. A shift to the left would result in an increased inflammatory response to a given bacterial challenge and potentially an exacerbation of disease. A shift to the right would have the opposite effect. *(Modified from Champagne CM, Buchanan W, Reddy MS, et al: Potential for gingival crevice fluid measures as predictors of risk for periodontal diseases.* Periodontol 2000 *31:167–180, 2003.)*

other mediators may increase in the tissues, thereby leading to the histopathologic changes described previously and a transition to periodontitis. Thus a threshold exists between stable and active disease, and this varies from person to person. The dose–response curve for any individual can shift to the left or the right according to environmental changes. A shift to the left would result in an increase in the quantities of inflammatory mediators produced for a given bacterial challenge and potentially an exacerbation of disease; a shift to the right would have the opposite effect. In all cases, an increase in the bacterial challenge would have the tendency to increase the production of inflammatory mediators, which may tip the balance from a stable to a progressing periodontal lesion.

These are, of course, simplistic models to explain a highly complex phenomenon, and it is clear that cytokines and inflammatory mediators function in complicated networks (see Fig. 7.5).[85,141] Therefore, although increases and decreases in the absolute levels of cytokines have been reported in disease states, it is clear that the dysregulation of cytokine networks and other mediators is the key determinant of disease progression. Thus the relative proportions of mediators within inflammatory networks are fundamental to determining disease progression, and changes in these proportions are driven by inflammatory challenges and the genetic and environmental factors that govern how the host responds to such challenges.[91,134] Schematic illustrations to explain the pathogenesis of periodontal disease, such as presented in Fig. 7.5, can be useful; however, given the complexity of the disease processes, they are inevitably simplistic. Earlier models were very simplistic indeed, being essentially linear and suggesting that periodontitis resulted directly from the microbial challenge.[91] This concept influenced periodontal treatment over the decades and resulted in treatment strategies that focused primarily on the biofilm. Modern concepts of periodontal pathogenesis describe a host response that transitions from being proportionate and proresolving (in terms of resolving inflammation) to one that is disproportionate and nonresolving and ultimately self-destructive as chronic inflammation develops. These changes occur in parallel with changes in the biofilm, the nature of which is influenced by the development of inflammation in the tissues, as it transitions from being health-promoting to dysbiosis, thus perpetuating the chronic inflammation.[116]

Increasing awareness of the importance of host factors in determining interindividual differences in disease progression has resulted in the realization that, although plaque bacteria initiate and perpetuate the inflammatory response, most of the tissue damage results from the host response, which is influenced by genetic factors, as well as environmental and acquired risk factors. Risk factors such as smoking alter the progression of the immune–inflammatory response and shift the balance toward increased periodontal breakdown.[80] This implies that the presence of plaque bacteria does not inevitably lead to tissue destruction, and this concept is supported by a large number of epidemiologic studies, which confirm that more advanced disease is usually confined to a minority of the population.[108]

Our improved understanding of the disease processes in periodontitis has led to the development of a biologic systems model for representing periodontal pathogenesis. This involves bacterial components, environmental factors, specific inflammatory mechanisms, and host–genetic variations that are associated with disease.[91] A biologic systems approach provides a framework for viewing the contributions and relative importance of all the components that contribute to the clinical presentation of disease. Thus, in the context of periodontal disease, such a system would include a person level, a genetic/epigenetic level, the biologic phenotype, and, ultimately, the clinical phenotype (Fig. 7.8).[127] Such systems provide a more comprehensive view of the disease as a complex regulatory network in which aspects of the specific genetic factors, environmental

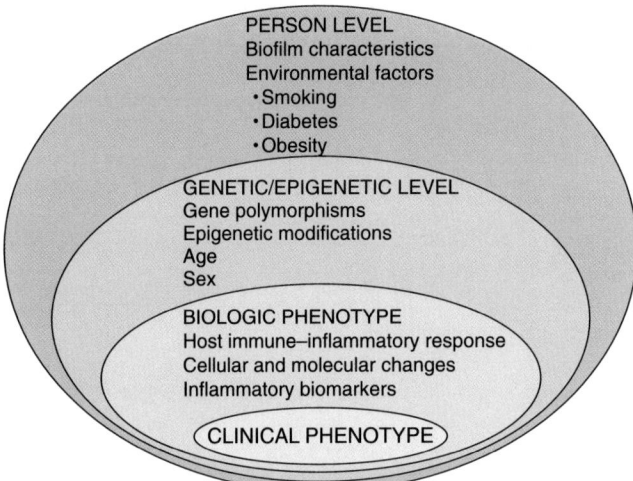

PERSON LEVEL
Biofilm characteristics
Environmental factors
• Smoking
• Diabetes
• Obesity

GENETIC/EPIGENETIC LEVEL
Gene polymorphisms
Epigenetic modifications
Age
Sex

BIOLOGIC PHENOTYPE
Host immune–inflammatory response
Cellular and molecular changes
Inflammatory biomarkers

CLINICAL PHENOTYPE

Fig. 7.8 A biologic systems model of periodontitis. The outermost level of this model is the *Person Level,* which represents an individual's unique characteristics as they are related to periodontitis. These include the compositional characteristics of the subgingival biofilm, as well as known risk factors and environmental exposures such as smoking and diabetes. The *Person Level* characteristics interact with the *Genetic/Epigenetic Level* characteristics, which include nonmodifiable factors such as age, sex, and genetic composition. Gene polymorphisms are known to be associated with periodontal disease, and epigenetics refers to changes in phenotype (i.e., clinical disease expression) caused by mechanisms other than changes in the underlying DNA sequence. Epigenetics can be defined as all the meiotically and mitotically inherited changes in gene expression that are not encoded in the DNA sequence itself. Epigenetic modifications are important permissive and suppressive factors for controlling the expressed genome through gene transcription. Two major epigenetic mechanisms are the posttranslational modification of histone proteins in chromatin and the methylation of DNA. The *Genetic/Epigenetic Level* characteristics influence the *Biologic Phenotype,* which is characterized by the specific immune–inflammatory responses (i.e., cellular and molecular events and the production of inflammatory mediators) that are associated with the *Clinical Phenotype* (i.e., the clinical presentation of the disease). This model reflects how different individuals with the same presentation (e.g., periodontitis) may have very different predisposing and risk factors. The model depicts the different biologic factors that underpin the development of periodontal disease in different individuals and that ultimately may be used to classify disease by the contribution provided to the clinical phenotype at each level. *(Modified from Offenbacher S, Barros SP, Beck JD: Rethinking periodontal inflammation.* J Periodontol *79:1577–1584, 2008.)*

exposures, and other modifying factors that an individual is exposed to determine the development of the disease state.

To summarize, it is clear that the subgingival bacteria initiate and perpetuate the immune–inflammatory responses in the periodontal tissues. These responses are characterized by classic signs of inflammation that are modified as a result of the unique anatomy of the periodontium and the dentogingival apparatus. The inflammatory events that develop in response to the bacterial challenge are protective by intent, but they result in the majority of tissue damage and breakdown that lead to the clinical signs of periodontitis. Individuals vary with regard to their susceptibility to periodontal disease and also in the threshold level at which a stable periodontal site progresses to an active site. Such variations are genetically determined, and they are also influenced by environmental risk factors (e.g., smoking), some of which are modifiable and some of which are not. The challenge for the future is to identify at-risk individuals who possess the hyperinflammatory trait so that disease can be prevented by careful management strategies before tissue loss has occurred.

 A Case Scenario is found on the companion website www.expertconsult.com.

References

 References for this chapter are found on the companion website www.expertconsult.com.

CHAPTER 8

Biofilm and Periodontal Microbiology

Wim Teughels | Isabelle Laleman | Marc Quirynen | Nicholas Jakubovics

CHAPTER OUTLINE

The Oral Cavity From a Microbe's
Perspective
Bacteria and Their Biofilm Mode of
Living
Characteristics of Biofilm Bacteria
(Life in "Slime City")

Bacterial Transmission and
Translocation
Nonbacterial Inhabitants of the Oral
Cavity
Microbiologic Specificity of
Periodontal Diseases

The Transition From Health to
Disease
Virulence Factors of
Periodontopathogens
Future Advances in Periodontal
Microbiology

 For additional content on the criteria for the identification of periodontopathogens, Videos 8.1 through 8.5, and expanded discussions of the structure of a mature dental plaque biofilm; the initial adhesion or attachment of bacteria; colonization and plaque maturation; and interactions among dental plaque bacteria, bacterial transmission and translocation, viruses, host susceptibility, adhesive surface proteins and fibrils, and tissue-destruction–promoting factors, please visit the companion website at www.expertconsult.com.

The human fetus inside the uterus is sterile, but as soon as it passes through the birth canal, it acquires vaginal and fecal microorganisms.[83,112] Within 2 weeks, a nearly mature *microbiota* is established in the gut of the newborn baby. After weaning (>2 years), the entire human microbiota is formed and comprises a very complex collection of hundreds of different types of bacteria with approximately 10^{14} microbial cells.[262] From this moment on, our body contains *1.3 to 10 times more bacteria* than human cells.[361] It has been estimated that, for a normal, healthy human being, the bacterial population comprises 2 kg of the total body weight. This is fascinating if one realizes that the average human brain weighs only about 1.4 kg.

The colonization of the oral cavity also starts close to the time of birth (Fig. 8.1). Within hours after birth, the sterile oral cavity is colonized by low numbers of mainly facultative and aerobic bacteria.[388] At that time, the oral microbiota of newborns closely resembles the mother's vaginal microbiota or, for newborns delivered by cesarean section, the mother's skin microbiota.[83] From the second day, anaerobic bacteria can be detected in the infant's edentulous mouth.[96,337] The number of oral bacteria increases gradually as a result of exposure to external environmental microbial sources.[189,288,337] *Streptococcus salivarius* and *Streptococcus mitis* (Fig. 8.2A) have been identified as the first and most dominant oral microbes to colonize the oral cavity of newborn infants.[187,188,210] *Veillonella* spp. (Fig. 8.2B), *Neisseria* spp., *Actinomyces* spp. (Fig. 8.2C and D), and *Staphylococcus* spp. are also among the first colonizers of the oral cavity. After tooth eruption, a more complex oral microbiota is established. The species that colonize the teeth after eruption include *Streptococcus sanguinis* (Fig. 8.2D), *Lactobacillus* spp. (Fig. 8.2E), and *Streptococcus oralis*. Oral streptococci, including *S. oralis*, *Streptococcus anginosus*, mutans streptococci (*Streptococcus mutans* and *Streptococcus sobrinus*), and *Streptococcus gordonii* (Fig. 8.2F) are commonly reported to be present after the first year of life.[49,53,230,288] In addition, anaerobes, including *Fusobacterium* spp. (Fig. 8.2G) and *Prevotella* spp. (Fig.

8.2H and I), can also be detected in young children.[49,189] In later childhood, the bacterial diversity and numbers in the oral cavity increase as more teeth erupt and provide more areas for the adherence and retention of bacteria.[33]

Because of the paucity of longitudinal studies, relatively little is known about the initial colonization of key microbes found in the oral cavity of children and adults.[210] It is estimated that the oral bacterial microbiome of adults encompasses approximately 700 commonly occurring species, approximately half of which can be present at any time in any individual.[25,281] When one thinks about bacteria, one almost immediately associates them with different pathologic conditions. However, most oral bacteria are harmless commensals under normal circumstances. This means that this microbiota lives in harmony with its host but that, under specific conditions (i.e., increased mass and/or pathogenicity, suppression of commensal or beneficial bacteria, and/or reduced host response), disease can occur. The importance of the commensal microbiota is clearly illustrated by the development of *Candida* infections when the normal oral microbiota is reduced, such as after a longer period of systemic antibiotic usage.[430] In addition, it has been shown that aggressive periodontitis is associated with a loss of colonization of *S. sanguinis*.[394] Conversely, investigators showed in mice that the commensal microbiota is required for *Porphyromonas gingivalis*–induced bone loss.[2,76]

It is obvious that the periodontal microbiota is extremely complex. Because it both affects and is affected by the host, the oral environment, and periodontal treatment, a profound knowledge of periodontal microbiology is necessary.

The Oral Cavity From a Microbe's Perspective

With the exception of those microorganisms that are present in feces and in secretory fluids, all bacteria maintain themselves within their

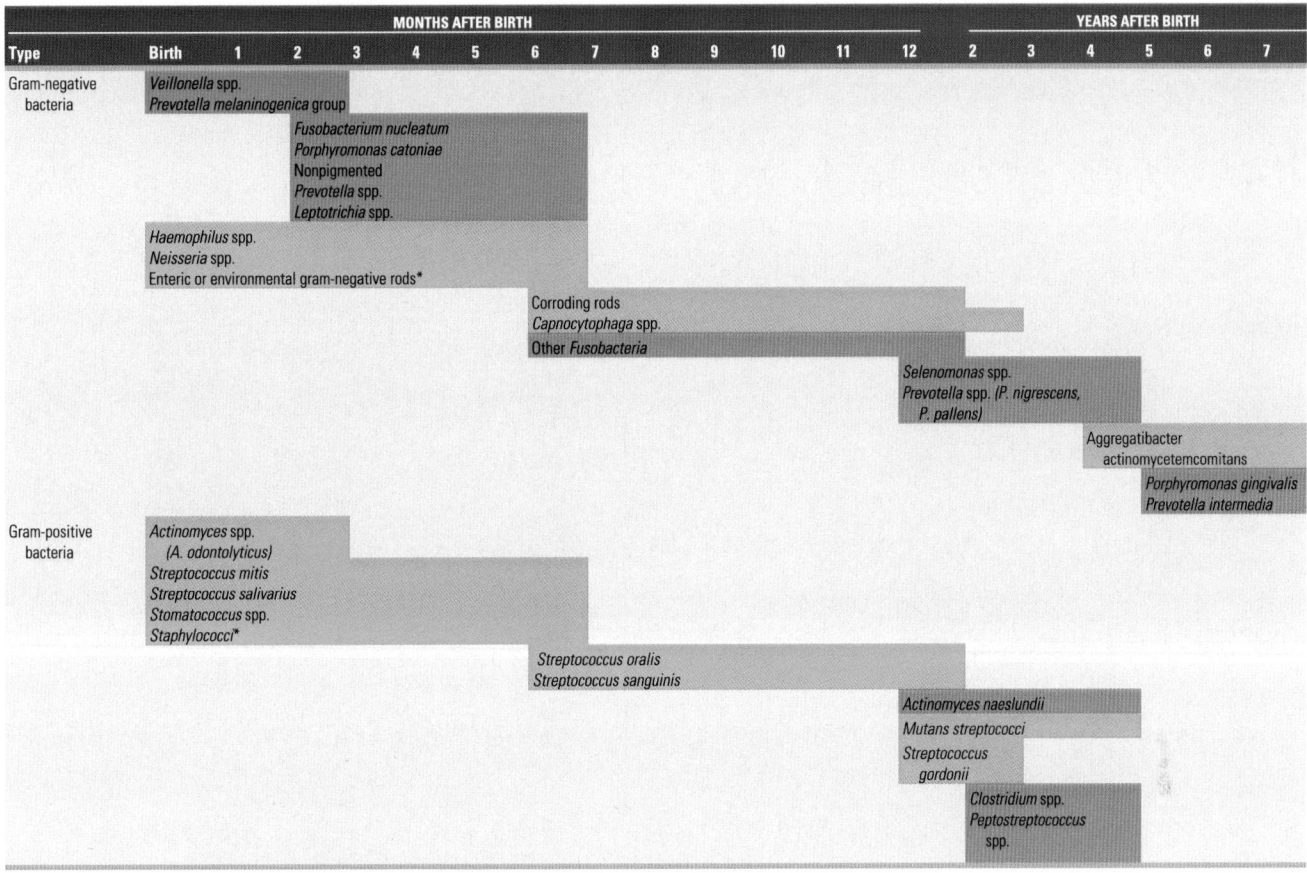

Type	Birth	1	2	3	4	5	6	7	8	9	10	11	12	2	3	4	5	6	7

(MONTHS AFTER BIRTH / YEARS AFTER BIRTH)

Gram-negative bacteria
Veillonella spp.
Prevotella melaninogenica group
Fusobacterium nucleatum
Porphyromonas catoniae
Nonpigmented Prevotella spp.
Leptotrichia spp.
Haemophilus spp.
Neisseria spp.
Enteric or environmental gram-negative rods*
Corroding rods
Capnocytophaga spp.
Other Fusobacteria
Selenomonas spp.
Prevotella spp. (P. nigrescens, P. pallens)
Aggregatibacter actinomycetemcomitans
Porphyromonas gingivalis
Prevotella intermedia

Gram-positive bacteria
Actinomyces spp. (A. odontolyticus)
Streptococcus mitis
Streptococcus salivarius
Stomatococcus spp.
Staphylococci*
Streptococcus oralis
Streptococcus sanguinis
Actinomyces naeslundii
Mutans streptococci
Streptococcus gordonii
Clostridium spp.
Peptostreptococcus spp.

Fig. 8.1 Colonization of the oral cavity. Amenable periods for the establishment of the most frequent bacterial species or groups (prevalence, >25%) in infants' mouths. Anaerobic bacteria are indicated in green, and aerobic or facultative bacteria are indicated in orange. *Asterisk,* The prevalence of these bacteria decrease with age. *(Adapted from Kononen E: Oral colonization by anaerobic bacteria during childhood: role in health and disease. Oral Dis 5:278, 1999; and Kononen E: Development of oral bacterial flora in young children. Ann Med 32:107, 2000.)*

host by adhering to a surface. This principle also applies to the oral cavity. From an ecologic viewpoint, the oral cavity, which communicates with the pharynx, should be considered as an "open growth system" with an uninterrupted ingestion and removal of microorganisms and their nutrients.

KEY FACT

Most organisms can survive in the oropharynx only when they adhere to either the soft tissues or the hard surfaces. Otherwise, they may be removed by:
- Swallowing, mastication, or blowing the nose
- Tongue and oral hygiene implements
- The wash-out effect of the salivary, nasal, and crevicular fluid outflow
- The active motion of the cilia of the nasal and sinus walls

The ability of a bacterium to adhere to its host is crucial for the induction of infectious diseases, such as gingivitis or periodontitis.[327] Oral bacteria and especially pathogenic bacteria, such as *Porphyromonas gingivalis* (Fig. 8.2H and J) and *Aggregatibacter*

actinomycetemcomitans (Fig. 8.2K), have a large battery of virulence factors, one of which is the ability to adhere to hard intraoral surfaces and/or to the oral mucosae (Fig. 8.3).[56,58,110,377]

On the basis of physical and morphologic criteria, the oral cavity can be divided into *six major ecosystems* (also called *niches*), each with the following distinct ecologic determinants:
1. The intraoral and supragingival hard surfaces (teeth, implants, restorations, and prostheses)
2. Subgingival regions adjacent to a hard surface, including the periodontal/peri-implant pocket (characterized by the presence of crevicular fluid, the root cementum or implant surface, and the pocket epithelium)
3. The buccal palatal epithelium and the epithelium of the floor of the mouth
4. The dorsum of the tongue
5. The tonsils
6. The saliva

In health, a core set of microorganisms is almost universally present in these ecosystems. This core microbiome includes members of the phyla Firmicutes (*Streptococcus* spp., *Veillonella* spp., and *Granulicatella* spp.), Proteobacteria (*Neisseria* spp., *Campylobacter* spp., and *Haemophilus* spp.), Actinobacteria (*Corynebacterium* spp., *Rothia* spp., and *Actinomyces* spp.), Bacteroidetes (*Prevotella* spp., *Capnocytophaga* spp., and *Porphyromonas* spp.), and Fusobacteria (*Fusobacterium* spp.).[156,211,457]

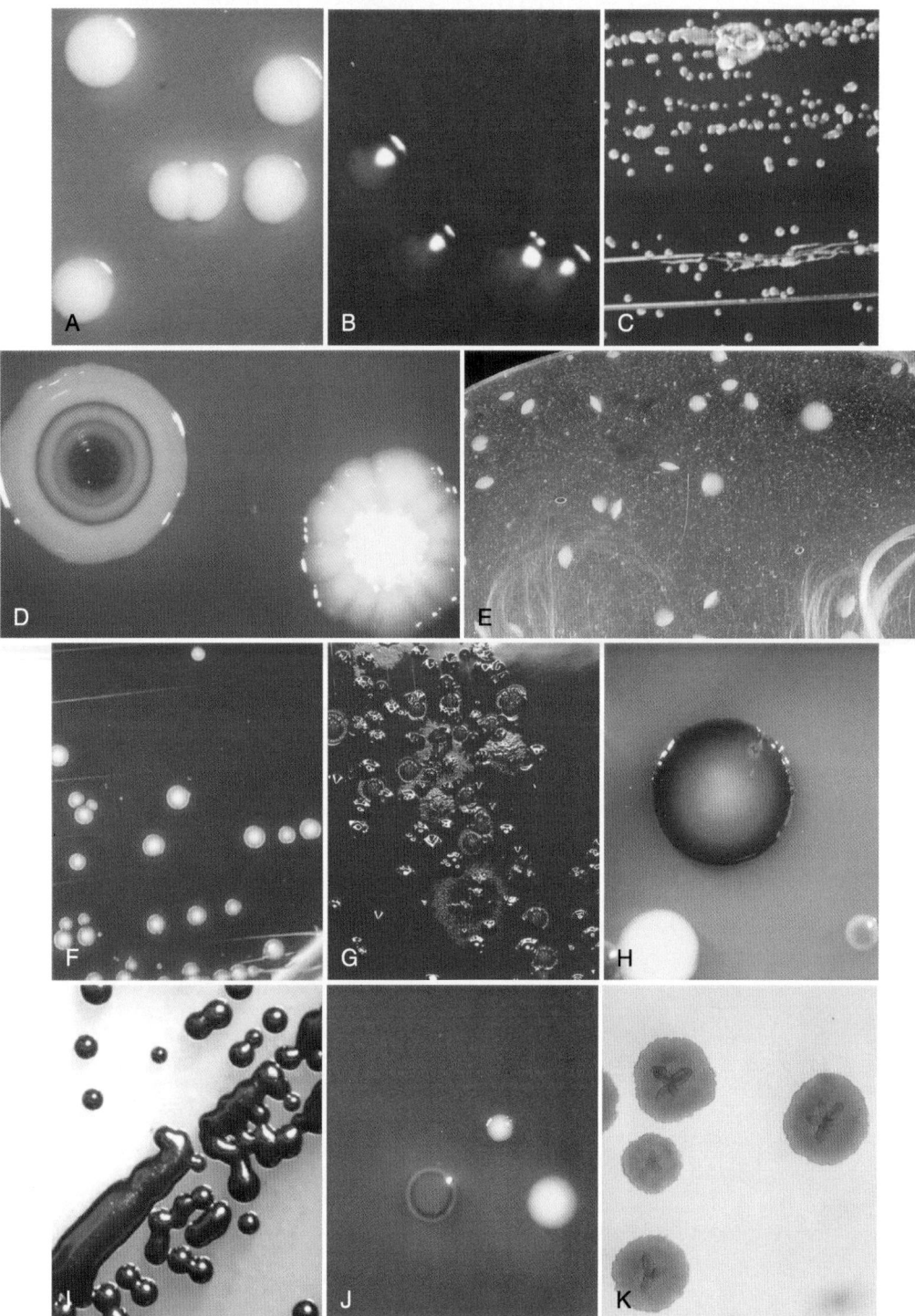

Fig. 8.2 Various periodontal and cariogenic species grown on agar plates. (A) *Streptococcus mitis* are gram-positive, fast-growing, facultatively anaerobic bacteria that are easy to culture on a blood-agar plate. A clear halo surrounding the colonies appears through hemolytic activity. (B) *Veillonella parvula* are anaerobic, gram-negative, small cocci. They form small transparent colonies (<1.0 mm) after 48 hours of incubation. (C) *Actinomyces viscosus* are microaerophilic to anaerobic gram-positive rods with possible branches (pseudomycelium). They form slimy, white, spherical colonies in 48 hours. (D) The typical colony morphology of *Streptococcus sanguinis (right)* and *Actinomyces odontolyticus (left)*. (E) *Lactobacillus* spp. typically grow on Rogosa agar as a sesame seed. (F) *Streptococcus gordonii* are facultative, anaerobic, gram-positive cocci. On a blood plate, colonies of 1 to 3 mm are formed within 48 hours. These bacteria are α-hemolytic, which results in the formation of a clear halo surrounding the colony. (G) This selective agar plate, which contains crystal violet and erythromycin (i.e., a CVE-agar plate), will allow *Fusobacterium nucleatum* to grow as a round, flat rhizoid, opaque purple colony. (H) A detailed picture of *Porphyromonas gingivalis* (green-brown colony) and *Prevotella intermedia* (black colony) on a classic nonspecific blood-agar plate. (I) *Prevotella nigrescens* forms like *P. intermedia*, a black pigmented colony on a blood agar plate. It is a strictly anaerobic bacterium with growth that is limited to an oxygen-free environment. (J) A detailed picture of *Parvimonas micra* (small white colony) next to *Porphyromonas gingivalis* (green-brown colony) on a classic nonspecific blood-agar plate. (K) A detailed picture of *Aggregatibacter actinomycetemcomitans* grown on a selective agar plate that contains tryptic soy, horse serum, bacitracin, and vancomycin (i.e., a TSBV-agar plate).

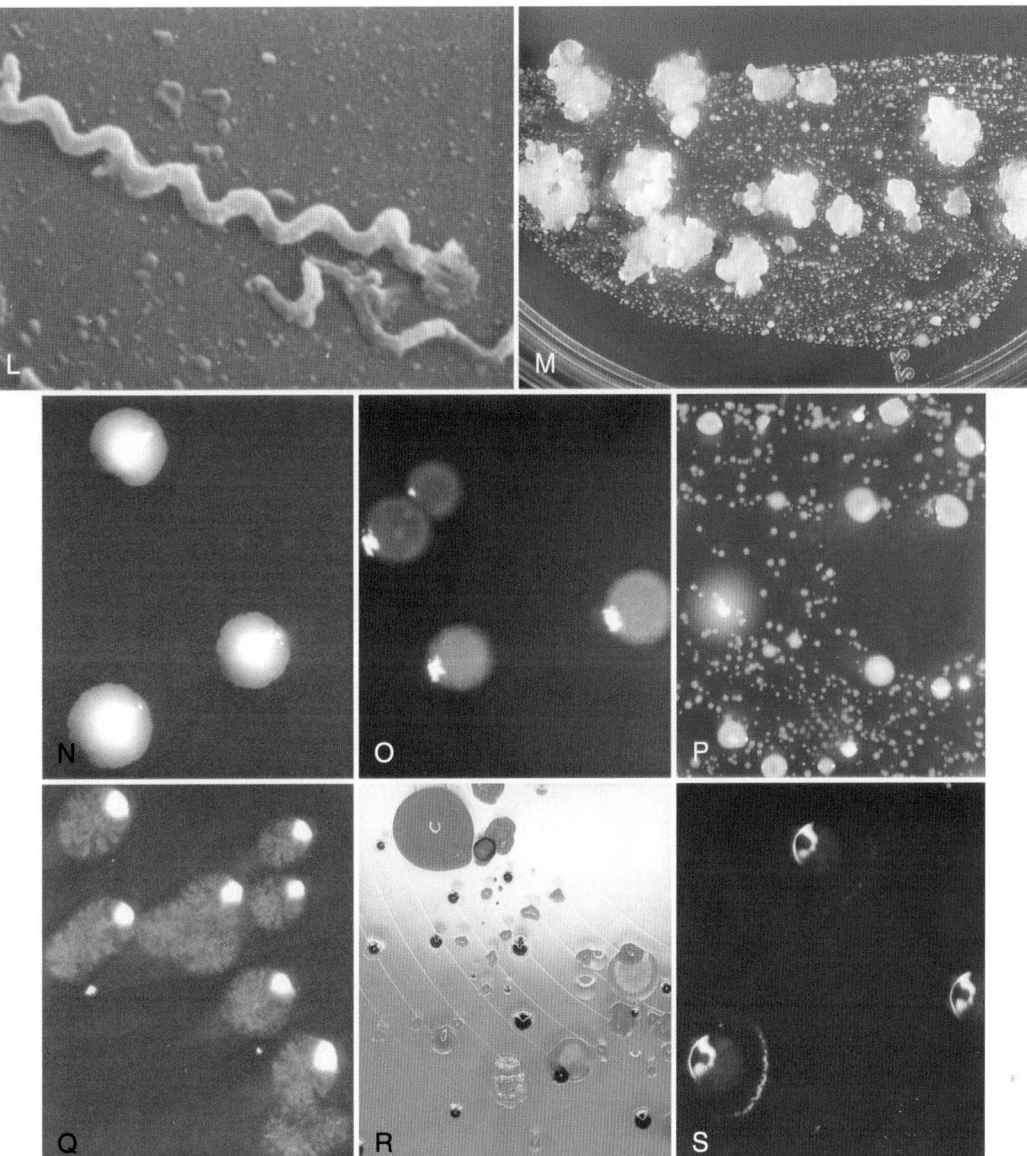

Fig. 8.2, cont'd (L) It is extremely difficult to culture *Treponema denticola* (spirochete) on an agar plate and therefore not possible to identify this bacteria with classic culture. A phase-contrast microscope, a dark-field microscope, or an electron microscope is often used to visualize this bacterium. Identification and quantification are possible only through DNA analysis. (M) On a selective agar plate that contains trypticase yeast extract, cystine, sucrose, and bacitracin (i.e., a TYCSB agar plate), *Streptococcus mutans* will grow as a sugar cube. (N) *Eubacterium nodatum* colony morphology strongly depends on its substrate. Its growth is very slow, and it is an obligate anaerobic gram-positive rod. (O) *Tannerella forsythia* organisms are fastidious bacteria that are therefore difficult to culture. This organism grows on a blood-agar plate as a smooth white colony with a faded edge. The bacteria are strictly anaerobic. (P) The typical colony morphology of *Streptococcus sobrinus* on TYCSB agar (colony with a white halo). (Q) *Capnocytophaga* are slowly growing bacteria that require an elevated carbon dioxide concentration for their growth. They are facultative anaerobic rods. (R) *Campylobacter rectus* grows on a Hammond plate as small, smooth, opaque, round colonies that are black. (S) *Eikenella corrodens* has a variable colony morphology and shows different biochemical and serologic reactions. Because of the difficult determination with classic culture, identification and quantification through DNA techniques are very suitable for this organism. *E. corrodens* cells are facultative, anaerobic, gram-negative rods. ([A] to [C], [F], [I], [L], [N], [O], [Q], and [S] Courtesy ADD Clinident, Malden, the Netherlands.)

Table 8.1 summarizes several publications that discuss the detection frequency of periodontopathogens in these different niches. Most species (with the exception of spirochetes) (Fig. 8.2L) are able to colonize all of them. Some periodontopathogens (e.g., *Fusobacterium nucleatum* [see Fig. 8.2G] and *Prevotella intermedia* [see Fig. 8.2H]) are involved in the etiology of tonsillitis, and most periodontopathogens are able to colonize the maxillary sinus.[37,426]

The soft tissue surfaces are actively involved in the process of bacterial adhesion and colonization.[153] They use a variety of mechanisms to prevent the adhesion of pathogenic organisms, with shedding being one of the most important.

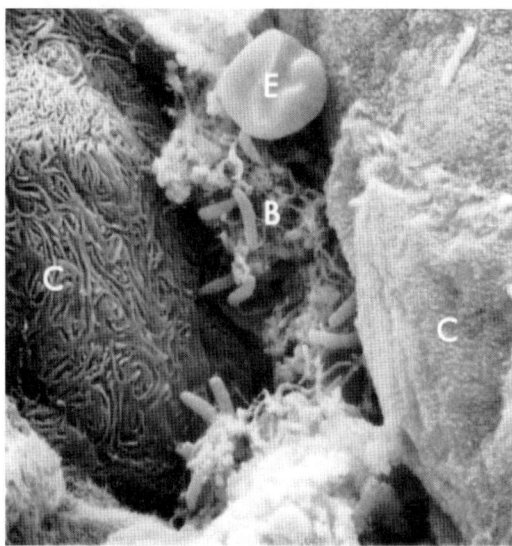

Fig. 8.3 Epithelial intercellular spaces containing plaque. Scanning electron micrograph of epithelial intercellular spaces that contain bacterial plaque *(B)* enmeshed in a fibrin-like material. *C,* Epithelial cells; *E,* erythrocyte. The cells to the *left* show signs of necrosis. ×4000.

CLINICIAN'S CORNER

Is it necessary to brush the gums?

In essence, not. The epithelial cells are shed twice a day in a process known as *desquamation*, which is considered to be a natural cleansing mechanism. However, due to the morphology of the tongue and under removable prostheses, desquamated epithelial cells will not be flushed away by removal forces within the oral cavity. Brushing of these areas may therefore be recommended.

The host vaginal epithelial cells, for example, supply glucose for the colonized lactobacilli, which in turn produce acid. A lowering of the pH prevents the growth of many other species that have deleterious effects on the vaginal environment.[334] As such, these endogenous bacteria and their products can be considered necessary and beneficial components of a healthy body.

In periodontal pockets, studies have shown high numbers of bacteria attached to pocket epithelial cells in vivo. Areas of gingival inflammation are characterized by an increased number of adhering bacteria.[86,420] These adhering bacteria can also infiltrate the pocket wall in relatively large numbers and reach the underlying stroma (Fig. 8.4).[104,244,345] In general, a positive correlation exists between the adhesion rate of pathogenic bacteria to different epithelia and the susceptibility of the affected patient to certain infections.[277]

Women prone to urinary tract infections, for example, harbor five times more bacteria per cell in adhesion assays of *Escherichia coli* to different epithelial cells of their urogenital tract (periurethral, vaginal, or uroepithelial cells). Similar observations have been made regarding the adhesion of *Streptococcus pneumoniae* to nasopharyngeal epithelial cells of children prone to recurrent otitis media infections, as well as regarding the adhesion of *Haemophilus influenzae* to buccal cells of subjects prone to acute bronchitis.[71,403]

Some indications exist that the same may be true for periodontal infections. Isogai and coworkers[162] reported a significantly lower adherence rate of *P. gingivalis* and *P. intermedia* strains to gingival epithelial cells in rats that were resistant to gingivitis compared with susceptible rats. An in vitro study of cultured human pocket epithelial cells (Fig. 8.5) showed a similar tendency when patients who were resistant to periodontitis were compared with patients with severe periodontal breakdown.[314]

Bacteria also adhere to hard tissues. In the human body, teeth and nails are the only naturally occurring nonshedding surfaces. Artificial nonshedding surfaces of medical importance include prosthetic devices such as catheters, artificial joints, dental implants, and heart valves. From a microbiologic viewpoint, teeth and implants are unique for two reasons: (1) they provide a hard, nonshedding surface that allows for the development of extensive structured bacterial deposits; and (2) they form a unique ectodermal interruption. A special seal of epithelium (junctional epithelium) and connective tissue is present between the external environment and the internal parts of the body. The accumulation and metabolism of bacteria on these hard surfaces are considered the primary causes of caries, gingivitis, periodontitis, peri-implantitis, and, sometimes, bad breath.

In the periodontal pocket, different strategies contribute to bacterial survival, such as adhesion to the pocket epithelium and, when dentin is encountered, the colonization of the dentinal tubules.[305] The crevicular fluid with its constant outflow does not favor the maintenance of unattached bacteria in the periodontal pocket.

Investigators have suggested that teeth are the primary habitat for periodontopathogens because soon after a full-mouth tooth extraction in patients with severe periodontitis, key pathogens such as *A. actinomycetemcomitans* and *P. gingivalis* disappeared from the oral cavity, as determined by bacterial culturing techniques.[73] *P. intermedia* and other black-pigmented *Prevotella* spp. remained, but at lower detection frequencies and numbers (see Table 8.1).

The same applies to edentulous infants and wearers of full dentures in whom significant proportions of periodontopathogens have been recorded, with the exception of *A. actinomycetemcomitans* and *P. gingivalis*.[72,189] Therefore, teeth were considered as a "porte d'entrée" for periodontopathogens.

However, studies involving the use of molecular tools to detect and quantify oral bacteria seem to indicate that *A. actinomycetemcomitans* and *P. gingivalis* are not entirely eradicated after full-mouth extraction. They may remain colonizers of the oral cavity, but when teeth are lost, the relative numbers of these bacteria decrease.[318,320]

KEY FACT

Hard surfaces such as teeth and dental implants are very important habitats for oral pathogens. However, they are by far not the only habitats.

Alternatively, cariogenic species were thought to be relatively restricted to solid surfaces (see Table 8.1). Therefore, *S. mutans* (Fig. 8.2M) was often considered an *obligate periphyte*.[402] In some studies, this species was detected only from the time that the deciduous teeth erupted in the oral cavity.[50] In a longitudinal observation of adults with severe dental caries, the cariogenic species fell below detection level after full-mouth extraction but reappeared a few days after denture insertion.[51] On the basis of these reports and on their own observations, Caufield and Gibbons[54] concluded that most of the *S. mutans* cells in the saliva or on the tongue are derived from the biofilm present on the teeth and that the mucosae could not act as a reservoir for the infection of teeth by those organisms. These investigators suggested a "window of infectivity" for the acquisition of *S. mutans* at a mean age of 26 months (range, 9 to 44 months).[53] This observation has been supported by a few clinical studies, which showed that the initial colonization of *S. mutans* varied between 7 to 36 months, which is the time period that coincides with the eruption of the primary teeth.[7,49,106] Conversely, longitudinal studies by Wan and coworkers[431,432] and Law and Seow[209] showed that *S. mutans* colonization increased with the age of children, without any discrete

TABLE 8.1   Intraoral Habitats (Periodontal Pockets, Buccal Mucosa, Tongue, Saliva, Tonsils, and Supragingival Plaque) for Periodontopathogenic and Cariogenic Species

Authors	Infection	Age Group (n)	Species	No. of Positive Patients	DIFFERENT INTRAORAL NICHES					
					Periodontal Pockets	Buccal Mucosa	Tongue	Saliva	Tonsils	Supragingival Plaque
Asikainen et al, 1991	Periodontitis	Adult	A. a.	—	100%[a]	—	56%	72%	—	—
Petit et al, 1994	—	Child (45)	A. a.	5	4[b]	3	1	3	2	—
			P. g.	1	0	1	0	1	1	—
			P. i.	34	23	18	25	31	22	—
			Spi	13	6	0	7	3	1	—
Petit et al, 1994	Periodontitis	Adult (24)	A. a.	13	13[c]	11	11	11	5	—
			P. g.	18	18	14	7	10	11	—
			P. i.	24	24	22	23	23	23	—
			Spi	22	22	0	2	5	1	—
von Troil-Lindén et al, 1995	Periodontitis	Adult (10)	A. a.	—	6[c]	—	—	6	—	—
			P. g.	—	7	—	—	4	—	—
			P. i.	—	10	—	—	9	—	—
Danser et al, 1994	Periodontitis/E	Adult (8)	A. a.	2	2/—[d]	2/0	2/0	2/0	2/0	1/0
			P. g.	6	6/—	2/0	4/0	4/0	3/0	2/0
			P. i.	8	8/—	4/1	6/3	6/4	5/3	6/1
			Prev.	8	3/—	4/5	7/6	7/5	4/6	5/4
Danser et al, 1996	Periodontitis/R	Adult (15)	A. a.	11	9/4[e]	10/9	—	5/2	—	2/0
			P. g.	10	6/5	9/7	—	4/1	—	6/0
			P. i.	15	11/1	15/15	—	14/13	—	11/1
Gibbons and van Houte, 1975	—[f]	—[f]	S. m.	—	?	<1[e]	<1	<1	—	0–50
			L.		?	<0.1	<0.1	<1	—	0–1

[a]Percentage of "specific" positive sites in positive patients.

[b]Number of "specific" positive sites in positive patients.

[c]Number of "specific" positive sites in patients with advanced periodontitis.

[d]Number of "specific" positive sites in positive patients before/after full-mouth extraction (e.g., two patients tested positive for A. a. before extraction, and no patients tested positive for A. a. after full-mouth extraction).

[e]Number of "specific" positive sites in positive patients before/after periodontal therapy including surgery (e.g., nine patients tested positive for A. a. before periodontal therapy as compared with only four patients after periodontal therapy).

[f]Percentage of total flora cultivable in anaerobically incubated agar in nonspecific patients as estimated from several studies.

A. a., Aggregatibacter actinomycetemcomitans; E, full-mouth extraction; L., Lactobacillus spp.; P. g., Porphyromonas gingivalis; P. i., Prevotella intermedia; Prev., Prevotella spp. (e.g., P. melaninogenica, P. denticola, P. loescheii, P. veroralis); R, periodontal therapy including surgery; S. m., Streptococcus mutans; Spi, spirochetes.

window of infectivity. Clinical evidence now shows that *S. mutans* can be detected in the mouths of predentate children, before the eruption of the first tooth.[256,431,433]

Bacteria and Their Biofilm Mode of Living

The importance of surfaces for microbial growth was recognized as early as the 1920s, when a number of workers independently noted that bacteria growing on glass slides submerged in soil were different from bacteria that could be cultured in broth.[208] However, it was not until around 50 years later that sessile microbial populations were considered to be sufficiently different from free-living microorganisms to merit their own name, and the term *biofilms* was coined (Fig. 8.6 and Fig. 8.7B and C). Biofilms are composed of microbial cells encased within a matrix of extracellular polymeric substances, such as polysaccharides, proteins, and nucleic acids.

Biofilm bacteria are often up to 1000 times more resistant to antimicrobial agents than their planktonic counterparts.[9,96] Bacteria that grow in multispecies biofilms interact closely with neighboring cells. Sometimes these interactions are mutually beneficial, as is the case when one organism removes another's waste products and uses them as an energy source.

In other instances, bacteria compete with their neighbors by secreting antibacterial molecules such as inhibitory peptides (bacteriocins) or hydrogen peroxide (H_2O_2) (Video 8.1). In addition, the biofilm mode of growth facilitates cell–cell signaling and deoxyribonucleic acid (DNA) exchange between bacteria. It is clear that microbial ecology within biofilm communities is highly complex and that, in many cases, knowledge is only emerging at this point.

Biofilms are heterogeneous: variations in biofilm structure exist within individual biofilms, between different types of biofilms, and between individuals[321] (Fig. 8.8). However, some structural features that are common to many biofilms have been noted. For example, biofilms frequently contain microcolonies of bacterial cells. Water channels are commonly found in biofilms, and these can form a primitive circulatory system that removes waste products and brings fresh nutrients to the deeper layers of the film. Surface structures, such as fronds, can dissipate the energy of fluid flowing over the biofilm and lead to the rapid blockage of vessels.[85] Mixed-species biofilms often have heterogeneity in the distribution of different

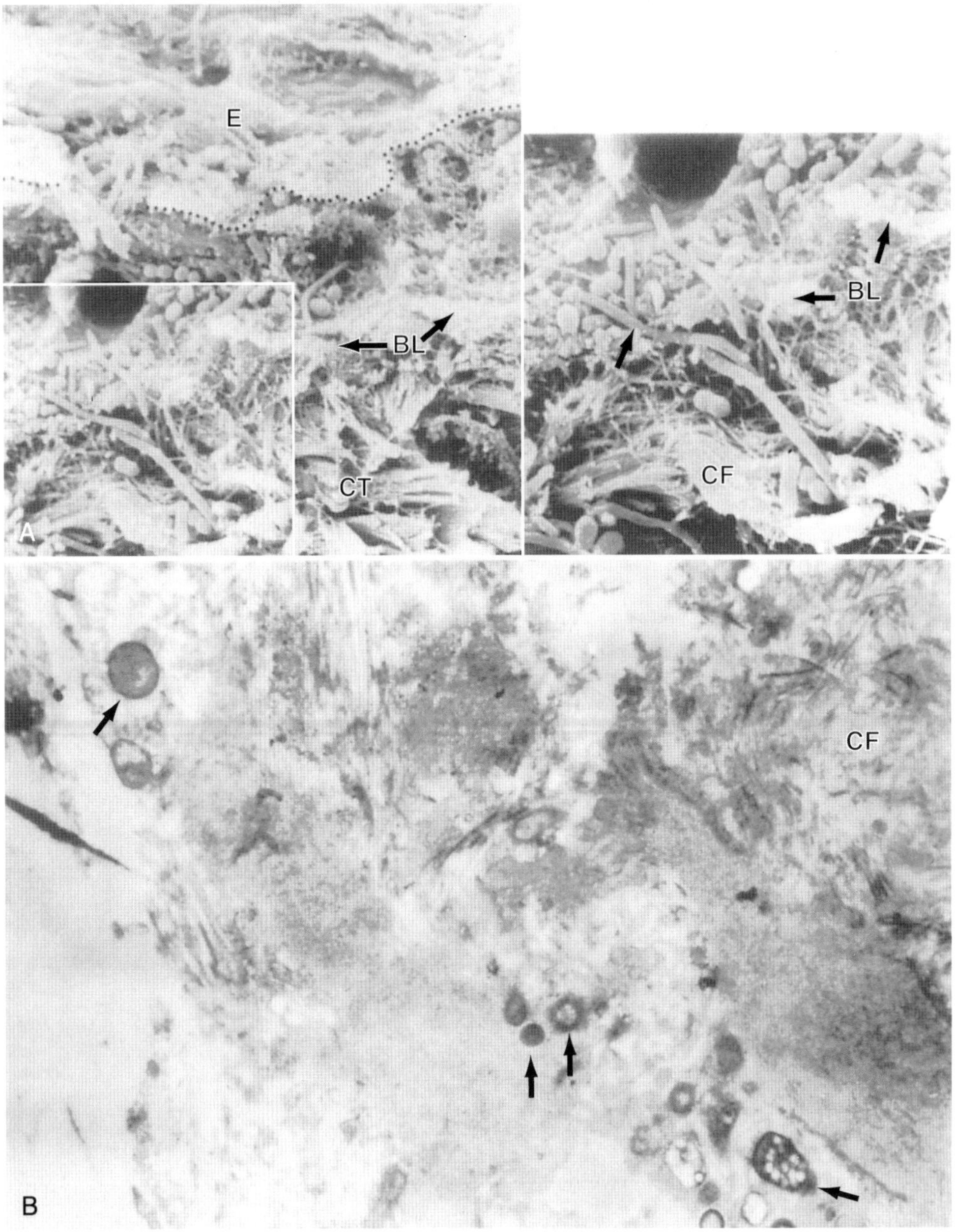

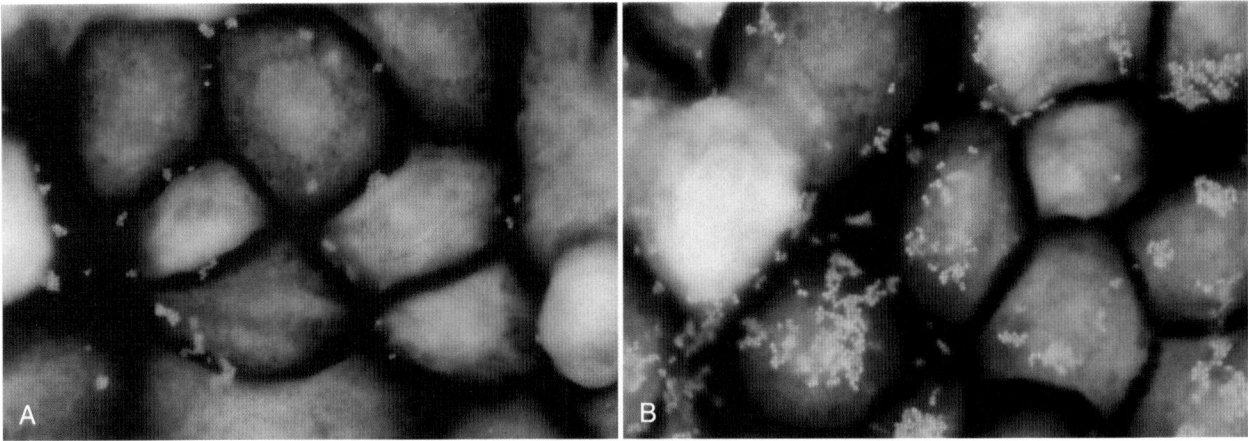

Fig. 8.4 Bacterial penetration into the pocket wall with advanced periodontitis. (A) Penetration through the pocket epithelium *(E)* and the basement lamina *(BL)* into the connective tissue *(CT) (arrows). CF,* Collagen fibers. (B) Connective-tissue–associated bacteria *(arrows)* in a patient with advanced periodontitis. *([A] Courtesy Dr. R. Saglie. [A] and [B] From Nissengard RJ, Newman MG: Oral microbiology and immunology, ed 2, Philadelphia, 1994, Saunders.)*

Fig. 8.5 *Porphyromonas gingivalis* adhesion capacity differences. Microscopic confirmation of significant differences in the adhesion capacity of *P. gingivalis (small green dots)* to epithelial cells from (A) a resistant patient as compared with (B) a patient with severe periodontitis.

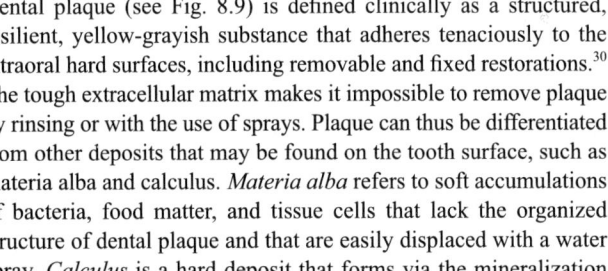

Fig. 8.6 Vertical section through a 4-day human plaque sample. An intraoral device designed for the *in vivo* generation of plaque biofilms on enamel was used. Confocal microscopy enabled the visualization of the section of plaque without the dehydration steps used in conventional histologic preparations. Notice the open fluid-filled channels *(arrows)* that traverse from the plaque surface through the bacterial mass *(M;* gray-white areas) to the enamel surface. An area in which the bacterial mass appears to attach to the enamel surface *(A)* is indicated. Scale bar = 25 μm. *(From Wood SR, Kirkham J, Marsh PD, et al: Architecture of intact natural human plaque biofilms studied by confocal laser scanning microscopy. J Dent Res 79:21, 2000.)*

species. Steep chemical gradients exist, such as those of oxygen or pH, and these produce distinct microenvironments within the biofilm.

Microbial populations on the surfaces of teeth (dental plaque) are excellent examples of biofilm communities (Fig. 8.9). The architecture of a dental plaque biofilm has many features in common with other biofilms. It is heterogeneous in structure, with clear evidence of open fluid-filled channels running through the plaque mass[64,65,449] (see Fig. 8.6). Nutrients make contact with the sessile (attached) microcolonies by diffusion from the water channels to the microcolony, rather than from the matrix. The bacteria exist and proliferate within the intercellular matrix through which the channels run. The matrix confers a specialized environment that distinguishes the bacteria that exist within the biofilm from those that are free floating; this is the so-called planktonic state in solutions such as saliva or crevicular fluid. The biofilm matrix functions as a barrier. Substances produced by bacteria within the biofilm are retained and concentrated, which fosters metabolic interactions among the different bacteria.

The intercellular matrix consists of organic and inorganic materials derived from saliva, gingival crevicular fluid, and bacterial products.

Organic constituents of the matrix include polysaccharides, proteins, glycoproteins, lipid material, and DNA.[226] Albumin, which probably originates from crevicular fluid, has been identified as a component of the plaque matrix. The lipid material consists of debris from the membranes of disrupted bacterial and host cells, bacterial vesicles, and possibly food debris. *Glycoproteins* from the saliva are important components of the pellicle that initially coats a clean tooth surface, but they also become incorporated into the developing plaque biofilm. Polysaccharides produced by bacteria also contribute to the organic portion of the matrix. They play a major role in maintaining the integrity of the biofilm.

The *inorganic components* of plaque are predominantly calcium and phosphorus, with trace amounts of other minerals such as sodium, potassium, and fluoride. The source of inorganic constituents of supragingival plaque is primarily saliva. As the mineral content increases, the plaque mass becomes calcified to form calculus (Fig. 8.10). Calculus is frequently found in areas of the dentition adjacent to salivary ducts (e.g., the lingual surface of the mandibular incisors and canines, the buccal surface of the maxillary first molars), and this reflects the high concentration of minerals available from saliva

in those regions. The inorganic components of subgingival plaque are derived from crevicular fluid (a serum transudate). The calcification of subgingival plaque also results in calculus formation (Fig. 8.11). Subgingival calculus is typically dark green or dark brown, which probably reflects the presence of blood products that are associated with subgingival hemorrhage.

The importance of these biofilms for oral diseases, such as dental caries and periodontitis—together with the relative ease with which tooth surface biofilms can be accessed—has caused dental plaque to be one of the most highly studied biofilm systems. It is anticipated that, by understanding the mechanisms involved in the accumulation of dental plaque and the transition from health to disease, it will be possible to improve our control over these processes and to restrict plaque-associated oral diseases further.

Structure of a Mature Dental Plaque Biofilm

Dental plaque (see Fig. 8.9) is defined clinically as a structured, resilient, yellow-grayish substance that adheres tenaciously to the intraoral hard surfaces, including removable and fixed restorations.[30] The tough extracellular matrix makes it impossible to remove plaque by rinsing or with the use of sprays. Plaque can thus be differentiated from other deposits that may be found on the tooth surface, such as materia alba and calculus. *Materia alba* refers to soft accumulations of bacteria, food matter, and tissue cells that lack the organized structure of dental plaque and that are easily displaced with a water spray. *Calculus* is a hard deposit that forms via the mineralization of dental plaque and that is generally covered by a layer of unmineralized plaque (Table 8.2).

Dental plaque is composed primarily of microorganisms. One gram of plaque (wet weight) contains approximately 10^{11} bacteria.[358,380] The number of bacteria in supragingival plaque on a single tooth surface can exceed 10^9 cells. In a periodontal pocket, counts can range from 10^3 bacteria in a healthy crevice to more than 10^8 bacteria in a deep pocket. With the use of highly sensitive molecular techniques for microbial identification, it has been estimated that more than 750 distinct microbial phylotypes can be present as natural inhabitants of dental plaque.[1]

Any individual may harbor hundreds of different species. Next to bacteria, nonbacterial organisms can also be found in the dental plaque biofilm, including archaea, yeasts, protozoa, and viruses.[62,217]

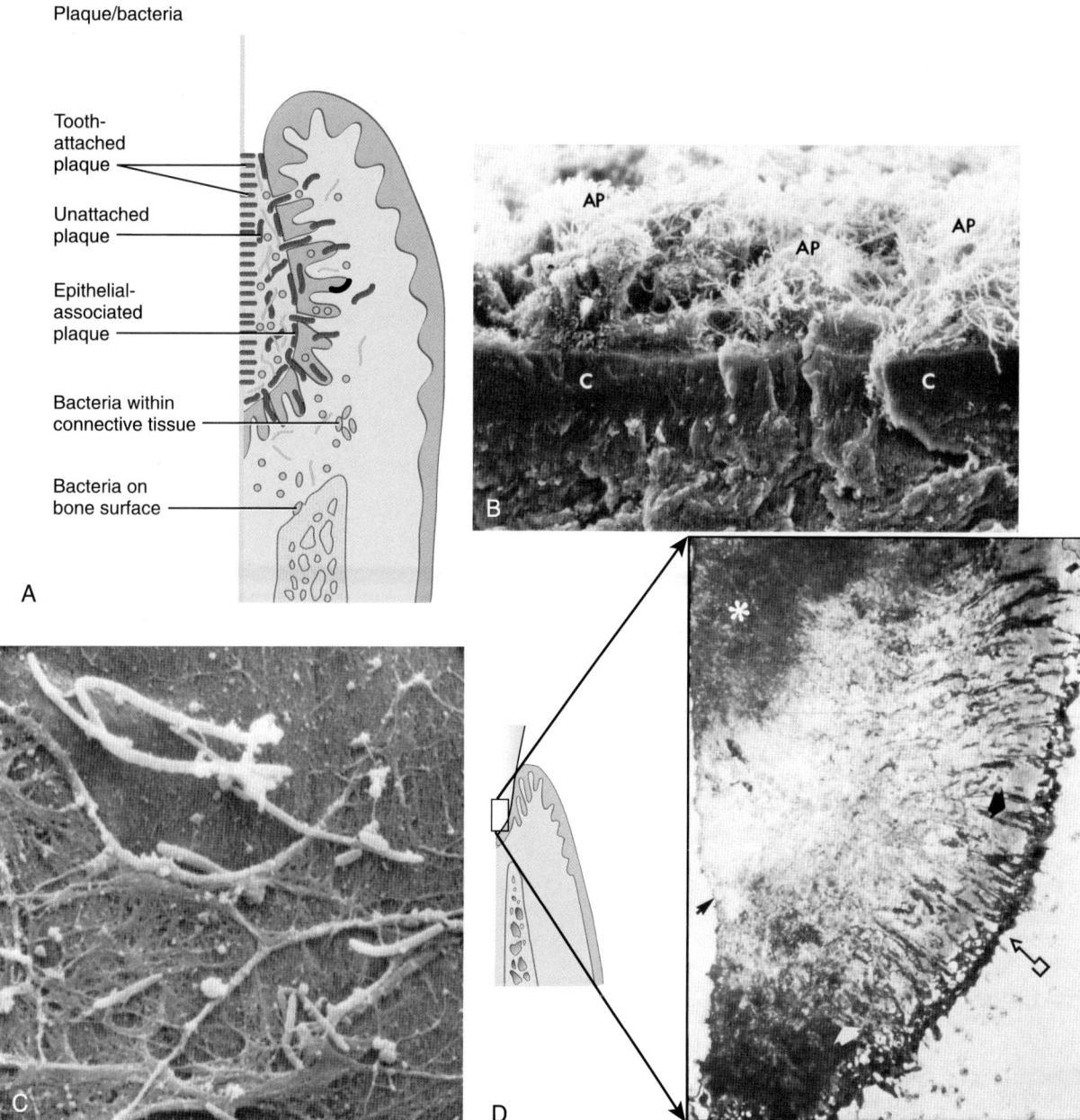

Fig. 8.7 Subgingival plaque. (A) Diagram depicting the plaque–bacteria association between the tooth surface and the periodontal tissues. (B) Scanning electron photomicrograph of a cross-section of cementum *(C)* with attached subgingival plaque *(AP).* The area shown is within a periodontal pocket. (C) Scanning electron micrograph of cocci and filaments associated with the surface of pocket epithelium in a case of marginal gingivitis. ×3000. (D) *Left,* Diagrammatic representation of the histologic structure of subgingival plaque. *Right,* Histologic section of subgingival plaque. *Arrow with box,* Sulcular epithelium. *White arrow,* Predominantly gram-negative unattached zone. *Black arrow,* Tooth surface. *Asterisk,* Predominantly gram-positive attached zone. *(B, Courtesy Dr. J. Sottosanti, La Jolla, Calif.)*

CLINICIAN'S CORNER

Is it possible to remove dental plaque by rinsing?
The biofilm nature of dental plaque means that it tenaciously adheres to surfaces. Therefore it cannot be removed by rinsing or sprays.

Dental plaque is broadly classified as supragingival or subgingival on the basis of its position on the tooth surface toward the gingival margin.

- *Supragingival plaque* is found at or above the gingival margin; when in direct contact with the gingival margin, it is referred to as *marginal plaque.*
- *Subgingival plaque* is found below the gingival margin, between the tooth and the gingival pocket epithelium.

  Supragingival plaque typically demonstrates the stratified organization of a multilayered accumulation of bacterial morphotypes (Fig. 8.12).[462] Gram-positive cocci and short rods predominate at the tooth surface, whereas gram-negative rods, filaments, and spirochetes predominate in the outer surface of the mature plaque mass.

Subject 1   Subject 2   Subject 3

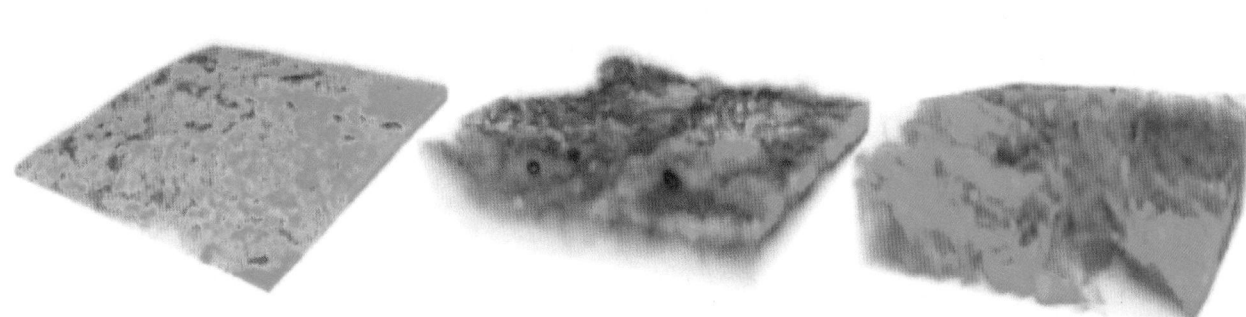

Fig. 8.8 Architecture of oral biofilms formed on enamel discs in situ in three subjects. Biofilms were allowed to develop on the enamel surfaces mounted on healing abutments in the oral cavity for 7 days. The abutments were then removed, stained with BacLight Live/Dead (ThermoFisher Scientific, Waltham, Mass.) staining, and visualized using confocal laser scanning microscopy. *(Adapted from Rabe P, Twetman S, Kinnby B, et al: Effect of fluoride and chlorhexidine digluconate mouthrinses on plaque biofilms.* Open Dent J *31:106–11, 2015.)*

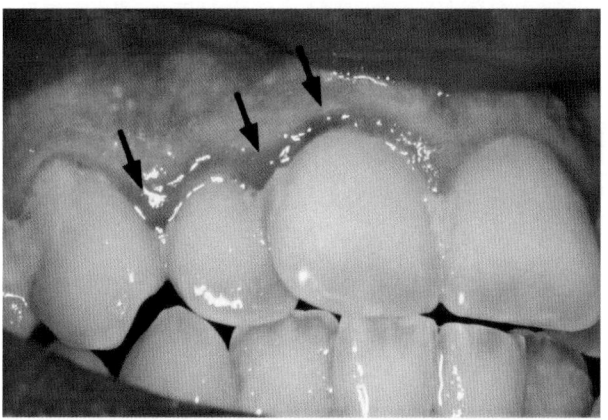

Fig. 8.9 Clinical picture of 10-day-old supragingival plaque. The first signs of gingival inflammation *(arrows)* are becoming visible.

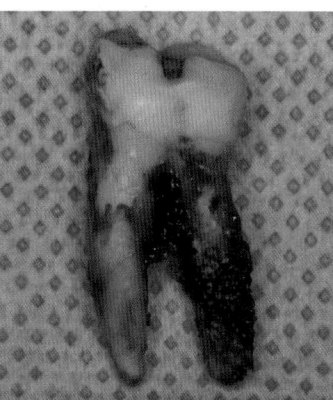

Fig. 8.11 Dark-pigmented deposits of subgingival calculus on the distal root of an extracted lower molar.

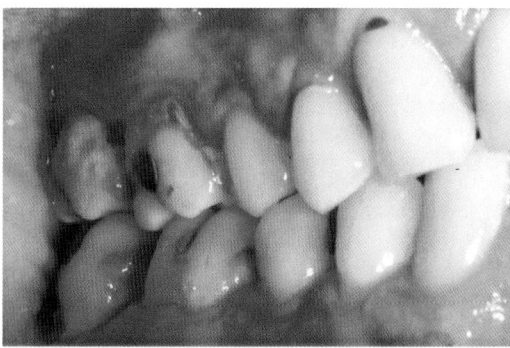

Fig. 8.10 Supragingival calculus is depicted on the buccal surface of the maxillary molars adjacent to the orifice of the parotid duct.

In general, the subgingival microbiota differs in composition from the supragingival plaque, primarily because of the local availability of blood products and a low reduction–oxidation (redox) potential, which characterizes the anaerobic environment.

The environmental parameters of the subgingival region differ from those of the supragingival region. The gingival crevice or pocket is bathed by the flow of crevicular fluid, which contains many substances that bacteria may use as nutrients. Host inflammatory cells and mediators are likely to have considerable influence on the establishment

and growth of bacteria in the subgingival region. Both morphologic and microbiologic studies of subgingival plaque reveal distinctions between the tooth-associated regions and the soft tissue–associated regions of subgingival plaque (see Fig. 8.7A to C).[222,268]

KEY FACT

The specific microbial composition and structure of dental biofilms are highly dependent on the region of the tooth and the local environmental parameters.

The tooth-associated cervical plaque that adheres to the root cementum does not markedly differ from that observed in gingivitis. At this location, filamentous microorganisms dominate, but cocci and rods also occur. This plaque is dominated by gram-positive rods and cocci, including *S. mitis, S. sanguinis, Actinomyces oris, Actinomyces naeslundii,* and *Eubacterium* spp. (see Fig. 8.2N). However, in the deeper parts of the pocket, the filamentous organisms become fewer in number; in the apical portion, they seem to be virtually absent. Instead, the microbiota is dominated by smaller organisms without a particular orientation.[222] The apical border of the plaque mass is separated from the junctional epithelium by a layer of host leukocytes, and the bacterial population of this apical-tooth–associated region shows an increased concentration of gram-negative rods (see Fig. 8.7D).

TABLE 8.2 Differences Between Tooth Deposits

Materia Alba	Dental Plaque	Calculus
• White, cheeselike accumulation	• Resilient clear to yellow-grayish substance	• Hard deposit that forms via the mineralization of dental plaque
• Soft accumulation of salivary proteins, some bacteria, many desquamated epithelial cells, and occasional disintegrating food debris	• Primarily composed of bacteria in a matrix of salivary glycoproteins and extracellular polysaccharides	• Generally covered by a layer of unmineralized dental plaque
• Lacks an organized structure and is therefore not as complex as dental plaque	• Considered to be a biofilm	
• Easily displaced with a water spray	• Impossible to remove by rinsing or with the use of sprays	

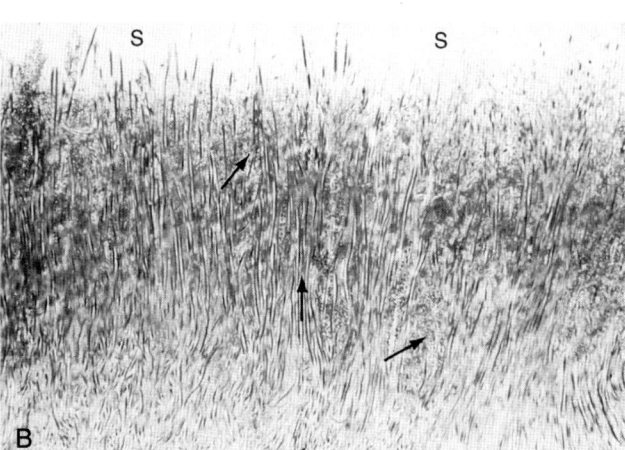

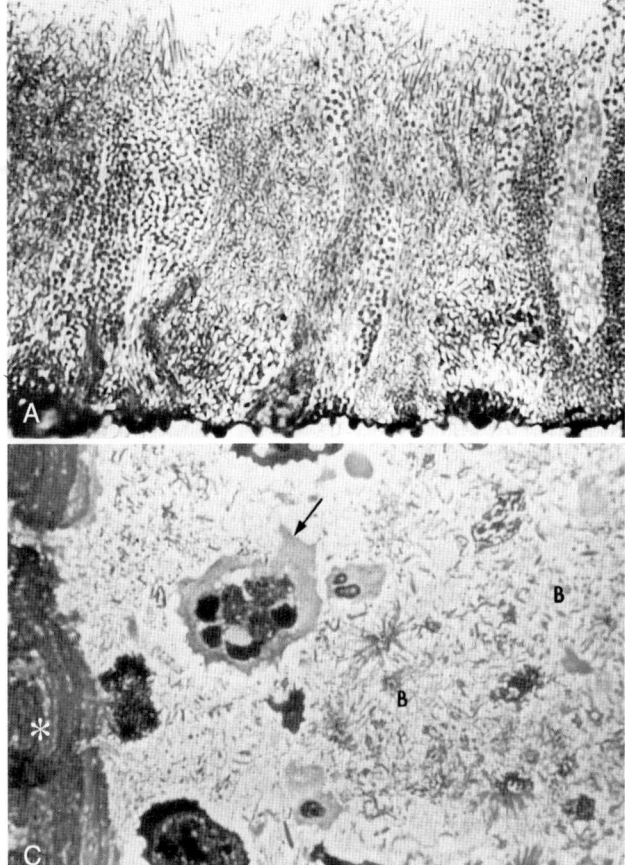

Fig. 8.12 Plaque formation. (A) One-day-old plaque. Microcolonies of plaque bacteria extend perpendicularly away from the tooth surfaces. (B) Developed supragingival plaque showing the overall filamentous nature and the microcolonies *(arrows)* that extend perpendicularly away from the tooth surface. The saliva–plaque interface is shown *(S)*. (C) A histologic section of plaque showing nonbacterial components such as white blood cells *(arrow)* and epithelial cells *(asterisk)* interspersed among bacteria *(B)*. *(Courtesy Dr. Max Listgarten, Philadelphia, Pa.)*

The layers of microorganisms that face the soft tissue lack a definite intermicrobial matrix and contain primarily gram-negative rods and cocci, as well as large numbers of filaments, flagellated rods, and spirochetes. Studies of plaque associated with crevicular epithelial cells indicate a predominance of species such as *S. oralis, S. intermedius, Parvimonas micra* (formerly *Micromonas micra* and *Peptostreptococcus micros*), *P. gingivalis, P. intermedia, Tannerella forsythia* (see Fig. 8.12), and *F. nucleatum*.[81,86] Host-tissue cells (e.g., white blood cells, epithelial cells) may also be found in this region (see Fig. 8.12C). Bacteria are also found within the host tissues, such as in the soft tissues (see Fig. 8.4), and within epithelial cells (Fig. 8.13), as well as in the dentinal tubules (Fig. 8.14).[344,345]

The composition of the subgingival plaque depends on the pocket depth. The apical part is more dominated by spirochetes, cocci, and rods, whereas in the coronal part more filaments are observed.

The site specificity of plaque is significantly associated with diseases of the periodontium. Marginal plaque, for example, is of prime importance during the initiation and development of gingivitis. Supragingival plaque and tooth-associated subgingival plaque are critical in calculus formation and root caries, whereas tissue-associated subgingival plaque is important in the tissue destruction that characterizes different forms of periodontitis. Biofilms also establish on artificial surfaces exposed to the oral environment, such as prostheses and implants.

Accumulation of a Dental Plaque Biofilm

The process of plaque formation can be divided into several phases: (1) the formation of the pellicle on the tooth surface, (2) the initial adhesion/attachment of bacteria, and (3) colonization/plaque maturation.

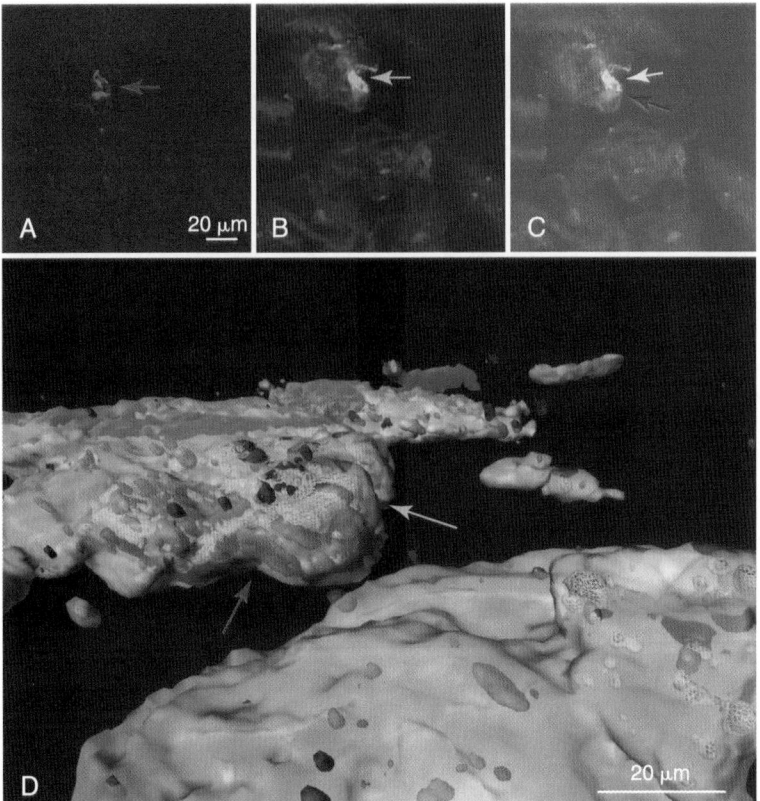

Fig. 8.13 Bacteria in epithelial cells. (A) to (C) Images of z-section no. 39 from a stack of 74 0.2-μm z-sections (×600; the scale bar in [A] also applies to [B] and [C]). Buccal epithelial cells in this field were double-labeled with (A) the EUB338 universal probe and (B) the *Aggregatibacter actinomycetemcomitans*–specific probe. The cell in the center of (A) contained a large mass of brightly fluorescent intracellular bacteria *(red arrow)*. Other cells in the field contained smaller bacterial masses (not marked). (B) A portion of the large mass labeled with the universal probe also hybridized with the *A. actinomycetemcomitans*–specific probe *(green arrow)*. Images from (A) and (B) were superimposed in (C) to confirm that bacteria labeled with both probes *(yellow arrow)* were adjacent to other bacteria labeled only with the universal probe *(red arrow)*. (D) Three-dimensional reconstruction of the same field. Bacteria recognized only by the universal probe are shown in solid red, whereas the colocalization of the *A. actinomycetemcomitans* and universal probes is depicted by a green wireframe over a red interior. Reconstructed buccal epithelial cell surfaces are presented in blue. The red and green colors are muted when bacterial masses are intracellular and brighter when bacteria appear to project out of the surface. The angle of view was rotated along the z-axis, and the image was zoomed. The large mass that appeared to have a lobular structure in z-section no. 39 was seen to be a cohesive unit that contained *A. actinomycetemcomitans* in direct proximity to other species *(red and green arrows)*. *(From Rudney JD, Chen R, Sedgewick GJ:* Actinobacillus actinomycetemcomitans, Porphyromonas gingivalis, *and* Tannerella forsythensis *are components of a polymicrobial intracellular flora within human buccal cells.* J Dent Res *84:59–63, 2005.)*

Formation of the Pellicle

All surfaces in the oral cavity, including the hard and soft tissues, are coated with a layer of organic material known as the acquired pellicle. The pellicle on tooth surfaces consists of more than 180 peptides, proteins, and glycoproteins, including keratins, mucins, proline-rich proteins, phosphoproteins (e.g., statherin), histidine-rich proteins, and other molecules that can function as adhesion sites (receptors) for bacteria.[366,367,453] The salivary pellicle can be detected on clean enamel surfaces within 1 minute after their introduction into the mouths of volunteers.[143] By 2 hours, the pellicle is essentially in equilibrium between adsorption and detachment, although further pellicle maturation can be observed for several hours.

Transmission electron microscopy shows the pellicle to be composed of two layers: a thin basal layer that is very difficult to remove, even with harsh chemical and mechanical treatments, and a thicker globular layer, up to 1 μm or more, that is easier to detach.[143,144] From these observations, it can be concluded that dental

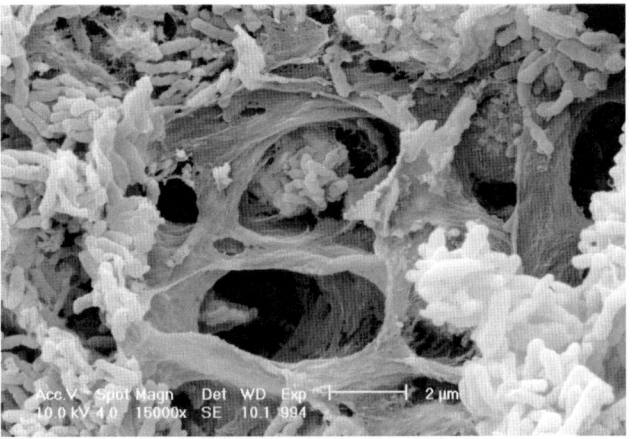

Fig. 8.14 Scanning electron micrograph of bacteria within dentinal tubules.

enamel is permanently covered with an acquired pellicle from the moment that teeth erupt.

Consequently, bacteria that adhere to tooth surfaces do not contact the enamel directly but interact with the acquired enamel pellicle. However, the pellicle is not merely a passive adhesion matrix. Many proteins retain enzymatic activity when they are incorporated into the pellicle, and some of these, such as peroxidases, lysozyme, and α-amylase, may affect the physiology and metabolism of adhering bacterial cells.[138,140–142]

In addition, a close ecologic relationship between the pellicle and its associated microbiology seems to exist. Walker and coworkers[429] reported that dental plaque samples produced in vitro biofilms only if the surface on which they were grown contained a salivary pellicle belonging to the patient who donated the plaque sample. No biofilm could be grown on a pellicle that came from a different subject.[429]

 ### Initial Adhesion/Attachment of Bacteria

Colonization of a surface begins immediately after its introduction in the oral cavity. Colonizing bacteria can be detected within 3 minutes after the introduction of sterile enamel into the mouth.[139]

The initial steps of transport and interaction with the surface are essentially nonspecific (i.e., they are the same for all bacteria). The proteins and carbohydrates that are exposed on the bacterial cell surface become important when the bacteria are in loose contact with the acquired enamel pellicle. The specific interactions between microbial cell surface "adhesin" molecules and receptors in the salivary pellicle determine whether a bacterial cell will remain associated with the surface. Only a relatively small proportion of oral bacteria possess adhesins that interact with receptors in the host pellicle, and these organisms are generally the most abundant bacteria in biofilms on tooth enamel shortly after cleaning. Over the first 4 to 8 hours, the genus *Streptococcus* tends to dominate, usually accounting for >20% of bacteria present.[82,273,427] Other bacteria that commonly present at this time include species that cannot survive without oxygen (obligate aerobes), such as *Haemophilus* spp. and *Neisseria* spp., as well as organisms that can grow in the presence or absence of oxygen (facultative anaerobes), including *Actinomyces* spp. and *Veillonella* spp.[1,79] These species are considered the "primary colonizers" of tooth surfaces. The primary colonizers provide new binding sites for adhesion by other oral bacteria. The metabolic activity of the primary colonizers modifies the local microenvironment in ways that can influence the ability of other bacteria to survive in the dental plaque biofilm. For example, by removing oxygen, the primary colonizers provide conditions of low oxygen tension that permit the survival and growth of obligate anaerobes.

The initial steps in colonization of teeth by bacteria occur in three phases. Phase 1 is transport to the surface, phase 2 is initial reversible adhesion, and phase 3 is strong attachment.

 ### Colonization and Plaque Maturation

The primary colonizing bacteria (Table 8.3) adhered to the tooth surface provide new receptors for attachment by other bacteria as part of a process known as *coadhesion*.[185] Together with the growth of adherent microorganisms, coadhesion leads to the development of microcolonies (Fig. 8.15) and eventually to a mature biofilm.

Cell–cell adhesion between genetically distinct oral bacteria also occurs in the fluid phase (i.e., in saliva). In the laboratory, interactions between genetically distinct cells in suspension result in clumps or coaggregates that are macroscopically visible (Fig. 8.16).

Different species—or even different strains of a single species—have distinct sets of coaggregation partners (see eFig. 8.6 online). Fusobacteria coaggregate with all other human oral bacteria, whereas

TABLE 8.3 Overview of Primary and Secondary Colonizers in Dental Plaque

Primary colonizers	*Streptococcus gordonii*
	Streptococcus intermedius
	Streptococcus mitis
	Streptococcus oralis
	Streptococcus sanguinis
	Actinomyces gerencseriae
	Actinomyces israelii
	Actinomyces naeslundii
	Actinomyces oris
	Aggregatibacter actinomycetemcomitans serotype a
	Capnocytophaga gingivalis
	Capnocytophaga ochracea
	Capnocytophaga sputigena
	Eikenella corrodens
	Actinomyces odontolyticus
	Veillonella parvula
Secondary colonizers	*Campylobacter gracilis*
	Campylobacter rectus
	Campylobacter showae
	Eubacterium nodatum
	Aggregatibacter actinomycetemcomitans serotype b
	Fusobacterium nucleatum spp. *nucleatum*
	Fusobacterium nucleatum spp. *vincentii*
	Fusobacterium nucleatum spp. *polymorphum*
	Fusobacterium periodonticum
	Parvimonas micra
	Prevotella intermedia
	Prevotella loescheii
	Prevotella nigrescens
	Streptococcus constellatus
	Tannerella forsythia
	Porphyromonas gingivalis
	Treponema denticola

Veillonella spp., *Capnocytophaga* spp. (see Fig. 8.2Q), and *Prevotella* spp. bind with streptococci and/or actinomyces.[184,186,442] Each newly accreted cell becomes itself a new surface and therefore may act as a coaggregation bridge to the next potentially accreting cell type that passes by.

Many coaggregations among strains of different genera are mediated by lectin-like adhesins (proteins that recognize carbohydrates) and can be inhibited by lactose and other galactosides or by amino acids such as L-arginine. The significance of coaggregation in oral colonization has been documented in studies of biofilm formation in vitro as well as in animal model studies.[32,249]

Well-characterized interactions of secondary colonizers (see Table 8.3) with early colonizers include the coaggregation of *F. nucleatum* with *S. sanguinis*, *Prevotella loescheii* with *A. oris*, and *Capnocytophaga ochracea* with *A. oris*.[170,172,437–439] Streptococci show intrageneric coaggregation, which allows them to bind to the nascent monolayer of already bound streptococci.[155,181,274,368]

Secondary colonizers (see Table 8.3) such as *P. intermedia*, *P. loescheii*, *Capnocytophaga* spp., *F. nucleatum*, and *P. gingivalis* do not initially colonize clean tooth surfaces but rather adhere to bacteria that are already in the plaque mass.[184] The transition from early supragingival dental plaque to mature plaque growing below the

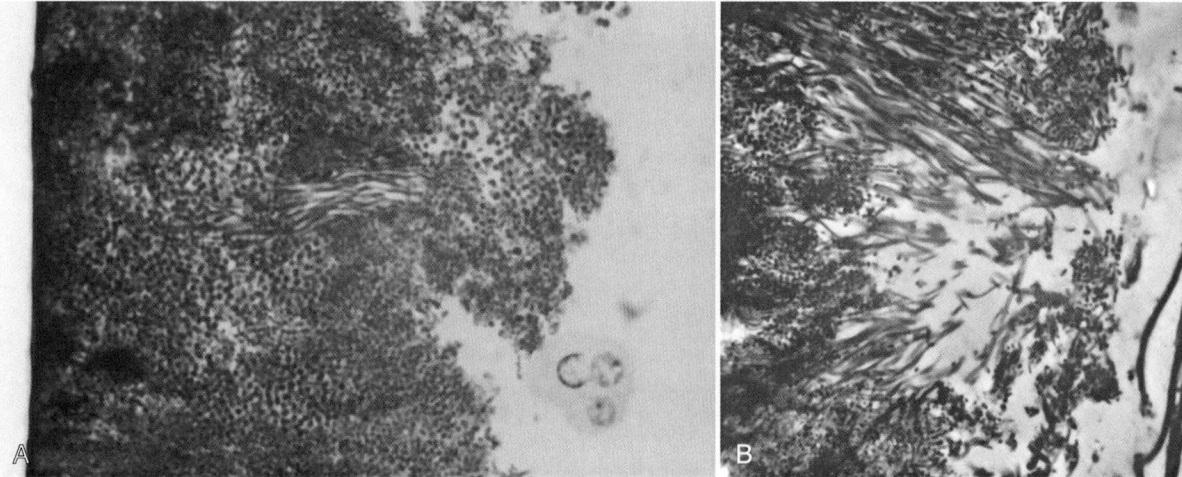

Fig. 8.15 Dental plaque. (A) and (B) When a single microorganism adheres to the tooth surface, it can start to multiply, and it slowly forms a microcolony of daughter cells. These views were taken after plaque formation on a plastic strip (e.g., as shown in Fig. 8.20) glued to a tooth surface.

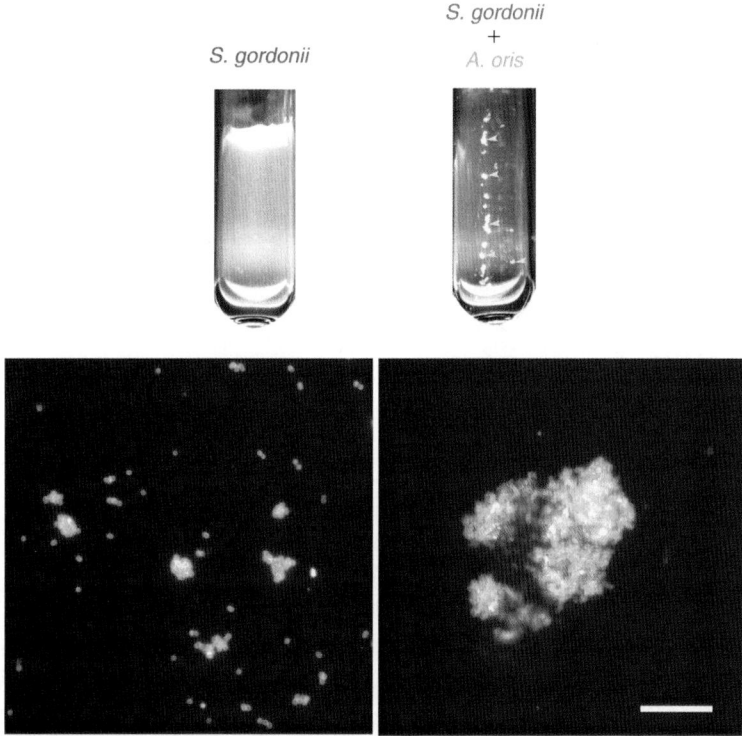

Fig. 8.16 Coaggregation. Coaggregation between *Streptococcus gordonii* DL1 and *Actinomyces oris* MG1 in vitro. A monoculture of *S. gordonii* appears uniformly turbid. Microscopically, cells labeled with specific anti-DL1 antibodies (green) are in small chains or clumps. After the addition of *A. oris,* cells clump together to form macroscopic coaggregates *(yellow arrowhead).* Under the microscope, *S. gordonii* (green) are evenly distributed throughout the coaggregates with *A. oris* (orange). Bar = 20 μm. *(Image reproduced in part from Jakubovics NS, Gill SR, Iobst SE, et al: Regulation of gene expression in a mixed-genus community: stabilized arginine biosynthesis in* Streptococcus gordonii *by coaggregation with* Actinomyces naeslundii. J Bacteriol 190:3646, 2008.)*

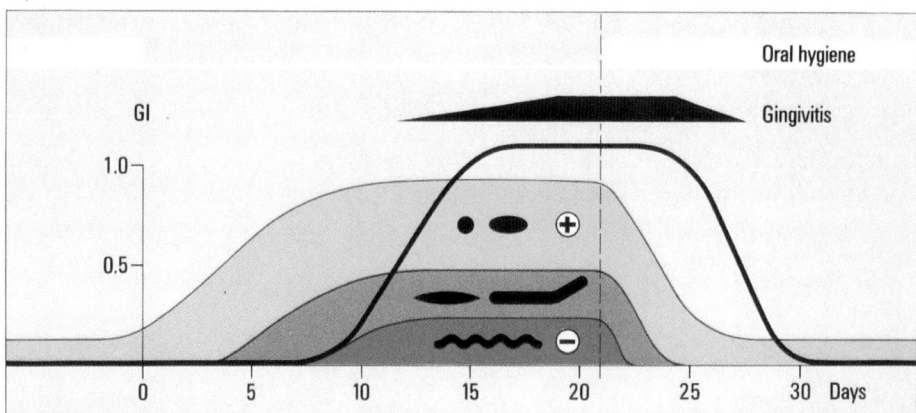

Fig. 8.17 Artistic impression of the 1965 published classic experimental proof of the bacterial etiology of gingivitis using the experimental gingivitis model. In plaque-free subjects with clinically noninflamed gingiva, plaque will slowly develop on the teeth when all mechanical plaque control is stopped. With time, the plaque composition changes. During the first few days, the plaque is mainly composed of gram-positive (+) cocci and rods. Later on, the composition is shifted toward more gram-negative species and more rods and filaments; finally, gram-negative (−) spirochetes appear (see morphotypes in *black*). Within a few days, mild gingivitis ensues (*black line;* gingival index [GI] of 1 according to Löe and Silness). From the moment that proper plaque control is reestablished *(vertical line)*, the plaque composition returns to the initial situation, and the symptoms of gingivitis disappear. *(From Löe H, Theilade E, Jensen SB: Experimental gingivitis in man.* J Periodontol *36:177, 1965.)*

gingival margin involves a shift in the microbial population from primarily gram-positive organisms to high numbers of gram-negative bacteria. Therefore, during the later stages of plaque formation, coaggregation among different gram-negative species is likely to predominate. Examples of these types of interactions are the coaggregation of *F. nucleatum* with *P. gingivalis* or *Treponema denticola* (see Fig. 8.2L).[173,180,186]

KEY FACT

Biofilm maturation is a highly specific event that involves a nonrandom aggregation of different bacteria.

Factors That Affect Supragingival Dental Plaque Formation

Clinically, early undisturbed plaque formation on teeth follows an exponential growth curve when measured planimetrically.[313] During the first 24 hours when starting with a clean tooth surface, plaque growth is negligible from a clinical viewpoint (i.e., <3% coverage of the vestibular tooth surface, which is an amount nearly undetectable clinically). This "lag time" is a result of the fact that the microbial population must reach a certain size before it can easily be detected by a clinician. During the following 3 days, coverage progresses rapidly to the point at which, after 4 days, an average of 30% of the total coronal tooth area will be covered with plaque (Video 8.2: Plaque growth).

Several reports have shown that the microbial composition of the dental plaque will change, with a shift toward a more anaerobic and a more gram-negative flora, including an influx of fusobacteria, filaments, spiral forms, and spirochetes (Fig. 8.17). This was clearly illustrated in experimental gingivitis studies.[398,409] For example, using next-generation sequencing, the microbiota was shown to shift from baseline to a significantly different community within 1 week of withdrawing oral hygiene.[175] With this ecologic shift within the biofilm, a transition occurs from the early aerobic environment, which is characterized by gram-positive facultative species, to a highly

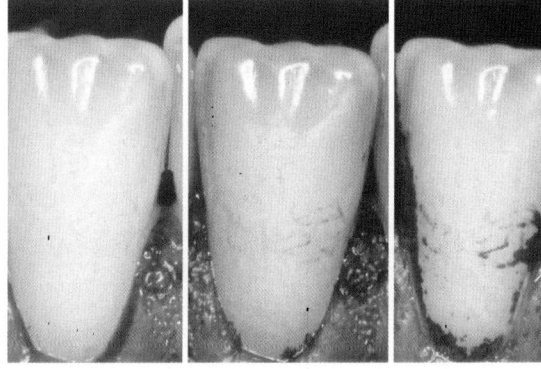

Fig. 8.18 Typical topography of plaque growth. Initial growth starts along the gingival margins and from the interdental spaces (i.e., areas protected from shear forces) to extend farther in a coronal direction. This pattern may fundamentally change, for example, if the tooth surface contains irregularities, such as those evident in Fig. 8.19.

oxygen-deprived environment, in which gram-negative anaerobic microorganisms predominate. Bacterial growth in older plaque is much slower than in newly formed dental plaque, presumably because nutrients become limiting for much of the plaque biomass.[436]

Topography of Supragingival Plaque

Early plaque formation on teeth follows a typical topographic pattern (Fig. 8.18), with initial growth along the gingival margin and from the interdental spaces (i.e., the areas protected from shear forces). Later, a further extension in the coronal direction can be observed.[254,317] This pattern may change severely when the tooth surface contains irregularities that offer a favorable growth path (Fig. 8.19). Plaque formation may also originate from grooves, cracks, perikymata, or pits. Scanning electron microscopy studies clearly revealed that the early colonization of the enamel surface starts from surface irregularities in which bacteria shelter from shear forces, thereby permitting them the time needed to change from reversible to irreversible binding.

KEY FACT

Dental plaque growth starts at areas that are protected from shear forces such as the gingival margin, the interdental space, and along grooves, cracks, pits, and fissures.

By multiplication, the bacteria subsequently spread out from these starting-up areas as a relatively even monolayer. Surface irregularities are also responsible for the so-called individualized plaque growth pattern (see Fig. 8.19), which is reproduced in the absence of optimal oral hygiene.[254,255] This phenomenon illustrates the importance of surface roughness in plaque growth, which should lead to proper clinical treatment options.

Surface Microroughness

Rough intraoral surfaces (e.g., crown margins, implant abutments, denture bases) accumulate and retain more plaque and calculus in terms of thickness, area, and colony-forming units.[305] Ample plaque also reveals an increased maturity or pathogenicity of its bacterial

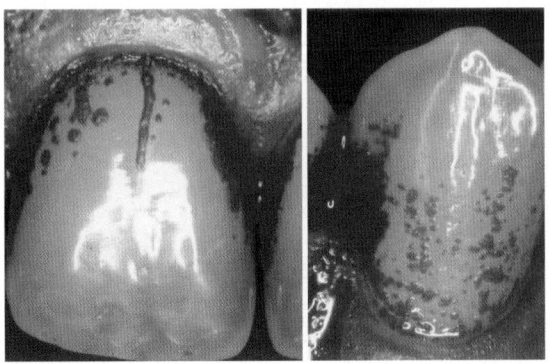

Fig. 8.19 Surface irregularities and plaque growth. Important surface irregularities (i.e., a crack on the central upper incisor, several small pits on the canine) are also responsible for the so-called individualized plaque growth pattern.

components, which is characterized by an increased proportion of motile organisms and spirochetes and/or a denser packing of them (Figs. 8.20 and 8.21). Smoothing an intraoral surface decreases the rate of plaque formation. Below a certain surface roughness (R_a < 0.2 μm), however, further smoothing does not result in an additional reduction in plaque formation.[28,306] There seems to be a threshold level for surface roughness (R_a ≈ 0.2 μm) above which bacterial adhesion will be facilitated.[27] Although surface free energy and surface roughness are two factors that influence plaque growth, the latter predominates (see Figs. 8.20 and 8.21).

Individual Variables That Influence Plaque Formation

The rate of plaque formation differs significantly among subjects, and these differences may overrule surface characteristics. A distinction is often made between "heavy" (fast) and "light" (slow) plaque formers (Video 8.3: Difference in plaque growth between heavy and light plaque formers).

A multiple regression analysis showed that the clinical wettability of the tooth surfaces, the saliva-induced aggregation of oral bacteria, and the relative salivary flow conditions around the sampled teeth explained 90% of the variation. Moreover, the saliva from light plaque formers reduced the colloidal stability of bacterial suspensions of, for example, *S. sanguinis*.[364]

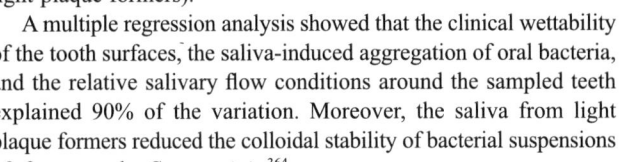

CLINICIAN'S CORNER

Do some patients form plaque faster than others?

Yes, so-called heavy and light plaque formers exist. However, in both cases it takes days before the plaque is clinically visible. Patients cannot justify poor oral hygiene by being heavy plaque formers.

In a study by Zee and colleagues,[459] de novo plaque formation was followed on small enamel blocks that were bonded onto the teeth of slow and heavy plaque formers. After 1 day, the heavy plaque formers showed more plaque with a more complex supra-gingival structure. However, from days 3 to 14, no discernible

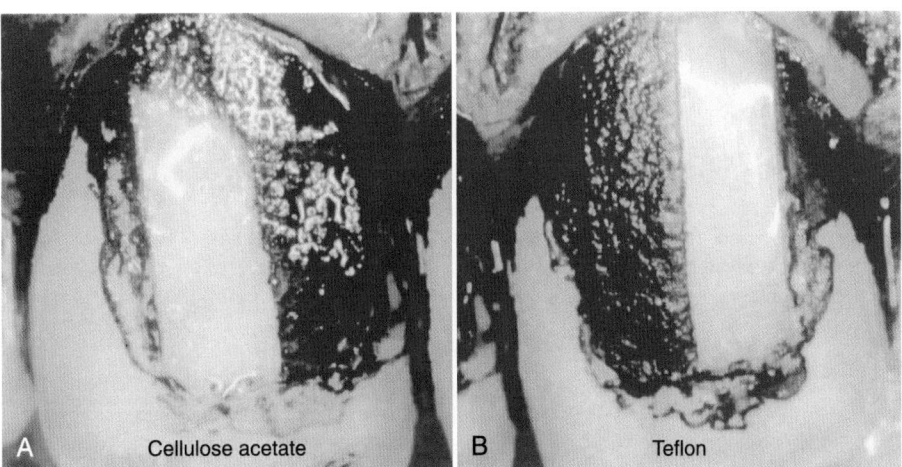

Fig. 8.20 Photographs showing the clinical impact of surface roughness and surface free energy on de novo plaque formation. (A) and (B) Two small strips were glued to the central upper incisors of a patient who refrained from oral hygiene for 3 days. Each strip was divided in two halves: a rough region (R_a 2.0 μm) located mesially and a smooth region (R_a 0.1 μm) located distally. (A) Cellulose acetate strip (medium surface free energy [sfe]: 58 ergcm^{-2}). (B) Teflon strip (low sfe: 20 ergcm^{-2}). Plaque was disclosed with 0.5% neutral red solution. The smooth regions show the decrease in biofilm formation because of the low sfe; the rough regions demonstrate the predominance of surface roughness (i.e., more plaque with no difference between the two surfaces), even with different sfe. *(From Quirynen M, Listgarten MA: Distribution of bacterial morphotypes around natural teeth and titanium implants ad modum Brånemark. Clin Oral Implants Res 1:8, 1990.)*

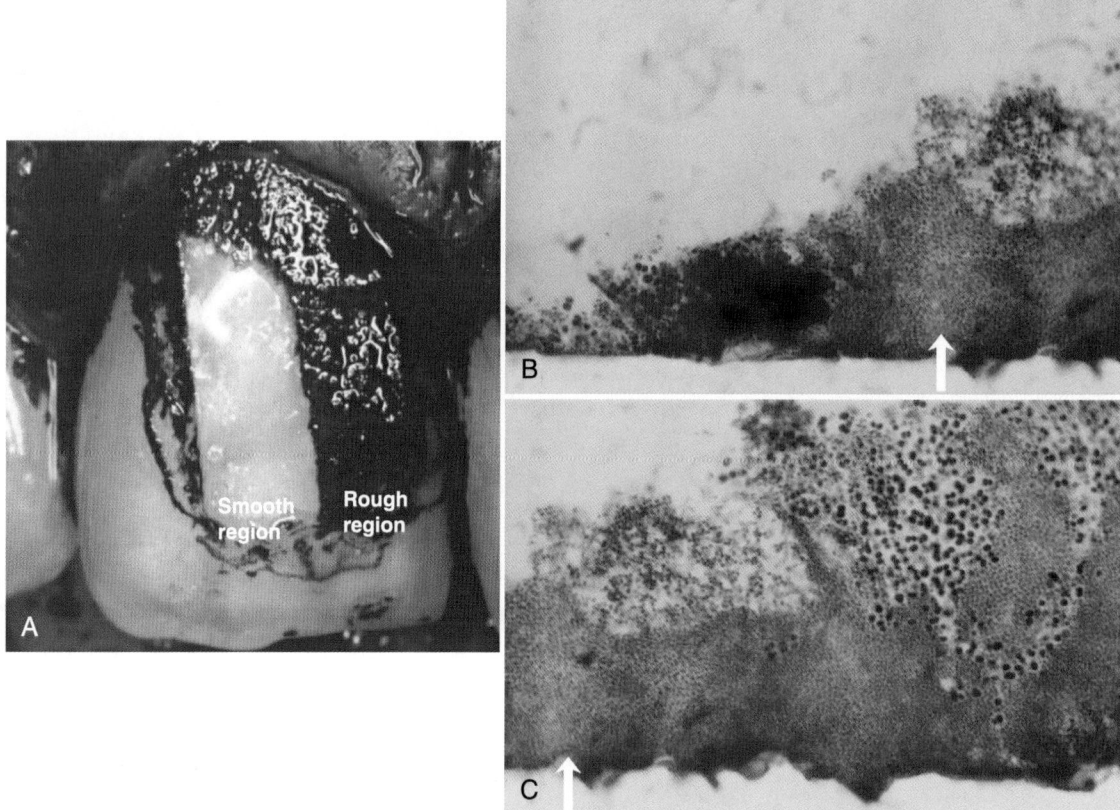

Fig. 8.21 Plaque formation and surface roughness. (A) A small plastic strip, divided in half (a rough region [R_a 2.0 μm] located mesially and a smooth region [R_a 0.1 μm] located distally), had been glued to the central upper incisors of a patient who refrained from oral hygiene for 3 days. (B) and (C) After removal, the strip had been cut into small slices for microscopic evaluation. It is obvious that the rough part (C) contains a thicker plaque layer than the smooth part (B). The *arrow* shows the border between the rough and smooth surfaces. *(From Quirynen M, Listgarten MA: Distribution of bacterial morphotypes around natural teeth and titanium implants ad modum Brånemark.* Clin Oral Implants Res *1:8, 1990.)*

differences were noted between both groups, except for a more prominent intermicrobial matrix in the group of fast growers. In another study by the same group of investigators, qualitative differences in the composition of the plaque between slow and rapid plaque formers were detected.[458] Rapid plaque formers demonstrated higher proportions of gram-negative rods (35% versus 17%) in 14-day-old plaque. The intersubject variation in plaque formation can also be explained by factors such as diet, chewing fibrous food, smoking, the presence of copper amalgam, tongue and palate brushing, the colloid stability of bacteria in the saliva, antimicrobial factors present in the saliva, the chemical composition of the pellicle, and the retention depth of the dentogingival area.*

Variation Within the Dentition

Within a dental arch, large differences in plaque growth rate can be detected. In general, early plaque formation occurs faster: in the lower jaw (as compared with the upper jaw); in molar areas; on the buccal tooth surfaces (as compared with palatal sites, especially in the upper jaw); and in the interdental regions (as compared with the buccal or lingual surfaces).[109,207,304]

Impact of Gingival Inflammation and Saliva

Several studies clearly indicate that early in vivo plaque formation is more rapid on tooth surfaces facing inflamed gingival margins

*References 3, 6, 16, 160, 164, 362, 364, 365.

than on those adjacent to healthy gingivae.[309,322,323] These studies suggest that the increase in crevicular fluid production enhances plaque formation. Probably some substances from this exudate (e.g., minerals, proteins, carbohydrates) favor both the initial adhesion and/or the growth of the early colonizing bacteria. In addition, it is known that, during the night, the plaque growth rate is reduced by some 50%.[317] This seems surprising because one would expect that reduced plaque removal and the decreased salivary flow at night would enhance plaque growth. The fact that the supragingival plaque obtains its nutrients mainly from the saliva appears to be of greater significance than the antibacterial activity of saliva.[47]

Impact of Patient's Age

Although older studies were contradictory, more recent reports clearly indicate that a subject's age does not influence de novo plaque formation. In a study by Fransson and colleagues,[105] no differences could be detected in de novo plaque formation between a group of young (20 to 25 years old) patients and a group of older (65 to 80 years old) subjects who abolished mechanical tooth cleaning measures for 21 days, neither in amount nor in composition.[105] This observation largely confirms data by Holm-Pedersen and colleagues[154] and data by Winkel and coworkers.[446] However, the developed plaque in the older patient group resulted in more severe gingival inflammation, which seems to indicate an increased susceptibility to gingivitis with aging.

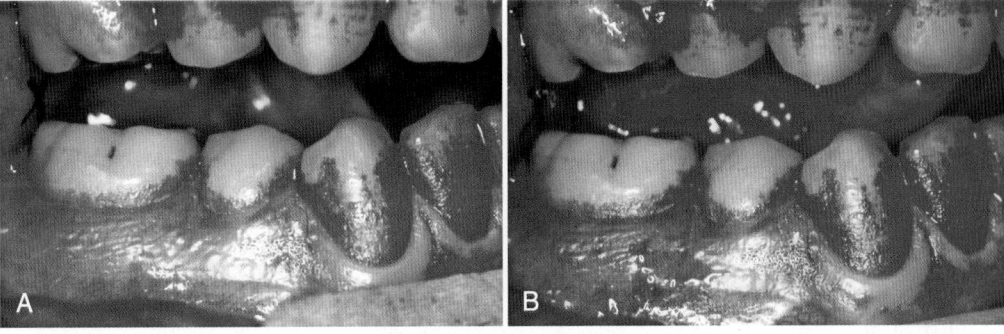

Fig. 8.22 Lower premolars and molars from a dental student who refrained from oral hygiene for 100 hours to evaluate undisturbed plaque formation. (A) Before dinner. (B) After dinner, which included fibrous foods. Nearly no reduction in plaque extension could be observed, thereby illustrating the absence of spontaneous plaque removal.

CLINICIAN'S CORNER

Do older people form more plaque?
No, the rate of de novo plaque formation is similar in young and old patients. However, older patients may have less dexterity, which could explain larger amounts of plaque.

Spontaneous Tooth Cleaning

Many clinicians still think that plaque is removed spontaneously from the teeth, such as during eating. However, on the basis of the firm attachment between the bacteria and the surface, this seems unlikely. Even in the occlusal surfaces of the molars, plaque remains, even after chewing fibrous food (e.g., carrots, apples, chips). The inefficiency of the spontaneous plaque removal is neatly illustrated by the clinical pictures in Fig. 8.22, which were taken before and after dinner starting from 4 days of undisturbed plaque formation. Only negligible differences in plaque extent could be observed.

De Novo Subgingival Plaque Formation

It is technically impossible to record the dynamics of subgingival plaque formation in an established dentition for the simple reason that one cannot sterilize a periodontal pocket. Some early studies involving the use of culturing techniques examined the changes within the subgingival microbiota during the first week after mechanical debridement and reported an only partial reduction of around 3 logs (from 10^8 bacterial cells to 10^5 cells), followed by rapid regrowth toward nearly pretreatment levels (–0.5 log) within 7 days.[118,145,242] The fast recolonization was explained by several factors. A critical review of the effectiveness of subgingival debridement, for instance, revealed that a high proportion of treated tooth surfaces (5% to 80%) still harbored plaque and/or calculus after scaling. These remaining bacteria were considered the primary source for the subgingival recolonization.[294] Some pathogens penetrate the soft tissues or the dentinal tubules and eventually escape instrumentation (see Fig. 8.14).[5,115,338] In a beagle dog study, Leknes and colleagues[214] studied the extent of subgingival colonization in 6-mm pockets with smooth or rough root surfaces. These investigators also observed that smooth surfaces harbored significantly less plaque and concluded that subgingival irregularities shelter submerged microorganisms. Moreover, biopsies of the soft tissues showed an elevated proportion of inflammatory cells in the junctional epithelium (and the underlying connective tissue) facing the rough surfaces.[215] Finally, the same group reported higher rates of attachment loss around teeth with grooves in the root surface.[213]

The introduction of oral implants, especially of the two-stage type, provided a new experimental setup. When the transmucosal part of the implant (the abutment) is inserted on top of the osseointegrated endosseous part, a new "pristine" surface is created on which the intraoral translocation of bacteria can be investigated.[306] It has been demonstrated that a complex subgingival microbiota, including most periodontopathogens, is established within 1 week after abutment insertion. This is followed by a slow increase in the number of periodontopathogens.[108,319,320] Oral implants have also been used as a model to study the impact of surface roughness on subgingival plaque formation.[28,43,125,306,316,333] Smooth abutments ($R_a <$ 0.2 μm) were found to harbor 25 times fewer bacteria than rough ones, with a slightly higher density of coccoid (i.e., nonpathogenic) cells. The subgingival microbiota was also largely dependent on the remaining presence of teeth and the degree of periodontitis in the remaining natural dentition (for a review, see reference 293). These observations highlight the importance of intraoral bacterial translocation for subgingival biofilms.

Characteristics of Biofilm Bacteria (Life in "Slime City")

Metabolism of Dental Plaque Bacteria

Most nutrients for dental plaque bacteria originate from saliva or gingival crevicular fluid, although the host diet provides an occasional but nevertheless important food supply. The transition from gram-positive to gram-negative microorganisms observed in the structural development of dental plaque is paralleled by a physiologic transition in the developing plaque.

The early colonizers (e.g., *Streptococcus* and *Actinomyces* spp.) use oxygen and lower the redox potential of the environment, which then favors the growth of anaerobic species.[80,428] Many of the gram-positive early colonizers use sugars as an energy source. The bacteria that predominate in mature plaque are anaerobic and asaccharolytic (i.e., they do not break down sugars), and they use amino acids and small peptides as energy sources.[231]

Laboratory studies have demonstrated many metabolic interactions among the different bacteria found in dental plaque (Fig. 8.23). For example, lactate and formate are byproducts of the metabolism of streptococci and *Actinomyces* spp.; they may be used in the metabolism of other plaque microorganisms, including *Veillonella* spp. and *A. actinomycetemcomitans*.[42,91] Interestingly, the commensal bacterium *S. gordonii* have also been shown to provide electron acceptors that promote respiratory growth of *A. actinomycetemcomitans* in vivo during abscess formation.[392] The importance of this cross-respiration in dental plaque biofilms is not yet clear.

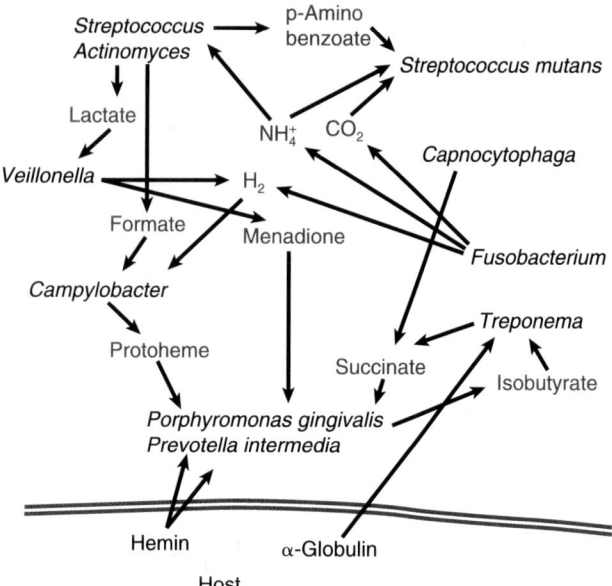

Fig. 8.23 Schematic illustration of metabolic interactions among different bacterial species found in plaque and between the host and the plaque bacteria. These interactions are likely to be important to the survival of bacteria in the periodontal environment. CO_2, Carbon dioxide; H_2, hydrogen; NH^+_4, ammonium. *(Data from Carlsson J: Microbiology of plaque associated periodontal disease. In Lindhe J, editor: Textbook of clinical periodontology, Munksgaard, 1983, Munksgaard International Publishers; Grenier D: Nutritional interactions between two suspected periodontopathogens,* Treponema denticola *and* Porphyromonas gingivalis. *Infect Immun 60:5298, 1992; Loesche WJ: Importance of nutrition in gingival crevice microbial ecology. Periodontics 6:245, 1968; and Walden WC, Hentges DJ: Differential effects of oxygen and oxidation-reduction potential on the multiplication of three species of anaerobic intestinal bacteria. Appl Microbiol 30:781, 1975.)*

The growth of *P. gingivalis* is also enhanced by metabolic byproducts produced by other microorganisms, such as succinate from *C. ochracea* or *T. denticola* and protoheme from *Campylobacter rectus* (see Fig. 8.2R).[121,122,248] In turn, *P. gingivalis* provides isobutyric acid that stimulates growth of *T. denticola*.[121] Overall, the total plaque population is more efficient than any one constituent organism at releasing energy from the available substrates.[443]

Metabolic interactions also occur between the host and the plaque microorganisms. The bacterial enzymes that degrade host proteins mediate the release of ammonia, which may be used by bacteria as a nitrogen source.[48] Hemin iron from the breakdown of host hemoglobin may be important in the metabolism of *P. gingivalis*.[34] Increases in steroid hormones are associated with significant increases in the proportions of *P. intermedia* found in subgingival plaque.[191] These nutritional interdependencies are probably critical to the growth and survival of microorganisms in dental plaque, and they may partly explain the evolution of the highly specific structural interactions observed among bacteria in plaque.

Communication Between Biofilm Bacteria

Bacterial cells do not exist in isolation. In a biofilm, bacteria have the capacity to communicate with each other. One example of this is quorum sensing, in which bacteria secrete a signaling molecule that accumulates in the local environment and triggers a response such as a change in the expression of specific genes once they reach a critical threshold concentration. The threshold concentration is reached only at a high cell density, and therefore bacteria sense that the population has reached a critical mass or quorum. Some evidence

indicates that intercellular communication can occur after cell–cell contact and that, in this case, communication may not involve secreted signaling molecules.[165] Two types of signaling molecules have been detected from dental plaque bacteria: peptides released by gram-positive organisms during growth and a "universal" signal molecule called *autoinducer 2* (AI-2).[182] Peptide signals are produced by oral streptococci; they are recognized by cells of the same strain that produced them and possibly also by different species of streptococci.[103] Responses are induced only when a threshold concentration of the peptide is attained, and thus the peptides act as cell density or quorum sensors. Local concentrations of signaling molecules may be enhanced in biofilms if the signals become trapped in the biofilm matrix. The streptococcal peptides are known as *competence-stimulating peptides* because the major response to these signals is the induction of competence, a physiologic state during which cells are primed for DNA uptake and incorporation.

In some species, such as *S. mutans*, a few of the cells in a population respond to competence-stimulating peptides by lysing.[292] Lysis is considered to be an altruistic behavior that helps to disseminate genetic information throughout the population of *S. mutans* cells.

In contrast to the strain-specific competence-stimulating peptides, AI-2 is produced and detected by many different bacteria. The detection of AI-2 produces wide-ranging changes in gene expression, in some cases affecting up to one-third of the entire genome.[399]

Little is known about the specific functions of AI-2 in oral biofilms. However, this molecule has been demonstrated to play a role in mutualistic interactions between *S. oralis* and *A. oris* (*A. naeslundii*).[332] Thus, in an in vitro model system, neither *S. oralis* nor *A. oris* formed biofilms in monoculture. When cultured together, these organisms grew abundantly on surfaces to form thick, confluent biofilms. This mutualistic behavior was observed only when AI-2 was present: disrupting the gene for AI-2 in *S. oralis* abrogated mutualistic growth. These data demonstrate that AI-2 is produced and sensed by oral bacteria and suggest that interbacterial communication is important for the development of dental plaque.

Quorum sensing therefore appears to play diverse roles in, for example, modulating the expression of genes for antibiotic resistance, encouraging the growth of beneficial species in the biofilm, and discouraging the growth of competitors.

Interactions Among Dental Plaque Bacteria

Some evidence indicates from laboratory studies that nonpathogenic organisms in subgingival dental plaque can modify the behavior of periodontal pathogens. For example, long and short fimbriae of *P. gingivalis* are required for adhesion and biofilm formation. The expression of long fimbriae is down-regulated in the presence of *Streptococcus cristatus*, and short fimbriae are down-regulated by *S. gordonii*, *S. mitis*, or *S. sanguinis*.[221,284] Changes in bacterial physiology after transitions from monoculture to mixed-species communities may be quite wide ranging.

With the use of a proteomics approach to probe the phenotype of *P. gingivalis*, it has been shown that the expression of almost 500 *P. gingivalis* proteins is changed in model oral microbial communities that contain *S. gordonii* and *F. nucleatum*.[197] At present, it is not clear how these changes affect the interaction between *P. gingivalis* and the host.

In multispecies biofilms in which many bacteria are juxtaposed to cells of different species, interactions among genetically distinct microorganisms can be mutually beneficial (see Fig. 8.5A). However, many examples of competitive interactions between different bacteria exist (Fig. 8.24). For example, *S. mutans* produces antimicrobial peptides that have broad activity against bacteria in vitro.[195] Other oral streptococci compete with *S. mutans* by excreting the strongly

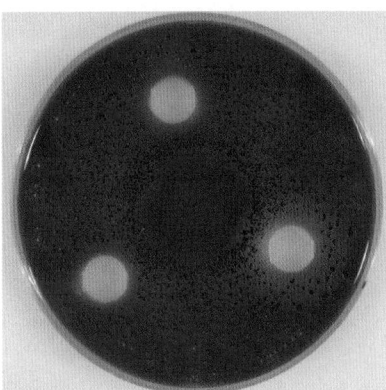

Fig. 8.24 Growth inhibition induced by streptococci. The growth of *Prevotella intermedia* (black colonies) is inhibited by the presence of *Streptococcus mitis, Streptococcus salivarius,* and *Streptococcus sanguinis* (in the white holes). This is represented by a zone of no growth (halo) around the white holes. This is a typical example of growth inhibition induced by streptococci.

oxidizing molecule H_2O_2.[195] In fact, *Streptococcus oligofermentans* can convert lactic acid produced by *S. mutans* into H_2O_2, which then kills the *S. mutans* cells.[411]

In subgingival biofilms, oxygen is scarce, and therefore H_2O_2 production by bacteria is lower. Oxidizing agents may be more important in the interaction between the host and the pathogen because reactive oxygen species are a major component of the neutrophil response to bacteria.

Another example of competitive interaction exists between streptococci and periodontopathogens. *S. sanguinis, S. salivarius,* and *S. mitis* have been shown to inhibit hard and soft tissue colonization of *A. actinomycetemcomitans* (Video 8.4: Colonization inhibition), *P. gingivalis,* and *P. intermedia* in vitro.[370,405,422]

Studies have shown that these interactions can also influence the host. Although in a study by Teughels and coworkers[406] no clinical effect was expected, a reduction in bleeding on probing was noted in pockets that received the streptococci. At that time, this observation was explained by the establishment of a more host-compatible microbiota. However, an interaction with the host via the immune system seems to be an additional interesting hypothesis. Oral streptococci have been shown to modulate bacteria–host interactions that involve both *F. nucleatum* and *A. actinomycetemcomitans*. Thus, *S. cristatus* and other oral streptococci attenuate the ability of *F. nucleatum* to stimulate interleukin-8 production by host oral epithelial cells.[460] Sliepen and coworkers[371] demonstrated similar results for the streptococci that were used in the study by Teughels and coworkers.

Another interesting example is the *S. gordonii*–induced increased expression of a complement resistance protein, ApiA, in *A. actinomycetemcomitans,* thereby resulting in a higher resistance to killing by host serum.[326]

Biofilms and Antimicrobial Resistance

Bacteria growing in microbial communities adherent to a surface do not "behave" the same way as bacteria growing suspended in a liquid environment (i.e., in a planktonic or unattached state). For example, the resistance of bacteria to antimicrobial agents is dramatically increased in the biofilm.[9,65,147,302] Almost without exception, organisms in a biofilm are 1000 to 1500 times more resistant as compared with antibiotics in their planktonic state. The mechanisms of this increased resistance differ from species to species, from antibiotic to antibiotic, and for biofilms growing in different habitats.

It is generally accepted that the resistance of bacteria to antibiotics is affected by their nutritional status, growth rate, temperature, pH, and prior exposure to subeffective concentrations of antimicrobial agents.[40,41,444] Variations in any of these parameters will lead to a varied response to antibiotics within a biofilm. An important mechanism of resistance appears to be the slower rate of growth of bacterial species in a biofilm, which makes them less susceptible to many but not all antibiotics.[18,38,65,452] The biofilm matrix, although not a significant physical barrier to the diffusion of antibiotics, does have certain properties that can retard antibiotic penetration. For example, strongly charged or chemically highly reactive agents can fail to reach the deeper zones of the biofilm because the biofilm acts as an ion-exchange resin that removes such molecules from solution.[113,400]

KEY FACT

The bacteria within biofilms are often up to 1000 times more resistant to antimicrobial agents than their planktonic counterparts.

In addition, extracellular enzymes such as β-lactamases, formaldehyde lyase, and formaldehyde dehydrogenase may become trapped and concentrated in the extracellular matrix, and as such inactivate some antibiotics (especially positively charged hydrophilic antibiotics).

Some antibiotics, such as the macrolides, which are positively charged but hydrophobic, are unaffected by this process.

"Superresistant" bacteria were identified within a biofilm. These cells have multidrug resistance pumps that can extrude antimicrobial agents from the cell.[38] Because these pumps place the antibiotics outside of the outer membrane, the process offers protection against antibiotics that target, for example, cell wall synthesis. The penetration and efficacy of antimicrobials against biofilm bacteria are critical issues for the treatment of periodontal infections.

Antibiotic resistance may be spread through a biofilm via the intercellular exchange of DNA. The high density of bacterial cells in a biofilm facilitates the exchange of genetic information among cells of the same species and across species and even across genera. Conjugation (i.e., the exchange of genes through a direct interbacteria connection formed by a sex pilus), transformation (i.e., the movement of small pieces of DNA from the environment into the bacterial chromosome), plasmid transfer, and transposon transfer have all been shown to occur in biofilms.

Bacterial Transmission and Translocation

The transmission of pathogens from one *locus* to another is an important aspect of infectious diseases. In theory, such transmission may jeopardize the outcome of periodontal therapy; in addition, the transmission of pathogens from one person to another may be important in terms of disease transmission. The significance of such an intraoral transmission or of a vertical or horizontal transmission is, however, difficult to prove or to quantify.

One of the first questions in this regard is, "Are oral bacteria transmissible between humans?" Molecular fingerprinting techniques have clearly illustrated that periodontal pathogens are transmissible within members of a family[455] (Fig. 8.25).

This bacterial transmission between subjects (and even between animals and human beings) should not be confused with contagion (with the term *contagious* referring to the likelihood that a microorganism will be transmitted from an infected to an uninfected host to create disease). Asikainen and coworkers[19] used a genetic fingerprinting method called *arbitrarily primed-polymerase chain reaction* to

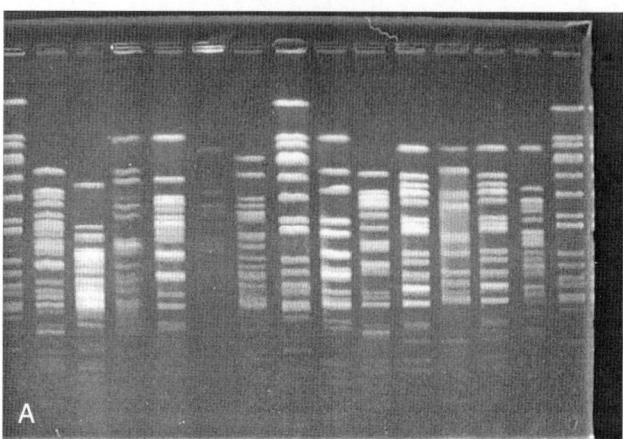

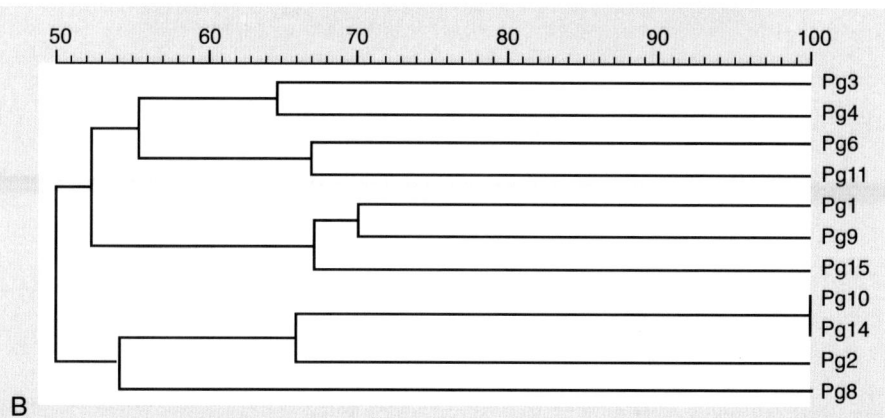

Fig. 8.25 *Porphyromonas gingivalis* strains. (A) Band pattern of DNA isolated from multiple *Porphyromonas gingivalis* strains after pulsed-field gel electrophoresis. Lanes 1, 8, and 15 contain a reference strain of DNA (*Staphylococcus aureus*) cut with SmaI (a restriction endonuclease) in lanes 2 through 7 and 9 through 14; 12 different *P. gingivalis* strains are compared for their genetic similarity. (B) The genetic similarity is expressed in a dendrogram. Bacteria are considered genetically similar when their band patterns are 80% similar.

genotype *A. actinomycetemcomitans* isolates from family members. In 11 of 12 families, these investigators found identical *A. actinomycetemcomitans* genotypes among family members. This finding suggests the transmission of this microorganism among family members. However, it was more often encountered that children carried a genotype identical to one of their parents than that spouses carried an identical genotype. This indicates that, in terms of *A. actinomycetemcomitans* transmission, vertical transmission is more important than horizontal transmission. Similar observations were made for the transmission of cariogenic species from mother to child.[177] The vertical or horizontal transmission of *P. gingivalis* has rarely been observed.[418]

The existence of an "intraoral" translocation of bacteria (i.e., from one niche to another) has been investigated more thoroughly. Intraoral transmission of bacteria was first examined in cariology. Loesche and coworkers[233] showed that streptomycin-resistant strains of *S. mutans* grown on a dental inlay were spontaneously transmitted to the neighboring teeth (probably via saliva) and could even reach the contralateral quadrant after transmission with a dental explorer. Previously, Edman and coworkers[89] had successfully implanted the previously mentioned species in two volunteers by means of inoculated dental flosses. Comparable observations have been made for periodontopathogens.

Christersson and coworkers[57] demonstrated a translocation of *A. actinomycetemcomitans* via periodontal probes in localized juvenile periodontitis patients. These investigators were able successfully to

colonize previously noninfected pockets with *A. actinomycetemcomitans* via a single course of probing with a probe that had been previously inserted in an infected pocket of the same patient. Although the colonization was only temporary, the question remained whether the colonization could not have been permanent if the site had offered more suitable growth conditions (e.g., a deep bleeding pocket, as frequently encountered immediately after initial periodontal therapy). It is well established that colonization of an already established microbial niche by a new species is difficult because it is hampered by a variety of microbial interactions. Therefore, intraoral translocation to and the colonization of sterile surfaces may be different from the translocation and colonization of already colonized surfaces. Within the oral cavity, such sterile surfaces are not naturally occurring. However, at the moment of abutment placement on a dental implant, a sterile subgingival pocket is created. A large series of articles compared the microbiota in pockets around teeth with that found in peri-implant pockets in partially edentulous patients and reported a striking similarity.* Several studies have investigated the subgingival colonization of such "sterile" peri-implant pockets in partially edentulous patients. Investigators have shown that translocation to and the colonization of these pockets is extremely fast. Periodontopathogens could already be detected in this niche 30 minutes after abutment placement.[108] The initial colonization of these pockets with periodontopathogens

---

*References 13, 158, 159, 176, 178, 212, 216, 250, 260, 283, 312, 352.

is completed within 1 week. After 2 weeks, only minor additional changes occur in this newly developed microbiota.[108,319,320] These additional changes mainly reflect changes in the numbers of species. On the basis of the previously mentioned similarities between the microbial populations associated with teeth and implants, it has been suggested that, at least in partially edentulous patients, teeth may act as a reservoir for the (re)colonization of the subgingival area around implants. This hypothesis was supported by Sumida and coworkers,[397] who detected similar intrasubject pulsed field gel electrophoresis patterns for *P. gingivalis* from teeth and implants (indicating that these locations contained precisely the same *P. gingivalis* strains) as compared with large intersubject variations.

Nonbacterial Inhabitants of the Oral Cavity

Oral microbiology is often reduced to "oral bacteriology." However, the oral cavity comprises a much more diverse microbiota than merely a bacterial one. Viruses, fungi, archaea, and protozoa can be encountered in the oral cavity of humans. Many of these species can reside in the oral cavity in harmony with the host as commensals, similar to oral bacteria, but they can also cause several oral diseases.

KEY FACT

In addition to bacteria, viruses can be present in the mouth. Herpesviruses, human papillomaviruses, picornaviruses, and retroviruses can all contribute to the development of oral ulcers, tumors, mononucleosis, Sjögren syndrome, osteomyelitis, osteonecrosis, oral leukoplakia, and oral lichen planus.

Viruses

Viral diseases of the oral mucosa and the perioral region are often encountered in dental practice. Viruses are important ulcerogenic and tumorigenic agents of the human mouth. The finding of an abundance of mammalian viruses in periodontitis lesions may suggest a role for viruses in more oral diseases than previously recognized.[360] A more in-depth review can be found in two articles by Slots.[375,376]

In contrast to most bacteria, viruses replicate only when they are present within eukaryotic (animals, plants, protists, and fungi) or prokaryotic (bacteria and archaea) cells and not on their own. The extracellular virion particle ranges in size from 20 to 300 nm and consists of either DNA or ribonucleic acid (RNA) contained within a protective protein coat or capsid (Fig. 8.26).

Some viruses have an additional envelope that comprises a lipid bilayer derived from the outer cellular membrane, the internal nuclear

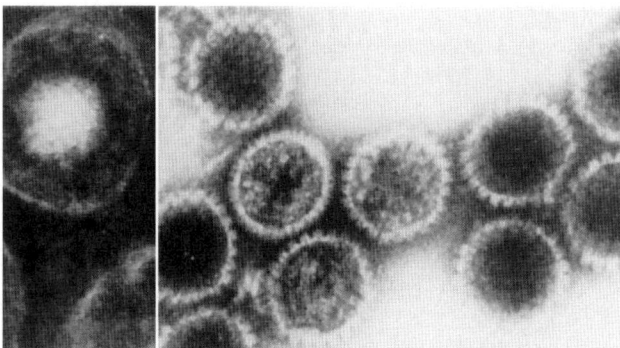

Fig. 8.26 Herpes simplex virus type 1. Electron micrographic picture of herpes simplex virus type 1, enveloped *(left)* and naked capsids *(right)*. ×198,000. *(From Fields BN, Knipe DM: In Fields BN, editors:* Virology, *New York, 1985, Raven Press.)*

membrane, or the endoplasmic reticulum membrane of the infected cell. In healthy individuals, most viruses in the oral cavity are bacteriophages.[10] Four major viral families are associated with the main viral oral diseases of adults:

1. The group of herpesviruses contains eight different members that are all enveloped double-stranded DNA viruses (Table 8.4). In the oral cavity, they are related to different ulcers, tumors, and other oral pathoses.
2. Human papillomaviruses are grouped within five genera and are nonenveloped double-stranded DNA viruses (Table 8.5). In the oral cavity, they are related to ulcers, tumors, and oral pathoses.
3. Picornaviruses are all nonenveloped, single-stranded RNA viruses (Table 8.6). In the oral cavity, they are related to ulcers and different oral pathoses.
4. Retroviruses are divided into seven genera of which two are human pathogens. All retroviruses are enveloped single-stranded RNA viruses (Table 8.7). In the oral cavity, they are related to different tumors and oral pathoses.

Clinical Manifestations of Oral Viral Diseases

Oral Ulcers

Ulcers or erosions are relatively common in the oropharyngeal mucosa.[356] Although oral ulcers can have a variety of causes, a viral cause of oral ulcers has been established for primary and recurrent herpetic gingivostomatitis (primarily herpes simplex virus-1 but also herpes simplex virus-2), varicella/herpes zoster outbreak (varicella-zoster virus), herpangina (coxsackievirus), and hand, foot, and mouth disease (enteroviruses). Viruses may also play a role in some cases of recurrent aphthous stomatitis (varicella-zoster virus, cytomegalovirus [CMV], other herpesviruses, adenoviruses, and measles virus) and in systemic diseases with an oral ulcerogenic component, such as erythema multiforme (herpes simplex virus), Behçet syndrome (herpes simplex virus and CMV), pemphigus vulgaris (herpes simples virus and CMV), and systemic lupus erythematosus (Epstein-Barr virus [EBV]).

Oral Tumors

Viruses can be connected to a single or a limited number of tumor types (e.g., hepatitis B virus) or to multiple tumor types (e.g., EBV), a difference that probably reflects the extent of tissue tropism of the viruses. Viruses may cause cell transformation and proliferation by directly expressing oncogenic genes in infected cells or by acting as a necessary or noncompulsory cofactor in the development of malignancy. However, even though most individuals harbor oncogenic viruses in the oral cavity, cancer that occurs as a result of infection with such viruses is relatively rare. Risk factors apart from the viral infection are obviously important for cancer development, including family history, age, tobacco smoking, and alcohol consumption. The most important oncoviruses of the human mouth are EBV, herpesvirus-8, and papillomaviruses; the most common virally related malignant diseases in the oral cavity are epithelial neoplasms, lymphomas, and Kaposi sarcoma.[348]

Other Oral Pathologies

In addition to oral ulcers and tumors, viruses have also been implicated in infectious mononucleosis (primary EBV infection and occasionally a primary CMV infection), Sjögren syndrome (hepatitis C virus, human T-lymphotropic virus type I, human immunodeficiency virus [HIV], and herpesviruses), osteomyelitis (herpes zoster virus and CMV), osteonecrosis (herpes zoster), oral leukoplakia (papillomaviruses, mainly types 16 and 18), and oral lichen planus (papillomaviruses and hepatitis C virus).

TABLE 8.4   Herpesviruses That Can Be Recovered in the Oral Cavity

Virus	Characteristics	Disease Association	Oral Pathoses
Herpes simplex virus-1	Latency in sensory ganglia Causes orolabial disease	Herpetic gingivostomatitis, recurrent orolabial lesions, herpetic whitlow, keratoconjunctivitis, eczema herpeticum, pharyngitis, mononucleosis-like syndrome, encephalitis, neonatal infections	Adult herpetic gingivostomatitis HIV/AIDS-related oral ulcers Recurrent oral aphthous stomatitis Behçet syndrome Oral pemphigus vulgaris Erythema multiforme Dry socket after tooth extraction
Herpes simplex virus-2	Latency in sensory ganglia Causes genital and newborn infections	Genital infection, aseptic meningitis, sacral autonomic nervous system dysfunction.	—
Varicella-zoster virus	Latency in sensory ganglia Only three major genotypes of the wild-type virus are known More than 90% are infected before adolescence in an unvaccinated population	Varicella (chickenpox), herpes zoster (shingles), central nervous system involvement, pneumonia, secondary bacterial infections, and death Available varicella vaccines (about 90% effectiveness) include a single-antigen vaccine and a combination vaccine against MMRV	Recurrent oral aphthous stomatitis Osteomyelitis Herpes zoster (Hunt syndrome)
EBV	Identified initially in 1964 from African Burkitt lymphoma Infects epithelial cells with a cytolytic infection and B lymphocytes with a latent infection	Infectious mononucleosis, hairy leukoplakia of the tongue, Burkitt lymphoma, B lymphoproliferative disease, Hodgkin lymphoma, X-linked lymphoproliferative disease, nasal T-cell lymphoma, nasopharyngeal carcinoma, gastric carcinoma, parotid carcinoma, and leiomyosarcoma	Recurrent oral aphthous stomatitis Erythema multiforme Various epithelial type tumors, such as lymphoepithelioma-like carcinoma, salivary gland lymphoepithelial carcinoma, Warthin tumor (cystadenolymphoma) of the parotid gland, oral squamous cell carcinoma, tonsillar carcinoma, oral undifferentiated carcinomas, and oral hairy leukoplakia Various lymphoid type tumors, such as Hodgkin lymphoma, T-cell/natural killer cell lymphoma, Burkitt lymphoma, cyclosporine-related posttransplant lymphoproliferative disorder, oral post-transplant lymphoproliferative disorder/B-cell lymphoma, follicular lymphoid hyperplasia, and plasmablastic lymphoma Infectious mononucleosis
hCMV	Infects mainly T lymphocytes and macrophages The gB protein in the virion envelope participates in the virus–cell interaction and is a major target of the immune response	Preterm birth, preeclampsia, transplant rejection, immunosenescence, hemorrhagic retinal necrosis (patients with HIV), encephalitis, infectious mononucleosis, atherosclerosis, gastrointestinal disease, pneumonia, and encephalitis	HIV/AIDS-related oral ulcers Recurrent oral aphthous stomatitis Behçet syndrome Oral pemphigus vulgaris Erythema multiforme Cyclosporine-steroid associated lymphoproliferative disorder Benign infantile hemangioendothelioma Kaposi sarcoma Occasionally infectious mononucleosis Sialadenitis Osteomyelitis
Human herpesvirus-6	Cell tropism for T lymphocytes and neural cells Frequently shed in the saliva of healthy donors	Roseola infantum (sixth disease), meningitis, encephalitis, and possibly multiple sclerosis	Uvulopalatoglossal junctional ulcers Oral squamous cell carcinoma Oral leukoplakia Oral lichen planus

TABLE 8.4   Herpesviruses That Can Be Recovered in the Oral Cavity—cont'd

Virus	Characteristics	Disease Association	Oral Pathoses
Human herpesvirus-7	Latency in macrophages and T lymphocytes Frequently shed in the saliva of healthy donors	Exanthema subitum, macular–papular rashes, and transplant–recipient pathogens	
Human herpesvirus-8	Six genetic subtypes with marked clustering to geographic areas B lymphocytes and monocytes serve as reservoirs	Kaposi sarcoma, multicentric Castleman disease, primary effusion lymphoma, mononucleosis-like illness, and aplastic anemia (Unlike EBV, herpesvirus-8 is not involved in epithelial tumors)	Recurrent oral aphthous stomatitis Kaposi sarcoma

EBV, Epstein-Barr virus; *hCMV,* human cytomegalovirus; *HIV,* human immunodeficiency virus; *AIDS,* acquired immunodeficiency syndrome; *MMRV,* measles, mumps, rubella, and varicella.
Adapted from Slots J: Oral viral infections of adults. *Periodontol 2000* 49:60, 2009.

TABLE 8.5   Papillomaviruses That Can Be Recovered in the Oral Cavity

Virus	Characteristics	Disease Association	Oral Pathoses
Papillomavirus (types 6, 11, 16, 18, 31, 36, and 42)	Epithelial cell proliferation with specificity principally in the anogenital area, the urethra, the skin, the larynx, tracheobronchial region, and the oral mucosa	Genital and cutaneous warts, cervical and anogenital cancers, condylomata acuminate (sexually transmitted disease), and recurrent respiratory papillomatosis	Unspecified oral ulcers Recurrent oral aphthous stomatitis Focal epithelial hyperplasia Oral squamous cell carcinoma/verrucous carcinoma Oral leukoplakia Oral lichen planus

Adapted from Slots J: Oral viral infections of adults. *Periodontol 2000* 49:60, 2009.

TABLE 8.6   Picornaviruses That Can Be Recovered in the Oral Cavity

Virus	Characteristics	Disease Association	Oral Pathoses
Coxsackievirus	Coxsackievirus A16 is closely related to enterovirus-71, and both belong to a discrete subgroup of type A enteroviruses that are prominently associated with hand, foot, and mouth disease	Uncomplicated hand, foot, and mouth disease (coxsackievirus A serotypes 10 and 16); herpangina (mostly coxsackievirus A); myocarditis; infectious type 1 diabetes (coxsackievirus B); and atherosclerosis	Herpangina Hand, foot, and mouth disease
Echovirus	Some echovirus replication occurs in the nasopharynx	Meningitis; pericarditis; myocarditis; herpangina; and Guillain-Barré syndrome	Herpangina
Enterovirus	Enterovirus-71 was first isolated in 1969 from a child with encephalitis Can cause large epidemics of acute disease Mutates readily	Hand, foot, and mouth disease (enterovirus-71); herpangina (enterovirus-71); poliomyelitis-like illness; meningoencephalitis (enterovirus-71); acute pulmonary edema (enterovirus-71); and hemorrhagic conjunctivitis	Herpangina Hand, foot, and mouth disease

Adapted from Slots J: Oral viral infections of adults. *Periodontol 2000* 49:60, 2009.

Periodontitis

Bacteria are recognized as indispensable for the development of periodontitis, and the current hypotheses regarding the pathogenic mechanisms of periodontitis emphasize the importance of assessing bacterial and host factors collectively. Sole bacterial–host interactions appear insufficient to explain the clinical characteristics of the disease.[374] The localized distribution and intermittent exacerbations of periodontal breakdown and other issues remain a riddle. In response, the involvement of herpesviruses in the etiology of periodontitis has been suggested on the basis of their increased presence in inflamed gingival tissue, crevicular fluid, and subgingival plaque in periodontally diseased sites and their potential to induce proinflammatory cytokines.[374,376] However, it remains unclear whether herpesvirus activation occurs spontaneously or as a result of concurrent infection, stress, or other immunosuppressive factors.[46] Several risk factors for periodontitis also have the potential to reactivate herpesviruses.[66] Bacterioviral synergism may play an important role in the onset and progression of periodontitis.[376] However, the hypothesis that herpesviruses are involved in the etiology of periodontitis is still

TABLE 8.7   Retroviruses That Can Be Recovered in the Oral Cavity

Virus	Characteristics	Disease Association	Oral Pathoses
HIV-1	Global infection Infects cells that contain CD4 receptors, such as T-helper lymphocytes and cells of the macrophage lineage	Rank order of AIDS-defining pathoses is as follows: _Pneumocystis_ pneumonia (43%) Esophageal candidiasis (15%) Wasting (11%) Kaposi sarcoma (11%) Disseminated _Mycobacterium avium_ infection (5%) _Mycobacterium tuberculosis_ infection (5%), cytomegalovirus disease (4%) HIV-associated dementia (4%) Recurrent bacterial pneumonia (3%) Toxoplasmosis (3%) Oral hairy leukoplakia	Plasmablastic lymphoma Kaposi sarcoma Xerostomia (Sjögren syndrome) Sialadenitis Osteomyelitis
HIV-2	Infection occurring mainly in West Central Africa (Guinea-Bissau)	HIV-2 is associated with similar types of diseases as HIV-1 but is generally less virulent	Oral hairy leukoplakia Plasmablastic lymphoma Kaposi sarcoma Xerostomia (Sjögren syndrome) Sialadenitis Osteomyelitis

AIDS, acquired immunodeficiency syndrome; _HIV,_ Human immunodeficiency virus.
Adapted from Slots J: Oral viral infections of adults. _Periodontol 2000_ 49:60, 2009.

controversial.[46] No doubt exists that herpesviruses are present in the periodontal pocket. Next to herpesviruses, many other viruses have been detected in periodontal pockets. Papillomaviruses, HIV, human T-lymphotropic virus type I, hepatitis B and C viruses, and torque teno virus can all inhabit periodontitis lesions.[375] In addition, the inflamed periodontium may constitute the major oral reservoir for EBV, CMV, papillomaviruses, and hepatitis C virus.[375]

Fungi

Many fungal species have been isolated from the oral cavity. Most isolates are _Candida,_ and the most prevalent species is _Candida albicans_ (Fig. 8.27). Together with _C. albicans,_ some of the most common opportunistic fungal candidal pathogens in humans are _C. tropicalis, C. glabrata, C. krusei, C parapsilosis, C. guilliermondii,_ and _C. dubliniensis. Candida_ spp. thrive in low-pH environments, and high _Candida_ loads are associated with the presence of relatively low-diversity dental plaque that contains aciduric and acidogenic species such as _Streptococcus_ spp. and _Lactobacillus_ spp.[193] In addition to _C. albicans, C. glabrata_ is now emerging as an important agent in both mucosal and bloodstream infections.[219,295]

Yeasts such as _Rhodotorula glutinis_ and _Saccharomyces cerevisiae_ are rarely found in the oral cavity and are not known to cause oral infections. _Cryptococcus neoformans_ is occasionally isolated from the mouth but usually from patients with pulmonary cryptococcosis.[393]

C. albicans is the species that is most frequently encountered in infected tissues, including the oral mucosal layers. It is also the predominant species found during vaginal and invasive bloodstream infections. Superficial _C. albicans_ infections are increasing in prevalence, especially among denture wearers and aging people; they may lead to invasive disease, which has a high mortality rate.[351]

In contrast to most other _Candida_ spp., _C. albicans_ is a pleomorphic fungus that exhibits different modes of growth. It can proliferate as unicellular budding yeast, and it may undergo morphologic switching when triggered by specific environmental conditions, thereby leading to elongated growth forms called _pseudohyphae_ and _hypha_ and collectively named _filamentous forms._[398] Hyphae are characterized as unconstricted filaments with parallel-sided walls. In contrast, pseudohyphae seem to represent a growth form between those of yeast and hyphae in which the cells remain attached to each other but can vary in shape from elongated ellipsoidal cells to forms that superficially closely resemble hyphae. The various growth forms are important for the establishment of _Candida_ infections, with specific roles proposed in the areas of adhesion, biofilm formation, tissue penetration, and organ colonization.[198] In addition, _C. albicans_ produces a cytolytic toxin, candidalysin, which damages epithelial barriers and is essential for virulence in animal models of mucosal infection.[266]

Some systemic mycotic diseases that were once considered exotic are now manifesting intraorally with increasing frequency as a result of the high prevalence of immunocompromised individuals in the community[239,347] (Table 8.8).

Protozoa

The mouth is the entry port for many parasites that have adapted to the human host. Only a few parasites affect the oral cavity, but an increasing body of literature indicates that oral protozoa are more common than previously appreciated.[24] Depending on the type of infection, the parasitic infectious agents can be divided into two categories: those that induce local infections and those that induce systemic infections with indirect effects on the oral cavity. The former group comprises saprophytes (e.g., _Entamoeba gingivalis, Trichomonas tenax_) (Fig. 8.28; Video 8.5: Phase contrast) that have the potential to turn into opportunistic pathogens or free-living amoebas that occasionally become invasive but that are seldom present clinically. Protozoa tend to be seen in cases of poor oral hygiene and poor periodontal health.

E. gingivalis is possibly less commonly found in the oral cavity than _T. tenax._ However, there are indications that _E. gingivalis_

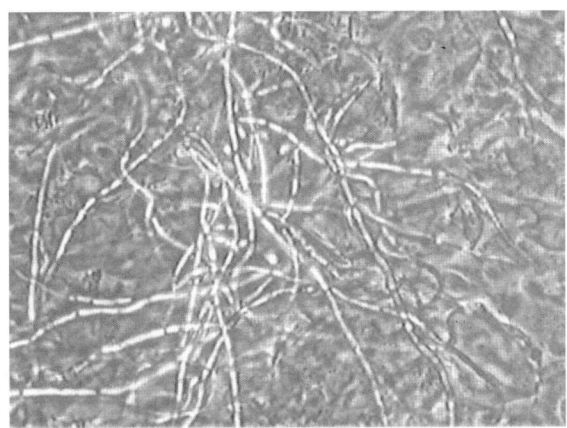

Fig. 8.27 Sample from the palate of a patient with denture stomatitis with clear candidal mycelia visualized under a phase-contrast microscope.

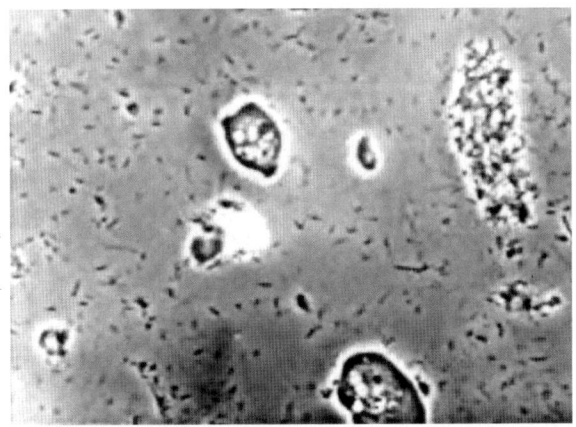

Fig. 8.28 *Trichomonas* in dental plaque visualized under a phase-contrast microscope.

TABLE 8.8   Etiologic Agents for Different Types of Oral Yeast Infections

Oral Mycoses	Etiologic Agent
Candidiasis	*Candida albicans, Candida glabrata, Candida tropicalis, Candida dubliniensis, Candida krusei,* and so on
Aspergillosis	*Aspergillus fumigatus*
Blastomycosis	*Blastomyces dermatitidis*
Coccidioidomycosis	*Coccidioides immitis*
Cryptococcosis	*Cryptococcus neoformans*
Fusariosis	*Fusarium moniliforme*
Geotrichosis	*Geotrichum candidum*
Histoplasmosis	*Histoplasma capsulatum*
Mucormycosis	*Order* Mucorales
Paracoccidiomycosis	*Paracoccidioides brasiliensis*
Penicilliosis	*Penicillium marneffei*
Sporotrichosis	*Sporothrix schenckii*

From Samaranayake LP, Keung LW, Jin L: Oral mucosal fungal infections. *Periodontol 2000* 49:39, 2009.

produces a particular progressive periodontal disease in immuno-compromised patients, who often present with a necrotic gingival infection.

This type of painful oral lesion often has an unclear etiology, but, during the late 1990s, a Swedish study not only showed its association with HIV-1 but also reported that this parasite association seemed to be exclusive for HIV-1 in that no other parasite was ever found with this type of immunodeficiency.[238]

Among systemic parasitic infections, only the protozoan flagellate *Leishmania* can produce clinical symptoms that affect the oral cavity.[24] This effect is indirect, and it is caused by disfigurations produced by infections with the mucocutaneous form of the infection, thereby resulting in granulomatous growth that involves the mouth and nose. Although the distribution of the local oral parasites is worldwide, leishmaniasis exists only in certain areas.

Archaea

Archaea are single-celled organisms that are as distinct from bacteria as they are from eukaryotes. The role of archaea in oral diseases is only beginning to be explored. Methanogenic archaea produce methane from hydrogen gas (H_2)/carbon dioxide (CO_2) and sometimes from formate, acetate, methanol, or methylamine. These organisms have been isolated from patients with periodontal disease via the enrichment of cultures with H_2 and CO_2. They mainly occur in the anaerobic part of the subgingival biofilm and in infected root canals.[22,424,425] In addition, although they were not identified in periodontally healthy subjects, archaea were identified in 37 out of 48 samples from periodontal disease sites with the use of molecular detection methods.[217] Methanogenic archaea were found to thrive better in diseased sites as compared with healthy sites in patients with aggressive periodontitis, and a clear correlation was established with pathogenic microbiota.[98,247] It is postulated that these archaea may favor the growth of periodontopathogens by modulating the subgingival biofilm constitution inherent in their metabolism. However, the precise clinical relevance of archaea remains a matter of conjecture.[246]

Microbiologic Specificity of Periodontal Diseases

Nonspecific Plaque Hypothesis

During the mid-1900s, periodontal diseases were thought to result from an accumulation of plaque over time, eventually in conjunction with a diminished host response and increased host susceptibility with age. This theory, which is called the *nonspecific plaque hypothesis*, was supported by epidemiologic studies that correlated both age and the amount of plaque with evidence of periodontitis.[237,340,355]

According to the nonspecific plaque hypothesis, periodontal disease results from the "elaboration of noxious products by the entire plaque flora."[232] When only small amounts of plaque are present, the noxious products are neutralized by the host. Similarly, large amounts of plaque would cause a higher production of noxious products, which would essentially overwhelm the host's defenses.

KEY FACT

Although the nonspecific plaque hypothesis has been discarded in favor of other etiologic hypotheses, most of the therapeutic interventions are still based on the principles of the nonspecific plaque hypothesis.

Several observations contradicted these conclusions. First, some individuals with considerable amounts of plaque and calculus, as well as gingivitis, never developed destructive periodontitis. Furthermore, individuals who did present with periodontitis demonstrated considerable site specificity with regard to the pattern of disease. Some sites were unaffected, whereas advanced disease was found in adjacent sites. In the presence of a uniform host response, these findings were inconsistent with the concept that all plaque was equally pathogenic. Recognition of the differences in plaque at sites of different clinical status (i.e., disease versus health) led to a renewed search for specific pathogens in periodontal diseases and a conceptual transition from the nonspecific to the specific plaque hypothesis.[230,373,380]

Inherent in the nonspecific plaque hypothesis is the concept that the control of periodontal disease depends on the reduction of the total amount of plaque. The current standard treatment of periodontitis by debridement (nonsurgical or surgical) and oral hygiene measures still focuses on the removal of plaque and its products. Although the nonspecific plaque hypothesis has been discarded in favor of other etiologic hypotheses, most of the therapeutic interventions are still based on the basic principles of the nonspecific plaque hypothesis.

Specific Plaque Hypothesis

The specific plaque hypothesis underlines the importance of the qualitative composition of the resident microbiota. The pathogenicity of dental plaque depends on the presence of or an increase in specific microorganisms.[232] This concept encapsulates that plaque that harbors specific bacterial pathogens may provoke periodontal disease because key organisms produce substances that mediate the destruction of host tissues. The association of specific bacterial species with disease came about during the early 1960s, when the microscopic examination of plaque revealed that different bacterial morphotypes were found in healthy versus periodontally diseased sites (see Video 8.5). At about the same time, major advances were made in the techniques used to isolate and identify periodontal microorganisms. These included improvements in procedures to sample subgingival plaque, in the handling of samples to prevent killing the bacteria, and in the media used to grow the bacteria in the laboratory.[382] The results were a tremendous increase in the ability to isolate periodontal microorganisms and considerable refinement in bacterial taxonomy.[196] Acceptance of the specific plaque hypothesis was spurred by the recognition of *A. actinomycetemcomitans* as a pathogen in localized aggressive periodontitis.[269,373] These advances led to a series of association studies focused on identifying specific periodontal pathogens by examining the microbiota associated with states of health and disease in cross-sectional and longitudinal studies.

The introduction of molecular methods for bacterial identification has greatly increased the power of association studies because we are no longer constrained to analyzing those bacteria that can be cultured (i.e., up to 50% of the total oral microbiota). For example, specific members of the phylum Synergistetes that have never been cultured in isolation show a clear association with periodontal disease.[423] Molecular identification techniques such as DNA checkerboard hybridization can identify and enumerate many different organisms simultaneously and are thus well suited to high-throughput studies (see eFig. 8.8 online). The association of Socransky's "red complex" bacteria (*P. gingivalis, T. forsythia,* and *T. denticola*) with periodontal disease was based on the analysis of 40 different bacteria in more than 13,000 plaque samples.[384] Nevertheless, disease association studies do not reveal whether the presence of specific bacteria *causes* or *correlates with* the presence of disease. In addition, these studies have shown that periodontal disease can occur even in the absence of defined "pathogens," such as red complex bacteria, and conversely that "pathogens" may be present in the absence of disease.

Ecologic Plaque Hypothesis

During the 1990s, Marsh and coworkers[245a] developed the "ecologic plaque hypothesis" as an attempt to unify the existing theories regarding the role of dental plaque in oral disease (Fig. 8.29). According to the ecologic plaque hypothesis, both the total amount of dental plaque and the specific microbial composition of plaque may contribute to the transition from health to disease. The health-associated dental plaque microbiota is considered to be relatively stable over time and in a state of dynamic equilibrium or "microbial homeostasis." The host controls subgingival plaque to some extent by a tempered immune response and low levels of gingival crevicular fluid flow. Perturbations to the host response may be brought about by an excessive accumulation of nonspecific dental plaque, by plaque-independent host factors (e.g., the onset of an immune disorder, changes in hormonal balance [e.g., during pregnancy]), or by environmental factors (e.g., smoking, diet).

Changes in the host status, such as inflammation, tissue degradation, and/or high gingival crevicular fluid flow, may lead to a shift in the microbial population in plaque. As a result of microenvironmental changes, the number of beneficial species may decrease, whereas the number of potentially pathogenic species increases. This gradual shift in the entire microbial community, known as *dysbiosis*, may

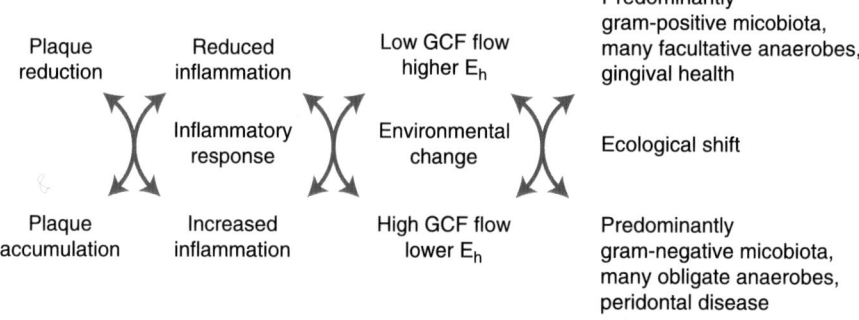

Fig. 8.29 Ecologic plaque hypothesis in relation to periodontal diseases: gingivitis and periodontitis. The accumulation of plaque causes the inflammation of adjacent tissues (gingivitis) and other environmental changes that favor the growth of gram-negative anaerobes and proteolytic species, including periodontopathogens. The increased proportions of such species result in the destruction of periodontal tissues (i.e., periodontitis). E_h, Redox potential; *GCF*, gingival crevicular fluid. (*Adapted from Marsh PD: Microbial ecology of dental plaque and its significance in health and disease.* Adv Dent Res 8:263, 1994.)

result in a chronic disease state such as periodontitis.[23] The ecologic plaque hypothesis is entirely consistent with observations that disease-associated organisms are minor components of the oral microbiota in health; these organisms are kept in check by interspecies competition during microbial homeostasis. Disease is associated with the overgrowth of specific members of the dental plaque biofilm when the local microenvironment changes, but it is not necessarily the same species in each case. An important consideration of the ecologic plaque hypothesis is that therapeutic intervention can be useful on a number of different levels. Eliminating the etiologic stimulus—whether it is microbial, host, or environmental—will help to restore microbial homeostasis. Targeting specific microorganisms may be less effective because the conditions for disease will remain.

Keystone Pathogen Hypothesis and Polymicrobial Synergy and Dysbiosis Model

The keystone pathogen hypothesis indicates that certain low-abundance microbial pathogens can orchestrate inflammatory disease by remodeling a normally benign microbiota into a dysbiotic one. It may provide a novel conceptual basis for the development of targeted diagnostic and treatment modalities for complex dysbiotic diseases.[131,133]

Some evidence indicates that certain pathogens may trigger the disruption of microbial homeostasis, thereby leading to the development of periodontal disease, even when they are present only in low numbers. For example, specific pathogen-free mice exposed to *P. gingivalis* developed periodontal bone loss even when the pathogen was present in less than 0.1% of the total microbiota. Disease did not occur in the absence of other bacteria (i.e., in germ-free mice) or in mice lacking the C3a or C5a complement receptors. These data indicated that *P. gingivalis* subverts the host immune system and changes the microbial composition of dental plaque, ultimately leading to periodontal bone loss. On this basis, *P. gingivalis* was labeled a "keystone" pathogen; this means that it is an organism that is central to the disease process, even when it is at a relatively low abundance.

The keystone pathogen hypothesis has been extended to include the concept of a disrupted homeostasis in addition to the important roles of keystone pathogens in the polymicrobial synergy and dysbiosis model of disease.[132] In this model, interspecies communication between keystone pathogens and other members of the community (known as *accessory pathogens*) is considered one important factor that leads to overgrowth of the more pathogenic microbiota and to a dysbiotic microbial community. This model is based on a number of observations of microbial synergy among species that are not considered periodontal pathogens such as the oral streptococci and more pathogenic organisms including *P. gingivalis* and *A. actinomycetemcomitans*.[132]

Complicating Factors

The identification of bacterial pathogens in periodontal diseases has been difficult because of a number of factors.[382] The periodontal microbiota is a complex community of microorganisms, many of which are still difficult or impossible to cultivate or identify. The chronic nature of periodontal disease has complicated the search for bacterial pathogens. It was previously thought that periodontal diseases progressed at a slow but steady rate.[228] However, epidemiologic studies established that the disease progresses at different rates, with alternating episodes of rapid tissue destruction and periods of remission (Fig. 8.30).[385] At this moment, by means of multilevel modeling, the linear and burst theories of periodontitis progression are considered to be manifestations of the same phenomenon: some sites improve, whereas others progress, and this occurs in a cyclic manner.[114] Identification of the microorganisms found during the

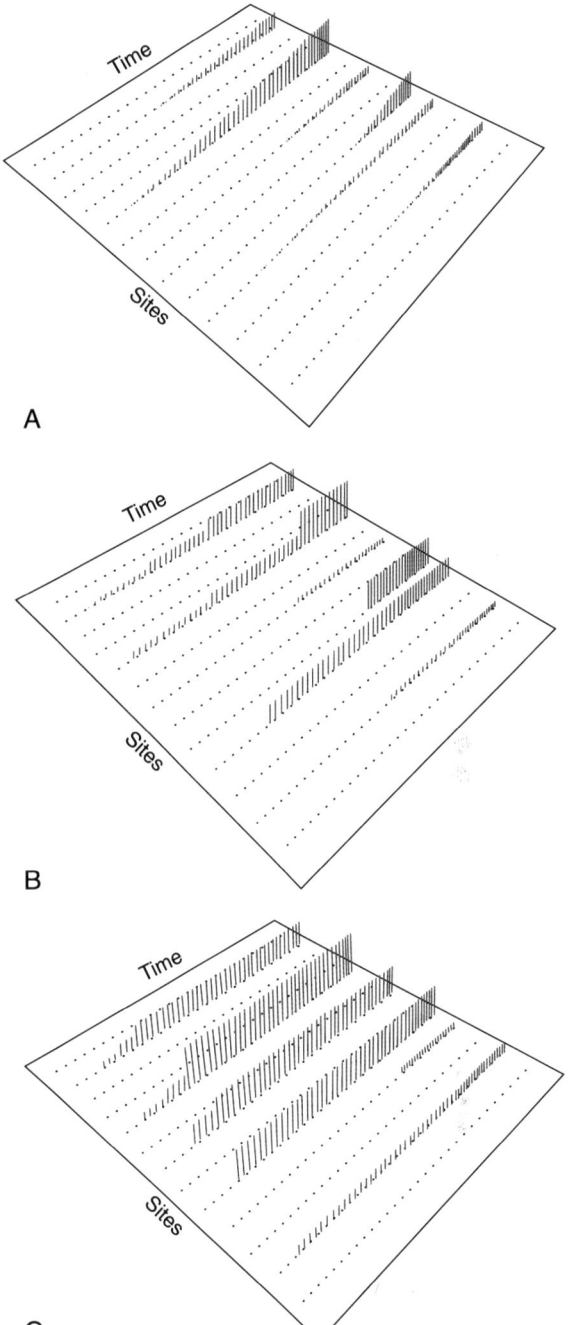

Fig. 8.30 Diagrammatic representation of possible modes of progression of chronic destructive periodontal diseases. Sites on the x-axis are plotted against time on the y-axis, and activity is shown on the z-axis. (A) Some sites show a progressive loss of attachment over time, whereas others show no destruction. The time of onset and the extent of destruction vary among sites. (B) Random burst model. Activity occurs at random in any site. Some sites show no activity, whereas others show one or several bursts of activity. The cumulative extent of destruction varies among sites. (C) Asynchronous multiple burst model. Several sites show bursts of activity over a finite period followed by prolonged periods of inactivity. Occasional bursts may occur infrequently at certain sites at later periods. Other sites show no periodontal disease activity at any time. The difference from the model shown in (B) is that in (C) the majority of destructive disease activity takes place within a few years of the individual's life. *(Courtesy Drs. S. Socransky, A. Haffajee, and M. Goodson, [Boston] and J. Lindhe [Göteborg, Sweden].)*

different phases of the disease progression is technically challenging. The interpretation of microbiologic data is further complicated by the clinical classification of the disease status, an area that has undergone revisions.[15,421] Previous and perhaps current classifications involve the grouping of potentially different disease states as a result of difficulties with accurately distinguishing them clinically. It is important to recognize that groupings such as this may obscure microbiologic associations.

Periodontitis is currently considered a mixed infection. This has significant implications for both the diagnosis and the treatment of periodontitis. For the diagnosis, some clinicians evaluate the presence of up to 40 species, but it still is unclear whether some combinations of species are more pathogenic than others. The treatment is directed toward the eradication or reduction of the number of key periodontopathogens. Because several species may be involved, the appropriate use of antimicrobials (especially antibiotics) is extremely difficult to define, given that not all expected periodontopathogens are equally susceptible to the same antibiotic.

Microbiologic diagnostic tests indicated that the presence of periodontopathogens alone is not sufficient for the development of periodontitis. Because of the high sensitivity of these tests, several pathogens have been detected in periodontitis-free patients. Thus, merely the presence of pathogens is not sufficient for disease, and the amount of the pathogens plays a key role in relation to disease.[339] These observations have major clinical implications. First, the specificity of microbial detection is dramatically reduced (specificity in the sense that the presence of a specific pathogen means periodontitis). In other words, even though the result of a microbiologic analysis is positive, the patient can be without disease.[236] In addition, the understanding of the etiology becomes more complicated, because the threshold level for periodontopathogens between health and disease is unknown and obviously subject dependent. Moreover, for several species, large intrastrain variations in genetic information have been detected (i.e., different genotypes), so that, in fact, genotypical information is necessary for pathogenicity assessment.[55,77,124,289] The quality of the host response also plays an essential role, but this cannot yet be correctly estimated. Finally, it may be questioned whether periodontopathogens are endogenous resident species or exogenous invaders. Indeed, the newer techniques have reported high detection frequencies of all pathogens in healthy subjects.[236,350] This has significant impact on the treatment strategies. For endogenous species, the endpoint of a therapy is the quantitative reduction of the species, whereas for exogenous species, the endpoints are eradication and the prevention of reinfection.

It is currently impossible to alter the susceptibility of the host, so periodontal therapy must be focused on the reduction or elimination of periodontopathogens in combination with the reestablishment, often by surgical pocket elimination, of a more suitable (i.e., less anaerobic) environment for a more beneficial microbiota. Several studies have indicated that the presence of the previously mentioned periodontopathogens (that persist or are reestablished after treatment) is associated with a negative clinical outcome of periodontal treatment.[127,328,329] Because several species may be involved, the use of antimicrobials (especially antibiotics) is extremely difficult because antibiotic susceptibility is very diverse among periodontopathogens and often depends on the geographic region.[315,419]

It is obvious that several key questions still remain unanswered. Some researchers question whether the presence of specific microorganisms in the periodontal pocket is a cause or a consequence of disease.[386] Because most periodontopathogens are fastidious strict anaerobes, they may contribute little to the initiation of disease in shallow gingival pockets and instead be found only in deep periodontal pockets, which is their preferred habitat.

The Transition From Health to Disease

The oral microbial ecology is dynamic. The presence and numbers of particular microorganisms, even as a part of a community colonizing a niche in a human being, are controlled by the type and quantity of nutrients present (nutritional determinant), their ability to tolerate the specific physicochemical factors (physicochemical determinants), and their ability to cope with antimicrobial compounds (biologic determinants) or mechanical removal forces (mechanical determinants).[445] Although these determinants are well defined from a theoretical point of view, in practice they overlap each other, especially in more complex environments (i.e., multispecies environments). Inherent to their biologic nature, bacteria interact with each other, with their environment, and vice versa. Therefore, the microbial ecology will change its composition or the composition of the microbial ecology will be changed when transitioning from a healthy status to a diseased status or vice versa. A change in the composition of a bacterial community as the result of external, nonmicrobial factors is termed *allogenic succession.* Smoking is a good example of such interaction. In *autogenic succession* (i.e., a change in the composition of a microbial community that arises from microbial activities), interbacterial and viral–bacterial interactions are involved.

🔑 KEY FACT

Transition from health to disease results from complex interplay among the host, pathogenic bacteria, and commensal bacteria.

Early microscopic studies clearly demonstrated that the number and proportions of different subgingival bacterial morphotypes differ between healthy and diseased sites (Figs. 8.31 and 8.32; see Video 8.5).[223,373,380] The total number of bacteria, which was determined by microscopic counts per gram of plaque, was twice as high in periodontally diseased sites as compared with healthy sites.[380] Because considerably more plaque is found at diseased sites, this suggests that, in general, the total bacterial load in diseased sites is greater than that of healthy sites. Fewer coccal cells and more motile rods and spirochetes are found in diseased sites as compared with healthy sites.[223] Although this morphologic criterion can be of diagnostic value, one should remember that nearly all key periodontal pathogens (except *C. rectus* and spirochetes) are immobile rods, which adds to the confusion regarding the bacterial etiology of periodontal diseases. Culturing has shown that the microbiota in periodontally healthy sites consists predominantly of gram-positive facultative rods and cocci (approximately 75%).[373] The recovery of this group of microorganisms is decreased proportionally in gingivitis (44%) and periodontitis (10% to 13%). These decreases are accompanied by increases in the proportions of gram-negative rods, from 13% in health to 40% in gingivitis and 74% in advanced periodontitis.

The current concept regarding the etiology of periodontal diseases considers three groups of factors that determine whether active periodontal destruction will occur in a subject: a susceptible host, the presence of pathogenic species, and the absence or small proportion of so-called beneficial bacteria.[12,379,382,389,448] The clinical manifestations of periodontal destruction will result from a complex interplay among these etiologic agents. In general, small amounts of bacterial plaque can be controlled by the body's defense mechanisms without destruction; however, when dysbiosis happens (e.g., as a result of increased susceptibility, high bacterial load, or pathogenic infections), periodontal destruction could occur.[23]

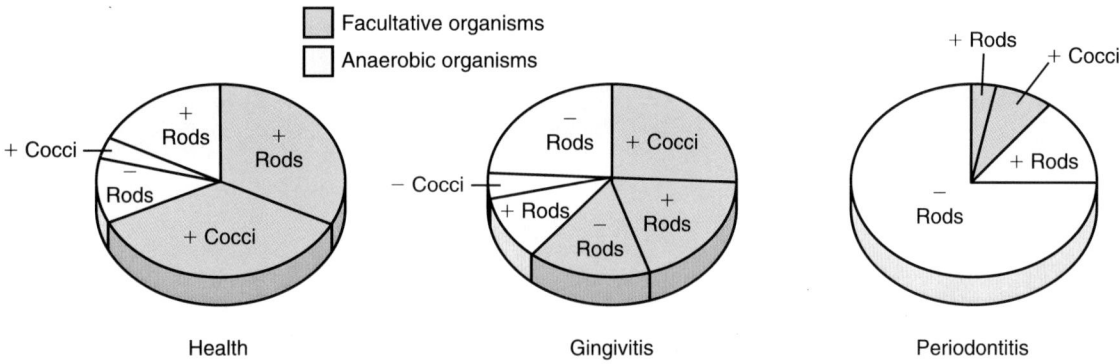

Fig. 8.31 Pie charts based on culturing studies that represent the relative proportion of different morphotypes in subgingival samples in cases of periodontal health, gingivitis, and periodontitis. A clear distinction is made between facultative species and obligate anaerobic species. Spirochetes are not included. +, Gram-positive; −, gram-negative.

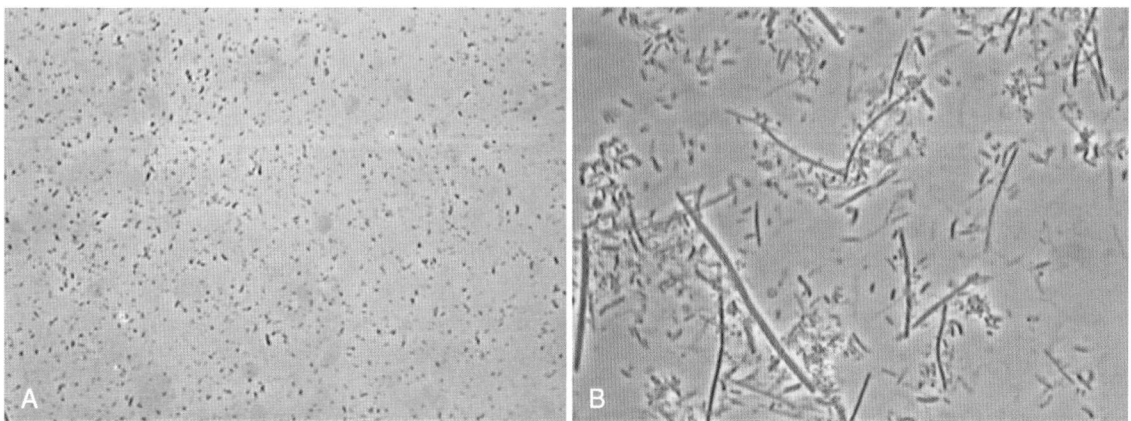

Fig. 8.32 Phase-contrast micrographs of plaque samples. Phase-contrast micrographs of plaque samples from (A) a healthy patient and (B) a patient with periodontitis. Note the large rods and spirochetes in the periodontitis plaque sample.

Host Susceptibility

The susceptibility of the host is determined by genetic factors, as well as by environmental and behavioral factors, such as smoking, stress, and viral infections.

Genetic factors seem important for patients with so-called early onset periodontitis, which is now referred to as aggressive periodontitis.[252] Reports regarding the familial nature of chronic forms of periodontitis are less conclusive. The aggregation of aggressive periodontitis within families is consistent with a genetic predisposition, although common environmental factors cannot be excluded (see Chapter 11).

Smoking is considered a behavioral factor and eventually an environmental factor. It dramatically increases host susceptibility to periodontal breakdown. Nevertheless, the exact nature of the relationship between periodontitis and smoking is unclear (see Chapter 12). Reports are conflicting regarding the effects of smoking on the oral microbiota. Some are in favor of an increased prevalence of *P. gingivalis, A. actinomycetemcomitans, T. forsythia, E. coli,* and *C. albicans* in smokers, whereas others report no difference.[29,129,303,398,413,417,456]

More recently, pyrosequencing revealed a lower subgingival taxonomic diversity in smokers as compared with nonsmokers.[26] Moreover, investigators showed that in smokers the ability to rebound from a dysbiotic state and reestablish a health-compatible community is impaired.[169] Smoking cessation, in contrast, can alter the subgingival biofilm and suggests a mechanism for improved periodontal health associated with smoking cessation.[107] Some evidence indicates that the epithelial cells of smokers are more prone to colonization by respiratory pathogens. Depending on the bacterial strain, the relative increase in the number of adhering pathogens in smokers versus nonsmokers ranged from 40% up to 150%.[97,342] Cigarette smoke has been shown to modify the expression of *P. gingivalis* genes directly, including several virulence-associated genes.[20] After exposure to cigarette smoke extract, *P. gingivalis* cells induce a lower proinflammatory response than unexposed *P. gingivalis* cells.

Viral infections have been added to the list of factors that modify host susceptibility. HIV and herpesviruses are often associated with periodontal infections.

With regard to periodontopathogen adhesion to virally infected cells, Teughels and coworkers[407] showed a 100% increase in *A. actinomycetemcomitans* colonization when epithelial cells were infected with human CMV (hCMV).

Increasing evidence suggests that emotional stress and negative life events can play an important role in the development and progression of periodontitis and that they may also modify the response to periodontal treatment. Stress associated with financial strain is a significant risk indicator for more severe periodontitis in adults (odds ratio: 2.24; confidence interval: 1.15 to 4.38).[111] Emotional and psychological loads can influence the immune system, and they will also alter oral health behaviors.[69] Both factors increase the susceptibility to periodontitis.

TABLE 8.9   Prevalence of Microbial Species Associated With Various Clinical Forms of Periodontitis

Species	FORMS OF PERIODONTITIS		
	Chronic Periodontitis (%)	Localized Aggressive Periodontitis (%)	Aggressive Periodontitis (%)
Aggregatibacter actinomycetemcomitans	28.2	81.8	40.9
Porphyromonas gingivalis	53.8	13.3	79.6
Prevotella intermedia/nigrescens	50.2	53.4	71.4
Tannerella forsythia	50.6	0	50.8
Campylobacter rectus	40.3	12.5	47.8

0, Occasionally isolated.
Adapted from Haffajee AD, Socransky SS: Microbial etiological agents of destructive periodontal diseases. *Periodontol 2000* 5:78, 1994; and Mombelli A, Casagni F, Madianos PN: Can presence or absence of periodontal pathogens distinguish between subjects with chronic and aggressive periodontitis? A systematic review. *J Clin Periodontol* 29(Suppl 3):10, 2002.

TABLE 8.10   Prevalence of Key Pathogens in Healthy Subjects and Patients With Periodontitis

Species	PREVALENCE		SIGNIFICANCE OF DIFFERENCE	
	Health (%)	Periodontitis (%)	P Value	Odds Ratio[a]
Aggregatibacter actinomycetemcomitans	12.8	31.0	0.002	3.1
Porphyromonas gingivalis	10.6	59.5	<0.001	12.3
Prevotella intermedia/nigrescens	69.1	87.9	0.001	3.3
Tannerella forsythia	47.9	90.5	<0.001	10.4
Fusobacterium nucleatum	85.1	95.7	0.014	3.9
Parvimonas micra	67	94	<0.001	7.7
Campylobacter rectus	13.8	20.7	NS	1.6

[a]The ratio of the probability of developing the disease to the probability of nonoccurrence. For example, "3" means a threefold increased chance that the disease will develop if that species is present.
NS, Not significant.
Adapted from Van Winkelhoff A, Loos BG, van der Reijden WA, et al: *Porphyromonas gingivalis, Bacteroides forsythus* and other putative periodontal pathogens in subjects with and without periodontal destruction. *J Clin Periodontol* 29:1023, 2002.

Racial factors have also been implicated in the differences in prevalence of early-onset periodontitis and in the frequency of detection of putative periodontopathogens.[21,229]

Pathogenic Bacteria

The second essential factor for disease initiation and progression is the presence of one or more pathogens of the appropriate clonal type and in sufficient numbers. Despite the difficulties inherent in characterizing the microbiology of periodontal diseases, a small group of pathogens is recognized because of their close association with disease. Obvious data support the designation of *A. actinomycetemcomitans, T. forsythia, T. denticola,* and *P. gingivalis* as key pathogens because they are strongly associated with periodontal disease status, disease progression, and unsuccessful therapy. For the following list of bacteria, moderate evidence for etiology has been reported, at least if their concentration passes a certain threshold level: *P. intermedia, Prevotella nigrescens* (see Fig. 8.2I), *C. rectus, P. micra* (see Fig. 8.2J), *F. nucleatum, Eubacterium nodatum* (see Fig. 8.2N), and various spirochetes.[12,379,382,389,448] The significance of the role of these key pathogens is largely based on epidemiologic data, the ability of these microorganisms to produce disease when inoculated in animals, and their capacity to produce virulence factors. However, the mere presence of putative periodontopathogens in the gingival crevice is not in itself sufficient to initiate or cause periodontal inflammation. An elevation in the relative proportion or number of these pathogens to reach a critical mass seems more crucial to mount an effective tissue-damaging process. Indeed, even in health, periodontopathogens are or can be present in the gingival crevice, albeit in low numbers, as members of the normal resident flora.[236] Table 8.9 gives a general overview of the detection frequency for most key pathogens in different forms of periodontal infections. It is immediately obvious that no black-and-white situation exists; there are no specific types of periodontitis for which any known pathogen is always present. This table also illustrates the difficulties with using the microbial composition to differentiate between different forms of periodontal infections. Table 8.10 further highlights the complexity of the microbiology of periodontitis. Most periodontopathogens can also be detected in healthy subjects, with frequencies that range from 10% to 85%. It is obvious that this automatically reduces the specificity of microbiologic testing in periodontology.

However, technologic advancements such as next-generation sequencing have lengthened the list of bacterial species associated with periodontitis. Moderate evidence in the literature is suggested to support the association of 17 species of phylotypes from the phyla Bacteroidetes, Candidatus Saccharibacteria, Firmicutes, Proteobacteria, Spirochaetes, and Synergistetes.[287] The phylum Candidatus Saccharibacteria and the Archaea domain also seem to be associated with disease.[287] For more information, see Table 8.11.

TABLE 8.11 Newly Identified Pathogens in the Etiology of Periodontitis for Which Three or More Studies Are Available

Phylum	Species	Gram	Culture Characteristics	No. of Studies
Bacteroidetes	*Bacteroidales* sp. oral taxon 274 HOT 274	–	a	3
	Porphyromonas endodontalis HOT 273	–	a	4
Firmicutes	*Eubacterium saphenum* HOT 759	+	a	5
	Mogibacterium timidum HOT 042	+	a	3
	Peptostreptococcus stomatis HOT 112	+	a	3
	Filifactor alocis HOT 539	+	a	5
	Anaeroblobus geminatus HOT 112	–	a	3
	Selenomonas sputigena HOT 151	–	a	5
	Enterococcus faecalis HOT 604	+	f	4
Proteobacteria	*Desulfobulbus* sp. oral taxon 041 HOT 041	/	/	3
Spirochaetes	*Treponema lecithinolyticum* HOT 653	–	a	4
	Treponema medium HOT 667	–	a	5
	Treponema vincentii HOT 029	–	a	3
Synergistetes	*Fretibacterium* sp. oral taxon 360 HOT 360	/	/	4
	Fretibacterium fastidiuosum HOT 363	–	a	3
Candidatus saccharibacteria	TM7 sp. oral taxon 356 HOT 356	/	/	3

/, Not yet cultivable; +, gram positive, – gram negative; *a*, anaerobic; *f*, facultative anaerobic.
Data from Pérez-Chaparro PJ, Gonçalves C, Figueiredo LC, et al: Newly identified pathogens associated with periodontitis: a systematic review. *J Dent Res* 93:846–58, 2014.

Beneficial Species

The role of "beneficial" species is less obvious in the development of periodontal diseases.[334,382] These bacteria can affect the pathogenic species in different ways and thus modify the disease process as follows: (1) by passively occupying a niche that may otherwise be colonized by pathogens, (2) by actively limiting a pathogen's ability to adhere to appropriate tissue surfaces, (3) by adversely affecting the vitality or growth of a pathogen, (4) by affecting the ability of a pathogen to produce virulence factors, or (5) by degrading the virulence factors produced by the pathogen. The often-used textbook example of such a beneficial action is the effect of *S. sanguinis* (formerly known as *S. sanguis*) on *A. actinomycetemcomitans*.[412] *S. sanguinis* produces H_2O_2, which either directly or by host enzyme amplification can kill *A. actinomycetemcomitans*.[151] However, interactions between oral streptococci and *A. actinomycetemcomitans* are not so simple and streptococci may actually promote the growth of *A. actinomycetemcomitans* by providing nutrients in the form of lactic acid and electron acceptors that enhance respiratory growth.[325,392] To obtain the benefits of oral streptococcal products without succumbing to H_2O_2, *A. actinomycetemcomitans* regulates the exopolysaccharide-degrading enzyme dispersin B to position itself at an optimal distance from streptococcal cells.[391] Although the so-called beneficial bacteria may be of importance for maintaining a healthy subgingival ecosystem, evidence is limited.[334] Despite rapidly increasing knowledge of periodontopathogen–host interactions, the role of beneficial microbiota in this crosstalk remains obscure. In periodontal microbiology, a bacterial strain is considered beneficial when its prevalence is high in periodontal health and low in diseased situations. It has been shown for other fields in microbiology that direct and indirect microbial interactions can suppress the emergence of pathogens.[36] The importance of the latter is evidenced within the oral cavity by the development of *Candida* infections when the normal oral flora is reduced, such as after a period of systemic antibiotic usage.[430]

Because it has so far been impossible to alter the susceptibility of the host, periodontal therapy is necessarily focused on the reduction or elimination of periodontopathogens in combination with the reestablishment, often by surgical pocket elimination, of a more suitable (e.g., less anaerobic) environment for a more beneficial microbiota. Several studies have indeed indicated that the presence of the previously mentioned periodontopathogens (that have persisted or been reestablished after treatment) is associated with a negative clinical outcome of periodontal treatment.[67,128,328,329,384]

Taking all of this together, it is clear that the periodontal microbiota will shift when going from a periodontally healthy situation toward a periodontally diseased situation (Fig. 8.33).

When comparing the microbiota among conditions of health, gingivitis, and periodontitis, the following microbial shifts can be identified as health progresses to periodontitis:
- From gram-positive to gram-negative
- From cocci to rods (and, at a later stage, to spirochetes)
- From nonmotile to motile organisms
- From facultative anaerobes to obligate anaerobes
- From fermenting to proteolytic species

Periodontal Health

The recovery of microorganisms from periodontally healthy sites is lower as compared with diseased sites (Table 8.12). The bacteria associated with periodontal health are primarily gram-positive facultative species and members of the genera *Streptococcus* and *Actinomyces* (e.g., *S. sanguinis*, *S. mitis*, *A. oris*, *Actinomyces israelii*, *Actinomyces gerencseriae*, *Actinomyces viscosus* [see Fig. 8.2C], *A. naeslundii*). Small proportions of gram-negative species are also found, most frequently *P. intermedia*, *F. nucleatum*, *F. nucleatum* spp. polymorphum, *F. periodonticum*, *Capnocytophaga* spp. (*C. gingivalis*, *C. ochracea*, and *C. sputigena*), *Neisseria* spp., and *Veillonella* spp. Microscopic analyses indicate that a few spirochetes and motile rods may also be present. On the basis of checkerboard DNA–DNA hybridization data, *Eubacterium saburreum*, *Propionibacterium acnes*, *S. anginosus*, *S. gordonii*, and *S. oralis* can also be considered as health-associated bacteria.[98,404,450,451]

Certain bacterial species have been proposed to be protective or beneficial to the host, including *S. sanguinis*, *Veillonella parvula*

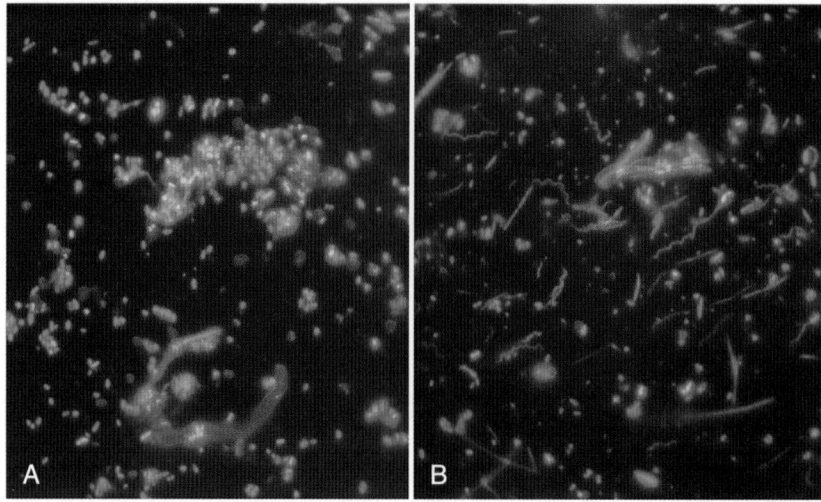

Fig. 8.33 Vitality stain of subgingival plaque. (A) Plaque derived from a healthy patient that primarily consists of cocci. (B) Plaque derived from a patient with periodontitis. Note the important morphologic differences from (A). Green bacteria are alive; red bacteria are dead.

TABLE 8.12   Summary of Bacterial Species Significantly Associated With Different Clinical Conditions Based on Culture, Polymerase Chain Reaction, and Checkerboard Data

Bacterial Species	Health	Gingivitis	Chronic Periodontitis	Localized Aggressive Periodontitis	Aggressive Periodontitis	Necrotizing Periodontal Diseases	Abscesses of the Periodontium	Peri-implantitis
Actinomyces gerencseriae	X							
Actinomyces israelii	X							
Actinomyces naeslundii 1	X	X						
Actinomyces oris	X							
Actinomyces viscosus	X	X						
Aggregatibacter actinomycetemcomitans								X
Aggregatibacter actinomycetemcomitans high (leukotoxin clone)				X				
Aggregatibacter actinomycetemcomitans serotype a			X					
Aggregatibacter actinomycetemcomitans serotype b			X		X			
Campylobacter concisus			X					
Campylobacter gracilis					X			
Campylobacter rectus		X	X	X				X
Campylobacter showae					X			
Capnocytophaga gingivalis	X							
Capnocytophaga ochracea	X							
Capnocytophaga spp.	X	X		X				X
Capnocytophaga sputigena	X							
Eikenella corrodens		X	X	X				
Enterobacter spp.			X					X
Eubacterium nodatum		X	X	X	X			

TABLE 8.12 Summary of Bacterial Species Significantly Associated With Different Clinical Conditions Based on Culture, Polymerase Chain Reaction, and Checkerboard Data—cont'd

Bacterial Species	Health	Gingivitis	Chronic Periodontitis	Localized Aggressive Periodontitis	Aggressive Periodontitis	Necrotizing Periodontal Diseases	Abscesses of the Periodontium	Peri-implantitis
Eubacterium saburreum	X							
Fusobacterium nucleatum		X	X	X		X	X	X
Fusobacterium periodonticum	X							
Fusobacterium polymorphum	X							
Haemophilus spp.		X						
Leptotrichia buccalis			X	X				
Neisseria spp.	X							
Parvimonas micra		X	X				X	X
Prevotella intermedia			X	X	X	X	X	X
Prevotella intermedia spirochetes		X						
Porphyromonas gingivalis			X	X	X		X	X
Prevotella nigrescens			X		X			
Propionibacterium acnes	X							
Pseudomonas aeruginosa								X
Selenomonas noxia			X					
Spirochetes			X	X	X	X	X	X
Staphylococcus aureus								X
Staphylococcus epidermidis								X
Streptococcus anginosus	X	X						
Streptococcus gordonii	X							
Streptococcus intermedius		X						
Streptococcus mitis	X	X						
Streptococcus oralis	X	X						
Streptococcus sanguinis	X	X						
Tannerella forsythia			X	X	X			X
Treponema denticola			X	X	X			X
Treponema spp.		X	X	X	X	X		X
Veillonella parvula	X	X						

(see Fig. 8.2B), and *C. ochracea*. They are typically found in high numbers at periodontal sites that do not demonstrate attachment loss (inactive sites) but in low numbers at sites where active periodontal destruction occurs.[88,382] These species probably function to prevent the colonization or proliferation of pathogenic microorganisms. Clinical studies have shown that sites with high levels of *C. ochracea* and *S. sanguinis* are associated with a greater gain in attachment after therapy, thereby further supporting this concept.[382] A better understanding of plaque ecology and the interactions between bacteria and their products in plaque will undoubtedly reveal many other examples.

Gingivitis

The development of gingivitis has been extensively studied in a model system referred to as *experimental gingivitis* and initially described by Löe and coworkers.[230,409] Periodontal health is first established in human subjects via cleaning and rigorous oral hygiene measures that are followed by abstinence from oral hygiene for 21 days. After 8 hours without oral hygiene, bacteria may be found at concentrations of 10^3 to 10^4 per square millimeter of tooth surface, and they will increase in number by a factor of 100 to 1000 during the next 24-hour period.[387] After 36 hours, the plaque becomes clinically visible (see Video 8.2). The initial microbiota of experimental gingivitis (see Fig. 8.17) consists of gram-positive rods, gram-positive cocci, and gram-negative cocci. The transition to gingivitis is evidenced by inflammatory changes; it is accompanied first by the appearance of gram-negative rods and filaments and then by spirochetal and motile microorganisms.[409]

The subgingival microbiota of dental-plaque–induced gingivitis (chronic gingivitis) differs from that of both health and chronic periodontitis (see Table 8.11).[174] It consists of roughly equal proportions of gram-positive (56%) and gram-negative (44%) species as well as facultative (59%) and anaerobic (41%) microorganisms.[373] It should be noted that the majority of predominant species in chronic periodontitis are already present in the gingivitis state, but mostly in small numbers.

Predominant gram-positive species include Streptococcus spp. *(S. sanguinis, S. mitis, S. intermedius, S. oralis, S. anginosus), Actinomyces* spp. *(A. oris, A. naeslundii), E. nodatum,* and *P. micra.* The gram-negative microorganisms are predominantly *Capnocytophaga* spp., *Fusobacterium* spp., *Prevotella* spp., *Campylobacter gracilis, Campylobacter concisus, V. parvula, Haemophilus* spp., and *Eikenella corrodens.* Both groups are commonly associated with gingivitis. The following gram-negative species are commonly found in periodontitis, and they are also associated with gingivitis but in fewer numbers: *P. gingivalis, T. forsythia, P. intermedia, C. rectus, Treponema* spp., and *A. actinomycetemcomitans* serotype a.[258,264,373] Pyrosequencing has identified additional taxa that are associated with gingivitis, including *Leptotrichia* spp. and *Selenomonas* spp.[157] In this study, *Streptococcus* spp. were more strongly associated with health than with gingivitis.

Pregnancy-associated gingivitis is an acute inflammation of the gingival tissues that is associated with pregnancy. This condition is accompanied by increases in steroid hormones in the crevicular fluid and dramatic increases in the levels of *P. intermedia* and *C. rectus,* which use the steroids as growth factors.[191,454]

Studies of gingivitis support the conclusion that disease development is associated with selected alterations in the microbial composition of dental plaque and not just the result of an accumulation of plaque. Gingivitis was generally thought to precede the development of chronic periodontitis; however, many individuals demonstrate long-standing gingivitis that never advances to the destruction of the periodontal attachment.[39,227]

Chronic Periodontitis

Numerous forms of periodontal disease are found in adult populations, and they are characterized by different rates of progression (see Fig. 8.30) and different responses to therapy.[15] Studies in which untreated populations were examined over long time intervals indicate disease progression at mean rates that range from 0.05 mm to 0.3 mm of attachment loss per year (i.e., the gradual model).[39] When populations are examined over short time intervals, individual sites demonstrated short phases of attachment destruction interposed by periods of no disease activity (i.e., the burst model).[119] At this moment, by means of multilevel modeling, the linear and burst theories of periodontitis progression are considered to be manifestations of the same phenomenon: some sites improve whereas others progress, and this occurs in a cyclic manner.[114]

Microbiologic examinations of chronic periodontitis have been carried out in both cross-sectional and longitudinal studies; the latter have been conducted with and without treatment. These studies support the concept that chronic periodontitis is associated with specific bacterial agents. The microscopic examination of plaque from sites with chronic periodontitis has consistently revealed elevated proportions of spirochetes (see Video 8.5).[223,234] The cultivation of plaque microorganisms from sites of chronic periodontitis reveals high percentages of anaerobic (90%) gram-negative (75%) bacterial species[372,373] (see Fig. 8.23 and Table 8.12).

In patients with chronic periodontitis, the bacteria that are most often detected at high levels include *P. gingivalis, T. forsythia, P. intermedia, P. nigrescens, C. rectus, E.a corrodens* (see Fig. 8.2S), *F. nucleatum, A. actinomycetemcomitans* (often serotype b), *P. micra, E. nodatum, Leptotrichia buccalis, Treponema (T. denticola),*

Selenomonas spp. *(S. noxia),* and *Enterobacter* spp.* The introduction of pyrosequencing techniques for microbial community analysis has provided additional sensitivity for detecting periodontal pathogens, although the broad picture has not changed. Unculturable organisms such as Synergistetes appear to correlate with periodontal disease, whereas high proportions of *Actinomyces* spp., *Rothia* spp., and *Streptococcus* spp. are correlated with health.[2,123] When periodontally active sites (i.e., with recent attachment loss) were examined in comparison with inactive sites (i.e., with no recent attachment loss), concentrations of *C. rectus, P. gingivalis, P. intermedia, F. nucleatum,* and *T. forsythia* were found to be elevated in the active sites.[87] Furthermore, detectable levels of *P. gingivalis, P. intermedia, T. forsythia, C. rectus,* and *A. actinomycetemcomitans* are associated with disease progression, and their elimination via therapy is associated with an improved clinical response.[59,87,127,378,440] Both *P. gingivalis* and *A. actinomycetemcomitans* are known to invade host tissue cells, which may be significant in aggressive forms of periodontitis.[52,56,345]

Studies have documented an association between chronic periodontitis and viral microorganisms of the herpesviruses group, most notably EBV-1 and hCMV.[62] Furthermore, the presence of subgingival EBV-1 and hCMV are associated with high levels of putative bacterial pathogens, including *P. gingivalis, T. forsythia, P. intermedia,* and *T. denticola.* These data support the hypothesis that viral infection may contribute to periodontal pathogenesis, but the potential role of viral agents remains to be determined.

Localized Aggressive Periodontitis

Several forms of periodontitis are characterized by rapid and severe attachment loss that occurs in individuals during or before puberty. Localized aggressive periodontitis, which was previously referred to as localized juvenile periodontitis, develops around the time of puberty. It is observed in females more often than in males, and it typically affects the permanent first molars and incisors (Fig. 8.34). This condition is almost uniformly seen in individuals who demonstrate some systemic defect in immune regulation, and often affected individuals demonstrate defective neutrophil function. Without treatment, the local form often extends to a more generalized form that involves severe attachment loss around many teeth. The first symptoms of localized juvenile periodontitis are already detectable in the deciduous dentition, especially via periodontal destruction around the canines and the second molars.[48]

The microbiota associated with localized aggressive periodontitis is predominantly composed of gram-negative, capnophilic (i.e., CO_2-requiring), anaerobic rods[269,270,373] (see Table 8.12). Microbiologic studies indicate that almost all localized juvenile periodontitis sites harbor *A. actinomycetemcomitans,* which may comprise as much as 90% of the total cultivable microbiota.[192,261] Other organisms found in significant levels include *P. gingivalis, E. corrodens, C. rectus, F. nucleatum, B. capillus, Eubacterium brachy,* and *Capnocytophaga* spp. and spirochetes.[192,253,261,263] Checkerboard DNA–DNA hybridization studies have also shown high proportions of *E. nodatum, P. intermedia, Treponema* spp. *(T. denticola), L. buccalis,* and *T. forsythia.*[98,450] In addition, herpesviruses, including EBV-1 and hCMV, have also been associated with localized aggressive periodontitis.[62,253,410]

A. actinomycetemcomitans is generally accepted as the primary etiologic agent in most but not all cases of localized aggressive periodontitis.[190,382] A high leukotoxic clone, known as JP2, is uniquely associated with aggressive forms of periodontitis. However, the finding that not all patients with aggressive periodontitis show this feature points to the possibility that several other factors may provoke

---

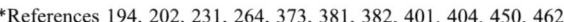

*References 194, 202, 231, 264, 373, 381, 382, 401, 404, 450, 462.

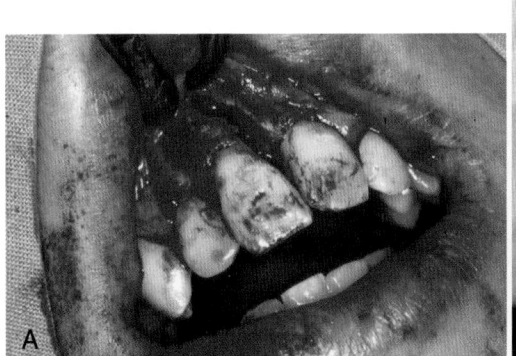
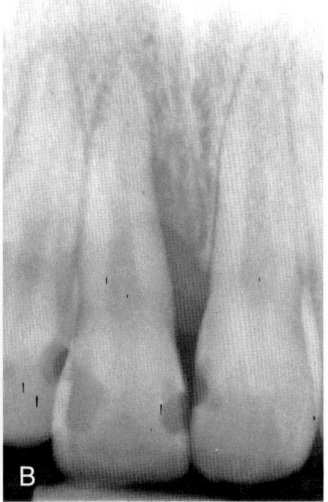

Fig. 8.34 Localized aggressive periodontitis. (A) Clinical photograph and (B) intraoral radiograph of dramatic bone destruction in an adolescent patient with localized aggressive periodontitis.

this disease.[257] Studies of therapy indicate that mechanical debridement in combination with systemic antibiotic treatment is necessary to control the levels of *A. actinomycetemcomitans* associated with this disease.[192,330,331] The failure of mechanical therapy alone may relate to the ability of this organism to invade host tissues.[52,56,345]

Aggressive Periodontitis

Aggressive periodontitis, which is also known as generalized aggressive periodontitis, early-onset periodontitis, and rapidly progressive periodontitis, is a severe form of periodontitis that occurs at a relatively young age (i.e., between 20 and 40 years). It is characterized by severe gingivitis, a large number of deepened pockets, and a high tendency for bleeding on probing. In relation to the patient's age, bone destruction is extensive. It is sometimes considered a generalized form of localized aggressive periodontitis. From a microbiologic point of view, it has many similarities with localized aggressive periodontitis (see Table 8.12). However, aggressive periodontitis is clearly dominated more by *P. gingivalis, P. intermedia, T. forsythia,* and *Treponema* spp. *(T. denticola)* and less by *A. actinomycetemcomitans.* Checkerboard DNA–DNA hybridization studies also indicate high proportions of *E. nodatum, Campylobacter gracilis, Campylobacter showae,* and *P. nigrescens.*[98,450]

Necrotizing Periodontal Diseases

Necrotizing periodontal diseases (Fig. 8.35) manifest as acute inflammation of the gingival and periodontal tissues that is characterized by the necrosis of the marginal gingival tissue and the interdental papillae. Clinically, these conditions are often associated with stress or HIV infection. They may be accompanied by malodor and pain and possibly systemic symptoms, including lymphadenopathy, fever, and malaise. Microbiologic studies indicate that high levels of *P. intermedia* and especially of spirochetes and *F. nucleatum* are present in necrotizing ulcerative gingivitis lesions. Spirochetes are found to penetrate necrotic tissue and apparently unaffected connective tissue.[224,225]

Abscesses of the Periodontium

Periodontal abscesses (Fig. 8.36) are acute lesions that may result in the very rapid destruction of the periodontal tissues. They often occur in patients with untreated periodontitis, but they also may be found in patients during maintenance or after the scaling and root

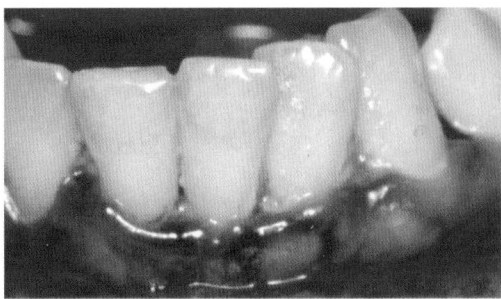

Fig. 8.35 Clinical picture of lower front teeth with necrotizing gingivitis.

planing of deep pockets. Periodontal abscesses may also occur in the absence of periodontitis; for example, they may be associated with the impaction of a foreign object (e.g., a popcorn kernel, dental floss) or with endodontic problems.[150] Typical clinical symptoms of periodontal abscesses include pain, swelling, suppuration, bleeding on probing, and mobility of the involved tooth. Signs of systemic involvement may be present, including cervical lymphadenopathy and an elevated white blood cell count.[149] Investigations reveal that bacteria that are recognized as periodontal pathogens are commonly found in significant numbers in periodontal abscesses. These microorganisms include *F. nucleatum, P. intermedia, P. gingivalis, P. micra,* and *T. forsythia.*[130,149,269] Periradicular lesions, which arise as a consequence of endodontic infections, appear to have a similar microbial composition, with a microbiota that is dominated by anaerobes. In addition, *Streptococcus* spp. can also be detected.[343]

Peri-implantitis

The term *peri-implantitis* refers to an inflammatory process that affects the tissues around an already osseointegrated implant and that results in the loss of supporting bone.[15] Originally this inflammatory process was thought to be associated (e.g., in animal studies, in cross-sectional and longitudinal observations in man) with a microbiota comparable to that of periodontitis (i.e., a high proportion of anaerobic gram-negative rods, motile organisms, and spirochetes), but this association does not necessarily prove a causal relationship.[310] Evidence suggests a lower degree of bacterial complexity in the peri-implant crevice.[199] Healthy peri-implant pockets are characterized

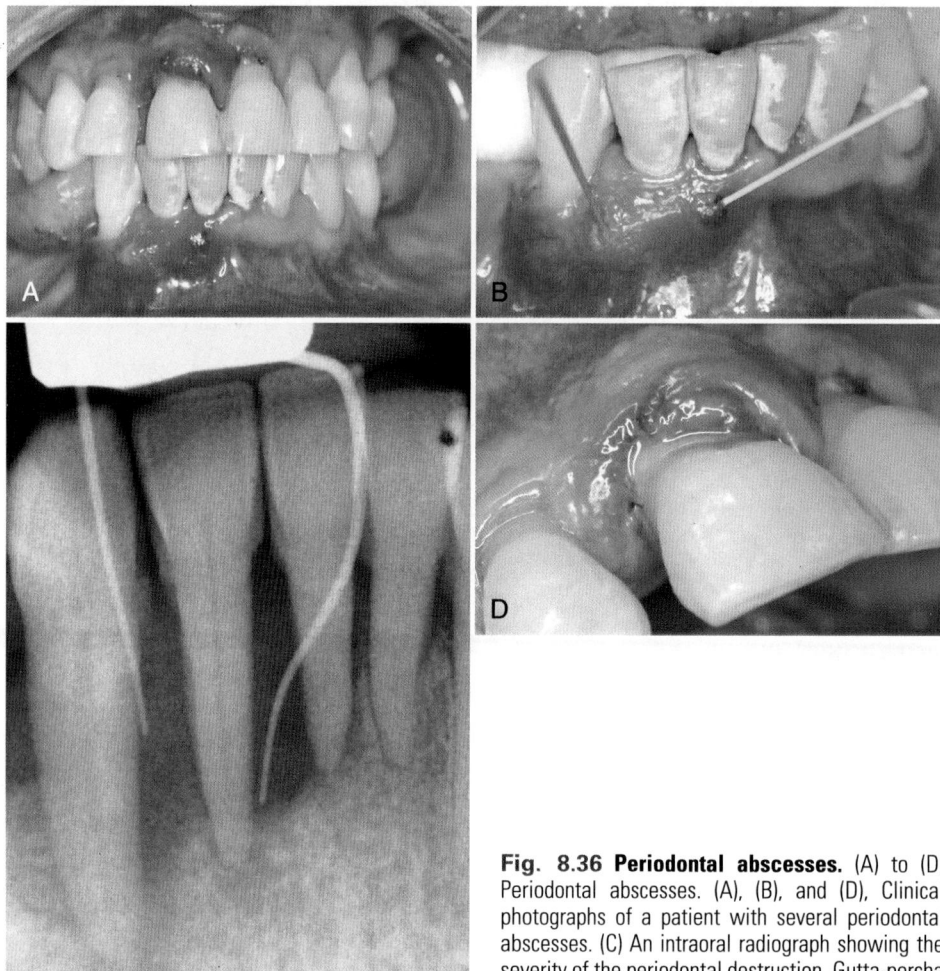

Fig. 8.36 Periodontal abscesses. (A) to (D) Periodontal abscesses. (A), (B), and (D), Clinical photographs of a patient with several periodontal abscesses. (C) An intraoral radiograph showing the severity of the periodontal destruction. Gutta-percha points (B) and (C) are inserted in the fistulas to show their course.

by high proportions of coccoid cells, a low ratio of anaerobic-to-aerobic species, a low number of gram-negative anaerobic species, and low detection frequencies for periodontopathogens.[4,31,212,278] Implants with peri-implantitis reveal a microbiota that encompasses conventional periodontal pathogens (see Table 8.12), as well as the cariogenic bacterium *S. mutans*.[199,293] Species such as *A. actinomycetemcomitans, P. gingivalis, T. forsythia, P. micra, C. rectus, F. nucleatum, P. intermedia, T. denticola,* and *Capnocytophaga* are often isolated from failing sites, but they can also be detected around healthy peri-implant sites.[363] Other species, such as *Pseudomonas aeruginosa, Enterobacter* spp., *C. albicans,* and staphylococci, are also frequently detected around implants.[8] These organisms are uncommon in the subgingival area, but they have been associated with refractory periodontitis.[379] High proportions of *Staphylococcus aureus* and *S. epidermidis* on oral implants have been reported.[324] The relative resistance of these organisms to commonly used antibiotics suggests that their presence may represent an opportunistic colonization that is caused by systemic antibiotic therapy.[378]

However, some studies using open-ended microbial techniques suggest that the microbiota associated with peri-implantitis is not as similar as thought to that associated with periodontitis.[68,70,99,200,390,461] Some large-scale clinical follow-up studies seem to indicate that implant failures cluster within patients, with increased odd ratios for a second implant failure in patients who have already lost one implant.[416,441] These observations indicate that, within patients,

systemic factors are important for the characterization of implant losses.

Virulence Factors of Periodontopathogens

It is clear that some organisms, such as *P. gingivalis, A. actinomycetemcomitans,* spirochetes, and *P. intermedia,* are strongly associated with a number of periodontal diseases. However, periodontal disease never occurs in the absence of a complex microbiota, and it is often difficult (if not impossible) to determine precisely how different organisms contribute to an individual case of disease. In fact, the contributions of specific bacteria to disease may be unimportant according to the ecologic plaque hypothesis.

KEY FACT

The best-known virulence factors of periodontopathogens are adhesive surface proteins and fibrils, tissue destruction–promoting factors, and host immunity–evading strategies.

Targeting one or more "pathogens" will not necessarily cure disease because other organisms with similar activities may take their place. Therefore, it may make sense to focus on the specific molecules that contribute to disease (virulence factors), rather than on the microorganisms that produce them. In fact, it is often difficult to separate the virulence determinants from the organisms that produce them. For example, adhesins are produced by commensal organisms, as well as by pathogens, yet only those adhesins that promote the attachment of a pathogenic organism could be considered virulence determinants. With this in mind, some of the known or putative virulence factors for periodontal disease are described in the following sections. The following are important:

1. Only a proportion of periodontal bacteria has ever been isolated, and almost certainly many other virulence factors are currently unknown.
2. Most of our understanding of virulence factors has come from studies of a very limited number of bacterial species and strains. It is far from clear that the molecules that have been studied in the greatest detail are truly representative of their classes.

Virulence factors of periodontal microorganisms can be subdivided as follows: (1) factors that promote colonization (adhesins), (2) toxins and enzymes that degrade host tissues, and (3) mechanisms that protect pathogenic bacteria from the host.

 ## Adhesive Surface Proteins and Fibrils

To colonize the periodontal pocket, bacteria must adhere to cells or tissues in the region, such as teeth, the existing microbial biofilm, or the pocket epithelium. Bacterial cell surface structures provide the points of contact. Often these structures extend some distance from the cell surface. Fimbriae or pili are polymeric fibrils that are composed of repeating subunits that can extend several micrometers from the cell membrane. Pili were once thought to be unique to gram-negative bacteria, but they have now been identified in several gram-positive organisms, including streptococci and actinomyces.[243] Strains of *P. gingivalis* produce two types of fimbriae, which are known as the major fimbriae and the minor fimbriae.[135]

The major fimbriae are single-stranded filaments approximately 5 nm in diameter and up to 3 μm in length. The backbone of major fimbriae is a chain of repeating subunits of the 43-kDa FimA protein. Minor fimbriae are composed of a 67-kDa protein, Mfa1, and they extend approximately 0.1 to 0.5 μm from the cell surface.[14] Major and minor fimbriae interact with oral streptococci such as *S. gordonii*. *P. gingivalis* FimA binds to glyceraldehyde-3-phosphate dehydrogenase, whereas Mfa1 interacts with the *S. gordonii* cell surface adhesin B.[241,285] Major fimbriae have also been shown to bind host extracellular matrix proteins fibronectin and type I collagen, salivary proline-rich proteins and statherin, and epithelial cells.[11,136,271] Extensive variation in the *fimA* gene that encodes the FimA fimbrial subunit has been observed, and six different genotypes have been designated (i.e., genotypes I, Ib, II, III, IV, and V).[95] Of these, genotypes II and IV are associated with periodontitis.[10,94] However, at present, no evidence indicates that fimbriae of genotypes II and IV are functionally distinct from other major fimbriae.

 ## Tissue Destruction–Promoting Factors

Many bacterial proteins that interact with host cells are recognized by the immune system, and they may trigger immune responses. Fimbriae of *P. gingivalis* and *A. actinomycetemcomitans* are highly antigenic. Inflammation is a major contributor to tissue destruction in periodontal disease; this is considered separately in Chapter 7. However, some bacterial products directly promote tissue destruction in addition to modulating host immunity, with extracellular proteolytic enzymes being the most notable. Most of the tissue destruction in periodontal pockets is actually caused by host matrix metalloproteinases (MMPs), but bacterial proteases play important roles in activating the host enzymes.[120]

Bacterial proteolytic activity in dental plaque—and, in particular, trypsin-like protease activity—is closely correlated with clinical markers of periodontal disease.[276]

However, the bulk of the host tissue–degrading activity is restricted to a small number of these enzymes. In the case of *P. gingivalis*, three enzymes known as gingipains are responsible for at least 85% of the total proteolytic activity of the bacterium.[299]

The gingipains belong to the cysteine protease family, and they use an active-site cysteine residue for catalysis. Gingipains are classed as "Arg-gingipains" (RgpA and RgpB) or "Lys-gingipains" (Kgp) on the basis of their ability to cleave Arg-Xaa or Lys-Xaa peptide bonds (Xaa represents any amino acid). Gingipains are multifunctional proteins that play important roles in adhesion, tissue degradation, and the evasion of host responses.

Proteases are produced by *A. actinomycetemcomitans,* but these appear to be less important for the virulence of this organism than the leukotoxin (LtxA). LtxA is a member of the repeats-in-toxin family of proteins. These toxins act by delivering an adenylate cyclase domain into cells, which catalyzes the uncontrolled conversion of adenosine triphosphate to cyclic adenosine monophosphate.

Most strains of *A. actinomycetemcomitans* produce low levels of LtxA. However, some strains are regarded as hyperleukotoxic because they express high levels of the transcript from the *ltxA* gene, thereby encoding LtxA. Hyperleukotoxic strains include the JP2 clone of *A. actinomycetemcomitans*, which is uniquely associated with localized aggressive periodontitis.[146,257] Two distinct mechanisms that give rise to high levels of *ltxA* expression have been described.[354] The JP2 clone contains a deletion in a regulatory gene, designated *orfA*, that is upstream of the *ltxCABD* gene locus. Hyperleukotoxic *A. actinomycetemcomitans* strains isolated in Japan were not found to contain deletions in *orfA* but instead harbored a mobile genetic element (transposon), IS*1301*, that was upstream of the *orfA* gene. The sequence of IS*1301* contains elements that direct the enhanced transcription of the *orfA-ltxCABD* operon. From a diagnostic point of view, it is important to consider that simply detecting *A. actinomycetemcomitans*, LtxA, or both in the periodontal biofilm is by no means indicative of disease. However, the detection of a hyperleukotoxic strain of *A. actinomycetemcomitans* may be significant.

Strategies for Evading Host Immunity

Pathogenic bacteria have many and varied strategies for evading or subverting the host immune system, including the following: (1) the production of an extracellular capsule, (2) the proteolytic degradation of host innate or acquired immunity components, (3) the modulation of host responses by binding serum components on the bacterial cell surface, and (4) the invasion of gingival epithelial cells. A detailed description of bacteria–host interactions is given in Chapter 9. Selected examples of factors that mediate these processes are given in the following paragraphs.

Strains of *P. gingivalis* produce polysaccharide capsules (Fig. 8.37) that surround the outer membrane. Six different antigenic capsule types have been described on the basis of the differences in the polysaccharide K antigen.[204] In a mouse model, capsular strains of *P. gingivalis* produced a spreading type of infection, whereas acapsular strains tended to form more localized abscesses.[205] Most *P. gingivalis* isolates from periodontitis patients are encapsulated.[203] It is hypothesized that the capsule protects cells from the host immune system. However, protection against the complement system appears to be mediated primarily by a branched phosphomannan polysaccharide that is independent of the K antigen.[369]

Several periodontopathogens are resistant to complement-mediated phagocytosis, and it is thought that the proteolysis of complement components contributes to resistance to some extent. *P. gingivalis*

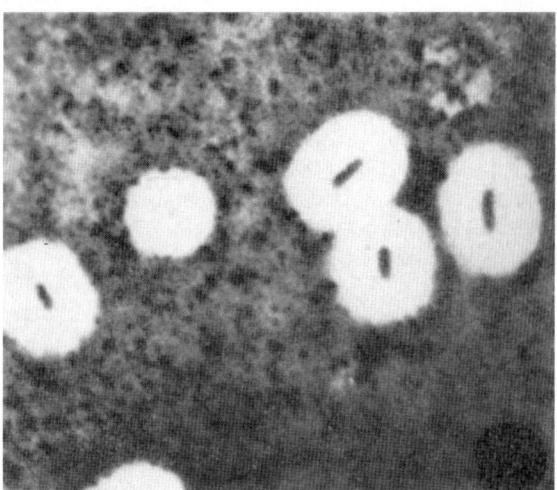

Fig. 8.37 Glycocalyx or polysaccharide capsule of *Porphyromonas gingivalis* visualized with East Indian ink staining (clear halo).

gingipains have been shown to degrade complement components C3, C4, C5, and factor B.[298] More recently, a cysteine protease of *P. intermedia* called interpain A has also been shown to degrade C3.[300] In vitro, interpain A acts synergistically with gingipains to decrease the deposition of complement C3b.[300] These data fit with the hypothesis that periodontal disease processes are mediated by polymicrobial consortia rather than by individual periodontopathogens.

A novel mechanism for complement evasion has been identified in *A. actinomycetemcomitans*. This organism produces a 100-kDa protein on the outer membrane, Omp100 or ApiA, which mediates adhesion to and the invasion of host cells.[17,218] Mutants lacking ApiA were sensitized to killing by human serum: wild-type cells were almost completely resistant to 30% or 50% normal human serum, whereas 90% of ApiA mutant cells were killed. ApiA was shown to bind factor H, which is an inhibitor of the complement cascade. H_2O_2 produced by *S. gordonii* induces the expression of ApiA and enhances the serum resistance of *A. actinomycetemcomitans*.[326] It has been proposed that H_2O_2 derived from oral streptococci may stimulate the immune response and that the early detection of H_2O_2 by *A. actinomycetemcomitans* may provide an ecologic advantage under these conditions.[327] Alternatively, the ability of *A. actinomycetemcomitans* to detect streptococcal H_2O_2 may be a fortuitous consequence of a system that has evolved primarily to detect and respond to the neutrophil oxidative burst.

Periodontal pathogens are notoriously difficult to eradicate completely. Despite aggressive antibacterial attacks from the host defenses and from clinical treatments, it is often impossible to prevent reinfection. One potential reservoir for periodontopathogens is inside gingival epithelial cells. *P. gingivalis* and *A. actinomycetemcomitans*, for example, can invade epithelial cells in vitro.[206,251] In vivo, *P. gingivalis*, *T. forsythia*, *P. intermedia*, *T. denticola*, and *A. actinomycetemcomitans* can be detected within the gingival epithelial cells of patients with periodontitis before and after periodontal therapy.[168] Adhesion to host cells is critical for invasion. However, it has been suggested that some factors may specifically control the ability of bacteria to invade cells. In *A. actinomycetemcomitans*, a screen for invasion-associated genes identified two loci, encoding ApiA (see previous paragraph) and ApiBC, which are related to known bacterial invasion proteins (invasins).[218] The ability of bacteria to invade cells may be influenced by their interactions with other organisms in the gingival sulcus. Thus, the coinfection of an epithelial cell line with *P. gingivalis* and a coaggregating strain of *F. nucleatum* resulted in increased invasion by *P. gingivalis* as compared with a monoculture control.[346] Coaggregation with *F. nucleatum* is mediated by the *P. gingivalis* capsular polysaccharide and lipopolysaccharide; therefore, these molecules may indirectly contribute to invasion.[335]

Future Advances in Periodontal Microbiology

Scientific progress at the end of the 20th century, particularly in the field of molecular biology, has led to significant advances in our understanding of periodontal microbiology. DNA-based methodologies for the identification and detection of specific bacteria and viruses offer remarkable time and cost advantages as compared with culturing techniques. A dramatic increase in the number of samples that can be examined and the number of microorganisms enumerated is now possible. Perhaps even more relevant is the present ability to detect microorganisms that cannot be cultivated so far, which has underscored the limitations of our knowledge of this complex ecologic niche. Greater awareness of the role of the host response in periodontal disease will further improve the understanding of the severity and therapy of periodontal infections. Finally, the recognition of the beneficial activity of several groups of commensal species may open new strategies for the treatment of periodontal disease, such as the use of probiotics or microbial replacement therapy.[408]

 Case Scenarios are found on the companion website www.expertconsult.com.

References

 References for this chapter are found on the companion website www.expertconsult.com.

CHAPTER 9

Practical Molecular Biology of Host–Microbe Interactions

Chad M. Novince | Carlos Rossa, Jr. | Keith L. Kirkwood

CHAPTER OUTLINE

Microbe-Associated Molecular Patterns
Toll-Like Receptors

NOD-Like Receptors
Complement System

Antimicrobial Peptides
Immunomodulatory Therapies

The periodontium is a dynamic remodeling tissue that is continuously challenged by bacterial biofilms colonizing proximal odontogenic and mucosal surfaces. Periodontal disease pathogenesis has classically been associated with specific "periopathogenic" bacteria, initially identified as the prominent culturable bacteria isolated from periodontal pocket disease sites.[154,155] Although early empiric thought dictated that periopathogenic bacteria had direct catabolic actions on periodontal tissue matrices, extensive molecular research has elucidated that the host immune response is the primary mediator of periodontal tissue destruction.[8,37,91,169] Experimental periodontitis investigations in animal models deficient in specific immune cell subsets,[9,82] receptors,[20,26,72,86,126] and cytokines[4,42,145,192] have begun to delineate the immunopathophysiology of periodontal disease. Clinical observations and studies in immunocompromised persons demonstrating increased susceptibility and greater severity of periodontal disease further underscore the significance of the host immune response to the oral bacterial challenge.[39,104]

This chapter focuses on molecular aspects of host–microbe interactions in periodontal disease. To avoid redundancy with other chapters addressing the pathophysiology of periodontitis, we emphasize the direct recognition of microbe-associated molecular patterns (MAMPs) at pattern-recognition receptors (PRRs). PRRs that predominantly recognize bacteria, including Toll-like receptors (TLRs) and nucleotide-binding oligomerization domain–like receptors (NLRs), are discussed in detail, along with their associated signal transduction pathways. Complement and antimicrobial peptides are covered briefly, highlighting their influence on PRR signaling. Finally, immunomodulatory therapeutic interventions targeting host–microbe molecular interactions in periodontitis are examined mechanistically.

Microbe-Associated Molecular Patterns

Considering the oral microbiome as a diverse microbial community consisting of more than 600 known bacterial species[33] and knowing that classically defined periopathogenic bacteria are present in both health and disease[170,178] implies that the vigilance and the tolerance mechanisms are used by the host to mount an appropriate immune defense response. Tolerance mechanisms modulate the host response to commensal (nonpathogenic) bacteria to establish a balanced or homeostatic relationship, whereas vigilance mechanisms protect

against periopathogenic bacteria–associated opportunistic infections. The host is capable of discerning among commensal and pathogenic bacteria, and appropriately modulating the immune response, by the direct recognition of MAMPs at PRRs.[21,81,165]

MAMPs, which are evolutionary-conserved molecular motifs present in microorganisms, are not found in higher eukaryotes. MAMPs include microbial cell wall macromolecules, nucleic acids, and flagellin, which function as ligands having specificity for corresponding PRRs, expressed by host cells.[21,81,165] The host immune system discriminates between self and the resident oral flora by direct recognition of MAMPs at PRRs (Table 9.1). MAMP recognition by the corresponding PRR induces host cell signaling, leading to the expression of cytokines and enzymes (Table 9.2) that drives the immune response. MAMP signaling immunomodulation plays a critical role in the homeostatic regulation of colonizing commensal microbes in health, and it also contributes to pathophysiologic tissue destruction in chronic inflammatory disease states such as periodontitis.

 KEY FACT

In periodontal health, pattern-recognition receptor (PRR) signaling is effectively modulated to regulate the oral commensal microbiota (tolerance) and protect against periopathogenic bacteria (vigilance), thus supporting periodontal tissues homeostasis. Conversely, failed tolerance and vigilance mechanisms in periodontal disease states lead to shifts in the oral microbiota that drive supraphysiologic PRR signaling–induced proinflammatory periodontal tissue destruction.

The periodontal innate immune response functions as the first line of defense against the colonizing oral microbiota. Although the innate immune response was formerly perceived as nondiscriminate and crude, the discovery of PRRs led to the realization that the innate immune response is specific and calculated. Recognition of MAMPs by innate immune cells stimulates the secretion of proinflammatory cytokines (e.g., interleukin-1 beta [IL-1β], IL-6, and tumor necrosis factor [TNF]) and type I interferons (IFN-α, IFN-β), critical for mounting an appropriate innate immune response to colonizing or invading microorganisms (see Table 9.2). Furthermore, MAMP

TABLE 9.1 Host Cell Pattern-Recognition Receptor Ligand Binding of Periodontal Bacteria-Derived Microbe-Associated Molecular Patterns

Host Cells	PRRs	MAMPs	Periodontal Bacteria	References
Neutrophils, monocytes, macrophages, epithelial cells, fibroblasts, cementoblasts, osteoblasts, dendritic cells, T and B lymphocytes	TLR-2	Lipoproteins	*Porphyromonas gingivalis*	61, 66, 115
		Lipoproteins	*Tannerella forsythia*	60, 105
		Lipoproteins	*Actinomyces viscosus*	152
		Peptidoglycan	*Actinomyces naeslundii*	146
		Lipoproteins, lipoteichoic acid, peptidoglycan	*Streptococcus gordonii*	24, 101
	TLR-4	LPS	*Porphyromonas gingivalis*	13, 67, 117, 147
		LPS	*Aggregatibacter actinomycetemcomitans, Fusobacterium nucleatum*	63, 137, 156, 190
	TLR-9	CpG-DNA	*Porphyromonas gingivalis, Tannerella forsythia*	28, 44, 86, 110, 143
	NOD1	iE-DAP	*Porphyromonas gingivalis, Aggregatibacter actinomycetemcomitans, Fusobacterium nucleatum*	107, 119, 157, 162, 175–177, 182
	NOD2	MDP		

iE-DAP, Gamma-D-glutamyl-mesodiaminopimelic acid; *LPS,* lipopolysaccharide; *MAMP,* microbe-associated molecular pattern; *NOD,* nucleotide-binding oligomerization domain; *PRR,* pattern-recognition receptor; *TLR,* Toll-like receptor.

TABLE 9.2 Periopathogenic Bacteria Microbe-Associated Molecular Pattern Induction of Biologic Mediators in Host Periodontal Tissue Cells

Host Cells	MAMPs	Biologic Mediators	References
Epithelial cells	LPS, fimbriae, bacteria cell wall extracts, gingipains	IL-8, G-CSF, GM-CSF, β-defensin-2, MMPs-3/9/13, MIP-1α, IL-1β	27, 32, 49, 57, 63–65, 112, 120, 141, 144, 159, 163, 183
Dendritic cells	LPS, CpG-DNA, fimbriae	IFN-α, IL-6, IL-8, IL-10, IL-12, TNF-α, GM-CSF	68, 77, 78, 128, 158
Endothelial cells	LPS	IL-6, GM-CSF, ICAM-1	31, 40, 63, 75, 98
Gingival fibroblasts	LPS, CpG-DNA, gingipains, peptidoglycan	IL-1β, IL-6, IL-8, TNF-α, PGE₂, MCP-1, MMP-2	5, 15, 35, 62, 63, 110, 112, 116, 118, 131, 164, 171, 183, 184
PDL fibroblasts	LPS	IL-6, IL-8, MMP-13, RANKL	62, 63, 138, 139, 189
Cementoblasts	LPS	OPN, OCN, RANKL, IL-6	107, 109
Macrophages	LPS, CpG-DNA, leukotoxin	IL-1α/1β, IL-6, IL-12, TNF-α, MMP-1, NO	63, 83, 87, 103, 110, 116, 168, 187
Osteoblasts	LPS	IL-1β, IL-6, TNF-α, RANKL, PGE₂, NO, MMP-2, MMP-9	63, 85, 124, 161, 185–188, 196
Neutrophils	LPS, CpG-DNA	IL-8, MIP-1α	141, 172, 173
Monocytes	LPS, CpG-DNA, fimbriae	IFN-γ, IL-1α/1β, IL-6, IL-8, IL-12, TNF-α, LIF, RANKL, PGE₂	10, 11, 16, 31, 34, 40, 51, 59, 63, 71, 94, 97, 106, 131, 134
B lymphocytes	CpG-DNA, cell sonicate extracts	IL-6, IL-10, IL-12, TNF-α	23, 114, 181, 193
T lymphocytes	LPS, CpG-DNA, peptidoglycan	IFN-γ, IL-4, IL-10, IL-13	43, 99, 100, 128, 166, 193

G-CSF, Granulocyte colony-stimulating factor; *GM-CSF,* granulocyte-macrophage colony-stimulating factor; *ICAM,* intercellular adhesion molecule; *IFN,* interferon; *IL,* interleukin; *LIF,* leukocyte inhibitory factor; *LPS,* lipopolysaccharide; *MAMP,* microbe-associated molecular pattern; *MCP,* monocyte chemoattractant protein; *MMP,* matrix metalloproteinase; *NO,* nitric oxide; *OCN,* osteocalcin; *OPN,* osteopontin; *PDL,* periodontal ligament; *PGE₂,* prostaglandin E₂; *RANKL,* receptor activator of nuclear factor-κB ligand; *TNF,* tumor necrosis factor.

signaling at innate immune cells up-regulates the production of co-stimulatory molecules that are critical for the activation of adaptive immunity. For this reason, PRRs are considered the bridge between the innate and adaptive immune systems.[69,113]

In addition to innate immune cells (neutrophils, monocytes, macrophages, dendritic cells, natural killer cells), investigators have realized that PRRs are also expressed by epithelial cells, extracellular matrix cells (fibroblasts, cementoblasts, osteoblasts), and adaptive immune cells (T lymphocytes, B lymphocytes) (see Table 9.1). Although innate immune cells were formerly perceived to derive

solely from the hematopoietic lineage, MAMP-PRR recognition at epithelial cells and tissue extracellular matrix cells revealed that both hematopoietic and mesenchymal cells are central to innate immune defense mechanisms regulating colonizing or invading microorganisms. The realizations that MAMPs are directly recognized by adaptive immune cells and do not require innate immune cell processing or priming provided insight demonstrating that the innate and adaptive immune systems act more as a continuum than as separate entities. Notably, the identification of PRRs has significantly advanced our understanding of innate and adaptive immunity.

The two major families of PRRs that have been most extensively studied in the periodontium are the TLRs and the NLRs.[21,81,165] TLRs are transmembrane receptors, and NLRs are cytosolic receptors, which recognize a broad range of MAMPs derived from the oral microbiota (see Table 9.1). In addition to recognizing MAMPs, more recently it has been realized that PRRs also recognize immunostimulatory by-products derived from damaged host tissues, known as *damage-associated molecular patterns* (DAMPs).[21,81,165] Although PRR recognition of MAMPs and DAMPs is essential for the host immune defense and normal tissue remodeling, the chapter focuses on MAMPs studied in the context of periodontal bacteria (see Table 9.1).

Toll-Like Receptors

The TLR family currently consists of 10 known functional TLRs in humans, of which TLR-10 is the only member having an unclear biologic role.[80,113] TLR-1 through TLR-9 have been reported to be expressed in the periodontium, in both health and disease.[12] TLR family members are generally subdivided into two groups according to their localization at the plasma membrane (TLR-1, TLR-2, TLR-4, TLR-5, TLR-6, TLR-10) or endolysosomal membrane (TLR-3, TLR-7,

TLR-8, TLR-9).[80] Notably, TLR-4 is unique in that it has the ability to localize to both the plasma membrane and the endolysosomal membrane.[80,113] Plasma membrane TLR signaling induces the expression of proinflammatory cytokines, whereas endosomal TLR signaling predominantly induces the expression of type I IFNs.[81,165]

TLRs localized to the plasma membrane recognize extracellular microbial cell wall components (TLR-1, TLR-2, TLR-4, TLR-6) or flagellin (TLR-5), whereas TLRs localized to the endolysosomal membrane recognize microbial nucleic acids (TLR-3, TLR-7, TLR-8, TLR-9).

The chapter focuses on MAMP ligand recognition at TLR-2, TLR-4, and TLR-9 because these TLR family members have been studied most extensively in the context of sensing periopathogenic bacteria (see Table 9.1). TLR-2 and TLR-4 are discussed in the context of recognizing extracellular bacterial cell wall components at the cell surface, and TLR-9 is addressed with regard to recognizing bacterial nucleic acids within endosomes (Fig. 9.1).

The TLRs are single-pass transmembrane proteins (see Fig. 9.1) characterized by an N-terminal leucine-rich recognition domain and an intracellular C-terminal Toll/IL-1 receptor signaling domain (TIR). On MAMP ligand recognition at the N-terminal domain and subsequent formation of a sustainable homodimer or heterodimer, TIR

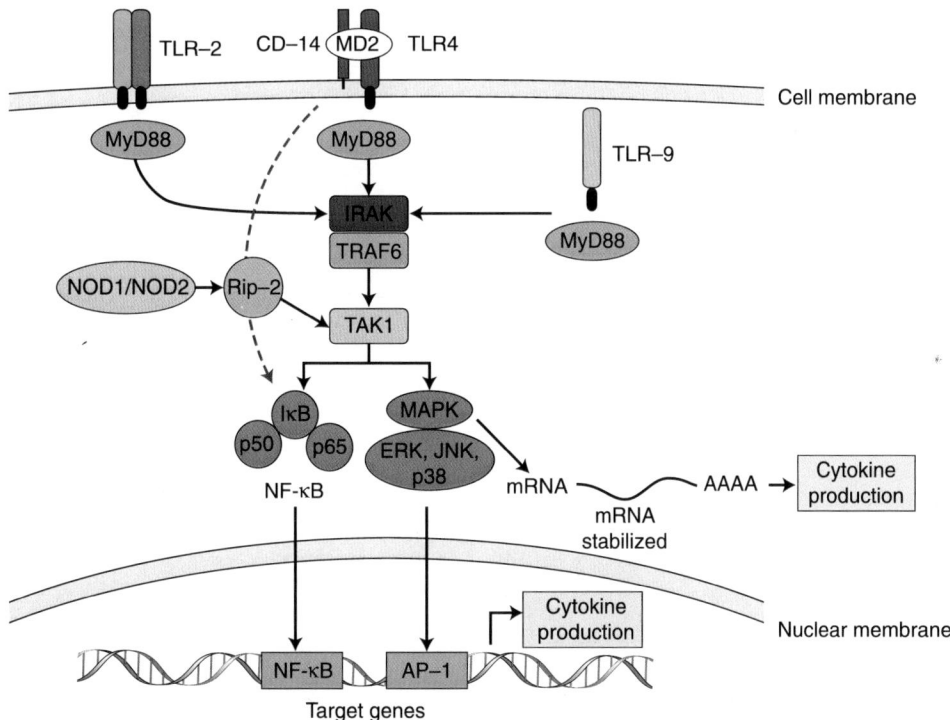

Fig. 9.1 Pattern-recognition receptor (PRR)/microbe-associated molecular pattern (MAMP) signaling.
Toll-like receptor 2 (TLR-2), TLR-4, and TLR-9 are depicted as examples of TLRs expressed in cells of the periodontal tissues. After ligand binding, all TLRs (except TLR-3) recruit myeloid differentiation primary response gene 88 (MyD88) adaptor protein and activate the common upstream activator (interleukin-1 receptor-associated kinase [IRAK]/tumor necrosis factor receptor-associated factor-6 [TRAF6] and transforming growth factor-β activated kinase 1 [TAK1]) of nuclear factor-kappa B (NF-κB) and mitogen-activated protein kinases (MAPKs). TLR-4 may also activate NF-κB independently of MyD88, with delayed kinetics *(red dashed arrow)*. Nucleotide-binding oligomerization domain 1 (NOD1) and NOD2 are cytosolic PRRs that recognize peptidoglycan fragments of the bacterial cell wall, and they may amplify the TLR-induced activation of signaling pathways. Activated NF-κB and MAP kinases translocate to the nucleus and bind to their motifs (NF-κB and activator protein 1 [AP-1]) in the promoters of target genes (including early-response and inflammatory genes) and induce their transcription into mRNA, which will ultimately lead to increased cytokine production. p38 MAPK is also involved after the transcriptional regulation of proinflammatory genes (e.g., interleukin-6 [IL-6], cyclooxygenase-2 [COX-2]) via the modulation of mRNA stability in the cytoplasm. *CD14,* cluster of differentiation 14 molecule; *ERK,* extracellular signal-regulated kinase; *I-κB,* inhibitor of NF-κB; *JNK,* c-Jun N-terminal kinase; *MD2,* myeloid differentiation protein-2, *RIP-2,* serine/threonine kinase adapter protein.

domains of TLRs act as a scaffold to recruit various TIR domain-containing adaptor proteins: myeloid differentiation primary-response protein 88 (MYD88) and MYD88-adaptor-like protein (MAL), or TIR domain-containing adaptor protein inducing IFN-β (TRIF) and TRIF-related adaptor molecule (TRAM).[81,165] With the exception of TLR-3, all TLRs engage the MyD88 adapter protein. TLR-3 and endosomal TLR-4 uniquely interact with the TRIF adapter protein.[80,113] Engagement of the adapter proteins at the TIR domain of TLRs initiates signal transduction (see Fig. 9.1) that involves interactions between the adaptor molecules, IL-1 receptor–associated kinases (IRAKs) and TNF receptor–associated factors (TRAFs). In the case of TLR-2 and TLR-4 localized to the plasma membrane, MyD88-dependent downstream activation of transforming growth factor-beta (TGF-β)–activated kinase 1 (TAK-1) simultaneously induces mitogen-activated protein kinase (MAPK) and nuclear factor-κB (NF-κB) signaling. NF-κB translocates to the nucleus, and MAPK cascades activate activator protein 1 (AP-1), ultimately resulting in the expression of proinflammatory cytokine genes. When TLR-4 translocates to endosomes, TRIF-dependent signaling leads to the activation of NF-κB and IFN-regulatory factor (IRF)-3, resulting in the expression of proinflammatory cytokine and type I IFN genes. Concerning TLR-9 localized to the endolysosomal membrane, MyD88-dependent signaling leads to the activation of IRF-7, which up-regulates the expression of type I IFN genes.[81,165] The notable crosstalk of the TLR signaling pathways (see Fig. 9.1) highlights the potential for synergy or amplification effects modulating the host immune response.

Toll-like Receptor-4–Lipopolysaccharide Recognition

Knowledge of the molecular architecture of gram-positive versus gram-negative bacterial cell walls is central to a conceptual understanding of MAMP recognition by the host. Oral bacterial interactions with host TLRs are largely dependent on the exposed macromolecules making up the outer membrane of bacterial cell walls. Whereas lipopolysaccharide (LPS) is unique to the outer membrane of gram-negative bacteria, lipoteichoic acid (LTA) and peptidoglycan are distinct to the outer membrane of gram-positive bacteria. Importantly, lipoproteins are common constituents of the outer membranes of both gram-negative and gram-positive bacteria.[130]

LPS is the major macromolecule composing the outer surface envelope of gram-negative bacteria, critical to the bacterium for maintaining structural integrity, selective permeability, and proper folding and insertion of outer membrane proteins. LPS is typically made up of three domains (lipid A, a short core oligosaccharide, and an O-antigen), and it induces a host immune response through recognition of lipid A.[108,129] Mammalian cells recognize LPS through a TLR-4 homodimer protein complex consisting of TLR-4, the coreceptor myeloid differentiation factor 2 (MD2), and accessory proteins CD14 and lipopolysaccharide-binding protein (LBP) (see Fig. 9.1). LBP processes and delivers LPS to CD14, which sensitizes cells for LPS binding by the MD2-TLR-4 receptor.[80,113]

Toll-like Receptor-2–Lipoprotein/Lipoteichoic Acid/Peptidoglycan Recognition

Different from the TLR-4 homodimer protein complex that is specific for LPS, TLR-2 has the capacity to recognize diverse microbial macromolecules due to forming heterodimer protein complexes with other TLR family members (TLR-1, TLR-6).[80,113] TLR-2 ligands highly relevant to oral flora interactions with host cells include lipoproteins, LTA, and peptidoglycan (see Table 9.1). Lipoproteins, ubiquitously expressed in the outer cell membranes of all bacteria, are anchored to the bacterial cell membrane by lipid chains covalently attached to conserved N-terminal cysteines.[130] Triacylated lipoproteins

commonly expressed by gram-negative bacteria are recognized by TLR-2/TLR-1 heterodimer complexes, whereas diacylated lipoproteins primarily expressed by gram-positive bacteria or mycoplasmas are recognized by TLR-2/TR-6 heterodimer complexes.[80,113] Unique to the outer membranes of gram-positive bacteria, LTA and peptidoglycan are recognized by incompletely characterized TLR-2/TLR-6 heterodimer complexes.[81] Not as well understood as LPS–TLR-4 signaling (reviewed in the previous paragraph), differences in extracellular accessory or coreceptor proteins (CD14, CD36) and intracellular adaptor proteins associated with TLR-2/TLR-1 versus TLR-2/TLR-6 signal transduction appear to regulate TLR-2–mediated host immune response mechanisms critically.[80,113]

Toll-like Receptor-9–CpG-DNA Recognition

Different from TLR-2 and TLR-4 localized to the plasma membrane, which recognize MAMPs at the cell surface, TLR-9 recognizes MAMPs in endosomes (see Fig. 9.1). TLR-9 is the endosomal TLR family member that has been studied most extensively with regard to the recognition of intracellular microbial nucleic acids. During infection, microbe-derived nucleic acids are sensed by endosomal TLRs, and this sensing facilitates mounting a host immune response to clear the invading microorganisms. Although TLR-9 recognizes both viral and bacterial CpG-DNA,[81,165] periodontal research has focused on TLR-9 because CpG motifs are abundant in bacterial DNA (see Table 9.1). CpG-DNA localized within lysosomal compartments induces the trafficking of TLR-9 from the endoplasmic reticulum to the endolysosome, which activates TLR-9 signal transduction.[81,165]

Role of Toll-like Receptors in Periodontitis

TLRs are expressed in the periodontium in health, and they notably have been reported to be expressed at supraphysiologic levels in periodontal tissues afflicted by severe disease states.[12] Both commensal and pathogenic periodontal bacteria stimulate TLR-2 signaling,[84,191] a finding that speaks to the importance of vigilance and tolerance mechanisms in the host immune defense regulation of the colonizing oral microbiota. The fact that lipoproteins derived from gram-positive versus gram-negative bacteria are differentially recognized by TLR-2/TLR-6 and TLR-2/TLR-1 heterodimer complexes[80,113] highlights the complexity of a single TLR receptor in the modulation of the host immune defense response. Considering that the resident periodontal flora shifts from a predominantly gram-positive microbiota in health to a predominantly gram-negative microbiota in periodontal disease states, gram-negative periopathogenic bacteria–induced periodontal destruction could be mediated through differential TLR-2 signal transduction associated with increased activation of TLR-2/TLR-1 versus TLR-2/TLR-6 heterodimer complexes.

Current knowledge of TLR signaling suggests that gram-negative periopathogenic bacteria–induced catabolic actions are due to differential signaling at the TLR-2 receptor, as well as the concomitant activation of TLR-4 receptor by LPS.[84,115] *Porphyromonas gingivalis* has been most extensively investigated in its ability to stimulate TLR signal transduction through various MAMPs. Early investigations assessing *P. gingivalis* LPS induced up-regulation of proinflammatory cytokine expression in various human and murine cells were controversial in terms of whether the actions of LPS were mediated through TLR-2– versus TL-R4–dependent recognition. Understanding that LPS recognition is specific to the lipid A domain, definitive evidence that *P. gingivalis* LPS activates only TLR-4 was elucidated through chemically synthesized *P. gingivalis* lipid A analogues which activated TLR-4, not TLR-2.[92,147,195] Research demonstrating that a *P. gingivalis*–derived lipoprotein that specifically activates TLR-2 can be co-isolated with LPS[115] implies that early contradictory reports concerning *P. gingivalis* LPS recognition at TLR-2 versus TLR-4 were due to lipoprotein contamination. Highlighting the importance of periopathogenic bacteria–induced activation of concomitant TLR receptors in periodontal tissue destruction, studies using TLR-2 or TLR-4 knockout mice have shown that *P. gingivalis* coactivation of TLR-2 and TLR-4 is critical in stimulating host immune response mechanisms driving alveolar bone loss.[20]

Relative to TLR-2 and TLR-4, investigations delineating the role of TLR-9 in the pathogenesis of periodontal disease have been scarce. Similar to TLR-2 and TLR-4, TLR-9 expression has been reported to be up-regulated in clinical periodontitis tissues when compared with gingivitis tissues[79] and healthy gingival biopsy samples.[136] Notably, an experimental periodontitis investigation assessing *P. gingivalis*–challenged TLR-9–deficient mice provides evidence indicating that TLR-9 contributes to periodontal bone loss.[86] TLR-9 knockout versus wild-type mice were resistant to *P. gingivalis*–induced alveolar bone loss, which correlated with lower levels of IL-6, TNF, and receptor activator of NF-κB ligand (RANKL) in the gingival tissues of knockout mice. Ex vivo studies performed in the aforementioned report, demonstrating that TLR-2 or TLR-4 agonist challenge resulted in significantly lower cytokine production in TLR-9 knockout versus wild-type cells, highlight the possibility of TLR-9 crosstalk with TLR-2 and TLR-4 signaling in periodontal pathogenesis.[86]

Nucleotide-Binding Oligomerization Domain–Like Receptors

Currently, 22 family members comprise the intracellularly expressed NLRs in humans.[21,81,165] NLRs are localized to the cytosol, and they play a critical role in sensing invading microorganisms and prompting the immune response. NLRs are characterized by C-terminal leucine-rich repeats that act as a sensing domain, a central nucleotide-binding and oligomerization domain (i.e., a NOD), and an N-terminal effector domain that mediates downstream signaling.[21,81,165] This discussion is limited to NOD1 and NOD2, which are specialized NLRs that recognize bacterial peptidoglycan structures of invading pathogens in the cytoplasm, and NLRP3, which is an example of how NLRs function as a component of inflammasome complexes.

NOD1/NOD2–Peptidoglycan Recognition

NOD1 recognizes gamma-D-glutamyl-mesodiaminopimelic acid (iE-DAP), a component of peptidoglycan present in most gram-negative and some gram-positive bacteria, whereas NOD2 recognizes muramyl dipeptide (MDP), which is found in peptidoglycan from all gram-negative and gram-positive bacteria.[3,165] Peptidoglycan binding at NOD1 and NOD2 receptors causes their oligomerization, which results in recruitment of a serine/threonine kinase adapter protein, RIP-2/RICK, to a caspase activation and recruitment domain (CARD) at the N-terminus. RIP-2/RICK recruitment at the N-terminus activates NF-κB and MAPK-dependent up-regulation of proinflammatory cytokine genes (see Fig. 9.1).[3,165]

NLRP3–Inflammasome Complex

Inflammasomes are multiprotein complexes that recognize diverse inflammation-inducing stimuli, including exogenous MAMPs and endogenous DAMPs, to control the production of proinflammatory cytokines and regulate pyroptosis (an inflammatory form of cell death).[48,160] Several PRR families act as components in the inflammasome complex, including the cytosolic NLRs. The NLR proteins represent the "core" of the multiprotein inflammasome complex and are reflected in the name of the inflammasome. NLRP3, the most extensively investigated inflammasome complex and the focus of this chapter, plays a critical role in the terminal processing and secretion of the proinflammatory cytokines IL-1β and IL-18.[48,160]

Recognition of cytosolic MAMPs and DAMPs induces NLRP3 to acts as a recruiting scaffold for the inactive zymogen pro-caspase-1. Pro-caspase-1 (which has a CARD) is recruited to the inflammasome complex through homotypic binding of CARD via a pyrin domain (PYD) and the adaptor apoptosis-associated specklike protein containing a CARD (ASC). Oligomerization of pro-caspase-1 proteins in the inflammasome leads to their autoproteolytic cleavage into active caspase-1. Activated caspase-1 subsequently functions to cleave pro–IL-1β and pro–IL-18 into their biologically active forms.[48,160]

Pattern-Recognition Receptor–Microbe-Associated Molecular Pattern Ligand Recognition in Periodontitis

PRRs	Localization	MAMP Ligand	Ligand Origin
TLR-2/ TLR-1	Plasma membrane	Triacylated lipoproteins	G− bacteria
TLR-2/ TLR-6	Plasma membrane	Diacylated lipoproteins	G+ bacteria
		Lipoteichoic acid (LTA)	G+ bacteria
		Peptidoglycan	G+ bacteria
TLR-4	Plasma membrane Endolysosome	Lipopolysaccharide (LPS)	G− bacteria
TLR-9	Endolysosome	CpG-DNA	Bacterial and viral
NOD1	Cytoplasm	Gamma-D-glutamyl-mesodiaminopimelic acid (iE-DAP)	G+ bacteria G− bacteria
NOD2	Cytoplasm	Muramyl dipeptide (MDP)	G+bacteria G− bacteria

G+, Gram positive; G−, gram negative; MAMP, microbe-associated molecular pattern; NOD, nucleotide-binding oligomerization domain; PRR, pattern-recognition receptor; TLR, Toll-like receptor.

Role of NOD-like Receptors in Periodontitis

Clinical investigations of NOD1 and NOD2 receptor expression in oral tissues biopsies and isolated cultured cells have demonstrated that both NOD1 and NOD2 are expressed in human oral epithelium,[162] gingival fibroblast cells,[95,177] and periodontal ligament fibroblast cells.[95,167] Interestingly, no reports show that periodontal disease states alter NOD1 or NOD2 expression levels in the human periodontium.

Experimental periodontitis investigations in NLR-deficient mice have provided limited insight into the critical role of NOD1 and NOD2 in periodontal pathogenesis. Although study methodologies were not consistent across investigations, intriguingly no consistency has been found in reported study outcomes. The initial experimental periodontitis investigation using the NOD1 and NOD2 knockout mouse models, which induced periodontitis via applying ligatures, found that mice deficient in NOD2 showed comparable levels of alveolar bone resorption, whereas mice deficient in NOD1 demonstrated reduced levels of alveolar bone loss when compared with wild-type control mice.[72] Corresponding with the blunted alveolar bone loss findings, NOD1 knockout mice had fewer osteoclasts and lower proinflammatory cytokine expression levels in gingival tissue isolates.[72] A subsequent experimental periodontitis investigation in the NOD1 knockout mouse model, which induced periodontitis via intragingival injection of heat killed gram-negative or gram-positive bacteria, reported contradictory findings.[26] NOD1 knockout mice had exacerbated alveolar bone loss, increased osteoclast numbers, and up-regulated proinflammatory cytokine expression levels in cultured bone marrow macrophages.[26] In light of the aforementioned conflicting study outcomes concerning NOD1, and an additional experimental periodontitis report showing that *P. gingivalis* inoculation induced less alveolar bone loss in NOD2 knockout versus wild-type mice,[126] it is unclear whether NOD1 or NOD2 critically regulates periodontal bone loss.

Although ongoing research is indicated to delineate whether NOD1 and NOD2 receptor signaling is required for periodontitis-associated tissue destruction, investigations highlighting that NOD1 and NOD2 and TLR receptor signaling have crosstalk provide novel insight into the role of NOD1 and NOD2 in the pathogenesis of periodontitis. MAMPs that are present in the biofilm can simultaneously activate TLRs and NOD1/2 signaling, which converge at the MAPK and NF-κB signaling pathways. Downstream synergistic signaling effects may enhance the host immune response to the colonizing oral biofilm. A seminal report demonstrating that NOD1 and NOD2 activation has synergistic effects with TLR signaling to enhance the production of proinflammatory cytokines in cultured human periodontal ligament fibroblast (IL-1β, IL-6, IL-8)[167] provides early evidence that periopathogenic biofilms may induce a destructive host immune response via concomitant activation of diverse PRRs.

With regard to NLR family inflammasome complexes, periodontitis investigations have predominantly focused on NLRP3. The expressions of NLRP3 and its endogenous antagonist NLRP2 were found to be increased in human gingival tissues afflicted by various forms of periodontal disease versus gingival biopsy samples from periodontally healthy sites.[17] The aforementioned clinical study also demonstrated that IL-1β and IL-18 mRNA expression levels were increased in gingival tissues affected by periodontal disease states,[17] a finding consistent with prior periodontitis gene expression studies assessing IL-1β and IL-18 levels.[38,76,121] The realization that NLRP3 levels were positively correlated with the IL-1β and IL-18 expression levels in periodontal disease–affected versus healthy gingival biopsy samples[17] provides indirect evidence implying a role for the NLRP3 inflammasome in the pathogenesis of periodontal diseases states. In vitro studies showing that microorganisms from the dental biofilm modulated the expression of the NLRP3 inflammasome, which correlated with the production of IL-1β and IL-18, provide additional support for the NLRP3 inflammasome in periodontitis-associated catabolic effects.[18]

KEY FACT

Diverse pattern-recognition receptor (PRR) signaling pathways commonly converge downstream, resulting in crosstalk that has the potential for synergy or amplification effects modulating the periodontal immune response. Considering that individual periopathogenic bacteria express a multitude of heterogeneous microbe-associated molecular patterns recognized at several distinct Toll-like receptors and nucleotide-binding oligomerization domain–like receptors, which commonly activate nuclear factor-κB and mitogen-activated protein kinase signal transduction pathways, downstream signaling synergy or amplification likely contributes to the supraphysiologic expression of proinflammatory cytokines driving periodontal tissue destruction. Although current research has focused on elucidating the biologic actions of individual PRRs in the periodontium, future research is necessary to delineate the role of PRR signaling crosstalk in orchestrating immune responses supporting periodontal health versus causing disease.

Complement System

Complement is addressed briefly in the current chapter due to its role in PRR signaling and the periodontal host immune defense. The periodontal host immune response is dependent on a functional complement system, which notably coordinates the recruitment and activation of immune cells, bacterial opsonization, phagocytosis, and lysis.[55,132]

Complement–Pattern-Recognition Receptor Signaling

In addition to PRR localization in plasma membranes (TLRs) and the cytoplasmic compartment (NLRs), some soluble PRR families are also secreted into the plasma as humoral proteins. Soluble PRRs include pentraxins, mannose-binding lectin (MBL), ficolins, and properdin, which represent the functional ancestors of antibodies. Soluble PRRs interact with circulating MAMPs and DAMPS to activate the complement system, ultimately resulting in the opsonization, phagocytosis, and lysis of microbes.[132,133] Notably, complement interactions can amplify the host immune response through synergy with TLRs, another example of crosstalk among diverse PRR signaling pathways.[53]

Classical/Lectin/Alternative Pathways

The activation of the complement cascade involves the sequential activation and proteolytic cleavage of a series of serum proteins by three distinct mechanisms, namely, the classical, lectin, and alternative pathways (Fig. 9.2).[132,133] Classical pathway activation occurs in response to antigen–antibody complexes that are recognized by the C1q subunit of C1. C1q activates complement by functioning as a PRR to recognize distinct MAMPs and DAMPs, or alternatively through other soluble PRRs such as pentraxins (i.e., C-reactive protein). The lectin pathway is similarly triggered through soluble PRRs, including MBL and ficolins, which predominantly recognize carbohydrate groups. Both the classical and the lectin pathways then proceed through C4 and C2 cleavage for the generation of the classical/lectin C3 convertase (C4bC2b) (see Fig. 9.2). The alternative pathway is initiated by the hydrolysis of C3 to C3(H2O), which is a C3b analogue that forms the initial alternative pathway for C3 convertase. The alternative pathway also possesses a PRR-based initiation mechanism via properdin, which recognizes MAMPs and DAMPs. The alternative pathway also serves as a positive feedback loop for the classical and lectin pathways. All three pathways converge at the third component of complement (C3), which on activation by pathway-specific C3 convertases leads to the generation of key effector molecules. These include the C3a and C5a anaphylatoxins, which activate specific G-protein–coupled receptors and mediate the mobilization and activation of leukocytes. Also important are the C3b opsonins, which promote phagocytosis through complement receptors, and the C5b-9 membrane attack complex, which can lyse targeted pathogens (see Fig. 9.2).[132,133]

Role of Complement in Periodontitis

In the context of periodontal inflammation, complement subversion appears to play a major role in periodontal pathogenesis.[54,96] The dysregulation of complement activities may lead to a failure to protect the host against pathogens and amplify inflammatory tissue damage.[55,132] Activated complement components are found at higher levels in the gingival crevicular fluid of periodontitis patients as compared with healthy subjects.[7,123,148] Furthermore, virtually all of the complement components have been detected in chronically inflamed gingiva, whereas complement is nondetectable or not present at lower levels in healthy gingival biopsy specimens.[50,55] Local

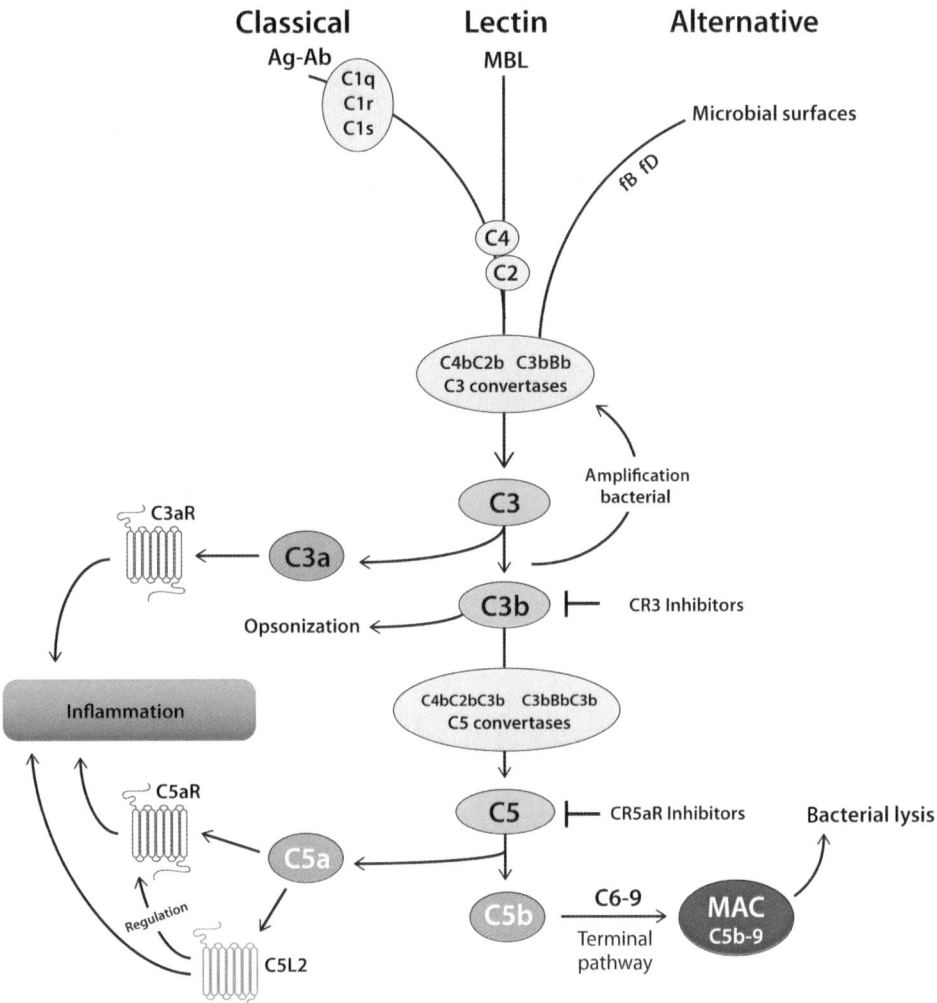

Fig. 9.2 Activation and therapeutic blockade of the complement system. All three pathways converge at the third component of complement (C3). The classical pathway is activated by antigen–antibody (Ag–Ab) complexes, and it requires C1, C2, and C4 components. Mannose-binding lectin (MBL) activates the lectin pathway through MBL-associated serine proteases (MASPs) and C2 and C4 cleavage. The alternative pathway is propagated through hydrolyzed C3 by complexing with factor B (fB) and via the fB cleavage of factor D (fD). The alternative pathway can also be activated via bacterial lipopolysaccharide in a properdin-dependent manner. Downstream from C3, proteolytic cleavage generates C3a and C5a anaphylatoxins, which activate the receptors C3aR and C5aR. C5aR can also be activated via C5L2. C5b initiates the assembly of C5b-9 membrane attack complex (MAC), which can induce bacterial lysis. Therapeutic blockage is depicted with the C3 and C5 components. *C5L2,* C5a receptor-like-2.

complement activation may promote periodontal inflammation predominantly via C5a-induced vasodilation, increased vascular permeability and flow of inflammatory exudate, and chemotactic recruitment of inflammatory cells, especially neutrophils.[50,55]

Antimicrobial Peptides

Antimicrobial peptides are components of the innate immune response in eukaryotes, thus providing defense against a wide spectrum of gram-positive and gram-negative bacteria, viruses, and fungi.[58,185,194] In the oral cavity, at least 45 different antimicrobial peptides belonging to different biochemical classes are found in the saliva and the gingival crevicular fluid.[45,46] The discussion of antimicrobial peptides in this chapter focuses on defensins and the cathelicidin LL-37, to highlight another molecular variable that affects PRR signaling and the periodontal host immune response.

Defensins and Cathelicidin LL-37

Defensins and cathelicidin LL-37, the most thoroughly studied antimicrobial peptides,[47,74] are cationic peptides that bind to negatively charged molecules on the microbial cell surface (e.g., LPS in gram-negative bacteria and lipoteichoic acid in gram-positive bacteria) that ultimately depolarize the cell membrane and render it permeable, with resulting bacterial cell death. In addition to their primary antimicrobial function, defensins are modulated by immune response mediators and also have immunomodulatory functions of their own.[90,151]

Defensins can be classified into α-defensins and β-defensins, based on structural distinctions in the connecting patterns of three disulfide bonds and in the spacing of cysteine residues.[74] Six human α-defensins and four human β-defensins have been extensively characterized. α-Defensins 1 to 4, known as human neutrophil peptides due to their expression in neutrophils, are present in the oral cavity, whereas α-defensins 5 and 6 are localized to the mucosal Paneth cells of the small intestine. β-Defensins 1 to 4, which are produced by a variety of epithelial cells throughout the body,[29,30] are abundantly produced by epithelial tissues within the oral cavity and are found in the gingival crevicular fluid and saliva.[30,36,47,142,149] Cathelicidin LL-37 is another important human defense peptide residing in neutrophils, and it can be found in the gingival epithelium.[47]

Role of Antimicrobial Peptides in Periodontitis

In the periodontium, the expression of β-defensins 1, 2, and 3 is observed at the mRNA level, in both clinically healthy and diseased tissues; the expression of these epithelium-derived peptides appears to be correlated with periodontal health, thereby suggesting a protective role.[14,19,180] Specific β-defensins are located in different anatomic regions of the periodontal epithelium: β-defensins 1 and 2 are observed in the upper layers of the gingival and sulcular epithelium, adjacent to the microbial biofilm and external environment, consistent with the innate immune "barrier" function of the epithelium. Interestingly, neither β-defensin 1 nor β-defensin 2 is found in the junctional epithelium. Protection in the junctional epithelium may be provided by the higher concentration of α-defensins and LL-37 produced by granulocytes migrating toward the gingival sulcus.[29,30,102]

Although the role of defensins and LL-37 in periodontal disease is currently not well understood, the expression of neutrophil derived α-defensins 1 to 3 and LL-37 has been reported to be significantly elevated in the gingival crevicular fluid of patients with chronic periodontitis.[127,174] The expression of defensins induced by whole periopathogenic bacteria such as *Fusobacterium nucleatum*, *P. gingivalis*, *A. actinomycetemcomitans,* and *T. denticola* is largely dependent on TLR signaling,[70,125,153,179] a property that reinforces the complexity of host–microbe interactions and the periodontal immune defense.

Antimicrobial Peptides in the Periodontium

Antimicrobial Peptides	Cellular Expression	Periodontitis Presentation
α-defensins 1, 2, 3, 4	Neutrophils	Elevated in GCF
β-defensins 1, 2, 3, 4	Epithelial cells	Elevated in gingival / crevicular epithelium
Cathelicidin LL-37	Neutrophils	Elevated in GCF

GCF, Gingival crevicular fluid.

Immunomodulatory Therapies

Various treatment strategies have been developed to target the host response to LPS-mediated tissue destruction.[88] Matrix metalloproteinase (MMP) inhibitors (e.g., low-dose formulations of doxycycline)

have been used in combination with scaling and root planing[22] or surgical therapy.[41] In addition, high-risk patient populations (e.g., diabetic patients, patients with refractory periodontal disease) have benefited from the systemic administration of MMP inhibitors.[25,111,140] Encouraging results have been shown with the use of soluble antagonists of TNF-α and IL-1β delivered locally to periodontal tissues in nonhuman primates.[6] Other therapeutic strategies that are being explored are aimed at inhibiting the signal transduction pathways involved in inflammation. Pharmacologic inhibitors of NF-κB and p38 MAPK pathways are actively being developed to manage rheumatoid arthritis and inflammatory bone diseases,[2,73,93] and they have been applied in periodontal disease models with noteworthy accomplishments.[89,135] With the use of this novel strategy, inflammatory mediators including proinflammatory cytokines (e.g., IL-1, TNF, IL-6), MMPs, and others would be inhibited at the level of the cell-signaling pathways required for the transcription factor activation necessary for inflammatory gene expression or mRNA stability. Indeed, the targeting of RNA-binding proteins that mediate the effects of inflammatory cytokines does have therapeutic value in small animal models of periodontal disease progression.[122] These therapies may provide the next wave of adjuvant chemotherapeutics that may be used to manage chronic periodontitis.

Regarding the complement system, therapeutic strategies are evolving that target either CR3 or CR5 (see Fig. 9.2). Because C3 is a central component of all three activation pathways, blockade at this level is a reasonable approach to treating complement-associated diseases, including periodontitis. CR3 antagonism through topical small molecule inhibitors has been shown to reduce *P. gingivalis*–induced alveolar bone loss.[52,56] The complement-generated fragment C5a functions as a potent mediator of complement signaling and neutrophil recruitment that may protect but also mediate excessive neutrophil activation, and it has the potential to augment tissue damage during periodontal disease progression. As such, C5aR inhibitor use in preclinical models indicate that the potential to inhibit C5aR may be a viable option for the treatment and management of periodontal diseases.[1]

The antimicrobial and immunomodulatory roles of defensins also have obvious attractiveness for therapeutic applications. However, the biochemical purification process is cost inefficient, and the synthesis process is complicated by the size and tridimensional structure of the peptides. Novel analogues of defensins have shown even higher antibacterial activity than the endogenous β-defensins 1 and 3, without any cytotoxic effects on host cells,[150] thus indicating the promise of this approach.

References

 References for this chapter are found on the companion website www.expertconsult.com.

CHAPTER 10

Resolution of Inflammation

Marcelo Freire

CHAPTER OUTLINE

 For additional content on systemic links, including type 2 diabetes, cardiovascular diseases, cancer, and pregnancy outcomes, please visit the companion website at www.expertconsult.com.

Inflammation has protective functions that are regulated by multiple endogenous interactions with the host cells and microbiome. Acute inflammation is temporally and spatially controlled to maintain homeostasis. Four specialized lipid mediator families activate resolution signals (lipoxins, resolvins, protectins, and maresins). Understanding the crosstalk of resolution signals in tissue response to injury has the potential to prevent and treat chronic diseases. The therapeutic applications of inflammation resolution include prevention, maintenance, and regeneration of periodontal tissues. This chapter presents fundamental concepts of resolution as an active biochemical mechanism regulated by endogenous/therapeutic lipid mediators. Novel concepts of resolution mediators in tissue regeneration and potential therapeutic applications are also discussed.

Inflammation

Inflammation is an essential biologic response observed across species with particular importance to human health and disease. The first description of a localized response to injury and infection that resembled signs of inflammation was recorded by the ancient Egyptian and Greek cultures. Four cardinal signs describing inflammation were identified: *rubor et tumor cum calore et dolore* (redness and swelling with heat and pain).[93] In 1958 Virchow's investigations led to the understanding of the cellular basis of inflammation as a pathologic condition, and his observations led to the addition of a new cardinal sign, functio laesa (loss of organ/tissue function).[93]

More recently, advanced cellular and molecular mechanisms governing the fate of inflammation have been identified. The initiation of acute response is accepted to be a physiologic response occurring in vascularized tissues to defend the host and maintain homeostasis. Inflammation, or "set on fire," response is an active cellular and molecular response that aims to control challenge.[61] When activated, inflammation is protective to host tissues against stimuli, such as pathobions, foreign bodies, toxic chemicals, and trauma.

Innate immunity, characterized by the local inflammatory response, is the early response to identifying and eliminating infectious agents or damaged tissues. As an initial and protective response to challenges presented by host tissues, inflammation is characterized by increased blood flow, vascular dilation, increased vascular permeability, and cellular recruitment. This response requires four biologic components: inflammation inducers, detecting sensors, downstream mediators, and target tissues. The type and degree of an inflammatory response are dependent on the nature of the trigger (e.g., bacterial, viral, parasitic, or chemical) and its duration.[60] With specific cellular and molecular cues, inducers will be detected by antigen first line of response and activate a cascade of events that are tightly regulated.

The major sensors for the inflammatory response are epithelial cells and innate immune cells that migrate to the injured site and resident stromal cells. Polymorphonuclear leukocytes (PMNs) or neutrophils (named for their staining characteristics with hematoxylin and eosin) constitute the cellular arm of the first line of defense of the innate immune system. PMNs are phagocytes with potent oxidative and nonoxidative killing mechanisms that combat bacteria.[10] PMN infiltration is followed by the entry of mononuclear cells, monocytes, and activated macrophages into the inflammatory site that clears cellular debris, bacteria, and apoptotic PMNs by phagocytosis without prolonging inflammation. Together, innate cells trigger production of mediators that modulate the fate of inflammation. Neutrophils, macrophages, dendritic cells, and mast cells produce low-molecular-weight proteins called cytokines that control initiation, maintenance, and regulation of the amplitude and duration of the inflammatory response.

In response to bacteria conserved receptors, expressed in innate immune cells, Toll-like receptors (TLRs) sense molecules expressed on pathogens, such as pathogen-associated molecular patterns (PAMPs). Binding of TLRs to specific pathogen molecules induces a signal that activates downstream events. In consequence, the production of communicating molecules such as inflammatory cytokines, interleukins (ILs), chemokines (CXCs), and inflammatory lipid mediators (LMs) is key to signal an effective response.[13,14] The inflammatory mediators are communicators establishing the "language" responsible to signal bacterial clearance. A didactical, and hopefully functional, classification of mediators categorized the inflammatory molecules according to their functions in the context of activation (pro-) or inhibition (anti-) of inflammation. It is important to note the binary terminologies of pro- and anti-inflammatory are more dynamic than first described. This complex relationship is controlled by the molecule concentration, the interaction with its receptors and other interactants, and finally the time of production and activity. The binary view of a molecule's activity is still the convention and the accepted terminology, but it is crucial to contextualize these concepts. Pro-inflammatory mediators, for example, are produced locally in the tissues or systemically in the bloodstream (e.g., IL-1β, IL-6, tumor necrosis factor alpha [TNF-α], and PGE2). In response to the direct challenge or to the production of pro-inflammatory molecules, anti-inflammatory cytokines control the response and maintain the reaction in check (e.g., IL-10, IL13, TGF-β, IL1RA).[82]

The regulation leading to transcription of pro-inflammatory cytokine genes, their translation, and secretion from a variety of cells is dependent on nuclear factor kappa-light-chain-enhancer of activated B cells (NF-κB). NF-κB gene clusters and proteins function as dimeric transcription factors that regulate a broad range of biologic processes, including innate and adaptive immunity, inflammation, stress responses, B-cell development, lymphoid organogenesis, and cytokine production. Cytokines are low-molecular-weight proteins that modulate inflammation positively or negatively. Cytokines are released by local cells, such as epithelial cells and fibroblasts, and phagocytes in the acute inflammation phase, and by immune cells in adaptive immunity (please refer to Chapters 7 and 9 for more details on inflammation).

Although the inflammatory response is protective, unresolved inflammation is detrimental to tissue function, promoting dysbiosis. Failure to resolve inflammation leads to chronic diseases including inflammatory bowel syndrome, type 2 diabetes, cardiovascular diseases, Alzheimer disease, cancer, and periodontal diseases. Resolution of inflammation is an active biochemical mechanism regulated by mediators that switch gene expression, protein functions, and cells to return to homeostasis. Among the mediators that regulate this process, specialized lipid mediators (SPMs) activate cells to start resolution. Thus, beneficial acute inflammation is spatially and temporally regulated by SPMs.[9,20,67,74,86]

 KEY FACTS

Pro-resolution Versus Anti-inflammation

Pro-resolution lipid mediators are fatty acids that are expressed endogenously to activate cells and tissues to control inflammation. Initiation of inflammation requires external and internal cellular signals, which in turn activates pro-resolution enzymes to produce lipid ligand signals. Upon interaction with a cellular receptor with lipid ligands, cells are activated to produce pro-resolution or anti-inflammation. The stereospecificity guides the cell function to either suppress and/or pro-resolve. In anti-inflammation, blocking and suppressing pathways that activate inflammation are the usual mechanism. In pro-resolution, specific lipids are able to activate cell switching from pro-inflammation to pro-resolution. For example, the endogenous mediators are able to enhance deficient phagocytosis seen in type 2 diabetes, increase chemotaxis in localized aggressive periodontitis, and prevent gingivitis. Thus, stimulating resolution either endogenously or therapeutically activates protective signals that prevent collateral damage and limit acute or continuous inflammation.

Acute Inflammation Is Self-Limited

To maintain homeostasis, a class switch activity of enzymes from pro-inflammation to pro-resolution controls temporal regulation of acute inflammation.[26,31] For many years, our understanding of inflammation was mostly on initiation as an active process, whereas termination (a.k.a. resolution) was thought to be a passive process with

decay of inflammation (Fig. 10.1) until basic and translational studies from Drs. Charles Serhan and Thomas Van Dyke came to light that proved otherwise. Contrary to old belief, they showed that resolution is an active process and can only be initiated when enzymes produce bioactive pro-resolution lipids.[31,77,88]

In the context of acute inflammation initiation, locally produced lipid mediators, such as prostaglandins, prostacyclin, leukotrienes, and thromboxanes, regulate major processes and act as autacoids (short-lived molecules that act at the site of synthesis). These lipid mediators are synthesized in a sequence of enzymatic activation when arachidonic acid (AA) is released from the cell membrane due to trauma or via cell-cell communication. Structurally, most of the lipids of inflammation are eicosanoids (20-carbon chains) and act as endogenous precursors for biosynthesis of a chain of several molecules. In fact, the enzyme phospholipase A2 releases AA from the phospholipid membrane. This release constitutes the rate-determining step in the generation of eicosanoids produced by most phagocytic and immune cells.[54] AA is rapidly converted into various potent lipid mediators with specific functions in a cell-specific manner by cyclooxygenases (COXs), lipoxygenases (LOs), or epoxygenases to yield prostaglandins, leukotrienes, and endoperoxides, respectively.

Arachidonic acids are metabolized mostly by two major enzyme pathways: COXs and LOs. Whereas COX-1 (constitutively expressed COX) is responsible for basal levels of prostaglandin synthesis, COX-2 (inducible COX) catalyzes the conversion of AA to lipid mediators during inflammation. Prostaglandins have ten subclasses, of which, D, E, F G, H, and I are the most important in inflammation. Specifically, PGE2 is generated via PGE synthase in leukocytes, whereas PGI2 is generated by prostacyclin synthase in endothelial cells and thromboxanes (TXA) are generated via TXA synthase in platelets.[16,32]

Lipoxygenases catalyze the formation of hydroxyeicosatetraenoic acids (HETEs) from AA leading to the formation of leukotrienes (LTs) and other biologically active compounds.[94] LTs are predominantly produced by inflammatory cells, including polymorphonuclear leukocytes, macrophages, and mast cells. There are three distinct lipoxygenases (LOs) that are cell specific; 5-LO in myeloid cells, 12-LO in platelets, and 15-LO in epithelial/endothelial cells. Cellular activation by pathogens and immune complexes results in activation of a sequential enzymatic reaction that includes cPLA2 and 5-LO. 5-LO converts released AA to the epoxide LTA4, which undergoes transformation by distinct pathways—one to generate LTB4, which is a potent regulator of neutrophil chemotaxis and leukocyte adhesion to endothelial cells.[32] The end products of 12- and 15-LO are 12- and 15-HETE, which are further metabolized. Excessive production of inflammatory mediators such as prostaglandins and leukotrienes with an exacerbated sensing response to inflammatory triggers is correlated with progression from acute inflammation to chronic inflammation in many diseases. Favorable inflammatory processes are self-limiting, which implies the existence of termination signals that regulate acute inflammation. Endogenous pro-resolution lipids are produced by enzymatic pathways that switch inflammation to resolution.[75] In addition to pro-inflammatory mediators that turn on inflammation, there is a separate set of lipid mediators that act as endogenous agonists to activate termination of inflammation by stimulating resolution.[72] The following sections provide a more detailed look at specific lipid mediators (SLMs) in the resolution of acute inflammation.

Specialized Lipid Mediators

Pro-resolution signals are activated mostly by resolvins, lipoxins, maresins, and protectins. Lipid mediator class-switches biosynthesize

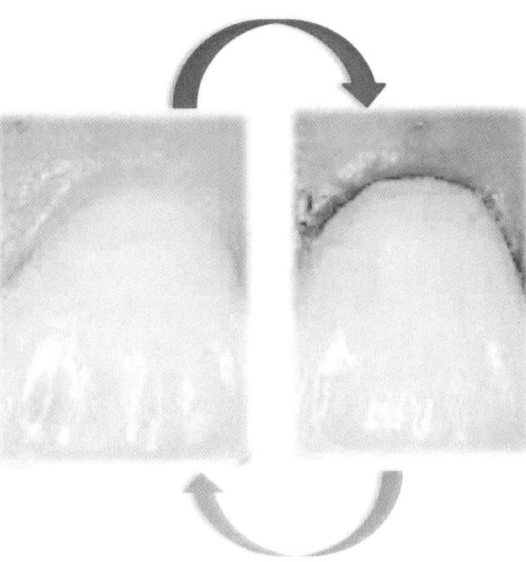

Pro-Inflammation

- Cellular Function -
Chemotaxis
Diapedesis
NF-κB activation
Cytokine
Production
Apoptosis

- Mediators -
TNF-α
IL-1
IL- 6
CCL2
CXCL8
Histamine
Prostaglandins
Leukotrienes

- Tissue Response -
Vasodilation
Swelling
Heat
Pain

**Acute
Inflammation**

Pro-Resolution

- Cellular Function -
Phagocytosis
Decrease chemotaxis
NF-κB inhibition
Class switch of enzymes
Efferocyotsis

- Mediators -
TGF-β
IL-1r
IL-10
CXCR4
Resolvins
Lipoxins
Protectins
Maresins

- Tissue Response -
Vasoconstriction
Non fever
Analgesic
Return to Homeostasis

**Resolution
of Inflammation**

Fig. 10.1 Acute inflammation is self-limited. In clinical scenarios of health, resident cells, molecular mediators, and tissues respond to injure effectively and return to homeostasis. If acute inflammation is unresolved, chronic inflammation and disease will establish. Tissue healing is effective when a class switch from pro-inflammation to pro-resolution is activated. *CXC motif*, Chemokine; *IL*, interleukin; *NF-κB*, nuclear factor kappa-B; *TNF-α*, tumor necrosis factor-α.

pro-resolution lipid mediators, such as lipoxin A4, eicosapentaenoic acid (EPA)–derived resolvins (i.e., RvE1, RvE2), and docosahexaenoic acid (DHA)–derived lipid mediators including D-series resolvins, protectins, and maresins (Fig. 10.2).[92] More details on the key pro-resolution mediators are given next.

Lipoxins

Derived from AA, lipoxins are natural pro-resolving molecules produced from endogenous fatty acids. Lipoxins have strong dual anti-inflammatory and pro-resolution actions. Lipoxins A4 and B4 were first isolated and identified as inhibitors of PMN infiltration and stimulators of nonphlogistic (non fever) recruitment of macrophages.[27,35,71] Three main pathways of lipoxin synthesis have been identified. In humans, sequential oxygenation of AA-derived lipids by 15-lipoxygenase and 5-lipoxygenase, followed by enzymatic hydrolysis, leads to LXA4, and LXB4 occurs in the mucosal tissues including the oral cavity, gastrointestinal tract, and airways. While in blood vessels, 5-lipoxygenase biosynthesizes LXA4 and 12-lipoxygenase in platelets produce LXB4. Lipoxin receptors are ubiquitously expressed by many cells, including neutrophils and monocytes. Aspirin triggers a third synthetic pathway. Aspirin promotes acetylation of COX-2 leading to a change in COX-2 activity and the chirality of the products, which are termed *aspirin triggered lipoxins* (ATLs).[34] Cells that express COX-2 include vascular endothelial cells, epithelial cells, macrophages, and neutrophils.[81] In addition to the synthesis of lipoxin, aspirin also blocks prostaglandin synthesis by acetylation of COX-2 inhibiting inflammation.[66]

Resolvins

Resolvins are endogenous lipid mediators induced during the resolution phase of inflammation. These lipid mediators are biosynthesized from the essential ω-3 polyunsaturated fatty acids (EPA and DHA) derived from the diet. The two primary groups of the resolvin family have distinct chemical structures: E-series, obtained from EPA, and D-series, derived from DHA. Vascular endothelium produces E-series resolvins via aspirin-modified COX-2 that converts EPA to 18R-hydroperoxyeicoapentaenoic acid (18R-HPEPE) and 18S-hydroperoxyeicoapentaenoic acid (18S-HPEPE). Neutrophils are rapidly taken up by human monocytes and metabolized to RvE1 and RvE2 by 5-lipoxygenase. Resolvin E1 production increases in plasma of individuals taking aspirin or EPA, resulting in amelioration of clinical signs of inflammation.[58] Similarly, DHA-derived D-series resolvins have been shown to reduce inflammation by decreasing platelet–leukocyte adhesion, and aspirin-triggered DHA conversion produces molecules with dual anti-inflammatory and pro-resolution function.[79]

The interaction between resolvins and specific receptors modulates the fate of innate immune cells and counterregulates active inflammation. Selective target sites for resolvins are G-protein coupled receptors (GPCRs).[80] ERV1 receptor (also known as ChemR23 or CMKLR1) is a GPCR expressed on monocytes and dendritic cells. BLT1, a leukotriene receptor, is the resolvin E1 receptor on neutrophils. Upon selective binding to the receptors, RvE1 attenuates NF-κB signaling and production of pro-inflammatory cytokines including TNF-α.[12,65] D-series resolvins target GPR32 and ALX

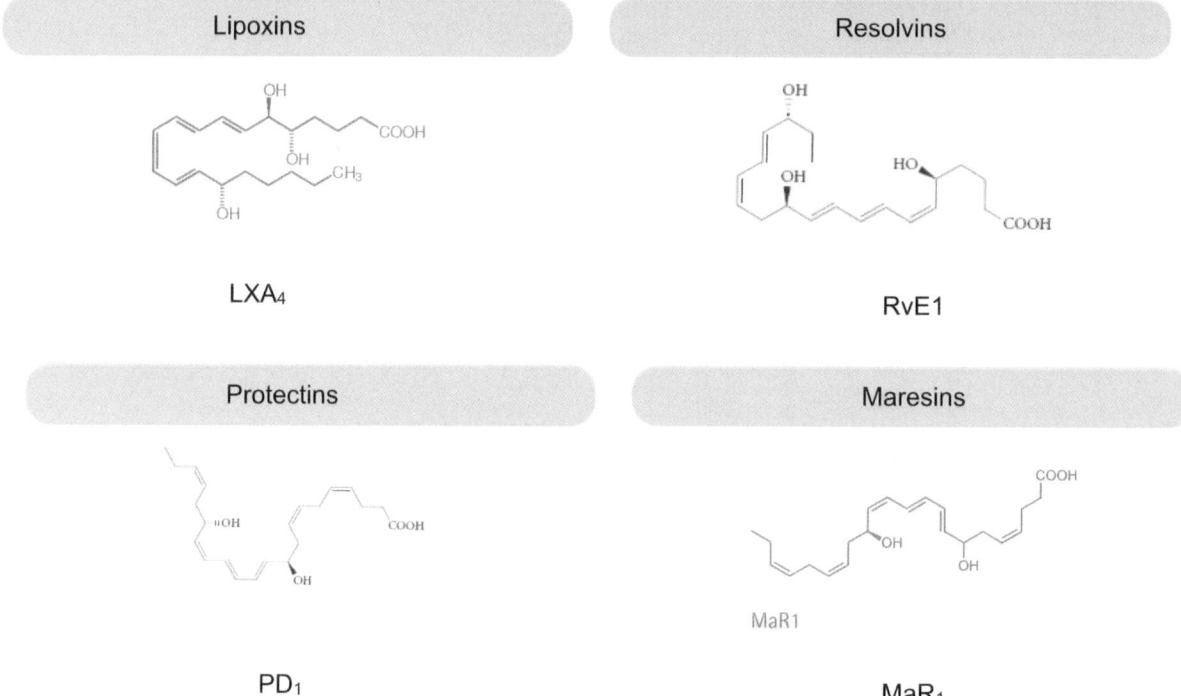

Fig. 10.2 Chemical structure of pro-resolution lipid mediators. Lipid mediator class switches yield lipoxins, eicosapentaenoic acid–derived E-series resolvins, and docosahexaenoic-acid derived D series resolvins, protectins, and maresins. *LXA₄*, Lipoxin A4; *MaR₁*, maresin 1; *PD₁*, protectin D1; *RvE₁*, resolvin E1.

receptors[97] expressed on platelets and PMN. Activation of CB2 leads to inhibition of P-selectin expression, decreasing PMN chemotaxis. Resolvins induce hallmark functions of resolution of inflammation, including decreasing neutrophil migration, phagocytosis of apoptotic cells, and increasing clearance of infection to activate tissue healing.[80]

Protectins

Protectins are also biosynthesized via a lipoxygenase-mediated pathway. The pathway converts DHA into a 17S-hydroxyperoxide-containing intermediate that is taken up by leukocytes and converted into 10,17-diHDHA, known as protectin D1 or neuroprotectin.[11] The name accounts for the protective actions observed in neural tissues and within the immune system. Human peripheral blood lymphocytes produce protectin D1 with a Th2 phenotype, thereby reducing TNF-α and interferon-γ secretion, blocking T-cell migration, and promoting T-cell apoptosis.[59] A novel protectin synthesis pathway was found that utilizes aspirin-triggered COX-2 to synthesize epimeric 17R-hydroxyperoxide from DHA, called AT-PD1, and has shown a positive interaction with CB2 and peroxisome proliferator-activated receptor (PPAR) family receptors. Protectins reduce PMN transmigration through endothelial cells and enhance clearance (efferocytosis) of apoptotic PMN by human macrophages.[84]

Maresins

Macrophage mediators in resolving inflammation (maresins, or MaR) have been identified as primordial molecules produced by macrophages with homeostatic functions. Metabololipidomic approaches in peritonitis models led to the identification of a novel pathway of DHA metabolism.[1] Macrophage phagocytosis of apoptotic cells triggers biosynthesis of RvE1, PD1, LXA4, and MaR1. Conversion of DHA into 14-hydroxy diHA was identified via the 14-lipoxygenase

cascade. MaR1 effectively stimulates efferocytosis of human cells and also has regenerative functions.[21]

In sum, the local lipid mediators constitute a new genus of pro-resolving endogenous compounds with potent actions in treating immune-metabolic human diseases. Lipoxin A4/ATL and resolvin E1 have been shown to inhibit neutrophil recruitment, attenuate pro-inflammatory gene expression, and reduce the severity of colitis in a murine model. PMN infiltration and lymphatic removal of phagocytes were observed when resolvin E1, D2, protectin D1, lipoxin, and maresin were used to ameliorate colitis.[3,44]

KEY FACTS

- Resolution of inflammation is an active biochemical process regulated by a class switch of enzymes and lipid mediators.
- A novel class of lipid mediators is known to modulate the resolution of inflammation; it consists of lipoxins, resolvins, maresins, and protectins.

Unresolved Chronic Inflammation in Periodontal Diseases

The oral microbiome modulates oral and systemic immune development, and a physiologic interaction maintains the homeostatic response. Periodontal diseases are chronic inflammatory diseases initiated by dybiosis and microbial biofilms.[17] In the case of gingivitis, acute inflammation is self-limited and reversible. When the etiologic factor and modifiers are "removed," the host returns to health. When stimuli persist, unresolved inflammation causes chronic lesions, loss of attachment, disease progression, and tissue loss. The host immune response functions as a protective mechanism, but continuous or exacerbated response risks the tissue integrity.[64]

The presence of plaque bacteria is highly prevalent in humans; in fact, 90% of the adult dentate population presents with some form of gingivitis.[22] Through co-evolution host-microbiota interactions results in host benefits including, nutrient utilization, colonization resistance and immune development. Altered balance either from the microbiota or the host response (or both) allows the disease initiation and progression.[17,36]

Although plaque is an evident etiologic factor in gingivitis, in periodontitis the specificity or number of the pathogens has not explained the variability in individual host response. Despite abundant microbial deposits in most people, the prevalence of moderate periodontitis is only around 40% of the population.[51] It is therefore possible that bacteria are not the primary factor of gingivitis-periodontitis transition. Whereas "plaque" is a traditional concept in etiology, the host presents multiple variations that provide increased susceptibility changing taxonomic composition of the plaque and metabolomic functions.[90] Resolution failure is a plausible explanation of this pathologic transition.

Host modifiers, including genetic, behavioral, anatomic, metabolic, and environmental, modulate the magnitude of the disease. These factors influence the disease severity, progression, and response to therapy. Classic studies in the 1980s showed that intake of antiinflammatory medications prevented the progression of periodontal disease.[43a] Although this was promising, it is now clear that inflammation is an important biologic process, and complete suppression of its cascade influences the host entirely. Instead of suppressing the system, resolution aims to enhance "good" inflammation to terminate the disease process.[52,68] In fact, deficient phagocytosis is seen in aggressive forms of periodontitis and is reversed by resolution mediators.[29,37] Thus, host-derived etiology is now well accepted and is a target for future therapies.

In a clinical trial of patients with moderate to severe periodontitis, the actions of dietary supplementation of ω-3 polyunsaturated fatty acid (PUFA) and aspirin were evaluated. In patients taking the preceding supplements, in addition to scaling and root planing, significant improvements were noted in pocket depth reduction and clinical attachment level gain, with lower levels of inflammatory mediators in saliva compared to patients who underwent scaling and root planing alone.[23] Lipid mediators are considered excellent candidates for the prevention and treatment of periodontal diseases.

Bacteria have been recognized for years as the main etiologic factor for periodontal diseases. With advances in molecular immunology and genetics, inflammation and resolution pathways have shown to play an integral part in the multifactorial pathogenesis of periodontal diseases.

Therapeutic Actions of Resolution Mediators

Periodontal diseases, including gingivitis and periodontitis, are leukocyte-driven inflammatory conditions characterized by soft-tissue and osteoclasts-mediated bone loss.[51,64,83] Resolution mediators are needed to control and treat periodontal diseases. In animal models, restoration of tissue health by resolution lipids is initiated after acute response generates classic eicosanoids, prostanoids, and prostacyclins and leukotrienes. The synthesis of immune-resolvents by key enzymes that induce a class switch is partially known.[73] Thus,

return to homoeostasis is highly regulated by resolution pathways (Table 10.1).

Evidence from animal studies demonstrated that overexpression of 15-lipoxygenase type I in rabbits increased endogenous levels of LXA4 protecting the host from developing periodontal disease. While no animal model is a perfect fit for humans, as proof-of principle, these concepts could be translated. Also, RvE1 when topically applied to the tissues ameliorates signs of disease activity, decreasing bone loss by 95% and significantly reducing the number of tissue neutrophils. Leukocyte infiltration was also reduced when RvE1 was applied in a murine dorsal air pouch model.[46] Similarly, in human cells obtained from localized aggressive periodontitis (LAP), RvE1 and LXA4 treatment decreased neutrophil superoxide production in response to TNFα and the bacterial surrogate peptide marker N-formyl-methionyl-leucyl-phenylalanine by 80%.[29,87,98]

The potential for treatment of periodontal diseases with one or a combination of specialized lipid mediators is clear and requires further investigation clinically. In one trial, scaling and root planing (SRP) with dietary supplementation of ω-3 PUFA and lower dose of aspirin reduced pocket depths and increased clinical attachment levels significantly when compared to SRP alone.[24] The clinical benefits were accompanied by lower levels of inflammatory mediators in saliva compared to scaling and root planing alone.[23]

Failure to remove pathobions and inefficient clearance of the innate immune cells (mainly dead neutrophils) characterize the progression to chronic pathologic lesion. In susceptible individuals, periodontal inflammation fails to resolve, and chronic inflammation becomes periodontal pathology. In periodontitis, primed neutrophils can mediate destruction and feed forward destruction of the extracellular matrix, bone, scarring, and loss of periodontal tissue function.[17] In an inflammatory model, resolvin D1 has been associated with the regulation of miRNAs and target genes and the reduction of LTB4, PGD2, TXA2, PGF2α, and TXA2 in peritoneal exudates.

- Inflammation is a biologic protective mechanism against injury.
- Acute inflammation seen in gingivitis is reversible and self-limited.
- Chronic inflammation in periodontitis has a failure of signals that activate resolution and return to homeostasis.
- Inflammation and resolution are connecting links with systemic disease (e.g., type 2 diabetes, cancer, and cardiovascular diseases) and periodontal diseases.

Tissue regeneration has also being a target of specialized resolution mediators. Treatment with maresin 1 has been demonstrated to stimulate tissue regeneration in system models, including planaria models.[78] Consistently in periodontal disease models, lipoxin A4/ATL prevented connective tissue and bone loss. Treatment of experimental periodontitis with lipid mediators completely resolved inflammation and rescued tissue loss with the regeneration of periodontal tissues.[89,91] It has been suggested that defective endogenous resolution of inflammation underlies the inflammatory phenotype presented in chronic diseases and that exogenous therapeutic molecules rescue this phenotype. Pro-resolution lipid mediators play a role as natural molecules in the maintenance of homeostasis with promising potential as therapeutic agents in human diseases.[28,31]

Final Remarks

The role of acute inflammation is protection of the host and development of tissue integrity. The fate of this process is determined by

TABLE 10.1 Therapeutic Actions of Pro-resolution Lipid Mediators

Disease Models	Lipid Mediator Therapeutic Actions	References
Periodontitis	**Lipoxin A4/ATL** Rescues attachment loss Enhances tissue healing Promotes periodontal regeneration Ceases infiltration of neutrophils	Van Dyke et al. (2008) Serhan et al. (2003) Van Dyke et al. (2015) Van Dyke et al. (2015)
	Resolvin E1 Decreases bone loss Lowers number of osteoclasts	Hasturk et al. (2005) Hasturk et al. (2007)
Type 2 diabetes	**Resolvin E1** Increases cell counts Increases chemotaxis Rescues phagocytosis	Herrera et al. (2015) Tang et al. (2013) Freire et al. (2016)
	Resolvin D1 Increases monocyte recruitment Decreases inflammation in adipocytes	Spite et al. (2014) Spite et al. (2014)
Colitis	**Lipoxin A4/ATL** Decreases severe colitis Pro-inflammatory gene expression is down expressed Reduces immune dysregulation	Aliberti et al. (2002) Gewirtz et al. (2002) Gewirtz et al. (2002) Wallace et al. (2003)
	Resolvin E1 Improves animal survival rate Reduces weight loss Activates LPS detoxification Inhibits neutrophil recruitment	Arita et al. (2005) Arita et al. (2005) Campbell et al. (2010) Ishida et al. (2010)
	AT-Resolvin D1 Reduces diseases activity index Attenuates pro-inflammatory mediators' gene expression Attenuates neutrophil recruitment	Bento et al. (2011) Bento et al. (2011) Bento et al. (2011)
	Resolvin D-2 Ameliorates disease activity index Reduces colonic PMN infiltration	Bento et al. (2011) Bento et al. (2011)
Retinopathy	**Protectin D1** Protects against neovascularization	Connor et al. (2007)
Calvaria defects	**Resolvin E1** Promotes bone regeneration in calvaria defects	Gao et al. (2012)

the balance and magnitude of mediators and sensors that amplify the inflammatory process or control the restoration to normal health. It is now evident that the resolution of inflammation is modulated by protective mediators, such as AA-derived lipoxins and ATLs, ω3- EPA-derived resolvins of the E-series, DHA-derived resolvins of the D series, protectins, and maresins. The selective interaction of the lipid mediators with GPCR receptors of innate immune cells induces the cessation of leukocyte infiltration; the return to normal levels of vascular permeability/edema; PMN death (mostly via apoptosis); and nonphlogistic infiltration of monocyte/macrophages and macrophage removal of apoptotic PMN, foreign agents (bacteria), and necrotic debris from the site. These cellular events lead to resolution with a return to predisease homeostasis. Unresolved inflammation is a hallmark of various human diseases including diabetes, ulcerative colitis, rheumatoid arthritis, cancer, cardiovascular diseases, and periodontitis. The fate of acute inflammation determines the restoration to homeostasis versus disease establishment. Diseases associated with uncontrolled acute inflammation are characterized by a continuous release of histotoxic substances that results in local tissue damage, prolonged inflammatory response, and loss of function. In contrast, in health, the fate of inflammation is influenced by endogenous mediators, cells, tissue, and scaffolds to resolve the acute process and reestablish homeostasis, thereby promoting tissue healing and regeneration (Fig. 10.3).[6]

A localized inflammatory response to an injury or infection is a spatially defined and temporally regulated process that ideally should be self-limited as previously described. If the lesion does not resolve and becomes chronic, the acquired immune system is stimulated, including broad activation of lymphocytic pathways as well as cell-mediated and humoral immunity. The local infection or injury, if sustained, becomes systemic, defined as an extended response that

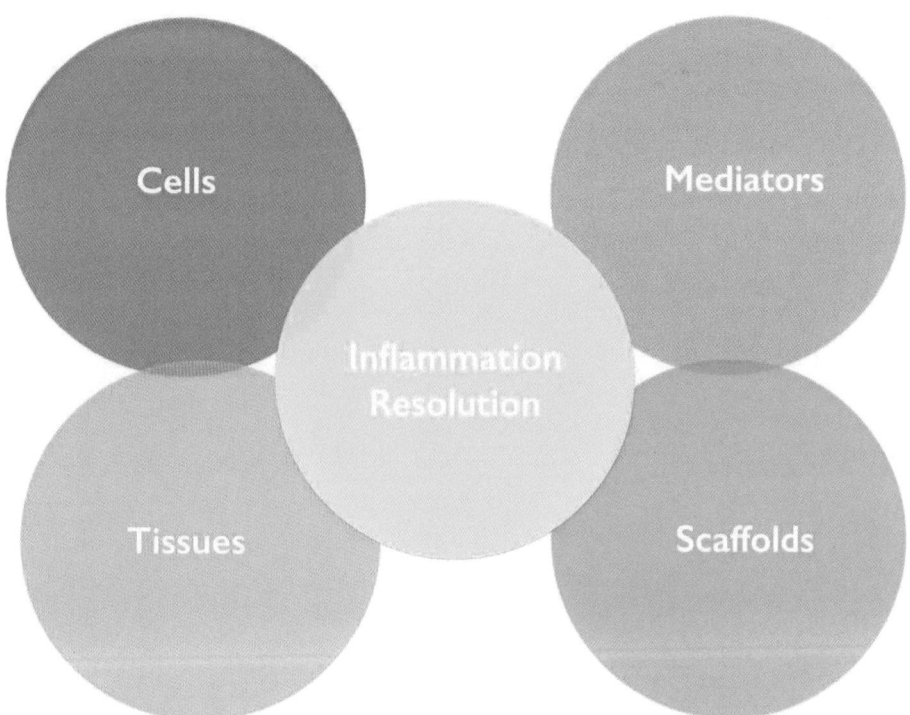

Fig. 10.3 Inflammation resolution is a key component of tissue healing and regeneration. Upon antigenic challenge, cells, tissue, vasculature, and mediators have to synchronize the host response to adequately remove triggers and protect the host prior to regeneration. Resolution of inflammation has main functions in the activation of cells to promote clearance, return to homeostasis, and together with the factors described promote tissue regeneration..

goes beyond the confined localization of one tissue. The chronicity of the lesion alters molecular, cellular, and overall tissue responses in remote regions of the body having a transient or permanent impact on overall health.

 A Case Scenario is found on the companion website www.expertconsult.com.

References

 References for this chapter are found on the companion website www.expertconsult.com.

CHAPTER 11

Precision Dentistry: Genetics of Periodontal Disease Risk and Treatment

Scott R. Diehl | Chih-Hung Chou | Fengshen Kuo | Ching-Yu Huang | Olga A. Korczeniewska

CHAPTER OUTLINE

Genomic Advances in the 21st Century
Genetic Basis for Individual Differences in Disease Risk
Precision Dentistry: Using Genetics for Personalized Treatment

 eTable 11.1, which is a comprehensive table about independent gene association reports for aggressive and chronic periodontitis, can be accessed on the companion website at www.expertconsult.com.

It is now widely accepted that differences among individuals who are at risk for the development of most diseases have a substantial inherited component. Factors in the environment (e.g., diet, smoking, preventive care, exposure to pathogens) interact with each person's genetic predisposition to determine his or her health outcomes. This complex combination of variables determines if and when a disease affects the person, how fast and how severely symptoms of the disease progress, and how the person responds to different treatments in terms of both side effects and the success of alternative therapies. Sometimes—and particularly with diseases such as cystic fibrosis and muscular dystrophy—the genetic component of risk predominates, and differences in environment play only a minor role. With other diseases, factors in the environment are most important, and variation inherited in the person's deoxyribonucleic acid (DNA) has only an infrequent or minor influence on disease susceptibility or progression. Examples of the latter include infectious diseases such as human immunodeficiency virus/acquired immunodeficiency syndrome (HIV/AIDS) as well as cancers such as mesothelioma, which is strongly associated with asbestos exposure. The majority of human diseases fall about halfway between these two extremes, with genes and the environment both playing important roles.

Most cases of periodontitis appear to fit this complex gene and environment model. With the exception of a handful of rare syndromes caused by mutations of single genes, evidence indicates that inherited variation in DNA has a role roughly equal to that of the environment in determining who remains periodontally healthy versus who is affected by this disease. Beyond this broad generalization, however, and despite more than 800 association studies of periodontitis and genetic polymorphisms reported to date, knowledge of which specific genes are most important remains extremely limited. We know virtually nothing about the role that inherited genetic differences are likely to have in determining how patients respond to alternative treatments. This knowledge is necessary for the development of "personalized" or "individualized" periodontal treatment strategies, an approach that is playing an increasingly important role in improving virtually all other areas of health care today.

This chapter reviews the challenges and barriers that have thus far limited progress in advancing our knowledge of the complex genetics of periodontitis. This requires a basic understanding of not only the architecture of the human genome and the complexity of genetic susceptibility but also of the critical roles that statistical power and sample size play in the process of discovery. These latter issues are important for all areas of research but especially for situations in which a large number of variables need to be evaluated. In genetic studies, about 20,000 genes need to be considered as potential hypotheses or "candidates" for influencing disease risk. Depending on the gene's size and the frequency of genetic recombination in the gene's chromosomal region, scientists need to evaluate a handful or up to several hundred inherited DNA variants in each gene as potential "biomarkers" of disease risk. Each one of these variants essentially amounts to a test of the hypothesis as to whether the variant is associated with disease risk. Furthermore, many complex diseases have been found to be strongly associated with DNA variation in parts of the human genome where no genes are known to exist but where the genetic material may have important functional effects nonetheless. Therefore to fully evaluate the entire human genome, the number of hypotheses that needs to be tested is truly enormous and involves roughly the equivalent of 1 million independent statistical tests. Only since the early 2000s have laboratory and computational tools been available that make this scale of work technically feasible at an affordable cost, and thus far only a few studies have reported results for a whole genome analysis for periodontitis genetic risk.

Opportunities for advanced study designs and next-generation DNA sequencing and other genomic technologies to improve the understanding of the inherited basis of periodontitis make it likely (although by no means certain) that genetic variation will become an important variable to be routinely considered by practicing dentists within the careers of dental students today, and this is already starting to occur. Therefore it is essential that dentists learn how to access and interpret the information coded in the human genome so they can use this wisely to improve periodontal disease prevention, diagnosis, and treatment for their patients. Alternatively, new interdisciplinary teams will need to be established with dentists as key members working closely with experts in bioinformatics, genomics, and genetic counseling so that patients will be able to reap the potentially significant benefits of these scientific advances. However the process evolves, the genomics revolution will surely lead to major changes in both dental education and dental practice in the not-so-distant future.[8,30]

Genomic Advances in the 21st Century

Most health care professionals are aware of the many major advances in genetics accomplished during the decades since the Human Genome Project officially began in 1990.[51] Headlines and announcements of "breakthroughs" continue to appear regularly in print and television media. All too often, many of these stories seem to promise rapid and significant improvements in health care that are totally unrealistic.[11] Cautious assessments are usually not deemed newsworthy by the media, and understatement is not in the interest of private companies or of grant-awarding government agencies supporting basic research and clinical trials. Consequently, the public has too often received overly optimistic pictures of what the future of medical care based on genomic medicine really holds in store for them. Despite this all-too-common overstatement about rapid translation to clinical practice, the actual advances in technical capabilities for genomic data acquisition and the accumulation of knowledge in the field of genetics have been truly enormous. The eventual impact of this explosion of biologic knowledge on all areas of human health, including those concerning the field of dentistry, is certain to be substantial over the longer term.

Unfortunately, for reasons explored further in the next section, genomic advances have thus far contributed little to advance our understanding of the molecular–pathologic causes of periodontitis nor pointed toward ways to improve treatment through individualized approaches based on patients' inherited genetic variation. Genome-wide association studies (GWAS, pronounced "gee-wahs") and next-generation DNA sequencing techniques are now being used in periodontology research. For these strategies to be successful, however, they must be combined with further improvement in research definitions of periodontal disease and much larger sample sizes than have been used in the majority of previous genetic studies. To provide a refresher on basic concepts and to help improve understanding, some of the commonly used terms in genetics are explained in Table 11.1.

Patterns in Populations and Pedigrees

With all of the attention focused on silicon arrays, laser scanners, and the other "glamorous" gadgets of advanced genomic technologies, it is important to consider how much can be learned about the genetic basis of a disease before stepping into a DNA laboratory. In fact, a strong foundation of knowledge about a disease's frequency in different populations and its occurrence among closely and distantly related family members (i.e., pedigrees) is absolutely essential. Without this foundation, endless gigabytes of DNA sequence data will not enable scientist–clinicians to develop a solid understanding of the causes of a disease. The human genome has not evolved in a test tube nor inside a supercomputer; rather, it has existed for millennia in natural populations and been transmitted from generation to generation, from parents to children. Only by carefully studying the genetics of a disease in populations and pedigrees can we hope to begin to unearth the complex interactions between genes and the environment that underlie individual differences in disease susceptibility. This field of research is known as *genetic epidemiology.*

Genetic epidemiologists often first look at whether a disease occurs more often in some human populations than others. These comparisons can include both populations in different geographic areas as well as racial or ethnic groups living in the same region. Does the disease have more severe symptoms, more rapid rates of progression, or an earlier age of onset in some populations? Such findings suggest (but do not prove) that genetic differences that are important for the disease may exist among the populations.

Before the massive human migrations in recent centuries, most human populations existed in semi-isolation from other populations around the globe. As a consequence of natural selection (i.e., differential survival and reproduction), populations sometimes adapted genetically to their local environments. The most famous example of adaptation is the sickle cell hemoglobin variant that protects an individual against the infectious disease malaria. This variant is common among populations who live in areas where this mosquito-borne parasite has long been endemic, because it provides strong protection against the severe symptoms of this disease. The variant persists at high frequency in these populations, although persons who inherit two copies of the mutation (i.e., one from mother and one from father) are severely affected by the disease sickle cell anemia. A balance between the benefit of malaria resistance in persons who inherit only one copy of the variant versus the disadvantage of sickle cell disease keeps the variant at relatively high frequencies among populations where malaria is present. Another example of population differentiation by natural selection is the ability to digest the milk sugar lactose as an adult that evolved in Europeans in conjunction with the domestication of dairy cattle more than 8000 years ago. In addition to differentiation driven by natural selection, as is seen in these examples, a random process called *genetic drift* also causes populations with little or no migration between them to differentiate genetically over time. Thus one cannot assume that every population difference observed has a functional biologic basis.

Regrettably, the comparison of periodontitis in different populations across the globe is extremely challenging because of the lack of calibrated examiners and standardized disease definitions.[6] One of the most dramatic population differences in which data quality is not an issue is the observation that both localized and generalized forms of early-onset aggressive periodontitis occur about ten times more frequently among African Americans as compared with Caucasians.[38] Human racial and ethnic groups often differ dramatically with regard to the frequency of mutations at genes that have major effects on disease risk. For example, cystic fibrosis is caused exclusively by recessive mutations in the CFTR gene, and it varies in frequency from 1 in 3000 Caucasians to 1 in 15,000 African Americans in the United States, whereas only 1 in 350,000 Japanese individuals are affected.[57] It is possible that the tenfold higher prevalence of early-onset aggressive periodontitis in African Americans is caused by the elevated frequency of high-risk gene variants in this population. However, additional evidence is needed before such a conclusion can be drawn. Although comparative studies of different populations may provide clues as to possible genetic mechanisms underlying a disease, the environments of the populations may also be dissimilar in important ways. It is possible that variations in diet, exposure to pathogenic oral bacteria, or some unknown and unmeasured environmental factors could entirely explain the observed differences in the frequency of aggressive periodontitis among population groups. Until solid data confirm a genetic basis for population differences, we need to wait before drawing firm conclusions.

The comparison of disease occurrence or severity in identical (monozygotic) versus nonidentical (dizygotic) twins is a powerful method for distinguishing between effects caused by variation in genes versus factors in the environment. This requires us to make what is usually a reasonable assumption that the environments of pairs of identical twins are no more or less similar than the

TABLE 11.1   Glossary of Terms Relevant to the Genetics of Periodontal Disease

Allele	One of several possible alternative forms of a gene caused by small or large differences in the DNA sequence within or near the gene. These differences arise by mutation, and some may affect the function of the gene product (i.e., a protein) or its abundance in different kinds of cells.
Autosomal dominant	DNA variation in a gene located on an autosome that has a dominant effect over other forms of variation at this location within the gene. When the dominant DNA sequence is present in combination with some other sequence, the gene's function is entirely or nearly entirely determined by the dominant sequence, whereas the alternative sequence that occurs on the person's other chromosome is essentially silent.
Autosomal recessive	DNA variation in a gene located on an autosome that has an effect on the gene's function only when the person has inherited two copies: one from the mother and the other from the father. For example, if an individual has two copies of an abnormal gene that is autosomal recessive, he or she will be subject to the effects of that gene.
Autosome	A chromosome that is not a sex chromosome.
Chromosome	A nuclear structure that contains genetic information. Humans have 46 chromosomes that are arranged in 23 pairs. There are 22 pairs of autosomes and one pair of sex chromosomes (either XX or XY).
Concordance	The probability that a pair of individuals (e.g., twins) both have a certain characteristic (e.g., periodontal disease), given that one of the pair has the characteristic. Presented as a number from 0 to 1 or as a percentage.
Dizygotic twins	Twins that have resulted from the fertilization of two separate eggs. They are no more similar to each other (from a genetic perspective) than are nontwin siblings. Nonidentical twins.
Epigenetics	Term used to describe the changes in phenotype or gene expression that result from mechanisms other than changes in the underlying DNA sequences (i.e., changes in which the gene is expressed rather than a change in the DNA sequence itself). Nongenetic factors cause the organism's genes to be expressed differently.
Exon	Protein coding regions of DNA.
Frameshift mutation	A mutation that results from the insertion or deletion of one or more nucleotides into a gene, thereby causing the coding regions to be read in the wrong frame and usually causing the protein produced to be defective in function.
Gene	The basic unit of heredity that occupies a specific position (locus) on a chromosome and that has specific effect(s) on the phenotype of the organism. A piece of DNA that is transcribed into a molecule of RNA and then translated into a protein.
Gene expression	The process by which the information in a gene is used via transcription and translation, thereby leading to the production of protein. Differences in gene expression can affect the phenotype of the organism, including the risk of disease.
Genetic code	In RNA and DNA, the consecutive nucleotide triplets (codons) that specify the sequence of amino acids for protein synthesis (translation).
Genome	The entire hereditary information of an organism. This term refers to all of the genes and other nongene portions of DNA carried by an individual cell.
Genotype	The genetic makeup of an organism or cell as distinct from its expressed features or phenotype.
Haplotype	A contraction of the term *haploid genotype*. This word refers to a combination of alleles at multiple loci, which are usually transmitted together on the same region of a chromosome.
Heredity	The passing of traits to offspring from parents or ancestors. In biology, the study of heredity is referred to as *genetics*. As a result of heredity, variation among individuals allows species to evolve by natural selection in response to changes in their environment or by random change over long periods of time.
Heterozygous	The presence of two different alleles at a specific position in a gene.
Homozygous	The presence of identical alleles at a specific position in a gene.
Intron	A DNA region within a gene that is not translated into protein. These intervening (noncoding) portions of DNA or RNA are removed during RNA processing.
Isoform	Any of several different forms of the same protein. Isoforms may be produced from related genes, or they may arise from the same gene via alternative splicing. Many isoforms are caused by single nucleotide polymorphisms.
Ligand	A molecule that binds to another molecule (usually a cellular receptor molecule).
Linkage	The tendency for certain genes to be transmitted from parent to child together because they are located close to each other on the same chromosome.
Linkage disequilibrium	The occurrence of specific alleles at different locations in the DNA that are relatively close to each other (linked) more often than would be expected by chance alone (disequilibrium).
Locus	The physical location that a gene occupies within a chromosome. (Plural: loci.)
Monozygotic twins	Twins with identical genetic makeup (i.e., identical twins) as a result of the fertilization of a single egg that then splits into two embryos.

TABLE 11.1 Glossary of Terms Relevant to the Genetics of Periodontal Disease—cont'd

Mutation	Changes in the DNA sequence of the genome can result from errors that occur during DNA replication or meiosis and can be caused by radiation, viruses, and mutagenic chemicals. Most mutations have little or no measurable effect on the gene's function; some are harmful, and a rare few may be advantageous.
Nucleotide	Molecules that, when linked, make up the structural units of RNA and DNA. They are composed of a phosphate group; the bases adenine, cytosine, guanine, and thymine; and a pentose sugar. In RNA, the thymine base is replaced by uracil.
Penetrance	The proportion of individuals who have a particular allele/genotype who express an associated trait (phenotype). Genotypes with a high penetrance result in a larger number of individuals in the population with the associated phenotype as compared with genotypes with a low penetrance.
Phenotype	The observable characteristics displayed by an organism (e.g., morphology, development, gender, eye color, physiologic properties, behavior). Phenotype results from the expression of the organism's genes as well as from the influence of environmental factors and interactions between the two.
Polymorphism	Polymorphism exists when two or more different phenotypes exist within different individuals of the same population. In the context of genetics, it refers to a region of the genome that varies between individual members of the population in such proportions that the rarest of them cannot be maintained just by recurrent mutation. Polymorphism may be actively maintained in populations by natural selection and also by random drift.
Sequencing	Determining in the laboratory the linear arrangement of nucleotides (in RNA or DNA) or amino acids (in proteins).
Signal transduction	A cascade of intracellular events that occurs after the binding of an extracellular signal (e.g., a hormone, a cytokine) to a receptor on the cell surface. The intracellular cascade can result in changes in gene expression in the nucleus and hence an altered phenotype of the cell (e.g., as a result of different protein production).
Single nucleotide polymorphism (SNP)	A polymorphism in a gene caused by a change in a single nucleotide in the DNA sequence. A large number of protein isoforms result from SNPs. SNPs occur frequently; approximately every 100 to 1000 base pairs occur as a result of deletions, insertions, and substitutions. There are estimated to be more than 10 million SNPs in the human genome. Many SNPs that occur in genes have no effect on the encoded protein, but some SNPs do influence the function of the protein that the gene produces. An SNP initially arises as a rare mutation, but it is considered to be an SNP if it occurs in at least 1% of the population.
Splicing	The removal of introns from transcribed RNA. The process of removal can vary, and some exons are skipped or excluded from splicing. This causes the production of "splice variants" or "alternatively spliced" protein isoforms, thereby resulting in the formation of different proteins from the same initial RNA.
Transcription	RNA synthesis. The process of creating an RNA copy of an equivalent section of DNA is the first step of gene expression, and it occurs in the nucleus. The RNA copy that is produced is called *messenger RNA* (mRNA).
Translation	The first stage of protein synthesis. mRNA produced during transcription is decoded to produce an amino acid chain that will later fold into an active protein. Translation occurs in the cytoplasm: ribosomes bind to the mRNA and then facilitate decoding via the binding of transfer RNAs (tRNAs) that have complementary anticodon sequences to those of mRNA. The tRNAs carry specific amino acids that are joined to form a polypeptide as the mRNA passes through the ribosome.

DNA, Deoxyribonucleic acid; *RNA,* ribonucleic acid.

environments shared by pairs of nonidentical twins. If variation among individuals in disease susceptibility or severity is caused entirely by factors in the environment, then we expect pairs of identical twins to be no more similar to each other in terms of disease risk than pairs of nonidentical twins. All twins (whether identical or nonidentical) are expected to be more similar to their co-twins, on average, than to unrelated members of their local population because they were raised in the same family environment, with similar diets, microbial exposures, and so on. However, if genetic variation plays an important role in determining a certain trait, then genetically identical twin pairs will be more similar to each other than nonidentical twin pairs. This is because identical twins share 100% of the same genes, whereas nonidentical twin pairs share only 50% of their parents' genes on average. Genetic epidemiologists calculate a measure called *heritability* that is based on these correlations and that estimates the portion of all variation in the trait attributable to inherited genetic variation. Traits with variation that is determined entirely by differences in environmental exposures have heritabilities of 0.0, whereas traits with variation attributable solely to inherited genetic differences without any environmental influence have heritabilities of 1.0.

Heritabilities are sometimes reported as a percentage that ranges from 0% to 100%.

Most human diseases and nondisease traits fall in the middle of this range, with heritability ranging between 0.25 and 0.75. For example, in one study, type 2 diabetes was estimated to have a heritability of 0.26, and abnormal glucose tolerance had a heritability of 0.61.[58] For it to be feasible to use the twin method with adequate statistical power, the disease has to be fairly common so that the researcher can recruit enough twin pairs in which at least one of the twins is affected by the disease. Not surprisingly, with regard to periodontal disease, only chronic periodontitis occurs frequently enough to have been studied using the twin design. Two twin studies of modest size (i.e., 110 and 117 pairs) have been reported, and these estimate the heritability of measures of chronic periodontitis range between 40% and 80%, thereby clearly implicating genetic variation in disease risk.[48,49] Interestingly, a study of bacteria associated with periodontitis found no difference between identical versus nonidentical twins.[50] This suggests (at least for these twins, most of whom did not have severe periodontitis) that inherited variation in risk is not mediated by genes that influence the presence of specific bacteria in subgingival plaque. Another review also failed to find an association between single nucleotide polymorphisms (SNPs; pronounced "snips") at interleukin-1 or other host genes and the presence or counts of subgingival bacteria.[52] These studies were performed before today's high-throughput DNA sequencing technologies were fully available to study the microbiome in depth, however, and it remains to be seen whether sharing specific strains of the hundreds of oral microbial species may be related to host genetics.

Another method used by genetic epidemiologists to understand and distinguish different mechanisms of transmission of diseases through families is called *segregation analysis.* This is relatively straightforward for traits in which mutation in a single gene causes the disease to develop with nearly 100% certainty in carriers, whereas persons who do not inherit the mutation are at little or no risk. For example, carriers of a single copy of the Huntington disease gene mutation or carriers of two copies of a cystic fibrosis gene mutation always develop these diseases if they reach the ages at which symptoms of these conditions normally emerge. By tracking the transmission of these diseases in families, it is obvious, for example, that Huntington disease is a dominant single-gene disorder: it is transmitted with 50% probability to offspring of affected individuals, and thus it is often found occurring across many generations of large pedigrees. By contrast, parents of children with cystic fibrosis are rarely affected themselves, and 25% of siblings are affected by cystic fibrosis when the disease is present in a nuclear family. This pattern of transmission is expected if a disease is recessive (i.e., it requires the inheritance of a mutated gene copy from both parents, who themselves have one normal and one mutated copy and so are not affected). For most common "complex" diseases, however, having a high-risk gene does not automatically lead to development of the disease; this phenomenon is called *reduced penetrance.* Furthermore, several genes or even dozens or more different genes may influence disease susceptibility; this is known as *oligogenic inheritance* and *genetic heterogeneity.* Environmental exposures are also important modifiers of disease risk. Such highly complex combinations of multiple genetic and environmental risk factors make the challenge of deciphering genetic mechanisms by merely observing transmission patterns in families using the segregation analysis approach unfeasible. The limitations of this approach were humorously illustrated in an analysis that facetiously presented evidence of a recessive gene controlling the trait of attending medical school.[44] "Risk" for this outcome among first-degree relatives of a doctor was elevated 61 times above that of the general population. More recently, a robust quantitative analysis of the family histories of characters in the Harry Potter series suggested that a dominant gene controls the inheritance of magic abilities.[62] Because the etiology of periodontitis is likely to be highly complex, segregation analyses of this disease that have been reported in the literature should be viewed with considerable skepticism. Unfortunately, the simplifying assumptions required for this method make the results unreliable and potentially misleading. For highly complex diseases, such as most cases of periodontitis, assays at the DNA level need to be combined with careful evaluations of clinical measures among related individuals to derive robust conclusions about a disease's genetic architecture. Some of the key features of the different techniques for studying the genetics of periodontal disease are explained in Table 11.2.

Searching for Answers in the DNA

In theory, a *genetic marker* can be any type of biomolecule or assay that allows us to read inherited differences among individuals in their DNA sequences. Blood groups, protein isozymes, and human leukocyte antigens (HLAs) were among the first developed markers,

but even simple traits that are controlled by single genes (e.g., eye color) can also serve this purpose. Genomic methods have made these methods obsolete, because researchers can now determine a person's inherited variation directly at the DNA level for a much lower cost and with greater speed and accuracy. So-called next-generation DNA sequencing methods are projected to enable researchers and clinicians to obtain nearly the entire 3 billion–DNA base human genetic blueprint for less than $1000.[20,76] At present, most genetic studies use a combination of whole genome arrays that can evaluate up to 1 million variable DNA sites in a single assay in combination with lower-throughput methods that are used for the fine mapping of chromosome regions of special interest.[61] These regions are said to contain *candidate genes* of high priority for further investigation either because of the genes' known biologic functions or because results of previous genome-wide surveys indicate strong statistical chances that disease susceptibility genes are located in certain regions of one or more chromosomes. Types of variation include SNPs in which one DNA base is substituted for another; small insertions and deletions ("in/dels") of one or more DNA bases; and larger structural changes in the DNA, such as inversions (in which a piece of DNA of hundreds or thousands of bases in size is cut out and sewn back into the chromosome in the opposite orientation) and copy number changes (in which a given segment of DNA is either missing or occurs in more than the usual two copies inherited as one copy from each parent).

Equipped with these powerful tools for rapidly measuring DNA variation, the next question to address is what kinds of study designs are most powerful for identifying the dozen or more variants that influence the risk of disease from among the millions of DNA differences that exist between any two individuals in a typical population. One method that has been highly successful for finding molecular defects related to simple genetic diseases caused by the mutation of a single gene, such as cystic fibrosis and Huntington disease, is *linkage analysis.*[1,7] This gene-mapping strategy requires families with one or more members affected by the disease to be recruited and clinically and molecularly evaluated for a relatively small number of genetic markers. Depending on the type of marker used, as few as 500 markers or up to 10,000 markers distributed evenly across the genome are needed. Investigators usually try to recruit families with two or more close relatives, such as sibling pairs, who are affected by the disease as well as parents and other siblings who may be unaffected. With a *null hypothesis* that suggests that a region of the chromosome does *not* contain genetic variation that influences disease risk, siblings share identical genetic material inherited from their parents an average of 50% of the time. However, if the region of the chromosome being evaluated contains a gene that has a substantial effect on disease risk (i.e., increases the risk by tenfold or more), then pairs of siblings who are both affected by the disease will share the chromosome region that contains the disease gene substantially more often than 50% of the time, and the null hypothesis of 50% sharing will be statistically rejected if the study has an adequately large enough sample of such families. This simple example illustrates how linkage analysis is performed. In practice, both small and large extended families are studied; this will include the simultaneous evaluation of the sharing of genetic material among both affected and unaffected relatives. Sophisticated mathematical algorithms and computer programs are used to carry out the huge number of calculations required for data analyses.

After achieving many successes with the use of linkage analysis for "simple" diseases caused by the mutation of a single gene, this method was extended to complex diseases caused by combinations of multiple susceptibility genes and environmental risk factors. Unfortunately, these conditions proved to be beyond the reach of

TABLE 11.2 Techniques for Studying the Genetics of Periodontal Disease

Candidate gene approach	A gene-mapping approach that tests whether one allele of a gene occurs more often in patients with the disease than in subjects without the disease. These methods are also referred to as *association analyses,* and they aim to identify which genes are associated with the disease. Candidate genes are chosen on the basis of their known or presumed function (i.e., they have some plausible role in the disease process, such as producing a protein that is important in the disease pathogenesis). Conceptually this makes sense, but it requires some knowledge of the candidate gene to look for it.
Case–control studies	Studies in which the genetic makeup is compared between cases (who have the disease in question) and controls (who do not). The populations need to be carefully matched, otherwise apparent observed differences between cases and controls could arise because of ethnic or geographic variation, for example.
Twin studies	Comparisons of traits—including diseases in monozygotic, dizygotic, or usually both types of twins—aimed at determining whether variation in the trait among members of a population is caused by genetic variation in inherited DNA sequences, environmental exposures in the subjects' lives, or some combination of both of these processes. Twin studies often measure the *concordance rates* of twins with regard to a particular trait or disease of interest. Monozygotic (identical) twins are nearly identical in their DNA, whereas dizygotic (nonidentical) twins share an average of half of their DNA as identical sequences inherited from their parents. If a disease has high heritability, identical twins will be more likely to be either both affected or both unaffected (concordant). However, this assumption is complicated in many diseases. A genetic mutation may not have complete *penetrance,* and environmental conditions may contribute to the development of the disease (e.g., one twin may smoke and the other may not). Furthermore, many diseases are polygenic (i.e., caused by alterations in multiple genes).
Familial aggregation and relative risk	Many diseases run in families, and the degree of clustering within the family can be estimated by comparing the number of disease cases in relatives of patients to the risk of disease in the general population. Difficulties with this approach relate to the fact that, in addition to having many genes in common, family members also share many aspects of a common environment (e.g., diet, nutrition, smoking, infectious organisms, shared socioeconomic factors).
Segregation analyses	Statistical analyses of the patterns of transmission of a disease in families in an attempt to determine the relative likelihood that the disease is caused by a single gene with dominant or recessive inheritance, by multiple genes, or entirely by variation in exposure to risk factors. The observed proportions of offspring who have the trait or disease being evaluated (i.e., the phenotype) are compared with the proportions expected to be found in the general population.
Linkage analysis	A technique used to map a gene responsible for a trait to a specific location on a chromosome. These studies are based on the fact that genes that are located close to each other on the chromosome tend to be inherited together as a unit. As such, these genes are said to be "linked." Because linkage analysis initially requires the use of expensive DNA markers, this was originally only considered justified after finding strong evidence of a genetic basis for a trait with the use of segregation analyses or family aggregation studies. One difficulty with linkage analyses is that many diseases are not caused by a single gene of "major" effect but rather by multiple genes of "minor" effect. In the latter situation, multiple genes each contribute a small amount to the phenotype, disease, or trait. The linkage study approach has little power for detection, whereas association analysis methods may still be quite powerful.
Genome-wide analyses	A genome-wide association study (GWAS) investigates genetic variation across the entire genome simultaneously, with the aim of identifying genetic associations related to a trait or disease of interest. The completion of the Human Genome Project in 2003 and the development of microarray technologies capable of assaying more than half a million single nucleotide polymorphisms have made GWASs possible. This method has the potential to identify the genetic contributions to common diseases. Because the entire genome is analyzed, an important advantage of this approach is that the technique permits the genetics of a disease to be investigated in a nonhypothesis-driven way. In other words, it is not necessary to correctly guess which candidate genes are most interesting to evaluate. A GWAS requires that well-characterized cases and controls be identified. A disadvantage of GWASs is that large clinical sample sizes are required to reduce the likelihood of differences between the cases and controls being observed simply by chance as a result of the hundreds of thousands of multiple statistical tests required to search the entire human genome.

linkage analysis in most instances. In numerous studies conducted during the 1990s, either researchers failed to find any genes or initially positive findings failed to replicate. Linkage studies of large numbers of carefully diagnosed families for complex diseases (e.g., orofacial clefting, in which twin studies had firmly established heritability of 70%) identified at most a tiny fraction of this genetic variation. Mathematical analyses have subsequently shown that the linkage analysis gene-mapping strategy has extremely low statistical power for complex diseases in which each individual susceptibility gene has a relatively small effect on risk (e.g., twofold or less) and in

which there is extensive heterogeneity among different families that have different combinations of susceptibility genes and environmental exposures.[64] Consequently, it is not surprising that linkage analysis has been successfully applied only to syndromic forms of periodontitis (summarized later in this book).

Disappointment over this setback in human disease mapping caused by the initially unrecognized limitations of linkage analysis was short lived. An alternative approach called *association analysis* was also available, although this had been relegated to studies of HLA and a few other markers of special interest during the prime

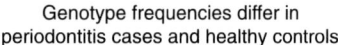

Genotype frequencies differ in
periodontitis cases and healthy controls

8% AA 33% AC 59% CC   50% AA 33% AC 17% CC

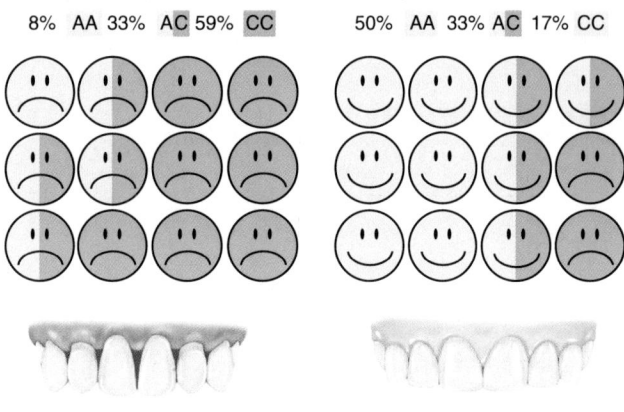

Periodontitis cases   Healthy controls

Fig. 11.1 Case–control design for a genetic association study. Periodontitis cases shown on the left have frequencies for a hypothetic genetic marker of 8% AA, 33% AC, and 59% CC, which are substantially different from genotype frequencies found in healthy periodontal controls of 50% AA, 33% AC, and 17% CC. In this example, the CC genotype is associated with increased risk, because it occurs at a much higher frequency in the disease cases; alternatively, the AA allele is protective, because this variant is much more common in the healthy controls.

time of linkage approaches.[1,7] Mathematical analyses indicated that if we make some reasonable assumptions about the nature of genetic factors in human disease, this method could provide adequate statistical power for finding genes of small to modest effect on risk while requiring only moderately large sample sizes that would be feasible to recruit.[64] There was, however, one major catch: to search the entire genome using the GWAS method, the number of genetic markers needed was several orders of magnitude greater (i.e., 500,000 to 1 million assays needed per subject). Fortunately, advances in molecular assay technologies converged at this time period, and several methods of array-based genotyping provided this capability at an acceptable cost.[61]

How association studies are used to find disease susceptibility genes is illustrated for the case–control design in Fig. 11.1. Association analyses are sometimes referred to as *case–control studies,* although this is only one of several sampling methods that can be used (including studies of families). Genotype frequencies of an inherited DNA variant for a group of periodontitis cases are statistically compared with the frequencies of the variant in a matched group of periodontally healthy control subjects. If the genotype frequencies differ so greatly that the results are unlikely to occur by chance, then we conclude that the genotype that is more common in the cases as compared with the controls is "associated with" increased disease risk. In Fig. 11.1, 59% of the cases have the CC genotype (having inherited a C allele from both of their parents), whereas only 17% of the healthy controls inherited the CC genotype. Therefore this DNA variant could be used to predict periodontitis risk (but not until after the finding was validated in additional independent studies). Conversely, we can also say that the AA genotype is "protective" against disease because it occurs much more often in the healthy controls (50%) as compared with periodontitis cases (8%). Ideally, the cases and healthy controls are matched as closely as possible for race/ethnicity, smoking behavior, age, gender, and so on, so that differences in genotype frequency are likely to be caused by real biologic effects on disease development or progression rather than as artifacts of some kind. For example, it is well known that races and ethnic groups sometimes differ dramatically with regard to genotype frequencies as a result

of their historic isolation in different geographic regions. Consider, for example, a study that had mostly Swedish cases and mostly Italian controls. We know that there are thousands of DNA variants that differ substantially among these populations because of their geographic isolation throughout human history. Few if any of these variants have anything to do with differences in disease risk, but they could falsely appear to be associated because of the failure to carefully match ethnicity in cases and controls. In practice, this is usually not a problem, provided that investigators take reasonable precautions with regard to how cases and controls are selected. It is also now routine practice to use several statistical methods to check for mismatching and then adjust for this during data analysis if it occurs.

The good news is now clearly in: association studies have been a boon for the discovery of inherited genetic variation important for a wide range of complex diseases, including diabetes, cardiovascular disease, metabolic disorders, obesity, and mental illnesses. Reviews show that dozens of genes have been identified with unquestionable statistical confidence for type 2 diabetes alone, and the list continues to grow.[18,73] Most of these genetic polymorphisms with elevated risk are common in the population (i.e., from 5% up to >50%). Although each variant only increases risk slightly (i.e., twofold or less), because the risk alleles are so common they can account for a nontrivial proportion of the occurrence of disease in the population; this is a measure that epidemiologists call *attributable risk.*

An especially attractive aspect of the GWAS approach is that because the entire human genome is searched, we no longer have to depend on prior hypotheses about the disease's molecular pathology. In most GWAS studies, about half of the statistically definitive findings point to genes that experts in the field had no suspicion whatsoever were involved in the disease's etiology. This allows researchers to open up entirely new pathways for investigation that may lead to insights about the disease's biologic mechanism and suggest novel molecular strategies for pharmaceutical or other therapeutic interventions. In more than a few cases, robust GWAS findings implicate regions of the human genome in which no genes appear to be present, thereby highlighting the limitations of our current knowledge of basic genome functions.

Although great progress has been made toward understanding the etiology of many complex human diseases by using GWAS methods, the approach has nevertheless usually failed to account for most of the heritability known to exist for these conditions.[12,43] One study found that well-established nongenetic diabetes risk factors (e.g., gender, smoking, family history, body mass index, blood lipid and glucose levels) were better predictors of risk than a combination of the top 20 genetic markers for this disease.[74] To improve gene-based risk estimates, the missing heritability needs to be found. The emergence of next-generation DNA-sequencing tools may help advance this search. In theory, data from the entire human genome of more than 3 billion bases may enable researchers to identify the less common (i.e., 1% to 5%) genetic variants that are predicted to have individual gene effects of greater magnitude on disease risk (i.e., greater than twofold but less than tenfold) that cannot readily be found with the use of either GWAS or linkage analysis methods.

Genetic Basis for Individual Differences in Disease Risk

As a result of the appropriate focus on the role of bacterial infections in the disease pathogenesis of periodontitis, inherited human genetic variation is often referred to as *host defense* or, somewhat more broadly, *host response.* However, these terms cover only a small portion of the range of gene functions that may be important for

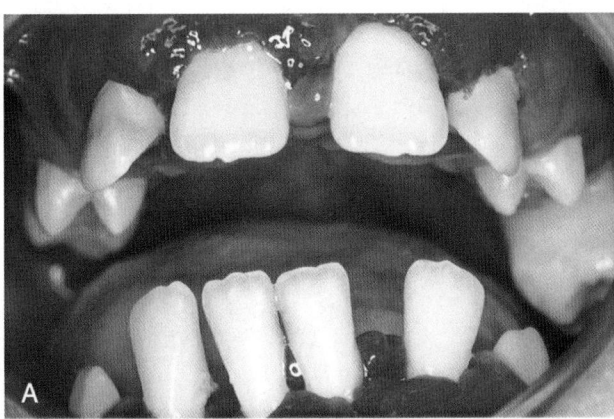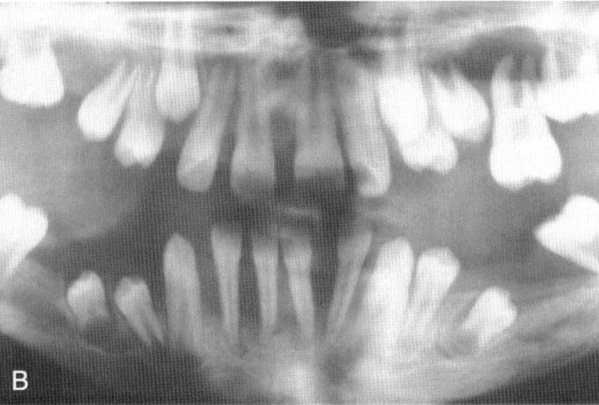

Fig. 11.2 Oral (A) and radiographic (B) appearance of a patient with leukocyte adhesion deficiency. The child was deficient in CD18 (i.e., leukocyte adhesion deficiency type I), which results in absent or severely reduced levels of the β2 integrin molecule. The patient suffered from recurrent infections of the middle ear, the tongue, and the perirectal areas as well as of the periodontium. *(B, From Majorana A, Notarangelo LD, Savoldi E, et al: Leukocyte adhesion deficiency in a child with severe oral involvement.* Oral Surg Oral Med Oral Pathol Oral Radiol Endod *87:691–694, 1999.)*

periodontitis risk. Many additional biologic processes that are not directly related to defenses against or responses to infection by microbial pathogens are also likely to play important roles in determining an individual's susceptibility to this disease.

Periodontitis in Genetic Syndromes and Other Diseases

A number of extremely rare conditions consistently include periodontitis among the array of clinical manifestations that define a syndrome. Many genetic syndromes involve mutations of single genes or larger chromosomal regions. However, a number of syndromes, such as fetal alcohol syndrome, are purely environmental in origin. Some of the syndromes that include periodontitis are caused by mutations in specific genes. For example, mutations in the cathepsin C gene have been shown to cause both Papillon–Lefèvre syndrome and Haim–Munk syndrome as well as some forms of nonsyndromic prepubertal periodontitis, and they may also be associated with a risk of aggressive periodontitis.[55] Periodontitis frequently occurs with some subtypes of Ehlers–Danlos syndrome, Kindler syndrome, Down syndrome (trisomy 21), leukocyte adhesion deficiencies (Fig. 11.2), hypophosphatasia, two types of neutropenia, and aplasia of the lacrimal and salivary glands. A large triracial extended family demonstrated evidence of a single gene that caused both early-onset aggressive periodontitis and dentinogenesis imperfecta.

The gene has been mapped with the use of linkage to a chromosomal region that contains a dentin matrix protein gene.[42] Many of these conditions are so rare that few periodontists see even a single case during a lifetime of practice. However, dentists should be aware that these single-gene conditions exist; they need to be prepared to extend clinical evaluations to close relatives and to seek the assistance of or to refer to appropriately trained genetic counselors or specialists if a patient's medical history or the presentation of multiple symptoms raises the possibility that he or she may be affected. Clinicians can obtain updated information about these conditions by accessing the publicly available Online Mendelian Inheritance in Man database and typing in "periodontitis OR periodontal disease" as the query term.[2] Further research is necessary to determine whether inherited variation in the genes that cause these rare syndromes may also influence the risk of nonsyndromic forms of aggressive or chronic periodontitis.

Genetic Disorders Associated With Periodontitis

Genetic Syndrome With Periodontitis as an Oral Manifestation	Mutated Gene/Genes	Functions of Affected Genes
Chédiak–Higashi syndrome	LYST	LYST encodes for lysosomal trafficking regulator that aids in intracellular transport of materials into lysosomes.
Ehlers–Danlos syndrome, Periodontal types, 1 and 2; EDSPD1 and EDSPD2 (formerly type VIII)	C1R and C1S	Genes C1r and C1s encode serine proteases that are major constituents of human complement subcomponent C1. Complement is part of the innate immune system and is involved in inflammation.
Papillon–Lefèvre syndrome	CTSC	CTSC encodes for cathepsin C, which is a key activator of serine proteases in immune cells, regulating their function.

Nonsyndromic Aggressive and Chronic Periodontitis

In this section, evidence for the association of inherited genetic variation with aggressive and chronic periodontitis will be considered for cases that present without the co-occurrence of anomalies or disorders of other parts of the body or of the affected individual's behavior. Such cases are appropriately classified as *nonsyndromic periodontitis*. This terminology is similar to the way that other human diseases, such as orofacial clefting, have long been recognized as occurring in both syndromic and nonsyndromic forms. The elevated risk of periodontitis that is associated with metabolic conditions (e.g., diabetes, which is addressed elsewhere in this book) is more appropriately considered a comorbidity rather than cause for the designation of a syndrome.

> *"A finding of no statistical significance in a well designed, conceptually sound, adequately powered study testing an important hypothesis is likely to provide more useful information than significance in a study that does not meet these criteria."*[5]

As described previously, twin studies have shown that chronic periodontitis has substantial heritability, and we know that aggressive periodontitis aggregates strongly in families. Because aggressive periodontitis occurs so rarely, it is not feasible to perform a twin study to confirm the heritability of this condition. Neither segregation analyses nor gene-mapping linkage studies are capable of providing reliable information about the genetic etiology of a highly complex disease such as periodontitis. However, large numbers of susceptibility genes have been identified for complex disorders, such as diabetes and cardiovascular disease, using association analysis. It seems reasonable to expect that similar successes could be achieved for periodontitis using this approach. In fact, since the early 2000s several hundred papers have reported associations of nonsyndromic aggressive and chronic periodontitis with polymorphisms in a number of candidate genes. Certain classes of genes (e.g., cytokines) that have long been a focus of attention by immunologists and cell biologists studying pathogenic mechanisms associated with periodontitis have received the most attention. Early reports of relatively weak associations with variation in interleukin-1 (IL-1) genes led to a large number of attempts to replicate and extend these findings. Unfortunately, with few exceptions, association studies of periodontitis have been inadequately powered to detect genetic variation with modest effects on disease risk or progression (i.e., sample sizes that are much too small). In addition, inconsistency with regard to the methods used to classify subjects as periodontal cases versus controls or to quantitatively measure disease severity and extent greatly limit our ability to draw sound conclusions by comparing results reported in different studies.

 KEY FACT

Oral Manifestations of Chédiak–Higashi Syndrome

This autosomal recessive condition occurs due to a mutation of the LYST gene that encodes for a lysosomal trafficking regulator protein. The phagocytosis function of immune cells is drastically affected in these patients, making them significantly prone to infections. As a result, severe forms of periodontitis and early exfoliation of both deciduous and permanent teeth are common findings in these patients.

The reason why association studies of periodontitis have largely failed will be challenging to fully address. The first issue is straightforward and simply a matter of numbers. It is noteworthy that the successes achieved for many complex diseases (e.g., diabetes) with the use of the GWAS mapping approach were based on sample sizes involving thousands of cases and controls, with multiple replications by *independent* teams of investigators. Statistical theory shows that to detect genes of modest effect, these large sample sizes are absolutely

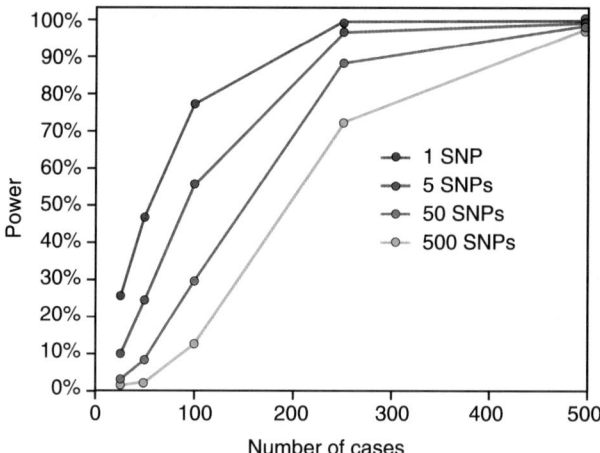

Fig. 11.3 Statistical power estimates are shown for a situation in which we hypothesize that a dominantly transmitted disease susceptibility gene that increases risk twofold and that has an allele frequency in the population of 25% is being mapped by a case–control association study. The lines illustrate the loss of statistical power caused by the requirement to adjust for multiple comparisons when a research study involves the evaluation of not just a single genetic marker but as many as 5, 50, or 500 independent genetic polymorphisms. Although only 100 cases (and 100 controls) may provide sufficient power if only a single marker is being tested, 250 cases and 250 controls are needed if 5 or 50 single nucleotide polymorphisms are assayed; a minimum of 500 cases and 500 controls will be necessary if a study investigates 500 independent genetic markers.

essential. With the use of a statistical power calculator developed for case–control studies,[60] sample sizes required for 80% power are shown in Fig. 11.3 for a study that involves only a single genetic marker as well as for studies that evaluate 5, 50, or 500 independent genetic markers in which the effects of multiple comparisons need to be accommodated. In this example, we assume that the risk gene acts in a dominant manner, with the high-risk allele occurring at a frequency of 25% in the population, and that this allele causes risk among carriers to increase twofold (i.e., a greater effect on risk than observed for many susceptibility alleles found in GWAS studies of other complex diseases).

Many periodontitis association studies reported in the literature involved multiple markers in each publication, and often the same research team reported positive findings for other genes in subsequent papers. Furthermore, because of the difficulties of publishing negative findings (i.e., when no association is found), many research teams working in this area may assay 50 or more genetic markers over the course of their work over several years. Results shown in Fig. 11.3 demonstrate that to obtain 80% power, a study of 50 markers would require more than 200 cases and 200 controls. Even if a research team assays only five SNPs, its study would still require 100 cases and 100 controls to achieve adequate power.

Our search of PubMed in early 2010 using the search term "(periodontal disease OR periodontitis) AND (SNP OR SNPs OR polymorphism OR polymorphisms OR linkage)" identified 311 periodontitis gene association tests with a *P* value of 0.05 or less for at least one statistical test reported. These results are summarized in Fig. 11.4, in which the x-axis indicates the number of cases included in the study; the *P* value for the strongest finding is plotted on the y-axis. When more than one statistical test was reported, only the one with the smallest *P* value is shown in this figure. In some cases, this inflated the actual statistical significance, because investigators rarely adjust their findings for these multiple tests when the findings are reported in a publication. This analysis shows clearly that most

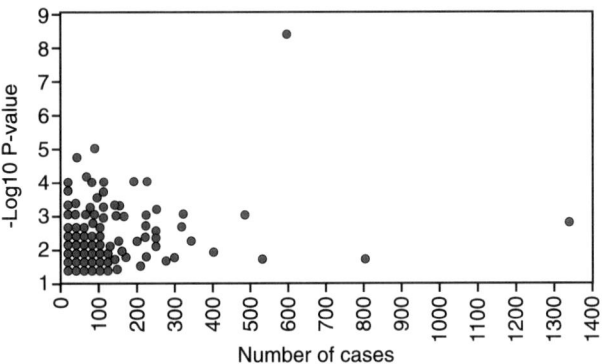

Fig. 11.4 Number of cases and the *P* values reported for 307 gene association tests for aggressive or chronic periodontitis reported in the literature. Only findings with *P* values of 0.05 or less are included. When multiple tests were performed, the strongest association (i.e., the smallest *P* value) is the one used for this presentation.

association findings have been drastically underpowered if periodontitis is assumed to be a complex disease. The majority (66%) of these association reports for chronic and aggressive periodontitis are based on samples of 100 cases or fewer, and 41% are based on fewer than 60 cases. As shown in Fig. 11.3, studies of such small sample size have little power to detect a susceptibility gene that increases risk twofold. Given the added concern about publication bias (i.e., that positive findings are more likely to be accepted for publication), we can have little confidence that even the more statistically significant findings are valid and likely to be independently replicated if they are based on such inadequate samples sizes. With only a few exceptions from GWAS, which are noted later in this chapter, publications since 2010 have continued to involve small numbers of cases and to provide marginal statistical support for association.

Aside from important lessons about how *not* to carry out association studies of a complex disease, there are some tentative conclusions that can be drawn from the data available thus far. Detailed results of our review and manual curation of 298 publications reporting association findings for periodontitis are presented in eTable 11.1 (www.expertconsult.com), and key findings are condensed in Table 11.3.

This summary includes a total of 41 genes plus a combination of the IL-1A and IL-1B genes analyzed jointly. Only genes that had at least two findings classified as "weak" or one finding of association with a "moderate" or "strong" level of support are included in this summary. The technical criteria for these designations are based on a combination of each study's sample size (assuming larger studies are less likely to produce false positives) and the study's *P* value (statistical significance or type I error) as described in the Table 11.3 footnotes and in online supplementary documentation.

Genes in Table 11.3 have usually been evaluated in multiple independent studies for association with either aggressive or chronic periodontitis or both. Occasionally these subtypes of the disease have been pooled together, so it is not possible to determine from the publication whether the association involves primarily one subtype or both. With the exception of only the one GWAS study that has been published for this disease, all association tests reported to date involve the evaluation of candidate genes that were selected on the basis of known or postulated mechanisms of disease pathogenesis.

Ehlers–Danlos Syndromes

Ehlers–Danlos syndromes (EDSs) are connective tissue disorders characterized by joint laxity and skin hyperextensibility, scarring, and bruising. Periodontal EDS (EDSPD; previously EDS VIII) is a subtype with autosomal dominant inheritance with severe periodontal inflammation. Children exhibit extensive gingivitis followed by early-onset periodontitis in teen years leading to attachment and tooth loss. Serious complications including arterial or gastrointestinal ruptures have also been reported.

For example, when bacteria challenge gingival tissue, CD14 binds lipopolysaccharide, and TLR4 plays a key role in pathogen recognition and the activation of innate immunity.[36] Lactotransferrin (LTF) plays an antimicrobial role as the first line of host defense, and it can also neutralize endotoxin and inhibit the induction of nuclear factor-κβ (NF-κβ) in monocytes in response to lipopolysaccharides.[31,75] Myeloperoxidase (MPO) is an oxidative enzyme expressed in polymorphonuclear leukocytes. It is involved in the defense against periodontal bacteria and is also able to mediate inflammatory tissue destruction in periodontal disease.[45] Glutathione S-transferase mu 1 (GSTM1)[10] and *N*-acetyltransferase 2 (NAT2)[34] genes are responsible for the detoxification of a wide range of chemicals, including tobacco carcinogens. HLA complex genes[72] play a central role in the immune system by presenting extracellular peptides that are important for either self-recognition or initiating immune responses to foreign pathogens. The Fcγ receptor genes (FcγRS) encode receptors for the Fc portion of immunoglobulin G, and they are involved in the removal of antigen–antibody complexes from the circulation as well as other antibody-dependent responses.[40] Formyl peptide receptor (FPR1) is a G-protein–coupled receptor of phagocytic cells that interacts with bacterial peptides and that mediates chemotaxis, degranulation, and superoxide production involved in inflammation.[22] Cytokines such as the interleukins (IL-1, IL-2, IL-4, IL-6, IL-10), tumor necrosis factor (TNF), and lymphotoxin-alpha (LTA) play a number of important roles in the immunopathology of periodontal disease.[54] Prostaglandin-endoperoxide synthase (PTGS2), which is also known as *cyclooxygenase-2*, is the key enzyme in prostaglandin biosynthesis. It is regulated by specific stimulatory events, which suggests that it is responsible for the prostanoid biosynthesis involved in inflammation.[25] S100 calcium binding protein A8 (S100A8), which is the light subunit of calprotectin, is also associated with inflammatory diseases, including periodontitis.[37] Fibrinogen (FBG) is an acute-phase protein; FBG levels are elevated during inflammation, and the substance has been associated with cardiovascular disease risk.[65] Vitamin D receptor (VDR)[24] and estrogen receptor (ESR1)[77] are hormone receptors involved in skeletal muscle metabolism, including calcium absorption and bone loss. The matrix metalloproteinases (MMPs) are a group of endogenous proteinases that contribute to the degradation of extracellular and basement membrane components.[23] CDKN2B antisense RNA (CDKN2BAS) is a nonprotein coding gene of unknown function that has also been reported to be associated with coronary heart disease.[68] The one GWAS reported for periodontitis, which is described in detail later in this chapter, revealed a strong association of a glycosyltransferase gene (GLT6D1) with aggressive periodontitis,[70] but there is no clear functional relationship of this gene with periodontal disease pathogenesis.

With few exceptions, there are just as many or more reports in Table 11.3 in which no significant association was found for the gene as there were reports with positive findings. For example, HLA-B has 9 negative reports and 6 weak positive findings. IL-1B has 45 negative reports, 20 weak associations, and 3 moderately supportive

TABLE 11.3   Number of Independent Gene Association Reports for Aggressive Periodontitis and Chronic Periodontitis[a]

Gene Symbol[b]	AGGRESSIVE PERIODONTITIS				CHRONIC PERIODONTITIS		
	None[c]	Weak	Moderate	Strong	None	Weak	Moderate
CD14	3				7	5	
CDKN2BAS		1	1				
ESR1	1	1				2	
FCGR2A	8	1			12	3	
FCGR2B	2	1			2	1	
FCGR3A	7	1			7	3	
FCGR3B	3	8			11	2	2
FGB	1				1	2	
FPR1	4	4	1		2		
GLT6D1				1			
GSTM1			1			2	
HLA-A	3	11			2	5	
HLA-B	8	2			1	4	
HLA-C	8				1	2	
HLA-DQ	1	1			1	1	
HLA-DQB1	3	3			2		
HLA-DR	3	2			2	1	
HLA-DRB1	3	2			2	2	
HLA-DRB3/4/5	1	1			1	1	
IL-10	10	2			10	4	2
IL-1A	17	5			23	5	3
IL-1A.IL-1B	3	1			9	8	4
IL-1B	16	9	1		29	11	2
IL-1RN	10	2	1		10	3	1
IL-2	2				2	2	
IL-4	2	2			7	1	
IL-6	4	3	1		8	11	
IL-6R		1				1	
LTA					1	2	
LTF	1	3				1	
MMP1	2	1			5	3	
MMP9	1	1			1	3	
MPO						2	
NAT2						2	1
NOS3		1				1	
PTGS2			1			2	1
S100A8	1	2				1	
SERPINE1	1					2	1
TGFB1	1				4	3	
TLR4	6	1			12	1	1
TNF	13	1			17	6	
VDR	3	6			7	12	

[a]Only genes with two or more reports of association are included.
[b]Full gene names and a summary of knowledge about the gene's function can be found by typing the gene symbol into the search box at http://www.ncbi.nlm.nih.gov/gene.
[c]Strength of association is defined as follows: weak (P value of <0.05 but ≥0.001; if <50 cases are in the study, then the finding is considered weak, regardless of the P value); moderate (P value of <0.001 but ≥0.0001 or if <101 cases are in the study regardless of P value); strong (P value <0.0001 and >250 cases in the study).

findings. The inconsistency among these findings requires a much deeper analysis to understand what may be going on. One possibility is that genetic variation at the candidate gene is *not* associated with periodontitis. When a large number of studies are performed using a multitude of alternative ways of classifying small numbers of cases versus controls, when multiple alternative statistical analyses are run for the same small data sets, and when there may be a bias against the publication of negative results, then a substantial portion of studies should report positive findings, even if no real association exists. Then again, heterogeneity among studies may be real. The negative studies may differ in terms of the racial or ethnic composition of the subjects, and the findings may be valid for some human populations but not others. Different genetic polymorphisms in the candidate gene may be evaluated in the different studies, and only some of these may actually be associated with disease risk. Different clinical definitions or sources of information (e.g., clinical attachment loss versus bone loss measured from radiographs) may be used to define cases or various quantitative measures may be employed, and these sources of variation may also influence the outcome of association tests. With data limited to mostly small studies, it is not currently possible to definitively determine which of these potential explanations applies to most of the findings shown in Table 11.3.

CLINICAL CORRELATION

Papillon–Lefèvre Syndrome and Dental Implants

Caused by a mutation in the cathepsin C gene, this syndrome is characterized by advanced periodontitis affecting both deciduous and permanent dentition and palmar plantar hyperkeratosis affecting palms and soles. Patients become edentulous very early in life. Limited scientific evidence in the form of case reports indicates that edentulous patients with this syndrome can be successfully treated with dental implant–supported restorations.

Fig. 11.4 shows that a handful of periodontitis association studies have been reported that approach the sample size needed for complex diseases with more than 400 cases.[17,39,46,47,68,69] This includes the GWAS in which more than 322,825 SNP genetic markers were evaluated for association with the risk of aggressive periodontitis.[70] In the GWAS, statistical testing was performed in sequence for three independent sets of samples with a total of 438 cases and 1320 controls. Interestingly, this relatively powerful analysis failed to yield significant support for the usual suspect candidate genes shown in Table 11.3, after adjusting for the large number of hypotheses tested in the analysis. Instead, several novel chromosomal regions and candidate genes were implicated, with among the strongest being a glycosyltransferase gene (GLT6D1), one of several glycosyltransferases in the human genome. This had an unadjusted P value of 0.000000006. However, the P value was reduced by three orders of magnitude to 0.000006 after accounting for the effects of gender, smoking, and diabetes. The adjusted P value indicates that we should expect to see a difference in genotype frequency of this magnitude by chance alone about 1 out of 166,666 times under the null hypothesis of no association with disease risk. This may seem to be strong evidence for rejection of the null hypothesis, but this adjusted finding is actually only a marginal statistical significance in the context of a GWAS. In fact, this sometimes occurs by chance alone in the absence of a valid association, because this study involved testing more than 300,000 genetic markers. Because there is no obvious functional connection of this gene with what we currently know about the pathogenesis of periodontitis (the protein is thought to play a role in signaling in development), it may be tempting to further downplay

the finding's significance. However, experience with GWAS studies of other complex diseases has shown that, quite often, valid gene associations are discovered in pathways that experts in the field did not previously realize were even related to the disease's biology. This makes such discoveries all the more valuable, assuming that they are definitively and independently replicated, because they offer the potential of revealing completely new avenues for further exploration at the cellular and molecular levels and because they potentially may also provide novel targets for therapeutic interventions.

During the years since the report of a strong association of aggressive periodontitis with GLT6D1, it has been interesting that no replications of this finding have been reported. The first genome-wide study that focused on chronic periodontitis included 4504 European Americans, with 43% having moderate chronic periodontitis and 17% having severe chronic periodontitis.[16] No genome-wide significant associations were found in this large sample, with no support whatsoever for the much-studied periodontitis candidate genes IL-1A, IL-1B, IL-1RN, IL-4, IL-6, IL-10, CD14, FCGR2A, MMP1, TLR4, TNF, and VDR. However, intriguing suggestive evidence was found supporting the role of cellular immune response, nervous system, and cytokine signaling pathways. By broadening the phenotype, a subset of these subjects were also analyzed using genome-wide SNP data for periodontal pathogen colonization, but again only statistically suggestive results were obtained with this smaller sample.[15] A large-scale replication analysis of 23 much-studied candidate genes in 600 aggressive periodontitis cases and 1448 control subjects of German ethnicity found support only for SNPs in IL-10, but this association was not replicated in 1437 chronic periodontitis cases of German ethnicity.[67] Several GWAS of periodontitis have now been completed for moderately large sample sizes, and the results are sobering.[53,66] No statistically strong, replicated associations have been found in any of these studies. Furthermore, in two large cohort studies, DNA sequencing of the coding regions of nearly all genes (exome sequencing) also failed to reveal any rare variants with a statistically significant association with chronic periodontitis.[33]

It is clear from these findings that large-scale association studies, possibly involving family-based designs and searches for rare high-risk variants, will be needed to more fully elucidate the role of genetics in periodontal disease. From what we now know, it appears increasingly likely that the high heritability estimated for chronic periodontitis is likely attributable to a large number of inherited DNA variations in more than 100 or possibly 500 or more different genes. This is the genetic architecture that we know underlies other highly heritable traits such as height, and this discovery has important implications and places limitations on the use of genetic variation for tests to predict risk, as will be addressed later in this chapter.

Challenges and Opportunities for the Future

The classification of disease used for research studies is an especially difficult challenge to be faced if we are to benefit fully from the opportunities offered by the genomics revolution.[59] If we cannot agree which subjects in a study are affected by disease, by a particular subtype of disease, how severely they are affected, or how quantitative measures related to disease should be obtained and analyzed, then the chances of making progress will be low, regardless of how advanced our molecular or bioinformatics technologies become. This problem is important for all kinds of research, not only genetics, and the issue of diagnosis is addressed elsewhere in this book. However, genetics may have a unique role to contribute toward solving this dilemma. This may best be illustrated by an example from the early 1980s, in which medical geneticists and oncologists could not agree about the classification of the disease neurofibromatosis

(NF). "Splitters" argued for up to a dozen different etiologic subtypes, whereas "lumpers" suggested that there may be only a single disease with a lot of variation among individuals as a result of differences in environmental exposures and variation in "genetic background" (a term that encompasses the cumulative influence of all other genes distributed throughout the genome in addition to the "major gene"). It had been discovered in research conducted during earlier decades that NF was transmitted in families as a single dominant gene, but the question remained as to how many different genes were involved (locus heterogeneity). Furthermore, even if only one gene was involved, it was possible that different mutations caused unique patterns of signs and symptoms (allelic heterogeneity). The controversy was largely resolved by the discovery of the NF1[41] and NF2[71] genes. After these genes were identified, DNA testing could distinguish individual patients, and the diagnostic classification controversies were resolved. In hindsight, it became clear that the clustering of signs and symptoms fell into two major categories among different types of families and depended on which NF1 or NF2 mutation was involved and on what kind of gene mutation was involved. Although such gene-based clarity is unlikely for a complex multigenic condition such as periodontitis, the potential exists that subtypes of patients may eventually be classified more effectively by examining their DNA to see what kinds of susceptibility genes they inherited.

To move toward this desired outcome, however, we need to use the best strategies available today to classify research subjects into categories such as cases versus controls. Alternatively, we can attempt to use quantitative measures of bone loss or attachment loss to classify research subjects along a more continuous gradient that ranges from persons with extremely healthy periodontium with little or no signs of disease to those with tooth loss and high measures of pocket depth and attachment loss in remaining teeth. Family studies have numerous advantages in genetics; for these designs, the use of a quantitative measures approach is especially attractive. When searching for gene associations in unrelated cases and controls, we can decide to select only subjects who are clearly affected as cases and compare them with control subjects who clearly are periodontally healthy. When studying families, however, one has to assign a disease status to all of the family members to fully make use of all of the information in the biologic unit. We may initially recruit the family on the basis of an unambiguous case known as the *proband* (i.e., the subject who makes the family eligible for inclusion in the study), but the handling of parents, siblings, and other close relatives who may be neither clearly periodontally healthy nor clearly diseased is not easy to determine. For example, if we establish a threshold and require that two or more teeth have a minimum of 4 mm of attachment loss for subjects to be classified as affected, then how we handle family members who are borderline becomes the challenge. For example, siblings of the proband may have several teeth with 3 mm of attachment loss in addition to one tooth with 6 mm of loss. Such subjects are close to but not quite over the threshold. They are neither clearly healthy nor clearly diseased, and this makes them problematic for categorical data analyses that require them to be classified as cases versus controls.

One aspect of the diagnosis challenge that is especially poorly understood is how and why different teeth are affected by periodontitis. Dentists have long recognized that incisors and first molars are more likely to be affected during early-onset disease, but it is not straightforward to incorporate this information into threshold disease definitions. One way to begin to address the problem of variation among teeth is to apply multivariate methods, such as principal components analysis, as was done in a study of aggressive periodontitis.[14] This method maximizes the proportion of the total variation in attachment loss among all 28 teeth explained by a limited number of master

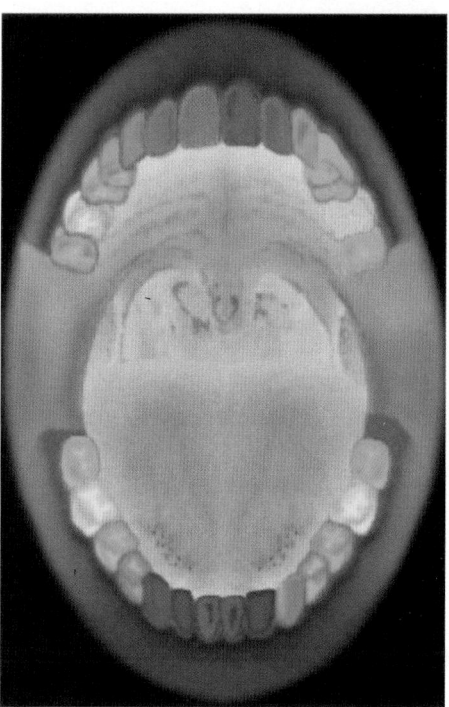

Fig. 11.5 Illustration of the similarities and differences among different kinds of teeth with regard to the frequency and severity of attachment loss observed in early-onset aggressive periodontitis patients and their unaffected family members with the use of the principal components analysis method.[14]

variables called *principal components.* In this study, three principal components explained 77.8% of the total variance. The results are displayed in Fig. 11.5, with color intensities being used to help visualize the patterns of correlation among different tooth types. Mixtures of red, green, and blue are "painted" onto the teeth, with each color's intensity adjusted according to the tooth's relative "weight" calculated for each of the principal components. This quantitative analysis shows how attachment loss is correlated among different kinds of teeth. First molar teeth are consistently painted yellow by their principal components scores; these teeth are very different from all of the other teeth with regard to their patterns of attachment loss. There is a gradual change in the patterns of attachment loss for the other teeth that extend out from the central incisors (magenta) to the lateral incisors (purple), the cuspids (blue), the premolars (blue green), and the second molars (green). In addition to generally exploring patterns of periodontal disease dispersed in the geography of the mouth, because these are studies conducted in families, we can also use genetic epidemiologic methods to validate and compare alternative measures of disease.

Specifically, we can calculate heritability for different quantitative variables (e.g., simple mean attachment loss averaged across all teeth or averaged for specific groups of teeth) as well as for more complex variables like these principal components. In the study of aggressive periodontitis illustrated in Fig. 11.5, the principal component most heavily weighted on the first molars had a heritability of 30%, which was actually slightly higher than the 26% heritability estimated for a simple mean of attachment loss in the first molars. By using heritability and other genetic measures such as association with specific inherited polymorphisms, it may be possible to refine diagnostic and disease classification systems by aligning these according to subgroups of subjects that share homogeneous etiologies. Another example of moving beyond simply classifying subjects as cases versus controls but using principal component analysis to

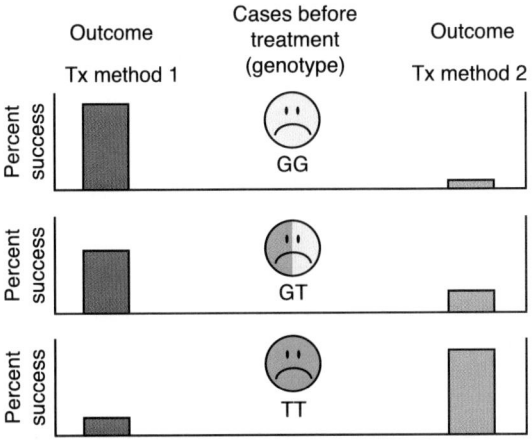

Outcome of different treatment methods predicted by genotype

Outcome
Tx method 1

Cases before
treatment
(genotype)

Outcome
Tx method 2

GG

GT

TT

Fig. 11.6 Inherited genetic variation determines treatment success. Individuals who inherited the GG or GT genotypes at a gene involved in a biologic pathway related to either the underlying disease susceptibility mechanisms or to the body's response to the therapy have very good chances for success with treatment method 1 *(Tx method 1)* but poor prognoses with treatment method 2 *(Tx method 2),* whereas individuals with the TT genotype respond positively to treatment method 2 only.

combine multiple measures of disease such as levels of pathogens and inflammatory markers was reported using a GWAS design.[56] The results of this more complex approach to the phenotype pointed to several novel genes of potential interest that now require independent replication.

Learning from the experience of other complex diseases, Sir Isaac Newton famously remarked in 1676: "What Descartes did was a good step. You have added much several ways ... If I have seen a little further it is by standing on the shoulders of Giants."

Although there remains some enthusiasm for further GWAS studies, as noted previously, even the most successful GWAS results (e.g., those that have been obtained for type 2 diabetes) have failed to identify most of the genetic variation responsible for the disease. The discovery of so many gene associations related to risk of type 2 diabetes accounts for a small fraction of the disease's heritability.[12] To track down the missing genetic variation, a great deal of attention is now turning to whole genome DNA-sequencing methods that will be available at low cost in the coming years. Sequencing methods also expand the ability to measure gene expression in various tissues. These data, in combination with the ever-increasing availability of proteomic assays, will challenge investigators with huge quantities of information. Aside from generating the many gigabytes of data involved in this technology, the greatest challenges of "systems biology" may lie in developing the bioinformatics tools needed to sift through and identify the key bits of information that are important for advancing our knowledge from among the vast rising sea of biologic data pouring out of our laboratories.[4]

Strategies for improving our understanding of the genetics of periodontitis as well as for increasing the possibilities for the translation of this knowledge to benefit patients in the clinic are being mapped out today by teams of geneticists, clinicians, and information scientists who are currently focused on major medical conditions. By continuing to learn from the experiences of these early genomic explorers, it is reasonable to hope that dental researchers will be able to avoid some of their mistakes and follow the quickest path to advances in knowledge about diseases of interest.

Precision Dentistry: Using Genetics for Personalized Treatment

Pharmacogenomics and Individualized Dentistry

If individuals differ in susceptibility to a disease, especially if underlying the superficial signs and symptoms of a disease there really are etiologically distinct subtypes of disease pathogenesis, then the traditional medical model of "one size fits all" treatment may not be optimal. As shown in Fig. 11.6, cases of disease (as illustrated by circles with unhappy faces) may differ with regard to genotype for a gene that determines which treatment works best for each individual. Some cases inherited G alleles from both their mother and their father and thus have a GG genotype, whereas others have a GT or TT genotype.

The gene may distinguish between different subtypes of disease etiology or pathogenesis, or it might code for an enzyme, transporter, or receptor important for the metabolism of a therapeutic drug and have nothing directly to do with disease susceptibility. In the example illustrated in this figure, treatment method 1 *(Tx method 1)* has a high success rate when it is provided to subjects with the GG or GT genotypes, but it usually fails for cases with the TT genotype. TT genotypes experience much better outcomes when provided with treatment method 2 *(Tx method 2),* but this method often fails for subjects with the GG and GT genotypes. Sometimes concerns about severe side effects that limit the use of a therapy rather than differences in efficacy and risk of side effects can also be genetically determined. If clinicians are not aware of the relationships between these genotypes and treatment success or side effects, it would appear that neither treatment is consistently effective. Clinicians would be forced to use a trial-and-error approach, first trying one method and then switching to the other if the first method fails. At best, this causes unnecessary expense and does not provide an optimal quality of care. Furthermore—and especially for deadly diseases such as cancer—precious time may be lost in halting the advance of the disease; by the time the clinician discovers an individual's best treatment, it may be too late. This strategy of individualized medicine is already being practiced for an increasing number of diseases.[9,21]

In dentistry, a test based on inherited genetic variation at the interleukin-1 alpha (IL-1α) and IL-1β cytokine genes was proposed as being able to predict the risk, progression, and severity of periodontitis. The test has been commercialized and has gone through multiple versions (PST, PerioPredict, and today's version is called ILUSTRA). Although specific numbers are not available, the test does not appear to be widely used yet. A number of reviews of the large number of studies of the IL-1 gene polymorphisms (see eTable 11.1 [online] and Table 11.3) indicate that genetic variation at these loci may be associated with, at most, a modest effect on disease risk.[26,54] In 2007 Huynh-Ba and colleagues concluded that "there is insufficient evidence to establish if a positive IL-1 genotype status contributes to progression of periodontitis or treatment outcomes."[26] A similar lack of supporting evidence for the use of IL-1 genetic testing to predict implant success has also been reported.[3,27] A more recent meta-analysis of the available data suggested that these much-studied IL-1 polymorphisms have a small (odds ratio, ≈1.5) but significant effect on periodontitis risk, although only for chronic periodontitis in white populations.[32] However, it is essential to emphasize that because heritability for chronic periodontitis is estimated to be 50%,[49] the small effect of the IL-1 polymorphisms makes up at most a tiny fraction of the genetic component of risk for this disease (which remains missing, as discussed previously).

Candidate Genes Possibly Related to Risk of Chronic or Aggressive Periodontitis

- Interleukin (IL)-1 gene cluster (IL-1A, IL-1B, IL-1 receptor antagonist), IL-4, IL-6, and IL-10.
- TNF-alpha
- Leukocyte receptors for the constant (Fc) part of immunoglobulin (FcγR)
- Vitamin D receptor
- Pattern recognition receptor genes (TLRs, cluster of differentiation [CD]-14)
- Matrix metalloproteinase (MMP)-1

As the benefits of individualized or personalized treatments that are optimally matched to the genome of each patient have been demonstrated for cancer and increasing numbers of other human diseases, interest has grown in applying this approach to dentistry.[35,63] The first major study that attempted to develop guidelines for individualized treatment has been reported.[19] This study involved 5117 adults between the ages of 34 and 55 years with no prior diagnosis of early periodontitis who were followed retrospectively for 16 years. The aim was to evaluate whether only a subset of high-risk patients really benefits from two versus only one preventive visit per year to avert tooth loss. The risk factors that were tested were smoking, diabetes, and the IL-1 composite genotype. The authors of the study concluded that all three risk factors predict which patients benefit from two preventive visits. They proposed the use of the IL-1 genetic test[28] to detect the IL-1 composite genotype, which along with smoking and diabetic status was looked at as a risk factor for progressive periodontitis. The study claimed that by reducing the preventive dental visits to one per year in so-called low-risk patients, $4.8 billion would be saved annually. However, an independent reanalysis of the findings[13] showed that of the three assessed risk factors, only diabetes and smoking had statistically significant effects on tooth extraction risk. This conclusion was supported by an independent critical commentary by a leading expert in the field of epidemiology.[29] Therefore it is clear that we lack consistent evidence to demonstrate the scientific validity or clinical utility, of the IL-1 genetic test that is commercially available as a periodontitis risk prediction tool.[28] This first major attempt to use a genetic test in mainstream dentistry continues to be an area of great controversy, and dentists will need to remain aware of the scientific consensus regarding such tests as these emerge in the future so that they can accurately advise patients on their use and limitations.

As genetic testing becomes widespread, especially if it is marketed through direct-to-consumer models, increasing responsibility will fall on dentists to fully understand and counsel their patients about the implications of test results for their treatment options and their risk of developing various dental diseases in the future. Tests for diseases of the oral cavity may likely combine inherited polymorphisms with oral microbial profiles, and they might also include assays of gene expression or proteomic data measured in saliva or other oral tissues. Few dentists practicing today have been educated to prepare themselves for these future challenges. This major shortfall of knowledge urgently needs to be addressed. This can be done by continually educating today's dental professionals about advances in knowledge of human genetics and the uses and potential misuses of genetic testing; by establishing multidisciplinary teams of health practitioners in which dentists work closely with genetics counselors and medical geneticists; or by combining these approaches.

Acknowledgments

We acknowledge the support provided by the National Institutes of Health's National Institute of Dental and Craniofacial Research grants 5R01DE016057 and 5R01DE018635 and the Foundation of the University of Medicine and Dentistry of New Jersey.

 A Case Scenario is found on the companion website www.expertconsult.com.

References

 References for this chapter are found on the companion website www.expertconsult.com.

CHAPTER 12

Smoking and Periodontal Disease

Philip M. Preshaw | Leandro Chambrone | Richard Holliday

The Smoking Epidemic

Smoking is highly prevalent and can be considered an epidemic in both developed and developing nations. Smoking rates, however, have seen marked declines since the 1980s. Global estimated daily tobacco smoking prevalence rates (in individuals >15 years old) reduced from 41.2% in 1980 to 31.1% in 2012 for men and from 10.6% (1980) to 6.2% (2012) for women.[96] Despite this development, with population growth, the number of daily smokers worldwide has actually increased to just short of a billion people in 2012, upholding tobacco smoking's position as a major public health threat. Developed countries had their highest prevalence rates in those aged 30 to 34 years, whereas in developing countries the greatest prevalence was among those aged 45 to 49 years. The highest prevalence rates (male) are now often seen in developing countries (e.g., Bangladesh [44.4%], China [40.1%], Indonesia [57%]), although several developed countries also have similarly high rates (e.g., Russia [50.1%], Greece [40.8%], Japan [35.3%]).[96] The overall daily smoking prevalence rates for the United States were 15.5% in 2012 (17.2% for males, 14.3% for females) and for the United Kingdom were 21.6% (23% for males, 20.1% for females).[96] Canada, Iceland, Mexico, and Norway all achieved reductions of greater than 50% in male and female smoking prevalence rates between 1980 and 2012.[96] Interestingly, Sweden is the only country with more female than male smokers (males, 12.3%; females, 14.8%) which can likely be attributed to snus (oral tobacco) use.[96]

> **A Global Perspective**
> - As many as 6.25 trillion cigarettes are smoked annually across the globe.[96]
> - Tobacco kills 6 million people each year.[147]
> - Only 15% of people worldwide have access to smoking cessation services.[147]
> - About 18% of people worldwide are protected by smoke-free laws.[147]

Smoking is harmful to almost every organ in the body and is associated with multiple diseases that reduce life expectancy and quality of life. Diseases associated with smoking include lung cancer, heart disease, stroke, emphysema, bronchitis, and cancers of the oral cavity, bladder, kidney, stomach, liver, and cervix. Approximately half of long-term smokers will die early as a result of smoking, and those who die before the age of 70 years will lose an average of 20 years of life.[37] Most deaths from smoking are due to lung cancer, chronic obstructive pulmonary disease, and coronary heart disease.

Tobacco smoke contains thousands of noxious chemicals, and it comprises a gaseous phase and a solid (particulate) phase. The gas phase contains carbon monoxide, ammonia, formaldehyde, hydrogen cyanide, and many other toxic and irritant compounds, including more than 60 known carcinogens such as benzo(a)pyrene and dimethylnitrosamine. The particulate phase includes nicotine, "tar" (itself made up of many toxic chemicals), benzene, and benzo(a)-pyrene. Tar is inhaled with the smoke. In its condensate form, it is the sticky brown substance that stains fingers and teeth yellow and brown. Nicotine, which is an alkaloid, is found within the tobacco leaf and evaporates when the cigarette is lighted. It is quickly absorbed in the lungs, and it reaches the brain within 10 to 19 seconds. Nicotine is highly addictive. It causes a rise in blood pressure, increased heart and respiratory rates, and peripheral vasoconstriction.

CLINICIAN'S CORNER

Smokeless Tobacco

Smokeless tobacco products are becoming increasingly popular and exist in many different forms. Tobacco can be ground/grated and presented with salt and water as "moist snuff," which is usually delivered as a small tea-bag-like sachet placed under the lip. Alternatively, tobacco can be ground to a powder ("dry snuff") that is inhaled into the nasal cavity. Finally, tobacco can be coarsely cut (chewing tobacco) and placed into the cheek. Numerous smokeless tobacco varieties are popular in South Asian communities. The International Agency for Research on Cancer classifies smokeless tobacco as a cause of mouth, esophageal, and pancreatic cancer.[64]

Snus (or Swedish snuff) is a special type of smokeless tobacco that is popular in Sweden and increasingly the United States. It is banned across the rest of Europe. The manufacturers claim to use a special process to lower the levels of carcinogens in the product. Studies have shown a link to pancreatic cancer but not to mouth or lung cancer.[81]

All dental patients must be asked about their smoking status or tobacco usage. Current smoking status is the minimal information that must be recorded (e.g., "Patient is currently smoking *X* cigarettes per day"), but the importance of cumulative exposure to cigarette smoke means that it is more appropriate to record pack-years of

BOX 12.1   Challenge of Assessing Smoking Status

Current Smokers

Ask about current smoking and past smoking. Many smokers are trying to quit, and therefore simply asking how many cigarettes they are smoking today may not give an accurate assessment of their lifetime exposure (e.g., a patient who is currently smoking 5 cigarettes per day may have been smoking 40 cigarettes per day until yesterday, when he or she decided to cut down). Try to get an indication of the patient's approximate level of smoking (e.g., the average number of cigarettes per day for a certain number of years). It can also be useful to calculate the number of pack-years:

$$\text{Pack-years} = \text{Number of packs smoked per day} \times \text{Number of years of smoking}$$

In other words, 1 pack-year is the cumulative exposure that corresponds with the smoking of 1 pack of 20 cigarettes per day for 1 year. For example, a smoker who has smoked 20 cigarettes per day for 15 years has 15 pack-years of smoking.

Former Smokers

Ask patients about their past smoking. Patients with periodontitis may have a significant smoking history that has had an impact on their periodontal status, even if they no longer smoke. Former smokers should always be congratulated for their achievement in quitting, but it is also very important to document the following:
- How much they used to smoke
- How many years they smoked
- When they quit

Is the Patient's Response Accurate?

The inaccurate or false reporting of smoking status is common; patients will tell you what they think you want to hear, or they may be embarrassed because they have not managed to cut down yet. Many patients report smoking 20 cigarettes per day, because this is the number of cigarettes in a pack in most countries, so 20 may be a convenient response rather than an accurate response. Cultural factors may also influence responses.[128]

When Is a Smoker Not a Smoker?

- Smokers have smoked ≥100 cigarettes in their lifetime and currently smoke.
- Former smokers have smoked ≥100 cigarettes in their lifetime and do not currently smoke.
- Nonsmokers have not smoked ≥100 cigarettes in their lifetime and do not currently smoke.

It must be noted that many periodontal research studies have not used these definitions, and this can sometimes make it difficult to interpret the studies, particularly in the context of what constitutes a former smoker. For example, from an exposure point of view, there is a big difference between someone who smoked 5 cigarettes per day for 10 years and who quit 30 years ago as compared with someone who smoked 40 cigarettes per day for 20 years and quit 6 months ago. It is always best in clinical practice to gather full information about each patient's smoking history.

TABLE 12.1   Effects of Smoking on Gingivitis and Periodontitis

Periodontal Disease	Effects of Smoking
Gingivitis	↓ Gingival inflammation and bleeding on probing
Periodontitis	↑ Prevalence and severity of periodontal destruction ↑ Pocket depth, attachment loss, and bone loss ↑ Rate of periodontal destruction ↑ Prevalence of severe periodontitis ↑ Tooth loss ↑ Prevalence with increased number of cigarettes smoked per day ↓ Prevalence and severity with smoking cessation

↓, Decreased; ↑, increased.

and saliva cotinine concentrations of less than 2 ng/mL, unless they are passive smokers. Biochemical validation of nonsmoking uses cotinine levels of 1 to 6 ng/mL to confirm nonsmoking status depending on race/ethnicity.[11]

Smoking is a major risk factor for periodontitis, and it affects the prevalence, extent, and severity of disease. In addition, smoking has an adverse impact on the clinical outcome of nonsurgical and surgical therapy as well as the long-term success of implant placement. With 41.9% of periodontitis cases in the United States reported as being *attributable* to smoking (discussed next),[139] it is essential to understand the impact of smoking on the initiation, progression, and management of the disease. This chapter discusses the effects of smoking on the prevalence, severity, etiology, and pathogenesis of periodontal disease as well as its impact on treatment. The reader is referred to several excellent reviews of the topic for detailed results of specific studies.[1,27,54,70,71,97,98,112,140,145]

Effects of Smoking on the Prevalence and Severity of Periodontal Diseases

Gingivitis

Controlled clinical studies have demonstrated that, in human models of experimental gingivitis, the development of inflammation in response to plaque accumulation is reduced in smokers as compared with nonsmokers (Table 12.1).[19,33] In addition, cross-sectional studies have consistently demonstrated that smokers present with less gingival inflammation than nonsmokers.[12,13,17,105,106] These data suggest that smokers have a decreased expression of clinical inflammation in the presence of plaque accumulation as compared with nonsmokers. The microbiologic, immunologic, and physiologic factors that may account for this observation are discussed later.

Periodontitis

Although gingival inflammation in smokers appears to be reduced in response to plaque accumulation as compared with nonsmokers, an overwhelming body of evidence points to smoking as a major risk factor for increasing the prevalence and severity of periodontal destruction. Multiple cross-sectional and longitudinal studies have demonstrated that pocket depth, attachment loss, and alveolar bone loss are more prevalent and severe in patients who smoke as compared with nonsmokers.[70,71,112,140] An assessment of the relationship between cigarette smoking and periodontitis was performed in more than 12,000 dentate individuals who were more than 18 years old as part of the Third National Health and Nutrition Examination Survey.[139] Periodontitis was defined as one or more sites with clinical attachment loss of 4 mm or greater and pocket depth of 4 mm or greater. Smoking

smoking (Box 12.1). Biochemical tests can also be used to assess smoking status, including exhaled carbon monoxide and the measurement of cotinine (the major metabolite of nicotine) in serum, saliva, or urine. Cotinine is measured in preference to nicotine because the half-life of nicotine is short (≈1 to 2 hours),[104] whereas that of cotinine is approximately 20 hours.[67] Plasma and saliva cotinine concentrations in smokers are approximately 100 ng/mL[11,39] and the urine concentration is approximately 1200 ng/mL.[76] Nonsmokers usually have plasma status was defined with the use of criteria established by the Centers for Disease Control and Prevention (see Box 12.1). Of the more than 12,000 individuals studied, 9.2% had periodontitis; this represented approximately 15 million cases of periodontitis in the United States. On average, smokers were four times as likely to have periodontitis as compared with persons who had never smoked after adjusting for age, gender, race/ethnicity, education, and income/poverty ratio. Former smokers were 1.7 times more likely to have periodontitis than persons who had never smoked. This study also demonstrated a dose–response relationship between cigarettes smoked per day and the odds of having periodontitis. In subjects smoking 9 or fewer cigarettes per day, the odds for having periodontitis were 2.8, whereas subjects who smoked 31 or more cigarettes per day were almost six times more likely to have periodontitis. In former smokers, the odds of having periodontitis declined with the number of years since quitting. These data indicated that approximately 42% of periodontitis cases (6.4 million cases) in the U.S. adult population were attributable to current smoking and that approximately 11% (1.7 million cases) were attributable to former smoking. These data highlight the serious threat to dental public health posed by cigarette smoking and raise questions about the best methods for managing periodontitis in patients who smoke (Box 12.2).

These data are consistent with the findings of other cross-sectional studies performed in the United States and Europe. The odds ratio for periodontitis in current smokers has been estimated to range from as low as 1.5 to as high as 7.3 compared to nonsmokers, depending on the observed severity of periodontitis.[98] A meta-analysis of data from six such studies involving 2361 subjects indicated that current smokers were almost three times more likely to have severe periodontitis than nonsmokers.[97] The detrimental impact of long-term smoking on the periodontal and dental status of older adults has been clearly demonstrated. Older adult smokers are approximately three times more likely to have severe periodontal disease,[10,80] and the number of years of tobacco use is a significant factor in tooth loss, coronal root caries, and periodontal disease.[68,69]

Smoking has also been shown to affect periodontal disease severity in younger individuals. Cigarette smoking is associated with increased severity of generalized aggressive periodontitis in young adults,[127] and those who smoke are 3.8 times more likely to have periodontitis as compared with nonsmokers.[48] Longitudinal studies have demonstrated that young individuals who smoke more than 15 cigarettes per day showed the highest risk for tooth loss.[60] In addition, smokers are more than six times as likely as nonsmokers to demonstrate continued attachment loss.[65] Over a 10-year period, bone loss has been reported to be twice as rapid in smokers as in nonsmokers[20] and to proceed more rapidly even in the presence of excellent plaque control.[14] Less information is available about the effects of cigar and pipe smoking, but it appears that effects similar to those of cigarette smoking are observed with these forms of tobacco use.[5,40,41,78] The prevalence of moderate and severe periodontitis and the percentage of teeth with more than 5 mm of attachment loss were most severe in current cigarette smokers, but cigar and pipe smokers showed a severity of disease that was intermediate between that of current cigarette smokers and nonsmokers.[5] Tooth loss is also increased among cigar and pipe smokers as compared with nonsmokers.[78]

Former smokers have less risk for periodontitis than current smokers but more risk than nonsmokers, and the risk for periodontitis decreases with the increasing number of years since quitting smoking.[139] This suggests that the negative effects of smoking on the host are reversible with smoking cessation and therefore that smoking cessation programs must be an integral component of periodontal education and therapy (Box 12.3, Table 12.2). Several tobacco intervention approaches can be used when helping the patient deal with the physiologic factors (i.e., nicotine withdrawal symptoms) and the psychological factors associated with smoking cessation (Box 12.4).[99,116] Electronic cigarettes have also emerged and are being used by many smokers to help them quit (Box 12.5). However, the effects on oral health are yet to be established.

BOX 12.2   Should We Change How We Manage Periodontal Disease?

Fact 1: Smoking is a major risk factor for periodontal disease.
Fact 2: According to the literature, smoking may be responsible for more than half of periodontitis cases among adults in the United States.[139]
Fact 3: Depending on the study, approximately 10% to 15% of adults in most populations examined have advanced periodontitis.

Questions

- Would there be a benefit at the population level for periodontal health if all smokers in the population quit smoking today?
- Would dental professionals be able to more successfully manage periodontitis in smokers if we focused more on smoking cessation as a primary treatment strategy for managing peripdontitis?

These questions are intended to be controversial. It is clear that smoking has a huge deleterious impact on periodontal status, and smoking cessation *must* be a core part of periodontal treatment in patients with periodontitis who smoke. The answer to the first question is almost certainly a resounding yes, but this probably will never be able to be tested. The answer to the second question is more difficult. Certainly smokers with periodontitis must be educated about the harm that they are causing to their periodontal tissues, and they must be encouraged and helped to quit smoking. Treatment outcomes are improved among smokers who quit as compared with those who continue to smoke.[109]

Two Final Points (These Are Contentious and Designed to Stimulate Discussion.)

- If more than half of the cases of periodontitis are attributable to smoking, then patients who smoke may be better served if dental professionals put more than half of their efforts into treating these patients via smoking cessation treatments (as opposed to other forms of periodontal therapy). Discuss!
- It is absurd for smokers in the Western world to worry about anything except stopping smoking.[103]

Beyond E-Cigarettes

The popularity of e-cigarettes took most people by surprise. But what's next?

"Heat-Not-Burn" Tobacco Products

These products heat tobacco to ~500°C, producing an inhalable aerosol.[24] Although not a new idea, they have received recent attention. One manufacturer introduced a product into the Japanese market in 2015, which has been popular, with the media reporting sales outstripping demand.

Water Pipes (Hookah, Shisha)

Popular in some communities, these are likely to carry significant negative health risks. A good summary is produced by the National Center for Smoking Cessation and Training (NCSCT).[94]

Nicotine Gels

These gels allow nicotine to be absorbed through the skin. Currently they are not very popular.

BOX 12.3 Helping Your Patients to Quit Smoking

Smoking cessation is a public health priority for governments around the world. Excellent online resources are available to provide information about the harmful effects of smoking and to help people to quit, including the following:

- http://www.cdc.gov/tobacco
- http://www.ash.org.uk
- http://smokefree.nhs.uk

Smoking cessation must be an integral part of the management of dental patients who smoke, and it is the responsibility of all dental health professionals to address this issue with their patients. The dental team is well placed to provide this treatment, because they see patients on a regular basis as part of ongoing routine dental management. Furthermore, interventions to help patients quit smoking in dental practices are effective, with quit rates of 15% to 20% as compared with approximately 5% in control groups.[119] The whole dental team should therefore be involved in smoking cessation, but this is not always the case. Why? Some of the barriers to providing smoking cessation counseling in the dental practice are shown in Table 12.2.

Various methods for helping patients to quit smoking in the dental environment have been described, and these are typically referred to as *brief intervention programs*. One such program[12] is known as the 5 A's:

ASK Ask the patient about his or her smoking status (see Box 12.1). This should be part of the medical history.

ADVISE Advise smokers of the associations between oral disease and smoking.

Be informative, honest, and helpful but not judgmental. The patient's response to this information will reveal his or her interest in quitting.

ASSESS Assess the patient's interest in and readiness to attempt smoking cessation.

Patients may not yet be in an action phase when it comes to quitting smoking, which is why it is always important to make these assessments every time you see the patient.

ASSIST Assist the patient with his or her quit attempt.

If you are trained, there are many techniques that can be used (see Box 12.4). Alternatively, assist the patient with seeking the help that he or she needs.

ARRANGE Arrange for a follow-up visit or a referral to professional smoking cessation services.

The most important aspect of this strategy is to keep in regular contact, particularly around the quit date and during the immediate period after the patient quits.

A simplified version of this is the 3 A's. This is a *very brief intervention* and can be particularly useful for the dental team.[95,111] The intervention is designed to be used at every clinical contact, and its very brief nature may help overcome some of the barriers presented by dental practices (the duration is <30 seconds). The focus is taken away from advising smokers to stop and shifts to offering support. The "advise" step deliberately leaves out the health benefits of stopping smoking or the harms of smoking. This minimizes the duration of the intervention and helps to avoid a defensive reaction or developing anxiety in the patient. The 3 A's technique is as follows:

ASK and record smoking status.

ADVISE how to stop.

ACT on the patient's response (prescribe, monitor, or refer).

Clearly, for the patient undergoing a comprehensive course of periodontal therapy, over several visits, there may be more opportunity to focus on the harms of smoking and the personal benefits of quitting.

TABLE 12.2 Barriers Against and Stimuli for the Provision of Smoking Cessation Advice by the Dental Team in Dental Practice

	Barriers	Stimuli
Professional Characteristics	Perceived lack of efficacy or lack of confidence in giving the advice	Self-efficacy
	Concerns about disturbing the patient–dentist relationship	Positive attitude toward giving advice as part of health care provider role
	Lack of knowledge about how to give the correct advice	Training
	Belief that counseling is unnecessary or perception that advising patients is frustrating and has a low success rate	Self-belief
	Dental team member may be a smoker himself or herself	Dental team member needs to quit!
Practice Organization	Lack of time	Task delegation
	No organizational support in the practice to deliver advice	Focus on helping smokers quit
Health Care System	No reimbursement	Health care system changes to encourage healthier lifestyles
	No referral options for further help	Local availability of smoking cessation services

Adapted from Rosseel JP, Jacobs JE, Hilberink SR, et al: What determines the provision of smoking cessation advice and counselling by dental care teams? *Br Dent J* 206:E13, 2009.[119]

Effects of Smoking on the Etiology and Pathogenesis of Periodontal Disease

The increased prevalence and severity of periodontal destruction associated with smoking suggests that the host–bacterial interactions normally seen with chronic periodontitis are altered, resulting in more extensive periodontal breakdown (Table 12.3). This imbalance between bacterial challenge and host response may be caused by changes in the composition of the subgingival biofilm (e.g., increases in the numbers and virulence of pathogenic organisms), changes in the host response to the bacterial challenge, or a combination of both.

Microbiology

Several studies have explored the possible changes in the subgingival microbiome caused by smoking. Earlier studies tended to show little difference between smokers and nonsmokers. For example, Preber and colleagues (1992) took plaque samples from deep pockets (i.e.,

BOX 12.4   Methods of Smoking Cessation

Willpower Alone
This is the least effective method of smoking cessation, with only 3% of smokers managing to quit after 12 months.[2]

Self-Help Materials
The provision of self-help materials can increase quit rates compared to no intervention, although only by a small amount.[53] When included with any other intervention, there was no additional benefit.

Brief Intervention Program in Primary Care
A brief advice intervention delivered by a physician or dentist can increase the rate of quitting (12 months) by 40% to 90%.[25,132] Assuming an unassisted quit rate of 3%, a brief intervention by a dentist could increase the quit rates to 4.5% to 6%. Although this cessation rate may seem low, if the dental team gave this brief advice to most of their smoking patients, a significant number of smokers in the whole population would be assisted to quit each year.

Nicotine Replacement Therapy
Nicotine replacement therapy (NRT) can increase the rate of quitting (12 months) by 50% to 70%.[133] For example, in primary care settings in which brief advice is given, 12-month success rates can increase from around 5% to around 8% if NRT is also used. In an intensive setting such as a smoker's clinic, success rates increase from around 10% to up to 16%. NRT is not a magic cure, but it helps with cravings and withdrawal when a person quits smoking. Although NRT products do contain nicotine, they do not contain the toxic products such as tar and carbon monoxide that are found in cigarette smoke. NRT products include the following:

- Patches (available in different doses and worn for 16 to 24 hours per day)
- Lozenges and gum (available in different flavors; should be chewed slowly to allow the nicotine to be absorbed through the mouth)
- Nasal spray (delivers nicotine solution via the nasal passages)
- Inhalator (a plastic mouthpiece with a supply of nicotine cartridges that fit on the end; nicotine is absorbed in the mouth by drawing on the inhalator like a cigarette).

Varenicline
A course of varenicline, at standard dose, can increase the rate of quitting (12 months) by 100% to 150%.[22] Varenicline is a nicotine receptor partial agonist, and it aims to reduce both withdrawal symptoms and the pleasure people usually experience when they smoke.

Bupropion
Bupropion can increase the rate of quitting (12 months) by 50% to 80%.[62] This medication is used as an antidepressant at higher doses, but it is effective for smoking cessation at lower doses. It is usually prescribed to be started 1 to 2 weeks before the quit date. There are serious potential drug interactions and unwanted effects.

Other Methods
Whatever works for the patient is good! In addition to combinations of the methods listed here, techniques for smoking cessation can include intensive counseling, motivational interviewing, cognitive behavioral therapy, hypnosis, and acupuncture. Many smokers are now also using e-cigarettes to help to quit smoking (see Box 12.5).

BOX 12.5   Electronic Cigarettes

Electronic cigarettes (e-cigarettes) are electronic devices that produce an aerosol that the user inhales. The e-cigarette contains a solution, often called an "e-liquid," which is drawn through a heating element to produce the aerosol. The process of using an e-cigarette (often referred to as *vaping*) closely resembles tobacco smoking, making e-cigarettes a particularly attractive alternative to smokers. In contrast, this similarity to cigarette smoking has produced much of the controversy and concerns around e-cigarettes.

What Is in the E-liquid?
The e-liquid usually comprises three main components: diluents, nicotine, and flavorings. The diluents account for the majority of the solution and are usually propylene glycol or vegetable glycerin. Nicotine is included at a wide range of concentrations, the most popular strength in Great Britain being 13 to 18 mg/ml.[3] Nicotine-free e-liquids are available and used by approximately 10% of users (Great Britain).[3] Flavorings are often added, as both nicotine and the diluents are largely tasteless. The large range of flavors can generally be divided into three main groups: tobacco, fruit, and menthol/mint.

Are E-cigarettes a Useful Smoking Cessation Aid?
E-cigarettes are a modern phenomenon introduced to the U.S. and European markets in 2006, with their popularly taking off in around 2011. The evidence base is continually growing with several ongoing clinical trials. A Cochrane Collaboration systematic review concluded that e-cigarettes helped smokers to stop smoking and showed particular promise in reducing cigarette consumption in smokers unwilling to quit (although further studies are needed to confirm this conclusion).[88]

Are E-cigarettes Safe?
This has been the topic of many debates, and controversy still exists. Two substantial reports concluded that the hazard to health from long-term e-cigarette vapor inhalation was unlikely to exceed 5% of the harm from smoking tobacco.[87,120]

What Are the Oral Health Effects?
Very little has been published in this field. A handful of in vitro cell line studies have shown a variety of effects including cytotoxicity and DNA damage.[125,146,148] As with all in vitro studies, the clinical relevance is difficult to interpret, and unfortunately some of these studies are of questionable quality.[59] From a clinical perspective, e-cigarette vapor is likely to have different effects on the oral tissues when compared with the well-known effects of tobacco smoke. Interestingly, nicotine has been shown to be angiogenic[66] with wound-healing properties[85] and with potential intraoral applications.[114,115] Well-conducted clinical studies are required to enable us to appropriately inform patients about e-cigarette use.

How Are E-cigarettes Regulated?
A range of regulatory approaches have been taken across the globe, from e-cigarettes being completely prohibited to being classified under general consumer product regulations.[24]

What Is the Bottom Line?
E-cigarettes are a consumer led bottom-up public health initiative that has taken the realms of research, public health, regulation, and industry by surprise. They are extremely popular with users (smokers/former smokers), with probably only a fraction of the health hazard of tobacco smoking. From a public health perspective they have the potential to significantly reduce tobacco-related morbidity and mortality. The oral health risks are currently unknown but are likely to be less than those associated with tobacco smoking.

TABLE 12.3   Effects of Smoking on the Etiology and Pathogenesis of Periodontal Disease

Etiologic Factor	Effects of Smoking
Microbiology	Increased complexity of the microbiome and colonization of periodontal pockets by periodontal pathogens
Immune–inflammatory response	Altered neutrophil chemotaxis, phagocytosis, and oxidative burst ↑ Tumor necrosis factor-α and prostaglandin E$_2$ in gingival crevicular fluid ↑ Neutrophil collagenase and elastase in gingival crevicular fluid ↑ Production of prostaglandin E$_2$ by monocytes in response to lipopolysaccharide
Physiology	↓ Gingival blood vessels with ↑ inflammation ↓ Gingival crevicular fluid flow and bleeding on probing with ↑ inflammation ↓ Subgingival temperature ↑ Time needed to recover from local anesthesia

↓, Decreased; ↑, increased.

≥6 mm) in 142 patients and found no differences in the counts of *Aggregatibacter actinomycetemcomitans*, *Porphyromonas gingivalis*, and *Prevotella intermedia*.[108] In a similar study of 615 patients involving the use of immunoassay, the prevalence of *A. actinomycetemcomitans*, *P. gingivalis*, *P. intermedia*, and *Eikenella corrodens* was not found to be significantly different between smokers and nonsmokers.[134]

By contrast, other studies have demonstrated differences in the microbial composition of subgingival biofilm of smokers and nonsmokers. A study of 798 subjects with different smoking histories found that smokers had significantly higher levels of *Tannerella forsythia* and that smokers were 2.3 times more likely to harbor *T. forsythia* as compared with nonsmokers and former smokers.[149] Of interest were observations that smokers did not respond to mechanical therapy as well as nonsmokers did; this was associated with increased levels of *T. forsythia*, *A. actinomycetemcomitans*, and *P. gingivalis* remaining in the pockets after therapy in the smoking group as compared with nonsmokers.[45,46,49,113]

Many discrepancies between the findings of microbiologic studies are a function of the methodology involved, including bacterial counts versus proportions or prevalence of bacteria, the number of sites sampled and the pocket depths selected, the sampling technique, the disease status of the subject, and the methods of bacterial identification and data analysis. In an attempt to overcome some of these problems, one study sampled subgingival biofilm from all teeth with the exception of third molars in 272 adult subjects, including 50 current smokers, 98 former smokers, and 124 nonsmokers.[51] Using checkerboard DNA–DNA hybridization technology to screen for 29 different subgingival species, it was found that members of the orange and red complex species—including *Eikenella nodatum*, *Fusobacterium nucleatum* ss *vincentii*, *P. intermedia*, *Peptostreptococcus micros*, *Prevotella nigrescens*, *T. forsythia*, *P. gingivalis*, and *Treponema denticola*—were significantly more prevalent in current smokers than in nonsmokers and former smokers. The increased prevalence of these periodontal pathogens was caused by an increased colonization of shallow sites (pocket depth ≤4 mm), with no differences among smokers, former smokers, and nonsmokers in pockets 4 mm or greater. In addition, these pathogenic bacteria were more prevalent in the

maxilla than the mandible. These data suggest that smokers have a greater extent of colonization by periodontal pathogens than nonsmokers or former smokers, which may increase the risk of periodontal disease progression. Contemporary studies have drawn similar conclusions, with next generation sequencing analysis of periodontally healthy smokers demonstrating a highly diverse, pathogen-rich, commensal-poor, anaerobic microbiome that is more similar to the microbiome observed in patients with advanced periodontitis than that observed in periodontally healthy nonsmokers, and which is primed for future development of periodontitis given appropriate ecologic and environmental changes.[86]

Immune–Inflammatory Responses

The immune response of the host to biofilm accumulation is essentially protective. In periodontal health, a balance exists between the bacterial challenge of the biofilm and the immune–inflammatory responses in the gingival tissues, with no resulting loss of periodontal support. By contrast, periodontitis is associated with an alteration in the host–bacterial balance that may be initiated by changes in the bacterial composition of the subgingival biofilm, changes in the host responses, other environmental changes, or a combination of these.

Smoking exerts a major effect on the immune–inflammatory response that results in an increase in the extent and severity of periodontal destruction. The deleterious effects of smoking appear to result from alterations in the immune-inflammatory response to bacterial challenge. The neutrophil is an important component of the host response to the bacterial challenge, and alterations in neutrophil number or function may result in localized and systemic infections. Critical functions of neutrophils include *chemotaxis* (directed locomotion from the bloodstream to the site of infection), *phagocytosis* (internalization of foreign particles such as bacteria), and *killing* via oxidative and nonoxidative mechanisms.

Neutrophils obtained from the peripheral blood, oral cavity, or saliva of smokers or exposed in vitro to whole tobacco smoke or nicotine have demonstrated functional alterations in chemotaxis, phagocytosis, and the oxidative burst.[38,74] In vitro studies of the effects of tobacco products on neutrophils have shown detrimental effects on cell movement as well as on the oxidative burst.[32,73,79,123,129] In addition, levels of antibody to the periodontal pathogens essential for phagocytosis and killing of bacteria, specifically immunoglobulin G$_2$, have been reported to be reduced in smokers as compared with nonsmokers with periodontitis,[23,47,49,136] thereby suggesting that smokers may have reduced protection against periodontal bacteria. By contrast, elevated levels of tumor necrosis factor–α have been demonstrated in the gingival crevicular fluid of smokers,[21] and elevated levels of prostaglandin E$_2$, neutrophil elastase, and matrix metalloproteinase-8 have also been found.[131] In vitro studies have also shown that exposure to nicotine increases the secretion of prostaglandin E$_2$ by monocytes in response to lipopolysaccharide.[101]

These data suggest that smoking alters the response of neutrophils to the bacterial challenge such that there are increases in the release of tissue-destructive enzymes, causing increased periodontal tissue destruction. However, the exact changes in the immunologic mechanisms involved in the rapid tissue destruction seen in smokers are not yet fully understood, and more research in this area is indicated.

Physiology

Previous studies have shown that certain clinical signs of inflammation (e.g., gingival redness, gingival bleeding) are less pronounced in smokers than in nonsmokers.[13,33] This may result from alterations in the vascular response of the gingival tissues. Although no significant differences in the vascular density of healthy gingiva have been observed between smokers and nonsmokers,[102] the response of the microcirculation to biofilm accumulation appears to be altered in smokers as compared with nonsmokers. With developing inflammation, increases in gingival crevicular fluid flow, bleeding on probing,[19] and gingival blood vessels[18] are lower in smokers than in nonsmokers. In addition, the oxygen concentration in healthy gingival tissues appears to be lower in smokers than in nonsmokers, although this condition is reversed in the presence of moderate inflammation.[52] Subgingival temperatures are lower in smokers than nonsmokers,[35] and recovery from the vasoconstriction caused by local anesthetic administration takes longer in smokers.[75,142] These data suggest that significant alterations are present in the gingival microvasculature of smokers as compared with nonsmokers and that these changes lead to decreased blood flow and decreased clinical signs of inflammation. This explains the long-observed phenomenon of a transient increase in gingival bleeding when a smoker quits; patients need to be warned about this phenomenon.

Is Nicotine the Bad Guy?

The role of nicotine in the detrimental health effects seen in smokers has never been more relevant with the increasing popularity of novel nicotine delivery devices (e.g., e-cigarettes). Nicotine is not carcinogenic,[55,63] and it is now largely accepted that nicotine has likely been unfairly blamed. A classic quote, with reference to lung cancer, is "smokers smoke for nicotine but are killed by tar."[121] The potential role of nicotine in periodontitis development is less clear. Nicotine has been the subject of many in vitro investigations with oral cells. These studies often present conflicting results with regard to cellular viability and functions. For example, with regard to cellular viability, overall the studies show that the harsher the conditions (e.g., higher concentrations of nicotine and longer durations of exposure), the more significant the detrimental effects of the nicotine on cell culture systems. Cellular viability has generally been shown to be unaffected[44,93,130] by nicotine concentrations in the range found in blood plasma (~36 ng/ml)[122] or the saliva of smokers (906 ng/ml).[42] Much higher nicotine concentrations can be found in the saliva of smokeless tobacco users (70–1560 μg/ml),[58] and studies with these nicotine concentrations demonstrate significant cellular toxicity in vitro.[6,31,138] Interestingly, cells derived from smokers and older donors demonstrated less sensitivity to nicotine.[31]

Clinical studies are required to determine the clinical relevance of these in vitro results.

Effects of Smoking on the Response to Periodontal Therapy

Nonsurgical Therapy

Numerous studies have indicated that current smokers do not respond as well to periodontal therapy as nonsmokers or former smokers do (Table 12.4). Most clinical research supports the observation that probing depth reductions are generally greater in nonsmokers than in smokers after nonsurgical periodontal therapy.[4,45,46,49,72,107,113] In addition, gains in clinical attachment as a result of nonsurgical treatment are less pronounced in smokers than in nonsmokers. In a study of patients with previously untreated advanced periodontal disease, nonsurgical therapy resulted in significantly greater mean reductions in probing depth and bleeding on probing in nonsmokers than in smokers when evaluated 6 months after the completion of therapy.[113] Mean probing depth reductions of 2.5 mm for nonsmokers and 1.9 mm for smokers were observed in pockets that averaged 7 mm or more before treatment. In another study, the nonsurgical

TABLE 12.4   Effects of Smoking on the Response to Periodontal Therapy

Therapy	Effects of Smoking
Nonsurgical	↓ Clinical response to root surface debridement ↓ Reduction in probing depth ↓ Gain in clinical attachment levels ↓ Negative impact of smoking with ↑ level of plaque control
Surgery and implants	↓ Probing depth reduction and ↓ gain in clinical attachment levels after access flap surgery ↑ Deterioration of furcations after surgery ↓ Gain in clinical attachment levels, ↓ bone fill, ↑ recession, and ↑ membrane exposure after guided tissue regeneration ↓ Root coverage after grafting procedures for localized gingival recession ↓ Probing depth reduction after bone graft procedures ↑ Risk for implant failure and periimplantitis
Maintenance care	↑ Probing depth and attachment loss during maintenance therapy ↑ Disease recurrence in smokers ↑ Need for retreatment in smokers ↑ Tooth loss in smokers after surgical therapy

↓, Decreased; ↑, increased.

management of pockets of 5 mm or greater showed that smokers had less probing depth reduction than nonsmokers after 3 months (1.29 mm versus 1.76 mm) as well as less gain in clinical attachment levels.[45] When a higher level of oral hygiene was achieved as part of nonsurgical care, the differences in the resolution of 4- to 6-mm pockets between nonsmokers and smokers became clinically less significant.[107]

It can be concluded that smokers respond less well to nonsurgical therapy than do nonsmokers. With excellent plaque control, these differences may be minimized, but the emphasis is on truly excellent plaque control. When comparing current smokers with former smokers and nonsmokers, the former and nonsmoking subjects appear to respond equally well to nonsurgical care,[45] thereby reinforcing the need for patients to be informed of the benefits of smoking cessation.

Surgical Therapy and Implants

The less favorable response of the periodontal tissues to nonsurgical therapy that is observed in current smokers is also observed after surgical therapy. In a longitudinal comparative study of the effects of four different treatment modalities (coronal scaling, root planing, modified Widman flap surgery, and osseous resection surgery), smokers (with "heavy" defined as ≥20 cigarettes/day and "light" defined as ≤19 cigarettes/day) consistently showed less pocket reduction and less gain in clinical attachment as compared with nonsmokers or former smokers.[72] These differences were evident immediately after the completion of therapy and continued throughout 7 years of supportive periodontal therapy. During the 7 years, deterioration at furcation areas was greater in heavy and light smokers than in former smokers and nonsmokers. Smoking has also been shown to have a negative impact on the outcomes of guided tissue regeneration[141,143] and the treatment of infrabony defects by bone grafts.[118] By 12 months after guided tissue regeneration therapy at deep infrabony defects, smokers demonstrated less than half the attachment gain that was observed in nonsmokers (2.1 mm versus 5.2 mm).[141] In a second study, 73 smokers also showed less attachment gain than nonsmokers (1.2 mm versus 3.2 mm), more gingival recession, and less bone infill of the defect. Similarly, after the use of bone grafts for the treatment of infrabony defects, smokers showed less reduction in probing depths as compared with nonsmokers.[118]

Open flap access surgery without regenerative or grafting procedures is a common surgical procedure used for accessing the root and bone surfaces. By 6 months after this procedure, smokers showed significantly less reduction of deep pockets (≥7 mm) than nonsmokers (3 mm for smokers versus 4 mm for nonsmokers) and significantly less gain in clinical attachment (1.8 mm for smokers versus 2.8 mm for nonsmokers), even though all of the patients received supportive periodontal therapy every month for 6 months.[126]

Tobacco smoking also affects the outcomes of periodontal plastic surgery.[27,30] For instance, a systematic review assessed the influence of smoking on the outcomes achieved by root coverage procedures.[27] This review identified that significantly greater root coverage and greater gains in clinical attachment levels were recorded for nonsmokers as compared with smokers after the treatment of gingival recession defects by subepithelial connective-tissue grafts. Furthermore, smokers showed significantly fewer sites with complete root coverage than were seen in the nonsmokers.[30]

Several meta-analyses have investigated the influence of smoking on the short- and long-term outcomes of implant therapy and have identified that smoking increases the risk of implant failure.[28,57,77,90,135] These studies used various definitions to define implant failure, including implant loss, implant bone loss, mobility, pain, and periimplantitis. Overall, the risk for implant failure in smokers appears to be approximately double the risk for failure in nonsmokers, and the risks appear to be higher in maxillary implants and when implants are placed in poor-quality bone. Smoking has also been shown to be a risk factor for periimplantitis, with a majority of studies showing a significant increase in periimplant bone loss as compared with nonsmokers.[56] Collectively, these data indicate that implant failure is more common among smokers than nonsmokers. However, because numerous factors can influence implant success, further controlled clinical trials are needed to address the role of smoking as an independent variable in implant failure. Given the current evidence, all patients who are considering implant therapy should be informed about the benefits of smoking cessation and the risks of smoking for the development of periimplantitis and implant failure.

Maintenance Therapy

The detrimental effect of smoking on treatment outcomes appears to be long lasting and independent of the frequency of maintenance therapy. After four modalities of therapy (scaling, scaling and root planing, modified Widman flap surgery, and osseous surgery), maintenance therapy was performed by a hygienist every 3 months for 7 years.[72] Smokers consistently had deeper pockets than nonsmokers and less gain in attachment when evaluated each year for the 7-year period. Even with more intensive maintenance therapy given every month for 6 months after flap surgery,[126] smokers had deeper and more residual pockets than nonsmokers, although no significant differences in plaque or bleeding on probing scores were found. These data suggest that the effects of smoking on the host response and the healing characteristics of the periodontal tissues may have a long-term effect on pocket resolution in smokers, possibly requiring more intensive management during the maintenance phase. Smokers also tend to experience more periodontal breakdown than nonsmokers after therapy.[82,84] In studies of patients who failed to respond to

periodontal therapy, approximately 90% of these poorly responding patients were smokers.[82,83]

A systematic review that assessed the potential predictors of tooth loss during long-term periodontal maintenance care demonstrated that, although oral health and the prevention of tooth loss were achieved in the majority of patients, the long-term outcomes were also influenced by smoking.[26] Tobacco smoking was positively associated with tooth loss even when regular recall maintenance care was performed (overall, smokers had a risk of losing their teeth that was up to 380% higher than that of nonsmokers).[26] Similarly, smoking has a detrimental effect on periimplant tissue status, even when patients are under strict periimplant preventive maintenance care.[34] It has been also demonstrated in a practice-based study that the smoking status may be highly associated with periimplant tissue loss around 10-mm implants restored with single crowns.[34] For instance, when comparing nonsmokers and light smokers (i.e., subjects who smoked <10 cigarettes per day), it was found that the majority of patients who experienced bone loss were smokers (88.9%), with an odds ratio of 39.64 (95% confidence interval, 8.62 to 182.27) for increased risk of bone loss.[34]

It is clear from these studies that (1) smokers may present with periodontal disease at an early age; (2) they may be difficult to treat effectively with conventional therapeutic strategies; (3) they may continue to have progressive or recurrent periodontitis; and (4) they may be at an increased risk of tooth loss or periimplant bone loss, even when adequate maintenance control is established. For these reasons, smoking cessation counseling must be a cornerstone of periodontal therapy in smokers.

Effects of Smoking Cessation on Periodontal Treatment Outcomes

The effect of smoking cessation on periodontal status has been studied in a large number of cross-sectional and cohort observational studies, in which the periodontal status of smokers, former smokers, and nonsmokers is compared.[8,9,14-16,20,36,48,50,69,100,137,139] Similarly, periodontal treatment outcomes have been assessed in smokers, former smokers, and nonsmokers.[46,61,72,89,110,124] Collectively, these studies have demonstrated that smokers have significantly worse periodontal status (i.e., deeper probing depths, more attachment loss and bone loss) than either former smokers or nonsmokers and usually have poorer treatment outcomes. The periodontal status of former smokers is intermediate to that of current smokers and nonsmokers, and it appears to usually be closer to that of nonsmokers.

There are very few intervention studies of the effect of smoking cessation on periodontal treatment outcomes (i.e., studies in which smokers were helped to quit and in which the effect on periodontal status was then assessed). Two short-term studies have indicated that smoking has a negative impact on the gingival vasculature and that these changes are reversible with smoking cessation.[91,92] Two interventional studies have assessed the impact of smoking cessation on outcomes after nonsurgical periodontal treatment.[109,117] The first study employed dental hygienists who were trained as smoking cessation advisers and who achieved a 20% quit rate at 12 months in a population of smokers who also had periodontitis. The hygienists used a variety of strategies to assist these smokers, including counseling, nicotine replacement therapy, and bupropion. All of the patients received nonsurgical therapy as treatment for their periodontitis in addition to smoking cessation counseling. Those individuals who successfully quit smoking for the entire 12 months of the study had the best response to the periodontal treatment. The treatment responses in the nonquitters and the failed quitters (i.e., the "oscillators" who initially quit but who then resumed smoking) were significantly poorer than those seen in the quitters, and they did not differ significantly from each other. The second study was a 12-month prospective single-blinded study in which smoking cessation advice, nicotine replacement therapy, and medication were provided at four consecutive appointments, once a week, by a multidisciplinary team that included doctors, psychologists, and a dentist, in addition to nonsurgical treatment of periodontitis.[117] The confirmed continuous quit rate at 12 months was 18.3%. At the end of the 12-month follow-up period, it was identified that the quitters had improved clinical attachment gain as compared with the nonquitters. In addition, a supplementary study that described a set of meta-analyses performed with individual patient data from these two trials reported a highly significant beneficial impact of quitting smoking, with quitters demonstrating 30% more sites with probing depth reductions of 2 mm or more as compared with nonquitters.[29] Equally, quitters had 22% fewer sites with residual probing depths of 4 mm or greater as compared with nonquitters at the end of the 12-month follow-up period.[29]

The benefit of smoking cessation on the periodontium is likely to be mediated through various pathways, such as a shift toward a less pathogenic microbiome, the recovery of the gingival microcirculation, and improvements in certain aspects of the immune–inflammatory responses. In support of this observation, in the interventional study described previously,[109] plaque samples were collected as the study progressed. It became clear that subgingival microbial profiles differed significantly between smokers and quitters at 6 and 12 months after smoking cessation.[43] At 6 and 12 months after treatment, the microbial community in smokers was similar to that observed at baseline (i.e., before periodontal treatment/smoking cessation counseling), whereas the quitters demonstrated significantly divergent profiles; changes in bacterial levels contributed to this shift. These data suggest a critical role for smoking cessation in the alteration of the subgingival biofilm. Further research is necessary to investigate the impact of quitting smoking on the immune–inflammatory mechanisms that drive tissue destruction in the periodontium.

In conclusion, smoking is a major risk factor for periodontitis, and smoking cessation should be an integral part of periodontal therapy among patients who smoke. Smoking cessation should be considered a priority for the management of periodontitis in smokers.

 A Case Scenario is found on the companion website www.expertconsult.com.

References

 References for this chapter are found on the companion website www.expertconsult.com.

CHAPTER 13

The Role of Dental Calculus and Other Local Predisposing Factors

James E. Hinrichs | *Vivek Thumbigere-Math*

CHAPTER OUTLINE

Calculus
Other Predisposing Factors

The primary cause of gingival inflammation is bacterial plaque. Other predisposing factors include calculus, faulty restorations, complications associated with orthodontic therapy, self-inflicted injuries, and the use of tobacco. These will be discussed in turn.

Calculus

Calculus consists of mineralized bacterial plaque that forms on the surfaces of natural teeth and dental prostheses.

Supragingival and Subgingival Calculus

Supragingival calculus is located coronal to the gingival margin and therefore is visible in the oral cavity. It is usually white or whitish yellow in color; hard, with a claylike consistency; and easily detached from the tooth surface. After removal, it may rapidly recur, especially in the lingual area of the mandibular incisors. The color is influenced by contact with substances such as tobacco and food pigments. It may be localized on a single tooth or group of teeth, or it may be generalized throughout the mouth.

KEY FACT

Mechanical removal of subgingival plaque and calculus is considered the fundamental cornerstone to the treatment of chronic periodontitis.

The two most common locations for the development of supragingival calculus are the buccal surfaces of the maxillary molars (Fig. 13.1) and the lingual surfaces of the mandibular anterior teeth (Fig. 13.2).[37]

Saliva from the parotid gland flows over the facial surfaces of the upper molars via the parotid duct, whereas the submandibular duct and the lingual duct empty onto the lingual surfaces of the lower incisors from the submaxillary and sublingual glands, respectively. In extreme cases, calculus may form a bridge-like structure over the interdental papilla of adjacent teeth or cover the occlusal surface of teeth that are lacking functional antagonists.

Subgingival calculus is located below the crest of the marginal gingiva and therefore is not visible on routine clinical examination. The location and the extent of subgingival calculus may be evaluated by careful tactile perception with a delicate dental instrument such as an explorer. Clerehugh and colleagues[34] assessed the validity of the World Health Organization no. 621 probe to detect and score subgingival calculus. Following clinical detection of subgingival calculus, teeth were extracted and microscopically scored for subgingival calculus. An agreement of 80% was found between the two scoring methods. Subgingival calculus is typically hard and dense; it frequently appears to be dark brown or greenish black in color (Fig. 13.3), and it is firmly attached to the tooth surface. Supragingival calculus and subgingival calculus generally occur together, but one may be present without the other. Microscopic studies demonstrate that deposits of subgingival calculus usually extend nearly to the base of periodontal pockets in individuals with chronic periodontitis but do not reach the junctional epithelium.

When the gingival tissues recede, subgingival calculus becomes exposed and is therefore reclassified as supragingival (Fig. 13.4A). Thus, supragingival calculus can be composed of both the initial supragingival calculus and previous subgingival calculus. A reduction in gingival inflammation and probing depths with a gain in clinical attachment can be observed after the removal of subgingival plaque and calculus (see Fig. 13.4B; see Chapter 50).

CLINICAL CORRELATION

A reduction in gingival inflammation and probing depths accompanied by a gain in clinical attachment can be expected following thorough removal of subgingival plaque and calculus.

Prevalence

Anerud and colleagues[4] observed the periodontal status of a group of Sri Lankan tea laborers and a group of Norwegian academicians for a 15-year period. The Norwegian population had ready access to preventive dental care throughout their lives, whereas the Sri Lankan tea laborers did not. The formation of supragingival calculus was observed early in life in the Sri Lankan individuals, probably shortly after the teeth erupted. The first areas to exhibit calculus deposits were the facial aspects of maxillary molars and the lingual surfaces of mandibular incisors. The deposition of supragingival calculus continued as individuals aged, and it reached a maximal calculus score when the affected individuals were 25 to 30 years old.

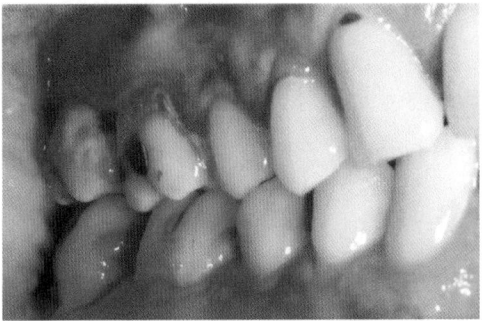

Fig. 13.1 Supragingival calculus is depicted on the buccal surfaces of maxillary molars adjacent to the orifice for the parotid duct.

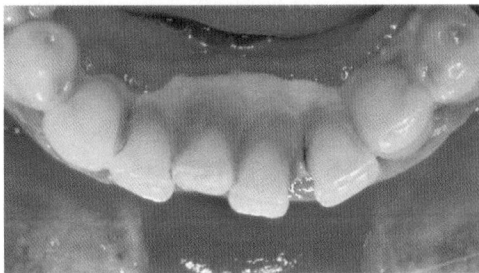

Fig. 13.2 Extensive supragingival calculus is present on the lingual surfaces of the lower anterior teeth.

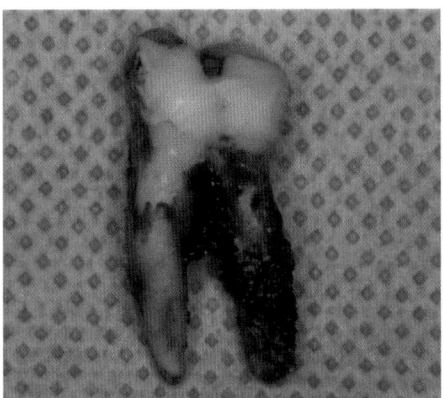

Fig. 13.3 Dark pigmented deposits of subgingival calculus are shown on the distal root of an extracted lower molar.

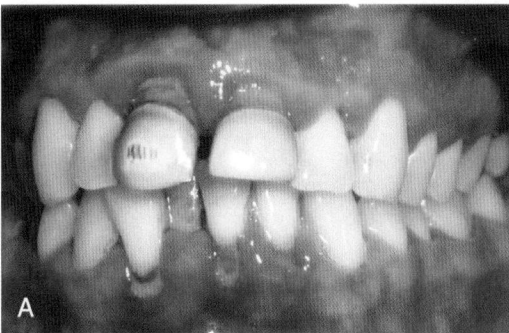

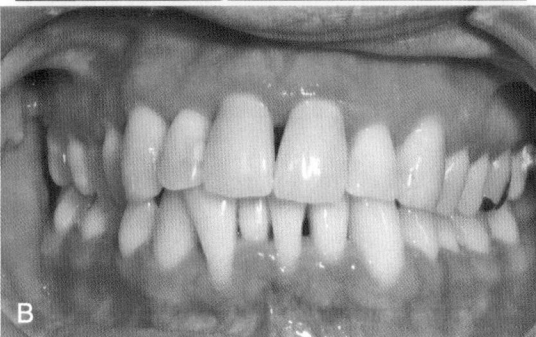

Fig. 13.4 (A) A 31-year-old white man with extensive supragingival and subgingival calculus deposits throughout his dentition is shown. (B) One year after receiving thorough scaling and root planing to remove supragingival and subgingival calculus deposits, followed by restorative care. Note the substantial reduction in gingival inflammation.

Both supragingival calculus and subgingival calculus may be seen on radiographs (see Chapter 33). Highly calcified interproximal calculus deposits are readily detectable as radiopaque projections that protrude into the interdental spaces (Fig. 13.5).

However, the sensitivity level of detecting calculus by radiographs is inconsistent.[27] The location of calculus does not indicate the bottom of the periodontal pocket, because the most apical plaque is not sufficiently calcified to be visible on radiographs.

 FLASH BACK

Whereas the presence of subgingival calculus can be observed on dental radiographs, the sensitivity of such detection is inconsistent.

At this time, most of the teeth were covered by calculus, although the facial surfaces had less calculus than the lingual or palatal surfaces. Calculus accumulation appeared to be symmetric, and by the age of 45 years, these individuals had only a few teeth (typically the premolars) without calculus deposits. Subgingival calculus appeared first either independently or on the interproximal aspects of areas where supragingival calculus already existed.[4] By the age of 30 years, all surfaces of all teeth had subgingival calculus without any pattern of predilection.

In contrast to the Sri Lankan group, the Norwegian academicians who received oral hygiene instructions and frequent preventive dental care throughout their lives exhibited a marked reduction in the accumulation of calculus. Approximately 80% of teenagers formed limited supragingival calculus on the facial surfaces of the upper first molars and the lingual surfaces of lower incisors. However, no additional calculus formation occurred on other teeth, and its presence did not increase with the individual's age.[4]

Composition

Inorganic Content

Dental calculus is primarily composed of inorganic components (70% to 90%[59]) and the organic components constitute the rest. The major inorganic proportions of calculus are approximately 76% calcium phosphate ($Ca_3[PO_4]_2$), 3% calcium carbonate ($CaCO_3$), 4% magnesium phosphate ($Mg_3[PO_4]_2$), 2% carbon dioxide, and traces of other elements such as sodium, zinc, strontium, bromine, copper, manganese, tungsten, gold, aluminum, silicon, iron, and fluorine.[132,206] The percentage of inorganic constituents in calculus is similar to that of other calcified tissues of the body (Table 13.1).

At least two-thirds of the inorganic component is crystalline in structure.[103] The four main crystal forms and their approximate percentages are as follows: hydroxyapatite, 58%; magnesium whitlockite, 21%; octacalcium phosphate, 12%; and brushite, 9%.

Two or more crystal forms are typically found in a sample of calculus. Hydroxyapatite and octacalcium phosphate are detected

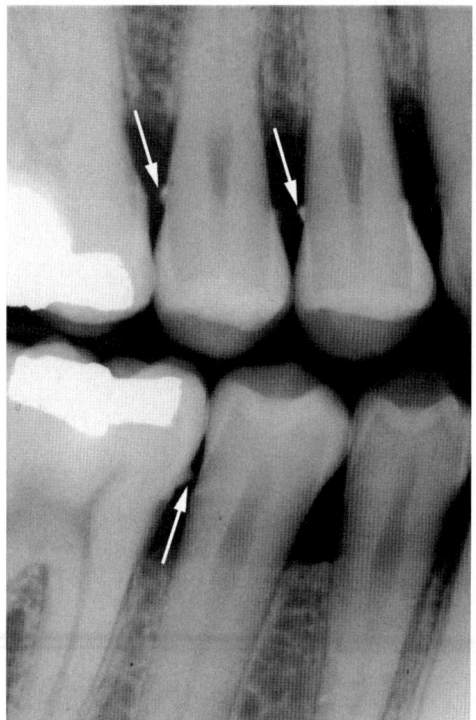

Fig. 13.5 A bitewing radiograph illustrating subgingival calculus deposits that are depicted as interproximal spurs *(arrows)*.

TABLE 13.1 Calculus versus Other Oral Hard Tissues

Structure	Inorganic Content (%)*
Dental Calculus	70–90
Enamel	96
Dentin	45
Bone	60–70

*Organic components and water constitute the rest.

most frequently (i.e., in 97% to 100% of all supragingival calculus) and constitute the bulk of the specimen. Brushite is more common in the mandibular anterior region, and magnesium whitlockite is found in the posterior areas. The incidence of the four crystal forms varies with the age of the deposit.[17]

FLASH BACK

The four main crystalline inorganic forms of calculus are hydroxyapatite, magnesium whitlockite, octacalcium phosphate, and brushite.

Organic Content

The organic component of calculus consists of a mixture of protein–polysaccharide complexes, desquamated epithelial cells, leukocytes, and various types of microorganisms.[116]

Between 1.9% and 9.1% of the organic component is carbohydrate, which consists of galactose, glucose, rhamnose, mannose, glucuronic acid, galactosamine, and sometimes arabinose, galacturonic acid, and glucosamine.[109,115,186] All of these organic components are present in salivary glycoprotein, with the exception of arabinose and rhamnose. Salivary proteins account for 5.9% to 8.2% of the organic component

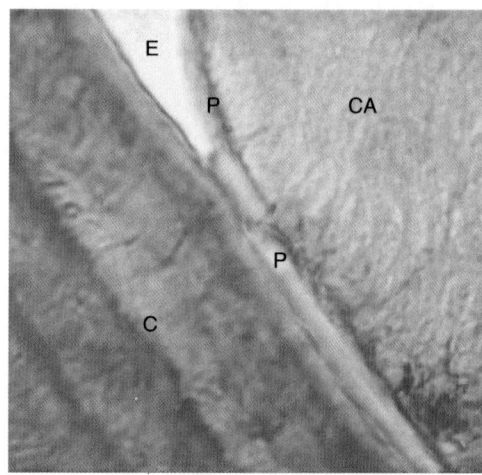

Fig. 13.6 Calculus attached to the pellicle on the enamel surface and the cementum. An enamel void *(E)* has been created during the preparation of the specimen. *C,* Cementum; *CA,* calculus; *P,* pellicle.

of calculus and include most amino acids. Lipids account for 0.2% of the organic content in the form of neutral fats, free fatty acids, cholesterol, cholesterol esters, and phospholipids.[110]

The composition of subgingival calculus is similar to that of supragingival calculus, with some differences. It has the same hydroxyapatite content but more magnesium whitlockite and less brushite and octacalcium phosphate.[167,191] The ratio of calcium to phosphate is higher in subgingival calculus, and the sodium content increases with the depth of periodontal pockets.[111] These altered compositions may be attributed to fact that the origin of subgingival calculus is plasma, whereas supragingival calculus is partially composed of salivary constituents. Salivary proteins present in supragingival calculus are not found in subgingival calculus.[12] Dental calculus, salivary duct calculus, and calcified dental tissues are similar in inorganic composition.

Attachment to the Tooth Surface

Differences in the manner in which calculus is attached to the tooth surface affect the relative ease or difficulty encountered during its removal. Four modes of attachment have been described.[94,175,180,214] (1) Attachment by means of an organic pellicle on cementum is depicted in Fig. 13.6, and attachment on enamel is shown in Fig. 13.7. (2) Mechanical locking into surface irregularities, such as caries lesions or resorption lacunae, is illustrated in Fig. 13.8. (3) Close adaptation of the undersurface of calculus to depressions or gently sloping mounds of the unaltered cementum surface[186] is shown in Fig. 13.9. (4) Penetration of bacterial calculus into cementum is shown in Figs. 13.10 and 13.11.

FLASH BACK

Four modes by which calculus may attach to cementum are (1) organic pellicle, (2) mechanical locking into surface irregularities, (3) close adaption to gentle depression or sloping mounts of unaltered cementum, and (4) bacterial penetration into cementum surface.

Formation

Calculus is *mineralized dental plaque.* The soft plaque is hardened by the precipitation of mineral salts, which usually starts between the 1st and 14th days of plaque formation. Calcification has been reported to occur within as little as 4 to 8 hours.[192] Calcifying plaques

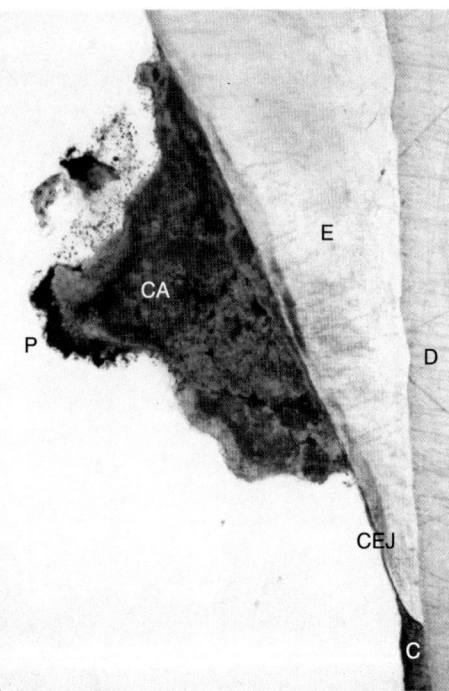

Fig. 13.7 Non-decalcified specimen with calculus *(CA)* attached to enamel *(E)* surface just coronal to the cementoenamel junction *(CEJ)*. Note plaque *(P)* on the surface of the calculus; dentin *(D)* and cementum *(C)* are also identified. *(Courtesy Dr. Michael Rohrer, Minneapolis, MN.)*

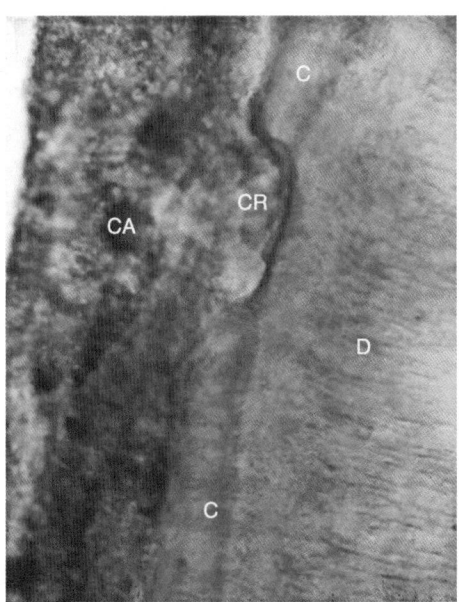

Fig. 13.8 Calculus *(CA)* attached to a cemental resorption area *(CR)* with cementum *(C)* adjacent to dentin *(D)*.

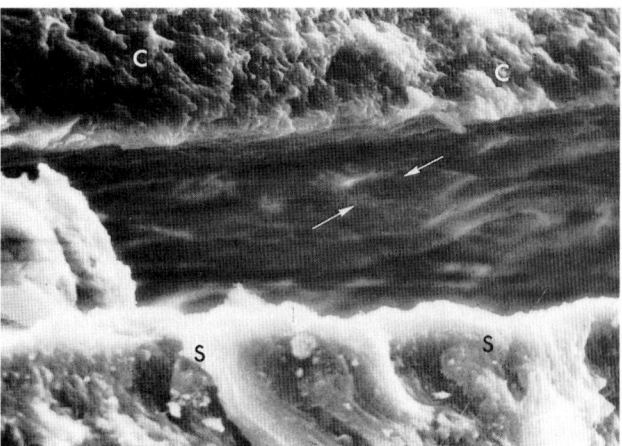

Fig. 13.9 Undersurface of subgingival calculus *(C)* previously attached to the cementum surface *(S)*. Note the impression of cementum mounds in the calculus *(arrows)*. *(Courtesy Dr. John Sottosanti, La Jolla, CA.)*

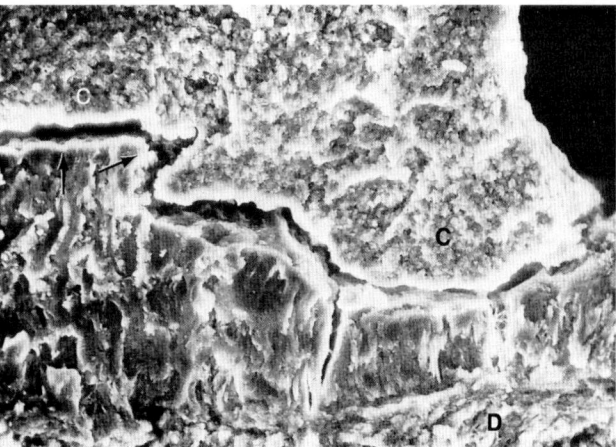

Fig. 13.10 Subgingival calculus *(C)* embedded beneath the cementum surface *(arrows)* and penetrating to the dentin *(D)*, thereby making removal difficult. *(Courtesy Dr. John Sottosanti, La Jolla, CA.)*

KEY FACT

Calculus by itself does not contribute directly to gingival inflammation. Like other retentive factors such as open crown margin or an overhanging restoration, calculus retains dental plaque, which contributes to gingival inflammation.

---

may become 50% mineralized in 2 days and 60% to 90% mineralized in 12 days.[131,170,179] All plaque does not necessarily undergo calcification. Early plaque contains a small amount of inorganic material, which increases as the plaque develops into calculus. Plaque that does not develop into calculus reaches a plateau of maximal mineral content within 2 days.[169] Microorganisms are not always essential in calculus formation, because calculus readily occurs in germ-free rodents.[66]

Saliva is the primary source of mineralization for supragingival calculus, whereas the serum transudate called *gingival crevicular fluid* furnishes the minerals for subgingival calculus.[80,188] The calcium concentration or content in plaque is 2 to 20 times higher than in saliva.[17] Early plaque of heavy calculus formers contains more calcium, three times more phosphorus, and less potassium than that of non-calculus formers, suggesting that phosphorus may be more critical than calcium for plaque mineralization.[116] Calcification entails the binding of calcium ions to the carbohydrate–protein complexes of the organic matrix and the precipitation of crystalline calcium phosphate salts.[114] Crystals form initially in the intercellular matrix and on the bacterial surfaces and finally within the bacteria.[60,215]

The calcification of supragingival plaque and the attached component of subgingival plaque begins along the inner surface

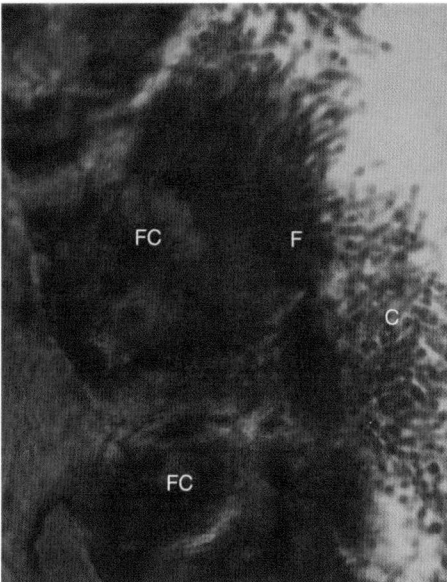

Fig. 13.11 Plaque and calculus on the tooth surface. Note the spherical areas of focal calcification *(FC)* and the perpendicular alignment of the filamentous *(F)* organisms along the inner surface of plaque and cocci *(C)* on the outer surface.

adjacent to the tooth structure. Separate foci of calcification increase in size and coalesce to form solid masses of calculus (see Fig. 13.11). For the initial mineralization process to occur, calcium phosphate supersaturation, certain membrane-associated components, and regulation of nuclear inhibitors are required.[82] Calcification may be accompanied by alterations in the bacterial content and staining qualities of the plaque. As calcification progresses, the number of filamentous bacteria increases, and the foci of calcification change from basophilic to eosinophilic. There is a reduction in the staining intensity of groups that exhibit a positive periodic acid–Schiff reaction.

Sulfhydryl and amino groups are also reduced and instead stain with toluidine blue, which is initially orthochromatic but becomes metachromatic and disappears.[202] Calculus is formed in layers, which are often separated by a thin cuticle that becomes embedded in the calculus as calcification progresses.[118]

The initiation of calcification and the rate of calculus accumulation vary among individuals, among tooth variety in the same dentition, and at different times in the same person.[132,195] On the basis of these differences, persons may be classified as *heavy, moderate,* or *slight* calculus formers or as noncalculus formers. The average daily increment in calculus formers is from 0.10% to 0.15% of dry weight calculus.[179,195] Calculus formation continues until it reaches a maximum, after which it may be reduced in amount. The time required to reach the maximal level has been reported to be between 10 weeks[35] and 6 months.[200]

The decline from maximal calculus accumulation, which is referred to as the *reversal phenomenon,* may be explained by the vulnerability of bulky calculus to mechanical wear from food and from the cheeks, lips, and tongue movement.

Theories Regarding the Mineralization of Calculus

The theoretical mechanisms by which plaque becomes mineralized can be stratified into two categories.[133]

1. Mineral precipitation results from a local rise in the degree of saturation of calcium and phosphate ions, which may be brought about in several ways:

- *A rise in the pH of the saliva causes the precipitation of calcium phosphate salts by lowering the precipitation constant.* The pH may be elevated by the loss of carbon dioxide and the formation of ammonia by dental plaque bacteria or by protein degradation during stagnation.[16,74]
- *Colloidal proteins in saliva bind calcium and phosphate ions and maintain a supersaturated solution with respect to calcium phosphate salts.* With the stagnation of saliva, colloids settle out, and the supersaturated state is no longer maintained, thereby leading to the precipitation of calcium phosphate salts.[152,171]
- *Phosphatase liberated from dental plaque, desquamated epithelial cells, or bacteria precipitates calcium phosphate by hydrolyzing organic phosphates in saliva, thereby increasing the concentration of free phosphate ions.*[205] *Esterase* is another enzyme that is present in the cocci and filamentous organisms, leukocytes, macrophages, and desquamated epithelial cells of dental plaque.[10] Esterase may initiate calcification by hydrolyzing fatty esters into free fatty acids. The fatty acids form soaps with calcium and magnesium that are later converted into the less-soluble calcium phosphate salts.

2. Seeding agents induce small foci of calcification that enlarge and coalesce to form a calcified mass.[135] This concept has been referred to as the *epitactic concept* or, more appropriately, as *heterogeneous nucleation.* The seeding agents in calculus formation are not known, but it is suspected that the intercellular matrix of plaque plays an active role.[117,131,215] The carbohydrate–protein complexes may initiate calcification by removing calcium from the saliva (chelation) and binding with it to form nuclei that induce the subsequent deposition of minerals.[114,201]

Role of Microorganisms in the Mineralization of Calculus

Mineralization of plaque generally starts extracellularly around both gram-positive and gram-negative organisms, but it may also start intracellularly.[99] Filamentous organisms, diphtheroids, and *Bacterionema* and *Veillonella* species have the ability to form intracellular apatite crystals (see Fig. 13.11). Mineralization spreads until the matrix and the bacteria are calcified.[60,216]

Bacterial plaque may actively participate in the mineralization of calculus by forming phosphatases, which change the pH of the plaque and induce mineralization,[43,114] but the prevalent opinion is that these bacteria are only passively involved[60,162,205] and are simply calcified with other plaque components. The occurrence of calculus-like deposits in germ-free animals supports this opinion.[66] However, other experiments suggest that transmissible factors are involved in calculus formation and that penicillin in the diets of some of these animals reduces calculus formation.[11]

Etiologic Significance

Distinguishing between the effects of calculus and plaque on the gingiva is difficult, because calculus is always covered with a nonmineralized layer of plaque.[169] A positive correlation between the presence of calculus and the prevalence of gingivitis exists,[156] but this correlation is not as great as that between plaque and gingivitis.[62] The initiation of periodontal disease in young people is closely related to plaque accumulation, whereas calculus accumulation is more prevalent in chronic periodontitis found in older adults.[62,106]

The incidence of calculus, gingivitis, and periodontal disease increases with age. It is extremely rare to find periodontal pockets in adults without at least some subgingival calculus being present, although the subgingival calculus may be of microscopic proportions.

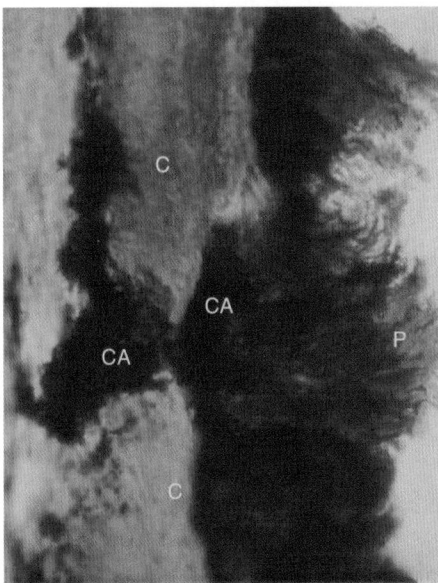

Fig. 13.12 Calculus *(CA)* penetrates the tooth surface and is embedded within the cementum *(C)*. Note the plaque *(P)* attached to the calculus.

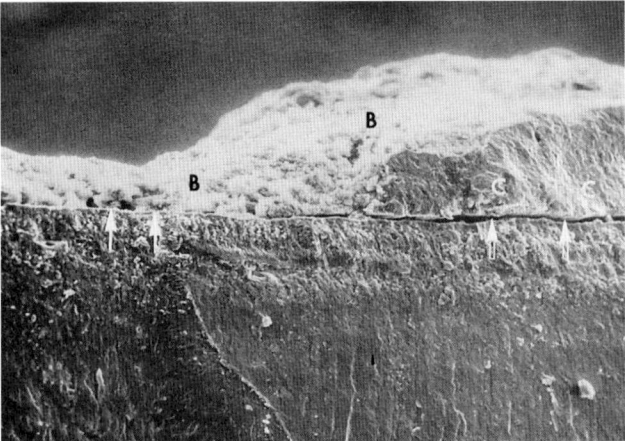

Fig. 13.13 Scanning electron microscope view of an extracted human tooth showing a cross-section of subgingival calculus *(C)* separated *(arrows)* from the cemental surface during processing of the specimen. Note the bacteria *(B)* attached to the calculus and the cemental surfaces. *(Courtesy Dr. John Sottosanti, La Jolla, CA.)*

Calculus does not contribute directly to gingival inflammation, but it provides a fixed nidus for the continued accumulation of bacterial plaque and its retention in close proximity to the gingiva (Fig. 13.12). Periodontal pathogens such as *Aggregatibacter actinomycetemcomitans*, *Porphyromonas gingivalis*, and *Treponema denticola* have been found within the structural channels and lacunae of supragingival and subgingival calculus.[136,137]

Subgingival calculus is likely to be the product rather than the cause of periodontal pockets. Plaque initiates gingival inflammation, which leads to pocket formation, and the pocket in turn provides a sheltered area for plaque and bacterial accumulation. The increased flow of gingival crevicular fluid associated with gingival inflammation provides the minerals that mineralize the continually accumulating plaque, resulting in the formation of subgingival calculus (Fig. 13.13). Over a 6-year period, Albandar and colleagues observed 156 teenagers with aggressive periodontitis.[2] They noted that areas with detectable subgingival calculus at the initiation of the study were much more

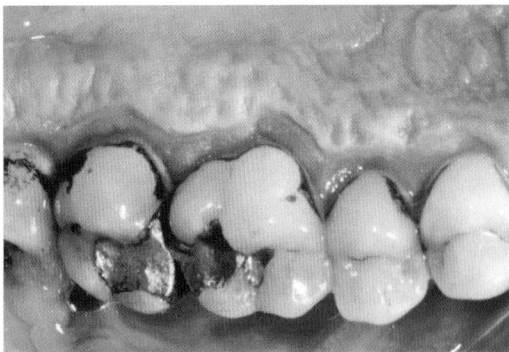

Fig. 13.14 Tobacco stains on the apical third of the clinical crown caused by cigarette smoking.

likely to experience a loss of periodontal attachment than sites that did not initially exhibit subgingival calculus.

Although the bacterial plaque that coats the teeth is the main etiologic factor in the development of periodontal disease, the removal of subgingival plaque and calculus constitutes the cornerstone of periodontal therapy. Calculus plays an important role in maintaining and accentuating periodontal disease by keeping plaque in close contact with the gingival tissue and by creating areas where plaque removal is impossible. Therefore, the clinician must not only possess the clinical skill to remove the plaque and calculus, but he or she must also be very conscientious about performing this task.

Materia Alba, Food Debris, and Dental Stains

Materia alba is an accumulation of microorganisms, desquamated epithelial cells, leukocytes, and a mixture of salivary proteins and lipids, with few or no food particles; it lacks the regular internal pattern observed in plaque.[172] It is a yellow or grayish-white, soft, sticky deposit, and it is somewhat less adherent than dental plaque. The irritating effect of materia alba on the gingiva is caused by bacteria and their products.

Most food debris is rapidly liquefied by bacterial enzymes and cleared from the oral cavity by salivary flow and the mechanical action of the tongue, cheeks, and lips. The rate of clearance from the oral cavity varies with the type of food and the individual. Aqueous solutions are typically cleared within 15 minutes, whereas sticky foods may adhere for more than 1 hour.[101,199] Dental plaque is not a derivative of food debris, and food debris is not an important cause of gingivitis.[42,86]

Pigmented deposits on the tooth surface are called *dental stains*. Stains are primarily an aesthetic problem and do not cause inflammation of the gingiva. The use of tobacco products (Fig. 13.14), coffee, tea, certain mouthrinses, and pigments in foods can contribute to stain formation.[112,187]

Other Predisposing Factors

Iatrogenic Factors

Deficiencies in the quality of dental restorations or prostheses are contributing factors to gingival inflammation and periodontal destruction. Inadequate dental procedures that contribute to the deterioration of the periodontal tissues are referred to as *iatrogenic factors*. Iatrogenic endodontic complications that can adversely affect the periodontium include root perforations, vertical root fractures, and endodontic failures that may necessitate tooth extraction.[211,214] Immediate implant placement in conjunction with extraction can contribute to an excessive labial and apical position of the implant, whereby the blood supply of surrounding osseous and gingival tissues

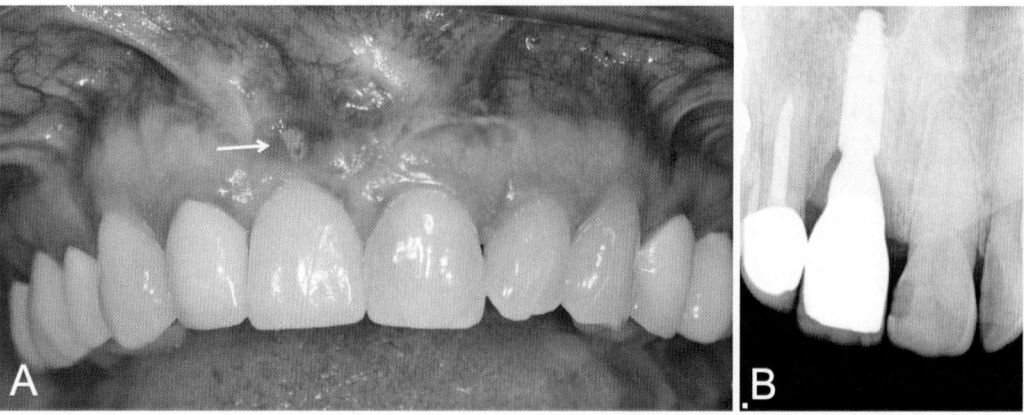

Fig. 13.15 (A) A fenestration defect *(arrow)* is noted after placement of a dental implant too far labial and apical, yielding inadequate bone and blood supply to support the surrounding gingiva. (B) Radiograph of the malpositioned dental implant.

is compromised, yielding to gingival fenestration or dehiscence[193] (Fig. 13.15). In order to mitigate the risk of dental implant complications, evidence-based clinical guidelines encourage practitioners to consider cone-beam computed tomography (CBCT) for dental implant treatment planning while taking into account the cost, acceptable radiation dose, and risks versus benefits.[196]

Characteristics of dental restorations and removable partial dentures that are important to the maintenance of periodontal health include the location of the gingival margin for the restoration, the space between the margin of the restoration and the unprepared tooth, the contour of the restorations, the occlusion, the materials used in the restoration, the restorative procedure itself, and the design of the removable partial denture. These characteristics are described in this chapter as they relate to the etiology of periodontal disease. A more comprehensive review with special emphasis on the interrelationship between restorative procedures and the periodontal status is presented in Chapter 70.

Margins of Restorations

Overhanging margins of dental restorations contribute to the development of periodontal disease by (1) changing the ecologic balance of the gingival sulcus to an area that favors the growth of disease-associated organisms (predominantly gram-negative anaerobic species) at the expense of the health-associated organisms (predominantly gram-positive facultative species)[101] and (2) inhibiting the patient's access to remove accumulated plaque.

The frequency of overhanging margins on proximal restorations has varied in different studies from 16.5% to 75%.[19,58,79,142] A highly significant statistical relationship has been reported between marginal defects and reduced bone height.[19,67,79] Gilmore and Sheiham noted that persons with overhanging posterior restorations had an average of 0.22 mm reduced alveolar bone support adjacent to the surfaces with overhangs.[58] The removal of overhangs allows for the more effective control of plaque, thereby resulting in a reduction of gingival inflammation and a small increase in radiographic alveolar bone support[61,71,183] (Fig. 13.16).

The location of the gingival margin of a restoration is directly related to the health status of the adjacent periodontal tissues.[181] Numerous studies have shown a positive correlation between restoration margins located apical to the marginal gingiva and the presence of gingival inflammation.[58,76,85,159,183] Subgingival margins are associated with large amounts of plaque, more severe gingivitis, deeper pockets, and a change in the composition of the subgingival microflora that closely resembles the microflora noted in chronic periodontitis.[98]

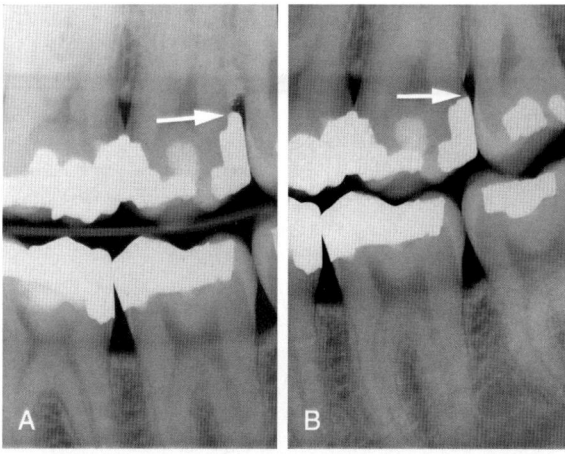

Fig. 13.16 (A) Radiograph of an amalgam overhang on the distal surface of the maxillary second molar that is a source of plaque retention and gingival irritation. (B) Radiograph depicts the removal of excessive amalgam.

Even high-quality restorations with clinically perfect margins, if placed subgingivally, will increase plaque accumulation, gingival inflammation,[98,101,129,134,160,182] and the rate of gingival crevicular fluid flow.[13,63] Margins placed at the level of the gingival crest induce less severe inflammation, whereas supragingival margins are associated with a degree of periodontal health similar to that seen with nonrestored interproximal surfaces.[52,181]

Roughness in the subgingival area is considered to be a major contributing factor to plaque buildup and subsequent gingival inflammation.[181] The subgingival zone is composed of the margin of the restoration, the luting material, and the prepared and unprepared tooth surfaces. Sources of marginal roughness include grooves and scratches in the surface of acrylic resin, porcelain, or gold restorations (Fig. 13.17); separation of the restoration margin and the luting material from the cervical finish line, thereby exposing the rough surface of the prepared tooth (Fig. 13.18); dissolution and disintegration of the luting material between the preparation and the restoration, thereby leaving a space; and inadequate marginal fit of the restoration.[181] Subgingival margins typically have a gap of 20 to 40 μm between the margin of the restoration and the unprepared tooth.[178] Colonization of this gap by bacterial plaque undoubtedly contributes to the detrimental effect of margins placed in a subgingival environment (Fig. 13.19).

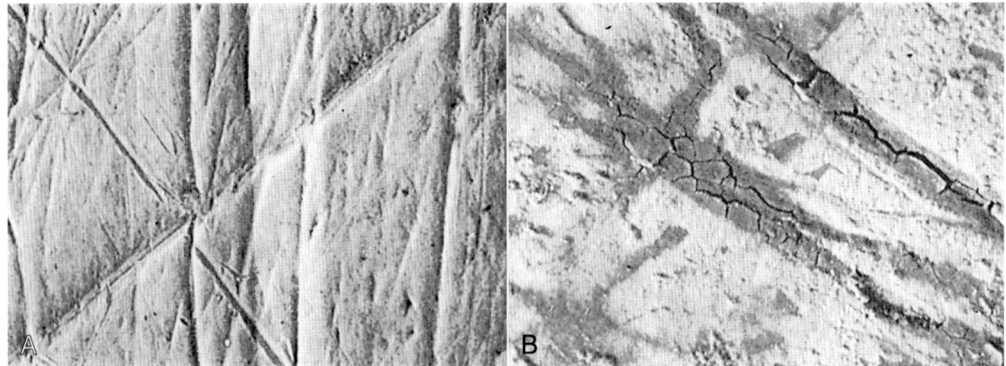

Fig. 13.17 (A) Polished gold alloy crown demonstrating surface scratches. (B) Gold alloy crown that had been in the patient's mouth for several years has scratches filled with deposits. *(From Silness J: Fixed prosthodontics and periodontal health.* Dent Clin North Am *24:317–329, 1980.)*

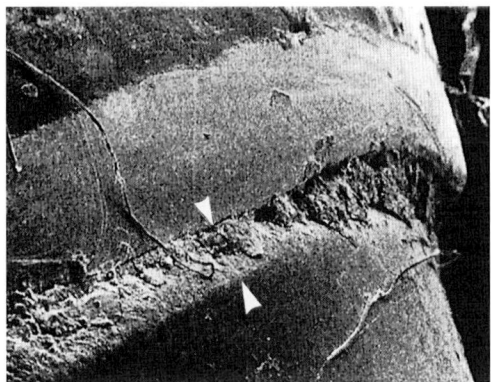

Fig. 13.18 After cementation, luting material prevents the approximation of the crown margin and the finishing line, thereby leaving part of the prepared tooth uncovered *(area between arrowheads). (From Silness J: Fixed prosthodontics and periodontal health.* Dent Clin North Am *24:317–329, 1980.)*

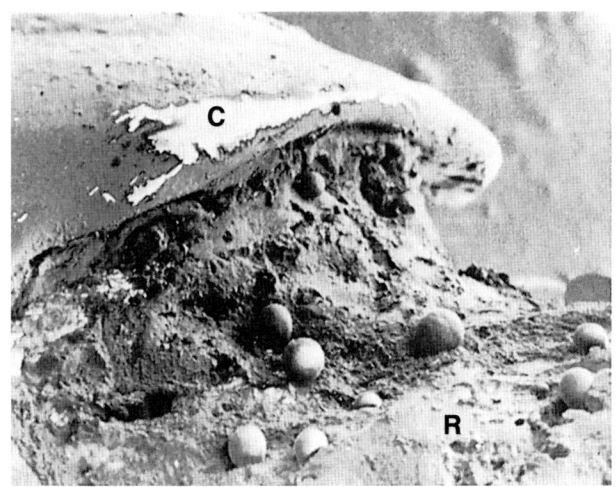

Fig. 13.19 A void has developed after dissolution and disintegration of the luting material. Spherical bodies are not identified. *C,* Crown; *R,* root. *(From Silness J: Fixed prosthodontics and periodontal health.* Dent Clin North Am *24:317–329, 1980.)*

Retained Cement and Periimplantitis

Periimplantitis is an inflammatory disease of the tissues around dental implants resulting in progressive bone loss (Fig. 13.20A and B), whereas periimplant mucositis is a reversible inflammatory change of the soft tissues around implants without bone loss.[107] The prevalence of periimplantitis among implant-supported prostheses/restorations ranges from 28% to 56%.[218] The early diagnosis of this condition and its proper management are critical to the longevity of the implant and the supported prosthesis.

Complex microbiota colonize pristine periimplant crevices within a week after implant placement, and the microbiota associated with failing implants is significantly different from that of healthy implants.[22,75,102,154,168] Classic studies that explored the composition of the periimplant biofilm in disease have shown that periimplantitis is an infection that is dominated by gram-negative bacteria with many similarities to the microbiota that is responsible for the development of periodontal diseases, including *Aggregatibacter actinomycetemcomitans, Porphyromonas gingivalis, Tannerella forsythia,* and *Fusobacterium* species.[154,161,168] The application of new microbiologic approaches has allowed for a broader characterization of the periimplant microbiome, which has led to the identification of periimplant-specific microbial lineages such as *Streptococcus mutans* and *Butyrivibrio fibrisolvens.*[97,127,168]

« FLASH BACK

Periimplantitis is frequently associated with crowns exhibiting retained excessive luting cement.

A larger proportion of black-pigmented bacteria are found at periimplantitis sites in dentate patients as compared with edentulous patients. Presumably these periimplantitis infectious organisms arise from the sulcular microbiota of the natural dentition.[7] Consequently, it is critical that practitioners evaluate the patient's periodontal status and provide appropriate periodontal therapy in conjunction with implant rehabilitation.

Local factors such as retained residual cement or inadequate seating of the implant abutment or prosthesis can lead to bone loss around an implant (see Fig. 13.20C–E). In a retrospective study, Wilson found that 81% of the implants diagnosed with periimplantitis had residual cement associated with their cement-retained restorations.[208] The surgical removal of the residual cement resolved the infection and halted the periimplantitis in 74% of the implants. A deeper crown margin makes it more difficult to

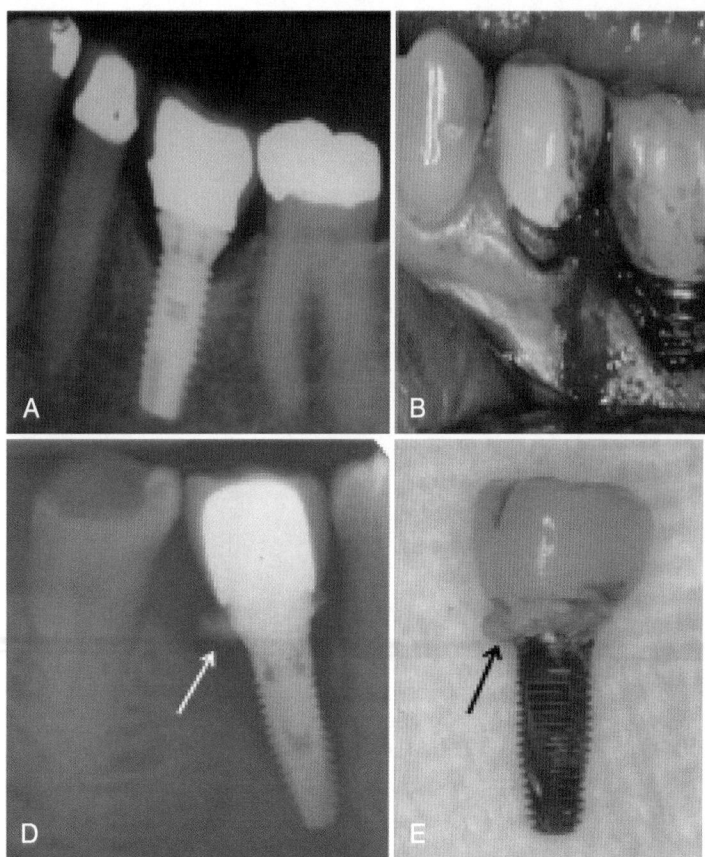

Fig. 13.20 (A) Radiograph of a moat-like bony defect at a periimplantitis site associated with retained cement and a crown that is not fully seated. (B) Moat-like bony defect and retained excessive cement. (C) The *arrow* points to visibly retained excessive cement between the crown margin and the abutment that prevents the full seating of the crown and leads to hyperocclusion. *(Courtesy Dr. Emilie Vachon, Minneapolis, MN.)* (D) Radiograph of a periimplantitis site shows bone loss associated with retained excessive cement *(arrow).* (E) Retrieved implant restoration shows excessive cement remnants *(arrow)* on implant surface.

remove excess cement. The greatest amount of residual cement was noted when the crown margin was 2 or 3 mm below the gingival margin.[108]

 CLINICAL CORRELATION

The deeper a subgingival crown margin is placed, the higher the likelihood of poorer marginal integrity with accompanying gingival inflammation.

The possible adverse effect of traumatic occlusion on implants has been correlated with early implant failures.[125] However, the relationship between traumatic occlusion and periimplantitis is, to date, a controversial issue. In vivo experiments have shown that, in the absence of periimplant inflammation, the application of excessive occlusal stress leads to only minor alterations in the marginal bone level.[92] Alternatively, the application of excessive occlusal forces in the presence of plaque-induced inflammation can significantly increase the rate of bone loss around implant-supported restorations.[32]

Contours and Open Contacts

Overcontoured crowns and restorations tend to accumulate plaque and handicap oral hygiene measures in addition to possibly preventing the self-cleaning mechanisms of the adjacent cheek, lips, and tongue[6,95,130,209] (Fig. 13.21). Restorations that fail to reestablish adequate interproximal embrasure spaces are associated with papillary inflammation. Undercontoured crowns that lack a protective height of contour do not retain as much plaque as overcontoured crowns and therefore may not be as detrimental during mastication as once thought.[209]

 CLINICAL CORRELATION

Overcontoured crowns are more detrimental to periodontal health than undercontoured crowns.

The contour of the occlusal surface as established by the marginal ridges and related developmental grooves normally serves to deflect food away from the interproximal spaces. The optimal cervico-occlusal location for a posterior contact is at the longest mesiodistal diameter of the tooth, which is generally just apical to the crest of the marginal ridge. The integrity and location of the proximal contacts along with the contour of the marginal ridges and developmental grooves typically prevent interproximal food impaction. *Food impaction* is the forceful wedging of food into the periodontium by occlusal forces. As the teeth wear down, their originally convex proximal surfaces become flattened, and the wedging effect of the opposing cusp is exaggerated. Cusps that tend to forcibly wedge food into interproximal embrasures are known as *plunger cusps.* The interproximal plunger cusp effect may also be observed when missing teeth are not replaced and the relationship between the proximal contacts of adjacent teeth is altered. An intact proximal contact precludes the forceful wedging of food into the interproximal embrasure space, whereas a light or open contact is conducive to impaction.

 FLASH BACK

Posterior teeth with open contact and food impaction exhibit greater probing depth and clinical attachment loss than contralateral control sites without food impaction.

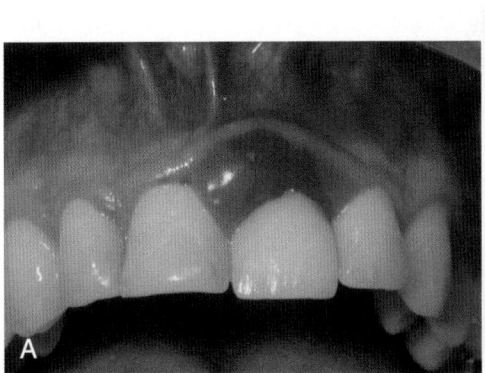
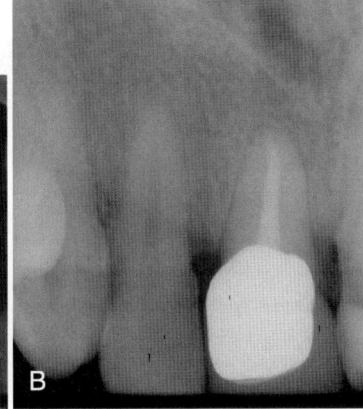

Fig. 13.21 (A) Inflamed marginal and papillary gingiva adjacent to an overcontoured porcelain-fused-to-metal crown on the maxillary left central incisor. (B) Radiograph of an ill-fitting porcelain-fused-to-metal crown.

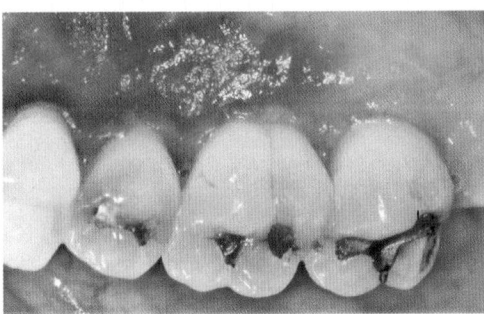

Fig. 13.22 Inflamed palatal gingiva associated with a maxillary provisional acrylic partial denture. Note the substantial difference in color of the inflamed gingiva adjacent to the premolars and the first molar as compared with the gingiva adjacent to the second molar.

The classic analysis of the factors that lead to food impaction was made by Hirschfeld,[73] who recognized the following factors: uneven occlusal wear, opening of the contact point as a result of loss of proximal support or from extrusion, congenital morphologic abnormalities, and improperly constructed restorations.

The presence of the previously mentioned abnormalities does not necessarily lead to food impaction and periodontal disease. A study of interproximal contacts and marginal ridge relationships[101] in three groups of periodontally healthy males revealed that 4.9% to 62.5% of the proximal contacts were defective and that 33.5% of adjacent marginal ridges were uneven.[140] However, greater probing depth and a loss of clinical attachment have been reported for sites that exhibited both an open contact and food impaction as compared with contralateral control sites without open contacts or food impaction.[81] Excessive anterior overbite is a common cause of food impaction on the lingual surfaces of the maxillary anterior teeth and the facial surfaces of the opposing mandibular teeth. These areas may be exemplified by attachment loss with gingival recession.

Materials

In general, restorative materials are not in themselves injurious to the periodontal tissues.[6,88] One exception to this may be self-curing acrylics[203] (Fig. 13.22).

Plaque that forms at the margins of restorations is similar to that found on adjacent nonrestored tooth surfaces. The composition of plaque formed on all types of restorative materials is similar, with the exception of that formed on silicate.[135] Although surface textures of restorative materials differ with regard to their capacity to retain plaque,[206] all can be adequately cleaned if they are polished and accessible to methods of oral hygiene.[138,184] The undersurface of pontics in fixed bridges should barely touch the mucosa. Access for oral hygiene is inhibited with excessive pontic-to-tissue contact, thereby contributing to plaque accumulation that will cause gingival inflammation and possibly the formation of pseudopockets.[50,181]

Design of Removable Partial Dentures

Several investigations have shown that, after the insertion of partial dentures, mobility of the abutment teeth, gingival inflammation, and periodontal pocket formation all increase.[18,29,174] This is because partial dentures favor the accumulation of plaque, particularly if they cover the gingival tissue. Partial dentures that are worn during both night and day induce more plaque formation than those worn only during the daytime.[18] These observations emphasize the need for careful and personalized oral hygiene instruction to avoid the harmful effects of partial dentures on the remaining teeth and the periodontium.[13] The presence of removable partial dentures induces not only quantitative changes in dental plaque[57] but also qualitative changes, thereby promoting the emergence of spirochetal microorganisms.[56]

Restorative Dentistry Procedures

The use of rubber dam clamps, matrix bands, and burs in such a manner as to lacerate the gingiva results in varying degrees of mechanical trauma and inflammation. Although such transient injuries generally undergo repair, they are needless sources of discomfort to the patient. The forceful packing of a gingival retraction cord into the sulcus to prepare the subgingival margins of a tooth or for the purpose of obtaining an impression may mechanically injure the periodontium and leave behind impacted debris that is capable of causing a foreign body reaction.

Malocclusion

The irregular alignment of teeth as found in cases of malocclusion may facilitate plaque accumulation and make plaque control more difficult. Several authors have found a positive correlation between crowding and periodontal disease,[28,145,190] whereas other investigators did not find such a correlation.[55] Uneven marginal ridges of contiguous posterior teeth have been found to have a low correlation with pocket depth, loss of attachment, plaque, calculus, and gingival inflammation.[90]

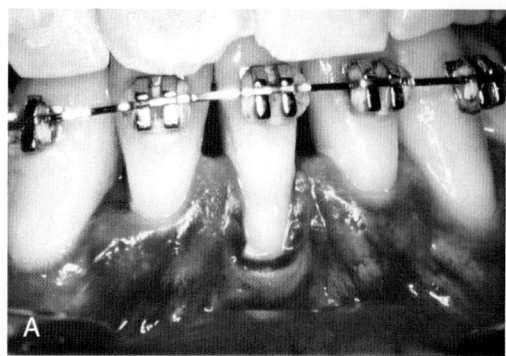
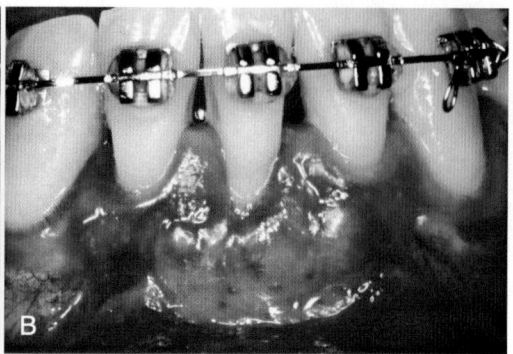

Fig. 13.23 (A) Lower incisor showing a prominent root with gingival recession and a lack of attached gingiva. (B) Appearance 3 months after the placement of a free gingival graft, which resulted in a gain in attached gingiva and a reduction in gingival recession.

Roots of teeth that are prominent in the arch (Fig. 13.23)—such as in a buccal or lingual version or that are associated with a high frenal attachment and small quantities of attached gingiva—frequently exhibit recession.[1,124]

The failure to replace missing posterior teeth may have adverse consequences on the periodontal support for the remaining teeth.[31] The following hypothetical scenario illustrates the possible ramifications of not replacing a missing posterior tooth. When the mandibular first molar is extracted, the initial change is a mesial drifting and tilting of the mandibular second and third molars with extrusion of the maxillary first molar. As the mandibular second molar tips mesially, its distal cusps extrude and act as plungers. The distal cusps of the mandibular second molar wedge between the maxillary first and second molars and open the contact by deflecting the maxillary second molar distally. Subsequently, food impaction may occur and may be accompanied by gingival inflammation with the eventual loss of the interproximal bone between the maxillary first and second molars. This example does not occur in all cases in which mandibular first molars are not replaced. However, the drifting and tilting of the remaining teeth with an accompanying alteration of the proximal contacts is generally a consequence of not replacing posterior teeth that have been extracted.

Tongue thrusting exerts excessive lateral pressure on the anterior teeth, which may result in the spreading and tilting of the anterior teeth (Fig. 13.24). Tongue thrusting is an important contributing factor to tooth migration and the development of an anterior open bite.[30] Mouth breathing may be observed in association with a habit of tongue thrusting and an anterior open bite. Marginal and papillary gingivitis is frequently encountered in the maxillary anterior sextant in cases that involve an anterior open bite with mouth breathing. However, the role of mouth breathing as a local causative factor is unclear, because conflicting evidence has been reported.[3,77,78,190]

Restorations that do not conform to the occlusal pattern of the mouth result in occlusal disharmonies that may cause injury to the supporting periodontal tissues. More issues involving deeper initial probing depths, worse prognoses, and greater mobility have been observed for teeth with occlusal discrepancies as compared with teeth without initial occlusal discrepancies.[69,139] Histologic features of the periodontium for a tooth that has been subjected to traumatic occlusion include a widened subcrestal periodontal ligament space, a reduction in the collagen content of the oblique and horizontal fibers, an increase in vascularity and leukocyte infiltration, and an increase in the number of osteoclasts on bordering alveolar bone.[15] However, these observations are generally apical and separate from the bacteria-induced inflammation that occurs at the base of the sulcus. On the basis of current human trials, it is still impossible to definitively answer the question, "Does occlusal trauma modify the progression of periodontal attachment loss that is associated with periodontal inflammation?"[176] (See Chapter 55 for a more detailed explanation of periodontal trauma from occlusion and the periodontal response to external forces.)

Periodontal Complications Associated With Orthodontic Therapy

Orthodontic therapy may affect the periodontium by favoring plaque retention, by directly injuring the gingiva as a result of overextended bands, and by creating excessive forces, unfavorable forces, or both on the tooth and its supporting structures.

Plaque Retention and Composition

Orthodontic appliances tend to retain bacterial plaque and food debris, thereby resulting in gingivitis (Fig. 13.25), and they are also capable of modifying the gingival ecosystem. Scanning electron microscopic examination of the orthodontic bracket–tooth junction shows that excess bonding composite around the bracket base creates a critical site for plaque accumulation due to its rough surface texture and the presence of a distinct gap at the composite–enamel interface. A complex community of bacterial plaque may be noted on the excess composite material within 2 to 3 weeks after bonding.[189] An increase in *Prevotella melaninogenica, Prevotella intermedia,* and *Actinomyces odontolyticus* and a decrease in the proportion of facultative microorganisms was detected in the gingival sulcus after the placement of orthodontic bands.[40] More recently, *A. actinomycetemcomitans* was found in at least one site in 85% of children who were wearing orthodontic appliances.[143] By contrast, only 15% of unbanded control subjects were positive for *A. actinomycetemcomitans.*

 KEY FACT

Orthodontic treatment should not be commenced in the presence of uncontrolled periodontal disease because it will worsen the periodontal condition.

Gingival Trauma and Alveolar Bone Height

Orthodontic treatment is often started soon after the eruption of the permanent teeth, when the junctional epithelium is still adherent to the enamel surface. Orthodontic bands should not be forcefully placed beyond the level of attachment, because this will detach the gingiva from the tooth and result in the apical proliferation of

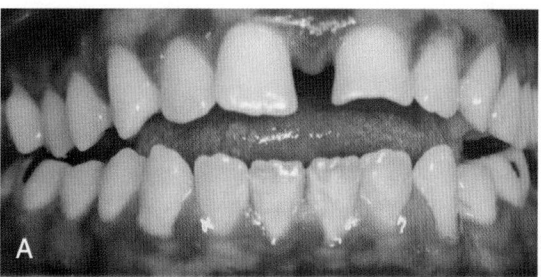

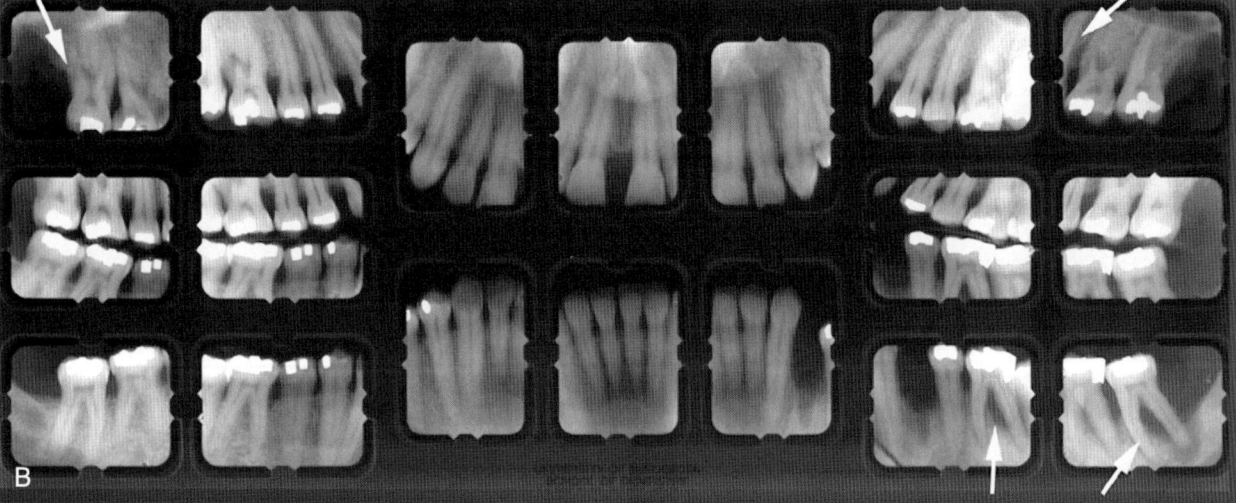

Fig. 13.24 (A) Anterior open bite with flared incisors as observed in association with a habit of tongue thrusting. (B) Radiographs show severe periodontal destruction *(arrows)* in the molar regions.

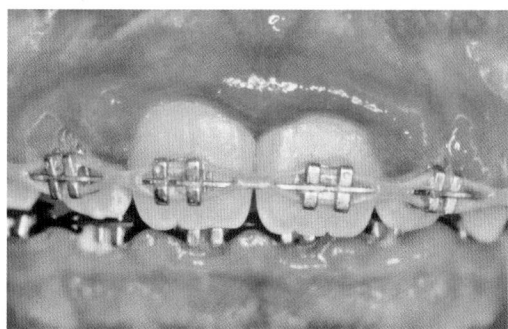

Fig. 13.25 Gingival inflammation and enlargement associated with an orthodontic appliance and poor oral hygiene.

the junctional epithelium with an increased incidence of gingival recession.[146]

 KEY FACT

Adult patients planning to undergo orthodontic care should undergo pretreatment assessment for their periodontal status and potential risk for root resorption.

The mean alveolar bone loss per patient for adolescents who underwent 2 years of orthodontic care during a 5-year observation period ranged between 0.1 and 0.5 mm.[21] This small magnitude of alveolar bone loss was also noted in the control group and therefore is considered to be of little clinical significance. However, the degree of bone loss during adult orthodontic care may be higher than that observed in adolescents,[113] especially if the periodontal condition is

not treated before the initiation of orthodontic therapy. Orthodontic treatment in adults with active periodontitis (evidenced by deep pockets and bleeding on probing) has been shown to accelerate the periodontal disease process.[8,45,212]

Tissue Response to Orthodontic Forces

Orthodontic tooth movement is possible because the periodontal tissues are responsive to externally applied forces.[158,173] Alveolar bone is remodeled by osteoclasts that induce bone resorption in areas of pressure and by osteoblasts that form bone in areas of tension. Although moderate orthodontic forces ordinarily result in bone remodeling and repair, excessive force may produce necrosis of the periodontal ligament and the adjacent alveolar bone.[149-151] Excessive orthodontic forces also increase the risk of apical root resorption.[25,26] The prevalence of severe root resorption (i.e., resorption of more than one-third of the root length) during orthodontic therapy in adolescents has been reported to be 3%.[83] The incidence of moderate to severe root resorption for incisors among adults aged 20 to 45 years has been reported to be 2% before treatment and 24.5% after treatment.[113] Risk factors associated with root resorption during orthodontic treatment include the duration of treatment, the magnitude of the force applied, the direction of the tooth movement, and the continuous versus intermittent application of forces[148] (Fig. 13.26).

 KEY FACT

It is important to avoid excessive force and too-rapid tooth movement during orthodontic treatment to prevent injury to the periodontium.

The use of elastics to close a diastema may result in severe attachment loss with possible tooth loss as the elastics migrate apically

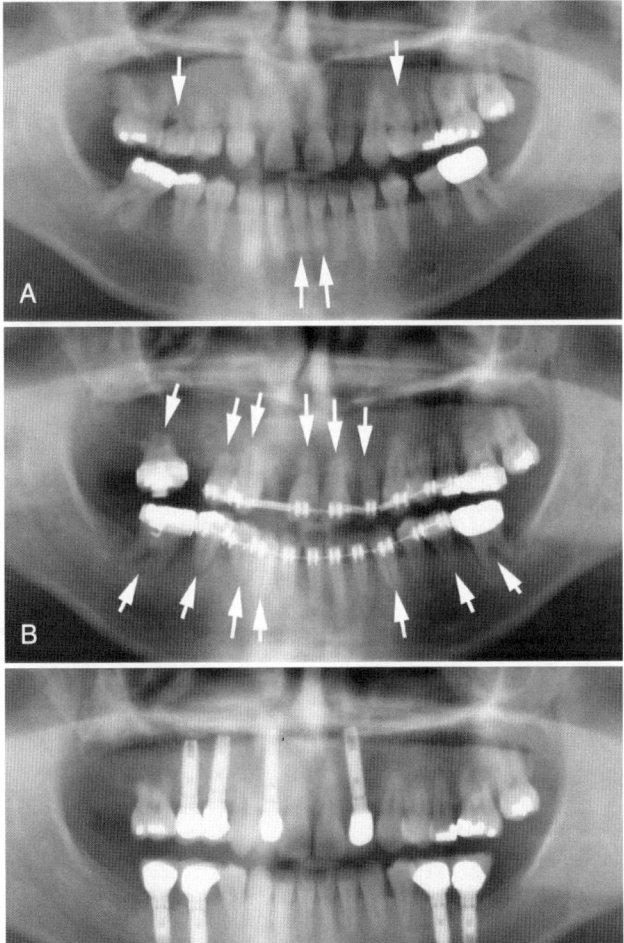

Fig. 13.26 (A) Panoramic radiograph illustrating that a limited degree of pretreatment root resorption *(arrows)* existed before orthodontic care. (B) Note that several roots have undergone severe resorption *(arrows)* during 4 years of intermittent orthodontic treatment. (C) The teeth that developed extensive root resorption with accompanying hypermobility have been extracted and replaced with implant-supported crowns.

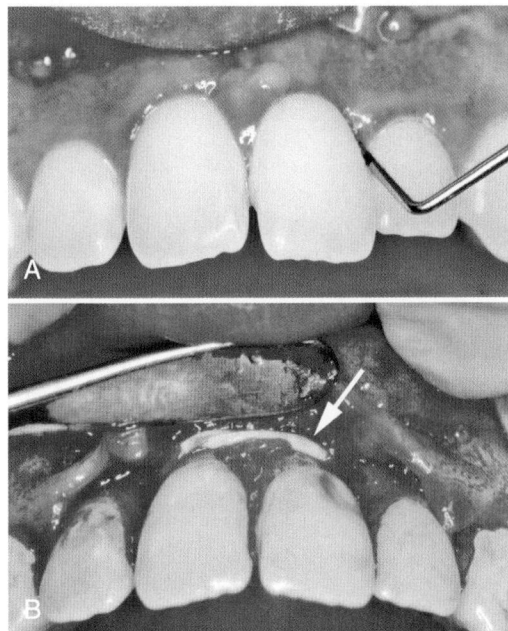

Fig. 13.27 (A) Maxillary central incisors for which an elastic ligature was used to close a midline diastema. Note the inflamed gingiva and the deep probing depths. (B) Reflection of a full-thickness mucoperiosteal flap reveals elastic ligature *(arrow)* and angular intrabony defects around the central incisors.

along the root surface (Fig. 13.27). The surgical exposure of impacted teeth and orthodontic-assisted eruption has the potential to compromise periodontal attachment on adjacent teeth (Fig. 13.28). However, the majority of impacted teeth that are surgically exposed and aided in their eruption by orthodontic treatment subsequently exhibited more than 90% of their attachment as being intact.[72]

It has been reported that the dentoalveolar gingival fibers that are located within the marginal and attached gingiva are stretched when teeth are rotated during orthodontic therapy.[41] The surgical severing or removal of these gingival fibers in combination with a brief period of retention may reduce the incidence of relapse after orthodontic treatment that is intended to realign rotated teeth.[24,126]

Extraction of Impacted Third Molars

Numerous clinical studies have reported that the extraction of impacted third molars often results in the creation of vertical defects distal to the second molars.[9,96,121] This iatrogenic effect is unrelated to flap design,[153] and it appears to occur more often when third molars are extracted from individuals who are more than 25 years old.[9,96,121] Other factors that appear to play a role in the development

of lesions on the distal surface of second molars—particularly in those who are more than 25 years old—include the presence of visible plaque, bleeding on probing, root resorption in the contact area between the second and third molars, the presence of a pathologically widened follicle, the inclination of the third molar, and the close proximity of the third molar to the second molar (Fig. 13.29).[96] Other potential iatrogenic adverse consequences of the removal of third molars include permanent paresthesia (i.e., numbness of the lip, tongue, and cheek), damage to adjacent teeth, mandibular fracture, maxillary tuberosity fracture, displacement of third molars and root tips, oro-antral communications or fistula, and temporomandibular joint complications.[23] Permanent paresthesia occurs at a frequency of approximately 1 of every 100,000 wisdom teeth removed in the United States.[53] The incidence of damage to second molar as a consequence of third molar extraction has been estimated to be 0.3% to 0.4%.[33] Although the incidence of mandibular fracture during or after third molar removal is low (0.003% to 0.005%),[105] it may pose important medicolegal and patient care implications. Iatrogenic displacement of a maxillary third molar into the maxillary sinus[144,210] and displacement of a mandibular third molar into the sublingual, submandibular, pterygomandibular, and lateral pharyngeal spaces[47,210] have been reported with unknown incidence rates.

 FLASH BACK

Preoperative use of three-dimensional radiographs in conjunction with extraction of impacted third molars has the potential to minimize the risk of inferior alveolar nerve paresthesia or damage to the adjacent second molar.

For several decades, panoramic radiography has been the standard of choice to assess the state of third molar impaction, including angulation of the tooth, root morphology, root development, related

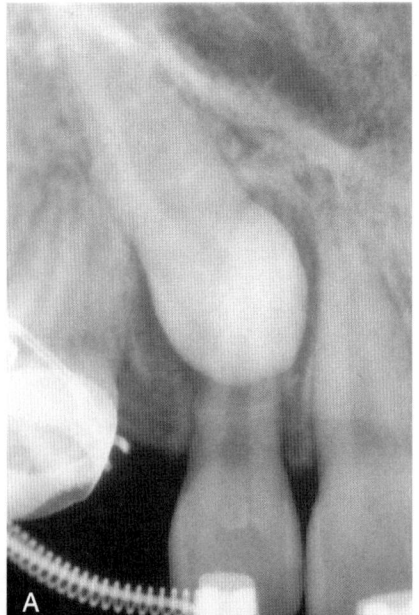

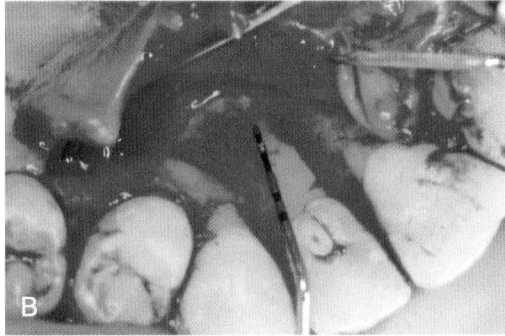

Fig. 13.28 (A) Radiograph of an impacted maxillary canine that required surgical exposure and orthodontic assistance to erupt. (B) A palatal flap is reflected to reveal bony dehiscence on the maxillary lateral incisor after orthodontic therapy.

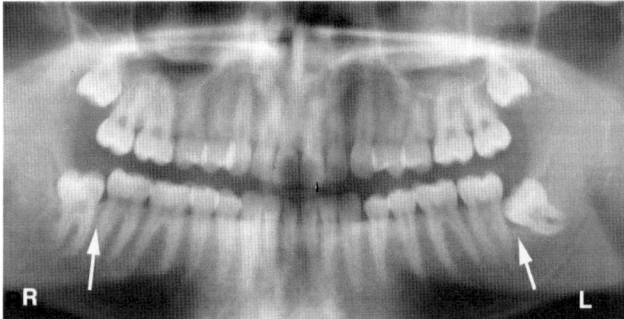

Fig. 13.29 Panoramic radiograph illustrating a mesially impacted lower left third molar with a widened follicle and no apparent bone on the distal interproximal surface of the second molar. Alternatively, the lower right third molar is vertically impacted and exhibits interproximal bone distal to the second molar and mesial to the third molar.

pathology, and, most importantly, the relation between the tooth or roots and the mandibular canal. However, when an overprojection is observed between the impacted third molar and the mandibular canal, or when specific signs suggest a close contact between the third molar and the mandibular canal, CBCT is recommended to be more beneficial in proper treatment planning[123] (Fig. 13.30).

Habits and Self-Inflicted Injuries

Patients may not be aware of their self-inflicted injurious habits that may be important to the initiation and progression of their periodontal disease. Mechanical forms of trauma can stem from the improper use of a toothbrush, the wedging of toothpicks between the teeth, the application of fingernail pressure against the gingiva (Fig. 13.31), pizza burns, and other causes.[20] Sources of chemical irritation include the topical application of caustic medications such as aspirin or cocaine, allergic reactions to toothpaste or chewing gum, the use of chewing tobacco, and concentrated mouthrinses.[177] Accidental and iatrogenic gingival injuries may be caused by a variety of chemical, physical, and thermal sources, yet they are generally self-limited. Iatrogenic injuries are often acute, whereas factitious injuries tend to be more chronic in nature.[157]

 FLASH BACK

Sources of self-inflicted injuries include improper use of toothbrushes, wedging toothpicks between teeth, application of fingernail pressure against gingiva, and pizza burn. Chemical sources include topical application of caustic medications such as aspirin or cocaine, allergic reaction to toothpaste or chewing gum, use of chewing tobacco, and concentrated mouthrinses.

Trauma Associated With Oral Jewelry

The use of piercing jewelry in the lip or tongue has become more common among teenagers and young adults (Fig. 13.32A). However, piercings are associated with potential complications including gingival injury or recession[70,100,104,213,217]; damage to teeth, restorations, and fixed porcelain prostheses[48,54,70,104]; increased salivary flow[54,197]; interference with speech, mastication, or deglutition[84,198]; scar tissue formation[197]; and development of metal hypersensitivities.[93]

 FLASH BACK

Use of tongue or lip piercing jewelry is associated with localized gingival recession and periodontitis.

Whittle and Lamden[207] surveyed 62 dentists and found that 97% had seen patients with either lip- or tongue-piercing jewelry within the previous 12 months. The incidence of lingual recession with pocket formation (Fig. 13.32B) and radiographic evidence of bone loss (Fig. 13.32C) was 50% among subjects with a mean age of 22 years who wore lingual "barbells" for 2 years or longer.[38] Chipped lower anterior teeth were noted in 47% of the patients who wore tongue-piercing jewelry for 4 years or longer. Patients need to be informed of the risks of wearing oral jewelry and cautioned against such practices.

Toothbrush Trauma

Abrasions of the gingiva as well as alterations in tooth structure may result from aggressive toothbrushing in a horizontal or rotary fashion. The deleterious effect of excessively forceful brushing is accentuated when highly abrasive dentifrices are used. The gingival changes that are attributable to toothbrush trauma may be acute or chronic. The acute changes vary with regard to their appearance and duration, from scuffing of the epithelial surface to denudation of the underlying connective tissue with the formation of a painful gingival ulcer (Fig. 13.33). Diffuse erythema and denudation of the attached gingiva throughout the mouth may be a striking result of overzealous

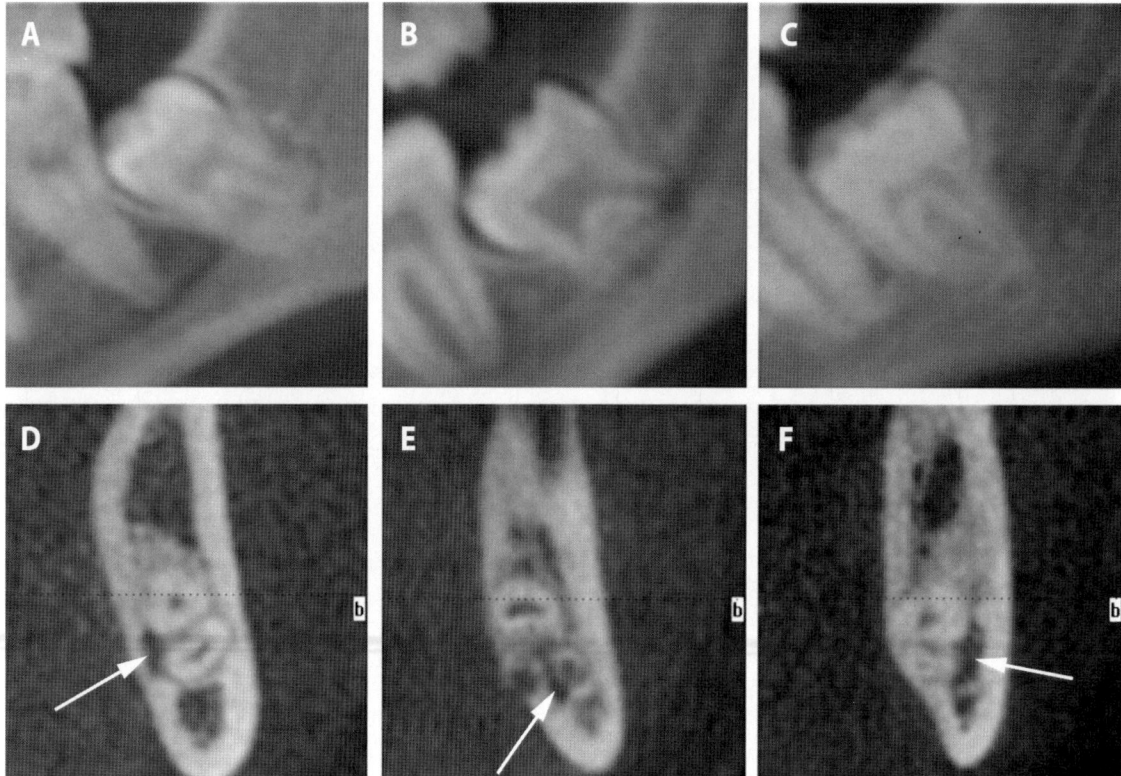

Fig. 13.30 Segmented panoramic images. (A and B) Overprojection between the impacted third molar and the mandibular canal. (C) Signs of close contact between the third molar and the mandibular canal. (D through F) Corresponding core-beam computed tomographic images (axial views) of the impacted third molars reveal the path of the inferior alveolar nerve *(arrow)* (D) lingual to the root, (E) surrounded by three segments of the root, and (F) buccal to the root. *(Courtesy Dr. Mansur Ahmad, Minneapolis, MN.)*

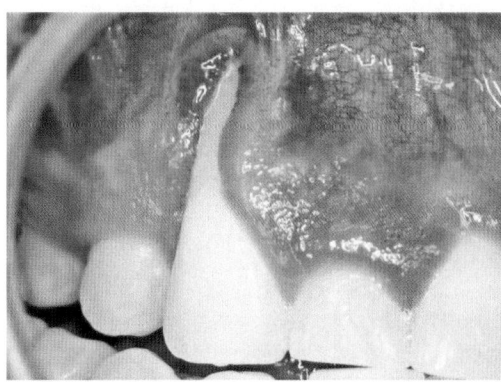

Fig. 13.31 Gingival recession on a maxillary canine caused by self-inflicted trauma from the patient's fingernail.

brushing. Signs of acute gingival abrasions are frequently noted when the patient first uses a new brush. Puncture lesions may be produced when heavy pressure is applied to firm bristles that are aligned perpendicular to the surface of the gingiva. A forcibly embedded toothbrush bristle can be retained in the gingiva and cause an acute gingival abscess.

Chronic toothbrush trauma results in gingival recession with denudation of the root surface. Interproximal attachment loss is generally a consequence of bacteria-induced periodontitis, whereas buccal and lingual attachment loss is frequently the result of toothbrush abrasion.[185] The improper use of dental floss may result in lacerations of the interdental papilla.

Chemical Irritation

Acute gingival inflammation may be caused by chemical irritation that results from either sensitivity or nonspecific tissue injury. In allergic inflammatory states, the gingival changes range from simple erythema to painful vesicle formation and ulceration. Severe reactions to ordinarily innocuous mouthwashes, dentifrices, and denture materials are often explainable on this basis.

Acute inflammation with ulceration may be produced by the nonspecific injurious effect of chemicals on the gingival tissues. The indiscriminate use of strong mouthwashes, the topical application of corrosive drugs such as aspirin (Fig. 13.34) or cocaine, and accidental contact with drugs such as phenol or silver nitrate are common examples of chemical exposures that cause irritation of the gingiva. A histologic view of an aspirin-induced chemical burn shows vacuoles with serous exudates and an inflammatory infiltrate in the connective tissue (Fig. 13.35).

Smokeless Tobacco

Snuff and chewing tobacco constitute the two main forms of smokeless tobacco. Snuff is a fine-cut form of tobacco that is available loosely packed or in small sachets. Chewing tobacco is a more coarse-cut tobacco that is available in the form of loose leaves, a solid block, a plug, or a twist of dried leaves. Chewing tobacco is typically placed in the mandibular buccal vestibule for several hours, during which time saliva and dilute tobacco are periodically expectorated.[204] The nicotine uptake of smokeless tobacco is similar to that of smoking cigarettes in that the consumption of a 34-gram container of smokeless tobacco is approximately equal to 1.5 packs of cigarettes.[64] Many professional baseball players use chewing tobacco. The perceived

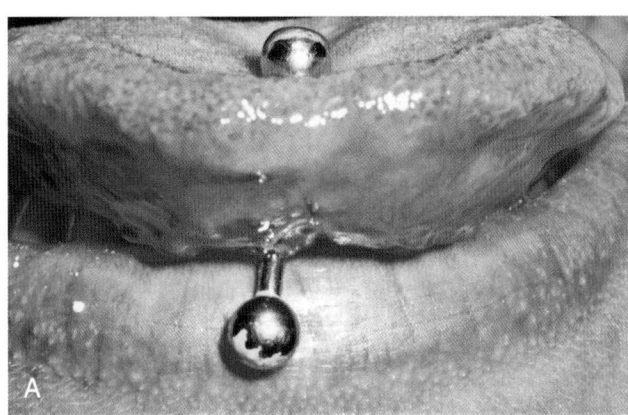

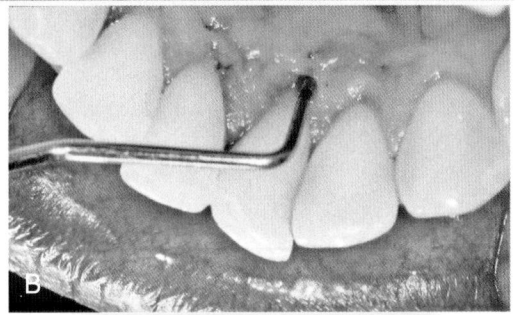

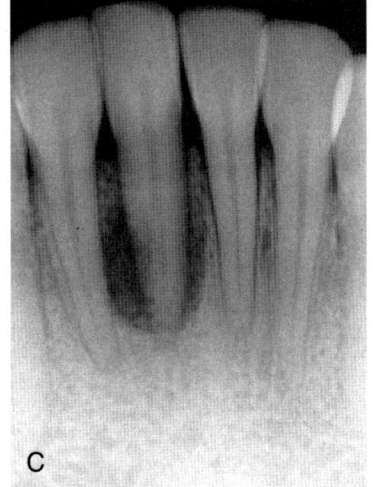

Fig. 13.32 (A) Tongue pierced with oral jewelry. (B) Probing depth of 8 mm with 10 mm of clinical attachment loss on the lingual surface of the lower central incisor adjacent to the oral jewelry in the pierced tongue. The central incisor was found to be vital. (C) Bone loss associated with a tongue pierced by oral jewelry. *(B, Courtesy Dr. Leonidas Batas, Thessaloniki, Greece.)*

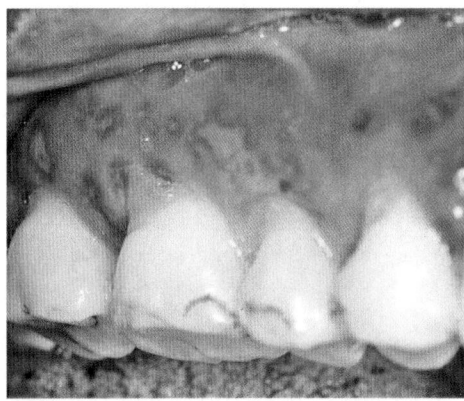

Fig. 13.33 The overzealous use of a toothbrush resulted in denudation of the gingival epithelial surface and exposure of the underlying connective tissue as a painful ulcer.

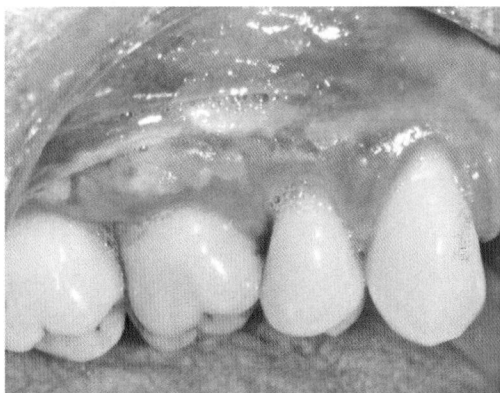

Fig. 13.34 Chemical burn caused by aspirin; note the sloughing gingival tissue and the resultant recession.

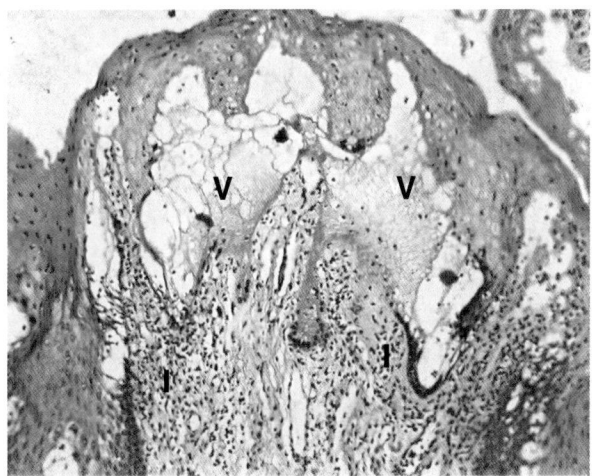

Fig. 13.35 Biopsy of an aspirin-induced chemical burn. Note the intraepithelial vesicles *(V)* and inflammatory infiltrate *(I)* within the underlying connective tissue.

benefits of chewing tobacco are those derived from nicotine, including improved mental alertness, diminished reaction time, muscle relaxation, and reduced anxiety and appetite.[65,163] A 1990 survey of 1109 professional baseball players in the United States reported that 39% of the players used smokeless tobacco, with 46% of the users exhibiting leukoplakia within the gingiva or the mucosa (Fig. 13.36).[46] Histologic features of oral leukoplakia associated with smokeless tobacco include (1) a chevron-like pattern of hyperkeratosis with focal areas of inflammation and (2) hyperplasia in the basal cell layer (Fig. 13.37). Increased incidences of gingival recession, cervical root abrasion, and root caries have been reported with the use of smokeless tobacco (Fig. 13.38).[141,164,165,194]

The incidence of gingival recession among adolescents who use smokeless tobacco has been reported to be 42%, compared with 17% among nonusers.[36,122,124,128] The Third National Health and Nutrition Examination Survey (NHANES III) investigated the adverse effect of smokeless tobacco on the periodontium and found double the incidence of severe periodontitis (odds ratio, 2.1; 95% confidence interval, 1.2 to 3.7) among 12,932 adults who used smokeless tobacco but who never smoked cigarettes.[49] However, Bergstrom and colleagues found similar incidences of severe periodontitis among both smokeless tobacco users and nonusers.[14] It can be concluded that the use of smokeless tobacco is associated with at least localized gingival recession, clinical attachment loss, leukoplakia, and possibly enhanced susceptibility to severe periodontitis.

Radiation Therapy

Radiation therapy has cytotoxic effects on both normal cells and malignant cells. A typical total dose of radiation for head and neck tumors is in the range of 5000 to 8000 centigray (cGy); 1 cGy is equal to 1 radiation absorbed dose (rad) and equivalent to 50 to 80 Sieverts (Sv).[147] The total dose of radiation is usually given in partial incremental doses, and this is referred to as *fractionation*. Fractionation helps to minimize the adverse effects of radiation while maximizing the death rate for the tumor cells.[51] Fractionated doses are typically administered in the range of 100 to 1000 cGy or 1 to 10 Sv per week.

Radiation treatment induces an obliterative endarteritis that results in soft tissue ischemia and fibrosis; irradiated bone becomes hypovascular and hypoxic.[119] Adverse effects of head and neck radiation therapy include dermatitis and mucositis of the irradiated area as well as muscle fibrosis and trismus, which may restrict access to the oral cavity.[166] The mucositis typically develops 5 to 7 days after radiation therapy is initiated. The severity of the mucositis can be reduced by asking the patient to avoid secondary sources of irritation (e.g., smoking, alcohol, spicy foods) to the mucous membrane. The use of a chlorhexidine digluconate mouthrinse may help to reduce the mucositis.[155] However, most chlorhexidine mouthrinses currently available in the United States have a high alcohol content that may act as an astringent, which dehydrates the mucosa and thus intensifies the pain. Saliva production is permanently impaired when salivary glands that are located within the portal of radiation receive 6000 cGy (60 Sv) or more.[120] Xerostomia results in greater plaque accumulation and a reduced buffering capacity of saliva. Effective oral hygiene, professional dental prophylactic cleanings, fluoride applications, and frequent dental examinations are essential to control caries and periodontal disease. The use of customized trays appears to be a more effective method for fluoride application compared with the toothbrush.[89]

Among cancer patients who were treated with high-dose unilateral radiation, periodontal attachment loss and tooth loss were reported to be greater on the irradiated site compared with the nonradiated control side of the dentition.[44] Patients who are diagnosed with oral cancer and who require radiation therapy should ideally be assessed for dental needs (i.e., mucositis, xerostomia, faulty restorations, periapical lesion, coronal and cervical decay, and periodontal status) before the initiation of radiation treatment.[68] The treatment and prevention of trismus, oral fungal infections, odontogenic infections, osteoradionecrosis, decay, and periodontal disease are critical to minimize oral morbidity for these patients. Dental and periodontal infections have the potential to be severe risks for patients who have been treated with head and neck radiation. The risk of

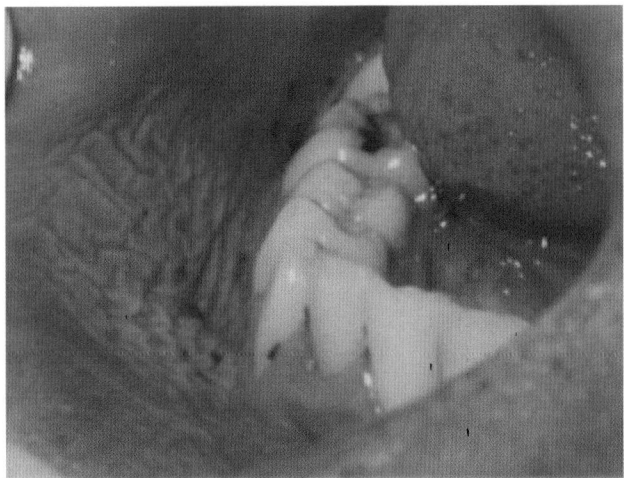

Fig. 13.36 Oral leukoplakia in the vestibule associated with the use of smokeless tobacco.

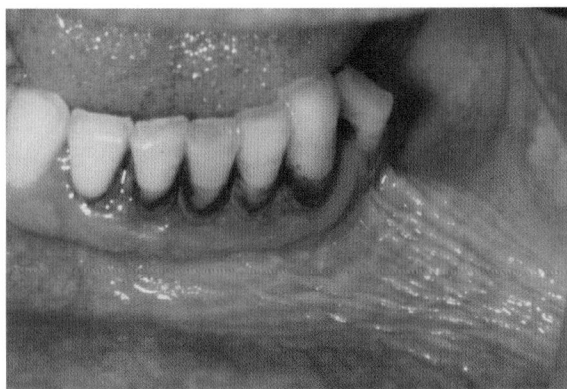

Fig. 13.38 Oral leukoplakia, recession, and clinical attachment loss associated with the use of smokeless tobacco.

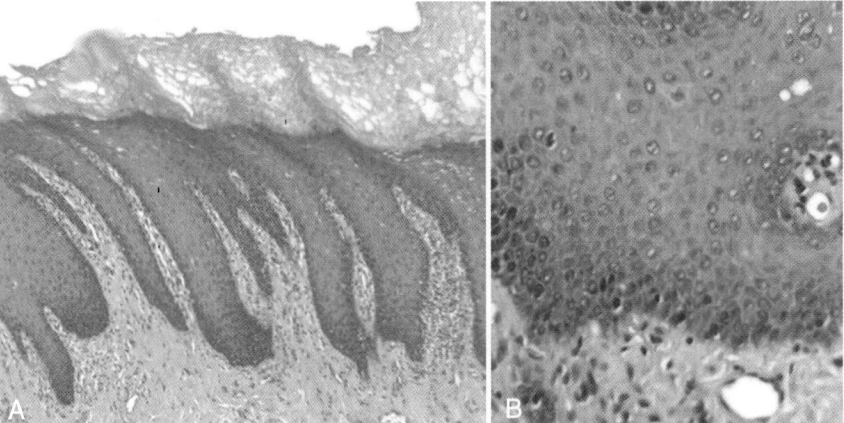

Fig. 13.37 (A) Histologic features of oral leukoplakia associated with smokeless tobacco. Note the chevron-like pattern of hyperkeratosis with focal areas of inflammation. (B) Hyperplasia in the basal cell layer.

osteoradionecrosis for oncology patients can be minimized by evaluating their oral status, providing dental care, and allowing time for tissue repair before the commencement of radiotherapy.[91]

Oral conditions that increase the risk of osteoradionecrosis for patients about to undergo radiation therapy for oral malignancies include periodontal probing depths of more than 5 mm, dental plaque score of more than 40%, and alveolar bone loss of more than 60%.[87] Nonrestorable teeth and teeth with significant periodontal problems should be extracted before radiation therapy to reduce the risk of postradiotherapy osteoradionecrosis.[91] (See Chapter 39 for more detail regarding the periodontal management of medically compromised patients.)

The risk of osteoradionecrosis must be evaluated before the performance of atraumatic extractions or limited periodontal surgical procedures in previously irradiated sites. Therefore, the dentist may choose to consult with the patient's oncologist before the initiation of dental therapy. A randomized multicenter clinical trial questioned the merit of using hyperbaric oxygen therapy to treat osteoradionecrosis because, at 1 year after treatment, only 19% of test subjects had responded to hyperbaric oxygen therapy, compared with 32% of placebo subjects.[5] The administration of the combination of pentoxifylline with vitamin E as antioxidant therapy currently shows the greatest promise for revascularization and treatment of osteoradionecrosis sites.[39]

CLINICAL CORRELATION

Use of smokeless tobacco has been associated with localized gingival leukoplakia, recession, clinical attachment loss, and increased susceptibility to severe periodontitis.

 A Case Scenario is found on the companion website www.expertconsult.com.

References

 References for this chapter are found on the companion website www.expertconsult.com.

CHAPTER 14

Influence of Systemic Conditions

Perry R. Klokkevold | Brian L. Mealey

CHAPTER OUTLINE

Endocrine Disorders and Hormonal
  Changes
Hematologic Disorders and Immune
  Deficiencies

Genetic Disorders
Stress and Psychosomatic
  Disorders
Nutritional Influences

Medications
Other Systemic Conditions
Conclusion

 For expanded discussions on female sex hormones, genetic disorders, and nutritional influences on periodontal disease as well as online-only content on hyperparathyroidism, anemia, thrombocytopenia, antibody deficiency disorders, and other systemic conditions, please visit the companion website at www.expertconsult.com.

Many systemic diseases, disorders, and conditions have been implicated as risk indicators or risk factors in periodontal disease. Clinical and basic science research over the past several decades has led to an improved understanding of and appreciation for the complexity and pathogenesis of periodontal diseases.[193] Although there is clear evidence for a bacterial etiology and there are specific bacteria (periodontal pathogens) associated with destructive periodontal disease, the presence of these pathogens does not invariably cause disease. Their absence, on the other hand, appears to be consistent with periodontal health. The role of bacteria in disease etiology and pathogenesis is discussed in Chapters 7 and 8.

Perhaps the most significant advance in our understanding of the pathogenesis of periodontitis is that the host response varies among individuals and that an altered, deficient, or exaggerated host immune response to bacterial pathogens may lead to more severe forms of the disease. In other words, the individual host immune response to periodontal pathogens is very important and likely explains many of the differences in disease severity observed from one individual to the next. Furthermore, systemic diseases, disorders, and conditions alter host tissues and physiology, which may impair the host's barrier function and immune defense against periodontal pathogens, thereby creating the opportunity for destructive periodontal disease to progress.

Evidence also suggests that periodontal infections can adversely affect systemic health with manifestations such as coronary heart disease, stroke, diabetes, preterm labor, low-birth-weight delivery, and respiratory disease.[171] The role of periodontal infections on these systemic health conditions is discussed in Chapter 15.

The relationships between periodontal infections and host defense are complex. A number of environmental, physical, and psychosocial factors have the potential to alter periodontal tissues and the host immune response, thereby resulting in more severe periodontal disease expression. It is important to recognize that the systemic diseases, disorders, or conditions themselves do not cause periodontitis; rather, they may predispose, accelerate, or otherwise increase the disease's progression. This chapter discusses important systemic diseases, disorders, and conditions that have the potential to influence periodontal health.

Endocrine Disorders and Hormonal Changes

Endocrine diseases such as diabetes and hormonal fluctuations that are associated with puberty and pregnancy are well-known examples of systemic conditions that adversely affect the condition of the periodontium. Endocrine disturbances and hormone fluctuations affect the periodontal tissues directly, modify the tissue response to local factors, and produce anatomic changes in the gingiva that may favor plaque accumulation and disease progression. This section describes the evidence that supports the relationships among endocrine disorders, hormonal changes, and periodontal disease.

Diabetes Mellitus

Diabetes mellitus is an extremely important disease from a periodontal standpoint. It is a complex metabolic disorder characterized by chronic hyperglycemia. Diminished insulin production, impaired insulin action, or a combination of both result in the inability of glucose to be transported from the bloodstream into the tissues, which in turn results in high blood glucose levels and the excretion of sugar in the urine. Lipid and protein metabolism are altered in diabetes as well. Uncontrolled diabetes (chronic hyperglycemia) is associated with several long-term complications, including microvascular diseases (retinopathy, nephropathy, or neuropathy), macrovascular diseases (cardiovascular and cerebrovascular conditions), increased susceptibility to infections, and poor wound healing. An estimated 25.8 million individuals (both children and adults)—8.3% of the US population—have diabetes.[43] Approximately 7 million of these individuals are unaware that they have the disease.

There are two major types of diabetes, type 1 and type 2, with several less common secondary types. *Type 1 diabetes mellitus,* which was formerly known as *insulin-dependent diabetes mellitus,* is caused by a cell-mediated autoimmune destruction of the insulin-producing beta cells of the islets of Langerhans in the pancreas, which results in insulin deficiency. Type 1 diabetes accounts for 5% to 10% of all cases of diabetes and most often occurs in children and young adults. This type of diabetes results from a lack of insulin production, and it is very unstable and difficult to control. It has a marked tendency toward ketosis and coma, it is not preceded by obesity, and it requires the injection of insulin to be controlled. Patients with type 1 diabetes mellitus present with the symptoms that are traditionally associated with diabetes, including polyphagia, polydipsia, polyuria, and predisposition to infections.

Type 2 diabetes mellitus, which was formerly known as *non–insulin-dependent diabetes mellitus,* is caused by peripheral resistance to insulin action, impaired insulin secretion, and increased glucose production in the liver. The insulin-producing beta cells in the pancreas are not destroyed by cell-mediated autoimmune reaction. It typically begins as insulin resistance, which leads to the reduced pancreas production of insulin as the demand increases. Type 2 diabetes is the most common form of diabetes, and it accounts for 90% to 95% of all diagnosed cases in adults. Individuals are often not aware they have the disease until severe symptoms or complications occur. Type 2 diabetes generally occurs in obese individuals, and it can often be controlled by diet and oral hypoglycemic agents. Ketosis and coma are uncommon. Type 2 diabetes can manifest with the same symptoms as type 1 diabetes but typically in a less severe form.

An additional category of diabetes is *hyperglycemia* secondary to other diseases or conditions. A prime example of this type of hyperglycemia is gestational diabetes associated with pregnancy. *Gestational diabetes* develops in 2% to 10% of all pregnancies but disappears after delivery. Women who have had gestational diabetes are at increased risk of developing type 2 diabetes. Other secondary types of diabetes are those associated with diseases that involve the pancreas and the destruction of the insulin-producing cells. Endocrine diseases (e.g., acromegaly, Cushing syndrome), tumors, pancreatectomy, and drugs or chemicals that cause altered insulin levels are included in this group. Experimentally induced types of diabetes generally belong in this category rather than in the categories of type 1 or 2 diabetes mellitus.

KEY FACT

Diabetes mellitus is an extremely important disease that impacts multiple systems including periodontal health. It is a complex metabolic disorder characterized by chronic hyperglycemia. Uncontrolled diabetes is associated with long-term complications, including microvascular diseases (retinopathy, nephropathy, or neuropathy), macrovascular diseases (cardiovascular and cerebrovascular conditions), increased susceptibility to infections, and poor wound healing. An estimated 25.8 million individuals (both children and adults)—8.3% of the US population—have diabetes.[43] Approximately 7 million of these individuals are unaware that they have the disease.

Oral Manifestations

Numerous oral changes have been described in patients with diabetes, including cheilosis, mucosal drying and cracking, burning mouth and tongue, diminished salivary flow, and alterations in the flora of the oral cavity, with greater predominance of *Candida albicans,* hemolytic streptococci, and staphylococci.[1,23,103,166] An increased rate of dental caries has also been observed in patients with poorly controlled diabetes.[77,87] It is important to note that these changes are not always present, that they are not specific, and that they are not pathognomonic for diabetes.[169] Furthermore, these changes are less likely to be observed in patients with well-controlled diabetes. Individuals with controlled diabetes have a normal tissue response, a normally developed dentition, a normal defense against infections, and no increase in the incidence of caries.[246]

The influence of diabetes on the periodontium has been thoroughly investigated. Although it is difficult to make definitive conclusions

about the specific effects of diabetes on the periodontium, a variety of changes have been described, including a tendency toward an enlarged gingiva, sessile or pedunculated gingival polyps, polypoid gingival proliferations, abscess formation, periodontitis, and loosened teeth[116] (Fig. 14.1). Perhaps the most striking changes in patients with uncontrolled diabetes are the reductions in the defense mechanisms and the increased susceptibility to infections, which lead to destructive periodontal disease. In fact, periodontal disease is considered to be the sixth complication of diabetes.[152] Periodontitis in patients with type 1 diabetes appears to start after the age of 12 years, and it has a fivefold increased prevalence in teenagers.[50] The prevalence of periodontitis has been reported as 9.8% in 13- to 18-year-old patients, and it increases to 39% in those who are 19 years old and older.

The extensive literature on this subject and the overall impression of clinicians indicate that *periodontal disease in patients with diabetes follows no consistent or distinct pattern.* Severe gingival inflammation, deep periodontal pockets, rapid bone loss, and frequent periodontal abscesses often occur in patients with poorly controlled diabetes and poor oral hygiene[3] (Figs. 14.2 and 14.3). Children with type 1 diabetes tend to have more destruction around the first molars and incisors, but this destruction becomes more generalized at older ages.[49] In patients with juvenile diabetes, extensive periodontal destruction often occurs as a consequence of having more severe disease at a younger age.

Other investigators have reported that the rate of periodontal destruction appears to be similar for those with diabetes and those without diabetes up to the age of 30 years.[93,240] Older patients with diabetes have a greater degree of periodontal destruction, possibly related to more disease destruction over time. Patients who have had overt diabetes for more than 10 years have a greater loss of periodontal support than those with a diabetic history of less than 10 years.[93] This destruction may also be related to the diminished tissue integrity, which continues to deteriorate over time (see Altered Collagen Metabolism).

Although some studies have not found a correlation between the diabetic state and the periodontal condition, the majority of well-controlled studies show a higher prevalence and severity of periodontal disease in individuals with diabetes compared with nondiabetic persons with similar local factors.[15,23,40,52,113,183,185,187,243] Findings include a greater loss of attachment, increased bleeding on probing, and increased tooth mobility. A study of risk indicators for a group of 1426 patients between the ages of 25 and 74 years revealed that individuals with diabetes were twice as likely to exhibit attachment loss as nondiabetic individuals.[110] The lack of consistency across studies is most likely related to the different degrees of diabetic involvement, variations in the level of disease control and the diversity of indices, and patient sampling from one study to another.

Studies have suggested that uncontrolled or poorly controlled diabetes is associated with an increased susceptibility to and severity of infections, including periodontitis.[17,217] Adults who are 45 years of age or older with poorly controlled diabetes (i.e., with a glycated hemoglobin level >9%) were 2.9 times more likely to have severe periodontitis than those without diabetes. The likelihood was even greater (4.6 times) among smokers with poorly controlled diabetes.[43] As with other systemic conditions associated with periodontitis, diabetes mellitus does not cause gingivitis or periodontitis, but evidence indicates that it alters the response of the periodontal tissues to local factors, thereby hastening bone loss and delaying postsurgical healing. Frequent periodontal abscesses appear to be an important feature of periodontal disease in patients with diabetes.

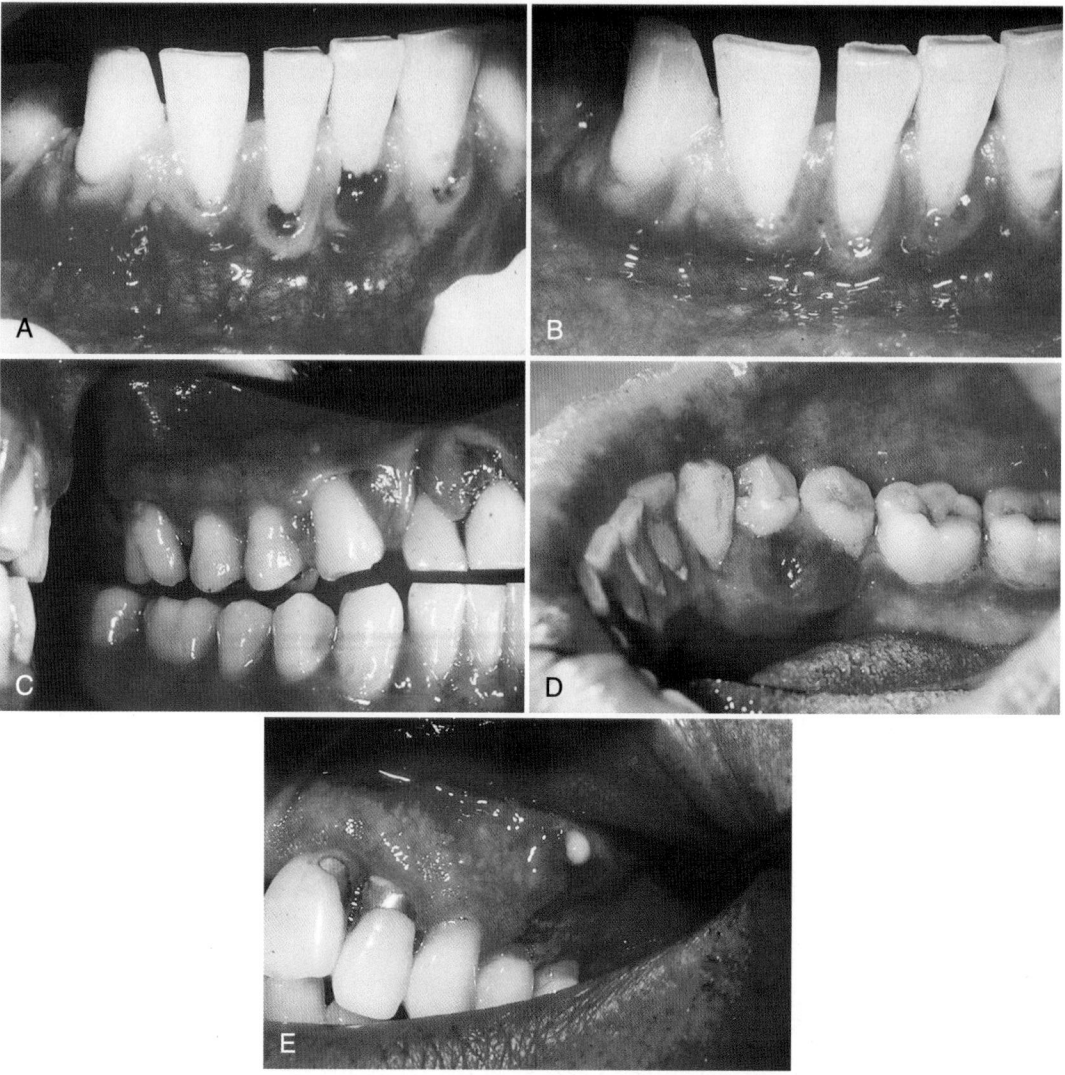

Fig. 14.1 Periodontal condition in patients with diabetes. (A) Adult with diabetes (blood glucose level >400 mg/dL). Note the gingival inflammation, spontaneous bleeding, and edema. (B) The same patient as shown in A. Improved control of diabetes was noted after 4 days of insulin therapy (blood glucose level <100 mg/dL). The clinical periodontal condition has improved without local therapy. (C) Adult patient with uncontrolled diabetes. Note the enlarged, smooth, erythematous gingival margins and papilla in the anterior area. (D) The same patient as shown in C. This is a lingual view of the right mandibular area. Note the inflamed and swollen tissues in the anterior and premolar areas. (E) Adult patient with uncontrolled diabetes. There is a suppurating abscess on the buccal surface of the maxillary premolars.

Approximately 40% of adult Pima Indians in Arizona have type 2 diabetes. A comparison of individuals with and without diabetes in this Native American tribe showed a clear increase in the prevalence of destructive periodontitis as well as a 15% increase in edentulousness among patients with diabetes.[229] The risk of developing destructive periodontitis was increased threefold in these individuals.[74]

Bacterial Pathogens

The glucose content of gingival fluid and blood is higher in individuals with diabetes than in those without diabetes with similar plaque and gingival index scores.[80] The increased glucose in the gingival fluid and blood of patients with diabetes could change the environment of the microflora, thereby inducing qualitative changes in bacteria that may contribute to the severity of periodontal disease observed in those with poorly controlled diabetes.

Patients with type 1 diabetes mellitus and periodontitis have been reported to have a subgingival flora that is composed mainly of *Capnocytophaga*, anaerobic vibrios, and *Actinomyces* species. *Porphyromonas gingivalis*, *Prevotella intermedia*, and *Aggregatibacter actinomycetemcomitans*, which are common in periodontal lesions of individuals without diabetes, are present in low numbers in those with the disease.[112,167] However, other studies have found scarce *Capnocytophaga* and abundant *A. actinomycetemcomitans* and black-pigmented *Bacteroides* as well as *P. intermedia*, *Prevotella melaninogenica*, and *Campylobacter rectus*.[166,220] Black-pigmented species—especially *P. gingivalis*, *P. intermedia*, and *C. rectus*—are prominent in severe periodontal lesions of Pima Indians with type 2 diabetes.[90,275] Although these results may suggest an altered flora in the periodontal pockets of patients with diabetes, the exact role of these microorganisms has not been determined. To date, there is insufficient evidence to support the role of a specific altered microflora

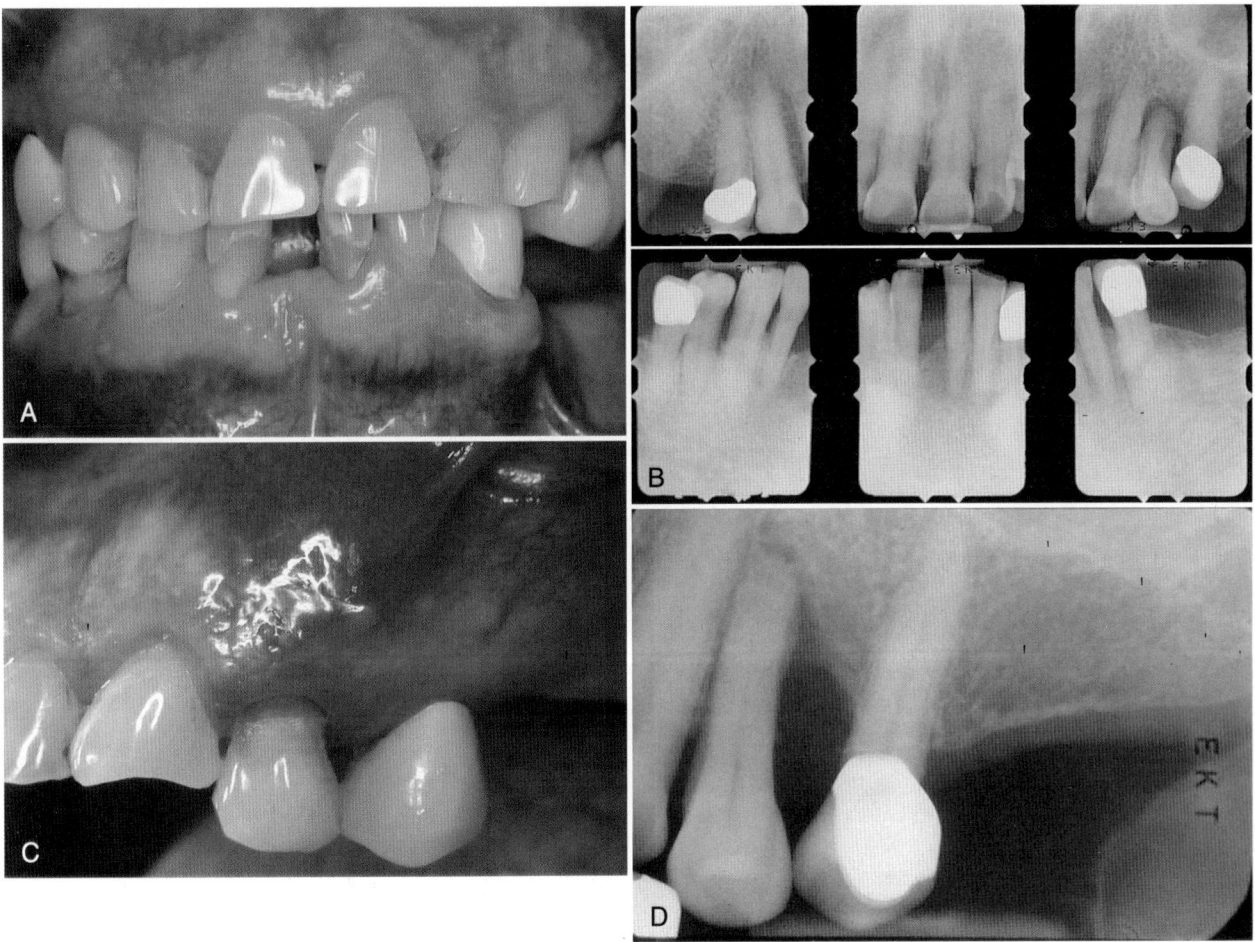

Fig. 14.2 A 60-year-old patient with a long-term history of type 2 diabetes. (A) Anterior retracted view of the patient's dental and periodontal condition. Note the missing posterior teeth, the supereruption of the premolars, and the mild generalized gingival inflammation. (B) Periapical radiographs of the remaining teeth. Note the mild generalized bone loss with localized areas of severe bone loss. The failure to replace the posterior teeth adds to the occlusal burden of the remaining dentition. (C) Clinical photograph of the maxillary premolar area presenting with abscess. Notice the diffuse erythema and inflammation surrounding the abscess area. (D) Periapical radiograph of the maxillary premolar showing extensive bone loss associated with abscess.

that is responsible for periodontal disease destruction in patients with diabetes.

Polymorphonuclear Leukocyte Function

The increased susceptibility of patients with diabetes to infection has been hypothesized as being caused by polymorphonuclear leukocyte (PMN) deficiencies that result in impaired chemotaxis, defective phagocytosis, or impaired adherence.[170,243] In patients with poorly controlled diabetes, the functions of PMNs, monocytes, and macrophages are impaired.[120] As a result, the primary defense mounted by PMNs against periodontal pathogens is diminished, and bacterial proliferation is more likely. No alteration of immunoglobulin A (IgA), G (IgG), or M (IgM) has been found in patients with diabetes.[210]

Altered Collagen Metabolism

Chronic hyperglycemia impairs collagen structure and function, which may directly impact the integrity of the periodontium. Decreased collagen synthesis, osteoporosis, and a reduction in alveolar bone height have been demonstrated in diabetic animals.[94,224] Chronic hyperglycemia adversely affects the synthesis, maturation, and maintenance of collagen and extracellular matrix. In the hyperglycemic state, numerous proteins and matrix molecules undergo a nonenzymatic

glycosylation, thereby resulting in *accumulated glycation end-products* (AGEs). The formation of AGEs occurs at normal glucose levels as well; however, in hyperglycemic environments, AGE formation is excessive. Many types of molecules are affected, including proteins, lipids, and carbohydrates. Collagen is cross-linked by AGE formation, which makes the collagen less soluble and less likely to be normally repaired or replaced. Cellular migration through cross-linked collagen is impeded, and, perhaps more importantly, tissue integrity is impaired as a result of damaged collagen that remains in the tissues for longer periods (i.e., collagen is not renewed at a normal rate).[110] As a result, collagen in the tissues of patients with poorly controlled diabetes is older and more susceptible to pathogenic breakdown (i.e., less resistant to destruction by periodontal infections).

AGEs and receptors for AGEs (RAGEs) play a central role in the classic complications of diabetes,[34] and they may play a significant role in the progression of periodontal disease as well. Poor glycemic control, with the associated increase in AGEs, renders the periodontal tissues more susceptible to destruction.[223] The cumulative effects of altered cellular response to local factors, impaired tissue integrity, and altered collagen metabolism undoubtedly play a significant role in the susceptibility of patients with diabetes to infections and destructive periodontal disease.

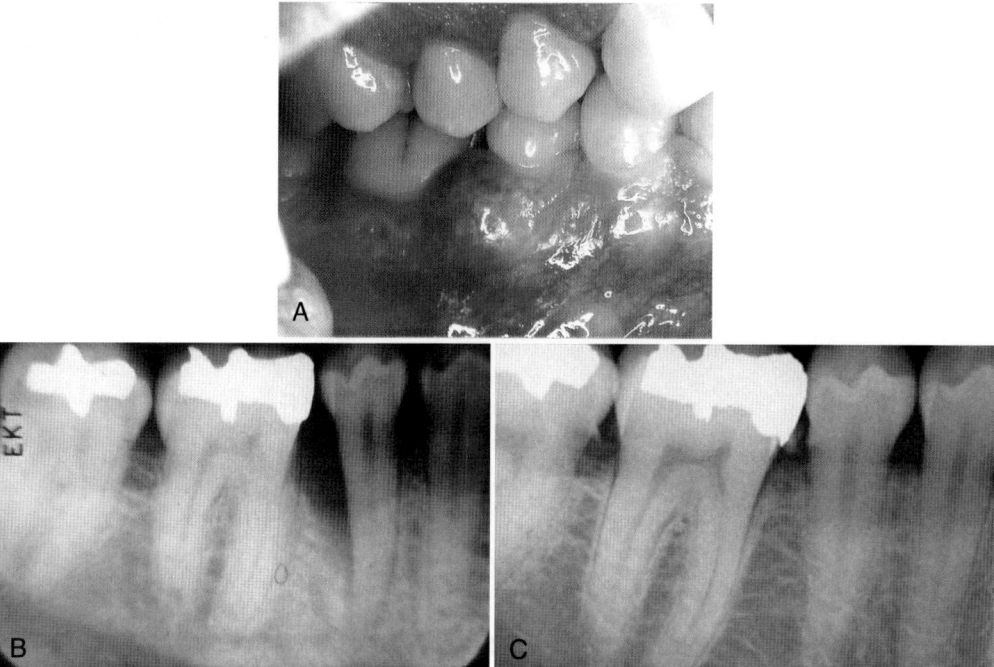

Fig. 14.3 Periodontal abscess in a 28-year-old patient with poorly controlled type 1 diabetes. (A) The patient presented with pain and abscess a few weeks after scaling and root planing of the area. (B) Radiograph of the mandibular right premolar area demonstrating severe localized destruction of bone in the area of periodontal abscess. (C) Radiograph of the mandibular right premolar area taken 2 months before the presentation of the abscess. Note the presence of calculus and the level of interproximal bone before the abscess occurred.

CLINICAL CORRELATION

Chronic hyperglycemia impairs collagen structure and function. Chronic hyperglycemia causes proteins and matrix molecules to undergo a non-enzymatic glycosylation, thereby resulting in accumulated glycation end-products (AGEs). AGEs and receptors for AGEs (RAGEs) play a central role in the classic complications of diabetes, and they most likely play a significant role in the progression of periodontal disease as well.

Metabolic Syndrome

Obesity is a global concern with serious health consequences including diabetes mellitus and cardiovascular disease. It is believed that the condition of excess adipose tissue contributes to an increased systemic proinflammatory response in these individuals. Metabolic syndrome is a term used to describe a condition of abdominal obesity combined with two or more of the following metabolic disturbances: hypertension, dyslipidemia, and hyperglycemia. Individuals diagnosed with metabolic syndrome are at increased risk for developing type 2 diabetes mellitus[221] and cardiovascular disease.

Recent evidence suggests that obesity, obesity-related characteristics, and metabolic syndrome in particular may be risk indicators for the severity and progression of periodontitis.[10,142,182,266] Previous studies have documented the relationship between obesity and periodontitis as well as obesity-related characteristics such as body mass index and future progression of periodontal disease.[102] A systematic review that included the results from five prospective studies evaluating the association between weight gain and the incidence of periodontitis in adults found a clear positive relationship: subjects who became overweight and obese had a higher risk of developing periodontitis when compared with those who did not

gain weight.[181] The authors cautioned that the evidence was limited and that more prospective, longitudinal research is needed to establish obesity as a risk factor for periodontitis.

The association between periodontitis and metabolic syndrome is thought to be the result of systemic oxidative stress and an increased inflammatory response.[142] It may be explained by common risk factors such as obesity and obesity-related habits including diet, exercise, and poor oral hygiene.[136] Obesity is associated with increased cytokine production as well as T-cell and monocyte/macrophage dysfunction, factors known to contribute to periodontitis. The proinflammatory cytokines interleukin-6 (IL-6) and tumor necrosis factor alpha (TNF-α), which are elevated in obese individuals, are thought to be produced by activated macrophages that have infiltrated adipose tissue.[136] Although these associations are highly suggestive, the specific mechanisms and relationship between metabolic syndrome and periodontitis remain unknown. More well-designed studies are needed to better understand this relationship.

Female Sex Hormones

Gingival alterations during puberty, pregnancy, and menopause are associated with physiologic hormonal changes in the female patient. During puberty and pregnancy, these changes are characterized by nonspecific inflammatory reactions with a predominant vascular component, which leads clinically to a marked hemorrhagic tendency. Oral changes during menopause may include thinning of the oral mucosa, gingival recession, xerostomia, altered taste, and burning mouth.

The changes associated with each phase of the female life cycle from puberty to menopause are briefly addressed in the online materials associated with this book. See Chapter 41 for a detailed description of these changes, including management considerations for the periodontal manifestations of hormonal changes in the female patient.

Hematologic Disorders and Immune Deficiencies

All blood cells play an essential role in the maintenance of a healthy periodontium. White blood cells (WBCs) are involved in inflammatory reactions, and they are responsible for cellular defense against microorganisms as well as for proinflammatory cytokine release. Red blood cells (RBCs) are responsible for gas exchange and nutrient supply to the periodontal tissues and platelets, and they are necessary for normal hemostasis as well as for the recruitment of cells during inflammation and wound healing. Consequently, disorders of any blood cells or blood-forming organs can have a profound effect on the periodontium.

Certain oral changes (e.g., hemorrhage) may suggest the existence of a blood dyscrasia. However, a specific diagnosis requires a complete physical examination and a thorough hematologic study. Comparable oral changes occur in more than one form of blood dyscrasia, and secondary inflammatory changes produce a wide range of variation in the oral signs.

Gingival and periodontal disturbances associated with blood dyscrasias must be viewed in terms of fundamental interrelationships among the oral tissues, the blood cells, and the blood-forming organs rather than in terms of a simple association of dramatic oral changes with hematologic disease. Hemorrhagic tendencies occur when the normal hemostatic mechanisms are disturbed. Abnormal bleeding from the gingiva or other areas of the oral mucosa that is difficult to control is an important clinical sign that suggests a hematologic disorder. Petechiae (Fig. 14.4) and ecchymosis (Fig. 14.5), observed

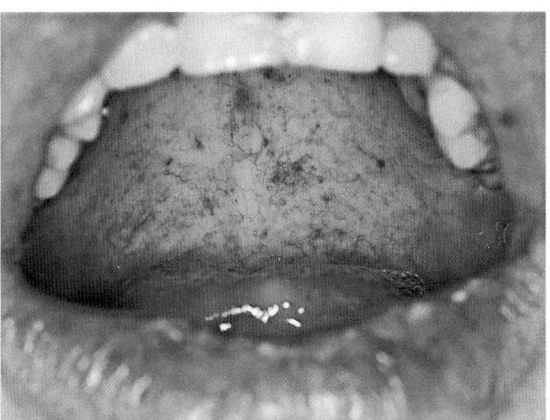

Fig. 14.4 Petechiae evident on the soft palate of a patient with an underlying bleeding disorder (thrombocytopenia).

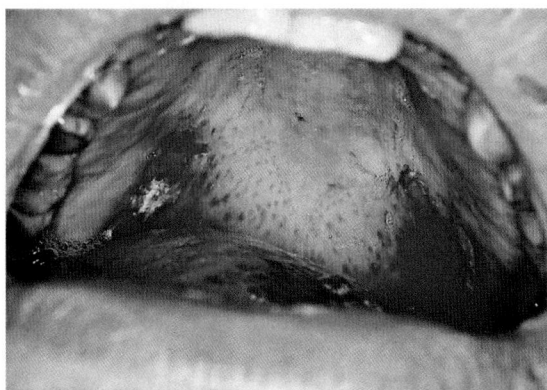

Fig. 14.5 Ecchymosis that is evident on the lateral aspects of the soft palate and tonsillar pillars of a patient with chemotherapy-induced thrombocytopenia.

most often in the soft palate area, are signs of an underlying bleeding disorder. It is essential to diagnose the specific etiology to appropriately address any bleeding or immunologic disorder.

Deficiencies in the host immune response may lead to severely destructive periodontal lesions. These deficiencies may be primary (inherited) or secondary (acquired) and may be caused by either immunosuppressive drug therapy or the pathologic destruction of the lymphoid system. Leukemia, Hodgkin disease, lymphomas, and multiple myeloma may result in secondary immunodeficiency disorders. This section discusses common hematologic and certain immunodeficiency disorders that are not related to the human immunodeficiency virus or acquired immunodeficiency syndrome. See Chapter 30 for a detailed discussion of patients with human immunodeficiency virus infection.

KEY FACT

Clinicians must be aware that certain oral manifestations (e.g., hemorrhage, ecchymosis) can suggest the existence of a systemic disorder. Atypical gingival and periodontal findings should be assessed in terms of the interrelationships among oral tissues, blood cells, and blood-forming organs rather than in terms of a simple association of dramatic oral changes with hematologic disease. Determining a specific systemic diagnosis requires a complete physical examination and a thorough hematologic study. Patients should be referred to a medical doctor for comprehensive workup.

Leukocyte (Neutrophil) Disorders

Disorders that affect the production or function of leukocytes may result in severe periodontal destruction. PMNs (i.e., neutrophils) in particular play a critical role in bacterial infections, because PMNs are the first line of defense (see Chapter 7). A quantitative deficiency of leukocytes (e.g., neutropenia, agranulocytosis) is typically associated with a more generalized periodontal destruction that affects all teeth.

Neutropenia

Neutropenia is a blood disorder that results in low levels of circulating neutrophils. It is a serious condition that may be caused by diseases, medications, chemicals, infections, idiopathic conditions, or hereditary disorders. It may be chronic or cyclic and severe or benign. It affects as many as one in three patients who are receiving chemotherapy for cancer. An absolute neutrophil count (ANC) of 1000 to 1500 cells/µL is diagnostic for mild neutropenia. An ANC of 500 to 1000 cells/µL is considered moderate neutropenia, and an ANC of <500 cells/µL indicates a severe neutropenia. Infections are sometimes difficult to manage and may be life threatening, particularly with severe neutropenia.

Agranulocytosis

Agranulocytosis is a more severe neutropenia that involves not only neutrophils but also basophils and eosinophils. It is defined as an ANC of <100 cells/µL. It is characterized by a reduction in the number of circulating granulocytes, and it results in severe infections, including ulcerative necrotizing lesions of the oral mucosa, the skin, and the gastrointestinal and genitourinary tracts. Less severe forms of the disease are called *neutropenia* or *granulocytopenia.*

Drug idiosyncrasy is the most common cause of agranulocytosis, but, in some cases, its cause cannot be explained. Agranulocytosis has been reported after the administration of drugs such as aminopyrine, barbiturates and their derivatives, benzene ring derivatives, sulfonamides, gold salts, and arsenical agents.[140,157,174,203] It generally

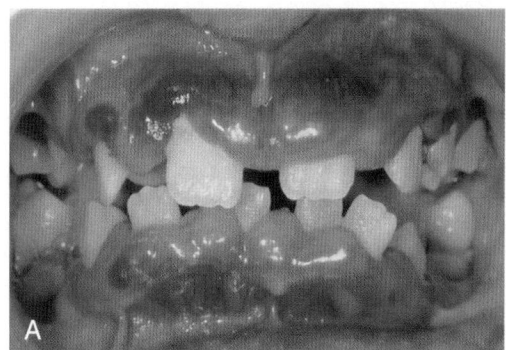

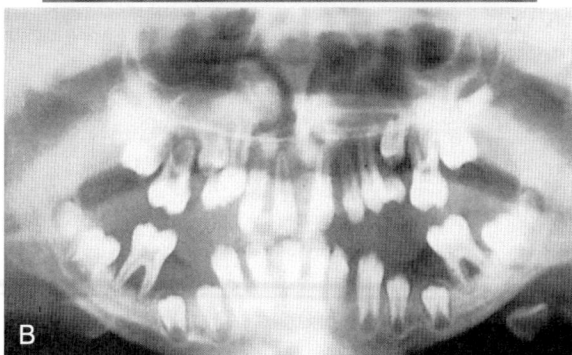

Fig. 14.6 Aggressive periodontitis in 10-year-old boy with cyclic neutropenia and agammaglobulinemia. (A) Clinical presentation of the periodontal condition. Note the severe swelling and inflammation of the marginal and papillary gingiva. There is gross migration of teeth caused by a loss of bone support. (B) Panoramic radiograph demonstrating severe bone loss around all permanent teeth that have erupted into the oral cavity.

occurs as an acute disease. It may be chronic or periodic, with recurring neutropenic cycles (e.g., cyclic neutropenia).[244]

The onset of disease is accompanied by fever, malaise, general weakness, and sore throat. Ulceration in the oral cavity, the oropharynx, and the throat is characteristic. The mucosa exhibits isolated necrotic patches that are black and gray and that are sharply demarcated from the adjacent uninvolved areas.[130,161] The absence of a notable inflammatory reaction caused by a lack of granulocytes is a striking feature. The gingival margin may or may not be involved. Gingival hemorrhage, necrosis, increased salivation, and fetid odor are accompanying clinical features. With cyclic neutropenia, the gingival changes recur with recurrent exacerbation of the disease.[53] The occurrence of generalized aggressive periodontitis has been described in patients with cyclic neutropenia[227] (Fig. 14.6).

Because infection is a common feature of agranulocytosis, the differential diagnosis involves consideration of such conditions as necrotizing ulcerative gingivitis, noma, acute necrotizing inflammation of the tonsils, and diphtheria. Definitive diagnosis depends on the hematologic findings of pronounced leukopenia and the almost complete absence of neutrophils.

Leukemia

Leukemia is an important disease to understand and appreciate because of its seriousness and its periodontal manifestations. The leukemias are malignant neoplasias of WBC precursors that are characterized by the following: (1) diffuse replacement of the bone marrow with proliferating leukemic cells; (2) abnormal numbers and forms of immature WBCs in the circulating blood; and (3) widespread infiltrates in the liver, spleen, lymph nodes, and other body sites.[209]

According to the cell type involved, leukemias are classified as *lymphocytic* or *myelogenous*. A subgroup of the myelogenous

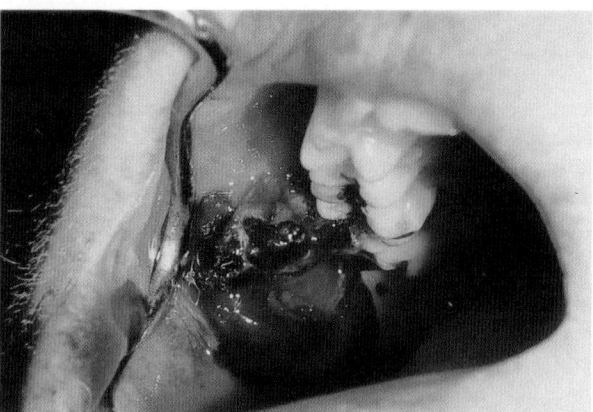

Fig. 14.7 Spontaneous bleeding from the gingival sulcus in a patient with thrombocytopenia. Normal coagulation is evident by the appearance of the large clot that forms in the mouth. However, platelets are inadequate to establish hemostasis at the site of hemorrhage.

leukemias are the *monocytic* leukemias. The term *lymphocytic* indicates that the malignant change occurs in cells that normally form lymphocytes. The term *myelogenous* indicates that the malignant change occurs in cells that normally form red blood cells (RBCs), some types of WBCs, and platelets. According to their evolution, leukemias can be *acute* (which is rapidly fatal), *subacute,* or *chronic*. In acute leukemia, the primitive blast cells released into the peripheral circulation are immature and nonfunctional; in chronic leukemia, the abnormal cells tend to be more mature and to have normal morphologic characteristics and functions when released into the circulation.

All leukemias tend to displace normal components of the bone marrow elements with leukemic cells, thereby resulting in the reduced production of normal RBCs, WBCs, and platelets, which leads to anemia, *leukopenia* (a reduction in the number of *nonmalignant* WBCs), and thrombocytopenia. Anemia results in poor tissue oxygenation, which makes tissues more friable and susceptible to breakdown. A reduction of normal WBCs in the circulation leads to a poor cellular defense and an increased susceptibility to infections. *Thrombocytopenia* leads to bleeding tendency, which can occur in any tissue but which in particular affects the oral cavity, especially the gingival sulcus (Fig. 14.7). Some patients may have normal blood counts while leukemic cells reside primarily in the bone marrow. This type of disease is called *aleukemic leukemia*.[100]

The Periodontium in Leukemic Patients

Oral and periodontal manifestations of leukemia may include leukemic infiltration, bleeding, oral ulcerations, and infections. The expression of these signs is more common with acute and subacute forms of leukemia than with chronic forms.

Leukemic Infiltration

Leukemic cells can infiltrate the gingiva and, less frequently, the alveolar bone. Gingival infiltration often results in *leukemic gingival enlargement* (see Chapter 19).

A study of 1076 adult patients with leukemia showed that 3.6% of the patients with teeth had leukemic gingival proliferative lesions, with the highest incidence seen in patients with acute monocytic leukemia (66.7%), followed by those with acute myelocytic–monocytic leukemia (18.7%) and acute myelocytic leukemia (3.7%).[66] It should be noted, however, that monocytic leukemia is an extremely rare form of the disease. Leukemic gingival enlargement is not found in edentulous patients or in patients with chronic leukemia, suggesting that it represents the accumulation of immature leukemic blast cells in the gingiva adjacent to tooth surfaces with bacterial plaque. Leukemic gingival enlargement consists of a basic infiltration of the gingival corium by leukemic cells that increases the gingival thickness and creates gingival pockets in which bacterial plaque accumulates, thereby initiating a secondary inflammatory lesion that contributes to the enlargement of the gingiva. It may be localized to the interdental papilla area (Fig. 14.8), or it may expand to include the marginal gingiva and partially cover the crowns of the teeth (Fig. 14.9C

and D). Clinically, the gingiva appears bluish red and cyanotic, with a rounding and tenseness of the gingival margin. The abnormal accumulation of leukemic cells in the dermal and subcutaneous connective tissue is called *leukemia cutis,* and it forms elevated and flat macules and papules[66,209] (see Fig. 14.9A and B).

Microscopically, the gingiva exhibits a dense, diffuse infiltration of predominantly immature leukocytes in the attached and marginal gingiva. Occasionally, mitotic figures indicative of ectopic hematopoiesis may be seen. The normal connective tissue components of the gingiva are displaced by the leukemic cells (Fig. 14.10). The nature of the cells depends on the type of leukemia. The cellular accumulation is denser in the entire reticular connective tissue layer. In almost all cases, the papillary layer contains comparatively few leukocytes. The blood vessels are distended and contain predominantly leukemic cells, and the RBCs are reduced in number. The epithelium shows a variety of changes, and it may be thinned or hyperplastic. Common findings include degeneration associated with intercellular and intracellular edema and leukocytic infiltration with diminished surface keratinization.

The microscopic picture of the marginal gingiva differs from that of other gingival locations in that it usually exhibits a notable inflammatory component in addition to the leukemic cells. Scattered foci of plasma cells and lymphocytes with edema and degeneration are common findings. The inner aspect of the marginal gingiva is usually

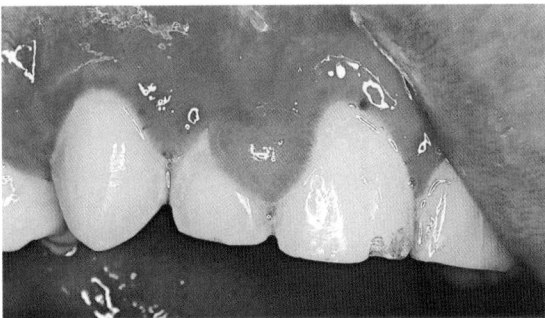

Fig. 14.8 Leukemic infiltration that causes localized gingival swelling of the interdental papillae between the maxillary lateral and central incisors. Note the tense induration of the area.

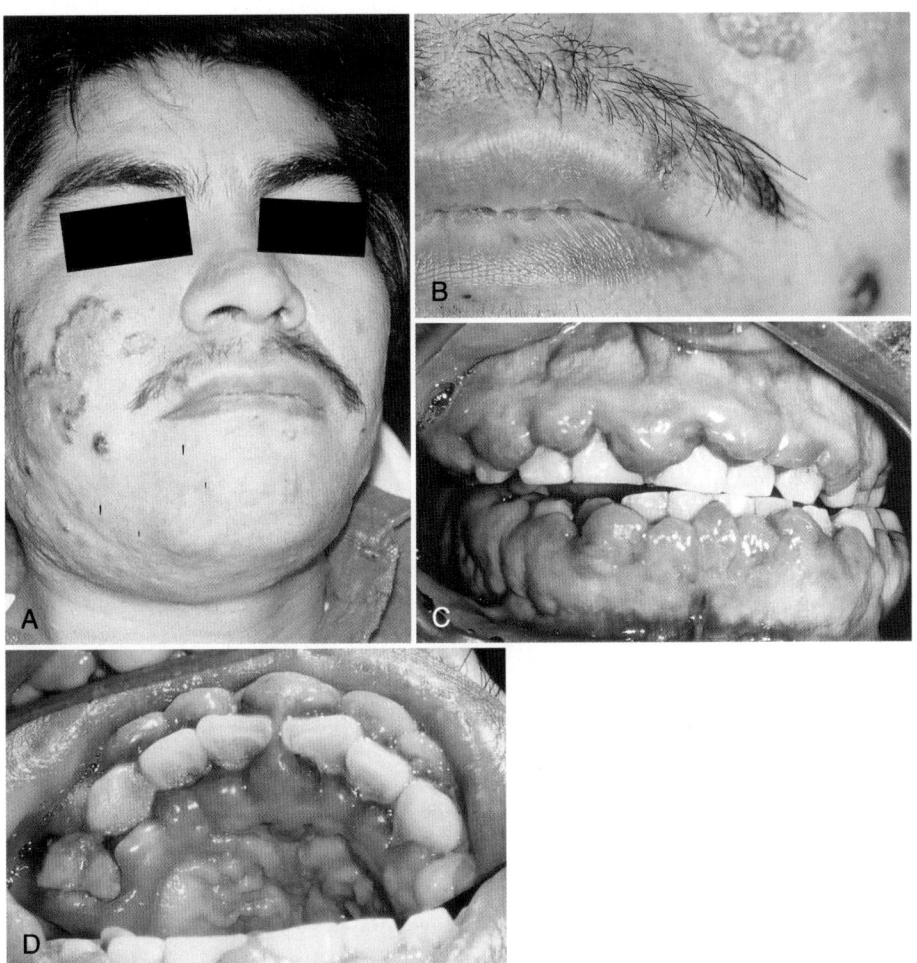

Fig. 14.9 Adult male with acute myelocytic leukemia. (A) A view of the patient's face. Note the elevated, flat macules and papules (leukemia cutis) on the right cheek. (B) Close-up view of skin lesions. (C) An intraoral view showing pronounced gingival enlargements of the entire gingival margin and interdental papilla areas of both arches. (D) Occlusal view of the maxillary anterior teeth. Note the marked enlargement in both the facial and the palatal aspects. *(Courtesy Dr. Spencer Woolfe, Dublin, Ireland.)*

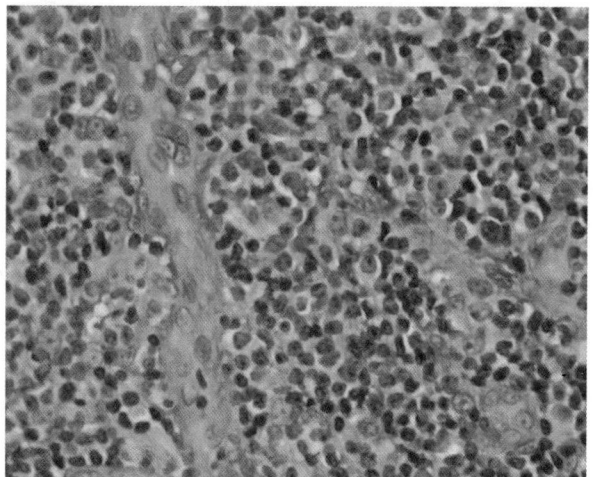

Fig. 14.10 Human histologic appearance of leukemic infiltrate with dense diffuse infiltration of predominantly immature leukocytes. The normal connective tissue components of the gingiva are displaced by the leukemic cells. The cellular accumulation is denser in the entire reticular connective tissue layer. *(Courtesy Dr. Russell Christensen, University of California, Los Angeles, CA.)*

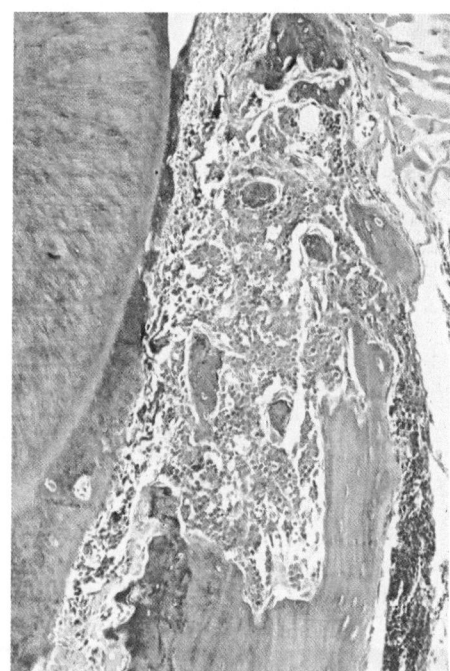

Fig. 14.11 Leukemic infiltrate in alveolar bone in a leukemic mouse. Note the leukemic infiltrate causing destruction of the bone and a loss of the periodontal ligament.

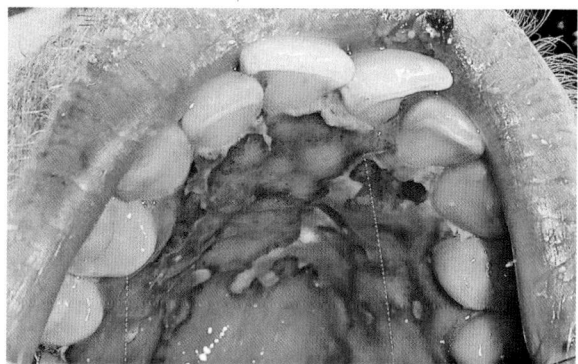

Fig. 14.12 Large ulcerations on the palate of a patient with granulocytopenia secondary to leukemia. These atypical ulcerations are caused by a herpesvirus opportunistic infection. Notice the smaller, discrete, round ulcerations that have coalesced into the larger lesion.

ulcerated, and marginal necrosis with pseudomembrane formation may also be seen.

The periodontal ligament and alveolar bone may also be involved in acute and subacute leukemia. The periodontal ligament may be infiltrated with mature and immature leukocytes. The marrow of the alveolar bone exhibits a variety of changes, such as localized areas of necrosis, thrombosis of the blood vessels, infiltration with mature and immature leukocytes, occasional RBCs, and the replacement of the fatty marrow with fibrous tissue.

In leukemic mice, the presence of infiltrate in marrow spaces and the periodontal ligament results in osteoporosis of the alveolar bone with destruction of the supporting bone and disappearance of the periodontal fibers[32,41] (Fig. 14.11).

Bleeding

Gingival hemorrhage is a common finding in leukemic patients (see Fig. 14.7), even in the absence of clinically detectable gingivitis. Bleeding gingiva can be an early sign of leukemia. It is caused by the thrombocytopenia that results from the replacement of bone marrow cells with leukemic cells and from the inhibition of normal stem cell function by leukemic cells or their products.[209] This bleeding tendency can also manifest in the skin and throughout the oral mucosa, where petechiae are often found, with or without leukemic infiltrates. A more diffuse submucosal bleeding manifests as ecchymosis (see Fig. 14.5). Oral bleeding has been reported as a presenting sign in 17.7% of patients with acute leukemia and in 4.4% of patients with chronic leukemia.[156] Bleeding may also be a side effect of the chemotherapeutic agents used to treat leukemia.

Oral Ulceration and Infection

In patients with leukemia, the response to bacterial plaque or other local irritation is altered. The cellular component of the inflammatory exudate differs both quantitatively and qualitatively from that found in nonleukemic individuals in that there is a pronounced infiltration of immature leukemic cells in addition to the usual inflammatory cells. As a result, the normal inflammatory response may be diminished.

Granulocytopenia (diminished WBC count) results from the displacement of normal bone marrow cells by leukemic cells, which increases the host susceptibility to opportunistic microorganisms and leads to ulcerations and infections. Discrete, punched-out ulcers that penetrate deeply into the submucosa and are covered by a firmly attached white slough can be found on the oral mucosa.[16] These lesions occur in sites of trauma (e.g., the buccal mucosa) in relation to the line of occlusion or on the palate. Patients with a history of herpesvirus infection may develop recurrent herpetic oral ulcers (often in multiple sites) and large atypical forms, especially after chemotherapy is instituted[106] (Fig. 14.12).

A gingival (bacterial) infection in leukemic patients can be the result of an exogenous bacterial infection or an existing bacterial infection (e.g., gingival or periodontal disease). Acute gingivitis and lesions that resemble necrotizing ulcerative gingivitis are more frequent and more severe in patients with terminal cases of acute leukemia[22] (Figs. 14.13 and 14.14). The inflamed gingiva in patients with leukemia differs clinically from that found in nonleukemic individuals. The gingiva is a peculiar bluish red, it is spongelike and friable, and it

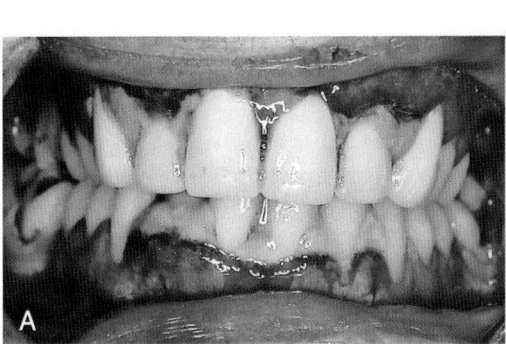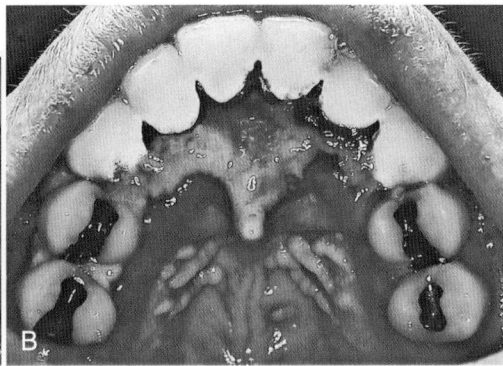

Fig. 14.13 Adult female with acute myelocytic leukemia. (A) Anterior view of a patient with acute myelocytic leukemia. The interdental papillae are necrotic, with highly inflamed and swollen gingival tissue at the base of the lesions. (B) Palatal view demonstrating extensive necrosis of the interdental and palatal tissues behind the maxillary incisors.

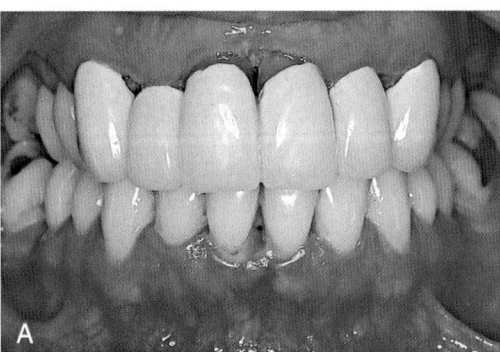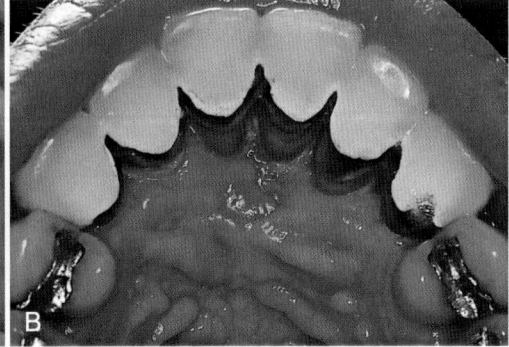

Fig. 14.14 The same patient as shown in Fig. 14.13 after chemotherapy that resulted in the remission of her leukemia. (A) An anterior view reveals dramatic improvement in gingival health after the remission of leukemia. Note the loss of interdental papillae as well as gingival recession in the anterior areas. (B) A palatal view shows the extensive loss of gingival tissue around the maxillary incisors.

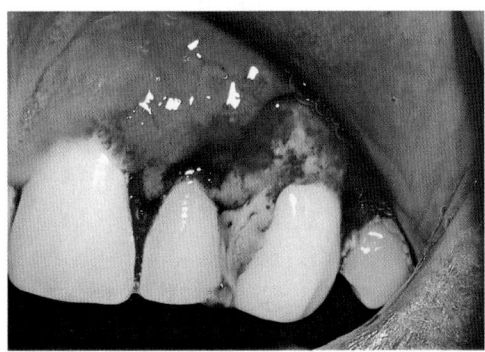

Fig. 14.15 An opportunistic bacterial infection of the gingiva in a patient who has been hospitalized with leukemia. The gingival tissue is highly inflamed, bleeding, and necrotic, with pseudomembrane formation.

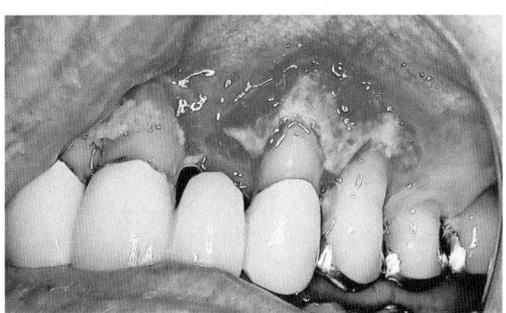

Fig. 14.16 An opportunistic bacterial infection in an immunosuppressed patient caused the complete destruction of the gingiva, thus exposing the underlying alveolar bone.

bleeds persistently on the slightest provocation or even spontaneously in leukemic patients. This greatly altered and degenerated tissue is extremely susceptible to bacterial infection, which can be so severe as to cause acute gingival necrosis with pseudomembrane formation (Fig. 14.15) or bone exposure (Fig. 14.16). These are secondary oral changes that are superimposed on the oral tissues that have been altered by the blood dyscrasia. They produce associated disturbances that may be a source of considerable difficulty to the patient, such as systemic toxic effects, loss of appetite, nausea, blood loss from persistent gingival bleeding, and constant gnawing pain. Eliminating

or reducing local factors (e.g., bacterial plaque) can minimize the severe oral changes associated with leukemia. In some patients with severe acute leukemia, symptoms may be relieved only by treatment that leads to the remission of the disease.

In those with chronic leukemia, oral changes that suggest a hematologic disturbance are rare. The microscopic changes of chronic leukemia may consist of replacing the normal fatty marrow of the jaws with islands of mature lymphocytes or lymphocytic infiltration of the marginal gingiva without dramatic clinical manifestations.

The existence of leukemia is sometimes revealed by a gingival biopsy performed to clarify the nature of a troublesome gingival condition. In such cases, the gingival findings must be corroborated by medical examination and hematologic study. In patients with diagnosed leukemia, gingival biopsy may indicate the extent to which leukemic infiltration is responsible for the altered clinical appearance of the gingiva. *Although such findings are of interest, their benefit to the patient is insufficient to warrant routine gingival biopsy studies in patients with leukemia.* Furthermore, it is important to note that the absence of leukemic involvement in a gingival biopsy specimen does not rule out the possibility of leukemia. A gingival biopsy in a patient with chronic leukemia may reveal typical gingival inflammation without any suggestion of a hematologic disturbance.

 See the online material for discussion of additional blood dyscrasias and their influence on periodontal health.

Genetic Disorders

Systemic conditions that are associated with or that predispose an individual to periodontal destruction include genetic disorders that result in an inadequate number or reduced function of circulating neutrophils. This underscores the importance of the neutrophil in the protection of the periodontium against infection. Severe periodontitis has been observed in individuals with primary neutrophil disorders such as neutropenia, agranulocytosis, Chédiak–Higashi syndrome, and lazy leukocyte syndrome. In addition, severe periodontitis has been observed in individuals who exhibit secondary neutrophil impairment, such as those with Down syndrome, Papillon–Lefèvre syndrome, and inflammatory bowel disease.

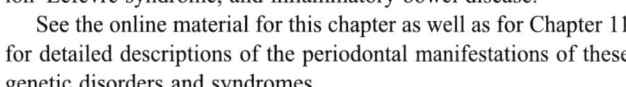 See the online material for this chapter as well as for Chapter 11 for detailed descriptions of the periodontal manifestations of these genetic disorders and syndromes.

Stress and Psychosomatic Disorders

Psychologic conditions, particularly psychosocial stress, have been implicated as risk indicators for periodontal disease.[88] The most notable example is the documented relationship between stress (e.g., experienced by soldiers at war or by students during examinations) and acute necrotizing ulcerative gingivitis (see Chapters 20 and 29). The presence of necrotizing ulcerative gingivitis among soldiers stressed by wartime conditions in the trenches led to one of the early diagnostic terms used to describe this condition: "trench mouth." Despite this well-known association between stress and necrotizing ulcerative gingivitis, confirming the connection between psychologic conditions and other forms of periodontal disease (e.g., chronic periodontitis) has been elusive. These relationships are difficult to elucidate, because, as with many common diseases, the etiology and pathogenesis of periodontal disease is multifactorial, and the role of individual risk factors is difficult to define.

Some studies have failed to recognize a relationship between psychologic conditions and periodontal disease despite specific efforts to identify them. In a study of 80 patients (40 with aggressive periodontitis and 40 with chronic periodontitis), Monteiro da Silva and colleagues failed to find a relationship between psychologic factors and periodontal disease.[180] The researchers were able to identify depression and smoking as marginally significant in the aggressive periodontitis group. Their inability to find a relationship may be attributed to a lack of significant differences in psychologic characteristics between the two groups in the study. In an earlier study, the same researchers identified depression and loneliness as significant factors associated with aggressive periodontal disease in 50 patients as compared with 50 periodontally healthy individuals and 50 individuals with chronic periodontitis.[179] Another challenge when defining the relationship between psychosocial status and periodontitis is the myriad confounding factors and the difficulty of controlling for them.[68]

Psychosocial Stress, Depression, and Coping

Several clinical studies and a systematic review of the subject have documented a positive relationship between psychosocial stress and chronic forms of periodontal disease.[200] In case–control studies, individuals with stable lifestyles (based on family structure and employment status) and minimal negative life events had less periodontal disease destruction than individuals with less stable lifestyles (e.g., unmarried, unemployed) and more negative life events.[59] It is now becoming apparent that the effect is not simply a matter of the presence or absence of stress; rather, the type of stress and the ability of the individual to cope with stress correlate with destructive periodontal disease.

All individuals experience stress, but these events do not invariably result in destructive periodontitis. The types of stress that lead to periodontal destruction appear to be more chronic or long term and less likely to be controlled by the individual. Life events such as the loss of a loved one (e.g., spouse, family member), a failed relationship, loss of employment, and financial difficulties are examples of stressful life events that are typically not controllable by the individual or not perceived by the individual as being under his or her control, thereby resulting in a feeling of helplessness. The duration of the stressful life event also has an influence on the total impact of the stress-induced disease destruction.

Financial stress is an example of a long-term, constant pressure that may exacerbate periodontal destruction in susceptible individuals. Genco and colleagues[89] found that individuals with high levels of financial stress and poor coping skills had twice as much periodontal disease as those with minimal stress and good coping skills. Psychologic tests were used to identify and weigh the causes of stress (e.g., children, spouse, finances, single life, work) and to measure individual coping skills. Individuals with problem-focused (practical) coping skills fared better than individuals with emotion-focused (avoidance) coping skills with respect to periodontal disease. As part of their analysis, the researchers also found that chronic stress and inadequate coping could lead to changes in daily habits, such as poor oral hygiene, clenching, and grinding, as well as physiologic changes such as decreased saliva flow and suppressed immunity.

When comparing 89 patients with periodontal disease to 63 periodontally healthy individuals, Wimmer and colleagues[267] found that patients with defensive (emotional) coping skills were more likely to refuse responsibility and to downplay their condition. All patients completed a comprehensive stress assessment questionnaire (given in German) to evaluate their coping behavior. Patients with periodontal disease were less likely to use active coping skills (i.e., situation control) and more likely to cope with stress by averting blame (emotional) than were periodontally healthy individuals.

These studies support the concept that one of the most important aspects related to the influence of stress on periodontal disease destruction is the manner in which the individual copes with the stress. Emotional coping methods appear to render the host more susceptible to the destructive effects of periodontal disease than do practical coping methods. Furthermore, emotional coping is more common in situations that must be accepted and among individuals who feel helpless in the situation.

 KEY FACT

The effect of psychosocial stress on the manifestation of disease (i.e., periodontitis) is not simply a matter of the presence or absence of stress; rather, the type of stress and the ability of the individual to cope with stress correlate with destructive periodontal disease.

Stress-Induced Immunosuppression

Stress and psychosomatic disorders most likely impact periodontal health via changes in the individual's behavior and through complex interactions among the nervous, endocrine, and immune systems. Individuals under stress may have poorer oral hygiene; they may start or increase the clenching and grinding of their teeth; and they may smoke more frequently. All of these behavioral changes increase their susceptibility to periodontal disease destruction. Likewise, individuals who are under stress may be less likely to seek professional care.

In addition to the many behavioral changes that may influence periodontal disease destruction, psychosocial stress may also impact the disease through alterations in the immune system. The influence of stress on the immune system and systemic health conditions (e.g., cardiovascular disease) is well known. Stress-related immune system changes clearly have the potential to affect the pathogenesis of periodontal disease as well. One possible mechanism involves the production of cortisol. Stress increases cortisol production from the adrenal cortex by stimulating an increase in the release of adreno-corticotropic hormone from the pituitary gland. Increased cortisol suppresses the immune response directly through the suppression of neutrophil activity, immunoglobulin G production, and salivary IgA secretion. All of these immune responses are critical for the normal immunoinflammatory response to periodontal pathogens (see Chapter 7). The resulting stress-induced immunosuppression increases the potential for destruction by periodontal pathogens. Stress may also affect the cellular immune response directly through an increased release of neurotransmitters, including epinephrine, norepinephrine, neurokinin, and substance P, which interact directly with lymphocytes, neutrophils, monocytes, and macrophages via receptors that cause an increase in their tissue-destructive function. Thus, in a manner similar to cortisol production, the stress-induced release of these neurotransmitters results in an upregulated immune response that increases the potential for destruction by the cellular response to periodontal pathogens.

It is important to remember that, although stress may predispose an individual to more destruction from periodontitis, the presence of periodontal pathogens remains as the essential etiologic factor. In other words, stress alone does not cause or lead to periodontitis in the absence of periodontal pathogens.

Influence of Stress on Periodontal Therapy Outcomes

Psychologic conditions such as stress and depression may also influence the outcome of periodontal therapy. In a large-scale retrospective study of 1299 dental records from a health maintenance organization database, 85 individuals with depression had posttherapy outcomes that were less favorable (below median) than the outcomes of individuals without depression.[73] More than half of these records (697) were complete enough for a comprehensive evaluation that included both periodontal diagnosis and psychologic profiles. The authors concluded that depression might have a negative effect on periodontal treatment outcomes.

A study investigating the relationship between psychologic stress and wound repair in patients after routine surgery (in this case, inguinal hernia open incision repair) revealed that stress impairs the inflammatory response and matrix degradation.[31] Forty-seven adults were given a standardized questionnaire to assess their psychologic stress before surgery. Wound fluids were collected during the first 20 hours after surgery to measure inflammatory markers: IL-1, IL-6, and matrix metalloproteinase-9 (MMP-9). Greater psychologic stress was significantly associated with lower levels of IL-1 and MMP-9

as well as with a significantly more painful, poorer, and slower recovery.

Another study compared the psychiatric characteristics of individuals with different outcomes to periodontal therapy.[11] Two groups were compared to evaluate the psychologic characteristics of 11 individuals who were responsive to periodontal treatment compared with 11 individuals who were not responsive to periodontal treatment. The members of the responsive group had more rigid personalities, whereas those in the nonresponsive group had more passive, dependent personalities. Furthermore, the nonresponsive group reported more stressful life events having occurred in their past.

These studies suggest that both stressful life events and the individual's personality and coping skills are factors to consider when assessing the risk of periodontal disease destruction and the potential for successful periodontal therapy. If patients with emotional or defensive coping skills are identified, care should be taken to ensure that they receive information in a manner that does not elicit a defensive reaction.

Psychiatric Influence of Self-Inflicted Injury

Psychosomatic disorders may result in harmful effects to the health of tissues in the oral cavity through the development of habits that are injurious to the periodontium. Neurotic habits such as grinding or clenching the teeth, nibbling on foreign objects (e.g., pencils, pipes), nail biting, and excessive use of tobacco are all potentially injurious to the teeth and the periodontium. Self-inflicted gingival injuries, such as gingival recession, have been described in both children and adults (Fig. 14.17). However, these types of self-inflicted, factitious injuries do not appear to be common among psychiatric patients.[219]

Nutritional Influences

Some clinicians enthusiastically adhere to the theory in periodontal disease that assigns a key role to nutritional deficiencies and imbalances. Previous research did not support this view, but numerous problems in experimental design and data interpretation could be responsible for making these research findings inadequate.[5,218] The majority of opinions and research findings regarding the effects of nutrition on oral and periodontal tissues point to the following:

1. *There are no nutritional deficiencies that by themselves can cause gingivitis or periodontitis.* However, nutritional deficiencies can

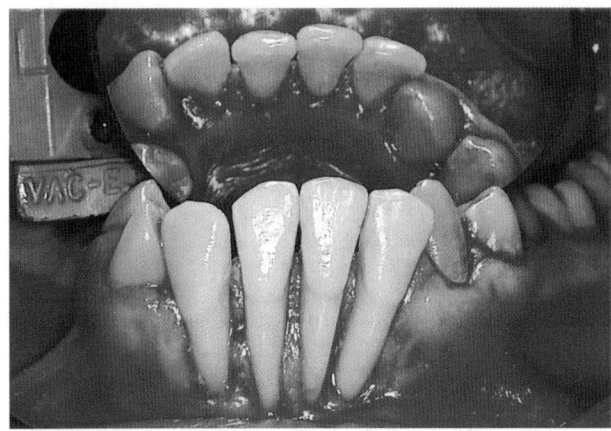

Fig. 14.17 Severe gingival recession localized to the labial surface of all mandibular incisors. This finding was discovered in an uncooperative, institutionalized adult with mental disorders who had been placed under general anesthesia. The patient was known to pace around the home with all four fingers inside his lower lip.

affect the condition of the periodontium and thereby may accentuate the deleterious effects of plaque-induced inflammation in susceptible individuals. Theoretically, one may presume that an individual with a nutritional deficiency is less able to defend against a bacterial challenge as compared with a nutritionally competent individual.

2. *There are nutritional deficiencies that produce changes in the oral cavity.* These changes include alterations of the tissues of the lips, oral mucosa, gingiva, and bone. These alterations are considered to be the periodontal and oral manifestations of nutritional disease.

The role of nutrition in periodontal disease may be related to the effect of nutrition on inflammation. A 2009 review of the literature evaluating the effect of nutritional factors on inflammation demonstrated that subtle shifts in nutritional status are associated with the prevalence of periodontitis.[46] More specifically, the authors reported that the results of contemporary animal and human studies have demonstrated the role of specific micronutrients in the modulation of the host's inflammatory response by reducing inflammatory biomarkers, which may in turn be responsible for periodontal destruction. The evidence for the effect of nutrition on inflammation is significant. Data suggest that diets that contain foods rich in antioxidants are beneficial, whereas foods that contain high levels of refined carbohydrates are detrimental to the inflammatory process.[46]

See the online material for a review of the existing knowledge of the effects of vitamin and protein deficiencies on changes in the periodontium.

Medications

Some medications that are prescribed to cure, manage, or prevent diseases may have adverse effects on periodontal tissues, wound healing, or the host immune response. Bisphosphonates are a class of medications widely prescribed for the treatment of osteoporosis and various types of cancer. They have recently been implicated in osteonecrosis of the jaw (ONJ), a serious condition that is characterized by non-healing and often painful exposure of nonvital and often sequestrating bone in the jaws. Corticosteroids have long been prescribed to suppress the immune system for the control and management of autoimmune disease, during cancer treatment, and as an antirejection medication after organ transplantation. This section discusses the effect of bisphosphonates and corticosteroids on the periodontium. Readers are referred to Chapter 39 for additional information about these and other important medications.

Bisphosphonates

Bisphosphonate medications are primarily used to treat cancer (via intravenous [IV] administration) and osteoporosis (via oral administration). They act by inhibiting osteoclastic activity, which leads to less bone resorption, less bone remodeling, and less bone turnover.[216] The use of bisphosphonates in cancer treatment is aimed at preventing the often lethal imbalance of osteoclastic activity. During the treatment of osteoporosis, the goal is simply to harness osteoclastic activity to minimize or prevent bone loss and, in many cases, to increase bone mass by creating an advantage for osteoblastic activity. The major differences in the use of bisphosphonates for cancer versus osteoporosis are the potency and route of administration of the specific bisphosphonate medication used. Potency is influenced by the chemical properties as well as by the binding and release pharmacokinetic properties of these agents as they apply to bone. Specifically, the strength of binding and the ease of release of bisphosphonates with hydroxyapatite make these drugs more or less potent.

Pyrophosphate

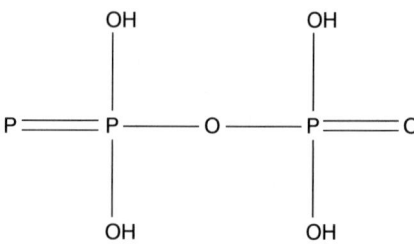

Generic bisphosphonate

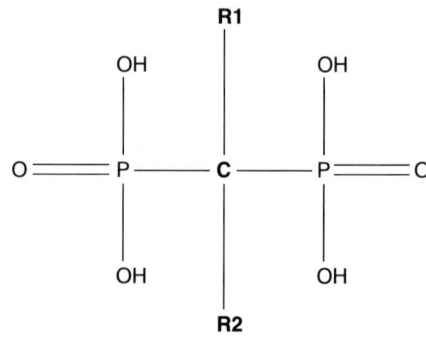

R1 Enhances binding to hydroxyapatite
-C- Enhances chemical stability
R2 Determines antiresorptive potency

Fig. 14.18 Chemical structure of a bisphosphonate molecule. Two phosphate groups are covalently bonded with a central carbon. The carbon also has two side chains, R1 and R2.

Bisphosphonates were first synthesized during the 1950s as a substitute for pyrophosphate, a compound used in detergent. The ability of bisphosphonates to increase bone mass was discovered after animal studies that took place in 1966, but the potential advantage of using bisphosphonates in humans with low bone mass was not appreciated until 1984.[257] The US Food and Drug Administration approved the use of alendronate for osteoporosis in 1995.

The chemical structure of bisphosphonate consists of two phosphate groups covalently bonded to a central carbon (Fig. 14.18). In addition to the two phosphate groups, the central carbon also has two side chains, R1 and R2. Both the short R1 side chain and the long R2 side chain influence the chemical properties and pharmacokinetics. The long R2 side chain also influences the mode of action and determines the strength or potency of the medication. Bisphosphonates inhibit osteoclasts by two mechanisms that depend on whether the R2 side chain contains nitrogen. Nonaminobisphosphonates are metabolized by osteoclasts to form an adenosine triphosphate analog that interferes with energy production and causes osteoclast apoptosis. Aminobisphosphonates (i.e., risedronate, zoledronate, ibandronate, and alendronate) are more potent and have multiple effects on osteoclasts, including the following: (1) inactivation of adenosine triphosphate; (2) osteoclast cytoskeletal disruption; (3) impairment of osteoclast recruitment; and (4) induction of osteoblasts to produce osteoclast-inhibiting factor.[190] Bisphosphonates also inhibit bone metabolism via antiangiogenic activity.[35]

Table 14.1 lists some of the common bisphosphonate medications used for osteoporosis and cancer treatment that are currently available in the United States.

There is growing evidence that bisphosphonates also affect soft tissues and that they may contribute to ONJ via inhibition of soft

TABLE 14.1   Current Nonaminobisphosphonate and Aminobisphosphonate Medications and Common Therapeutic Uses

Generic Name	Commercial Name	Route of Administration	Therapeutic Use	Nitrogen-Containing R2 Side Chain	Relative Antiresorptive Potency
Etidronate	Didronel	PO	Paget disease	No	1
Tiludronate	Skelid	PO	Paget disease	No	10
Risedronate	Actonel	PO	Osteoporosis, Paget disease	Yes	5,000
Ibandronate	Boniva	PO	Osteoporosis	Yes	10,000
Alendronate	Fosamax	PO	Osteoporosis, Paget disease	Yes	1000
Pamidronate	Aredia	IV	Paget disease, cancer	Yes	100
Zoledronate	Zometa	IV	Cancer	Yes	10,000+

IV, Intravenous; *PO*, by mouth.

tissue healing.[143] An in vitro study by Kim and colleagues suggested that bisphosphonates may act on oral keratinocytes to impair wound healing by inhibiting epithelial migration and wound closure.[133] Interestingly, the effects of bisphosphonates on oral mucosal cells and bone cells share the common mechanism of interference with products of the mevalonate pathway, which may be more significant to the overall problem than the reported apoptosis effects on osteoclasts. The inhibition of farnesyl pyrophosphate synthase leads to inhibition of the mevalonate pathway end product, geranylgeranyl pyrophosphate (Fig. 14.19). This bisphosphonate-inhibited pathway is required for many essential cellular functions in a variety of tissues. In the case of soft tissues, the bisphosphonate-induced senescence of human oral keratinocytes was found to be mediated, at least in part, by inhibition of the mevalonate pathway. Similarly, Fisher and colleagues reported that bisphosphonates inhibit bone resorption via prevention of protein prenylation in osteoclasts that is caused by the inhibition of farnesyl pyrophosphate synthase, resulting in interference with the production of geranylgeranyl pyrophosphate.

Bisphosphonates have a high affinity for hydroxyapatite. They are rapidly absorbed in bone, especially in areas of high activity, which may help to explain why bisphosphonate-induced osteonecrosis is found only in the jaws.[257] The bisphosphonate molecule gets incorporated into bone without being metabolized or modified. During the osteoclastic resorption of bone, the trapped bisphosphonate is released and able to affect osteoclasts again. As a result, the half-life of bisphosphonates in the bone is estimated to be 10 years or longer.

ONJ associated with bisphosphonates was first described in 2003 by Marx in a report of 36 patients with avascular necrosis of the jaw who had been treated with IV bisphosphonate for malignant tumors.[163] Several case series reporting an association between bisphosphonates and ONJ were published subsequently.[165,214] Various terms have been used to describe this type of ONJ, including *avascular necrosis, bisphosphonate-associated ONJ, bisphosphonate-induced ONJ,* and *bisphosphonate-related ONJ (BRONJ).*[257] Today, with the widespread recognition of BRONJ, it is important to remember that necrotic bone exposure of the jaw (ONJ) is a condition with multiple possible etiopathogenic factors, including systemic medications, radiation, infection, trauma, direct chemical toxicity, and other idiopathic mechanisms; clinicians should carefully consider all factors before making a diagnosis of BRONJ.[8]

The condition of BRONJ has been defined as the exposure and necrosis of portions of the jaw bone in patients who have been exposed to bisphosphonates that has persisted for longer than 8 weeks with no history of radiation therapy to the jaws.[212] The stage of osteonecrosis is used to categorize patients and to make treatment decisions.[2,164,165,212] Stage 0 patients are patients at risk who have been treated with IV or oral bisphosphonates but who have no apparent exposed or necrotic bone. Stage 1 involves exposed or necrotic bone in patients who are asymptomatic with no infection. Stage 2 involves exposed or necrotic bone in patients with pain and clinical evidence of infection. Stage 3 involves exposed or necrotic bone in patients with pain, infection, and one or more of the following: pathologic fracture, extraoral fistula, or osteolysis that extends to the inferior border.

Clinically, BRONJ manifests as exposed alveolar bone that occurs spontaneously or after a traumatic event such as a dental procedure (Figs. 14.20 and 14.21). The sites may be painful, with surrounding soft tissue induration and inflammation. Infection with drainage may be present. Radiographically, lesions appear radiolucent, with sclerosis of the lamina dura, a loss of the lamina dura, or a widening of the periodontal ligament in areas where teeth are present. Histologically, bone appears necrotic, with empty lacunae demonstrating a lack of living osteocytes. In advanced cases, pathologic fracture may be present through the area of exposed or necrotic bone.

The high potency of nitrogen-containing bisphosphonates— especially those administered intravenously for cancer treatment (e.g., zoledronate)—may explain the high incidence of BRONJ in these patients compared with osteoporotic patients taking oral bisphosphonates. The incidence among patients who are being treated for cancer has been reported to range from 2.5% to 5.4%[261] or from 1% to 10%.[35] Estimating the incidence among patients who are taking oral bisphosphonates for osteoporosis is more difficult due to the large number of patients taking this prescription medication and a lack of good reporting or documentation for these patients. Some reports estimate the incidence of BRONJ from oral bisphosphonates to range from 0.007% to 0.04%,[257] whereas other reports suggest a slightly higher incidence that ranges from 0.004% to 0.11%.[233] Clearly, the incidence among patients taking oral bisphosphonates appears to be low.

It has been observed that BRONJ lesions occur most often in areas with dense bone and thin overlying mucosa, such as tori, bony exostoses, and the mylohyoid ridge.[165,213,214] Lesions are found more commonly in the mandible than in the maxilla at a 2 : 1 ratio.[212] Work by Schaudinn and colleagues suggests that there may be a toxic threshold of accumulated bisphosphonate in the bone that leads to the induction of BRONJ lesions and that measuring or calculating the concentration in bone may be a means of assessing an individual's risk for the development of BRONJ.[222]

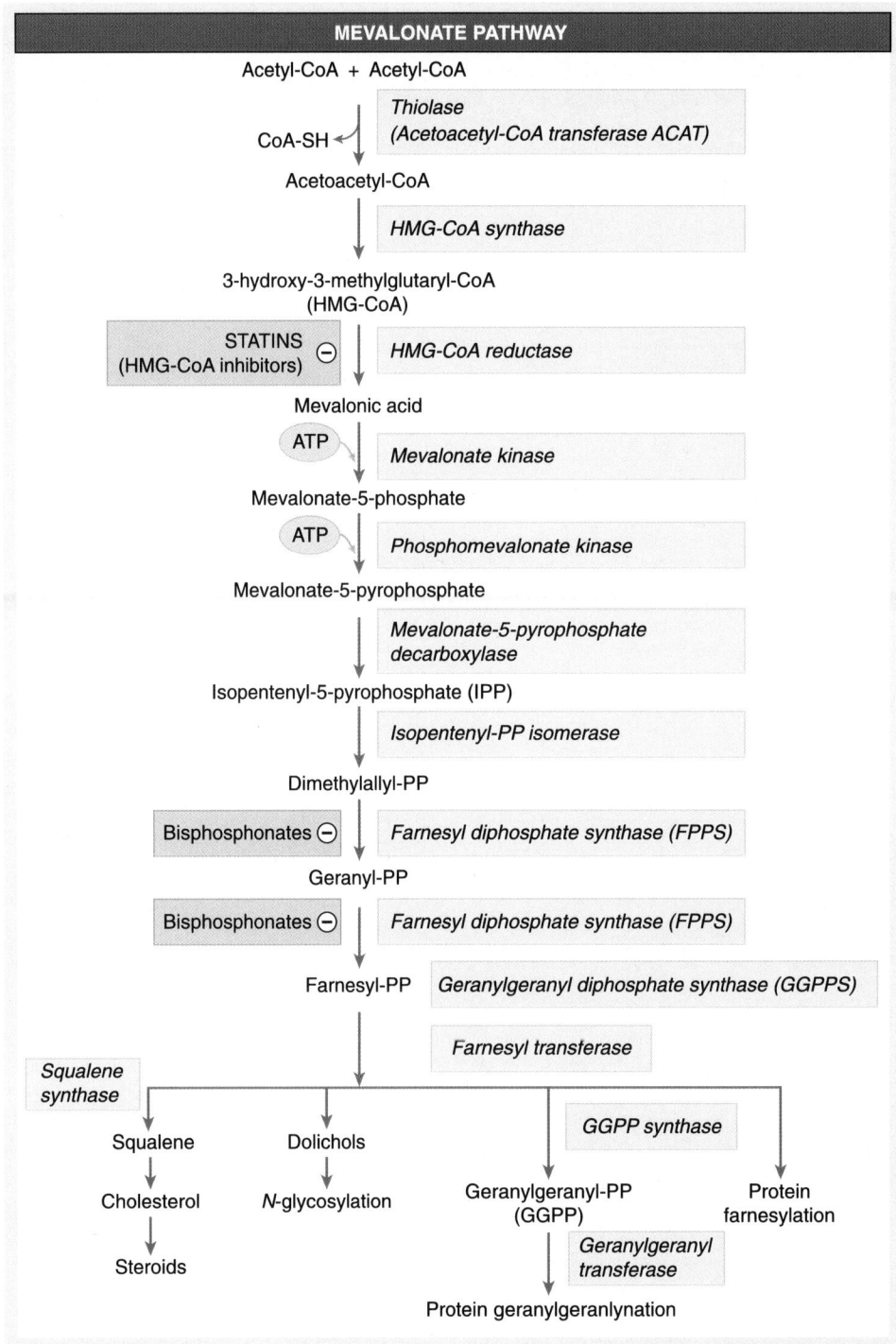

Fig. 14.19 Mevalonate pathway. Bisphosphonates interfere with the farnesyl pyrophosphate synthase enzyme, which leads to the inhibition of geranylgeranyl pyrophosphate, an important end product for cellular functions.

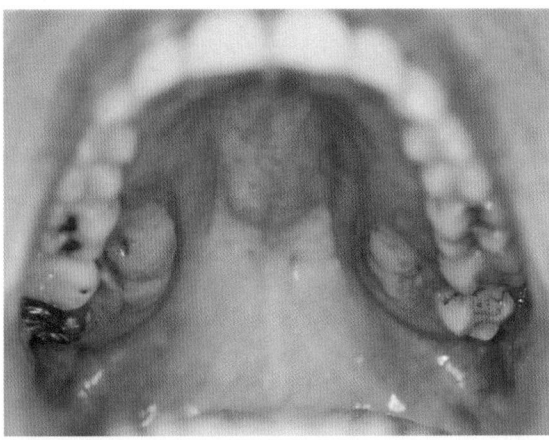

Fig. 14.20 Clinical photograph of exposed bone on the palatal surface of the maxilla adjacent to the molar root in a 60-year-old female with bisphosphonate-induced osteonecrosis of the bone (maxilla). The bone exposures were noted after about 1 year of treatment with bisphosphonate (Aredia and Zometa). *(Courtesy Drs. Eric S. Sung and Evelyn M. Chung, University of California, Los Angeles, CA.)*

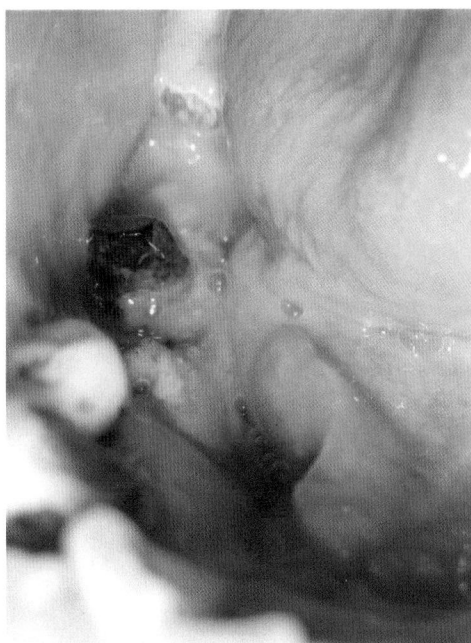

Fig. 14.21 Clinical photograph of exposed bone on the lingual surface of the posterior mandible of a 70-year-old male with bisphosphonate-induced osteonecrosis of the bone (mandible). The bone exposure was noted after 3 years of bisphosphonate treatment (Aredia and Zometa) for multiple myeloma. *(Courtesy Drs. Eric S. Sung and Evelyn M. Chung, University of California, Los Angeles, CA.)*

In addition to bisphosphonate therapy, other factors are thought to increase individual susceptibility to BRONJ. Potential risk factors that may contribute to BRONJ include systemic corticosteroid therapy, smoking, alcohol, poor oral hygiene, chemotherapy, radiotherapy, diabetes, and hematologic disease.[29] The precipitating factors or trauma-inducing events that lead to BRONJ are reported to include extractions, root canal treatment, periodontal infections, periodontal surgery, and dental implant surgery; however, some cases appear to be idiopathic, with spontaneous exposures.[165] In a retrospective evaluation of patients treated with IV bisphosphonates for metastatic bone cancer from 1996 to 2006, Estilo and colleagues[76] found that

the type of cancer, the duration of bisphosphonate therapy, sequential IV bisphosphonate treatment with pamidronate followed by zoledronate, comorbid osteoarthritis, rheumatoid arthritis, and benign hematologic conditions were significantly associated with an increased likelihood of ONJ. In their study, the systemic administration of corticosteroids was not found to be associated with an increased risk of BRONJ.[76]

As stated previously, patients who are being treated for cancer with IV bisphosphonates are at greater risk than patients being treated for osteoporosis with oral bisphosphonates. Dental health care providers should evaluate patients carefully, consider the risks, communicate with medical health care providers, inform patients, and consider treatment options and risks carefully.

KEY FACT

The effects of bisphosphonates on oral hard and soft tissue cells share the common mechanism of interference with products of the mevalonate pathway, which may be more significant to the overall problem than the reported apoptosis effects on osteoclasts. The inhibition of farnesyl pyrophosphate synthase leads to the inhibition of the mevalonate pathway end product, geranylgeranyl pyrophosphate (see Fig. 14.19). This bisphosphonate-inhibited pathway is required for many essential cellular functions in a variety of tissues.

Bisphosphonates and Periodontal Bone Loss

Not surprisingly, the bone-preserving action of bisphosphonates has been studied and advocated for use in the prevention of bone loss from periodontal disease.[245] Several animal studies have shown that bisphosphonates, either applied topically or administered systemically, have the potential to prevent the alveolar bone loss caused by periodontitis.[44,105,173,175,191,231,264] The use of bisphosphonates for bone regeneration has been proposed as well.[245] Although some studies have demonstrated bone preservation with low doses of bisphosphonate, higher doses and longer administration may have a neutral or detrimental effect on bone loss caused by periodontitis.[36,44] In a 2- to 3-year follow-up report of four female patients with periodontitis treated with etidronate (200 mg daily for periods of 2 weeks with 10-week off-drug periods), the potential of this agent to prevent periodontal bone loss was reported.[242] In a 2-year, randomized, placebo-controlled clinical trial of 335 patients treated with alendronate (70 mg once weekly), no significant difference in alveolar bone loss or alveolar bone density was found.[124] Interestingly, alendronate was found to significantly reduce bone loss relative to controls in a subset of this group (i.e., patients with low mandibular bone mineral density [BMD] at baseline), suggesting that the effect may be more perceptible in cases with less bone mass or less bone density. In another clinical trial of 24 patients (12 experimental and 12 control), alendronate was shown to have a significant positive (bone-preserving) effect on bone density in jaws.[71] The BMD of the maxilla and mandible was measured for all patients with the use of dual-energy x-ray absorptiometry (DEXA) at baseline and after 6 months of treatment (10 mg daily for 6 months).

Corticosteroids

In humans, the systemic administration of cortisone and adrenocorticotropic hormone appears to have no effect on the incidence or severity of gingival and periodontal disease. However, renal transplantation patients receiving immunosuppressive therapy (either prednisone or methylprednisone combined with either azathioprine or cyclophosphamide) have significantly less gingival inflammation than control subjects with similar amounts of plaque.[21,129,141,189,249]

Exogenous cortisone may have an adverse effect on bone quality and physiology. The systemic administration of cortisone in experimental animals resulted in the osteoporosis of alveolar bone.[98] There was capillary dilation and engorgement with hemorrhage into the periodontal ligament and gingival connective tissue, degeneration and a reduction in the number of collagen fibers in the periodontal ligament, and increased destruction of the periodontal tissues associated with inflammation.[98]

Stress increases circulating endogenous cortisol levels through stimulation of the adrenal glands (i.e., the hypothalamic–pituitary–adrenal axis). This increased exposure to endogenous cortisol may have adverse effects on the periodontium by diminishing the immune response to periodontal bacteria (see the section about Psychosocial Stress, Depression, and Coping).

 See the online material for discussion of additional systemic conditions and their influence on periodontal health.

 A Case Scenario is found on the companion website www.expertconsult.com.

Conclusion

Today, we have a better appreciation for the complexity and significance of interrelationships between periodontal infections and host defense. Genetic, environmental, physical, and psychosocial factors have the potential to alter periodontal tissues and the host immune response, thereby resulting in more severe periodontal disease. It is important to recognize that the systemic diseases, disorders, or conditions themselves do not cause periodontitis; rather, they may predispose, accelerate, or otherwise increase disease progression. This chapter reviewed important systemic diseases, disorders, and conditions that influence periodontal health.

References

 References for this chapter are found on the companion website www.expertconsult.com.

CHAPTER 15

Impact of Periodontal Infection on Systemic Health

Brian L. Mealey | Perry R. Klokkevold

CHAPTER OUTLINE

 For online-only content on periodontal disease and pregnancy outcome, periodontal disease and chronic obstructive pulmonary disease, and periodontal disease and acute respiratory infections, please visit the companion website at www.expertconsult.com.

Knowledge of the pathogenesis of periodontal diseases has evolved markedly over the last 50 years.[82] Periodontal disease is an inflammatory disease initiated by bacterial pathogens. Environmental, physical, social, and host stresses may affect and modify disease expression through a multitude of pathways. Certain systemic conditions can affect the initiation and progression of gingivitis and periodontitis (see Chapter 14). Systemic disorders that affect neutrophil, monocyte, macrophage, and lymphocyte function result in the altered production or activity of host inflammatory mediators.[82,125] These alterations may manifest clinically as the early onset of periodontal destruction or as a more rapid rate of destruction than would occur in the absence of such disorders.

Evidence has also shed light on the converse side of the relationship between systemic health and oral health: the potential effects of inflammatory periodontal diseases on a wide range of organ systems. This field of periodontal medicine addresses the following important questions:

- Can the inflammatory response to bacterial infection of the periodontium have an effect that is remote from the oral cavity?
- Is periodontal infection a risk factor for systemic diseases or conditions that affect human health?

Pathobiology of Periodontitis

Our understanding of the pathogenesis of periodontitis has changed remarkably over the last 30 years.[82,125,131] The nonspecific accumulation of bacterial plaque was once thought to be the cause of periodontal destruction, but it is now recognized that periodontitis is an infectious disease associated with a small number of predominantly gram-negative microorganisms that exist in a subgingival biofilm.[54] Furthermore, the importance of the host in disease initiation and progression is clearly recognized. Although pathogenic bacteria are necessary for periodontal disease, they are not sufficient alone to

cause the disease. A susceptible host is also imperative. In a host who has relatively low susceptibility to disease, bacterial pathogens may have no clinical effect. This may be due to a particularly effective host immunoinflammatory response that eliminates pathogenic organisms while minimizing destruction of native tissues. Conversely, in a host with relatively high disease susceptibility, marked destruction of periodontal tissues may result.

KEY FACT

Whereas pathogenic bacteria are necessary for periodontal disease, bacteria alone are not sufficient to cause disease. A susceptible host is imperative. In a host with relatively low susceptibility, bacterial pathogens may have little or no clinical effect.

Recognizing the importance of host susceptibility opens a door to understanding the differences in the onset, natural history, and progression of periodontitis seen throughout the scientific literature. Because of differences in host susceptibility, not all individuals are equally vulnerable to the destructive effects of periodontal pathogens and the immunoinflammatory response to those organisms. Thus, patients may not necessarily have similar disease expression despite the presence of similar bacteria. Likewise, the response to periodontal treatment may vary depending on the wound-healing capacity and susceptibility of the host to further disease progression. The importance of host susceptibility is clearly evident in the medical literature. For example, respiratory tract pathogens may have a minimal effect on many individuals, but in a susceptible host such as an elderly patient, these same pathogens may cause life-threatening respiratory tract illnesses.

There are many systemic conditions that can modify the host's susceptibility to periodontitis. For example, patients with immune suppression may not be able to mount an effective host response to subgingival microorganisms, thereby resulting in more rapid and severe periodontal destruction. Conversely, individuals with a significant increase in the production of proinflammatory mediators may respond to periodontal pathogens with an exuberant inflammatory response that results in the destruction of periodontal tissues. Although the potential impact of many systemic disorders on the periodontium is well documented, evidence suggests that periodontal infection may significantly enhance the risk for certain systemic diseases or alter the natural course of systemic conditions.[90,110,121,133,150,173] Although more than 50 different systemic conditions have been associated with periodontal diseases, the evidence base is quite large for many of these conditions and small for others. For example, conditions in which the influences of periodontal infection are well documented include coronary heart disease (CHD) and CHD-related events such as angina, infarction, atherosclerosis, and other vascular conditions; stroke; diabetes mellitus; preterm labor, low-birth-weight delivery, and preeclampsia; and respiratory conditions such as chronic obstructive pulmonary disease[90,110,132] (Box 15.1). A smaller but growing evidence base supports an association between poor oral health, tooth loss, or periodontitis and conditions such as chronic kidney disease and renal insufficiency[20,43,44,84,85,153]; certain forms of cancer[2,45,118,119,160] affecting the liver, pancreas, and colorectal region;

rheumatoid arthritis[29,30]; and altered cognitive function, dementia, and Alzheimer disease.[75,76,90,157,159,178] This chapter focuses on those conditions with the strongest evidence base, recognizing that ongoing research will further elucidate relationships between inflammatory periodontal diseases and systemic health.

Focal Infection Theory Revisited

Research in the area of periodontal medicine marks a resurgence in the concept of focal infection. In 1900, British physician William Hunter first developed the idea that oral microorganisms were responsible for a wide range of systemic conditions that were not easily recognized as being infectious in nature.[123,173] He claimed that restoration of carious teeth, instead of extraction, resulted in the trapping of infectious agents under restorations. In addition to caries, pulpal necrosis, and periapical abscesses, Hunter identified gingivitis and periodontitis as foci of infection. He advocated the extraction of teeth with these conditions to eliminate the source of sepsis. Hunter thought that teeth were prone to septic infection primarily because of their structure and their relationship to alveolar bone. He stated that the degree of systemic effect produced by oral sepsis depended on the virulence of the oral infection and the individual's degree of resistance. He also thought that oral organisms had specific actions on different tissues and that these organisms acted by producing toxins, thereby resulting in low-grade "subinfections" that produced systemic effects over prolonged periods. Finally, Hunter thought that the connection between oral sepsis and resulting systemic conditions could be shown via removal of the causative sepsis through tooth extraction and observation of the improvement in systemic health. Because it explained a wide range of disorders for which there was no known explanation at the time, Hunter's theory became widely accepted in Britain and eventually in the United States, leading to the wholesale extraction of teeth.

The focal infection theory fell into disrepute during the 1940s and 1950s, when widespread extraction—often of the entire dentition—failed to reduce or eliminate the systemic conditions to which the supposedly infected dentition had been linked.[173] The theory, while offering a possible explanation for perplexing systemic disorders, had been based on very little (if any) scientific evidence. Hunter and other advocates of the theory were unable to explain how focal oral sepsis produced these systemic maladies. They were also unable to elucidate possible interactive mechanisms between oral and systemic health. Furthermore, the suggested intervention of tooth extraction often had no effect on the systemic conditions for which patients sought relief. However, Hunter's ideas did encourage extensive research in the areas of microbiology and immunology.

FLASH BACK

The focal infection theory fell into disrepute during the 1940s and 1950s, when widespread extraction—often of the entire dentition—failed to reduce or eliminate the systemic conditions. The theory, while offering a possible explanation for perplexing systemic disorders, had been based on very little (if any) scientific evidence.

Evidence-Based Clinical Practice

Many of the precepts of the focal infection theory are being revived today in light of recent research demonstrating links between oral and systemic health. However, as expressed by Newman, for the "hypothesis not to fall into disrepute for a second time, there must be no unsubstantiated attributions, no theories without evidence."[123]

BOX 15.1 Organ Systems and Conditions Possibly Influenced by Periodontal Infection

Cardiovascular and Cerebrovascular Systems
Atherosclerosis
Coronary heart disease
Angina
Myocardial infarction
Cerebrovascular accident (stroke)
Erectile dysfunction
Anemia

Endocrine System
Metabolic syndrome
Diabetes mellitus

Reproductive System
Preterm and low-birth-weight infants
Preeclampsia

Respiratory System
Chronic obstructive pulmonary disease
Acute bacterial pneumonia

Kidney Diseases
Renal insufficiency
Chronic kidney disease
End-stage kidney disease

Autoimmune Diseases
Rheumatoid arthritis
Ankylosing spondylitis

Cognitive Function
Dementia
Alzheimer disease

Cancers
Colorectal
Pancreatic
Hepatocellular
Others

TABLE 15.1 Evaluation of Evidence

Type of Evidence	Strength of Evidence	Description
Case report	+/−	• Provides relatively weak retrospective anecdotal evidence • May suggest that further study is needed
Cross-sectional study	+	• Compares groups of subjects at a single point in time • Stronger than a case report • Fairly easy to conduct • Relatively inexpensive to conduct
Longitudinal study	++	• Follows groups of subjects over time • Stronger than a cross-sectional study • Studies with a control group much stronger than studies without controls • More difficult and expensive to conduct
Intervention trial	+++	• Examines the effects of some intervention • Studies with a control group (i.e., placebo) much stronger than studies without controls • Strongest form of evidence is the randomized controlled intervention trial • Difficult and expensive to conduct
Systematic review	++++	• Systematically evaluates evidence from multiple studies, especially randomized controlled trials • Uses clearly defined guidelines for the selection of evidence to be included or excluded from the review • Examines for heterogeneity in the overall data to indicate variations in study design, sample populations, and assessment methodologies

Today's era of evidence-based medicine and dentistry provides an excellent environment in which to examine the possible relationships between oral infection and systemic disorders. To establish a relationship between conditions A and B, different levels of evidence must be examined. All scientific evidence is not given the same weight.[64,114,124] The stronger the evidence, the more likely it is that a true relationship exists between the conditions. Table 15.1 describes these various levels of evidence.

For example, when examining the relationship between elevated cholesterol levels and CHD-related events, the literature might initially consist entirely of *case reports* or similar anecdotal information in which individual patients with recent myocardial infarction (MI) are found to have elevated cholesterol levels. These anecdotal reports suggest a possible relationship between elevated cholesterol and MI, but the evidence is weak. The case reports may lead to *cross-sectional studies,* in which a large subject population is examined to determine whether those individuals who had an MI have higher cholesterol levels than other individuals (control subjects) who did not have an MI. Ideally, these cross-sectional studies are controlled for other potential causes or factors associated with MI, such as age, gender, and smoking history. In other words, the subjects with a previous MI would be retrospectively matched with subjects of similar age, gender, and smoking history, and their cholesterol levels would then be examined for similarities or differences. Significantly higher cholesterol levels in subjects with a previous MI compared with those without MI offer stronger evidence than case reports; such evidence further substantiates a possible link between elevated cholesterol and MI.

Even stronger evidence is provided by *longitudinal studies,* in which subject populations are examined over time. For example, a group of subjects might periodically have their cholesterol levels evaluated over several years. If individuals with elevated cholesterol levels have a significantly higher rate of MI over time compared with subjects with normal cholesterol levels, then even stronger evidence is available to substantiate the link between cholesterol and MI. Finally, *intervention trials* may be designed to alter the potentially causative condition and to determine the effect of this change on the resultant condition. For example, patients with elevated cholesterol levels may be divided into two groups: a group that uses a cholesterol-lowering drug or diet and a control group that uses no intervention. These two groups might also be compared with a third group of subjects with normal cholesterol levels. Over time, the rate of MI in each group would be determined. If the group receiving the cholesterol-lowering regimen has a significantly lower rate of MI than the group with continued elevations in cholesterol level, strong evidence of a link between cholesterol and MI is established.

Finally, the highest level of evidence is the *systematic review.* A systematic review is not a standard literature review in which the articles selected for review are based on the desires and search methods chosen by the author, often for convenience. In a systematic review, the topic in question is selected before the review begins. For example, the authors may state the question as follows: "As compared with subjects not taking cholesterol-lowering medications, do subjects taking such medications demonstrate a difference in the rate of myocardial infarction?" A specific search strategy is then determined to reveal as much potential data as possible to answer the stated question. The authors state specifically why research papers were included or excluded from the review. If possible, the data are subjected to meta-analysis, a statistical method that combines the results of multiple studies that address a similar research hypothesis. This provides a more robust evaluation of the overall data than one can glean from individual research articles.

At each level of evidence, it is important to determine whether a biologically plausible link exists between conditions A and B. For example, if case reports, cross-sectional studies, longitudinal studies, and intervention trials all support a link between cholesterol levels and MI, the following questions remain:

• How is cholesterol related to MI?
• What are the mechanisms by which cholesterol affects the cardiovascular system and thus increases the risk for MI?

These studies evaluate the mechanisms by which conditions A and B might be linked and provide explanatory data that further substantiate the association between the two conditions.

The focal infection theory, as proposed and defended during the early part of the 20th century, was based on almost no evidence. Only the occasional case report and other anecdotes were available to substantiate the theory. Although explanatory mechanisms were proposed, none were validated with scientific research. This theory predated current concepts of evidence-based clinical practice and led to the unnecessary extraction of millions of teeth. Currently, when reexamining the potential associations between oral infections and systemic conditions, it is important (1) to determine what evidence is available; (2) to determine what evidence is still needed to substantiate the associations; and (3) to validate the possible mechanisms of association. This chapter reviews current knowledge that relates periodontal infection to overall systemic health.

Subgingival Environment as a Reservoir for Bacteria

The subgingival microbiota in patients with periodontitis provides a significant and persistent gram-negative bacterial challenge to the host that is met with a potent immunoinflammatory response.[126] These organisms and their products, such as *lipopolysaccharides* (LPSs), have ready access to the periodontal tissues and to the circulation via the sulcular epithelium, which is frequently ulcerated and discontinuous. Even with treatment, complete eradication of these organisms is difficult, and their reemergence is often rapid. The total surface area of pocket epithelium in contact with subgingival bacteria and their products in a patient with generalized moderate periodontitis has been estimated to be approximately the size of the palm of an adult hand, with even larger areas of exposure in cases of more advanced periodontal destruction.[131] Bacteremias are common after mechanical periodontal therapy, and they also occur frequently during normal daily function and oral hygiene procedures.[39,92,109] Just as the periodontal tissues mount an immunoinflammatory response to bacteria and their products, systemic challenge with these agents also induces a major vascular response.[35,59,139] This host response may offer explanatory mechanisms for the interactions between periodontal infection and a variety of systemic disorders.

KEY FACT

The subgingival microbiota in patients with periodontitis provides a significant and persistent gram-negative bacterial challenge to the host. These organisms and their products, such as LPSs, have access to the periodontal tissues and to the circulation via ulcerations in the sulcular epithelium.

Periodontal Disease and Mortality

The ultimate medical outcome measure is mortality. A number of studies suggest that an increased mortality rate from various causes is associated with inflammatory periodontal diseases.[2,20,37,46,71,89,142] The Normative Aging Study examined 2280 healthy men every 3 years for longer than 30 years after baseline clinical, radiographic, laboratory, and electrocardiographic examinations. A subset of this population was examined in the Veterans Affairs Dental Longitudinal Study to determine age-related changes in the oral cavity and identify risk factors for oral disease. Clinical examinations were performed, and alveolar bone level measurements were determined from full-mouth radiographs. The mean percentage of alveolar bone loss and mean probing depth were determined for each subject. From the original sample of 804 dentate, medically healthy subjects, a total of 166 died during the study.[46] Periodontal status at the baseline

examination was a significant predictor of mortality independent of other factors such as smoking, alcohol use, cholesterol levels, blood pressure, family history of heart disease, education level, and body mass. For those subjects with the most alveolar bone loss (>21% alveolar bone loss at baseline), the risk of dying during the follow-up period was 70% higher than for all other subjects. Interestingly, alveolar bone loss increased the risk of mortality more than smoking (52% increased risk), which is a well-known risk factor for mortality. A later evaluation of these same subjects confirmed a higher incidence of CHD-related events such as MI and unstable angina among men younger than 60 years of age with alveolar bone loss compared with those without bone loss.[37]

In a prospective cohort study of 1400 dentate men from Northern Ireland, subjects were divided into thirds (tertiles) based on average periodontal attachment loss.[89] Those with the highest levels of periodontal attachment loss has a significantly higher risk of death compared with those with the least attachment loss. The mortality rate over a 9-year period was 15.7% in those with the greatest attachment loss and 7.9% in those with the lowest level of periodontal attachment loss. In these studies, periodontitis preceded and increased the risk of mortality. However, this finding only establishes an association; it does not confirm causation. It is possible that periodontal disease reflects other health behaviors not evaluated in this study rather than acting as a specific cause of mortality. In other words, patients with poor periodontal health may also have other risk factors that increase mortality rate (e.g., smoking).

When examining research that suggests oral health status is a possible risk factor for systemic conditions, it is important to recognize when other known risk factors for those systemic conditions have been accounted for in the analysis. Host susceptibility factors that place individuals at risk for periodontitis may also place them at risk for systemic diseases such as cardiovascular disease. In these patients, the association may actually be among the risk factors rather than among the diseases. For example, periodontitis and cardiovascular disease share such risk factors as smoking, age, race, male gender, and stress. Genetic risk factors may also be shared.[83] In the Veterans Affairs Dental Longitudinal Study, smoking was an independent risk factor for mortality. When the data were examined to determine whether periodontal status was a risk factor, smoking status and other known risk factors for mortality were removed from the equation to allow for the independent evaluation of periodontal status. Other studies support an association between poor oral health and an increased risk of mortality.[142] In a prospective longitudinal study of subjects with type 2 diabetes, those with severe periodontitis had 3.2 times the risk of death from ischemic heart disease or kidney disease as subjects without periodontitis or with only slight periodontitis, after adjusting for other risk factors, including age, sex, duration of diabetes, glycemic control, macroalbuminuria, body mass index, serum cholesterol concentration, hypertension, and current smoking.[142]

Periodontal Disease, Coronary Heart Disease, and Atherosclerosis

To further explore the association between periodontal disease and CHD or atherosclerosis, investigators have studied specific systemic disorders and medical outcomes to determine their relationship to periodontal status. The proceedings of the first international Workshop on Periodontitis and Systemic Disease held by the American Academy of Periodontology (AAP) and the European Federation of Periodontology (EFP) were published in 2013, a major focus of which was the relationship between periodontitis and atherosclerotic cardiovascular disease.[32,38,136,147] CHD-related events are a major cause of death. MI has been associated with acute systemic bacterial and viral infections and is sometimes preceded by influenza-like symptoms.[102,158] Is it possible that oral infection is similarly related to MI? Traditional risk factors such as smoking, dyslipidemia, hypertension, and diabetes mellitus do not explain the presence of coronary atherosclerosis in a large number of patients. Localized infection that results in a chronic inflammatory reaction has been suggested as a mechanism underlying CHD in these individuals.[113]

In cross-sectional studies of patients with acute MI or confirmed CHD who were compared with age- and gender-matched control patients, patients with MI had significantly worse dental health (e.g., periodontitis, periapical lesions, caries, pericoronitis) than controls.[70,103,104] This association between poor dental health and MI was independent of known risk factors for heart disease, such as age, cholesterol levels, hypertension, diabetes, and smoking. Because atherosclerosis is a major determinant of CHD-related events, dental health has also been related to coronary atheromatosis. Mattila and colleagues[105] performed oral radiographic examinations and diagnostic coronary angiography on men with known CHD and found a significant correlation between the severity of dental disease and the degree of coronary atheromatosis. This relationship remained significant after accounting for other known risk factors for coronary artery disease. Similarly, Malthaner and colleagues[101] found an increased risk of angiographically defined coronary artery disease in subjects with greater bone loss and attachment loss; however, after adjusting for other known cardiovascular risk factors, the relationship between periodontal status and coronary artery disease was no longer statistically significant. There is evidence that the extent of periodontal disease may be associated with CHD. For example, there may be a greater risk for CHD-related events, such as MI, in subjects who have periodontitis affecting a greater number of teeth in the mouth compared with those who have periodontitis involving fewer teeth.[7]

Cross-sectional studies thus suggest a possible link between oral health and CHD; however, such studies cannot determine causality in this relationship. Rather, dental diseases may be indicators of general health practices. For example, periodontal disease and CHD are both related to lifestyle and share numerous risk factors, including smoking, diabetes, and low socioeconomic status. Bacterial infections have significant effects on endothelial cells, blood coagulation, lipid metabolism, and monocytes and macrophages.

Longitudinal studies provide compelling data regarding this relationship. In a 7-year follow-up study of the patients from the study by Mattila and colleagues, dental disease was significantly related to the incidence of new fatal and nonfatal coronary events as well as overall mortality.[106] In a prospective study of a national sample of adults, subjects with periodontitis had a 25% increased risk for CHD compared with those with no or minimal periodontal disease, after adjusting for other known risk factors.[36] Among males between the ages of 25 and 49 years, periodontitis increased the risk of CHD by 70%. The level of oral hygiene was also associated with heart disease. Patients with poor oral hygiene, as indicated by higher debris and calculus scores, had a twofold increased risk for CHD.

In another large prospective study, 1147 men were followed for 18 years.[11] During that time, 207 men (18%) developed CHD. When periodontal status at baseline was related to the presence or absence of CHD-related events during the follow-up period, a significant relationship was found. Subjects with more than 20% mean bone loss had a 50% increased risk of CHD compared with those with <20% bone loss. The extent of sites with probing depths >3 mm was strongly related to the incidence of CHD. Subjects with probing depths >3 mm on at least half of their teeth had a twofold increased risk, whereas those with probing depths of >3 mm on all of their

teeth had more than a threefold increased risk of CHD. This study and others in which the periodontal condition was known to have preceded the CHD-related events have supported the concept that periodontal disease is a risk factor for CHD, independent of other classic risk factors. Not all studies, however, support this concept; some show little independent effect of periodontal status on the risk for CHD after adjusting for commonly accepted cardiovascular risk factors.[65,66] It is particularly difficult to control for smoking as a confounding variable in these studies, because it is such an important risk factor for both periodontal disease and cardiovascular disease. This confounding influence of smoking makes it difficult to clarify the significance of the relationship between the diseases.

Perhaps the best evidence available comes from systematic reviews of studies examining the relationship between periodontal infection and cardiovascular disease. A systematic review and meta-analysis of data from 15 studies showed a significant 14% to 222% increase in the risk of CHD-related events in patients with periodontal disease as compared with those without periodontal disease.[9] A similar systematic review of longitudinal cohort and case–control studies showed a significant increase in the risk of incident MI, angina, or CHD-related death in subjects with periodontitis in five of the six studies reported.[38] This increased risk was noted mainly in younger subjects (i.e., <65 years old). Janket and colleagues[69] performed a meta-analysis of periodontal disease as a risk factor for future cardiovascular events and found an overall 19% increased risk of such events among individuals with periodontitis. The increase in risk was greater (44%) among people younger than 65 years of age. Although this increased risk is fairly modest, the extensive prevalence of periodontal disease in the population may increase the significance of the risk from a public health perspective. Extensive systematic reviews by Scannapieco and colleagues[143] and by an American Heart Association working group[91] concluded that a moderate degree of evidence exists to support an association between periodontal disease and atherosclerosis, MI, and cardiovascular disease independent of known confounders; however, causality is unclear. The results of the 2103 AAP/EFP Workshop on Periodontitis and Systemic Diseases concluded that "there is consistent and strong epidemiologic evidence that periodontitis imparts increased risk for future cardiovascular disease," but whereas many studies support multiple biologic mechanisms to explain this relationship, "intervention trials to date are not adequate to draw further conclusions."[169] That is, insufficient evidence exists to show that the treatment of periodontal disease has any impact on the risk of heart disease.

KEY FACT

There is consistent and strong epidemiologic evidence that periodontitis imparts increased risk for future cardiovascular disease.

Effects of Periodontal Infection

There are numerous mechanisms—both direct and indirect—through which periodontal infection may affect the onset or progression of atherosclerosis and CHD.[77,136,147] Periodontitis and atherosclerosis both have complex etiologic factors that combine genetic and environmental influences. In addition to smoking, the diseases share many risk factors and have distinct similarities with regard to their basic pathogenic mechanisms.

Ischemic Heart Disease

Ischemic heart disease is associated with the processes of atherogenesis and thrombogenesis (Fig. 15.1). Damage to the vascular endothelium, with a subsequent inflammatory reaction, plays a major role in

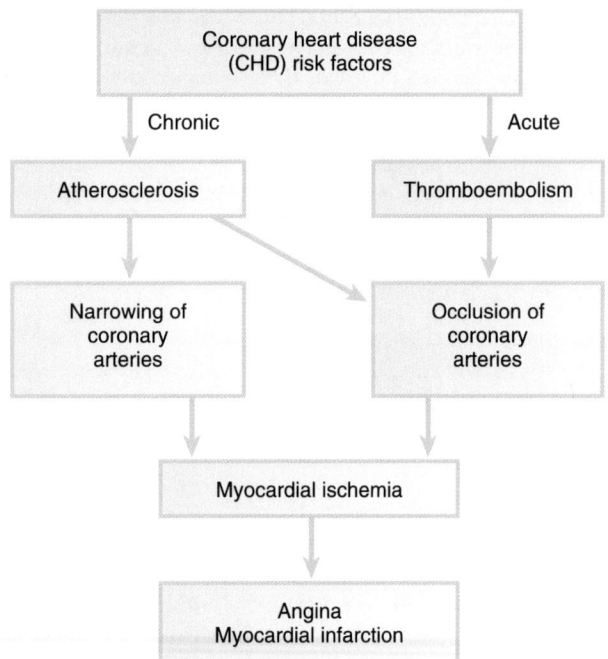

Fig. 15.1 Acute and chronic pathways to ischemic heart disease. Coronary heart disease–related events, such as angina and myocardial infarction, may be precipitated by either pathway or both pathways.

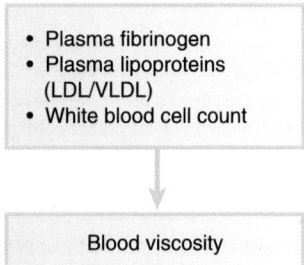

Fig. 15.2 Factors that affect blood viscosity in health. *LDL,* Low-density lipoprotein; *VLDL,* very-low-density lipoprotein.

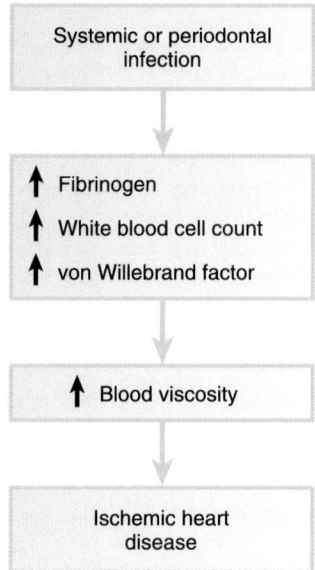

Fig. 15.3 The effect of infection on blood viscosity. Increased plasma fibrinogen and von Willebrand factor cause hypercoagulability. When they are combined with an increased white blood cell count, the blood viscosity increases, thereby increasing the risk of coronary ischemia.

atherosclerosis and ischemic organ damage.[169] Increased viscosity of blood may promote major ischemic heart disease and cerebrovascular accident (stroke) by increasing the risk of thrombus formation.[98] Fibrinogen is a major factor in the promotion of this hypercoagulable state. *Fibrinogen* is the precursor to fibrin, and increased fibrinogen levels increase blood viscosity. Increased plasma fibrinogen is a recognized risk factor for cardiovascular events and peripheral vascular disease[97] (Fig. 15.2). An elevated white blood cell count is also a predictor of heart disease and stroke, and circulating leukocytes may promote the occlusion of blood vessels. Coagulation factor VIII (von Willebrand factor) has likewise been associated with a risk of ischemic heart disease.[137]

Systemic Infections

Systemic infections are known to induce a hypercoagulable state and increase blood viscosity (Fig. 15.3). Fibrinogen levels and white blood cell counts are often increased in patients with periodontal disease.[22,88] Individuals with poor oral health may also have significant elevations in coagulation factor VIII/von Willebrand factor antigen, thereby increasing the risk of thrombus formation. Thus, periodontal infection may also promote increased blood viscosity and

thrombogenesis, which leads to an increased risk for central and peripheral vascular disease.

Daily Activity

Routine daily activities such as mastication and oral hygiene procedures result in frequent bacteremia with oral organisms.[92] Periodontal disease may predispose the patient to an increased incidence of bacteremia, including the presence of virulent gram-negative organisms associated with periodontitis. There is a greater risk of bacteremia after toothbrushing in patients with higher levels of plaque, calculus, and gingivitis as compared with those with minimal plaque and gingival inflammation.[93] In fact, subjects with generalized gingival bleeding after brushing showed an almost eightfold increase in their incidence of bacteremia as compared with those with minimal gingival bleeding. An estimated 8% of all cases of infective endocarditis are associated with periodontal or dental disease without a preceding dental procedure.[39] The periodontium, when affected by periodontitis, also acts as a reservoir of *endotoxins* (LPSs) from gram-negative organisms. Endotoxins can pass readily into the systemic circulation during normal daily function, thereby inducing damage to the vascular endothelium and precipitating many negative cardiovascular effects. In a study of the incidence of endotoxemia after simple chewing, subjects with periodontitis were four times more likely to have endotoxin present in the bloodstream than subjects without periodontitis. Furthermore, the concentration of endotoxin in the bloodstream was more than fourfold greater in those with periodontitis as compared with healthy subjects.[47]

Thrombogenesis

Platelet aggregation plays a major role in thrombogenesis, and most cases of acute MI are precipitated by thromboembolism. Oral organisms may be involved in coronary thrombogenesis. Platelets selectively bind some strains of *Streptococcus sanguinis,* which is a common component of supragingival plaque, and *Porphyromonas gingivalis,* which is a pathogen closely associated with periodontitis.[60,61] The aggregation of platelets is induced by the *platelet aggregation–associated protein* (PAAP) expressed on some strains of these bacteria.[140] In animal models, intravenous infusion of PAAP-positive

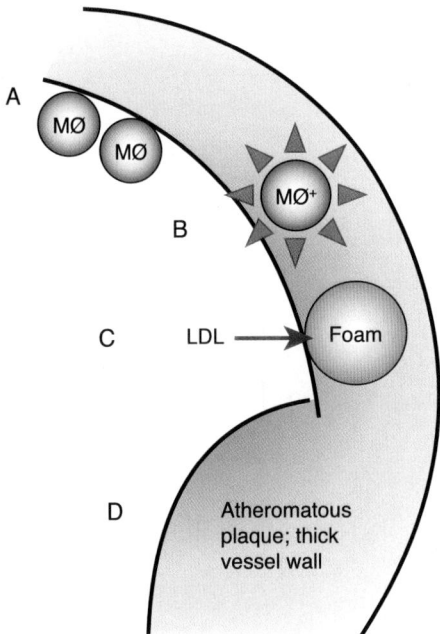

Fig. 15.4 Pathogenesis of atherosclerosis. (A) Monocytes and macrophages *(MØ)* adhere to the vascular endothelium. (B) Monocytes and macrophages penetrate into the arterial media and produce proinflammatory cytokines and growth factors. (C) The ingestion of oxidized low-density lipoprotein *(LDL)* enlarges monocytes to form foam cells. (D) Smooth muscle proliferation and plaque formation thicken vessel walls and narrow the lumen. *MØ⁺,* Hyperinflammatory monocyte/macrophage phenotype.

bacterial strains resulted in alterations of heart rate, blood pressure, cardiac contractility, and electrocardiogram readings consistent with MI. Platelet accumulation also occurred in the lungs and led to tachypnea. No such changes were seen with the infusion of PAAP-negative strains. PAAP-positive bacteria caused aggregation of circulating platelets, which resulted in the formation of thromboemboli and resultant cardiac and pulmonary changes. Thus, periodontitis-associated bacteremia with certain strains of *S. sanguinis* and *P. gingivalis* may promote acute thromboembolic events via interaction with circulating platelets.

Atherosclerosis

Atherosclerosis is a focal thickening of the arterial *intima,* the innermost layer lining the vessel lumen, and the *media,* the thick layer under the intima that consists of smooth muscle, collagen, and elastic fibers (Fig. 15.4).[140] The formation of atherosclerotic plaques is precipitated by damage to vascular endothelium that results in an inflammatory response in which circulating monocytes adhere to the vascular endothelium. Damage to vascular endothelium can occur because of the presence of intravascular microorganisms and their products; chemical damage, often resulting from elements of tobacco and other exogenous toxins; and increased shear force along the vascular lining, such as that occurring in hypertension. The adherence of monocytes to the damaged vascular endothelium is mediated by several adhesion molecules on the endothelial cell surface, including intercellular adhesion molecule-1 (ICAM-1), endothelial leukocyte adhesion molecule-1 (ELAM-1), and vascular cell adhesion molecule-1 (VCAM-1).[12,80] These adhesion molecules are up-regulated by a number of factors, including bacterial LPSs, prostaglandins, and proinflammatory cytokines. After binding to the endothelial cell lining, monocytes penetrate the endothelium and migrate under the arterial intima. The monocytes ingest circulating low-density

lipoprotein in its oxidized state and become engorged, thereby forming the foam cells that are characteristic of atheromatous plaque. After entering the arterial media, monocytes may also transform to macrophages.

A host of proinflammatory cytokines such as interleukin-1 (IL-1), tumor necrosis factor alpha (TNF-α), and prostaglandin E_2 (PGE_2) are then produced, and they propagate the atheromatous lesion. Mitogenic factors such as fibroblast growth factor and platelet-derived growth factor stimulate smooth muscle and collagen proliferation within the media, thereby thickening the arterial wall.[97] Atheromatous plaque formation and thickening of the vessel wall narrow the lumen and dramatically decrease blood flow through the vessel.[140] Arterial thrombosis often occurs after an atheromatous plaque ruptures. Plaque rupture exposes circulating blood to arterial collagen and tissue factor from monocytes and macrophages that activate platelets and the coagulation pathway. Platelet and fibrin accumulation forms a thrombus that may occlude the vessel and result in an ischemic event such as angina or MI. The thrombus may separate from the vessel wall and form an embolus, which may also occlude vessels, again leading to an acute event such as MI or cerebral infarction (stroke).

Role of Periodontal Disease in Atherosclerotic Myocardial or Cerebral Ischemia

In animal models, gram-negative bacteria and associated LPSs cause infiltration of inflammatory cells into the arterial wall, proliferation of arterial smooth muscle, and intravascular coagulation. These changes are identical to those seen with naturally occurring athero-matosis. There is strong evidence that periodontal bacteria disseminate from the oral cavity to the systemic vasculature, can be found within distant tissues, and can live within those affected tissues.[136] Further-more, in animal models, dissemination of periodontal bacteria can induce atherosclerosis in distant vessels. Patients with periodontitis are at increased risk for thickening of the walls of the major coronary arteries.[11] In several studies of atheromas obtained from humans during endarterectomy, more than half of the lesions contained periodontal pathogens, and many atheromas contained multiple different periodontal species.[21,57,180] Periodontal diseases result in chronic systemic exposure to products of these organisms. Low-level bacteremia may initiate host responses that alter coagulability, endothelial and vessel wall integrity, and platelet function, thereby resulting in atherogenic changes and possible thromboembolic events (Fig. 15.5).

> ### CLINICAL CORRELATION
>
> There is strong evidence that periodontal bacteria disseminate from the oral cavity to the systemic vasculature, can be found within distant tissues, and can live within those affected tissues.

Research has clearly shown a wide variation in host response to bacterial challenge. Some individuals with heavy plaque accumulation and high proportions of pathogenic organisms appear relatively resistant to bone and attachment loss. Others develop extensive periodontal destruction in the presence of small amounts of plaque and low proportions of putative pathogens. Patients with an abnormally exuberant inflammatory response often have a hyperinflammatory monocyte and macrophage phenotype (MØ⁺). Monocytes and macrophages from these individuals secrete significantly increased levels of proinflammatory mediators (e.g., IL-1, TNF-α, PGE_2) in response to bacterial LPSs compared with patients with a normal monocyte and macrophage phenotype. Patients with aggressive periodontitis, refractory periodontitis, and type 1 diabetes mellitus

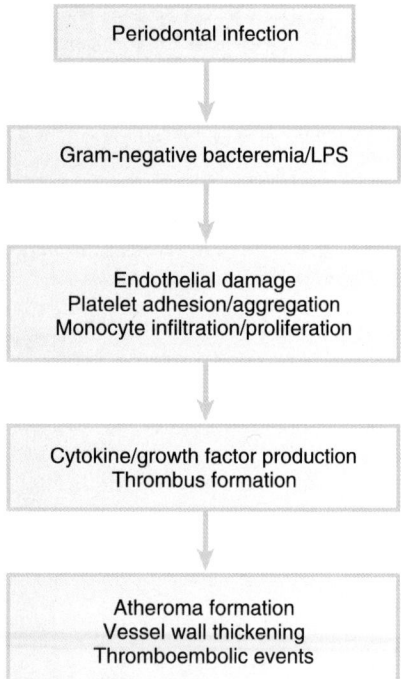

Fig. 15.5 The influence of periodontal infection on atherosclerosis. Periodontal pathogens and their products result in damage to the vascular endothelium. Monocytes and macrophages enter the vessel wall and produce cytokines that further increase the inflammatory response and propagate the atheromatous lesion. Growth factor production leads to smooth muscle proliferation in the vessel wall. Damaged endothelium also activates platelets, thereby resulting in platelet aggregation and potentiating thromboembolic events. *LPS*, Lipopolysaccharide.

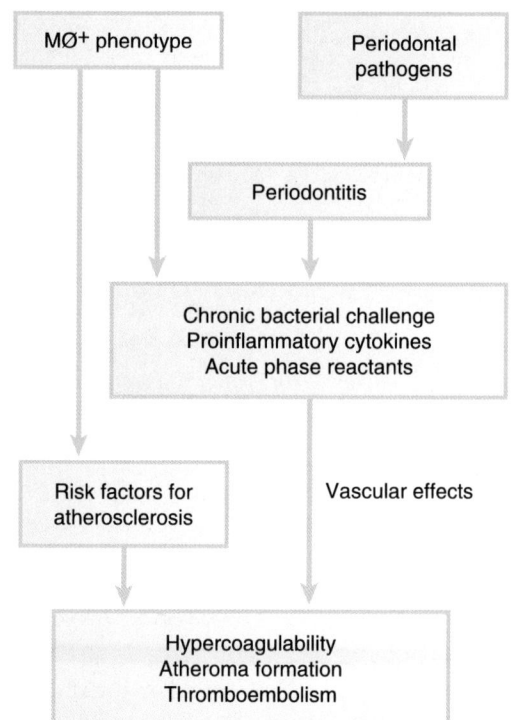

Fig. 15.6 The cardiovascular and periodontal consequences of the hyper-responsive monocyte/macrophage phenotype *(MØ⁺)*. In combination with other risk factors, the MØ⁺ phenotype predisposes individuals to both atherosclerosis and periodontitis. Bacterial products and inflammatory mediators associated with periodontitis affect vascular endothelium, monocytes and macrophages, platelets, and smooth muscle and may increase blood coagulability. This may further increase atherosclerosis and may result in thromboembolism and ischemic events.

often possess the MØ⁺ phenotype,[13] which appears to be under both genetic and environmental control.

The monocyte and macrophage cell line is intimately involved in the pathogenesis of both periodontal disease and atherosclerosis. Diet-induced elevations in serum low-density lipoprotein levels up-regulate monocyte and macrophage responsiveness to bacterial LPSs. Thus, elevated low-density lipoprotein levels, which is a known risk factor for atherosclerosis and CHD, may increase the secretion of destructive and inflammatory cytokines by monocytes and macrophages. This may result not only in the propagation of atheromatous lesions, but also in enhanced periodontal destruction in the presence of pathogenic organisms. This is one example of a potential shared mechanism in the pathogenesis of cardiovascular and periodontal diseases. The presence of an MØ⁺ phenotype may place patients at risk for both CHD and periodontitis (Fig. 15.6). Periodontal infections may contribute to atherosclerosis and thromboembolic events by repeatedly challenging the vascular endothelium and arterial wall with bacterial LPSs and proinflammatory cytokines. Vascular monocytes and macrophages in patients with an MØ⁺ phenotype meet this challenge with an abnormally elevated inflammatory response that may directly contribute to atherosclerosis and may precipitate thromboembolic events.[110]

Cardiovascular diseases are increasingly recognized as having a major systemic inflammatory component, further emphasizing possible similarities with inflammatory periodontal diseases.[140] As such, the detection of systemic inflammatory markers plays an increasingly important role in risk assessment for vascular events such as MI and cerebral infarction. Acute-phase proteins such as *C-reactive protein* (CRP) and fibrinogen are produced in the liver in response to inflammatory or infectious stimuli and act as inflammatory markers.[139]

CRP induces monocytes and macrophages to produce tissue factor, which stimulates the coagulation pathway and increases blood coagulability. Increased fibrinogen levels may contribute to this process. CRP also stimulates the complement cascade, further exacerbating inflammation.

Elevations in serum CRP and fibrinogen levels are well-accepted risk factors for cardiovascular disease.[138,139] Research has focused on periodontitis as a potential trigger for systemic inflammation. Serum CRP and fibrinogen levels are often elevated in subjects with periodontitis as compared with subjects without periodontitis.[27,94,175] These acute-phase proteins may act as intermediary steps in the pathway from periodontal infection to cardiovascular disease (see Figs. 15.5 and 15.6). Thus, periodontal diseases may have both direct effects on the major blood vessels (e.g., atheroma formation) and indirect effects that stimulate changes in the cardiovascular system (e.g., elevation of systemic inflammatory responses).

Interesting supportive evidence for these mechanisms can be derived from intervention trials in which serum levels of inflammatory mediators and markers are assessed before and after treatment that is aimed at decreasing periodontal inflammation. For example, in subjects with chronic periodontitis, serum levels of IL-6 and CRP are reduced after scaling and root planing.[33] A systematic review and meta-analysis of 25 intervention studies examining periodontitis patients with and without periodontal treatment demonstrated that periodontal treatment was associated with a significant reduction in serum levels of CRP, IL-6, fibrinogen, and TNF-α.[164] Inflammatory periodontal disease (compared with periodontal health) is also associated with altered vascular endothelial function.[34] Altered vascular endothelial function is a major risk factor for acute thrombotic events.

After scaling and root planing with a resultant decrease in periodontal inflammation, markers of vascular health improve significantly over time.[34,168] The functional assessment of vascular endothelial function also returns to normal after scaling and root planing.[148,168] These results suggest that periodontal inflammation adversely affects the health of the vascular endothelium, whereas a reduction in inflammation improves endothelial health. Whether these changes directly impact the risk of acute cardiovascular events remains to be determined in prospective controlled clinical intervention trials over long periods; such studies do not currently exist.

Role of Periodontal Disease in Erectile Dysfunction

Erectile dysfunction (ED) is associated with endothelial dysfunction, and elevated levels of oxidative stress and systemic inflammation are common to both periodontal disease and ED. Studies have shown a relationship between ED and periodontitis. In a large case–control study of almost 200,000 subjects in Taiwan, those with ED were significantly more likely to have chronic periodontitis than those without ED, with an overall significant odds ratio of 3.35 after adjusting for confounding variables.[78] Other studies have supported these findings in smaller populations in other countries,[129,152,179] and a systematic review of four studies found a significant association between periodontitis and ED, with an odds ratio of 3.07.[171] An intervention trial was conducted in 120 subjects with ED and chronic periodontitis; 60 subjects received scaling and root planing, and 60 control subjects received no periodontal treatment.[1] Three months later, the treatment group had significant improvement in ED, whereas the control group had no change. These preliminary studies suggest a relationship between periodontitis and ED, but more research is needed to understand the mechanisms of interaction.

Periodontal Disease and Stroke

Ischemic cerebral infarction, or stroke, is often preceded by systemic bacterial or viral infection. In one study, patients with cerebral ischemia were five times more likely to have had a systemic infection within 1 week before the ischemic event than nonischemic control subjects.[52] Recent infection was a significant risk factor for cerebral ischemia; it was independent of other known risk factors such as hypertension, history of a previous stroke, diabetes, smoking, and CHD. Interestingly, the presence of systemic infection before the stroke resulted in significantly greater ischemia and a more severe postischemic neurologic defect than stroke not preceded by infection.[53] Stroke patients with a preceding infection had slightly higher levels of plasma fibrinogen and significantly higher levels of CRP compared with those without infection.

Periodontal Infection Associated With Stroke

Stroke is classified as either hemorrhagic or nonhemorrhagic. Nonhemorrhagic stroke, or ischemic stroke, is usually caused by thromboembolic events and cerebrovascular atherosclerosis, whereas hemorrhagic stroke often results from a vascular bleed such as an aneurysm. Periodontal disease has been associated primarily with an increased risk of nonhemorrhagic stroke. Numerous studies have shown that periodontal disease is associated with an increased risk of stroke. In a case–control study, subjects with severe periodontitis had a 4.3 times higher risk of stroke than subjects with mild or no periodontitis.[51] Severe periodontitis was a risk factor in men but not women, and in those younger but not older than 65 years of age. In a longitudinal study of 1137 dentate men who were followed for a mean of 24 years, subjects with >20% mean radiographic bone loss at baseline were more than three times as likely to have a stroke

than subjects with <20% bone loss.[74] There was a stronger effect of periodontitis on the risk for stroke among men younger than 65 years of age compared with older subjects. Both large epidemiologic studies and systematic reviews of the evidence have suggested an approximate threefold increased risk of stroke in subjects with periodontitis.[69,176]

As previously discussed, periodontal infection may contribute directly to the pathogenesis of atherosclerosis by providing a persistent bacterial challenge to the arterial endothelium, thereby contributing to the monocyte- and macrophage-driven inflammatory process that results in atheromatosis and narrowing of the vessel lumen. Furthermore, periodontal infection may stimulate a series of indirect systemic effects, such as elevated production of fibrinogen and CRP, which increases the risk of stroke (see Figs. 15.5 and 15.6). Finally, bacteremia with PAAP-positive bacterial strains from supragingival and subgingival plaque can increase platelet aggregation, thereby contributing to thrombus formation and subsequent thromboembolism, which is the leading cause of stroke.[110]

! CLINICAL CORRELATION

Periodontal infection may contribute directly to the pathogenesis of atherosclerosis by providing a persistent bacterial challenge to the arterial endothelium, thereby contributing to the monocyte- and macrophage-driven inflammatory process that results in atheromatosis and narrowing of the vessel lumen.

Periodontal Disease and Diabetes Mellitus

The relationship between diabetes mellitus and periodontal disease has been extensively examined. It is clear from epidemiologic research that diabetes increases the risk for and severity of periodontal diseases.[112] The biologic mechanisms through which diabetes influences the periodontium are discussed in Chapter 14. The increased prevalence and severity of periodontitis typically seen in patients with diabetes—especially those with poor metabolic control—has led to the designation of periodontal disease as the "sixth complication" of diabetes.[99] In addition to the five "classic" complications of diabetes (Box 15.2), the American Diabetes Association has officially recognized that periodontal disease is common among patients with diabetes, and its Standards of Care include taking a history of current or past dental infections as part of the physician's examination.[4] Since 2009, the American Diabetes Association's Standards of Medical Care in Diabetes have specifically recommended that physicians refer patients with diabetes to a dentist for a comprehensive dental and periodontal examination.[5]

Many studies have examined the effects of diabetes on the periodontium, whereas others have examined the effect of periodontal infection on the control of diabetes.[112] Such studies are difficult to

---

BOX 15.2 Complications of Diabetes Mellitus

1. Retinopathy
2. Nephropathy
3. Neuropathy
4. Macrovascular disease
5. Altered wound healing
6. Periodontal disease

From Löe H: Periodontal disease: the sixth complication of diabetes mellitus. *Diabetes Care* 16(Suppl 1):329, 1993.

perform because of the influence of ongoing medical management of diabetes during the study. The following questions remain:

- Does the presence or severity of periodontal disease affect the metabolic state of diabetic patients?
- Does periodontal treatment aimed at reducing the bacterial challenge and minimizing inflammation have a measurable effect on glycemic (blood glucose) control?

A review of four studies including more than 22,000 subjects found that the incidence of type 2 diabetes (i.e., new diagnoses) was significantly greater in individuals with periodontal disease than in those without periodontal disease.[15] In a longitudinal study of patients with type 2 diabetes, severe periodontitis was associated with the significant worsening of glycemic control over time.[161] Individuals with severe periodontitis at the baseline examination had a greater incidence of worsening glycemic control over a 2- to 4-year period as compared with those without periodontitis at baseline. In this study, periodontitis was known to have preceded the worsening of glycemic control. Periodontitis has also been associated with the classic complications of diabetes. Diabetic adults with severe periodontitis at baseline had a significantly greater incidence of kidney and macrovascular complications over the subsequent 1 to 11 years than did diabetic adults with only gingivitis or mild periodontitis.[167] This was true despite both groups' having similar glycemic control. One or more cardiovascular complications occurred in 82% of patients with severe periodontitis versus 21% of patients without severe periodontitis. Again, severe periodontitis preceded the onset of clinical diabetic complications in these subjects.

Among diabetic patients with periodontitis, periodontal therapy may have beneficial effects on glycemic control.[41,112,151,154,163] This may be especially true for patients with relatively poor glycemic control and more advanced periodontal destruction before treatment. A large number of studies, starting as far back as 1960,[174] have examined the impact of periodontal therapy on glycemic control in patients with diabetes. Most of these studies compared scaling and root planing (with or without adjunctive systemic antibiotics) with no periodontal therapy and followed patients for several months to assess changes in glycemic control measured by glycated hemoglobin (HbA1c) values. Others included in the treatment regimen not only scaling and root planing but also extraction of periodontally hopeless teeth and even periodontal surgery. Many of these studies showed a significant improvement in glycemic control, as determined by reductions in HbA1c values, in the periodontal treatment group compared with the nontreatment group.[55,81,120] Other studies showed minimal change in glycemic control in periodontally treated patients.[3,23,42,156]

When studies of similar treatment regimens demonstrate conflicting results, systematic reviews with meta-analyses of the data are essential to aid the clinician in evaluating the evidence. Numerous systematic reviews and meta-analyses have consistently shown that periodontal therapy is associated with a statistically significant and clinically relevant improvement in glycemic control in patients with diabetes and periodontitis.[41,151,163] However, clinicians must understand that individual patients may or may not have outcomes similar to the average outcome in any given study or systematic review. That is, treatment results vary from patient to patient, and clinicians should not expect the same result in all patients. These studies suggest that periodontal therapy is most likely to result in short-term improvement in glycemia in those diabetic patients with severe periodontitis and poor metabolic control who demonstrate marked reduction in periodontal inflammation after treatment. Conversely, individuals with moderately well-controlled or well-controlled diabetes and periodontitis who have less reduction in

inflammation may demonstrate no or only minimal changes in glycemic control.

FLASH BACK

Periodontal disease was designated as the "sixth complication" of diabetes because of the increased prevalence and severity of periodontitis typically seen in patients with diabetes, especially those with poor metabolic control.

Most of the studies evaluating the treatment of periodontal disease and its impact on glycemic control have been performed in subjects with type 2 diabetes. However, research suggests that periodontal therapy may have a smaller impact on glycemic control in patients with type 1 diabetes than in those with type 2 disease.[16] In a study of subjects with type 1 and type 2 diabetes with periodontitis, periodontal therapy was associated with a significant improvement in glycemic control overall in those with type 2 diabetes but not in those with type 1 disease, despite improvement in the periodontal condition of both groups.[16]

It is common to observe wide interindividual variability in responses to various medical management approaches in patients with type 1 diabetes. Similarly, wide variability in the impact of periodontal therapy on glycemic control can be expected in the type 1 diabetic population. For example, a study of periodontal therapy in 65 people with type 1 diabetes and chronic periodontitis showed highly variable responses.[166] Although there was an overall improvement in periodontal health after therapy, approximately 35% of subjects had an improvement in glycemic control after treatment, 37% had no significant change, and 28% showed a worsening of glycemic control. In this study, subjects were divided into those with better baseline glycemic control (i.e., glycated hemoglobin values <8.5%) and those with poorer glycemic control (i.e., glycated hemoglobin values ≥8.5%). Interestingly, twice as many subjects showed improved glycemic control among those whose glycemic control before periodontal treatment was poor compared with those among whom baseline glycemic control was good. Therefore, the clinician may anticipate a greater glycemic response to periodontal therapy among those patients with type 1 diabetes whose glycemic control is relatively poor than among those whose glycemic control is already good before periodontal treatment.

Although the routine use of systemic antibiotics for treatment of chronic periodontitis is not justified, patients with poorly controlled diabetes and severe periodontitis may constitute one patient group for whom such therapy is appropriate. Antibiotics remain an adjunct to the necessary mechanical removal of plaque and calculus. The mechanisms by which adjunctive antibiotics may induce positive changes in glycemic control when they are combined with mechanical debridement are unknown at this time. Systemic antibiotics may eliminate residual bacteria after scaling and root planing, thereby further decreasing the bacterial challenge to the host. Tetracyclines are also known to suppress the glycation of proteins and decrease the activity of tissue-degrading enzymes such as matrix metalloproteinases. These changes may contribute to improvements in the metabolic control of diabetes.

Periodontal Infection Associated With Glycemic Control in Diabetes

An understanding of the effects of other infections is useful to delineate the mechanisms by which periodontal infection influences glycemia. It is well known that systemic inflammation plays a major role in insulin sensitivity and glucose dynamics. As discussed previously, periodontal diseases can induce or perpetuate an elevated systemic chronic inflammatory state, which is reflected in increased serum CRP, IL-6, and fibrinogen levels seen in many people with periodontitis.[33,94,162] Inflammation induces insulin resistance, and such resistance often accompanies systemic infections. For example, acute nonperiodontal bacterial and viral infections have been shown to increase insulin resistance and aggravate glycemic control.[141,177] This occurs in individuals either with or without diabetes. Systemic infections increase tissue resistance to insulin through a variety of mechanisms, thereby preventing glucose from entering target cells, causing elevated blood glucose levels, and requiring increased pancreatic insulin production to maintain normoglycemia. Insulin resistance may persist for weeks or even months after the patient has recovered clinically from the illness. In an individual with type 2 diabetes who already has significant insulin resistance, further tissue resistance to insulin as a result of infection may considerably exacerbate poor glycemic control.

It is possible that chronic gram-negative periodontal infections may also result in increased insulin resistance and poor glycemic control.[54,162] In patients with periodontitis, persistent systemic challenge with periodontopathic bacteria and their products results in an up-regulation of the immunoinflammatory response, with elevation in serum levels of proinflammatory mediators such as IL-1β, TNF-α, and IL-6, similar to well-recognized systemic infections but on a more persistent, chronic basis (Fig. 15.7). Increased serum levels of several cytokines, including TNF-α and IL-6, are associated with increased insulin resistance. This mechanism would explain the worsening of glycemic control associated with severe periodontitis. Periodontal treatment designed to decrease the bacterial insult and reduce inflammation may result in decreased systemic inflammation, restoring insulin sensitivity over time and thereby resulting in improved metabolic control. The improved glycemic control seen in many studies of periodontal therapy would support such a hypothesis. This mechanism may also explain differences in the glycemic response to periodontal therapy between individuals with type 1 and type 2 diabetes.[16] Because type 2 diabetes is strongly associated with insulin resistance, periodontal therapy that reduces systemic inflammation may improve insulin sensitivity and result in improved glycemic control. Conversely, type 1 diabetes is not strongly associated with insulin resistance, so reduced inflammation after periodontal therapy may not have a major effect on insulin sensitivity in patients with type 1 disease, which would minimize the impact of periodontal treatment in these patients.

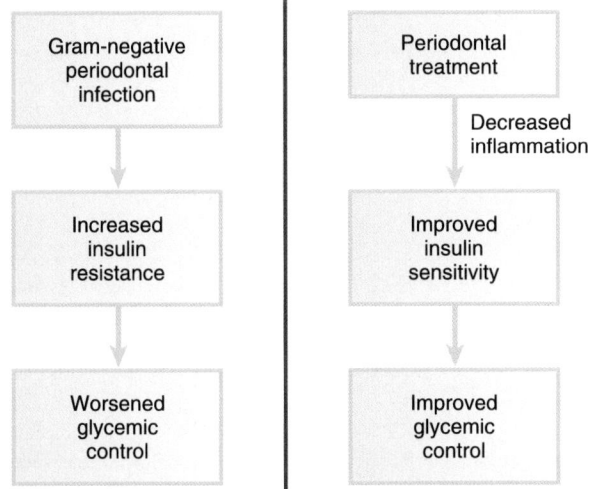

Fig. 15.7 Potential effects of periodontal infection and periodontal therapy on glycemia in patients with diabetes.

Periodontal Disease and Asthma

Evidence evaluating the relationship between periodontal disease and asthma is relatively sparse. The largest study has been a case–control study of 220 adults, half with severe asthma and half without asthma.[50] After adjusting for age, smoking habit, education level, and body mass index, people with periodontitis were 4.8 times more likely to have severe asthma than those without periodontitis. Although this study does not demonstrate causation, it suggests a possible link between inflammatory periodontal disease and asthma in adults.

Periodontal Medicine in Clinical Practice

The concept of periodontal diseases as localized entities that affect only the teeth and the supporting apparatus is oversimplified. Rather than being confined to the periodontium, inflammatory periodontal diseases may have wide-ranging systemic effects. In most people, these effects are relatively inconsequential, or at least not clinically evident. In susceptible individuals, however, periodontal infection may act as an independent risk factor for systemic disease, and it may be involved in the basic pathogenic mechanisms of these conditions. Furthermore, periodontal infection may exacerbate existing systemic disorders.

Periodontal Disease and Systemic Health

Proper use of the knowledge of potential relationships between periodontal disease and systemic health requires the dental professional to recognize the oral cavity as one of many interrelated organ systems. A palm-sized infection on the leg of a pregnant woman would be of major concern to the patient and her health care provider, given the potential negative consequences of this localized infection on fetal and maternal health. Similarly, a suppurating infection on the foot of a person with diabetes would be cause for immediate evaluation and aggressive treatment, considering the effects of such infections on the metabolic control of diabetes.

Periodontal infection must be viewed in a similar manner. Periodontitis is a gram-negative infection that often results in severe inflammation, and it potentially involves the intravascular dissemination of microorganisms and their products throughout the body. However, periodontitis tends to be a "silent" disease until destruction results in acute oral symptoms. Most patients—and many medical professionals—do not recognize the potential infection that may exist within the oral cavity.

Patient Education

Patient education is a priority. Only 30 years ago, the factors involved in CHD were unclear. At present, however, it would be difficult to find an individual who was unfamiliar with the link between cholesterol and heart disease. This change was precipitated by research that clearly demonstrated the increased risk for heart disease among individuals with high cholesterol levels, followed by intensive education efforts to spread the message from the scientific community to the public at large. It is important to recognize that high cholesterol levels have not been shown to *cause* heart disease in all individuals; rather, they significantly *increase the risk* of disease. Cholesterol has also been demonstrated to have a biologically plausible role in the pathogenesis of CHD.

Similarly, patient education efforts in the realm of periodontal medicine must emphasize the inflammatory nature of periodontal infections, the increased risk for systemic disease associated with the infection, and the biologically plausible role that periodontal infection may play in systemic disease. Few individuals had their cholesterol levels evaluated until knowledge of the link between cholesterol and heart disease became widespread. Likewise, an increased appreciation of the potential effects of periodontal infection on systemic health may result in increased patient demand for periodontal evaluation.

Enhanced community awareness may be derived from newspapers, magazines, and other lay sources. However, the most reliable origin of information should be dental and medical professionals, through daily contact with patients. A pregnant woman usually knows that infections may adversely affect her pregnancy. Individuals with diabetes generally know that infections impair glycemic control. However, many of these patients do not know that occult periodontal infections can have the same effect as more clinically evident infections. The dentist is responsible for diagnosing periodontal infections, providing appropriate treatment, and preventing disease recurrence or progression. Because many medical professionals are unfamiliar with the oral cavity and oral health research, dentists must reach out to the medical community to improve patient care through education and communication.[111] Likewise, patients must be educated about disease prevention. Just as patients know that lowering their cholesterol levels may decrease their risk for heart disease, similar knowledge regarding the prevention of periodontal infection should be emphasized. A physician would be remiss if he or she did not provide education about decreasing cholesterol level, losing weight, and ceasing a smoking habit to a patient at risk for CHD. Likewise, controlling the risk factor of periodontal infection requires the dentist to emphasize personal and professional preventive measures that are focused on oral hygiene and regular recall.

Conclusions

Does periodontal disease *cause* CHD, COPD, or adverse pregnancy outcomes? This question may be answered only by use of the evidence that is currently available, with the full knowledge that conclusions may change as future evidence dictates. Periodontal disease may increase the risk for many systemic disorders. Biologically plausible mechanisms support the role of periodontal infection in these conditions, but it should not be presented as the cause of such systemic diseases, any more than cholesterol should be said to cause heart disease. Periodontal infection is one of many potential risk factors for a number of systemic conditions. Fortunately, it is a readily modifiable risk factor, unlike age, gender, and genetic influences.

The focal infection theory of the early 20th century was widely and appropriately discredited when treatment based on the theory, which consisted almost solely of tooth extraction, had no effect on the underlying diseases that oral sepsis supposedly caused. Similarly, the clinical utility of our current knowledge base is only now evolving. Future research will further delineate the role of periodontal infection in systemic health. The associations between periodontal infection and conditions such as LBW delivery, diabetes, cardiovascular and cerebrovascular diseases, and respiratory diseases may be further substantiated. Longitudinal studies and intervention trials are needed before any causative role can be assigned.

The field of periodontal medicine offers new insights into the concept of the oral cavity as one system that is interconnected with the whole human body. For many years, the dental profession has recognized the effects of systemic conditions on the oral cavity. Only now, however, are dental professionals beginning to understand more fully the impact of the periodontium on systemic health.

Finally, it is important to appreciate the differences between the science and the art of dental practice as they relate to periodontal medicine. Science is based, in general, on means and standard deviations or standard errors. Thus, science may determine that, on average, diabetic patients with periodontal disease have poorer glycemic control than diabetic patients who are periodontally healthy. However, the patient who is sitting in the dental chair at any given time may or may not be a "mean" patient: in other words, she may or may not demonstrate the same relationship that science has determined to exist as an average within the population. She may lie somewhere within or outside the standard deviation. She may have extremely poor glycemic control that is directly related to her extensive periodontal inflammation; she may have average glycemic control; or she may have good glycemic control. The clinical practice of periodontal medicine recognizes that, while using an evidence-based approach is absolutely key to modern dentistry, each patient is an individual, and he or she may not always fit the average determined by science.

 Case Scenarios are found on the companion website www.expertconsult.com.

References

 References for this chapter are found on the companion website www.expertconsult.com.

Defense Mechanisms of the Gingiva

Marcelo Freire | Jaime Bulkacz | Fermin A. Carranza

CHAPTER OUTLINE

Sulcular Fluid
Leukocytes in the Dentogingival Area
Saliva

The gingival tissue is continuously subjected to challenge, influencing the host response type. The epithelial surface, immune response, crevicular fluid, and saliva provide active responses to maintain gingival health. Chapter 3 reviews the role of the epithelium, including its degree of keratinization and its turnover rate. This chapter describes important mechanisms of the gingival response repertoire, including the role of sulcular fluid, junctional epithelium, permeability, sulcular epithelia, sulcular fluid, saliva, and leukocytes.

Sulcular Fluid

Sulcular fluid, or *gingival crevicular fluid* (GCF), contains an array of biologic mediators, cells, and bacteria. Recognized since the 19th century, its possible role in oral defense was first elucidated by the pioneering work of Waerhaug[110] and Brill and Krasse[14] during the 1950s. The latter investigators applied filter paper to the gingival sulci of dogs that had previously been injected intramuscularly with fluorescein; within 3 minutes, the fluorescent material was recovered on the paper strips. This indicated the passage of fluid from the bloodstream through the tissues and the exiting of fluid via the gingival sulcus.

In subsequent studies, Brill[11,13] confirmed the presence of GCF in humans and considered it as "transudate." However, others[66,111] demonstrated that GCF is an inflammatory exudate rather than a continuous transudate. In strictly normal gingiva, little or no fluid can be collected.

More recently, interest in the development of tests for the detection or prediction of periodontal disease has resulted in numerous research papers about the components, origin, and function of GCF.[19] Potential markers from crevicular fluid are now used as diagnostic tools for the activity of periodontal diseases and a return to homeostasis, with potential for the evaluation of systemic markers.

Methods of Collection

The most difficult hurdle to overcome when collecting GCF is the scarcity of material that can be obtained from the sulcus. Many collection methods have been tried.[10,12,54,57,68,70,95] These methods include the use of absorbing paper strips, the placement of twisted threads around and into the sulcus, and techniques involving micropipettes and intracrevicular washings. There are limitations to the techniques, including fluid collection, collection time, flow rate, contamination, and reproducibility.

The absorbing paper strips are placed within the sulcus (intrasulcular method) or at its entrance (extrasulcular method) (Fig. 16.1). Placement of the filter paper strip in relation to the sulcus or pocket is important. The Brill technique involves inserting it into the pocket until resistance is encountered (Fig. 16.1A). This method produces some degree of irritation of the sulcular epithelium that by itself can trigger the flow of fluid.

To minimize this irritation, Löe and Holm-Pedersen[66] placed the filter paper strip just at or over the pocket entrance (Fig. 16.1B–C). In this way, fluid that seeps out is picked up by the strip, but the sulcular epithelium is not in contact with the paper.

Weinstein and colleagues[111] used preweighed twisted threads. The threads were placed in the gingival crevice around the tooth, and the amount of fluid collected was estimated by weighing the sample thread.

The use of micropipettes permits the collection of fluid by capillarity. Capillary tubes of standardized length and diameter are placed in the pocket, and their contents are later centrifuged and analyzed.[10-12]

Crevicular washings can be used to study GCF from clinically normal gingiva. One method involves the use of an appliance that consists of a hard acrylic plate that covers the maxilla, with soft borders and a groove that follows the gingival margins; it is connected to four collection tubes. Washings are obtained by rinsing the crevicular areas from one side to the other with the use of a peristaltic pump.[20]

A modification of the previous method involves the use of two injection needles that have been fitted one within the other so that, during sampling, the inside (ejection) needle is at the bottom of the pocket and the outside (collecting) needle is at the gingival margin. The collection needle is drained into a sample tube via continuous suction.[95]

Permeability of Junctional and Sulcular Epithelia

The initial studies by Brill and Krasse[14] involving the use of fluorescein were later confirmed with substances such as India ink[89] and saccharated iron oxide.[20] Substances that have been shown to penetrate the sulcular epithelium include albumin,[88] endotoxin,[87,92] thymidine,[45] histamine,[25] phenytoin,[105] and horseradish peroxidase.[72] These findings indicate permeability to substances with a molecular weight of up to 1000 kD.

Squier and Johnson[104] reviewed the mechanisms of penetration through an intact epithelium. The intercellular movement of molecules and ions along intercellular spaces appears to be a possible mechanism. Substances that take this route do not traverse the cell membranes.

Amount

The amount of GCF collected on a paper strip can be studied in multiple ways. The wetted area can be made more visible by staining with Ninhydrin; it is then measured planimetrically on an enlarged photograph or with a magnifying glass or a microscope.

An electronic method has been devised for measuring the fluid collected on a "blotter" (Periopaper) with the use of an electronic transducer (Periotron, Harco Electronics, Winnipeg, Manitoba, Canada) (Fig. 16.2). The wetness of the paper strip affects the flow of an electric current and provides a digital readout. A comparison between the Ninhydrin-staining method and the electronic method performed in vitro revealed no significant differences between the two techniques.[107]

The amount of GCF collected is extremely small. Measurements performed by Cimasoni[20] showed that a strip of paper 1.5-mm wide and inserted 1 mm within the gingival sulcus of a slightly inflamed gingiva absorbs about 0.1 mg of GCF in 3 minutes. Challacombe[18] used an isotope dilution method to measure the amount of GCF present in a particular space at any given time. His calculations for human volunteers with mean gingival indices of less than 1 showed that the mean GCF volume in the proximal spaces from the molar teeth ranged from 0.43 to 1.56 μL.

Composition

The components of GCF are characterized by individual proteins, metabolites,[66,79,96] specific antibodies, antigens,[32,86] and enzymes of several specificities.[15] The GCF also contains cellular elements.[25,28,113]

Multiple research efforts have attempted to use GCF components to detect or diagnose active disease or to predict which patients are at risk for periodontal disease (Table 16.1).[3] So far, more than 40 compounds found in GCF have been analyzed,[83] but their origin is not known with certainty. These compounds can be derived from the host or produced by bacteria in the gingival crevice, but their source can be difficult to elucidate; examples include β-glucuronidase, which is a lysosomal enzyme, and lactic acid dehydrogenase, which is a cytoplasmic enzyme. The sources of collagenases may be fibroblasts or polymorphonuclear leukocytes (PMNs [neutrophils]),[5,81] or collagenases may be secreted by bacteria.[32] Phospholipases are lysosomal and cytoplasmic enzymes, but they are also produced by

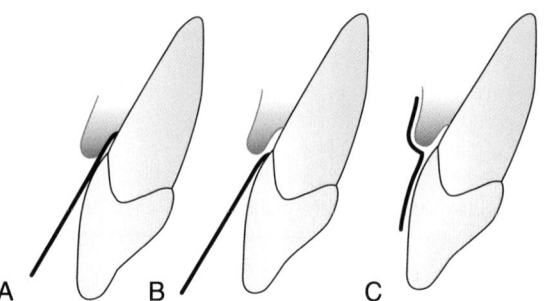

Fig. 16.1 Placement of a filter strip in the gingival sulcus for the collection of fluid. (A) Intrasulcular method. (B–C) Extrasulcular methods.

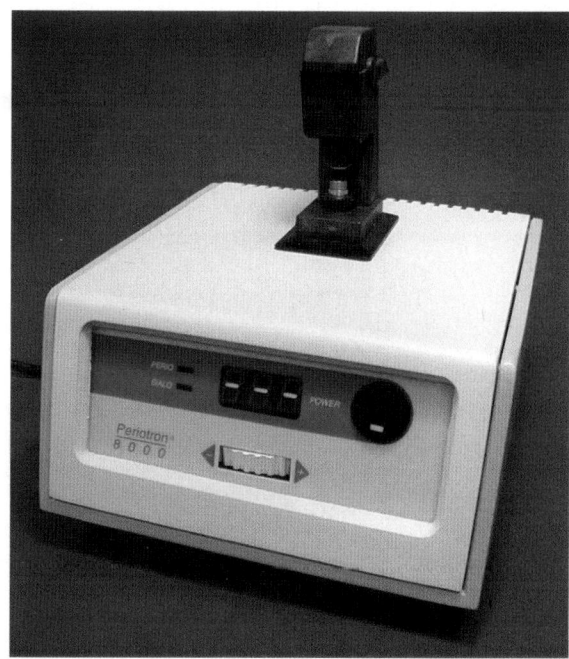

Fig. 16.2 Electronic device for measuring the amount of fluid collected on filter paper.

TABLE 16.1   Gingival Crevicular Fluid Diagnostic Tests

Test Name	Target	References
Periocheck	Proteinases	Page RC: Host response tests designed for diagnosing periodontal disease. *J Periodontol* 63(4 Suppl):356–366, 1992.
Prognostik	Elastase	http://www.ncbi.nlm.nih.gov/pmc/articles/PMC3118084/
Biolise	Elastase	https://www.ncbi.nlm.nih.gov/pmc/articles/PMC3118084/
MMP dipstick	MMPs	Mäntylä P, Stenman M, Kinane DF, Tikanoja S, Luoto H, Salo T, Sorsa T: Gingival crevicular fluid collagenase-2 (MMP-8) test stick for chair-side monitoring of periodontitis. *J Periodontal Res* 38(4):436–439, 2003.
TOPAS	Bacterial toxins and proteases	http://www.ncbi.nlm.nih.gov/pmc/articles/PMC3118084/
Pocket watch	AST	Mäntylä P, Stenman M, Kinane DF, Tikanoja S, Luoto H, Salo T, Sorsa T: Gingival crevicular fluid collagenase-2 (MMP-8) test stick for chair-side monitoring of periodontitis. *J Periodontal Res* 38:436–439, 2003.

MMP, Mucous membrane pemphigoid.

microorganisms.[15] The majority of GCF elements detected thus far have been enzymes, but there are nonenzymatic substances as well.

Cellular Elements

Cellular elements found in GCF include bacteria, desquamated epithelial cells, and leukocytes (i.e., PMNs, lymphocytes, and monocytes/macrophages), which migrate through the sulcular epithelium.[25,28]

Electrolytes

Potassium, sodium, and calcium have been studied in the GCF. Most studies have demonstrated a positive correlation of calcium and sodium concentrations with the sodium/potassium ratio seen with inflammation.[51-53] (For more information, see references 51 and 52.)

Organic Compounds

Both carbohydrates and proteins have been investigated. Glucose hexosamine and hexuronic acid are two compounds that are found in GCF.[43] Blood glucose levels do not correlate with GCF glucose levels; glucose concentration in GCF is three to four times greater than that in serum.[43] This is interpreted not only as a result of the metabolic activity of adjacent tissues but also as a function of the local microbial flora.

The total protein content of GCF is much less than that of serum.[12,14] No significant correlations have been found between the concentration of proteins in GCF and the severity of gingivitis, pocket depth, or extent of bone loss.[8] Metabolic and bacterial products identified in GCF include lactic acid,[44] urea,[38] hydroxyproline,[85] endotoxins,[101] cytotoxic substances, hydrogen sulfide,[103] and antibacterial factors.[24] Many enzymes have also been identified.

The methodology used to analyze GCF components is as varied as the diversity of those components. Examples include fluorometry to detect metalloproteinases,[25] enzyme-linked immunosorbent assays to detect enzyme levels and interleukin-1β (IL-1β),[64] radioimmunoassays to detect cyclooxygenase derivatives[80] and procollagen III,[108] high-pressure liquid chromatography to detect timidazole,[61] and direct and indirect immunodot tests to detect acute-phase proteins.[100]

Cellular and Humoral Activity in Gingival Crevicular Fluid

Monitoring periodontal disease is a complicated task, because few noninvasive procedures can follow the initiation and progress of the disease. Analyzing GCF constituents in health and disease may be extremely useful as a result of GCF's simplicity and because GCF can be obtained with noninvasive methods.

The analysis of GCF has identified cell and humoral responses in both healthy individuals and those with periodontal disease.[59] The cellular immune response includes the appearance of cytokines in GCF, but there is no clear evidence of a relationship between cytokines and disease. However, IL-1α and IL-1β are known to increase the binding of PMNs and monocytes/macrophages to endothelial cells, to stimulate the production of prostaglandin E_2 and the release of lysosomal enzymes, and to stimulate bone resorption.[62] Preliminary evidence also indicates the presence of interferon-α in GCF,[59] which may have a protective role in periodontal disease because of its ability to inhibit the bone resorption activity of IL-1β.[40]

Because the amount of fluid recoverable from gingival crevices is small, only the use of very sensitive immunoassays permits the analysis of the specificity of antibodies.[24,26,27] A study that compared antibodies in different crevices with serum antibodies directed at specific microorganisms did not provide any conclusive evidence regarding the significance of the presence of antibodies in GCF among individuals with periodontal disease.[59]

Although the role of antibodies in the gingival defense mechanisms is difficult to ascertain, the consensus is that in a patient with periodontal disease, a reduction in antibody response is detrimental, and an antibody response plays a protective role.[58]

Clinical Significance

As an exudate, GCF is a biologic fluid that has potential in diagnostics and disease management.[66] Its presence in clinically normal sulci can be explained, because gingiva that appears clinically normal invariably exhibits inflammation when it is examined microscopically. Commercially available kits for diagnosis are now available (see Table 16.1).

> ## ! CLINICAL CORRELATION
>
> - Novel diagnostics tools allow evaluations of biomarkers from tissue and oral biofluids.
> - Drug delivery targeting oral tissues has optimal absorption and bioavailability.
> - Gingival fluid and saliva are biologic fluids that can provide information on human genomics and metagenomics (microbiome, transcriptome, metabolome and proteome).
> - Oral immunity is activated through rapid response from innate immune components (fluids, mucosal surfaces, epithelium, cell mediators, molecules, host-bacterial interactions).

The amount of GCF is greater when inflammation is present,[31,98] and it is sometimes proportional to the severity of inflammation.[82] GCF production is not increased by trauma from occlusion,[71] but it is increased by the mastication of coarse foods, toothbrushing and gingival massage, ovulation,[64] hormonal contraceptives,[65] prosthetic appliances,[77] and smoking.[73] Other factors that influence the amount of GCF are circadian periodicity and periodontal therapy.

Circadian Periodicity

There is a gradual increase in the amount of GCF from 6 a.m. to 10 p.m. and a decrease thereafter.[9]

Sex Hormones

Female sex hormones increase GCF flow, probably because they enhance vascular permeability.[62] Pregnancy, ovulation,[61] and hormonal contraceptives[63] all increase GCF production.

Mechanical Stimulation

Chewing[11] and vigorous gingival brushing stimulate the flow of GCF. Even minor stimuli represented by intrasulcular placement of paper strips increases the production of fluid.

Smoking

Smoking produces an immediate transient but marked increase in GCF flow but, in the long term, a decrease of salivary and GCF flow.[73]

Periodontal Therapy

There is an increase in GCF production during the healing period after periodontal surgery.[4]

Drugs in Gingival Crevicular Fluid

Drugs that are excreted through the GCF may be used advantageously in periodontal therapy. Bader and Goldhaber[7] demonstrated in dogs that tetracyclines are excreted through the GCF; this finding triggered extensive research that showed a concentration of tetracyclines in

GCF as compared with serum.[39] Metronidazole is another antibiotic that has been detected in human GCF[29] (see Chapter 52).

Leukocytes in the Dentogingival Area

Leukocytes have been found in clinically healthy gingival sulci in humans and experimental animals. The leukocytes found are predominantly PMNs. They appear in small numbers extravascularly in the connective tissue adjacent to the apical portion of the sulcus; from there, they travel across the epithelium[17,41] to the gingival sulcus, where they are expelled (Figs. 16.3 and 16.4).

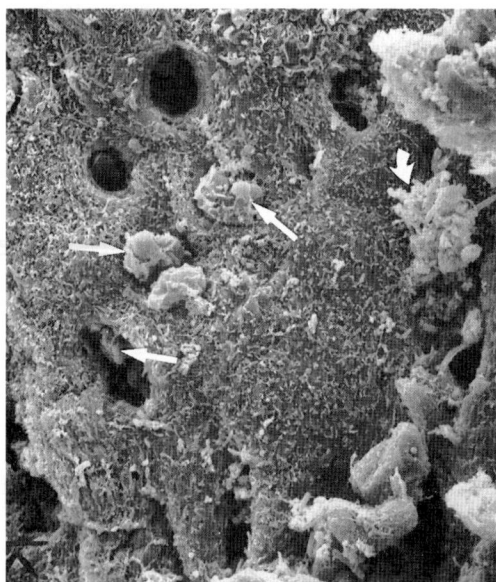

Fig. 16.3 Scanning electron microscope view of the periodontal pocket wall. Several leukocytes are emerging *(straight arrows)*, some of which are partially covered by bacteria *(curved arrow)*. Empty holes correspond to tunnels through which leukocytes have emerged.

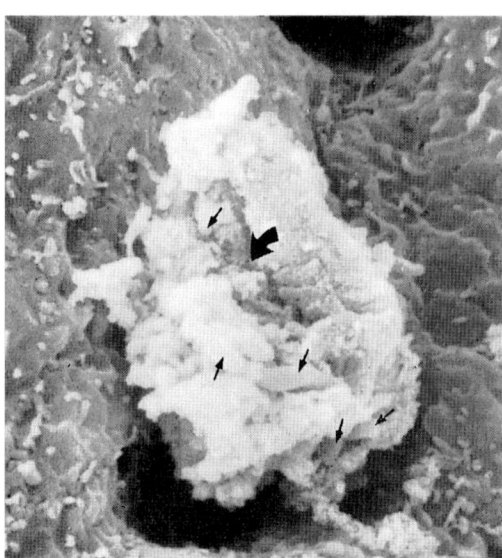

Fig. 16.4 Scanning electron microscope view at higher magnification than shown in Fig. 16.3. A leukocyte emerging from the pocket wall is covered with bacteria *(small arrows)*. The *large curved arrow* points to a phagosomal vacuole through which bacteria are being engulfed.

Leukocytes are present in sulci even when histologic sections of adjacent tissue are free of inflammatory infiltrate.[90] Differential counts of leukocytes from clinically healthy human gingival sulci have shown 91.2% to 91.5% PMNs and 8.5% to 8.8% mononuclear cells.[102,113]

Mononuclear cells were identified as 58% B lymphocytes, 24% T lymphocytes, and 18% mononuclear phagocytes. The ratio of T lymphocytes to B lymphocytes was found to be reversed from the normal ratio of about 3:1 found in peripheral blood to about 1:3 in GCF.[113]

Leukocytes are attracted by different plaque bacteria,[49,112] but they can also be found in the dentogingival region of germ-free adult animals.[67,94] Leukocytes were reported in the gingival sulcus in nonmechanically irritated (resting) healthy gingiva, thereby indicating that their migration may be independent of an increase in vascular permeability.[6] The majority of these cells are viable and have phagocytic and killing capacity.[56,84,91] Therefore leukocytes constitute a major protective mechanism against the extension of plaque into the gingival sulcus.

Live and dead leukocytes are found in saliva; this is discussed later in this chapter. The main port of entry of leukocytes into the oral cavity is the gingival sulcus.[97]

Saliva

Saliva has protective functions and maintains the oral tissues in a physiologic state (Table 16.2). Saliva exerts a major influence on plaque by mechanically cleansing the exposed oral surfaces, buffering acids produced by bacteria, and modulating bacterial activity with immune mediators.[78] Saliva is now considered a main biologic fluid for diagnosis of human health and diseases. Systemic and local disease markers are available through saliva. Available tests allow the individual to measure multi-omics outputs.[22] Functional and static assays are now available as biosensors of health and disease.

TABLE 16.2 Role of Saliva in Oral Health

Function	Salivary Components	Probable Mechanism
Lubrication	Glycoproteins, mucoids	Coating similar to gastric mucin
Physical protection	Glycoproteins, mucoids	Coating similar to gastric mucin
Cleansing	Physical flow	Clearance of debris and bacteria
Buffering	Bicarbonate and phosphate	Antacids
Tooth integrity maintenance	Minerals	Maturation, remineralization
	Glycoprotein pellicle	Mechanical protection
Antibacterial action	Immunoglobulin A	Control of bacterial colonization
	Lysozyme	Breaking of bacterial cell walls
	Lactoperoxidase	Oxidation of susceptible bacteria

Antibacterial Factors

Saliva carries inorganic and organic factors that influence bacteria and their products in the oral environment. Inorganic factors include ions and gases, bicarbonate, sodium, potassium, phosphates, calcium, fluorides, ammonium, and carbon dioxide. Organic factors include lysozyme, lactoferrin, myeloperoxidase, lactoperoxidase, defensins, peptides, and agglutinins such as glycoproteins, mucins, β2-macroglobulins, fibronectins,[108] and antibodies.

Lysozyme is a hydrolytic enzyme that cleaves the linkage between structural components of the glycopeptide muramic acid–containing region of the cell wall of certain bacteria in vitro. Lysozyme works on both gram-negative and gram-positive organisms[46]; its targets include *Veillonella* species and *Actinobacillus actinomycetemcomitans.* It works on the molecular level, protecting the oral cavity and repelling transient bacterial invaders.[48]

The *lactoperoxidase–thiocyanate system* in saliva has been shown to be bactericidal to some strains of *Lactobacillus* and *Streptococcus*[75,93] by preventing the accumulation of lysine and glutamic acid, both of which are essential for bacterial growth. Another antibacterial finding is lactoferrin, which is effective against *Actinobacillus* species.[50]

Myeloperoxidase, an enzyme that is similar to salivary peroxidase, is released by leukocytes; it is bactericidal for *Actinobacillus,*[74] but it has the added effect of inhibiting the attachment of *Actinomyces* strains to hydroxyapatite.[21]

Human alpha and beta-defensins (hBD)-1,-2,-3 are a family of low-molecular-weight antimicrobial peptides. Produced by a number of cells, including neutrophils, they amplify and combat bacterial[1] infections important to homeostasis.

Salivary Antibodies

As with GCF, saliva contains antibodies that are reactive with indigenous oral bacterial species. Although immunoglobulins G (IgG) and M (IgM) are present, the preponderant immunoglobulin found in saliva is *immunoglobulin A* (IgA), whereas IgG is more prevalent in GCF.[106] Major and minor salivary glands contribute all of the secretory IgA and lesser amounts of IgG and IgM. GCF contributes most of the IgG, complement, and PMNs that, in conjunction with IgG or IgM, inactivate or opsonize bacteria.

Salivary antibodies appear to be synthesized locally, because they react with bacteria that are indigenous to the mouth but not with organisms that are characteristic of the intestinal tract.[33,35] Bacteria found in saliva are frequently associated with IgA, and the bacterial deposits on teeth contain both IgA and IgG in quantities that are greater than 1% of their dry weight.[34] It has been shown that IgA antibodies present in parotid saliva can inhibit the attachment of oral *Streptococcus* species to epithelial cells.[30,110] Gibbons and colleagues[33-35] suggested that antibodies in secretions may impair the ability of bacteria to attach to mucosal or dental surfaces.

FLASH BACK

Saliva was known to have protective actions against infection through immunoglobulins only. Now it is clear that enzymes, cytokines, nucleotides, and live cells are part of the host armamentarium.

Enzymes

The *enzymes* that are normally found in saliva are derived from the salivary glands, bacteria, leukocytes, oral tissues, and ingested substances; the major enzyme is parotid amylase. Certain salivary enzymes have been reported in increased concentrations in periodontal disease: hyaluronidase and lipase,[16] β-glucuronidase and chondroitin sulfatase,[37] aspartate aminotransferase and alkaline phosphatase,[109] amino acid decarboxylases,[37] catalase, peroxidase, and collagenase.[55]

Proteolytic enzymes in the saliva are generated by both the host and oral bacteria. These enzymes have been recognized as contributors to the initiation and progression of periodontal disease.[45,69] To combat these enzymes, saliva contains antiproteases that inhibit cysteine proteases such as cathepsins[47] and antileukoproteases that inhibit elastase.[81] Another antiprotease, which has been identified as a tissue inhibitor of matrix metalloproteinase, has been shown to inhibit the activity of collagen-degrading enzymes.[23]

High-molecular-weight mucinous glycoproteins in saliva bind specifically to many plaque-forming bacteria. The glycoprotein–bacteria interactions facilitate bacterial accumulation on the exposed tooth surface.[30,33-35,112] The specificity of these interactions has been demonstrated. The interbacterial matrix of human plaque appears to contain polymers that are similar to salivary glycoproteins and may aid in maintaining the integrity of plaque. In addition, these glycoproteins selectively adsorb to the hydroxyapatite to make up part of the acquired pellicle. Other salivary glycoproteins inhibit the sorption of some bacteria to the tooth surface and to epithelial cells of the oral mucosa. This activity appears to be associated with the glycoproteins that possess blood group reactivity.[2,30,33,35,110] Another effect of mucin is the deletion of bacterial cells from the oral cavity via aggregation with mucin-rich films.

Glycoproteins and a glycolipid that is present on mammalian cell surfaces appear to serve as receptors for the attachment of some viruses and bacteria. Thus the close similarity between the glycoproteins of salivary secretions and the components of the epithelial cell surface suggests that the secretions can competitively inhibit antigen sorption and that they therefore may limit pathologic alterations.

Salivary Buffers and Coagulation Factors

The maintenance of physiologic hydrogen ion concentration (pH) at the mucosal epithelial cell surface and tooth surface is an important function of salivary buffers. The primary effect action of buffers has been investigated with relationship to dental caries. In saliva, the most important buffer is the bicarbonate–carbonic acid system.[68]

Saliva also contains coagulation factors (i.e., factors VIII, IX, and X; plasma thromboplastin antecedent; and Hageman factor) that hasten blood coagulation and protect wounds from bacterial invasion.[60] An active fibrinolytic enzyme may also be present.

Leukocytes

In addition to desquamated epithelial cells, saliva contains all forms of leukocytes, of which the principal cells are PMNs. Whole-blood PMNs are naïve and not activated, whereas the cells found in saliva have interacted with multiple antigens from the microbiome. The number of PMNs varies from person to person at different times of the day, and it is increased in the presence of gingivitis. PMNs reach the oral cavity by migrating through the lining of the gingival sulcus. Living PMNs in saliva are sometimes referred to as *orogranulocytes,* and their rate of migration into the oral cavity is termed the *orogranulocytic migratory rate.* Novel investigation presents the positive correlation between rate of PMN migration and the severity of gingival inflammation, and it is therefore a reliable index for the assessment of gingivitis.[102] In a high-throughput methods, distinct subsets of neutrophils were found in oral mucosa, including naïve, parainflammatory, and proinflammatory cells.[76]

What is the clinical importance of saliva?

Saliva has several important properties, including mechanical, chemical, biologic, and immunologic.[22] It is a viscous, clear, watery fluid secreted from salivary glands. It is a major biologic fluid for diagnosis and "omics" research. Diagnosing local and systemic conditions is possible through salivary markers. Low saliva is a risk factor for caries and periodontal disease. Xerostomia is defined as dry mouth resulting from reduced or absent saliva flow. Xerostomia is a symptom of various medical conditions, and it is a side effect of radiation to the head and neck and a wide variety of medications.

Role in Periodontal Pathology

Saliva modulates plaque initiation, maturation, and metabolism. Salivary flow and composition also influence calculus formation, periodontal disease, and caries. The removal of the salivary glands in experimental animals significantly increases the incidence of dental caries[36] and periodontal disease[42] in addition to delaying wound healing.[99]

In humans, increases of inflammatory gingival conditions, dental caries, rapid tooth destruction, and cervical or cemental caries are associated, at least partially, with decreased salivary gland secretion (xerostomia; Box 16.1). Xerostomia may result from sialolithiasis, sarcoidosis, Sjögren syndrome, Mikulicz disease, irradiation, surgical removal of the salivary glands, and other factors (see Chapters 37 and 26).

BOX 16.1 Hallmarks of Xerostomia

Features	Healthy	Xerostomia
Flow rate	1–2 mL	< 0.1 mg/mL
Sensation	Normal	Dry mouth
Consistency and texture	Resilient and lubricated	Erythematous, sticky

FLASH BACK

- Gingival tissue is constantly challenged by external factors.
- Epithelial surface, crevicular fluid, saliva, epithelial surfaces, immune cells, and mediators provide oral immunity.
- Oral diseases, including caries and periodontal diseases, benefit from oral immune components.

A Case Scenario is found on the companion website www.expertconsult.com.

References

References for this chapter are found on the companion website www.expertconsult.com.

CHAPTER 17

Gingival Inflammation

Joseph P. Fiorellini | David M. Kim | Marcelo Freire | Panagiota G. Stathopoulou | Hector L. Sarmiento

CHAPTER OUTLINE

Stage I Gingival Inflammation: The Initial Lesion
Stage II Gingival Inflammation: The Early Lesion
Stage III Gingival Inflammation: The Established Lesion
Stage IV Gingival Inflammation: The Advanced Lesion

Local innate and specific immunity will maintain gingival health. Components from the innate immune response include epithelial cells and nonspecific cells within the epithelium, mucins, lysozyme, lactoferrin, lactoperoxidase, and various antimicrobial peptides such as histatins, beta-defensins, and protease inhibitors. Epithelial cells (keratinocytes) themselves are reactive and express a variety of receptors, including Toll-like receptors, and produce a variety of cytokines on activation.

The pathologic changes of gingivitis are initiated by a host response to oral microorganisms attached to the tooth and perhaps in or near the gingival sulcus. These organisms are capable of synthesizing products (e.g., collagenase, hyaluronidase, protease, chondroitin sulfatase, endotoxin) that cause damage to epithelial and connective tissue cells as well as to intercellular constituents such as collagen, ground substance, and glycocalyx (cell coat). The resultant widening of the spaces between junctional epithelial cells during early gingivitis may permit injurious agents derived from bacteria or bacteria themselves to gain access to the connective tissue.[10,44,48] Microbial products activate cells, including monocytes and macrophages, to produce vasoactive substances such as prostaglandin E2, interferon, tumor necrosis factor, and interleukin-1.[25,38] In addition, interleukin-1β alters the properties of gingival fibroblasts by delaying their death via mechanism-blocking apoptosis. This stabilizes the gingival fibroblast population during inflammation.[54]

Morphologic and functional changes in the gingiva during plaque accumulation have been thoroughly investigated, especially in beagle dogs and humans.[36] A useful framework for the organization and consideration of these data has been devised on the basis of histopathologic, radiographic, and ultrastructural features and biochemical measurements.[37,39] The sequence of events that culminates in clinically apparent gingivitis is categorized as the *initial, early,* and *established stages* of disease, with periodontitis designated as the *advanced stage*[38] (Table 17.1). One stage evolves into the next, with no clear-cut dividing lines.

Despite extensive research, we still cannot definitively distinguish between normal gingival tissue and the initial stage of gingivitis.[36] Most biopsies of clinically normal human gingiva contain inflammatory cells; these consist predominantly of T cells, with very few B cells or plasma cells.[36,49,50] These cells do not create tissue damage, but they appear to be important in the day-to-day host response to bacteria and other substances to which the gingiva is exposed.[36] Therefore, under normal conditions, a constant stream of neutrophils is migrating from the vessels of the gingival plexus through the junctional epithelium, to the gingival margin, and into the gingival sulcus and the oral cavity.[43]

Stage I Gingival Inflammation: The Initial Lesion

The first manifestations of gingival inflammation are vascular changes that consist of dilated capillaries and increased blood flow. These initial inflammatory changes occur in response to the microbial activation of resident leukocytes and the subsequent stimulation of endothelial cells. Clinically, this initial response of the gingiva to bacterial plaque (i.e., subclinical gingivitis[26]) is not apparent.

> Microscopically, some classic features of acute inflammation can be seen in the connective tissue beneath the junctional epithelium. Changes in blood vessel morphologic features (e.g., the widening of small capillaries or venules) and the adherence of neutrophils to vessel walls (margination) occur within 1 week and sometimes as early as 2 days after plaque has been allowed to accumulate[18,41] (Fig. 17.1). The etiopathogenesis of gingival diseases is linked to local or systemic immune response, to innate or adaptive immunity, and to cellular or secretory factors. Leukocytes—mainly polymorphonuclear neutrophils (PMNs)—leave the capillaries by migrating through the walls via diapedesis and emigration[25,50,51] (Fig. 17.2). They can be seen in increased quantities in the connective tissue, the junctional epithelium, and the gingival sulcus[2,3,24,34,41,45,46] (Figs. 17.3 and 17.4). Exudation of fluid from the gingival sulcus[18] and extravascular proteins is present.[20,21]

However, these findings are not accompanied by manifestations of tissue damage that are perceptible at the light microscopic or ultrastructural level; they do not form an infiltrate, and their presence is not considered to indicate pathologic change.[36]

Subtle changes can also be detected in the junctional epithelium and perivascular connective tissue at this early stage. For example, the perivascular connective tissue matrix becomes altered, and there

TABLE 17.1   Stages of Gingivitis

Stage	Time (Days)	Blood Vessels	Junctional and Sulcular Epithelia	Predominant Immune Cells	Collagen	Clinical Findings
I. Initial lesion	2 to 4	Vascular dilation Vasculitis	Infiltration by PMNs	PMNs	Perivascular loss	Gingival fluid flow
II. Early lesion	4 to 7	Vascular proliferation	Same as stage I Rete pegs Atrophic areas	Lymphocytes	Increased loss around infiltrate	Erythema Bleeding on probing
III. Established lesion	14 to 21	Same as stage II, plus blood stasis	Same as stage II but more advanced	Plasma cells	Continued loss	Changes in color, size, texture, and so on

PMNs, Polymorphonuclear leukocytes (neutrophils).

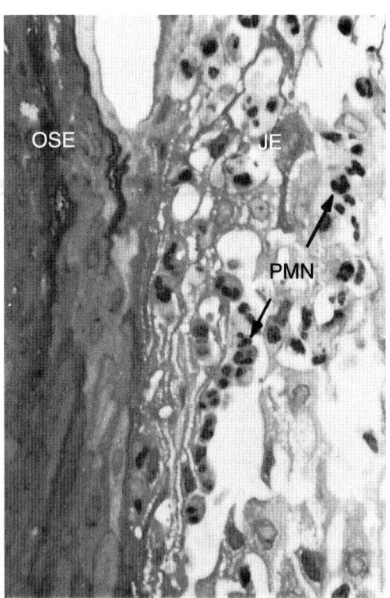

Fig. 17.1 Human biopsy sample, experimental gingivitis. After 4 days of plaque accumulation, the blood vessels immediately adjacent to the junctional epithelium are distended and contain polymorphonuclear leukocytes (neutrophils) (PMNs). Neutrophils have also migrated between the cells of the junctional epithelium (JE). *OSE*, Oral sulcular epithelium (magnification, ×500). *(From Payne WA, Page RC, Ogilvie AL, et al: Histopathologic features of the initial and early stages of experimental gingivitis in man. J Periodontal Res 10:51, 1975.)*

is exudation and deposition of fibrin in the affected area.[36] In addition, lymphocytes soon begin to accumulate (see Fig. 17.2D). The increased migration of leukocytes and their accumulation within the gingival sulcus may be correlated with an increased flow of gingival fluid into the sulcus.[4]

The character and intensity of the host response determine whether this *initial lesion* resolves rapidly, with restoration of the tissue to a normal state; alternatively, it may evolve into a chronic inflammatory lesion. If the latter occurs, an infiltrate of macrophages and lymphoid cells appears within a few days.

Stage II Gingival Inflammation: The Early Lesion

The *early lesion* evolves from the *initial lesion* within about 1 week after the beginning of plaque accumulation.[35,41] Clinically, the early lesion may appear as early gingivitis, and it overlaps with and evolves from the initial lesion with no clear-cut dividing line. As time goes on, clinical signs of erythema may appear, mainly because of the proliferation of capillaries and the increased formation of capillary loops between rete pegs or ridges (Fig. 17.5). Bleeding on probing may also be evident.[1] Gingival fluid flow and the numbers of transmigrating leukocytes reach their maximum between 6 and 12 days after the onset of clinical gingivitis.[26]

> Microscopic examination of the gingiva reveals leukocyte infiltration in the connective tissue beneath the junctional epithelium, which consists mainly of lymphocytes (75%, with the majority being T cells)[41,47] but also includes some migrating neutrophils as well as macrophages, plasma cells, and mast cells. All of the changes seen in the initial lesion continue to intensify with the early lesion.[15,28,30,35,47] The junctional epithelium becomes densely infiltrated with neutrophils, as does the gingival sulcus, and may begin to show the development of rete pegs or ridges.

The amount of collagen destruction also increases[12,28,47]; 70% of the collagen is destroyed around the cellular infiltrate. The main fiber groups that are affected appear to be the circular and dentogingival fiber assemblies. Alterations in blood vessel morphologic features and vascular bed patterns have also been described.[18,19]

PMNs that have left the blood vessels in response to chemotactic stimuli from plaque components travel to the epithelium and cross the basement lamina; they are found in the epithelium, emerging in the pocket area (see Fig. 17.3). PMNs are attracted to bacteria and engulf them during the process of phagocytosis (Fig. 17.6). PMNs release their lysosomes in association with the ingestion of bacteria.[23] Fibroblasts show cytotoxic alterations,[40] with a decreased capacity for collagen.

Meanwhile, on the opposite side of molecular events, collagen degradation is related to matrix metalolproteinases (MMPs). Different MMPs are responsible for extracellular matrix remodeling within 7 days of inflammation, which is directly related to MMP-2 and MMP-9 production and activation.[54]

Stage III Gingival Inflammation: The Established Lesion

Over time, the *established lesion* evolves. It is characterized by a predominance of plasma cells and B lymphocytes, and it is probably in conjunction with the creation of a small gingival pocket lined with a pocket epithelium.[46] The B cells that are found in the established

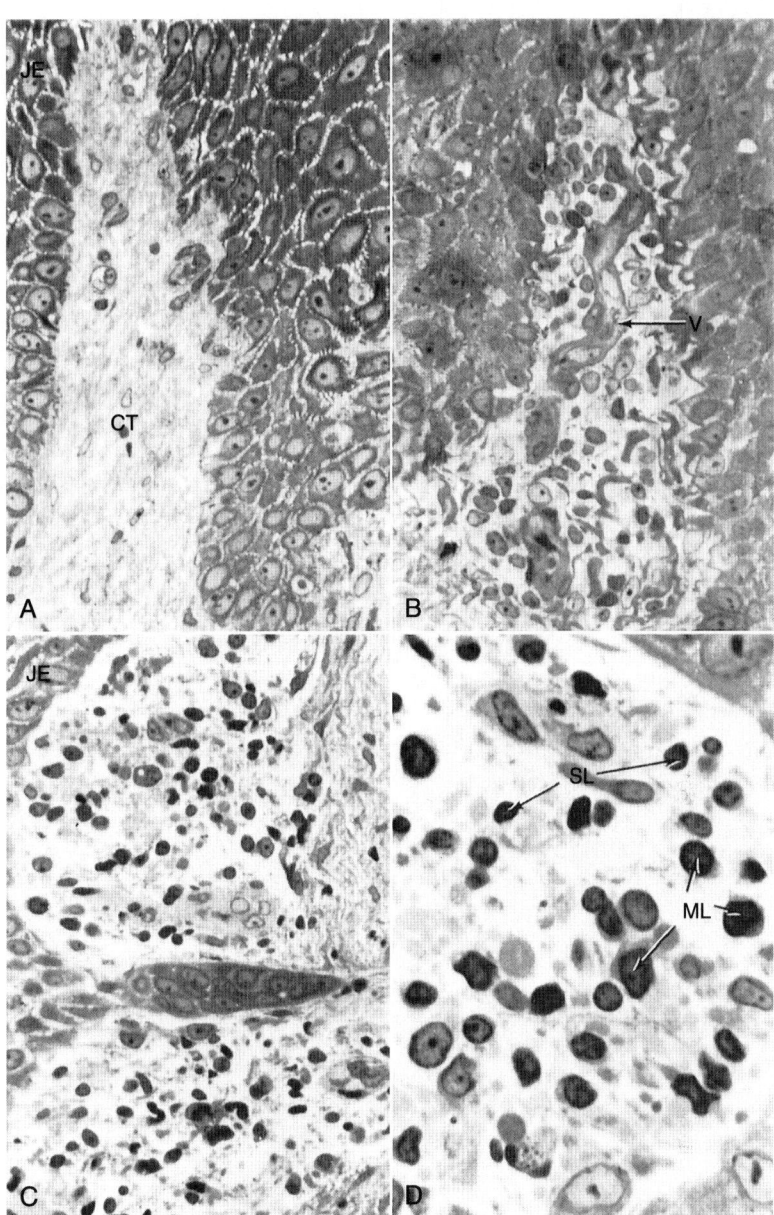

Fig. 17.2 Human biopsy, experimental gingivitis. (A) Control biopsy specimen from a patient with good oral hygiene and no detectable plaque accumulation. The junctional epithelium is on the left. The connective tissue (CT) shows few cells other than fibroblasts, blood vessels, and a dense background of collagen fibers (magnification, ×500.) (B) Biopsy specimen taken after 8 days of plaque accumulation. The connective tissue is infiltrated with inflammatory cells, which displace the collagen fibers. A distended blood vessel (V) is seen in the center (magnification, ×500). (C) After 8 days of plaque accumulation, the connective tissue next to the junctional epithelium at the base of the sulcus shows a mononuclear cell infiltrate and evidence of collagen degeneration (i.e., clear spaces around the cellular infiltrate (magnification, ×500). (D) The inflammatory cell infiltrate at higher magnification (×1250). After 8 days of plaque accumulation, numerous small (SL) and medium-sized (ML) lymphocytes are seen within the connective tissue. Most of the collagen fibers around these cells have disappeared, presumably as a result of enzymatic digestion. *(From Payne WA, Page RC, Ogilvie AL, et al: Histopathologic features of the initial and early stages of experimental gingivitis in man. J Periodontal Res 10:51, 1975.)*

lesion are predominantly of the immunoglobulin G1 and G3 subclasses.[36]

With chronic gingivitis, which occurs 2 to 3 weeks after the beginning of plaque accumulation, the blood vessels become engorged and congested, venous return is impaired, and the blood flow becomes sluggish (Fig. 17.7). The result is localized gingival *anoxemia,* which superimposes a somewhat bluish hue on the reddened gingiva.[17] The extravasation of erythrocytes into the connective tissue and the breakdown of hemoglobin into its component pigments can also deepen the color of the chronically inflamed gingiva. The established lesion can be described as moderately to severely inflamed gingiva.

In histologic sections, an intense and chronic inflammatory reaction is observed. Several detailed cytologic studies have been performed on chronically inflamed gingiva.[13-15,40,46,49,53] A key feature that differentiates established lesions is the increased number of plasma cells, which become the preponderant inflammatory cell type. Plasma cells invade the connective tissue not only immediately below the junctional epithelium but also deep into the connective tissue, around the blood vessels, and between the bundles of collagen fibers.[6] The junctional epithelium reveals widened intercellular spaces that are filled with granular cellular debris, including lysosomes derived from disrupted neutrophils, lymphocytes, and monocytes (Fig. 17.8). The lysosomes contain acid hydrolases that can destroy tissue components. The junctional epithelium develops rete pegs or ridges that protrude into the connective tissue, and the basal lamina is destroyed in some areas. In the connective tissue, collagen fibers are destroyed around the infiltrate of intact and disrupted plasma cells, neutrophils, lymphocytes, monocytes, and mast cells (Fig. 17.9).

The predominance of plasma cells is thought to be a primary characteristic of established lesions. However, several studies of human experimental gingivitis have failed to demonstrate plasma cell predominance in the affected connective tissues,[7,8,49] including one study of 6 months' duration.[1] An increase in the proportion of plasma cells was evident with longstanding gingivitis, but the

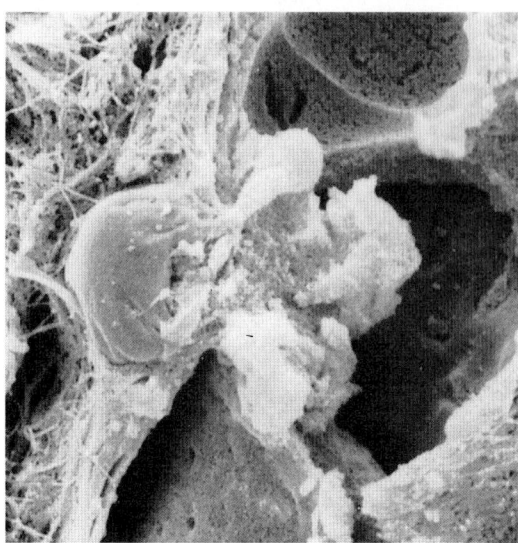

Fig. 17.3 Scanning electron micrograph showing a leukocyte traversing the vessel wall to enter into the gingival connective tissue.

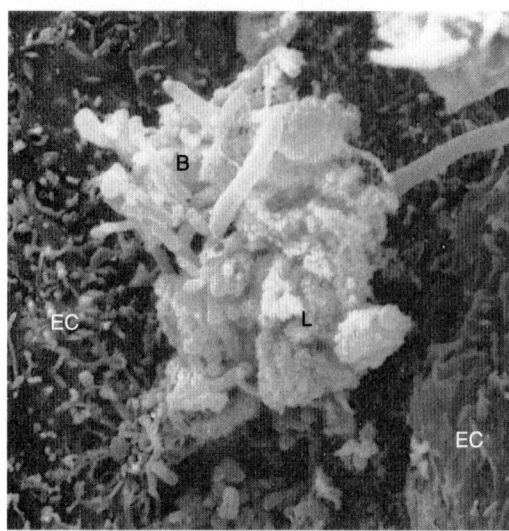

Fig. 17.6 Scanning electron micrograph of a leukocyte emerging to the pocket wall and covered with bacteria and extracellular lysosomes. *B,* Bacteria; *EC,* epithelial cells; *L,* lysosomes.

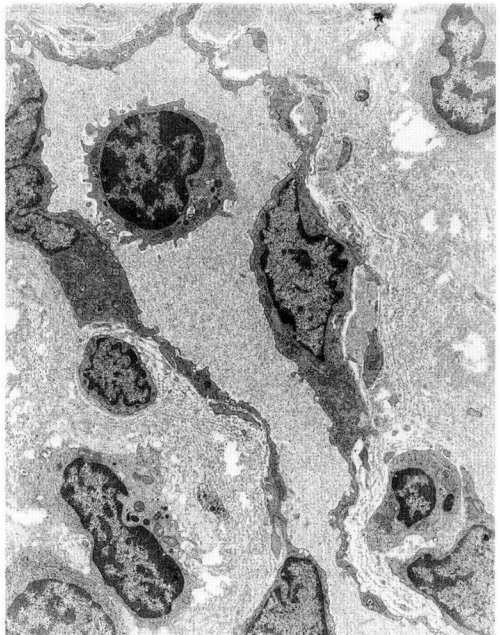

Fig. 17.4 Early human gingivitis lesion. There is an area of lamina propria subjacent to the crevicular epithelium that shows a capillary with several extravascular lymphocytes and one lymphocyte within the lumen. The specimen also exhibits a considerable loss of perivascular collagen density (magnification, ×2500). *(Courtesy Dr. Charles Cobb, Kansas City, Missouri.)*

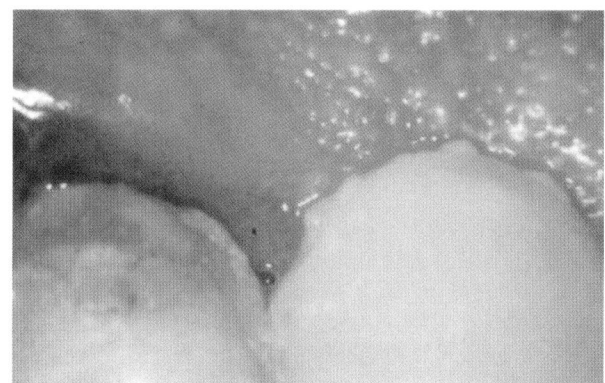

Fig. 17.7 Marginal supragingival plaque and gingivitis.

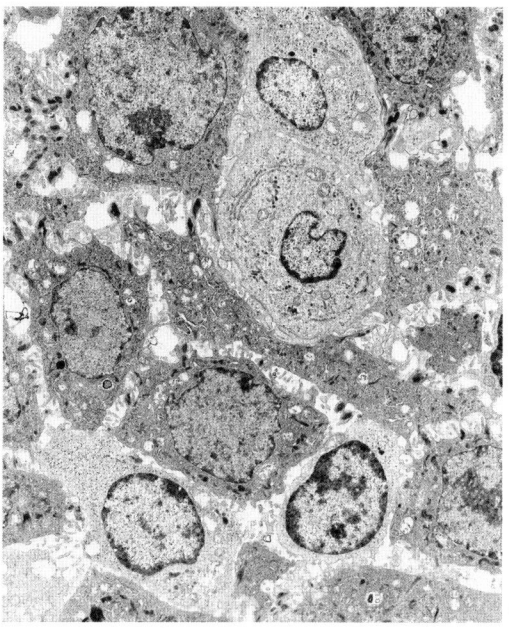

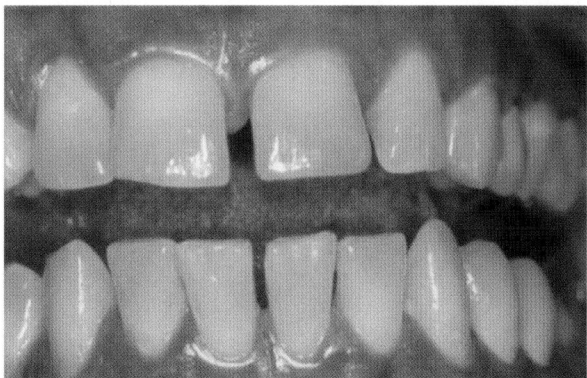

Fig. 17.5 Marginal gingivitis and irregular gingival contour.

Fig. 17.8 Established gingivitis in a human subject. An area of crevicular epithelium exhibits enlarged intercellular spaces with numerous microvilli and desmosomal junctions. Several lymphocytes, both small and large, are seen migrating through the epithelial layer (magnification, ×3000).

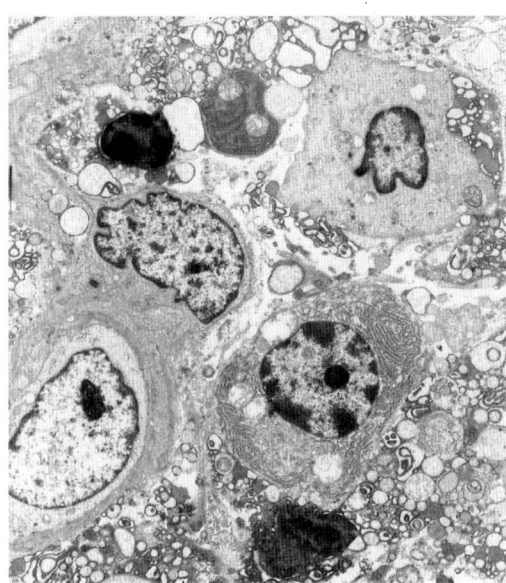

Fig. 17.9 Advanced gingivitis in a human subject. This specimen from the lamina propria exhibits plasma cell degeneration, with abundant cellular debris visible (magnification, ×3000). *(Courtesy Dr. Charles Cobb, Kansas City, Missouri.)*

of the sequence of events observed as gingivitis develops. As the flora reverts from that characteristically associated with destructive lesions to that associated with periodontal health, the percentage of plasma cells decreases greatly and the lymphocyte population increases proportionately.[27,31]

Stage IV Gingival Inflammation: The Advanced Lesion

The extension of the lesion into alveolar bone characterizes the fourth stage, which is known as the *advanced lesion*[40] or *phase of periodontal breakdown.*[26] This is described in detail in Chapter 21.

> Microscopically, fibrosis of the gingiva is present and there is widespread manifestation of inflammatory and immunopathologic tissue damage.[36] At the advanced stage, the presence of plasma cells dominates the connective tissue, and neutrophils continue dominating the junctional epithelium.

time for development of classic "established lesions" may exceed 6 months.

An inverse relationship appears to exist between the number of intact collagen bundles and the number of inflammatory cells.[51] Collagenolytic activity is increased in inflamed gingival tissue[16] by the enzyme collagenase. Collagenase is normally present in gingival tissues[5]; it is produced by some oral bacteria and by PMNs.

Enzyme histochemistry studies have shown that chronically inflamed gingivae have elevated levels of acid and alkaline phosphatase,[55] β-glucuronidase, β-glucosidase, β-galactosidase, esterases,[29] aminopeptidase,[33,42] and cytochrome oxidase.[9] Neutral mucopolysaccharide levels are decreased,[53] presumably as a result of degradation of the ground substance.

Established lesions of two types appear to exist; some remain stable and do not progress for months or years,[32,33,52] and others seem to become more active and convert to progressively destructive lesions. In addition, established lesions appear to be reversible, in that the sequence of events that occurs in the tissues as a result of successful periodontal therapy seems to be essentially the reverse

Patients with experimental gingivitis had significantly more plaque accumulation, higher interleukin-1β levels, and lower interleukin-8 concentrations at 28 days.[11]

Gingivitis will progress to periodontitis only in individuals who are susceptible. Patients who had sites with consistent bleeding (gingival index = 2) had 70% more attachment loss as compared with sites that were not consistently inflamed (gingival index = 0). Teeth with noninflamed sites consistently had a 50-year survival rate of 99.5%, whereas teeth with consistently inflamed gingiva had a 63.4% survival rate over 50 years. On the basis of this longitudinal study of the natural history of periodontitis in a well-maintained male population, persistent gingivitis represents a risk factor for periodontal attachment loss and tooth loss.[22] However, whether periodontitis can occur without a precursor of gingivitis is not known at this time.

References

 References for this chapter are found on the companion website www.expertconsult.com.

CHAPTER 18

Clinical Features of Gingivitis

Joseph P. Fiorellini | Hector L. Sarmiento | David M. Kim | Yu-Cheng Chang

CHAPTER OUTLINE

Course and Duration
Description
Clinical Findings

Experimental gingivitis studies provided the first empiric evidence that the accumulation of microbial biofilm on clean tooth surfaces results in the development of an inflammatory process in gingival tissue.[42,69] Research also shows that local inflammation persists as long as the microbial biofilm is present adjacent to the gingival tissues and that the inflammation resolves after meticulous removal of the biofilm.[69]

The prevalence of gingivitis is evident worldwide. Epidemiologic studies indicate that more than 82% of adolescents in the United States have overt gingivitis and signs of gingival bleeding. A similar or higher prevalence of gingivitis is reported for children and adolescents in other parts of the world.[4] A significant percentage of adults also show signs of gingivitis; more than half of the US adult population is estimated to exhibit gingival bleeding, and other populations have even higher levels of gingival inflammation.[3,5,6,8,66] Plaque remains the primary etiologic factor that causes gingivitis, but other factors can affect the development of periodontal disease. Experimental gingivitis studies suggest an important role of the host response in the development and degree of gingival inflammation.[82]

Clinical features of gingivitis can be characterized by any of the following clinical signs: redness and sponginess of the gingival tissue, bleeding on provocation, changes in contour, and the presence of calculus or plaque with no radiographic evidence of crestal bone loss.[10] Histologic examination of inflamed gingival tissue reveals ulcerated epithelium. Inflammatory mediators negatively affect epithelial function as a protective barrier. Repair of this ulcerated epithelium depends on the proliferative or regenerative activity of the epithelial cells, and removal of the etiologic agents that triggered gingival breakdown is essential.

Course and Duration

Gingivitis can develop with sudden onset and have a short duration, and it can be painful. A less severe phase of this condition can also occur.

Chronic gingivitis develops slowly and has a long duration. It is painless, unless it is complicated by acute or subacute exacerbations, and it is the type that is most often encountered (Fig. 18.1). Chronic gingivitis is a fluctuating disease in which inflammation persists or resolves and normal areas become inflamed.[30,36]

Recurrent gingivitis reappears after having been eliminated by treatment or after disappearing spontaneously.

Description

Localized gingivitis is confined to the gingiva of a single tooth or group of teeth. *Generalized gingivitis* involves the entire mouth.

Marginal gingivitis involves the gingival margin, and it can include a portion of the contiguous attached gingiva. *Papillary gingivitis* involves the interdental papillae, and it often extends into the adjacent portion of the gingival margin. Papillae are involved more frequently than the gingival margin, and the earliest signs of gingivitis often occur in the papillae. *Diffuse gingivitis* affects the gingival margin, the attached gingiva, and the interdental papillae. Gingival disease in individual cases is described by combining the preceding terms as follows:

- *Localized marginal gingivitis* is confined to one or more areas of the marginal gingiva (Fig. 18.2).
- *Localized diffuse gingivitis* extends from the margin to the mucobuccal fold in a limited area (Fig. 18.3).
- *Localized papillary gingivitis* is confined to one or more interdental spaces in a limited area (Fig. 18.4).
- *Generalized marginal gingivitis* involves the gingival margins in relation to all the teeth. The interdental papillae are usually affected (Fig. 18.5).
- *Generalized diffuse gingivitis* involves the entire gingiva. Because the alveolar mucosa and attached gingiva are affected, the mucogingival junction is sometimes obliterated (Fig. 18.6). Systemic conditions can be involved in the case of generalized diffuse gingivitis and should be evaluated if they are suspected as an etiologic cofactor.

Hallmarks of Gingivitis

Feature	Healthy Gingiva	Gingivitis
Color	Coral pink	Red
Contour	Knife-edged and scalloped	Rolled with bulbous papillae
Consistency and texture	Firm and resilient with stippling of the attached gingiva	Edematous and with loss of stippling

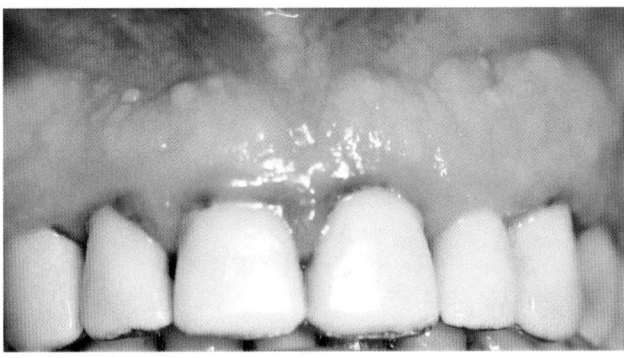

Fig. 18.1 Chronic gingivitis. The marginal and interdental gingivae are smooth, edematous, and discolored. Isolated areas of acute response are seen.

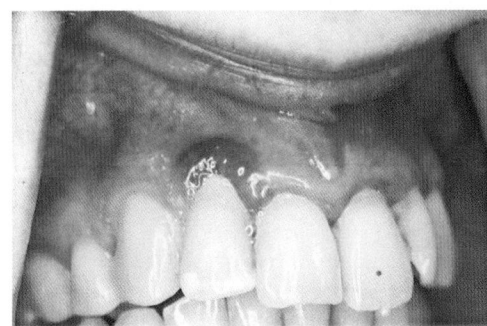

Fig. 18.2 Localized diffuse, intensely red area on the facial surface of tooth #7 and dark pink marginal changes in the remaining anterior teeth.

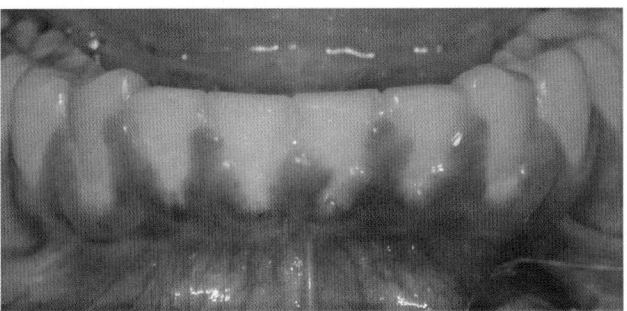

Fig. 18.3 Generalized marginal gingivitis in the lower jaw with areas of diffuse gingivitis.

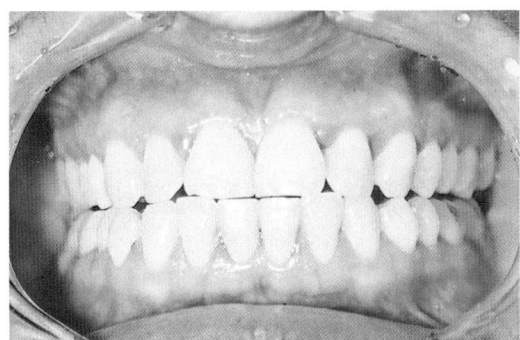

Fig. 18.4 Generalized papillary gingivitis.

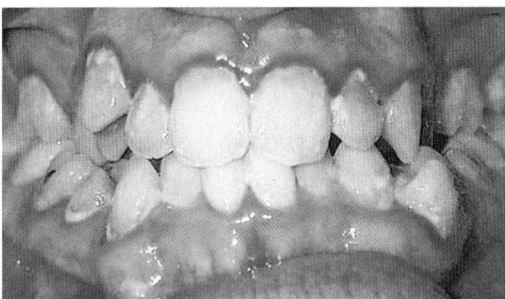

Fig. 18.5 Generalized marginal and papillary gingivitis.

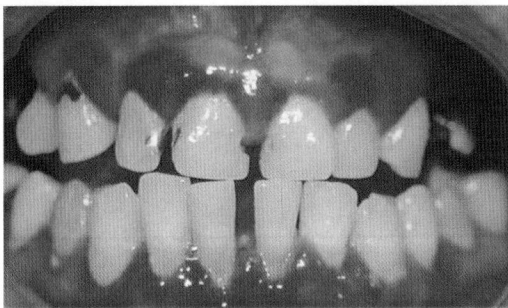

Fig. 18.6 Generalized diffuse gingivitis involves the marginal, papillary, and attached gingivae.

Clinical Findings

A systematic approach is required for the evaluation of the clinical features of gingivitis. The clinician should focus on subtle tissue alterations because they may have diagnostic significance. A systematic clinical approach requires an orderly examination of the gingiva for color, contour, consistency, position, and ease and severity of bleeding and pain. This section discusses these clinical characteristics and the microscopic changes that are responsible for each.

Gingival Bleeding on Probing

The two earliest signs of gingival inflammation that precede established gingivitis are increased gingival crevicular fluid production and bleeding from the gingival sulcus on gentle probing (Fig. 18.7). Chapter 16 discusses gingival crevicular fluid in detail.

Gingival bleeding varies in severity, duration, and ease of provocation. Bleeding on probing (BOP) is easily detected clinically and therefore is of value for early diagnosis and for prevention of more advanced gingivitis. BOP appears earlier than a change in color or other visual signs of inflammation.[36,37,46] The use of bleeding rather than color changes to diagnose early gingival inflammation is advantageous, in that bleeding is a more objective sign that requires less subjective estimation by the examiner.

An estimated 53.2 million (50.3%) US adults who are 30 years of age or older exhibit gingival bleeding.[5] Probing pocket depth measurements by themselves are of limited value in assessing the extent and severity of gingivitis. For example, gingival recession may result in a reduction of probing depth and cause inaccurate assessment of the periodontal status.[7] BOP is widely used by clinicians and epidemiologists to measure disease prevalence and progression, measure outcomes of treatment, and motivate patients to perform necessary home care.[24] See Chapter 6 for several gingival indices that are based on bleeding[2,16,53] and for more information on probing.

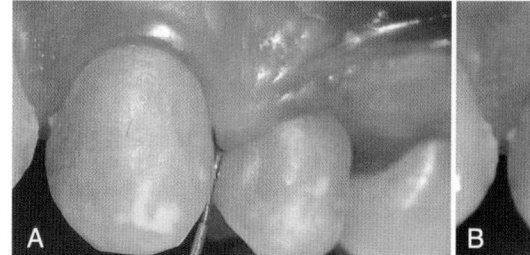
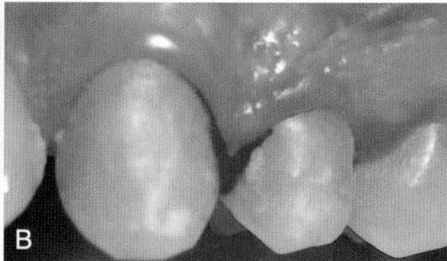

Fig. 18.7 Bleeding on probing. (A) To explore mild edematous gingivitis, a probe is introduced to the bottom of the gingival sulcus. (B) Bleeding appears after a few seconds.

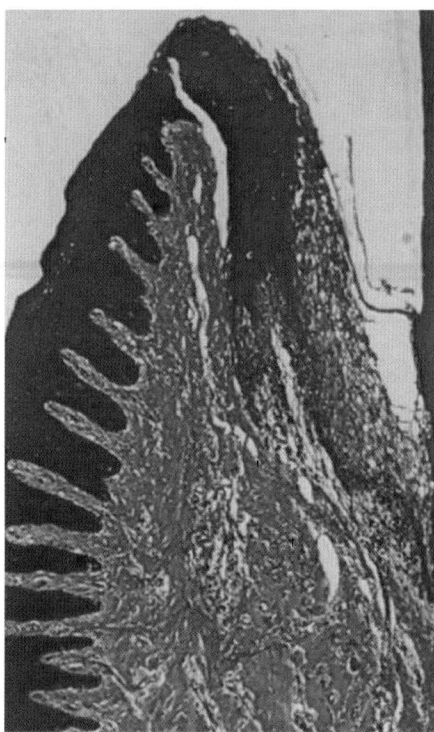

Fig. 18.8 Microscopic view of the interdental space in a human autopsy specimen. Note the inflammatory infiltrate and thinned epithelium in the area adjacent to the tooth and the collagenous tissue in the outer half of the section.

Gingival BOP indicates an inflammatory lesion in the epithelium and the connective tissue that exhibits specific histologic differences compared with healthy gingiva.[25] Although gingival BOP may not be a good diagnostic indicator of clinical attachment loss, its absence is an excellent negative predictor of future attachment loss.[34] The absence of gingival BOP is desirable and implies a low risk of future clinical attachment loss. Longitudinal findings revealed that sites with consistent bleeding (gingival index = 2) had 70% more attachment loss than sites that were noninflamed over a 26-year period in 565 male patients. Persistent gingivitis can be considered a risk factor for periodontal attachment loss that may lead to tooth loss.[35]

Numerous studies have shown that current cigarette smoking suppresses the gingival inflammatory response, and smoking was found to exert a strong, chronic, dose-dependent suppressive effect on gingival BOP in the Third National Health and Nutrition Examination Survey (NHANES III).[19] Research has revealed an increase in gingival BOP in patients who quit smoking,[54] and people who are committed to a smoking cessation program should be informed about the possibility of an increase in gingival bleeding associated with smoking cessation.

Gingival Bleeding Caused by Local Factors

Factors that contribute to plaque retention and may lead to gingivitis include anatomic and developmental tooth variations, caries, frenum pull, iatrogenic factors, malpositioned teeth, mouth breathing, overhangs, partial dentures, lack of attached gingiva, and recession. Orthodontic treatment and fixed retainers are associated with increased plaque retention and increased BOP.[38,78]

Chronic and Recurrent Bleeding

The most common cause of abnormal gingival BOP is chronic inflammation.[50] The bleeding is chronic or recurrent, and it is provoked by mechanical trauma (e.g., toothbrushing, toothpicks, food impaction) or by biting into solid foods (e.g., apples).

In gingival inflammation, histopathologic alterations that result in abnormal gingival bleeding include dilation and engorgement of the capillaries and thinning or ulceration of the sulcular epithelium (Fig. 18.8). Because the capillaries are engorged and closer to the surface and because the thinned, degenerated epithelium is less protective, stimuli that are normally innocuous cause rupture of the capillaries, and gingival bleeding occurs. Sites that bleed on probing have a greater area of inflamed connective tissue (i.e., cell-rich, collagen-poor tissue) than sites that do not bleed. In most cases, the cellular infiltrate of sites that bleed on probing is predominantly lymphocytic, which is a characteristic of stage II (early) gingivitis.[9,17,25]

Histologic evaluations of animal specimens have revealed that during the early stages of gingivitis, expression of the cytokines (i.e., matrix metalloproteinases [MMPs]) that are responsible for connective tissue breakdown is ubiquitous. Different MMPs play roles in this breakdown at different stages (e.g., a decrease of MMP-14 activity at day 7 of inflammation; immediate increase in MMP-2, especially with fibroblastic stimulation). MMP-9 expression peaked 5 days after gingivitis occurrence, which was also regulated by macrophages and neutrophils. Extracellular matrix remodeling was regulated with MMP-2 and MMP-9 production and activation by the host inflammatory response.[39]

CLINICAL CORRELATION

Medications and Gingival Bleeding

- Drugs such as antiplatelet medications (e.g., aspirin) or anticoagulants (e.g., warfarin) that are prescribed for specific medical indications also increase the bleeding tendencies of gingival tissues.
- Women taking oral contraceptives are significantly more prone to gingivitis and therefore to gingival bleeding.

The severity of bleeding and the ease of its provocation depend on the intensity of inflammation. After the vessels are damaged and ruptured, interrelated mechanisms induce hemostasis.[73] The vessel walls contract, blood flow diminishes, blood platelets adhere to the edges of the tissue, and a fibrous clot is formed that contracts and results in approximation of the edges of the injured area. Bleeding recurs when the area is irritated.

In cases of moderate or advanced periodontitis, BOP is considered a sign of active tissue destruction. Acute episodes of gingival bleeding are caused by injury, and they can occur spontaneously in patients with gingival disease. Laceration of the gingiva by toothbrush bristles during aggressive toothbrushing or by sharp pieces of hard food can cause gingival bleeding, even in the absence of gingival disease. Gingival burns from hot foods or chemicals increase the ease of gingival bleeding.

Spontaneous bleeding or bleeding on slight provocation can occur with acute necrotizing ulcerative gingivitis. With this condition, engorged blood vessels in the inflamed connective tissue are exposed by ulceration of the necrotic surface epithelium.

Gingival Bleeding Associated With Systemic Changes

With some systemic disorders, gingival hemorrhage occurs spontaneously or after irritation (usually generalized), and it is excessive and difficult to control. These hemorrhagic diseases represent a wide variety of conditions that vary with regard to etiologic factors and clinical manifestations. Such conditions have the common feature of a hemostatic mechanism failure that results in abnormal bleeding in the skin, internal organs, and other tissues, including the oral mucosa.[71]

Hemorrhagic disorders in which abnormal gingival bleeding is encountered include vascular abnormalities (e.g., vitamin C deficiency, allergy such as Henoch–Schönlein purpura), platelet disorders[27] (e.g., thrombocytopenic purpura), hypoprothrombinemia (e.g., vitamin K deficiency), other coagulation defects (e.g., hemophilia, leukemia, Christmas disease), deficient platelet thromboplastic factor as a result of uremia,[47] multiple myeloma,[12] and postrubella purpura.[30] The effects of hormonal replacement therapy, oral contraceptives, pregnancy, and the menstrual cycle are also reported to affect gingival bleeding.[43,65,79,80] In women, long-term depression-related stress exposure may increase concentrations of interleukin-6 in gingival crevicular fluid and worsen periodontal conditions, producing elevated levels of gingival inflammation and increased pocket depths.[32]

CLINICAL CORRELATION

Pregnancy Gingivitis
Pregnancy gingivitis affects many pregnant women and is primarily caused by the hormonal imbalances associated with pregnancy. It is characterized by mild to severe gingival inflammation along with pain and, in some cases, significant hyperplasia and bleeding. In most patients, the condition normally resolves by itself after delivery, when the hormonal levels return to normal.

Changes in sex hormones have long been established as significant modifying factors in gingivitis, especially among adolescents. Several reports have shown notable effects of fluctuating estrogen and progesterone levels on the periodontium, starting as early as puberty.[1,55] Diabetes is an endocrine condition with a well-characterized effect on gingivitis.[78] In diabetes, marked inflammation affects both epithelial and connective tissues, leading to degeneration of the dermal papilla,

an increase in the number of inflammatory cells, the destruction of reticulin fibers, and an accumulation of dense collagen fibers that causes fibrosis.[70]

Several medications have also been found to have adverse effects on the gingiva. For example, anticonvulsants, antihypertensive calcium channel blockers, and immunosuppressive drugs cause gingival enlargement (see Chapter 19), which can cause gingival inflammation and bleeding. The American Heart Association has recommended over-the-counter aspirin as a prophylactic and therapeutic agent for cardiovascular disease, and aspirin is often prescribed for other conditions such as rheumatoid arthritis, osteoarthritis, rheumatic fever, and other inflammatory joint diseases.[28] It is important to consider aspirin's effect on bleeding during a routine dental examination to avoid false-positive readings that could result in an inaccurate diagnosis.[67] Chapter 19 discusses periodontal involvement in hematologic disorders.

Color Changes in the Gingiva

The color of the gingiva is determined by several factors, including the number and size of blood vessels, the epithelial thickness, the quantity of keratinization, and the pigments in the epithelium.

Color Changes With Gingivitis

Change in color is an important clinical sign of gingival disease. The normal gingival color is coral pink, and it is produced by the tissue's vascularity and modified by the overlying epithelial layers. The gingiva becomes red when vascularization increases or the degree of epithelial keratinization is reduced or disappears. The color becomes pale when vascularization is reduced (in association with fibrosis of the corium) or epithelial keratinization increases. Chronic inflammation intensifies the red or bluish red color as a result of vascular proliferation and a reduction of keratinization. Venous stasis contributes a bluish hue. The gingival color changes with increasing chronicity of the inflammatory process. The changes start in the interdental papillae and gingival margin and then spread to the attached gingiva.

Proper diagnosis and treatment depend on understanding the tissue changes that alter the color of the gingiva at the clinical level. Color changes in acute gingival inflammation differ in both nature and distribution from those in patients with chronic gingivitis. The color changes can be marginal, diffuse, or patchlike, depending on the underlying acute condition. With acute necrotizing ulcerative gingivitis, the involvement is marginal; with herpetic gingivostomatitis, it is diffuse; and with acute reactions to chemical irritation, it is patchlike or diffuse.

CLINICAL CORRELATION

Mouth Breathing and Gingival Inflammation
Gingivitis in the maxillary buccal area of the oral cavity is a common finding in patients who are mouth breathers. The affected gingiva typically appears red, shiny, and edematous, which is thought to be related to the surface dehydration caused by mouth breathing.

Color changes vary with the intensity of inflammation. Initially, there is an increase in erythema. If the condition does not worsen, this is the only color change until the gingiva reverts to normal. With severe acute inflammation, the red color gradually becomes a dull, whitish gray. The gray discoloration produced by tissue necrosis is demarcated from the adjacent gingiva by a thin, sharply defined erythematous zone. Chapter 14 provides detailed descriptions of the

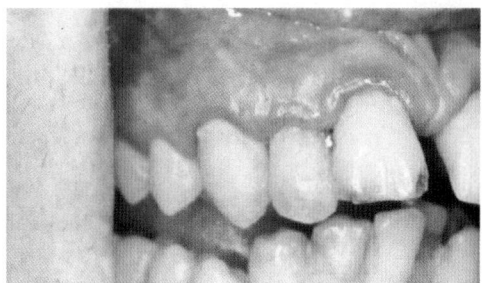

Fig. 18.9 Bismuth gingivitis. Note the linear black discoloration of the gingiva in a patient who is receiving bismuth therapy.

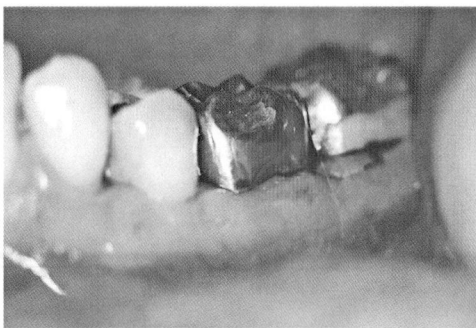

Fig. 18.10 Discoloration of the gingiva is caused by embedded metal particles (i.e., amalgam).

clinical and pathologic features of the various forms of acute gingivitis.

Metallic Pigmentation

Heavy metals (i.e., bismuth, arsenic, mercury, lead, and silver) that are absorbed systemically as a result of therapeutic use or occupational or household exposures can discolor the gingiva and other areas of the oral mucosa.[45] These changes are rare, but they should be ruled out in suspected cases.

Metals typically produce a black or bluish line in the gingiva that follows the contour of the margin (Fig. 18.9). The pigmentation may also appear as isolated black blotches involving the interdental marginal and attached gingiva. This is different from the tattooing produced by the accidental embedding of amalgam or other metal fragments[15] (Fig. 18.10).

Gingival pigmentation from systemically absorbed metals results from the perivascular precipitation of metallic sulfides in the subepithelial connective tissue. Gingival pigmentation is not a result of systemic toxicity. It occurs only in areas of inflammation in which the increased permeability of irritated blood vessels permits the seepage of metal into the surrounding tissue. In addition to inflamed gingiva, mucosal areas that are irritated by biting or abnormal chewing habits (e.g., inner surface of lips, cheek at the level of the occlusal line, lateral border of the tongue) are common sites of pigmentation. Pigmentation can be eliminated by treating the inflammatory changes without necessarily discontinuing the metal-containing medication.

Color Changes Associated With Systemic Factors

Many systemic diseases can cause color changes in the oral mucosa, including the gingiva.[22] In general, these abnormal pigmentations are nonspecific, and they should stimulate further diagnostic efforts or referral to the appropriate specialist.[68]

Endogenous oral pigmentation can be caused by melanin, bilirubin, or iron.[45] *Melanin* oral pigmentation can be normal, and

is often found in highly pigmented ethnic groups (see Chapter 18). Diseases that increase melanin pigmentation include the following:

- Addison disease is caused by adrenal dysfunction, and it produces isolated patches of discoloration that vary from bluish black to brown.
- Peutz–Jeghers syndrome produces intestinal polyposis and melanin pigmentation in the oral mucosa and lips.
- Albright syndrome (i.e., polyostotic fibrous dysplasia) and von Recklinghausen disease (i.e., neurofibromatosis) produce areas of oral melanin pigmentation.

The skin and mucous membranes can also be stained by *bile pigments.* Jaundice is best detected by examination of the sclera, but the oral mucosa may also acquire a yellowish color. The deposition of *iron* in hemochromatosis may produce blue-gray pigmentation of the oral mucosa. Several endocrine and metabolic disturbances, including diabetes and pregnancy, can result in color changes. Blood dyscrasias such as anemia, polycythemia, and leukemia also can induce color changes.

Exogenous factors that are capable of producing color changes in the gingiva include atmospheric irritants, such as coal and metal dust, and coloring agents in food and lozenges. Tobacco causes hyperkeratosis of the gingiva, and it can induce a significant increase in melanin pigmentation of the oral mucosa.[56] Localized bluish black areas of pigment are often caused by amalgam implanted in the mucosa (see Fig. 18.10).

The need for aesthetics in dentistry has increased, with a growing demand for a pleasing smile. This has made many individuals more aware of their gingival pigmentation, which may be apparent when smiling and speaking.[20,21] Traditionally, gingival depigmentation has been carried out with the use of nonsurgical and surgical procedures, including chemical, cryosurgical, and electrosurgical techniques. However, those techniques were met with skepticism because of their various degrees of success.

Lasers have been used to ablate cells that produce the melanin pigment; a nonspecific laser beam destroys the epithelial cells, including those at the basal layer. Selective ablation using a laser beam with a wavelength that is specifically absorbed by melanin effectively destroys the pigmented cells without damaging the nonpigmented cells. In both cases, radiation energy is transformed into ablation energy, resulting in cellular rupture and vaporization with minimal heating of the surrounding tissue.[76]

Changes in Gingival Consistency

Chronic and acute inflammations produce changes in the normal firm and resilient consistency of the gingiva. In patients with chronic gingivitis, destructive (i.e., edematous) and reparative (i.e., fibrotic) changes coexist, and the consistency of the gingiva is determined by their relative predominance (Figs. 18.11 and 18.12). Table 18.1 summarizes the clinical alterations in the consistency of the gingiva and the microscopic changes that produce them.

Calcified Masses in the Gingiva

Calcified microscopic masses may be found in the gingiva.[14,52] They can occur alone or in groups, and they vary with regard to size, location, shape, and structure. Such masses may be calcified material that was removed from the tooth and traumatically displaced into the gingiva during scaling,[52] root remnants, cementum fragments, or cementicles. Chronic inflammation and fibrosis, an occasional foreign body, and giant-cell activity occur in reaction to the masses, which are sometimes enclosed in an osteoid-like matrix. Crystalline foreign bodies have also been described in the gingiva, but their origin has not been determined.[60]

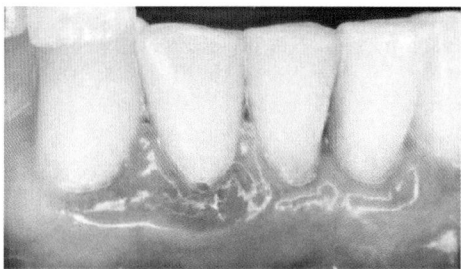

Fig. 18.11 Chronic gingivitis. Swelling, loss of stippling, and discoloration occur when inflammatory exudate and edema are the predominant microscopic changes. The gingiva is soft and friable and bleeds easily.

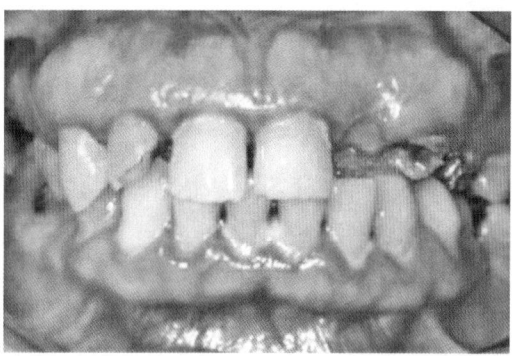

Fig. 18.12 Chronic gingivitis. Firm gingiva is produced when fibrosis predominates in the inflammatory process.

TABLE 18.1 Clinical and Histopathologic Changes in Gingival Consistency

Clinical Changes	Underlying Microscopic Features
Chronic Gingivitis	
1. Soggy puffiness that pits on pressure	1. Infiltration by fluid and cells of inflammatory exudate
2. Marked softness and friability, with ready fragmentation on exploration with probe and pinpoint surface areas of redness and desquamation	2. Degeneration of connective tissue and epithelium associated with injurious substances that provoke inflammation and inflammatory exudate; change in the connective tissue–epithelium relationship, with inflamed, engorged connective tissue expanding to within a few epithelial cells of the surface; thinning of epithelium and degeneration associated with edema and leukocyte invasion, separated by areas in which rete pegs are elongated to connective tissue
3. Firm, leathery consistency	3. Fibrosis and epithelial proliferation associated with long-standing chronic inflammation
Acute Gingivitis	
1. Diffuse puffiness and softening	1. Diffuse edema of acute inflammatory origin; fatty infiltration in xanthomatosis
2. Sloughing with grayish, flakelike particles of debris adhering to eroded surface	2. Necrosis with formation of pseudomembrane composed of bacteria, polymorphonuclear leukocytes, and degenerated epithelial cells in fibrinous meshwork
3. Vesicle formation	3. Intercellular and intracellular edema with degeneration of nucleus and cytoplasm and rupture of cell wall

Toothbrushing

Toothbrushing has various effects on the consistency of the gingiva, such as promoting keratinization of the oral epithelium, enhancing capillary gingival circulation, and thickening alveolar bone.[44,49,77] In animal studies, mechanical stimulation by toothbrushing was found to increase the proliferative activity of the junctional basal cells in dog gingiva by 2.5 times compared with the use of a scaler.[31] These findings may indicate that toothbrushing causes an increased turnover rate and desquamation of the junctional epithelial surfaces. This process may repair small breaks in the junctional epithelium and prevent direct access to the underlying tissue by periodontal pathogens.[81]

Changes in Gingival Surface Texture

The surface of normal gingiva usually exhibits numerous small depressions and elevations that give the tissue an orange-peel appearance referred to as *stippling*.[13] Stippling is restricted to the attached gingiva and is predominantly localized to the subpapillary area, but it extends to various degrees into the interdental papilla.[61] Although the biologic significance of gingival stippling is not known, some investigators conclude that the loss of stippling is an early sign of gingivitis.[33,61] However, clinicians must take into consideration that its pattern and extent vary in different mouth areas, among patients, and with age.

In patients with chronic inflammation, the gingival surface is smooth and shiny or firm and nodular, depending on whether the dominant changes are exudative or fibrotic. A smooth surface texture is also produced by epithelial atrophy in atrophic gingivitis, and peeling of the surface occurs with chronic desquamative gingivitis. Hyperkeratosis results in a leathery texture, and drug-induced gingival overgrowth produces a nodular surface.

CLINICAL CORRELATION

Stippling and Its Clinical Importance
Healthy, attached gingiva has a pitted orange-peel appearance on its surface. This surface feature, called *stippling*, is an external reflection of the underlying connective tissue projections into the overlying epithelium. Presence of stippling in the attached gingiva is indicative of gingival health, and this surface feature is usually lost when the tissue is edematous.

Changes in Gingival Position
Traumatic Lesions

A feature of gingival disease classification is the recognition of non–plaque-induced traumatic gingival lesions as distinct gingival conditions.[11] Traumatic lesions—whether chemical, physical, or thermal—are among the most common lesions in the mouth. Sources of chemical injuries include aspirin, hydrogen peroxide, silver nitrate, phenol, and endodontic materials. Physical injuries can include lip, oral, and tongue piercings, which can result in gingival recession. Thermal injuries can result from hot drinks and foods.

In acute cases, the appearance of slough (i.e., necrotizing epithelium), erosion, or ulceration and accompanying erythema are common features. In chronic cases, permanent gingival defects usually take the form of gingival recession. Typically, the localized nature of the lesions and lack of symptoms readily eliminate them from the differential diagnosis of systemic conditions that may exist with erosive or ulcerative oral lesions.[64]

Gingival Recession

Gingival recession is a common finding. The prevalence, extent, and severity of gingival recession increase with age, and this condition is more prevalent among males.[5]

Positions of the Gingiva

By clinical definition, recession is exposure of the root surface by an apical shift in the position of the gingiva. To understand recession, it helps to distinguish between the actual and apparent positions of the gingiva. The *actual position* is the level of the coronal end of the epithelial attachment on the tooth, whereas the *apparent position* is the level of the crest of the gingival margin (Fig. 18.13). The severity of recession is usually determined by the apparent position of the gingiva. However, the actual gingival position is used to determine the clinical attachment loss. For example, in periodontal disease, the inflamed pocket wall covers part of the denuded root; some of the recession is hidden, and some maybe visible. The total amount of clinical attachment loss is the sum of the two.

Recession refers to the location of the gingiva rather than to its condition. Receded gingiva can be inflamed, but it may be normal except for its position (Fig. 18.14). Recession can be localized to one tooth or a group of teeth, or it may be generalized throughout the mouth.

Gingival recession increases with age; the incidence varies from 8% among children to 100% after 50 years of age.[84] This has led some investigators to assume that recession might be a physiologic process related to aging. However, no convincing evidence has been presented for a physiologic shift of the gingival attachment.[40]

The gradual apical shift most likely results from the cumulative effect of minor pathologic involvement and repeated minor direct trauma to the gingiva. In some populations without access to dental care, however, recession can result from increasing periodontal disease.[29,41]

The following etiologic factors have been implicated in gingival recession: faulty toothbrushing technique (i.e., gingival abrasion), tooth malposition, friction from the soft tissues (i.e., gingival ablation),[72] gingival inflammation, abnormal frenum attachment, and iatrogenic dentistry. Trauma from occlusion has been suggested in the past, but its mechanism of action has never been demonstrated. For example, a deep overbite has been associated with gingival inflammation and recession. Excessive incisal overlap may result in a traumatic injury to the gingiva. Orthodontic movement in a labial direction in monkeys has been shown to result in the loss of marginal bone and connective tissue attachment and in gingival recession.[74]

Standard oral hygiene procedures, including toothbrushing and flossing, frequently lead to transient and minimal gingival injury.[18,62] Although toothbrushing is important for gingival health, faulty technique or brushing with hard bristles can cause significant injury. This type of injury can manifest as lacerations, abrasions, keratosis, or recession, with the facial marginal gingiva being affected most often.[57] In these cases, recession tends to be more frequent and more severe in patients with clinically healthy gingiva, little bacterial plaque, and good oral hygiene.[23,58,59]

> ### CLINICAL CORRELATION
>
> #### Biologic Width and Gingival Inflammation
> Biologic width is the circumferential rim of space around teeth where the junctional epithelium and the underlying connective tissue of the gingiva attach to the teeth. When restoring teeth, if the margins of the restorations violate the biologic width, gingival inflammation ensues. If left untreated, it can lead to bone loss. Crown lengthening is a surgical procedure that is performed clinically (i.e., before restoration delivery) to intentionally create space for the biologic width to reestablish.

Susceptibility to recession is influenced by the position of teeth in the arch,[83] the root–bone angle, and the mesiodistal curvature of the tooth surface.[51] On rotated, tilted, or facially displaced teeth, the bony plate is thinned or reduced in height. Pressure from mastication or moderate toothbrushing damages the unsupported gingiva and produces recession. The effect of the angle of the root in the bone with recession is often observed in the maxillary molar area. If the lingual inclination of the palatal root is prominent or the buccal roots

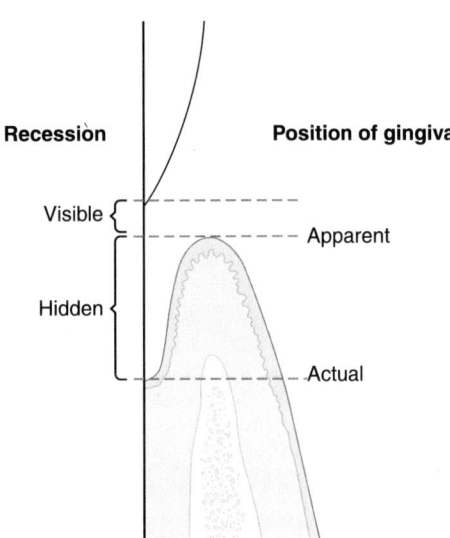

Fig. 18.13 Diagram of apparent and actual positions of the gingiva and visible and hidden recession.

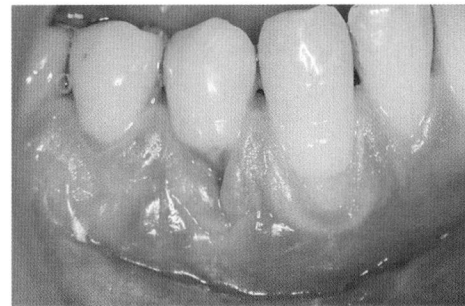

Fig. 18.14 Degrees of recession. Recession is slight in teeth #26 and #29 and marked in teeth #27 and #28. The change in gingival contour and the recession, as seen in tooth #28, are referred to as *Stillman clefts.*

flare outward, the bone in the cervical area is thinned or shortened, and recession results from repeated trauma of the thin marginal gingiva.

The health of the gingival tissue also depends on properly designed and placed restorative materials. Pressure from a poorly designed partial denture, such as an ill-fitting denture clasp, can cause gingival trauma and recession.[85] Overhanging dental restorations have long been viewed as a contributing factor to gingivitis because of plaque retention. In addition, there is general agreement that placing restorative margins within the biologic width frequently leads to gingival inflammation, clinical attachment loss, and eventually bone loss. Clinically, the violation of biologic width typically manifests as gingival inflammation, deepened periodontal pockets, and gingival recession.

A relationship may exist between smoking and gingival recession (see Chapter 12). The multifactorial mechanisms probably include reduced gingival blood flow and an altered immune response, but current evidence is not conclusive.[26,63]

Clinical Significance

Several aspects of gingival recession make it clinically significant. Exposed root surfaces are susceptible to caries. Abrasion or erosion of the cementum exposed by recession leaves an underlying dentinal surface that can be sensitive. Hyperemia of the pulp and associated symptoms can result from excessive exposure of the root surface.[48] Interproximal recession creates oral hygiene problems results in plaque accumulation.

Changes in Gingival Contour

Changes in gingival contour are primarily associated with gingival enlargement (see Chapter 19), but changes may also occur with other conditions. Of historical interest are descriptions of indentations of the gingival margin referred to as Stillman clefts (see Fig. 18.14)[75] and McCall festoons. The term *Stillman cleft* has been used to describe a specific type of gingival recession that consists of a narrow, triangular-shaped gingival recession. As the recession progresses apically, the cleft becomes broader, thereby exposing the cementum of the root surface. When the lesion reaches the mucogingival junction, the apical border of oral mucosa is usually inflamed because of the difficulty in maintaining adequate plaque control at this site.

The term *McCall festoon* has been used to describe a rolled, thickened band of gingiva that is usually seen adjacent to the cuspids when recession approaches the mucogingival junction. Initially, Stillman clefts and McCall festoons were attributed to traumatic occlusion, and the recommended treatment was occlusal adjustment. However, this association was never proved, and the indentations merely represent peculiar inflammatory changes of the marginal gingiva.[14]

Case Scenarios are found on the companion website www.expertconsult.com.

References

References for this chapter are found on the companion website www.expertconsult.com.

CHAPTER 19

Gingival Enlargement

Alpdogan Kantarci | Fermin A. Carranza | Eva Hogan

Enlargement of gingiva has many causes and can manifest with various clinical characteristics. A change in the dimensions of gingival tissue is always a pathologic event. Gingival enlargement can be transient and reversible or can be chronic and irreversible. As in other pathologic processes, inflammation of the periodontal tissues typically results in three outcomes: complete resolution of inflammation and restoration of tissue integrity (i.e., homeostasis), destruction of periodontal tissues and loss of attachment (i.e., chronic periodontitis), or fibrosis.

Fibrosis is a component of the defense mechanism against progression of periodontal inflammation. During this process, fibroblasts play a major role by generating excessive amounts of collagen and noncollagenous proteins of the extracellular matrix. Increased matrix deposition is not sufficiently balanced by the enzymatic degradation of the matrix composition (e.g., collagen), resulting in fibrotic changes in soft tissues. Fibrosis of gingival tissues is commonly referred to as *gingival hyperplasia*. In contrast to other tissues in which fibrosis is observed, gingival lesions are usually inflamed due to accumulation of bacteria and reduced oral care. Gingival overgrowth lesions are unique in their pathogenetic mechanisms.

Pathologic enlargements of gingival tissues were recognized in ancient civilizations and were linked to systemic conditions as early as the 18th century. Most common forms of gingival enlargement result from systemic use of various medications. The first scientific report on drug-induced gingival overgrowth was published in 1939, when the anticonvulsant diphenylhydantoinate was associated with gingival enlargement.[59] Later studies provided significant insights into the complex molecular and cellular mechanisms underlying gingival enlargement. Because many forms of gingival enlargement are associated with systemic factors and conditions, understanding the exact pathogenesis of lesions is essential for designing better approaches to treatment.

This chapter focuses on the clinical, etiologic, and pathologic aspects of gingival enlargement that are used to develop novel and targeted approaches to therapy. Neoplastic enlargement of gingival tissues associated with benign or malignant oral cancers is not covered in depth because this emerging field of oral pathology has evolved beyond the scope of this chapter and can be found in oral pathology textbooks that provide extensive coverage of oral tumors.

Terminology and Classification

Gingival enlargement and *gingival overgrowth* are terms used interchangeably with *hyperplasia*, *hypertrophy*, and *fibrosis*. *Hyperplasia* is an increase in the number of cells in tissues that results in increased tissue volume. *Hypertrophy* refers to increased tissue size and volume resulting from increased cell size. Although their pathogenetic mechanisms are different, hyperplasia and hypertrophy usually occur simultaneously when cellular involvement in hyperplasia most likely triggers the overgrowth.

The two processes are closely linked. *Fibrosis* refers to a pathologic process in which disrupted wound healing is associated with defective cell proliferation, cell-to-cell interactions, cell-to-matrix interactions, and matrix deposition and with an impaired immune system response. In this regard, fibrosis can be defined as a pathologic lesion, whereas hyperplasia and hypertrophy can be viewed as pathologic processes.

All of these terms refer to different pathogenetic states. In gingival tissues, they are associated with various phases of inflammation. Hyperplastic, hypertrophic, and fibrotic changes are observed during gingival enlargement and cannot be accurately differentiated. This chapter therefore uses *gingival overgrowth* (GO) or *gingival enlargement* to refer to all pathologic forms in periodontal tissues.

Classification of GO is based on etiologic factors. The most common form results from systemic use of medications and is called *drug-induced gingival overgrowth* (DIGO). Three families of drugs can lead to DIGO: anticonvulsants, calcium channel blockers, and immunosuppressants. GO also is associated with severe systemic diseases such as leukemia and with genetic factors. Any form that cannot be classified among these GO forms is known as *idiopathic GO*. GO can also be the result of inflammatory changes due to gingivitis. GO cases are classified as follows:
- Inflammatory enlargement due to chronic gingivitis
- Drug-induced enlargement
- GO associated with systemic conditions
- GO associated with systemic diseases
- Gingival fibromatosis

Enlargement of the gingiva can be indirectly associated with changes in the dimensions of underlying osseous structures. Although not covered in depth in this chapter, neoplastic lesions in the oral cavity can manifest with fibrotic lesions and can appear clinically similar to other forms of GO. Regardless of the cause, all forms of gingival enlargement have distinct pathologic characteristics that should be carefully considered during treatment. It is important to identify the cause and confounding etiologic factors that lead to different forms of GO.

Diagnosis

Because GO is frequently associated with systemic conditions, the general health of the patient and his or her drug use should be carefully managed. GO is one of the most serious pathologies in periodontal medicine, and it requires a meticulous differential diagnosis for selecting a therapeutic approach tailored to the patient's systemic status.

Accurate diagnosis requires a thorough review of the medical history of the patient. Gingival enlargement should be distinguished as localized or generalized. Generalized GO can affect marginal gingiva; localized forms can be confined to papillae. Previous classifications also distinguished between diffuse and discrete enlargements, which are sometimes difficult to differentiate. However, these categorizations can be critical for determining the correct cause of the pathology.

In periodontal tissues, indices are important for quantification of the extent and severity of GO. Various indices have been proposed. For example, the degree of gingival enlargement can be scored as follows:
- Grade 0: no signs of gingival enlargement
- Grade I: enlargement confined to interdental papilla
- Grade II: enlargement involves papilla and marginal gingiva
- Grade III: enlargement covers three-fourths or more of the crown

In addition to clinical determination of the degree of severity, a more accurate assessment of GO can be made by models cast on the impressions. A technique developed by Seymour and colleagues has been validated by others and can be a valuable tool for precise determination of the severity and extent of GO, especially for research purposes and long-term follow-up.[23,35,56,95,102] Other indices used to assess the severity of GO include those developed by Angelopoulos and Goaz[4] and Pernu and coworkers.[81] Three-dimensional scanning can be used to measure GO and compare the treatment outcomes with baseline values.[111]

Regardless of the method used for measuring the extent and severity of GO lesions, an accurate assessment is critical for identifying the inflammatory and fibrotic components. Indices should be chosen based on practicality of the data acquired to allow clinicians to select the method of therapy (e.g., gingivectomy and gingivoplasty vs. nonsurgical treatment measures) and plan the maintenance phase.

Types of Gingival Enlargement

Inflammatory Enlargement of Gingiva Due to Gingivitis

Clinical Manifestations

All changes in gingival tissues manifest with some degree of inflammation. In some cases, gingival enlargement is a direct outcome of gingivitis without any complicating factors or involvement of systemic conditions. When a patient with gingival enlargement is seen, the initial assessment is made by careful visual examination of abnormalities of gingival contours, texture, and color, which are compared with normal standards. Visual inspection is accompanied by a detailed medical history to exclude potential systemic factors and conditions. Dental irregularities, dysfunctional habits, and oral care efficiency should be considered in the evaluation, and clinical measurements should be recorded.

Inflammatory GO originates as a slight ballooning of the interdental papilla and marginal gingiva. In the early stages, it produces swelling around the involved teeth, which can increase in size until it covers part of the crowns. Gingival enlargement may be localized or generalized. It progresses slowly and painlessly unless it is complicated by acute infection or trauma (Figs. 19.1 and 19.2). Occasionally, chronic inflammatory GO occurs as a discrete sessile or pedunculated mass that resembles a tumor. It can be interproximal or located on the marginal or attached gingiva. Painful ulceration sometimes occurs in the fold between the mass and the adjacent gingiva.

Etiology

Acute inflammatory enlargement of the gingiva usually is caused by a mechanical, chemical, or physical irritation and can be resolved by removal of the irritant. Mouth breathing, impacted food items, and poor oral hygiene are usually responsible for acute inflammatory reactions in gingival tissues. Acute lesions are usually localized to marginal or papillary gingiva.

The main etiologic factor for acute inflammatory gingival enlargement is trauma. Traumatic lesions occur when a foreign substance (e.g., toothbrush bristle) is forcefully embedded in the gingiva and complicated by resident microbes. Trauma-induced injuries result in a chronic process characterized by granulation tissue formation and fibrosis. Because nerve tissue does not proliferate, pain is uncommon.

> **KEY FACT**
>
> The main etiological factor for acute inflammatory gingival enlargement is trauma. Traumatic lesions occur when a foreign substance (e.g., toothbrush bristle) is forcefully embedded into the gingiva and the situation is complicated by the presence of microbial pathogens. Trauma-induced injuries result in a chronic process characterized by granulation tissue formation and fibrosis. Because nerve tissue does not proliferate, pain is uncommon.

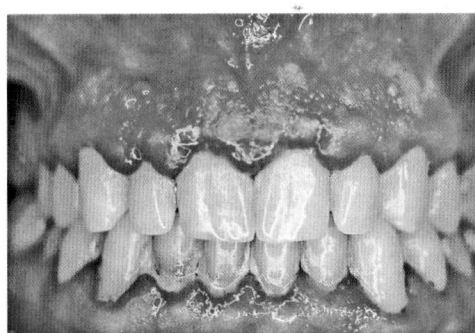

Fig. 19.1 Chronic inflammatory gingival enlargement localized to the anterior region.

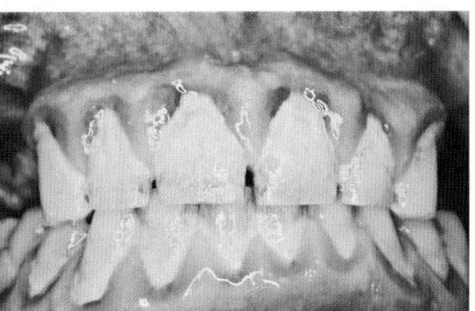

Fig. 19.2 Chronic inflammatory gingival enlargement.

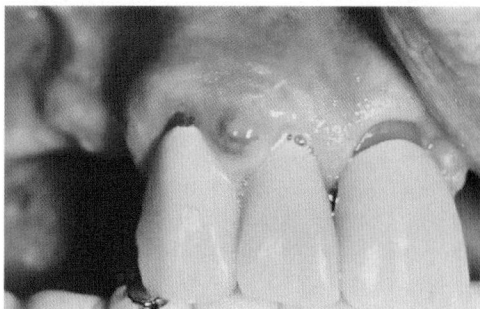

Fig. 19.3 Gingival abscess on the facial gingival surface in the space between the cuspid and the lateral incisor, unrelated to the gingival sulcus.

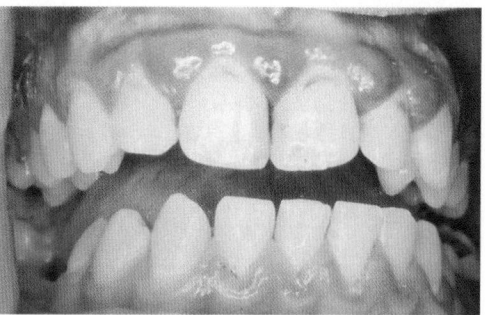

Fig. 19.4 Gingival enlargement in a mouth breather. The lesion is sharply circumscribed in the anterior marginal and papillary areas.

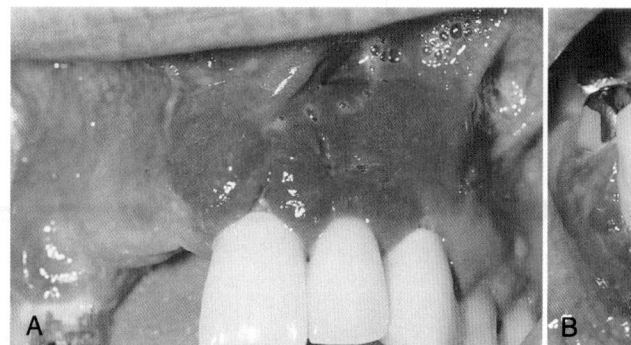
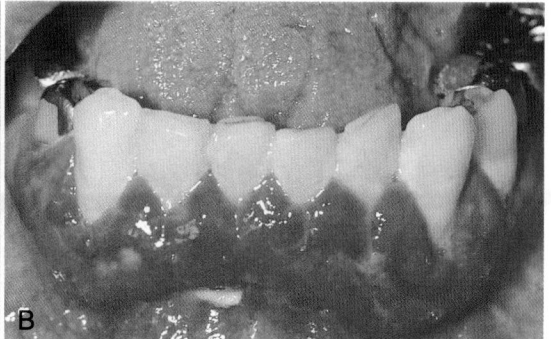

Fig. 19.5 Plasma cell gingivitis. (A) Diffuse lesions on the facial surface of the anterior maxilla. (B) Mandibular lesions. *(Courtesy Dr. Kim D. Zussman, Thousand Oaks, CA.)*

Acute inflammatory enlargement can lead to the formation of gingival abscess. Gingival abscess is a localized, painful, and rapidly expanding lesion (Fig. 19.3). It is typically limited to the marginal gingiva or the interdental papilla. In its early stages, it appears as a red swelling with a smooth, shiny surface. The lesion usually becomes fluctuant and pointed, with a surface orifice and a purulent exudate in 24 to 48 hours. Adjacent teeth may become sensitive to percussion. The lesion usually ruptures spontaneously. Because of an acute inflammatory process, the gingival abscess consists of a purulent exudate of a diffuse infiltration of polymorphonuclear leukocytes, edematous tissue, and vascularization. The surface epithelium has various degrees of intracellular and extracellular edema, invasion by leukocytes, and sometimes ulceration. The lesion is confined to the gingiva, and it should be distinguished from periodontal abscess.

Chronic inflammatory GO is commonly associated with microbial biofilm. Biofilm can be linked to a lack of proper oral hygiene, orthodontic appliances, faulty restoration margins, misaligned teeth, oral habits, an open bite, or other factors. Factors that favor plaque accumulation and retention include poor oral hygiene, irritation by anatomic abnormalities, and improper restorative and orthodontic appliances. Gingivitis and gingival enlargement are often seen in patients who are mouth breathers. The gingiva appears red and edematous, with a diffuse surface shininess of the exposed area. The maxillary anterior region is commonly involved. In many cases, the altered gingiva is clearly demarcated from the adjacent, unexposed normal gingiva (Fig. 19.4). Irritation from surface dehydration is attributed to mouth breathing. However, comparable changes could not be reproduced by air-drying the gingiva of experimental animals, suggesting that the pathogenesis of mouth breathing–associated gingival changes is far more complex.

Plasma cell gingivitis sometimes manifests as a mild marginal gingival enlargement that extends to the attached gingiva. The gingiva appears red, friable, and sometimes granular, and it bleeds easily; usually, gingivitis does not cause the loss of attachment (Fig. 19.5). The lesion is located on the oral aspect of the attached gingiva and is different from plaque-induced gingivitis.

In addition to the acute and chronic forms of gingival enlargements associated with gingivitis, inflammatory lesions can be observed in other forms of GO. Systemic conditions also cause inflammatory changes in gingiva. The distinction should be made very early in treatment planning, and the involvement of drugs, systemic conditions, and neoplastic lesions should be carefully ruled out.

Histopathology

Inflammatory enlargement of the gingiva typically follows the sequence of the inflammatory process. Chronic inflammatory GO lesions show the exudative and proliferative features of chronic inflammation (Fig. 19.6). Lesions that are deep red or bluish red are soft and friable with a smooth, shiny surface, and they bleed easily. They also have a preponderance of inflammatory cells and fluid, along with vascular engorgement, new capillary formation, and associated degenerative changes. Lesions that are relatively firm, resilient, and pink have a greater fibrotic component, with an abundance of fibroblasts and collagen fibers.

In patients with plasma cell gingivitis, the oral epithelium shows spongiosis and infiltration with inflammatory cells. Ultrastructurally, there are signs of damage in the lower spinous layers and the basal layers. The underlying connective tissue contains a dense infiltrate of plasma cells that also extends to the oral epithelium, producing a dissecting type of injury. Associated cheilitis and glossitis have been reported.[91]

Plasma cell gingivitis is thought to be allergic in origin and possibly a reaction to components of chewing gum, dentifrices, or various dietary items. Cessation of exposure to the allergen brings resolution of the lesion. In rare instances, marked inflammatory gingival enlargements with a predominance of plasma cells can appear; they are associated with aggressive periodontitis.[78] A solitary plasma cell tumor (i.e., plasmocytoma) has been described in the nasopharynx and rarely in the oral mucosa.[10] It is a slow-growing, pedunculated tumor with a pink and smooth surface, and it is composed of normal plasma cells. It is usually benign, but in rare cases it can be an oral manifestation of multiple myeloma, which is a malignant B-cell tumor of the bone marrow.

Treatment

Chronic enlargement of the gingiva due to gingivitis is reversible and can be resolved by removal of the etiologic factors, including the biofilm, and correction of environmental factors. In severe forms of inflammatory enlargement, surgical approaches may be required.

Drug-Induced Overgrowth of Gingiva

Most common forms of DIGO are caused by the use of anticonvulsants, calcium channel blockers, and immunosuppressants prescribed to patients for serious health concerns. The prevalence of DIGO substantially varies for different medications and among studies. Three drugs associated with DIGO are phenytoin, nifedipine, and cyclosporine. About 20 other medications have been linked to DIGO. An estimated 30% to 80% of the patients using these medications are at risk for overgrowth lesions. Genetic factors, drug dosage, and local factors can affect the development and severity of DIGO.[93,105]

DIGO frequently results in impaired oral hygiene, biofilm accumulation, and gingival inflammation. Increased prevalence of gingival infection and inflammation among patients with DIGO poses risk for their general health.[20,24,70] The inciting drugs are being replaced with alternatives, but they remain the drugs of choice in many countries for the treatment of specific conditions. Alternatives have also been linked to DIGO, and GO associated with medication use continues to be a clinical problem in dentistry and medicine.

DIGO lesions usually develop fast and become chronic over time (Fig. 19.7). The first signs of overgrowth can be observed as early as 3 months of drug use as a localized nodular enlargement of the interdental papilla. Because most of the medications associated with DIGO are prescribed for an extended time, the lesions expand and in some cases cover the crowns of the teeth. Severe forms of DIGO may result in complete coverage of dental surfaces (Fig. 19.8). Clinically, there are subtle differences in how the lesions manifest depending on the type of medication used. Dental biofilm and bacterial infection frequently lead to inflamed tissues characterized by edema and bleeding (Fig. 19.9). The degree of fibrosis and inflammation depend on the dose, duration, and type of drug; oral hygiene; individual susceptibility, including genetic factors; and environmental influences.[104,106]

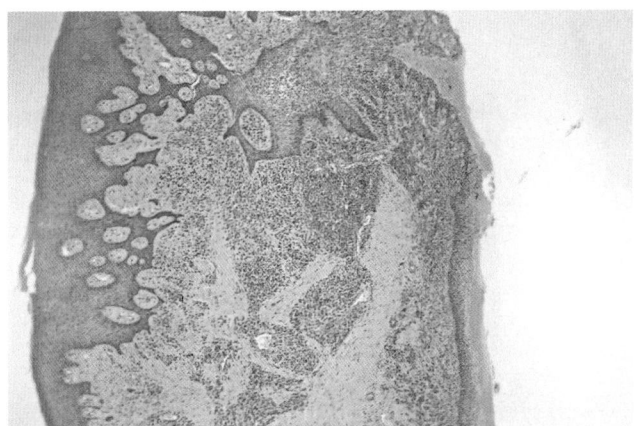

Fig. 19.6 Survey section of chronic inflammatory gingival enlargement shows the inflamed connective tissue core and strands of proliferating epithelium.

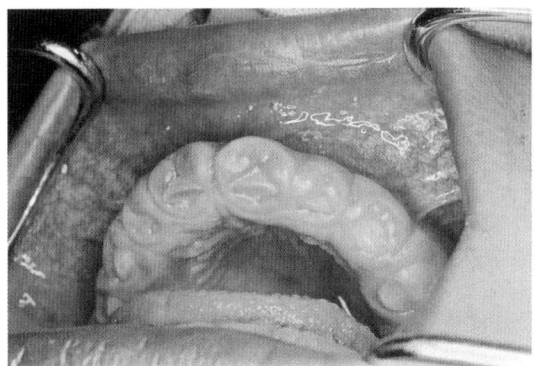

Fig. 19.8 Phenytoin-induced gingival enlargement.

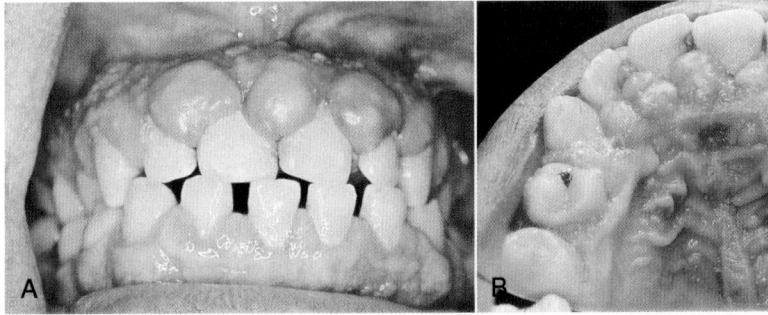

Fig. 19.7 Gingival enlargement associated with phenytoin therapy. (A) Facial view. (B) Occlusal view of the maxillary arch.

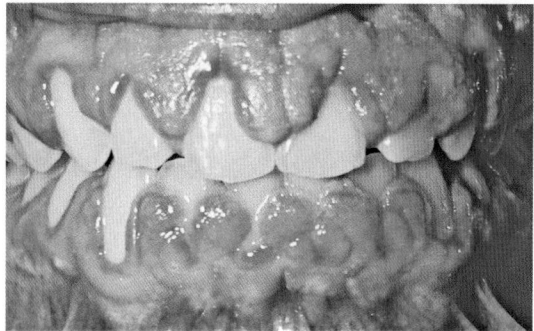

Fig. 19.9 Combined gingival enlargement resulted from the inflammatory involvement of a phenytoin-induced overgrowth.

Anticonvulsants

Phenytoin (diphenylhydantoinate) is the drug of choice for the treatment of grand mal, temporal lobe, and psychomotor seizures, and it has been linked to GO for more than 70 years.[68] Other anticonvulsant agents such as phenobarbital and valproic acid have been associated with GO less often than phenytoin.[62,87] The estimated prevalence of phenytoin-induced GO is about 50%.[22] Clinical onset occurs as early as 1 month, and increasing severity is seen in 12 to 18 months.[1,14,29]

Phenytoin-induced GO lesions frequently occur on the anterior buccal maxilla and mandible, and the entire dentition can be covered in severe cases.[19,63] Phenytoin-induced GO is characterized by enlargement of interdental papillae and increased thickening of the marginal tissues,[4] causing aesthetic and functional problems, such as malpositioning of teeth, difficulty in speech, and impaired oral hygiene.[82]

Calcium Channel Blockers

Calcium channel blockers are a group of drugs commonly used to treat hypertension, angina pectoris, coronary artery spasm, and cardiac arrhythmia.[68] Benzothiazepine derivatives (e.g., diltiazem), phenylalkylamine derivatives (e.g., verapamil), and dyhydropyridines (e.g., amlopidine, felodipine, isradipine, nicardipine, nifedipine, nitrendipine, oxodipine, nimodipine, nisoldipine) are different types of calcium channel blockers that have been associated with some degree of DIGO.[13,15,17,28,64,71,94]

The first case of GO associated with the calcium channel blocker nifedipine was reported in 1984.[85] Among patients taking the medication, the prevalence of nifedipine-induced GO is highly variable, ranging from 6% to 83%.[7,36,37,98] Clinically, interdental papillae are affected, and overgrowth is limited to attached and marginal gingiva, which usually is observed on the anterior segments.[92] Nifedipine-induced GO can coexist with periodontitis and attachment loss that is different from other forms of DIGO.

Immunosuppressants

Cyclosporin A has been the immunosuppressant of choice for preventing rejection of solid organ and bone marrow transplants and for treatment of autoimmune conditions.[45] The prevalence of cyclosporin A–induced GO has been reported to be about 30% but it can be much higher, especially for pediatric populations.[58]

The first case of cyclosporin A–induced GO was reported in 1983.[86] Clinically, the lesions are more inflamed and bleed more than other forms of DIGO, and they commonly are limited to buccal surfaces. Severity of the lesions can be similar to those of phenytoin and nifedipine. They affect the entire dentition and interfere with occlusion, mastication, and speech.[38]

Histopathology

Lesions from different types of DIGO demonstrate significant histologic variations.[106] GO biopsies from patients undergoing treatment with phenytoin show a thick, stratified squamous epithelium with long, thin rete pegs extending deep into the connective tissue.[3,19,33] Fibrosis with minimal inflammatory cell infiltration is a common finding.[105] The histologic characteristics of GO induced by calcium channel blockers are similar to phenytoin-induced lesions, including epithelial thickness, rete peg formation, and excessive matrix accumulation (Fig. 19.10).

Cyclosporin A induced–GO also manifests with a thickened epithelium, rete peg formation, and irregular collagen fibers. These lesions, however, are characterized with more inflammatory infiltration and vascularization compared with phenytoin and calcium channel blockers (Fig. 19.11; see Fig. 19.10).[86]

KEY FACT

Different types of DIGO lesions demonstrate a thick, stratified squamous epithelium with long, thin rete pegs extending deep into the connective tissue. Fibrosis is a common finding in patients with phenytoin-induced GO. Histologic characteristics of GO induced by calcium channel blockers are similar to those of phenytoin-induced lesions, including epithelial thickness, rete peg formation, and excessive matrix accumulation. Cyclosporin A–induced GO lesions have more inflammatory infiltration and increased vascularization compared with GO caused by phenytoin or calcium channel blockers.

Pathogenesis of Drug-Induced Gingival Overgrowth

The pathogenesis of DIGO is complex. The main mechanism is mediated through defective function of gingival fibroblasts. Because gingival fibroblasts are responsible for the matrix deposition of gingival tissues, extensive research has focused on these key cells and their function. Study findings vary, some pathways have not been validated in humans, and data are limited to in vitro and animal studies, but collectively the findings suggest that DIGO-associated medications affect the extracellular matrix metabolism by decreasing collagenase activity and increasing the production of matrix proteins.

Gingival fibroblasts from phenytoin-induced GO are characterized by elevated levels of collagen synthesis.[46] It has been suggested that fibroblasts may be susceptible to the development of DIGO.[46] Gingival fibroblasts from nifedipine-induced GO lesions have defective collagen production due to decreased levels of collagenase activity, which can result in collagen deposition.[103] Through interference with calcium metabolism, calcium channel blockers decrease calcium levels in gingival fibroblasts and T cells, thereby affecting T-cell proliferation or activation and collagen biosynthesis.[7,103]

Cyclosporin A directly impairs collagen synthesis by gingival fibroblasts,[67] with a concomitant rise in the levels of type I collagen.[90] Cyclosporin A also decreases expression of matrix metalloproteinase-1 (MMP-1) and MMP-3.[12] In addition to collagen, which is the major extracellular matrix component of gingival tissues, noncollagenous matrix is affected by the medications that result in DIGO. Glycosaminoglycan metabolism is impaired in patients with phenytoin-induced GO[32] and in response to cyclosporin A treatment of gingival fibroblasts.[76]

In addition to fibroblast metabolism and function, inflammatory regulation of tissue turnover is a major factor in DIGO pathogenesis. Fibroblast functions such as proliferation, differentiation, and production of extracellular matrix are affected by levels of cytokines and

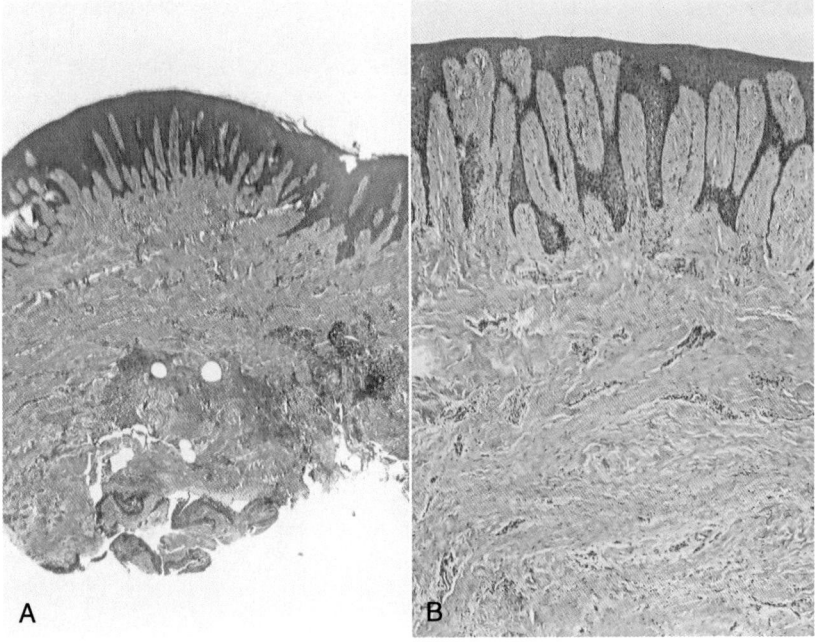

Fig. 19.10 Microscopic view of gingival enlargement associated with phenytoin therapy. (A) Hyperplasia and acanthosis of the epithelium and densely collagenous connective tissue are seen with evidence of inflammation in the area adjacent to the gingival sulcus. (B) High-power view shows extension of deep rete pegs into the connective tissue.

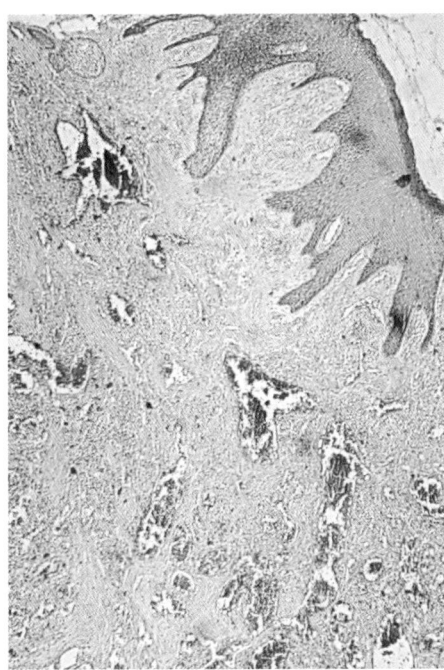

Fig. 19.11 Microscopic view of cyclosporine-associated gingival enlargement.

growth factors. GO lesions are characterized by increased levels of interleukin-6 (IL-6), IL-1β, platelet-derived growth factor subunit B (PDGFB), fibroblast growth factor 2 (FGF2), transforming growth factor-β (TGF-β), and connective tissue growth factor (CTGF).[6,16,31,48,50,73,75,83,88,89,106,108] Macrophages are the main source of these cytokines.[18,23,30,34,80]

The TGF-β1–CTGF axis has been characterized in detail and is an essential mechanism leading to DIGO. TGF-β1 regulates cell proliferation and differentiation and can activate gene expression for the synthesis of extracellular matrix components, including collagen in cyclosporin A–induced GO.[53,88] TGF-β1 induces CTGF mRNA and protein expression in human gingival fibroblasts; the TGF-β1–CTGF pathway directly regulates fibrosis, gingival fibroblast lysyl oxidase, and collagen generation.[48] CTGF expression is increased in all forms of DIGO, with the highest levels occurring in phenytoin-induced GO, which also has the highest levels of fibrosis.[106]

CTGF expression is not limited to the connective tissue. It also is demonstrated in the gingival epithelium, predominantly in the basal epithelial cells close to the connective tissue border.[55] In vitro studies showed that CTGF could be produced by gingival epithelial cells,[55] illustrating a possible mechanism of fibrosis in gingiva, which may be related to crosstalk between epithelial and connective tissue cells. Studies revealed a unique mechanism for TGF-β1–induced CTGF expression in gingival fibroblasts regulated by prostaglandin E₂, cAMP, mitogen-activated protein kinases (MAPKs), and activation of Jun N-terminal kinases (JNKs).[11]

A key event in the pathogenetic mechanism of DIGO is some degree of epithelial-mesenchymal transition induced by medications. Highly fibrotic tissues are characterized by increased epithelial-mesenchymal transition, through which epithelial cells in the gingiva acquire fibroblast function, and the process is regulated by CTGF.[100] The molecular pathways of DIGO have been reviewed elsewhere.[105]

Treatment

DIGO cannot be prevented by conventional approaches, but it can be ameliorated by elimination of local factors, plaque control, and regular periodontal maintenance. The most effective treatment of DIGO is withdrawal or substitution of medications. A case report showed resolution of gingival lesions in 1 to 8 weeks after discontinuing the medication.[57] For example, changing nifedipine to another antihypertensive drug, isradipine, caused regression of gingival enlargement.[107] Tacrolimus, used as an alternative for cyclosporin A, resulted in regression of gingival enlargement.[52] However, most alternatives have also been linked to DIGO in recent years.

In addition to withdrawal or substitution of medication, scaling and root planing have given relief to patients with GO.[99] Nonsurgical treatment can eliminate the inflammatory component of DIGO, which can account for 40% of tissue enlargement.[56]

Because the anterior labial gingiva is frequently affected, surgery is commonly performed to solve aesthetic problems. Surgical elimination of DIGO lesions involves gingivectomy and gingivoplasty.[51] However, the recurrence rate is high; the recurrence rate for GO among patients taking cyclosporin A or nifedipine was approximately 40% 18 months after the surgery.[51]

Patients should be given oral hygiene instructions, and periodontal prophylaxis and removal of calculus should be done as needed during recall visits. New pharmacologic strategies, especially using animal models, are being explored.[5]

! CLINICAL CORRELATION

DIGO cannot be prevented, but it can be ameliorated by elimination of local factors, plaque control, and regular periodontal maintenance. The most effective treatment for drug-induced gingival overgrowth is withdrawal or substitution of the medication. Nonsurgical treatment results in elimination of the inflammatory component of DIGO. Surgical elimination of DIGO lesions involves gingivectomy and gingivoplasty. The recurrence rate is high. Maintenance should include oral hygiene instructions, periodontal prophylaxis, and removal of calculus as needed.

Gingival Overgrowth Associated With Systemic Conditions

Changes in systemic conditions can lead to gingival enlargement. The causes and clinical features of GO associated with systemic conditions are diverse and usually manifest with amplification of existing inflammation due to bacterial inflammation. These gingival pathologies are referred as *conditioned enlargements* and include lesions associated with hormonal and nutritional etiologic factors. Gingival inflammation due to microbial factors is a prerequisite that hormonal and nutritional changes modify, and some researchers classify these lesions as gingivitis-associated pathologies. However, pregnancy and puberty have been established as causes for hormonal changes. Nutritional factors are rare but have historically included deficits such as vitamin C deficiency. Likewise, allergic reactions may be linked to GO.

Pregnancy-Associated Gingival Overgrowth
Clinical Manifestations

GO is a common pathology in pregnancy. Clinically, it manifests as a single mass or multiple tumor-like masses at the gingival margin. Marginal gingival enlargement during pregnancy results from the aggravation of previous inflammation, and its incidence has been reported as 10% to 70%. Sometimes, the lesions can be observed as single enlargements, which are referred to as *pregnancy tumors*. Pregnancy tumors are not neoplasms; they represent an inflammatory response to microbial plaque modified by the patient's condition. It usually appears after the third month of pregnancy, but it may occur earlier. The reported incidence is 1.8% to 5%.[65]

Overall, pregnancy-associated GO manifests with a highly varied clinical picture. Enlargement is usually generalized, but it tends to be more prominent interproximally than on the facial and lingual surfaces. The enlarged gingiva is bright red or magenta, soft, and friable, and it has a smooth, shiny surface. Bleeding occurs spontaneously or on slight provocation. The lesion appears as a discrete, mushroom-like, flattened spherical mass that protrudes from the gingival margin or, more often, from the interproximal space, and

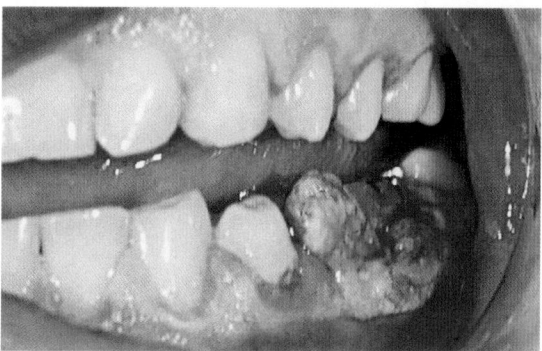

Fig. 19.12 Localized gingival enlargement in a 27-year-old, pregnant patient.

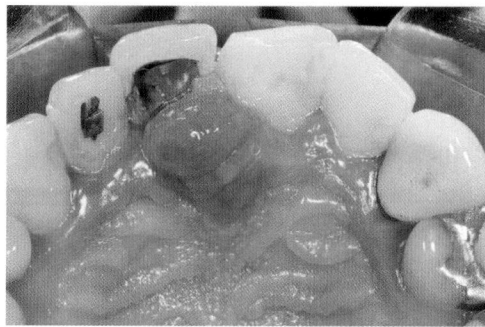

Fig. 19.13 Pyogenic granuloma. *(Courtesy Dr. Silvia Oreamuno, San Jose, Costa Rica.)*

it is attached by a sessile or pedunculated base (Fig. 19.12). It tends to expand laterally, and pressure from the tongue and the cheek perpetuates its flattened appearance. It is dusky red or magenta; it has a smooth, glistening surface that often exhibits numerous deep red, pinpoint markings.

The superficial lesion of pregnancy-associated GO usually does not invade the underlying bone. The mass is usually firm, but it may have various degrees of softness and friability. It is usually painless unless its size and shape foster the accumulation of debris under its margin or interfere with occlusion, in which case painful ulceration may occur. Although the microscopic findings are characteristic of gingival enlargement during pregnancy, they are not pathognomonic.

Pyogenic granuloma is similar in clinical and microscopic appearance to the gingival enlargement seen during pregnancy. This lesion manifests as a tumor-like gingival enlargement that is considered to be an exaggerated response to minor trauma (Fig. 19.13). The exact nature of the systemic conditioning factor has not been identified. The differential diagnosis is based on the patient's history.[9]

Etiology

Hormonal changes have always been linked to pathology in periodontal tissues. For example, progesterone and estrogen levels increase 10 to 30 times by the end of the third trimester compared with the menstrual cycle.[2] Although mechanistic evidence is lacking, it is hypothesized that these hormonal changes induce an increased vascular permeability, which leads to gingival edema and an increased inflammatory response to dental plaque. During this process, the impaired vascular response and inflammatory milieu can lead to modification of the subgingival microbiota. Although not specific, an increased presence of *Prevotella intermedia, Prevotella melaninogenica,* and *Porphyromonas gingivalis* has been linked to pregnancy-associated GO in vivo and in vitro,[60,61,84] demonstrating that the lesions have strong infectious associations.

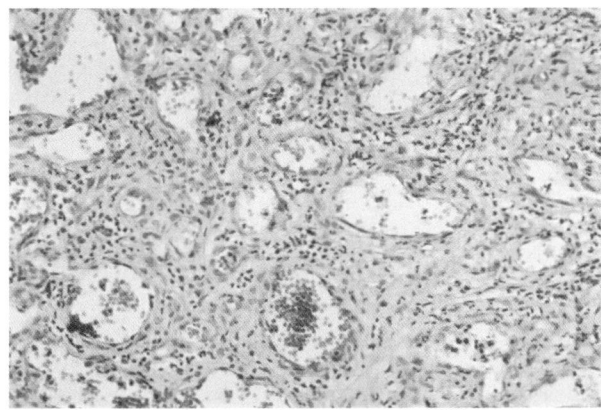

Fig. 19.14 Microscopic view of gingival enlargement in a pregnant patient.

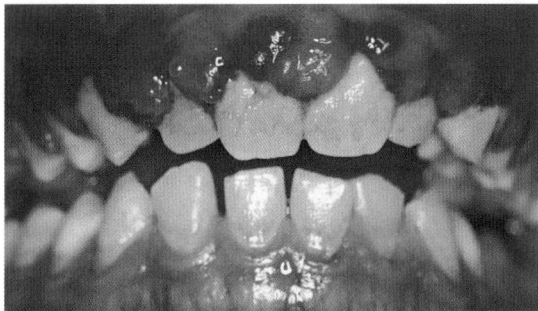

Fig. 19.15 Conditioned gingival enlargement during puberty.

Histopathology

Gingival enlargement in pregnancy is called *angiogranuloma,* referring to its strong clinical presentation with vascular changes and fibrotic process. Marginal and tumor-like enlargements consist of a central mass of connective tissue, with numerous diffusely arranged, newly formed, and engorged capillaries lined by cuboid endothelial cells (Fig. 19.14) and of a moderately fibrous stroma with various degrees of edema and chronic inflammatory infiltrate. The stratified squamous epithelium is thickened, with prominent rete pegs and some degree of intracellular and extracellular edema, prominent intercellular bridges, and leukocytic infiltration.

Treatment

Similar to other forms of gingival changes associated with hormonal variations during pregnancy, GO lesions can be prevented by good oral hygiene. Oral care in pregnant women should be meticulous, and patients should be treated by removal of plaque and calculus. Severe cases may require removal during the second trimester; however, removal of the GO lesions without establishment of an optimal oral hygiene regimen ensures recurrence of gingival enlargement. Although spontaneous reduction in the size of gingival enlargement typically follows the termination of pregnancy, complete elimination of the residual inflammatory lesion and GO requires removal of all plaque deposits, elimination of factors that favor its accumulation, and in some fibrotic cases, surgical intervention.

Treatment of pyogenic granuloma consists of the removal of the lesions and the elimination of irritating local factors. The recurrence rate of pyogenic granuloma is about 15%.

Puberty-Associated Gingival Overgrowth

Clinical Manifestations

Enlargement of the gingiva is sometimes seen during puberty. The lesions are not specific to female gender; they occur in male and female adolescents. Clinically, there is a strong association with plaque accumulation. The lesions are usually marginal and interdental, and they are characterized by prominent bulbous interproximal papillae (Fig. 19.15). Often, only the facial gingivae are enlarged, and the lingual surfaces are relatively unaltered. The mechanical action of the tongue and the excursion of food prevent a heavy accumulation of local irritants on the lingual surface.

Etiology

Gingival enlargement during puberty has all of the clinical features that are associated with chronic inflammatory gingival disease. The degree of enlargement and its tendency to recur in the setting of relatively scant plaque deposits distinguish puberty-associated GO from purely gingivitis-associated lesions, suggesting a profound impact by the hormonal changes. The incidence of puberty-associated GO lesions decline with age,[101] further supporting the role of hormonal changes during puberty.

Studies of the subgingival microbiota of children between the ages of 11 and 14 years and their association with clinical parameters implicated *Capnocytophaga* species in the initiation of pubertal gingivitis.[40,72] Other studies have reported that hormonal changes coincide with an increase in the proportion of *Prevotella intermedia* and *Prevotella nigrescens.*[74,110] The etiologic role of the changes in microbiota, however, is not clear. It is not known whether changes in inflammatory conditions predispose to a shift in microbial species.

Histopathology

The microscopic appearance of gingival enlargement during puberty is one of chronic inflammation with prominent edema. It cannot be distinguished from other forms of gingivitis-associated GO lesions.

Treatment

After puberty, enlargement undergoes spontaneous reduction, but it does not disappear completely until the plaque and calculus are removed.

Nutrition-Associated Gingival Overgrowth

Malnutrition has been historically associated with several oral lesions. GO has been observed in cases of chronic vitamin C deficiency in patients with scurvy. These lesions are no longer common, but GO is still considered a part of the classic description of scurvy.

Clinical Manifestations

Gingival enlargement with vitamin C deficiency is marginal. The gingiva is bluish red, soft, and friable, and it has a smooth, shiny surface. Hemorrhage that occurs spontaneously or on slight provocation and surface necrosis with pseudomembrane formations are common features.

Etiology

Acute vitamin C deficiency alone does not cause gingival inflammation, but it does cause hemorrhage, collagen degeneration, and edema of the gingival connective tissue. These changes modify the response of the gingiva to plaque to the extent that the normal defensive delimiting reaction is inhibited and the extent of the inflammation is exaggerated, thereby resulting in the massive gingival enlargement seen in patients with scurvy (Fig. 19.16).

Histopathology

In patients with vitamin C deficiency, the gingiva has a chronic inflammatory cellular infiltration with a superficial acute response. There are scattered areas of hemorrhage with engorged capillaries.

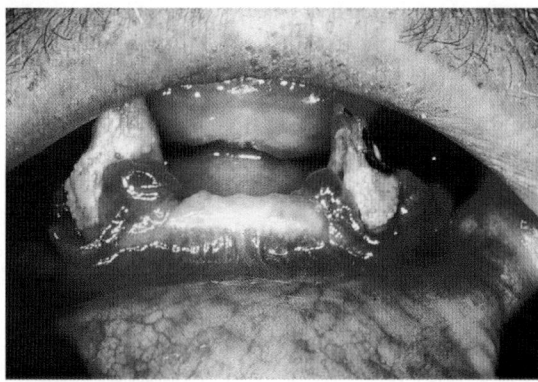

Fig. 19.16 Gingival enlargement in a patient with vitamin C deficiency. *(Courtesy Dr. Gerald Shklar, Boston, MA.)*

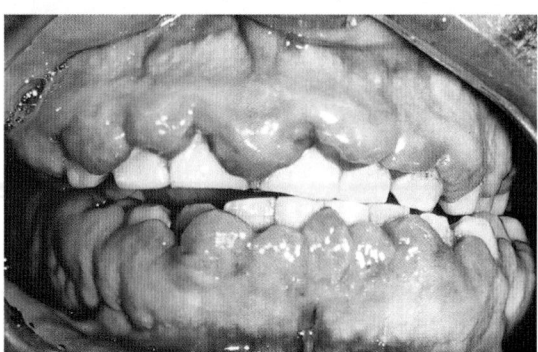

Fig. 19.17 Leukemia-associated gingival enlargement *(Courtesy Dr. Spencer Wolfe, Dublin, Ireland.)*

Marked diffuse edema, collagen degeneration, and a scarcity of collagen fibrils and fibroblasts are striking findings.

Treatment

Nutrition-associated GO lesions are rare. Changes in nutrition accompanied by nonsurgical treatment and good oral hygiene usually result in complete resolution of the pathology. In rare cases, surgical removal may be indicated.

Gingival Overgrowth Associated With Systemic Diseases

GO may be linked to various systemic diseases. Although uncommon and occurring with different etiopathogenetic mechanisms, the GO associated with systemic diseases can be linked to serious issues in clinical management. These lesions should be carefully diagnosed.

Leukemia-Associated Gingival Overgrowth

Clinical Manifestations

Leukemic gingival enlargement can be diffuse or marginal and localized or generalized. It can appear as a diffuse enlargement of the gingival mucosa, an oversized extension of the marginal gingiva (Fig. 19.17), or a discrete tumor-like interproximal mass. In patients with leukemic enlargement, the gingiva is bluish red, and it has a shiny surface. The consistency is moderately firm, but there is a tendency toward friability and hemorrhage that occur spontaneously or with slight irritation.

Acute painful necrotizing ulcerative inflammatory involvement can occur in the crevice formed at the junction of the enlarged gingiva and the contiguous tooth surfaces. Patients with leukemia may also have a simple chronic inflammation without the involvement of leukemic cells, and they can have the same clinical and microscopic features seen in patients without the systemic disease. Most cases,

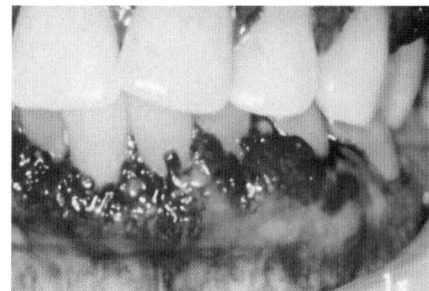

Fig. 19.18 Wegener granulomatosis affecting the gingival tissue.

however, have features of simple chronic inflammation and leukemic infiltrate. True leukemic enlargement often occurs with acute leukemia, but it may also be seen with subacute leukemia. It seldom occurs with chronic leukemia.

Histopathology

Gingival enlargements in leukemic patients show various degrees of chronic inflammation. Mature leukocytes are seen along with areas of connective tissue that are infiltrated with a dense mass of immature and proliferating leukocytes, the specific nature of which varies with the type of leukemia. Engorged capillaries, edematous and degenerated connective tissue, and epithelium with various degrees of leukocytic infiltration and edema are found. Isolated surface areas of acute necrotizing inflammation with a pseudomembranous meshwork of fibrin, necrotic epithelial cells, polymorphonuclear leukocytes, and bacteria are often seen.

Wegener Granulomatosis

Clinical Manifestations

Wegener granulomatosis is a rare disease that is characterized by acute granulomatous necrotizing lesions of the respiratory tract, including nasal and oral defects. Renal lesions develop, and acute necrotizing vasculitis affects the blood vessels. The initial manifestations of Wegener granulomatosis can involve the orofacial region and include oral mucosal ulceration, gingival enlargement, abnormal tooth mobility, exfoliation of teeth, and a delayed healing response. The granulomatous papillary enlargement is reddish purple and bleeds easily on stimulation (Fig. 19.18).

Etiology

The cause of Wegener granulomatosis is unknown, but the condition is considered an immunologically mediated tissue injury. At one time the usual outcome for patients with this condition was death from kidney failure within a few months, but more recently the use of immunosuppressive drugs has produced prolonged remissions in more than 90% of patients.

Histopathology

Chronic inflammation involves scattered giant cells, foci of acute inflammation, and microabscesses covered by a thin, acanthotic epithelium. Vascular changes have not been described with gingival enlargement in patients with Wegener granulomatosis, probably because of the small size of the gingival blood vessels.

Sarcoidosis

Clinical Manifestations

Sarcoidosis is a granulomatous disease of unknown etiology. It starts in individuals during their 20s or 30s, it predominantly affects blacks, and it can involve almost any organ, including the gingiva, in which a red, smooth, painless enlargement may appear.

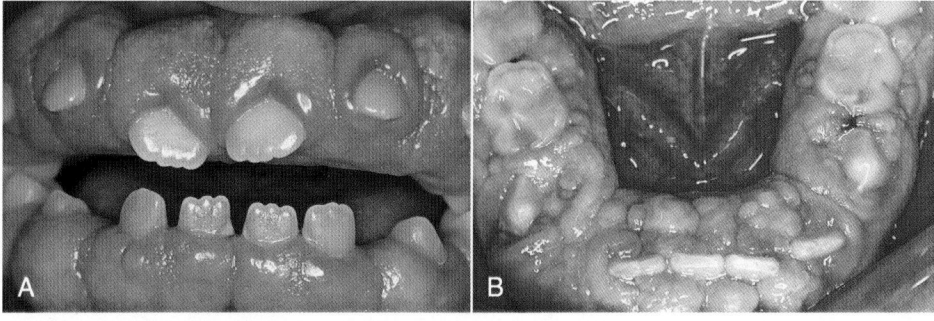

Fig. 19.19 Idiopathic gingival enlargement. (A) Facial view. (B) Occlusal view of the mandibular arch.

Histopathology

Sarcoid granulomas consist of discrete epithelioid cells and multinucleated, foreign body–type giant cells with peripheral mononuclear cells.

Gingival Fibromatosis

Clinical Manifestations

Gingival fibromatosis can be hereditary or idiopathic. These lesions are rare and occur in highly fibrotic forms of GO.[39,109] Hereditary gingival fibromatosis is the most common form, and it has been linked to several genetic loci.[8,26,42,43,96,112,113] Idiopathic gingival enlargement is a rare condition of undetermined cause.

The enlargement affects the attached gingiva, the gingival margin, and the interdental papillae. The facial and lingual surfaces of the mandible and maxilla usually are affected, but the involvement may be limited to either jaw. The enlarged gingiva is pink, firm, and almost leathery in consistency, and it has a characteristic minutely pebbled surface (Fig. 19.19). In severe cases, the teeth are almost completely covered, and the enlargement projects into the oral vestibule. The jaws appear distorted because of the bulbous enlargement of the gingiva. Secondary inflammatory changes are common at the gingival margin.

Etiology

The genetic basis of hereditary gingival fibromatosis is well established, with different populations having different genetic loci and specific genes.[27,41,44,49,69,77,79,97,114,115] In some families, gingival enlargement is linked to the impairment of physical development. Other syndromes are sometimes colocalized with gingival fibromatosis.[47,66] Idiopathic forms of gingival fibromatosis have not been linked to specific genes, and the condition is designated as idiopathic.

KEY FACT

The genetic basis of hereditary gingival fibromatosis is well established. In some families, gingival enlargement is linked to impairment of physical development. Other syndromes can coexist with gingival fibromatosis. Idiopathic forms of gingival fibromatosis have not been linked to any specific genes.

Although the genes associated with lesions of hereditary forms have been identified, the pathogenetic mechanisms linked to these genetic factors are not fully understood. Enlargement usually begins with the eruption of the primary or secondary dentition, and it may regress after extraction, which suggests that the teeth or the plaque attached to them may be initiating factors. The presence of bacterial plaque is a complicating factor. Gingival enlargement has been described in tuberous sclerosis, which is an inherited condition

characterized by the triad of epilepsy, mental deficiency, and cutaneous angiofibromas.

Histopathology

In cases of GO with fibromatosis, the lesions are highly fibrotic, with a bulbous increase in connective tissue that is relatively avascular and consists of densely arranged collagen bundles and numerous fibroblasts. The surface epithelium is thickened and acanthotic, with elongated rete pegs.[21,54,55] Histopathology is similar to phenytoin-induced GO with low levels of inflammatory infiltration. However, collagen bundle formation, dominance, and orientation are distinctive in areas where cellular structures are reduced.[21]

Treatment

Treatment of GO lesions manifesting as gingival fibromatosis requires gingivectomy and gingivoplasty. Clinical management is difficult because of the high recurrence rate, and the severity of lesions usually results in extreme crowding and misalignment of teeth. After removal of the fibromatosis lesions, patients may require orthodontic treatment.[25]

Other Forms of Gingival Enlargement

Multiple forms of gingival enlargement have various causes. In addition to the types of GO previously discussed in this chapter, the gingiva can be enlarged due to increases in the size of the underlying osseous and dental tissues. These *false enlargements* usually have no abnormal clinical features except for the massive increase in the size of the area. For example, enlargement of the bone subjacent to the gingival area occurs most often with tori and exostoses, but it can also occur with Paget disease, fibrous dysplasia, cherubism, central giant cell granuloma, ameloblastoma, osteoma, and osteosarcoma.

The gingival tissue can appear normal, or it can have unrelated inflammatory changes. Likewise, during the various stages of eruption, particularly of the primary dentition, the labial gingiva can have a bulbous marginal distortion caused by superimposition of the bulk of the gingiva on the normal prominence of the enamel in the gingival half of the crown. This enlargement is called *developmental enlargement,* and it often persists until the junctional epithelium has migrated from the enamel to the cementoenamel junction.

In a strict sense, developmental gingival enlargements are physiologic, and they usually present no problems for patients. However, when the enlargement is complicated by marginal inflammation, the composite picture gives the impression of extensive gingival enlargement (Fig. 19.20).

Neoplastic formations in gingival tissues can be clinically confused with fibrotic enlargements of gingiva. Oral cancer accounts for less than 3% of all malignant tumors in the body, but it is the 6th most common cancer in males and the 12th most common in females. The gingiva is not a common site of oral malignancy, accounting for only 6% of oral cancers.

Epulis is a generic term that is used to clinically designate all discrete tumors and tumor-like masses of the gingiva. It serves to locate the tumor but does not describe it. Most lesions referred to by this term are inflammatory rather than neoplastic. For example, fibromas arise from the gingival connective tissue or from the periodontal ligament. They are slow-growing, spherical tumors that tend to be firm and nodular but that may be soft and vascular. Fibromas are usually pedunculated. Hard fibromas of the gingiva are rare; most of the lesions that are diagnosed clinically as fibromas are inflammatory enlargements.

Histopathologic review of fibromas demonstrates bundles of well-formed collagen fibers with scattered fibrocytes and various degrees of vascularity. The so-called giant cell fibroma contains multinucleated fibroblasts. In another variant, mineralized tissue (i.e., bone, cementum-like material, and dystrophic calcifications) can be found; this type of fibroma is called *peripheral ossifying fibroma.*

Similar to fibromas, papillomas are benign proliferations of surface epithelium that are in many cases associated with human papillomavirus (HPV) infection. Gingival papillomas appear as solitary wartlike or cauliflower-like protuberances (Fig. 19.21). They can be small and discrete, or they can be broad, hard elevations with minutely irregular surfaces. The lesions consist of finger-like projections of stratified squamous epithelium that are often hyperkeratotic, with central cores of fibrovascular connective tissue.

Peripheral giant cell granulomas of the gingiva arise interdentally or from the gingival margin. They occur most frequently on the labial surface, and they can be sessile or pedunculated. They vary in appearance from smooth, regularly outlined masses to irregularly shaped, multilobulated protuberances with surface indentations (Fig. 19.22). Ulceration of the margin is occasionally seen. The lesions are painless, vary in size, and can cover several teeth. They can be firm or spongy, and their color varies from pink to deep red or purplish blue.

Clinically, peripheral giant cell granulomas cannot be easily differentiated from other forms of gingival enlargement. Microscopic examination is required for definitive diagnosis. The word *peripheral* is needed to differentiate them from comparable lesions that originate within the jawbone (i.e., central giant cell granulomas). In some cases, the giant cell granuloma of the gingiva is locally invasive and causes destruction of the underlying bone (Fig. 19.23A). Complete removal leads to uneventful recovery. The lesion has numerous foci of multinuclear giant cells and hemosiderin particles in a connective tissue stroma (see Fig. 19.23B). Areas of chronic inflammation are

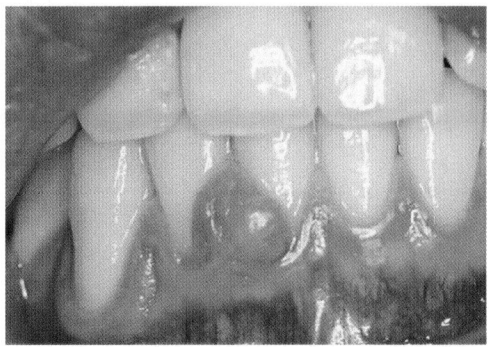

Fig. 19.21 Papilloma of the gingiva.

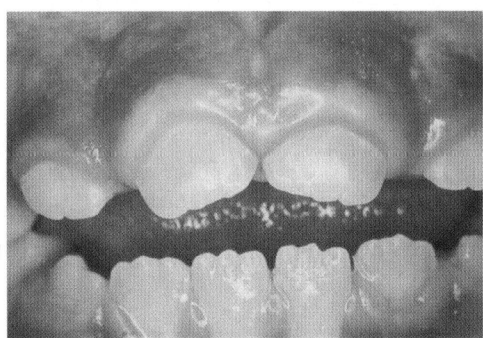

Fig. 19.20 Developmental gingival enlargement.

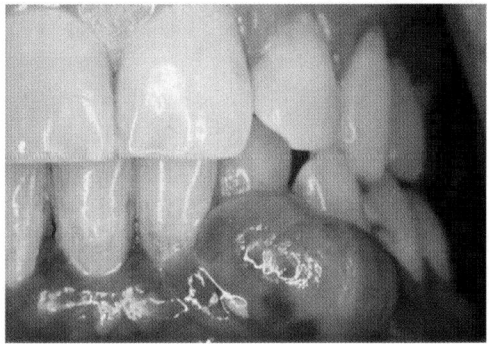

Fig. 19.22 Gingival giant cell granuloma.

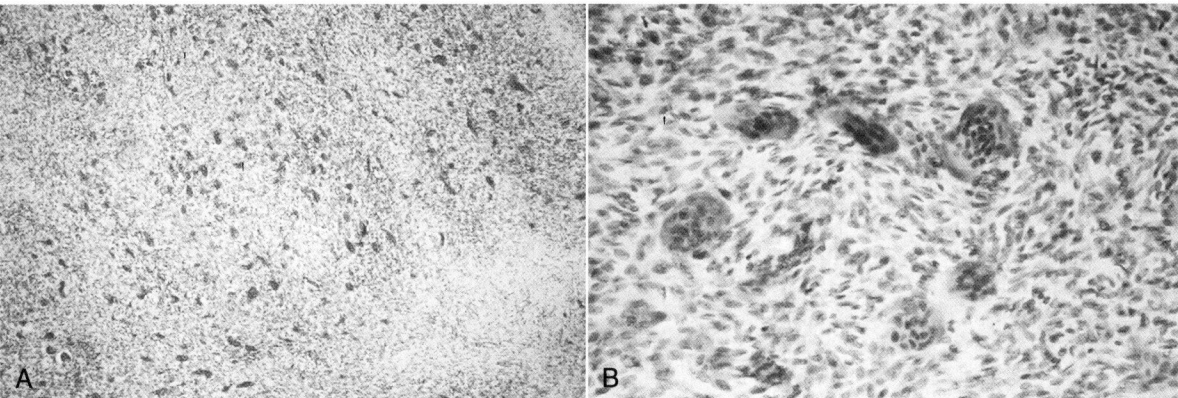

Fig. 19.23 (A) Microscopic survey of a peripheral giant cell granuloma. (B) High-power microscopic study of the lesion demonstrates the giant cells and the intervening stroma.

scattered throughout the lesion, with acute involvement occurring at the surface. The overlying epithelium is usually hyperplastic, with ulceration at the base. Bone destruction occasionally occurs within the lesion (Fig. 19.24).

Gingival cysts of microscopic proportions are common, but they seldom reach a clinically significant size. When they do, they appear as localized enlargements that may involve the marginal and attached gingiva. The cysts occur in the mandibular canine and premolar areas, most often on the lingual surface. They are painless, but with expansion they can cause erosion of the surface of the alveolar bone. The gingival cyst should be differentiated from the lateral periodontal cyst, which arises within the alveolar bone adjacent to the root and which is developmental in origin. Gingival cysts develop from odontogenic epithelium or from surface or sulcular epithelium traumatically implanted in the area. Removal is followed by uneventful recovery.

A gingival cyst cavity is lined by a thin, flattened epithelium with or without localized areas of thickening. Less frequently, the following types of epithelium can be found: unkeratinized stratified squamous epithelium, keratinized stratified squamous epithelium, and parakeratinized epithelium with palisading basal cells.

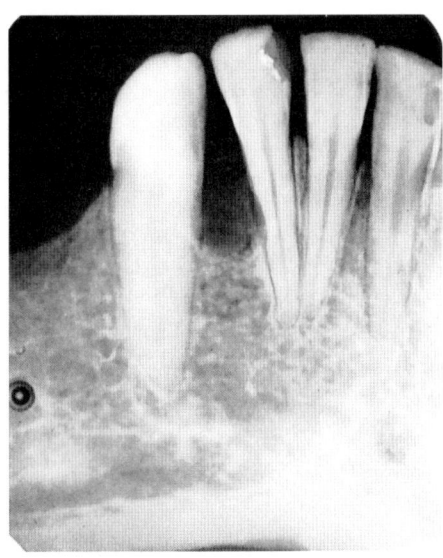

Fig. 19.24 Bone destruction in the interproximal space between the canine and the lateral incisor is caused by the extension of a peripheral giant cell reparative granuloma of the gingiva. *(Courtesy Dr. Sam Toll.)*

Squamous cell carcinoma is the most common malignant tumor of the gingiva. It may be *exophytic,* manifesting as an irregular outgrowth, or *ulcerative,* appearing as a flat, erosive lesion. It is often symptom free, going unnoticed until complicated by inflammatory changes that can mask the neoplasm but cause pain; it sometimes becomes evident after tooth extraction. These masses are locally invasive, and they involve the underlying bone and periodontal ligament of adjoining teeth and the adjacent mucosa (Fig. 19.25). Metastasis is usually confined to the region above the clavicle; however, involvement that is more extensive can include the lung, liver, or bone.

Malignant melanoma is a rare oral tumor that tends to occur in the hard palate and maxillary gingiva of older persons. It is usually darkly pigmented, and it is often preceded by localized pigmentation. It can be flat or nodular, and it is characterized by rapid growth and early metastasis. It arises from melanoblasts in the gingiva, cheek, or palate. Infiltration into the underlying bone and metastasis to cervical and axillary lymph nodes are common.

Fibrosarcoma, lymphosarcoma, and reticulum cell sarcoma of the gingiva are rare; only isolated cases have been described in the literature. Kaposi sarcoma often occurs in the oral cavity, particularly in the palate and the gingiva, of patients with acquired immunodeficiency syndrome. Tumor metastasis to the gingiva occurs infrequently.

The low incidence of oral malignancy should not mislead the clinician. Ulcerations that do not respond to therapy in the usual manner and all gingival tumors and tumor-like lesions must be biopsied and submitted for microscopic diagnosis.

In most clinical cases of GO, the clinical appearance is complicated by inflammation, bleeding, and swelling, which further creates difficulty in identifying the cause and pathologic process. A thorough knowledge of GO and the patient's systemic and oral medical histories are critical for designing the treatment and maintaining outcomes. Because some GO forms are linked to systemic and severe diseases, this approach is also essential for securing the patient's safety before treatment is initiated.

 A Case Scenario is found on the companion website www.expertconsult.com.

References

 References for this chapter are found on the companion website www.expertconsult.com.

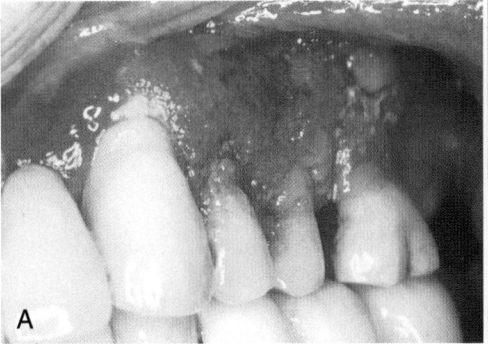
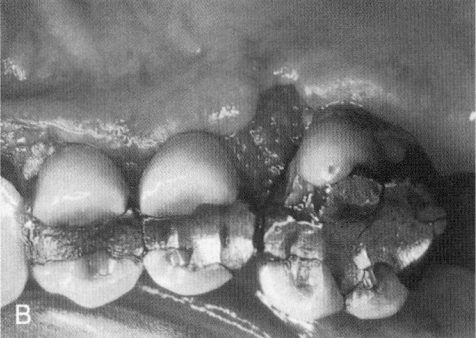

Fig. 19.25 Squamous cell carcinoma of the gingiva. (A) Facial view shows extensive verrucous involvement. (B) Palatal view shows mulberry-like tissue emerging between the second premolar and the first molar.

CHAPTER 20

Acute Gingival Infections

Perry R. Klokkevold | Fermin A. Carranza

CHAPTER OUTLINE

Necrotizing Ulcerative Gingivitis
Primary Herpetic Gingivostomatitis
Pericoronitis
Conclusions

Necrotizing Ulcerative Gingivitis

Necrotizing ulcerative gingivitis (NUG) is a microbial disease of the gingiva that most often occurs in an impaired host. It manifests with the characteristic clinical signs of necrosis and sloughing of the gingival tissues and may be accompanied by systemic symptoms.

Clinical Features

NUG has historically been identified as an acute disease. However, the term *acute* in this case is used as a clinical descriptor and not a diagnosis because chronic forms of the disease do not exist. Although the acronym *ANUG* is frequently used, it is a misnomer.[60] A summary of acute periodontal lesions advocated the more simplified term, *necrotizing gingivitis,* rather than *necrotizing ulcerative gingivitis,* but the latter term continues to be used in this chapter.[29] Involvement can be limited to a single tooth or group of teeth, or it can be widespread throughout the mouth (Fig. 20.1).

More advanced forms of necrotizing ulcerative disease can include destruction of the periodontal attachment apparatus, including bone,[41] especially in patients with long-standing disease or severe immunosuppression. When periodontal attachment loss and bone loss occurs, the condition is called *necrotizing ulcerative periodontitis* (NUP) (see Chapter 29).

History

NUG is characterized by a sudden onset of symptoms, sometimes occurring after an episode of debilitating disease or acute respiratory tract infection. A change in living habits, protracted work without adequate rest, poor nutrition, tobacco use, and psychological stress are common features of the patient's history.

Oral Signs

Characteristic lesions are punched-out, craterlike depressions at the crest of the interdental papillae that subsequently extend to the marginal gingiva and rarely to the attached gingiva and oral mucosa. The surface of the gingival crater is covered by a gray, pseudomembranous slough that is demarcated from the remainder of the gingival mucosa by a pronounced linear erythema (see Fig. 20.1A). In some cases, the lesions are denuded of the surface pseudomembrane, thereby exposing the gingival margin, which is red, shiny, and hemorrhagic.

The characteristic lesions can progressively destroy the gingiva and the underlying periodontal tissues (see Fig. 20.1B).

Spontaneous gingival hemorrhage and pronounced bleeding after the slightest stimulation are additional characteristic clinical signs (see Fig. 20.1B and C). Other common signs include a fetid odor and increased salivation.

NUG can occur in otherwise disease-free mouths, or it can be superimposed on chronic gingivitis or periodontitis with periodontal pockets. However, NUG does not usually lead to periodontal pocket formation because the necrotic changes involve the gingival and junctional epithelium; healthy epithelium is needed for periodontal pocket deepening (see Chapter 23). Although the numbers are much less, spirochetes and fusiform bacilli are found on normal edentulous mucosa.[59]

KEY FACT

Necrotizing ulcerative gingivitis can be superimposed on chronic periodontitis with pockets, but it does not usually lead to pocket formation because the necrotic changes involve the gingival and junctional epithelium.

Oral Symptoms

The lesions are extremely sensitive to touch, and the patient often complains of a constant radiating, gnawing pain that is intensified by eating spicy or hot foods and chewing. There is a metallic foul taste, and the patient is conscious of an excessive amount of pasty saliva.

Extraoral and Systemic Signs and Symptoms

Patients are usually ambulatory and have a minimum of systemic symptoms. Local lymphadenopathy and a slight elevation in temperature are common features of the mild and moderate stages of the disease. In severe cases, patients can have high fever, increased pulse rate, leukocytosis, loss of appetite, and general lassitude. Systemic reactions are more severe in children. Insomnia, constipation, gastrointestinal disorders, headache, and mental depression sometimes accompany the condition.

In rare cases, severe sequelae such as gangrenous stomatitis and noma have been described.[2,3,18,33] These patients are almost exclusively encountered in populations in developing countries, especially children with systemic disease or malnutrition.[18,29,60]

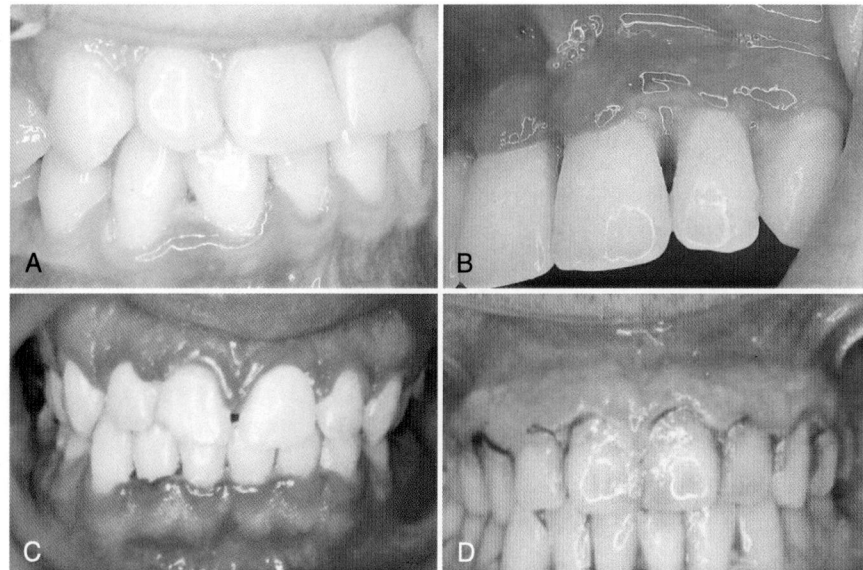

Fig. 20.1 Necrotizing ulcerative gingivitis. (A) Typical punched-out papilla between the mandibular canine and lateral incisor is covered by a grayish white pseudomembrane. (B) More advanced case shows the destruction of the papillae, which results in an irregular marginal contour. (C) Typical lesions with spontaneous hemorrhage. (D) Generalized involvement of the papillae and the marginal gingiva with whitish necrotic lesions.

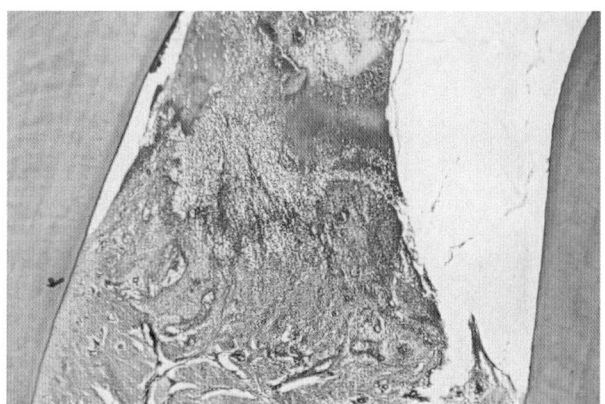

Fig. 20.2 In a survey section of interdental papilla in a patient with necrotizing ulcerative gingivitis, the necrotic tissue forms the gray marginal pseudomembrane *(top)*. Ulceration and the accumulation of leukocytes and fibrin replace normal epithelium *(bottom)*.

Clinical Course

The clinical course varies among individuals. The severity of NUG often diminishes without treatment, leading to a subacute stage with milder clinical symptoms. Some patients experience repeated remissions and exacerbations, and the condition can recur in previously treated patients. If untreated, especially in an immunocompromised host, NUG can lead to progressive destruction of the periodontium and gingival recession accompanied by an increase in the severity of systemic complications.[31,52]

Histopathology

Microscopically, the NUG lesion is a nonspecific acute necrotizing inflammation of the gingival margin that involves the stratified squamous epithelium and the underlying connective tissue. The surface epithelium is destroyed and replaced by a meshwork of fibrin, necrotic epithelial cells, polymorphonuclear leukocytes (PMNs, predominantly neutrophils), and various types of microorganisms (Fig. 20.2). This is the zone that appears clinically as the surface pseudomembrane. At the immediate border of the necrotic pseudomembrane, the epithelium is edematous, and the individual cells exhibit various degrees of hydropic degeneration. PMNs infiltrate the intercellular spaces.

The underlying connective tissue is markedly hyperemic, with numerous engorged capillaries and a dense infiltration of PMNs. This acutely inflamed zone appears clinically as the linear erythema beneath the surface pseudomembrane. Numerous plasma cells can appear in the periphery of the infiltrate; this is interpreted as an area of established chronic gingivitis on which the acute lesion became superimposed.[30] The epithelium and connective tissue alterations decrease as the distance from the necrotic gingival margin increases, blending gradually with the uninvolved gingiva.

The microscopic appearance of tissues in a NUG lesion is nonspecific. Comparable changes result from trauma, chemical irritation, or the application of caustic medications.

Relationship of Bacteria and the Necrotizing Ulcerative Gingivitis Lesion

Light and electron microscopy have been used to study the relationship of bacteria and the characteristic lesion of NUG. Light microscopy shows that the exudate on the surface of the necrotic lesion contains microorganisms that morphologically resemble cocci, fusiform bacilli, and spirochetes.[75] The layer between the necrotic and living tissue contains enormous numbers of fusiform bacilli and spirochetes in addition to leukocytes and fibrin. Spirochetes and other bacteria invade the underlying living tissue.[5,13,17,38]

Spirochetes have been found as deep as 300 μm from the surface. Most spirochetes in the deeper zones are morphologically different from cultivated strains of *Treponema microdentium*. They occur in nonnecrotic tissue before other types of bacteria, and they can achieve high intercellular concentrations in the epithelium and connective tissue adjacent to the ulcerated lesion.[37]

Smears from the lesions (Fig. 20.3) show scattered bacteria (predominantly spirochetes and fusiform bacilli), desquamated epithelial cells, and occasional PMNs. Spirochetes and fusiform bacteria are usually seen with other oral spirochetes, vibrios, and filaments.

Diagnosis

Diagnosis is based on clinical findings of gingival pain, ulceration, and bleeding. A bacterial smear is not necessary or definitive because the bacterial picture is not appreciably different from that of patients with marginal gingivitis, periodontal pockets, pericoronitis, or primary herpetic gingivostomatitis.[58] However, bacterial studies are useful for the differential diagnosis of NUG and specific infections of the oral cavity (e.g., diphtheria, thrush, actinomycosis, streptococcal stomatitis).

The microscopic examination of a biopsy specimen is not sufficiently specific to be diagnostic. It can be used to differentiate NUG from specific infections (e.g., tuberculosis) or from neoplastic disease, but it does not differentiate NUG from other necrotizing conditions of nonspecific origin, such as those produced by trauma or caustic medications.

KEY FACT

A bacterial smear or culture is not necessary or definitive in the diagnosis of NUG because the bacterial flora is not appreciably different from that of patients with other common inflammatory conditions (e.g., gingivitis, periodontitis). However, bacterial studies are useful for the differential diagnosis of NUG when specific infections of the oral cavity (e.g., diphtheria, thrush, actinomycosis, streptococcal stomatitis) are suspected.

Differential Diagnosis

NUG should be differentiated from other conditions that resemble it in some respects, such as herpetic gingivostomatitis (Table 20.1), chronic periodontitis, desquamative gingivitis (Table 20.2), streptococcal gingivostomatitis, aphthous stomatitis, gonococcal gingivostomatitis, diphtheritic and syphilitic lesions (Table 20.3), tuberculous gingival

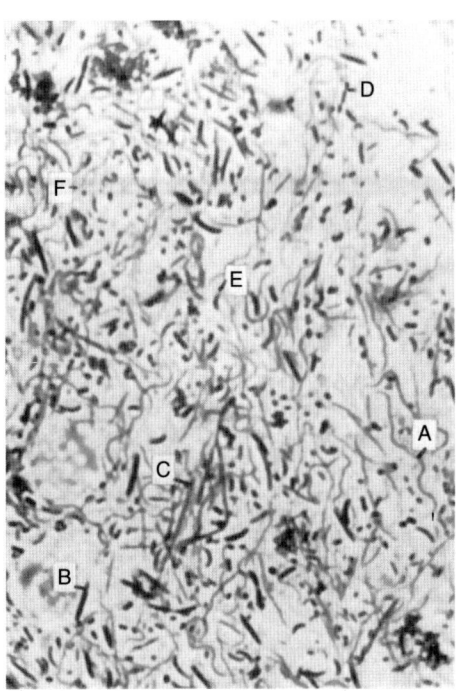

Fig. 20.3 A bacterial smear was obtained from a lesion in a patient with necrotizing ulcerative gingivitis. *A*, Spirochete. *B*, *Bacillus fusiformis*. *C*, Filamentous organism (i.e., *Actinomyces* or *Leptotrichia*). *D*, *Streptococcus*. *E*, *Vibrio*. *F*, *Treponema microdentium*.

TABLE 20.1 Differentiation of Necrotizing Ulcerative Gingivitis and Primary Herpetic Gingivostomatitis

Necrotizing Ulcerative Gingivitis	Primary Herpetic Gingivostomatitis
Caused by interaction between host and bacteria, most often fusospirochetes	Caused by specific viral infection
Necrotizing condition	Diffuse erythema and vesicular eruption
Punched-out gingival margin; pseudomembrane that peels off and leaves raw areas	Vesicles that rupture and leave slightly depressed oval or spherical ulcer
Marginal gingiva affected; other oral tissues rarely affected	Diffuse involvement of gingiva; may include buccal mucosa and lips
Uncommon in children	Occurs more frequently in children
No definite duration	Duration of 7 to 10 days
No demonstrated immunity	Acute episode results in some degree of immunity
Contagion not demonstrated	Contagion

TABLE 20.2 Differentiation of Necrotizing Ulcerative Gingivitis, Chronic Desquamative Gingivitis, and Chronic Periodontal Disease

Necrotizing Ulcerative Gingivitis	Desquamative Gingivitis	Chronic Destructive Periodontal Disease
Bacterial smears show fusospirochetal complex	Bacterial smears reveal numerous epithelial cells and few bacterial forms	Bacterial smears vary
Marginal gingiva affected	Diffuse involvement of marginal and attached gingivae and other areas of oral mucosa	Marginal gingiva affected
Acute history	Chronic history	Chronic history
Painful	May or may not be painful	Painless if uncomplicated
Pseudomembrane	Patchy desquamation of gingival epithelium	Usually no desquamation, but purulent material may appear from pockets
Papillary and marginal necrotic lesions	Papillae do not undergo necrosis	Papillae do not undergo noticeable necrosis
Affects adults of both genders and occasionally affects children	Affects adults, most often women	Usually found in adults, occasionally found in children
Characteristic fetid odor	No odor	Some odor but not strikingly fetid

TABLE 20.3   Differentiation of Necrotizing Ulcerative Gingivitis, Diphtheria, and Secondary Stage of Syphilis

Necrotizing Ulcerative Gingivitis	Diphtheria	Secondary Stage of Syphilis (Mucous Patch)
Caused by interaction between host and bacteria, typically fusospirochetes	Caused by *Corynebacterium diphtheriae*	Caused by *Treponema pallidum*
Affects marginal gingiva	Rarely affects marginal gingiva	Rarely affects marginal gingiva
Membrane removal easy	Membrane removal difficult	Membrane not detachable
Painful condition	Less painful	Minimal pain
Marginal gingivae affected	Throat, fauces, and tonsils affected	Any part of mouth affected
Serologic findings normal	Serologic findings normal	Serologic findings abnormal[a]
Immunity not conferred	Immunity conferred by an attack	Immunity not conferred
Doubtful contagiousness	Contagious	Only direct contact can communicate disease
Antibiotic therapy relieves symptoms	Antibiotic treatment is effective	Antibiotic therapy has excellent results

[a]Wassermann test, Kahn test, and Venereal Disease Research Laboratories (VDRL) test.

lesions, candidiasis, agranulocytosis, and dermatoses (e.g., pemphigus, erythema multiforme, lichen planus), and stomatitis venenata (see Chapter 22).

Treatment options for these diseases vary dramatically, and misdiagnosis and improper treatment can exacerbate the condition. In the case of primary herpetic gingivostomatitis, early diagnosis can result in treatment with antiviral drugs that would be ineffective for NUG, whereas the treatment of a case of herpes with the debridement required for NUG could exacerbate the herpes.

Streptococcal gingivostomatitis is a rare condition that is characterized by a diffuse erythema of the gingiva and other areas of the oral mucosa.[44] In some cases, it is confined as a marginal erythema with marginal hemorrhage. Necrosis of the gingival margin is not a feature of this disease, and there is no fetid odor. Bacterial smears show a preponderance of streptococcal forms, which were identified as *Streptococcus viridans,* but other studies report findings of group A β-hemolytic streptococci.[39]

Agranulocytosis is characterized by a marked decrease in the number of circulating PMNs, lesions of the throat and other mucous membranes, and ulceration and necrosis of the gingiva that can resemble that of NUG and that occurs most commonly after chemotherapy in cancer patients or in patients with leukemia. The oral condition of patients with agranulocytosis is primarily necrotizing, but it lacks the severe inflammatory reaction seen with NUG. Blood studies can differentiate between NUG and the gingival necrosis associated with agranulocytosis.

Vincent angina is a fusospirochetal infection of the oropharynx and throat that is distinguished from NUG, which affects the marginal gingiva. Patients with Vincent angina have a painful membranous ulceration of the throat, with edema and hyperemic patches breaking down to form ulcers that are covered with pseudomembranous material. The process can extend to the larynx and the middle ear.

NUG in leukemia patients results from the reduced host defense mechanisms that occur with the disease. NUG can be superimposed on the gingival tissue alterations caused by leukemia. The differential diagnosis does not require distinguishing between NUG and leukemic gingival changes; instead, it is determined whether leukemia is a predisposing factor in the mouth of a patient with NUG. For example, if a patient with necrotizing involvement of the gingival margin also has diffuse discoloration and generalized edema of the attached gingiva, the possibility of an underlying systemically induced gingival

change should be considered. Leukemia is one of the conditions that would need to be ruled out (see Chapter 14).

NUG in the patient with human immunodeficiency virus (HIV) infection has the same clinical features, although it often follows an extremely destructive course that leads to NUP, with a loss of soft tissue and bone and the formation of bony sequestra[26] (see Chapter 29).

CLINICAL CORRELATION

A serious systemic disease or condition such as leukemia or acquired immunodeficiency that renders the host immunocompromised can be the predisposing causative factor leading to acute gingival disease.

Etiology

Role of Bacteria

Plaut[54] in 1894 and Vincent[77] in 1896 postulated that NUG was caused by specific bacteria: fusiform bacilli and spirochetal organisms. Opinions still differ about whether bacteria are the primary causative factors of NUG. Several observations support this concept, including that spirochetal organisms and fusiform bacilli are always found in patients with the disease along with other organisms. Rosebury and colleagues[58] described a fusospirochetal complex that consists of *T. microdentium,* intermediate spirochetes, vibrios, fusiform bacilli, and filamentous organisms in addition to several *Borrelia* species.

Loesche and colleagues[40] described a predominant constant flora and a variable flora associated with NUG. The constant flora is composed of *Prevotella intermedia* in addition to *Fusobacterium, Treponema,* and *Selenomonas* species. The variable flora consists of a heterogeneous array of bacterial types.

Treatment with metronidazole results in a significant reduction of *Treponema* species, *Prevotella intermedia,* and *Fusobacterium,* with resolution of the clinical symptoms.[16,40] The antibacterial spectrum of this drug provides evidence for the anaerobic members of the flora as etiologic agents. These bacteriologic findings have been supported by immunologic data[9] that demonstrated increased immunoglobulin G and M antibody titers for medium-sized spirochetes and *P. intermedia* in patients with NUG compared with titers in patients with chronic gingivitis and healthy controls.

Role of the Host Response

Regardless of whether specific bacteria are implicated in the cause of NUG, the presence of these organisms without other predisposing factors appears to be insufficient to cause the disease. The fusospirochetal flora is frequently found in patients who do not have NUG. Exudates from NUG lesions produce fusospirochetal abscesses rather than typical NUG lesions when the exudates are inoculated subcutaneously into experimental animals.[57]

The role of an impaired host response in NUG has long been recognized. Even in the early descriptions of the disease, NUG was associated with physical and emotional stress[11,60] and decreased resistance to infection. NUG has not been produced experimentally in humans or animals, only by inoculation of bacterial exudates from the lesions. In the animal model, local or systemic immunosuppression with glucocorticoids (e.g., ketoconazole) results in more characteristic lesions of NUG in infected animals. Swenson and Muhler used scillaren B, an amorphous glucoside, which reduced tissue resistance to create oral fusospirochetal infections in dogs.[71,72]

NUG is not found in well-nourished individuals with a fully functional immune system. All of the predisposing factors for NUG are associated with immunosuppression. Cogen and colleagues[10] described depression of host defense mechanisms, particularly in PMN chemotaxis and phagocytosis, in patients with NUG. Host–bacteria interactions are described in Chapter 9.

It is essential for the clinician to determine the predisposing factors that lead to immunodeficiency in patients with NUG to address the continued susceptibility of the patient and to determine whether an underlying systemic disease exists. Immunodeficiency may be related to various levels of nutritional deficiency, fatigue caused by chronic sleep deprivation, other health habits (e.g., alcohol, drug abuse), psychosocial factors, or systemic disease. NUG can be the presenting symptom for patients with immunosuppression related to HIV infection.

Local Predisposing Factors

Preexisting gingivitis, injury to the gingiva, and smoking are important predisposing factors. Although NUG can appear in an otherwise disease-free mouth, it most often occurs superimposed on preexisting chronic gingival disease and periodontal pockets. Deep periodontal pockets and pericoronal flaps are particularly vulnerable areas because they offer a favorable environment for the proliferation of anaerobic fusiform bacilli and spirochetes. Areas of the gingiva that are traumatized by opposing teeth in malocclusion (e.g., palatal surface behind the maxillary incisors, labial gingival surface of the mandibular incisors) can predispose an individual to the development of NUG.

The relationship between NUG and smoking has often been mentioned in the literature. Pindborg[52] reported that 98% of his patients with NUG were smokers and that the increasing frequency of this disease correlates with increasing exposure to tobacco smoke. The effect of smoking on periodontal disease in general has been the subject of numerous studies during the past 2 decades,[1a,21a,22a,33a,35a,49a] and smoking has been established as a high-risk factor for disease (see Chapter 12).

Systemic Predisposing Factors

NUG is not found in a well-nourished individual with a fully functional immune system. It is therefore important for the clinician to determine the predisposing factors for immunodeficiency. Immunodeficiency can be related to various levels of nutritional deficiency, psychosocial stress, fatigue caused by chronic sleep deficiency, other health habits (e.g., alcoholism, drug abuse), and systemic disease (e.g., diabetes, debilitating infection).

Nutritional Deficiency

Necrotizing gingivitis has been produced in animals by giving them nutritionally deficient diets.[7,34,47,73,76] Several researchers found an increase in the fusospirochetal flora in the mouths of the experimental animals, but the bacteria were regarded as opportunists that proliferated only when the tissues were altered by the deficiency.

A poor diet has been cited as a predisposing factor for NUG and its sequelae in developing African countries, although the effects appear primarily to diminish the effectiveness of the immune response.[19,20,35] Nutritional deficiencies (e.g., vitamin C, vitamin B_2) accentuate the severity of the pathologic changes induced when the fusospirochetal bacterial complex is injected into animals.[70]

Debilitating Disease

Debilitating systemic disease can predispose patients to NUG. Systemic disturbances include chronic diseases (e.g., syphilis, cancer), severe gastrointestinal disorders (e.g., ulcerative colitis), blood dyscrasias (e.g., leukemia, anemia), and acquired immunodeficiency syndrome. Nutritional deficiency that results from debilitating disease can be an additional predisposing factor. Experimentally induced leukopenia in animals can produce ulcerative gangrenous stomatitis.[47,74,75] Ulceronecrotic lesions appear in the gingival margins of hamsters that are exposed to total body irradiation[43]; these lesions can be prevented with systemic antibiotics.[42]

Psychosomatic Factors

Psychological factors appear to be important in the cause of NUG. The disease often occurs in association with stressful situations (e.g., induction into the armed forces, academic examinations).[24] Psychological disturbances[25] and increased adrenocortical secretion[65] are common in patients with the disease.

A significant correlation between disease incidence and two personality traits—dominance and abasement—suggests a NUG-prone personality.[22] Data from a study evaluating the relationship between personality traits and stress with gingival inflammation and soft tissue pathology in military recruits found that gingival inflammation correlated significantly with personality traits (e.g., tolerance to change, anxiety).[48]

The mechanisms by which psychologic factors create or predispose an individual to gingival damage have not been established. However, alterations in digital and gingival capillary responses that suggest increased autonomic nervous activity have been demonstrated in patients with NUG.[23]

It can be concluded that opportunistic bacteria are the primary etiologic agents of NUG in patients who demonstrate immunosuppression. Stress, smoking, and preexisting gingivitis are common predisposing factors.

Epidemiology and Prevalence

The prevalence of NUG appears to have been rather low in the United States and Europe before 1914. During World Wars I and II, numerous epidemics broke out among the Allied troops, but German soldiers did not seem to have been similarly affected. Epidemic-like outbreaks have also occurred among civilian populations. A study at a dental clinic in Prague, Czech Republic, reported the incidence of NUG as 0.08% among patients 15 to 19 years old, 0.05% among those 20 to 24 years old, and 0.02% among those 25 to 29 years old.[68]

NUG occurs in individuals of all ages, with the highest incidence reported for patients between the ages of 15 and 30 years.[15,36,68,70] It is not common among children in the United States, Canada, and Europe, but it has been reported in children from low socioeconomic groups in underdeveloped countries.[33] In India, 54%[46] and 58%[53] of patients in two studies were younger than 10 years of age.

In a random school population in Nigeria, NUG occurred in 11.3% of children between the ages of 2 and 6 years.[66] In a Nigerian hospital population, it affected 23% of children who were younger than 10 years of age.[19] Studies of African populations typically report a higher prevalence of necrotizing periodontal disease among young children than in those older than 10 years.[1] NUG has been reported in several members of the same family in low socioeconomic groups. Twenty percent of households with children 2 to 6 years of age in a rural Nigerian city had one or more children with NUG.[66] NUG is more common among children with Down syndrome than among other children with mental deficiencies.[4]

Opinions differ with regard to whether NUG is more common during the winter,[36,50] summer, or fall[66] and whether there is a peak seasonal incidence.[14]

Communicability

NUG often occurs in groups in an epidemic pattern. At one time, NUG was considered contagious and required reporting to the community health department, but it was later concluded not to be communicable.[56,62]

A distinction must be made between communicability and transmissibility when referring to the characteristics of disease. The term *transmissible* denotes a capacity for the maintenance of an infectious agent in successive passages through a susceptible animal host.[56] The term *communicable* signifies a capacity for the maintenance of infection by natural modes of spread, such as direct contact through drinking water, food, and eating utensils; by the airborne route; or by arthropod vectors. A disease that is communicable is described as *contagious.* It has been demonstrated that disease associated with the fusospirochetal bacterial complex is transmissible; however, *it is not communicable or contagious.*

Attempts to spread NUG from human to human have been unsuccessful.[63] King[35] traumatized an area in his own gingiva and introduced debris from a patient with a severe case of NUG. There was no response until he happened to fall ill shortly thereafter. After his illness, he observed the characteristic lesion in the experimental area. It can be inferred with reservation from this experiment that systemic debility is a prerequisite for the contagion of NUG.

Because NUG often occurs among groups that use the same kitchen facilities, it is a common impression that the disease is spread by bacteria on eating utensils. However, the growth of fusospirochetal organisms requires carefully controlled conditions and an anaerobic environment; they do not ordinarily survive on eating utensils.[12,28]

The occurrence of NUG in epidemic-like outbreaks does not necessarily mean that it is contagious. The affected groups may be afflicted by the disease as a result of common predisposing factors rather than because of its spread from person to person. In all likelihood, a predisposed immunocompromised host and the presence of appropriate bacteria are necessary for the production of this disease.

KEY FACT

Although certain bacteria (e.g., fusospirochetal complex) are likely responsible for the lesions observed in necrotizing ulcerative gingivitis, immunocompromise appears to be a necessary predisposing condition for the disease.

Primary Herpetic Gingivostomatitis

Primary herpetic gingivostomatitis is an infection of the oral cavity caused by herpes simplex virus (HSV) type 1.[15,44,45,61] It occurs most often among infants and children who are younger than 6 years of age,[6,61,64] but it is also seen in adolescents and adults. It occurs with equal frequency in male and female patients. In most individuals, however, the primary infection is asymptomatic.

As part of the primary infection, the virus ascends through the sensory and autonomic nerves, where it persists as latent HSV in neuronal ganglia that innervate the site. In approximately one-third of the world's population, secondary manifestations result from various stimuli, such as sunlight, trauma, fever, and stress. Secondary manifestations include herpes labialis (Fig. 20.4), herpetic stomatitis, herpes genitalis, ocular herpes, and herpetic encephalitis. Secondary herpetic stomatitis can occur on the palate, on the gingiva (Fig. 20.5), or on the mucosa as a result of dental treatment that traumatizes or stimulates the latent virus in the ganglia that innervate the area. It may manifest as pain away from the site of treatment 2 to 4 days later. Careful inspection for characteristic vesicles can be diagnostic (see Fig. 20.4).

Clinical Features
Oral Signs

Primary herpetic gingivostomatitis appears as a diffuse, erythematous, shiny involvement of the gingiva and the adjacent oral mucosa, with various degrees of edema and gingival bleeding. During its initial stage, it is characterized by discrete, spherical, gray vesicles, which can occur on the gingiva, labial and buccal mucosae, soft palate,

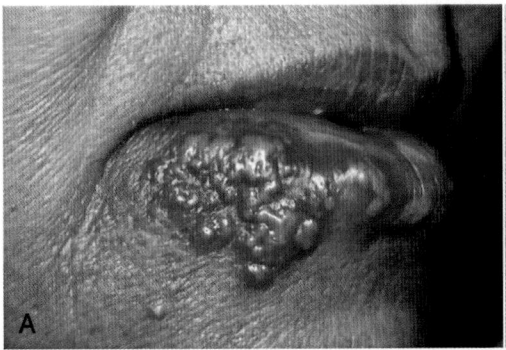
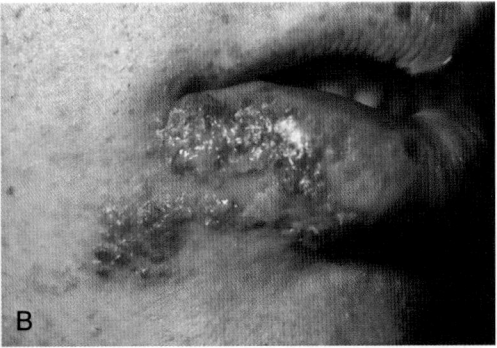

Fig. 20.4 Herpetic vesicles recurred in the lip. (A) Early stage. (B) Late stage, showing brownish, crusted lesions. *(From Sapp JP, Eversole LR, Wysocki GP: Contemporary oral and maxillofacial pathology. ed 2, St Louis, 2002, Mosby.)*

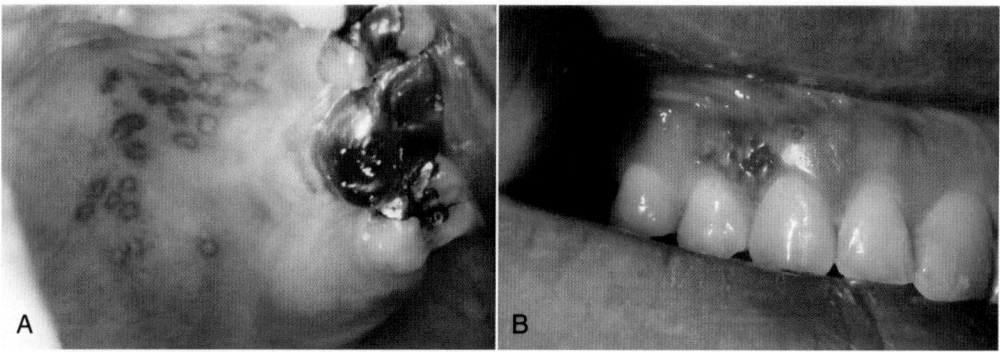

Fig. 20.5 Recurrent intraoral herpetic vesicles are seen (A) in the palate and (B) in the gingiva. The latter location is rare. *(From Sapp JP, Eversole LR, Wysocki GP:* Contemporary oral and maxillofacial pathology, *ed 2, St Louis, 2002, Mosby.)*

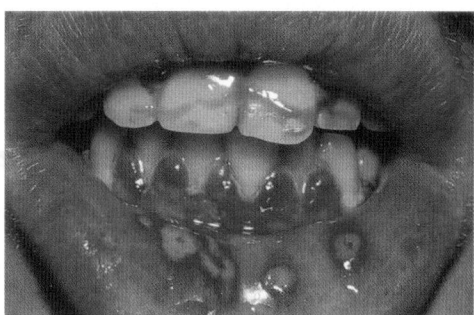

Fig. 20.6 Primary herpetic gingivostomatitis in a 12-year-old boy, who has diffuse erythematous involvement of the gingiva and a spherical, gray vesicle in the lip. *(Courtesy Dr. Heddie Sedano, University of California, Los Angeles, and University of Minnesota.)*

pharynx, sublingual mucosa, and tongue (Fig. 20.6). After approximately 24 hours, the vesicles rupture and form painful small ulcers with red, elevated, halo-like margins and depressed yellowish or grayish white central portions. They occur in widely separated areas or in clusters where confluence occurs (Fig. 20.7).

Occasionally, primary herpetic gingivitis occurs without overt vesiculation. The clinical picture consists of diffuse, erythematous, shiny discoloration and edematous enlargement of the gingivae with a tendency to bleed.

The course of the disease is limited to 7 to 10 days. The diffuse gingival erythema and edema that appear early during the course of the disease persist for several days after the ulcerative lesions have healed. Scarring does not occur in the areas of healed ulcerations.

Oral Symptoms

The disease is accompanied by generalized soreness of the oral cavity, which interferes with eating, drinking, and oral hygiene. The ruptured vesicles are the focal sites of pain; they are particularly sensitive to touch, thermal changes, foods such as condiments and fruit juices, and the action of coarse foods. In infants, the disease is marked by irritability and refusal to take food.

Extraoral and Systemic Signs and Symptoms

Cervical lymphadenitis, fever as high as 101° to 105° F (38° to 40.6° C), and generalized malaise are common.

History

Primary herpetic gingivostomatitis is the result of an acute infection by HSV. There is an acute onset of symptoms.

Histopathology

The virus targets the epithelial cells called *Tzanck cells*, which show ballooning degeneration that consists of acantholysis, nuclear clearing, and nuclear enlargement. Infected cells fuse to form multinucleated cells, and intercellular edema leads to the formation of intraepithelial vesicles that rupture and develop a secondary inflammatory response with a fibropurulent exudate[49] (Fig. 20.8). Discrete ulcerations that result from the rupture of the vesicles have a central portion of acute inflammation, with various degrees of purulent exudate surrounded by engorged blood vessels.

Diagnosis

It is critical to arrive at a diagnosis as early as possible for a patient with a primary herpetic infection. Treatment with antiviral medications can dramatically alter the course of the disease by reducing symptoms and potentially reducing recurrences. The diagnosis is usually established from the patient's history and the clinical findings. Material can be obtained from the lesions and submitted to the laboratory for confirmatory tests, including virus culture and immunologic tests that involve the use of monoclonal antibodies or deoxyribonucleic acid hybridization techniques.[6,55] This should not delay treatment if strong clinical evidence exists for primary gingivostomatitis.

Differential Diagnosis

Primary herpetic gingivostomatitis should be differentiated from several conditions. Lesions of recurrent aphthous stomatitis (RAS)[21] range from occasional small (0.5 to 1 cm in diameter), well-defined, round or ovoid, shallow ulcers with a yellowish gray central area surrounded by an erythematous halo, which heal in 7 to 10 days without scarring, to larger (1 to 3 cm in diameter), oval or irregular ulcers, which persist for weeks and heal with scarring (Fig. 20.9). The cause is unknown, although immunopathologic mechanisms appear to play a role.

RAS is a different clinical entity from primary herpetic gingivostomatitis. The ulcerations may look the same for the two conditions, but diffuse erythematous involvement of the gingiva and acute toxic systemic symptoms do not occur with RAS. A history of previous episodes of painful mucosal ulcerations suggests RAS rather than primary HSV.

Information about erythema multiforme, bullous lichen planus, and desquamative gingivitis can be found in Chapter 22.

Communicability

Primary herpetic gingivostomatitis is contagious.[8,39] Most adults have developed immunity to HSV as a result of infection during childhood,

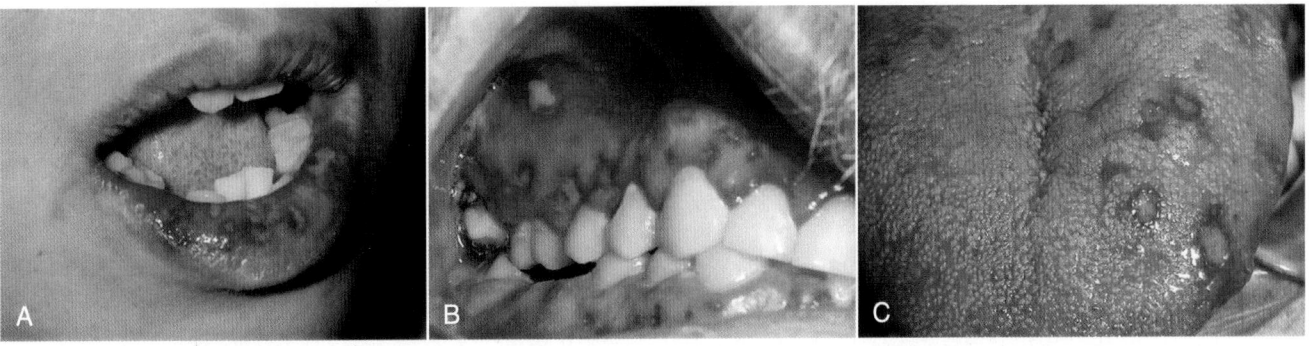

Fig. 20.7 Involvement of the lip (A), gingiva (B), and tongue (C) in primary herpetic gingivostomatitis. *(From Sapp JP, Eversole LR, Wysocki GP: Contemporary oral and maxillofacial pathology. ed 2, St Louis, 2002, Mosby.)*

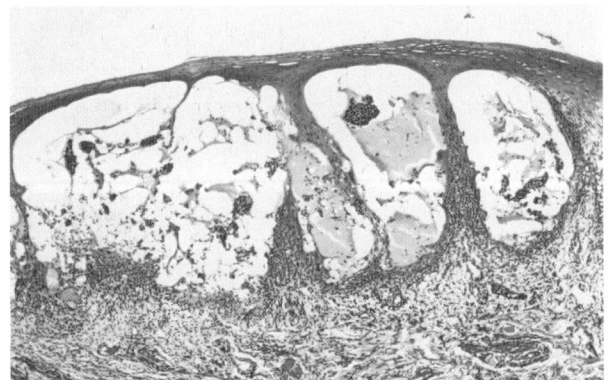

Fig. 20.8 Biopsy showing intraepithelial viral vesicles that contain fluid and debris, with a large number of viruses and virally altered epithelial cells (i.e., Tzanck cells). *(Courtesy Dr. Heddie Sedano, University of California, Los Angeles, and University of Minnesota.)*

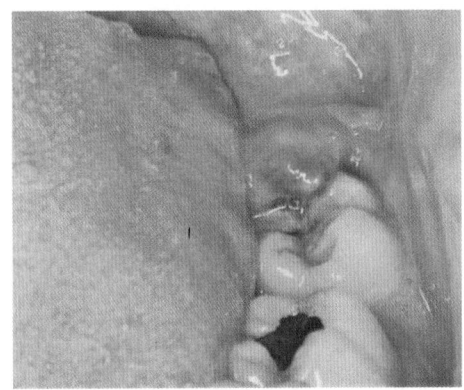

Fig. 20.10 Pericoronitis. An inflamed coronal flap covers the disto-occlusal surface of the impacted mandibular third molar. Note the swelling and redness. *(From Glickman I, Smulow J: Periodontal disease: clinical, radiographic and histopathologic features. Philadelphia, 1974, Saunders.)*

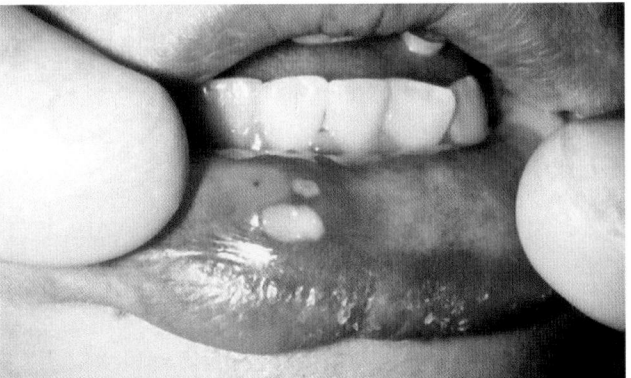

Fig. 20.9 Aphthous lesion in the lip. The depressed gray center is surrounded by an elevated red border. *(From Sapp JP, Eversole LR, Wysocki GP: Contemporary oral and maxillofacial pathology. ed 2, St Louis, 2002, Mosby.)*

which in most cases is subclinical. For this reason, acute herpetic gingivostomatitis usually occurs in infants and children. Recurrent herpetic gingivostomatitis has been reported,[27] although it is not often clinically significant unless immunity is destroyed by debilitating systemic disease. Studies that have demonstrated HSV in periodontal pockets suggest more recurrence of viral replication than has previously been recognized.[69] Secondary herpetic infection of the skin, such as herpes labialis, does recur.[67]

> ### CLINICAL CORRELATION
>
> Acute herpetic gingivostomatitis usually occurs in infants and children because most adults have developed immunity to herpes simplex virus from childhood exposure, often with mild or no symptoms.

Pericoronitis

The term *pericoronitis* refers to inflammation of the gingiva in relation to the crown of an incompletely erupted tooth (Fig. 20.10). It occurs most often in the mandibular third molar area. Pericoronitis can be acute, subacute, or chronic.

Clinical Features

The partially erupted or impacted mandibular third molar is the most common site of pericoronitis. The space between the crown of the tooth and the overlying gingival flap (i.e., operculum) is an ideal area for the accumulation of food debris and bacterial growth. Even in patients with no clinical signs or symptoms, the gingival flap is often chronically inflamed and infected, and it has various degrees of ulceration along its inner surface. Acute inflammatory involvement is a constant possibility; it may be exacerbated by trauma, occlusion, or a foreign body trapped underneath the tissue flap (e.g., popcorn husk, nut fragment).

Acute pericoronitis is identified by various degrees of inflammatory involvement of the pericoronal flap and adjacent structures and by systemic complications. The inflammatory fluid and cellular exudate increase the bulk of the flap, which can interfere with complete closure of the jaws. It also can be traumatized by contact with the opposing dentition, thereby aggravating the inflammatory involvement.

The resultant clinical picture is a red, swollen, suppurating lesion that is exquisitely tender, with radiating pains to the ear, throat, and floor of the mouth. The patient is extremely uncomfortable as a result of pain, a foul taste, and an inability to close the jaws. Swelling of the cheek in the region of the angle of the jaw and lymphadenitis are common findings. Trismus may be a presenting complaint. The patient can have systemic complications such as fever, leukocytosis, and malaise.

Complications

Involvement can be localized in the form of a pericoronal abscess. It may spread posteriorly into the oropharyngeal area and medially to the base of the tongue, making it difficult for the patient to swallow. Depending on the severity and extent of the infection, there may be involvement of the submaxillary, posterior cervical, deep cervical, and retropharyngeal lymph nodes.[32,51] Peritonsillar abscess formation, cellulitis, and Ludwig angina are infrequent but potential sequelae of acute pericoronitis.

Conclusions

Acute gingival diseases are similar in that they typically manifest with painful intraoral or perioral lesions and there is a need for urgent treatment to relieve symptoms. However, each case requires careful assessment and an accurate diagnosis, including identification of risk factors. In many cases, there are systemic risk factors that increase susceptibility to acute gingival disease.

 A Case Scenario is found on the companion website www.expertconsult.com.

References

 References for this chapter are found on the companion website www.expertconsult.com.

CHAPTER 21

Gingival Disease in Childhood

Daniela R. Silva | Clarice S. Law | Donald F. Duperon | Fermin A. Carranza

CHAPTER OUTLINE

Periodontal disease in adults is partly precipitated by gingival inflammation during the formative years of childhood and early adolescence. Without appropriate intervention, the nondestructive gingival inflammation of childhood may progress to the more significant periodontal diseases seen in the adult population.

After reviewing anatomic and physiologic changes in the periodontium and dentition, this chapter describes the gingival changes associated with childhood and adolescence. Periodontal diseases during these early periods of life are discussed in Chapters 14, 27, and 28.

Periodontium of the Primary Dentition

In the edentulous infant, the gingival tissues have thick gingival mucosa and segmentations that correspond with the primary buds (Fig. 21.1). A high labial frenum attachment is a normal finding in almost 85% of infants; it may diminish in size with normal development.[58] During the primary dentition stage, the normal gingiva continues to be somewhat different from that found in adults. The tissues are pale pink, but they are pink to a lesser degree than the attached gingiva of adults because the thinness of the keratinized layer allows the underlying vessels in children to be more visible.[42] Stippling appears at about 3 years of age and has been reported for 56% of children between 3 and 10 years of age, with little differences between maxillary and mandibular arches or between boys and girls throughout childhood[11] (Fig. 21.2).

The *interdental gingiva* is broad buccolingually and narrow mesiodistally, which is consistent with the morphology of the primary dentition. Its structure and composition are similar to those of the adult gingiva.

Gingival sulcular depth is shallower in the primary dentition than in the permanent dentition. Probing depths range from 1 to 2 mm, with increasing depth from anterior to posterior.[8,25,61]

The *attached gingiva* varies in width anteroposteriorly, with a range of 3 to 6 mm. On the buccal surfaces, the width decreases from anterior to posterior, with some data indicating a narrowing over the canines (Fig. 21.3). The lingual attached gingiva shows an inverse relationship, with an increase in width from anterior to posterior.[25] The gingival width normally increases with age as children transition from the primary to the permanent dentition.[5,8,15,61] The junctional epithelium is thicker in the primary dentition than in the permanent dentition,[10] which is thought to reduce the permeability of the tissues to bacterial toxins.

Radiographically, the lamina dura is prominent in the primary dentition, with a wider periodontal space than in the permanent dentition. The marrow spaces of the bone are larger, and the crests of the interdental bony septa are flat, with bony crests within 1 to 2 mm of the cementoenamel junction[26,54] (Fig. 21.4).

Periodontal Changes Associated With Normal Development

Significant changes occur in the periodontium as the dentition changes from the primary to the permanent teeth. Most of the changes are associated with eruption and are physiologic in nature. These changes should be distinguished from gingival disease, which can occur simultaneously.

Tooth Eruption

Before the eruption of a primary or permanent tooth, the gingiva reveals a bulge that is firm and pink or blanched as a result of the underlying tooth crown. An *eruption cyst* occasionally is evident. This fluctuant mass can be filled with blood, and it usually manifests as a bluish or deep red enlargement of the gingiva over the erupting tooth (Fig. 21.5A). The most common sites of these cysts are the primary first molars and the permanent first molars. Many resolve without treatment, but they can be marsupialized if they are painful or interfere with occlusion (see Fig. 21.5B).[14]

As a tooth erupts, the gingival margin and the sulcus develop. At this point, the margin is rounded, edematous, and reddened. During the period of active tooth eruption, it is normal for the marginal gingiva that surrounds partially erupted teeth to appear prominent; this is most evident in the maxillary anterior region. The prominence is caused by the height of the contour of the erupting tooth and mild inflammation from mastication. Poor oral hygiene can contribute to the development of significant gingivitis in unprotected gingival areas.

Teething

The effect of primary tooth eruption on infant health has been debated for centuries, but there is little scientific evidence regarding the diagnosis and management of the teething child. The period associated

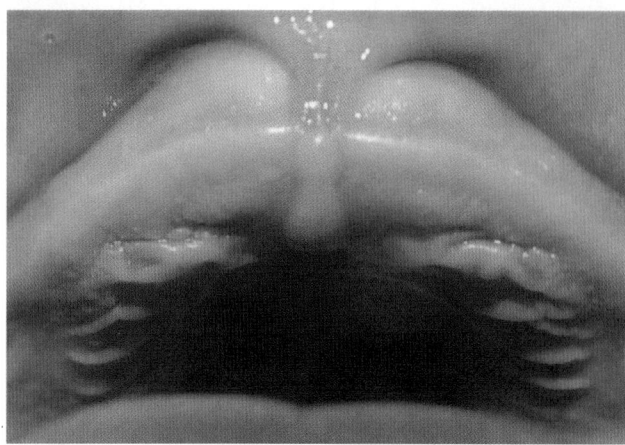

Fig. 21.1 Normal gingiva of an edentulous 1-month-old child shows a high labial frenulum and pink and healthy tissues. *(Copyright Dr. Daniela Silva. All rights reserved.)*

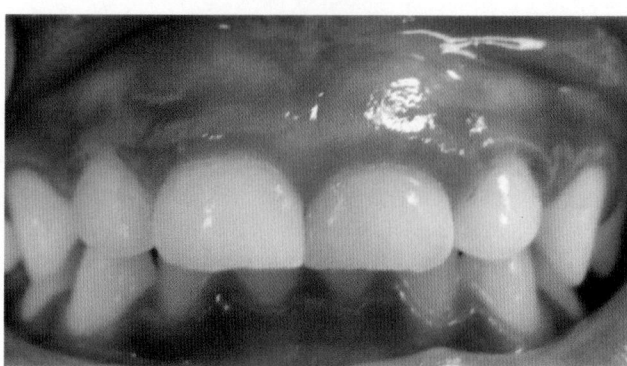

Fig. 21.3 Normal gingiva of a 4-year-old African-American child demonstrates the width of the attached gingiva, as illustrated by the pigmentation that occurs only in the attached area. *(Copyright Dr. Daniela Silva. All rights reserved.)*

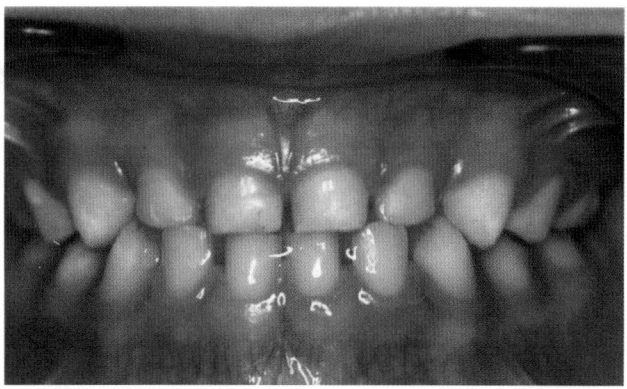

Fig. 21.2 Normal gingiva of a 4-year-old child shows light stippling and flattened interproximal gingiva in areas of physiologic spacing. *(Copyright Dr. Daniela Silva. All rights reserved.)*

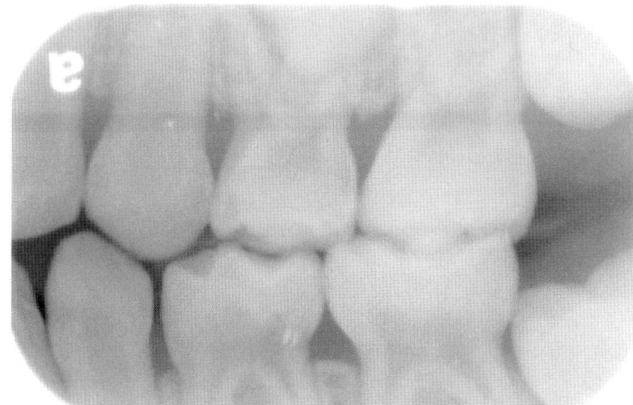

Fig. 21.4 Bitewing radiograph of a 6-year-old child shows the flattened interseptal bone and bony crests within 1 to 2 mm of the cementoenamel junction. *(Copyright Dr. Daniela Silva. All rights reserved.)*

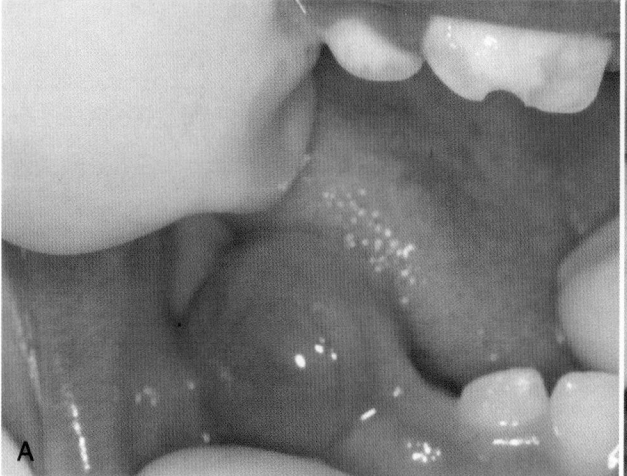
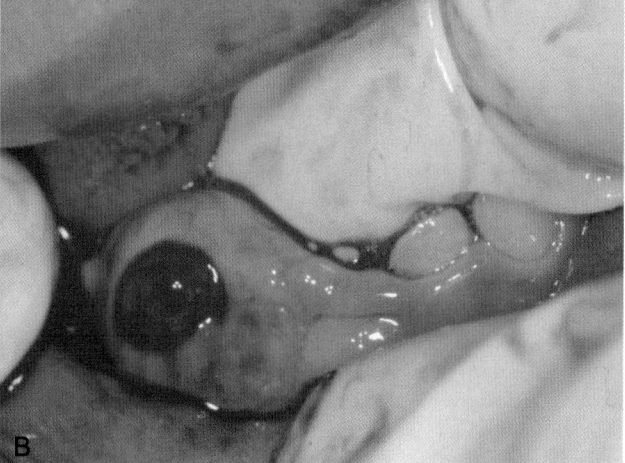

Fig. 21.5 (A) An eruption cyst is seen at the lower right first primary molar area of a 16-month-old child. With this condition, there is transparent, bluish, blue, or blue-black swelling of the alveolar mucosa over a tooth in eruption. (B) An eruption cyst is located at the lower right first primary molar area of a 16-month-old child. After a small incision of the mucosa, the hemorrhagic content was marsupialized. *(Copyright Dr. Daniela Silva. All rights reserved.)*

with the eruption of the primary teeth in infants can be difficult and stressful for the child and the parents. The timing of primary incisor eruption (i.e., 5 to 12 months of age) coincides with diminution of the passive humoral immunity conferred by the transfer of maternal antibodies through the placenta and establishment of the child's own immunity.[17,29,60] Pain is a common feature of teething as reported by parents and some health care providers. The tooth does not cause the pain; rather, the follicle, which is a rich source of eicosanoids, cytokines, and growth factors, stimulates a localized inflammatory response.[57,60]

Most medical and dental professionals agree that teething does not cause life-threatening illness, but they disagree about which symptoms are associated with tooth eruption. The studies and systematic reviews of symptoms related to teething most commonly include decreased appetite, biting, drooling, gum rubbing, irritability, sucking, and abnormal temperature.[24,28,29,38,39,46,53,57,60,67,68] However, there is no evidence that any of these symptoms can be diagnostic of teething in a child without excluding the possibility of other systemic diseases.

Primary Tooth Exfoliation

As with tooth eruption, the process of tooth exfoliation involves changes in the periodontium. The depth of the gingival sulcus increases as the junctional epithelium migrates down the resorbing root of an exfoliating tooth.[9,10] Microscopically, minor traumatic changes demonstrate compression, ischemia, and hyalinization of the periodontal ligament.[49] Changes in the permeability and integrity of the junctional epithelium can make the exfoliating tooth more susceptible to inflammation.[10]

During the process of exfoliation, teeth can change position, leading to changes in occlusion. Malalignment caused by spacing and changes in skeletal relationships related to erupting teeth can contribute to significant trauma of the periodontal structures. With more severe injury, crushing and necrosis of the periodontal ligament can occur. In most patients, these injuries spontaneously resolve as the teeth exfoliate, erupt, and align through the normal growth and development processes.

Other Developmental Issues
Relation of Periodontal Status to Malocclusion

Data indicate an association between abnormal tooth position and gingivitis.[20] Crowding in the mixed dentition can often make plaque and food removal more difficult, increasing the likelihood of gingivitis. Severe changes include gingival enlargement, discoloration, occasional ulceration, and formation of deep pockets or pseudopockets. Gingival health usually can be restored with orthodontic correction, but failure to align the teeth does not necessarily have an effect on periodontal disease later in life.[20]

Mucogingival Problems

The prevalence of mucogingival problems and recession in children ranges from 1% to 19%, depending on the criteria used to assess the condition.[33] Evidence suggests that some mucogingival problems start during the primary dentition as a consequence of developmental

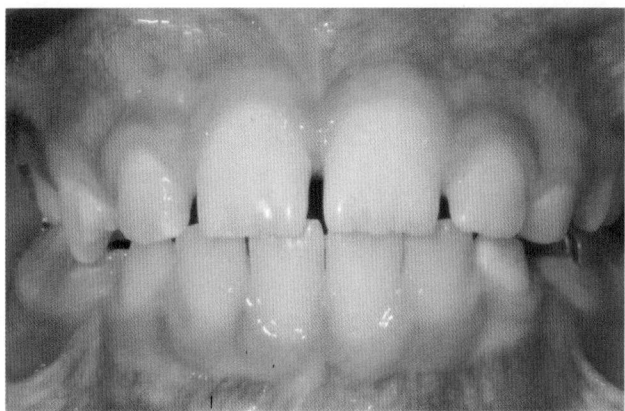

Fig. 21.6 Erupting permanent incisors have minimal attached gingiva. *(Copyright Dr. Daniela Silva. All rights reserved.)*

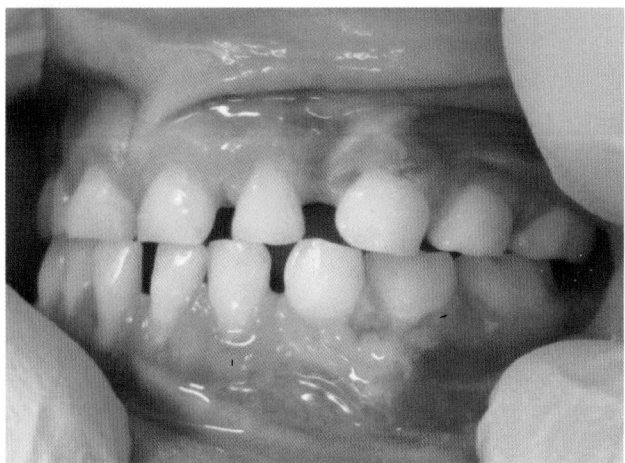

Fig. 21.7 Gingival recession on the maxillary and mandibular left primary canine areas is caused by self-inflicted trauma from the patient's fingernail. *(Copyright Dr. Daniela Silva. All rights reserved.)*

aberrations in eruption and deficiencies in the thickness of the periodontium.[42,43] A high frenum attachment may also be a factor in the development of mucogingival problems if there is excess tension at the marginal tissues.[52,62] During the mixed dentition, recession is most often found on the facial aspect of mandibular permanent incisors due to rotations or labial positioning related to space problems. Although erupting permanent lower incisors often show minimal attached gingiva, gingival width often increases as the teeth erupt and stimulate bone development[15] (Fig. 21.6).

The maxillary canine region is prone to localized gingival recession. Late-erupting canines in a crowded dentition can be displaced buccally, erupting into or near unattached gingiva or mucosa and increasing the risk of insufficient gingival tissue width and recession. Recession also can be associated with an anterior open bite as a result of the labial inclination of the teeth.[36] Orthodontic treatment and realignment may be necessary to protect the integrity of the attached gingiva.

Mucogingival problems can result from factitious habits, such as self-inflicted trauma from a fingernail (Fig. 21.7) or excessive toothbrushing by the parent or the child. Because the width of the attached gingiva increases with age, any of these problems may resolve spontaneously, suggesting a cautious approach to treatment with judicious monitoring instead of immediate surgical intervention.[15,54]

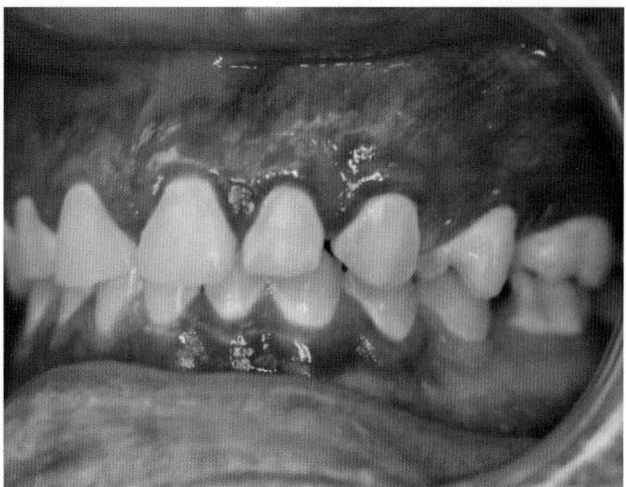

Fig. 21.8 Plaque-induced gingivitis is limited to the marginal gingiva in a 12-year-old girl. *(Copyright Dr. Daniela Silva. All rights reserved.)*

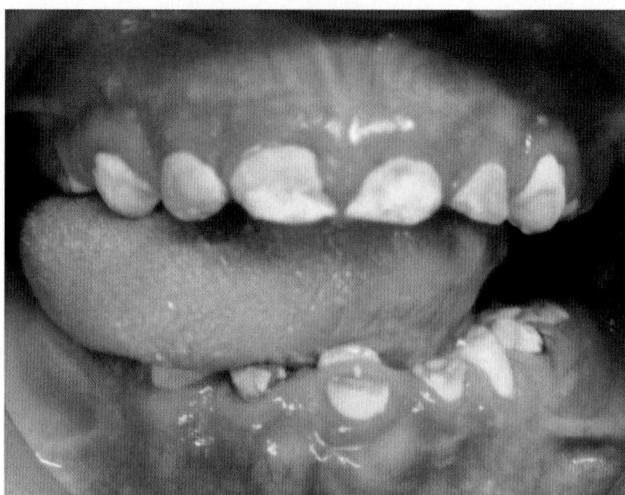

Fig. 21.9 A 5-year-old boy with a history of liver transplantation and gastric tube feeding has a generalized calculus deposit. *(Copyright Dr. Daniela Silva. All rights reserved.)*

Gingival Diseases of Childhood
Plaque-Induced Gingival Disease

Gingivitis is extremely common among children and adolescents, and it affects up to 70% of children who are more than 7 years old.[16,47] Inflammation is usually limited to the marginal gingiva (Fig. 21.8), with undetectable loss of bone or connective tissue attachment in most cases. Although gingivitis does not always progress to periodontitis, the management of gingival disease in children and adolescents is important, because periodontitis is always preceded by gingivitis.[47]

In children and adults, the primary cause of gingivitis is dental plaque, which is related to poor oral hygiene. The relationship between plaque and the gingival index, however, is weak and remains unclear.[9,37,38,41] Although gingivitis is highly prevalent among children, its severity usually is less intense than that found in adults.[10] Similar oral hygiene conditions produce less severe forms of disease in children compared with adults.[47]

As children age, their tendency to develop gingivitis increases.[10] The prevalence of disease is lowest during the preschool years and increases throughout childhood, peaking during puberty. However, increases in the degree of gingival inflammation do not fully correlate with the amount of plaque, which suggests the influence of other factors.

Clinical Features

The most prevalent type of gingival disease in childhood is *chronic marginal gingivitis* (see Fig. 21.8). The gingival tissues exhibit changes in color, size, consistency, and surface texture that are similar to those of chronic inflammation in the adult. Red, linear inflammation is accompanied by underlying chronic changes, including swelling, increased vascularization, and hyperplasia. Bleeding and increased pocket depth are not found as often in children as in adults, but they may be observed if severe gingival hypertrophy or hyperplasia occur.[9,47]

Chronic gingivitis in children is characterized by a loss of collagen in the area around the junctional epithelium and an infiltrate that consists mostly of lymphocytes, with small numbers of polymorphonuclear leukocytes, plasma cells, monocytes, and mast cells. Lesions typically have relatively few plasma cells, and they resemble the early nondestructive, nonprogressive lesions that are seen in adults. Unlike the adult inflammatory response, gingivitis in children is dominated by T lymphocytes, with few B lymphocytes and plasma cells in the infiltrate. This difference may explain why gingivitis in children rarely progresses to periodontitis.[34,35,41,55] Gingival histology in children also demonstrates other unique features that may decrease the tendency to progress to severe gingivitis. The junctional epithelium of the primary dentition tends to be thicker than in the permanent dentition,[10] which is thought to reduce the permeability of the gingival structures to bacterial toxins that initiate the inflammatory response.

Calculus

Calculus deposits are uncommon in infants and toddlers, but they can increase with age. About 9% of 4- to 6-year-old children exhibit calculus deposits. By the age of 7 to 9 years, 18% of children have calculus deposits, and by the age of 10 to 15 years, 33% to 43% have some calculus formation.[69] In the category of special needs patients, children with cystic fibrosis[69] or chronic kidney disease[40] have a higher incidence of calculus deposits, which can be caused by increased calcium and phosphate concentrations in saliva. Children who are fed exclusively with gastric or nasogastric tubes show significant calculus buildup as a result of a lack of function and increased oral pH (Fig. 21.9).[23]

Microbiology of Disease

Because the intensity of gingival disease increases as a child develops into adulthood, it is important to understand the microbiology of disease, which is discussed further in Chapter 8. The composition of the oral microflora changes as the child matures.[10] Yang and colleagues[70] analyzed samples of dental plaque in children and reported that 71% of 18- to 48-month-old children were infected with at least

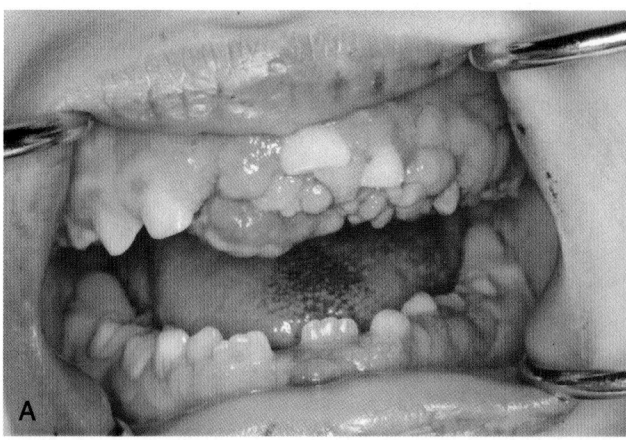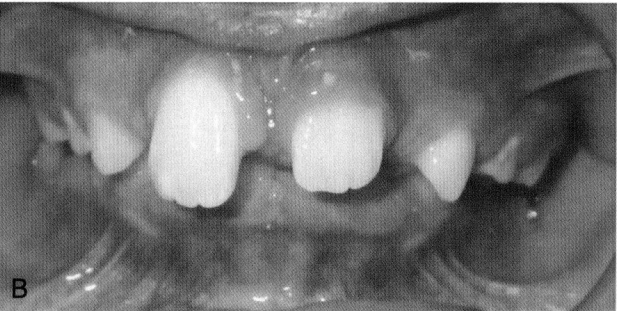

Fig. 21.10 (A) A 7-year-old boy with a history of aplastic anemia and cyclosporine-induced gingival hyperplasia. (B) The same patient 1 year after gingivectomy and 6 months after the dosage of cyclosporine was decreased to one-half of the initial dosage. *(Copyright Dr. Daniela Silva. All rights reserved.)*

one periodontal pathogen. Sixty-eight percent were infected with *Porphyromonas gingivalis,* and 20% had *Tannerella forsythia* (previously called *Bacteroides forsythus*).[70] A moderate correlation was found between *T. forsythia* in children and periodontal disease in their mothers. *T. forsythia* also has been associated with gingival bleeding in children.

In a similar study, 60% of children between the ages of 2 and 18 years had detectable levels of *P. gingivalis* in their plaque, and 75% showed similar levels of *Actinobacillus actinomycetemcomitans. P. gingivalis* was most strongly associated with the progression of gingivitis and the onset of periodontitis in otherwise healthy children.[45]

Pediatric gingivitis models have demonstrated increased subgingival levels of *Actinomyces, Capnocytophaga, Leptotrichia,* and *Selenomonas*[16]—pathogens usually not seen in adult gingivitis—thereby raising interest in their potential role in the cause of childhood gingivitis.

Eruption Gingivitis

Gingivitis associated with tooth eruption is so common that the term *eruption gingivitis* has come into frequent use. Although tooth eruption does not directly cause gingivitis, inflammation associated with plaque accumulation around erupting teeth, perhaps due to discomfort caused by brushing these friable areas, may contribute to gingivitis.[10] The gingiva around erupting teeth can appear reddened because gingival margins have not yet keratinized fully and sulcus development is incomplete.

Exfoliating and severely carious primary teeth often contribute to gingivitis caused by plaque accumulation as a result of pain during brushing or food impaction in areas of cavitation. As a normal part of exfoliation, the junctional epithelium migrates under the resorbing tooth, thereby increasing pocket depth and potentially creating a niche for pathogenic bacteria.[10] The discomfort of chewing on severely infected teeth often leads to unilateral chewing on the unaffected side.

Puberty Gingivitis

The incidence of marginal gingivitis increases as a child matures, peaking when he or she is 9 to 14 years old and then decreasing slightly after puberty.[10] Gingival disease that behaves in such a manner is often referred to as *pubertal* (or *puberty*) *gingivitis.* Chapters 19 and 41 continue the discussion of this condition.

The most frequent manifestation of puberty gingivitis is bleeding and inflammation in interproximal areas. Inflammatory gingival enlargement may also occur in males and females, but it typically subsides after puberty[44] (see Fig. 21.8). The altered gingival response during this developmental stage is thought to be the result of hormonal changes that magnify the vascular and inflammatory response to dental plaque[10,47] and that modify the reactions of dental plaque microbes.[22]

Drug-Induced Gingival Enlargement

Gingival enlargement (see Chapter 19) can result from the use of certain drugs. Cyclosporine, phenytoin, and calcium channel blockers, which are used to treat conditions that are encountered during childhood (e.g., organ transplantation, epilepsy, cardiac anomalies), increase the prevalence of gingival enlargement (Fig. 21.10). A randomized clinical trial found an interesting and significant decrease in the incidence (21%) of phenytoin-induced gingival hyperplasia in children with epilepsy taking oral folic acid supplementation (0.5 mg/day) compared with the control group[6] (88%).[6] Although complicated by the plaque levels along the gingival margin, this form of gingival disease has features that are not typical of chronic marginal gingivitis.[47]

LEARNING BOX 21.3

What are the most common drugs that cause gingival enlargement in children, and what conditions do they treat? Cyclosporine is an immunosuppressant drug used by patients who have undergone organ transplantation. Phenytoin is an antiepileptic medication, and calcium channel blockers are used to treat hypertension, abnormal heart rhythms, and Raynaud phenomenon.

Gingival Changes Related to Orthodontic Appliances

Gingival enlargement can be related to the presence of fixed orthodontic appliances, which complicate plaque removal (Fig. 21.11). Gingival changes can occur within 1 to 2 months of appliance placement. They usually are transient, and they only rarely produce long-term damage to periodontal tissues.[20] The fact that most orthodontic treatment is provided to individuals during puberty, when they are subject to the inflammatory changes associated with puberty gingivitis, may exacerbate the observed effect.

Mouth Breathing

Mouth breathing and lip incompetence, which are together referred to as an *open mouth posture,* are often associated with increased plaque and gingival inflammation.[20] The area of inflammation is often limited to the gingiva of the maxillary incisors. There is usually a clear line of demarcation where the gingiva is uncovered by the lip.

Non–Plaque-Induced Gingival Lesions

Intraoral soft tissue lesions can be encountered in the pediatric population as they are in the adult population. The six most common pediatric intraoral lesions are primary herpetic gingivostomatitis, recurrent herpes simplex, recurrent aphthous stomatitis, candidiasis, angular cheilitis, and geographic tongue.[47] Most of these lesions manifest without significant differences between the pediatric and adult populations, but two do have specific pediatric considerations.

Primary Herpetic Gingivostomatitis

Primary herpetic gingivostomatitis is an acute-onset viral infection that occurs early during childhood, with a heightened incidence

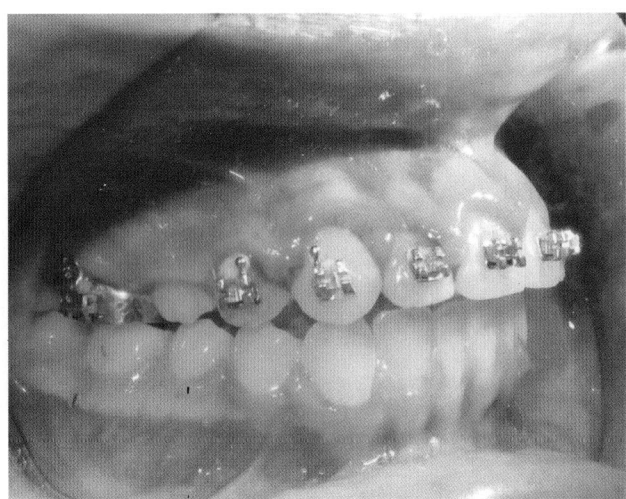

Fig. 21.11 Chronic marginal gingivitis was a result of orthodontic therapy and inadequate oral hygiene. *(Copyright Dr. Daniela Silva. All rights reserved.)*

between the ages of 1 and 3 years (see Chapter 20). Among children with primary herpetic infections, 99% are symptom free or have symptoms that are attributed to teething. The remaining 1% can develop significant gingival inflammation and ulceration of the attached gingiva, tongue, palate, and lips[28,47] (Fig. 21.12).

The most important therapeutic measure is to control the child's hydration with bland, nonacetic fluids. Hospitalization may be necessary in some severe cases.

Candidiasis

Candidiasis results from an overgrowth of *Candida albicans,* usually after a course of antibiotics or as a result of congenital or acquired immunodeficiency. It is far less common in children than in adults, and it rarely occurs in a healthy child.[13]

Localized Juvenile Spongiotic Gingival Hyperplasia

Another condition that appears to be unrelated to plaque accumulation is localized juvenile spongiotic gingival hyperplasia. This condition was identified only recently, and its pathogenesis is not well defined. The lesions are localized patches on the attached gingiva that manifest as bright red, raised overgrowths; they are usually painless and associated with easy bleeding. These lesions are most commonly seen on the anterior labial maxillary and mandibular gingiva.[18] Most of the patients with this condition are between 8 and 14 years of age (Fig. 21.13).

Periodontal Diseases of Childhood

Although gingivitis is considered to be almost universal among children who are older than 7 years of age,[16,47] frank periodontal disease with the loss of periodontal attachment and supporting bone is far less common in the pediatric population than in adults.[16] The incidence of disease begins increasing between the ages of 12 and 17 years, but the prevalence of severe attachment loss involving multiple teeth remains low at 0.2% to 0.5%.[16] Of the various manifestations of periodontal disease, chronic periodontitis is more prevalent among adults, and aggressive periodontitis is more common among children and adolescents.[16]

Oral hygiene habits should be imprinted early during life, with instructions about proper technique and directions regarding the frequency of plaque removal procedures. These will form a foundation

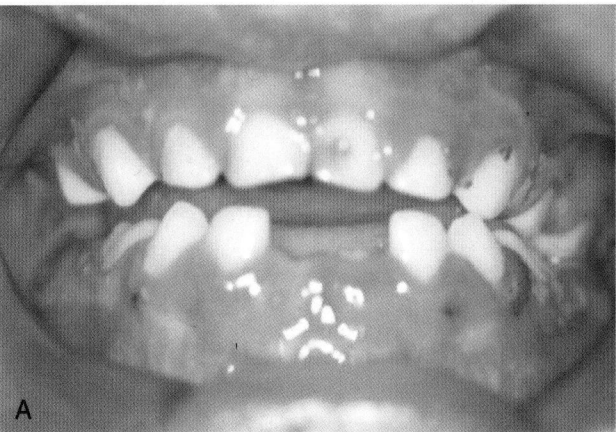 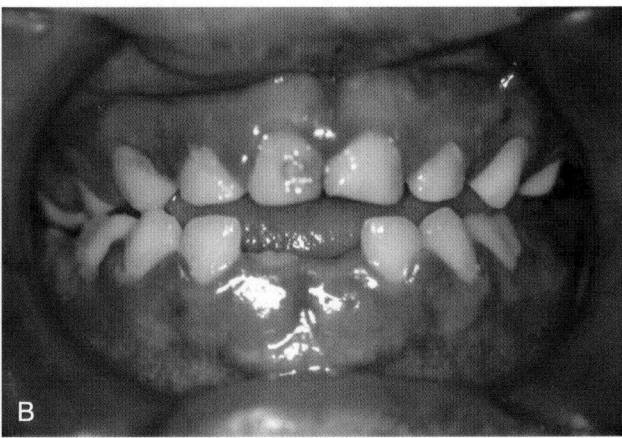

Fig. 21.12 (A) Acute herpetic gingivostomatitis in a 5-year-old girl produced spontaneous bleeding. The infection is mostly limited to the attached gingiva, tongue, palate, and lips. (B) In the same patient 1 week later, the attached gingiva demonstrates initial healing. *(Courtesy Dr. Thomas K. Barber, University of California, Los Angeles Pediatric Dentistry.)*

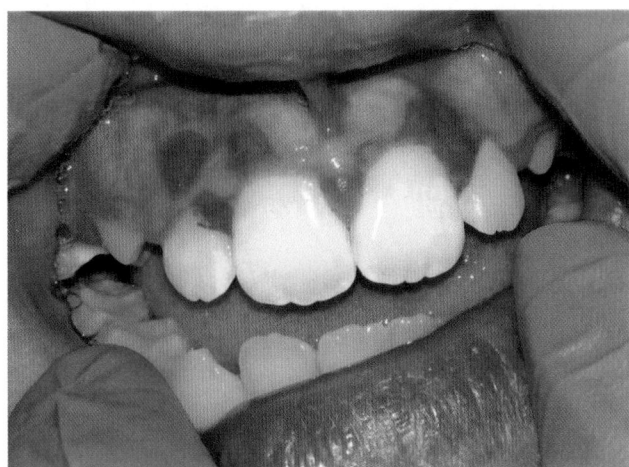

Fig. 21.13 Localized juvenile spongiotic gingival hyperplasia is seen in an 11-year-old girl. The papillary gingiva is red, and the gingival overgrowth is prone to easy bleeding. *(Courtesy Dr. Chanel McCreedy. All rights reserved.)*

for a lifetime of dedication to periodontal health. Clinicians should be aware of the specific periodontal needs of children with particular abnormalities, such as gingival hyperplasia associated with immunosuppression protocols used with organ transplantation, antiseizure medications, and increased severity of periodontal disease in diabetic children. Physically and mentally challenged children deserve special care to ensure that appropriate preventive techniques are available; techniques may include the use of electric toothbrushes and antibacterial mouth rinses. Chapters 27 to 29 describe the different types of periodontal disease.

Aggressive Periodontitis

Aggressive periodontitis is addressed in greater detail in Chapter 28. Because of the relatively early onset of disease, which occurs around the time of puberty, former classifications mention the developmental stage: early-onset periodontitis, prepubertal periodontitis, and juvenile periodontitis.[16,47] The currently accepted designation of aggressive periodontitis may be further broken down into two forms: localized and generalized. Localized aggressive periodontitis has been defined as "interproximal attachment loss on at least two permanent first molars and incisors, with attachment loss on no more than two teeth other than first molars and incisors."[16]

In young individuals, localized aggressive periodontitis is more common than the generalized form. Studies consistently show that among different geographic locations and racial groups, aggressive periodontitis is most prevalent in African populations and their descendants, ranging between 1% and 5%. The prevalence in whites residing in Europe is 0.1% to 0.5%, and in North America, the disease affects approximately 0.1% to 0.2% of whites, 0.5% to 1% of Hispanics, and 2.6% of African Americans.[2,15,56] Some studies suggest a higher prevalence among Asian children.[2,48,64] Of relevance to the pediatric population is the finding that the classic clinical presentation of localized aggressive periodontitis may be preceded by signs of bone loss around the teeth during the primary dentition.[16]

The generalized form of aggressive periodontitis, which is defined as a generalized interproximal attachment loss, including at least three teeth that are not first molars and incisors, is rare among children (Fig. 21.14). The onset of this form of periodontitis usually occurs after the initiation of adolescence. Overall prevalence is 0.13% among 14- to 17-year-old children[16]; however, the prevalence is higher among individuals with Down syndrome.[4,15,50] A purported genetic influence

in the disease process suggests that any signs of disease in a child with a family history of generalized aggressive periodontitis should be investigated further.

Several studies have suggested the involvement of *A. actinomycetemcomitans*[2,18,32,56,59] and *P. gingivalis*[2] in the pathogenesis of aggressive periodontitis, with the former found at higher levels in children with the localized form and the latter found at higher levels in those with the generalized form. Both of these pathogens are rare in healthy children, with a prevalence of 4.8%, but the rate is elevated for children with periodontitis, with a reported prevalence of 20%.[48] One study found a very strong association between localized aggressive periodontitis and the prevalence and abundance of *A. actinomycetemcomitans*. The study authors also observed *A. actinomycetemcomitans* as being very site specific; it was more prevalent and abundant in diseased sites compared with healthy sites in individuals with localized aggressive periodontitis.[56]

Chronic Periodontitis

Chronic periodontitis, which was formerly known as *adult periodontitis* or *chronic adult periodontitis*, is one of the most prevalent forms of periodontitis. It is characterized by a "slow to moderate rate of progression that may include periods of rapid destruction."[16] Although the disease can appear in children and adolescents as a result of retained plaque and calculus, it is far less prevalent in this population than it is in adults.[16]

Similar to the adult version, which is discussed in greater detail in Chapter 27, chronic periodontitis can occur in children in the localized form, in which less than 30% of the dentition is affected, and in the generalized form, in which more than 30% of the dentition is affected.

The microbiology of this disease is discussed in Chapters 8 and 9. Studies suggest the familial transmission of certain bacteria associated with chronic periodontitis. Strains such as *T. forsythia*, *Prevotella intermedia*, and *Prevotella nigrescens* are found more often in the children of individuals who harbor these types of bacteria.[66] *Fusobacterium nucleatum* and *P. gingivalis* have been identified at significant levels in children of similarly affected parents.[12,30] Levels of these strains increase with age, suggesting that *P. gingivalis* and *T. forsythia* may serve as early markers during screening for periodontal disease.[12,32,63] Although chronic periodontitis may not be highly prevalent among children, early colonization may underscore the importance of early detection, particularly for those at elevated risk for adult forms of the disease.

Gingival Manifestation of Systemic Disease in Children

Systemic diseases that result in periodontitis occur more frequently in children than adults.[2] Chapter 14 discusses some of the systemic diseases and disorders that affect periodontal health. However, many diseases are expressed differently in children than in adults and therefore merit special mention.

Acute necrotizing gingivitis is rarely seen, except in cases of primary or secondary immune suppression, Down syndrome, or severe malnutrition.[19,50] The child's breath is fetid, and he or she complains of pain and discomfort when eating (see Chapter 20).

Endocrine Disorders and Hormonal Changes
Diabetes Mellitus

Type 1 or insulin-dependent diabetes mellitus occurs more frequently in children and young adults than type 2 or non–insulin-dependent diabetes mellitus. As with diabetic adults, gingival inflammation and periodontitis are more prevalent in affected children than in

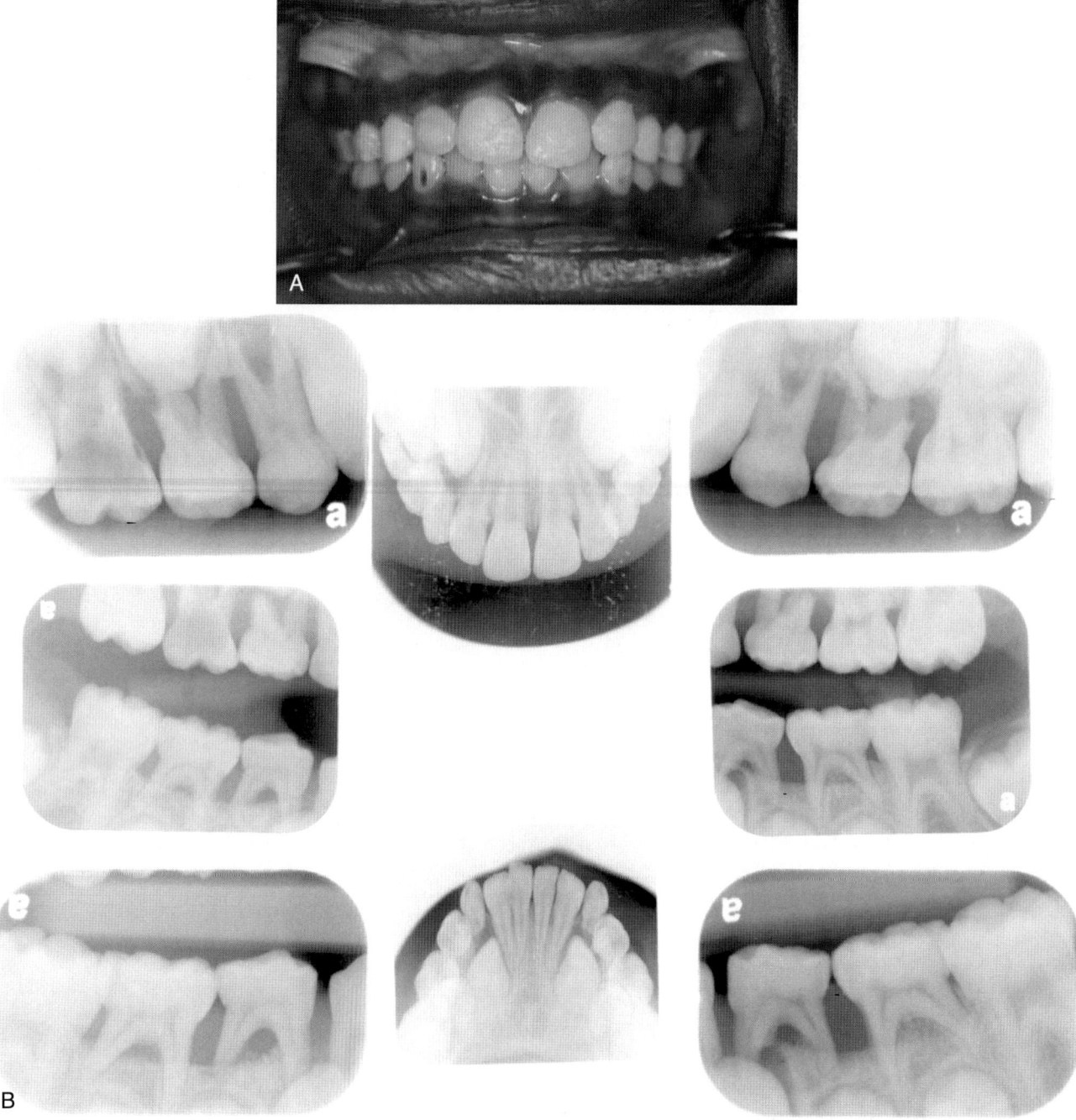

Fig. 21.14 (A) In an 8-year-old African-American girl with aggressive periodontitis, the clinical appearance of the mucosa is similar to normal tissue, but the primary canines and molars have mobility, bleeding on probing, and deep pockets. (B) In an 8-year-old African-American girl with aggressive periodontitis, radiographs show advanced bone loss at the primary canine and molar areas. *(Copyright Dr. Daniela Silva. All rights reserved.)*

unaffected individuals.[47,51] Clinical consequences include premature tooth loss and impaired immune response to the oral flora. The severity of periodontal disease is worse in children with poor metabolic control.

Although destructive changes are rare in healthy children, periodontal destruction can be observed in diabetic children, usually appearing around the time of puberty and becoming progressively worse as children mature into adulthood. Disease prevention and fastidious oral hygiene measures should be highly promoted.[31,32]

Hematologic Disorders and Immune Deficiencies
Leukemias

Leukemia is the most common type of cancer in children. Acute lymphocytic leukemia accounts for most cases among children who are younger than 7 years of age. Leukemia must be considered as part of the differential diagnosis for children who present with the hallmark features of acute gingival enlargement, ulceration, bleeding, and infection (Fig. 21.15).[1]

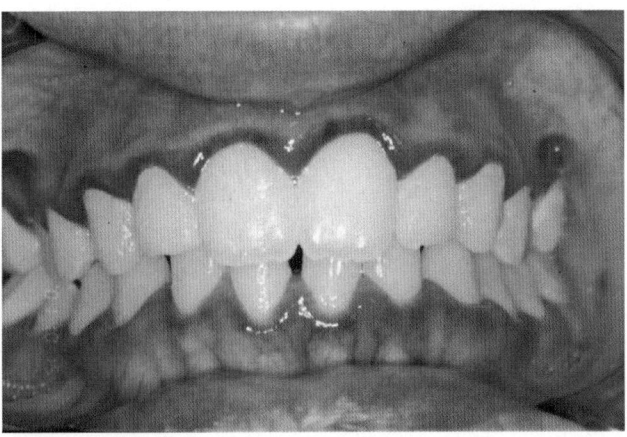

Fig. 21.15 In a 12-year-old boy with acute lymphoblastic leukemia, there is generalized redness of the marginal gingiva with spontaneous bleeding. *(Copyright Dr. Daniela Silva. All rights reserved.)*

Neutrophil Disorders

Neutrophil disorders impair defenses against infections, making afflicted individuals susceptible to severe periodontal destruction (see Chapter 14). Many neutrophil disorders are genetic, including some forms of neutropenia, such as familial and cyclic neutropenia, Chédiak–Higashi syndrome, leukocyte adhesion deficiency, Papillon–Lefèvre syndrome, and Cohen syndrome.[16,27] The diagnosis of the systemic disorder usually occurs before any signs of periodontal destruction appear.

Because periodontal changes are difficult to reverse in children with neutrophil disorders, disease management includes oral hygiene measures, mechanical debridement, antimicrobial therapy, and supportive care for any resultant tissue destruction or tooth loss. Treatment success is unpredictable because of the impact of systemic disease.[16,27]

Congenital Anomalies

Down syndrome is another congenital condition that is diagnosed before the expression of periodontal disease. People with Down syndome experience a high prevalence of severe aggressive periodontitis during early adulthood. The disease process likely reflects a host susceptibility that results in an exaggerated immune and inflammatory response rather than a reaction to a specific causative microbe.[3,4,19,27] Studies of people with Down syndrome uncovered defective neutrophil chemotaxis, which can lead to significant tissue loss and the progression of periodontitis.[27]

Oral Mucosa in Childhood Diseases

Some childhood diseases, such as rubeola (i.e., rubella or measles), varicella (i.e., chickenpox), diphtheria, and scarlatina (i.e., scarlet fever), cause alterations or lesions of the oral mucosa and the underlying tissues. These diseases are explored in textbooks that discuss oral and pediatric pathology.

Therapeutic Considerations for Pediatric Patients

The diagnostic process for pediatric patients follows the general outline described in Chapter 32. Medical and dental histories should be recorded for each child, with parents or legal guardians serving as the primary historians. However, differences between the primary and permanent dentition and aspects related to development warrant some differences in clinical practices that involve the care of children.

Periodontal indices do not need to be recorded during the primary dentition unless a child exhibits signs of aggressive periodontitis or other unusual disease processes. More explicit periodontal assessments should begin during mixed dentition, when children have permanent incisors and first molars. Rather than recording full-mouth probing depths, clinicians can focus on selected teeth. For example, a rudimentary assessment of teeth #3, #8, #14, #19, #24, and #30 has been suggested,[20] with notes made regarding gingival health, bleeding on probing, and degree of calculus. This quick screening usually is sufficient for children up to the age of 11 years. Between the ages 12 to 19 years, when most individuals have a full permanent dentition, clinicians should also record pocket depths of more than 4 mm. By this stage of dental development, full-mouth pocket-depth probing may be warranted on the basis of general indicators of each patient's gingival health or risk of disease.

In-office professional plaque control procedures can vary in accordance with a patient's stage of development. Calculus deposits are uncommon in infants and toddlers. Supragingival plaque removal with the use of simple rubber-cup coronal polishing or a toothbrush is usually sufficient during the primary dentition.[20] If calculus deposits are evident, selective supragingival scaling can be performed. As the permanent teeth erupt, the prevalence of calculus deposits increases, often necessitating targeted subgingival scaling in addition to supragingival plaque removal.[20]

Chapter 48 discusses plaque control for periodontal patients. In children, however, the dynamic process of developing manual dexterity affects the ability of a child to perform expected procedures. Each child requires an individualized home care program based on his or her ability to perform the requested activities. For young children, plaque control should be a shared responsibility between children and their parents or caregivers. Instruction in plaque control should be delivered to parents and children in language and terms that both understand.

For children who are younger than 7 years of age, parents or caregivers should be asked to assist with toothbrushing.[20] Children may be encouraged to take a turn brushing their teeth using a simple scrub technique. However, parents should also take a turn to ensure the proper removal of plaque. By 7 years old, children usually possess the manual dexterity to brush their teeth on their own and may require only limited adult supervision.[20] More refined brushing techniques can be introduced during adolescence.

The oral hygiene habits of parents and caregivers have a significant influence on children's oral health behavior. An extensive survey of parents in the United Kingdom found that children and parents place a large emphasis on the cosmetic benefit of toothbrushing. Parents who placed more emphasis on the short-term benefits of toothbrushing were more likely to miss brushing the child's teeth in the evening, but when brushing a child's teeth was habitual, there was a significantly higher chance of brushing twice each day.[64]

Mechanical toothbrushes with rotary heads are effective for plaque removal.[20] The use of these devices can be encouraged as soon as children are able to tolerate the vibrating sensation because many children initially dislike the feeling of the rotary movement. Mechanical toothbrushes are especially recommended for physically challenged children and individuals with fixed orthodontic appliances.[47]

Flossing is usually not indicated for children during the primary dentition stage because most children have interdental spacing throughout most of their arches. However, as interdental contacts develop, flossing should be added to the home care routine. Studies have demonstrated a decrease in gingival bleeding and the quantity of microbes associated with periodontal disease when tooth and tongue brushing are combined with flossing.[7,21] Limitations in manual dexterity may necessitate parental assistance with flossing during the mixed dentition stage. Adolescents with sufficient manual dexterity can be expected to floss on their own.[20]

Antimicrobial mouthrinses for chemical plaque control are not indicated for very young children because of the risk of ingestion of chemical agents.[20] However, rinses may be indicated for older children who demonstrate the ability to expectorate after rinsing.

Conclusions

The periodontium of the primary dentition is different from that of the permanent dentition. Normal development can result in changes to the periodontium. Plaque-induced gingivitis is very common in children, although it may be less intense than in adults. With the exception of localized aggressive periodontitis, children rarely show signs of periodontitis. Some systemic disorders that are commonly associated with periodontal disease manifest initially during childhood.

Recommendations regarding home plaque control routines should be individualized according to each patient's periodontal disease status and developmental stage. Because early diagnosis ensures the greatest chance for successful treatment, it is paramount that children receive a periodontal examination as part of their routine dental visits.

 A Case Scenario is found on the companion website www.expertconsult.com.

References

 References for this chapter are found on the companion website www.expertconsult.com.

CHAPTER 22

Desquamative Gingivitis

Alfredo Aguirre | Jose Luis Tapia Vazquez | Yasmin Mair

 For online-only content on miscellaneous conditions that mimic desquamative gingivitis, please visit the companion website at www.expertconsult.com.

Chronic Desquamative Gingivitis

Although the condition was first recognized and reported in 1894,[171] the term *chronic desquamative gingivitis* was not coined by Prinz[131] until 1932. It describes a reaction characterized by intense erythema, desquamation, and ulceration of the free and attached gingiva[54,106] (Fig. 22.1).

Patients can be asymptomatic, but when symptomatic, their complaints range from a mild burning sensation to intense pain. Approximately 50% of desquamative gingivitis cases are localized to the gingiva, although patients can have involvement of the gingiva plus other intraoral and extraoral sites.[59,121]

The cause was initially unclear, with a variety of possibilities suggested. Because most cases were diagnosed in women during the fourth and fifth decades of life (although desquamative gingivitis can occur as early as puberty or as late as the seventh or eighth decade), hormonal derangement was suspected. In 1960, McCarthy and colleagues[102] suggested that desquamative gingivitis was not a specific disease entity but was instead a *gingival response associated with a variety of conditions*. This concept has been supported by numerous immunopathologic studies.[82,90,123,142,162,172]

The use of clinical and laboratory parameters has revealed that approximately 75% of desquamative gingivitis cases have a dermatologic genesis. Lichen planus and cicatricial pemphigoid account for 84% of the desquamative gingivitis cases.[83,119] However, many other mucocutaneous autoimmune conditions (e.g., bullous pemphigoid, pemphigus vulgaris, linear immunoglobulin A [IgA] disease, dermatitis herpetiformis, lupus erythematosus, chronic ulcerative stomatitis, dermatomyositis, mixed connective tissue disease) can manifest as desquamative gingivitis.[83,152]

Other conditions that must be considered in the differential diagnosis of desquamative gingivitis include chronic bacterial, fungal, and viral infections and reactions to medications, mouthwashes, and chewing gum. Although less common, Crohn disease, sarcoidosis, some leukemias, and factitious lesions have also been reported to manifest clinically as desquamative gingivitis.[135,152,178]

It is important to ascertain the disease responsible for desquamative gingivitis to establish the appropriate therapeutic approach. To achieve this goal, a clinical examination is coupled with a thorough history and routine histologic and immunofluorescence studies.[24,90,166,178] Despite a systematic diagnostic approach, the cause of desquamative gingivitis cannot be elucidated in up to one-third of cases.[136]

Diagnosis of Desquamative Gingivitis: A Systematic Approach

Desquamative gingivitis is a clinical term and not a diagnosis. After the condition is identified, a series of laboratory procedures should be used to arrive at a final diagnosis. The success of any therapeutic approach depends on the establishment of an accurate final diagnosis. The following sections describe a systematic approach to determining the disease that is triggering desquamative gingivitis (Fig. 22.2).

Clinical History

A thorough clinical history is mandatory to begin the assessment of desquamative gingivitis.[90,122] Data regarding the symptoms associated with this condition and its historical aspects (e.g., lesion onset, whether it has worsened, habits that exacerbate it) provide the foundation for a thorough examination. Information about previous therapy to alleviate the condition should be documented.

Clinical Examination

The distribution pattern of the lesions (e.g., focal or multifocal, with or without confinement to gingival tissues) provides information that can begin to narrow the differential diagnosis.[24,90] A simple clinical maneuver such as the Nikolsky sign offers insight into the plausibility of a vesiculobullous disorder.[107]

CLINICAL CORRELATION

The Nikolsky sign is characterized by blister formation or peeling of skin or mucosa when horizontal tangential pressure is applied to the skin or mucosa in patients with vesiculobullous disorders.

Biopsy

Given the extent and number of lesions that may be present in an individual, an incisional biopsy is the best strategy for beginning the microscopic and immunologic evaluation.[24] An important consideration is the selection of the biopsy site. A perilesional incisional biopsy should avoid areas of ulceration because necrosis and epithelial denudation severely hamper the diagnostic process.[169]

After the tissue is excised from the oral cavity, the specimen can be bisected and then submitted for microscopic examination. Buffered formalin (10%) should be used to fix the tissue for conventional hematoxylin and eosin (H&E) evaluation. Michel's buffer (i.e., ammonium sulfate buffer, pH 7.0) is used as the transport solution for immunofluorescence assessment. An incisional biopsy of uninvolved (normal) mucosa typically shows the same immunofluorescent findings as the biopsy of the perilesional tissue. However, there are notable exceptions, such as lichen planus and chronic cutaneous lupus erythematosus, in which only the lesional tissue exhibits the corresponding immunologic markers (Table 22.1).[169]

Microscopic Examination

Sections of approximately 5 μm of formalin-fixed, paraffin-embedded tissue stained with conventional H&E are obtained for light microscopy examination.[169]

Immunofluorescence

For *direct* immunofluorescence, unfixed frozen sections are incubated with a variety of fluorescein-labeled, antihuman serum (i.e., anti-IgG, anti-IgA, anti-IgM, antifibrin, and anti-C3). For *indirect* immunofluorescence, unfixed frozen sections of oral or esophageal mucosa

from an animal such as a monkey are first incubated with the patient's serum to enable attachment of serum antibodies to the mucosal tissue. The tissue is then incubated with fluorescein-labeled antihuman serum. Immunofluorescence tests are positive if a fluorescent signal is observed in the epithelium, its associated basement membrane, or the underlying connective tissue (see Table 22.1).[169]

Management

After the diagnosis is established, the dentist must choose the optimal management strategy. The choice depends on the practitioner's experience, the systemic impact of the disease, and the systemic complications of the medications. A detailed consideration of these factors dictates three scenarios.

In the first scenario, the dental practitioner takes direct and exclusive responsibility for the treatment of the patient. This occurs with conditions such as erosive lichen planus, which is responsive to topical steroids (Fig. 22.3).

In the second scenario, the dentist collaborates with another health care provider to evaluate and treat a patient concurrently. The classic example is seen with cicatricial pemphigoid, in which dentists and ophthalmologists work together to provide treatment (Fig. 22.4). Although the dentist addresses the oral lesions, the ophthalmologist monitors the integrity of the ocular conjunctiva.

In the third scenario, the patient is immediately referred to a dermatologist for further evaluation and treatment. This occurs with conditions for which the systemic impact of the disease transcends the boundaries of the oral cavity and results in significant morbidity or mortality. Pemphigus vulgaris is an example of a condition that, after diagnosis by the dentist, requires immediate referral to a dermatologist (Fig. 22.5). The complications (e.g., diabetes mellitus, osteoporosis, methemoglobinemia) of chronically administered systemic medications that are indicated for the management of diseases such as pemphigus vulgaris or nonresponsive mucous membrane pemphigoid (MMP) warrant referral to a dermatologist or a specialist in internal medicine.

When oral treatment is provided, periodic evaluation is needed to monitor the response of the patient to therapy. Initially, the patient should be evaluated at 2 to 4 weeks after beginning treatment to ensure that the condition is under control. Observation should continue until the patient is free of discomfort. Appointments every 3 to 6 months are then appropriate. Medication dosages are usually adjusted during this interval.

Table 22.2 summarizes suggested contemporary therapeutic approaches that can be used to treat selected conditions that can manifest as desquamative gingivitis. Dentists play an important role in the diagnosis and management of desquamative gingivitis. The

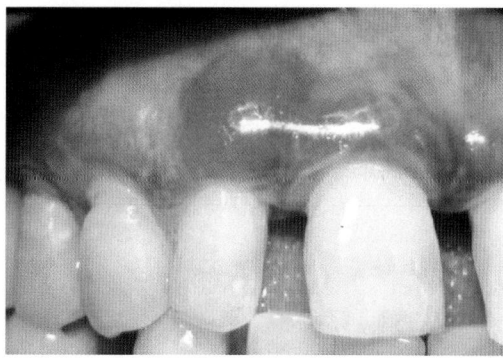

Fig. 22.1 In chronic desquamative gingivitis, irregular, conspicuous erythema involves the free and attached gingival tissues.

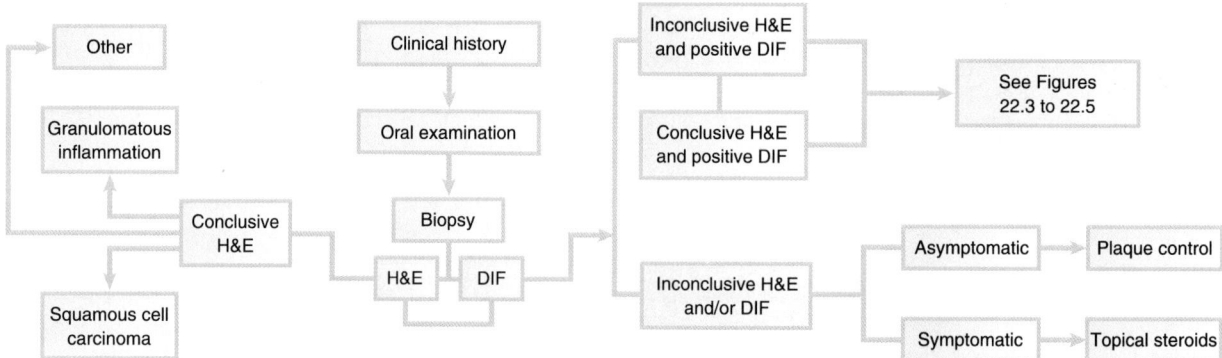

Fig. 22.2 The diagnostic approach for desquamative gingivitis includes hematoxylin and eosin (H&E) and direct immunofluorescence (DIF) evaluation of biopsy specimens.

TABLE 22.1   Diagnostic Findings for Conditions That Can Manifest as Desquamative Gingivitis

Disease	Histopathology	DIRECT IMMUNOFLUORESCENCE		INDIRECT IMMUNOFLUORESCENCE
		Biopsy of Perilesional Mucosa	Biopsy of Uninvolved Mucosa	Serum
Pemphigus	Intraepithelial clefting above the basal cell layer; basal cells have a characteristic tombstone appearance; acantholysis	Intercellular deposits in epithelium; IgG in all cases and C3 in most cases	Same as for perilesional mucosa	Intercellular antibodies (IgG) in ≥90% of cases
Cicatricial pemphigoid	Subepithelial clefting with epithelial separation from the underlying lamina propria, leaving an intact basal layer	Linear deposits of C3 with or without IgG at the basement membrane zone in most cases	Same as for perilesional mucosa	Basement membrane zone antibodies (IgG) in 10% of cases
Bullous pemphigoid	Subepithelial clefting with epithelial separation from the underlying lamina propria, leaving an intact basal layer	Linear deposits of C3 with or without IgG at the basement membrane zone in most cases	Same as for perilesional mucosa	Basement membrane zone in 40%–70% of cases
Epidermolysis bullosa acquisita	Similar to bullous and cicatricial pemphigoid	Linear deposits of IgG and C3 at the basement membrane zone in most cases	Same as for perilesional mucosa	Basement membrane zone antibodies (IgG) in 25% of cases
Lichen planus	Hyperkeratosis, hydropic degeneration of the basal layer, and sawtooth rete pegs; lamina propria exhibits dense, bandlike infiltrate, primarily of T lymphocytes; colloid bodies	Fibrillar deposits of fibrin at the dermal–epidermal junction	Negative	Negative
Chronic ulcerative stomatitis	Similar to erosive lichen planus; hyperkeratosis, acanthosis, basal cell layer liquefaction, subepithelial clefting, and lymphohistiocytic chronic infiltrate in a bandlike configuration	IgG deposits in the nuclei of the basal layer of epithelial cells	Same as for perilesional mucosa	ANA specific for basal cells of stratified squamous epithelium
Linear IgA disease	Similar to erosive lichen planus	Linear deposits of IgA at the basement membrane zone	Same as for perilesional mucosa	IgA basement membrane zone antibodies (IgA) in 30% of cases
Dermatitis herpetiformis	Collection of neutrophils, eosinophils, and fibrin in the connective tissue papillae	IgA deposits in the dermal papillae in 85% of cases	IgA deposits in dermal papillae in 100% of cases	IgA endomysial antibodies in 70% of cases; gliadin antibodies in 30% of cases
Systemic lupus erythematosus	Hyperkeratosis, basal cell degeneration, epithelial atrophy, and perivascular inflammation	IgG or IgM with or without C3 deposits at the dermal–epidermal junction	Same as for perilesional mucosa	ANA in >95% of cases; DNA and ENA antibodies in >50% of cases
Chronic cutaneous erythematosus	Hyperkeratosis, basal cell degeneration, epithelial atrophy, and perivascular inflammation	IgG or IgM with or without C3 deposits at the dermal–epidermal junction	Negative	Usually negative
Subacute lupus erythematosus	Less inflammatory cell infiltrate than systemic and chronic cutaneous forms but with similar microscopic features	IgG or IgM with or without C3 deposits at the dermal-epidermal junction in 60% of cases; granular IgG deposits in basal cell cytoplasm in 30% of cases	Same as for perilesional mucosa	ANA in 60% to 90% of cases; Ro (SSA) in 80% of cases; RF in 30% of cases; anti-RNP in 10% of cases

ANA, Antinuclear antibodies; *C3*, complement 3; *DNA*, deoxyribonucleic acid; *ENA*, extractable nuclear antigens; *IgA*, immunoglobulin A; *IgG*, immunoglobulin G; *IgM*, immunoglobulin M; *RF*, rheumatoid factor; *RNP*, ribonucleoprotein.
Adapted from Rinaggio J, Neiders ME, Aguirre A, Kumar V: Using immunofluorescence in the diagnosis of chronic ulcerative lesions of the oral mucosa. *Compend Contin Educ Dent* 20:943–944, 947–948, 950 passim, 1999.

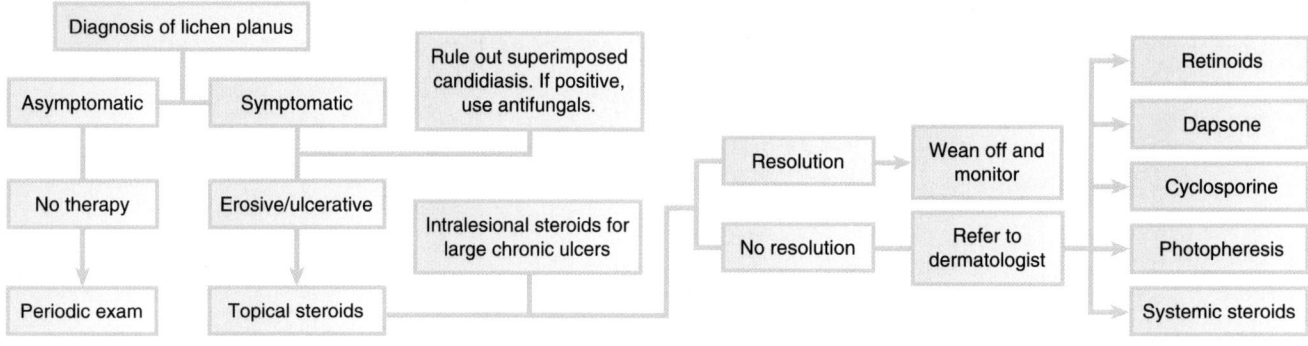

Fig. 22.3 Algorithm for the treatment of lichen planus.

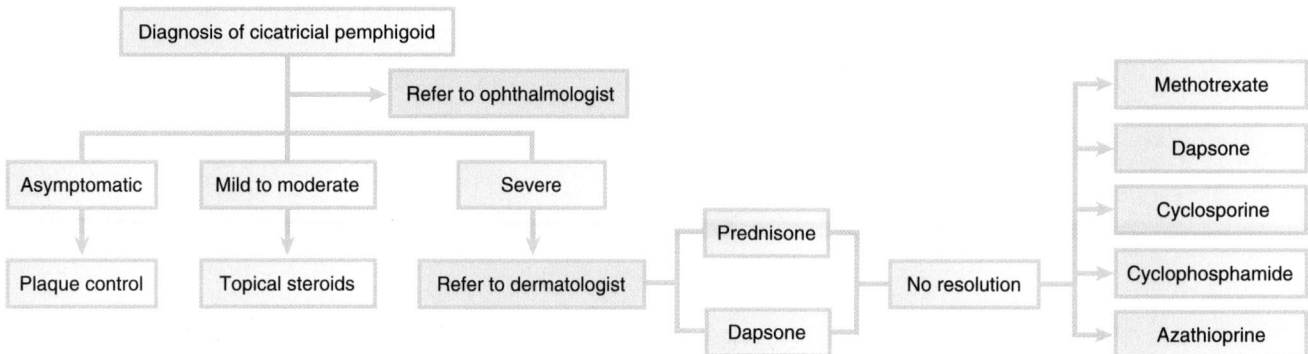

Fig. 22.4 Algorithm for the treatment of cicatricial pemphigoid.

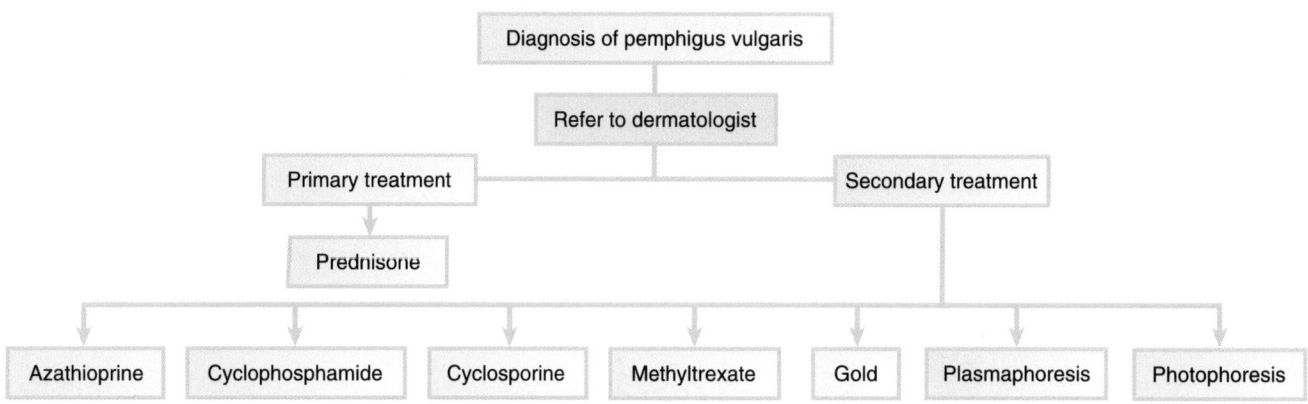

Fig. 22.5 Algorithm for the treatment of pemphigus vulgaris.

importance of recognizing and properly diagnosing this condition is accentuated by the fact that a serious and life-threatening disease (i.e., squamous cell carcinoma) can mimic desquamative gingivitis.[138]

Diseases That Can Manifest as Desquamative Gingivitis

Lichen Planus

Lichen planus is an inflammatory mucocutaneous disorder that can involve the mucosal surfaces (e.g., oral cavity, genital tract, other mucosae) and the skin, including the scalp and the nails.[141] Evidence suggests that lichen planus is an immunologically mediated mucocutaneous disorder in which host T lymphocytes play a central role.[11,68,76,100] Although the oral cavity can have lichen planus lesions with a distinct clinical configuration and distribution, the clinical presentation can simulate other mucocutaneous disorders. Oral lichen planus has a broad differential diagnosis.

Numerous epidemiologic studies have found that oral lichen planus occurs in 0.1% to 4% of the population.[146,153] Most patients with oral lichen planus are middle-aged or older women; the disorder occurs with a 2 : 1 ratio of women to men. Children are rarely affected. In a dental setting, cutaneous lichen planus is observed in about one-third of patients diagnosed with oral lichen planus.[97] Two-thirds of patients seen in dermatologic clinics exhibit oral lichen planus.[149]

KEY FACT

Lichen planus is a mucocutaneous disorder that classically manifests with bilateral, white striae on the buccal mucosae. The classic reticular subtype is asymptomatic, and no treatment is needed. Atrophic and erosive forms of oral lichen planus are associated with pain and a burning sensation, and topical corticosteroids are the mainstay of treatment. One percent of oral lichen planus cases may develop squamous cell carcinoma.

TABLE 22.2 Therapeutic Approaches for Treating Selected Conditions That Manifest as Desquamative Gingivitis

Disease	Mild Cases	Recalcitrant Cases	Severe or Refractory Cases
	THERAPY		
Erosive lichen planus	Delivery of therapeutic agent is enhanced with use of vacuum-formed custom trays **Rx:** Lidex (0.05% fluocinonide) gel **Disp:** One tube (15 g) **Sig:** Apply to affected area pc and hs Monitoring of patient's oral cavity warranted because candidiasis may develop after a few weeks of topical steroid use; concomitant use of antifungal may be necessary **Rx:** Clotrimazole 10-mg troches **Disp:** 90 **Sig:** Dissolve in mouth tid, then expectorate for 30 consecutive days	**Rx:** Protopic (0.1% tacrolimus) ointment **Disp:** One tube (15 g) **Sig:** Apply to affected area bid	Refer to dermatologist for management with systemic corticosteroids
Cicatricial pemphigoid	**Rx:** Lidex (0.05% fluocinonide) gel **Disp:** One tube (15 g) **Sig:** Apply to affected area pc and hs **Rx:** Temovate (0.05% clobetasol propionate) **Disp:** One tube (15 g) **Sig:** Apply to affected area qid		Refer to dermatologist for management with prednisone (20–30 mg/day); concomitant use of azathioprine may be needed; dapsone, sulfonamide, and tetracycline are other alternatives
Pemphigus	Refer to dermatologist for management with prednisone (20 to 30 mg/day); concomitant use of azathioprine may be needed		
Chronic ulcerative stomatitis	**Rx:** Lidex (0.05% fluocinonide) gel **Disp:** One tube (15 g) **Sig:** Apply to affected area qid **Rx:** Temovate (0.05% clobetasol propionate) **Disp:** One tube (15 g) **Sig:** Apply to affected area qid		

bid, Twice daily; *g,* grams; *hs,* at bedtime; *IU,* international units; *mg,* milligrams; *pc,* after meals; *qid,* four times daily.

Oral Lesions

Although there are several clinical forms of oral lichen planus (i.e., reticular, patch, atrophic, erosive, and bullous), the most common are the reticular and erosive subtypes. The typical reticular lesions are asymptomatic and bilateral, and they consist of interlacing white lines on the posterior region of the buccal mucosa. The lateral border and dorsum of the tongue, the hard palate, the alveolar ridge, and the gingiva may also be affected.[26] The reticular lesions can have an erythematous background, which is a feature associated with coexisting candidiasis. Oral lichen planus lesions follow a chronic course and have alternating, unpredictable periods of quiescence and flare-ups.

The erosive subtype of lichen planus is often associated with pain. It manifests as atrophic, erythematous, and often ulcerated areas. Fine, white radiating striations are observed bordering the atrophic and ulcerated zones. These areas may be sensitive to heat, acid, and spicy foods (Fig. 22.6).

Gingival Lesions

Approximately 7% to 10% of patients with oral lichen planus have lesions restricted to the gingival tissue.[109,149] They may occur as one or more types of the following four distinctive patterns:

1. *Keratotic lesions.* The raised, white lesions can manifest as groups of individual papules, linear or reticular lesions, or plaquelike configurations.

2. *Erosive or ulcerative lesions.* The extensive erythematous areas with a patchy distribution can manifest as focal or diffuse hemorrhagic areas. The lesions are exacerbated by slight trauma (e.g., toothbrushing) (Fig. 22.7).

3. *Vesicular or bullous lesions.* The raised, fluid-filled lesions are uncommon and short lived on the gingiva, quickly rupturing and leaving ulcerations.

4. *Atrophic lesions.* Atrophy of the gingival tissues with ensuing epithelial thinning results in erythema that is confined to the gingiva.

Histopathology

Microscopically, three main features characterize oral lichen planus: (1) hyperkeratosis or parakeratosis, (2) hydropic degeneration of the basal layer, and (3) a dense, bandlike infiltrate, consisting primarily of T lymphocytes, in the lamina propria (Fig. 22.8). Classically, the epithelial rete ridges have a sawtooth configuration. Hydropic degeneration of the basal layer of the epithelium can be sufficiently extensive that the epithelium becomes thin and atrophic or detaches from the underlying connective tissue and produces a subepithelial vesicle or an ulcer. Colloid bodies (i.e., Civatte bodies) are often seen at the epithelium–connective tissue interface.

The microscopic diagnosis of oral lichen planus is straightforward for the keratotic lesions, and biopsy specimens should be obtained from these areas if possible. However, classic histologic features may be obscured in areas of ulceration, making a conclusive diagnosis

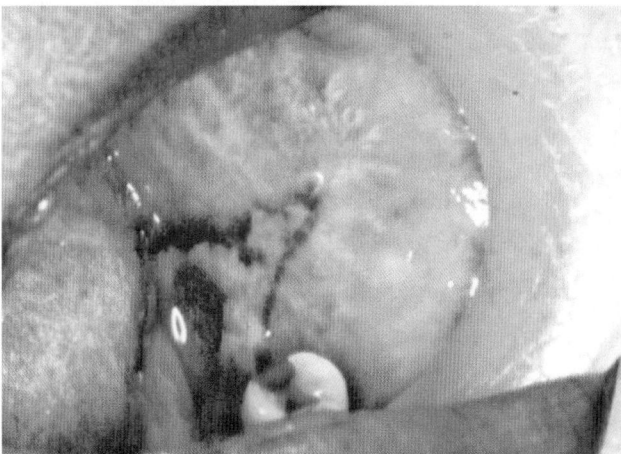

Fig. 22.6 In a case of erosive lichen planus, the large ulcerative lesion on the left buccal mucosa exhibits bordering erythema. The typical white striations of lichen planus are evident in the periphery of the ulcer.

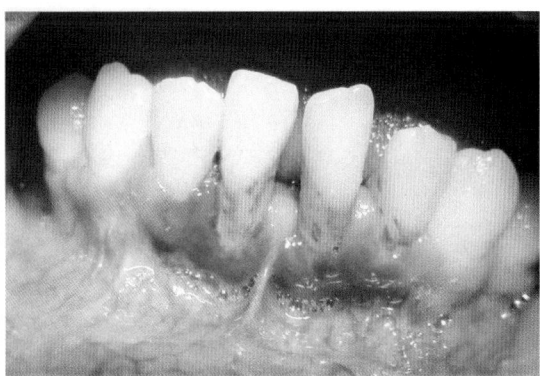

Fig. 22.7 Erosive lichen planus can manifest as desquamative gingivitis. The gingival tissues are erythematous, ulcerated, and painful. *(Courtesy Dr. Luis Gaitan, Oral Pathology Laboratory, Faculty of Odontology, National Autonomous University of Mexico, Mexico City, Mexico.)*

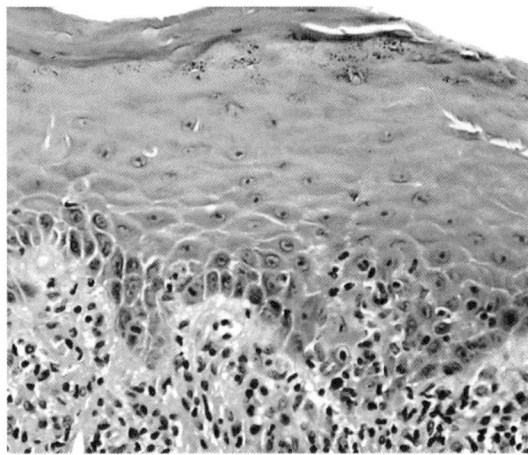

Fig. 22.8 Microscopic appearance of lichen planus. The biopsy specimen from a gingival lesion shows hyperkeratosis and mild hypergranulosis, along with focal basal cell degeneration, lymphocytic exocytosis, and thickening of the basement membrane. The rete pegs exhibit a slight serrated configuration. The papillary lamina propria shows a bandlike infiltrate of lymphohistiocytic chronic inflammatory cells. Hematoxylin and eosin stain; original magnification ×100.

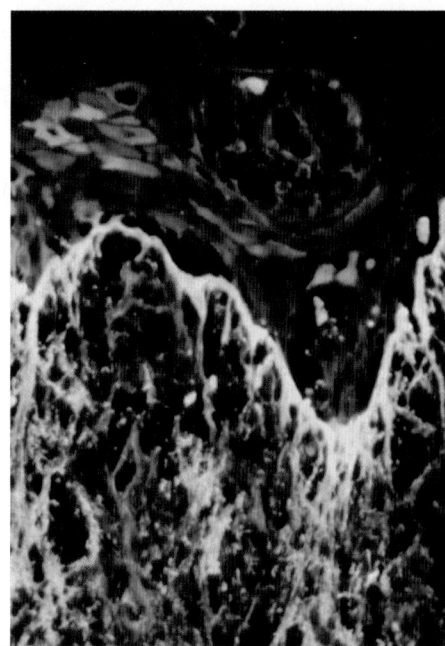

Fig. 22.9 Direct immunofluorescence staining of lichen planus. Fibrin deposits along the basement membrane of the epithelium exhibit a shaggy configuration.

of oral lichen planus difficult if it is based solely on conventional microscopy. Electron microscopy studies indicate that separation of the basal lamina from the basal cell layer is an early manifestation of lichen planus.[65]

KEY FACT

Civatte bodies are eosinophilic globules typically seen at the junction of epithelium and connective tissue in lichen planus. They are derived from keratinocytes that are undergoing apoptosis.

The pattern of oral lesions of lichen planus can change, and in unusual cases a second or third biopsy may be necessary to arrive at a definitive diagnosis. Controversy exists regarding the malignant potential of oral lichen planus. Some researchers posit that oral cancer emerges in up to 2% of patients with oral lichen planus.[45,66,67,91,161] Other researchers reject or question the connection between oral lichen planus and oral cancer.[46,70,95,133] Despite this controversy, biopsy and close follow-up are warranted for these patients.

Immunopathology

Direct immunofluorescence of lesional and perilesional oral lichen planus biopsy specimens reveals linear fibrillar (i.e., shaggy) deposits of fibrin in the basement membrane zone (Fig. 22.9), along with scattered immunoglobulin-staining cytoid bodies in the upper areas of the lamina propria (Fig. 22.10). Results of serum tests involving the use of indirect immunofluorescence are negative for patients with lichen planus (see Table 22.1).

Differential Diagnosis

The classic clinical presentation of oral lichen planus can be simulated by other conditions, mainly by lichenoid mucositis. If oral lichen planus is confined to the gingival tissues (i.e., erosive oral lichen planus), the identification of fine, white radiating striations bordering the erosive areas support a diagnosis of oral lichen planus. If the

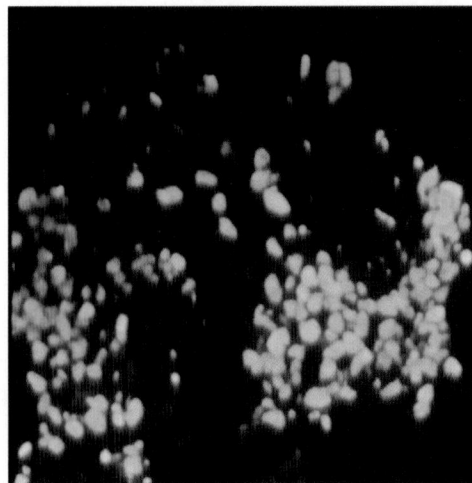

Fig. 22.10　Direct immunofluorescence staining of lichen planus. Clusters of cytoid bodies exhibit immunoglobulin M deposits in the lamina propria.

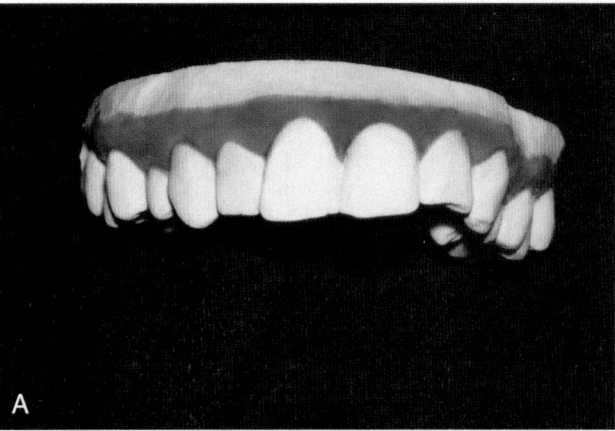
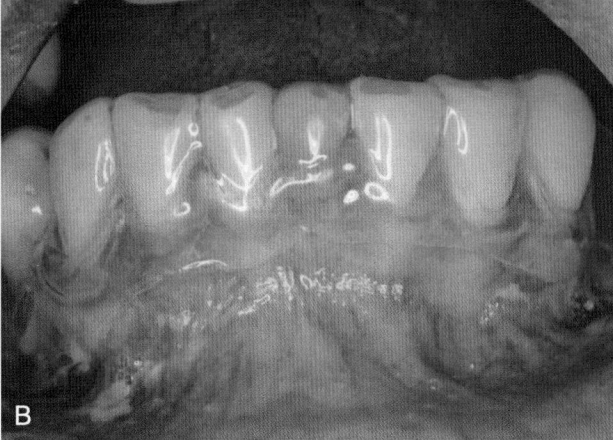

Fig. 22.11 (A) An alginate impression is obtained to create a stone model. A thin layer of block-out resin is applied on the gingival and alveolar mucosal areas with desquamative gingivitis to create a space to carry the medication. A trimmed maxillary stone model shows the block-out resin in place *(blue area)*. (B) A mandibular gingival tray is in place. Soft sheet material for vacuum-forming trays is prepared and trimmed to conform to the local anatomy.

white striations are absent, the differential diagnosis should primarily include MMP and pemphigus vulgaris. Less common possibilities include linear immunoglobulin A disease (LAD), lichen planus pemphigoides, and chronic ulcerative stomatitis.

Treatment

The keratotic lesions of oral lichen planus are asymptomatic and do not require treatment after the microscopic diagnosis has been established. However, evaluation of the patient every 6 to 12 months is warranted to monitor suspicious clinical changes and to look for the emergence of an erosive component.

The erosive, bullous, or ulcerative lesions of oral lichen planus are treated with high-potency topical steroids, such as 0.05% fluocinonide gel (Lidex, three times daily). Lidex can also be mixed 1 : 1 with carboxymethylcellulose (Orabase) paste or another adhesive ointment. A gingival tray can be used to deliver 0.05% fluocinonide ointment or gel or 0.05% clobetasol propionate with 100,000 IU/ml of nystatin in Orabase (Fig. 22.11).

Three 5-minute applications daily of the mixture appear to be effective for controlling erosive lichen planus.[60] Intralesional injections of triamcinolone acetonide (10 to 20 mg) or short-term regimens of 40 mg of prednisone daily for 5 days, followed by 10 to 20 mg daily for an additional 2 weeks, have also been used in more severe cases.[121] Because of the potential side effects, systemic steroids should be administered and monitored by a dermatologist.

Other treatment modalities (e.g., retinoids, hydroxychloroquine, cyclosporine, azathioprine, cyclophosphamide, free gingival grafts) have been used.[121,128] A promising therapeutic agent, tacrolimus (0.1% Protopic ointment, twice daily), is an immunosuppressant that is effective for controlling the lesions of erosive lichen planus.[77,99,113,155]

Because candidiasis is often associated with symptomatic oral lichen planus and because topical steroid therapy promotes fungal growth, treatment should also include a topical antifungal agent.[16,56,71]

Pemphigoid

The term *pemphigoid* applies to several cutaneous, immune-mediated, subepithelial bullous diseases that are characterized by a separation of the basement membrane zone, including bullous pemphigoid, MMP, and pemphigoid (herpes) gestationis.[127,147] Among these conditions, bullous pemphigoid and MMP (i.e., benign MMP or cicatricial pemphigoid) have received considerable attention.

Molecular findings for these two diseases indicate that they are separate entities.[147] However, considerable histologic and immunopathologic overlap exists between them, and differentiation may be impossible on the basis of the two criteria.[127]

In many cases, the clinical findings are probably the best way to discriminate between them. Accordingly, the term *bullous pemphigoid* is preferred when the disease is nonscarring and mainly affects the skin. The term *cicatricial pemphigoid* is favored when scarring occurs, and the disease is mainly confined to mucous membranes, although scarring may be absent with some subtypes of MMP.[174] Until more research allows a better understanding of this family of diseases, bullous pemphigoid and MMP are discussed separately.

Bullous Pemphigoid

Bullous pemphigoid is a chronic, autoimmune, subepidermal bullous disease with tense cutaneous bullae that rupture and become flaccid (Fig. 22.12). Oral involvement occurs in about a third of affected patients.[159] Although the skin lesions of bullous pemphigoid clinically resemble those of pemphigus, the microscopic picture is quite distinct.

Histopathology

There is no evidence of acantholysis in bullous pemphigoid, and the developing vesicles are subepithelial rather than intraepithelial. The

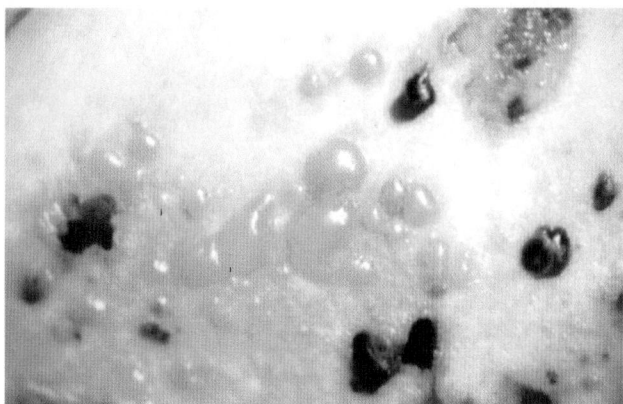

Fig. 22.12 Coalescing cutaneous bullae are seen in a case of bullous pemphigoid, and some of them are hemorrhagic. Rupture of the bullae leads to the formation of serpiginous ulcers.

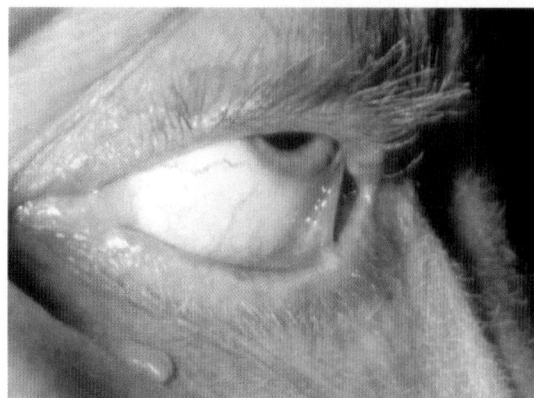

Fig. 22.13 In a patient with mucous membrane pemphigoid (i.e., cicatricial pemphigoid), the characteristic ocular lesion is a symblepharon, an adhesion of the eyelid to the eyeball. *(Courtesy Dr. Carl Allen, The Ohio State University, Columbus, OH.)*

epithelium separates from the underlying connective tissue at the basement membrane zone. Electron microscopic studies show horizontal splitting or replication of the basal lamina. The separating epithelium remains relatively intact, and the basal layer appears to be regular. The two major antigenic determinants of bullous pemphigoid are the 230-kDa protein plaque known as *bullous pemphigoid 1 (BP1)* and the 180-kDa collagen-like transmembrane protein known as *bullous pemphigoid 2 (BP2)*.[114,130,140]

Immunofluorescence

Immunologically, bullous pemphigoid is characterized by immunoglobulin G (IgG) and complement 3 (C3) immune deposits along the epithelial basement membranes and circulating IgG antibodies to the epithelial basement membrane.[75,118] Direct immunofluorescence studies are positive for 90% to 100% of these patients, whereas indirect immunofluorescence studies are positive for 40% to 70% of affected patients[119] (see Table 22.1).

Oral Lesions

Oral lesions of bullous pemphigoid have been reported to occur secondarily in up to 40% of cases. The clinical presentation includes an erosive or desquamative gingivitis and occasional vesicular or bullous lesions.[159]

Treatment

Because the etiologic factors of bullous pemphigoid are unknown, treatment is designed to control its signs and symptoms.[75,118] The primary treatment is a moderate dose of systemic prednisone. Steroid-sparing strategies (i.e., prednisone plus other immunomodulatory drugs) are used when high doses of steroids are needed or when the steroid alone fails to control the disease.[40] For localized lesions of bullous pemphigoid, high-potency topical steroids or tetracycline with or without nicotinamide can be effective.[121]

Mucous Membrane Pemphigoid

MMP (i.e., cicatricial pemphigoid) is a chronic vesiculobullous autoimmune disorder of unknown cause that predominantly affects women during the fifth decade of life. It has rarely been reported in young children.[22,115,147]

Cicatricial pemphigoid involves the oral cavity, the conjunctiva, and the mucosa of the nose, vagina, rectum, esophagus, and urethra. In about 20% of patients the skin may also be involved.

Investigations suggest that cicatricial pemphigoid encompasses a group of heterogeneous conditions with distinct clinical and molecular features.[38,110,144] An elaborate cascade of events is involved in the pathogenesis of cicatricial pemphigoid. Initially, antigen–antibody complexing occurs at the basement membrane zone, which is followed by complement activation and subsequent leukocyte recruitment. Proteolytic enzymes are then released and dissolve or cleave the basement membrane zone, usually at the level of the lamina lucida.[49]

The two major antigenic determinants for cicatricial pemphigoid are BP1 and BP2. Most cases of cicatricial pemphigoid are the result of an immune response directed against BP2; less often, this response is mounted against BP1, epiligrin (i.e., laminin 5, a lamina lucida protein in the basement membrane of stratified epithelium), and β_4 integrins.[8,21,38]

 KEY FACT

Mucous membrane pemphigoid (MMP) is an autoimmune disorder characterized by ocular and oral lesions. Symblepharon (i.e., scarring resulting in adhesion of the eyelid to the eyeball) is a significant complication of MMP. The diagnosis is made by using hematoxylin and eosin (H&E) and direct immunofluorescence studies, and the mainstay of treatment is corticosteroids.

There is strong evidence for the existence of at least five subtypes of cicatricial pemphigoid: oral pemphigoid, anti-epiligrin pemphigoid, anti-BP antigen mucosal pemphigoid, ocular pemphigoid, and multiple-antigen pemphigoid.[147] The sera of ocular pemphigoid patients recognize the β_4 integrin subunit, whereas the sera of patients with oral pemphigoid recognize the α_6 unit.[134]

Ocular Lesions

Among patients (mainly those with desquamative gingivitis) who first see a dentist, the eyes are affected in approximately 25%.[119] In contrast, among patients who first see a dermatologist, 66% have conjunctival lesions; in ophthalmic studies, 100% of patients have ocular involvement.[55,87,111,112]

The initial lesion is characterized by unilateral conjunctivitis that becomes bilateral within 2 years. Subsequently, adhesions of the eyelid to the eyeball (i.e. symblepharon) may form (Fig. 22.13). Adhesions at the edges of the eyelids (i.e., ankyloblepharon) may lead to a narrowing of the palpebral fissure. Small vesicular lesions may develop on the conjunctiva, which can eventually produce scarring, corneal damage, and blindness.

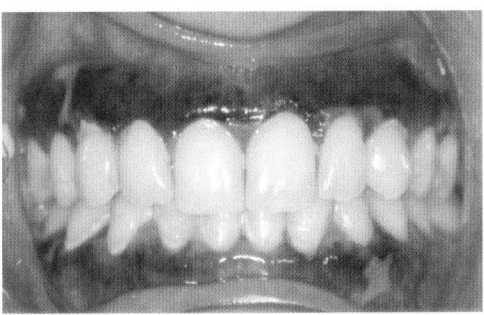

Fig. 22.14 In gingival mucous membrane pemphigoid, lesions are confined to the gingival tissues, where they produce the typical desquamative gingivitis appearance. *(Courtesy Dr. Stuart L. Fischman, State University of New York at Buffalo, Buffalo, NY.)*

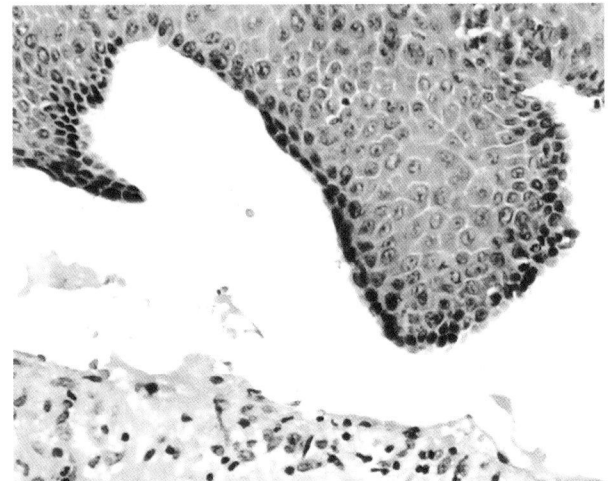

Fig. 22.15 Microscopic features of oral mucous membrane pemphigoid show a separation of the epithelium from the subjacent connective tissue (i.e., subepithelial clefting). An intact basal cell layer remains attached to the epithelium. Hematoxylin and eosin stain; original magnification ×100.

Oral Lesions

The most characteristic feature of oral involvement is desquamative gingivitis, typically with areas of erythema, desquamation, ulceration, and vesiculation of the attached gingiva[57,158] (Fig. 22.14). Vesiculobullous lesions can occur elsewhere in the mouth.[57] The bullae tend to have a relatively thick roof and rupture in 2 to 3 days after formation, leaving irregularly shaped areas of ulceration. Healing of these lesions can take 3 weeks or more.

Histopathology

The microscopic appearance of the oral lesions, although not completely diagnostic of MMP, is sufficiently distinctive that a tentative diagnosis can be considered. A striking subepithelial vesiculation with the epithelium separated from the underlying lamina propria leaves an intact basal layer (Fig. 22.15). Separation of the epithelium and the connective tissue occurs at the basement membrane zone. Electron microscopic studies demonstrate a split in the basal lamina.[167] A mixed inflammatory infiltrate (i.e., lymphocytes, plasma cells, neutrophils, and scarce eosinophils) is observed in the underlying fibrous connective tissue.

Immunofluorescence

Positive findings along the basement membrane area have been reported with the use of direct and indirect immunofluorescence.[39,74,81]

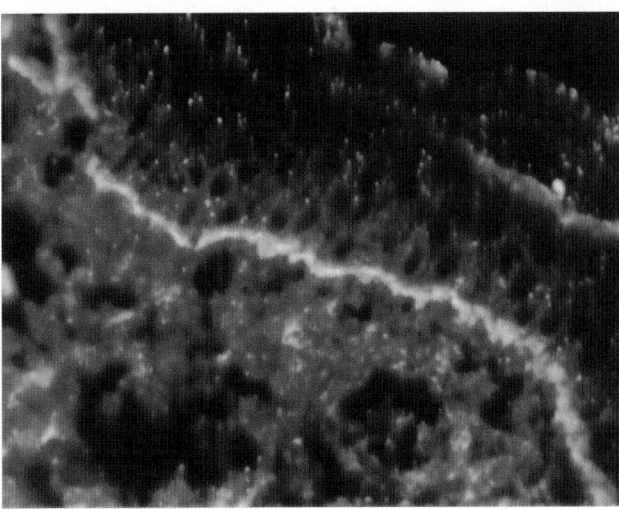

Fig. 22.16 Direct immunofluorescence staining of mucous membrane pemphigoid shows C3 deposits confined along the basement membrane.

In biopsy tests using direct immunofluorescence, the main immunoreactants are IgG and C3, which are confined to the basement membrane (Fig. 22.16). Some studies indicate that a positive indirect immunofluorescence result is rare (<25%) for these patients.[104] The lack of indirect immunofluorescence findings may reflect an earlier diagnosis of MMP, thereby resulting in the identification of patients with less extensive disease.[2,85] In any event, circulating autoantibodies do not appear to play a role in the pathogenesis of the disease.

Differential Diagnosis

Several disease entities manifest with similar clinical and histologic (i.e., subepithelial bulla) features.[44] They include bullous pemphigoid, bullous lichen planus, dermatitis herpetiformis, LAD, erythema multiforme, herpes gestationis, and epidermolysis bullosa acquisita.

Pemphigus may be confined to the oral cavity during its early stage, and the vesicular and ulcerative lesions may resemble those of MMP. An erosive or desquamative gingivitis also can be seen in pemphigus as a rare manifestation. Biopsy studies can quickly rule out pemphigus by revealing the absence or presence of acantholytic changes.

In erythema multiforme, there are obvious vesiculobullous lesions. However, the onset is usually acute rather than chronic, labial involvement is severe, and the gingivae are usually not affected. Desquamative gingivitis is an unusual finding in erythema multiforme, although occasional vesicular lesions can develop. A biopsy study of an oral lesion reveals an unusual degeneration of the upper stratum spinosum that is characteristically seen in oral erythema multiforme lesions.

Cicatricial pemphigoid must be differentiated from epidermolysis bullosa acquisita, which can manifest with similar histopathologic and immunopathologic features. When the biopsy is treated with salt to separate the dermis from the epidermis, basement membrane immunodeposits occur on the epidermal side with pemphigoid and on the dermal side with epidermolysis bullosa acquisita.[48]

Treatment

Topical steroids are the mainstay of treatment for MMP, particularly when lesions are localized. Fluocinonide (0.05%) and clobetasol propionate (0.05%) in an adhesive vehicle can be used three times daily for up to 6 months. When the oral lesions of MMP are confined to the gingival tissues, topical corticosteroids are effectively delivered with vacuum-formed custom trays or veneers.[147] Optimal oral hygiene is essential because local irritants on the tooth surface result in an exaggerated gingival inflammatory response. Gingival irritation from a dental prosthesis should be minimized.

If the disease is not severe and symptoms are mild, systemic corticosteroids may be omitted. If ocular involvement exists, systemic corticosteroids are indicated.

When lesions do not respond to steroids, systemic dapsone (4-4′-diaminodiphenylsulfone) has proved to be effective.[32,53,110,116] Because of the systemic side effects of dapsone, including hemolysis and methemoglobinemia (particularly in patients with glucose-6-phosphate dehydrogenase deficiency), referral to a dermatologist is often indicated.[124] Systemic steroids can be combined with azathioprine or cyclophosphamide.[7,150]

Biologic agents such as Rituximab (i.e., anti-CD20 monoclonal antibody) combined with an immunosuppressant (i.e., dapsone and/or sulfasalazine) have shown promising results in severe, refractory cases.[170] Some investigators advocate sulfonamides and tetracycline. Although surgery is not a treatment for MMP, it is used for some patients to prevent blindness and for esophageal and upper airways stenosis.[147] Connective tissue grafting to alleviate root surface sensitivity and to improve aesthetics has been used with success to manage gingival recession in a patient with cicatricial pemphigoid.[93]

Pemphigus Vulgaris

The pemphigus diseases are a group of autoimmune bullous disorders that produce cutaneous and mucous membranes blisters (Figs. 22.17 and 22.18). Pemphigus vulgaris is the most common of the pemphigus diseases, which also include pemphigus foliaceus, pemphigus vegetans, and pemphigus erythematosus.[139] Pemphigus vulgaris is a potentially lethal chronic condition with a 10% mortality rate and a worldwide annual incidence of 0.1 to 0.5 cases per 100,000 individuals.[12,139,148] A predilection for women, usually after the fourth decade of life, has been observed.[121] However, pemphigus vulgaris has also been reported in unusually young children and even in newborns.[30,139,154,176]

The epidermal and mucous membrane blisters occur when the cell-to-cell adhesion structures are damaged by the action of circulating autoantibodies and by the in vivo binding of the autoantibodies to the pemphigus vulgaris antigens, which are cell surface glycoproteins on keratinocytes. The pemphigus vulgaris glycoproteins are members of the desmoglein (DSG) subfamily of the cadherin superfamily of cell–cell adhesion molecules, which occur in desmosomes.[84] Whereas high levels of desmoglein 3 (DSG3) autoantibodies correlate with

the severity of oral disease in patients with pemphigus vulgaris, elevated levels of desmoglein 1 (DSG1) autoantibodies are associated with severity of cutaneous disease.[64] Evidence suggests that *DSG3*, which is the gene that codes for pemphigus vulgaris, is located on chromosome 18.[175]

KEY FACT

Pemphigus vulgaris (PV) is a severe autoimmune mucocutaneous disease that warrants immediate referral to a dermatologist or rheumatologist. This condition is potentially lethal if left untreated. Direct and indirect immunofluorescence studies along with H&E staining of biopsy specimens are used to diagnose PV. Systemic steroids are indicated to treat it.

Most cases of pemphigus vulgaris are idiopathic. However, medications such as penicillamine and captopril can produce drug-induced pemphigus, which is usually reversible after withdrawal of the causative drug. Paraneoplastic pemphigus is antigenically distinct from pemphigus vulgaris, and it is associated with underlying malignancies.[117]

In approximately 60% of patients with pemphigus vulgaris, the oral lesions are the first sign of the disease. The lesions may herald the dermatologic involvement by a year or more.[108,160]

Oral Lesions

Oral lesions can range from small vesicles to large bullae. When the bullae rupture, they leave extensive areas of ulceration (Fig. 22.19). Virtually any region of the oral cavity can be involved, but multiple lesions often develop at sites of irritation or trauma. The soft palate is most often involved (80%), followed by the buccal mucosa (46%), the ventral aspect or dorsum of the tongue (20%), and the lower labial mucosa (10%). Oral lesions of pemphigus vulgaris are confined less often to the gingival tissues.[80] In these patients, erosive gingivitis or desquamative gingivitis is the sole manifestation of oral pemphigus.

Histopathology

The lesions of pemphigus demonstrate a characteristic intraepithelial separation that occurs above the basal cell layer. The intraepithelial vesiculation begins as a microscopic alteration (Fig. 22.20) and gradually results in a grossly visible, fluid-filled bulla. Occasionally the entire superficial layers of epithelium are lost, leaving behind only the basal cells attached to the underlying lamina

Fig. 22.17 A patient with pemphigus vulgaris has a large bulla on the flexor surface of the wrist.

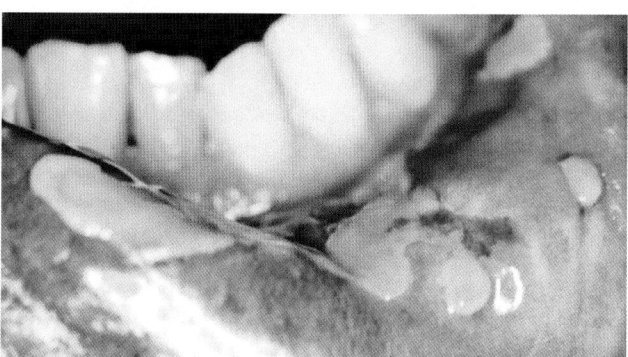

Fig. 22.18 In a patient with pemphigus vulgaris of the oral cavity, multiple and coalescent areas of ulceration are covered by pseudomembranes of necrotic epithelium. The patient had large ulcers on the labial mucosa, tongue, and soft palate.

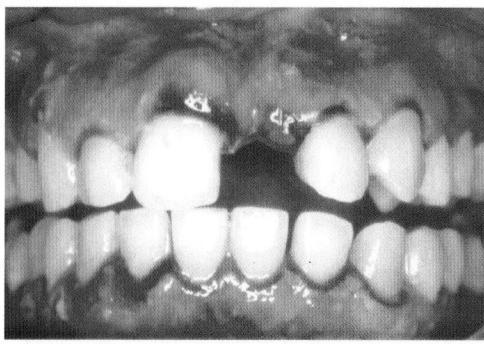

Fig. 22.19 In a patient with pemphigus vulgaris of the gingiva, oral lesions were confined to the gingivae and were clinically diagnosed as consistent with desquamative gingivitis. *(Courtesy Dr. Beatriz Aldape, Faculty of Odontology, National Autonomous University of Mexico, Mexico City, Mexico.)*

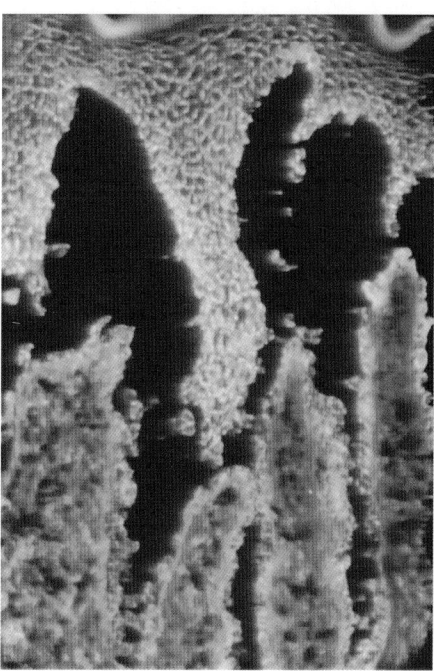

Fig. 22.21 Direct immunofluorescence staining of an oral pemphigus specimen shows the positive intercellular signal for immunoglobulin G deposits in keratinocytes of the stratified squamous epithelium.

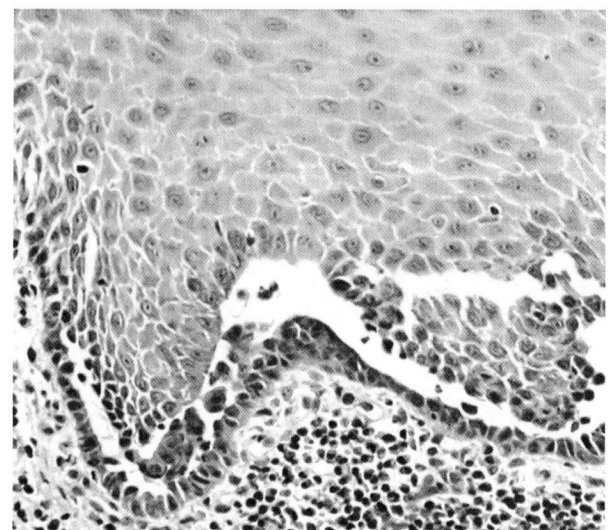

Fig. 22.20 Microscopic features of pemphigus vulgaris include typical intraepithelial clefting with a tombstone appearance of the basal cells, which remain attached to the subjacent basement membrane and fibrous connective tissue. Acantholysis of epithelial cells with the formation of Tzanck cells is seen in the intraepithelial cleft. (Hematoxylin and eosin stain; original magnification ×100.)

propria and conferring a characteristic tombstone appearance to the epithelial cells.

Acantholysis, which involves the separation of the epithelial cells of the lower stratum spinosum, takes place. It is characterized by round rather than polyhedral epithelial cells. The intercellular bridges are lost, and the nuclei are large and hyperchromatic.[36,86,179] The underlying connective tissue usually has a mild to moderate, chronic inflammatory cell infiltrate. As the vesicle or bulla ruptures, the ulcerated lesion becomes infiltrated with polymorphonuclear leukocytes, and the surface may show suppuration.

Immunofluorescence

Autoantibodies can be demonstrated in the oral mucosa of patients with oral pemphigus with the use of immunofluorescence techniques. For direct immunofluorescence, perilesional unfixed frozen sections are incubated with fluorescein-labeled human anti-IgG. For indirect immunofluorescence, unfixed frozen sections of oral or esophageal mucosa from an animal such as a monkey are first incubated with the patient's serum to allow attachment of serum antibodies to the mucosal tissue. The tissue is then incubated with fluorescein-labeled antihuman IgG serum. The test result is positive if immunofluorescence

is observed in the intercellular spaces of the stratified squamous epithelium of the mucosa (Fig. 22.21).

The indirect technique is less sensitive than the direct technique, and it may be negative during the early stages of the disease, particularly in its localized forms (see Table 22.1). In most cases, however, the indirect immunofluorescence titers are helpful for monitoring of disease activity, and they have prognostic value.

Differential Diagnosis

The oral lesions of pemphigus vulgaris may be similar to those seen in erythema multiforme. In patients with erythema multiforme, however, recurrent active episodes of comparatively short duration are followed by long intervals that are free of skin and oral lesions. Erythema multiforme affects the lips with considerable severity. Microscopic examination with conventional H&E and direct immunofluorescence can discriminate between the oral lesions of pemphigus and those of erythema multiforme. Pemphigus vulgaris shows characteristic intraepithelial clefting at the basal–spinous cell layers and interface with acantholysis, whereas erythema multiforme shows microvesiculation of the superficial epithelial layers and numerous necrotic keratinocytes. Pemphigus vulgaris shows an intercellular and intraepithelial signal with direct immunofluorescence; erythema multiforme exhibits negative immunofluorescence.

Pemphigoid may clinically resemble pemphigus. Microscopic examination and direct immunofluorescence studies are needed to establish a correct diagnosis. Bullous pemphigoid and MMP exhibit detachment of the epithelium from the underlying connective tissue (i.e., lifting off) rather than the acantholytic lesion characteristic of pemphigus.

Bullous lichen planus must also be considered during the differential diagnosis. The primary lesion of pemphigus may have a bullous character, and this may be followed by erosion, with its associated pain and discomfort. In patients with lichen planus, the characteristic reticular lesions are invariably associated with the bullae. Microscopic examination and direct immunofluorescence studies are necessary to differentiate this condition from pemphigus.

Bullous lichen planus shows separation of the epithelium from the underlying fibrous connective tissue, sawtooth rete pegs, and a band-like chronic inflammatory infiltrate in the lamina propria. Direct immunofluorescence reveals linear fibrillar deposits of fibrin in the basement membrane of bullous lichen planus, whereas pemphigus vulgaris has intercellular immunoglobulin deposition in the epithelium.

If the oral lesions of pemphigus vulgaris are restricted to the gingival tissues, erosive lichen planus, pemphigoid, LAD, and chronic ulcerative stomatitis should be ruled out.

Treatment

Guidelines for the treatment of pemphigus vulgaris are available.[105] The main therapy for pemphigus vulgaris is systemic corticosteroids with or without the addition of other immunosuppressive agents.[160] If the patient responds well to corticosteroids, the dosage can be gradually reduced, but a low maintenance dosage is usually necessary to prevent or minimize the recurrence of lesions. Many dermatologists monitor the dose of steroids by periodic evaluation of the titers of DSG3 and DSG1 antibodies. Increasing titers are often associated with an impending exacerbation and warrant an increase of the steroid dose. A decrease in titer justifies a reduction of the steroid dose.[25]

In patients who are not responsive to corticosteroids or who gradually adapt to them, steroid-sparing therapies are used. They are combinations of steroids plus other medications (e.g., azathioprine, cyclophosphamide, cyclosporine, dapsone, gold, methotrexate) and photoplasmapheresis and plasmapheresis.[121] The biologic Rituximab is used as an adjunct to treat pemphigus vulgaris.[27,47,151] However, when used in early stages of the disease, it may induce complete remission.[63]

The maintenance phase aims to control the disease with the lowest dose of medication. To minimize the risk of morbidity associated with the long-term use of steroids, alternate-day steroid therapy, steroid-sparing drugs, and topical steroids can be combined. Because topical steroids may promote the development of candidiasis, topical antifungal medication may also be needed.[98]

Minimization of oral irritation is important for patients with oral pemphigus vulgaris. Optimal oral hygiene is essential because there is usually widespread involvement of the marginal and attached gingivae and of other areas of the mouth, which can be exacerbated by plaque-associated gingivitis and periodontitis. Periodontal care is an important issue in the overall management of patients with pemphigus vulgaris. To prevent flare-ups, patients in the maintenance phase should receive prednisone before professional oral prophylaxis and periodontal surgery.[139] The fit and design of removable prosthetic appliances should receive special attention because even slight irritation from these prostheses can cause severe inflammation with vesiculation and ulceration.

Chronic Ulcerative Stomatitis

Chronic ulcerative stomatitis, which was first reported in 1990,[72] manifests with chronic oral ulcerations and has a predilection for women during the fourth decade of life. The erosions and ulcerations occur predominantly in the oral cavity, with only a few cases exhibiting cutaneous lesions.[29,88,177] Circulating specific IgG autoantibodies to ΔNp63α, an epithelial nuclear transcription factor that modulates epithelial cell growth, have been demonstrated.[20]

Oral Lesions

Painful solitary small blisters and erosions with surrounding erythema occur mainly on the gingiva and the lateral border of the tongue. Because of the magnitude and clinical features of the gingival lesions, a diagnosis of desquamative gingivitis is considered (Fig. 22.22). The buccal mucosae and hard palate also can have similar lesions.[163]

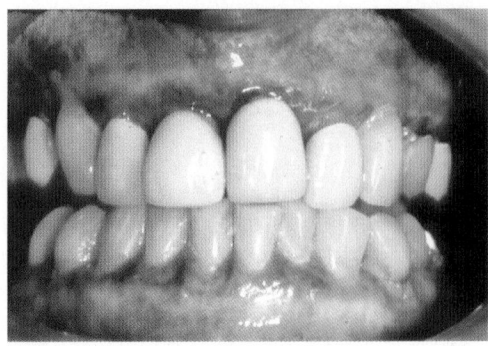

Fig. 22.22 Erythema and ulceration of the gingiva are consistent with a clinical diagnosis of chronic desquamative gingivitis. Direct and indirect immunofluorescence studies demonstrate stratified epithelium–specific antinuclear antibodies. *(Courtesy Dr. Douglas Damm, University of Kentucky, Lexington, KY.)*

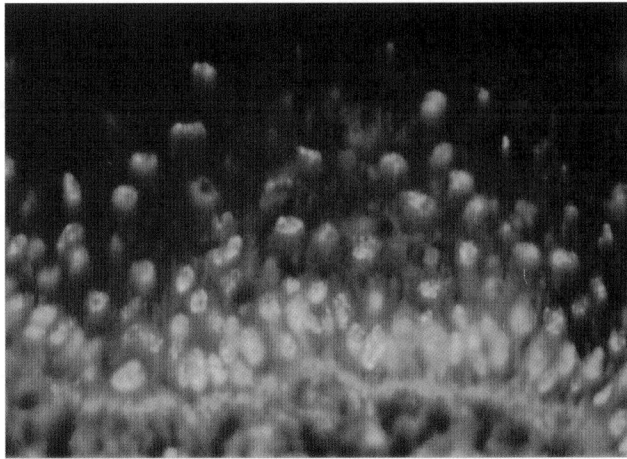

Fig. 22.23 Direct immunofluorescence study of chronic ulcerative stomatitis shows nuclear deposits of immunoglobulin G that are prominent in the basal cell layer and fade toward the superficial layers. *(Courtesy Dr. Douglas Damm, University of Kentucky, Lexington, KY.)*

Histopathology

The microscopic features of chronic ulcerative stomatitis are similar to those observed in erosive lichen planus. Hyperkeratosis, acanthosis, and liquefaction of the basal cell layer with areas of subepithelial clefting are prominent features of the epithelium. The underlying lamina propria exhibits a lymphohistiocytic chronic infiltrate in a bandlike configuration.

Immunofluorescence

Direct immunofluorescence of normal and perilesional tissues reveals typical stratified epithelium–specific antinuclear antibodies. They are nuclear deposits of IgG with a speckled pattern, and they are found mainly in the basal cell layer of the normal epithelium (Fig. 22.23). Fibrin deposits are visualized at the epithelial tissue–connective tissue interface. Indirect immunofluorescence studies involving the use of an esophageal substrate also reveal stratified epithelium–specific antinuclear antibodies.[164]

Diagnosis

Chronic ulcerative stomatitis is clinically similar to erosive lichen planus. Pemphigus vulgaris, MMP, LAD, bullous pemphigoid, and lupus erythematosus also have to be included in the differential diagnosis. Microscopic examination usually reduces the number of possibilities to chronic ulcerative stomatitis, LAD, and erosive lichen planus. Direct and indirect immunofluorescence studies are needed to arrive at the correct diagnosis.[132] An enzyme-linked immunosorbent assay (ELISA) has been developed that may allow correlation of antibody titers with treatment response.[165]

KEY FACT

Chronic ulcerative stomatitis is an autoimmune condition that mainly affects oral mucosa. Its clinical and histologic features are similar to those of oral lichen planus. Despite the similarities, severe cases of chronic ulcerative stomatitis do not respond to corticosteroid treatment, but they are responsive to hydroxychloroquine.

Treatment

For mild cases, topical steroids (e.g., fluocinonide, clobetasol propionate) and topical tetracycline can produce clinical improvement, but recurrences are common.[92] For severe cases, a high dose of a systemic corticosteroid is needed to achieve remission. Unfortunately, reduction of the corticosteroid dose results in relapse of the lesions. Hydroxychloroquine sulfate at a dosage of 200 to 400 mg per day seems to be the treatment of choice to produce complete, long-lasting remission.[13,31,69,72] However, a long-term follow-up study demonstrated that combined therapy (i.e., small doses of corticosteroids and chloroquine) might be required because the initial good response to chloroquine ceases after several months or years of treatment.[29]

Linear Immunoglobulin A Disease

LAD (i.e., linear IgA dermatosis) is an uncommon mucocutaneous disorder with a predilection for women. The etiopathogenic aspects of LAD are not fully understood, although drug-induced LAD triggered by angiotensin-converting enzyme inhibitors has been reported.[52]

LAD manifests as a pruritic vesiculobullous rash, usually during middle age or later, although younger individuals may be affected. Characteristic plaques or crops with an annular manifestation surrounded by a peripheral rim of blisters affect the skin of the upper and lower trunk, the shoulders, the groin, and the lower limbs. The face and perineum may also be affected. Mucosal involvement, including that of the oral mucosa, ranges from 50% to 100% of the cases published.[23,33,73]

LAD can mimic lichen planus clinically and histologically. Immunofluorescence studies are needed to establish the correct diagnosis.

Oral Lesions

Oral manifestations of LAD consist of vesicles, painful ulcerations or erosions, and erosive gingivitis or cheilitis. The hard and soft palates are affected more often; the tonsillar pillars, buccal mucosa, tongue, and gingiva follow in frequency. Rarely, oral lesions may be the only manifestation of LAD for several years before cutaneous lesions occur.[19] The oral lesions of LAD have been clinically reported as desquamative gingivitis[41,125,129,130] (Fig. 22.24).

Histopathology

The microscopic features of LAD are similar to those observed with erosive lichen planus.

Immunofluorescence

Linear deposits of IgA are observed at the epithelial tissue–connective tissue interface.[173] They are different from the granular pattern that is observed with dermatitis herpetiformis.

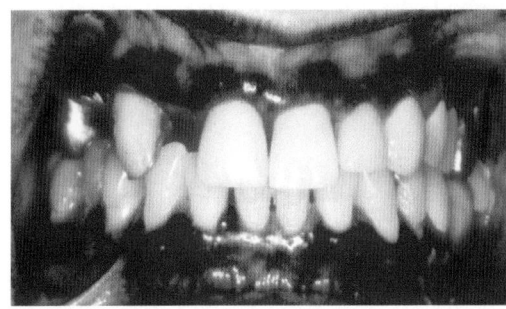

Fig. 22.24 In a patient with linear immunoglobulin A disease, intense erythema and ulceration of the gingiva are consistent with a diagnosis of desquamative gingivitis.

Differential Diagnosis

The differential diagnosis of LAD includes erosive lichen planus, chronic ulcerative stomatitis, pemphigus vulgaris, bullous pemphigoid, and lupus erythematosus. Microscopic examination and immunofluorescence studies are necessary to establish the correct diagnosis.

Treatment

The primary treatment of LAD involves a combination of sulfones and dapsone. Small amounts of prednisone (10 to 30 mg/day) can be added if the initial response is inadequate.[28] Alternatively, tetracycline (2 g/day) in combination with nicotinamide (1.5 g/day) has shown promising results.[126] Mycophenolate (1 g twice daily) in combination with prednisolone (30 mg/day) resulted in the resolution of the refractory ulcerations associated with LAD.[89]

Dermatitis Herpetiformis

Dermatitis herpetiformis is a chronic condition that usually develops in young adults between the ages of 20 and 30 years, and it has a slight predilection for men.[43] Evidence indicates that dermatitis herpetiformis is a cutaneous manifestation of celiac disease. Approximately 25% of patients with celiac disease have dermatitis herpetiformis. The cause of celiac disease is obscure, but tissue transglutaminase seems to be the predominant autoantigen in the intestine, the skin, and sometimes the mucosae.[35] Gluten enteropathy can be severe in about two-thirds of patients, and it is mild or subclinical in the remaining one-third. In severe cases, patients may complain of dysphagia, weakness, diarrhea, and weight loss.[101]

Clinically, dermatitis herpetiformis manifests with bilateral and symmetric pruritic papules or vesicles that are primarily restricted to the extensor surfaces of the extremities. The sacrum, the buttocks, and occasionally the face and oral cavity can be affected.[15,43]

The term *herpetic* is derived from the initial manifestation of the disease, in which clusters of vesicles or papules arise on the skin. These vesicles or papules eventually resolve and are followed by hyperpigmentation of the skin, which ultimately wanes. The oral lesions of dermatitis herpetiformis range from painful ulcerations preceded by the collapse of ephemeral vesicles or bullae to erythematous lesions.[120]

Histopathology

Microscopic examination of the initial lesions of dermatitis herpetiformis reveals focal aggregates of neutrophils and eosinophils among deposits of fibrin at the apices of the dermal pegs.[180]

Immunofluorescence

Direct immunofluorescence demonstrates IgA and C3 at the dermal papillary apices in both perilesional tissue and normal, uninvolved tissue. In contrast, biopsies taken from lesional sites may fail to exhibit IgA or C3, producing false-negative results.[180] Although no circulating autoantibodies to epithelial basement membrane occur in dermatitis herpetiformis, almost 80% of patients have anti-endomysial and gliadin antibodies.[14]

Treatment

A gluten-free diet is essential for the treatment of celiac disease and dermatitis herpetiformis. Oral dapsone is usually needed for patients with newly detected dermatitis herpetiformis to alleviate symptoms promptly.[19,35]

Lupus Erythematosus

Lupus erythematosus is an autoimmune disease with three clinical presentations: systemic, chronic cutaneous, and subacute cutaneous.

Systemic Lupus Erythematosus

Systemic lupus erythematosus (SLE) is a severe disease with a 10:1 predilection for women compared with men. SLE can affect the kidneys, heart, skin, and mucosa. The classic cutaneous lesions characterized by a rash on the malar area with a butterfly distribution are uncommon[37] (Fig. 22.25). The oral lesions of SLE are usually ulcerative or similar to those of lichen planus. Oral ulcerations occur in 36% of patients with SLE. In about 4% of patients, hyperkeratotic plaques reminiscent of lichen planus appear on the buccal mucosa and palate.[17]

Direct immunofluorescence of the perilesional and normal tissue reveals immunoglobulins and C3 deposits at the dermal-epidermal interface. Antinuclear antibodies are detected in more than 95% of cases, whereas deoxyribonucleic acid and extractable nuclear antigen antibodies are found in more than 50% of patients (see Table 22.1).

Chronic Cutaneous Lupus Erythematosus

Chronic cutaneous lupus erythematosus usually has no systemic signs or symptoms; lesions are limited to the skin or the mucosal surfaces. The skin lesions are referred to as *discoid lupus erythematosus* (DLE). DLE describes the chronic scarring, atrophy-producing lesion that may develop into hyperpigmentation or hypopigmentation of the healing area (Fig. 22.26). In the oral cavity, about 9% of patients with chronic cutaneous lupus erythematosus have lichen-planus–like plaques on the palate and the buccal mucosa.[5,17] The gingiva may be affected, and the condition can manifest as desquamative gingivitis (Fig. 22.27).

Histopathology

The histopathology of the oral lesions of chronic cutaneous lupus erythematosus consists of hyperkeratosis, alternating acanthosis and atrophy, and hydropic degeneration of the basal layer of the epithelium. The lamina propria exhibits a chronic inflammatory cell infiltrate similar to that observed with lichen planus. However, a more diffuse and deeper inflammatory infiltrate with a perivascular pattern is typically observed.[157]

Immunofluorescence

Direct immunofluorescence study of lesional tissue reveals immunoglobulins and C3 deposits at the dermal-epidermal junction of the lesional or perilesional tissue but not in normal tissue. This seems to differentiate SLE from DLE. The indirect immunofluorescence method reveals antinuclear antibodies in more than 95% of patients, whereas deoxyribonucleic acid and extractable nuclear antigen circulating antibodies are found in more than 50% of patients.

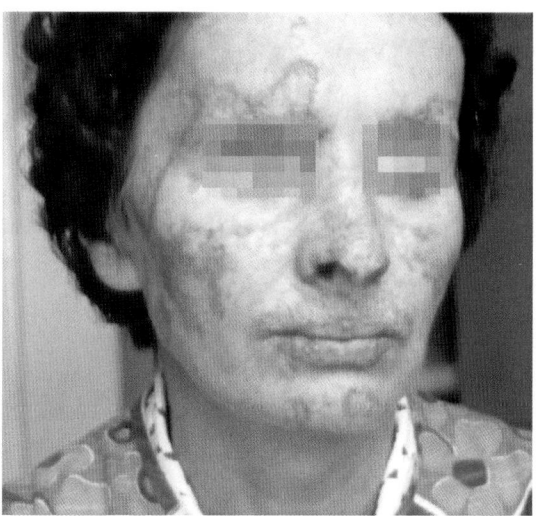

Fig. 22.26 In a patient with chronic cutaneous lupus erythematosus, there are multiple facial lesions with irregular hyperpigmented borders, some of which exhibit central scarring with cutaneous atrophy. Other lesions consist of hyperpigmented cutaneous patches.

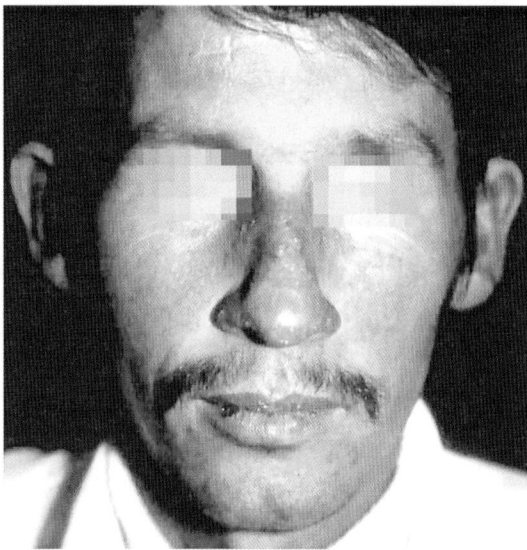

Fig. 22.25 Systemic lupus erythematosus produces erythema on the bridge of the nose with a butterfly pattern. *(Courtesy Department of Dermatology, Hospital General Manuel Gea González, Mexico City, Mexico.)*

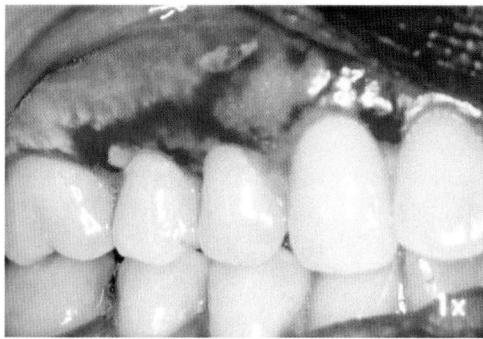

Fig. 22.27 Lupus erythematosus of the oral cavity can manifest as desquamative gingivitis. Intense erythema with ulceration is bordered by white radial lines. *(Courtesy Dr. Stuart L. Fischman, State University of New York at Buffalo, NY.)*

Subacute Cutaneous Lupus Erythematosus

Patients with subacute cutaneous lupus erythematosus have cutaneous lesions that are similar to those of DLE but that lack the development of scarring and atrophy.[18] Arthritis and arthralgia, low-grade fever, malaise, and myalgia can occur in up to 50% of patients with subacute cutaneous lupus erythematosus.[18,168]

Direct immunofluorescence reveals immunoglobulins and C3 deposits at the dermal-epidermal junction in 60% of cases and granular IgG deposits in the cytoplasm of basal cells in 30% of cases. About 80% of patients with subacute cutaneous lupus erythematosus have Ro (SSA) antibodies to nuclear antigens, whereas 25% to 30% have La (SSB) antibodies to nuclear antigens. The test result for rheumatoid factor is positive in about 30% of these patients, positive for antinuclear antibodies in 60% to 90%, and positive for anti-ribonucleoprotein antibodies to nuclear antigens in 10% (see Table 22.1).

Differential Diagnosis

Erosive lichen planus, erythema multiforme, and pemphigus vulgaris can simulate the lesions observed in patients with lupus erythematosus. The diagnosis of DLE confined to the oral cavity is difficult to make, but microscopic studies may suggest the characteristic histopathology.[4] Biopsy studies (i.e., H&E and direct immunofluorescence) help to differentiate lupus erythematosus from other erosive diseases.

Treatment

The therapy for SLE depends on the severity and extent of the disease. It can range from topical steroids to nonsteroidal antiinflammatory drugs to moderate to high doses of prednisone for severe systemic organ involvement. Immunosuppressive drugs (e.g., cytotoxic agents such as cyclophosphamide and azathioprine) and plasmapheresis alone or with steroids can be useful.[121] Rituximab has produced dramatic, long-term remissions.[37] For chronic cutaneous lupus erythematosus, topical steroids are effective to manage the cutaneous and oral lesions. For patients whose disease is resistant to topical therapy, systemic antimalarial drugs can be used with good results.[119]

Erythema Multiforme

Erythema multiforme is an acute bullous and macular inflammatory mucocutaneous disease that affects mainly young adults between the ages of 20 and 40 years; it is rarely seen in children (≤20%).[145] The genesis of the mucocutaneous lesions is thought to reside in the development of immune complex vasculitis. This is followed by complement fixation that leads to the leukocytoclastic destruction of vascular walls and small vessel occlusion. The culmination of these events produces ischemic necrosis of the epithelium and underlying connective tissue.[49]

Target (i.e., iris) lesions with central clearing are the hallmark of erythema multiforme. It can be a mild condition (i.e., erythema multiforme minor) or a severe and possibly life-threatening condition (i.e., erythema multiforme major or Stevens–Johnson syndrome). An underdiagnosed type of erythema multiforme is the oral form, with which most patients have chronic or recurrent oral lesions only.[6]

Erythema multiforme minor lasts approximately 4 weeks and exhibits moderate cutaneous and mucosal involvement. Stevens–Johnson syndrome can last a month or longer. It involves the skin, conjunctiva, oral mucosa, and genitalia, and it requires more aggressive therapy than erythema multiforme minor. Some researchers consider toxic epidermal necrolysis to be the most severe form of erythema multiforme, but other investigators think they are unrelated entities.[10]

The two most common etiologic factors for the development of erythema multiforme are herpes simplex infection and drug reactions.

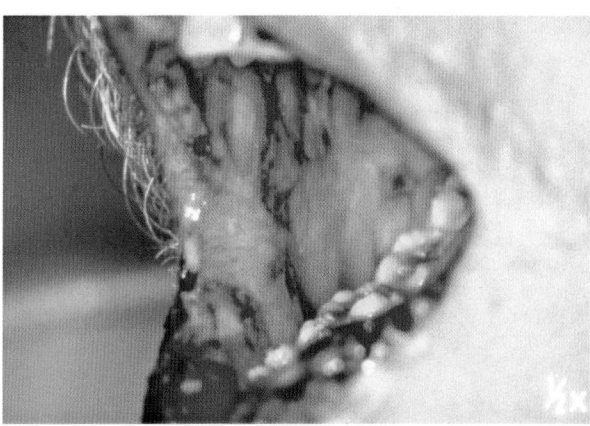

Fig. 22.28 In a patient with erythema multiforme, large, shallow, and painful ulcers involve the labial and buccal mucosae. Hemorrhagic crusting of the mandibular vermilion border of the lips is observed. *(Courtesy Dr. Stuart L. Fischman, State University of New York at Buffalo, NY.)*

The most common causative drugs are sulfonamides, penicillins, quinolones, chlormezanone, barbiturates, oxicam nonsteroidal antiinflammatory drugs, anticonvulsant drugs, protease inhibitors, and allopurinol.[50]

Oral lesions in patients with erythema multiforme are common, and they occur in more than 70% of patients with skin involvement.[51,96,103] In rare instances, erythema multiforme is confined to the mouth.[6,94,152] The oral lesions consist of multiple, large, shallow, painful ulcers with an erythematous border. They affect the entire oral mucosa in approximately 20% of patients with erythema multiforme. The lesions are so painful that chewing and swallowing are impaired (Fig. 22.28). The buccal mucosa and the tongue are the most frequently affected sites, followed by the labial mucosa. Areas that are less often affected include the floor of the mouth, the hard and soft palates, and the gingiva.[51] Erythema multiforme is rarely confined exclusively to the gingival tissues, prompting a clinical diagnosis of desquamative gingivitis.[9] Hemorrhagic crusting of the vermilion border of the lips may occur, which is helpful for arriving at a clinical diagnosis of erythema multiforme.

Histopathology

Common microscopic findings of erythema multiforme include the liquefaction degeneration of the upper epithelium and development of intraepithelial microvesicles without the acantholysis that occurs with pemphigus.[156] Acanthosis, pseudoepitheliomatous hyperplasia, and necrotic keratinocytes are observed in the epithelium. Degenerative changes also occur in the basement membrane. In some cases, the junction between the epithelium and the lamina propria is indistinct because of a dense inflammatory cell infiltrate. Edema of the lamina propria, vascular dilation, and congestion also occur. Deeper layers of the connective tissue stroma exhibit a perivascular chronic inflammatory cell infiltrate. However, neutrophils and eosinophils may also be seen.

Immunofluorescence

The immunofluorescence examination result is negative for patients with erythema multiforme. Its value resides in ruling out other vesiculobullous and ulcerative disorders.

Treatment

There is no specific treatment for erythema multiforme. For mild symptoms, systemic and local antihistamines, topical anesthetics, and debridement of lesions with an oxygenating agent are adequate. In patients with bullous or ulcerative lesions and severe symptoms, corticosteroids are considered the drug of choice, although their use is controversial and not completely accepted.[50]

Drug-Related Eruptions

An increase in the incidence of skin and oral manifestations of hypersensitivity to drugs occurred with the advent of sulfonamides, barbiturates, and various antibiotics. The cutaneous and oral lesions are attributed to the drug acting as an allergen that sensitizes the tissues.

Eruptions in the oral cavity that result from sensitivity to drugs that have been taken orally or parenterally are called *stomatitis medicamentosa*. The local reaction from the use of a medicament in the oral cavity (e.g., stomatitis resulting from topical penicillin use) is referred to as *stomatitis venenata* or *contact stomatitis*. In many cases, skin eruptions accompany the oral lesions.

Most drug eruptions in the oral cavity are multiform. Vesicular and bullous lesions occur most often, but pigmented or nonpigmented macular lesions are also frequently observed. Erosions, which are often followed by deep ulceration with purpuric lesions, can occur. The lesions are seen in different areas of the oral cavity, with the gingiva often being affected.[1,58]

The development of gingival lesions caused by contact allergy to the mercurial compounds in dental amalgam has been documented.[78] Because of financial considerations, biopsy and patch testing may be indicated before the indiscriminate replacement of dental amalgam restorations. Similarly, desquamative gingivitis has been reported with the use of tartar control toothpaste. Pyrophosphates and flavoring agents have been identified as the main causative agents of this unusual condition.[42] Oral reactions to cinnamon compounds (i.e., cinnamon oil, cinnamic acid, or cinnamic aldehyde) that are used to mask the taste of pyrophosphates in tartar control toothpaste include

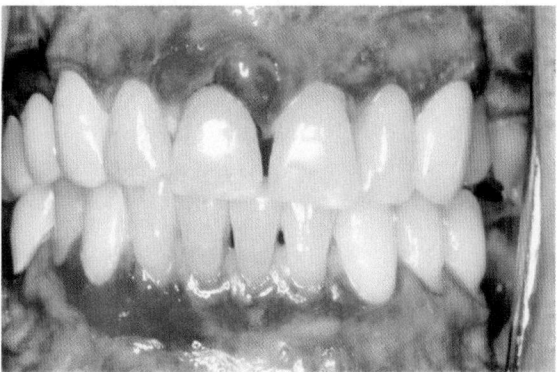

Fig. 22.29 Plasma cell gingivitis. The gingiva presents a band of moderate to severe inflammation that is reminiscent of desquamative gingivitis.

an intense erythema of the attached gingival tissues that is characteristic of plasma cell gingivitis[3,79] (Fig. 22.29).

A thorough clinical history usually discloses the source of gingival disturbance. Elimination of the offending agent (i.e., tartar control toothpaste) leads to resolution of the gingival lesions within a week, and challenge with the offending agent leads to recurrence of the oral lesions. If removal of the offending medication is not possible, topical corticosteroids and topical tacrolimus can be used to treat the lesions.[70]

 A Case Scenario is found on the companion website www.expertconsult.com.

References

 References for this chapter are found on the companion website www.expertconsult.com.

The Periodontal Pocket

Fermin A. Carranza | Satheesh Elangovan | Paulo M. Camargo

CHAPTER OUTLINE

The periodontal pocket, which is defined as a pathologically deepened gingival sulcus, is one of the most important clinical features of periodontal disease. All types of periodontitis, as outlined in Chapter 5, share histopathologic features, such as tissue changes in the periodontal pocket, mechanisms of tissue destruction, and healing mechanisms. However, they differ with regard to their etiology, natural history, progression, and response to therapy.[32]

Classification

Deepening of the gingival sulcus may occur as a result of coronal movement of the gingival margin, apical displacement of the gingival attachment, or a combination of the two processes (Fig. 23.1). Pockets can be classified as follows:

- *Gingival pocket* (also called "peudo-pocket") is formed by gingival enlargement without destruction of the underlying periodontal tissues. The sulcus is deepened because of the increased bulk of the gingiva (Fig. 23.2A).
- *Periodontal pocket* produces destruction of the supporting periodontal tissues, leading to the loosening and exfoliation of the teeth. The remainder of this chapter refers to this type of pocket. Based on the location of the base of the pocket in relation to the underlying bone, periodontal pockets can be classified into the following types:
  - *Suprabony* (*supracrestal* or *supraalveolar*) occurs when the bottom of the pocket is coronal to the underlying alveolar bone (Fig. 23.2B).
  - *Intrabony* (*infrabony, subcrestal,* or *intraalveolar*) occurs when the bottom of the pocket is apical to the level of the adjacent alveolar bone. With this second type, the lateral pocket wall lies between the tooth surface and the alveolar bone (Fig. 23.2C).

Pockets can involve one, two, or more tooth surfaces, and they can be of different depths and types on different surfaces of the same tooth and on approximal surfaces of the same interdental space.[30,38] Pockets can also be spiral (i.e., originating on one tooth surface and twisting around the tooth to involve one or more additional surfaces) (Fig. 23.3). These types of pockets are most common in furcation areas.

Clinical Features

Clinical signs that suggest the presence of periodontal pockets include a bluish red thickened marginal gingiva, a bluish red vertical zone from the gingival margin to the alveolar mucosa, gingival bleeding and suppuration, tooth mobility, diastema formation, and symptoms such as localized pain or pain "deep in the bone." The only reliable method of locating periodontal pockets and determining their extent is careful probing of the gingival margin along each tooth surface (Fig. 23.4 and Table 23.1). On the basis of depth alone, however, it is sometimes difficult to differentiate between a deep normal sulcus and a shallow periodontal pocket. In such borderline cases, pathologic changes in the gingiva distinguish the two conditions.

For a more detailed discussion of the clinical aspects of periodontal pockets, see Chapter 32.

KEY FACT

Sulcus Versus Periodontal Pocket
Gingival sulcus is the space between the neck of the tooth and the circumferential gingival tissue. Sulcus, when it deepens (as in periodontal disease) due to the apical migration of junctional epithelium, accompanied by attachment loss, it is referred to as a *periodontal pocket.*

Pathogenesis

The initial lesion in the development of periodontitis is the inflammation of the gingiva in response to a bacterial challenge. Changes involved in the transition from the normal gingival sulcus to the pathologic periodontal pocket are associated with different proportions of bacterial cells in dental plaque. Healthy gingiva is associated with few microorganisms, mostly coccoid cells and straight rods. Diseased gingiva is associated with increased numbers of spirochetes and motile rods.[40,41,43] However, the microbiota of diseased sites cannot be used as a predictor of future attachment or bone loss, because their presence alone is not sufficient for disease to start or progress.[35]

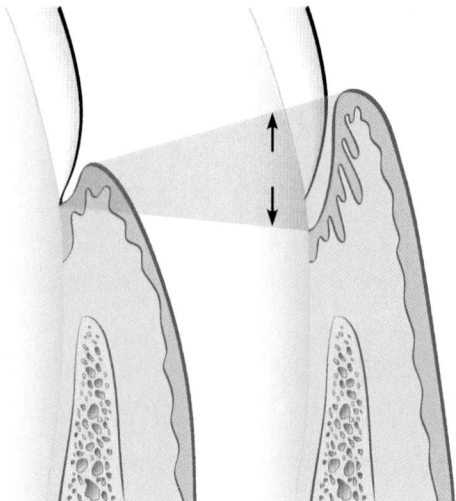

Fig. 23.1 Illustration of pocket formation that indicates expansion in two directions *(arrows)* from the normal gingival sulcus *(left)* to the periodontal pocket *(right).*

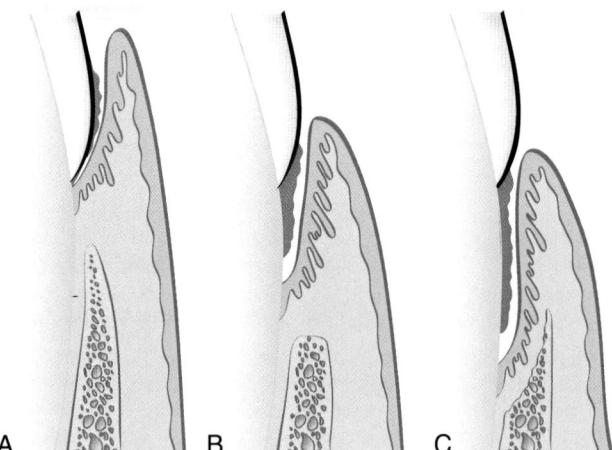

Fig. 23.2 Different types of periodontal pockets. (A) Gingival pocket. There is no destruction of the supporting periodontal tissues. (B) Suprabony pocket. The base of the pocket is coronal to the level of the underlying bone. Bone loss is horizontal. (C) Intrabony pocket. The base of the pocket is apical to the level of the adjacent bone. Bone loss is vertical.

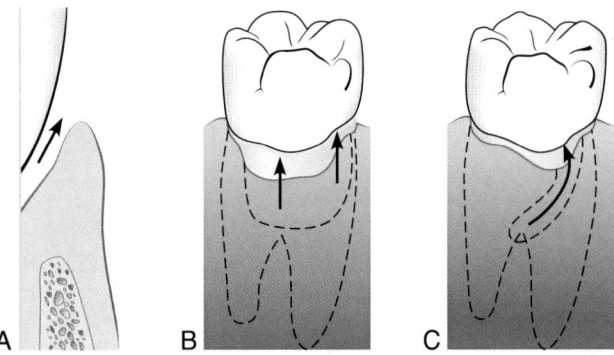

Fig. 23.3 Classification of pockets according to involved tooth surfaces. (A) Simple pocket. (B) Compound pocket. (C) Complex pocket.

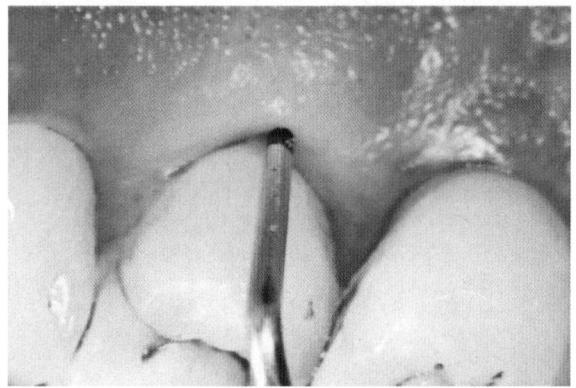

Fig. 23.4 Probing of a deep periodontal pocket. The entire length of the periodontal probe has been inserted to the base of the pocket in the palatal surface of the first premolar.

TABLE 23.1   Correlation of Clinical and Histopathologic Features of the Periodontal Pocket

Clinical Features	Histopathologic Features
1. The gingival wall of the pocket presents various degrees of bluish red discoloration; flaccidity; a smooth, shiny surface; and pitting on pressure.	1. The discoloration is caused by circulatory stagnation; the flaccidity by the destruction of gingival fibers and surrounding tissues; the smooth, shiny surface by atrophy of the epithelium and edema; and the pitting on pressure by edema and degeneration.
2. Less frequently, the gingival wall may be pink and firm.	2. In such cases, fibrotic changes predominate over exudation and degeneration, particularly in relation to the outer surface of the pocket wall. However, despite the external appearance of health, the inner wall of the pocket invariably presents some degeneration and is often ulcerated (see Fig. 23.15).
3. Bleeding is elicited by gently probing the soft-tissue wall of the pocket.	3. Ease of bleeding results from increased vascularity, the thinning and degeneration of the epithelium, and the proximity of engorged vessels to the inner surface.
4. When explored with a probe, the inner aspect of the pocket is generally painful.	4. Pain on tactile stimulation is caused by the ulceration of the inner aspect of the pocket wall.
5. In many cases, pus may be expressed with the application of digital pressure.	5. Pus occurs in pockets with suppurative inflammation of the inner wall.

The two mechanisms associated with collagen loss are as follows: (1) collagenases and other enzymes secreted by various cells in healthy and inflamed tissue, such as fibroblasts,[74] PMNs,[73] and macrophages,[53] become extracellular and destroy collagen (enzymes that degrade collagen and other matrix macromolecules into small peptides are called *matrix metalloproteinases*[75]); and (2) fibroblasts phagocytize collagen fibers by extending cytoplasmic processes to the ligament–cementum interface and degrading the inserted collagen fibrils and the fibrils of the cementum matrix.[20,21]

As a consequence of the loss of collagen, the apical cells of the junctional epithelium proliferate along the root surface and extend finger-like projections that are two or three cells in thickness (Fig. 23.6).

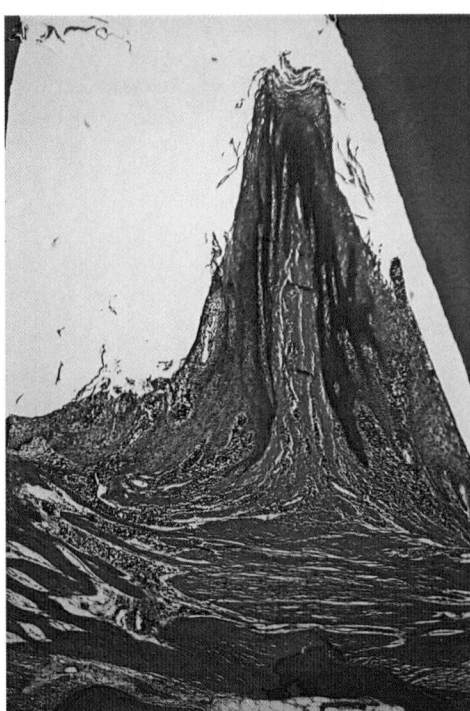

Fig. 23.5 Interdental papilla with suprabony pockets on proximal tooth surfaces. Note the densely inflamed connective tissue, with the infiltrate extending between the collagen fibers and the proliferating and ulcerated pocket epithelium.

> **KEY FACT**
>
> **Matrix Metalloproteinases and Tissue Inhibitors of Metalloproteinases**
>
> Matrix metalloproteinases (MMPs) are a group of proteases that play an important role in several biologic processes. Like any protease, they are involved in the degradation of proteins. Specifically, they are important players in extracellular matrix (ECM) degradation and are inhibited by tissue inhibitors of metalloproteinases (TIMPs). The balance between MMPs and TIMPs is critical for the maintenance of ECM remodeling in tissues, including the periodontium.

As a result of inflammation, PMNs invade the coronal end of the junctional epithelium in increasing numbers (Fig. 23.7). The PMNs are not joined to one another or to the epithelial cells by desmosomes. When the relative volume of PMNs reaches approximately 60% or more of the junctional epithelium, the tissue loses cohesiveness and detaches from the tooth surface. Thus the coronal portion of the junctional epithelium detaches from the root as the apical portion migrates, resulting in its apical shift; the oral sulcular epithelium gradually occupies an increasing portion of the sulcus (then a pocket) lining.[63]

> Pocket formation starts as an inflammatory change in the connective tissue wall of the gingival sulcus. The cellular and fluid inflammatory exudate causes degeneration of the surrounding connective tissue, including the gingival fibers. Just apical to the junctional epithelium, collagen fibers are destroyed,[20,61] and the area is occupied by inflammatory cells and edema (Fig. 23.5).

Early concepts assumed that after the initial bacterial attack, periodontal tissue destruction continued to be linked to bacterial action. More recently it was established that the host's immunoinflammatory response to the initial and persistent bacterial attack unleashes mechanisms that lead to collagen and bone destruction. These mechanisms are related to various cytokines, some of which are produced normally by cells in noninflamed tissue and others by cells that are involved in the inflammatory process, such as polymorphonuclear leukocytes (PMNs), monocytes, and other cells, thereby leading to collagen and bone destruction. This chapter describes the histologic aspects of gingival inflammation and tissue destruction. For further information about the molecular biology aspects of these mechanisms of tissue destruction, please see Chapter 9 and www.expertconsult.com.

Extension of the junctional epithelium along the root requires the presence of healthy epithelial cells. Marked degeneration or necrosis of the junctional epithelium impairs rather than accelerates pocket formation. (This occurs in necrotizing ulcerative gingivitis, which results in an ulcer rather than pocket formation.)

Degenerative changes seen in the junctional epithelium at the base of periodontal pockets are usually less severe than those in the epithelium of the lateral pocket wall (see Fig. 23.7). Because the migration of the junctional epithelium requires healthy, viable cells, it is reasonable to assume that the degenerative changes seen in this area occur after the junctional epithelium reaches its position on the cementum.

> The degree of leukocyte infiltration of the junctional epithelium is independent of the volume of inflamed connective tissue; thus this process may occur in gingiva with only slight signs of clinical inflammation.[61]
>
> With continued inflammation, the gingiva increases in bulk, and the crest of the gingival margin extends coronally. The apical cells of the junctional epithelium continue to migrate along the root, and its coronal cells continue to separate from it. The epithelium of the lateral wall of the pocket proliferates to form bulbous, cordlike extensions into the inflamed connective tissue. Leukocytes and edema from the inflamed connective tissue infiltrate the epithelium that lines the pocket, resulting in various degrees of degeneration and necrosis.

> **KEY FACT**
>
> Cytokines are proteins secreted by cells that interact with other cells and eventually lead to a specific cellular response. Cytokines can be proinflammatory or antiinflammatory in nature. Proinflammatory cytokines such as interleukin-1 (IL-1) and tumor necrosis factor-alpha (TNF-α) are implicated strongly in the pathogenesis of periodontal disease progression. Antiinflammatory cytokines such as IL-4 and IL-10 counteract the effects of proinflammatory cytokines.

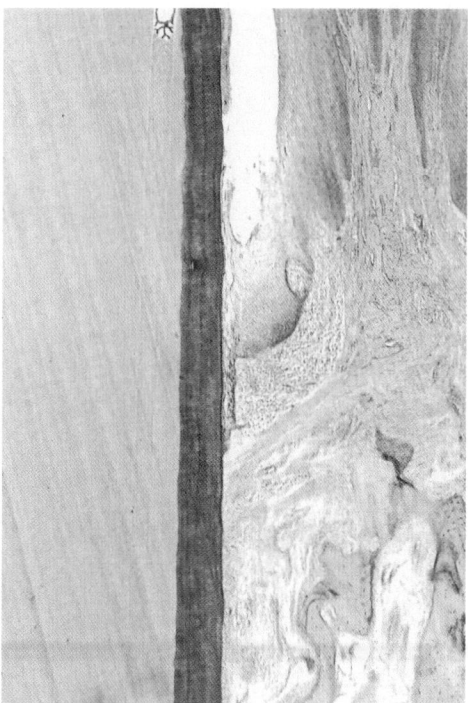

Fig. 23.6 Low-power view of the base of the periodontal pocket and apical area. Note the dense inflammatory infiltrate on the area of destroyed collagen fibers and the thin, finger-like extension of epithelium covering the cementum, which has been denuded of fibers.

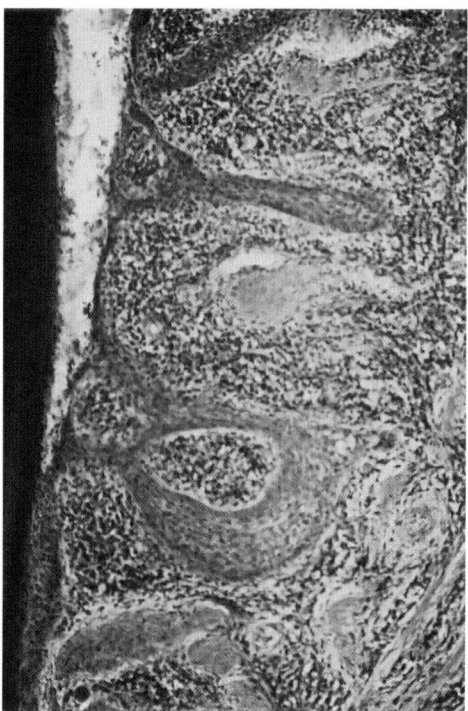

Fig. 23.7 Base of periodontal pocket showing extensive proliferation of lateral epithelium next to atrophic areas, dense inflammatory infiltrate, remnants of destroyed collagen fibers, and the junctional epithelium, which is apparently in a less altered state than the lateral pocket epithelium.

The transformation of a gingival sulcus into a periodontal pocket creates an area in which plaque removal becomes impossible, and a feedback mechanism is established. The rationale for pocket reduction is based on the need to eliminate areas of plaque accumulation.

Histopathology

Changes that occur during the initial stages of gingival inflammation are presented in Chapter 17. After the pocket is formed, several microscopic features are present, which are discussed in this section.

Soft-Tissue Wall

The connective tissue is edematous and densely infiltrated with plasma cells (approximately 80%), lymphocytes, and a scattering of PMNs.[82] The blood vessels are increased in number, dilated, and engorged, particularly in the subepithelial connective tissue layer.[10] The connective tissue exhibits varying degrees of degeneration. Single or multiple necrotic foci are occasionally present.[52] In addition to exudative and degenerative changes, the connective tissue shows proliferation of the endothelial cells, with newly formed capillaries, fibroblasts, and collagen fibers (see Fig. 23.5).

The junctional epithelium at the base of the pocket is usually much shorter than that of a normal sulcus. Although marked variations are found with regard to the length, width, and condition of the epithelial cells,[62] usually the coronoapical length of the junctional epithelium is reduced to only 50 to 100 μm.[14] The cells may be well formed and in good condition, or they may exhibit slight to marked degeneration (see Figs. 23.6 and 23.7).

The most severe degenerative changes in the periodontal pocket occur along the lateral wall (Fig. 23.8). The epithelium of the lateral wall of the pocket presents striking proliferative and degenerative changes. Epithelial buds or interlacing cords of epithelial cells project from the lateral wall into the adjacent inflamed connective tissue, and they may extend farther apically than the junctional epithelium (Figs. 23.7 and 23.9A). These epithelial projections, as well as the remainder of the lateral epithelium, are densely infiltrated by leukocytes and edema from the inflamed connective tissue. The cells undergo vacuolar degeneration and rupture to form vesicles. Progressive degeneration and necrosis of the epithelium lead to ulceration of the lateral wall, exposure of the underlying inflamed connective tissue, and suppuration. In some cases, acute inflammation is superimposed on the underlying chronic changes.

A comparative study of gingival changes in aggressive and chronic periodontitis revealed more pronounced degenerative changes in the epithelium of aggressive cases with more open intercellular spaces, including microclefts and necrotic areas.[35] The severity of the degenerative changes is not necessarily related to pocket depth. Ulceration of the lateral wall may occur in shallow pockets, and deep pockets are occasionally observed in which the lateral epithelium is relatively intact or shows only slight degeneration. The epithelium at the gingival crest of a periodontal pocket is generally intact and thickened, with prominent rete pegs.

For a detailed electron microscopic study of the pocket epithelium in experimentally induced pockets in dogs, see the article by Müller-Glauser and Schröder.[49]

Features of Junctional Epithelium

- It acts as a physical barrier against plaque bacteria.
- It is stratified squamous nonkeratinized in nature, which develops by the union of oral epithelium and reduced enamel epithelium during tooth eruption.
- It is attached to the tooth by internal basal lamina and to the connective tissue by external basal lamina.
- It exhibits higher permeability to cells, gingival fluid, and host-defense molecules to flow through.
- It has higher rate of cellular proliferation and turnover.

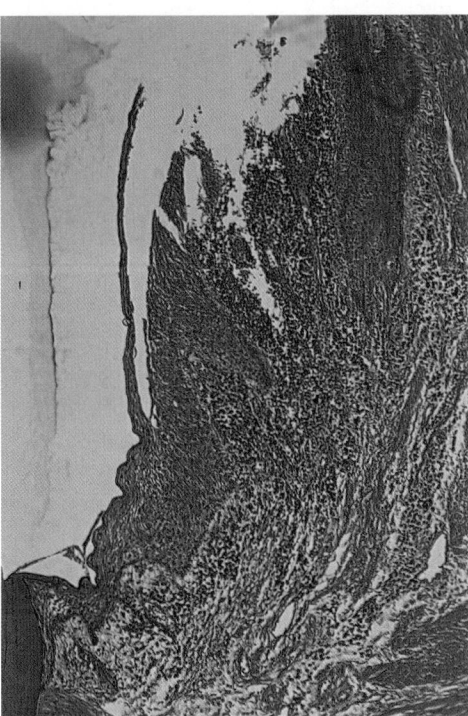

Fig. 23.8 View of the ulcerated lateral pocket wall of a periodontal pocket. Note the extension of epithelial cells and the dense accumulation of leukocytes within the epithelium and in the connective tissue.

Fig. 23.9 (A) Lateral wall of a periodontal pocket showing epithelial proliferative and atrophic changes as well as marked inflammatory infiltrate and the destruction of collagen fibers. (B) Slightly apical view of the same patient showing the shortened junctional epithelium.

Bacterial Invasion

Bacterial invasion of the apical and lateral areas of the pocket wall has been described in human chronic periodontitis. Filaments, rods, and coccoid organisms with predominant gram-negative cell walls have been found in intercellular spaces of the epithelium.[25,26] Hillmann and colleagues[35] have reported the presence of *Porphyromonas gingivalis* and *Prevotella intermedia* in the gingiva of aggressive periodontitis cases. *Aggregatibacter actinomycetemcomitans* has also been found in the tissues.[16,47,59]

Bacteria may invade the intercellular space under exfoliating epithelial cells, but they are also found between deeper epithelial cells as well as accumulating on the basement lamina. Some bacteria traverse the basement lamina and invade the subepithelial connective tissue[60] (Fig. 23.10 and 23.11).

The presence of bacteria in the gingival tissues has been interpreted by different investigators as bacterial invasion or as the "passive translocation" of plaque bacteria.[42] This important point has significant clinicopathologic implications and has not yet been clarified.[17,39,43]

Mechanisms of Tissue Destruction

The inflammatory response triggered by bacterial plaque unleashes a complex cascade of events aimed at destroying and removing bacteria, necrotic cells, and deleterious agents. However, this process is nonspecific; in an attempt to restore health, the host's cells (e.g., neutrophils, macrophages, fibroblasts, epithelial cells) produce proteinases, cytokines, and prostaglandins that can damage or destroy the tissues.

Chapter 9 describes in detail these aspects of inflammation and the mechanisms of tissue destruction at the molecular level.

Microtopography of the Gingival Wall

Scanning electron microscopy has permitted the description of several areas in the soft-tissue (gingival) wall of the periodontal pocket in which different types of activity take place.[56] These areas are irregularly oval or elongated and adjacent to one another, and they measure about 50 to 200 μm. These findings suggest that the pocket wall is constantly changing as a result of the interaction between the host and the bacteria. The following areas have been noted:

1. *Areas of relative quiescence,* showing a relatively flat surface with minor depressions and mounds and occasional shedding of cells (Fig. 23.12A).

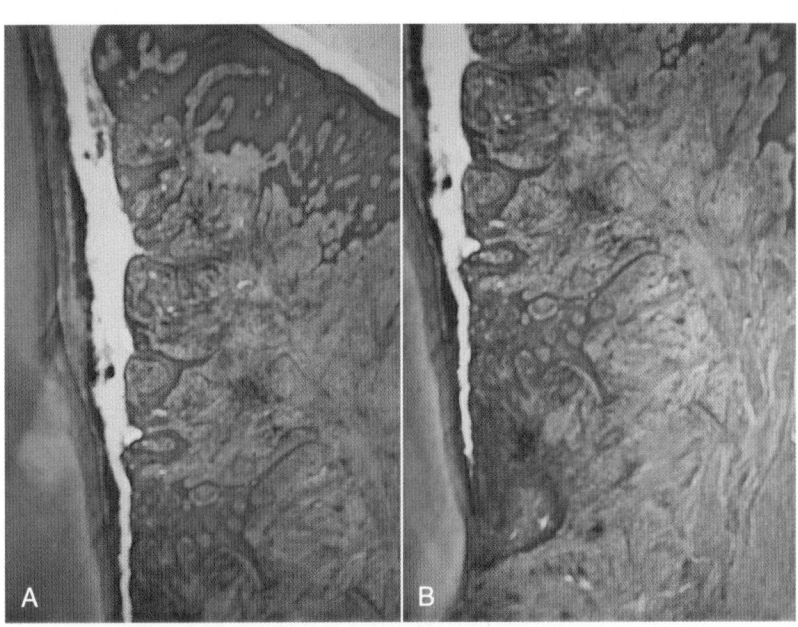

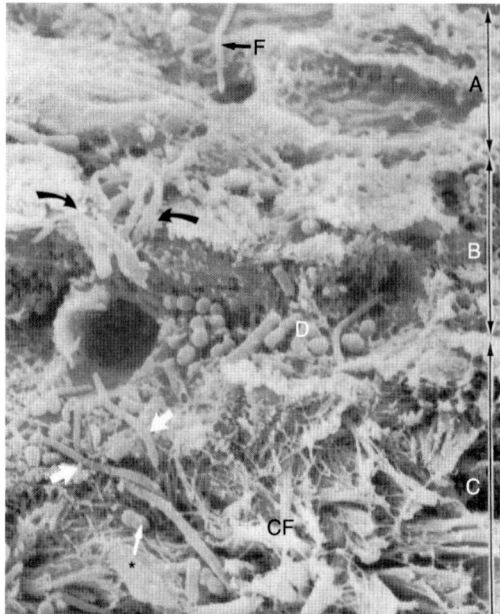

Fig. 23.10 Scanning electron micrograph of a section of pocket wall in advanced periodontitis in a human specimen showing bacterial penetration into the epithelium and connective tissue. Scanning electron microscope view of the surface of the pocket wall (A), sectioned epithelium (B), and sectioned connective tissue (C). Curved arrows point to areas of bacterial penetration into the epithelium. Thick white arrows point to bacterial penetration into the connective tissue through a break in the continuity of the basal lamina. *CF,* Connective tissue fibers; *D,* accumulation of bacteria (rods, cocci, and filaments) on the basal lamina; *F,* filamentous organism on the surface of the epithelium. The asterisk points to coccobacillus in the connective tissue.

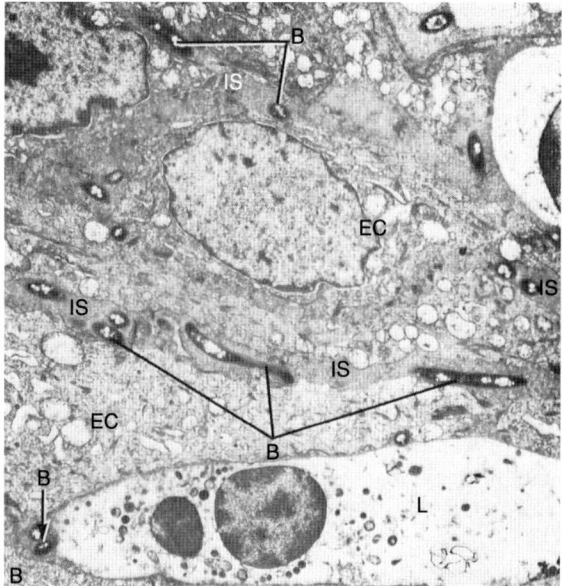

Fig. 23.11 Transmission electron micrograph of the epithelium in the periodontal pocket wall showing bacteria in the intercellular spaces. *B,* Bacteria; *EC,* epithelial cell; *IS,* intercellular space; *L,* leukocyte about to engulf bacteria. (×8000.)

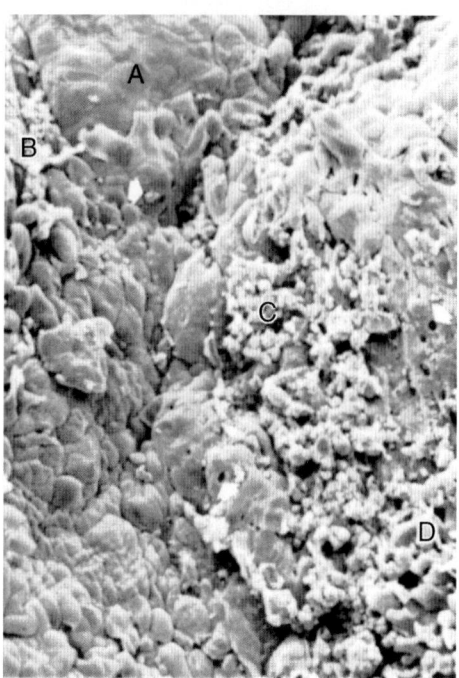

Fig. 23.12 Scanning electron frontal micrograph of the periodontal pocket wall. Different areas can be seen in the pocket wall surface. (A) Area of quiescence. (B) Bacterial accumulation. (C) Bacterial–leukocyte interaction. (D) Intense cellular desquamation. Arrows point to emerging leukocytes and holes left by leukocytes in the pocket wall. (Magnification ×800.)

2. *Areas of bacterial accumulation,* which appear as depressions on the epithelial surface, with abundant debris and bacterial clumps penetrating into the enlarged intercellular spaces. These bacteria are mainly cocci, rods, and filaments, with a few spirochetes (Fig. 23.12B).
3. *Areas of emergence of leukocytes,* in which leukocytes appear in the pocket wall through holes located in the intercellular spaces (Fig. 23.13).
4. *Areas of leukocyte–bacteria interaction,* in which numerous leukocytes are present and covered with bacteria in an apparent process of phagocytosis. Bacterial plaque associated with the epithelium is seen either as an organized matrix covered by a fibrin-like material in contact with the surface of cells or as bacteria penetrating into the intercellular spaces (Fig. 23.12C).
5. *Areas of intense epithelial desquamation,* consisting of semiattached and folded epithelial squames, which are sometimes partially covered with bacteria (Fig. 23.12D).
6. *Areas of ulceration,* with exposed connective tissue (Fig. 23.14).
7. *Areas of hemorrhage,* with numerous erythrocytes.

The transition from one area to another could result from bacteria accumulating in previously quiescent areas and triggering the emergence of leukocytes and the leukocyte–bacteria interaction. This would lead to intense epithelial desquamation and finally to ulceration and hemorrhage.

Periodontal Pockets as Healing Lesions

Periodontal pockets are chronic inflammatory lesions and thus are constantly undergoing repair. Complete healing does not occur because of the persistence of the bacterial attack, which continues to stimulate an inflammatory response, thereby causing degeneration of the new tissue elements formed during the continuous effort at repair.

The condition of the soft-tissue wall of the periodontal pocket results from the interplay of the destructive and constructive tissue changes. Their balance determines clinical features such as color, consistency, and surface texture of the pocket wall. If the inflammatory fluid and cellular exudate predominate, the pocket wall is bluish red, soft, spongy, and friable, with a smooth, shiny surface; at the clinical level, this is generally referred to as an *edematous pocket wall*. If there is a relative predominance of newly formed connective tissue cells and fibers, the pocket wall is more firm and pink and clinically referred to as a *fibrotic pocket wall* (see Table 23.1).

Edematous and fibrotic pockets represent opposite extremes of the same pathologic process rather than different disease entities.

They are subject to constant modification, depending on the relative predominance of exudative and constructive changes.

Fibrotic pocket walls may be misleading, because they do not necessarily reflect what is taking place throughout the pocket wall. The most severe degenerative changes in periodontal tissues occur adjacent to the tooth surface and the subgingival plaque. In some cases, inflammation and ulceration on the inside of the pocket are walled off by fibrous tissue on the outer aspect (Fig. 23.15). Externally the pocket appears pink and fibrotic, despite the inflammatory changes occurring internally.

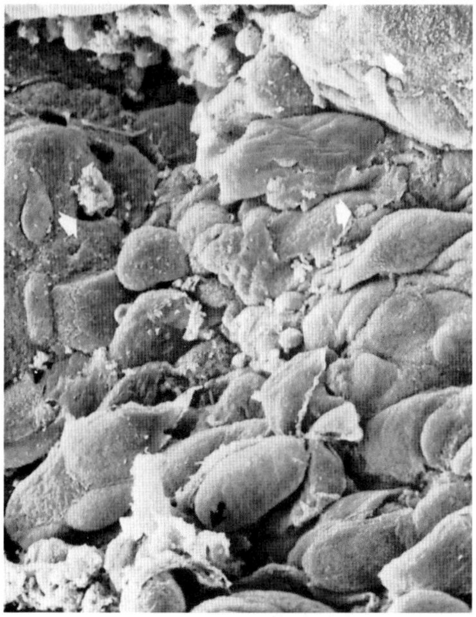

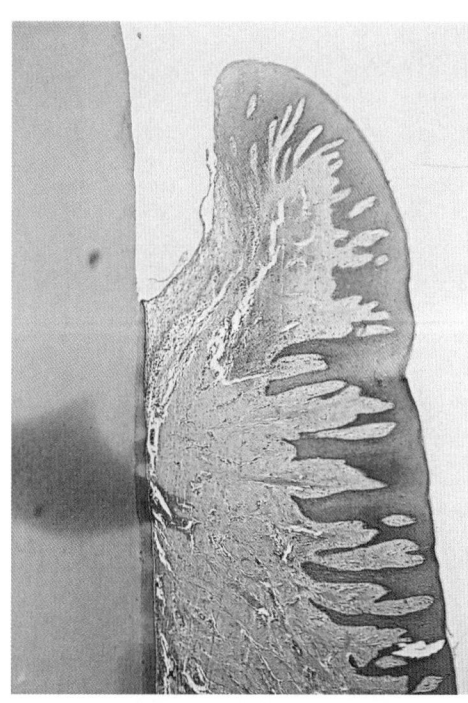

Fig. 23.13 Scanning electron micrograph of the periodontal pocket wall, frontal view, in a patient with advanced periodontitis. Note the desquamating epithelial cells and leukocytes *(white arrows)* emerging onto the pocket space. Scattered bacteria can also be seen *(black arrow)*. (Magnification ×1500.)

Fig. 23.15 Periodontal pocket wall. The inner half is inflamed and ulcerated; the outer half is densely collagenous.

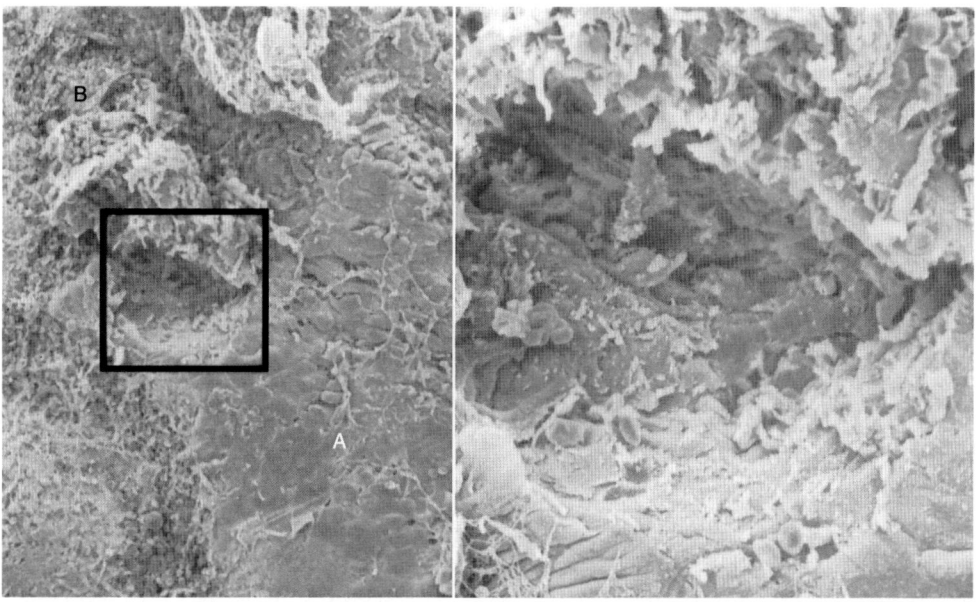

Fig. 23.14 Area of ulceration in the lateral wall of a deep periodontal pocket in a human specimen (magnification ×800) *(left)*. *A,* Surface of pocket epithelium in a quiescent state. *B,* Area of hemorrhage. Scanning electron microscopy (magnification ×3000) of the square on the left *(right)*. Connective tissue fibers and cells can be seen in the bottom of the ulcer.

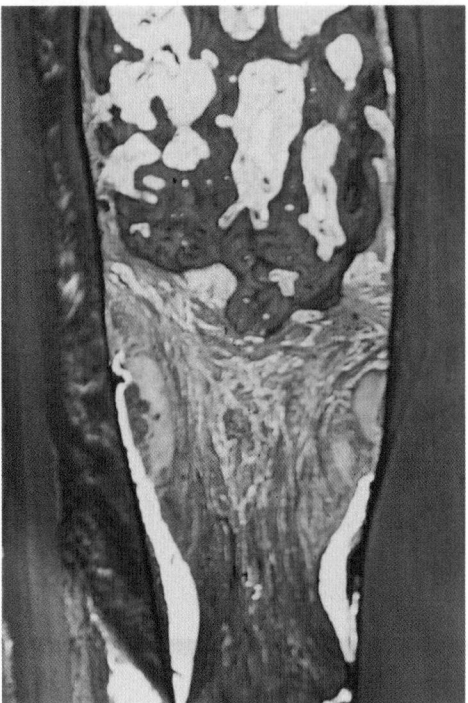

Fig. 23.16 Interdental papilla with ulcerated suprabony periodontal pockets on its mesial and distal aspects. Calculus is present on the approximal tooth surfaces and within the gingiva.

Pocket Contents

Periodontal pockets contain debris that consists principally of microorganisms and their products (enzymes, endotoxins, and other metabolic products), gingival fluid, food remnants, salivary mucin, desquamated epithelial cells, and leukocytes. Plaque-covered calculus usually projects from the tooth surface (Fig. 23.16). Purulent exudate, if present in the patient, consists of living, degenerated, and necrotic leukocytes; living and dead bacteria; serum; and a scant amount of fibrin.[46] The contents of periodontal pockets, when filtered free of organisms and debris, have been demonstrated to be toxic when injected subcutaneously into experimental animals.[31]

Pus is a common feature of periodontal disease, but it is only a secondary sign. The presence of pus or the ease with which it can be expressed from the pocket merely reflects the nature of the inflammatory changes in the pocket wall. It is not an indication of the depth of the pocket or the severity of the destruction of the supporting tissues. Extensive pus formation may occur in shallow pockets, whereas deep pockets may exhibit little or no pus. The localized accumulation of pus constitutes an abscess, which is discussed later in this chapter.

 KEY FACT

Gingival Crevicular Fluid
Gingival crevicular fluid (GCF) is an ultrafiltrate of blood, present in the gingival sulcus space, that contains several molecular components like bacterial degradation products, host tissue degradation products, and inflammatory mediators. Due to the location and ease of collection, several human clinical studies have been and are currently exploring and validating biomarkers of periodontal disease in GCF. The implant equivalent of GCF is commonly referred to as periimplant sulcular fluid (PISF).

Root Surface Walls

The root surface wall of periodontal pockets often undergoes changes that are significant because they may perpetuate the periodontal infection, cause pain, and complicate periodontal treatment.[11]

> As the pocket deepens, collagen fibers embedded in the cementum are destroyed, and cementum becomes exposed to the oral environment. Collagenous remnants of Sharpey fibers in the cementum undergo degeneration, creating an environment favorable to the penetration of bacteria. Viable bacteria have been found in the roots of 87% of periodontally diseased noncarious teeth.[2] Bacterial penetration into the cementum can be found as deep as the cementodentinal junction,[1,19] and it may also enter the dentinal tubules.[29,31] Penetration and the growth of bacteria lead to fragmentation and breakdown of the cementum surface and result in areas of necrotic cementum that are separated from the tooth by masses of bacteria.

Pathologic granules[9] have been observed with light and electron microscopy,[6,7] and they may represent areas of collagen degeneration or areas in which collagen fibrils have not been fully mineralized initially.

In addition, bacterial products (e.g., endotoxins[4,5]) have also been detected in the cementum wall of periodontal pockets. When root fragments from teeth with periodontal disease are placed in tissue culture, they induce irreversible morphologic changes in the cells of the culture. Such changes are not produced by normal roots.[33] Diseased root fragments also prevent the in vitro attachment of human gingival fibroblasts, whereas normal root surfaces allow the cells to attach freely.[3] When placed in the oral mucosa of the patient, diseased root fragments induce an inflammatory response, even if they have been autoclaved.[44]

 KEY FACT

Bacterial Endotoxin
Endotoxins are lipopolysaccharide (LPS) in nature and are associated with the cell walls of gram-negative bacteria. LPS is highly immunogenic, which the innate immune system recognizes via Toll-like receptors (TLRs), leading to an immune response. LPS from *Porphyromonas gingivalis*, a key pathogen in periodontal disease, plays an important role in both triggering and sustaining inflammation in the periodontium.

These changes manifest clinically as softening of the cementum surface; this is usually asymptomatic, but it can be painful when a probe or explorer penetrates the area. They also constitute a possible reservoir for reinfection of the area after treatment. During the course of treatment, these necrotic areas are removed by root planing until a hard, smooth surface is reached. Cementum is very thin in the cervical areas, and scaling and root planing often remove it entirely, exposing the underlying dentin. Sensitivity to cold may result until the pulp tissue forms secondary dentin.

Decalcification and Remineralization of Cementum
Areas of *increased mineralization*[65] are probably a result of an exchange of minerals and organic components at the cementum–saliva interface after exposure to the oral cavity. The mineral content of exposed cementum increases,[64] and the minerals that are increased in diseased root surfaces include calcium,[67] magnesium,[50,67] phosphorus,[50] and fluoride.[50] Microhardness, however, remains unchanged.[55,81] The

development of a highly mineralized superficial layer may increase the tooth's resistance to decay.[3]

The hypermineralized zones are detectable by electron microscopy, and they are associated with increased perfection of the crystal structure and organic changes that are suggestive of a subsurface cuticle.[64,65] These zones have also been seen in microradiographic studies[66] as a layer that is generally 10 to 20 mm thick, with areas as thick as 50 mm. No decrease in mineralization was found in deeper areas, indicating that increased mineralization does not come from adjacent areas. A loss of or reduction in the crossbanding of collagen near the cementum surface[27,28] and a subsurface condensation of organic material of exogenous origin[64] have also been reported.

Areas of demineralization are often related to root caries. Exposure to oral fluid and bacterial plaque results in proteolysis of the embedded remnants of Sharpey fibers; the cementum may be softened, and it may undergo fragmentation and cavitation.[34] Unlike enamel caries, root surface caries tend to progress around rather than into the tooth.[48] Active root caries lesions appear as well-defined yellowish or light brown areas; they are frequently covered by plaque, and they have a softened or leathery consistency on probing. Inactive lesions are well-defined darker lesions with a smooth surface and a harder consistency on probing.[24]

The dominant microorganism in root surface caries is *Actinomyces viscosus*,[72] although its specific role in the development of the lesion has not been established.[24] Other bacteria, such as *Actinomyces naeslundii, Streptococcus mutans, Streptococcus salivarius, Streptococcus sanguinis,* and *Bacillus cereus,* have been found to produce root caries in animal models. Quirynen and colleagues[54] reported that when plaque levels and pocket depths decrease after periodontal therapy (both nonsurgical and surgical), a shift in oral bacteria occurs, leading to a reduction in periodontal pathogens, an increase in *S. mutans,* and the development of root caries.

A prevalence rate study of root caries among 20- to 64-year-old individuals revealed that 42% had one or more root caries lesions and that these lesions tended to increase with age.[37]

The tooth may not be painful, but exploration of the root surface reveals the presence of a defect, and penetration of the involved area with a probe causes pain. Caries of the root may lead to pulpitis, sensitivity to sweets and thermal changes, or severe pain. Pathologic exposure of the pulp occurs in severe cases. Root caries may be the cause of toothache in patients with periodontal disease and no evidence of coronal decay.

Caries of the cementum requires special attention when the pocket is treated. The necrotic cementum must be removed by scaling and root planing until firm tooth surface is reached, even if this entails extension into the dentin.

Areas of cellular resorption of cementum and dentin are common in roots that are unexposed by periodontal disease.[68] These areas are of no particular significance because they are symptom free, and, as long as the root is covered by the periodontal ligament, they are likely to undergo repair. However, if the root is exposed by progressive pocket formation before repair occurs, these areas appear as isolated cavitations that penetrate into the dentin. These areas can be differentiated from caries of the cementum by their clear-cut outline and hard surface. They may be sources of considerable pain that require the placement of a restoration.

Surface Morphology of Tooth Wall[78]

The following zones can be found in the bottom of a periodontal pocket (Fig. 23.17):

1. *Cementum covered by calculus,* in which all of the changes described in the preceding paragraphs can be found.

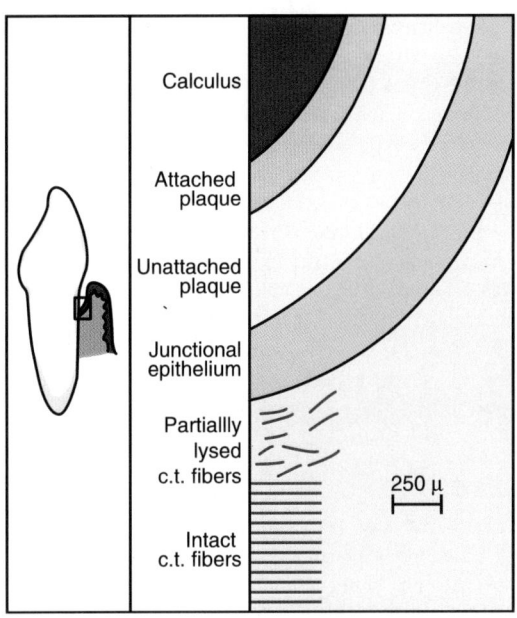

Fig. 23.17 Diagram of the area at the bottom of a pocket. *c.t.,* Connective tissue.

2. *Attached plaque,* which covers calculus and extends apically from it to a variable degree (typically 100 to 500 μm).
3. The zone of *unattached plaque* that surrounds attached plaque and extends apically to it.
4. The zone of *attachment of the junctional epithelium to the tooth.* The extension of this zone, which in normal sulci is more than 500 μm, is usually reduced in periodontal pockets to less than 100 μm.
5. A zone of *semidestroyed connective tissue fibers* may be apical to the junctional epithelium[60] (see the Pathogenesis section earlier in this chapter).

Zones 3, 4, and 5 make up the "plaque-free zone" seen in extracted teeth.[8,12,36,58,78] The total width of the plaque-free zone varies according to the type of tooth (i.e., it is wider in the molars than in the incisors) and the depth of the pocket (i.e., it is narrower in deeper pockets).[57] It is important to remember that the term *plaque-free zone* refers only to attached plaque, because unattached plaque contains a variety of gram-positive and gram-negative morphotypes, including cocci, rods, filaments, fusiforms, and spirochetes. The most apical zone contains predominantly gram-negative rods and cocci.[76]

Periodontal Disease Activity

For many years the loss of attachment produced by periodontal disease was thought to be a slow but continuously progressive phenomenon. More recently, as a result of studies of the specificity of plaque bacteria, the concept of periodontal disease activity has evolved.

According to this concept, periodontal pockets go through periods of exacerbation and quiescence as a result of episodic bursts of activity followed by periods of remission. *Periods of quiescence* are characterized by a reduced inflammatory response and little or no loss of bone and connective tissue attachment. A buildup of unattached plaque, with its gram-negative, motile, and anaerobic bacteria (see Chapter 8), starts a *period of exacerbation* during which bone and connective tissue attachment are lost and the pocket deepens. This period may last for days, weeks, or months, and it is eventually followed by a period of remission or quiescence during which gram-positive bacteria proliferate and a more stable condition is established. On the basis of a study of radioiodine[125]I absorptiometry, McHenry and colleagues[45] confirmed that bone loss in patients with untreated periodontal disease occurs in an episodic manner.

These periods of quiescence and exacerbation are also known as *periods of inactivity* and *periods of activity.* Clinically, active periods show bleeding, either spontaneously or with probing, and greater amounts of gingival exudate. Histologically, the pocket epithelium appears thin and ulcerated, and an infiltrate composed predominantly of plasma cells,[19] PMNs,[53] or both is seen. Bacterial samples from the pocket lumen that are analyzed with dark-field microscopy show high proportions of motile organisms and spirochetes.[43]

Methods to detect periods of activity or inactivity are currently being investigated (see www.expertconsult.com).

Site Specificity

Periodontal destruction does not occur in all parts of the mouth at the same time; rather it occurs on a few teeth at a time or even only on some aspects of some teeth at any given time. This is referred to as the *site specificity* of periodontal disease. Sites of periodontal destruction are often found next to sites with little or no destruction. Therefore the severity of periodontitis increases with the development of new disease sites and with the increased breakdown of existing sites.

Pulp Changes Associated With Periodontal Pockets

The spread of infection from periodontal pockets may cause pathologic changes in the pulp. Such changes may give rise to painful symptoms, or they may adversely affect the response of the pulp to restorative procedures. Involvement of the pulp in periodontal disease occurs through either the apical foramen or the lateral pulp canals after pocket infection reaches them. Atrophic and inflammatory pulpal changes occur in such cases (see Chapter 46).

Relationship of Attachment Loss and Bone Loss to Pocket Depth

The severity of the attachment loss in pocket formation is generally but not always correlated with the depth of the pocket. This is because the degree of attachment loss depends on the location of the base of the pocket on the root surface, whereas pocket depth is the distance between the base of the pocket and the crest of the gingival margin. Pockets of the same depth may be associated with different degrees of attachment loss (Fig. 23.18), and pockets of different depths may be associated with the same amount of attachment loss (Fig. 23.19).

The severity of bone loss is generally but not always correlated with pocket depth. Extensive attachment and bone loss may be associated with shallow pockets if the attachment loss is accompanied by recession of the gingival margin, and slight bone loss can occur with deep pockets.

Area Between Base of Pocket and Alveolar Bone

Normally, the distance between the apical end of the junctional epithelium and the alveolar bone is relatively constant. The distance between the apical extent of calculus and the alveolar crest in human periodontal pockets is most constant, having a mean length of 1.97 mm (±33.16%).[71,77]

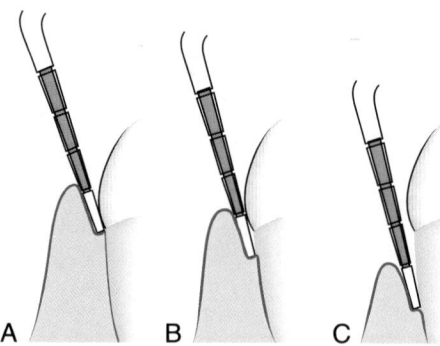

Fig. 23.18 Same pocket depth with different amounts of recession. (A) Gingival pocket with no recession. (B) Periodontal pocket of similar depth as shown in part A but with some degree of recession. (C) Pocket depth the same as shown in parts A and B but with still more recession.

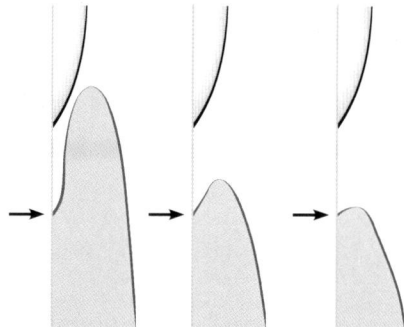

Fig. 23.19 Different pocket depths with the same amount of attachment loss. Arrows point to the bottom of the pocket. The distance between the arrow and the cementoenamel junction remains the same despite different pocket depths.

The distance from attached plaque to bone is never less than 0.5 mm and never more than 2.7 mm.[78-80] These findings suggest that the bone-resorbing activity induced by the bacteria is exerted within these distances. However, the finding of isolated bacteria or clumps of bacteria in the connective tissue[60] and on the bone surface[26] may modify these considerations.

Relationship of Pocket to Bone

In infrabony pockets, the base of the pocket is apical to the crest of the alveolar bone, and the pocket wall lies between the tooth and the bone. The bone loss is in most cases vertical. Alternatively, in suprabony pockets, the base is coronal to the crest of the alveolar bone, and the pocket wall lies coronal to the bone. The type of bone loss is always horizontal.

This creates some microscopic differences that have some therapeutic importance. They are the relationship of the soft-tissue wall of the pocket to the alveolar bone, the pattern of bone destruction, and the direction of the transseptal fibers of the periodontal ligament[15] (Figs. 23.20, 23.21, and 23.22).

In suprabony pockets, the alveolar crest gradually attains a more apical position in relation to the tooth, but it retains its general morphology and architecture. The interdental fibers that run over the bone from one tooth to the other maintain their usual horizontal direction. In infrabony pockets, the morphology of the alveolar crest changes completely, with the formation of an angular bony defect. The interdental fibers in this case run over the bone in an oblique direction between the two teeth of the interdental space.[15,80] This may affect the function of the area and also necessitate a modification in treatment

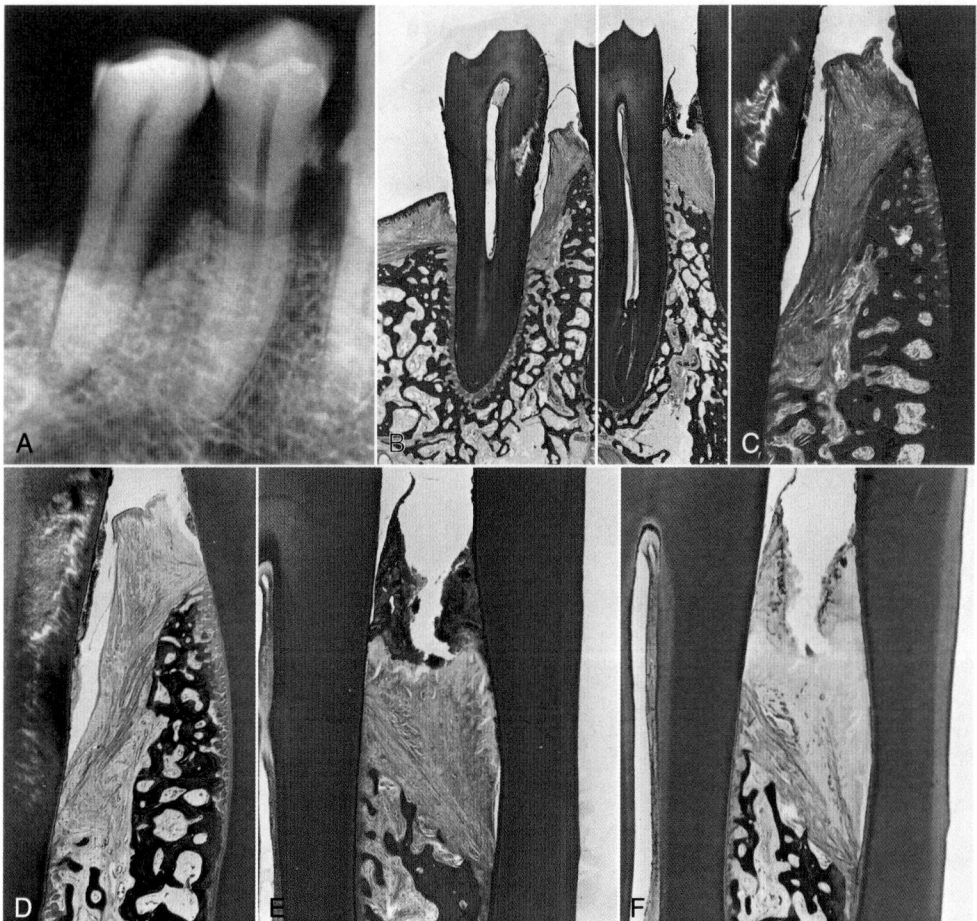

Fig. 23.20 Radiographic and microscopic features of intrabony pockets. (A) Radiograph of a mandibular canine and premolar area showing angular bone loss mesial to the second premolar. The type of bone loss between the first premolar and the canine is not radiographically apparent. (B) Mesiodistal histologic section of the teeth seen in A showing an intrabony pocket mesial to the second premolar as well as suprabony pockets distal to the second premolar and mesial and distal to the first premolar. The mesial suprabony pocket of the first premolar appears to be coronal to a vertical bone loss. (C) Higher-power view of the area between the premolars. Note the angular bone loss and the transseptal fibers that cover the bone. (D) Higher-power view of the area between the premolars stained with Mallory connective tissue stain, clearly showing the direction of transseptal fibers. (E) Higher-power view of the area between the first premolar and the canine. Note the abundant calculus, the dense leukocytic infiltration of the gingiva, and the angulation of the transseptal fibers and bone. The pocket is still suprabony. (F) Mallory stain of a similar area to the one shown in part E. Note the destruction of the gingival fibers caused by inflammation and the angular fibers formed over angular bone loss and less affected by the inflammation. Transseptal fibers extend from the distal surface of the premolar over the crest of the alveolar bone into the intrabony pocket. Note the leukocytic infiltration of the transseptal fibers. *(From Glickman I, Smulow J: Periodontal disease: clinical, radiographic and histopathologic features, Philadelphia, 1974, Saunders.)*

techniques (see Chapters 59 and 60).[13,15] Table 23.2 summarizes the distinguishing features of suprabony and infrabony pockets. The classification of infrabony pockets is discussed in Chapter 24.

⚠ CLINICAL CORRELATION

Pocket reduction surgeries

Pocket reduction surgeries are aimed at reducing the probing pocket depths in patients with periodontitis. Depending on the disease presentation, one can take a resective or regenerative approach. Suprabony pockets are primarily treated by resective procedures such as gingivectomy or osseous surgery, whereas infrabony defects with multiple walls (that are contained) are generally treated using regenerative approaches.

Periodontal Abscess

A periodontal abscess is a localized purulent inflammation in the periodontal tissues (Fig. 23.23). It is also known as a *lateral abscess* or a *parietal abscess*. Abscesses that are localized in the gingiva, that are caused by injury to the outer surface of the gingiva, and that do not involve the supporting structures are called *gingival abscesses*. Gingival abscesses may occur in the presence or absence of a periodontal pocket.

Periodontal abscess formation may occur in the following ways:
1. Extension of infection from a periodontal pocket deep into the supporting periodontal tissues and localization of the suppurative inflammatory process along the lateral aspect of the root.

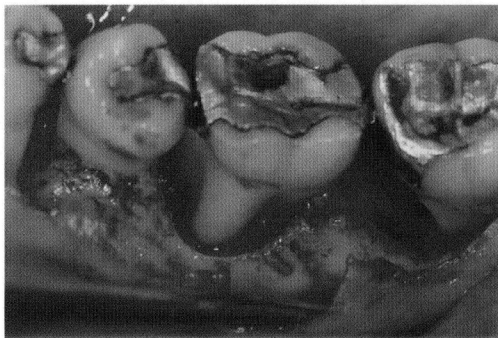

Fig. 23.21 After raising a flap for the treatment of the infrabony pockets, the vertical bone loss around the mesial roots of the mandibular first and second molars can be seen.

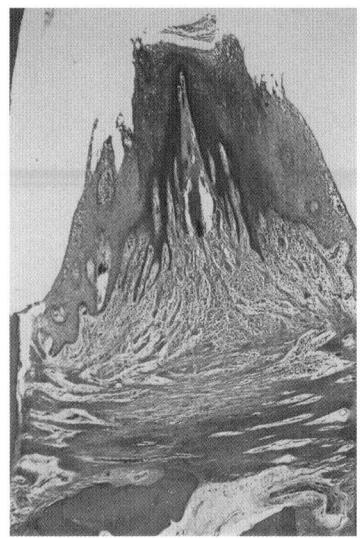

Fig. 23.22 Two suprabony pockets in an interdental space. Note the normal horizontal arrangement of the transseptal fibers.

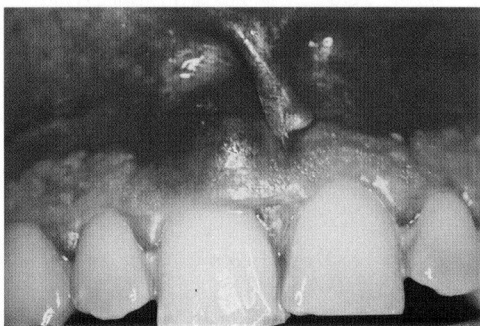

Fig. 23.23 Periodontal abscess on an upper right central incisor.

2. Lateral extension of inflammation from the inner surface of a periodontal pocket into the connective tissue of the pocket wall. Formation of the abscess results when drainage into the pocket space is impaired.
3. Formation in a pocket with a tortuous course around the root. A periodontal abscess may form in the cul-de-sac, the deep end of which is shut off from the surface.
4. Incomplete removal of calculus during treatment of a periodontal pocket. The gingival wall shrinks, thereby occluding the pocket orifice, and a periodontal abscess occurs in the sealed-off portion of the pocket.

TABLE 23.2 Distinguishing Features of Suprabony and Intrabony Periodontal Pockets

Suprabony Pocket	Intrabony Pocket
1. The base of the pocket is coronal to the level of the alveolar bone.	1. The base of the pocket is apical to the crest of the alveolar bone so that the bone is adjacent to the soft-tissue wall (see Fig. 23.2).
2. The pattern of destruction of the underlying bone is horizontal.	2. The pattern of bone destruction is vertical (angular) (see Figs. 23.20 and 23.21).
3. Interproximally, transseptal fibers that are restored during progressive periodontal disease are arranged horizontally in the space between the base of the pocket and the alveolar bone (see Fig. 23.22).	3. Interproximally, transseptal fibers are oblique rather than horizontal. They extend from the cementum beneath the base of the pocket along the alveolar bone and over the crest to the cementum of the adjacent tooth (see Fig. 23.20).
4. On the facial and lingual surfaces, periodontal ligament fibers beneath the pocket follow their normal horizontal–oblique course between the tooth and the bone.	4. On the facial and lingual surfaces, periodontal ligament fibers follow the angular pattern of the adjacent bone. They extend from the cementum beneath the base of the pocket along the alveolar bone and over the crest to join with the outer periosteum.

5. After trauma to the tooth or with perforation of the lateral wall of the root in endodontic therapy. In these situations, a periodontal abscess may occur in the absence of periodontal disease.

Periodontal abscesses are classified according to location as follows:

1. *Abscess in the supporting periodontal tissues along the lateral aspect of the root.* With this condition, a sinus generally occurs in the bone that extends laterally from the abscess to the external surface.
2. *Abscess in the soft-tissue wall of a deep periodontal pocket.*

> Microscopically, an abscess is a localized accumulation of viable and nonviable PMNs within the periodontal pocket wall. The PMNs liberate enzymes that digest the cells and other tissue structures, thereby forming the liquid product known as *pus,* which constitutes the center of the abscess. An acute inflammatory reaction surrounds the purulent area, and the overlying epithelium exhibits intracellular and extracellular edema and the invasion of leukocytes (Fig. 23.24).

The localized acute abscess becomes a chronic abscess when its purulent content drains through a fistula into the outer gingival surface or into the periodontal pocket and the infection that is causing the abscess is not resolved.

The bacterial invasion of tissues has been reported in abscesses; the invading organisms were identified as gram-negative cocci, diplococci, fusiforms, and spirochetes. Invasive fungi were also found and were interpreted as being "opportunistic invaders."[22] Microorganisms that colonize the periodontal abscess have been reported to be primarily gram-negative anaerobic rods.[51]

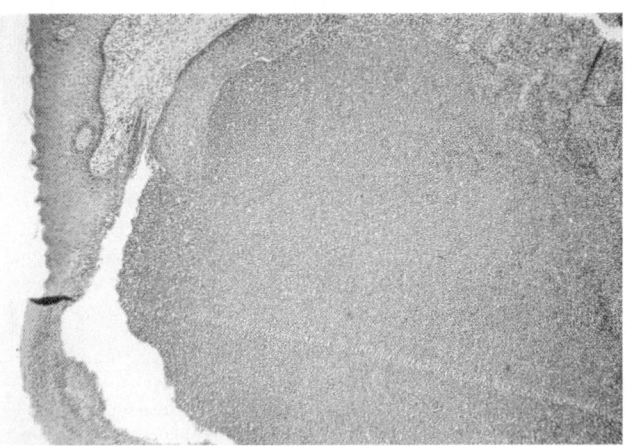

Fig. 23.24 Microscopic view of a periodontal abscess showing the dense accumulation of polymorphonuclear leukocytes covered by squamous epithelium.

Lateral Periodontal Cyst

The periodontal cyst, which is also called *lateral periodontal cyst,* is an uncommon lesion that produces localized destruction of the periodontal tissues along a lateral root surface, most often in the mandibular canine–premolar area.[23,70] It is considered to be derived from the rests of Malassez or other proliferating odontogenic rests.[69]

A periodontal cyst is usually asymptomatic, without grossly detectable changes, but it may present as a localized, tender swelling. Radiographically, an interproximal periodontal cyst appears on the side of the root as a radiolucent area bordered by a radiopaque line. Its radiographic appearance cannot be differentiated from that of a periodontal abscess.

Microscopically, the cystic lining may be (1) a loosely arranged, thin, nonkeratinized epithelium, sometimes with thicker proliferating areas, or (2) an odontogenic keratocyst.[23]

 A Case Scenario is found on the companion website www.expertconsult.com.

References

 References for this chapter are found on the companion website www.expertconsult.com.

CHAPTER 24

Bone Loss and Patterns of Bone Destruction

Paulo M. Camargo | Henry H. Takei | Fermin A. Carranza

CHAPTER OUTLINE

Bone Destruction Caused by the Extension of Gingival Inflammation
Bone Destruction Caused by Trauma From Occlusion
Bone Destruction Caused by Systemic Disorders
Factors Determining Bone Morphology in Periodontal Disease
Bone Destruction Patterns in Periodontal Disease
Conclusion

Editors' Note: An animation (slide show) has been added by the editors as a supplement to the chapter. It was produced by My Dental Hub as a patient education tool and covers the basic elements in a conceptual manner. It is not intended to be a procedural guide for dental professionals.

Periodontitis is an inflammatory condition of the teeth and their supporting structures. The inflammatory process, which occurs as a response to the bacterial biofilm insult, has detrimental effects on the periodontal unit, which results in the destruction of periodontal ligament fibers and bone loss.

The height and density of the alveolar bone are normally maintained by an equilibrium, which is regulated by local and systemic influences, between bone formation and bone resorption.[12,14] When resorption exceeds formation, both bone height and bone density may be reduced (Video 24.1: Vertical Bone Loss).

Bone loss is the ultimate and last consequence of the inflammatory process observed in periodontitis. Therefore the existing bone level is the consequence of past pathologic episodes, whereas changes present in the soft tissue of the pocket wall reflect the presence of the inflammatory condition. Thus the degree of bone loss does not necessarily correlate with the depth of periodontal pockets, the severity of ulceration of the pocket wall, or the presence or absence of suppuration. As an example, a reduced periodontium may exist in areas where bone loss occurred in the past but that currently present with periodontal health (i.e., following periodontal treatment; Fig. 24.1).

Bone Destruction Caused by the Extension of Gingival Inflammation

The most common cause of bone destruction in periodontitis is the extension of inflammation from the marginal gingiva into the supporting periodontal tissues. The inflammatory migration of the bone surface and the initial bone loss that follows mark the transition from gingivitis to periodontitis.

Periodontitis is always preceded by gingivitis, but not all gingivitis progresses to periodontitis. Some cases of gingivitis apparently never become periodontitis, and other cases go through a brief gingivitis phase and rapidly develop into periodontitis. The factors responsible for the extension of inflammation to the supporting structures, thereby initiating the conversion of gingivitis to periodontitis, are not clearly understood and are likely to be related to individual susceptibility to the insult presented by the bacterial biofilm or microbiologic changes that occur in the pocket environment and surrounding tissues.

LEARNING BOX 24.1

In periodontitis, the loss of bone is the ultimate and last event of the inflammatory process. The existing bone level is the result of past episodes of bone loss from the effects of periodontitis, but the changes present in the soft tissue of the pocket wall during periodontitis is the result of the ongoing inflammatory process. The degree of bone loss does not necessarily correlate with the depth of the periodontal pockets, the severity of ulceration of the pocket wall, or the presence or absence of exudate.

As stated previously, the transition from gingivitis to periodontitis is associated with changes in the composition of the bacterial biofilm. In advanced stages of disease, the number of motile organisms and spirochetes increases, whereas the number of coccoid rods and straight rods decreases.[34] The cellular composition of the infiltrated connective tissue also changes with increasing severity of the lesion (see Chapter 7). Fibroblasts and lymphocytes predominate in stage 1 gingivitis, whereas the number of plasma cells and blast cells increases gradually as the disease progresses. Seymour and colleagues[58,59] have postulated a stage of "contained" gingivitis, in which T lymphocytes are preponderant; they suggest that, as the lesion becomes a B-lymphocyte lesion, it becomes progressively destructive.

Heijl and coworkers[22] were able to convert, in experimental animals, a confined, naturally occurring state of chronic gingivitis into progressive periodontitis by placing a silk ligature into the sulcus and tying it around the neck of the teeth. Placement of the ligature induced ulceration of the sulcular epithelium, a shift in the inflammatory infiltrate from predominantly plasma cells to polymorphonuclear leukocytes, and osteoclastic resorption of the alveolar crest. The recurrence of episodes of acute destruction over time may be one mechanism that leads to progressive bone loss in individuals with chronic periodontitis.

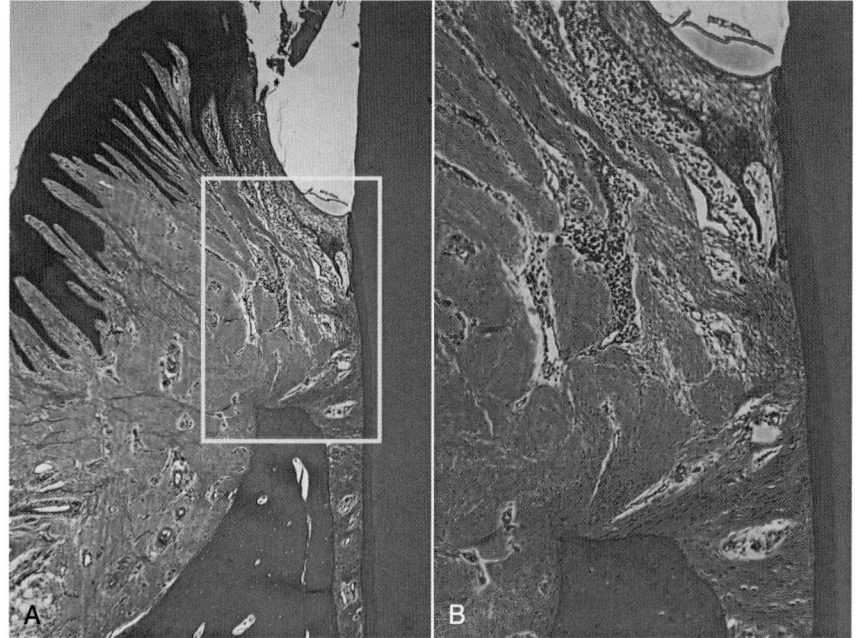

Fig. 24.1 (A) An area of inflammation extending from the gingiva into the suprabony area. (B) Extension of inflammation along the blood vessels and between collagen bundles.

The extension of the inflammatory process into the supporting structures of a tooth may be modified by the pathogenic potential of biofilm and the susceptibility/resistance of the host. The latter includes immunologic activity and other tissue-related mechanisms, such as the degree of fibrosis of the gingiva, probably the width of the attached gingiva, and the reactive fibrogenesis and osteogenesis that occur peripheral to the inflammatory lesion.[52] Some studies suggest that the quality of the host response to a similar bacterial insult varies, resulting in some individuals being more susceptible to the destructive aspects of periodontitis than others.

Histopathology

Gingival inflammation extends along the collagen fiber bundles and follows the course of the blood vessels through the loosely arranged tissues around them into the alveolar bone[67] (see Fig. 24.1). Although the inflammatory infiltrate is concentrated in the marginal periodontium, the reaction is a much more diffuse one, often reaching the bone and eliciting a response before evidence of crestal resorption or loss of attachment exists.[41] In the upper molar region, inflammation can extend to the maxillary sinus, resulting in thickening of the sinus mucosa.[40]

Interproximally, inflammation spreads to the loose connective tissue around the blood vessels, through the fibers, and then into the bone through vessel channels that perforate the crest of the interdental septum at the center of the crest (Fig. 24.2), toward the side of the crest (Fig. 24.3), or at the angle of the septum. In addition, inflammation may enter the bone through more than one channel. Less frequently, the inflammation spreads from the gingiva directly into the periodontal ligament and from there into the interdental septum[1] (Fig. 24.4).

Facially and lingually, inflammation from the gingiva spreads along the outer periosteal surface of the bone (see Fig. 24.4) and penetrates into the marrow spaces through vessel channels in the outer cortex.

Along its course from the gingiva to the bone, the inflammation destroys the gingival and transeptal fibers, reducing them to disorganized granular fragments interspersed among the inflammatory

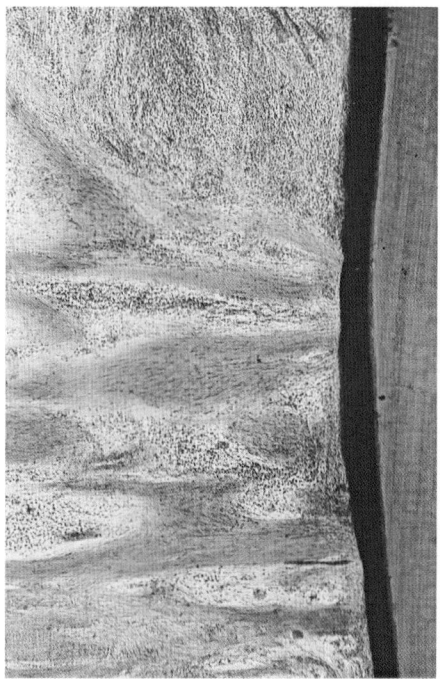

Fig. 24.2 Inflammation that extends from the pocket area *(top)* between the collagen fibers, which are partially destroyed.

cells and edema.[45] However, there is a continuous tendency to recreate transeptal fibers across the crest of the interdental septum farther along the root as the bone destruction progresses (Fig. 24.5). As a result, transeptal fibers are present, even in cases of extreme periodontal bone loss. The dense transeptal fibers form a firm covering over the bone that is encountered during periodontal flap surgery after the superficial granulation tissue is removed.[50]

After inflammation reaches the bone via extension from the gingiva (Fig. 24.6), it spreads into the marrow spaces and replaces the marrow

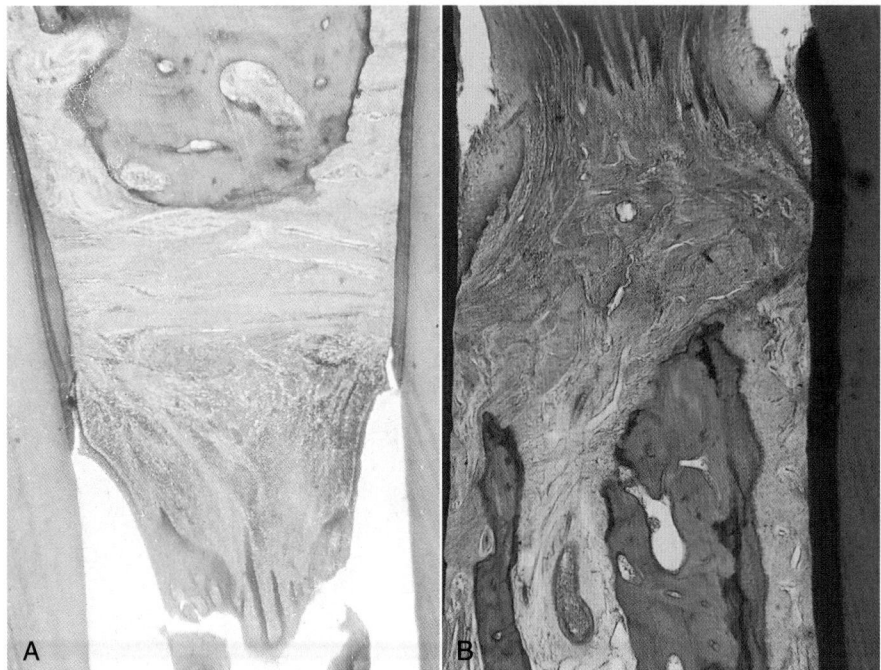

Fig. 24.3 (A) Extension of inflammation into the center of the interdental septum. Inflammation from the gingiva penetrates the transseptal fibers and enters the bone around the blood vessel in the center of the septum. (B) The cortical layer at the top of the septum has been destroyed, and the inflammation penetrates into the marrow spaces.

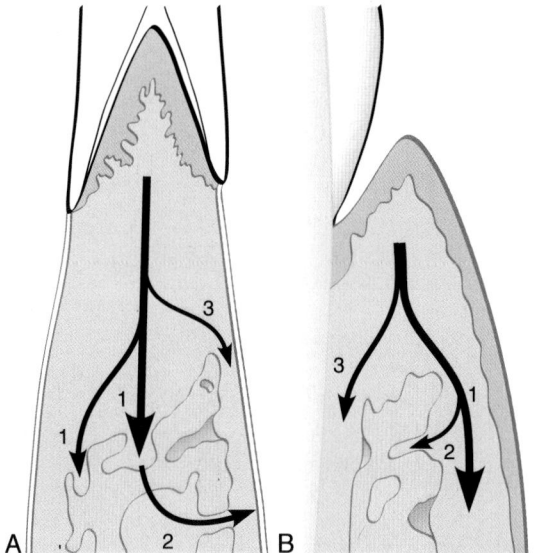

Fig. 24.4 Pathways of inflammation from the gingiva into the supporting periodontal tissues in a patient with periodontitis. (A) Interproximally, from the gingiva into the bone *(1)*, from the bone into the periodontal ligament *(2)*, and from the gingiva into the periodontal ligament *(3)*. (B) Facially and lingually, from the gingiva along the outer periosteum *(1)*, from the periosteum into the bone *(2)*, and from the gingiva into the periodontal ligament *(3)*.

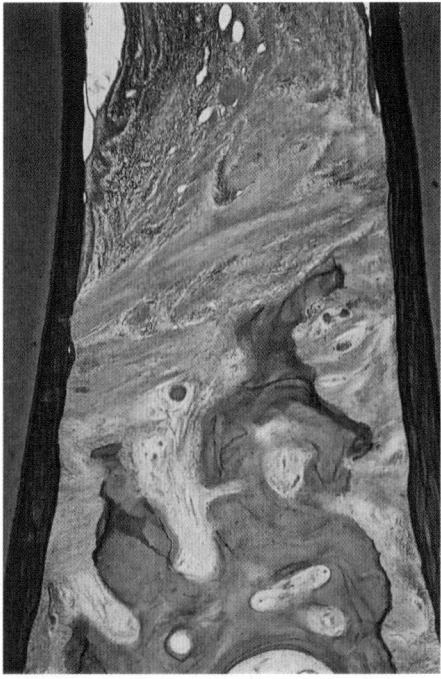

Fig. 24.5 Reformation of transseptal fibers. A mesiodistal section through the interdental septum shows gingival inflammation and bone loss. Recreated transseptal fibers can be seen above the bone margin, where they have been partially infiltrated by the inflammatory process.

with a leukocytic and fluid exudate, new blood vessels, and proliferating fibroblasts (Fig. 24.7). Multinuclear osteoclasts and mononuclear phagocytes increase in number, and the bone surfaces appear to be lined with Howship lacunae (Fig. 24.8).

In the marrow spaces, resorption proceeds from within and causes a thinning of the surrounding bony trabeculae and an enlargement of the marrow spaces; this is followed by the destruction of the bone

and a reduction in bone height. Normally, fatty bone marrow is partially or totally replaced by a fibrous type of marrow in the vicinity of the resorption.

Bone destruction in periodontal disease is not a process of bone necrosis.[27] It involves the activity of living cells along viable bone.

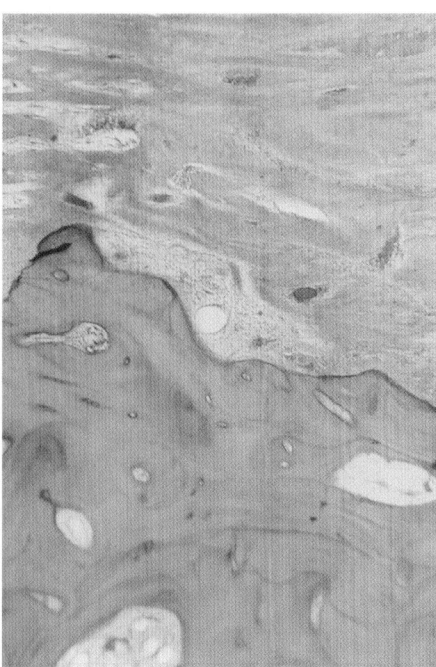

Fig. 24.6 Extension of inflammation has reached the crestal bone surface.

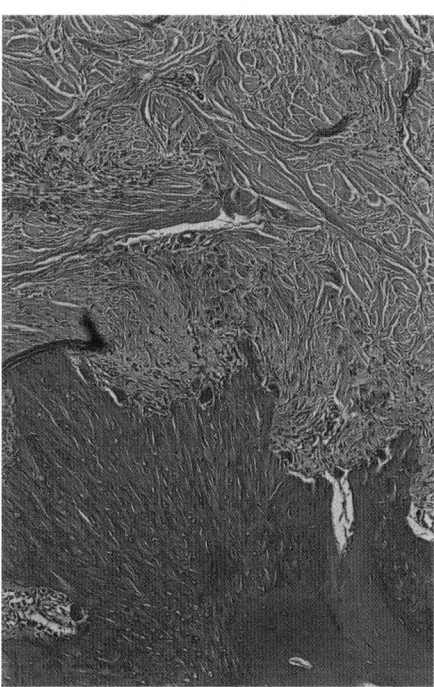

Fig. 24.8 Osteoclasts and Howship lacunae in the resorption of crestal bone.

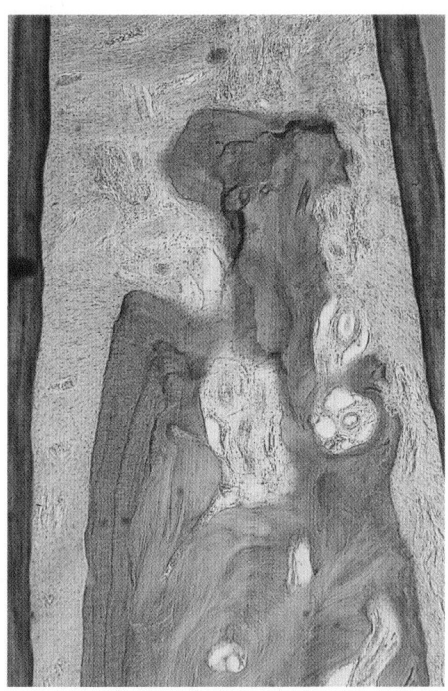

Fig. 24.7 Interdental septum in a human autopsy section. Extensive inflammatory infiltrate has invaded the marrow spaces, entering from both the mesial and distal aspects. Fatty bone marrow has been replaced by inflammatory cells and fibrous marrow.

With the exception of necrotic bone that is visible in distinct pathogenic processes such as necrotizing ulcerative periodontitis and bisphosphonate-related osteonecrosis of the jaws, all bone present in areas with periodontitis is viable, live bone. In periodontitis, bone resorption may be related to the analogy of the bone attempting to run away from the infectious/inflammatory process; this may be seen as a host protection mechanism.

The amount of inflammatory infiltrate correlates with the degree of bone loss but not with the number of osteoclasts. However, the distance from the apical border of the inflammatory infiltrate to the alveolar bone crest correlates with both the number of osteoclasts on the alveolar crest and the total number of osteoclasts.[51] Similar findings have been reported in experimentally induced periodontitis in animals.[32]

Radius of Action

Garant and Cho[10] suggested that locally produced bone resorption factors may need to be present in the proximity of the bone surface to exert their action. Page and Schroeder,[49] on the basis of Waerhaug's measurements made on human autopsy specimens,[64,65] postulated a range of effectiveness of about 1.5 mm to 2.5 mm in which bacterial biofilm can induce loss of bone. Beyond 2.5 mm, there is little or no effect; interproximal angular defects can appear only in spaces that are wider than 2.5 mm, because narrower spaces would end up with horizontal bone loss. Tal[61] corroborated this concept with measurements in human patients.

Large defects that greatly exceed a distance of 2.5 mm from the tooth surface (as described in aggressive types of periodontitis) may be caused by the presence of bacteria in the tissues.[6,10,54]

Rate of Bone Loss

In a study of Sri Lankan tea laborers with no oral hygiene and no dental care, Löe and colleagues[36] found the rate of bone loss averages about 0.2 mm per year for facial surfaces and about 0.3 mm per year for proximal surfaces when periodontal disease was allowed to progress untreated.

However, the rate of bone loss may vary, depending on the type of disease present. Löe and colleagues[35] also identified the following three subgroups of patients with periodontal disease on the basis of the interproximal loss of attachment and tooth mortality (loss of attachment can be equated with loss of bone, although attachment loss precedes bone loss by about 6 to 8 months[17]):

1. Approximately 8% of persons had a rapid progression of periodontal disease that was characterized by a yearly loss of attachment of 0.1 mm to 1 mm.

2. Approximately 81% of individuals had moderately progressive periodontal disease with a yearly loss of attachment of 0.05 mm to 0.5 mm.
3. The remaining 11% of persons had minimal or no progression of destructive disease with a yearly loss of attachment of 0.05 mm to 0.09 mm.

Periods of Destruction

Periodontal destruction occurs in an episodic, intermittent manner, with periods of inactivity or quiescence that alternate with destructive periods that result in the loss of collagen and alveolar bone and the deepening of the periodontal pocket.

Periods of destructive activity are associated with subgingival ulceration and an acute inflammatory reaction that results in the rapid loss of alveolar bone[49,56]; it has been hypothesized that this coincides with the conversion of a predominantly T-lymphocyte lesion to one with a predominantly B-lymphocyte–plasma cell infiltrate.[59] Microbiologically, these lesions are associated with an increase in the loose, unattached, motile, gram-negative, anaerobic pocket flora, whereas periods of remission coincide with the formation of a dense, unattached, nonmotile, gram-positive flora with a tendency to mineralize.[43]

It has also been suggested that the onset of periods of destruction coincide with tissue invasion by one or several bacterial species and that this is followed by an advanced local host defense that controls the attack.[54]

LEARNING BOX 24.2

The dense network transseptal fiber that is attached interdentally from tooth to tooth is one of the barriers that protects the interdental bone from the inflammatory process. Even after these fibers are initially destroyed, they continually re-form and are the fibers found during periodontal flap surgery.

Mechanisms of Bone Destruction

The factors involved in bone destruction in periodontal disease are bacterial and host mediated. The bacterial biofilm products induce the differentiation of bone progenitor cells into osteoclasts and stimulate gingival cells to release mediators that have the same effect.[21,57] Bacterial biofilm products and inflammatory mediators can also act directly on osteoblasts or their progenitors, thereby inhibiting their action and reducing their numbers.

In addition, in patients with rapidly progressing diseases (e.g., aggressive periodontitis), bacterial microcolonies or single bacterial cells have been found between collagen fibers and over the bone surface, suggesting a direct effect.[6,9,57]

Several host factors released by inflammatory cells are capable of inducing bone resorption in vitro, and they play a role in periodontal disease. These include host-produced prostaglandins and their precursors, interleukin-1α, interleukin-β, and tumor necrosis factor alpha.

When injected intradermally, prostaglandin E$_2$ induces the vascular changes that are seen with inflammation; when injected over a bone surface, prostaglandin E$_2$ induces bone resorption in the absence of inflammatory cells, with few multinucleated osteoclasts.[18,26] In addition, nonsteroidal antiinflammatory drugs (e.g., flurbiprofen, ibuprofen) inhibit prostaglandin E$_2$ production, thereby slowing bone loss in naturally occurring periodontal disease in beagle dogs and humans. This effect disappears 6 months after the cessation of drug administration.[25,68] (For more information about the host-mediated mechanisms of bone destruction, see Chapters 7 and 14.)

Bone Formation in Periodontal Disease

Areas of bone formation are also found immediately adjacent to sites of active bone resorption and along trabecular surfaces at a distance from the inflammation in an apparent effort to reinforce the remaining bone (i.e., buttressing bone formation). This estrogenic response is clearly found in experimentally produced periodontal bone loss in animals.[7] In humans, it is less obvious, but it has been confirmed by histometric[4,5] and histologic studies.[13]

Autopsy specimens from individuals with untreated disease occasionally show areas in which bone resorption has ceased and new bone is being formed on previously eroded bone margins. This confirms the intermittent character of bone resorption in periodontitis, and it is consistent with the varied rates of progression observed clinically in individuals with untreated periodontal disease.

The periods of remission and exacerbation (or inactivity and activity, respectively) appear to coincide with the quiescence or exacerbation of gingival inflammation as manifested by changes in the extent of bleeding, the amount of exudate, and the composition of bacterial biofilm (see Chapters 17 and 18).

The presence of bone formation in response to inflammation, even in those with active periodontal disease, has an effect on the outcome of treatment. The basic aim of periodontal therapy is the elimination of inflammation to inhibit the stimulus for bone resorption and therefore to allow the inherent constructive tendencies to predominate.

Bone Destruction Caused by Trauma From Occlusion

Another cause of periodontal bone destruction is trauma from occlusion, which can occur in the absence or presence of inflammation (see Chapter 25).

In the absence of inflammation, the changes caused by trauma from occlusion vary from increased compression and tension of the periodontal ligament and increased osteoclasis of alveolar bone to necrosis of the periodontal ligament and bone and the resorption of bone and tooth structure. These changes are reversible in that they can be repaired if the offending forces are removed. However, persistent trauma from occlusion results in funnel-shaped widening of the crestal portion of the periodontal ligament with resorption of the adjacent bone.[33] These changes, which may cause the bony crest to have an angular shape, represent adaptation of the periodontal tissues aimed at "cushioning" increased occlusal forces; however, the modified bone shape may weaken tooth support and cause tooth mobility.

When it is combined with inflammation, trauma from occlusion may aggravate the bone destruction caused by the inflammation[33] and results in bizarre bone patterns.

Bone Destruction Caused by Systemic Disorders

Local and systemic factors regulate the physiologic equilibrium of bone. When a generalized tendency toward bone resorption exists, bone loss initiated by local inflammatory processes may be magnified.

This systemic influence on the response of alveolar bone, as envisioned by Glickman[12] during the early 1950s, considers a systemic regulatory influence in all cases of periodontal disease. In addition to the virulence of biofilm bacteria, the nature of the systemic component rather than its presence or absence influences the severity of the periodontal destruction. This concept of a role played by systemic defense mechanisms has been validated by the studies of

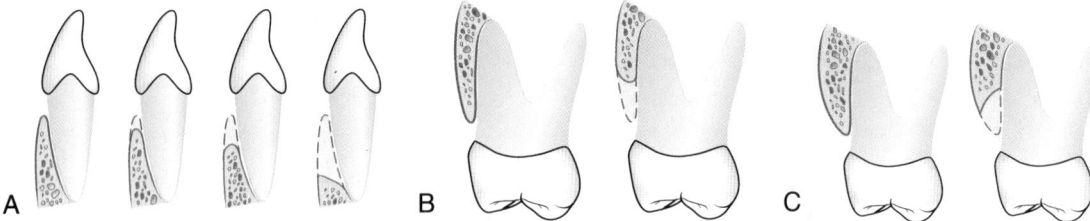

Fig. 24.9 (A) Lower incisor with thin labial bone. Bone loss can become vertical only when it reaches thicker bone in apical areas. (B) Upper molars with thin facial bone, where only horizontal bone loss can occur. (C) Upper molar with a thick facial bone that allows for vertical bone loss.

immune deficiencies and host modulation in severely destructive types of periodontitis.

Interest has increased concerning the possible relationship between periodontal bone loss and osteoporosis.[11] Osteoporosis is a physiologic condition of postmenopausal women that results in the loss of bone mineral content as well as structural bone changes. Periodontitis and osteoporosis share a number of risk factors (e.g., aging, smoking, certain diseases, medications that interfere with healing). Some studies show a relationship between skeletal density and oral bone density; between crestal height and residual ridge resorption; and among osteopenia and periodontitis, tooth mobility, and tooth loss.[19,23,24,55,63]

Periodontal bone loss may also occur with generalized skeletal disturbances (e.g., hyperparathyroidism, leukemia, histiocytosis X) via mechanisms that may be totally unrelated to the more common biofilm-induced, inflammatory periodontal lesion.

LEARNING BOX 24.3

In the absence of inflammation, the localized bone loss caused by trauma from occlusion is reversible (can be repaired) if the offending forces are removed.

Factors Determining Bone Morphology in Periodontal Disease

Normal Variation in Alveolar Bone

Considerable normal variation exists within the morphologic features of alveolar bone, and this affects the osseous contours produced by periodontal disease. The anatomic features that substantially affect the bone-destructive pattern of periodontal disease include the following:

- Thickness, width, and crestal angulation of the interdental septa
- Thickness of the facial and lingual alveolar plates
- Presence of fenestrations and dehiscences
- Alignment of the teeth
- Root and root trunk anatomy
- Root position within the alveolar process
- Proximity with another tooth surface

For example, angular osseous defects cannot form in thin facial or lingual alveolar plates, which have little or no cancellous bone between the outer and inner cortical layers. In such cases, the entire crest of the plate is destroyed, and the height of the bone is reduced in a horizontal fashion (Fig. 24.9).

Exostoses

Exostoses are outgrowths of bone of varied size and shape. Palatal exostoses have been found in 40% of human skulls.[46] They can occur as small nodules, large nodules, sharp ridges, spikelike projections, or any combination of these examples (Fig. 24.10).[42] Exostoses have

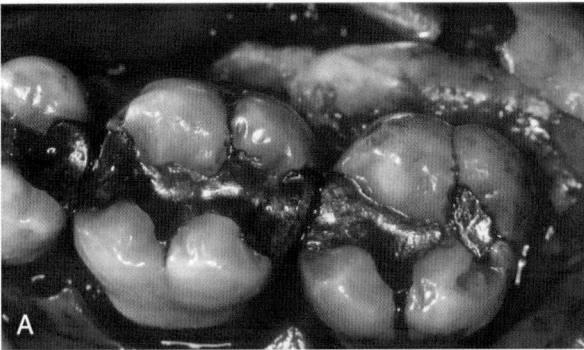

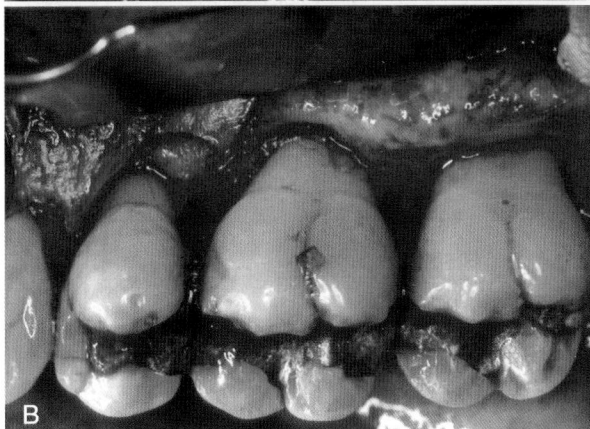

Fig. 24.10 Occlusal (A) and palatal (B) views of exostosis on the first and second molars.

been described in rare cases as developing after the placement of free gingival grafts.[46]

Trauma From Occlusion

Trauma from occlusion may be a factor in determining the dimension and shape of bone deformities. It may cause a thickening of the cervical margin of alveolar bone or a change in bone morphology (e.g., funnel-like crestal bone, buttressing bone) on which inflammatory changes may later be superimposed.

LEARNING BOX 24.4

Angular osseous defects—as often seen in the interdental areas of the posterior dentition—cannot form in thin radicular, facial, or lingual alveolar bone. These areas have little or no cancellous bone between the outer and inner cortical layers. In these anatomic areas, the entire crest of the plate is destroyed, and the height of the bone is reduced in a horizontal fashion.

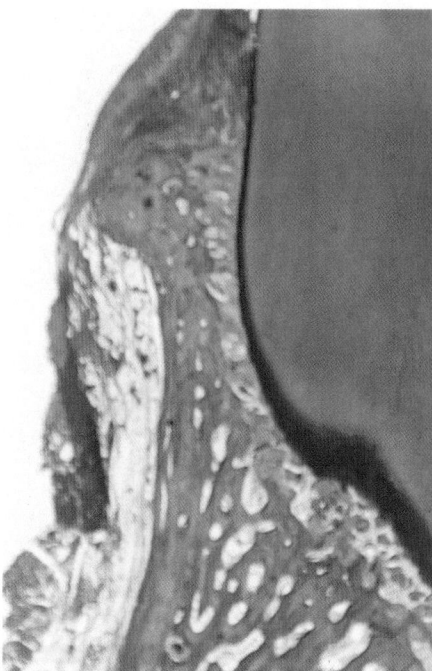

Fig. 24.11 Lipping of facial bone. There is a peripheral buttressing bone formation along the external surface of the facial bony plate and at the crest. Note the deformity in the bone produced by the buttressing bone formation and the bulging of the mucosa.

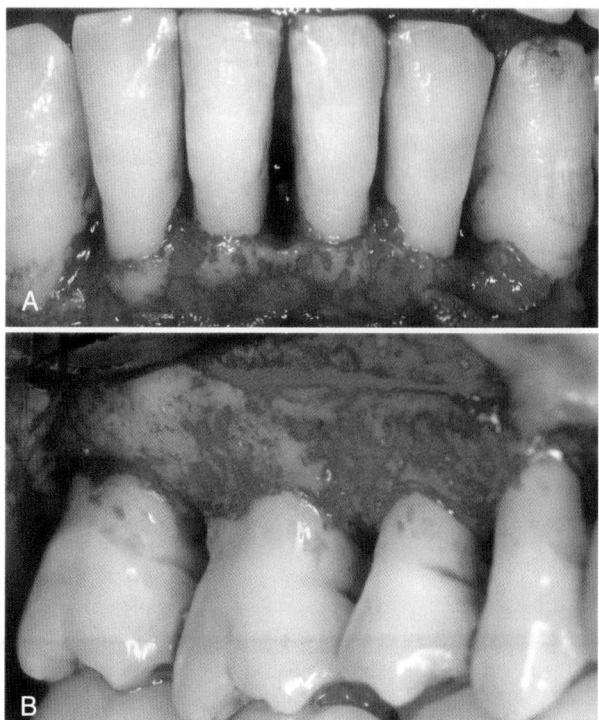

Fig. 24.12 Horizontal bone loss in the anterior (A) and posterior (B) areas. Notice the increased distance between the marginal bone and the cementoenamel junction; yet the overall bone contour is scalloped, indicating that bone resorption has affected the buccal and interproximal surfaces to a similar degree.

Buttressing Bone Formation

Bone formation sometimes occurs in an attempt to buttress bony trabeculae that are weakened by resorption. When this occurs within the jaw, it is termed *central buttressing bone formation*. When it occurs on the external surface, it is referred to as *peripheral buttressing bone formation*.[13] The latter may cause bulging of the bone contour, which sometimes accompanies the production of osseous craters and angular defects (Fig. 24.11).

Food Impaction

Interdental bone defects often occur where the proximal contact is light or absent. Physical pressure and the additional collection of bacteria from food impaction contribute to interproximal resorption and the development of reverse bone architecture. In some cases, the poor proximal relationship may result from a shift in tooth position as a result of extensive bone destruction that precedes food impaction. In patients with this condition, food impaction is a complicating factor rather than the cause of the bone defect.

Aggressive Periodontitis

Aggressive periodontitis usually results in attachment and bone loss around incisors and first molars, particularly in cases where the disease is observed in teenagers. Although such bone loss is usually horizontal in nature around incisors, a vertical or angular pattern of alveolar bone destruction is found around the first molars in aggressive periodontitis. The cause of the localized bone destruction associated with this type of periodontal disease is unknown (see Chapter 28).

Bone Destruction Patterns in Periodontal Disease

Periodontal disease alters the morphologic features of the bone in addition to reducing bone height. An understanding of the nature and pathogenesis of these alterations is essential for effective diagnosis and treatment.[48]

Horizontal Bone Loss

Horizontal bone loss is the most common pattern of bone loss in periodontal disease (Fig. 24.12A–B). The bone is reduced in height, but the bone margin remains approximately perpendicular to the tooth surface. The interdental septa and the facial and lingual plates are affected but not necessarily to an equal degree around the same tooth.

Vertical or Angular Defects

Different types of bone deformities can result from periodontal disease. These usually occur in adults, but they have also been reported in human skulls with deciduous dentitions.[28] Their presence may be suggested on radiographs, but careful probing and surgical exposure of the areas are required to determine their exact conformation and dimensions.

Vertical or angular defects are those that occur in an oblique direction, leaving a hollowed-out trough in the bone alongside the root; the base of the defect is located apical to the surrounding bone (Figs. 24.13A–B and 24.14). In most instances, angular defects have accompanying infrabony periodontal pockets; infrabony pockets, on the other hand, must always have an underlying angular defect.

Goldman and Cohen classified angular defects on the basis of the number of osseous walls.[16] Angular defects may have one, two, or three walls (Figs. 24.15 and 24.16). Continuous defects that involved more than one surface of a tooth, in a shape that is similar to a trough, are called *circumferential defects* (Fig. 24.17). The number of walls in the apical portion of the defect is often greater than that

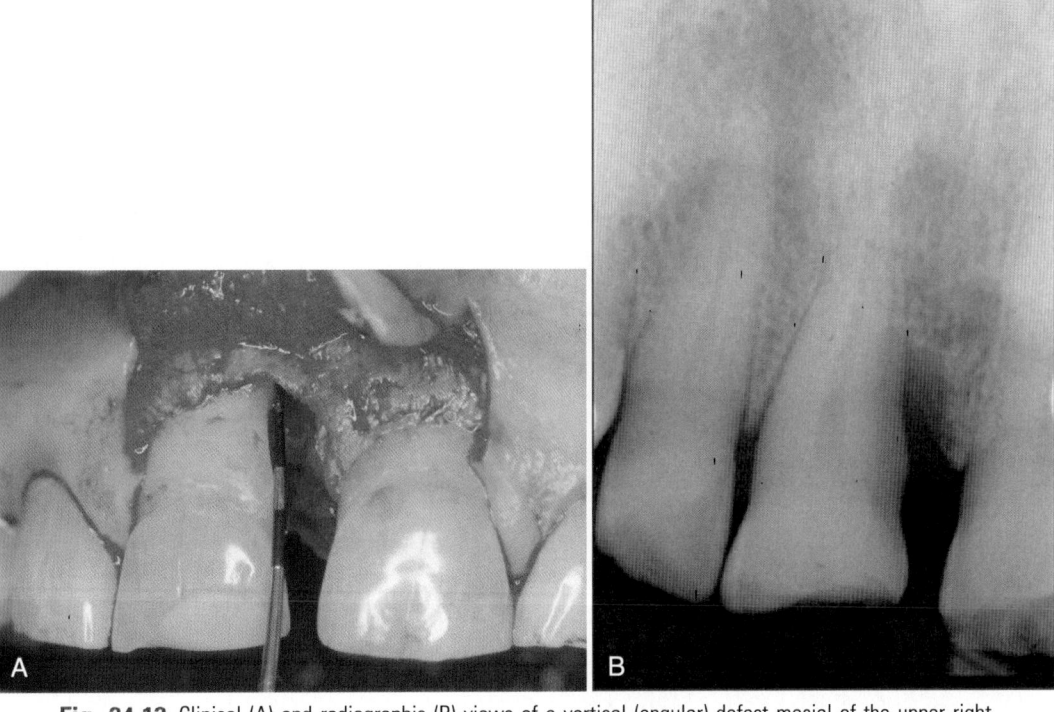

Fig. 24.13 Clinical (A) and radiographic (B) views of a vertical (angular) defect mesial of the upper right central incisor. Note the periodontal probe in a more apical position than the surrounding walls of the bony defect.

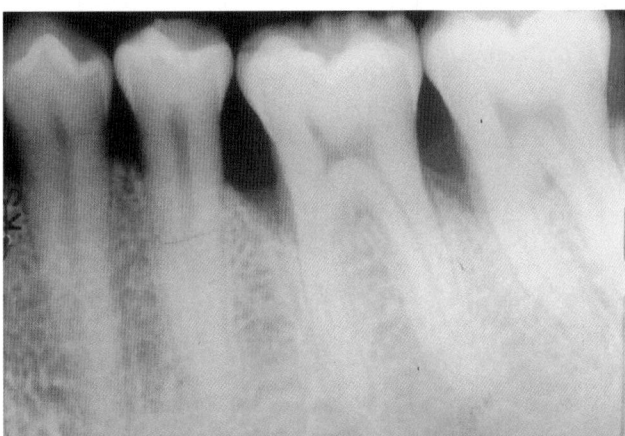

Fig. 24.14 Vertical (angular) defects mesial of the first and second molars.

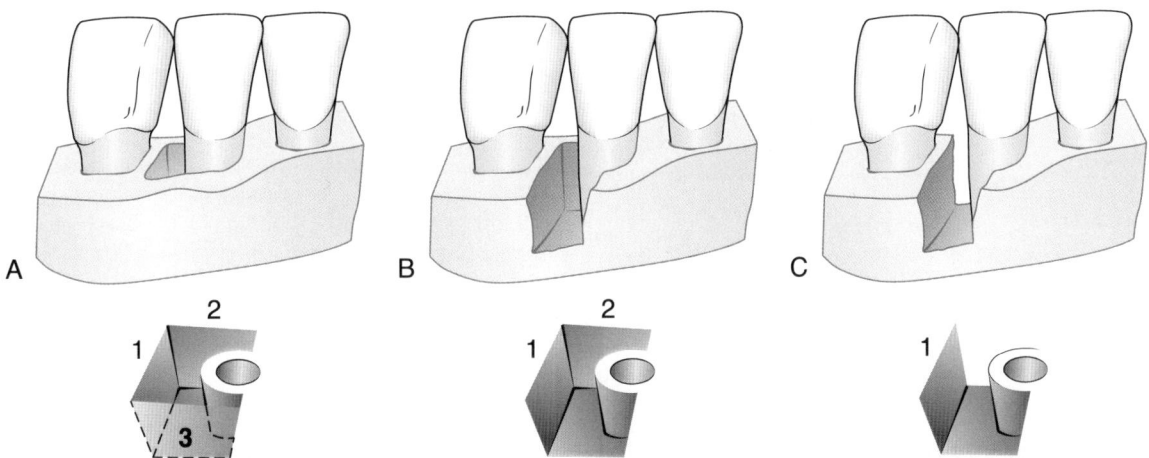

Fig. 24.15 Diagrammatic representation of one-, two-, and three-walled vertical defects on the right lateral incisor. (A) Three bony walls: distal *(1)*, lingual *(2)*, and facial *(3)*. (B) Two-wall defect: distal *(1)* and lingual *(2)*. (C) One-wall defect: distal wall only *(1)*.

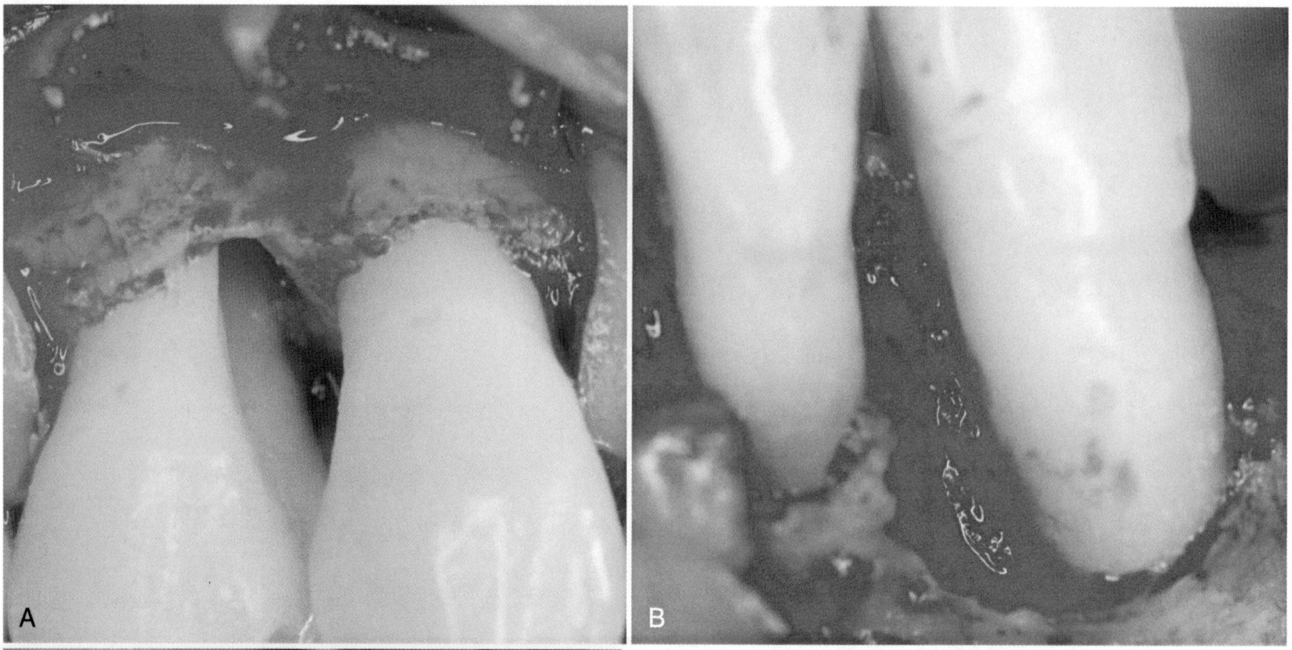

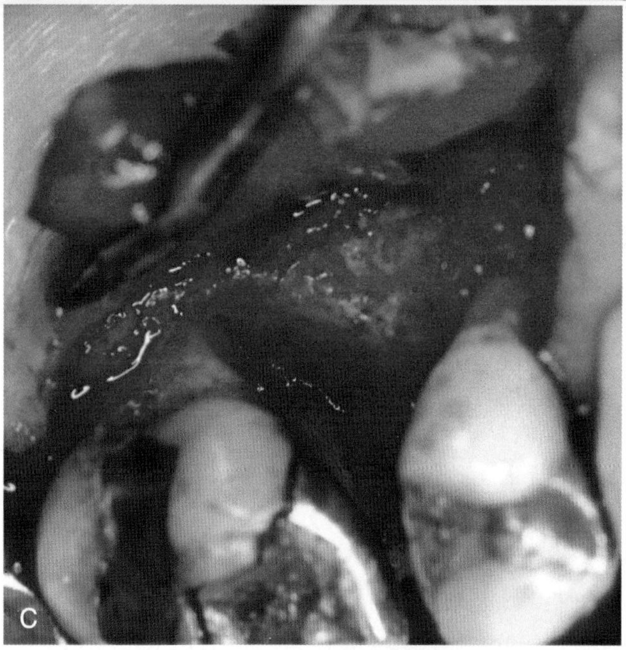

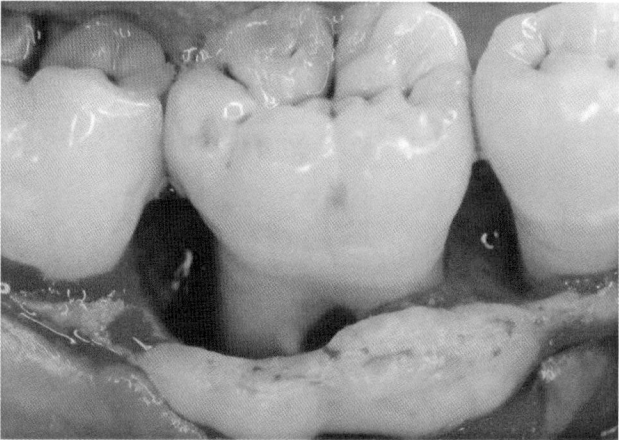

Fig. 24.16 Clinical examples of a three-wall defect mesial of the first bicuspid (A), two-wall defect mesial of the lower canine (buccal wall is missing) (B), and one-wall defect mesial of the first molar (buccal and lingual walls are missing) (C).

Fig. 24.17 Circumferential (troughlike) defect on the buccal and distal aspects of the first molar. Notice that the defect extends into the buccal furcation.

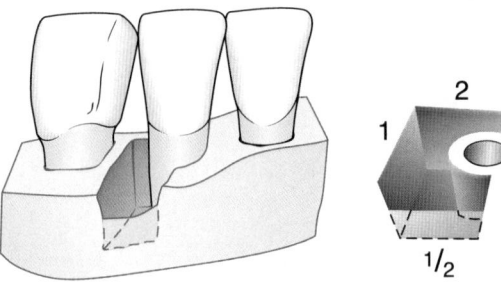

Fig. 24.18 Combined type of osseous defect. Because the facial wall is half the height of the distal *(1)* and lingual *(2)* walls, this is an osseous defect with three walls in its apical half and two walls in its occlusal half.

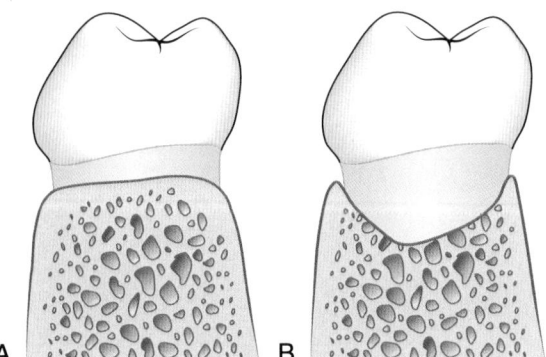

Fig. 24.19 (A) Diagrammatic representation of an osseous crater in a buccolingual section between two lower teeth. *Left,* Normal bone contour. *Right,* Osseous crater. (B) Clinical aspect of an osseous crater between the two bicuspids—notice the buccal and lingual bone walls.

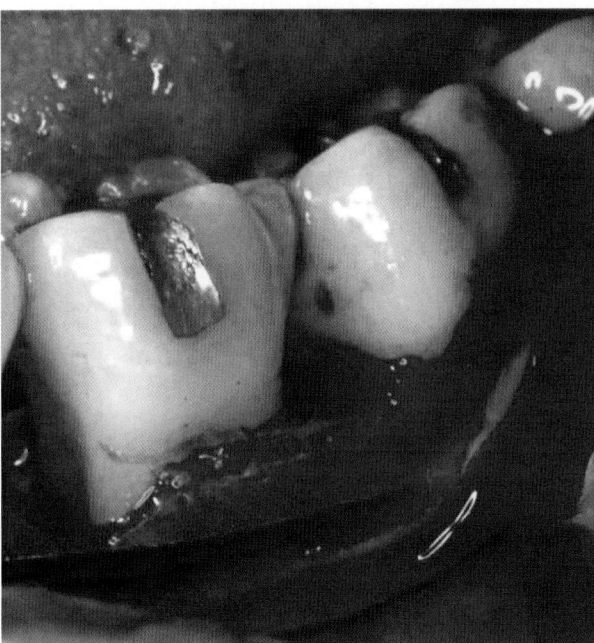

Fig. 24.20 Examples of positive (normal) and negative (reverse) osseous architecture on the lower left posterior segment. The interproximal bone level in the interdental space between the two bicuspids is more coronal than on the buccal aspect of both teeth, whereas the interproximal bone level in the interdental space between the second bicuspid and the first molar shows the bone level to be apical to the buccal bone.

in its occlusal portion, in which case the term *combined osseous defect* is used (Fig. 24.18).

Vertical defects that occur interdentally can generally be seen on the radiograph, although thick, bony plates may sometimes obscure them. Angular defects can also appear on facial and lingual or palatal surfaces, but these defects are more difficult to visualize on radiographs. Surgical exposure is the only sure way to determine the presence and configuration of vertical osseous defects.

Vertical defects increase with age.[44,47,69] Approximately 60% of people with interdental angular defects have only a single defect.[44] Vertical defects detected radiographically have been reported to appear most often on the distal[44] and mesial surfaces.[47] However, three-wall defects are more frequently found on the mesial surfaces of the upper and lower molars.[29]

Osseous Craters

Osseous craters are a specific type of two-wall defect; they present as concavities in the crest of the interdental bone that is confined within the facial and lingual walls (Fig. 24.19). Craters have been found to make up about one-third (35.2%) of all defects and about two-thirds (62%) of all mandibular defects; they occur twice as often in posterior segments as in anterior segments.[37,38]

The heights of the facial and lingual crests of a crater have been found to be identical in 85% of cases, with the remaining 15% being almost equally divided between higher facial crests and higher lingual crests.[53]

The following reasons for the high frequency of interdental craters have been suggested[37,38,53]:

- The interdental area collects biofilm and is difficult to clean.
- The normal flat or even slightly concave buccolingual shape of the interdental septum in the lower molars may favor crater formation.
- Vascular patterns from the gingiva to the center of the crest may provide a pathway for inflammation.

Bulbous Bone Contours

Bulbous bone contours are bony enlargements that are caused by exostoses (see Fig. 24.10), adaptation to function, or buttressing bone formation. They are found more frequently in the maxilla than in the mandible.

Reversed Architecture

Reverse (or negative) alveolar bone architecture is the result of a loss of interdental bone, without a concomitant loss of radicular (buccal or lingual/palatal) bone, thereby reversing the normal (or positive) architecture (Fig. 24.20). Negative architecture is more common in the maxilla of patients with periodontitis.[44]

Ledges

Ledges are plateau-like bone margins that are caused by the resorption of thickened bony plates (Fig. 24.21).

Furcation Involvement

The term *furcation involvement* refers to the invasion of the bifurcation and trifurcation of multirooted teeth by periodontitis. The prevalence

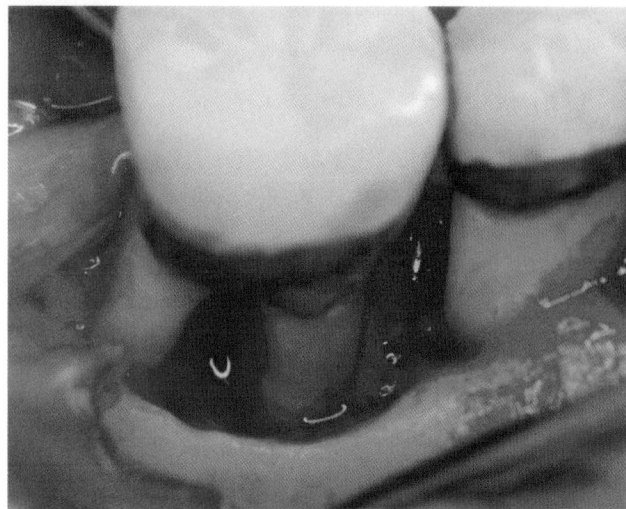

Fig. 24.21 Example of bone ledge on the lingual aspect of the bicuspid and molar.

of furcation-involved molars is not clear.[8,47] Although some reports indicate that the mandibular first molars are the most common sites and that the maxillary premolars are the least common,[30] other studies have found a higher prevalence in the upper molars.[69] The number of furcation involvements increases with age.[30,31]

The denuded furcation may be visible clinically or covered by the wall of the pocket. The extent of the involvement is determined by exploration with a periodontal or Nabers probe (Fig. 24.22A–B).

Furcation involvements have been classified as grades I through IV according to the amount of tissue destruction. Grade I involves incipient bone loss; grade II involves partial bone loss (cul-de-sac); and grade III involves total bone loss with a through-and-through opening of the furcation, but the opening of the furcation is not visible due to the gingiva, which covers the orifice. Grade IV is similar to grade III but includes gingival recession that exposes the furcation to view. (See Chapter 64 for further discussion on furcation classification.)

Microscopically, furcation involvement presents no unique pathologic features. It is simply the apical extension of the periodontal pocket along a multirooted tooth. During its early stages, widening of the periodontal space occurs with cellular and fluid inflammatory exudation, and this is followed by epithelial proliferation into the furcation area from an adjoining periodontal pocket. Extension of the inflammation into the bone leads to resorption and a reduction in bone height. The bone-destructive pattern may produce horizontal loss, but angular osseous defects associated with intrabony pockets may also exist (Fig. 24.23). Biofilm, calculus, and bacterial debris occupy the denuded furcation space.

The destructive pattern of a furcation involvement varies in different cases and with the degree of involvement. Bone loss around each individual root may be horizontal or angular, and frequently a crater develops in the interradicular area (Fig. 24.24A–B). Probing to determine the presence of these destructive patterns must be done horizontally and vertically around each involved root and in the crater area to establish the depth of the vertical component.

Furcation involvement is a stage of progressive periodontal disease, and it has its same etiology. The difficulty and sometimes the impossibility[2,3] of controlling biofilm in furcations are responsible for the presence of extensive lesions in this area.[66]

The role of trauma from occlusion in the etiology of furcation lesions is controversial. Some assign a key role to trauma, thinking

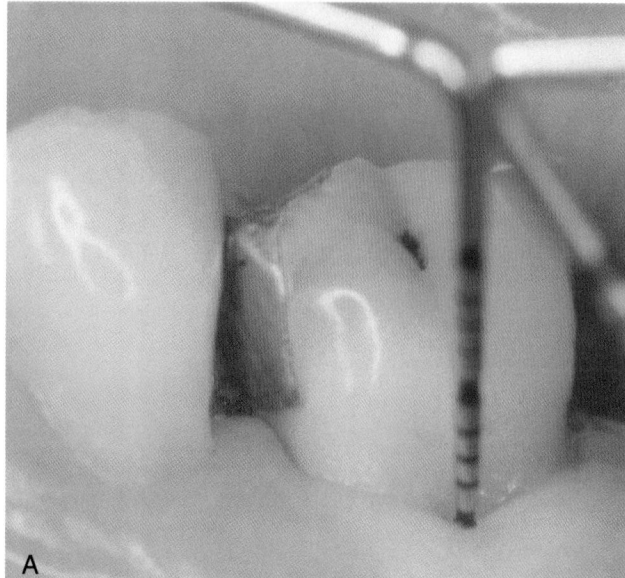

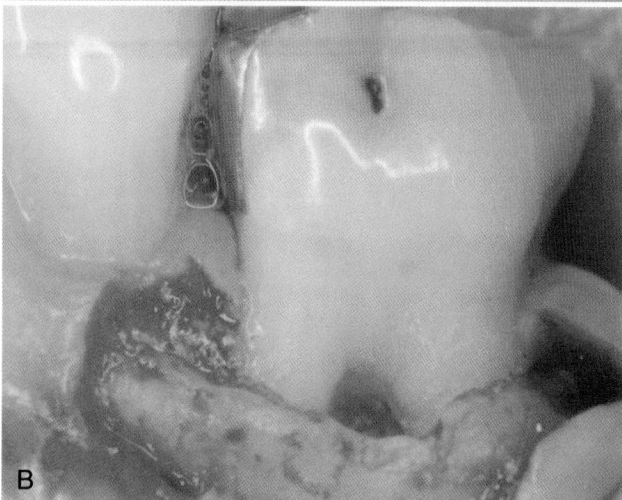

Fig. 24.22 Grade II furcation on the buccal aspect of the lower first molar. (A) Periodontal probe in place showing a 5-mm pocket. (B) After the flap was elevated, it revealed horizontal bone loss.

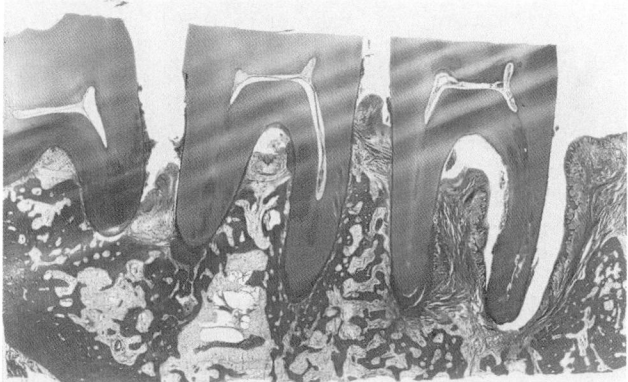

Fig. 24.23 Different degrees of furcation involvement in a human autopsy specimen. Furcation involvement is found in all three molars, with an advanced lesion in the second molar and an extremely severe lesion in the first molar that is combined with the exposure of the entire mesial root.

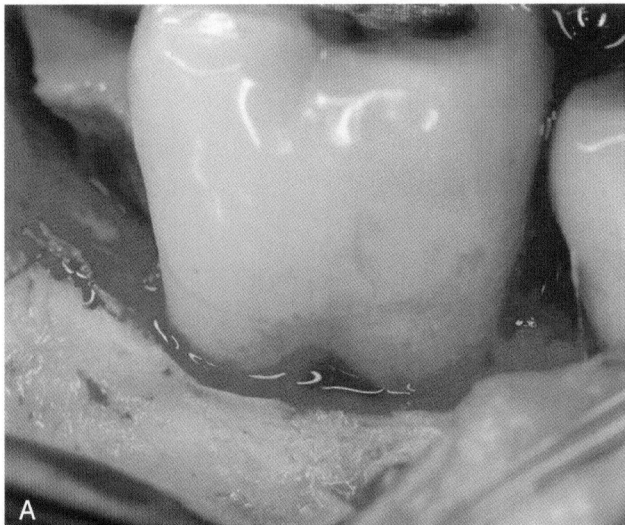

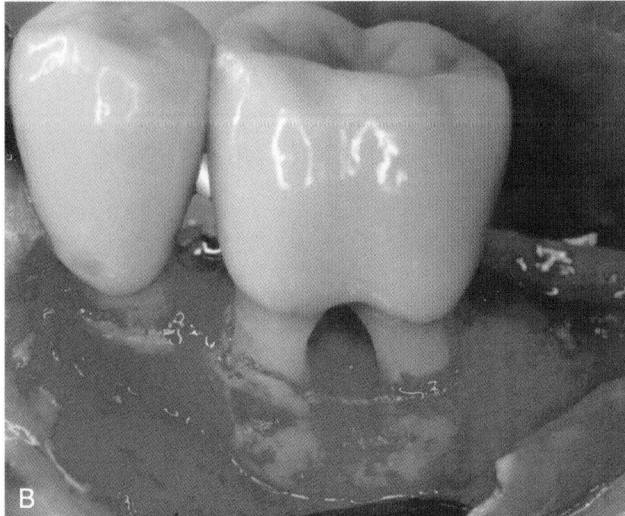

Fig. 24.24 Clinical examples of grade I furcation involvement (A) and grade II furcation involvement (B).

that furcation areas are most sensitive to injury from excessive occlusal forces.[15] Others deny the initiating effect of trauma and consider that inflammation and edema caused by biofilm in the furcation area tend to extrude the tooth, which then becomes traumatized and sensitive.[60,66]

Other factors that may play a role are the presence of enamel projections into the furcation,[39] which occurs in about 13% of multirooted teeth, and the proximity of the furcation to the cementoenamel junction, which occurs in about 75% of cases of furcation involvement.[31]

The presence of accessory pulpal canals in the furcation area may extend pulpal inflammation to the furcation.[20] This possibility should be carefully explored, particularly when mesial and distal bone retains its normal height. Accessory canals that connect the pulp chamber floor to the furcation have been found in 36% of maxillary first molars, 12% of maxillary second molars, 32% of mandibular first molars, and 24% of mandibular second molars.[62]

The diagnosis of furcation involvement is made by clinical examination and careful probing with a specially designed probe (see Chapters 32 and 64). Radiographic examination of the area is helpful, but lesions can be obscured by the angulation of the beam and the radiopacity of neighboring structures (see Chapter 33).

For more detailed clinical considerations involved with the diagnosis and treatment of furcation involvement, see Chapters 32, 33, and 64.

Conclusion

The understanding of the anatomy, histology, and pattern of bone loss for the diagnosis of and prognosis for periodontal disease is of major importance in determining the therapy that must be rendered. In the final analysis, it is the loss of bone that will determine the retention, maintenance, or loss of the dentition in periodontal disease.

 Case Scenarios are found on the companion website www.expertconsult.com.

References

 References for this chapter are found on the companion website www.expertconsult.com.

CHAPTER 25

Periodontal Response to External Forces

Flavia Q. Pirih | Paulo M. Camargo | Henry H. Takei | Fermin A. Carranza

CHAPTER OUTLINE

Adaptive Capacity of the
Periodontium to Occlusal Forces
Trauma From Occlusion
Stages of Tissue Response to
Increased Occlusal Forces

Effects of Insufficient Occlusal
Force
Reversibility of Traumatic Lesions
Effects of Excessive Occlusal Forces
on Dental Pulp

Relationship Between
Plaque-Induced Periodontal
Diseases and Trauma From
Occlusion
Pathologic Tooth Migration

Adaptive Capacity of the Periodontium to Occlusal Forces

The periodontal ligament has a cushioning effect on forces applied to teeth as means to accommodate forces exerted on the crown. Due to the elastic nature of the periodontal ligament, all teeth with normal bone support present with physiologic mobility in all directions. Physiologic tooth mobility varies among individuals and within the dentition of the same individual. In the absence of excessive occlusal forces or the absence of reduced bone support induced by inflammatory periodontal disease, tooth mobility remains unchanged due to the fact that physiologic forces are not able to induce changes to the periodontal tissues.[3]

When there is an increase in occlusal forces, changes occur in the periodontium in order to accommodate for such forces. Changes in the periodontium depend on the magnitude, direction, duration, and frequency of increased occlusal forces.

When the *magnitude* of occlusal forces is increased, the periodontium responds with a widening of the periodontal ligament space, an increase in the number and width of periodontal ligament fibers, and an increase in the density of alveolar bone.

Changing the *direction* of occlusal forces causes a reorientation of the stresses and strains within the periodontium (Fig. 25.1).[23] The principal fibers of the periodontal ligament are arranged so that they best accommodate occlusal forces along the long axis of the tooth. *Lateral* (horizontal) and *torque* (rotational) forces are more likely to injure the periodontium.

The response of alveolar bone is also affected by the *duration* and *frequency* of occlusal forces. Constant pressure on the bone is more injurious than intermittent forces. The more frequent the application of an intermittent force, the more injurious the force is to the periodontium.

Trauma From Occlusion

Trauma from occlusion is defined as microscopic alterations of periodontal structures in the area of the periodontal ligament that become manifest clinically in the elevation of tooth mobility. As mentioned earlier, an inherent "margin of safety" that is common to all tissues permits some variation in occlusion without adversely affecting the periodontium. However, when occlusal forces exceed the adaptive capacity of the tissues, tissue injury results.[43,44] The resultant injury is termed *trauma from occlusion,* which is also known as *occlusal trauma.*

Thus trauma from occlusion refers to the *tissue injury* rather than the *occlusal force.* An occlusion that produces such an injury is called a *traumatic occlusion.*[2] Excessive occlusal forces may also disrupt the function of the masticatory musculature and cause painful spasms, injure the temporomandibular joints, or produce excessive tooth wear. However, the term *trauma from occlusion* is generally used in connection with injury in the periodontium.

Classification of Trauma From Occlusion

Trauma from occlusion can be classified according to the injurious occlusal force(s) mode of onset (acute and chronic) or according to the capacity of the periodontium to resist to occlusal forces (primary and secondary).

Acute and Chronic Trauma From Occlusion

Acute trauma from occlusion refers to periodontal changes associated with an abrupt occlusal impact such as that produced by biting on a hard object (e.g., an olive pit). In addition, restorations or prosthetic appliances that interfere with or alter the direction of occlusal forces on the teeth may also induce acute trauma. Acute trauma results in tooth pain, sensitivity to percussion, and increased tooth mobility. If the force is dissipated by a shift in the position of the tooth or by

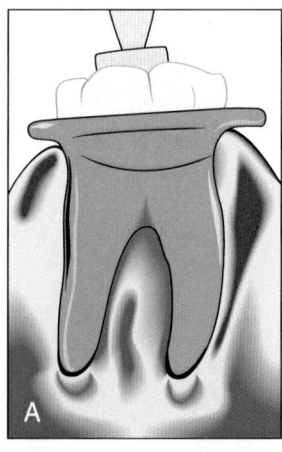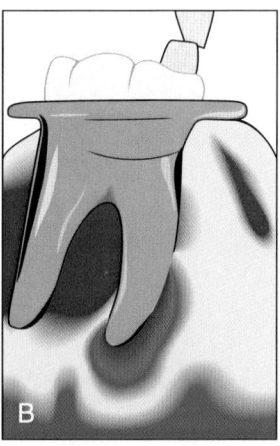

Fig. 25.1 Stress patterns around the roots changed by shifting the direction of occlusal forces (experimental model using photoelastic analysis). (A) Buccal view of an Ivorine molar subjected to an axial force. The shaded fringes indicate that the internal stresses are at the root apices. (B) Buccal view of an Ivorine molar subjected to a mesial tilting force. The shaded fringes indicate that the internal stresses are along the mesial surface and at the apex of the mesial root.

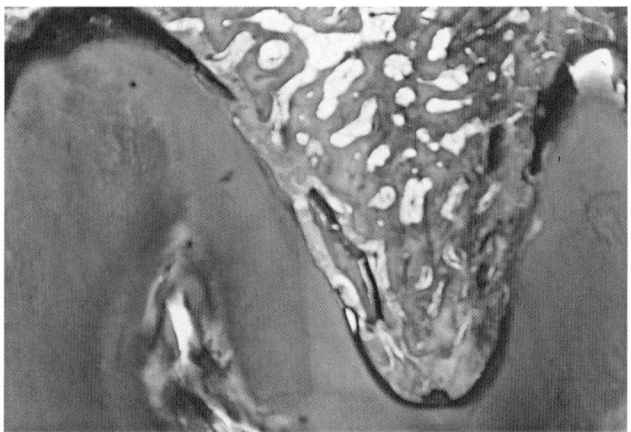

Fig. 25.2 Cemental tear, presumably caused by acute trauma from occlusion in a human autopsy specimen. Note the repair process depositing bone on the displaced, torn cementum and recreating a periodontal ligament.

the wearing away or correction of the restoration, then the injury heals, and the symptoms subside. Otherwise, periodontal injury may worsen and develop into necrosis accompanied by periodontal abscess formation, or it may persist as a symptom-free chronic condition. Acute trauma can also produce cementum tears (Fig. 25.2).

LEARNING BOX 25.3

Acute trauma from occlusion refers to periodontal changes associated with an abrupt occlusal impact such as that produced by biting on a hard object (e.g., an olive pit). In addition, restorations or prosthetic appliances that interfere with or alter the direction of occlusal forces on the teeth may also induce acute trauma. Acute trauma results in tooth pain, sensitivity to percussion, and increased tooth mobility.

Chronic trauma from occlusion refers to periodontal changes associated with gradual changes in occlusion produced by tooth wear, drifting movement, and extrusion of the teeth in combination with parafunctional habits (e.g., bruxism, clenching) rather than as a sequela of acute periodontal trauma. Chronic trauma from occlusion is more common than the acute form and of greater clinical

significance. The features of chronic trauma from occlusion and their significance are discussed in the following sections.

The criterion that determines if an occlusion is traumatic is whether it produces periodontal injury; the criterion is *not* based on how the teeth occlude. Any occlusion that produces periodontal injury is traumatic. Malocclusion is not necessary to produce trauma; periodontal injury may occur when the occlusion appears normal. The dentition may be anatomically and aesthetically acceptable but functionally injurious. Similarly, not all malocclusions are necessarily injurious to the periodontium. Traumatic occlusal relationships are referred to by such terms as *occlusal disharmony, functional imbalance,* and *occlusal dystrophy.* These terms refer to the effect of the occlusion on the periodontium rather than to the position of the teeth. Because trauma from occlusion refers to the tissue injury rather than the occlusion, an increased occlusal force is not traumatic if the periodontium can accommodate it.

LEARNING BOX 25.4

Chronic trauma from occlusion refers to periodontal changes associated with gradual changes in occlusion produced by tooth wear, drifting movement, and extrusion of the teeth in combination with parafunctional habits (e.g., bruxism, clenching) rather than as a sequela of acute periodontal trauma. Chronic trauma from occlusion is more common than the acute form and of greater clinical significance.

Primary and Secondary Trauma From Occlusion

As mentioned previously, trauma from occlusion can also be classified according to the capacity of the periodontium to resist occlusal forces into primary and secondary trauma from occlusion. In other words, trauma from occlusion may be caused by alterations in occlusal forces, a reduced capacity of the periodontium to withstand occlusal forces, or both. When trauma from occlusion is the result of alterations in occlusal forces, it is called *primary trauma from occlusion.* When it results from the reduced ability of the tissues to resist the occlusal forces, it is known as *secondary trauma from occlusion.*

Primary trauma from occlusion occurs if trauma from occlusion is considered the primary etiologic factor in periodontal destruction and if the only local alteration to which a tooth is subjected is a result of occlusion. Examples include periodontal injury produced around teeth with a previously healthy periodontium after the following: (1) the insertion of a "high filling"; (2) the insertion of a prosthetic replacement that creates excessive forces on abutment and antagonistic teeth; (3) the drifting movement or extrusion of the teeth into spaces created by unreplaced missing teeth; or (4) the orthodontic movement of teeth into functionally unacceptable positions. Most studies of the effect of trauma from occlusion involving experimental animals have examined the primary type of trauma. Changes produced by primary trauma do not alter the level of connective tissue attachment and do not initiate pocket formation. This is probably because the supracrestal gingival fibers are not affected and therefore prevent the apical migration of the junctional epithelium.[48]

LEARNING BOX 25.5

Primary trauma from occlusion occurs if trauma from occlusion is considered the primary etiologic factor in periodontal destruction and if the only local alteration to which a tooth is subjected is a result of occlusion.

Secondary trauma from occlusion occurs when the adaptive capacity of the tissues to withstand occlusal forces is impaired by

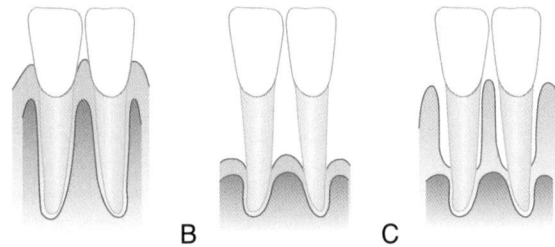

Fig. 25.3 Traumatic forces can occur on (A) normal periodontium with normal height of bone, (B) normal periodontium with reduced height of bone, or (C) marginal periodontitis with reduced height of bone.

bone loss that results from marginal inflammation. This reduces the periodontal attachment area and alters the leverage on the remaining tissues. The periodontium becomes more vulnerable to injury, and previously well-tolerated occlusal forces become traumatic.

Fig. 25.3 depicts three situations on which excessive occlusal forces can be superimposed:
1. Normal periodontium with normal height of bone
2. Normal periodontium with reduced height of bone
3. Marginal periodontitis with reduced height of bone

The first case is an example of primary trauma from occlusion, whereas the last two represent secondary trauma from occlusion. The effects of trauma from occlusion in these different situations are analyzed in the following discussion.

It has been found in experimental animals that systemic disorders can reduce tissue resistance and that previously tolerable forces may become excessive.[21,51,61] This could theoretically represent another mechanism by which tissue resistance to increased forces is lowered, thereby resulting in secondary trauma from occlusion.

Stages of Tissue Response to Increased Occlusal Forces

Tissue response occurs in three stages[4,8]: injury, repair, and adaptive remodeling of the periodontium.

Stage I: Injury

Tissue injury is produced by excessive occlusal forces. The body then attempts to repair the injury and restore the periodontium. This can occur if the forces are diminished or if the tooth drifts away from them. If the offending force is chronic, however, the periodontium is remodeled to cushion its impact. The ligament is widened at the expense of the bone, which results in angular bone defects without periodontal pockets, and the tooth becomes loose.

Under the forces of occlusion, a tooth rotates around a fulcrum or axis of rotation, which in single-rooted teeth is located in the junction between the middle third and the apical third of the clinical root and in multirooted teeth in the middle of the interradicular bone (Fig. 25.4). This creates areas of pressure and tension on opposite sides of the fulcrum. Different lesions are produced by different degrees of pressure and tension. If jiggling forces are exerted, these different lesions may coexist in the same area.

Slightly excessive pressure stimulates resorption of the alveolar bone, with a resultant widening of the periodontal ligament space. *Slightly excessive tension* causes elongation of the periodontal ligament fibers and the apposition of alveolar bone. In areas of increased pressure, the blood vessels are numerous and reduced in size; in areas of increased tension, they are enlarged.[67]

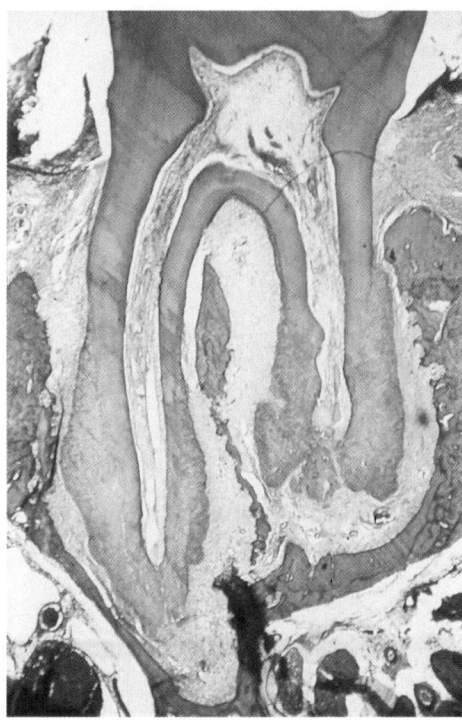

Fig. 25.4 Areas of tension and pressure in opposite sites of the periodontal ligament caused by experimentally induced orthodontic movement in a rat molar.

Greater pressure produces a gradation of changes in the periodontal ligament, starting with compression of the fibers, which produces areas of hyalinization.[54-56] Subsequent injury to the fibroblasts and other connective tissue cells leads to necrosis of areas of the ligament.[52,56] Vascular changes are also produced: within 30 minutes, impairment and stasis of blood flow occur; at 2 to 3 hours, blood vessels appear to be packed with erythrocytes, which start to fragment; and between 1 and 7 days, disintegration of the blood vessel walls and release of the contents into the surrounding tissue occur.[53,63] In addition, increased resorption of alveolar bone and resorption of the tooth surface occur.[29,34]

Severe tension causes widening of the periodontal ligament, thrombosis, hemorrhage, tearing of the periodontal ligament, and resorption of alveolar bone.

Pressure severe enough to force the root against bone causes necrosis of the periodontal ligament and bone. The bone is resorbed from viable periodontal ligament adjacent to necrotic areas and from marrow spaces; this process is called *undermining resorption.*[25,43]

The areas of the periodontium that are most susceptible to injury from excessive occlusal forces are the furcations.[22]

Injury to the periodontium produces a temporary depression in mitotic activity, in the rate of proliferation and differentiation of fibroblasts,[62] in collagen formation, and in bone formation.[29,58,60,62] These return to normal levels after the dissipation of the forces.

Stage II: Repair

Repair occurs constantly in the normal periodontium, and trauma from occlusion stimulates increased reparative activity. The damaged tissues are removed, and new connective tissue cells and fibers, bone, and cementum are formed in an attempt to restore the injured periodontium (Fig. 25.5). Forces remain traumatic only as long as the damage produced exceeds the reparative capacity of the tissues.

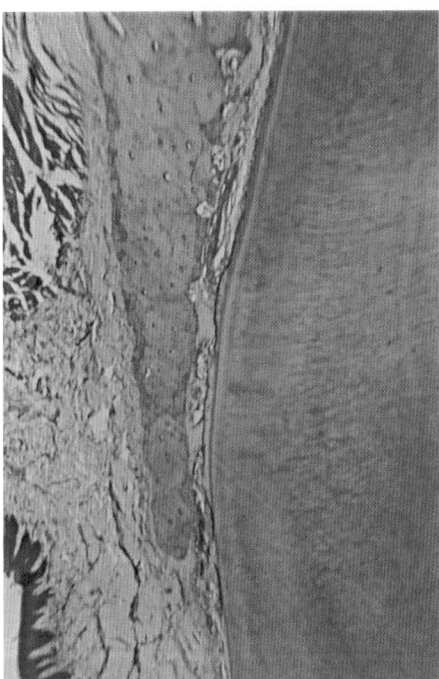

Fig. 25.5 Experimental occlusal trauma in rats. Note the area of necrosis of the marginal periodontal ligament and resorption and remodeling in the more apical periodontal sites.

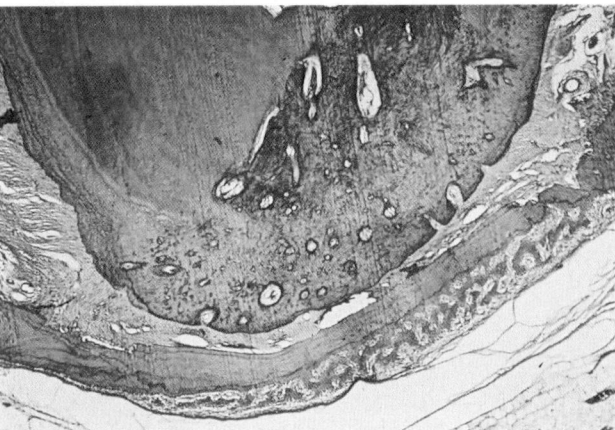

Fig. 25.6 Apical area of a premolar subjected to experimental occlusal trauma in a dog causing intrusion of the tooth and areas of necrosis in the periodontal ligament. Note the active bone formation on the outer aspect of the bone and the resorptive activity in the periphery of the necrotic site.

decrease in bone formation, whereas the repair phase demonstrates decreased resorption and increased bone formation. After adaptive remodeling of the periodontium, resorption and formation return to normal.

When bone is resorbed by excessive occlusal forces, the body attempts to reinforce the thinned bony trabeculae with new bone (Fig. 25.6). This attempt to compensate for lost bone is called *buttressing bone formation*, and it is an important feature of the reparative process associated with trauma from occlusion.[16] It also occurs when bone is destroyed by inflammation or osteolytic tumors.

Buttressing bone formation occurs within the jaw (central buttressing) and on the bone surface (peripheral buttressing). During *central buttressing*, the endosteal cells deposit new bone, which restores the bony trabeculae and reduces the size of the marrow spaces. *Peripheral buttressing* occurs on the facial and lingual surfaces of the alveolar plate. Depending on its severity, peripheral buttressing may produce a shelflike thickening of the alveolar margin, which is referred to as *lipping* (Fig. 25.7), or a pronounced bulge in the contour of the facial and lingual bone.[8,16]

Cartilage-like material sometimes develops in the periodontal ligament space as an aftermath of the trauma.[13] The formation of crystals from erythrocytes has also been demonstrated.[57]

Stage III: Adaptive Remodeling of the Periodontium

If the repair process cannot keep pace with the destruction caused by the occlusion, the periodontium is remodeled in an effort to create a structural relationship in which the forces are no longer injurious to the tissues.[18] *This results in a widened periodontal ligament, which is funnel shaped at the crest, and angular defects in the bone, with no pocket formation. The involved teeth become loose.*[67] Increased vascularization has also been reported.[9]

The three stages in the evolution of traumatic lesions have been differentiated histometrically by the relative amounts of periodontal bone surface undergoing resorption or formation[5,8] (Fig. 25.8). The injury phase shows an increase in areas of resorption and a

Effects of Insufficient Occlusal Force

Insufficient occlusal force may also be injurious to the supporting periodontal tissues.[6,36] Insufficient stimulation causes thinning of the periodontal ligament, atrophy of the fibers, osteoporosis of the alveolar bone, and a reduction in bone height. Hypofunction can result from an open-bite relationship, an absence of functional antagonists, or unilateral chewing habits that neglect one side of the mouth.

Reversibility of Traumatic Lesions

Trauma from occlusion is reversible. When trauma is artificially induced in experimental animals, the teeth move away or intrude into the jaw. When the impact of the artificially created force is relieved, the tissues undergo repair. Although trauma from occlusion is reversible under such conditions, it does not always correct itself, and therefore it is not always temporary or of limited clinical significance. The injurious force must be relieved for repair to occur.[22,49] If conditions in humans do not permit the teeth to escape from or adapt to excessive occlusal force, periodontal damage persists and worsens.

The presence of inflammation in the periodontium as a result of plaque accumulation may impair the reversibility of traumatic lesions.[30,49]

Effects of Excessive Occlusal Forces on Dental Pulp

The effects of excessive occlusal forces on the dental pulp have not been established. Some clinicians report the disappearance of pulpal symptoms after the correction of excessive occlusal forces. Pulpal reactions have been noted in animals subjected to increased occlusal forces,[7,35] but these did not occur when the forces were minimal and occurred over short periods.[35]

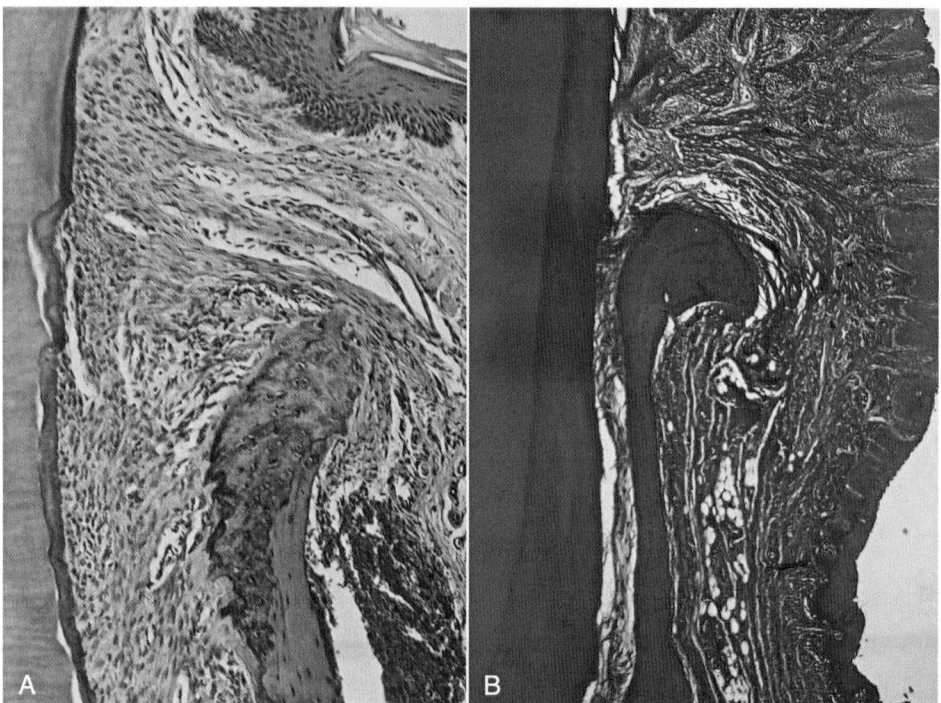

Fig. 25.7 (A) Widening of the periodontal ligament space in the cervical area and a change in the shape of the marginal alveolar bone as a result of chronic prolonged trauma from occlusion in rats. (B) Comparable changes in the shape of the marginal bone found in a human autopsy case.

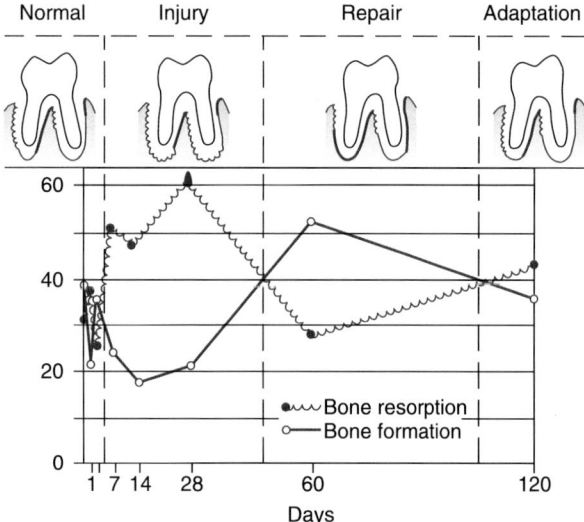

Fig. 25.8 Evolution of traumatic lesions as depicted experimentally in rats by variations in relative amounts of areas of bone formation and bone resorption in periodontal bone surfaces. The horizontal axis shows the number of days after the initiation of traumatic interference. The vertical axis shows the percentage of bone surface undergoing resorption or formation. The stages in the evolution of the lesions are represented in the top drawings, which show the average amount of bone activity for each group.[4]

LEARNING BOX 25.6

Secondary trauma from occlusion occurs when the adaptive capacity of the tissues to withstand occlusal forces is impaired by bone loss that results from marginal inflammation. This reduces the periodontal attachment area and alters the leverage on the remaining tissues. The periodontium becomes more vulnerable to injury, and previously well-tolerated occlusal forces become traumatic.

Relationship Between Plaque-Induced Periodontal Diseases and Trauma From Occlusion

The clinical impressions of early investigators and clinicians assigned an important role to trauma from occlusion in the etiology of periodontal lesions. Since then, numerous studies have been performed that have attempted to determine the mechanisms by which trauma from occlusion may affect periodontal disease.

Initial studies involved the placement of high crowns or restorations on the teeth of dogs or monkeys, thereby resulting in a continuous or intermittent force in one direction.[2,20] These investigations provided an orthodontic type of force and gave clear descriptions of changes that were occurring in pressure zones and tension zones. These procedures usually resulted in tooth displacement and consolidation in a new, nontraumatized position.

Trauma from occlusion in humans, however, is the result of forces that act alternatively in opposing directions. These were analyzed in experimental animals with "jiggling forces," which were usually produced by a high crown in combination with an orthodontic appliance that would bring the traumatized tooth back to its original position when the force was dissipated by separating the teeth. With another method, the teeth were separated by wooden or elastic material wedged interproximally to displace a tooth toward the opposite proximal side. After 48 hours, the wedge was removed, and the procedure was repeated on the opposite side.

These studies resulted in a combination of changes produced by pressure and tension on both sides of the tooth, with an increase in the width of the ligament and increased tooth mobility. None of these methods caused gingival inflammation or pocket formation, and the results essentially represented different degrees of functional adaptation to increased forces.[48,67] To mimic the problem in humans more closely, studies were then conducted on the effect produced by jiggling trauma and simultaneous plaque-induced gingival inflammation.

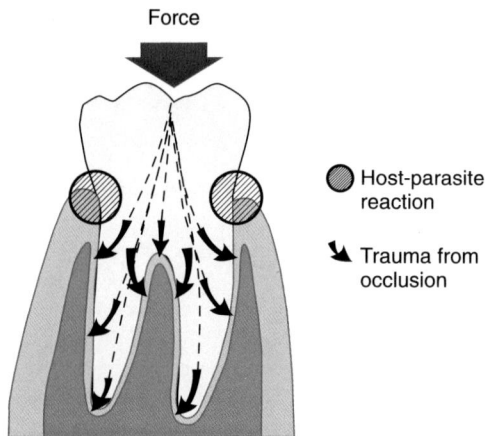

Force

Host-parasite reaction

Trauma from occlusion

Fig. 25.9 The reaction between dental plaque and the host takes place in the gingival sulcus region. Trauma from occlusion appears in the tissues that are supporting the tooth.

The accumulation of bacterial plaque that initiates gingivitis and results in periodontal pocket formation affects the marginal gingiva, but trauma from occlusion occurs in the supporting tissues and does not affect the gingiva (Fig. 25.9). The marginal gingiva is unaffected by trauma from occlusion because its blood supply is not affected, even when the vessels of the periodontal ligament are obliterated by excessive occlusal forces.[24] It has been repeatedly proved that trauma from occlusion does not cause pockets or gingivitis[2,20,50,65,66,68] and that it also does not increase gingival fluid flow.[27,33,36,41,42,50] Furthermore, experimental trauma in dogs does not influence the bacterial repopulation of pockets after scaling and root planing.[31] However, mobile teeth in humans harbor significantly higher proportions of *Campylobacter rectus* and *Peptostreptococcus micros* than do nonmobile teeth.[26]

As long as inflammation is confined to the gingiva, the inflammatory process is not affected by occlusal forces.[32] When inflammation extends from the gingiva into the supporting periodontal tissues (i.e., when gingivitis becomes periodontitis), plaque-induced inflammation enters the zone that is influenced by occlusion, which Glickman has called the *zone of co-destruction*.[14,15,17]

Two groups have studied this topic experimentally, with conflicting results, probably because of the different methods used. The Eastman Dental Center group in Rochester, New York, used squirrel monkeys, produced trauma by repetitive interdental wedging, and added mild to moderate gingival inflammation; experimental times were up to 10 weeks. They reported that the presence of trauma did not increase the loss of attachment induced by periodontitis.[42,45-47] The University of Gothenburg group in Sweden used beagle dogs, produced trauma by placing cap splints and orthodontic appliances, and induced severe gingival inflammation; experimental times were up to 1 year. This group found that occlusal stresses increase the periodontal destruction induced by periodontitis.[11,12,39]

When trauma from occlusion is eliminated, a substantial reversal of bone loss occurs, except in the presence of periodontitis. This indicates that inflammation inhibits the potential for bone regeneration.[30,38,48,49] Thus it is important to eliminate the marginal inflammatory component in cases of trauma from occlusion, because the presence of inflammation affects bone regeneration after the removal of the traumatizing contacts.[30] It has also been shown in experimental animals that trauma from occlusion does not induce progressive destruction of the periodontal tissues in regions that are kept healthy after the elimination of preexisting periodontitis.[11]

Trauma from occlusion also tends to change the shape of the alveolar crest. The change in shape consists of a widening of the marginal periodontal ligament space, a narrowing of the interproximal alveolar bone, and a shelflike thickening of the alveolar margin.[9,39,42] Therefore although trauma from occlusion does not alter the inflammatory process, it changes the architecture of the area around the inflamed site.[17,39] Thus in the absence of inflammation, the response to trauma from occlusion is limited to adaptation to the increased forces. In the presence of inflammation, however, the changes in the shape of the alveolar crest may be conducive to angular bone loss, and existing pockets may become intrabony.

Other theories that have been proposed to explain the interaction of trauma and inflammation include the following:

- Trauma from occlusion may alter the pathway of the extension of gingival inflammation to the underlying tissues. This may be favored by the reduced collagen density and the increased number of leukocytes, osteoclasts, and blood vessels in the coronal portion of increasingly mobile teeth.[3] Inflammation may then proceed to the periodontal ligament rather than to the bone. Resulting bone loss would be angular, and pockets could become intrabony.[1,17,19,40]
- Trauma-induced areas of root resorption uncovered by apical migration of the inflamed gingival attachment may offer a favorable environment for the formation and attachment of plaque and calculus and therefore may be responsible for the development of deeper lesions.[59]
- Supragingival plaque can become subgingival if the tooth is tilted orthodontically or if it migrates into an edentulous area, which results in the transformation of a suprabony pocket into an intrabony pocket.[10,12,17]
- Increased mobility of traumatically loosened teeth may have a pumping effect on plaque metabolites, thereby increasing their diffusion.[64]

Clinical and Radiographic Signs of Trauma From Occlusion Alone

The most common clinical sign of trauma to the periodontium is *increased tooth mobility.* During the injury stage of trauma from occlusion, the destruction of periodontal fibers occurs, which increases tooth mobility. During the final stage, the accommodation of the periodontium to increased forces entails a widening of the periodontal ligament, which also leads to increased tooth mobility. Although this tooth mobility is greater than the so-called normal mobility, it cannot be considered pathologic, because it is an adaptation and not a disease process. If it does become progressively worse, it can then be considered pathologic.

Other causes of increased tooth mobility include advanced bone loss, inflammation of the periodontal ligament of periodontal or periapical origin, and some systemic causes (e.g., pregnancy). The destruction of surrounding alveolar bone, such as occurs with osteomyelitis or jaw tumors, may also increase tooth mobility.

Radiographic signs of trauma from occlusion may include the following:

1. Increased width of the periodontal space, often with thickening of the lamina dura along the lateral aspect of the root, in the apical region, and in bifurcation areas. These changes do not *necessarily* indicate destructive changes, because they may result from thickening and strengthening of the periodontal ligament and alveolar bone, thereby constituting a favorable response to increased occlusal forces.
2. A vertical rather than horizontal destruction of the interdental septum.
3. Radiolucency and condensation of the alveolar bone.
4. Root resorption.

In summary, trauma from occlusion does not initiate gingivitis or periodontal pockets, but it may constitute an additional risk factor for the progression and severity of the disease. An understanding of the effect of trauma from occlusion on the periodontium is useful during the clinical management of periodontal problems.

Pathologic Tooth Migration

Pathologic migration refers to tooth displacement that results when the balance among the factors that maintain physiologic tooth position is disturbed by periodontal disease. Pathologic migration is relatively common. It may be an early sign of disease, or it may occur in association with gingival inflammation and pocket formation as the disease progresses.

Pathologic migration occurs most frequently in the anterior region, but posterior teeth may also be affected. The teeth may move in any direction, and the migration is usually accompanied by mobility and rotation. Pathologic migration in the occlusal or incisal direction is termed *extrusion*. All degrees of pathologic migration are encountered, and one or more teeth may be affected (Fig. 25.10). It is important to detect migration during its early stages and to prevent more serious involvement by eliminating the causative factors. Even during the early stage, some degree of bone loss occurs.

Pathogenesis

Two major factors play a role in maintaining the normal position of the teeth: the health and normal height of the periodontal attachment apparatus and the forces exerted on the teeth. The latter includes the forces of occlusion and pressure from the lips, cheeks, and tongue. Factors that are important in relation to the forces of occlusion include the following: (1) tooth morphologic features and cuspal inclination; (2) the presence of a full complement of teeth; (3) a physiologic tendency toward mesial migration; (4) the nature and location of contact point relationships; (5) proximal, incisal, and occlusal attrition; and (6) the axial inclination of the teeth. Alterations in any of these

factors start an interrelated sequence of changes in the environment of a single tooth or group of teeth that may result in pathologic migration. Thus pathologic migration occurs under conditions that weaken the periodontal support, that increase or modify the forces exerted on the teeth, or both.

Weakened Periodontal Support

The inflammatory destruction of the periodontium in patients with periodontitis creates an imbalance between the forces that maintain the tooth in position and the occlusal and muscular forces the tooth ordinarily needs to bear. The tooth with weakened support is unable to maintain its normal position in the arch and moves away from the opposing force unless it is restrained by proximal contact. The force that moves the weakly supported tooth may be created by factors such as occlusal contacts or pressure from the tongue.

It is important to understand that the abnormality of pathologic migration rests with the weakened periodontium; the force itself is not necessarily abnormal. Forces that are acceptable to an intact periodontium become injurious when periodontal support is reduced, as in the tooth with abnormal proximal contacts. Abnormally located proximal contacts convert the normal anterior component of force to a wedging force that causes occlusal or incisal movement of the tooth. The wedging force, which can be withstood by the intact periodontium, causes the tooth to extrude when the periodontal support is weakened by disease. *As its position changes, the tooth is subjected to abnormal occlusal forces, which aggravate the periodontal destruction and the tooth migration.*

Pathologic migration may continue after a tooth no longer contacts its antagonist. Pressures from the tongue, the food bolus during mastication, and the proliferating granulation tissue provide the force.

Pathologic migration is also an early sign of localized aggressive periodontitis. Weakened by the loss of periodontal support, the maxillary and mandibular anterior incisors drift labially and extrude, thereby creating diastemata between the teeth.

Changes in the Forces Exerted on the Teeth

Changes in the magnitude, direction, or frequency of the forces exerted on the teeth can induce the pathologic migration of a tooth or group of teeth. These forces do not have to be abnormal to cause migration if the periodontium is sufficiently weakened. Changes in the forces may result from unreplaced missing teeth or other causes.

Unreplaced Missing Teeth

The drifting of teeth into the spaces created by unreplaced missing teeth often occurs. Drifting differs from pathologic migration in that it does not result from the destruction of the periodontal tissues. However, it usually creates conditions that lead to periodontal disease,

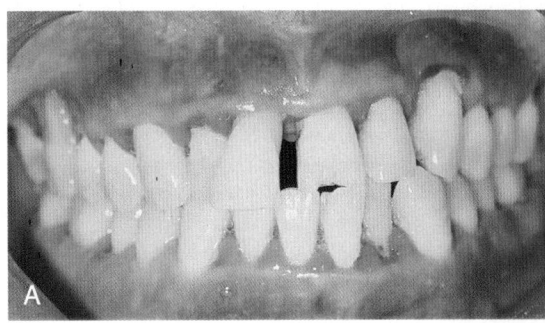
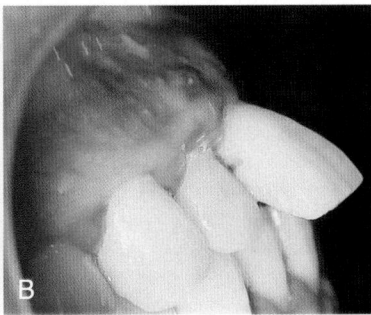

Fig. 25.10 Labial migration of the maxillary central incisors, especially the right incisor. (A) Frontal view. (B) Lateral view.

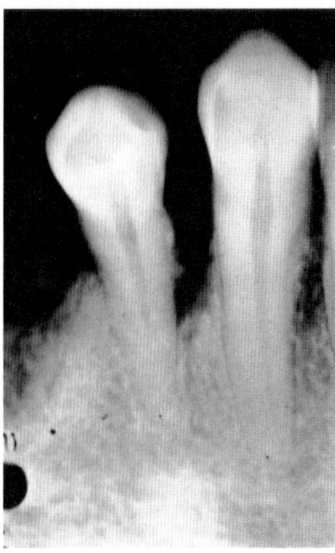

Fig. 25.11 Calculus and bone loss on the mesial surface of a canine that has drifted distally.

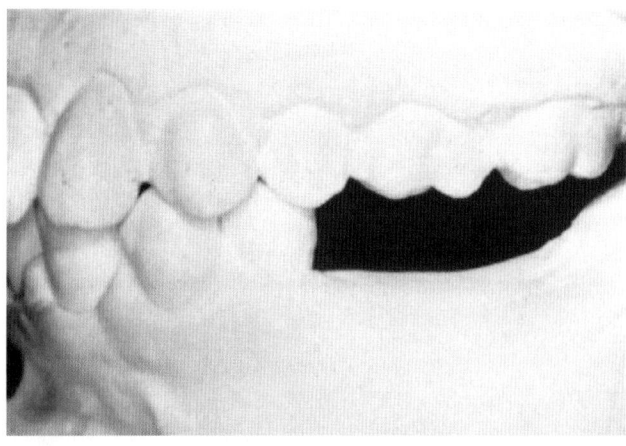

Fig. 25.13 No drifting or extrusion is present here, despite the 4-year absence of the mandibular teeth.

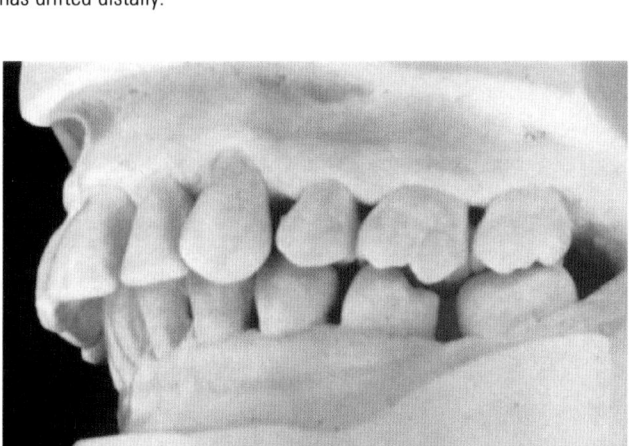

Fig. 25.12 Maxillary first molar that has tilted and extruded into the space created by a missing mandibular tooth.

and thus the initial tooth movement is aggravated by a loss of periodontal support (Fig. 25.11).

Drifting generally occurs in a mesial direction in combination with tilting or extrusion beyond the occlusal plane. The premolars frequently drift distally (Fig. 25.12). Although drifting is a common sequela when missing teeth are not replaced, it does not always occur (Fig. 25.13).

Failure to Replace First Molars

The pattern of changes that may follow the failure to replace missing first molars is characteristic. In extreme cases, it consists of the following:

1. The second and third molars tilt mesially, which results in a decrease in vertical dimension (Fig. 25.14).
2. The premolars move distally, and the mandibular incisors tilt or drift lingually. While drifting distally, the mandibular premolars lose their intercuspating relationship with the maxillary teeth, and they may tilt distally.
3. Anterior overbite is increased. The mandibular incisors strike the maxillary incisors near the gingiva or traumatize the gingiva.
4. The maxillary incisors are pushed labially and laterally (Fig. 25.15).

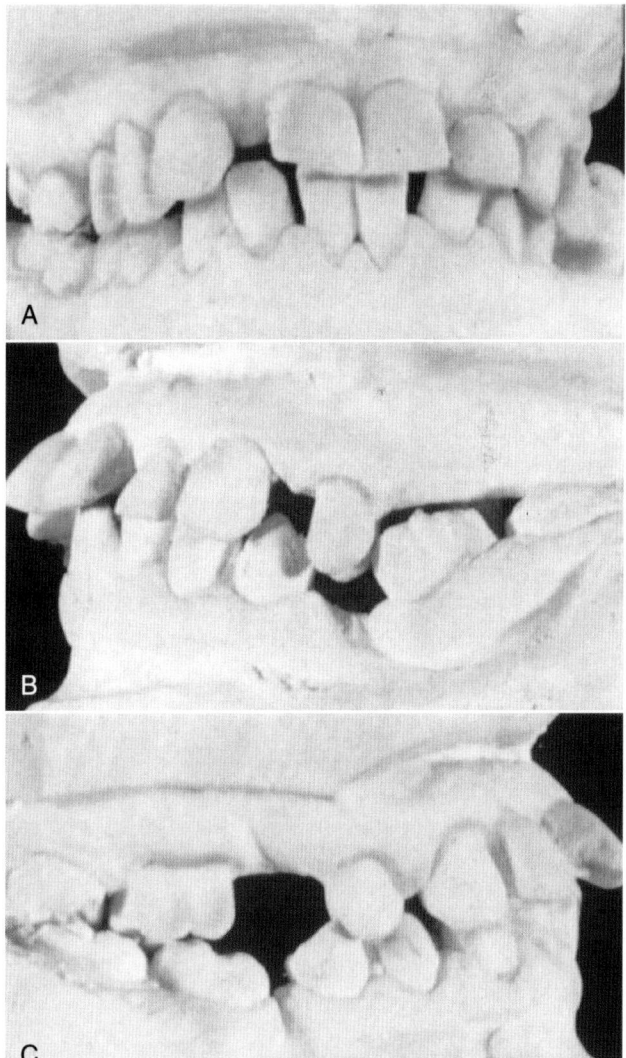

Fig. 25.14 Examples of the mutilation of occlusion associated with unreplaced missing teeth. Note pronounced pathologic migration, disturbed proximal contacts, and functional relationships with closing of the bite.

5. The anterior teeth extrude because the incisal apposition has largely disappeared.
6. Diastemata are created by the separation of the anterior teeth (see Fig. 25.14).

The disturbed proximal contact relationships lead to food impaction, plaque accumulation that results in gingival inflammation, and pocket formation, which are followed by bone loss and tooth mobility. Occlusal disharmonies created by the altered tooth positions traumatize the supporting tissues of the periodontium and aggravate the destruction caused by the inflammation. The reduction in periodontal support leads to the further migration of the teeth and the mutilation of the occlusion.

Other Causes

Trauma from occlusion may cause a shift in tooth position either by itself or in combination with inflammatory periodontal disease. The direction of movement depends on the occlusal force.

Pressure from the tongue may cause drifting of the teeth in the absence of periodontal disease, or it may contribute to the pathologic migration of teeth with reduced periodontal support (Fig. 25.16).

When tooth support has been weakened by periodontal destruction, *pressure from the granulation tissue of periodontal pockets* has been mentioned as contributing to pathologic migration.[28,37] The teeth may return to their original positions after the pockets are eliminated, but if more destruction has occurred on one side of a tooth than on the other, the healing tissues tend to pull in the direction of less destruction.

Summary

It is important to understand the etiology of the changes that occur in the periodontal tissues from both the clinical and histologic perspectives. Whatever the etiology, the periodontal tissues have a tremendous adaptive ability to accommodate both the microbial and the traumatic occlusal factors within a certain limit. It is the combination of both and the patient's ability to resist these factors that may complicate the diagnosis and treatment plan of the clinical cases that are presented.

 A Case Scenario is found on the companion website www.expertconsult.com.

References

 References for this chapter are found on the companion website www.expertconsult.com.

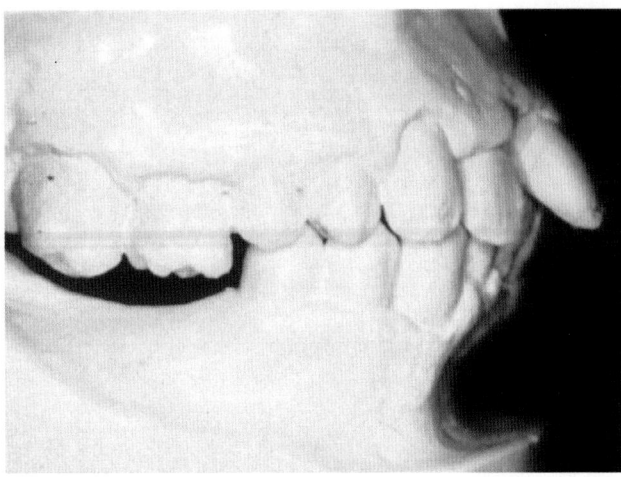

Fig. 25.15 Maxillary incisors pushed labially in a patient with bilateral unreplaced mandibular molars. Note the extrusion of the maxillary molars.

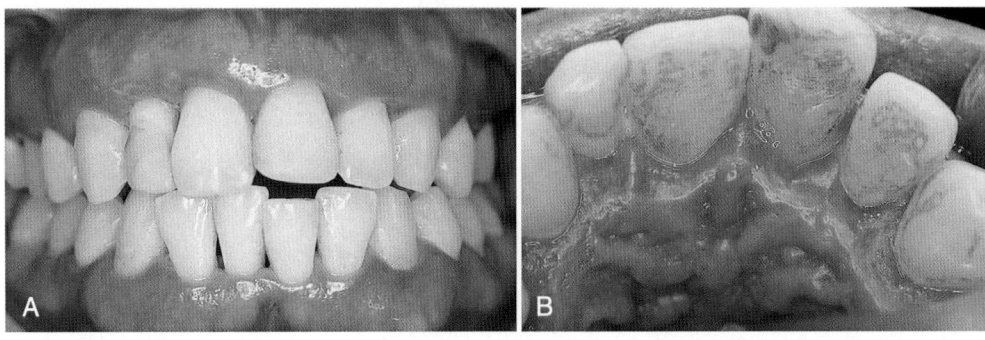

Fig. 25.16 Pathologic migration associated with tongue pressure. (A) Facial view. (B) Palatal view.

CHAPTER 26

Masticatory System Disorders That Influence the Periodontium

Michael J. McDevitt

 For online-only content about the biomechanics of the masticatory system as well as expanded discussions of the muscles and nerves of the masticatory system, dysfunction and deterioration, orofacial pain, and clinical examination, please visit the companion website at www.expertconsult.com.

The masticatory system consists of the temporomandibular joints (TMJs), the masticatory muscles, the teeth in occlusion, and the neurologic and vascular supplies that support all of these structures. Research suggests that masticatory system disorders include many varied conditions with multiple possible contributing factors rather than different manifestations of a single disease or syndrome.[2,85,131] The ability to understand the anatomy and function of the masticatory system and to correctly interpret relevant diagnostic information is a prerequisite to fulfilling comprehensive standards of care. Our diagnostic process must have a broad enough base and be inclusive enough to determine the most appropriate cause of masticatory dysfunction.[139]

Temporomandibular Joint

Harmonious function of the TMJs is a product of the coordination of the muscles of mastication by intricate mechanisms of neurologic control. Understanding the dynamics and the relationship of the TMJ to the associated muscles and nerves provides the working knowledge required for effective assessment and diagnosis.

The TMJ is one of the most complex joints in the human body. It is capable of providing both hinging (rotation) and gliding (translation) movements, and it is able to resist incredible forces of mastication. The TMJ is formed by the head of the condyle of the mandible as it fits into the articular fossa of the temporal bone (Fig. 26.1). The body of the mandible effectively connects both condyles so that neither condyle functions independently of the other. Interposed between the head of the condyle and the articular surface of the temporal bone is the articular disc, which consists of dense connective tissue; this results in a compound joint with two joint cavities (Fig. 26.2). The articulating surfaces of the osseous structures are essentially convex in a healthy situation, so the biconcave configuration of the articular disc compensates for the opposing convexities. The articular surfaces of the condyles and the temporal bones consist of fibrous connective tissue, which renders them resistant to breakdown and capable of repair. Deep to the superficial connective tissue layer, articular cartilage provides the cellular and structural basis for the response to the functional loading and movement of the TMJs.[85,139,191] The discal ligaments and attachments to the capsule, along with the disc itself, become the means of separating the joint into superior and inferior joint spaces (see Figs. 26.1 and 26.2). Synovial lubrication of the articular surfaces is a function of the production of synovial fluid by endothelial cells along the borders of each joint cavity and at the anterior extent of the retrodiscal tissues.[a]

Muscles and Nerves of the Masticatory System

The muscles and nerves of the masticatory system are extensively reviewed elsewhere. They are only briefly discussed here for the purpose of understanding the mechanisms involved. Appropriate references are provided for further reading.

Centric Relation

The mandible is suspended from the cranial base by ligaments and muscles. The understanding of mandibular movement begins with an initial reference point for each condyle, which is usually referred to as *centric relation;* this clinically determined relationship of the mandible to the maxilla occurs when both condyle–disc assemblies are in their most superior position in the maxillary (or glenoid) fossa and against the slope of the articular eminence of the temporal bone. Verification of centric relation is obtained by loading the TMJs bilaterally with the teeth apart via the bimanual mandibular manipulation technique advocated by Dawson and others.[43-46,176] When both condyles are in this relationship, rotation or hinging action occurs around an axis defined by the medial poles of each condyle (Fig. 26.3).

---

[a]References 43, 46, 85, 139, 185, 187, 191.

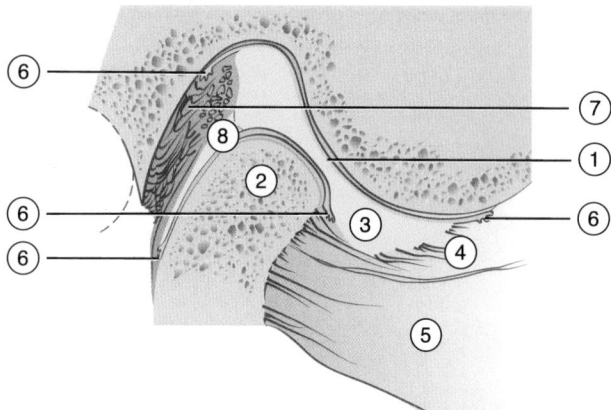

Fig. 26.1 Lateral view of a cross-section through the temporomandibular joint. *1,* Posterior slope of the articular eminence of the temporal bone; *2,* head of the condyle; *3,* articular disc (note the biconcave shape); *4,* superior lateral pterygoid muscle (note the attachment to both the head of the condyle and the articular disc); *5,* inferior lateral pterygoid muscle; *6,* synovial tissue; *7,* retrodiscal tissue; and *8,* discal ligament attachment to the posterior surface of the head of the condyle. *(Modified from Dawson PE: Evaluation, diagnosis, and treatment of occlusal problems, ed 2, St. Louis, 1989, Mosby.)*

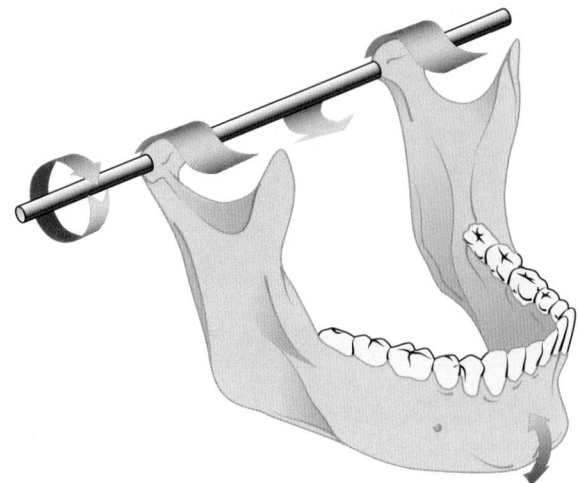

Fig. 26.3 When they are in centric relation, the condyles can rotate on a fixed axis. As long as the rotational axis stays fixed at the most superior position against the eminentiae, the mandible can open or close and still be in centric relation. If the condyle axis moves forward, it is no longer in centric relation. *(From Dawson PE: Evaluation, diagnosis, and treatment of occlusal problems, ed 2, St. Louis, 1989, Mosby.)*

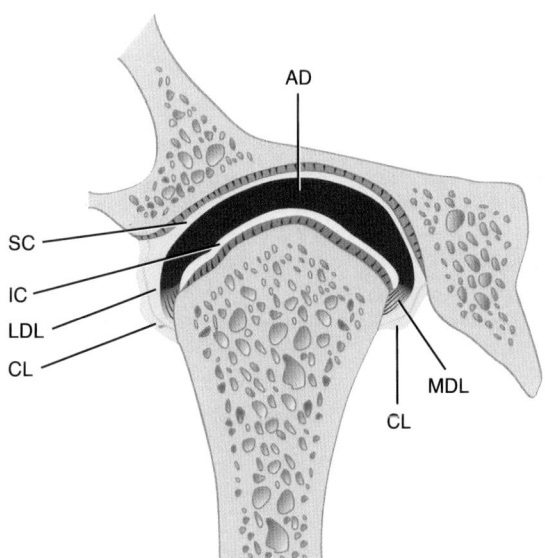

Fig. 26.2 Anterior view of the temporomandibular joint showing the collateral ligaments. *AD,* Articular disc; *CL,* capsular ligament; *IC,* inferior joint cavity; *LDL,* lateral discal ligament; *MDL,* medial discal ligament; *SC,* superior joint cavity. *(From Okeson JP: Management of temporomandibular joint disorders and occlusion, ed 4, St. Louis, 1998, Mosby.)*

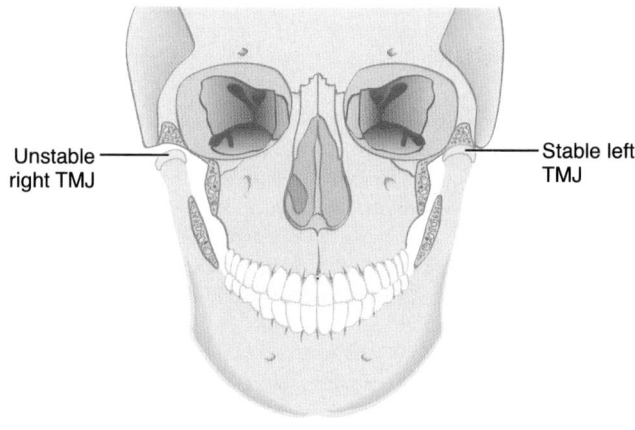

Stable occlusion

Fig. 26.4 Example of orthopedic instability. Note that, with the teeth in their stable position (i.e., maximum intercuspation), the left temporomandibular joint is in a stable relationship with the fossa. The right temporomandibular joint, however, is not in a stable position with the fossa. When the elevator muscles contract, the right condyle moves superiorly to seek a more stable relationship with the articular disc and fossa (i.e., the musculoskeletally stable position). This type of loading can lead to an intracapsular disorder. *(From Okeson JP: Management of temporomandibular joint disorders and occlusion, ed 4, St. Louis, 1998, Mosby.)*

The term *centric relation* is limited to the rotation axis through both condyles while they are seated in their respective glenoid fossae. The only occlusal consideration relative to centric relation occurs when rotation of the mandible initiates the first contact of opposing occlusal surfaces. The term *initial contact* in centric relation can be used to define this relationship (see Chapter 55). If the contraction of elevator muscles occurs at the point of initial occlusal contact and results in the distraction of one or both condyle–disc assemblies from their seated relationship, then centric relation is no longer occurring.[43,44,46]

For TMJs to maintain orthopedic stability, the condyles must remain fully seated in their respective fossae when the teeth occlude in maximal intercuspation. Orthopedic instability occurs when the occlusal relationships are such that the contraction of elevator muscles

is required to achieve stable occlusion in the maximal intercuspal position, which results in the unseating of one or both condyles from their respective fossae (Fig. 26.4).

The strain on the discal ligaments caused by a loaded joint being displaced from the fossa can lead to internal derangement of that joint, which will be described later in this chapter. Postural and parafunctional stress can also be a source of the orthopedic instability of a TMJ.

An individual's susceptibility to masticatory system disorders determines whether that person adapts with minimal consequence or develops dysfunction or degeneration.[26,43,46,139,176]

Dysfunction and Deterioration

Ideally, function never exceeds the integrity or adaptive limits of the structural elements of the masticatory system. Clinical experience shows that the tolerance of the components of the masticatory system can be exceeded by both acute trauma and chronic trauma. *Acute trauma* to the head and neck region can range from a distinct event, such as an accident or a blow to the face, to a sustained overuse experience, such as a long dental appointment. Acute trauma can serve as an initiating event that leads to a chronic condition, so accurate documentation and careful monitoring may prove extremely valuable should symptoms or dysfunction persist.[13,20,47]

Chronic trauma is defined as any experience that repeatedly exceeds the tolerances of the affected masticatory system structure. Postural stresses and parafunctional occlusal habits, with or without occlusal discrepancies, may produce musculoskeletal disharmony and orthopedic instability of the TMJ.

The general terms for occlusal parafunction used in this text include *bruxism*, which is the grinding of the teeth, and *clenching*, which is when a person holds the teeth firmly together with significant force. Bruxism is usually confirmed by the observation of excessive tooth wear. The clenching type of parafunction can be distinguished from the grinding of the teeth, and it seems to be more often associated with masticatory system disorders than does bruxism.[31,62,64,84,142,147] Sleep bruxism may include both tooth grinding and clenching, and it seems to occur primarily during stage 1 and stage 2 (i.e., non–rapid eye movement) sleep. These episodes often occur in association with short brain and cardiac reactivations called "microarousals." Rhythmic masticatory muscle activity is relatively common among nonbruxers, but the frequency and intensity of the muscle contraction is substantially greater for the sleep bruxer. The central pattern generator of the primate brain stem does not modulate or reduce muscle contraction during sleep as it does during waking hours. In addition, the amplification of oral parafunction has been reported in association with a patient's intake of selective serotonin reuptake inhibitors (e.g., Prozac).[11,43,46,139,150,178]

Discrimination between occlusal function–related and parafunction-related masticatory system disorders and those with other etiologies requires exacting standards of occlusal evaluation. If sufficient evidence exists to suspect that the occlusal relationships in function or parafunction may have exceeded the tolerances of that individual's masticatory system, responsible intervention or monitoring can be initiated.[46,67,142,149]

Disruption of the relationship or alignment of the condyle, the disc, and the articular surface of the temporal bone is typically called an *intracapsular disorder* or an *internal derangement of the TMJ*. The articular disc can be displaced as a result of an acute blow to the jaw, chronic trauma, or the uncoordinated contraction of the lateral pterygoid muscle. When the disc cannot return to its normal relationship to the condyle with full closure of the mouth, it is considered to be displaced or dislocated.

Orofacial Pain

Discomfort associated with masticatory system disorders falls under the larger umbrella of orofacial pain. Pain associated with TMJ dysfunction is most frequently muscular in origin,[43] and it may be amplified by both occlusal parafunction and stress.[65] Although pain itself is a complex entity,[172] a working knowledge of even the uncommon sources of pain perceived in the region of the masticatory system is essential to providing comprehensive diagnosis and treatment.

Sources of dental or periodontal pain should be identified by clinical, radiographic, and historic information. Nondental sources

---

BOX 26.1   Differential Diagnosis of Orofacial Pain

Intracranial Pain Disorders[71,77,85,123,138,144]
Neoplasm, aneurysm, abscess, hemorrhage, hematoma, edema

Primary Headache Disorders (Neurovascular Disorders)[93,126]
Migraine, migraine variants, cluster headache, paroxysmal hemicrania, cranial arteritis, carotidynia, tension-type headache[4,95,101,139]

Neurogenic Pain Disorders[123,126]
Paroxysmal neuralgias: Trigeminal, glossopharyngeal, nervus intermedius, and superior laryngeal neuralgias[166]
Continuous pain disorders: Deafferentation pain syndromes (peripheral neuritis, postherpetic neuritis, posttraumatic and postsurgical neuralgia, neuralgia-inducing cavitation osteonecrosis[17,18])
Sympathetically maintained pain[21]

Intraoral Pain Disorders
Dental pulp, periodontium, mucogingival tissues, tongue[14,111,123,189]

Temporomandibular Disorders
Masticatory muscle, temporomandibular joint, associated structures

Associated Structures[36,40,133,138,139]
Ears, eyes, nose, paranasal sinuses, throat, lymph nodes, salivary glands, neck

Axis II Mental Disorders
Somatoform disorders
Pain syndromes of psychogenic origin

Compiled by the American Academy of Orofacial Pain.

---

of pain include TMJ structures, muscles, cervical structures, neuropathies, vascular inflammation, all types of headache, sleep disorders, systemic disorders, and psychoimmune neurologic sources.[138] A survey of 45,700 American households revealed that 22% of respondents had experienced some type of orofacial pain during the previous 6 months, thereby establishing a meaningful probability that the periodontal patient's list of symptoms includes pain.[10]

Box 26.1 provides the current list of possible sources of orofacial pain. This list was prepared by the American Academy of Orofacial Pain.[138]

Headache pain is perceived primarily within the trigeminal nerve pathways, although other cranial and cervical nerves may offer painful sensory input.[85,138,162] Pain that originates in masticatory system structures, which are also innervated by the trigeminal nerve, requires diagnostic differentiation from headache pain.[163] Headache can present in myriad forms, and it can influence the perception of pain and the diagnosis of the origin of pain.[85,138]

Pain of dental and periodontal origin must be clearly defined and differentiated from heart attack, sinus pain, and myofascial pain.[138,139] Pain that originates in pulpal or periodontal nociceptors can be differentiated with a comprehensive clinical and radiographic evaluation. Orofacial pain that originates in the TMJs or the muscles of mastication can result from neoplasm, macrotrauma, repeated microtrauma, systemic disease, and anatomic predisposition.

Sleep-disordered breathing may also play a role in a patient's orofacial pain through various potential mechanisms.[8] Sleep bruxism has been associated with hypoxia and arousals during sleep disruption.[25,56,181,182] Pain tolerance appears to be diminished with sleep deprivation.[169] Oral appliances that have been prescribed for sleep-disordered breathing have the potential to cause at least

BOX 26.2   Examples of Questions About the Masticatory System to Include in the Patient History

Are you now experiencing or have you ever experienced:

1. Pain in either jaw joint or pain when opening or closing your mouth?[9]
2. Acute or direct trauma to the face, jaw, head, or neck, such as during an accident?
3. Any locking or restricted movement of either jaw joint?[50,170]
4. The inability to bite or close the teeth together completely without discomfort in one or both jaw joints?
5. Earache without infection, especially if it is recurring?
6. Ringing or rushing sounds in either ear?
7. Any type of neuralgia (nerve pain), especially with trigger points?[123,180]
8. Tooth pain without a diagnosed dental problem or after tooth removal?[124,125,173]
9. Fibromyalgia (muscle pain)?[42,146,152,168]
10. Sleep apnea or any sleep disturbance?
11. Any sounds, such as clicks or pops, in either jaw joint, especially when opening or while eating?
12. Chronic or frequently recurring headaches, especially migraines or cluster headaches?[4]
13. Shingles or any painful infection of the face or neck?
14. Having to "adjust" the jaw or manipulate the jaw joint with your hand to be able to open or close your mouth?
15. An occupation or activity that requires a regular stressful posture, such as cradling a telephone between the head and shoulder, working at a computer, playing a musical instrument, or scuba diving?[174,192]
16. An awareness of frequently keeping your teeth together, maintaining a clenched jaw, or holding your jaw in an assumed position, such as holding a pipe?
17. Lyme disease?[71]
18. Neck muscles that are often tired or sore?
19. A sleep position or posture that maintains pressure on your lower jaw?

transient symptoms of temporomandibular disorders as a result of the mandibular advancement that needs to be experienced for them to be effective.[41,51] Oral appliances prescribed for sleep bruxism may represent an additional airway obstruction for the patient with obstructive sleep apnea.[60] In the light of the increasing emphasis on the effects of sleep-disordered breathing in both medicine and dentistry, Chapter 40 has been developed for this text to serve as a reference for the reader.

Comprehensive Evaluation

Patient History and Interview

The written history and personal interview should be designed to invite open-ended responses and reflection by the patient on past experiences and the current condition. Standard dental or medical history forms may require modification to include questions about any history of limited or painful jaw movement, noise in either joint, and masticatory muscle symptoms (Box 26.2). These issues should be documented with regard to timing, duration, frequency, and relationship to any history of trauma.[138]

Clinical Examination

The clinical examination continues the interview process through the co-discovery of the patient's masticatory system status. The dentist

leads the patient to understand the meaning of signs and symptoms of dysfunction or deterioration and seeks opportunities to expand the patient's responses to questions.

The physical examination actually begins during the interview, when asymmetries in facial form, head posture, and mandibular movement patterns can be observed. The clinical evaluation of the various structures of the masticatory system, although individual to each practitioner, should afford the patient opportunities for understanding and include the following[11,43,139]:

1. The observation and measurement of the full range of motion of the mandible
2. The auscultation and light palpation of each TMJ in its full range of motion
3. The load testing of each TMJ
4. The palpation of each muscle of mastication and the related head and neck muscles
5. The evaluation of all of the soft tissues of the face, oral cavity, and oropharynx
6. Periodontal and dental examinations
7. Complete occlusal analysis, including accurately mounted diagnostic models

Imaging

When the clinical evaluation, panoramic radiographs, and patient history indicate the possibility of structural masticatory system disorders or the possible presence of pathology (especially neoplasm), appropriate imaging of the TMJ is warranted.[109] The state-of-the-art technique for the imaging of soft tissue, especially the articular disc, is magnetic resonance imaging. The current highest standard for the imaging of hard tissue, such as the condyle or the temporal bone, is computed tomography (CT). Cone-beam CT has become much more readily available to dentistry, with software systems able to display the data gathered as both anteroposterior and cross-sectional depictions of the condyle and cranial structures, with image quality that is the same as or better than spiral CT. Less radiation exposure and lower cost to the patient are both reasons to favor cone-beam CT over conventional CT. The interpretation of magnetic resonance and CT images usually requires specialized training for the clinician or access to a radiologist. Arthrography is still being used for certain diagnostic situations, such as the suspected perforation of the articular disc, and nuclear medicine has developed protocols to image the TMJ to determine if active deterioration is occurring.[j]

Although plain-film tomography is occasionally a feature of some of the newer radiographic equipment, the technique that is most readily available to a majority of practitioners is panoramic radiography. The image produced depicts only general relationships and gross anatomy, so the information provided should be used only for screening purposes. When pathology or marked deformation is suggested by a panoramic radiograph, further diagnostic imaging and procedures may be warranted.[19,85]

Diagnostic Decision Making

The complete evaluation of every patient's periodontal status must include the diagnostic components required to reveal any form of masticatory system disorder. The existence of factors that are responsible for the historical, current, or potential impairment of masticatory system function can be integrated into a comprehensive treatment plan. Patients who require substantial periodontal therapy or who have advanced periodontal disease may be at increased risk for masticatory system disorders, so diagnostic processes must remain consistently thorough and inclusive for all patients.[26,158] For the patient who presents with a symptomatic masticatory system disorder, the diagnostic strategy would logically begin with the inclusion of all potential sources of pain or dysfunction and be followed by the systematic exclusion of possible causative or contributing factors, beginning with the least likely. When no symptoms are reported, the history and clinical examination still need to be thorough, because some patients tend to tolerate modest dysfunction or mild transient discomfort. The diagnostic strategy for the patient who presents with minimal or no signs and symptoms of masticatory system disorders is to attempt to confirm a stable condition while identifying risk factors. The careful documentation of past or current trauma and disharmony provides the basis for the trend analysis and anticipation of possible future problems.[k]

Consistent professional maintenance care has been clearly demonstrated to be a key ingredient in the successful management

of a patient's periodontal condition.[74,126] By complementing any treatment sequence, these appointments afford dentists the opportunity at every stage of comprehensive care to provide continuing evaluation of the status of the entire masticatory system and to provide timely and appropriate intervention when needed (see Chapter 72).

Acknowledgments

I would like to acknowledge the encouragement and the recommendation of references provided by Dr. Henry Gremillion during the revision of this chapter.

 A Case Scenario is found on the companion website www.expertconsult.com.

References

 References for this chapter are found on the companion website www.expertconsult.com.

---

[k]References 32, 33, 49, 63, 74, 107, 126, 131, 132, 134, 177.

CHAPTER 27

Chronic Periodontitis

Henrik Dommisch | Moritz Kebschull

Chronic periodontitis is the most prevalent form of periodontitis, and it generally shows the characteristics of a slowly progressing inflammatory disease. Periodontitis belongs to the group of complex inflammatory diseases in humans. In this context, the word *complex* not only describes the fact that there are multiple clinical symptoms that account for the disease, but also explains the multiple factors that lead to and influence periodontal inflammation. Chronic periodontitis occurs most frequently in adults. Nonetheless, it may also be diagnosed in children and adolescents when associated with chronic plaque and calculus accumulation. Therefore chronic periodontitis should be understood as age-associated, but not age-dependent, complex chronic inflammation of the periodontal tissues. As described in this chapter, systemic or environmental factors (e.g., diabetes mellitus, smoking) modify the host immune response to the dental biofilm so that the periodontal destruction becomes more progressive.

Periodontitis is a highly prevalent progressing disease, and it affects approximately 10.5% to 12% of the world's population.[44] Periodontitis has been found to exert adverse effects on systemic health, and in this context, important pathologic interdependencies with, for example, diabetes mellitus have been identified.[9,32,55,73] Also, it is known that systemic inflammatory markers, such as the C-reactive protein (CRP), are elevated in patients with periodontitis.[69,96] In general, chronic periodontitis is considered as a slowly progressing disease, but in the presence of severe systemic conditions or environmental factors, such as smoking, this inflammatory disease progresses more rapidly.

The classic definition described chronic periodontitis as "an infectious disease resulting in inflammation within the supporting tissues of the teeth, progressive attachment loss, and bone loss."[24] The etiopathologic factors that lead to periodontal inflammation and, subsequently, destruction of periodontal tissues have been widely studied, and the interplay between the microbial environment and the individual host immune response has gained attention in the scientific community (discussed later).

Chronic periodontitis represents major clinical and etiologic characteristics such as (1) microbial biofilm formation (dental plaque), (2) periodontal inflammation (gingival swelling, bleeding on probing), and (3) attachment as well as alveolar bone loss.

Besides the local immune response to the dental biofilm, periodontitis may also be associated with a number of systemic disorders and defined syndromes. In most cases, patients with systemic diseases, which lead to impaired host immunity, may also show periodontal destruction. On the other hand, periodontitis is not only limited to the area of the oral cavity but may be associated with severe systemic diseases such as cardiovascular disease, stroke, and diabetes mellitus.[52,70,73,79]

This chapter discusses clinical features that have been described for chronic periodontitis, based on the consensus of the 1999 World Workshop in Periodontics. In addition, the etiology is summarized in categories explaining the known factors (microbiologic, immunologic, genetic, and environmental) involved in the pathology of chronic periodontitis.

At the time of writing of this chapter, a new World Workshop in Periodontics was jointly planned by the European Federation of Periodontology and the American Academy of Periodontology for November 2017, to further refine the classification of periodontal diseases.

Clinical Features

General Characteristics

Characteristic clinical findings in patients with untreated chronic periodontitis include the following symptoms (see the case presentation in Figs. 27.1 to 27.6):

- Supragingival and subgingival plaque (and calculus)
- Gingival swelling, redness, and loss of gingival stippling
- Altered gingival margins (rolled, flattened, cratered papillae, recessions)
- Pocket formation
- Bleeding on probing
- Attachment loss
- Bone loss (angular/vertical or horizontal)
- Root furcation involvement
- Increased tooth mobility
- Change in tooth position
- Tooth loss

Chronic periodontitis can be clinically revealed by means of periodontal screening and recording (PSR), diagnosed by an assessment of the clinical attachment level, and therewith the detection of inflammatory changes in the marginal gingiva (see Fig. 27.1). Measurements of periodontal probing pocket depth in combination with the location of the marginal gingiva allow conclusions regarding the loss of clinical attachment (see Figs. 27.3 and 27.6). Dental radiographs reveal the extent of bone loss indicated by the distance between the cemento-enamel-junction and the alveolar bone crest (Fig. 27.2).

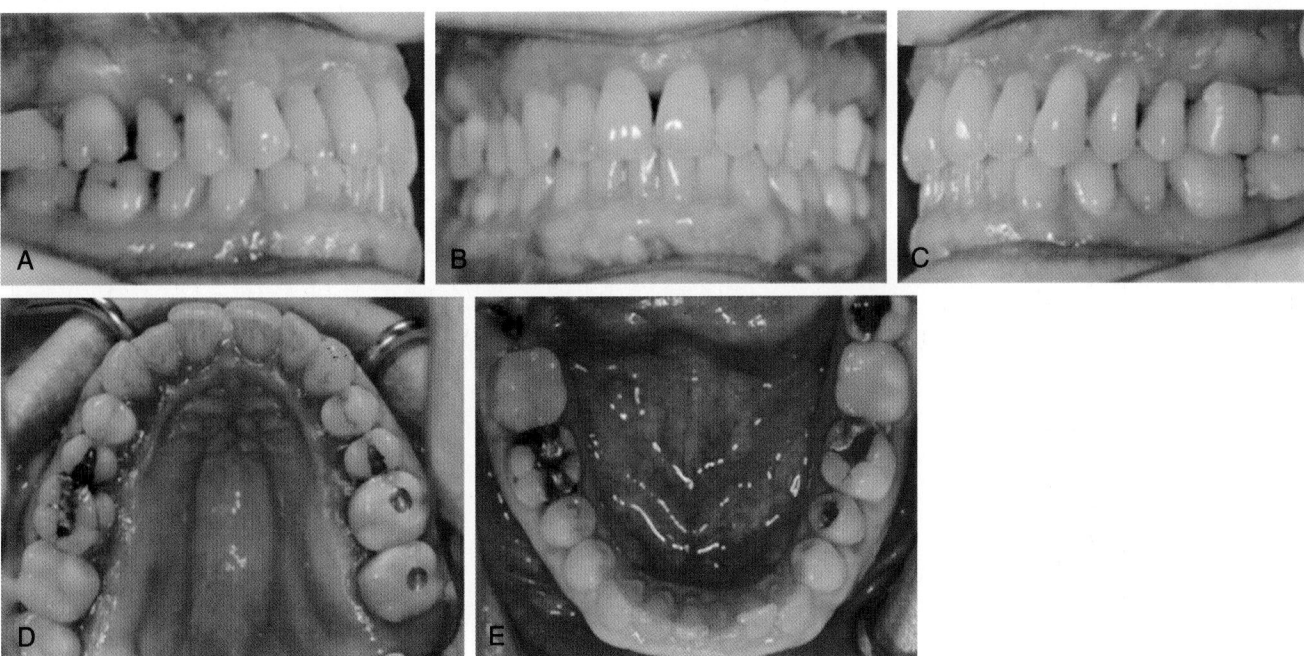

Fig. 27.1 Clinical features of generalized chronic periodontitis in a 49-year-old, medically healthy male patient who presented to the clinic for the first time. The patient reported smoking 15 cigarettes per day. Note the abundant dental plaque and calculus deposits, gingival redness and swelling, and alteration of the gingival texture (loss of gingival stippling). The patient noticed multiple recessions. In this case, recessions were the result from loss of clinical attachment and alveolar bone. (A) Right lateral view. (B) Frontal view. (C) Left lateral view. (D) Maxillary view. (E) Mandibular view. *(Reprinted from Kebschull M, Dommisch H: Resektive parodon-talchirurgie.* Zahnmedizin up-2-date. *2012; 525–545.)*

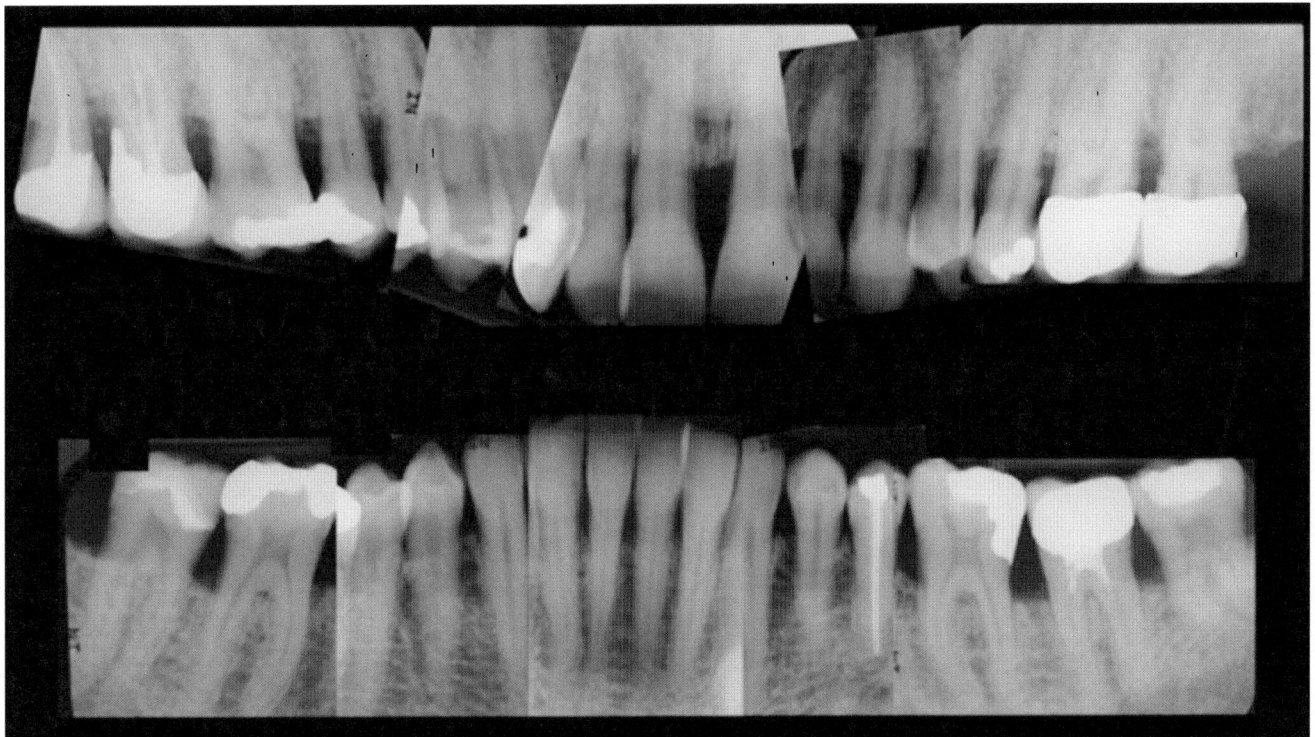

Fig. 27.2 Collage of the radiographic periodontal status (a total of 11 x-rays) at the time of diagnosis (compare Figs. 27.1 and 27.3). Generalized horizontal and localized angular, vertical bone loss on the mesial and distal sites of molars was noted. Radiographs present deep subgingival restorations (teeth #2 and #19), overhanging margins of restorations (teeth #14 and #15), carious lesion (tooth #14), and insufficient root canal treatment (tooth #18). *(Reprinted from Kebschull M, Dommisch H: Resektive parodontalchirurgie.* Zahnmedizin up-2-date. *2012; 525–545.)*

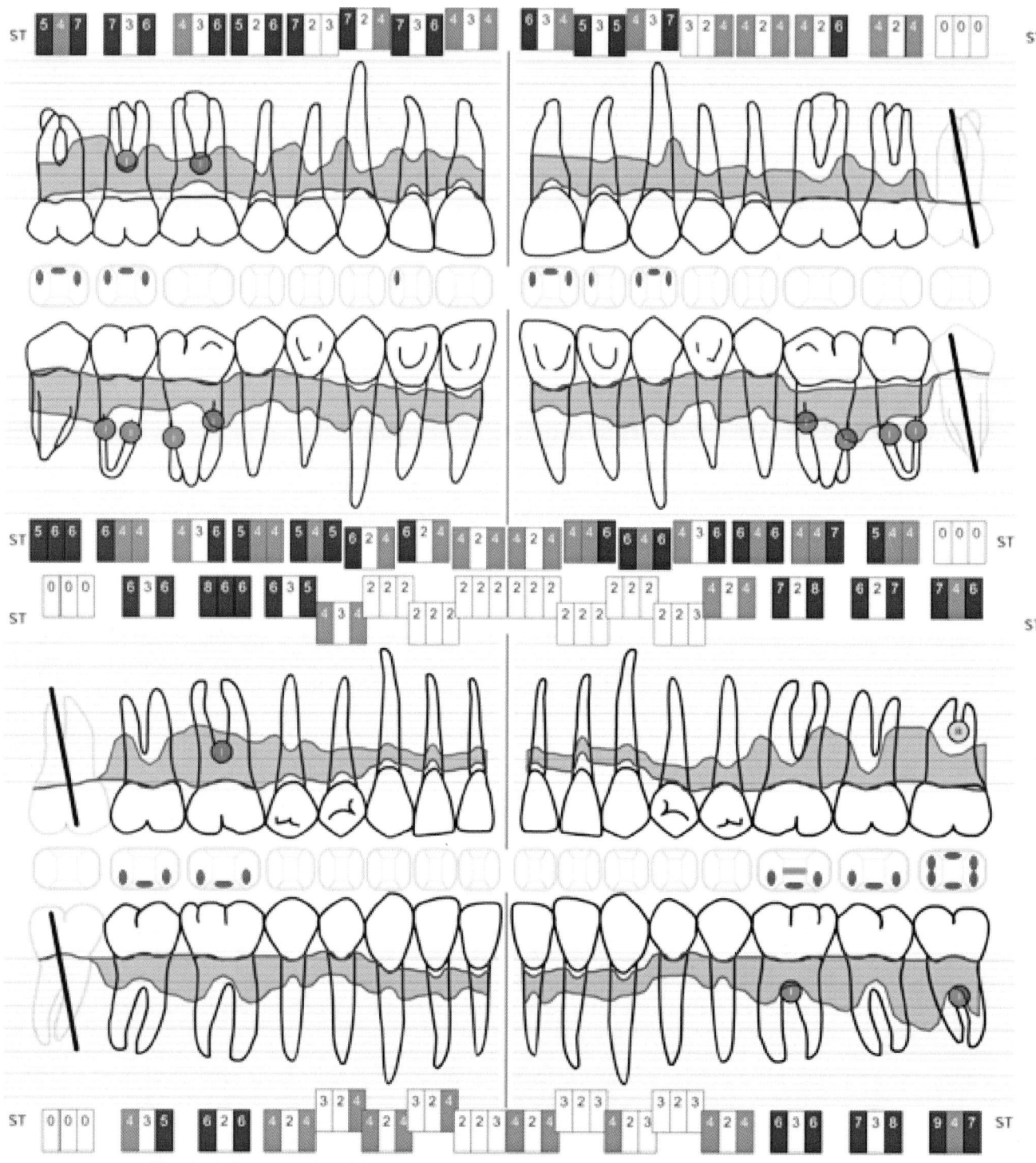

Fig. 27.3 Documentation of the periodontal attachment level in the same patient (see Fig. 27.1) at the time of the first visit. The red line displays the gingival margin reflecting recessions. Clinical attachment loss is illustrated by the filled (blue) area on the root surfaces. The deepest periodontal pocket measured was 9 mm. Class I (green) and class II (yellow) furcation involvement were documented. Bleeding upon periodontal probing (gingival inflammation) is reflected by orange dots. Due to the history of smoking, the bleeding on probing score was relatively low, although the patient presented advanced attachment loss. Tooth mobility is indicated by the green line (tooth #19). *(Reprinted from Kebschull M, Dommisch H: Resektive parodontalchirurgie. Zahnmedizin up-2-date. 2012; 525–545.)*

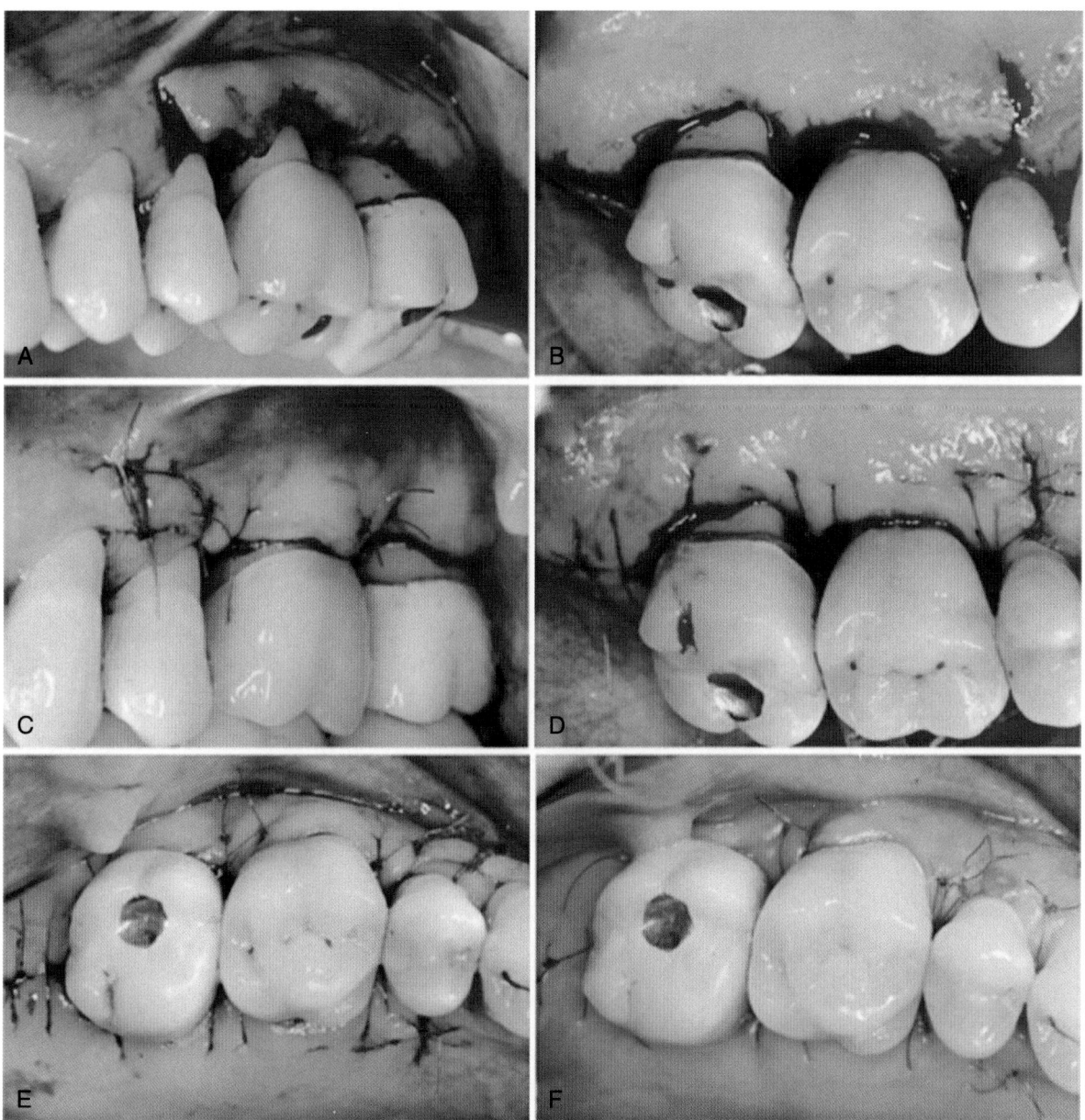

Fig. 27.4 Subsequent to the anti-infective therapy and periodontal reevaluation, resective periodontal surgery was performed in the patient introduced in Figs. 27.1, 27.2, and 27.3. Surgical method: apically repositioned flap. (A) Intrasulcular incision at buccal sites; notice class I furcation involvement on tooth #14. (B) Paramarginal incision at palatal sites, excision of a distal wedge. (C–D) Sutured using 5-0 Prolene, buccal and palatal view, respectively. (E) Occlusal view after suturing. (F) Occlusal view 1 week post surgery. Tooth #14 received endodontic therapy and crown restoration prior to periodontal surgery. *(Reprinted from Kebschull M, Dommisch H: Resektive parodontalchirurgie. Zahnmedizin up-2-date. 2012; 525–545.)*

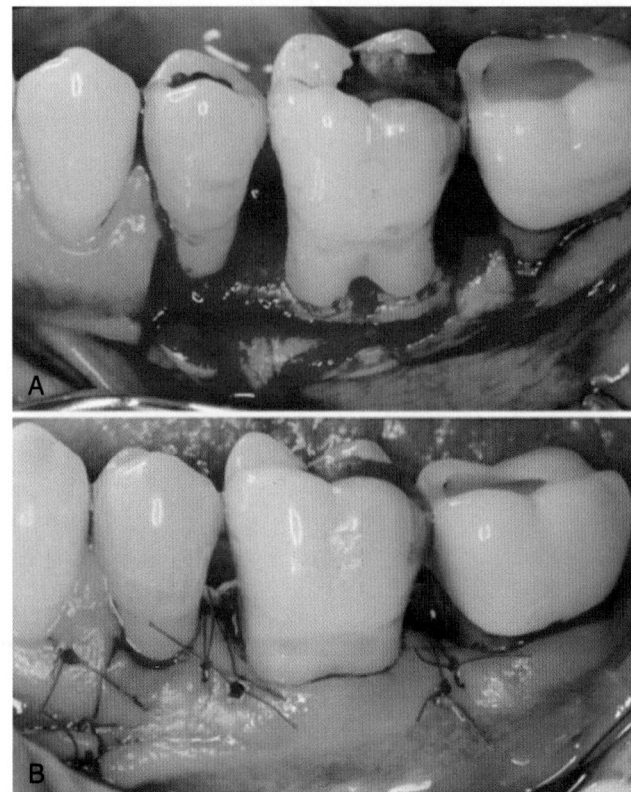

Fig. 27.5 Subsequent to the anti-infective therapy and periodontal reevaluation, resective periodontal surgery was performed in the patient introduced in Figs. 27.1 to 27.4. Surgical method: apically repositioned flap. (A) Intrasulcular incision at buccal sites; notice class I furcation involvement on tooth #19 and horizontal bone loss in teeth #18 to #20. (B) Sutured using 5-0 Prolene, buccal view. *(Reprinted from Kebschull M, Dommisch H: Resektive parodontalchirurgie.* Zahnmedizin up-2-date. *2012; 525–545.)*

The distinction between aggressive and chronic periodontitis is sometimes difficult, because the clinical features may be similar at the time of the first examination. At later time points during treatment, aggressive and chronic periodontitis may be differentiated by the rate of disease progression over time, familial nature of aggressive disease, and presence of local as well as systemic factors.

Disease Distribution

Chronic periodontitis exhibits a site-specific clinical picture, where attachment and bone loss are not equally distributed throughout the dentition as well as around teeth. Local inflammation, pocket formation, attachment loss, and bone loss are the sequelae of the direct exposure to the subgingival plaque (dental biofilm) and local inflammatory responses. Periodontal pocket formation, attachment, and bone loss may develop on one or more sites of a tooth, while other sites remain at a physiologic attachment level. Due to the site-specific nature and based on the number of teeth with clinical attachment loss, chronic periodontitis can be classified into the following categories:

- *Localized chronic periodontitis,* meaning that less than 30% of the teeth show attachment and bone loss
- *Generalized chronic periodontitis,* meaning that 30% or more of the teeth show attachment and bone loss

During chronic periodontitis, the local inflammatory response may lead to different patterns of bone loss, including vertical (angular) and horizontal bone destruction. Although vertical bone loss is associated with intrabony pocket formation, horizontal bone loss is usually associated with suprabony (supraalveolar) pockets.

Key Differences Between Gingivitis and Chronic Periodontitis

Plaque-Induced Gingivitis	Chronic Periodontitis
Inflammation of the gingiva without attachment/bone loss.	Inflammation of periodontal apparatus with attachment/bone loss.
With optimal oral hygiene, this condition can be resolved completely (reversible).	The attachment loss is irreversible, in spite of successfully controlling the inflammation.
Not all sites with gingivitis progress to periodontitis	All patients with chronic periodontitis must have experienced prior gingivitis
The dental implant counterpart of gingivitis is peri-implant mucositis.	The dental implant counterpart of periodontitis is peri-implantitis.

Disease Severity

With chronic periodontitis, severity and extent of periodontal destruction will occur over time in combination with systemic disorders impairing or enhancing host immune responses. Patients with chronic periodontitis experience a progression in attachment and bone loss as they become older. If untreated and oral hygiene behaviors remain unchanged, chronic periodontitis eventually leads to tooth loss and may negatively impact distant organs by the uncontrolled progression

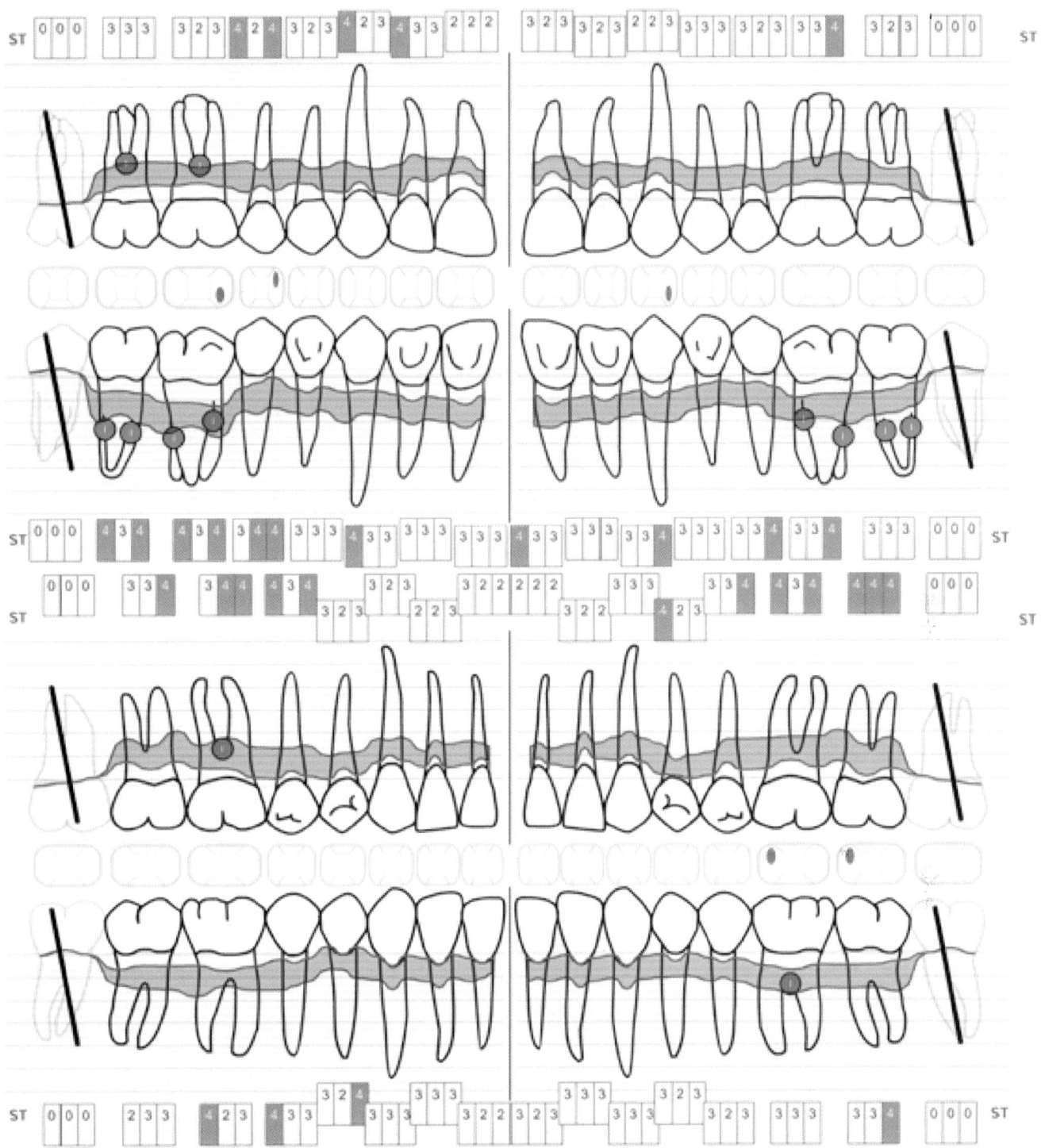

Fig. 27.6 Documentation of the periodontal attachment level in the same patient (see Figs. 27.1 to 27.5) after active periodontal therapy was completed and the supportive periodontal therapy was initiated. The red line displays the gingival margin reflecting recessions after therapy. Clinical attachment loss is illustrated by the filled (blue) area on the root surfaces. The deepest periodontal pocket measured was 4 mm. *(Reprinted from Kebschull M, Dommisch H: Resektive parodontalchirurgie. Zahnmedizin up-2-date. 2012; 525–545.)*

of periodontal inflammation and by the systemic spread of infection. Relative to the degree of attachment and bone loss, disease severity can be described as mild, moderate, or severe. These degrees are defined as follows:

- *Mild chronic periodontitis:* clinical attachment loss of 1 to 2 mm
- *Moderate chronic periodontitis:* clinical attachment loss of 3 to 4 mm

- *Severe chronic periodontitis:* clinical attachment loss of 5 mm or more

Symptoms

Chronic periodontitis is commonly a slowly progressing complex disease without a pain experience. Therefore most patients are unaware that they have developed a chronic disease. For the majority of patients, gingival bleeding during oral hygiene procedures or eating may be the first sign of disease occurrence. Areas with advanced periodontal inflammation may present with purulence emanating from the periodontal pocket. As a result of gingival recession, patients may notice black triangles between teeth or tooth sensitivity in response to temperature changes (cold and heat). In addition, food impaction may occur in the space of interdental triangles, leading to increased discomfort and bad breath. In cases with advanced attachment and bone loss, tooth mobility, tooth movement, fanned out or elongated front teeth, and, in rare occasions, tooth loss may be reported. In cases with advanced disease progression, areas of localized dull pain or pain sensations radiating to other areas of the mouth or head may occur.

KEY FACT

Site Specificity of Chronic Periodontitis

Not all sites in the mouth are equally prone to chronic periodontitis, and it exhibits site specificity. The progression of the disease occurs in certain sites but not uniformly. Interproximal sites, in general, are more prone to periodontal destruction, compared to buccal/facial sites.

Disease Progression

Chronic periodontitis may develop at any time in life. First clinical signs of inflammation may occur even during adolescence when the oral hygiene is neglected and dental plaque and calculus were allowed to accumulate. In general, the progression rate of chronic periodontitis is slow, so that symptoms of the disease appear around the age of 40 or later in life. Onset and the rate of disease progression, however, may be influenced by a number of modifiable (e.g., smoking, diet) and nonmodifiable (e.g., genetic disorders and risk issues) factors. In this context, patients who develop a metabolic disorder, such as diabetes mellitus, may exhibit a much higher progression rate of chronic periodontitis along with increased alveolar bone loss, periodontal bleeding, and pocketing.[73,95,100] Thus diabetes mellitus and the degree of blood sugar control belong to the most important systemic factors that are directly correlated with periodontal disease.

The progression pattern of chronic periodontitis does not show equal degrees of attachment loss on each affected site over time.

Although some sites exhibit more rapid periodontal breakdown over time, the attachment level remains static at other sites in the dentition for longer time periods.[58] Interestingly, disease progression is more rapid at interproximal sites compared to oral or buccal areas of neighboring teeth.[56,59] This phenomenon may be explained by the fact that these interproximal areas become wider along with disease progression, recession development, and the related increased probability of plaque accumulation and food impaction in those areas. Plaque control becomes more difficult, and interproximal furcation areas, interproximal caries, root caries, overhanging restoration margins, and tooth crowding may further promote interproximal attachment loss.

As chronic periodontitis exhibits individual and heterogeneous progression patterns throughout the dentition, three different models have been proposed to describe the rate of disease progression and determine the degree of attachment loss over time[17] as follows[92]:

- The continuous model:
  - Describes slow and continuous disease progression
  - Suggests that sites exhibit a constant progression rate of attachment loss throughout the duration of the disease
- The random or episodic-burst model:
  - Describes the episodic occurrence of short progressive bursts of periodontal destruction followed by periods of stagnation
  - Sites, teeth, and the chronology of bursts and stagnation are subject to random effects
- The asynchronous, multiple-burst model:
  - Describes the occurrence of periodontal destruction (bursts) during defined periods, which are asynchronously interrupted by periods of stagnation or remission for individual sites and teeth

Prevalence

Chronic periodontitis is considered to be one of the most common chronic diseases in humans, and the prevalence of the disease increases with age equally in both genders. In general, 40% of patients ≥50 years old and almost 50% of patients ≥65 years old show signs of mild to moderate periodontal destruction. The prevalence of severe forms of periodontitis also increases with age. From 11% to 30% of patients develop severe periodontitis at the age of 40 years or older (Figs. 27.7 and 27.8).[14,22,28,39,94] The worldwide prevalence for

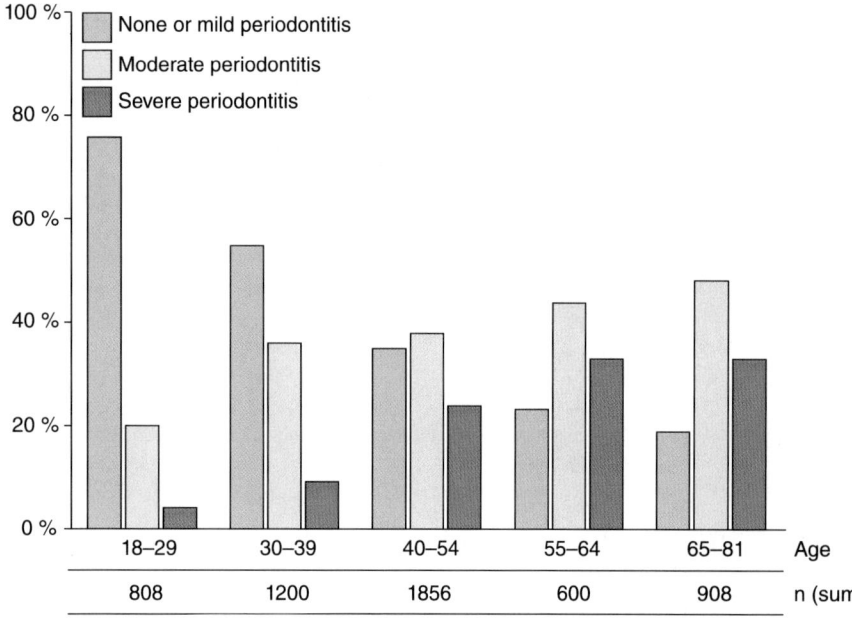

Fig. 27.7 Prevalence for periodontitis in the United States and Germany (2007–2009). *(Data from Genco et al., 2007,[28] and Holtfreter et al., 2009,[39] and reviewed in Demmer & Papapanou, 2010.[14])*

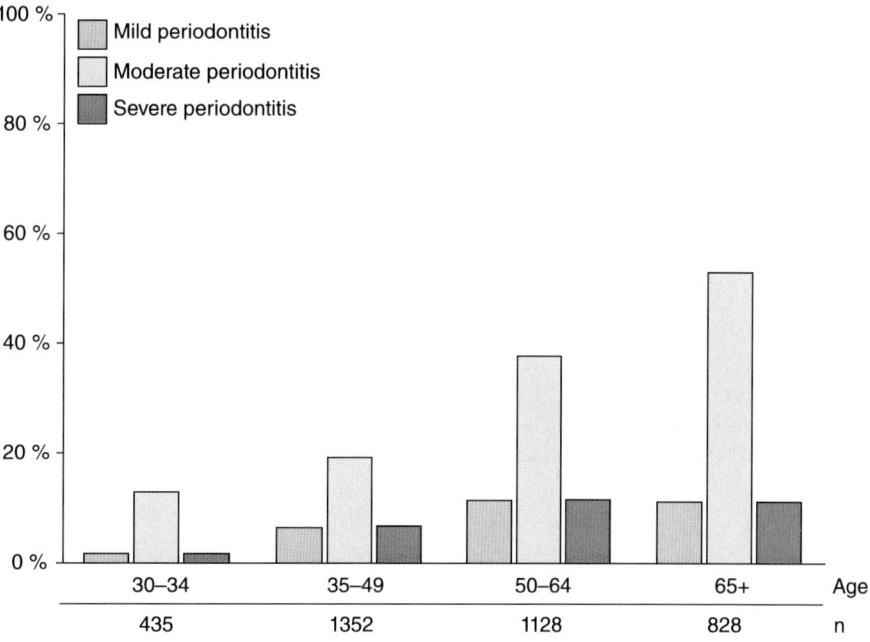

Fig. 27.8 Prevalence for periodontitis in the United States (2009–2010). *(Data from Eke PI, Dye BA, Wei L, et al: Prevalence of periodontitis in adults in the United States: 2009 and 2010. J Dent Res 91:914–920, 2012.)*

severe chronic periodontitis is estimated at 10.5% to 12% of the world's population.[44]

Risk Factors for Disease

A number of factors influence the etiopathogenesis of chronic periodontitis. The composition of the oral microflora and the amount of dental biofilm (plaque) are major etiologic factors. In this context, the extent of the periodontal destruction depends on the host immune competence as well as genetic predispositions influencing the individual susceptibility to disease. In addition, both systemic diseases and environmental factors interfere with the development and progression of chronic periodontitis. The risk factors described in the following sections (microbiological, local, systemic, immunologic, genetic, environmental, and behavioral) may occur simultaneously, or a selection of factors is present in patients with chronic periodontitis. The degree of the individual risk factor contribution differs among patients, so it is worthwhile to not only identify the risk factors but also to specify each risk factor's degree of contribution.

The prior history of gingivitis and periodontitis should be considered as general predictors for the development or progression of chronic periodontitis.[56] It is possible that the disease could not be successfully treated in the first place. The reason for an unsuccessful treatment outcome can be as simple as the patient's unwillingness (noncompliant patients) to understand the disease or perform proper oral hygiene. On the other hand, reasons for disease progression can also be more complex when nonmodifiable factors—such as genetic predispositions/syndromes, severe immunologic disorders, other therapies (e.g., organ transplantations) that affect the patient's immune status, lack of dexterity, or other systemic diseases—are present. This highlights the complexity of not only the development but also the progression/reoccurrence of chronic periodontitis. Several risk factors that contribute to the patient's susceptibility to chronic periodontitis are discussed next.

Microbiologic Aspects

Plaque accumulation on tooth and gingival surfaces (dental biofilm formation) at the dentogingival junction is considered the primary initiating agent in the etiology of gingivitis and chronic periodontitis.[56]

As the dental biofilm develops, early signs of an inflammatory reaction occur in the gingival margin (gingivitis) without attachment loss. Generally, optimal plaque control leads to the complete resolution of this early gingival inflammation.[62] With neglected oral hygiene on the other hand, inflammation will progress and eventually result in the loss of attachment around teeth.[56] Although not all patients with gingivitis develop periodontitis, it is known that all patients with periodontitis experienced prior gingivitis. The occurrence of periodontitis depends on the individual immune response that modifies the onset and progression of the disease.[56,68,70]

Attachment and bone loss are associated with an increase in the proportion of gram-negative organisms in the subgingival biofilm, with specific increases in organisms known to be pathogenic and virulent. *Porphyromonas gingivalis, Tannerella forsythia,* and *Treponema denticola,* otherwise known as the *red complex bacteria,* are frequently associated with ongoing attachment and bone loss in chronic periodontitis.[91] Development and progression of chronic periodontitis may not depend on the presence of one specific bacterium or bacterial complex alone. It is assumed that chronic periodontitis is the sequelae of a multispecies infection with a number of different bacteria that influence the proinflammatory immune response of the host.[46,82] Furthermore, the concept of host-microbial interactions has gained scientific attention. It has been found that increased numbers of periodontal pathogens contribute to the development of a dysbiotic microbial environment, which is triggered by the inflammatory milieu in the periodontal pocket.[2,36] This concept describes a shift from a symbiotic microbial environment to the development of dysbiosis within the biofilm involving so-called keystone pathogens, such as *P. gingivalis,* as a polymicrobial synergistic effect.[33–35] Periodontal pathogens like *P. gingivalis* may then invade the periodontal tissue and therewith induce further immune responses with increasing concentrations of proinflammatory mediators that may enhance periodontal breakdown. In addition, a number of periodontal pathogens are capable of producing proteases that directly affect the tissues and host immune responses.[70]

Local Factors

Plaque accumulation and biofilm development are the primary causes of periodontal inflammation and destruction. Therefore factors that facilitate plaque accumulation or prevent plaque removal by oral hygiene procedures can be detrimental to the patient. Plaque-retentive factors are important in the development and progression of chronic periodontitis because they retain microorganisms in proximity to the periodontal tissues, providing an ecologic niche for biofilm maturation. Calculus is considered the most important plaque-retentive factor because of its ability to retain and harbor plaque bacteria on its rough surface as well as inside.[42,89] As a consequence, calculus removal is essential for the maintenance of a healthy periodontium. In addition, the tooth morphology may influence plaque retention. Roots may show grooves or concavities, and in some instances, enamel projections on the surface or furcation entrances. Those morphologic variations may facilitate plaque retention, subgingival calculus formation, and disease progression.[29,40,78] In addition, subgingival and overhanging margins of restorations, carious lesions that extend subgingivally, and furcations exposed by loss of bone promote plaque retention.[50,101]

Common Retentive Local Factors That Contribute to Chronic Periodontitis
- Dental calculus
- Crown margins
- Restoration overhangs
- Furcation involvement
- Deep probing depths
- Anatomic grooves on the roots
- Subgingival caries or resorptive lesions

Systemic Factors

Chronic periodontitis is a complex disease that may not be limited to infection at local sites, but in several instances periodontitis is also associated with other systemic disorders, such as Haim–Munk syndrome, Papillon–Lefèvre syndrome, Ehlers–Danlos syndrome, Kindler syndrome, and Cohen syndrome. Patients who suffer from diseases that impair host immune responses (e.g., HIV/AIDS) may also show periodontal destruction. Further, it is also known that osteoporosis, severe unbalanced diet, and stress, as well as dermatologic, hematologic, and neoplastic factors, interfere with periodontal inflammatory responses. In addition to defined syndromes, periodontitis is also associated with severe systemic diseases, such as diabetes mellitus, cardiovascular disorders, stroke, and lung disorders.[1,9,45,67,70,98,99,102]

Periodontitis is now considered as the sixth complication of diabetes mellitus.[27,61] For diabetes mellitus and periodontitis, there is a known interaction during which both diseases mutually correlate to each other.[54] Patients with diabetes mellitus exhibit a higher risk to develop periodontitis, and the periodontal infection/inflammation may negatively interfere with the glycemic control of the diabetic patient.[73] A number of studies showed that prevalence, severity, and prognosis of periodontitis are associated with the incidence of diabetes mellitus. It was found that the average pocket depth as well as the clinical attachment loss was increased in patients with diabetes mellitus (independently from the type of diabetes mellitus).[15,47,73,81] Patients with poor glycemic control tend to experience more severe progression of periodontitis compared to patients with good glycemic control. Regarding the progression of severe periodontitis, no difference was found between patients with good glycemic control and nondiabetic patients.[100] With diabetes mellitus, advanced glycation end products (AGEs) may arise, which lead to the release of free oxygen and proinflammatory mediators (cytokines). AGEs may also promote

chemotaxis and adhesion of inflammatory cells to periodontal tissues, and increased apoptosis of fibroblasts and osteoblasts may occur.[31] Furthermore, patients with diabetes mellitus tend to show a higher body mass index, and therefore increased concentrations of adipokines that directly influence inflammatory responses were found.[74] Hyperglycemia per se leads to the release of proinflammatory mediators in the bloodstream, which in turn promote increased glucose concentration.[73] Periodontal therapy may contribute to glycemic control of the diabetic patient. It was shown that the systematic therapy of chronic periodontitis leads to an at least short-term reduction of glycated hemoglobin (HbA1c) of approximately 0.3% up to 0.6%.[7,9,41,57,90] Each therapy regimen that contributes to achieve reduction of glycated hemoglobin may decrease the risk of diabetes-related long-term consequences, such as myocardial infarction, microvascular complications, and many others.[73]

In the context of diabetes mellitus, a number of patients exhibit an increased body weight (obesity), which also correlates with the prevalence and severity of periodontal attachment and bone loss.[66] The negative effect of a high body mass index with regard to the outcome of periodontal therapy was comparable to the negative effect that has been described for smoking.[93]

Immunologic Factors

Chronic periodontitis is a disease induced by bacteria organized in the dental biofilm. Onset, progression, and severity of the disease depend, however, on the individual host immune response.[26,68] Patients may show alterations of peripheral monocytes, which relate to reduced reactivity of lymphocytes or enhanced B-cell response.[68,70] Not only B cells and macrophages, but also periodontal ligament cells, gingival fibroblasts, and epithelial cells synthesize proinflammatory mediators—such as interleukin-1 beta (IL-1 beta), IL-6, IL-8, prostaglandin-E2 (PGE2), tumor-necrosis factor alpha (TNF-alpha), and many others—that modify innate and adaptive immune responses at periodontal sites.[11,18–21,48,75] Proinflammatory mediators regulate synthesis and secretion of matrix-metalloproteinases (MMPs) and receptor-activator-of-NF-kappaB-ligand (RANKL). In periodontal lesions, MMPs contribute to soft and hard tissue degradation during active inflammatory processes.[26] RANKL binds to its receptor RANK on the cell surface of premature osteoclasts, and therewith it initiates osteoclast differentiation leading to degradation of alveolar bone.[26,48,75] Physiologically, osteoprotegerin (OPG) is an inhibitor of RANKL, and during periodontitis, an imbalance between OPG and RANKL promotes further bone degradation.[26]

In addition, reduced counts in neutrophils (polymorphonuclear neutrophils [PMNs]) influence the degree of periodontal inflammation. Congenital neutropenia (Kostmann syndrome) leads not only to an increased susceptibility to infection in general, but also to severe chronic periodontitis. Patients with Kostmann syndrome show reduced levels of antimicrobial peptides, such as the cathelicidin (LL-37) and neutrophil peptides (alpha defensins), which impair their innate immune response.[8,76] LL-37 is an effective antimicrobial peptide that is synthesized from inactive precursors, and mutations in the cathepsin C gene hinder cleavage, and therewith activation, of LL-37. Those genetic alterations contribute to the severity and progression of chronic periodontitis (Papillon–Lefèvre syndrome, Haim–Munk syndrome).[13,38]

Genetic Factors

Periodontitis is considered to be a complex inflammatory disease influenced by local, systemic, and immunologic factors (discussed earlier). Each factor is in turn directly related to individual genetic conditions. Several genetic disorders are known to show periodontal destruction as one of their major symptoms. For example,

Papillon–Lefèvre syndrome is a well-known genetic disorder (a defect on chromosome 11) that exhibits not only palmoplantar hyperkeratosis but also severe periodontitis.[23,37,51] Besides Papillon–Lefèvre syndrome, Haim–Munk syndrome, Ehlers–Danlos syndrome, Down syndrome, Kindler syndrome, Cohen syndrome, and congenital neutropenia (Kostmann syndrome) are other genetic disorders that have been related to periodontal disease. These genetic conditions are discussed extensively in Chapter 11.

Periodontal disease has been found in different family members (twins, siblings) and generations of one family. Early twin studies suggested the involvement of genetic susceptibility factors in the etiopathogenesis of periodontitis.[63] In a number of studies, the prevalence of aggressive and chronic periodontitis has been investigated in families with a history of one or more family members with periodontitis. The data from those studies showed variable results with a likelihood for heritability of up to 50%. Variations are mainly due to different study designs as well as the number of evaluated individuals.[3,60,64,83]

> ### Treatment of Chronic Periodontitis
> Chronic periodontitis can be treated effectively by a systematic periodontal therapy that includes optimal long-term plaque control, debridement of soft and hard deposits, or surgical pocket reduction (case-dependently either resective osseous surgery or regenerative surgery; Figs. 27.4 and 27.5). Depending on the individual periodontal risk, each patient should be remotivated, reinstructed, and retreated (if necessary) during a systematic supportive periodontal therapy regimen (revisits every 3, 6, or 12 months; Fig. 27.6).

In addition, other genetic variations (single nucleotide polymorphisms [SNPs], genetic copy number variations) that have so far not been identified as responsible for certain syndromes may also directly influence innate and adaptive immune responses as well as the structure of periodontal tissues. The identification of genes that are relevant to the development of periodontitis has led to new scientific concepts and findings. There are at least two different strategies (candidate genes and genome-wide associations) to identify genetic variances in relation to disease. In candidate gene studies, certain already known variances (SNPs) are correlated to a specific phenotype such as periodontitis. Therefore a hypothesis is required in order to choose specific SNPs in relevant genes. The data from those studies showed variable results, making it challenging to draw clear conclusions. In this context, studies on SNPs in the IL-1 gene led to the early conclusion that alterations in sequences of immunologically relevant genes may explain the heritability of periodontitis.[49] Conflicting data in the literature, however, indicate inconclusive knowledge regarding SNPs in the IL-1 gene and their potential role in the heritability and etiopathogenesis of periodontitis.[53] Also, it seems implausible that a single polymorphism in a specific gene sequence can cause a complex inflammatory disease, such as periodontitis, without causing any other symptoms relevant to one's systemic health. Thus genome-wide association studies (GWASs) have become more relevant. Here, a high number of DNA-sequence variances are evaluated at the same time. In contrast to candidate gene studies, no hypotheses are required for GWASs, so that there is no potential bias during analysis. In several GWASs, a number of new genes have been identified to be associated with periodontitis. One of the best replicated genes is called *ANRIL* (antisense RNA in the Inc locus). *ANRIL* is associated not only with periodontitis but

also with cardiovascular disease, which underlines potential systemic interactions.[12,85–87] The role of *ANRIL* during the development of periodontitis is subject to ongoing investigations. It is known that it represents a noncoding regulatory RNA, which is involved during the regulation of cell division and in affecting other genes that play a role in the glucose and lipid metabolism *(ADIPOR1, VAMP3, C11ORF10)*.[6,16,103] In addition to *ANRIL*, genetic variances (SNPs) in the sequences of the glucosyltransferase-6 domain containing 1 gene *(GLT6D1)*, the plasminogen gene *(PLA)*, and the neuropeptide Y gene *(NPY)* have been associated with periodontal disease.[25,84,88] Due to the current technical and scientific progress, it may be expected that more genes will be identified to be associated with periodontitis in the future.

Environmental and Behavioral Factors

In addition to microbial, immunologic, and genetic factors, the development and progression of chronic periodontitis is further influenced by environmental and behavioral factors such as smoking and psychological stress[68,70] Smoking is a major risk factor for the development and progression of generalized chronic periodontitis.[4] Periodontitis is influenced by smoking in a dose-dependent manner. The intake of more than 10 cigarettes per day tremendously increases the risk of disease progression when compared to nonsmokers and former smokers, respectively.[97]

Compared to nonsmokers, the following features are found in smokers[5,43,72,80]:

- Increased periodontal pocket depth with more than 3 mm
- Increased attachment loss
- More recessions
- Increased loss of alveolar bone
- Increased tooth loss
- Fewer signs of gingivitis (less bleeding upon probing)
- A greater incidence of furcation involvement

Due to the consumption of tobacco, reactive oxygen (radicals) is released that chemically irritates periodontal tissues by DNA damage, lipid peroxidation of cell membranes, damage of endothelial cells, and the induction of smooth muscle cell growth.[65]

Psychological factors, such as stress and depression, also negatively influence the progression of chronic periodontitis.[30] Patients with periodontitis often report the experience of family- or work-related stress.[71] Positive correlations between cortisol levels and periodontal indices (plaque index, gingival index), bone loss, and missing teeth were recorded.[17,30,77] In addition, stress as an etiologic factor was even strongly associated with periodontitis when patients were smokers compared to nonsmokers.[10]

> ### Stress and Periodontal Disease: Potential Mechanisms
> 1. Immunosuppression via cortisol secretion
> 2. Poor oral hygiene compliance in patients with chronic stress
> 3. Patients with stress are less likely to seek professional care
> 4. Patients with stress may smoke more frequently

 Case Scenarios are found on the companion website www.expertconsult.com.

References

 References for this chapter are found on the companion website www.expertconsult.com.

CHAPTER 28

Aggressive Periodontitis

Moritz Kebschull | Henrik Dommisch

Overview

Periodontitis is the pathologic manifestation of the host response against bacterial challenge that stems from a polymicrobial biofilm at the biofilm–gingival interface.[55] There are several subforms of the disease primarily defined by their clinical phenotype (i.e., the rate of disease progression and other features) rather than their (still partially unknown) etiology. This chapter addresses aggressive periodontitis, a clinically challenging subform of periodontitis featuring rapid loss of periodontal attachment and tooth supporting bone in otherwise healthy patients.

Historical Background

In 1923 Gottlieb reported on a patient with a fatal case of epidemic influenza and a disease that Gottlieb called "diffuse atrophy of the alveolar bone."[25] This disease was characterized by a loss of collagen fibers in the periodontal ligament and their replacement by loose connective tissue and extensive bone resorption, resulting in a widened periodontal space. The gingiva apparently was not involved. In 1928 Gottlieb attributed this condition to the inhibition of continuous cementum formation, which he considered essential for maintenance of the periodontal fibers.[26] He then termed the disease *deep cementopathia* and hypothesized that this was a "disease of eruption" and that cementum initiated a foreign body response. As a result, it was postulated that the host attempted to exfoliate the tooth, resulting in the observed bone resorption and pocket formation.

In 1938 Wannenmacher described incisor–first molar involvement and called the disease *parodontitis marginalis progressiva*.[85] Several explanations evolved for the etiology and pathogenesis of this type of disease. Many authors considered this to be a degenerative, noninflammatory disease process and therefore gave it the name *periodontosis*.[24,57,81] Other investigators denied the existence of a degenerative type of periodontal disease and attributed the changes observed to trauma from occlusion.[11,51] Finally, in 1966, the World Workshop in Periodontics concluded that the concept of "periodontosis" as a degenerative entity was unsubstantiated and that the term should be eliminated from periodontal nomenclature.[62] The committee did recognize that a clinical entity different from *adult periodontitis* might occur among adolescents and young adults.

The term *juvenile periodontitis* was introduced by Chaput and colleagues in 1967 and by Butler in 1969.[10] In 1971, Baer defined it

as "a disease of the periodontium occurring in an otherwise healthy adolescent which is characterized by a rapid loss of alveolar bone about more than one tooth of the permanent dentition. The amount of destruction manifested is not commensurate with the amount of local irritants."[6] In 1989 the World Workshop in Clinical Periodontics categorized this disease as *localized juvenile periodontitis (LJP)*, a subset of the broad classification of *early-onset periodontitis (EOP)*.[12] Under this classification system, age of onset and distribution of lesions were of primary importance when making a diagnosis of LJP.

In 1999 the World Workshop in Periodontics introduced a novel classification that was meant to eliminate the shortcomings of earlier endeavors in classifying periodontal disease. Importantly, the new 1999 classification sought "to discard classification terminologies that were age-dependent or required knowledge of rates of progression."[3] In the new classification scheme, several rapidly progressing periodontitis forms were united under the term *aggressive periodontitis*.

A new World Workshop in Periodontics was jointly planned by the European Federation of Periodontology and the American Academy of Periodontology for November 2017 in order to further refine the classification of periodontal diseases. Please check Expert Consult site for update.

Classification and Clinical Characteristics

Features

The 1999 international classification workshop defined the entity of aggressive periodontitis to be characterized by three primary features (Table 28.1)[43]:

1. *Rapid loss of attachment and tooth-supporting bone.* In aggressive periodontitis, as compared to the more common variant chronic periodontitis, the loss of attachment progresses significantly faster. To evaluate this rapid course of destruction, the evaluation of clinical or radiographic data from earlier points in time (allowing for making an estimate of the start of disease) is necessary.[56] Note that the age of the patient is per se no primary criterion for the diagnosis of aggressive periodontitis. Because earlier clinical records are often not available, many clinicians argue that severe loss of attachment in young patients conceivably must be due to a rapid course of disease progression. This is, however, not generally true—neglect of all oral hygiene in a

TABLE 28.1   Diagnostic Criteria to Distinguish Chronic and Aggressive Periodontitis

Criterion	Aggressive Periodontitis	Chronic Periodontitis
Rate of progression	Rapid	Slow; rapid episodes possible
Familiar aggregation	Typical	Can be present when families share imperfect oral hygiene habits
Presence of etiologic factors (plaque, calculus, overhanging restorations, etc.)	Often minimal	Often commensurate with observed periodontal destruction
Age	Often in young patients (<35 years) but can be found in all age groups	Often in older patients (>55 years) but can be found in all age groups
Clinical inflammation signs	Sometimes lacking (especially in localized aggressive periodontitis)	Commensurate with etiologic factors

TABLE 28.2   Diagnostic Criteria for Localized and Generalized Aggressive Periodontitis

Criterion	Localized Aggressive Periodontitis	Generalized Aggressive Periodontitis
Age of onset	Circumpubertal	Most often <30 years of age, but can occur in older individuals too
Serum antibody response against infecting agents	Robust	Poor
Destruction pattern	Localized attachment loss at incisors and first molars—interproximal attachment loss at ≥ 2 permanent teeth, one of which is a first molar, and involvement of ≤ 2 teeth, other than first molars and incisors	Generalized interproximal attachment loss at ≥3 permanent teeth other than first molars and incisors
Additional		Episodic nature of attachment loss

periodontitis-susceptible individual over a decade will lead to severe attachment loss, even with a slow rate of progression. On the other hand, severe attachment loss in an older individual is not necessarily the result of long-lasting, slowly progressing disease. It is therefore inappropriate to use the age of an individual as a primary diagnostic criterion for the distinction of aggressive and chronic periodontitis. Note that in chronic periodontitis, there are reportedly periods of rapid disease progression that can by themselves be misinterpreted as aggressive periodontitis.

2. *Subject is otherwise healthy (i.e., not suffering from any systemic disease or condition that could be responsible for the present periodontitis).* There are systemic diseases that lead to severely altered host defenses against periodontal pathogens, often resulting in rapid loss of attachment and tooth loss at an early age. This disease is designated "periodontitis as a manifestation of systemic disease" (see Chapter 14). Note that the specific properties or abnormalities of some types of immune cells listed here and reported to be often associated with the diagnosis of aggressive periodontitis do not themselves qualify for the aforementioned diagnosis.

3. *Familiar aggregation.* Familiar aggregation of aggressive periodontitis cases is a feature that can be evaluated by medical/dental history questionnaires and interviewing the patient. It is, however, advisable to verify similar cases in the family, if possible, as many individuals may not be fully aware of their diagnoses and not a few cases of "bad teeth that run in the family" turn out to be caries related or likely due to chronic periodontitis. In addition, the workshop defined several secondary features that are generally found in aggressive periodontitis cases

but that are not universally necessary to diagnose the disease entity:

a. Inconsistency of the low amounts of present etiologic factors and the observed pronounced tissue destruction
b. Strong colonization by *Aggregatibacter actinomycetemcomitans* and (in some populations) *Porphyromonas gingivalis*
c. Immunologic differences that do not entail the diagnosis "periodontitis as a manifestation of systemic disease":
   • Hyperresponsive macrophages
   • Abnormalities of neutrophil function
d. Self-limiting disease

Subgroups

Aggressive periodontitis can be subclassified into a localized and generalized form. The diagnosis of the subcategory is based on clinical, radiographic, and historical data. These include the age of onset, the involvement of teeth other than first molars and incisors (the first permanent teeth to erupt), and the presence of a systemic antibody response against periodontal pathogens (see Table 28.2).

Generalized Aggressive Periodontitis

Generalized aggressive periodontitis (GAP) is the subgroup of periodontal disease characterized by the highest severity and extent of disease, but also by its large heterogeneity. The diagnosis of GAP encompasses the diseases previously classified as *generalized juvenile periodontitis (GJP)* and *rapidly progressive periodontitis (RPP)*.

Two gingival tissue responses can be found in cases of GAP (Figs. 28.1 and 28.2). One is a severe, acutely inflamed tissue, often proliferating, ulcerated, and fiery red. Bleeding may occur

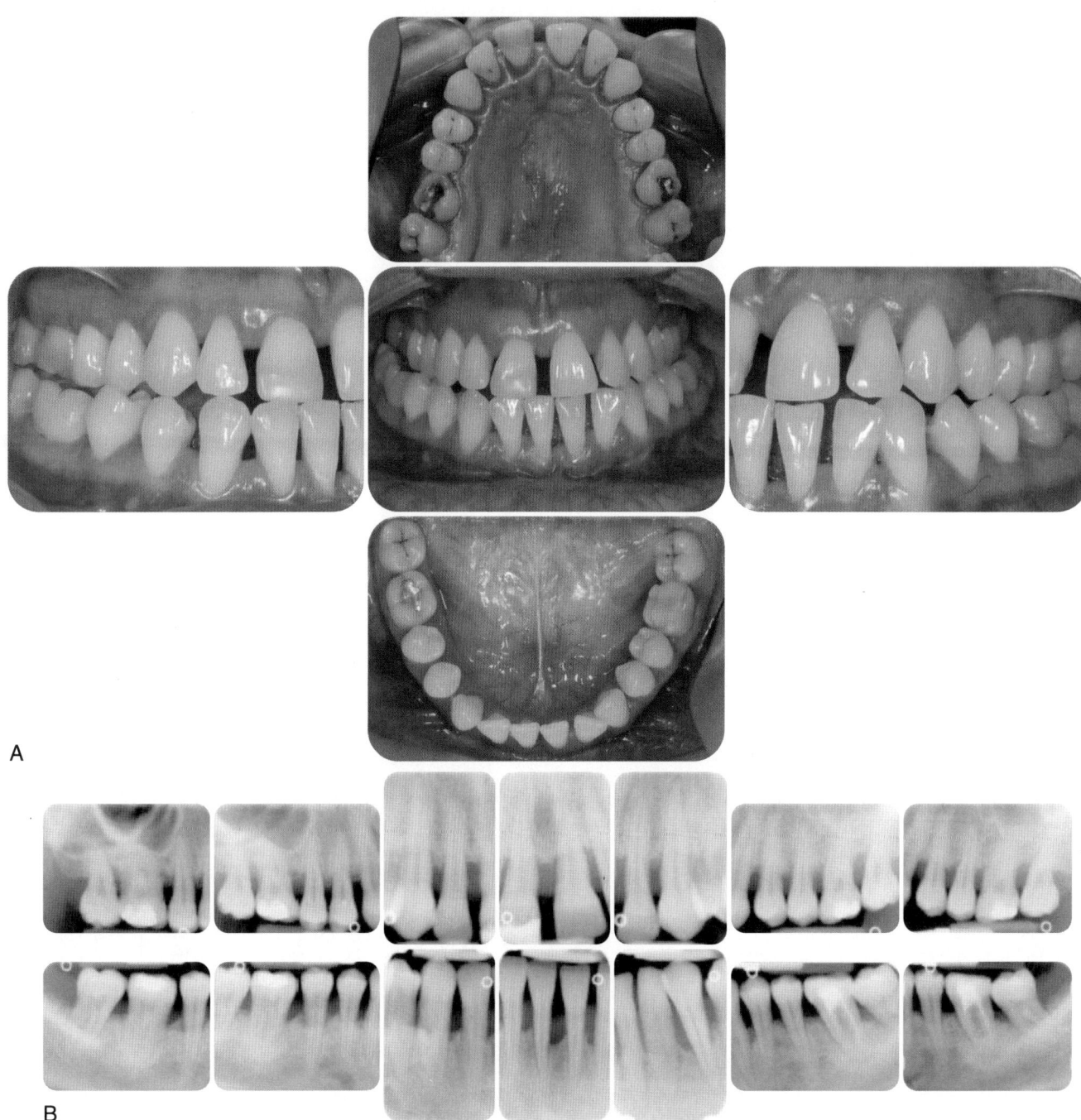

A

B

Fig. 28.1 Case Presentation: Generalized Aggressive Periodontitis Generalized aggressive periodontitis in a 28-year-old white female, nonsmoking patient. (A) Clinical views with minimal amounts of calculus and plaque. (B) Radiographically, bone loss ≥50% was present at all teeth.

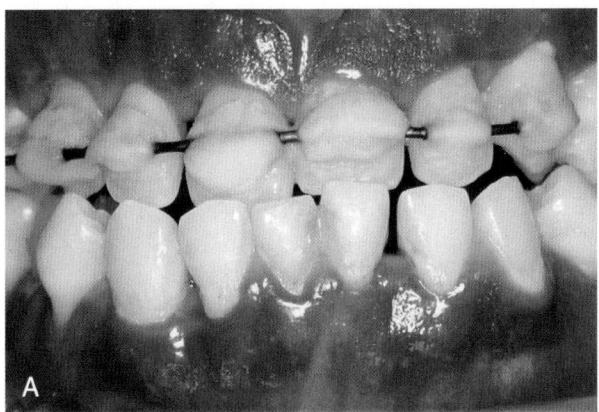
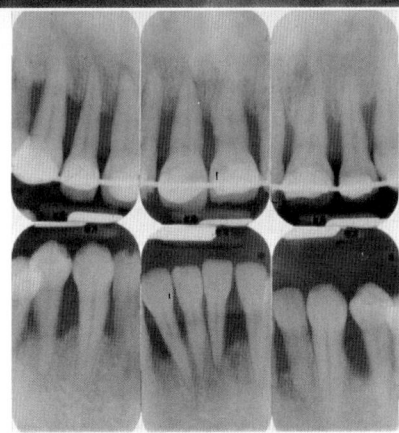
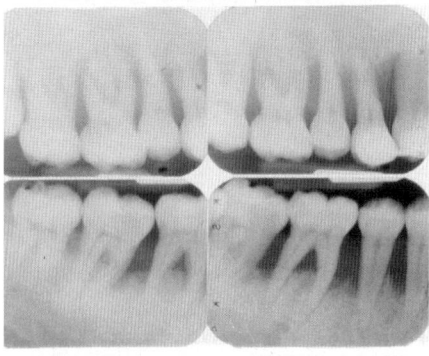
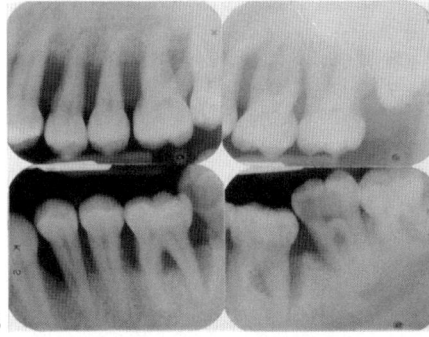

Fig. 28.2 Case Presentation: Generalized Aggressive Periodontitis Severe generalized aggressive periodontitis in a 22-year-old black male patient with a family history of early tooth loss through periodontal disease. (A) Clinical view showing minimal plaque and inflammation. A provisional wire-and-resin splint had been placed by the general-practice dentist to stabilize the teeth. (B) Radiographs showing the severe, generalized nature of the disease with all erupted teeth affected.

spontaneously or with slight stimulation. Suppuration may be an important feature. This tissue response is believed to occur in the destructive stage, in which attachment and bone are actively lost.

In other cases the gingival tissues may appear pink, free of inflammation, and occasionally with some degree of stippling, although stippling may be absent. However, despite the apparently mild clinical appearance, deep pockets can be demonstrated by probing. Page and Schroeder believed that this tissue response coincides with periods of quiescence in which the bone level remains stationary.[58]

Localized Aggressive Periodontitis

Localized aggressive periodontitis (LAP) is usually found in younger individuals than those affect by GAP (Figs. 28.3 and 28.4). It is characterized by more pronounced systemic antibody titers against periodontal pathogens than found in GAP patients. This could indicate that in individuals susceptible to disease, but with the ability to enact a robust response against pathogens, the disease might be limited in extent (i.e., LAP), whereas in individuals with a lesser humoral response, the disease would not be limited to the first permanent teeth (i.e., the patient would develop GAP). This would mean that LAP and GAP would merely be phenotypic variations of the same underlying disease. This assumption is backed by several reports that show a sequence of LAP and GAP in the same individuals over time.[9,31,74] On the other hand, several lines of evidence exist that support a claim that LAP constitutes a disease on its own, with dissimilar underlying molecular and cellular mechanisms.

Epidemiology

The question of the prevalence of aggressive periodontitis in different populations is complicated by the fact that the currently used classification[3] is relatively young and not easy to apply in epidemiologic studies. Therefore many available studies either (1) report on older, previously used entities of periodontitis that showed early onset or rapid progression but are not interchangeable with aggressive periodontitis or (2) report only on periodontitis severity, not on diagnosis (for detailed reviews, see Albandar[2] and Susin and Albandar[78]). The problem of a lacking universal case definition for epidemiologic research is critical, because different case definitions for periodontitis in adolescents described differences in prevalence of up to 10-fold.[47]

Case Definition

The diagnosis of aggressive periodontitis in epidemiologic studies is difficult, because all primary criteria for the disease—rapid progression, systemic health, and familiar aggregation—are difficult to reliably assess in the setting of such a study. The criteria of systemic health and familiar aggregation would require extensive interviews and thorough verification. The rapid progression of disease can consistently be documented only by following a subject longitudinally and performing at least two subsequent examinations within a reasonable time frame or (as noted previously) be extrapolated from older clinical or radiographic records. These, however, are frequently not available and would add extensive bias to the study, as prior providers of oral care were not calibrated. Radiographic examinations at the time of examination are, in the setting of an epidemiologic study, most often unfeasible.[2]

As a result, to date, methodologically sound epidemiologic studies investigating aggressive periodontitis as defined by the 1999 workshop are sparse (e.g., the study performed in a population of young Israeli army recruits).[44]

Therefore to be able to assess the prevalence of aggressive periodontitis in other populations, Demmer and Papapanou[16] proposed

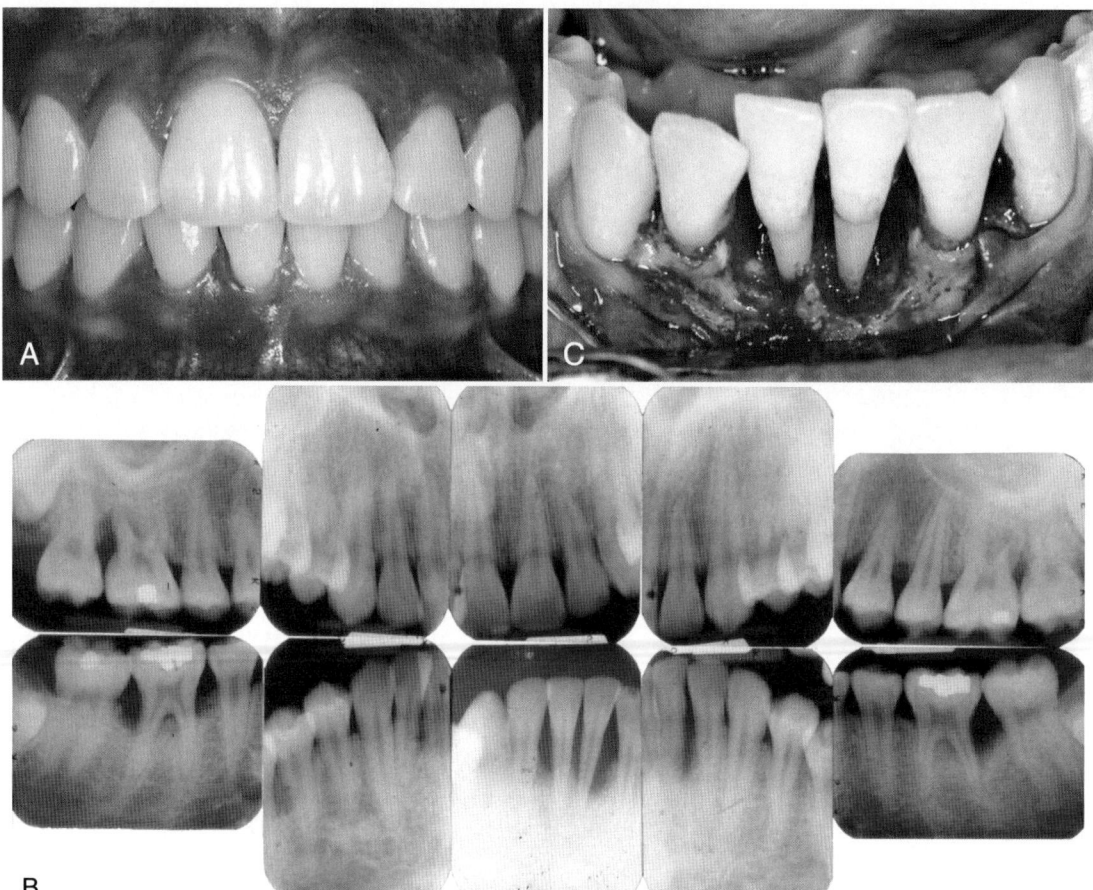

Fig. 28.3 Case Presentation: Localized Aggressive Periodontitis Localized aggressive periodontitis in a 15-year-old black female patient who had a twin with a similar disease. (A) Clinical view showing minimal plaque and inflammation except for localized inflammation on the distal side of the maxillary left central incisor and the mandibular right central incisor. (B) Radiographs showing localized, vertical, angular bone loss associated with the maxillary and mandibular first molars and the mandibular central incisors. The maxillary incisors show no apparent involvement. (C) Surgical appearance of the localized, vertical, angular bony defects affecting the mandibular incisors. Note the wide circumferential nature of the defects and the lack of calculus on the root surfaces.

to utilize the generally accepted case definition (see Chapter 6) for periodontitis proposed by a working group of the US Centers for Disease Control and Prevention (CDC) and the American Academy of Periodontology[17,59] in combination with the age of the study subject. Specifically, they assessed available studies for the proportion of subjects of ≤25 years of age who suffered from moderate or severe periodontitis according to the CDC definition, and the proportion of subjects 26 to 35 years of age who suffered from severe periodontitis (CDC definition). Similarly, Susin and Albandar[78] used a combination of diagnostic criteria to identify possible aggressive periodontitis cases in studies not designed following the 1999 classification.

Localized Aggressive Periodontitis

The prevalence of LAP in an Israeli army population ages 18 to 30 years was 4.3%. In this cohort, the presence of LAP was highly correlated with North African origin and current smoking.[44] A study of 830 Moroccan school students ages 12 to 25 years using the modified aggressive periodontitis definition of Albandar and coworkers[2] reported a prevalence of 4.9% for aggressive periodontitis, with approximately 70% exhibiting strong attachment loss at the molar sites.[37]

In addition to these data, several studies have examined the prevalence of LJP, the predecessor of LAP (however, not exactly

interchangeable), from diverse populations. The prevalence of this disease in geographically diverse adolescent populations was estimated at less than 1%. Most reports suggested a low prevalence of about 0.2%.[45] Two independent radiographic studies of 16-year-old adolescents, one in Finland[66] and the other in Switzerland,[39] followed the strict diagnostic criteria delineated by Baer[6] and reported a prevalence rate of 0.1%. A clinical and radiographic study of 7266 English adolescents 15 to 19 years old also showed a prevalence rate of 0.1%.[65] In the United States, a national survey of adolescents ages 14 to 17 reported that 0.53% had LJP.[45] Blacks were at much higher risk for LJP, and black male teenagers were 2.9 times more likely to have the disease than black female adolescents. In contrast, white female teenagers were more likely to have LJP than white male adolescents. Several other studies have found the highest prevalence of LJP among black males,[9,49,65] followed in descending order by black females, white females, and white males.[49]

JCP was reported to affect both males and females and is seen most frequently in the period between puberty and 20 years of age. Some studies have suggested a predilection for female patients, particularly in the youngest age groups,[31] whereas others reported no male–female differences in incidence when studies are designed to correct for ascertainment bias.[28]

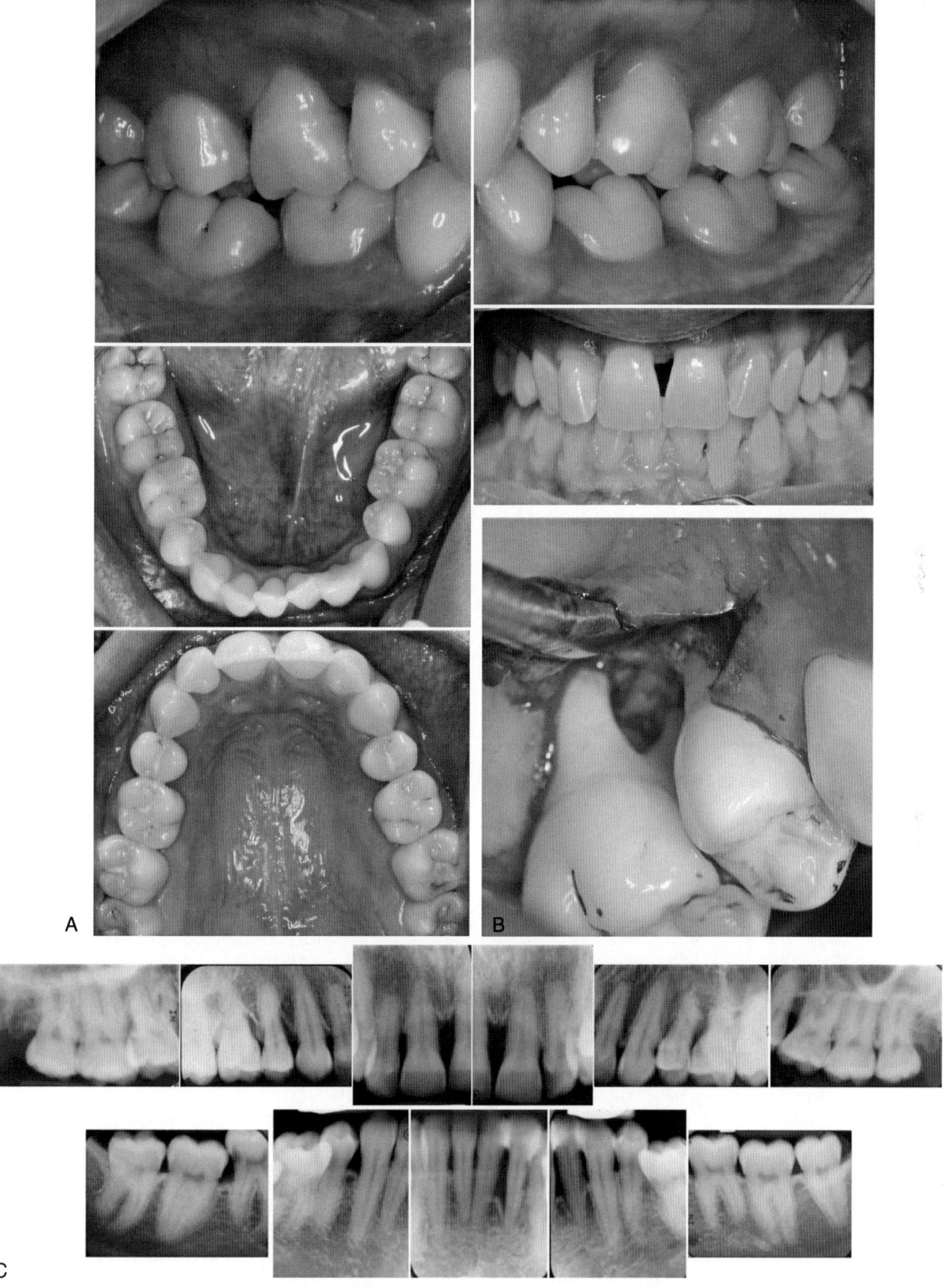

Fig. 28.4 Case Presentation: Localized Aggressive Periodontitis Localized aggressive periodontitis in an 18-year old white female, nonsmoking patient. Familiar aggregation was reported. (A) Clinical view showing recessions at incisors and first molars. (B) Intraoperative view showing massive localized, angular bony defect associated with a first molar. (C) Radiographs showing pronounced localized, angular bone loss. *(Courtesy Dr. Hendrik Schulze, Bonn, Germany.)*

Generalized Aggressive Periodontitis

Among young Israeli army recruits, 1.8% suffered from GAP.[44] When using extrapolation, as proposed by Demmer and Papapanou, a prevalence of about 1% to a maximum of 15% within the age range was found, depending on the study. Specifically, data from the German Study of Health in Pomerania indicate an extrapolated prevalence within the age group of 13% (≤29 years) and 7% (30–39 years), whereas the highest extrapolated prevalence was found in the Eerie County study, with up to 15% of the age group.

Note that, as indicated previously, using prior epidemiologic data for the heterogeneous predecessors of GAP, GJP, and RPP to assess GAP prevalence is not possible because these entities are not interchangeable with GAP. In contrast, LJP, although still different from LAP by definition, can be used as a surrogate for LAP.

Current Understanding

Taken together, these data primarily show that the discrimination of aggressive periodontitis and other forms of periodontitis is not always easy, especially when the patient is seen for only a single examination, as is the case in most epidemiologic studies. The prevalence of aggressive periodontitis of approximately 1% to 15% in subjects of ≤35 years of age, in combination with the severity and tendency for rapid progression of this disease, strongly suggests that all patients in this age group should be screened regularly for the presence of periodontal disease.

Pathobiology and Risk Factors

All forms of periodontitis share certain common pathobiologic principles as polymicrobial, biofilm-mediated chronic inflammatory diseases at the biofilm-gingival interface. These principles are addressed in detail in Chapters 7 to 9. Herein we focus on the biologic reasons for the rapid course of destruction in aggressive periodontitis, including work investigating the specific properties of aggressive periodontitis in periodontal microbiology, immunology, and genetics.

Microbiology

Periodontitis is caused by specific microorganisms in a susceptible host.[61] In the subgingival biofilm, up to 700 bacterial species have been identified,[40] some of which were identified to be causative.[14] Details on the current knowledge on different periodontal microorganisms are summarized in Chapters 8 and 9.

The observed higher rate of disease progression in aggressive versus chronic periodontitis could possibly be explained by the presence of specific microorganisms that cause and perpetuate tissue destruction. In addition, the reported familiar aggregation of aggressive periodontitis cases could also be, to a certain point, explained by an infection and within-family transmission of specific microorganisms.

Therefore several studies have sought to identify the specific microbial properties of aggressive periodontitis cases. However, when evaluating generalized and localized aggressive periodontitis as a single entity and solely focusing on a small number of "classic" pathogens, it has been concluded that microbiologic infection patterns could not reliably distinguish between this entity and chronic periodontitis cases.[52]

However, data from a limited number of studies using both classic microbiologic tools and more recent molecular techniques suggest that differences exist in the microbiologic composition between (1) localized aggressive periodontitis and both generalized aggressive and chronic periodontitis and (2) generalized aggressive and chronic periodontitis[20,23,41,63] (for a review, see Armitage[4]).

Specific Bacteria in Localized Aggressive Periodontitis

In localized aggressive periodontitis, the situation seems to be different. Here, several lines of evidence point to a strong role of specific microorganisms, most notably *A. actinomycetemcomitans*. For decades, this bacterial species has been associated with LAP[7,13,75] and could predict the development of LAP in two longitudinal studies.[21,30] Longitudinal studies are of critical importance for demonstrating a causal relationship, whereas cross-sectional studies can by definition only show correlations that cannot be used to infer causality.

In the first longitudinal study, age-, gender- and race-matched juvenile carriers and noncarriers of *A. actinomycetemcomitans* (serotypes a, b, c equally distributed, no JP2) were followed longitudinally. After 1 year of follow-up, 80% of the carriers, but only 10% of the noncarriers, had developed periodontitis.[21]

In the second, larger longitudinal study, the highly leukotoxic *A. actinomycetemcomitans* (serotype b) strain JP2, which has a 530-bp deletion in its leukotoxin gene operon that leads to a 10- to 20-fold higher production of leukotoxin,[29] was found to be directly related to the occurrence of LAP in children in northern Africa. Specifically, the OR for future attachment loss in carriers of the JP2 strain was 18.0, as compared to 3.0 for carriers of other, non-JP2 strains of *A. actinomycetemcomitans*.[30] Similar findings can be found in West African countries (e.g., Ghana[1]) in contrast to eastern parts of Africa where no studies have reported on JP2 clone strain in periodontitis patients.[18]

A recent study on the occurrence of JP2 clone strains in aggressive periodontitis patients shows a high incidence in both LAP and GAP, suggesting that both subclasses could be more related than initially thought.[19]

In addition, it needs to be noted that, as with all entities of periodontitis, LAP is clearly not a monoinfection with *A. actinomycetemcomitans* but features a polymicrobial biofilm. Supporting this notion are reports of confirmed cases of LAP that did not carry *A. actinomycetemcomitans*.[41,53]

Host Response to Bacterial Challenge

The inflammatory host response toward pathogens is generally attributed to be responsible for a larger proportion of the tissue destruction in periodontitis than the invading periodontal pathogens themselves. The rapid progression of aggressive periodontitis implies that, in addition to the aforementioned composition of the subgingival microbiologic flora, specific properties of this inflammatory response renders the individuals suffering from aggressive periodontitis both more susceptible to disease and more prone to lose more attachment in a shorter time.

Host Responses Specific to Aggressive Periodontitis

In generalized aggressive periodontitis, one review concluded that "there appears to be no difference between aggressive and chronic periodontitis in terms of their histopathology and immunopathology."[76] Still, it has to be acknowledged that this could mean that no differences exist or rather that "the differences between both disease entities only reflect variations in the degree of severity of susceptibility rather than actual different immune-pathologies."[22]

However, stronger activation of natural killer cells and natural killer T cells in aggressive periodontitis has been suggested to be causative for the observed more pronounced tissue destruction in aggressive periodontitis.[38,54] A distinction of chronic and aggressive periodontitis based on molecular markers (gingival tissue transcriptional signatures) using machine learning algorithms was possible with excellent sensitivity and specificity. At the same time, this work identified substantial diagnostic imprecision in the current classification.[33]

Abnormalities in Localized Aggressive Periodontitis

Earlier work has suggested that individuals suffering from LAP were characterized by an inherited defect of neutrophil function, leading to a dampened immune response against the microflora inhabiting the periodontal pocket.[84] Specifically, when challenged with periodontal pathogens, the LAP neutrophils were reported to show impaired chemotaxis, phagocytosis, and killing of bacteria. Alternatively, it was also hypothesized that these impaired defense properties were in fact acquired defects caused by prolonged exposure to an inflammatory microenvironment.

Today, the understanding of neutrophil biology is that neutrophils arriving at a site with uncontrolled periodontal inflammation are primed to attack the invading pathogens by releasing lytic enzymes. These enzymes may on the other hand accelerate tissue destruction. It is hypothesized that the observed dampened neutrophil function in deep aggressive periodontitis lesions is due to the heavy commitment of primed neutrophils to debridement, so that less potency remains for chemotaxis and defense.[64]

Genetics: Family Studies

A familiar aggregation of aggressive periodontitis cases is a secondary feature of the disease entity (i.e., it is often, but not always, found in aggressive periodontitis). To assess the familiar component of the disease, twin studies were performed[8,48] showing a strong genetic component with likely autosomal dominant inheritance mode and a 70% (African Americans) to 73% (Caucasians) penetrance.[48]

Genetics: Polymorphisms

Accordingly, there has been extensive work on the inherent genetic traits underlying this familiar aggregation.[42,77] First, it was suspected that an inherent susceptibility for periodontitis would likely be due to mutations of the DNA encoding for proteins of inflammatory mediators (candidate gene approach). DNA regions selected based on a priori knowledge of the disease pathobiology were assessed for sequence variations, most often single nucleotide polymorphisms (SNPs). Based on small sample sizes and often suboptimal study design, conceivably leading to false-positive results,[42,72] SNPs within genes encoding for cytokines such as interleukins (e.g., IL-1α, IL-1β, IL-6) were reported to be associated with aggressive periodontitis. However, with current knowledge, it has to be realized that these findings were possibly spurious or the result of confounding—all of the "classical" candidate gene associations could not be replicated in today's larger and better controlled cohorts.[68] Note that in the case of genetic association studies, meta-analyses are not generally suitable tools to overcome the problems of small, heterogeneous cohorts.

Use of the genome-wide association study (GWAS) has been made possible by technologic advances in the field of high-throughput analysis. Using a GWAS of a large number of aggressive periodontitis cases and controls, a number of common susceptibility loci for myocardial infarction and aggressive periodontitis could be identified and replicated in independent cohorts.[67,69–71]

Taken together, these data indicate that there is evidence for a strong genetic component in aggressive periodontitis. It is very likely that the low number of identified and replicated susceptibility loci for aggressive periodontitis are due to too few samples and issues in study design rather than to a lacking biologic association (for reviews, see Laine et al.[42] and Vaithilingam et al.[83]).

Environmental Factors Affecting Susceptibility

The amount and duration of smoking are important variables that can influence the extent of destruction seen in young adults.[82] Patients with GAP who smoke have more affected teeth and more loss of clinical attachment than nonsmoking patients with GAP.[27] However, smoking may not have the same impact on attachment levels in younger patients with LAP.[73]

Current Developments

Based on the aforementioned still incomplete current understanding of the specific microbiologic, immunologic, and genetic properties of the clinical symptom-based periodontitis entities aggressive and chronic periodontitis, research now focuses on the assessment of whether these entities are in fact sufficiently distinct with respect to their underlying pathobiology to form etiology-based clinical classes. For these analyses, novel unbiased high-throughput methodology such as microarrays and next-generation sequencing are employed.[32,34–36]

Therapeutic Considerations in Aggressive Periodontitis Patients

CLINICIAN'S CORNER

Aggressive periodontitis is defined by rapid attachment loss in clinically healthy individuals. There is considerable familiar aggregation. Aggressive periodontitis is most often found in younger individuals but can occur at any age. The entity is subdivided into two categories, localized and generalized aggressive periodontitis

Localized aggressive periodontitis (LAP) primarily affects first molars and incisor teeth in adolescents with deep pockets and advanced bone loss. It occurs in less than 1% of adolescents. There is a strong, hitherto only partially understood genetic component. In addition, the anaerobic gram-negative bacterium *Aggregatibacter actinomycetemcomitans* in the subgingival plaque biofilm was causally linked to LAP development in adolescents.

Generalized aggressive periodontitis (GAP) usually occurs first in young adults and may be present in some populations in up to 15% of the age group. Smoking may play a role because smokers with GAP have more teeth involved and more advanced pockets than nonsmokers.

Considerations for Anti-infective Therapy of Aggressive Periodontitis

Anti-infective therapy in patients with aggressive periodontitis seems to benefit strongly from the adjunctive use of systemic antibiotics[15] (see Chapter 52).

Considerations for Surgical Therapy of Aggressive Periodontitis

In general, individuals with aggressive periodontitis, especially LAP, have to undergo surgical therapy more often than the average periodontitis patient.[15] This is due to (1) the often much more pronounced loss of attachment with deep periodontal pockets that are challenging to instrument[5,46] and (2) the high prevalence of vertical defects, notably in LAP, that need to be resolved.[60]

Considerations for Supportive Periodontal Therapy of Aggressive Periodontitis Patients

Aggressive periodontitis patients are understood to suffer from an especially virulent microbiologic burden in combination with alterations in their host defense that render them more prone to rapid attachment loss, even in the absence of seemingly adequate numbers of etiologic factors. This suggests that during the maintenance phase, utmost care needs to be taken to optimize the self-performed oral hygiene in order to minimize the amount of plaque that could eventually lead to a new, rapid loss of attachment. Therefore many clinicians recommend performing supportive periodontal therapy, including regular assessments of periodontal parameters, at least every 3 months—even in subjects who show particularly high levels of oral hygiene proficiency and independent of the periodontal risk assessment (PRA) tool that seems to be of limited use in aggressive periodontitis.[50]

Considerations for Oral Rehabilitation and Implant Therapy in Aggressive Periodontitis Patients

Dental implants today allow for the routine, predictable, functional, and esthetic replacement of lost teeth. Still, there are concerns about the incidence of periimplantitis, an inflammatory condition of dental implants with parallels to periodontal disease for which no defined, predictable treatment protocols exist to date. Periimplantitis risk is linked to a history of periodontal disease in the individual treated with dental implants. Limited data exist that show an even stronger risk for developing the disease in patients suffering from aggressive periodontitis, as compared to chronic periodontitis patients or periodontally healthy controls.[79,80]

 Case Scenarios are found on the companion website www.expertconsult.com.

References

 References for this chapter are found on the companion website www.expertconsult.com.

CHAPTER 29

Necrotizing Ulcerative Periodontitis

Perry R. Klokkevold | Fermin A. Carranza

Necrotizing ulcerative periodontitis (NUP) may be an extension of *necrotizing ulcerative gingivitis (NUG)* into the periodontal structures that leads to periodontal attachment loss and bone loss. Alternatively, NUP and NUG may be different diseases. To date, there is little evidence to support the progression of NUG to NUP or to establish a relationship between the two conditions as a single disease entity. However, numerous clinical descriptions and case reports of NUP clearly demonstrate many clinical similarities between the two conditions. Until a distinction between NUG and NUP can be proved or disproved, it has been suggested that NUG and NUP be classified together under the broader category of *necrotizing periodontal diseases,* although with differing levels of severity.[1,15,20]

NUG has been recognized and described in the literature for centuries.[23] The features of NUG are presented in Chapter 20. The lesions of NUG are confined to the gingiva without a loss of periodontal attachment or alveolar bone support; this is the feature that distinguishes NUG from NUP.

The term *necrotizing ulcerative periodontitis* was first adopted at the 1989 World Workshop in Clinical Periodontics.[3] It was changed from the 1986 term *necrotizing ulcerative gingivoperiodontitis,* which represented the condition of recurrent NUG that progresses to a chronic form of periodontitis that includes attachment and bone loss. The adoption of NUP as a disease entity occurred in 1989 when there was a heightened awareness and an increase in the number of necrotizing periodontitis cases being diagnosed and described in the literature. Specifically, more cases of NUP were being described among immunocompromised patients, especially those who were human immunodeficiency virus (HIV) positive or who had acquired immunodeficiency syndrome (AIDS). In 1999, the subclassifications of NUG and NUP were included as separate diagnoses under the broader classification of "necrotizing ulcerative periodontal diseases."[1]

Clinical Features

Clinical cases of NUP are defined by necrosis and ulceration of the coronal portion of the interdental papillae and gingival margin, with a painful, bright-red marginal gingiva that bleeds easily. This is similar to the clinical features of NUG. The distinguishing feature of NUP is the *destructive progression* of the disease, which includes periodontal attachment and bone loss. Deep interdental osseous craters

typify periodontal lesions of NUP (Fig. 29.1). However, "conventional" periodontal pockets with deep probing depth are not found, because the ulcerative and necrotizing nature of the gingival lesion destroys the marginal epithelium and connective tissue, resulting in gingival recession. Periodontal pockets are formed because the junctional epithelial cells remain viable and can therefore migrate apically to cover areas of lost connective-tissue attachment. The necrosis of the junctional epithelium in patients with NUG and NUP creates an ulcer that prevents this epithelial migration, and a pocket cannot form. Advanced lesions of NUP lead to severe bone loss and tooth mobility, and may ultimately lead to tooth loss. In addition to these manifestations, as previously mentioned, patients with NUP may present with oral malodor, fever, malaise, or lymphadenopathy.

KEY FACT

Necrotizing ulcerative periodontitis (NUP) cases are defined by necrosis and ulceration of the coronal portion of the interdental papillae. Gingival margins are bright red and bleed easily. Lesions are painful. The feature that distinguishes NUP from NUG is the destructive progression of NUP, which includes periodontal attachment and bone loss.

Microscopic Findings

In a study involving the use of transmission electron microscopy and scanning electron microscopy of the microbial plaque overlying the necrotic gingival papillae, Cobb and colleagues[4] demonstrated striking histologic similarities between NUP in HIV-positive patients and previous descriptions of NUG in HIV-negative patients. Microscopic examination revealed a surface biofilm composed of a mixed microbial flora with different morphotypes and a subsurface flora with dense aggregations of spirochetes (i.e., the bacterial zone). Below the bacterial layers were dense aggregations of polymorphonuclear leukocytes (PMNs) (i.e., the neutrophil-rich zone) and necrotic cells (the necrotic zone). The biopsy technique used in this study did not allow for the observation of the deepest layer and thus was not able to identify the spirochetal infiltration zone, which is classically described in NUG lesions. In addition to the NUG-like microscopic features of NUP described in this study, high levels of yeasts and

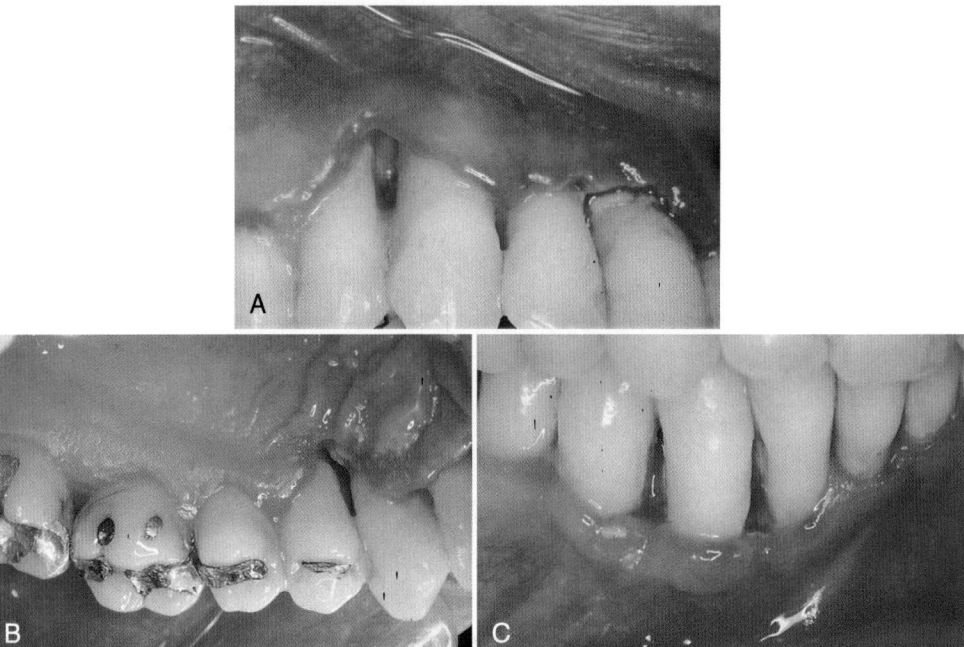

Fig. 29.1 Necrotizing ulcerative periodontitis in a 45-year-old, HIV-negative, white, male patient. (A) Buccal view of the maxillary cuspid–bicuspid area. (B) Palatal view of the same area shown in part A. (C) Buccal view of the mandibular anteriors. Note the deep craters associated with bone loss.

herpes-like viruses were observed. This latter finding is most likely indicative of the conditions afforded to opportunistic microbes in the immunocompromised host (i.e., HIV-positive patients).

Patients With HIV/AIDS

Gingival and periodontal lesions with distinctive features are frequently found in patients with HIV infection and AIDS. Many of these lesions are atypical manifestations of inflammatory periodontal diseases that arise during the course of HIV infection and as a result of the patient's concomitant immunocompromised state. Linear gingival erythema, NUG, and NUP are the most common HIV-associated periodontal conditions reported in the literature.[21] Chapter 30 provides detailed descriptions of these and other atypical periodontal diseases that occur in the patient with HIV.

NUP lesions found in patients with HIV or AIDS can present with features similar to those seen in HIV-negative patients. Alternatively, NUP lesions in patients with HIV or AIDS can be much more destructive and frequently result in complications that are extremely rare among patients without HIV or AIDS. For example, periodontal attachment and bone loss associated with NUP in an HIV-positive patient may be extremely rapid. Winkler and colleagues[31] described cases of NUP in HIV-positive patients with teeth that lost more than 90% of periodontal attachment and 10 mm of bone over a 3- to 6-month period. Ultimately, many of these lesions resulted in tooth loss. Other complications reported in this population included the progression of the lesions to involve large areas of soft-tissue necrosis, with the exposure of bone and the sequestration of bone fragments. This type of severe, progressive lesion with extension into the vestibular area and the palate is referred to as *necrotizing ulcerative stomatitis*.

The reported prevalence of NUP among patients with HIV infection varies.[6,13,21,23] Riley and colleagues[24] described only two cases of NUP in 200 HIV-positive patients (1%), whereas Glick and colleagues[13] found a prevalence of 6.3% for NUP cases in a prospective study

of 700 HIV-positive patients. Variations in reported findings may be related to differences in the populations studied (e.g., intravenous drug users versus homosexuals versus patients with hemophilia) and differences in the immune statuses of the study subjects.

Necrotizing forms of periodontitis appear to be more prevalent among patients with more severe immunosuppression.[21,22] Case reports have depicted NUP as a progressive extension of HIV periodontitis (i.e., chronic to necrotic progression).[25] Glick and colleagues[13,14] found a high correlation between the diagnosis of NUP and immunosuppression in HIV-positive patients. The patients who presented with NUP were 20.8 times more likely to have CD4+ counts of less than 200 cells/mm^3 as compared with HIV-positive patients without NUP. The authors consider a diagnosis of NUP to be a marker of immune deterioration and a predictor of the diagnosis of AIDS.[13] Others have suggested that NUP may be used as an indicator of HIV infection in undiagnosed patients. Shangase and colleagues[28] reported that a diagnosis of NUG or NUP in systemically healthy, asymptomatic South African patients was strongly correlated with HIV infection. Of patients presenting with NUG or NUP, 39 of 56 (69.6%) were subsequently found to be infected with HIV (see Chapter 30).

CLINICAL CORRELATION

Periodontal attachment and bone loss associated with NUP in an immunocompromised host (i.e., HIV-positive or AIDS) may be extremely rapid. NUP lesions in these patients are likely to be much more destructive and may also be associated with complications that are extremely rare among patients without HIV or AIDS.

Etiology of Necrotizing Ulcerative Periodontitis

The etiology of NUP has not been determined, although a mixed fusiform–spirochete bacterial flora appears to play a key role. Because bacterial pathogens are not solely responsible for causing the disease, some predisposing "host" factors may be necessary. Numerous predisposing factors have been attributed to NUG, including poor oral hygiene, preexisting periodontal disease, smoking, viral infections, immunocompromised status, psychosocial stress, and malnutrition. One case report attributed heavy tobacco use as the most significant contributing factor associated with NUP in a 21-year-old who had been smoking (>20 cigarettes/day) and chewing tobacco since the age of 7 years.[32]

NUG and NUP are more prevalent and more severe among patients with HIV. These patients require urgent treatment, because untreated lesions can progress rapidly; within a few days, severe bone loss around affected teeth can be seen.

Smoking, malnutrition, and high plaque levels all increase the risk of NUG and need to be changed so that treatment success is obtained.

Clinicians should check all patients who present with NUP to ascertain their HIV status. NUP can progress rapidly and lead to tooth exfoliation, so treatment should include local debridement, local antiplaque agents, and systemic antibiotics. The early diagnosis and treatment of NUP are crucial, because the osseous defects that occur during the late stages of the disease are extremely difficult to resolve.

Microbial Flora

Assessment of the microbial flora of NUP lesions is almost exclusively limited to studies involving patients with HIV or AIDS, with some conflicting evidence. Murray and colleagues[20] reported that cases of NUP in HIV-positive patients demonstrated significantly greater numbers of the opportunistic fungus *Candida albicans* and a higher prevalence of *Aggregatibacter actinomycetemcomitans*, *Prevotella intermedia*, *Porphyromonas gingivalis*, *Fusobacterium nucleatum*, and *Campylobacter* species as compared with HIV-negative controls. In addition, they reported a low or variable level of spirochetes, which is inconsistent with the flora associated with NUG. Citing differences in microbial flora, they refuted the notion that the destructive lesions seen in HIV-positive patients were related to NUG lesions; they suggested that the flora of NUP lesions in HIV-positive patients is comparable to that of chronic periodontitis lesions, thus supporting their concept that necrotizing periodontitis in the HIV-positive patient is an aggressive manifestation of chronic periodontitis in the immunocompromised host.

In contrast with these findings, Cobb and colleagues[4] reported that the microbial composition of NUP lesions in HIV-positive patients was very similar to that of NUG lesions, as discussed previously. Researchers used electron microscopy to describe a mixed microbial flora with various morphotypes in 81.3% of specimens. The subsurface microbial flora featured dense aggregations of spirochetes in 87.5% of specimens. The authors also reported opportunistic yeasts and herpes-like viruses in 65.6% and 56.5% of NUP lesions, respectively. The differences between these reports may be explained by the limitations of obtaining viable cultures of spirochetes[20] as compared with the more complete sample assessment with electron microscopic observation of spirochetes.[4]

In a review article, Feller and Lemmer suggested that spirochetes, herpesviruses, candida, and HIV all have potentially pathogenic roles in NUP lesions in the HIV-seropositive individual.[12] Spirochetes have the ability to modulate the host's innate and adaptive immune responses and to stimulate host inflammatory reactions,[8] which may reduce the local immune competence and facilitate the development of necrotizing disease.[12] Activated herpesviruses have the capacity to deregulate the host's immune system, which may lead to an increase in the colonization and activity of other pathogenic microorganisms.

Candida albicans has been reported to produce eicosanoids, leading to the release of proinflammatory mediators, which may facilitate spirochete colonization and invasion and promote the development of necrotizing periodontal diseases.[11,12]

KEY FACT

Patients with NUP are more likely to be immunocompromised. Although a mixed fusiform–spirochete bacterial infection appears to play a key role in the etiology of NUP, bacterial pathogens are not solely responsible. Predisposing "host" factors appear to be necessary. Factors that have been attributed to NUG include poor oral hygiene, preexisting periodontal disease, smoking, viral infections, immunocompromised status, psychosocial stress, and malnutrition.

Immunocompromised Status

Clearly, both NUG and NUP lesions are more prevalent among patients with compromised or suppressed immune systems. Numerous studies—particularly those evaluating patients with HIV or AIDS—support the concept that a diminished host response is present in those individuals who have been diagnosed with necrotizing ulcerative periodontal diseases.[31] Whereas a compromised immune system (i.e., "immune compromise") in the HIV-infected patient is driven by impaired T-cell function and altered T-cell ratios, evidence indicates that other forms of compromised immunity predispose individuals to NUG and NUP as well.

Cutler and colleagues[6] described the impaired bactericidal activity of PMNs in two children with NUP. In a comparative assay of PMNs and periodontal pathogens, two brothers who were 9 and 14 years old showed significant depression of PMN phagocytosis and killing function as compared with gender- and age-matched controls. Furthermore, Batista and colleagues[2] reported periodontal findings and NUP in an adolescent patient with a rare genetic disease (multifactorial congenital immunodeficiency) that causes the impaired secretion of immunoglobulin; the oral lesions resolved with the administration of intravenous immunoglobulin.

Psychologic Stress

Most studies evaluating the role of stress on necrotizing periodontal disease have involved subjects with NUG[7,16,29,30] and thus have not specifically addressed the role of stress on NUP. Patients with NUG have been found to have had significantly more anxiety, higher depression scores, a greater magnitude of recent stressful events, more overall distress and adjustments related to these events, and more negative life events.[5,14] Although the role of stress in the development of NUP has not been reported specifically, the many similarities between NUG and NUP would suggest that similar relationships to stress may exist.

The mechanisms that predispose an individual with stress to necrotizing ulcerative periodontal diseases have not been established. However, it is well known that stress increases the systemic cortisol levels, and sustained increases in cortisone have a suppressive effect on the immune response. In an investigation of 474 military personnel, Shannon and colleagues[29] found that urinary levels of 17-hydroxycorticosteroid were higher among subjects with NUG than in all other subjects who had been diagnosed with periodontal health, gingivitis, or periodontitis. Experimentally, noma-like lesions have been produced in rats by administering cortisone[27] and causing mechanical injury to the gingiva[26] and in hamsters via total body irradiation.[19] Thus stress-induced immunosuppression may be one mechanism that impairs the host response and leads to necrotizing periodontal disease. The scientific evidence supporting an etiologic role of stress in chronic periodontitis is not as clear (see Chapter 14).

Malnutrition

Direct evidence of the relationship between malnutrition and necrotizing periodontal disease is limited to descriptions of necrotizing infections in severely malnourished children. Lesions that resemble NUG but that progress to become *gangrenous stomatitis* or noma have been described in children with severe malnutrition in underdeveloped countries. Jimenez and Baer[18] reported cases of NUG among malnourished children and adolescents between the ages of 2 and 14 years in Colombia. In the advanced stages, NUG lesions extended from the gingiva to other areas of the oral cavity, becoming gangrenous stomatitis (noma) and causing exposure, necrosis, and sequestration of the alveolar bone. Later, Jimenez and colleagues reported that 44 of the 45 cases of necrotizing disease (NUG = 29, NUP = 7, and noma = 9) documented from 1965 to 2000 were from a low socioeconomic group and that malnutrition was associated with nearly all of the necrotizing conditions (29/29 NUG cases, 6/7 NUP cases, and 9/9 noma cases).[17] In a study of socioeconomically deprived Nigerian children with NUG (153 cases), Enwonwu and colleagues confirmed malnutrition by measuring circulating micronutrients.[10] As compared with neighborhood counterparts, the children with NUG and micronutrient deficiencies demonstrated dysregulated cytokine production with a complex interplay of elevated proinflammatory and antiinflammatory mediators.

KEY FACT

A fusiform–spirochete infection along with weakened host immune system seem to play a major role in the pathogenesis of necrotizing ulcerative periodontitis.

A possible explanation is that malnutrition, particularly when extreme, contributes to a diminished host resistance to infection and

necrotizing disease. It is well documented that many of the host defenses—including phagocytosis; cell-mediated immunity; and complement, antibody, and cytokine production and function—are impaired in malnourished individuals.[9] The depletion of nutrients to cells and tissues results in immunosuppression and increases disease susceptibility. Thus it is reasonable to conclude that malnutrition can predispose an individual to opportunistic infections or intensify the severity of existing oral infections.

Conclusion

NUP and NUG share many clinical and microbiologic features, but NUP is distinguished by a more severe condition with periodontal attachment and bone loss. Some individuals with NUP have severe and rapidly progressive disease. It appears that an impaired immune response and a lowered host resistance to infection are significant factors in the onset and progression of NUP. The best example of an immunocompromised host with a predisposition for NUP is the patient with HIV or AIDS. As with the other infection-related complications of HIV and AIDS, the immunocompromised status of affected patients renders them vulnerable to opportunistic periodontal infections, including NUP. Several predisposing factors have been identified in cases of NUG that may also play a role in NUP, including smoking, viral infections, psychosocial stress, and malnutrition. Although none of these factors alone is sufficient to cause necrotizing disease, when they occur together with an immunocompromised status, there is a potential to adversely influence the host response or resistance to infection.

 A Case Scenario is found on the companion website www.expertconsult.com.

References

 References for this chapter are found on the companion website www.expertconsult.com.

CHAPTER 30

Pathology and Management of Periodontal Problems in Patients With Human Immunodeficiency Virus Infection

Terry D. Rees

 For online-only content on pathogenesis, epidemiology and demographics, classification and staging, adverse drug effects, and necrotizing ulcerative stomatitis as well as expanded content about the oral and periodontal manifestations of human immunodeficiency virus infection and gingival and periodontal diseases, please visit the companion website at www.expertconsult.com. Some figures may be out of numeric order in this printed chapter.

Acquired immunodeficiency syndrome (AIDS) is characterized by profound impairment of the immune system. The condition was first reported in 1981, and a viral pathogen, the *human immunodeficiency virus (HIV)*, was identified in 1984.[221] The condition was originally thought to be restricted to male homosexuals. Subsequently, it was also identified in male and female heterosexuals and bisexuals who participated in unprotected sexual activities or who abused injected drugs.[187] Currently, sexual activity and drug abuse remain the primary means of transmission.

HIV has a strong affinity for cells of the immune system, most specifically those that carry the CD4 cell surface receptor molecule. Thus helper T lymphocytes (T4 cells) are most profoundly affected, but monocytes, macrophages, Langerhans cells, and some neuronal and glial brain cells may also be involved.[125] Viral replication occurs continuously in the lymphoreticular tissues of the lymph nodes, the spleen, the gut-associated lymphoid cells, and the macrophages.[282,283]

In 1986 a second type of HIV was isolated in Western Africa, and subsequently the two were named HIV-1 and HIV-2. Infection with HIV-2 was first reported in the United States in 1987 in an individual who had migrated from Western Africa. The two viruses apparently originated in different simian species. HIV-2 is very similar to HIV-1, but it appears to be less virulent and causes AIDS much more slowly. Infection with HIV-2 is rarely identified outside of Africa and countries that have been intimately associated with that area. During subsequent years, various subgroups of the viruses have been identified. HIV-1 consists of three named subgroups: M (main or major), N (new or non-M), and O (outlier). HIV-1 subgroup M is primarily responsible for the worldwide HIV epidemic. There are at least 10 subtypes of HIV-1 M, with subtype B being the most common. It has also been learned that coinfection with varying groups or subgroups can result in circulating recombinant forms of viral strains. There are also eight known HIV-2 subgroups. There is evidence that this growing plethora of viral mutations may play a role in the increasing resistance to antiretroviral therapy. It is known, for example, that HIV-2 possesses a natural resistance to nonnucleoside reverse transcriptase inhibitor antiretroviral drugs, and circulating recombinant forms may also develop resistance to drugs that are being used for treatment.[126,162,217]

Combined therapeutic regimens that consist of antiretroviral agents and protease-inhibiting drugs have resulted in marked improvement in the health status of HIV-infected individuals and occasionally a reduction in viral plasma bioloads to below detectable levels (i.e., <50 copies/mL), although the infection may still be transmissible.[79,108,114,290] Evidence indicates that the virus is never completely eradicated; rather, it is sequestered at low levels in resting CD4 cells, even in individuals with no detectable plasma viral ribonucleic acid (RNA).[49,78] These findings suggest that effective combination drug therapy may be necessary for the lifetime of infected individuals. Long-term control of the infection may be difficult, because the antiviral agents that are currently used have many adverse side effects and drug-resistant variant viral strains readily develop.[282] In addition, growing evidence suggests that oral pathogenic microorganisms (including putative periodontal pathogens) may help to induce HIV recrudescence by reactivating latently infected dendritic cells, macrophages, or T cells.[97,123,124]

Oral and Periodontal Manifestations of Human Immunodeficiency Virus Infection

Oral lesions are common in HIV-infected patients, although geographic and environmental variables may exist. Previous reports have indicated that most patients with AIDS have head and neck lesions,[223] whereas

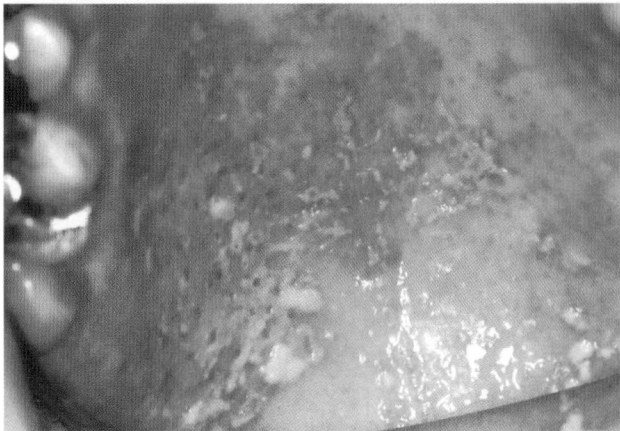

Fig. 30.1 Palatal pseudomembranous candidiasis.

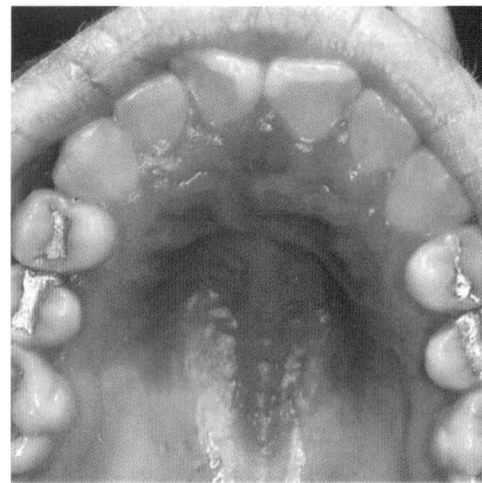

Fig. 30.2 Palatal erythematous candidiasis.

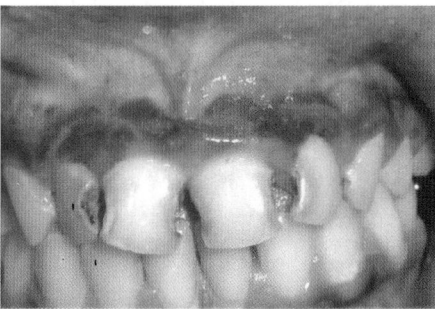

Fig. 30.3 Gingival erythematous candidiasis that is suggestive of desquamative gingivitis.

oral lesions are common among HIV-positive individuals who do not yet have AIDS.[16,93] Several reports have identified a strong correlation between HIV infection and oral candidiasis, oral hairy leukoplakia, atypical periodontal diseases, oral Kaposi sarcoma, and oral non-Hodgkin lymphoma.[68,71,153]

· Oral lesions less strongly associated with HIV infection include melanotic hyperpigmentation, mycobacterial infections, necrotizing ulcerative stomatitis (NUS), miscellaneous oral ulcerations, and viral infections (e.g., herpes simplex virus [HSV], herpes zoster, and condyloma acuminatum). Lesions that are seen in HIV-infected individuals with undetermined frequency include less common viral infections (e.g., CMV, molluscum contagiosum), recurrent aphthous stomatitis, and bacillary angiomatosis (epithelioid angiomatosis).[68]

The advent of HAART has resulted in a greatly diminished frequency of oral lesions associated with HIV infection and AIDS.[34,179,261]

Oral Candidiasis

Candidiasis is the most common oral lesion associated with HIV disease, and it has been found in approximately 90% of patients with AIDS.[194,246] It usually has one of four clinical presentations: pseudomembranous, erythematous, or hyperplastic candidiasis or angular cheilitis.[115,178]

Pseudomembranous candidiasis ("thrush") presents as painless or slightly sensitive, yellow-white, curdlike lesions that can be readily scraped and separated from the surface of the oral mucosa. This type is most common on the hard and soft palate and the buccal or labial mucosa, but it can occur anywhere in the oral cavity (Fig. 30.1).

Erythematous candidiasis may be present as a component of the pseudomembranous type, appearing as red patches on the buccal or palatal mucosa, or it may be associated with depapillation of the tongue. If the gingiva is affected, it may be misdiagnosed as desquamative gingivitis (Figs. 30.2, 30.3, and 30.4). Some evidence suggests that erythematous candidiasis is more common among HIV-positive individuals with CD4+ counts between 200 and 500 cells/μl, whereas the pseudomembranous form occurs in patient with less than 200 CD4+ cells/μl. Viral load is most often elevated to more than 100,000 copies/mL. However, it should be emphasized that any form of candidiasis can be found in individuals who are only minimally immunocompromised.[181]

Hyperplastic candidiasis is the least common form, and it may be seen in the buccal mucosa and the tongue. It is more resistant to removal than the other types (Figs. 30.5 and 30.6).

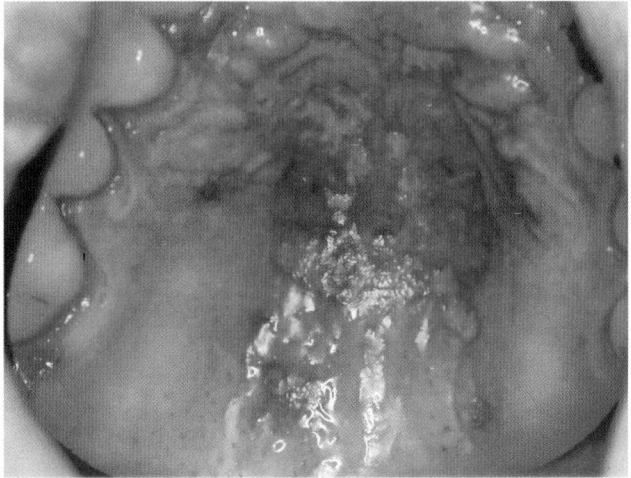

Fig. 30.4 Mixed erythematous and pseudomembranous candidiasis of the palate.

In *Candida*-related *angular cheilitis,* the commissures of the lips appear erythematous, with surface crusting and fissuring.

The diagnosis of candidiasis is made by clinical evaluation, culture analysis, or microscopic examination of a tissue sample or smear of material scraped from the lesion (oral cytology), which shows hyphae and yeast forms of the organisms (Fig. 30.7). When oral candidiasis appears in patients with no apparent predisposing cause, the clinician should be alerted to the possibility of HIV infection.[68] Many patients who are at risk for HIV infection who present with

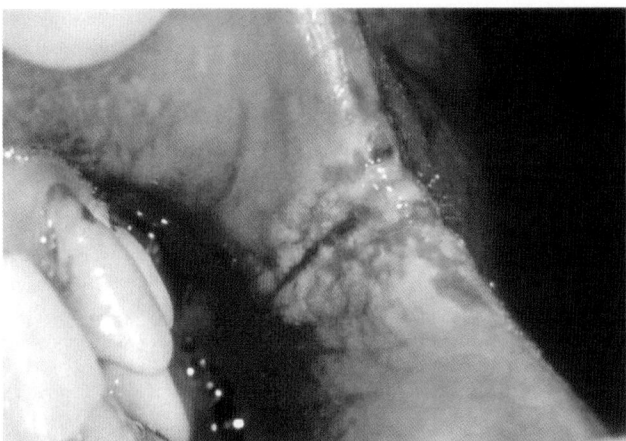

Fig. 30.5 Mixed erythematous and hyperplastic candidiasis of the corner of the mouth.

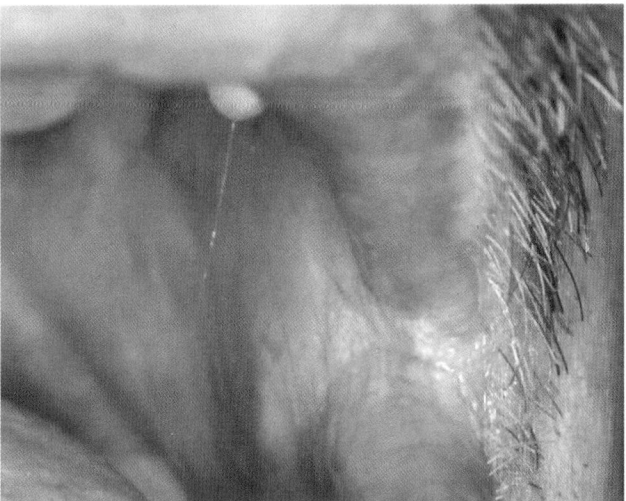

Fig. 30.6 Hyperplastic candidiasis in the corner of the mouth. The lesion persisted despite the use of systemic antifungal drugs.

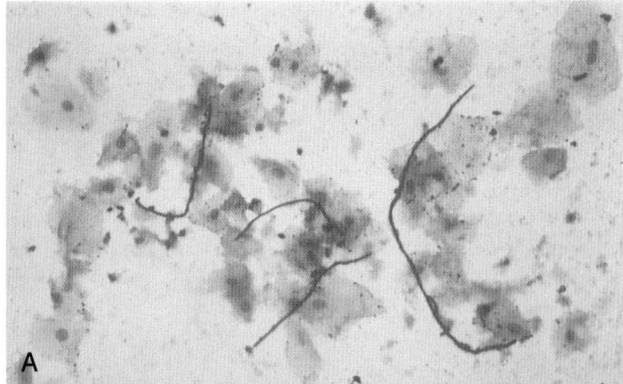

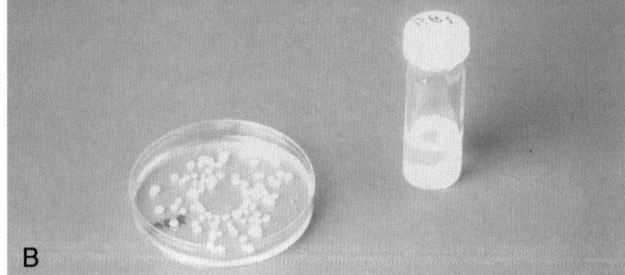

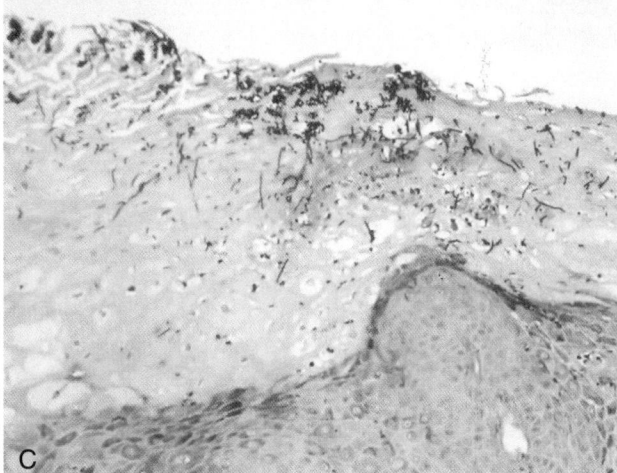

Fig. 30.7 Techniques for the diagnosis of candidiasis. (A) Candidal hyphae in a tissue smear after periodic acid–Schiff staining. (B) Culture media specific for *Candida* species. (C) Candidal hyphae in the epithelium of biopsied tissue.

oral candidiasis also have esophageal candidiasis, which is a diagnostic sign of AIDS.[263]

Oral Hairy Leukoplakia

Oral hairy leukoplakia (OHL) primarily occurs in persons with HIV infection.[101,104] It is found on the lateral borders of the tongue, it frequently has a bilateral distribution, and it may extend to the ventrum. OHL is caused by the Epstein–Barr virus (EBV), and it is the only EBV lesion with which viral shedding in saliva is common.[181] The lesion is characterized by an asymptomatic, poorly demarcated, keratotic area that ranges in size from a few millimeters to several centimeters (Fig. 30.8A). Often, characteristic vertical striations are present, and these impart a corrugated appearance; the surface may also be shaggy and appear hairy when dried. The lesion does not rub off, and it may resemble other keratotic oral lesions.

Kaposi Sarcoma and Other Malignancies

Oral malignancies occur more frequently in severely immuno-compromised individuals than in the general population. An HIV-positive individual with non-Hodgkin lymphoma (NHL) or Kaposi sarcoma (KS) is categorized as having AIDS (Fig. 30.9). Oral lesions are reported in approximately 4% of individuals with NHL, and the gingiva and palate are common sites. The incidence of oral squamous

cell carcinoma may also increase among HIV-infected individuals.[22] KS was a rare disease until the early 1980s. In its classic form, it is found in older men and occasionally in patients after organ transplants, and it is endemic in parts of Africa. An epidemic form has subsequently been described in HIV-positive individuals, and it is an AIDS-defining condition.[193]

KS is the most common oral malignancy associated with AIDS. This angioproliferative tumor is a rare, multifocal, vascular neoplasm; it was originally described in 1872 as occurring in the skin of the lower extremities of older men of Mediterranean origin. Today, it is closely associated with homosexual and heterosexual transmission, but it occurs 5 to 10 times more often among male homosexuals than in other groups at high risk for HIV. The causative agent has been identified as human herpesvirus-8 (HHV-8).

Microscopically, Kaposi sarcoma consists of four components: (1) endothelial cell proliferation with the formation of atypical vascular channels, (2) extravascular hemorrhage with hemosiderin deposition,

(3) spindle cell proliferation in association with atypical vessels, and (4) a mononuclear inflammatory infiltrate that consists mainly of plasma cells[99] (Fig. 30.10).

Non-Hodgkin Lymphoma

Lymphoma represents a heterogeneous malignancy that is characterized by the proliferation of lymphoid cells. It is broadly classified as Hodgkin disease (14%) or non-Hodgkin lymphoma (NHL). NHL in individuals with HIV infection is an AIDS-defining condition, and elevated cumulative viremia may be a strong predictor of AIDS-related lymphoma.[292]

Oral lesions usually appear as erythematous, painless enlargements that may become ulcerated as a result of traumatic injury

(Fig. 30.11). In some cases, bone involvement occurs, although this is rare in the United States. Lesions commonly affect the gingival, palatal, and alveolar mucosa, and they may mimic dental infections. Diagnosis is based on physical examination, complete blood count with differential, imaging studies, and lymph node and tissue biopsy.[172]

Bacillary (Epithelioid) Angiomatosis

Bacillary (epithelioid) angiomatosis (BA) is an infectious vascular proliferative disease with clinical and histologic features similar to those of KS. BA is caused by facultative intracellular gram-negative mobile bacilli of the genus *Bartonella* and the order Rickettsia (e.g., *Bartonella henselae, Bartonella quintana*).[68,211,230] Cats are the primary host of *B. henselae,* and the infection is usually transmitted to humans by bites, scratches, or fleas (i.e., cat-scratch fever). Humans are the primary reservoir for *B. quintana,* and it is usually transmitted by human lice. BA can occur in immunocompetent persons, but it is most commonly associated with AIDS. Skin lesions are similar to those associated with KS or cat-scratch disease.[57,254] Gingival BA manifests as red, purple, or blue edematous soft-tissue lesions that may cause the destruction of periodontal ligament and bone[91] (see Fig. 30.11).

Oral Hyperpigmentation

An increased incidence of *oral hyperpigmentation* has been described in HIV-infected individuals.[50,139,143,291] Oral pigmented areas often appear as spots or striations on the buccal mucosa, the palate, the

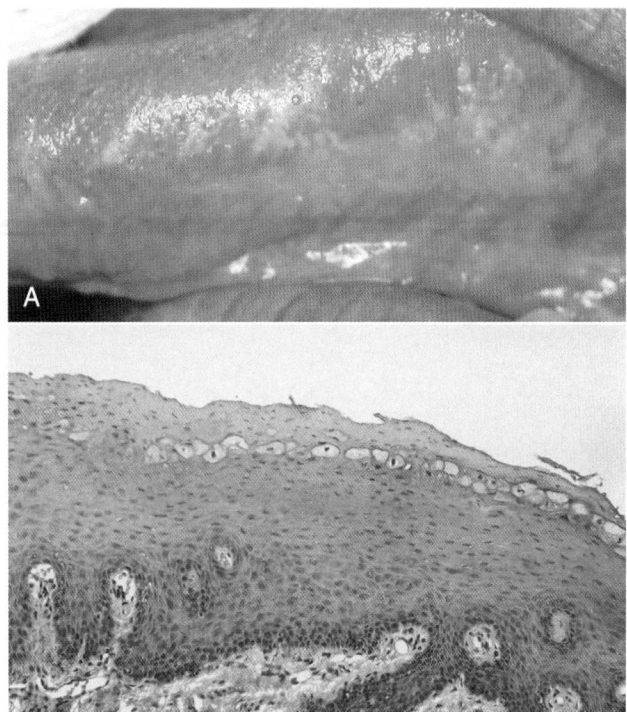

Fig. 30.8 Oral hairy leukoplakia on the left lateral border of the tongue. (A) Clinical view. (B) Biopsy confirmation of oral hairy leukoplakia. Note the ballooned epithelial cells near the surface of the epithelium.

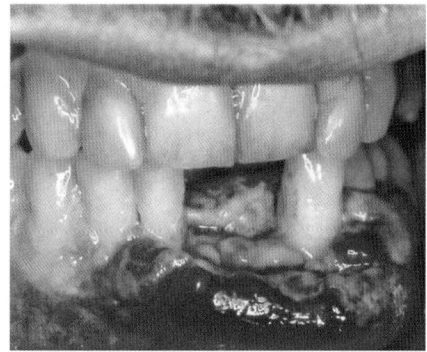

Fig. 30.9 Non-Hodgkin lymphoma of the anterior mandibular gingiva.

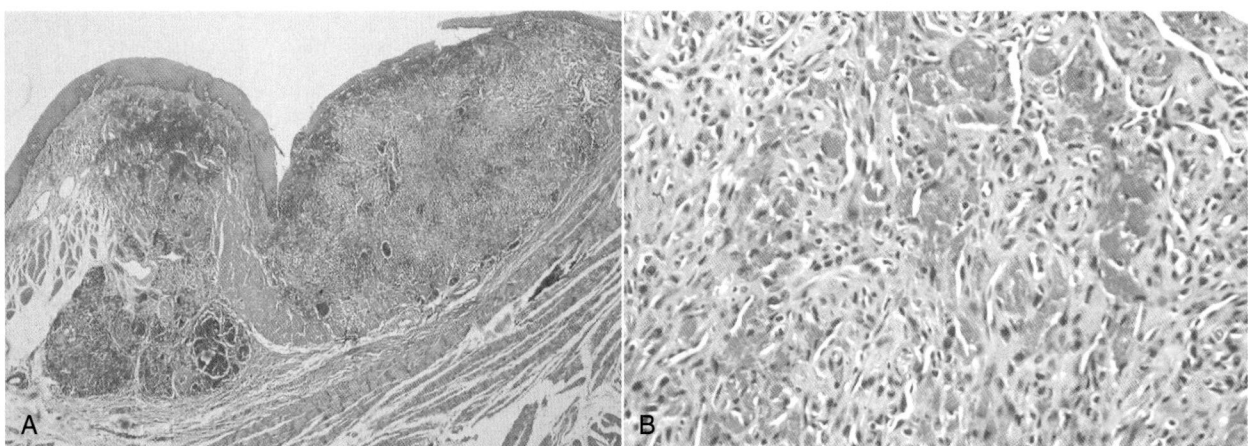

Fig. 30.10 (A) Histologic view of Kaposi sarcoma. This lesion is exophytic and only minimally inflamed (low magnification). (B) Note the sheets of endothelial cells and numerous small blood vessels (high magnification).

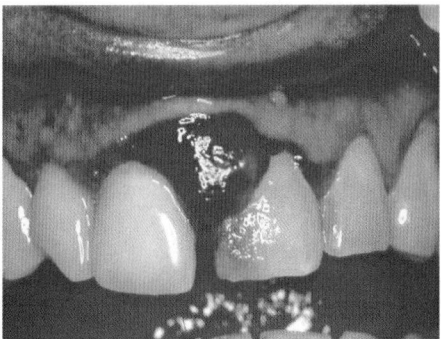

Fig. 30.11 Bacillary angiomatosis mimicking Kaposi sarcoma.

gingiva, or the tongue (Fig. 30.12). At present, most reports describing the oral features of HIV/AIDS or post-HAART HIV/AIDS come from areas of the world where racial pigmentation may be common. In these areas, oral evaluation may often be accomplished by non-dental health care workers. Consequently, it is not possible to accurately assess the degree of HIV-related oral hyperpigmentation before or after ART.

Atypical Ulcers

Atypical ulcers (nonspecific oral ulcerations) in HIV-infected individuals may have multiple etiologies that include neoplasms such as lymphoma, KS, and squamous cell carcinoma. HIV-associated neutropenia may also feature oral ulcerations.

HIV-infected patients have a higher incidence of recurrent herpetic lesions and aphthous stomatitis (Figs. 30.13 and 30.14). Approximately 10% of HIV-infected patients have herpes infection,[199] and multiple episodes are common. The CDC HIV classification system indicates that mucocutaneous herpes that lasts more than 1 month is diagnostic of AIDS in HIV-infected individuals.[39] Aphthae and aphthae-like lesions are common when patients are followed throughout the course of their immunosuppression.[93]

Salivary Gland Disorders and Xerostomia

Salivary gland hypofunction and xerostomia may be most common among HIV-infected men during both the early and advanced stages of HIV infection and immunosuppression. Salivary function does not appear to be affected by HAART, despite the fact that some individual antiretroviral medications are reported to induce xerostomia. However, it is clear that xerostomia is a relatively common condition among HIV-infected individuals and that up to 10% of these patients may be affected. Xerostomia appears to become more severe as immunosuppression worsens, and increased candidal carriage is associated with reduced salivary flow rate.[131]

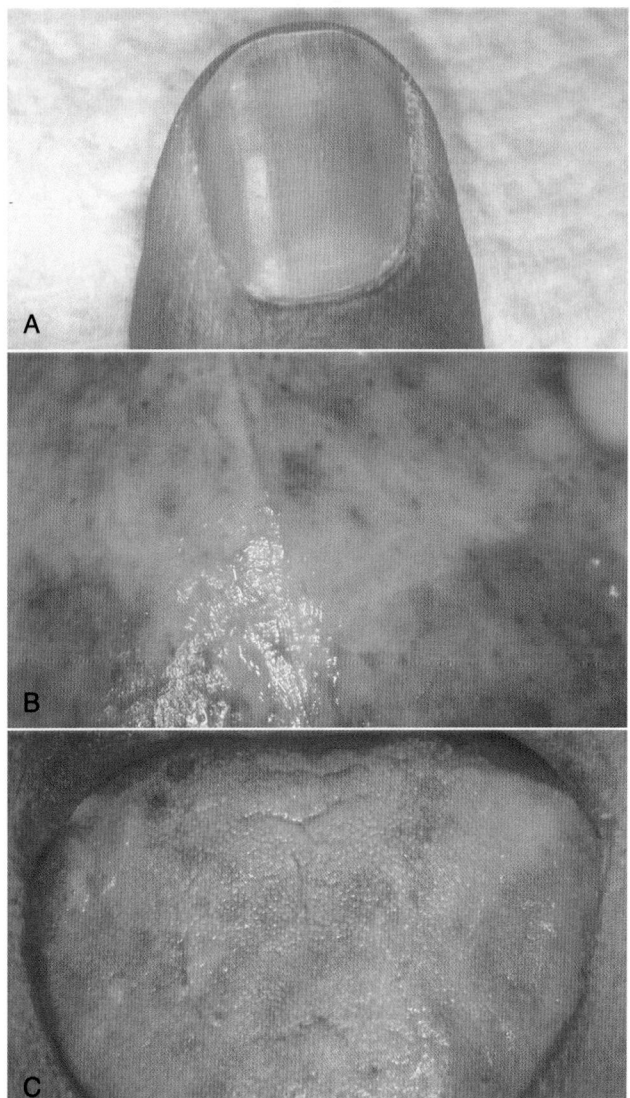

Fig. 30.12 Drug-induced hyperpigmentation as a result of zidovudine use. (A) Fingernail bed discoloration. (B) Palatal hyperpigmentation in the same patient. (C) Tongue hyperpigmentation in the same patient. Note the similarity between the oral lesions and those caused by adrenal cortex hypofunction (i.e., Addison disease).

immunocompromised individuals to minimize the risk of opportunistic infections (e.g., candidiasis), superinfection, and microorganism drug resistance.[169]

Dental Treatment Complications

Concerns have been expressed regarding the potential for postoperative complications (e.g., hemorrhage, infection, delayed wound healing) in individuals with HIV or AIDS. Medically compromised patients must be carefully managed in the dental office to avoid undue treatment complications.[60] However, *systematic reviews of the literature indicate that special precautions are usually not necessary based simply on the HIV status of patients when performing periodontal treatment procedures such as dental prophylaxis, scaling and root planing, periodontal surgery, extractions, and the placement of implants.* On occasion, the poor overall health status of an individual with AIDS may limit periodontal therapy to conservative, minimally invasive procedures, and antibiotic therapy may be required.[10,63,64,90,195] When possible, antibiotics should be avoided in significantly

Gingival and Periodontal Diseases

Considerable research has focused on the nature and incidence of periodontal diseases in HIV-infected individuals. Some studies suggest that chronic periodontitis is more common in this patient population, but others do not. Periodontal diseases are more common among HIV-infected users of injection drugs, but this may relate to poor oral hygiene and a lack of dental care rather than decreased CD4 cell counts. However, some unusual types of periodontal diseases do seem to occur with greater frequency among HIV-positive individuals.[12,106,142,199,213,259]

Linear Gingival Erythema

A persistent, linear, easily bleeding, erythematous gingivitis has been described in some HIV-positive patients. The intensity of the erythema

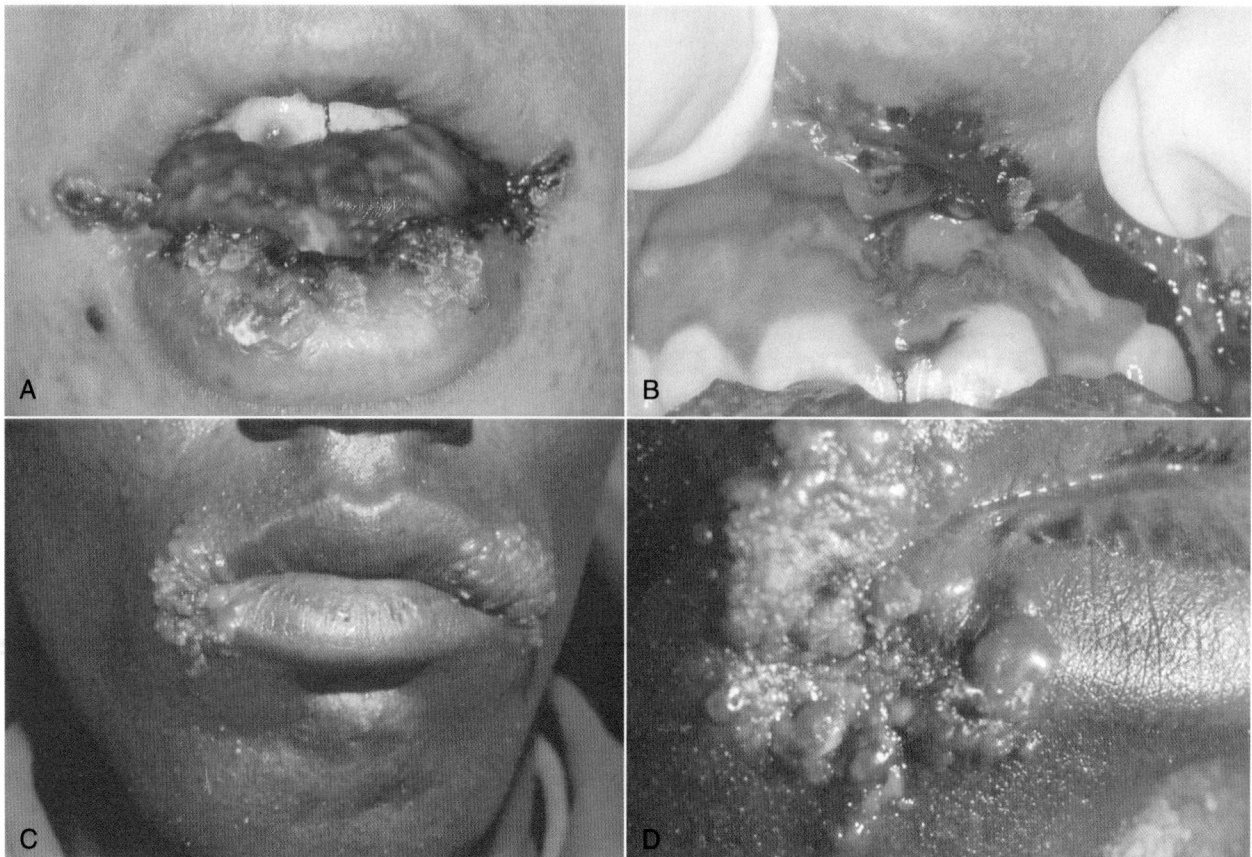

Fig. 30.13 Abnormal herpetic lesions in individuals with human immunodeficiency virus. (A) The lip crusting of primary herpetic gingivostomatitis. (B) Ulcerations of the gingiva, the alveolar mucosa, and the vestibule in the same patient. (C) Severe herpes labialis in the commissures of the lip. (D) A close-up view of herpes labialis. Note the fluid-filled vesicles.

is disproportionate to the amount of plaque present. There is no ulceration, pocketing, or attachment loss,[268] and the condition does not respond predictably to conventional periodontal therapy. Lesions that are clinically identical to linear gingival erythema were observed before the advent of HIV in association with severely immuno-compromised individuals or in those with NUG.

Linear gingival erythema (LGE) may or may not serve as a precursor to rapidly progressive NUP[92,94] (Figs. 30.15 and 30.16). The microflora of LGE may closely mimic that of periodontitis rather than gingivitis. However, *Candida* infection has been implicated as a major etiologic factor, and human herpesviruses have been proposed as possible triggers or cofactors.[7,53,226,250,268] Linear gingivitis lesions may be localized or generalized in nature. The erythematous gingivitis may be limited to marginal tissue, extend into attached gingiva in a punctate or diffuse erythema, or extend into the alveolar mucosa.

The diagnosis of LGE may be difficult, because it can be mistaken for conventional marginal gingivitis. This may be especially true in studies from undeveloped countries or countries with newly identified and largely untreated patients with HIV and AIDS. This makes it difficult to identify the true prevalence of LGE in HIV-infected and noninfected individuals. This prompted the report from the Fifth World Workshop on Oral Health and Disease in AIDS to limit the diagnosis of LGE only to individuals who do not respond to conventional periodontal debridement procedures.[268]

Although LGE may sometimes be unresponsive to corrective therapy, such lesions may undergo spontaneous remission. Concomitant oral candidiasis and LGE lesions have been identified, which

suggests a possible etiologic role for candidal species in LGE.[142] In one study, direct microscopic cultures from LGE lesions implicated *Candida dubliniensis* in four patients, all of whom experienced complete or partial remission after systemic antifungal therapy.[274] It is not yet known whether candidal infection is an etiologic factor in all LGE cases. A systematic review indicates that LGE is more common among HIV-infected populations but that most individuals who are HIV positive do not experience LGE.[194]

Others have reported that LGE is most often found in HIV-positive individuals whose CD4+ counts are depressed (200 to 500 cells/mm^3 or <200 cells/mm^3) or whose viral loads are elevated, suggesting that it may represent an early marker of progressive immunodeficiency or even the transition to outright AIDS.[194,251]

LGE-like lesions can sometimes be adequately managed by following the therapeutic principles associated with marginal gingivitis. However, as mentioned previously, it has been suggested that gingivitis lesions that respond to conventional therapy do not represent LGE.[264] The affected sites should be scaled and polished. Subgingival irrigation with chlorhexidine or 10% povidone–iodine may be beneficial. The patient should be carefully instructed regarding the performance of meticulous oral hygiene procedures. The condition should be reevaluated 2 to 3 weeks after initial therapy. If the patient is compliant with home care procedures and the lesions persist, the possibility of a candidal infection should be considered. It is doubtful that topical antifungal rinses will reach the base of the gingival crevices. Consequently, the treatment of choice may be the empiric administration of a systemic antifungal agent, such as fluconazole, for 7 to 10 days.[116]

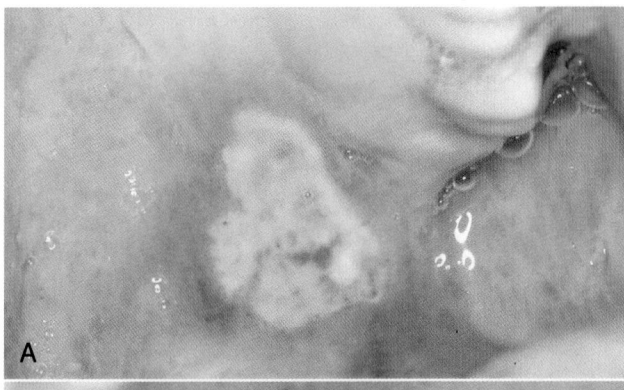

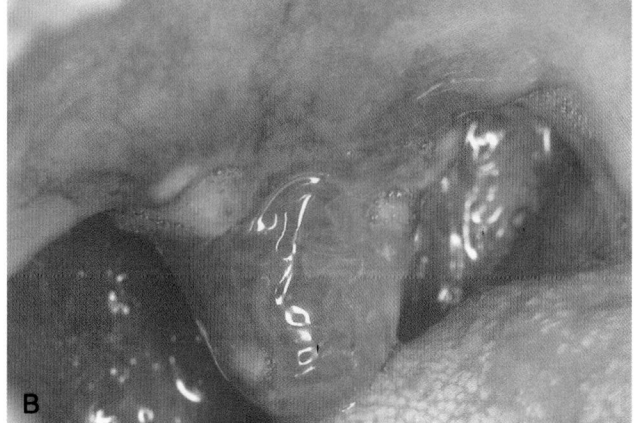

Fig. 30.14 Intraoral aphthous stomatitis in a patient with acquired immunodeficiency syndrome. (A) Major aphthous lesion in the left soft palate. (B) Ulcerations of the uvula in the same patient.

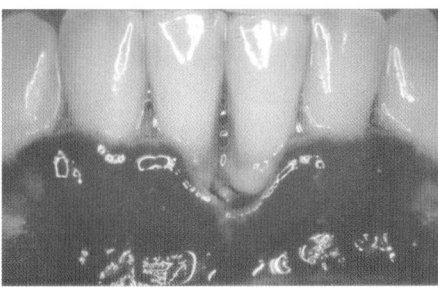

Fig. 30.15 Linear gingival erythema and necrotizing ulcerative gingivitis in a patient with acquired immunodeficiency syndrome.

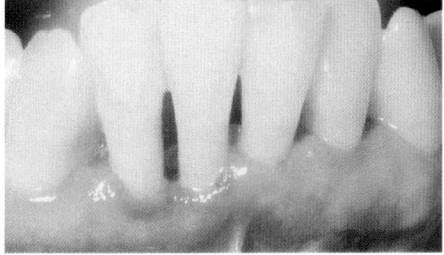

Fig. 30.16 Mild linear gingival erythema. The patient had a T4 count of 9 and a viral load that was too numerous to count.

It is important to remember that LGE is often refractory to treatment. If so, the patient should be carefully monitored for developing signs of more severe periodontal conditions (e.g., NUG, NUP, NUS). The patient should be placed on a 2- to 3-month recall maintenance interval and re-treated as necessary. As mentioned previously, despite

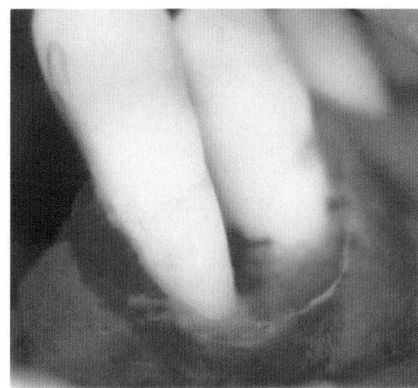

Fig. 30.17 Necrotizing ulcerative periodontitis. Note the adjacent linear gingival erythema.

the occasional resistance of LGE to conventional periodontal therapy, spontaneous remission may occur for reasons that are not yet known.

Necrotizing Ulcerative Gingivitis

Some reports have described an increased incidence of NUG among HIV-infected individuals, although this has not been substantiated by other studies.[66,93,94,120,228,256]

There is no consensus regarding whether the incidence of NUG increases in HIV-positive patients.[191,195,220,239] However, one study evaluated the HIV status of individuals who presented with necrotizing periodontal diseases, and 69% were found to be HIV seropositive.[239] The treatment of NUG in these patients does not differ from that in HIV-negative individuals (see Chapter 43).

Necrotizing Ulcerative Periodontitis

A necrotizing, ulcerative, rapidly progressive form of periodontitis occurs more frequently among HIV-positive individuals, although such lesions were described long before the onset of the AIDS epidemic. NUP appears to represent an extension of NUG in which bone loss and periodontal attachment loss occur.[182,239]

NUP is characterized by soft-tissue necrosis, rapid periodontal destruction, and interproximal bone loss[94,204] (Figs. 30.17, 30.18, and 30.19). Lesions may occur anywhere in the dental arches; they are usually localized to a few teeth, although generalized NUP is sometimes present after marked CD4+ cell depletion. Bone is often exposed, which results in necrosis and subsequent sequestration. NUP is severely painful at onset, and immediate treatment is necessary. Occasionally, however, patients undergo spontaneous resolution of the necrotizing lesions, which leave painless, deep, interproximal craters that are difficult to clean and that may lead to conventional periodontitis.[92]

Therapy for NUP includes local debridement; scaling and root planing; in-office irrigation with an effective antimicrobial agent such as chlorhexidine gluconate or povidone–iodine (Betadine); and the establishment of meticulous oral hygiene, including the home use of antimicrobial rinses or irrigation.[195,203,229] This therapeutic approach is based on reports that involved only a small number of patients.

In patients with severe NUP, antibiotic therapy may be necessary, but it should be used with caution in HIV-infected patients to avoid an opportunistic and potentially serious localized candidiasis or even candidal septicemia.[166] If an antibiotic is necessary, metronidazole (250 mg, with two tablets taken immediately and then two tablets taken four times daily for 5 to 7 days) is the drug of choice. The prophylactic prescription of a topical or systemic antifungal agent is prudent if an antibiotic is used.

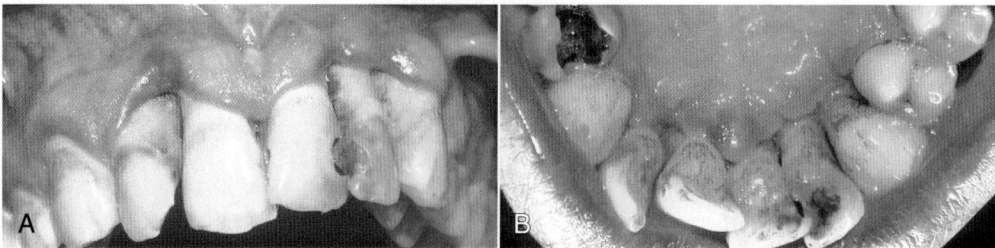

Fig. 30.18 Necrotizing ulcerative periodontitis in an otherwise healthy 19-year-old man without human immunodeficiency virus. (A) Anterior maxilla. (B) Palatal view.

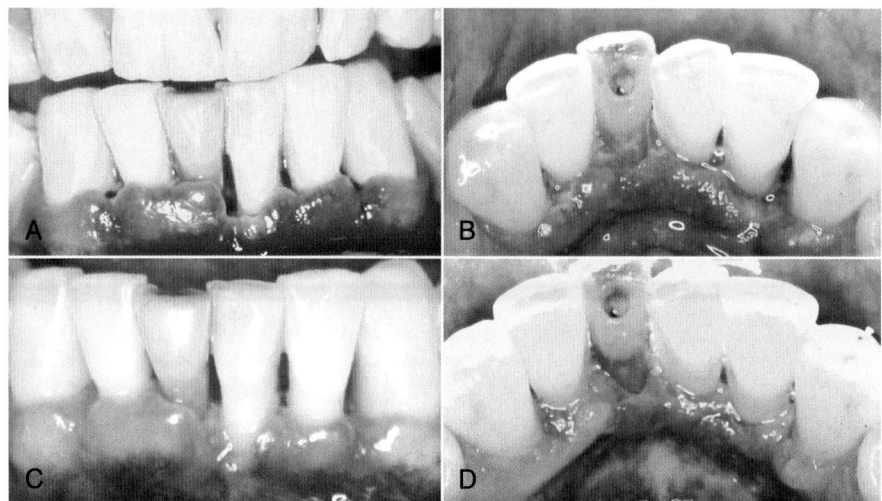

Fig. 30.19 Early necrotizing ulcerative periodontitis in a patient with acquired immunodeficiency syndrome. (A) Facial view. (B) Lingual view. (C) Facial view of the complete resolution of necrotizing ulcerative periodontitis after treatment. (D) Lingual view.

Chronic Periodontitis

A number of longitudinal studies and prevalence studies have suggested that HIV-positive individuals are more likely to experience chronic periodontitis than the general population.[12,163,174,214] Most studies, however, do not take into account the level of oral hygiene, the presence of preexisting gingivitis, poor diet, the age of the patient, smoking, other periodontal disease risk factors, the degree of immunodeficiency in the population studied, or whether the individuals in the study are injection drug users (IDUs); these confounding factors cloud the issue.

With proper home care and appropriate periodontal treatment and maintenance, HIV-positive individuals can anticipate reasonably good periodontal health throughout the course of their disease.[134] The median period between initial HIV infection and outright AIDS is approximately 15 years, and the life expectancy of persons living with AIDS has been significantly prolonged with current anti-HIV drug therapy.[23,42]

This indicates that HIV-infected patients are potential candidates for conventional periodontal treatment procedures, including surgery and implant placement. Treatment decisions should be based on the overall health status of the patient, the degree of periodontal involvement, and the motivation and ability of the patient to perform effective oral hygiene (Fig. 30.20).

Clearly, some less common periodontal diseases do occur more frequently in HIV-positive individuals, but these same conditions are also reported among HIV-negative persons. Consequently, definitions for these conditions and discussions of their management should not be construed as limiting them to individuals with HIV or AIDS.

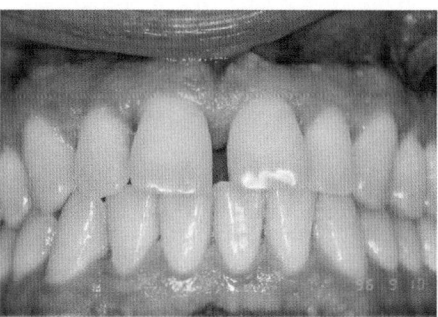

Fig. 30.20 Periodontal health in an individual with advanced acquired immunodeficiency syndrome.

Periodontal Treatment Protocol

It is imperative that medically compromised patients, including those with HIV or AIDS, be safely and effectively managed in dental practice.[240] Several universal treatment considerations are important to ensure that this goal is achieved.

Health Status

The patient's health status should be determined from the health history, the physical evaluation, and consultation with the patient's physician. Treatment decisions will vary, depending on the patient's state of health. For example, delayed wound healing and an increased risk of postoperative infection are possible complicating factors in patients with AIDS, but neither concern should significantly alter treatment planning for an otherwise healthy, asymptomatic, HIV-infected patient with a normal or near-normal CD4 count and a low viral bioload.[85,109,153,207]

It is important to obtain information about the patient's immune status with questions such as the following:

- What is the CD4+ T4 lymphocyte level?
- What is the current viral load?
- How do current CD4+ T4 cell and viral load counts differ from previous evaluations? How often are such tests performed?
- How long ago was the HIV infection identified? Is it possible to identify the approximate date of original exposure?
- Is there a history of drug abuse, sexually transmitted diseases, multiple infections, or other factors that may alter immune response? For example, does the patient have a history of chronic hepatitis B, hepatitis C, neutropenia, thrombocytopenia, nutritional deficiency, or adrenocorticoid insufficiency?
- What medications is the patient taking?
- Does the patient describe or present with possible adverse side effects from medications?

Infection Control Measures

The clinical management of HIV-infected periodontal patients requires strict adherence to established methods of infection control, which should be based on guidance from the American Dental Association and the CDC. Compliance, especially with universal precautions, will eliminate or minimize risks to both patients and the dental staff.[85,150,275] Immunocompromised patients are potentially at risk for acquiring as well as transmitting infections in the dental office and other health care facilities.[146,168,183]

Goals of Therapy

A thorough oral examination will determine the patient's dental treatment needs. The primary goal of dental therapy should be the restoration and maintenance of oral health, comfort, and function. At the very least, periodontal treatment goals should be directed toward the control of HIV-associated mucosal diseases, such as chronic candidiasis and recurrent oral ulcerations. Acute periodontal and dental infections should be managed, and the patient should receive detailed instructions regarding the performance of effective oral hygiene procedures.[90,116]

Conservative nonsurgical periodontal therapy should be a treatment option for virtually all HIV-positive patients, and the performance of elective surgical periodontal procedures, including implant placement, have been reported.[89,229] NUP or NUS can be severely destructive to periodontal structures, but a history of these conditions does not automatically dictate the extraction of involved teeth, unless the patient is unable to maintain effective oral hygiene in the affected

areas. Decisions regarding elective periodontal procedures should be made with the informed consent of the patient and after medical consultation, when possible.

Maintenance Therapy

It is imperative for the patient to maintain meticulous personal oral hygiene. In addition, periodontal maintenance recall visits should be conducted at short intervals (i.e., every 2 to 3 months), and any progressive periodontal disease should be treated vigorously.[288]

As mentioned previously, systemic antibiotic therapy should be administered with caution. Blood and other medical laboratory tests may be required to monitor the patient's overall health status, and close consultation and coordination with the patient's physician are necessary.

Psychological Factors

HIV infection of neuronal cells may affect brain function and lead to dementia. This may profoundly influence the responsiveness of affected patients to dental treatment. However, psychological factors are numerous in virtually all HIV-infected patients, even in the absence of neuronal lesions.

Patients may be greatly concerned with the maintenance of medical confidentiality, and such confidentiality must be upheld. Coping with a life-threatening disease may elicit depression, anxiety, and anger in such patients, and this anger may be directed toward the dentist and the staff. It is important to display concern and understanding for the patient's situation. Treatment should be provided in a calm, relaxed atmosphere, and stress to the patient must be minimized.[6]

The dentist should be prepared to advise and counsel patients regarding their oral health status. Dentists often encounter HIV-infected patients who are unaware of their disease status. The early diagnosis and treatment of HIV infection can have a profound effect on the patient's life expectancy and quality of life, and the dentist should be prepared to assist the patient with obtaining testing.[234,241] Any patient with oral lesions that are suggestive of HIV infection should be informed of the findings and, if appropriate, questioned about any previous exposure to HIV. If HIV testing is requested, it must be accompanied by patient counseling; therefore it may be best to obtain such tests through medical referral. However, if the dentist elects to request testing for the HIV antibody, the patient must be informed. In most circumstances, written informed consent is desirable before testing.

References

 References for this chapter are found on the companion website www.expertconsult.com.

CHAPTER 31

Levels of Clinical Significance

Philippe P. Hujoel

CHAPTER OUTLINE

Tangible Versus Intangible Benefits
Size of the Treatment Effect
Defining Four Levels of Clinical Significance
Summary

In one study of periodontal tissue regeneration, investigators reported that treatment that resulted in a gain of 1.2 mm in clinical attachment level and a reduction of 1 mm in probing pocket depth "may not have a great clinical impact."[5] In another study of a local antimicrobial, the investigators reported that a treatment that resulted in a gain of 0.0 mm in clinical attachment level and a reduction of 0.2 mm in probing depth had such clinical significance that it should "be used universally."[32] The American Dental Association defined a substantial effect as a mean change in attachment level greater than 0.6 mm.[28] These examples illustrate that different individuals will reach different decisions regarding what is meant by the term *clinical significance.* As a result, the term *clinically significant* has become more useful to marketers than to clinicians.

The term *clinically significant* could be made more relevant by recognizing (1) the nature of the benefits (tangible/intangible) and (2) the size of the treatment effect (large/small). The presence or absence of these two criteria can be used to classify clinical significance into four levels. Before doing so, each classification term is described.

Tangible Versus Intangible Benefits

Controversies remain as to whether outcomes tested in clinical trials designed for drug approval are tangible to the patient.[8,33] Some will argue that the clinical significance of a treatment should depend exclusively on whether the benefits identified are tangible or intangible to the patient who undergoes the procedure.

Tangible benefits are treatment outcomes that reflect how a patient feels, functions, or survives. The word *tangible* is defined as "capable of being precisely identified or realized by the mind." Examples of tangible benefits could include improved oral health–related quality of life,[15,16] a decrease in self-reported symptoms (e.g., bleeding) after brushing, prevention of tooth loss, or elimination of a painful periodontal abscess. These examples of treatment benefits can precisely be identified or realized by the *patient's mind*—that is, they are tangible. Tangible benefits can also

be referred to as "clinically relevant" or "clinically meaningful" benefits.

KEY FACT

The issues with surrogate endpoints were recognized when the first randomized controlled trial in periodontics was published.[4] Almost half a century later, these issues remain largely unaddressed.

Intangible benefits cannot be realized or perceived by the patient's mind. Changes in probing attachment level as a result of scaling, changes in enamel mineralization level as a result of fluoride application, and changes in the size of a periapical radiolucency as a result of root canal treatment are examples of changes that the patient's mind cannot identify or realize; thus they are described as intangible treatment benefits. Intangible treatment benefits can often be measured objectively by the clinician or by laboratory methods.

The first and most important step in assessing the clinical significance of a treatment is to determine whether the documented treatment benefits are tangible or intangible. This distinction is important because intangible benefits often do not translate into tangible benefits. A medication that lowers elevated blood lipid levels (an intangible-benefit) may shorten lifespan (a tangible patient harm). A treatment that increases bone density (an intangible benefit) can increase fracture risk (a tangible patient harm).[11] A treatment that provides extensive periodontal bone regeneration (an intangible benefit) may lead to tooth loss (a tangible harm).[14] A treatment that has been shown to provide tangible benefits has a higher level of clinical significance than a treatment for which only evidence of intangible benefits exists. The finding that implant-supported dentures improve quality of life[1] has a higher level of clinical significance than the finding that scaling increases probing attachment levels. The finding that an endodontic treatment reliably eliminates tooth pain has a higher level of clinical significance than the finding that chlorhexidine reduces *Streptococcus mutans* levels.

We do not have high-level evidence on all periodontal treatments. Obtaining such information will be helpful in documenting their treatment efficacy as we move into the 21st century, as future economic policies may channel limited health care resources to treatments with a proven tangible benefit.

Size of the Treatment Effect

A second important criterion for assessing clinical significance is the size of the treatment effect. The size of the treatment effect is a comparison of the success rates of the experimental treatment and the control treatment. This comparison can be a subtraction of the success rates, a division of the success rates, or some other mathematical operation. The size of the treatment effect, regardless of how it is calculated, has long been recognized as an important part of assessing clinical significance. The larger the likelihood of obtaining an expected benefit of a treatment (relative to a control treatment), the more clinically significant the treatment is. We suggest that the number needed to treat (NNT) may be a good measure to separate large and small treatment effects.

The likelihood of obtaining a treatment benefit (relative to the control) largely determines the methodological and analytic rigor required to establish treatment effectiveness. At one extreme, in all-or-none situations, reliable evidence may result from observations of a small number of patients. For example, no concurrent controlled trials were conducted to assess the effectiveness of general anesthesia. Determining the effectiveness of treatments that achieve a dramatic and immediate effect is straightforward, and only essential scientific principles (e.g., consistency of observations across different operators) are considered sufficient evidence of treatment effectiveness. Reportedly, the words "Gentleman, this is no humbug" were sufficient to convince an audience that general anesthesia was effective.

As in medicine, randomized controlled trials conducted in periodontics have primarily focused on surrogate endpoints. Having true endpoints in future randomized controlled trials will enhance the clinical applicability and relevance of their results.

At another extreme, if the likelihood of obtaining an expected treatment benefit is small, substantial rigor in both design and analysis of controlled clinical trials is required. The benefits of mammography screening for early detection of breast cancer, of one "clot-buster" drug over another after a myocardial event, and of local antibiotics in the treatment of periodontitis are all so small that large randomized controlled trials are required to provide reliable evidence as to whether small benefits indeed are associated with treatment.

The likelihood of obtaining a treatment benefit is a determinant of clinical significance; the larger the likelihood, the more confident a patient can feel that a treatment will be successful. Although it is possible to have a clear, unequivocal definition of what constitutes a tangible benefit associated with treatment, it is not possible to have a similar rigorous definition of what can be considered a large likelihood. We define a "large treatment effect" as an NNT of 5, which under fortuitous and very unusual

circumstances can be reliably identified with nonexperimental study designs.[7,29]

Many periodontal treatments result in small changes in clinical attachment levels or probing depths and consequently lead to questions regarding the clinical significance of periodontal therapy. For instance, one systematic review reported by the American Dental Association (ADA) indicated that the addition of metronidazole to scaling and root planing provided an additional gain of 0.18 mm in attachment level. The ADA refers to such an effect as a "zero effect."[28] Small to zero treatment effects are common in clinical trials in medicine.

Defining Four Levels of Clinical Significance

Based on the nature of the benefit (tangible/intangible) and the size of the treatment effect (large/small), four levels of clinical significance can be defined (Table 31.1). In order of decreasing levels of significance, these are numbered from 1 to 4.

Clinical Significance Level 1

Treatments of clinical significance level 1 are the "magic bullets" or "miracle cures," in which the treatment provides a tangible benefit and a large treatment effect. Examples include the use of vitamin C to treat scurvy, bone marrow transplantation to treat leukemia, and a very-low-carbohydrate diet to prevent all forms of dental decay. In all three examples, the benefits of the treatment are tangible and the size of the treatment effect is large.

Understanding the biologic mechanisms of a treatment is not required to establish that the treatment has clinical significance level 1. Lemon juice was identified as an effective method to prevent scurvy in 1601, but it was not until the beginning of the 20th century that vitamin C was isolated.[25] The dangers of carbohydrates in dental decay were recognized millennia before potential mechanisms of action were understood. Digitalis was discovered as a treatment for "dropsy" long before physicians became aware of the drug's cardiac effects.[31] Lithium is an effective drug for bipolar disorder, but its mechanism of action remains largely unknown.[27] In contrast, hormone replacement therapy (HRT), for which the biologic mechanisms explaining how the drug provided benefits were supposedly so well understood, resulted in more harm than good.[12]

TABLE 31.1   Definition of Levels of Significance Based on Size and Nature of the Benefit

		SIZE OF THE BENEFIT	
Clinical Significance		**Large[c]**	**Small[d]**
Nature of the Benefit	Tangible[a]	Level 1	Level 2
	Intangible[b]	Level 3	Level 4

[a]Tangible benefits are outcomes that directly measure how a patient feels, functions, or survives.
[b]Intangible benefits are outcomes that are not perceivable by the patient's mind.
[c]A large benefit is defined as one that can reliably be identified using epidemiologic methodology.
[d]A small benefit is defined as one that requires randomized controlled trials for reliable identification.

Treatments of clinical significance level 1 are not always immediately accepted or widely used. It took the British Navy 264 years from the time of the observations of Captain James until a universal preventive policy was established to prevent scurvy.[3] The lack of appreciation for this treatment of clinical significance level 1 was unfortunate:

> It is estimated that 5000 lives a year were needlessly lost from scurvy during this period: that is a total of nearly 800,000. In the 200 years from 1600 to 1800 nearly 1,000,000 men died of an easily preventable disease. There are in the whole of human history few more notable examples of official indifference and stupidity producing such disastrous consequence to human life.[24]

Although it is easy to determine clinical significance level 1 in retrospect, it may be difficult to recognize at the time of discovery.

Clinical Significance Level 2

Treatments of clinical significance level 2 are those that have demonstrated a tangible benefit but for which the likelihood of obtaining the benefit from treatment is small. As the size of the benefit of one therapy over another decreases, randomized controlled trials (RCTs), large in size and rigorous in execution and analysis, are required to provide unequivocal evidence that the treatment provides tangible patient benefits. Examples of such treatments include the advantage of tissue plasminogen activator (t-PA) over streptokinase[30] and the benefits of penciclovir in the treatment of herpetic lesions.[12]

Determining the clinical relevance of treatments of clinical significance level 2 is an individual choice in which issues such as cost and side effects often play a more important role. For example, administering antibiotics to 25 individuals could prevent 1 person from experiencing early implant loss.[6] Is a 4% increased survival probability of dental implants worth the potential side effects of antibiotics? Different individuals, different governments, and different health insurance companies may decide differently on this important question.

The use of penciclovir in the treatment of herpetic lesions provides another example of a drug of clinical significance level 2. When applying a 1% penciclovir cream, 70% of patients reported lesion healing by day 6. When applying placebo cream, 59% of patients reported lesion healing by day 6.[21] Is an 11% increased probability of lesion healing (NNT of 9) by day 6 of sufficient magnitude to refer to the treatment as "clinically relevant"? Once again, the answer to this question is highly subjective; the cream might be worth its weight in gold to a teenager when prom night is approaching, but it may be clinically irrelevant to an adult. By using the terminology "clinical significance level 2," the concept of small, tangible patient benefit can quickly be communicated without becoming trapped in meaningless discussions regarding the clinical relevance of small benefits.

experienced the tangible adverse outcome before the treatment became available but none now experience it. All-or-none situations reflect the highest level of evidence.[19]

Clinical Significance Level 3

Treatments of clinical significance level 3 are the magic bullets or miracle cures in the surrogate world, in which the beneficial but intangible effects are so convincing that the need for RCTs may appear unethical. Examples of such treatments include highly active antiretroviral therapy (HAART) in patients with acquired immunodeficiency syndrome (AIDS),[18] imatinib (Gleevec) in the treatment of chronic myeloid leukemia,[31] and chlorhexidine varnish in the prevention of caries.[26] In periodontics, examples of treatments of clinical significance level 3 could be complete restoration of periodontal attachment and bone around teeth that had extensive destruction of the periodontal apparatus, and reconstruction of voluminous amounts of bone on an atrophic mandible for the purpose of placing dental implants.

With a treatment that has the label "clinical significance level 3," there is always uncertainty as to whether the intangible benefits translate into real, tangible patient benefits. For instance, bone marrow transplantation to the periodontal defect indeed resulted in regenerating prodigious amounts of bone, but about 50% of the teeth were lost due to root resorption.[14] Nonetheless, the larger the effect size observed on the surrogate, the more likely the surrogate benefit translates into a real, tangible patient benefit.[9]

For certain treatments, such as HAART for AIDS or Gleevec for chronic leukemia, the opportunity may exist to avoid RCTs, and treatments of clinical significance level 3 can become those of level 1 by means of epidemiologic studies in which large secular changes are observed in the incidence of true endpoints since the introduction of the novel treatment. For example, drastic changes in the viral load of human immunodeficiency virus (HIV) have been shown to lead to large reductions in the risk of AIDS and death. Using historical controls, it was shown that HAART treatment reduced AIDS risk by 38% and mortality risk by 34%.[17] A large surrogate benefit (clinical significance level 3) translated into a large survival benefit (clinical significance level 1).

However, assuming that large, intangible treatment benefits invariably translate into tangible benefits remains dangerous, no matter how large the effect on the surrogate endpoint. A 40% chlorhexidine varnish used for the prevention of caries was reported to result in a 99.9% reduction in mutans streptococci counts in all 20 subjects treated, and the counts stayed below detectable levels for at least 4 weeks in 9 subjects. In contrast, the placebo varnish sealant led to only a 32% mutans streptococci reduction, and none of the 20 subjects had mutans streptococci below detectable levels for 4 weeks.[19] Based on these data, it was reported that "Chlorzoin will wipe out dental decay much like smallpox." A subsequent RCT in 1240 children at high risk for caries did not translate into a reduction of large cavities in the teeth: the Chlorzoin group had 6.8 D3 lesions (standard deviation, 6.2), and the placebo group had 6.4 D3 lesions (standard deviation, 6.4)—in other words, fewer lesions.[29] It has become clear since then that most forms of chlorhexidine are contraindicated in the treatment of caries.[10] A large treatment effect on a surrogate in this instance did not translate into a tangible benefit.

Clinical Significance Level 4

Treatments of clinical significance level 4 are those that have reliable evidence on small, intangible treatment benefits. Because the treatment effects are small, epidemiologic studies are incapable of identifying treatments of clinical significance level 4. In other words, rigorously conducted RCTs are necessary to reliably identify a small surrogate benefit. Examples of treatments of clinical significance level 4 include those that cause a small decrease in lipid level, a small drop in blood pressure, or a small decrease in pocket depth. A large leap of faith is often required to jump from the observation that small changes in surrogate endpoints translate into real, tangible benefits.

Clofibrate, used to lower lipid levels, is an example of a drug of clinical significance level 4. Clofibrate reduced mean cholesterol levels from 324 mg to 224 mg and mean triglyceride levels from 271 to 125 (which can be argued are "not so small" mean changes).[2] Clofibrate was the most widely prescribed lipid-lowering agent in the United States, but uncertainty remained as to whether it actually provided a tangible patient benefit. Advertisements that were widely used in medical journals accurately reflected the clinical uncertainty surrounding use of this drug. A textbox within the advertisements stated, "It has not been established whether the drug-induced lowering of serum cholesterol or lipid levels has a detrimental, beneficial, or no effect on the mortality and the morbidity due to atherosclerosis or coronary heart disease. Several years will be required before current investigations will yield an answer to this question." A subsequent World Health Organization (WHO) cooperative trial on clofibrate revealed the wisdom of this disclaimer. The trial outcome showed that clofibrate resulted in excess mortality of 47%, providing yet another example of a misleading surrogate.[22]

Treatment of clinical significance level 4 may cause more harm than good.[20] This observation has significant consequences in periodontics, because approved periodontal therapies are commonly of clinical significance level 4 and information on their long-term safety and lack of harm is minimal.

Summary

Two important determinants of clinical significance are the nature of benefit (tangible versus intangible) and the likelihood of obtaining the benefit (when compared to the control treatment). These two characteristics can be used to define four hierarchic levels of clinical significance. Treatments that provide a tangible patient benefit (levels 1 and 2) are of greater value and should correspond to a higher level of clinical significance than treatments with evidence of only intangible benefits (levels 3 and 4). Similarly, treatments with a large likelihood of clinical improvement (levels 1 and 3) are clinically more significant than treatments with a small likelihood of clinical improvement (levels 2 and 4). Providing four hierarchical levels of clinical significance may help clinicians and patients communicate more effectively regarding the clinical significance of a treatment. In particular, dental clinicians should inform their periodontal patients that no unequivocal evidence is available showing that periodontal treatments provide tangible patient benefit. We hope that we provide tangible benefits to our patients, but the RCTs are lacking to ensure that we really do.

References

 References for this chapter are found on the companion website www.expertconsult.com.

CHAPTER 32

Periodontal Examination and Diagnosis

Jonathan H. Do | Henry H. Takei | Fermin A. Carranza

CHAPTER OUTLINE

 For online-only content on periodontal probing, periodontal charting, clinical indices, periodontal pockets, and periodontal, gingival, and periapical abscesses, please visit the companion website at www.expertconsult.com.

Proper diagnosis is essential to intelligent treatment. Periodontal diagnosis should first determine whether disease is present. It should then identify the disease, and its severity and extent. Finally, it should provide an understanding of the underlying pathologic processes and their causes. Part 2 of this book provide detailed descriptions of the different diseases that can affect the periodontium.

The periodontal diagnosis is determined after careful analysis of the case history and evaluation of the clinical signs and symptoms as well as the results of various diagnostic procedures (e.g., probing, mobility assessment, radiographs, blood tests, and biopsies).

The interest should be in the patient who has the disease and not simply the disease itself. Diagnosis must therefore include a general evaluation of the patient and a consideration of the oral cavity.

Diagnostic procedures must be systematic and organized for specific purposes. It is not enough to assemble facts. Findings must be pieced together so that they provide a meaningful explanation of the patient's periodontal problem. The following is a recommended sequence of procedures for the diagnosis of periodontal diseases.

Overall Appraisal of the Patient

From the first meeting, the clinician should attempt an overall appraisal of the patient. This includes consideration of the patient's mental and emotional status, temperament, attitude, and physiologic age.

Health History

Most of the health history is obtained at the first visit, and it can be supplemented by pertinent questioning at subsequent visits. The health history can be obtained verbally by questioning the patient and recording his or her responses in the patient chart or by means of a questionnaire that the patient completes prior to the appointment. Fig. 32.1 shows the health history form recommended by the American Dental Association.

The importance of the health history should be clearly explained, because patients often omit information that they cannot relate to their dental problems. The patient should be made aware of the following: (1) the possible impact of certain systemic diseases, conditions, behavioral factors, and medications on periodontal disease, its treatment, and treatment outcomes; (2) the presence of conditions that may require special precautions or modifications of the treatment procedure (see Chapter 39); and (3) the possibility that oral infections may have a powerful influence on the occurrence and severity of a variety of systemic diseases and conditions (see Chapter 15).

The health history should include reference to the following:

1. The date of the last physical exam and the frequency of physical exams and physician visits. If the patient is under the care of a physician, the nature and duration of the problem and its therapy should be discussed. The name, address, and telephone number of the physician should be recorded, because direct communication with him or her may be necessary.
2. Details regarding hospitalizations and operations, including the diagnosis, the type of operation, and any untoward events (e.g., anesthetic, hemorrhagic, or infectious complications) should be obtained.
3. All medical problems (e.g., cardiovascular, hematologic, endocrine), including infectious diseases, sexually transmitted diseases, high-risk behavior for human immunodeficiency virus infection, and possible occupational disease, should be inquired.
4. Abnormal bleeding tendencies, such as nosebleeds, prolonged bleeding from minor cuts, spontaneous ecchymosis, a tendency toward excessive bruising, and excessive menstrual bleeding, should be cited. These symptoms should be correlated with the medications that the patient is taking.
5. Information is needed for females regarding the onset of puberty, menopause, menstrual disorders, hysterectomy, pregnancies, and miscarriages.
6. A list of all medications being taken and whether they were prescribed or obtained over the counter should be included. All of the possible effects of these medications should be carefully

Health History Form

AD>A.
American Dental Association
www.ada.org

E-mail: _____   Today's Date: _____

As required by law, our office adheres to written policies and procedures to protect the privacy of information about you that we create, receive or maintain. Your answers are for our records only and will be kept confidential subject to applicable laws. Please note that you will be asked some questions about your responses to this questionnaire and there may be additional questions concerning your health. This information is vital to allow us to provide appropriate care for you. This office does not use this information to discriminate.

Name: _____   Home Phone: *Include area code* ( )   Business/Cell Phone: *Include area code* ( )

   Last   First   Middle

Address: _____   City: _____   State: _____   Zip: _____

   Mailing address

Occupation: _____   Height: _____   Weight: _____   Date of birth: _____   Sex: M F

SS# or Patient ID: _____   Emergency Contact: _____   Relationship: _____   Home Phone: ( )   Cell Phone: ( )

   Include area codes

If you are completing this form for another person, what is your relationship to that person? _____

Your Name   Relationship

Do you have any of the following diseases or problems: *(Check DK if you Don't Know the answer to the question)*   **Yes No DK**

Active tuberculosis... ☐ ☐ ☐

Persistent cough greater than a 3 week duration... ☐ ☐ ☐

Cough that produces blood... ☐ ☐ ☐

Been exposed to anyone with tuberculosis... ☐ ☐ ☐

If you answer yes to any of the 4 items above, please stop and return this form to the receptionist.

Dental Information *For the following questions, please mark (X) your responses to the following questions.*

	Yes	No	DK		Yes	No	DK
Do your gums bleed when you brush or floss?	☐	☐	☐	Do you have earaches or neck pains?	☐	☐	☐
Are your teeth sensitive to cold, hot, sweets or pressure?	☐	☐	☐	Do you have any clicking, popping or discomfort in the jaw?	☐	☐	☐
Does food or floss catch between your teeth?	☐	☐	☐	Do you brux or grind your teeth?	☐	☐	☐
Is your mouth dry?	☐	☐	☐	Do you have sores or ulcers in your mouth?	☐	☐	☐
Have you had any periodontal (gum) treatments?	☐	☐	☐	Do you wear dentures or partials?	☐	☐	☐
Have you ever had orthodontic (braces) treatment?	☐	☐	☐	Do you participate in active recreational activities?	☐	☐	☐
Have you had any problems associated with previous dental treatment?	☐	☐	☐	Have you ever had a serious injury to your head or mouth?	☐	☐	☐
Is your home water supply fluoridated?	☐	☐	☐	Date of your last dental exam:			
Do you drink bottled or filtered water?	☐	☐	☐	What was done at that time?			
If yes, how often? Circle one: DAILY / WEEKLY / OCCASIONALLY							
Are you currently experiencing dental pain or discomfort?	☐	☐	☐	Date of last dental x-rays:			

What is the reason for your dental visit today? _____

How do you feel about your smile? _____

Medical Information *Please mark (X) your response to indicate if you have or have not had any of the following diseases or problems.*

	Yes	No	DK		Yes	No	DK
Are you now under the care of a physician?	☐	☐	☐	Have you had a serious illness, operation or been hospitalized in the past 5 years?	☐	☐	☐
Physician Name: Phone: *Include area code* ( )				If yes, what was the illness or problem?			
Address/City/State/Zip:				Are you taking or have you recently taken any prescription or over the counter medicine(s)?	☐	☐	☐
Are you in good health?	☐	☐	☐	If so, please list all, including vitamins, natural or herbal preparations and/or diet supplements:			
Has there been any change in your general health within the past year?	☐	☐	☐	_____			
If yes, what condition is being treated?				_____			
Date of last physical exam:				_____			

Fig. 32.1 Medical history form from the American Dental Association. *(From © American Dental Association. Reprinted with permission.)*   *Continued*

Medical Information
Please mark (X) your response to indicate if you have or have not had any of the following diseases or problems.

(Check DK if you Don't Know the answer to the question) Yes No DK

Do you wear contact lenses? ☐ ☐ ☐

Joint Replacement. Have you had an orthopedic total joint (hip, knee, elbow, finger) replacement? ☐ ☐ ☐
Date: _____ If yes, have you had any complications? _____

Are you taking or scheduled to begin taking either of the medications, alendronate (Fosamax®) or risedronate (Actonel®) for osteoporosis or Paget's disease? ☐ ☐ ☐

Since 2001, were you treated or are you presently scheduled to begin treatment with the intravenous bisphosphonates (Aredia® or Zometa®) for bone pain, hypercalcemia or skeletal complications resulting from Paget's disease, multiple myeloma or metastatic cancer? ☐ ☐ ☐
Date Treatment began: _____

Allergies - Are you allergic to or have you had a reaction to: Yes No DK
To all **yes** responses, specify type of reaction.
Local anesthetics _____ ☐ ☐ ☐
Aspirin _____ ☐ ☐ ☐
Penicillin or other antibiotics _____ ☐ ☐ ☐
Barbiturates, sedatives, or sleeping pills _____ ☐ ☐ ☐
Sulfa drugs _____ ☐ ☐ ☐
Codeine or other narcotics _____ ☐ ☐ ☐

Do you use controlled substances (drugs)? ☐ ☐ ☐
Do you use tobacco (smoking, snuff, chew, bidis)? ☐ ☐ ☐
If so, how interested are you in stopping?
(Circle one) VERY / SOMEWHAT / NOT INTERESTED
Do you drink alcoholic beverages? ☐ ☐ ☐
If yes, how much alcohol did you drink in the last 24 hours? _____
If yes, how much do you typically drink in a week? _____

WOMEN ONLY Are you:
Pregnant? ☐ ☐ ☐
Number of weeks: _____
Taking birth control pills or hormonal replacement? ☐ ☐ ☐
Nursing? ☐ ☐ ☐

Yes No DK
Metals _____ ☐ ☐ ☐
Latex (rubber) _____ ☐ ☐ ☐
Iodine _____ ☐ ☐ ☐
Hay fever/seasonal _____ ☐ ☐ ☐
Animals _____ ☐ ☐ ☐
Food _____ ☐ ☐ ☐
Other _____ ☐ ☐ ☐

Please mark (X) your response to indicate if you have or have not had any of the following diseases or problems.

Yes No DK
Artificial (prosthetic) heart valve ☐ ☐ ☐
Previous infective endocarditis ☐ ☐ ☐
Damaged valves in transplanted heart ☐ ☐ ☐
Congenital heart disease (CHD)
  Unrepaired, cyanotic CHD ☐ ☐ ☐
  Repaired (completely) in last 6 months ☐ ☐ ☐
  Repaired CHD with residual defects ☐ ☐ ☐

Except for the conditions listed above, antibiotic prophylaxis is no longer recommended for any other form of CHD.

Yes No DK
Cardiovascular disease. ☐ ☐ ☐
Angina ☐ ☐ ☐
Arteriosclerosis ☐ ☐ ☐
Congestive heart failure ☐ ☐ ☐
Damaged heart valves ☐ ☐ ☐
Heart attack ☐ ☐ ☐
Heart murmur ☐ ☐ ☐
Low blood pressure ☐ ☐ ☐
High blood pressure ☐ ☐ ☐
Other congenital heart
  defects ☐ ☐ ☐

Yes No DK
Mitral valve prolapse ☐ ☐ ☐
Pacemaker ☐ ☐ ☐
Rheumatic fever ☐ ☐ ☐
Rheumatic heart disease ☐ ☐ ☐
Abnormal bleeding ☐ ☐ ☐
Anemia ☐ ☐ ☐
Blood transfusion ☐ ☐ ☐
  If yes, date: _____
Hemophilia ☐ ☐ ☐
AIDS or HIV infection ☐ ☐ ☐
Arthritis ☐ ☐ ☐

Yes No DK
Autoimmune disease ☐ ☐ ☐
Rheumatoid arthritis ☐ ☐ ☐
Systemic lupus erythematosus ☐ ☐ ☐
Asthma ☐ ☐ ☐
Bronchitis ☐ ☐ ☐
Emphysema ☐ ☐ ☐
Sinus trouble ☐ ☐ ☐
Tuberculosis ☐ ☐ ☐
Cancer/Chemotherapy/
  Radiation Treatment ☐ ☐ ☐
Chest pain upon exertion ☐ ☐ ☐
Chronic pain ☐ ☐ ☐
Diabetes Type I or II ☐ ☐ ☐
Eating disorder ☐ ☐ ☐
Malnutrition ☐ ☐ ☐
Gastrointestinal disease ☐ ☐ ☐
G.E. Reflux/persistent
  heartburn ☐ ☐ ☐
Ulcers ☐ ☐ ☐
Thyroid problems ☐ ☐ ☐
Stroke ☐ ☐ ☐
Glaucoma ☐ ☐ ☐

Yes No DK
Hepatitis, jaundice or
  liver disease ☐ ☐ ☐
Epilepsy ☐ ☐ ☐
Fainting spells or seizures ☐ ☐ ☐
Neurological disorders ☐ ☐ ☐
  If yes, specify: _____
Sleep disorder ☐ ☐ ☐
Mental health disorders ☐ ☐ ☐
  Specify: _____
Recurrent infections ☐ ☐ ☐
  Type of infection: _____
Kidney problems ☐ ☐ ☐
Night sweats ☐ ☐ ☐
Osteoporosis ☐ ☐ ☐
Persistent swollen glands
  in neck ☐ ☐ ☐
Severe headaches/
  migraines ☐ ☐ ☐
Severe or rapid weight loss ☐ ☐ ☐
Sexually transmitted disease ☐ ☐ ☐
Excessive urination ☐ ☐ ☐

Has a physician or previous dentist recommended that you take antibiotics prior to your dental treatment? ☐ ☐ ☐

Name of physician or dentist making recommendation: _____   Phone: _____

Do you have any disease, condition, or problem not listed above that you think I should know about? ☐ ☐ ☐
Please explain:

NOTE: Both doctor and patient are encouraged to discuss any and all relevant patient health issues prior to treatment.
I certify that I have read and understand the above and that the information given on this form is accurate. I understand the importance of a truthful health history and that my dentist and his/her staff will rely on this information for treating me. I acknowledge that my questions, if any, about inquiries set forth above have been answered to my satisfaction. I will not hold my dentist, or any other member of his/her staff, responsible for any action they take or do not take because of errors or omissions that I may have made in the completion of this form.

Signature of Patient/Legal Guardian: _____   Date: _____

FOR COMPLETION BY DENTIST
Comments: _____

Fig. 32.1, cont'd

analyzed to determine their effect, if any, on the oral tissues and also to avoid administering medications that would interact adversely with them. Special inquiry should be made regarding the dosage and duration of therapy with anticoagulants and corticosteroids. Patients who are taking any of the family of drugs called bisphosphonates (e.g., Actonel, Fosamax, Boniva, Aredia, Zometa), which are often prescribed for osteoporosis, should be cautioned about possible problems related to osteonecrosis of the jaw after undergoing any form of oral surgery involving bone.

7. The patient's allergy history should be taken, including that related to hay fever, asthma, sensitivity to foods, sensitivity to drugs (e.g., aspirin, codeine, barbiturates, sulfonamides, antibiotics, procaine, laxatives), and sensitivity to dental materials (e.g., latex, eugenol, acrylic resins).

8. A family history should be taken, including that of bleeding disorders, cardiovascular disease, diabetes, or periodontal diseases.

9. Detailed information on current and history of alcohol, recreational drugs, and tobacco use, and desire to quit should be elicited.

As part of the overall patient appraisal, baseline vitals—at minimum, blood pressure—should be obtained. For patients who are on medications such as bisphosphonates, anticoagulants, or antiplatelets or patients who do not know the control of their systemic disease, such as diabetes, hypertension, or immunodeficiency, a medical consultation is required before any treatment can be rendered.

Dental History

Chief Complaint and Current Illness

Some patients may be unaware of any problems. However, many may report bleeding gums, loose teeth, spreading of the teeth with the appearance of spaces where none existed before, foul taste in the mouth, or an itchy feeling in the gums that is relieved by digging with a toothpick. There may also be pain of varied types and duration, including constant, dull, gnawing pain; dull pain after eating; deep radiating pain in the jaws; acute throbbing pain; sensitivity when chewing; sensitivity to hot and cold; burning sensation in the gums; or extreme sensitivity to inhaled air.

The dental history should include reference to the following:

1. Visits to the dentist should be listed, including their frequency, the date of the most recent visit, the nature of the treatment, and dental prophylaxis, periodontal maintenance, or scaling and root planing by a dentist or hygienist, including the frequency of cleaning and date of the most recent cleaning.

2. The patient's oral hygiene regimen should be described, including toothbrushing frequency, time of day, method, type of toothbrush and dentifrice, and interval when brushes are replaced. Other methods for mouth care, such as mouthwashes, interdental brushes, other devices, water irrigation, and dental floss, should also be listed.

3. Any orthodontic treatment, including its duration and the approximate date of termination, should be noted.

4. If the patient is experiencing pain in the teeth or in the gingiva, the manner in which the pain is provoked, its nature and duration, and the manner in which it is relieved should be described.

5. Note the presence of any gingival bleeding, including when it first occurred; whether it occurs spontaneously, on brushing or eating, at night, or with regular periodicity; whether it is associated with the menstrual period or other specific factors; and its duration of the bleeding and the manner by which it is stopped.

6. A bad taste in the mouth and areas of food impaction should be mentioned.

7. Assess whether the patient's teeth feel "loose" or insecure, if he or she has any difficulty chewing, and whether there is any tooth mobility.

8. Note the patient's general dental habits, such as grinding or clenching of the teeth during the day or at night. Do the teeth or jaw muscles feel "sore" in the morning? Are there other habits to address, such as tobacco smoking or chewing, nail biting, or biting on foreign objects?

9. Discuss the patient's history of previous periodontal problems, including the nature of the condition and, if it was previously treated, the type of treatment received (surgical or nonsurgical) and the approximate period of termination. If, in the opinion of the patient, the present problem is a recurrence of previous disease, what does he or she think caused it?

10. Note whether the patient wears a removable prosthesis. Does the prosthesis enhance or is it a detriment to the existing dentition or the surrounding soft tissues?

11. Does the patient have implants to replace any missing teeth?

LEARNING BOX 32.1

Periodontal examination and diagnosis must include obtaining a thorough health and dental history.

Photographic Documentation

An important part of periodontal examination and diagnosis is the documentation of clinical findings. Digital photographic documentation is important and useful for record-keeping, education of both the clinician and the patient, communication with referrals and colleagues, and planning and treatment of high aesthetic demand cases. Photographs can provide details that a clinician may not otherwise remember and allow the clinician to evaluate the mouth after the patient leaves and to monitor changes in the tissue over time. If possible, at the beginning of the clinical examination, a set of intraoral photos (Fig. 32.2) should be taken before the tissue is probed and manipulated to obtain an undisturbed baseline of the patient's mouth with gingiva and biofilm intact. These initial photos, when presented to the patient on a large-screen monitor, can be extremely powerful in educating and helping the patient to understand the conditions of his or her mouth; the presence and location of biofilm, inflammation, and any tissue abnormality; and the need for improvement in oral hygiene or treatment (Fig. 32.3).

LEARNING BOX 32.2

Initial photographs should be taken before the tissue is probed and manipulated to obtain an undisturbed baseline of the patient's mouth with gingiva and biofilm intact.

Clinical Examination

Examination of Extraoral Structures

Clinical examination should begin with an evaluation of the extraoral structures for abnormalities. The temporomandibular joints should be assessed for pain, crepitus, clicking, and range of motion. The muscles of mastication should be palpated for pain and tenderness.

Because periodontal, periapical, and other oral diseases may result in lymph node changes, the clinician should routinely examine and evaluate the lymph nodes of the head and neck. Lymph nodes can become enlarged or indurated as a result of an infectious episode, malignant metastases, or residual fibrotic changes.

Inflammatory nodes become enlarged, palpable, tender, and fairly immobile. The overlying skin may be red and warm. Patients are often aware of the presence of "swollen glands." Primary herpetic gingivostomatitis, necrotizing ulcerative gingivitis, and acute periodontal abscesses may produce lymph node enlargement. After successful therapy, lymph nodes return to normal in a matter of days to weeks.

Examination of the Oral Cavity

The entire oral cavity should be carefully examined, beginning with oral hygiene. The cleanliness of the oral cavity is appraised in terms of the extent of accumulated food debris, biofilm, calculus, and tooth surface stains, as well as biofilm coating of the dorsum of the tongue (Fig. 32.4). Oral malodor, which is also termed *fetor ex ore, fetor oris,* or *halitosis,* is a foul or offensive odor that emanates from the oral cavity. When present, mouth odors may be of diagnostic significance, and their origin may be either oral or extraoral (remote).[63] Chapter 49 discusses in detail the problems related to oral malodor.

The lips, the floor of the mouth, the tongue, the palate, the vestibule, and the oropharyngeal region should be evaluated for abnormalities and pathologies. The oral mucosa in the lateral and apical areas of the tooth may be palpated for tenderness to detect periapical and periodontal abscesses.

Although not all findings are related to periodontal problems, the dentist should detect all pathologic changes that are present in the mouth and, if necessary, make the appropriate dental or medical referral.

Examination of the Periodontium

The periodontal examination should be systematic and should not immediately begin with insertion of the periodontal probe into the gingival crevice, which can be uncomfortable and traumatic for a patient and may induce bleeding that may make visualization of inflammatory changes in the soft tissue challenging. Periodontal disease occurs as a result of biofilm accumulating on the tooth surface and the adjacent tissue responding to it. Therefore the periodontal examination should begin with a thorough and careful visual evaluation of the gingival margin to assess biofilm and calculus accumulation as well as inflammatory changes in the soft tissue (Fig. 32.5). Once a thorough visual periodontal assessment has been completed, the gingiva, the gingival crevice, and the subgingival tooth surface are carefully probed. Thorough probing of the gingival crevice and the surrounding tissue provides a wealth of valuable information beyond probing depth and bleeding on probing that is essential to the diagnosis and treatment of periodontal disease.

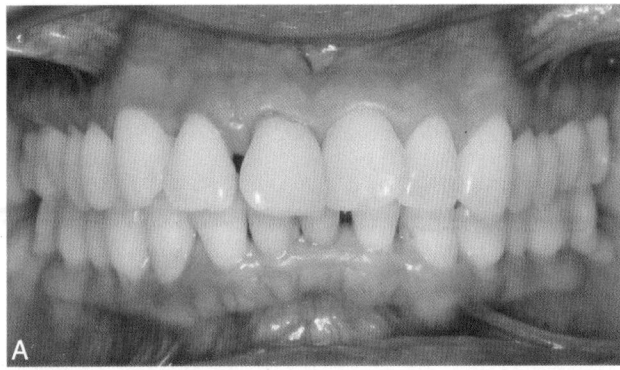

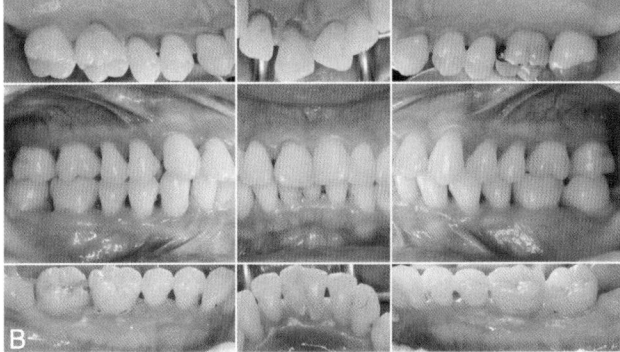

Fig. 32.2 At minimum, an initial set of photographs for a periodontal patient contains nine images. (A) The retracted frontal image is a direct shot, whereas the remaining eight images are mirror shots. (B) The two buccal shots are flipped horizontally and compiled with the remaining seven images to create a composite of the whole dentition. *(Copyright Jonathan H. Do, DDS. All rights reserved.)*

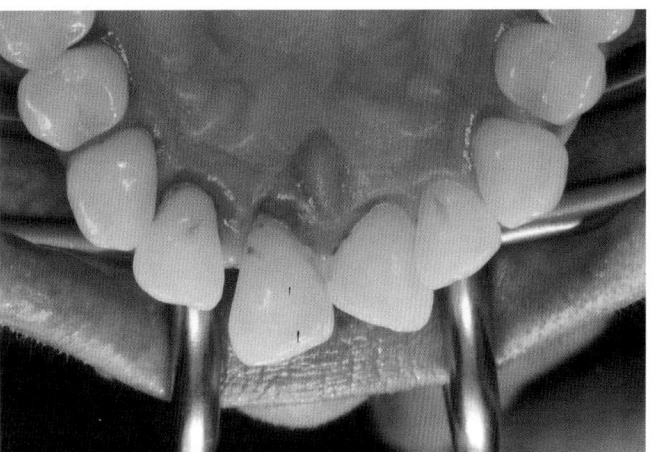

Fig. 32.3 An image capturing the palatal surfaces of the anterior maxilla is presented on a 27-inch computer screen to help a patient understand her periodontal disease. *(Copyright Jonathan H. Do, DDS. All rights reserved.)*

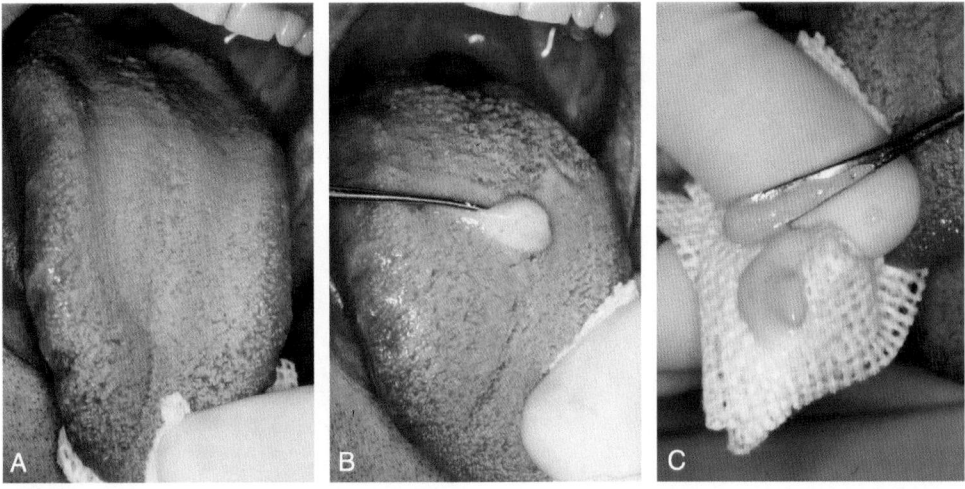

Fig. 32.4 A biofilm coating of the dorsum surface of the tongue (A) can be a source of oral malodor. When the tongue is heavily coated, the biofilm may need to be scraped off with a spatula (B and C).

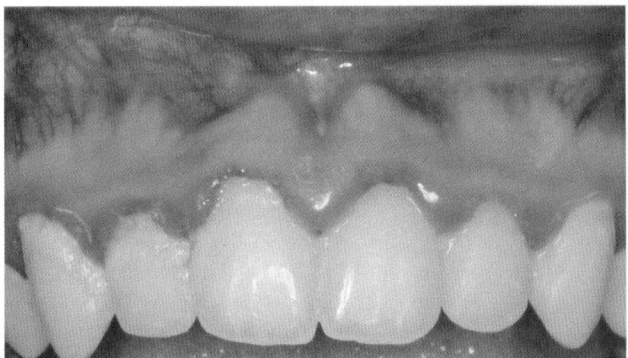

Fig. 32.5 The inflammatory response in the marginal gingiva is a result of biofilm accumulation on the tooth surface along the gingival margin. *(Copyright Jonathan H. Do, DDS. All rights reserved.)*

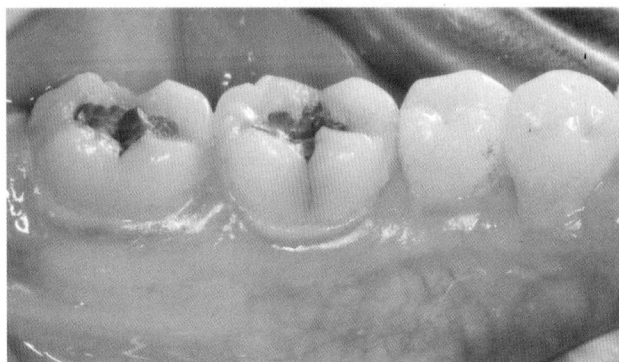

Fig. 32.6 Biofilm frequently accumulates on tooth surfaces in concavities along the gingival margin and interproximal spaces. *(Copyright Jonathan H. Do, DDS. All rights reserved.)*

Visual Periodontal Examination

Visual examination begins with drying the tissue and taking a survey of biofilm and calculus accumulation to assess oral hygiene as well as clinical signs of inflammation (erythema, edema, etc.) and recession to assess the presence and severity of disease.

Visual Examination of Biofilm and Calculus

There are many methods available for assessing biofilm and calculus accumulation.[19] The presence of biofilm and supragingival calculus can be observed directly. Biofilm frequently accumulates in concavities along the gingival margins and in embrasure spaces, especially in difficult-to-reach places, such as the distal surface of the distal-most tooth in the quadrant and the lingual surfaces of the mandibular molars (Fig. 32.6). Supragingival calculus commonly accumulates on the lingual surfaces of the mandibular anterior teeth and the buccal surfaces of the maxillary molars due to the presence of the respective Wharton and Stensen salivary ducts and ineffective biofilm removal. The amount and location of biofilm and supragingival calculus may provide insights into the effectiveness of the patient's biofilm control as well as possible inflammatory changes in the tissue. Biofilm on the buccal and facial surfaces of teeth closest to the midline are most accessible for removal. The presence of biofilm in these areas may suggest inadequate oral hygiene (see Fig. 32.5). The absence of biofilm may not necessarily indicate that the patient practices good oral hygiene at home or that the disease is absent, as

many patients, out of courtesy, brush their teeth thoroughly before seeing a dentist. The presence or absence of biofilm should be correlated to the presence and severity or absence of gingival inflammation.

The presence of subgingival calculus may not be easily detected. Sometimes shallow subgingival calculus may be visible along the gingival margin or through the soft tissue if the soft tissue is thin (Fig. 32.7). Most of the time, subgingival calculus will need to be detected by careful probing of the root surface. The presence of inflammatory changes in the soft tissue may provide clues to the location of the subgingival calculus.

Although radiographs may sometimes reveal heavy calculus deposits interproximally and even on the facial and lingual surfaces, they cannot be relied on for thorough detection of calculus.

Visual Examination of the Gingiva

The gingiva is the keratinized collar of masticatory mucosa around the teeth. It extends from the gingival margin to the mucogingival junction. On the palate, where the mucogingival junction is absent, the gingiva extends apically from the mucogingival junction and merges seamlessly with the mucosa of the hard palate.

The width of the gingiva is the distance from the mucogingival junction to the gingival margin. The mucogingival junction can be determined by stretching the lip and cheek or by placing a probe horizontally in the vestibule and rolling to the mucosa coronally. The mucogingival junction is where the mucosa stops rolling or

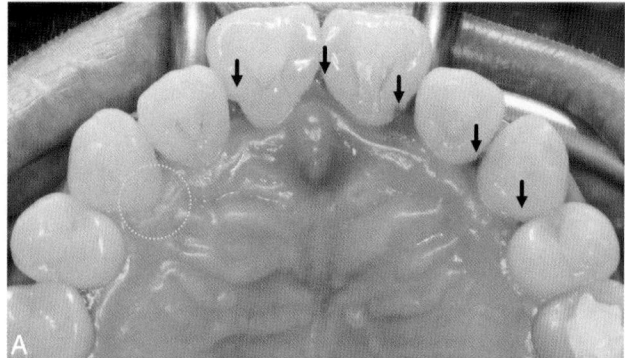

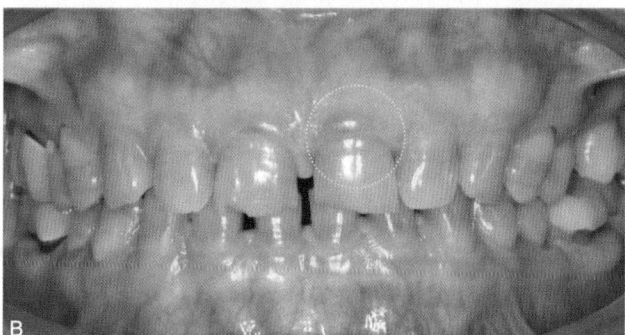

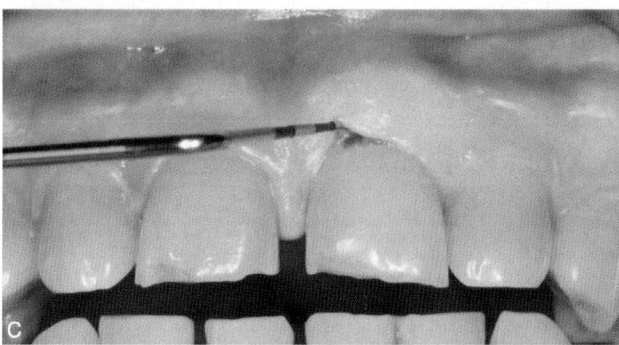

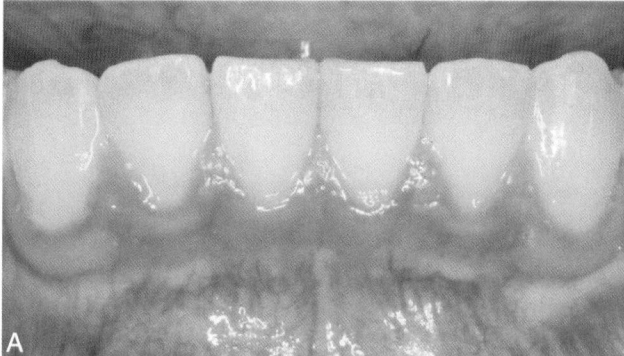

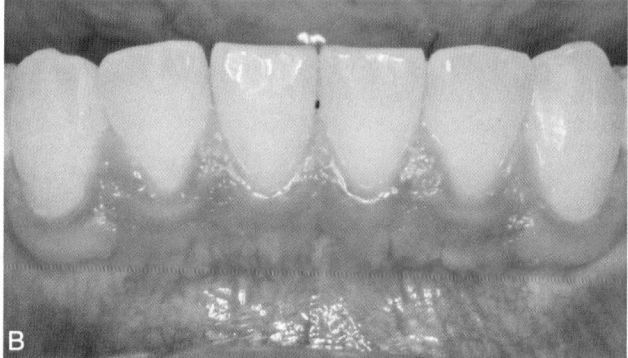

Fig. 32.8 Saliva obscures details. (A) The gingiva appears smooth when covered in saliva. (B) Once dried, stippling is visible, and erythema and edema become more obvious. *(Copyright Jonathan H. Do, DDS. All rights reserved.)*

Fig. 32.7 (A) Subgingival calculus can be visible on the tooth surface *(arrows)* along the gingival margin. Its presence is associated with inflammatory changes in the tissue. Where biofilm and calculus are absent, the gingiva is pink, firm, and stippled (circle). (B) Subgingival calculus may be visible through the marginal gingiva. (C) Retraction of the gingiva confirms its presence. *(Copyright Jonathan H. Do, DDS. All rights reserved.)*

moving. It is common for teeth to be surrounded by gingiva. However, there may be sites where keratinized tissue is absent and the gingival margin is lined by nonkeratinized mucosa.

Evaluation of the gingiva requires the tissue to be dried before accurate observations can be made. The presence of saliva can obscure details (Fig. 32.8). Once the gingiva is thoroughly dried with gauze, it is evaluated and assessed for inflammatory changes. Subtle inflammatory changes in the marginal gingiva may be best detected by comparing the marginal gingiva to the gingival tissue 2 or 3 mm away from the gingival margin, where the tissue is likely to be healthy (Fig. 32.9). Inflammatory changes at each site are correlated with the presence and severity of biofilm and calculus. If biofilm and supragingival calculus are insignificant, inflammatory changes may suggest the presence of subgingival calculus or other contributing factors.

The appearance of the soft tissue adjacent to a tooth may vary from patient to patient, and from tooth to tooth within the same patient, depending on the location and the anatomy of the area. Generally, healthy gingiva is coral pink or salmon pink in color. The

gingival contour consists of sharp, thin, knife-edge margins with scalloped gingival architecture and sharp papillae. The surface texture of healthy gingiva is matte and stippled. The presence of stippling can vary between individuals and sites within the same individual. The absence of stippling does not necessarily imply inflammatory changes in the tissue.

In the presence of inflammatory periodontal disease, the color of the gingiva may be erythematous or cyanotic. Instead of having knife-edge margins and sharp papillae gingival contours, inflamed gingiva may have rolled margins and bulbous papillae. The surface texture in the presence of inflammation may be smooth and shiny, and the gingiva may appear swollen and edematous. Table 32.1 summarizes clinical findings of healthy and inflamed gingiva. Chapter 18 further discusses the clinical features of gingival inflammation.

In individuals with physiologic pigmentation, the gingiva may be pigmented and dark in color. Even so, if healthy, it should exhibit the other features associated with gingival health. Likewise, in the presence of inflammation and disease, it should exhibit many of the characteristics of gingival inflammation (Fig. 32.10).

Gingival Recession

The location of the gingival margin around teeth should be evaluated and recorded, especially when recession is present. In the absence of attachment loss, the gingival margin is located coronal to the cementoenamel junction. The exact location of the gingiva with respect to the cementoenamel junction is difficult to ascertain, as the detection of a subgingival cementoenamel can be challenging. When the cementoenamel junction is supragingival, recession is the distance from the cementoenamel junction to the gingival margin. The presence of recession indicates that attachment loss has occurred, but not necessarily that inflammation is present. At sites with recession, the amount of recession should be recorded, and the presence of

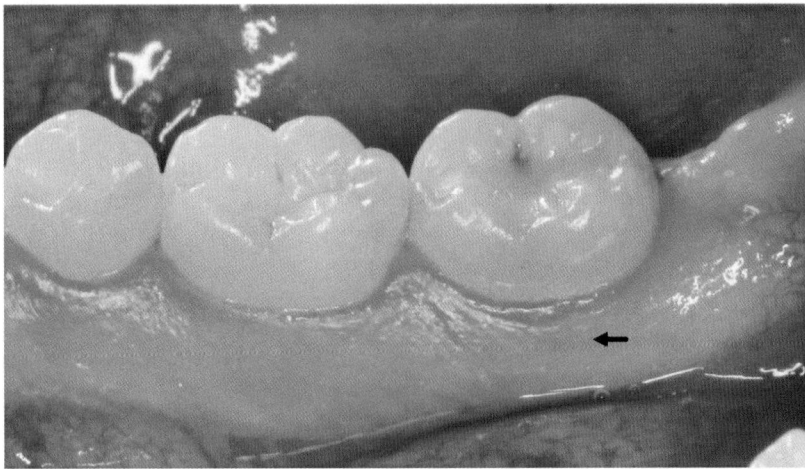

Fig. 32.9 When the marginal gingiva is compared to the gingiva 2 to 3 mm away from the gingival margin *(arrow)*, it is obvious that the marginal gingiva is erythematous and edematous. *(Copyright Jonathan H. Do, DDS. All rights reserved.)*

TABLE 32.1

Gingiva: Healthy	Gingiva: Inflammation
• Color: coral pink or salmon pink	• Color: erythematous, cyanotic
• Consistency: firm/tight, well adapted	• Consistency: edematous, spongy, loosely adapted
• Contour: scalloped, sharp papillae, knife-edge margin	• Contour: bulbous, swollen papillae, rolled margin
• Surface texture: matte, stippled	• Surface texture: smooth, shiny
• Marginal bleeding: absent or slight	• Marginal bleeding: moderate or severe
• Probing depth: 2–3 mm	• Probing depth: >3 mm
• Tissue resistance: present to probe penetration	• Tissue resistance: minimal to probe penetration
• Bleeding on probing: absent or slight	• Bleeding on probing: moderate to severe
• Pain on probing: absent or slight	• Pain: moderate to severe

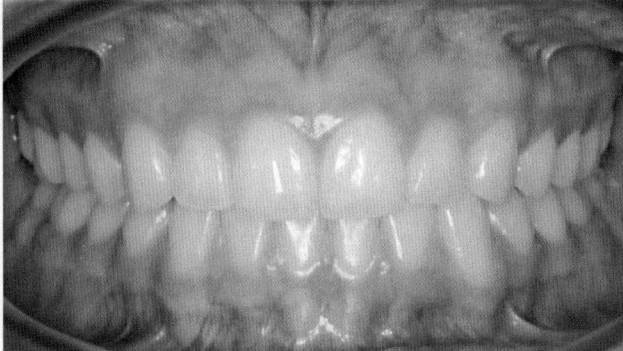
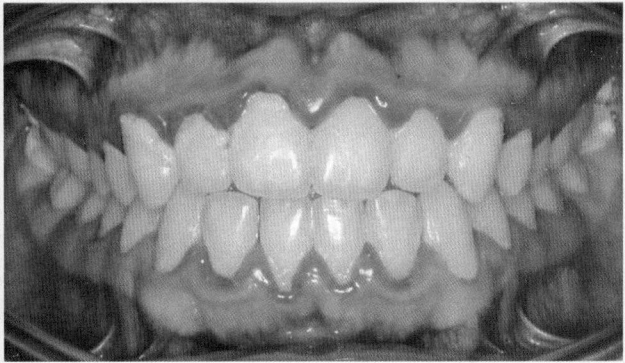

biofilm and calculus, the inflammatory changes in the gingiva, and the width of the keratinized tissue should be carefully evaluated (Fig. 32.11).

LEARNING BOX 32.4

Periodontal examination begins with the visual evaluation of the gingival margin for the presence of tooth surface accretion and inflammatory changes in the gingiva.

Tactile Periodontal Examination

Tactile periodontal examination begins with the evaluation of the consistency of the gingiva and its adaptation to the tooth as well as

the presence of marginal bleeding and suppuration. The gingival crevice is then probed to evaluate the subgingival environment. The tooth surface is carefully probed for aberrations, concavities, furcation, and subgingival calculus. The response of the gingival tissue to probing is appraised in terms of resistance to probe penetration, depth of probe penetration, bleeding on probing, and pain on probing.

Tactile Examination of the Marginal Gingiva

The marginal gingiva is palpated with a periodontal probe to assess its consistency and adaptation to the tooth. Healthy gingiva is firm, resilient, and well adapted to the tooth due to the presence of dense collagen fiber bundles in the lamina propria of the gingiva. When inflamed, the gingiva is edematous, spongy, and loosely adapted to the tooth surface due to the degradation of collagen and the influx of cells and fluid into the lamina propria (Fig. 32.12). In cases of

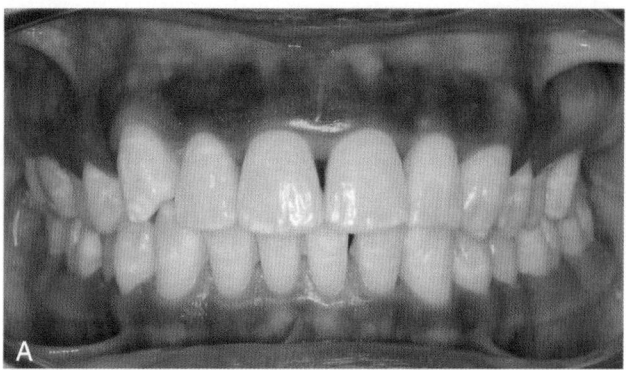

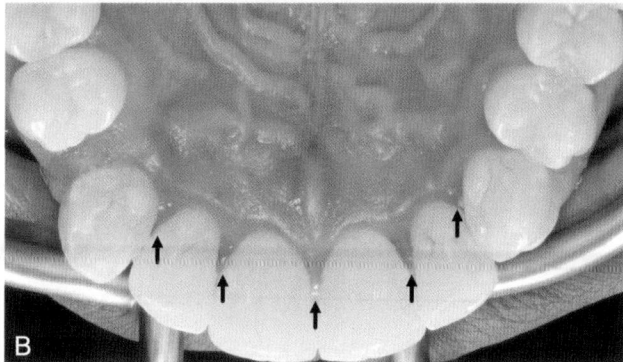

Fig. 32.10 Papillary *(arrows)* and marginal erythema and edema in a patient with physiologic pigmentation. *(Copyright Jonathan H. Do, DDS. All rights reserved.)*

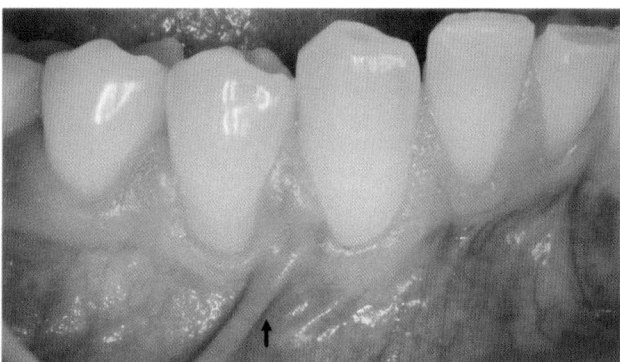

Fig. 32.11 The canine and first premolar exhibit gingival recession and minimal keratinized tissue. Both teeth are at risk of further recession due to the presence of gingival inflammation and a frenum pull *(arrow)*. *(Copyright Jonathan H. Do, DDS. All rights reserved.)*

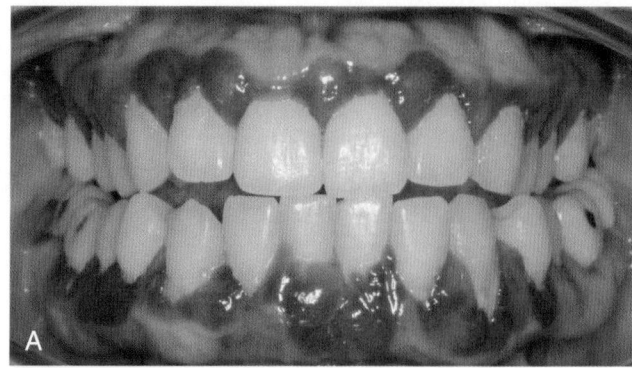

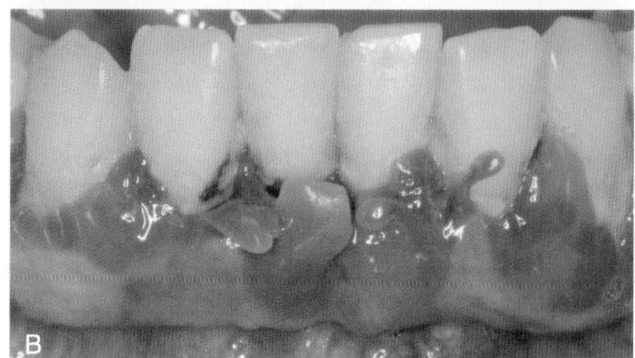

Fig. 32.12 The severely inflamed gingiva is loosely adapted to the tooth. The marginal gingiva is easily retracted to reveal heavy subgingival biofilm and calculus. *(Copyright Jonathan H. Do, DDS. All rights reserved.)*

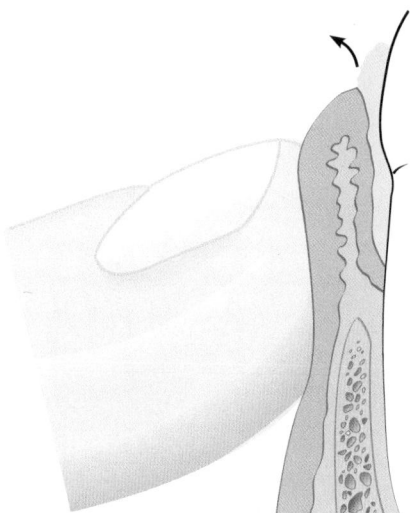

Fig. 32.13 Purulent exudate expressed from a periodontal pocket by digital pressure.

chronic inflammation and in smokers, the gingival tissue may be fibrotic.

Marginal Bleeding

Marginal bleeding is associated with inflammatory changes in the marginal gingiva. Marginal bleeding can be evaluated by running an instrument such as a probe or rubber tip along the gingival margin. Under pressure, healthy gingival tissue will blanch and not bleed, whereas in the presence of gingival inflammation, marginal bleeding may be observed. The ease and severity of marginal bleeding are correlated with the severity of gingival inflammation.

Suppuration

Palpation of the marginal gingiva with a probe, or digitally by placing the ball of the index finger on the gingiva apical to the margin, and pushing coronally toward the gingival margin (Fig. 32.13) may squeeze a white-yellowish exudate from the gingival crevice. The presence of an abundance of neutrophils in the gingival fluid transforms it into a purulent exudate.[5] Suppuration does not occur in all periodontal pockets, but pressure often reveals it in pockets where its presence is not suspected. Several studies[10,11,15,31] have evaluated the association between suppuration and the progression of periodontitis and have reported that this sign is present in a very low percentage of diseased sites (i.e., 3% to 5%).[5] Therefore, absence of suppuration does not indicate absence of disease.

Tactile Examination of the Gingival Crevice

The probe is inserted into the gingival crevice vertically with the tip of the probe touching and sliding down along the tooth surface to the bottom of the crevice. The probe is "walked" circumferentially around each surface of each tooth to detect the areas of deepest penetration. As the probe tip slides down along the tooth surface, attention is paid to the tactile feel of the gingival tissue and the tooth surface. Healthy gingival tissue will feel tight and resist probe penetration. The tightness of the tissue will increase and the probe will come to a stop. In fact, it is the adhesion of the junctional epithelium to the tooth surface that stops probe penetration in healthy tissue. If the gingival tissue is severely inflamed, the probe may not have any resistance at all as it "falls" to the depth of the gingival crevice.

As the probe tip slides along the tooth surface, if there is no irregularity or subgingival calculus, the tooth surface will feel smooth. If the tooth surface feels rough or if the probe tip stops on a hard surface, its path may be impeded by the presence of subgingival calculus. The probe may need to be moved axially away from the tooth to navigate around the calculus in order for it to penetrate to depth. The presence of subgingival calculus is usually associated with inflammatory changes in the gingival tissue (see Fig. 32.7), the absence of gingival tightness, and the presence of bleeding on probing.

LEARNING BOX 32.5

When probing, the probe tip should be in contact with the tooth surface as it slides down along the tooth surface to get to the bottom of the gingival crevice. This allows for detection of tooth surface irregularities, furcation invasion, and subgingival calculus.

Additionally, attention should be directed to detecting the presence of periodontal defects, interdental craters, root surface concavities, and furcation invasion. Periodontal defects tend to be associated with deep probing depths and gingival inflammation. To detect an *interdental crater*, the probe should be placed obliquely from both the facial and lingual surfaces to explore the deepest point of the pocket located beneath the contact point. The root surface should be carefully explored and probed to detect concavities and *furcation invasion*. The use of specially designed probes (e.g., Nabers probes) allows for an easier and more accurate exploration of the horizontal component of furcation lesions.

Tactile detection of inflammatory changes in the soft tissue is just as valuable as, if not more valuable than, measuring probing depth and evaluating bleeding on probing. The detection of inflammatory changes in the tissue, subgingival concavities, furcation invasion, and subgingival calculus via probing is instrumental in accurate diagnosis, prognosis, and treatment.

LEARNING BOX 32.6

Thorough probing of the gingival crevice and the surrounding tissue provides a wealth of valuable information beyond probing depth and bleeding on probing that is essential to the diagnosis and treatment of periodontal disease.

Probing Around Implants

Because implants are susceptible to biofilm-induced inflammatory diseases, probing around them becomes part of the examination and diagnosis. A traditional periodontal probe may be used under light force (e.g., 0.25 N) without damaging the peri-implant mucosal seal.[18] Peri-implant evaluation and probing of implants are further discussed in Chapter 86.

When Not to Probe

Thorough probing of the periodontal pocket and accurate probing depth measurement before, during, and after treatment are essential for diagnosing and monitoring periodontal disease. In the presence of severe gingival inflammation (see Figs. 32.5 and 32.12), accurate probing depth measurement is difficult to obtain without anesthesia due to the pain and discomfort inflicted on the patient with insertion of the periodontal probe into the inflamed periodontal pocket. Therefore, when periodontal disease is overt and obvious clinically and radiographically, thorough probing of the periodontal pocket and accurate probing depth measurement should only occur once the tissue is anesthetized. In cases that require scaling and root planing with anesthesia, accurate probing depth measurement should be delayed until the scaling and root planing appointment. After anesthesia has been administered and before root instrumentation occurs, the periodontal pocket should be thoroughly probed for subgingival calculus, root surface concavities, furcation invasions, and probing pocket depths. Furthermore, in moderate and advanced cases, probing depths will change dramatically with improvement in biofilm control and scaling and root planing (Fig. 32.14). As such, obtaining accurate probing depths at the reevaluation following nonsurgical therapy is much more important than obtaining accurate probing depth at the pretreatment periodontal examination.

LEARNING BOX 32.7

In the presence of overt and obvious periodontal disease, it may be best to delay accurate probing depth measurement until the scaling and root planing appointment, when the tissue is anesthetized.

Probing Depth

There are two different pocket depths: (1) the biologic or histologic depth and (2) the clinical or probing depth[29] (Fig. 32.15).

Biologic depth is the distance between the gingival margin and the base of the gingival crevice (i.e., the coronal end of the junctional epithelium). This can be measured only in carefully prepared and adequately oriented histologic sections.

Probing depth is the distance from the gingival margin to the bottom of the probeable crevice (i.e., where the probe tip stops). Probes that are presently used are described in Chapter 50.

Probe penetration can vary depending on the force of introduction, the shape and size of the probe tip, the direction of penetration, the resistance of the tissues, the convexity of the crown, and the degree of tissue inflammation.[5] Probing depth is generally ≤3 mm in gingival health and >3 mm in the presence of gingival inflammation. Several studies have been done to determine the depth of penetration of a probe in a sulcus or pocket. Armitage and colleagues[8] used beagle dogs to evaluate the penetration of a probe with the use of a standardized force of 25 g. They reported that in healthy gingiva, the probe penetrated the junctional epithelium to about two-thirds of its length; in gingivitis cases, it stopped 0.1 mm short of its apical end; and in cases of periodontitis, the probe tip consistently went past the most apical cells of the junctional epithelium (Fig. 32.16).

In human periodontal pockets, the probe tip penetrates to the most coronal intact fibers of the connective tissue attachment.[38,72] The depth of penetration of the probe in the connective tissue apical to the junctional epithelium in a periodontal pocket is about

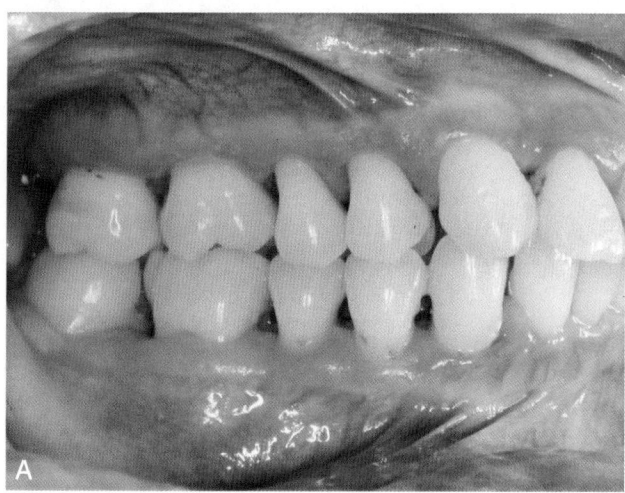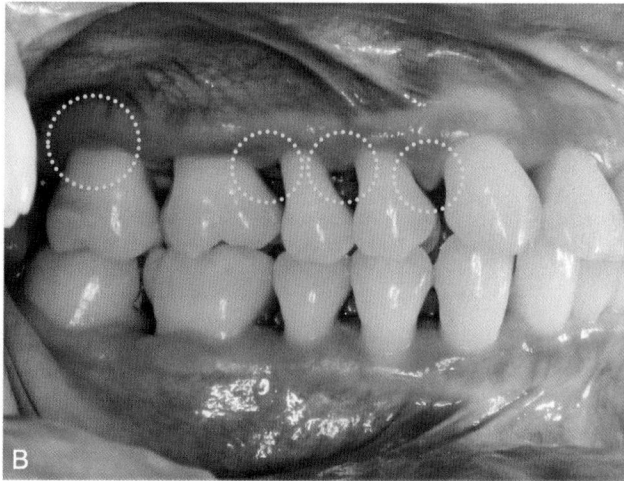

Fig. 32.14 Clinical presentation prior to scaling and root planing (A). Note the presence of supra- and subgingival calculus along the gingival margin. Following scaling and root planing, at the 6-week reevaluation (B), resolution of gingival inflammation resulted in dramatic gingival shrinkage *(circles)*. *(Copyright Jonathan H. Do, DDS. All rights reserved.)*

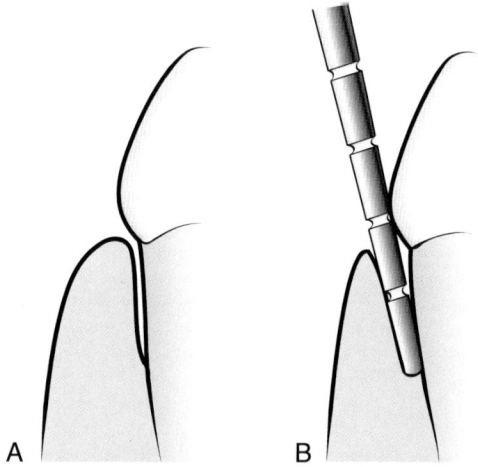

Fig. 32.15 (A) The biologic or histologic pocket depth is the actual distance between the gingival margin and the attached tissues (i.e., the bottom of the pocket). (B) The probing or clinical pocket depth is the depth of probe penetration.

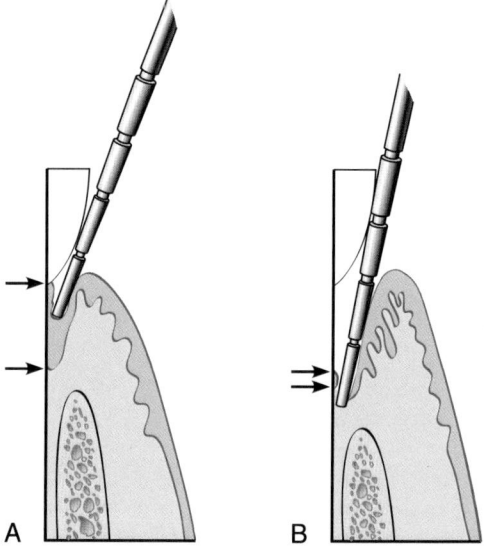

Fig. 32.16 (A) In a normal sulcus, the probe penetrates about one-third to half the length of the junctional epithelium *(between arrows)*. (B) In an inflamed periodontal pocket, the probe penetrates beyond the apical end of the junctional epithelium *(between arrows)*.

0.3 mm.[38,66,72] This is important when evaluating differences in probing depth before and after treatment, because the reduction in probe penetration may be a result of reduced inflammatory response rather than a gain in attachment.[37,40]

Probing depth may change from time to time, even in patients with untreated periodontal disease, as a result of changes in the position of the gingival margin. Therefore it may be unrelated to the existing attachment of the tooth.

Bleeding on Probing

The insertion of a probe to the bottom of the pocket elicits bleeding if the gingiva is inflamed and if the pocket epithelium is atrophic or ulcerated. Noninflamed sites rarely bleed. In most cases, bleeding on probing is an earlier sign of inflammation than gingival color changes[45] (see Chapter 18). However, color changes may be present without bleeding on probing.[26] Depending on the severity of inflammation, bleeding can vary from a tenuous red line along the gingival sulcus to profuse bleeding.[1] If periodontal treatment is successful, bleeding on probing will cease.[3]

To test for bleeding after probing, the probe is carefully introduced to the bottom of the pocket and gently moved laterally along the pocket wall. Sometimes bleeding appears immediately after the removal of the probe; other times it may be delayed for a few seconds. Therefore the clinician should recheck for bleeding 30 to 60 seconds after probing.

As a single test, bleeding on probing is not a good predictor of progressive attachment loss; however, its absence is an excellent predictor of periodontal stability.[5] When bleeding is present in multiple sites of advanced disease, bleeding on probing is a good indicator of progressive attachment loss.[5,22] Armitage analyzed the literature on this subject up to 1996; he performed a meta-analysis of the various papers and concluded that the presence of bleeding on probing in a "treated and maintained patient population" is an important risk predictor for increased loss of attachment.[5]

LEARNING BOX 32.9

The absence of bleeding on probing is an excellent predictor of periodontal stability.

Pain on Probing

Pain is a cardinal sign of inflammation. Gingival inflammation and periodontal disease in general are painless. However, periodontal probing of the gingival crevice can elicit pain in the gingival tissue. The presence of pain suggests that the gingival tissue is inflamed, and the level of pain is usually related to the severity of gingival inflammation. Unless gingival inflammation is generalized and severe, patients will not feel the same level of pain at every site. Probing of healthy sites will not produce pain, and probing of sites with inflammation will produce pain. Sites that do not exhibit bleeding or obvious clinical signs of inflammation can exhibit pain on probing. Although the clinician cannot directly measure pain on probing, it is useful to make the patient aware that pain indicates inflammation and to ask the patient to pay attention to its presence.

Attachment Loss

Attachment loss is the apical migration of the dentogingival junction—the periodontal attachment apparatus—as a result of the inflammatory response. The dentogingival junction consists of the epithelial attachment and the connective tissue attachment. The dimension of the dentogingival junction is called the biologic width and averages 2.04 mm.[21] In healthy conditions, without attachment loss, the connective tissue attachment of the dentogingival junction begins coronally at the cementoenamel junction, and the epithelial attachment exists coronal to the connective tissue attachment. With attachment loss, the cementoenamel junction becomes exposed. *Clinical attachment loss* measures the *amount* of attachment loss that has occurred, with the cementoenamel junction as the reference point. Clinical attachment loss is measured as the distance from the cementoenamel junction to the bottom of the probeable crevice.

When the *gingival margin is located on the anatomic crown,* clinical attachment loss is determined by subtracting the distance from the gingival margin to the cementoenamel junction from the probing depth. If both are the same, clinical attachment loss is zero.

When the gingival margin coincides with the cementoenamel junction, clinical attachment loss is equal to probing depth.

When the gingival margin is located apical to the cementoenamel junction, clinical attachment loss is greater than probing depth. Therefore clinical attachment loss, or the distance between the cementoenamel junction and the bottom of the probeable crevice, is the sum of gingival recession and probing depth. Drawing the gingival margin on the chart where probing depths are entered helps to clarify this important point.[70]

Clinical attachment loss is automatically calculated in many dental practice management software programs as the sum of probing depth and recession. This calculation is accurate only when both probing depth and recession are entered into the software correctly. However, when recession is not entered, many software programs assume the cementoenamel junction is at the level of the gingival margin and equate clinical attachment loss to probing depth. This is not necessarily correct, as many clinicians do not enter a value for recession when the cementoenamel junction is subgingival and not visible. As such, automatically calculated clinical attachment loss values must be scrutinized before they are used to help make a diagnosis.

Attachment Level

Attachment level describes the location *where* the dentogingival junction begins coronally on a tooth. For example, the attachment level of a tooth can be on the coronal third of the root or the apical third of the root. *Clinical attachment level* measures the distance between the attachment level and a reference point on a tooth, such as the cementoenamel junction. For example, the attachment level is 3 mm apical to the cementoenamel junction. Changes in the attachment level can be the result of a gain or a loss of attachment, and they can provide a better indication of the degree of periodontal destruction or gain. *Shallow pockets attached at the level of the apical third of the root connote more severe destruction than deep pockets attached at the coronal third of the root* (see Chapter 23).

LEARNING BOX 32.10

Clinical attachment loss measures *how much* attachment loss has occurred using the cementoenamel junction as the reference point. Clinical attachment level measures the distance between *where* the periodontal attachment apparatus begins coronally on a tooth and a fixed reference point.

Attached Gingiva

It is important to establish the relationship between the bottom of the pocket and the mucogingival junction, especially at sites with gingival recession and narrow gingival width (see Fig. 32.11). The width of the attached gingiva is the distance between the mucogingival junction and the projection on the external surface of the bottom of the gingival sulcus or the periodontal pocket. It should not be confused with the width of the gingiva, because the latter also includes the marginal gingiva (see Fig. 32.17).

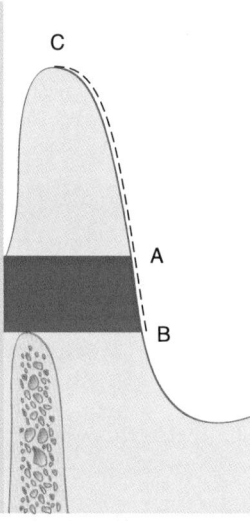

Fig. 32.17 The shaded area shows the attached gingiva, which extends between the projection on the external surface of the bottom of the pocket (A) and the mucogingival junction (B). The keratinized gingiva may extend from the mucogingival junction (B) to the gingival margin (C).

The width of the attached gingiva is determined by subtracting the sulcus or pocket depth from the total width of the gingiva (i.e., the gingival margin to the mucogingival line). The amount of attached gingiva is generally considered to be insufficient when the stretching of the lip or cheek induces the movement of the free gingival margin.

Other methods that are used to determine the amount of attached gingiva include pushing the adjacent mucosa coronally with a dull instrument and painting the mucosa with Schiller's potassium iodide solution, which stains keratin.

Examination of the Teeth and Implants

The teeth are examined for caries, poor restorations, developmental defects, anomalies of tooth form, wasting, hypersensitivity, and proximal contact relationships. The stability, position, and number of implants and their relationship to the adjacent natural dentition are also examined.

Wasting Disease of the Teeth

Wasting is defined as any gradual loss of tooth substance, which is characterized by the formation of smooth, polished surfaces without regard to the possible mechanism of this loss. The forms of wasting are erosion, abrasion, attrition, and abfraction.[47,65]

Erosion, which is also called *corrosion,* is a sharply defined wedge-shaped depression in the cervical area of the facial tooth surface.[55] The long axis of the eroded area is perpendicular to the vertical axis of the tooth. The surfaces are smooth, hard, and polished. Erosion generally affects a group of teeth. During the early stages, it may be confined to the enamel, but it generally extends to involve the underlying dentin as well as the cementum.

The etiology of erosion is not known. Decalcification by acidic beverages[44] or citrus fruits in combination with the effect of acid salivary secretion is a suggested cause. Sognnaes[71] refers to these lesions as *dentoalveolar ablations* and attributes them to forceful frictional action between the oral soft tissues and the adjacent hard tissues. In patients with erosion, the salivary pH, the buffering capacity, and the calcium and phosphorus content have been reported as normal, and the mucin level is elevated.[43]

Abrasion refers to the loss of tooth substance that is induced by mechanical wear other than that of mastication. Abrasion results in saucer-shaped or wedge-shaped indentations with a smooth, shiny surface (Fig. 32.18). Abrasion starts on exposed cementum surfaces rather than on the enamel, and it extends to involve the dentin of the root. A sharp "ditching" around the cementoenamel junction appears to be the result of the softer cemental surface as compared with the much harder enamel surface.

Continued exposure to the abrasive agent in combination with decalcification of the enamel by locally formed acids may result in a loss of enamel followed by a loss of the dentin of the crown.

Toothbrushing[26] with an abrasive dentifrice and the action of clasps are frequently mentioned, but aggressive toothbrushing with an abrasive dentifrice is the most common cause.[34] Tooth position (facial) is also a major factor in the abrasive loss of the root surface. The degree of tooth wear from toothbrushing depends on the abrasive effect of the dentifrice and the angle of brushing.[41,42] Horizontal brushing at right angles to the vertical axis of the teeth results in the severest loss of tooth substance. Occasionally, abrasion of the incisal edges occurs as a result of habits such as holding objects (e.g., bobby pins, tacks) between the teeth.

Attrition is occlusal wear that results from functional contact with opposing teeth. Such physical wear patterns may occur on incisal, occlusal, or approximal tooth surfaces. A certain amount of tooth wear is physiologic, but accelerated wear may occur when abnormal anatomic or unusual functional factors are present.

Occlusal or incisal surfaces worn by attrition are called *facets*. When active tooth grinding occurs, the enamel rods are fractured and become highly reflective to light.[79] Thus shiny, smooth, and curviplanar facets are usually the best indicators of ongoing frictional activity (Fig. 32.19). If dentin is exposed, a yellowish brown discoloration is frequently present. Facets vary with regard to size and location, depending on whether they are produced by physiologic or abnormal wear.[14,77] At least one significant wear facet has been reported in 92% of adults,[68] and facet prevalence approaches universality.[11,78] Facets are usually not sensitive to thermal or tactile stimulation.

Facets generally represent functional or parafunctional wear as well as iatrogenic dental treatment through coronoplasty (occlusal adjustment). However, coronoplasty does not appear to contribute to higher ratings of wear.[69] Excessive wear may result in the obliteration of the cusps and the formation of either a flat or cuneiform (cupped-out) occlusal surface. Contrary to earlier thought, attrition in young adults from modern societies is not age related.[17,69] This suggests that a significant amount of attrition, when present in young adults, is unlikely to occur as a result of functional wear,[36] and it is probably the result of bruxing activity.[69] Attrition has been correlated with age when older adults are considered.[9,67]

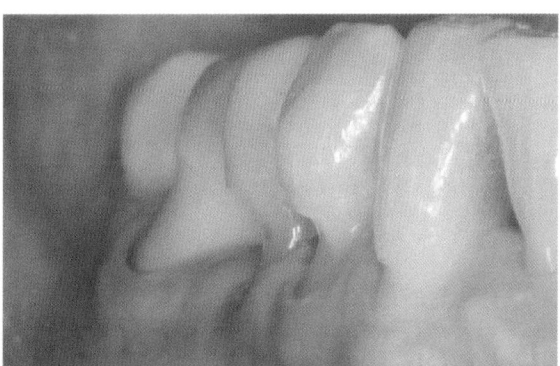

Fig. 32.18 Noncarious cervical lesions are attributed to a combination of abrasion, abfraction, and erosion. *(Copyright Jonathan H. Do, DDS. All rights reserved.)*

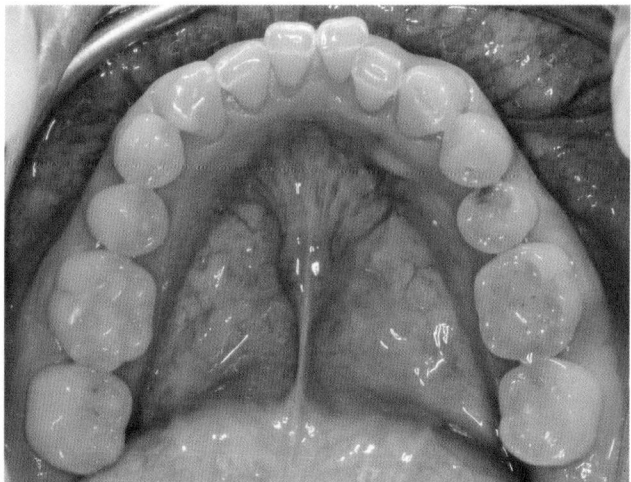

Fig. 32.19 Flat, shiny, discolored surfaces produced by occlusal wear.

The angle of the facet on the tooth surface is potentially significant to the periodontium. Horizontal facets tend to direct forces on the vertical axis of the tooth to which the periodontium can adapt most effectively. Angular facets direct occlusal forces laterally and increase the risk of periodontal damage. However, gradual attrition may be compensated for by continuous tooth eruption without alveolar bone growth, and it is characterized by a lack of inflammatory changes on the alveolar bone surfaces.[74]

Another mechanism of tooth wear that has been studied is called *abfraction,* and it results from occlusal loading surfaces causing tooth flexure and mechanical microfractures the cervical area.[28] Mechanical microfractures from abfraction weakens the cervical tooth structure and makes it much more susceptible to loss of tooth structure via abrasion (see Fig. 32.18).

These four mechanisms of tooth wear (corrosion, abrasion, attrition, and abfraction) can combine to increase the degree of tooth wear.

Dental Stains

Dental stains are pigmented deposits on the teeth. They should be carefully examined to determine their origin (see Chapter 13).

Hypersensitivity

Root surfaces exposed by gingival recession may be hypersensitive to thermal changes or tactile stimulation. Patients often direct the clinician to the sensitive areas. These may be located by gentle exploration with a probe or cold air.

Proximal Contact Relations

Open contacts allow for food impaction. The tightness of contacts should be checked by means of clinical observation and with dental floss. Abnormal contact relationships may also initiate occlusal changes, such as a shift in the median line between the central incisors with labial flaring of the maxillary canine, buccal or lingual displacement of the posterior teeth, and an uneven relationship of the marginal ridges. Teeth opposite an edentulous site may supererupt, thereby opening the proximal contacts.

Tooth Mobility

All teeth have a slight degree of physiologic mobility, which varies for different teeth and at different times of the day.[52,56] It is greatest when arising in the morning, and it progressively decreases. The increased mobility in the morning is attributed to slight extrusion of the tooth as a result of limited occlusal contact during sleep. During the waking hours, mobility is reduced by chewing and swallowing forces, which intrude the teeth in the sockets. These 24-hour variations are less marked in persons with a healthy periodontium than in those with occlusal habits such as bruxism and clenching.

Single-rooted teeth have more mobility than multirooted teeth, with incisors having the most mobility. Mobility occurs primarily in a horizontal direction, although some axial mobility occurs to a lesser degree.[54]

Tooth mobility occurs in the following two stages:
1. The initial or intrasocket stage occurs when the tooth moves within the confines of the periodontal ligament. This is associated with viscoelastic distortion of the ligament and the redistribution of the periodontal fluids, interbundle content, and fibers.[35] This initial movement occurs with forces of about 100 lb, and it is on the order of 0.05 mm to 0.10 mm (50 μm to 100 μm).[48]
2. The secondary stage occurs gradually and entails elastic deformation of the alveolar bone in response to increased horizontal forces.[50] When a force of 500 g is applied to the crown, the resulting displacement is about 100 μm to 200 μm for incisors,

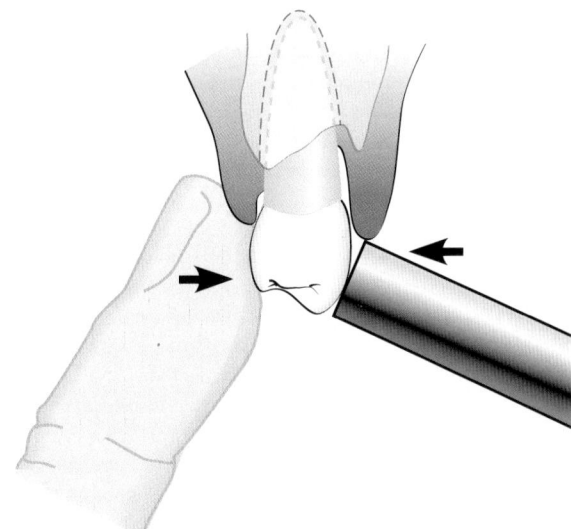

Fig. 32.20 Tooth mobility is checked with a metal instrument and one finger.

50 μm to 90 μm for canines, 8 μm to 10 μm for premolars, and 40 μm to 80 μm for molars.[48]

When a force such as that applied to teeth in occlusion is discontinued, the teeth return to their original position in two stages: the first is an immediate, springlike elastic recoil; the second is a slow, asymptomatic recovery movement. The recovery movement is pulsating, and it is apparently associated with the normal pulsation of the periodontal vessels, which occurs in synchrony with the cardiac cycle.[49]

Many attempts have been made to develop mechanical or electronic devices for the precise measurement of tooth mobility.[49,53,55,68] Although standardization of grading mobility would be helpful for the diagnosis of periodontal disease and for evaluating treatment outcomes, these devices are not widely used. As a general rule, mobility is graded clinically by holding the tooth firmly between the handles of two metallic instruments or with one metallic instrument and one finger (Fig. 32.20). An effort is then made to move it in all directions. Abnormal mobility most often occurs faciolingually. Mobility is scored according to the ease and extent of tooth movement according to the Miller Index[46] as follows:
- Mobility no. 1: first distinguishable sign of movement greater than "normal"
- Mobility no. 2: movement of the crown up to 1 mm in any direction
- Mobility no. 3: movement of the crown more than 1 mm in any direction or vertical depression or rotation of the crown in its socket

Physiologic mobility is movement up to 0.2 mm horizontally and 0.02 mm axially. Mobility beyond the physiologic range is termed *abnormal* or *pathologic.* It is pathologic in that it exceeds the limits of normal mobility values; however, the periodontium is not *necessarily* diseased at the time of examination.

Increased mobility is caused by one or more of the following factors:
1. *Loss of tooth support (bone loss)* can result in mobility. The amount of mobility depends on the severity and distribution of bone loss at individual root surfaces, the length and shape of the roots, and the root size as compared with that of the crown.[55] A tooth with short, tapered roots is more likely to loosen than one

with normal-size or bulbous roots with the same amount of bone loss. One should carefully evaluate postorthodontic cases for possible apical shortening of the root, which may lead to excessive mobility. Because bone loss usually results from a combination of factors and does not occur as an isolated finding, the severity of tooth mobility does not necessarily correspond to the amount of bone loss.

2. *Trauma from occlusion* (i.e., injury produced by excessive occlusal forces or incurred as a result of abnormal occlusal habits such as bruxism and clenching) is a common cause of tooth mobility. Mobility is also increased by hypofunction. Mobility produced by trauma from occlusion occurs initially as a result of resorption of the cortical layer of bone, which leads to reduced fiber support, and later as an adaptation phenomenon that results in a widened periodontal space.

3. *Extension of inflammation* from the gingiva or the periapex into the periodontal ligament results in changes that increase mobility. The spread of inflammation from an acute periapical abscess may increase tooth mobility in the absence of periodontal disease.

4. *Periodontal surgery* temporarily increases tooth mobility immediately after the intervention and for a short period.[58-61]

5. Tooth mobility is increased during *pregnancy,* and it is sometimes associated with the *menstrual cycle* or the use of *hormonal contraceptives.* This is unrelated to periodontal disease, and it occurs presumably because of physicochemical changes in the periodontal tissues.

6. *Pathologic processes of the jaws* that destroy the alveolar bone or the roots of the teeth can also result in mobility. Osteomyelitis and tumors of the jaws belong in this category.

One study[24] has suggested that pockets around mobile teeth harbor higher proportions of *Campylobacter rectus* and *Peptostreptococcus micros* and possibly *Porphyromonas gingivalis* as compared with nonmobile teeth. This hypothesis requires further verification.

LEARNING BOX 32.11

The three main etiologic factors of tooth mobility are periodontal inflammation, attachment loss, and occlusal trauma.

Trauma From Occlusion

Trauma from occlusion refers to *tissue injury* produced by occlusal forces rather than to the occlusal forces themselves (see Chapter 25). The criterion that determines that an occlusion is traumatic is whether it causes damage in the periodontal tissues; therefore the diagnosis of trauma from occlusion is made from the condition of the periodontal tissues. The periodontal findings are then used as a guide for locating the responsible occlusal relationships.

Periodontal findings that suggest the presence of trauma from occlusion include excessive tooth mobility, particularly in teeth that show radiographic evidence of a widened periodontal space; vertical or angular bone destruction; infrabony pockets; and pathologic migration, especially of the anterior teeth. These are discussed in more detail in the following sections.

Pathologic Migration of the Teeth

Alterations in tooth position should be carefully noted, particularly with a view toward identifying abnormal forces, a tongue-thrusting habit, or other habits that may be contributing factors (Fig. 32.21; see Chapter 25). Premature tooth contacts in the posterior region that deflect the mandible anteriorly contribute to the destruction of the periodontium of the maxillary anterior teeth and to pathologic migration (see also Chapter 25). The loss of posterior teeth can lead

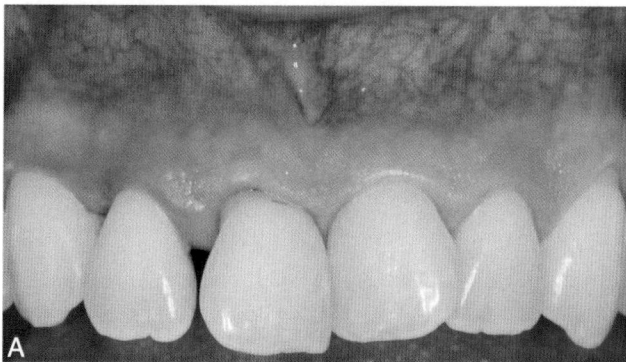

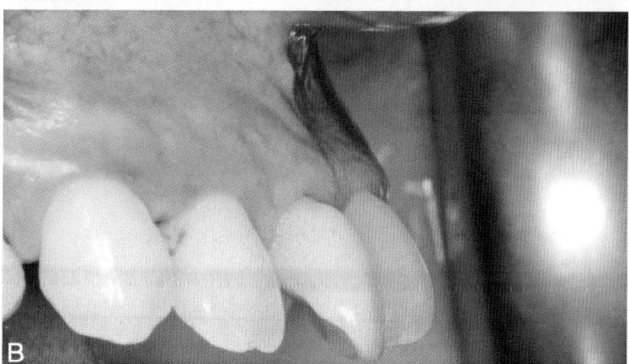

Fig. 32.21 Facial flaring and supraeruption of the right central incisor and spacing between the lateral and central incisors result from pathologic migration due to chronic periodontitis. *(Copyright Jonathan H. Do, DDS. All rights reserved.)*

to facial "flaring" of the maxillary anterior dentition. This is due to the increased trauma that the mandibular anterior dentition places against the palatal surface of the maxillary anterior dentition. Pathologic migration of the anterior teeth in young persons may be a sign of localized aggressive (juvenile) periodontitis.

Sensitivity to Percussion

Sensitivity to percussion is a feature of acute inflammation of the periodontal ligament. Gentle percussion of a tooth at different angles to the long axis often helps with the localization of the site of inflammatory involvement.

Dentition With the Jaws Closed

Examination of the dentition with the jaws closed can detect conditions such as irregularly aligned teeth, extruded teeth, improper proximal contacts, and areas of food impaction, all of which may favor plaque accumulation.

Excessive *overbite,* which is seen most often in the anterior region, may cause impingement of the teeth on the gingiva and food impaction, followed by gingival inflammation, gingival enlargement, and pocket formation. The real significance of the detrimental effect of an excessive anterior overbite on gingival health is still controversial.[2]

In *open-bite* relationships, abnormal vertical spaces exist between the maxillary and mandibular teeth. The condition occurs most often in the anterior region, although posterior open bite is occasionally seen. Reduced mechanical cleansing by the passage of food may lead to accumulation of plaque and debris, calculus formation, and extrusion of teeth.

With *crossbite,* the normal relationship of the mandibular teeth to the maxillary teeth is reversed, with the maxillary teeth being lingual to the mandibular teeth. Crossbite may be bilateral or unilateral, or may affect only a pair of antagonists. Trauma from occlusion, food impaction, spreading of the mandibular teeth, and associated gingival and periodontal disturbances may be caused by crossbite.

Functional Occlusal Relationships

The examination of functional occlusal relationships is an important part of the diagnostic procedure. Dentitions that appear to be normal when the jaws are closed may present marked functional abnormalities. Systematic procedures for the detection and correction of functional abnormalities are presented in Chapter 55.

Radiographic Examination

The radiographic survey should consist of a minimum of 14 intraoral films and 4 posterior bitewing films (Fig. 32.22). Panoramic radiographs are a simple and convenient method of obtaining a survey view of the dental arch and the surrounding structures (Fig. 32.23). They are helpful for the detection of developmental anomalies, pathologic lesions of the teeth and jaws, and fractures, as well as dental screening examinations of large groups. They provide an informative overall radiographic picture of the distribution and severity of bone destruction with periodontal disease, but *a complete intraoral series is required for periodontal diagnosis and treatment planning.* Chapter 33 gives a detailed description of radiographic interpretation in periodontics.

Laboratory Aids to Clinical Diagnosis

When unusual gingival or periodontal problems are detected that cannot be explained by local causes, the possibility of contributing systemic factors must be explored. The signs and symptoms of oral manifestations of systemic disease have to be clearly understood and analyzed and their presence discussed with the patient's physician. Chapter 14 presents discussions of many of these problems, and the reader is also directed to standard texts that discuss medical diagnoses for more detailed descriptions of the necessary tests and their interpretation.

Numerous laboratory tests aid in the diagnosis of systemic diseases that may contribute to periodontal and oral diseases; these tests will also be needed to make treatment decisions when dealing with medically compromised patients (see Chapter 39). Analyses of blood smears, blood cell counts, white blood cell differential counts, and erythrocyte sedimentation rates are used to evaluate the presence of blood dyscrasias and generalized infections. Determinations of coagulation time, bleeding time, clot retraction time, prothrombin time, and capillary fragility as well as bone marrow studies may be required at times. The reader is referred to books about medical diagnoses for a consideration of this subject.

Periodontal Diagnosis

Once the patient history has been obtained and clinical, radiographic, and other necessary examinations have been performed, the information acquired is synthesized and interpreted to answer three basic diagnostic questions[6] to derive the periodontal diagnosis:
1. What is the disease?
2. How severe is the disease?
3. What is the extent of the disease?

Diseases that can affect the periodontium are listed in the Classification of Periodontal Diseases and Conditions. Severity of periodontal disease is classified based on a three-tier system: slight,

mild, early, or initial; moderate; and severe or advanced. The extent of the disease is classified as generalized or localized. When localized, the extent can be specified to the quadrant, teeth, and even tooth surfaces.

Biofilm-induced inflammatory periodontal diseases are diagnosed based on the presence of inflammation and attachment loss (Table 32.2). In periodontal health, both inflammation and attachment loss are absent. When only inflammation is present, the diagnosis is biofilm-induced gingivitis. When both inflammation and attachment loss are present, the diagnosis is chronic periodontitis. It is possible that when both inflammation and attachment loss are present, biofilm-induced gingivitis is superimposed over a history of chronic periodontitis. However, it is prudent to diagnose the presence of both inflammation and attachment loss as chronic periodontitis due to the following reasons: progression of chronic periodontitis is sporadic, sites with previous attachment loss are susceptible to further attachment loss, and attachment loss is driven by the inflammatory response. Finally, when inflammation is absent and attachment is present, the diagnosis is healthy with a reduced periodontium or with a history of chronic periodontitis.

LEARNING BOX 32.12

Diagnosis of biofilm-induced inflammatory periodontal diseases is based on the presence of periodontal inflammation and attachment loss.

Currently, the severity of chronic periodontitis is characterized on a three-tier system based on clinical attachment loss (CAL): slight = 1 or 2 mm CAL, moderate = 3 or 4 mm CAL, and severe ≥5 mm CAL. This system is inadequate for two reasons: (1) chronic periodontitis is diagnosed based on the presence of both inflammation and attachment loss, not attachment loss alone, and (2) the link in the relationship between periodontitis and systemic disease is inflammation, not attachment loss. Therefore an ideal classification system should take into consideration the severity of inflammation as well. Furthermore, for cases with mild attachment loss or where the cementoenamel junction is subgingival, an accurate determination of clinical attachment loss is challenging as it is difficult to accurately determine the location of the cementoenamel junction. As such, the severity of attachment loss may depend on the interpretation of radiographic bone loss. Table 32.3 correlates severity of periodontitis to clinical attachment loss and the distance from the alveolar crest to the cementoenamel junction (CEJ) on radiographs.

LEARNING BOX 32.13

Severity of periodontitis is characterized based on clinical attachment loss.

TABLE 32.2 Diagnosis of Biofilm-Induced Inflammatory Periodontal Diseases

Periodontal Diagnosis	Inflammation	Attachment Loss
Healthy	No	No
Biofilm-induced gingivitis	Yes	No
Chronic periodontitis	Yes	Yes
Healthy with a reduced periodontium/ with a history of chronic periodontitis	No	Yes

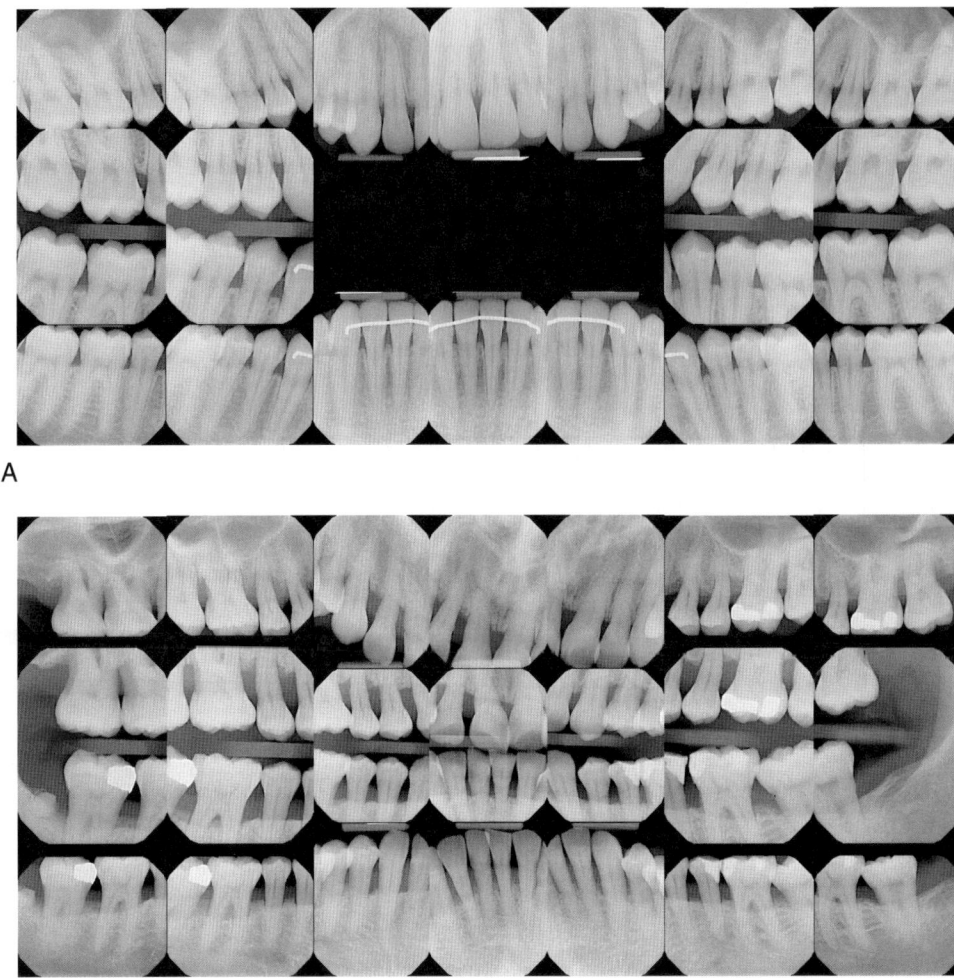

A

B

Fig. 32.22 A complete intraoral radiographic is an essential adjunct to periodontal diagnosis. (A) Intraoral radiographs of a patient with gingivitis. Note the radiopaque fixed lingual orthodontic retainer. (B) Intraoral radiographs of a patient with generalized moderate to severe chronic periodontitis. Vertical bitewing radiographs are useful to evaluate crestal bone loss. *(Copyright Jonathan H. Do, DDS. All rights reserved.)*

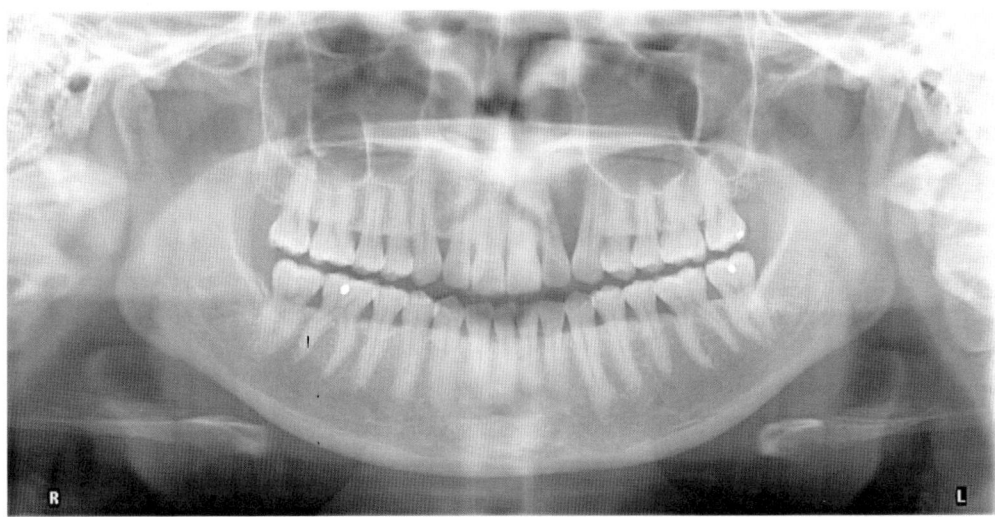

Fig. 32.23 Panoramic radiograph provides an overview of the dental arch and the surrounding structures.

TABLE 32.3 Clinical and Radiographic Guidelines for Determining Severity of Periodontitis

Severity of Periodontitis	Clinical Attachment Loss (mm)	Distance From Alveolar Crest to CEJ (mm)	Radiographic Findings
Health	0	<2	
Mild	1–2	3–4	
Moderate	3–4	5–6	
Severe	≥5	≥7	

CEJ, Cementoenamel junction.

Severity of biofilm-induced gingivitis can also be characterized based on a three-tier system of slight, moderate, and severe. However, this can be subjective.

The extent of chronic periodontitis is delineated based on the 30% threshold. Localized chronic periodontitis is defined as chronic periodontitis with a clear pattern of distribution, such as distal surfaces of second molars or ≤30% of teeth are affected.[4] Generalized chronic periodontitis is defined as periodontitis without a clear pattern of distribution or >30% of teeth are affected.[4] The extent of biofilm-induced gingivitis can also be characterized based on the 30% threshold similar to the extent of chronic periodontitis.

When biofilm-induced gingivitis and chronic periodontitis are present simultaneously, if the extent of both is generalized, the diagnosis is simply generalized chronic periodontitis, as the chronic periodontitis is the more advanced progression of the disease. Furthermore, biofilm-induced gingivitis by definition is inflammation without attachment loss, whereas chronic periodontitis is defined as inflammation with attachment loss. A diagnosis of both generalized biofilm-induced gingivitis and generalized chronic periodontitis is contradictory. Biofilm-induced gingivitis may be diagnosed together with chronic periodontitis if the periodontitis is localized. In this situation, the diagnosis is generalized biofilm-induced gingivitis with localized chronic periodontitis. Similarly, if the extent of mild and moderate chronic periodontitis is >30%, the diagnosis is simply generalized moderate chronic periodontitis, as moderate is the more severe of the two types of disease severity.

Assessment of Biofilm Control and Patient Education

Patients presenting for periodontal consultations typically expect to find out the problems they have and the treatments they need. By the end of the periodontal consultation, it may not be possible to determine the prognosis and formulate a complete treatment plan, as a careful analysis of the information obtained, more diagnostic information, or consultation with other dental and medical professionals may be required. However, the patient should be educated on the problems in his or her mouth, the need for further diagnostics, and the etiologies and prevention of these problems. Clinical photographs, radiographs, and models may be useful to help the patient to better understand the condition of his or her mouth. The patient may be presented with a preliminary treatment plan that may include emergency and palliative treatments and nonsurgical periodontal therapy to control infections.

Although patient education and biofilm control are part of nonsurgical periodontal therapy and not the focus of this chapter, a preventive approach to oral health care demands behavior modification, which requires time, effort, and repetition. As such, every opportunity should be seized to educate patients and alter their behavior. Patients should be given personalized oral hygiene instructions to control biofilm and to improve their oral health and the conditions of the periodontium. It is not uncommon for patients to report brushing and flossing multiple times daily, while having poorly controlled periodontal disease in their mouths. For that reason, the effectiveness of the patient's biofilm control must be evaluated. The patient should be asked to demonstrate biofilm control (toothbrushing, flossing, etc.,) in front of a mirror so that both the patient and the clinician can see his or her oral hygiene techniques. The patient should then be taught proper biofilm control techniques with a demonstration in his or her own mouth in front of a mirror. Detailed biofilm control is presented in Chapter 48.

Ideally, unless emergency treatment is required, patients should be given at least 1 or 2 weeks to improve their oral hygiene, to control biofilm and reduce periodontal inflammation, and to appreciate how they can impact their oral health with meticulous biofilm control before any periodontal treatment is rendered.

Conclusion

Periodontal examination and diagnosis begins with obtaining a thorough health and dental history. Although the periodontal examination presented in this chapter is divided into two parts, visual examination and tactile examination, in practice both visual and tactile assessments overlap and occur simultaneously, as do the evaluations of teeth and periodontium. Nevertheless, the examination should begin with an overall survey of biofilm and calculus, clinical signs of inflammation, and other obvious signs of disease to obtain insights into the patient's oral hygiene and disease status. As the examination progresses, it becomes more invasive and more specific information is acquired. Once a detailed patient history has been obtained and a thorough clinical examination has been completed, the information collected is analyzed and synthesized to arrive at a diagnosis. The periodontal examination is the basis from which the diagnosis, prognosis, and treatment plan are derived and from which treatment is ultimately rendered. Therefore a thorough and accurate periodontal examination is of the utmost importance.

LEARNING BOX 32.14

Examination → Diagnosis → Prognosis ↔ Treatment
- Diagnosis requires thorough and careful examination.
- Prognosis is based on accurate diagnosis.
- Treatment decisions are based on prognosis.
- Treatment decisions are made to improve prognosis.
- Diagnosis and prognosis will change with treatment.

 A Case Scenario is found on the companion website www.expertconsult.com.

References

 References for this chapter are found on the companion website www.expertconsult.com.

CHAPTER 33

Radiographic Aids in the Diagnosis of Periodontal Disease

Sotirios Tetradis | Sanjay M. Mallya | Henry H. Takei

Radiographs are valuable for the diagnosis of periodontal disease, estimation of severity, determination of prognosis, and evaluation of treatment outcome.[6,14,19] *However, radiographs are an adjunct to the clinical examination, not a substitute for it.* Radiographs demonstrate changes in calcified tissue; they do not reveal current cellular activity but rather reflect the effects of past cellular experience on the bone and roots.

LEARNING BOX 33.1

Radiographs provide a static view of the current available periodontal bone. Radiographic information must be considered as one of the elements of the diagnostic workup in conjunction with clinical and historical findings.

Normal Interdental Bone

Evaluation of bone changes in periodontal disease is based mainly on the appearance of the interdental bone, because the relatively dense root structure obscures the facial and lingual bony plates. The interdental bone normally is outlined by a thin, radiopaque line adjacent to the periodontal ligament (PDL) and at the alveolar crest, referred to as the *lamina dura* (Fig. 33.1). Because the lamina dura represents the cortical bone lining the tooth socket, the shape and position of the root and changes in the angulation of the x-ray beam produce considerable variations in its appearance.

The width and shape of the interdental bone and the angle of the crest normally vary according to the convexity of the proximal tooth surfaces and the level of the cementoenamel junction (CEJ) of the approximating teeth. The faciolingual diameter of the bone is related to the width of the proximal root surface. The angulation of the crest of the interdental septum is generally parallel to a line between the CEJs of the approximating teeth (see Fig. 33.1). When there is a difference in the level of the CEJs, the crest of the interdental bone appears angulated rather than horizontal.

Radiographic Techniques

In conventional radiographs, periapical and bitewing projections offer the most diagnostic information and are most commonly used in the evaluation of periodontal disease. To properly and accurately depict periodontal bone status, proper techniques of exposure and processing are required. The bone level, pattern of bone destruction, and PDL space width, as well as the radiodensity, trabecular pattern, and marginal contour of the interdental bone, vary by modifying exposure and development time, type of film, and x-ray angulation.[20] Standardized, reproducible techniques are required to obtain reliable radiographs for pretreatment and posttreatment comparisons.

Prichard[15] established the following four criteria to determine adequate angulation of periapical radiographs:
1. The radiograph should show the tips of molar cusps with little or none of the occlusal surface showing.
2. Enamel caps and pulp chambers should be distinct.
3. Interproximal spaces should be open.
4. Proximal contacts should not overlap unless teeth are out of line anatomically.

For periapical radiographs, the long-cone paralleling technique most accurately projects the alveolar bone level (Fig. 33.2). The bisection-of-the-angle technique elongates the projected image, making the bone margin appear closer to the crown; the level of the facial bone is distorted more than that of the lingual. Inappropriate horizontal angulation results in tooth overlap, changes the shape of the interdental bone image, alters the radiographic width of the PDL space and the appearance of the lamina dura, and may distort the extent of furcation involvement (see Fig. 33.2).

Periapical radiographs frequently do not reveal the correct relationship between the alveolar bone and the CEJ.[9] This is particularly true in cases in which a shallow palate or floor of the mouth does not allow ideal placement of the periapical film. Bitewing projections offer an alternative method that better images periodontal bone levels. For bitewing radiographs, the film is placed behind the crowns of the upper and lower teeth parallel to the long axis of the teeth. The x-ray beam is directed through the contact areas of the teeth and perpendicular to the film. Thus the projection geometry of the bitewing

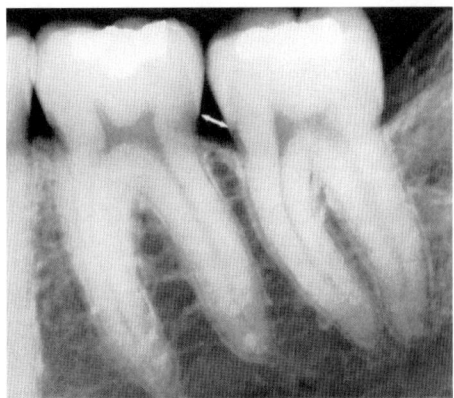

Fig. 33.1 Crest of interdental bone normally parallel to a line drawn between the cementoenamel junction of adjacent teeth *(arrow).* Note also the radiopaque lamina dura around the roots and interdental bone.

films allows the evaluation of the relationship between the interproximal alveolar crest and the CEJ without distortion[17] (Figs. 33.3 and 33.4). If the periodontal bone loss is severe and the bone level cannot be visualized on regular bitewing radiographs, films can be placed vertically to cover a larger area of the jaws (Fig. 33.5). More than two vertical bitewing films might be necessary to cover all of the interproximal spaces in the area of interest.

Bone Destruction in Periodontal Disease

Early destructive changes of bone that do not remove sufficient mineralized tissue cannot be captured on radiographs. Therefore slight radiographic changes of the periodontal tissues suggest that the disease has progressed beyond its earliest stages.[4] The earliest signs of periodontal disease must be detected clinically.

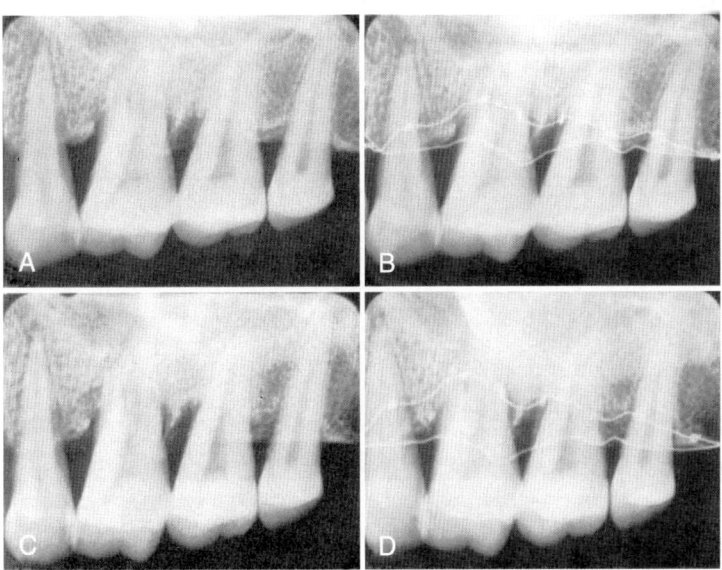

Fig. 33.2 Comparison of long-cone paralleling and bisection-of-the-angle techniques. (A) Long-cone paralleling technique, radiograph of dried specimen. (B) Long-cone paralleling technique, same specimen as shown in part A. Smooth wire is on the margin of the facial plate and knotted wire is on the lingual plate to show their relative positions. (C) Bisection-of-the-angle technique, same specimen as in parts A and B. (D) Bisection-of-the-angle technique, same specimen. Both bone margins are shifted toward the crown, the facial margin (smooth wire) more than the lingual margin (knotted wire), creating the illusion that the lingual bone margin has shifted apically. *(Courtesy Dr. Benjamin Patur, Hartford, Connecticut.)*

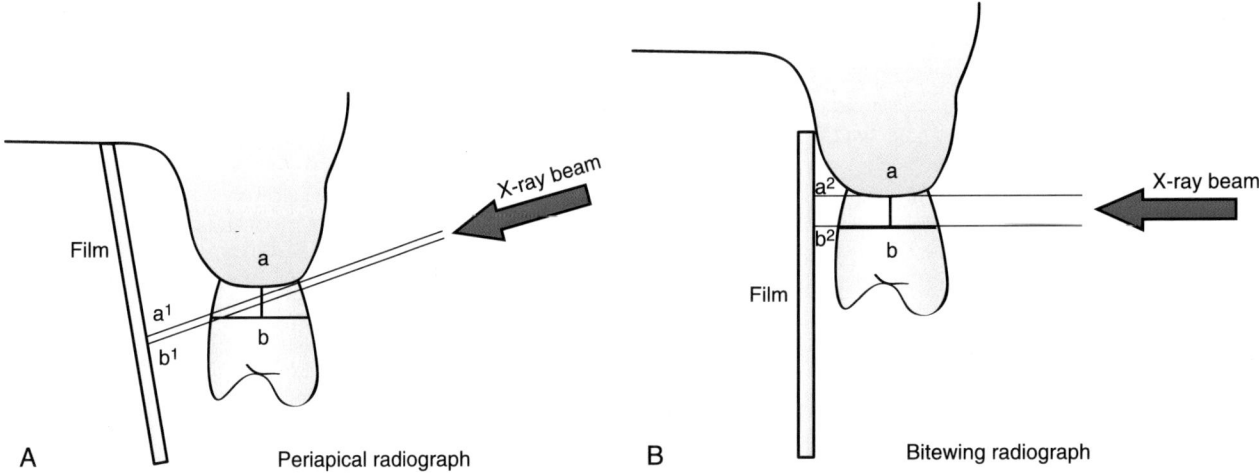

Fig. 33.3 Schematic diagram of periapical (A) and bitewing (B) radiographs. Angulation of the x-ray beam and the film on the periapical radiograph distort the distance between the alveolar crest and the cementoenamel junction (CEJ) (compare a–b versus a^1–b^1). In contrast, the projection geometry of the bitewing radiograph allows a more accurate depiction (a^2–b^2) of the distance between the alveolar crest and the CEJ (a–b).

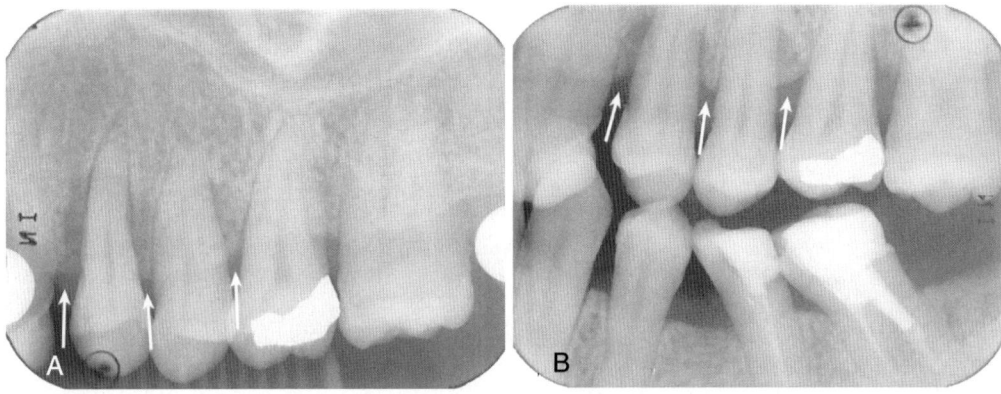

Fig. 33.4 Periapical (A) and bitewing (B) radiographs from a full-mouth series of a patient with periodontitis. The periapical film clearly underestimates the amount of bone loss *(white arrows)*. Because of appropriate projection geometry, the alveolar crest height is accurately depicted on the bitewing radiograph *(white arrows)*.

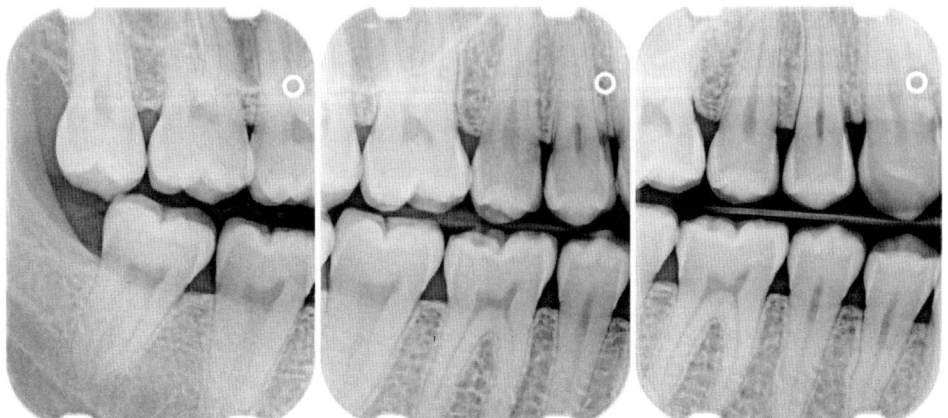

Fig. 33.5 Vertical bitewing films can be used to cover a larger area of the alveolar bone.

Bone Loss

The radiographic image tends to underestimate the severity of bone loss. The difference between the alveolar crest height and the radiographic appearance ranges from 0 to 1.6 mm, mostly accounted for by x-ray angulation.

Amount

Radiographs are an indirect method for determining the amount of bone loss in periodontal disease; they show the amount of remaining bone rather than the amount lost. The amount of bone lost is estimated to be the difference between the physiologic bone level and the height of the remaining bone.

Several investigators have analyzed the distance from the CEJ to the alveolar crest.[8,11,13] Most studies, conducted in adolescents, suggest a distance of 2 mm to reflect normal periodontium; this distance may be greater in older patients.

Distribution

The distribution of bone loss is an important diagnostic sign. It points to the location of destructive local factors in different areas of the mouth and in relation to different surfaces of the same tooth.

Pattern of Bone Destruction

In periodontal disease the interdental bone undergoes changes that affect the lamina dura, crestal radiodensity, size and shape of the

medullary spaces, and height and contour of the bone. The height of interdental bone may be reduced, with the crest perpendicular to the long axis of the adjacent teeth (*horizontal* bone loss; Fig. 33.6), or angular or arcuate defects (*angular,* or *vertical,* bone loss; Fig. 33.7) could form.

Radiographs do not indicate the internal morphology or depth of crater-like defects. Also, radiographs do not reveal the extent of involvement on the facial and lingual surfaces. Bone destruction of facial and lingual surfaces is masked by the dense root structure, and bone destruction on the mesial and distal root surfaces may be partially hidden by superimposed anatomy, such as a dense mylohyoid ridge (Fig. 33.8). In most cases, it can be assumed that bone loss seen interdentally continues in either the facial or lingual aspect, creating a troughlike lesion.

Dense cortical facial and lingual plates of interdental bone obscure destruction of the intervening cancellous bone. Thus a deep, craterlike defect between the facial and lingual plates might not be depicted on conventional radiographs. To record destruction of the interproximal cancellous bone radiographically, the cortical bone must be involved. A reduction of only 0.5 to 1 mm in the thickness of the cortical plate is sufficient to permit radiographic visualization of the destruction of the inner cancellous trabeculae.

Interdental bone loss may continue facially or lingually to form a troughlike defect that could be difficult to appreciate radiographically. These lesions may terminate on the radicular surface or may

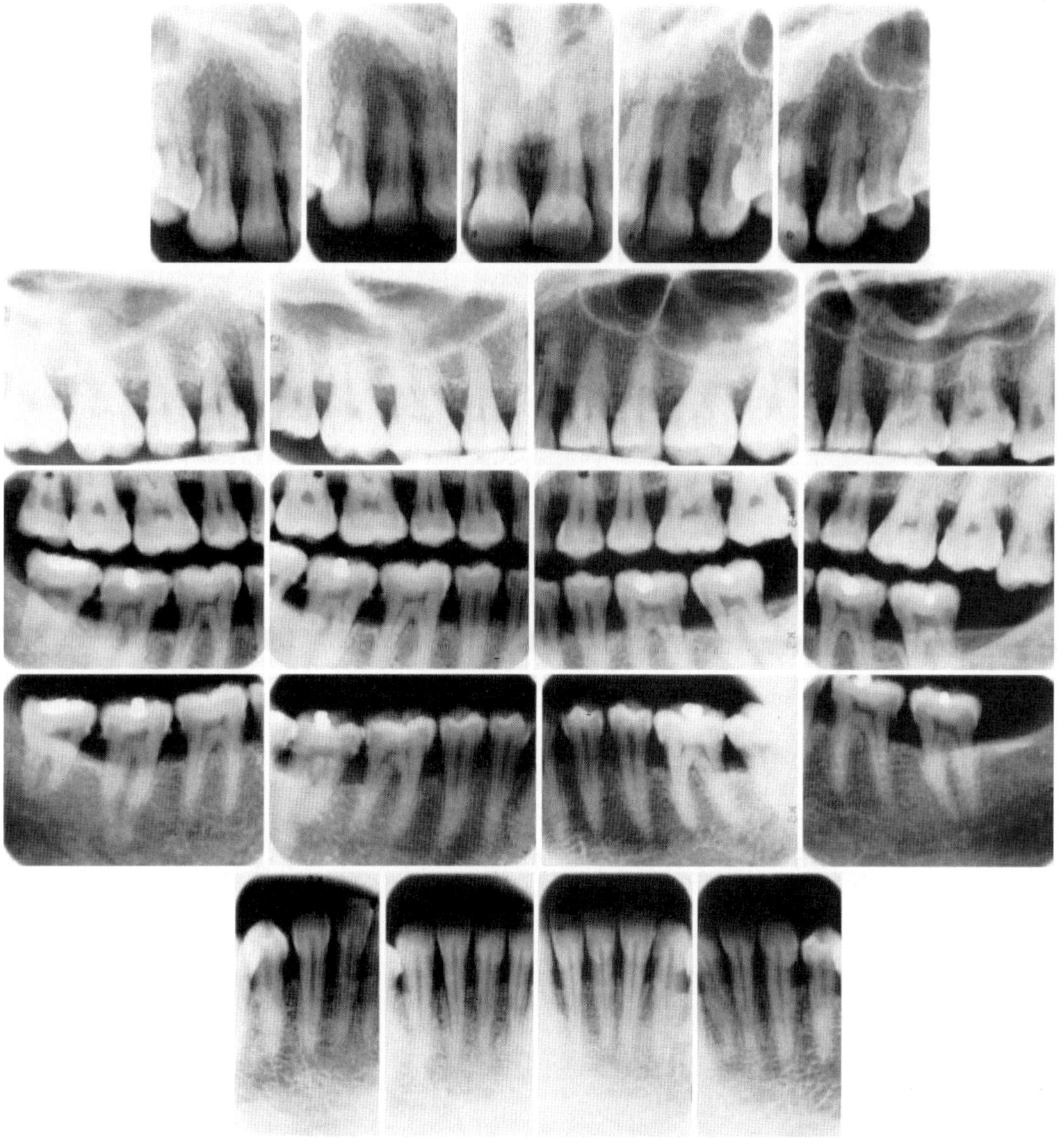

Fig. 33.6 Generalized horizontal bone loss.

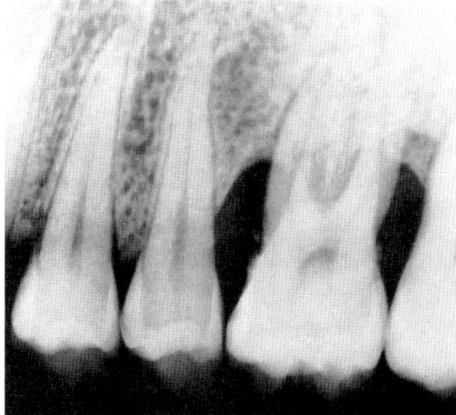

Fig. 33.7 Angular bone loss on first molar with involvement of the furcation.

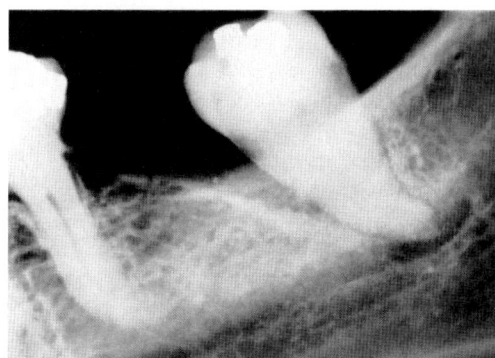

Fig. 33.8 Angular bone loss on mandibular molar partially obscured by a dense mylohyoid ridge.

communicate with the adjacent interdental area to form one continuous lesion (Fig. 33.9).

Fig. 33.10 shows two adjacent interdental lesions connecting on the radicular surface to form one interconnecting osseous lesion. Along with clinical probing of these lesions, the use of a radiopaque pointer placed in these radicular defects will demonstrate the extent of the bone loss.

Periodontal bone loss should be differentiated from normal anatomy or anatomic variants that can resemble disease. For example, nutrient canals in the alveolar bone can appear as linear and circular radiolucent areas (Fig. 33.11). These canals can be seen more frequently in the anterior mandible, although they can be present throughout the alveolar ridge.

Finally, it should be emphasized that radiographs can only assess the amount of periodontal bone that is present and deduce the extent of bone loss. However, it is sometimes necessary to determine whether the reduced bone level is the result of periodontal disease that is no longer destructive (usually after treatment and proper maintenance) or whether destructive periodontal disease is present. Differentiation between treated versus active periodontal disease can only be achieved

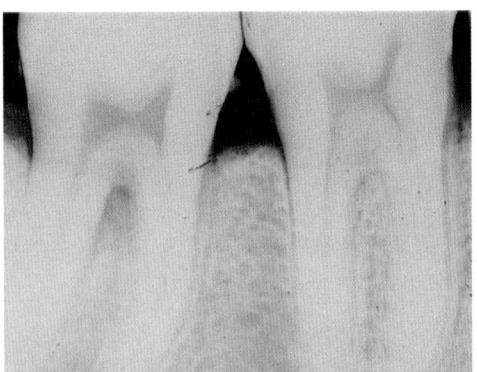
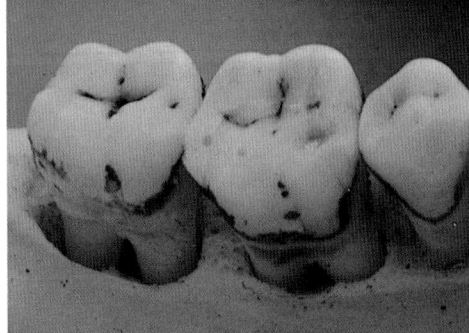

Fig. 33.9 Interdental lesion that extends to the facial or lingual surfaces in a troughlike manner.

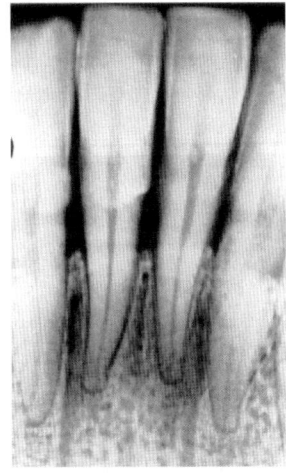

Fig. 33.11 Prominent nutrient canals in the mandible.

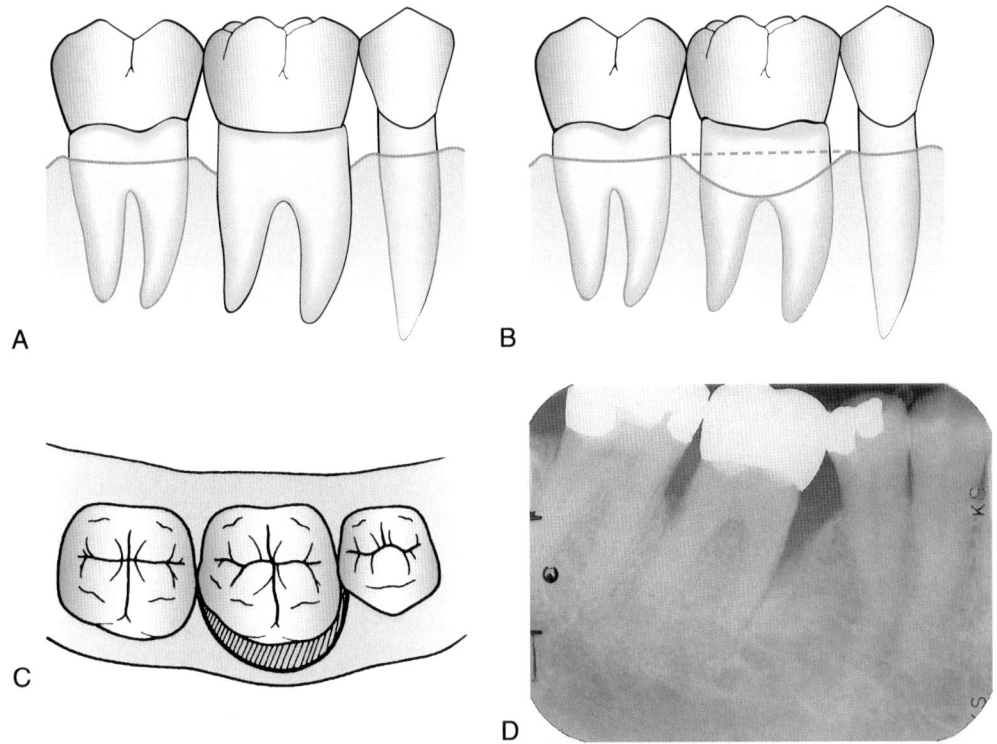

A

B

C

D

Fig. 33.10 (A) Interdental mesial and distal lesions. (B) Facial or lingual outlines of the actual lesion. (C) Occlusal view of the lesion. (D) Radiograph of mesial and facial lesions.

clinically. Radiographically detectable changes in the normal cortical outline of the interdental bone are corroborating evidence of destructive periodontal disease.

Radiographic Appearance of Periodontal Disease

Periodontitis

Radiographic changes in periodontitis follow the pathophysiology of periodontal tissue destruction and include the following:

1. *Fuzziness and disruption of lamina dura* crestal cortication continuity is the earliest radiographic change in periodontitis (Fig. 33.12A–B) and results from bone resorption activated by extension of gingival inflammation into the periodontal bone.

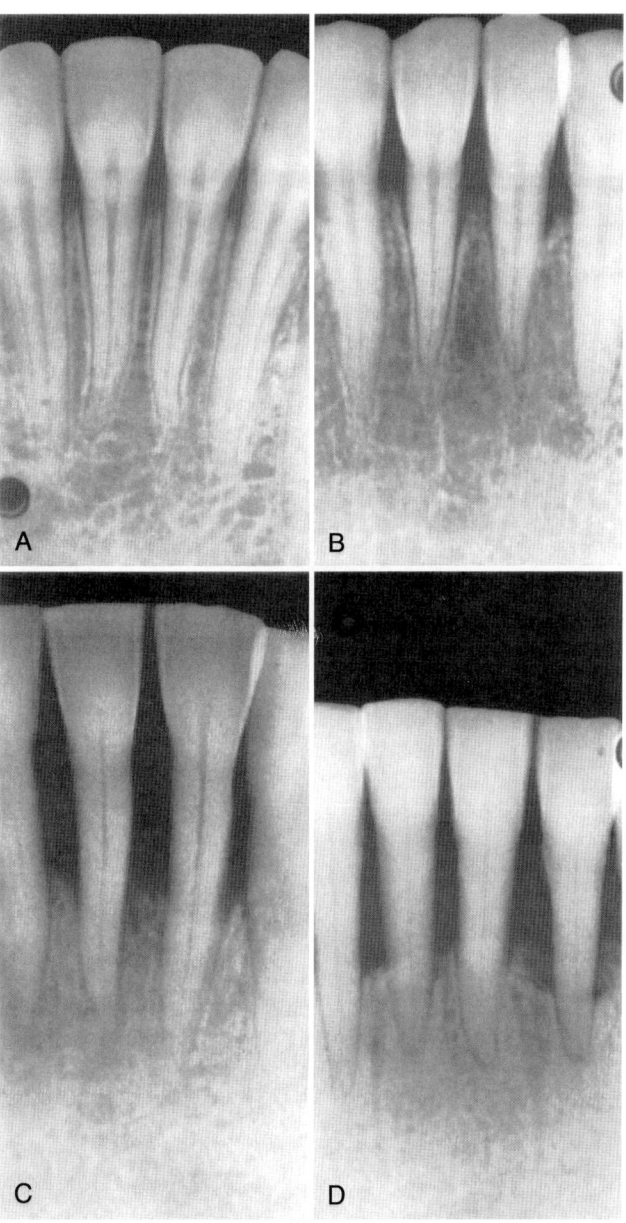

Fig. 33.12 Radiographic changes in periodontitis. (A) Normal appearance of interdental bone. (B) Fuzziness and a break in the continuity of the lamina dura at the crest of the bone distal to the central incisor *(left)*. There are wedge-shaped radiolucent areas at the crest of the other interdental bone. (C) Radiolucent projections from the crest into the interdental bone indicate extension of destructive processes. (D) Severe bone loss.

Depicting these early changes depends greatly on the radiographic technique, as well as on anatomic variations (thickness and density of interdental bone, position of adjoining teeth). No correlation has been found between crestal lamina dura in radiographs and the presence or absence of clinical inflammation, bleeding on probing, periodontal pockets, or loss of attachment.[16] Therefore it can be concluded that the presence of an intact crestal lamina dura may be an indicator of periodontal health, whereas its absence lacks diagnostic relevance.[1,3]

2. Continued periodontal bone loss and widening of the periodontal space results in a wedge-shaped radiolucency at the mesial or distal aspect of the crest (Fig. 33.12B). The apex of the area is pointed in the direction of the root.

3. Subsequently, the destructive process extends across the alveolar crest, thus reducing the height of the interdental bone. As increased osteoclastic activity results in increased bone resorption along the endosteal margins of the medullary spaces, the remaining interdental bone can appear partially eroded (Fig. 33.12C).

4. The height of the interdental septum is progressively reduced by the extension of inflammation and the resorption of bone (Fig. 33.12D).

5. Frequently a radiopaque horizontal line can be observed across the roots of a tooth. This opaque line demarcates the portion of the root where the labial or lingual bony plate has been partially or completely destroyed from the remaining bone-supported portion (Fig. 33.13).

LEARNING BOX 33.3

The earliest changes of periodontal disease often do not manifest on radiographs. Even when radiographic changes are evident, radiographic examination may underestimate the extent of bone loss. Thus assessment of periodontal bone level should be based on combined clinical-radiographic evaluation.

Interdental Craters

Interdental craters are seen as irregular areas of reduced density on the alveolar bone crests. Craters are generally not sharply demarcated

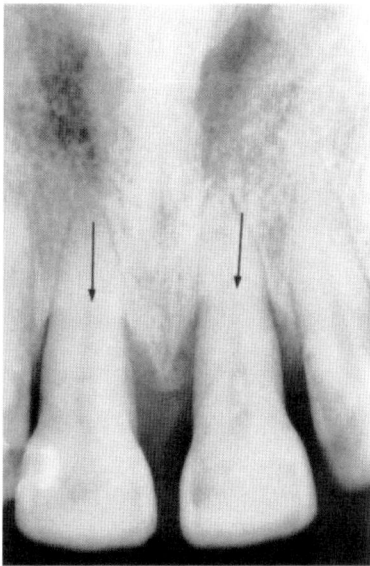

Fig. 33.13 Horizontal lines across the roots of the central incisors *(arrows)*. The area of the roots below the horizontal lines is partially or completely denuded of the facial and lingual bony plates.

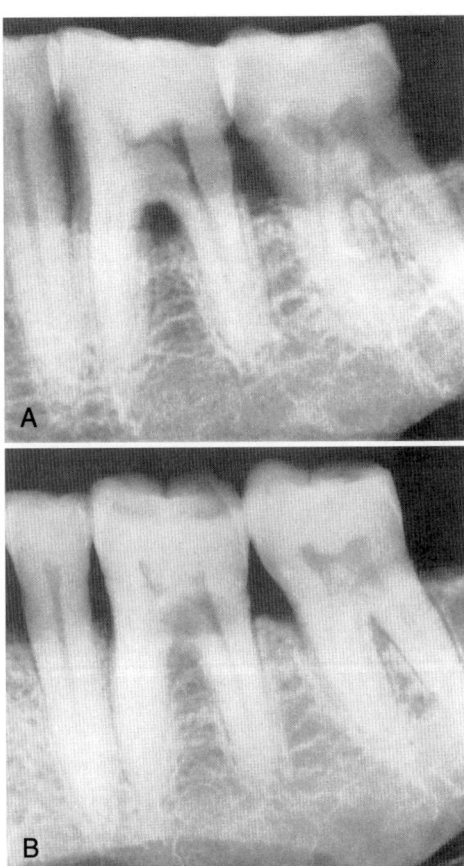

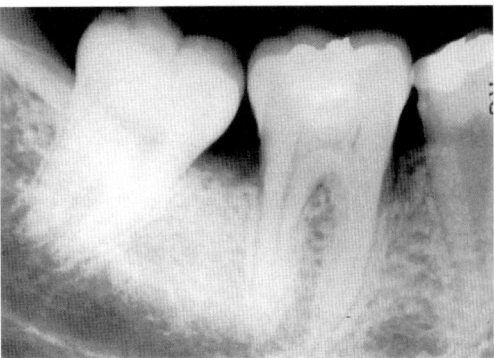

Fig. 33.15 Early furcation involvement suggested by fuzziness in the bifurcation of the mandibular first molar, particularly when associated with bone loss on the roots.

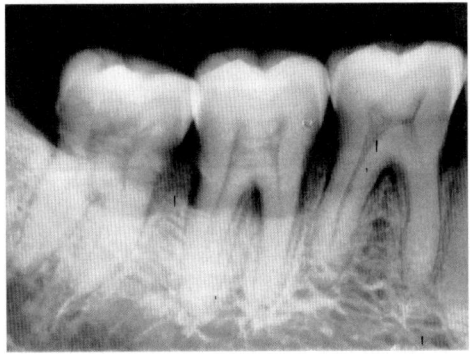

Fig. 33.14 (A) Furcation involvement indicated by triangular radiolucency in the bifurcation area of mandibular first molar. The second molar presents only a slight thickening of the periodontal space in the bifurcation area. (B) Same area as in A with different angulation. The triangular radiolucency in the bifurcation of the first molar is obliterated, and involvement of the second molar bifurcation is apparent.

Fig. 33.16 Furcation involvement of mandibular first and second molars indicated by thickening of the periodontal space in the furcation area. The furcation of the third molar is also involved, but the thickening of the periodontal space is partially obscured by the external oblique line.

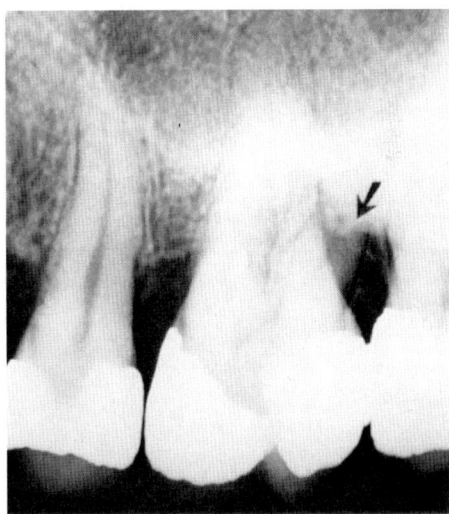

but gradually blend with the rest of the bone. Conventional radiographs do not accurately depict the morphology or depth of interdental craters, which sometimes appear as vertical defects.

Furcation Involvement

Definitive diagnosis of furcation involvement is made by clinical examination, which includes careful probing with a specially designed probe (e.g., Nabers). Radiographs are helpful, but root superimposition, caused by anatomic variations or improper technique, can obscure radiographic representation of furcation involvement. As a general rule, bone loss is greater than it appears in the radiograph. A tooth may present marked bifurcation involvement in one film (Fig. 33.14A) but appear to be uninvolved in another (Fig. 33.14B). Radiographs should be taken at different angles to reduce the risk of missing furcation involvement.

A large, clearly defined radiolucency in the furcation area is easy to identify (see Fig. 33.14A), but less clearly defined radiographic changes are often overlooked. To assist in the radiographic detection of furcation involvement, the following diagnostic criteria are suggested:

1. The slightest radiographic change in the furcation area should be investigated clinically, especially if there is bone loss on adjacent roots (Fig. 33.15).
2. Diminished radiodensity in the furcation area in which outlines of bony trabeculae are visible suggests furcation involvement (Fig. 33.16).

Fig. 33.17 Furcation involvement of the first molar partially obscured by the radiopaque lingual root. The horizontal line across the distobuccal root demarcates the apical portion *(arrow),* which is covered by bone, from the remainder of the root, where the bone has been destroyed.

3. Whenever there is marked bone loss in relation to a single molar root, it may be assumed that furcation is also involved (Fig. 33.17).

Periodontal Abscess

The typical radiographic appearance of a periodontal abscess is a discrete area of radiolucency along the lateral aspect of the root

(Figs. 33.18 and 33.19). However, the radiographic picture is often not characteristic (Fig. 33.20). This can be due to the following:

1. *The stage of the lesion.* In the early stages an acute periodontal abscess is extremely painful but presents no radiographic changes.
2. *The extent of bone destruction and the morphologic changes of the bone.*
3. *The location of the abscess.* Lesions in the soft tissue wall of a periodontal pocket are less likely to produce radiographic changes than those deep in the supporting tissues. Abscesses on the facial or lingual surface are obscured by the radiopacity of the root; interproximal lesions are more likely to be visualized radiographically.

Therefore radiographs alone cannot provide a final diagnosis of a periodontal abscess but need to be accompanied by careful clinical examination.

Clinical Probing

Regenerative and resective flap designs and incisions require prior knowledge of the underlying osseous topography. Careful probing of these pocket areas after scaling and root planing often requires local anesthesia and definitive radiographic evaluation of the osseous lesions. Radiographs taken with periodontal probes, gutta-percha points, or other indicators (e.g., Hirschfeld pointers) placed into the anesthetized pocket show the true extent of the bone lesion. As indicated previously, the attachment level on the radicular surface or interdental lesions with thick facial or lingual bone cannot be visualized in the radiograph. The use of radiopaque indicators is an efficient and necessary diagnostic aid (Fig. 33.21).

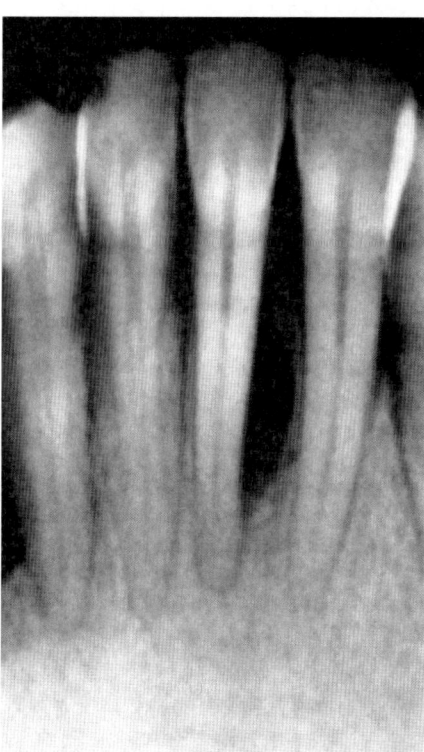

Fig. 33.18 Radiolucent area on lateral aspect of root with chronic periodontal abscess.

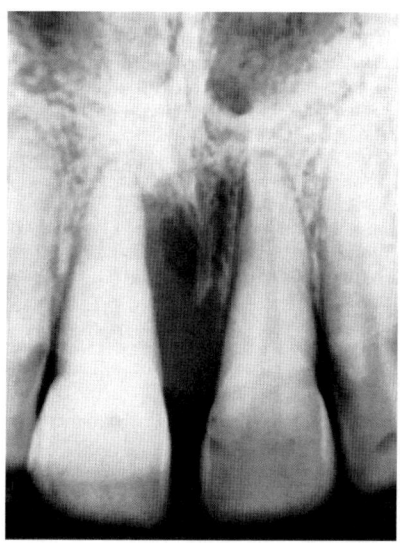

Fig. 33.19 Typical radiographic appearance of periodontal abscess on right central incisor.

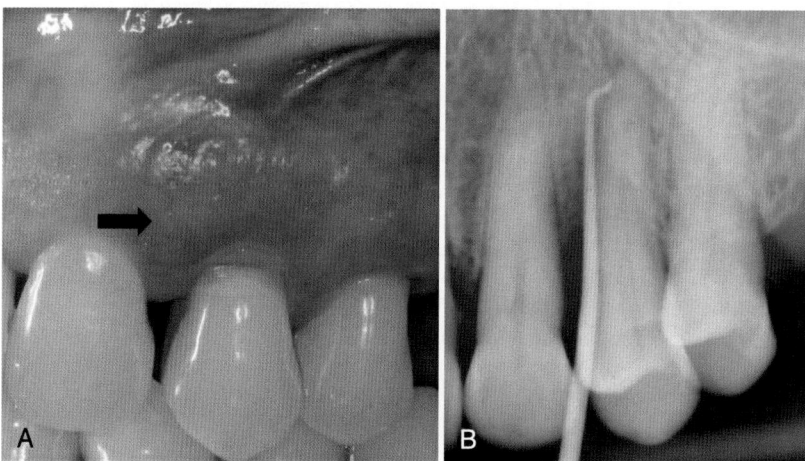

Fig. 33.20 Chronic periodontal abscess. (A) Periodontal abscess in the left maxillary first premolar area. (B) Extensive bone destruction on the mesial surface of the first premolar. Gutta-percha point traces to the root apex.

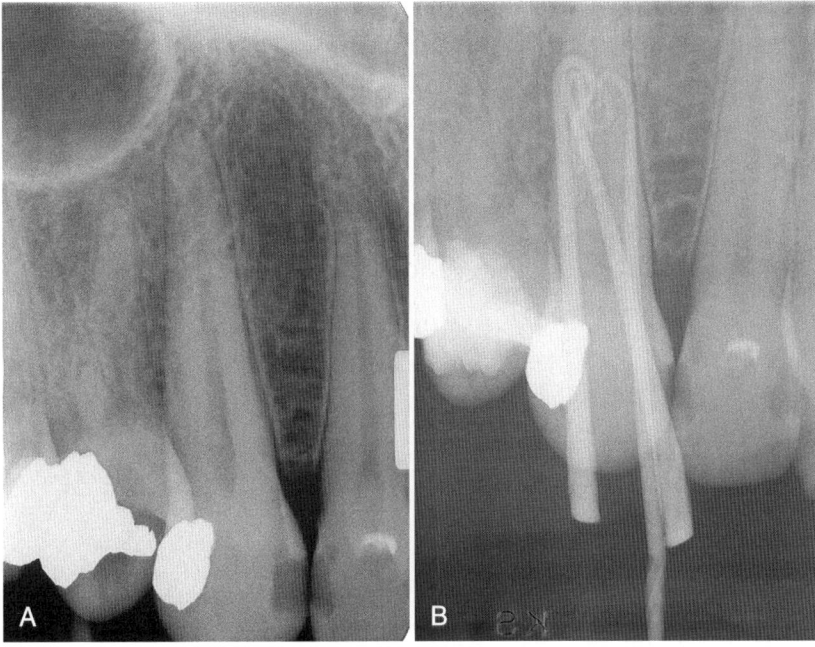

Fig. 33.21 (A) Radiograph of maxillary cuspid. This view does not show facial bone loss. (B) Radiograph of same maxillary cuspid as in part A, with gutta-percha points placed in the facial pocket to indicate bone loss.

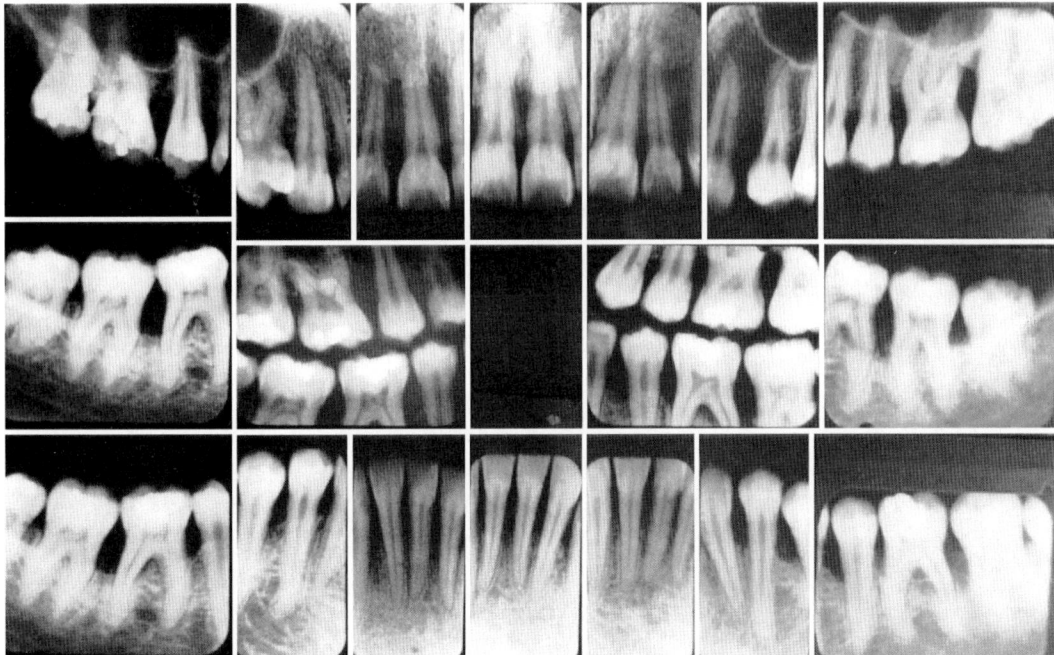

Fig. 33.22 Localized aggressive periodontitis. The accentuated bone destruction in the anterior and first molar areas is considered to be characteristic of this disease.

Localized Aggressive Periodontitis

Localized aggressive (formerly "localized juvenile") periodontitis is characterized by the following:
1. Initially, there is bone loss in the maxillary and mandibular incisor or first molar areas, usually bilaterally, resulting in a vertical, arclike destructive pattern (Fig. 33.22).
2. As the disease progresses, loss of alveolar bone may become generalized but remains less pronounced in the premolar areas.

Trauma From Occlusion

Trauma from occlusion can produce radiographically detectable changes in the thickness of the lamina dura, morphology of the alveolar crest, width of the PDL space, and density of the surrounding cancellous bone.[5]

Traumatic lesions manifest more clearly in faciolingual aspects because mesiodistally, the tooth has added stability provided by the contact areas with adjacent teeth. Therefore slight variations in the

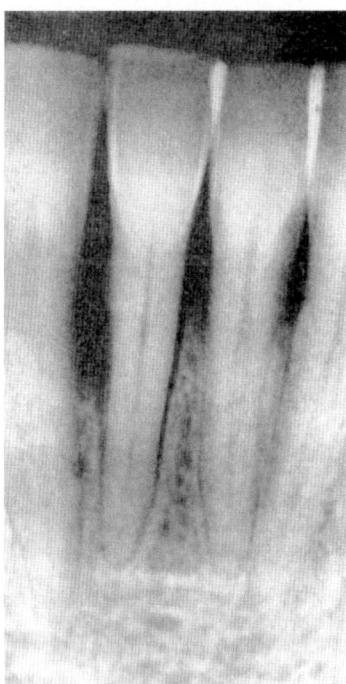

Fig. 33.23 Widened periodontal space caused by trauma from occlusion. Note the increased density of the surrounding bone caused by new bone formation in response to increased occlusal forces.

proximal surfaces may indicate greater changes in the facial and lingual aspects. *The radiographic changes listed next are not pathognomonic for trauma from occlusion and must be interpreted in combination with clinical findings,* particularly tooth mobility, presence of wear facets, pocket depth, and analysis of occlusal contacts and habits.

The *injury phase* of trauma from occlusion produces a loss of the lamina dura that may be noted in apices, furcations, and marginal areas. This loss of lamina dura results in widening of the PDL space (Fig. 33.23). The *repair phase* of trauma from occlusion results in an attempt to strengthen the periodontal structures to better support the increased loads. Radiographically, this is manifested by a widening of the PDL space, which may be generalized or localized.

Although microscopic measurements have determined normal variations in the PDL space width along the root surface, these are generally not detected radiographically. Thus, when seen on radiographs, variations in PDL space width suggest that the tooth is being subjected to increased forces. Successful attempts to reinforce the periodontal structures by widening the PDL space can be accompanied by increased width of the lamina dura and sometimes by condensation of the perialveolar cancellous bone.

More advanced traumatic lesions may result in deep angular bone loss, which, when combined with marginal inflammation, may lead to intrabony pocket formation. In terminal stages, these lesions extend around the root apex, producing a wide, radiolucent periapical image (cavernous lesions).

Root resorption may also result from excessive forces on the periodontium, particularly those caused by orthodontic appliances. Although trauma from occlusion produces many areas of root resorption, these areas are usually of a magnitude insufficient to be detected radiographically.

Digital Intraoral Radiography

Advances in digital imaging technology have driven rapid growth of digital intraoral radiography as a convenient alternative to conventional film-based radiography.[10,12,14,23] These technologies have been integrated into patient management systems, enabling dental offices to maintain fully electronic patient records (Fig. 33.24A). The digital records can be easily shared among dentists and other health care providers, enabling telediagnosis and facilitating transmission to third parties for reimbursement.

Digital intraoral radiographic systems use either solid-state detectors or photostimulable phosphor (PSP) plates.[21-23] Systems with solid-state detectors use either charge-coupled devices (CCDs) or complementary metal oxide semiconductor (CMOS) chips as image receptors. These receptors are typically wired and connected to a computer using a Universal Serial Bus (USB) connection. Wireless sensors are also available and require the use of disposable batteries. With CCD/CMOS-based receptors, images are recorded and displayed on a computer monitor virtually in real time. These sensors are bulkier than film, and the active image-recording area is slightly smaller than that of film. A second technology for intraoral radiography is PSP plates. These receptors are the same size as intraoral radiographic film. Unlike CCD/CMOS receptors, PSP plates do not provide a real-time display of the radiographic image. On interaction with x-ray photons, PSP crystals in the plate store energy, creating a latent radiographic image. The stored energy is then released by stimulating the plate with an appropriate wavelength of light. With PSP systems, the workflow is somewhat similar to that with silver halide emulsion film. Following radiographic exposure, the PSP plate is scanned by a laser beam, converting the latent radiographic image into a digital image.

Following capture, digital radiographic images can be enhanced to augment radiographic diagnosis. The brightness and contrast of the image can be altered to highlight specific anatomic regions, depending on the diagnostic task. The images can be magnified to allow closer examination of a specific area of interest. Importantly, a variety of image enhancement filters can be applied—for example, to sharpen images (enhance edges). Some software programs have preprogrammed algorithms that can be applied for specific diagnostic tasks—for example, to enhance interproximal caries, periodontal bone, pulp canals, and so forth (Fig. 33.24B). However, it is important to recognize that such image manipulations can produce artifacts that may be misinterpreted as disease. Clinicians should be aware of such artifacts produced by digital image manipulation. In addition to the image manipulation features, digital radiographic images facilitate patient education, allow for easy storage and sharing with other health care providers, and can be easily integrated into electronic patient records.

Advanced Imaging Modalities

Cone-beam computed tomography (CBCT) has revolutionized the field of oral and maxillofacial imaging. CBCT technology and its use in evaluating the implant patient are discussed in Chapter 76. However, CBCT finds application in almost every diagnostic task of clinical dentistry, including the evaluation of periodontal and periapical structures.[18] CBCT offers many advantages over conventional radiography, including accurate three-dimensional imaging of teeth and supporting structures. Although not recommended for every dental patient, CBCT avoids the problems of geometric superimposition and unpredictable magnification and can provide valuable diagnostic information in periodontal evaluation.

As discussed earlier, periapical and bitewing radiographs provide information mostly for interdental bone. However, a three-wall defect that preserves the buccal or lingual cortices can be difficult to diagnose, and the buccal, lingual, and furcational periodontal bone levels are hard to evaluate in conventional radiographs. When clinical

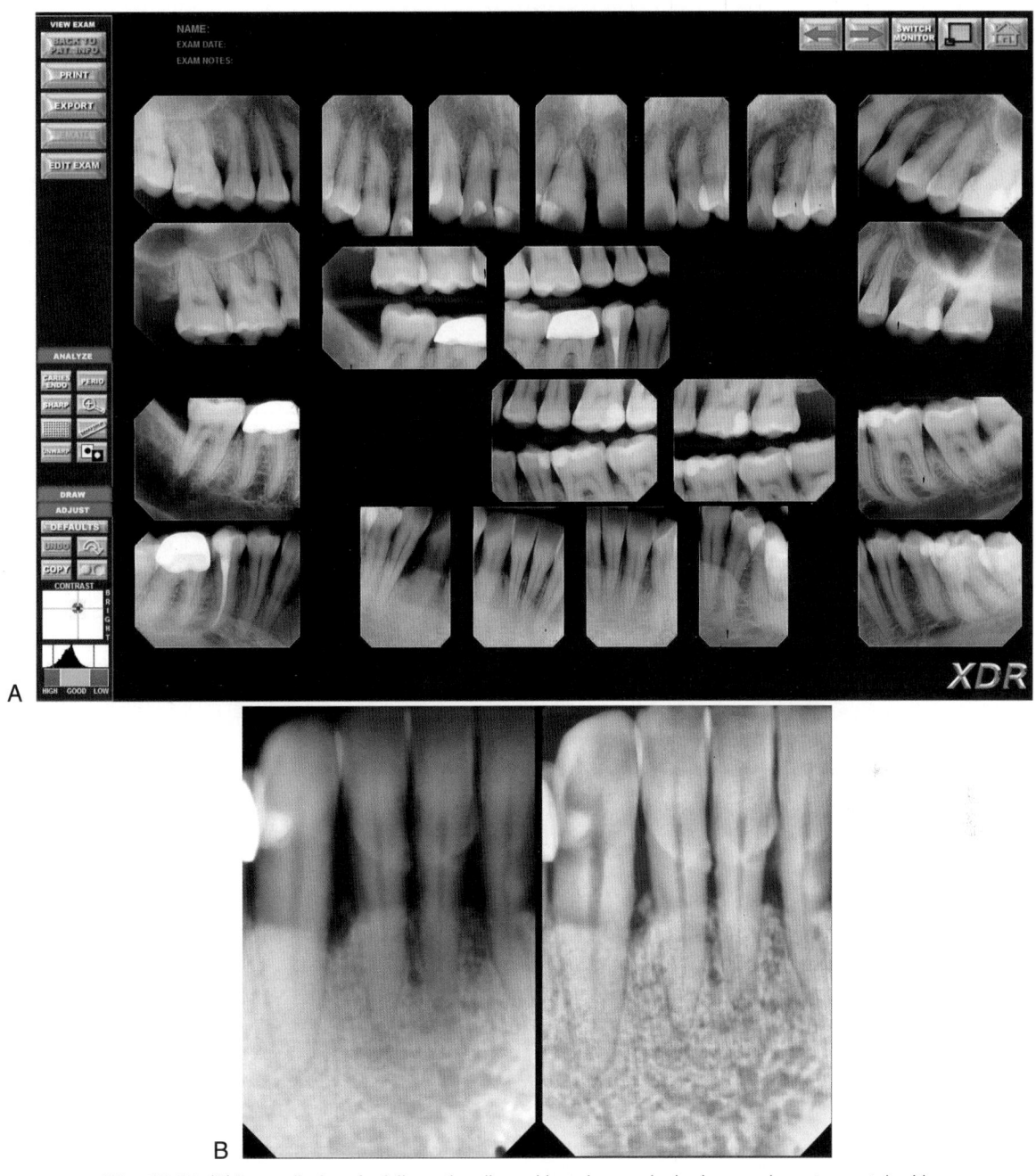

Fig. 33.24 (A) Image display of a full-mouth radiographic series acquired using complementary metal oxide semiconductor (CMOS) receptors. Specific features of the software program allow for image manipulation, measurements, and annotations. (B) The "perio" image enhancement filter applied to highlight the contrast of alveolar bone. Note the presence of calculus and better depiction of the alveolar crestal bone.

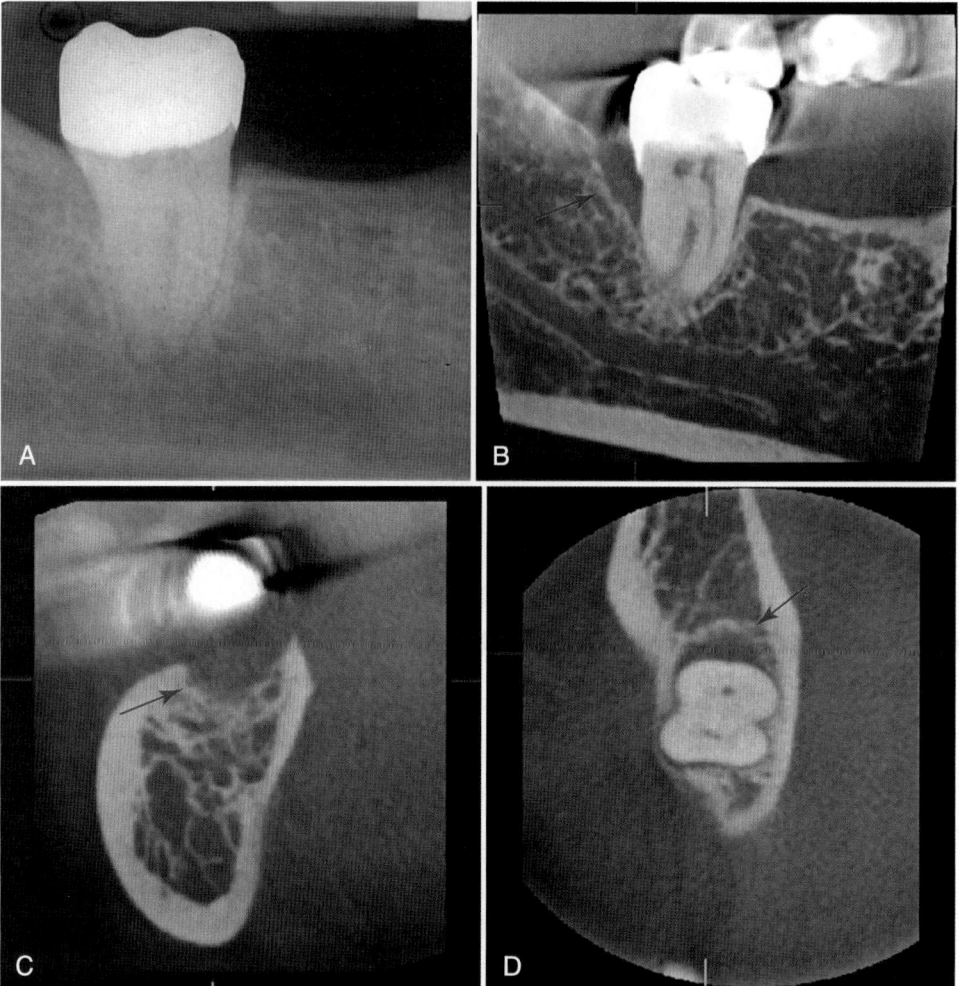

Fig. 33.25 Periapical radiograph (A) and sagittal (B), cross-sectional (C), and axial (D) cone-beam computed tomography (CBCT) sections of the mandibular right second molar. No pathology is detected on the periapical radiograph. However, CBCT images clearly illustrate a deep, vertical, three-wall defect on the distal surface of the mandibular right second molar *(red arrow).*

examination raises concerns for such areas, CBCT imaging can add diagnostic value. Indeed, when compared to periapical radiographs, CBCT was able to depict the buccal and lingual/palatal surfaces and offered improved visualization of the morphology of the periodontal defect.[7] Furthermore, for assessment of periodontal bone loss, CBCT performed better than digital radiographs in the detection of early furcational defects, three-wall defects, fenestrations, and dehiscence, but not in advanced furcation involvement or one- or two-wall and troughlike defects.[2]

Fig. 33.25 illustrates the diagnostic advantage of CBCT in the evaluation of a three-wall defect in the distal surface of tooth #32. A periapical radiograph (Fig. 33.25A) presents normal bone height at the mesial and distal surfaces of #32. CBCT sections (Fig. 33.25A–C) clearly demonstrate a three-wall defect on the distal surface of #32. Note that the buccal and lingual cortical plates are well preserved. For this reason, the periodontal defect is not depicted in the periapical radiograph. Similarly, Fig. 33.26 depicts a vertical defect in the interproximal area between the two right maxillary premolars extending from the alveolar crest to the apical third of the roots toward the palatal aspect of the alveolar ridge. This defect cannot be appreciated on the periapical radiograph.

CBCT imaging provides three-dimensional information and overcomes many of the limitations of conventional two-dimensional (2D) radiography. However, CBCT imaging is a higher-dose procedure relative to bitewing radiography, and is also more expensive. CBCT imaging for periodontal bone evaluation should be considered only for select cases where 2D information is insufficient for diagnostic or treatment planning needs, and it is not recommended for routine evaluation of periodontal bone loss.

Conclusion

Periapical radiographic examination should be part of every patient's periodontal evaluation and coupled with a detailed recording of pocket depths, gingival margin location, and bleeding on probing. Radiographic evaluation should be updated every 2 years. Periapical radiographs often underestimate the amount of periodontal bone loss, and early changes are usually not detected. Significant interdental bone loss can occur and may not be detectable on periapical

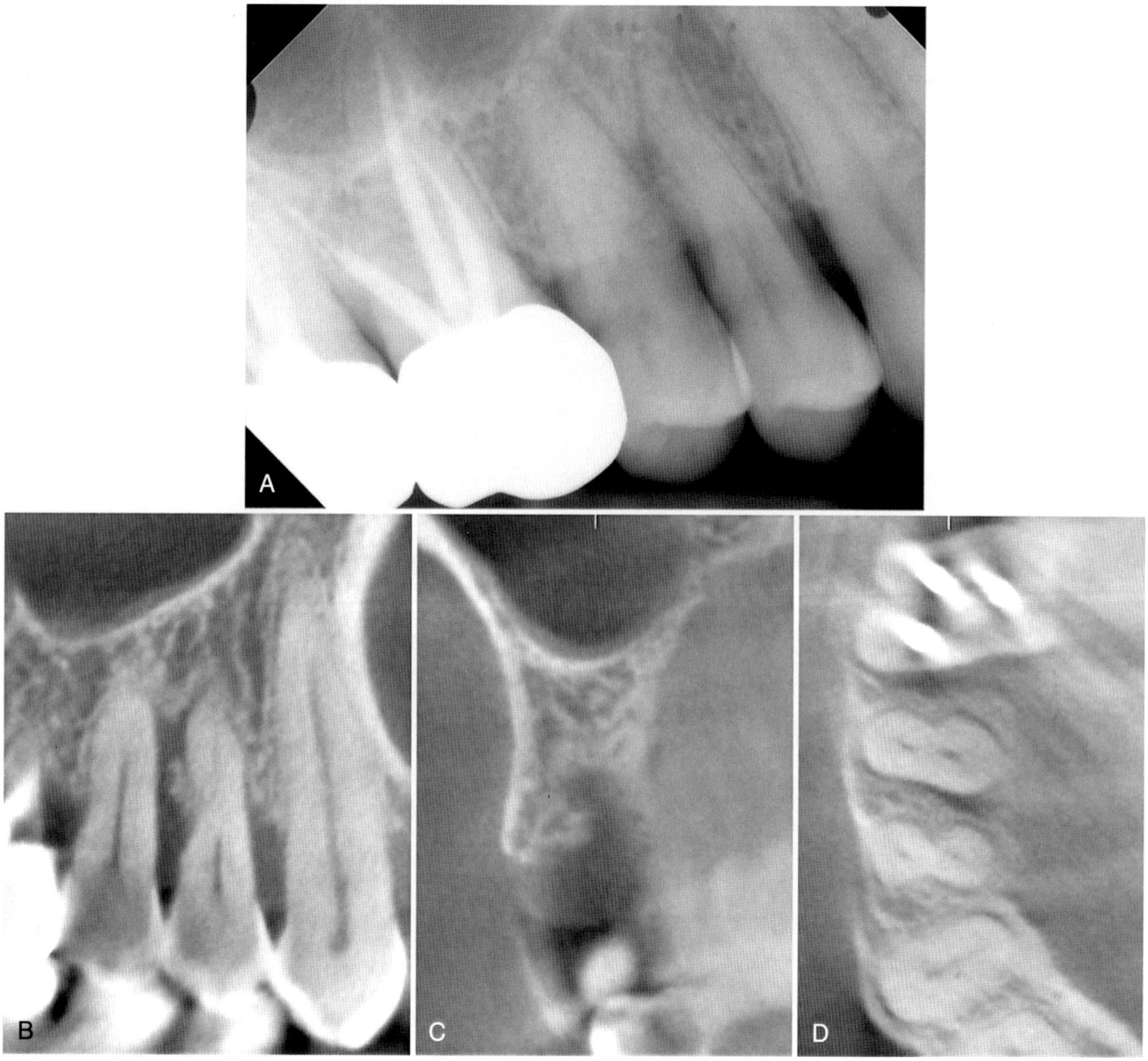

Fig. 33.26 Periapical radiograph (A) and sagittal (B), cross-sectional (C), and axial (D) cone-beam computed tomography (CBCT) sections of the maxillary premolar region. The periapical radiograph demonstrates horizontal bone loss. The CBCT images reveal the presence of a vertical defect between the premolars that extends from the palatal crest to the apical third of the roots. The extent of bone loss is underestimated on the periapical radiograph.

radiographs because the density of the intact buccal and lingual or palatal bone plates obscure changes that occur as a result of periodontitis. Comparing periapical radiographs of the same area taken at different times will only be reliable for documenting dramatic changes in bone levels, because variations in angulation of the beam, placement of the film, and development of the image make accurate measurements taken over time difficult and unreliable.

Three-dimensional radiographic techniques with CBCT give a much more accurate picture of periodontal bone loss than two-dimensional radiographs and will be more widely used as this technology becomes available in more clinics.

Case Scenarios are found on the companion website www.expertconsult.com.

References

References for this chapter are found on the companion website www.expertconsult.com.

CHAPTER 34

Clinical Risk Assessment

Satheesh Elangovan | Karen F. Novak | M. John Novak

 For online-only content on risk indicators, risk markers/predictors, and clinical risk assessment for periodontal disease, please visit the companion website at www.expertconsult.com.

Definitions

Risk assessment is defined by numerous components.[2,33] Disease risk is the probability that an individual will develop a specific disease in a given period. The risk of developing the disease will vary from individual to individual.

Risk factors may be environmental, behavioral, or biologic factors that, when present, increase the likelihood that an individual will develop the disease. Risk factors are identified through longitudinal studies of patients with the disease of interest. Exposure to a risk factor or factors may occur at a single point in time, over multiple separate points in time, or continuously. However, to be identified as a risk factor, the exposure must occur before disease onset. Interventions often can be identified and, when implemented, can help modify risk factors.

The term *risk determinant/background characteristic*, which is sometimes substituted for the term *risk factor*, should be reserved for risk factors that cannot be modified. *Risk indicators* are *probable* or *putative* risk factors that have been identified in cross-sectional studies but not confirmed through longitudinal studies. *Risk predictors/markers*, although associated with increased risk for disease, do not cause the disease. These factors also are identified in cross-sectional and longitudinal studies. Box 34.1 lists elements of these categories of risk for periodontal disease.

⚠ CLINICAL CORRELATION

Lack of bleeding on probing does appear to serve as an excellent indicator of periodontal health, but the presence of bleeding on probing alone is not a good predictor of future attachment loss.

Risk Factors for Periodontal Disease

Tobacco Smoking

Tobacco smoking is a well-established risk factor for periodontitis.[2,10] A direct relationship exists between smoking and the prevalence of periodontal disease (see Chapter 12). This association is independent of other factors such as oral hygiene or age.[20] Studies comparing the response to periodontal therapy in smokers, previous smokers, and nonsmokers have shown that smoking has a negative impact on the response to therapy. However, former smokers respond similarly to nonsmokers.[3] These studies demonstrate the therapeutic impact of intervention strategies on patients who smoke (see Chapter 12).

Diabetes

Diabetes is a clear risk factor for periodontitis.[2] Epidemiologic data demonstrate that the prevalence and severity of periodontitis are significantly higher in patients with type 1 or type 2 diabetes mellitus than in those without diabetes and that the level of diabetic control is an important variable in this relationship (see Chapter 14).

Pathogenic Bacteria and Microbial Tooth Deposits

It is well documented that the accumulation of bacterial plaque at the gingival margin results in the development of gingivitis and that the gingivitis can be reversed with the implementation of oral hygiene measures.[27] These studies demonstrate a causal relationship between the accumulation of bacterial plaque and gingival inflammation. However, a causal relationship between *plaque accumulation* and *periodontitis* has been more difficult to establish. Often patients with severe loss of attachment have minimal levels of bacterial plaque on the affected teeth, indicating that the *quantity* of plaque is not of major importance in the disease process. However, although quantity may not indicate risk, there is evidence that the composition, or *quality,* of the complex plaque biofilm is important.

In terms of quality of plaque, three specific bacteria have been identified as etiologic agents for periodontitis: *Aggregatibacter actinomycetemcomitans* (formerly *Actinobacillus actinomycetemcomitans*), *Porphyromonas gingivalis,* and *Tannerella forsythia* (formerly *Bacteroides forsythus*).[12] *Porphyromonas gingivalis* and *T. forsythia* are often found in chronic periodontitis, whereas *A. actinomycetemcomitans* is often associated with aggressive periodontitis. Cross-sectional and longitudinal studies support the delineation of these three bacteria as risk factors for periodontal

Risk Factors

Tobacco smoking

Diabetes

Pathogenic bacteria and microbial tooth deposits

Risk Determinants/Background Characteristics

Genetic factors

Age

Gender

Socioeconomic status

Stress

Risk Indicators

Human immunodeficiency virus (HIV)/acquired immunodeficiency syndrome (AIDS)

Osteoporosis

Infrequent dental visits

Risk Markers/Predictors

Previous history of periodontal disease

Bleeding on probing

disease. Additional evidence that these organisms are causal agents includes the following[17]:

1. Their elimination or suppression impacts the success of therapy.
2. There is a host response to these pathogens.
3. Virulence factors are associated with these pathogens.
4. Inoculation of these bacteria into animal models induces periodontal disease.

Although not completely supported by these criteria for causation, moderate evidence also suggests that *Campylobacter rectus, Eubacterium nodatum, Fusobacterium nucleatum, Prevotella intermedia, Prevotella nigrescens, Peptostreptococcus micros, Streptococcus intermedius,* and *Treponema denticola* are etiologic factors in periodontitis.[12]

It is becoming clear from investigations that the plaque composition shifts from a more symbiotic microbial community to one that is more dysbiotic (an imbalance in the relative abundance of microbes leading to disease), composed primarily of anaerobes, as we go from periodontal health to periodontal disease. Certain pathogens (termed *keystone pathogens*) such as *Porphyromonas gingivalis* play a major role in inducing such a shift, converting commensals into disease-provoking microbes (termed *pathobionts*).[18] Therefore the quantity of plaque present may not be as important as the quality of the plaque in determining risk for periodontitis.

Anatomic factors, such as furcations, root concavities, developmental grooves, cervical enamel projections, enamel pearls, and bifurcation ridges, may predispose the periodontium to disease as a result of their potential to harbor bacterial plaque and present a challenge to the clinician during instrumentation. Similarly, the presence of subgingival and overhanging margins in restorations can result in increased plaque accumulation, increased inflammation, and increased bone loss. Although not clearly defined as risk factors for periodontitis, anatomic factors and *restorative factors* that influence plaque accumulation may play a role in disease susceptibility for specific teeth.[7]

The presence of *calculus,* which serves as a reservoir of bacterial plaque, has been suggested as a risk factor for periodontitis. Although the presence of some calculus in healthy individuals receiving routine dental care does not result in a significant loss of attachment, the presence of calculus in other groups of patients, such as those not receiving regular care and those with poorly controlled diabetes, can have a negative impact on periodontal health.[33]

Risk Determinants/Background Characteristics for Periodontal Disease

Genetic Factors

Evidence indicates that genetic differences between individuals may explain why some patients develop periodontal disease and others do not. Studies conducted in twins have shown that genetic factors influence clinical measures of gingivitis, probing pocket depth, attachment loss, and interproximal bone height.[29-31] The familial aggregation seen in localized and generalized aggressive periodontitis also indicates genetic involvement in these diseases (see Chapter 11).

Kornman and colleagues[23] demonstrated that alterations (*polymorphisms*) in specific genes encoding inflammatory cytokines such as interleukin-1α (IL-1α) and interleukin-1β (IL-1β) were associated with severe chronic periodontitis in nonsmoking subjects.[23] However, results of other studies have shown a limited association between these altered genes and the presence of periodontitis. Overall, it appears that changes in the IL-1 genes may be only one of several genetic changes involved in the risk for chronic periodontitis. Therefore, although alteration in the IL-1 genes may be a valid marker for periodontitis in defined populations, its usefulness as a genetic marker in the general population may be limited.[22]

Immunologic alterations, such as neutrophil abnormalities,[19] monocytic hyperresponsiveness to lipopolysaccharide stimulation in patients with localized aggressive periodontitis,[40] and alterations in the monocyte/macrophage receptors for the Fc portion of antibody,[22,50] also appear to be under genetic control. In addition, genetics plays a role in regulating the titer of the protective immunoglobulin G2 (IgG2) antibody response to *A. actinomycetemcomitans* in patients with aggressive periodontitis[16] (see Chapter 28).

Age

Both the prevalence and severity of periodontal disease increase with age.[8,10,35] It is possible that degenerative changes related to aging may increase susceptibility to periodontitis. However, it is also possible that the attachment loss and bone loss seen in older individuals are the result of prolonged exposure to other risk factors over a person's life, creating a cumulative effect over time. In support of this theory, studies have shown minimal loss of attachment in aging subjects enrolled in preventive programs throughout their lives.[36,37] Therefore it is suggested that periodontal disease is not an inevitable consequence of the aging process and that aging alone does not increase disease susceptibility. However, it remains to be determined whether changes related to the aging process, such as medication intake, decreased immune function, and altered nutritional status, interact with other well-defined risk factors to increase susceptibility to periodontitis.

Evidence of loss of attachment may have more consequences in younger patients. The younger the patient, the longer the time for exposure to causative factors. In addition, aggressive periodontitis in young individuals is often associated with unmodifiable risk factors, such as a genetic predisposition to disease.[10] Therefore young individuals with periodontal disease may be at greater risk for continued disease as they age.

Gender

Gender plays a role in periodontal disease.[2] Surveys conducted in the United States since 1960 demonstrate that men have more loss of attachment than women.[45,47,48] In addition, men have poorer oral hygiene than women, as evidenced by higher levels of plaque and calculus.[1,46,48] Therefore gender differences in the prevalence and severity of periodontitis appear to be related to preventive practices rather than any genetic factor.

Socioeconomic Status

Gingivitis and poor oral hygiene can be related to lower socioeconomic status (SES).[2,45,47] This most likely can be attributed to decreased dental awareness and decreased frequency of dental visits compared with more educated individuals with higher SES. After adjusting for other risk factors, such as smoking and poor oral hygiene, lower SES alone does not result in increased risk for periodontitis (see Chapter 6).

Stress

The incidence of necrotizing ulcerative gingivitis increases during periods of emotional and physiologic stress, suggesting a link between the two.[11,41] Emotional stress may interfere with normal immune function[6,43] and may result in increased levels of circulating hormones, which can affect the periodontium.[39] Stressful life events, such as bereavement and divorce, appear to lead to a greater prevalence of periodontal disease,[14] and an apparent association exists between psychosocial factors and risk behaviors such as smoking, poor oral hygiene, and chronic periodontitis.[9] Adult patients with periodontitis who are resistant to therapy are more stressed than those who respond to therapy.[5] Individuals with financial strain, distress, depression, or inadequate coping mechanisms have more severe loss of attachment.[13] Although epidemiologic data on the relationship between stress and periodontal disease are limited, stress may be a putative risk factor for periodontitis.[10]

CLINICAL CORRELATION

The ultimate goal of performing periodontal risk assessment is to develop a more personalized treatment plan for a specific patient, taking into account the periodontal risk profile of that patient. Once an at-risk patient is identified and a diagnosis is made, the treatment plan may be modified accordingly.

Conclusion

Risk assessment involves identifying elements that either may predispose patients to developing periodontal disease or may influence the progression of disease that already exists. In either case, these patients may require modification of their prognosis and treatment plan. In addition to an evaluation of the factors contributing to their risk, these patients should be educated concerning their risk, and, when appropriate, suitable intervention strategies should be implemented.

 A Case Scenario is found on the companion website www.expertconsult.com.

References

 References for this chapter are found on the companion website www.expertconsult.com.

CHAPTER 35

Determination of Prognosis

Jonathan H. Do | Henry H. Takei | Karen F. Novak

Definitions

A *prognosis* is a prediction of the probable course, duration, and outcome of a disease based on a general knowledge of the pathogenesis of the disease and the presence of risk factors for the disease. It is established after the diagnosis is made and before the treatment plan is established. The prognosis is based on specific information about the disease and the manner in which it can be treated, but it also can be influenced by the clinician's previous experience with treatment outcomes (successes and failures) as they relate to the particular case. It is important to note that determination of prognosis is a dynamic process. As such, the prognosis initially assigned should be reevaluated after completion of all phases of therapy, including periodontal maintenance.

Prognosis is often confused with the term *risk*. Risk generally deals with the likelihood that an individual will develop a disease in a specified period (see Chapter 7). *Risk factors* are characteristics that put an individual at increased risk for developing a disease (see Chapter 6). In contrast, *prognosis* is the prediction of the course or outcome of a disease. *Prognostic factors* are characteristics that predict the outcome once the disease is present. In some cases, risk factors and prognostic factors are the same. For example, patients with diabetes or patients who smoke are more at risk for acquiring periodontal disease, and once they have it, they generally have a worse prognosis.

Types of Prognosis

Although some factors may be more important than others when assigning a prognosis[34,35] (Box 35.1), it may benefit the clinician to consider each factor. Historically, prognosis classification schemes have been designed based on studies evaluating tooth mortality.[2,3,25,33,34] One scheme[25,34] assigns the following classifications:

Good prognosis: Control of etiologic factors and adequate periodontal support ensure the tooth will be easy to maintain by the patient and clinician.
Fair prognosis: Approximately 25% attachment loss or grade I furcation invasion (location and depth allow proper maintenance with good patient compliance).
Poor prognosis: 50% attachment loss, grade II furcation invasion (location and depth make maintenance possible but difficult).

Questionable prognosis: >50% attachment loss, poor crown-to-root ratio, poor root form, grade II furcation invasion (location and depth make access difficult) or grade III furcation invasion; mobility no. 2 or no. 3; root proximity.
Hopeless prognosis: Inadequate attachment to maintain health, comfort, and function.

It should be recognized that good, fair, and hopeless prognoses in this classification system can be established with a reasonable degree of accuracy. However, poor and questionable prognoses are likely to change to other categories because they depend on a large number of factors that can interact in an unpredictable number of ways.[8,14,47]

In contrast to schemes based on tooth mortality, Kwok and Caton[25] proposed a scheme based on "the probability of obtaining stability of the periodontal supporting apparatus." This scheme is based on the probability of disease progression as related to local and systemic factors (see Box 35.1). Although some of these factors may affect disease progression more than others, consideration of each factor is important in assigning a prognosis. This scheme is as follows:

Favorable prognosis: Comprehensive periodontal treatment and maintenance will stabilize the status of the tooth. Future loss of periodontal support is unlikely.
Questionable prognosis: Local or systemic factors influencing the periodontal status of the tooth may or may not be controllable. If controlled, the periodontal status can be stabilized with comprehensive periodontal treatment. If not, future periodontal breakdown may occur.
Unfavorable prognosis: Local or systemic factors influencing the periodontal status cannot be controlled. Comprehensive periodontal treatment and maintenance are unlikely to prevent future periodontal breakdown.
Hopeless prognosis: The tooth must be extracted.

Because periodontal stability is assessed on a regular basis using clinical measures, it may be more useful in making treatment decisions and prognosis predictions than in trying to determine the likelihood that the tooth will be lost.

In many of these cases, it may be advisable to establish a *provisional prognosis* until phase I therapy is completed and evaluated. The provisional prognosis allows the clinician to initiate treatment of teeth that have a doubtful outlook in the hope that a favorable

BOX 35.1   Factors to Consider When Determining a Prognosis

Overall Clinical Factors
Patient age
Disease severity
Biofilm control
Patient compliance

Systemic and Environmental Factors
Smoking
Systemic disease or condition
Genetic factors
Stress

Local Factors
Biofilm and calculus
Subgingival restorations

Anatomic Factors
Short, tapered roots
Cervical enamel projections
Enamel pearls
Bifurcation ridges
Root concavities
Developmental grooves
Root proximity
Furcation invasion
Tooth mobility
Caries
Tooth vitality
Root resorption

Prosthetic and Restorative Factors
Abutment selection

response may tip the balance and allow teeth to be retained. The reevaluation phase in the treatment sequence allows the clinician to examine the tissue response to scaling, oral hygiene, and root planing, as well as to the possible use of chemotherapeutic agents where indicated. The patient's compliance with the proposed treatment plan also can be determined.

LEARNING BOX 35.1

A prognosis based on whether periodontal stability can be achieved with periodontal therapy and maintenance is as follows: favorable—likely, questionable—maybe, unfavorable—unlikely.

Overall Versus Individual Tooth Prognosis

Prognosis can be divided into overall prognosis and individual tooth prognosis. The *overall prognosis* is concerned with the dentition as a whole. Factors that may influence the overall prognosis include patient age; current severity of disease; systemic factors; smoking; the presence of biofilm, calculus, and other local factors; patient compliance; and prosthetic possibilities (see Box 35.1). The overall prognosis answers the following questions:

- Should treatment be undertaken?
- Is treatment likely to succeed?
- When prosthetic replacements are needed, are the remaining teeth able to support the added burden of the prosthesis?

The *individual tooth prognosis* is determined after the overall prognosis and is affected by it.[33] For example, in a patient with a

poor overall prognosis, the dentist likely would not attempt to retain a tooth that has a questionable prognosis because of local conditions. Many of the factors listed under local factors and prosthetic and restorative factors in Box 35.1 have a direct effect on the prognosis for individual teeth, in addition to any overall systemic or environmental factors that may be present.

Factors in Determination of Prognosis

Overall Clinical Factors

Patient Age

For two patients with comparable levels of remaining connective tissue attachment and alveolar bone, the prognosis is generally better for the older of the two. For the younger patient, the prognosis is not as good because of the shorter time frame in which the periodontal destruction has occurred; the younger patient may have an aggressive type of periodontitis, or disease progression may have increased because of systemic disease or smoking. In addition, although the younger patient would ordinarily be expected to have a greater reparative capacity, the occurrence of so much destruction in a relatively short period would exceed any naturally occurring periodontal repair.

Disease Severity

Studies have demonstrated that a patient's history of previous periodontal disease may be indicative of their susceptibility to future periodontal breakdown (see Chapter 6). Therefore the following variables should be carefully recorded because they are important in determining the patient's past history of periodontal disease: probing pocket depth, level of attachment, amount of bone loss, and type of bony defect. These factors are determined by clinical and radiographic evaluation (see Chapters 32 and 33).

Determining clinical attachment loss reveals the approximate extent of root surface that is devoid of periodontal ligament; the radiographic examination shows the amount of root surface still invested in bone. Probing pocket depth is less important than level of attachment because it is not necessarily related to bone loss. In general, a tooth with deep probing depths and little attachment and bone loss has a better prognosis than one with shallow pockets and severe attachment and bone loss. However, a biofilm in deep pockets is difficult to control and may contribute to disease progression.

Prognosis is adversely affected if the base of the pocket (level of attachment) is close to the root apex. The presence of apical disease as a result of endodontic involvement also worsens the prognosis. However, surprisingly good apical and lateral bone repair can sometimes be obtained by combining endodontic and periodontal therapy (see Chapter 46).

The prognosis also can be related to the height of remaining bone. Assuming bone destruction can be arrested, is there enough bone remaining to support the teeth? The answer is readily apparent in extreme cases—that is, when there is so little bone loss that tooth support is not in jeopardy (Fig. 35.1) or when bone loss is so severe that the remaining bone is obviously insufficient for proper tooth support (Fig. 35.2). Most patients, however, do not fit into these extreme categories. The height of remaining bone is usually somewhere in between, making bone level assessment alone insufficient for determining the overall prognosis.

The type of defect also must be determined. The prognosis for horizontal bone loss depends on the height of the existing bone because it is unlikely that clinically significant bone height regeneration will be induced by therapy. In the case of angular,

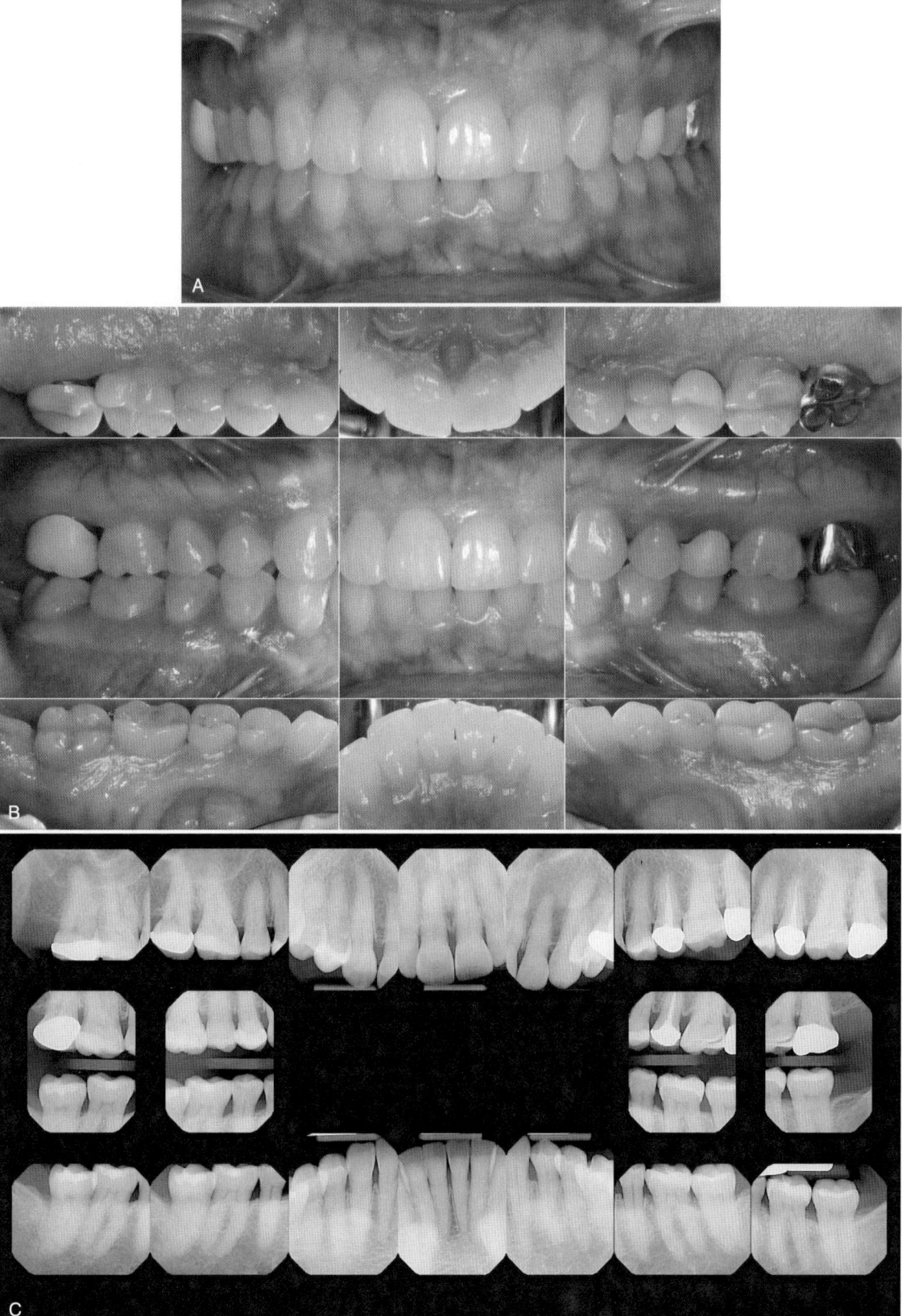

Fig. 35.1 Generalized mild chronic periodontitis in a healthy, nonsmoking 67-year-old female. Minimal clinical biofilm and gingival inflammation (A and B) and radiographic bone loss (C). Overall prognosis is favorable. *(Copyright Jonathan H. Do, DDS. All rights reserved.)*

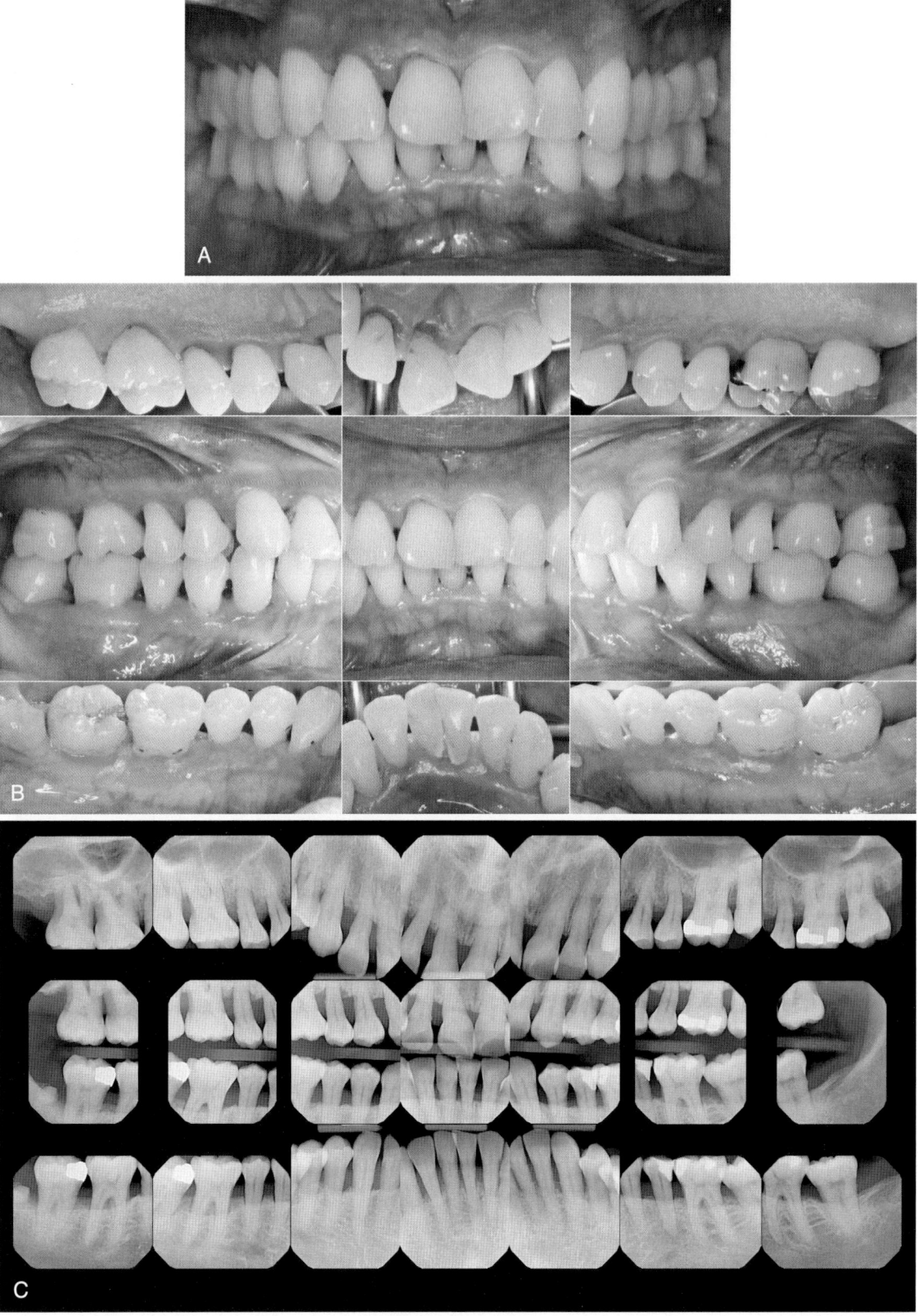

Fig. 35.2 Generalized moderate-to-severe chronic periodontitis in a healthy, nonsmoking 49-year-old female. (A and B) Moderate clinical biofilm, calculus, and gingival inflammation. (C) Moderate to severe radiographic bone loss. Overall prognosis is questionable/unfavorable. *(Copyright Jonathan H. Do, DDS. All rights reserved.)*

intrabony defects, if the contour of the existing bone and the number of osseous walls are favorable, there is an excellent chance that therapy could regenerate bone to approximately the level of the alveolar crest.[45]

When greater bone loss has occurred on one surface of a tooth, the bone height on the less involved surfaces should be taken into consideration when determining the prognosis. Because of the greater height of bone in relation to other surfaces, the center of rotation of the tooth will be nearer the crown (Fig. 35.3). This results in a more

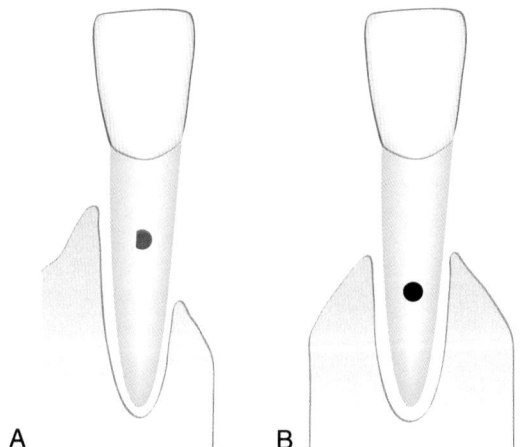

A   B

Fig. 35.3 Prognosis for tooth A is better than for tooth B, despite less bone on one of the surfaces of A. Because the center of rotation of tooth A is closer to the crown, the distribution of occlusal forces to the periodontium is more favorable than in B.

favorable distribution of forces to the periodontium and less tooth mobility.[49]

In dealing with a tooth that has a questionable prognosis, the chances of successful treatment should be weighed against any benefits that would accrue to the adjacent teeth if the tooth under consideration were extracted. Strategic extraction of teeth was first proposed as a means of improving the overall prognosis of adjacent teeth or enhancing the prosthetic treatment plan.[9] It has now been expanded to include the extraction of teeth with a questionable prognosis to enhance the likelihood of partial restoration of the bone supporting of the adjacent teeth (Fig. 35.4A–D) or successful implant placement. With the growing evidence of the long-term success of dental implants, it is proposed that a "watch and wait" approach may allow an area to deteriorate to the point that placing an implant is no longer a viable option. This means that the practitioner should weigh the potential success of one treatment option (extraction and implant placement) versus the other (periodontal therapy and maintenance) carefully when assigning a questionable prognosis to teeth.[20]

Biofilm Control

Bacterial biofilm is the primary etiologic factor associated with periodontal disease (see Chapter 8). Therefore effective removal of

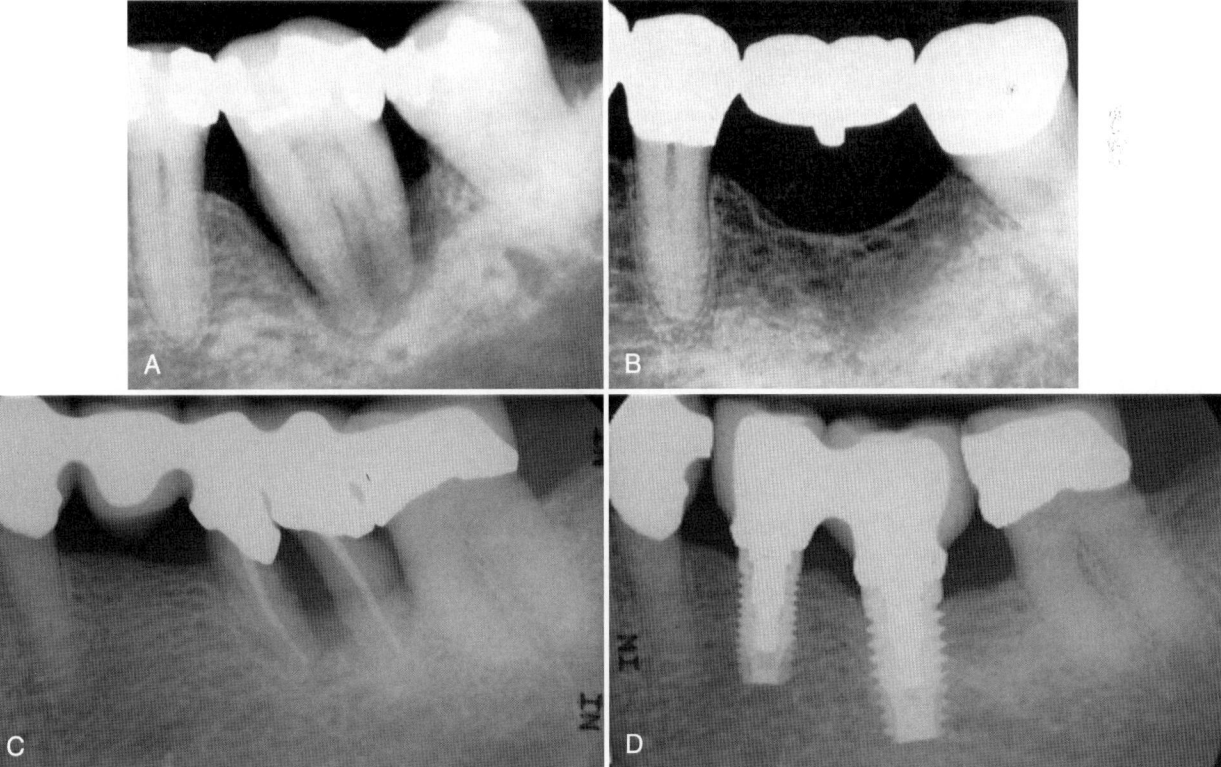

Fig. 35.4 Extraction of severely involved tooth to preserve bone on adjacent teeth. (A) Extensive bone destruction around the mandibular first molar. (B) Radiograph made years after extraction of the first molar and replacement by a prosthesis. Note the excellent bone support. (C) Extraction of periodontally involved bicuspid and molar. (D) Implant replacement of both teeth. *(Courtesy Dr. S. Angha, University of California, Los Angeles.)*

biofilm on a daily basis by the patient is critical to the success of periodontal therapy and the prognosis.

Patient Compliance and Cooperation

The prognosis for patients with gingival and periodontal disease is critically dependent on the patient's attitude, desire to retain the natural teeth, and willingness and ability to effectively control biofilm. Without these, treatment cannot succeed. Patients should be educated on the etiology and prevention of dental caries and periodontal diseases, and they should be clearly informed of the important role they must play for treatment to succeed. If a patient is unwilling to perform adequate biofilm control and receive the timely periodic maintenance checkups and treatments that the dentist deems necessary, the dentist can refuse to accept the patient for treatment. The dentist should make it clear to the patient and in the patient record that further treatment is needed but will not be performed because of a lack of patient cooperation.

Systemic and Environmental Factors

Smoking

Epidemiologic evidence suggests that smoking may be the most important environmental risk factor impacting the development and progression of periodontal disease (see Chapter 12). Therefore it should be made clear to patients that a direct relationship exists between smoking and the prevalence and incidence of periodontitis. In addition, patients should be informed that smoking affects not only the severity of periodontal destruction but also the healing potential of the periodontal tissues. As a result, patients who smoke do not respond as well to conventional periodontal therapy as patients who have never smoked.[43,44] Therefore the prognosis in patients who smoke and have slight to moderate chronic periodontitis is generally questionable. In patients with severe chronic periodontitis, the prognosis may be unfavorable or hopeless.

However, it should be emphasized that smoking cessation can affect the treatment outcome and therefore the prognosis.[5,17] As such, for patients who stop smoking, the prognosis can improve to favorable in those with slight to moderate chronic periodontitis and to questionable in those with severe chronic periodontitis.

Systemic Disease or Condition

The patient's systemic background affects the overall prognosis in several ways. For example, evidence from epidemiologic studies clearly demonstrates that the prevalence and severity of chronic periodontitis are significantly higher in patients with poorly controlled diabetes than in those whose diabetes is well controlled or those who do not have diabetes (see Chapter 6). Therefore patients at risk for diabetes should be identified as early as possible and informed of the relationship between periodontitis and diabetes. Similarly, patients diagnosed with diabetes must be informed of the impact of diabetic control on the development and progression of periodontitis. It follows that the prognosis in these cases depends on patient compliance relative to both medical and dental status. Patients with well-controlled diabetes and slight to moderate periodontitis who comply with their recommended periodontal treatment should have a favorable prognosis. Similarly, in patients with other systemic disorders that could affect disease progression, prognosis improves with correction of the systemic problem.

The prognosis is questionable when surgical periodontal treatment is required but cannot be provided because of the patient's health (see Chapter 39). Incapacitating conditions that limit the patient's performance of oral procedures (e.g., Parkinson disease) also adversely affect the prognosis. Newer "automated" oral hygiene devices, such as electric toothbrushes, may be helpful for these patients and may improve their prognosis (see Chapter 48).

Genetic Factors

Periodontal diseases represent a complex interaction between a microbial challenge and the host's response to that challenge, both of which may be influenced by environmental factors such as smoking. In addition to these external factors, evidence also indicates that genetic factors may play an important role in determining the nature of the host response.[18] Evidence for this type of genetic influence exists for patients with both chronic and aggressive periodontitis. Genetic polymorphisms in the interleukin-1 (IL-1) genes, resulting in increased production of IL-1β, have been associated with a significant increase in risk for severe, generalized, and chronic periodontitis.[24,37] It has been demonstrated that knowledge of the patient's IL-1 genotype and smoking status can aid the clinician in assigning a prognosis.[36] Genetic factors also appear to influence serum immunoglobulin G2 (IgG2) antibody titers and the expression of FcγRII receptors on neutrophils, both of which may be significant in aggressive periodontitis.[18] Other genetic disorders, such as leukocyte adhesion deficiency type 1, can influence neutrophil function, creating an additional risk factor for aggressive periodontitis.[18] Finally, the familial aggregation that is characteristic of aggressive periodontitis indicates that additional, as yet unidentified, genetic factors may be important in one's susceptibility to this form of disease (see Chapter 28).

The influence of genetic factors on prognosis is not simple. Although microbial and environmental factors can be altered through conventional periodontal therapy and patient education, genetic factors currently cannot be altered. However, detection of genetic variations linked to periodontal disease can potentially influence the prognosis in several ways. First, early detection of patients at risk because of genetic factors can lead to early implementation of preventive and treatment measures for these patients. Second, identification of genetic risk factors later in the disease or during the course of treatment can influence treatment recommendations, such as the use of adjunctive antibiotic therapy or increased frequency of maintenance visits. Third, identification of young individuals who have not been evaluated for periodontitis but who are recognized as being at risk because of the familial aggregation seen in aggressive periodontitis can lead to the development of early intervention strategies. In each of these cases, early diagnosis, intervention, and alterations in the treatment regimen may lead to an improved prognosis for the patient.

Stress

Physical and emotional stress, as well as substance abuse, may alter the patient's ability to respond to the periodontal treatment performed (see Chapter 6). These factors must be realistically faced when attempting to establish a prognosis.

Local Factors

Biofilm and Calculus

The microbial challenge presented by bacterial biofilm and calculus is the most important local factor in periodontal diseases. Therefore in most cases, having a favorable prognosis depends on the ability of the patient and the clinician to remove these etiologic factors (see Chapters 8 and 13).

LEARNING BOX 35.3

Periodontal prognosis depends on the ability of the patient and clinician to effectively remove bacterial biofilm and resolve inflammation.

Subgingival Restorations

Subgingival margins may contribute to increased biofilm accumulation, increased inflammation, and increased bone loss[4,40,48] when compared with supragingival margins. Furthermore, discrepancies in these margins (e.g., overhangs) can negatively impact the periodontium (see Chapter 13). The size of these discrepancies and duration of their presence are important factors in the amount of destruction that occurs. In general, however, a tooth with a discrepancy in its subgingival margins has a worse prognosis than a tooth with well-contoured supragingival margins.

Anatomic Factors

Anatomic factors that may predispose the periodontium to disease and therefore affect the prognosis include short, tapered roots with large crowns, cervical enamel projections and enamel pearls, intermediate bifurcation ridges, root concavities, and developmental grooves. The clinician must also consider root proximity and the location and anatomy of furcations when assigning a prognosis.

Prognosis is less favorable for teeth with short, tapered roots and relatively large crowns (Fig. 35.5). Because of the disproportionate crown-to-root ratio and the reduced root surface available for periodontal support,[21] the periodontium may be more susceptible to injury by occlusal forces.

Cervical enamel projections (CEPs) are flat, ectopic extensions of enamel that extend beyond the normal contours of the cementoenamel junction.[32] CEPs extend into the furcation of 28.6% of mandibular molars and 17% of maxillary molars.[32] CEPs are most likely to be found on buccal surfaces of maxillary second molars.[16,50] Enamel pearls are larger, round deposits of enamel that can be located in furcations or other areas on the root surface.[39] Enamel pearls are seen less frequently (1.1% to 5.7% of permanent molars; 75% appearing in maxillary third molars[39]) than CEPs. An intermediate bifurcation ridge has been described in 73% of mandibular first molars, crossing from the mesial to the distal root at the midpoint of the furcation.[10] The presence of these enamel projections on the root surface interferes with the attachment apparatus and may prevent regenerative procedures from achieving their maximum potential. Therefore their presence may have a negative effect on the prognosis for an individual tooth.

Scaling with root planing is a fundamental procedure in periodontal therapy. Anatomic factors that decrease the efficiency of this procedure can have a negative impact on the prognosis. Therefore the morphology of the tooth root is an important consideration when discussing prognosis. Root concavities exposed through loss of attachment can vary from shallow flutings to deep depressions. They appear more marked on maxillary first premolars, the mesiobuccal root of the maxillary first molar, both roots of mandibular first molars, and the mandibular incisors[6,7] (Figs. 35.6 and 35.7). Any tooth, however, can have a proximal concavity.[13] Although these concavities increase the attachment area and produce a root shape that may be more resistant to torquing forces, they also create areas that can be difficult for both the dentist and the patient to clean.

Other anatomic considerations that present accessibility problems are developmental grooves, root proximity, and furcation involvement. The presence of any of these can worsen the prognosis. Developmental grooves, which sometimes appear in the maxillary lateral incisors (palatogingival groove[51]; Fig. 35.8) or in the lower incisors, create an accessibility problem.[11,15] They initiate on enamel and can extend a significant distance on the root surface, providing a plaque-retentive area that is difficult to instrument. These palatogingival grooves are found on 5.6% of maxillary lateral incisors and 3.4% of maxillary

central incisors.[23] Similarly, root proximity can result in interproximal areas that are difficult for the clinician and patient to access. Finally, access to the furcation area is usually difficult to obtain. In 58% of maxillary and mandibular first molars, the furcation entrance diameter is narrower than the width of conventional periodontal curettes[7] (Fig. 35.9). Maxillary first premolars present the greatest difficulty, and therefore their prognosis is usually unfavorable when the lesion reaches the mesiodistal furcation. Maxillary molars also present some difficulty; sometimes their prognosis can be improved by resecting one of the buccal roots (see Chapter 64), thereby improving access to the area. When mandibular first molars or buccal furcations of maxillary molars offer good access to the furcation area, the prognosis is usually better.

Tooth Mobility

The principal causes of tooth mobility are loss of alveolar bone, inflammatory changes in the periodontium, and trauma from occlusion. Tooth mobility caused by inflammation and trauma from occlusion may be correctable.[38] However, tooth mobility resulting from loss of alveolar bone is not likely to be corrected. The likelihood of restoring tooth stability is inversely proportional to the extent to which mobility is caused by the loss of supporting alveolar bone. A longitudinal study of the response to treatment of teeth with different degrees of mobility revealed that pockets on clinically mobile teeth do not respond as well to periodontal therapy as pockets on nonmobile teeth exhibiting the same initial disease severity.[12] Another study, however, in which ideal plaque control was attained, found similar healing in both hypermobile and firm teeth.[45] The stabilization of tooth mobility through the use of splinting may have a beneficial impact on the overall and individual tooth prognosis.

Caries, Tooth Vitality, and Root Resorption

For teeth mutilated by extensive caries, the feasibility of adequate restoration and endodontic therapy should be considered before undertaking periodontal treatment. Extensive idiopathic root resorption or root resorption resulting from orthodontic therapy jeopardizes the stability of teeth and adversely affects the response to periodontal treatment. The periodontal prognosis of treated nonvital teeth does not differ from that of vital teeth. New attachment can occur to the cementum of both nonvital and vital teeth.

Prosthetic and Restorative Factors

The overall prognosis requires a general consideration of bone levels (evaluated radiographically) and attachment levels (determined clinically) to establish whether enough teeth can be saved either to provide functional and aesthetic dentition or to serve as abutments for a useful prosthetic replacement of the missing teeth.

At this point, the overall prognosis and individual tooth prognosis overlap because the prognosis for key individual teeth may affect the overall prognosis for prosthetic rehabilitation. For example, saving or losing a key tooth may determine whether other teeth are saved or extracted or whether the prosthesis is fixed or removable (see Fig. 35.4). When few teeth remain, the prosthodontic needs become more important, and sometimes periodontally treatable teeth may

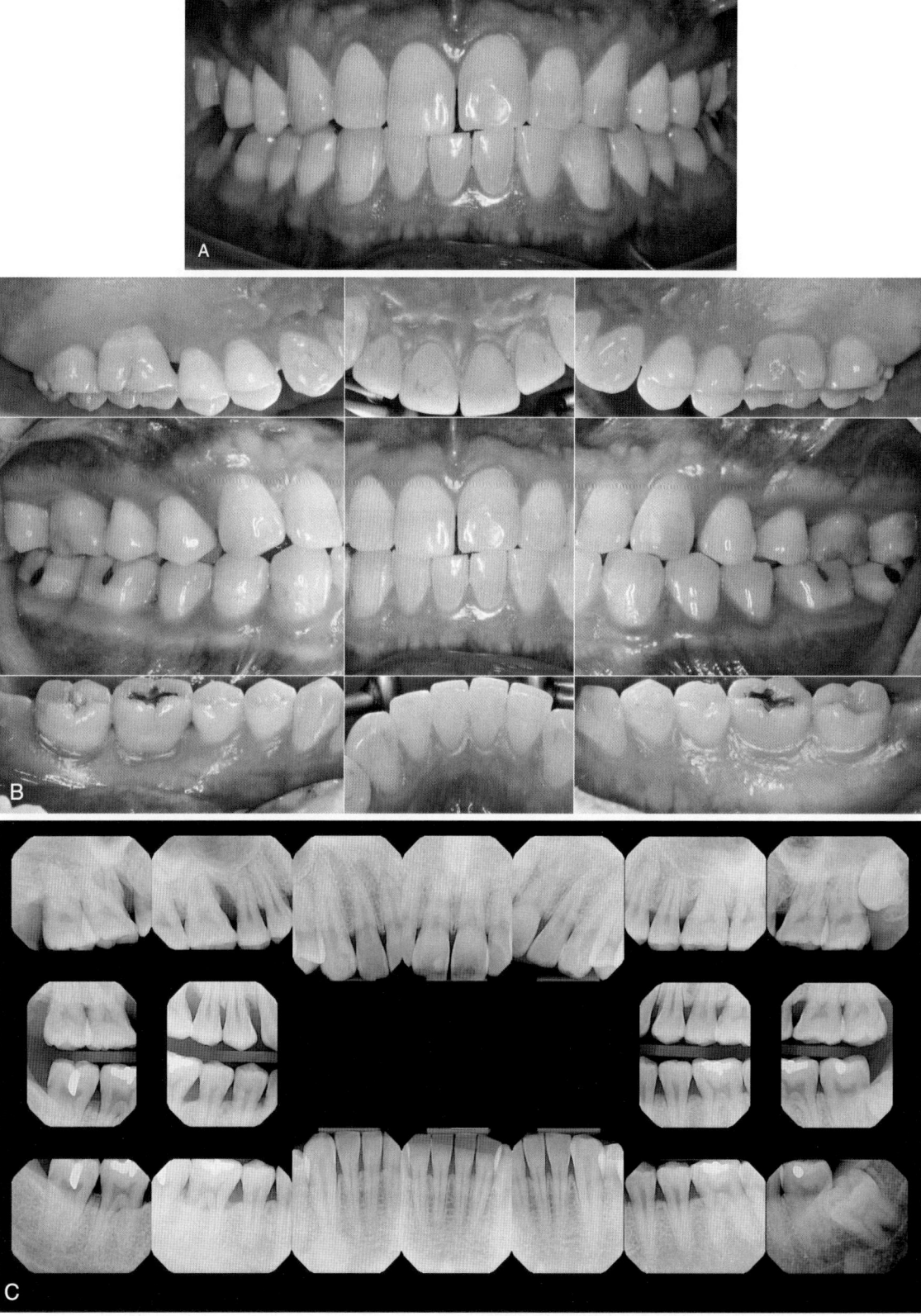

Fig. 35.5 Localized moderate-to-severe chronic periodontitis in a healthy, nonsmoking 32-year-old male. (A and B) Mild clinical biofilm and gingival inflammation. Localized moderate-to-severe radiographic bone loss and localized heavy subgingical calculus. (C) This patient likely had localized aggressive periodontitis that became chronic periodontitis as he aged. Overall prognosis is favorable; questionable for the maxillary right first molar. *(Copyright Jonathan H. Do, DDS. All rights reserved.)*

have to be extracted if they are not compatible with the design of the prosthesis.

Teeth that serve as abutments are subjected to increased functional demands. More rigid standards are required when evaluating the prognosis of teeth adjacent to edentulous areas. A tooth with a post that has undergone endodontic treatment is more likely to fracture when serving as a distal abutment supporting a distal removable partial denture. Additionally, special oral hygiene measures must be instituted in these areas.

Prognosis of Specific Periodontal Diseases

Many of the criteria used in the diagnosis and classification of the different forms of periodontal disease[1] (see Chapter 5) are also used in developing a prognosis (see Box 35.1). Factors such as patient age, severity of disease, genetic susceptibility, and presence of systemic disease are important criteria in the diagnosis of the condition and in developing a prognosis. These common

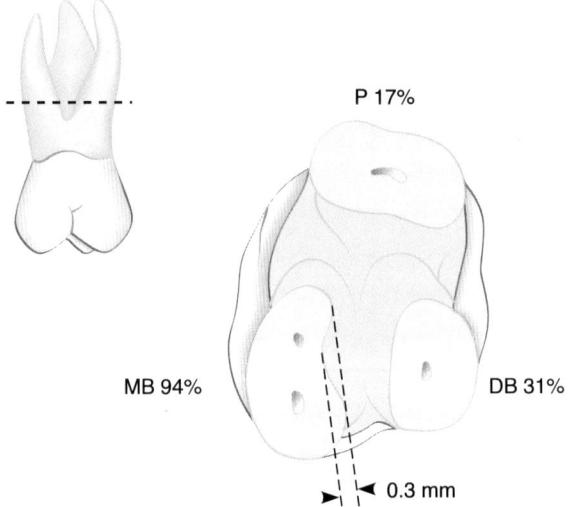

Fig. 35.6 Root concavities in maxillary first molars sectioned 2 mm apical to the furca. The furcal aspect of the root is concave in 94% of the mesiobuccal (MB) roots, 31% of the distobuccal (DB) roots, and 17% of the palatal (P) roots. The deepest concavity is found in the furcal aspects of the mesiobuccal roots (mean concavity, 0.3 mm). The furcal aspect of the buccal roots diverges toward the palate in 97% of teeth (mean divergence, 22 degrees). *(Redrawn from Bower RC: Furcation morphology relative to periodontal treatment–furcation root surface anatomy. J Periodontol 50:366, 1979.)*

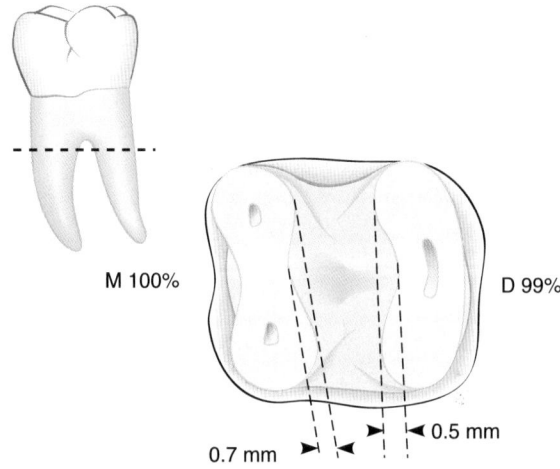

Fig. 35.7 Root concavities in mandibular first molars sectioned 2 mm apical to the furca. Concavity of the furcal aspect was found in 100% of mesial (M) roots and 99% of distal (D) roots. Deeper concavity was found in the mesial roots (mean concavity, 0.7 mm). *(Redrawn from Bower RC: Furcation morphology relative to periodontal treatment–furcation root surface anatomy. J Periodontol 50:366, 1979.)*

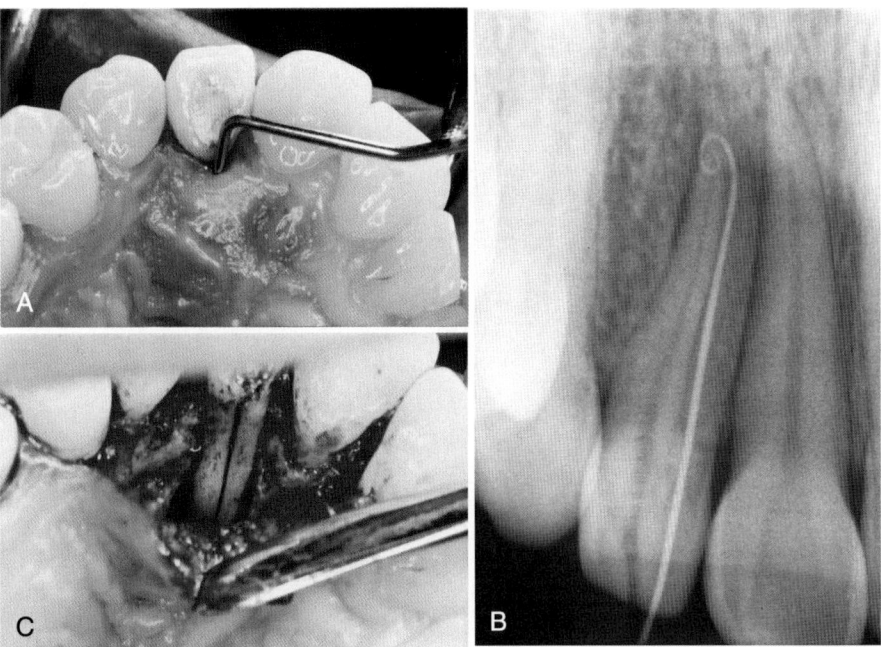

Fig. 35.8 Palatogingival groove. (A) Probe in place to indicate a deep pocket along the palatogingival groove. (B) Radiograph with a gutta-percha point placed in the pocket. (C) The area is surgically opened. Note the palatogingival groove along the entire palatal portion of the root. *(Courtesy Dr. Nadia Chugal, University of California, Los Angeles.)*

factors suggest that for any given diagnosis, there should be an expected prognosis under ideal conditions. This section discusses potential prognoses for the various periodontal diseases outlined in Chapter 5.

Prognosis for Patients With Gingival Disease
Biofilm-Induced Gingival Diseases
Gingivitis Associated With Dental Plaque Only

Biofilm-induced gingivitis is a reversible disease that occurs when bacterial biofilm accumulates at the gingival margin.[29,31] This disease

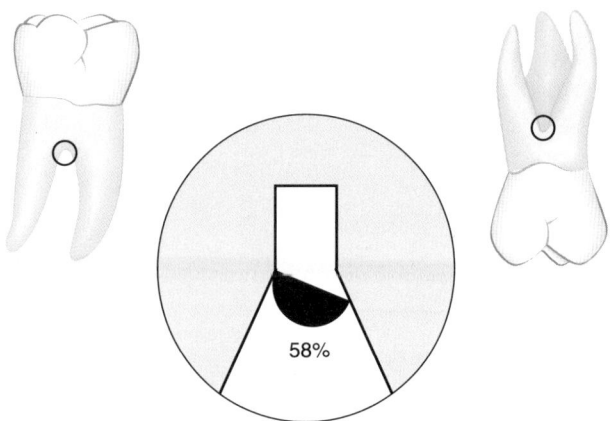

Fig. 35.9 The furcation entrance is narrower than a standard curette in 58% of first molars. *(Redrawn from Bower RC: Furcation morphology relative to periodontal treatment–furcation root surface anatomy. J Periodontol 50:366, 1979.)*

can occur on a periodontium that has experienced no attachment loss or on a periodontium with nonprogressing attachment loss. In either case, the prognosis is good for patients with gingivitis associated with bacterial biofilm only favorable, provided that all local irritants are eliminated, other local factors contributing to biofilm retention are eliminated, gingival contours conducive to the preservation of health are attained, and the patient cooperates by maintaining good oral hygiene.

Biofilm-Induced Gingival Diseases Modified by Systemic Factors

The inflammatory response to bacterial biofilm at the gingival margin can be influenced by systemic factors, such as endocrine-related changes associated with puberty, menstruation, pregnancy, and diabetes, and the presence of blood dyscrasias. In many cases, the frank signs of gingival inflammation that occur in these patients are seen in the presence of relatively small amounts of bacterial biofilm. Therefore the long-term prognosis for these patients depends not only on control of bacterial biofilm but also on control or correction of the systemic factors.

Biofilm-Induced Gingival Diseases Modified by Medications

Gingival diseases associated with medications include drug-influenced *gingival enlargement,* often seen with phenytoin, cyclosporine, and nifedipine and in oral contraceptive–associated gingivitis.

In drug-influenced gingival enlargement, the severity of the lesions is associated with inflammation, which is usually induced by bacterial biofilm. Inflammation may also be induced by repeated trauma (Fig. 35.10). Eliminating the source of inflammation, either trauma or biofilm, can limit the severity of the gingival overgrowth. However,

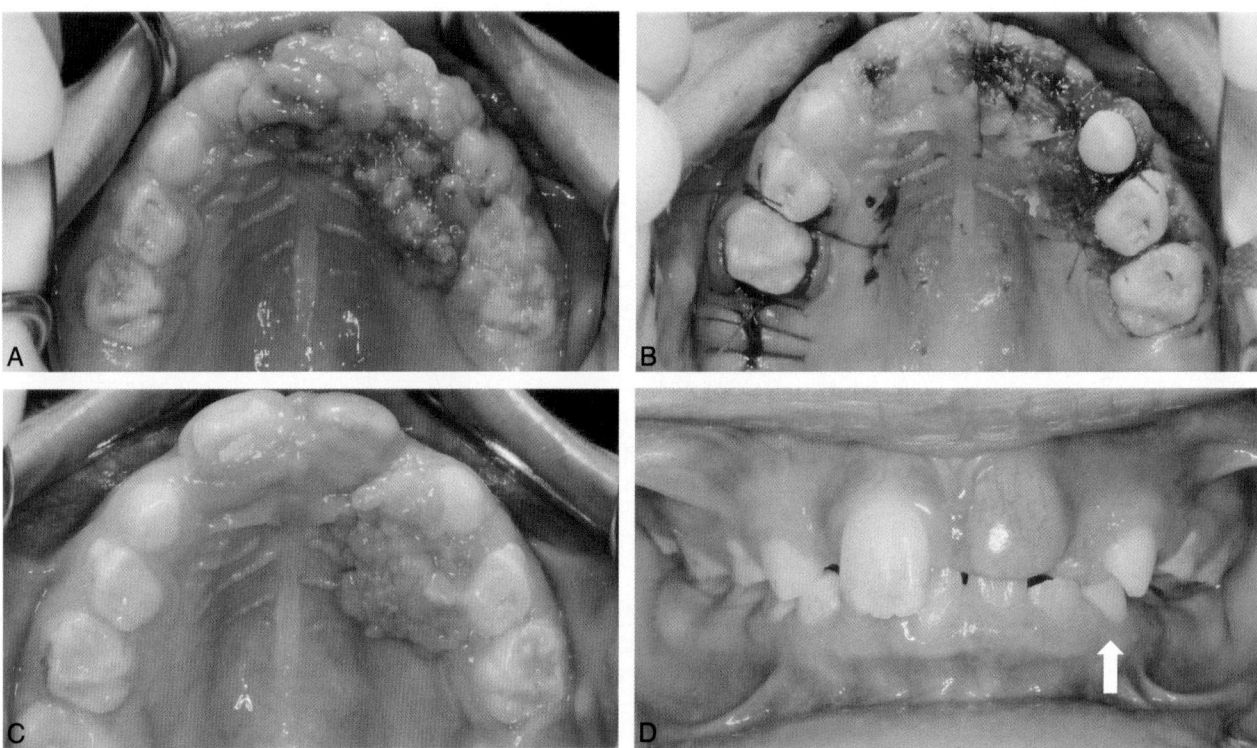

Fig. 35.10 (A) Gingival overgrowth in a 5-year-old male patient who was taking cyclosporine for the management of aplastic anemia. (B) The gingival overgrowth was resected surgically. (C) Recurrence of gingival overgrowth on the maxillary left quadrant at 1 year postop due to trauma from the opposing mandibular teeth occluding on the maxillary left palatal tissue (D). *(Copyright Jonathan H. Do, DDS. All rights reserved.)*

surgical intervention is usually necessary to correct the alterations in gingival contour. Continued use of the drug and persistence of inflammation usually result in recurrence of the enlargement, even after surgical intervention (see Chapter 19). Therefore the long-term prognosis depends on whether the etiology of the inflammation can be completely eliminated or the patient's systemic problem can be treated with an alternative medication that does not have gingival enlargement as a side effect.

In oral contraceptive–associated gingivitis, frank signs of gingival inflammation can be seen in the presence of relatively little biofilm. Therefore, as seen in biofilm-induced gingival diseases modified by systemic factors, the long-term prognosis in these patients depends not only on the control of bacterial biofilm but also on the likelihood of continued use of oral contraceptives.

Gingival Diseases Modified by Malnutrition

Although malnutrition has been suspected to play a role in the development of gingival diseases, most clinical studies have not shown a relationship between the two. One possible exception is severe vitamin C deficiency. In early experimental vitamin C deficiency, gingival inflammation and bleeding on probing were independent of the biofilm levels present. The prognosis in these patients may depend on the severity and duration of the deficiency and on the likelihood of reversing the deficiency through dietary supplementation.

Non–Biofilm-Induced Gingival Lesions

Non–biofilm-induced gingivitis can be seen in patients with a variety of bacterial, fungal, and viral infections.[19] Because the gingivitis in these patients is not usually attributed to biofilm accumulation, prognosis depends on elimination of the source of the infectious agent. Dermatologic disorders such as lichen planus, pemphigoid, pemphigus vulgaris, erythema multiforme, and lupus erythematosus also can manifest in the oral cavity as atypical gingivitis (see Chapter 22). Prognosis for these patients is linked to management of the associated dermatologic disorder. Finally, allergic, toxic, and foreign-body reactions, as well as mechanical and thermal trauma, can result in gingival lesions. Prognosis for these patients depends on the elimination of the causative agent.

Prognosis for Patients With Periodontitis
Chronic Periodontitis

Chronic periodontitis is a slowly progressive disease associated with well-known local environmental factors.[27] It can present in a localized or generalized form (see Chapter 27). In cases in which the clinical attachment loss and bone loss are not advanced (slight to moderate periodontitis), the prognosis is generally favorable, provided the inflammation can be controlled through good oral hygiene and the removal of local biofilm-retentive factors (see Fig. 35.1). In patients with more severe disease, as evidenced by furcation invasion and tooth mobility, or in patients who are noncompliant with oral hygiene practices, the prognosis may be questionable or unfavorable, and even hopeless.

Aggressive Periodontitis

Aggressive periodontitis can present in a localized or generalized form.[26] Two common features of both forms are (1) rapid attachment

loss and bone destruction in an otherwise clinically healthy patient and (2) a familial aggregation. These patients often present with limited microbial deposits that seem inconsistent with the severity of tissue destruction. However, the deposits that are present often have elevated levels of *Aggregatibacter actinomycetemcomitans* or *Porphyromonas gingivalis*. These patients also may present with phagocyte abnormalities and a hyperresponsive monocyte/macrophage phenotype. These clinical, microbiologic, and immunologic features would suggest that patients diagnosed with aggressive periodontitis would have an unfavorable prognosis.

However, the clinician should consider additional specific features of the localized form of disease when determining the prognosis (see Fig. 35.5). Localized aggressive periodontitis usually occurs around the age of puberty and is localized to first molars and incisors. The patient often exhibits a strong serum antibody response to the infecting agents, which may contribute to localization of the lesions (see Chapter 28). When diagnosed early, these cases can be treated conservatively with oral hygiene instruction and systemic antibiotic therapy,[42] resulting in a favorable prognosis. When more advanced disease occurs, the prognosis can still be favorable if the lesions are treated with debridement, local and systemic antibiotics, and regenerative therapy.[30,52]

In contrast, although patients with generalized aggressive periodontitis are young (usually under age 30), they present with generalized interproximal attachment loss and a poor antibody response to infecting agents. Secondary contributing factors, such as cigarette smoking, are often present. These factors, coupled with the alterations in host defense seen in many of these patients, may result in a case that does not respond well to conventional periodontal therapy (scaling with root planing, oral hygiene instruction, and surgical intervention). Therefore these patients often have a questionable or unfavorable prognosis, and the use of systemic antibiotics should be considered to help control the disease (see Chapter 52).

Periodontitis as a Manifestation of Systemic Diseases

Periodontitis as a manifestation of systemic diseases can be divided into the following two categories[22,28]:

1. Periodontitis associated with hematologic disorders such as leukemia and acquired neutropenias
2. Periodontitis associated with genetic disorders such as familial and cyclic neutropenia, Down syndrome, Papillon-Lefèvre syndrome, and hypophosphatasia

Although the primary etiologic factor in periodontal diseases is bacterial plaque, systemic diseases that alter the ability of the host to respond to the microbial challenge may affect the progression of disease and therefore the prognosis for the case. For example, decreased numbers of circulating neutrophils (as in acquired neutropenia) may contribute to widespread destruction of the periodontium. Unless the neutropenia can be corrected, these patients present with a fair to poor prognosis. Similarly, genetic disorders that alter the way the host responds to bacterial plaque (as in leukocyte adhesion deficiency [LAD] syndrome) also can contribute to the development of periodontitis. Because these disorders generally manifest early in life, the impact on the periodontium may be clinically similar to generalized aggressive periodontitis. The prognosis in these cases will be questionable or unfavorable.

Other genetic disorders do not affect the host's ability to combat infections but still affect the development of periodontitis. Examples include (1) hypophosphatasia, in which patients have decreased levels of circulating alkaline phosphatase, severe alveolar bone loss, and premature loss of deciduous and permanent teeth, and (2) Ehlers-Danlos syndrome, a connective tissue disorder, in which patients may present with clinical characteristics of aggressive periodontitis. In both examples the prognosis is questionable or unfavorable.

Necrotizing Periodontal Disease

Necrotizing periodontal disease can be divided into necrotic diseases that affect the gingival tissues exclusively (necrotizing ulcerative gingivitis [NUG]) and necrotic diseases that affect deeper tissues of the periodontium, resulting in a loss of connective tissue attachment and alveolar bone (necrotizing ulcerative periodontitis [NUP]).[41,46] In NUG, the primary predisposing factor is bacterial plaque. However, this disease is usually complicated by the presence of secondary factors such as acute psychologic stress, tobacco smoking, and poor nutrition, all of which can contribute to immunosuppression. Therefore superimposition of these secondary factors on preexisting gingivitis can result in the painful, necrotic lesions characteristic of NUG. With control of both the bacterial plaque and the secondary factors, the prognosis for a patient with NUG is favorable. However, the tissue destruction in these cases is not reversible, and poor control of the secondary factors may make these patients susceptible to recurrence of the disease. With repeated episodes of NUG, the prognosis may worsen to questionable.

The clinical presentation of NUP is similar to that of NUG, except the necrosis extends from the gingiva into the periodontal ligament and alveolar bone. In systemically healthy patients, this progression may have resulted from multiple episodes of NUG, or the necrotizing disease may occur at a site previously affected with periodontitis. In these patients, the prognosis depends on alleviating the biofilm and secondary factors associated with NUG. However, many patients presenting with NUP are immunocompromised by systemic conditions such as human immunodeficiency virus (HIV) infection. In these patients the prognosis depends not only on reducing local and secondary factors but also on dealing with the systemic problem (see Chapter 43).

Determination and Reassessment of Prognosis

Determination of prognosis of a tooth or teeth requires a careful and thorough assessment of the presence of disease and its severity and extent. An accurate prognosis cannot be made without an accurate diagnosis. Once disease has been properly and accurately diagnosed, determining the prognosis can still be difficult, particularly for teeth with disease. Many factors can influence disease progression and the response to therapy, and the specific influence of any one factor is unknown and likely different from one patient to another. In addition, each patient can respond differently at different times. Moreover, the outcome of therapy significantly depends on the treatment to be rendered, the quality of the treatment, the skills and knowledge of the treating clinician, and patient home care. For these reasons, determining an accurate prognosis can be challenging.

Prognosis of teeth with minimal disease is favorable and by far the easiest to assign with accuracy and precision. As disease develops and severity increases, prognosis becomes progressively harder to assign correctly and accurately, especially for teeth with moderate to advanced disease that have a questionable or unfavorable prognosis. Once disease progresses to a point that teeth are no longer functional or treatable, the prognosis is again easy to determine. These teeth are assigned a hopeless prognosis and the treatment is extraction. However, the treatability of a tooth can be easily skewed by the skills and expertise of the treating clinician, or lack thereof. It is also easier for a clinician

to make a diagnosis, determine a prognosis, and create a treatment plan that aligns with his or her expertise. For example, a prosthodontist may assign mandibular incisors with moderate attachment loss and mobility no. 2 a hopeless prognosis and develop a treatment plan that involves replacement of these teeth with a removable partial denture or dental implants. However, with the proper periodontal treatment and effective patient biofilm control, the health and function of these mandibular anterior teeth may be restored and maintained for many years.

It is not always possible to accurately determine the prognosis prior to initiating periodontal treatment. During the periodontal examination, due to the lack of anesthesia, it may not be possible to accurately and carefully probe a tooth to determine the true extent of bone loss and severity of disease. During scaling and root planing under anesthesia, it is possible to probe to the depth of the periodontal pocket. However, the anatomy of the osseous defect may not be determined until a periodontal flap has been elevated and all the granulation tissue removed. As such, the prognosis may change as more specific diagnostic information is discovered.

Prognosis may also change and improve with periodontal treatment or disease progression. During therapy, the patient's motivation and commitment, acknowledged as critical in all forms of periodontal therapy, can be determined, as well as the host response and the healing capacity of the patient. Clearly, enhancing the host response to a microbial biofilm challenge will significantly and positively influence the periodontal prognosis. Likewise, an *inability* to enhance the host response will negatively influence the prognosis. Either outcome, however, will allow the clinician to determine a more accurate prognosis.

A frank reduction in probing depth and inflammation after therapy indicates a favorable response to treatment and may suggest a better prognosis than previously assumed (Fig. 35.11). If the inflammatory changes cannot be controlled or reduced by therapy, the overall prognosis may be unfavorable. In these patients, the prognosis can be directly related to the severity of inflammation. Given two patients with comparable bone destruction, the prognosis may be better for the patient with the greater degree of inflammation because a larger component of that patient's bone destruction may be attributable to local etiologic factors. In addition, therapy allows the clinician an opportunity to work with the patient and the patient's physician to control systemic and environmental factors such as diabetes and smoking, which may have a positive effect on prognosis if adequately controlled.

The progression of periodontitis generally occurs in an episodic manner, with alternating periods of quiescence and shorter destructive stages (see Chapter 23). No methods are available at present to accurately determine whether a given lesion is in a stage of remission or exacerbation. Advanced lesions, if active, may progress rapidly to a hopeless stage, whereas similar lesions in a quiescent stage may be maintainable for long periods. Stable lesions in a patient in periodontal maintenance may also break down and advance due to changes in biofilm control, stress level, or systemic health. For these reasons, prognosis along with diagnosis must be carefully evaluated and reassessed throughout the course of treatment and over time during supportive maintenance therapy.

LEARNING BOX 35.6

Due to the dynamic nature of patients and periodontal disease, prognosis must be reevaluated during all phases of treatment.

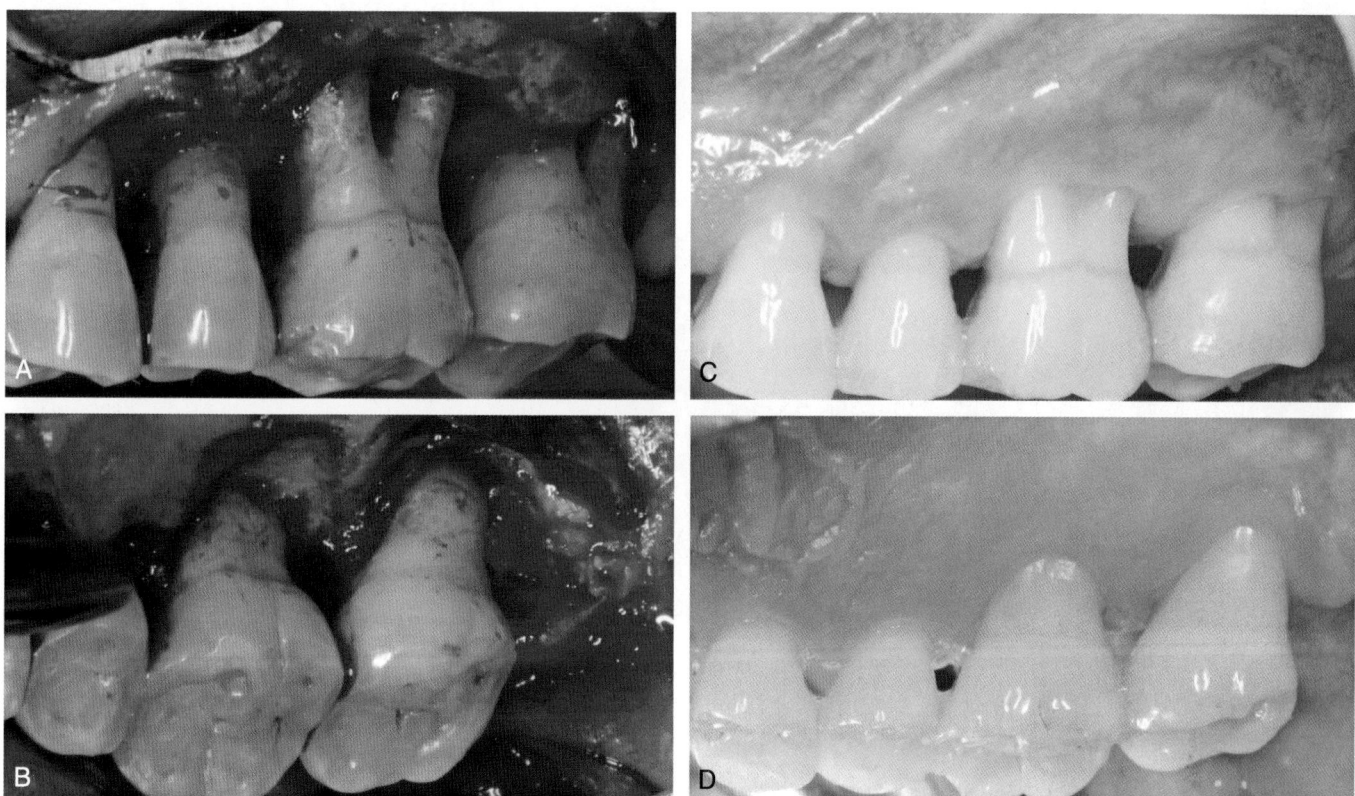

Fig. 35.11 Prognosis changes with treatment. The maxillary left first and second molars were initially assigned an unfavorable prognosis due to advanced bone loss and deep grade II furcation invasion (A, B). The clinician contemplated extraction of both teeth. However, both teeth were vital, stable, and did not require any restorative treatment, and the patient wanted to keep them and was willing to effectively control biofilm. Both teeth were treated with periodontal surgery. After 5 years, they remain healthy and functional, and the prognosis improved to favorable (C, D). *(Copyright Jonathan H. Do, DDS. All rights reserved.)*

Conclusion

The periodontal prognosis plays a pivotal role in therapy, as treatment decisions are made based on prognosis and to improve prognosis. Teeth with a hopeless diagnosis are extracted, whereas teeth with more favorable prognoses are treated, with the intent of restoring health and stability and ultimately improving the prognosis. A hopeless prognosis is perhaps the easiest prognosis to assign, because hopeless teeth usually have overt and severe disease. The hopeless prognosis is also perhaps the easiest to be erroneously assigned, due to clinical bias or lack of training and expertise. Therefore the hopeless prognosis must be assigned with caution, as the consequences are irreversible. It must also be recognized that patients and diseases are dynamic. As such, a prognosis will change and must be reevaluated over time.

References

 References for this chapter are found on the companion website www.expertconsult.com.

CHAPTER 36

The Treatment Plan

Jonathan H. Do | Henry H. Takei | Fermin A. Carranza

CHAPTER OUTLINE

Overall Treatment Plan
Sequence of Therapy
Explaining the Treatment Plan to the Patient
Conclusion

After the diagnosis and prognosis have been established, the treatment is planned. The plan should encompass immediate, intermediate, and long-term goals.

The *immediate goals* are the elimination of all infectious and inflammatory processes that cause periodontal and other oral problems that may hinder the patient's general health. Basically, the immediate goals are to bring the oral cavity to a state of health. This may require patient education on infectious oral diseases and disease prevention, periodontal procedures, endodontics, caries control, oral surgery, and treatment of oral mucous membrane pathologies. Referral to other dental and medical specialties may be necessary.

From a periodontal viewpoint, the immediate goals are important, because they consist of the elimination of gingival inflammation and the correction of conditions that cause and perpetuate it. These include not only elimination of root surface accretions but also pocket reduction and the establishment of good gingival contours and mucogingival relationships conducive to periodontal health. Extraction of hopeless teeth, restoration of carious lesions, and correction of poor existing restorations may be necessary.

The *intermediate goals* are the reconstruction of a healthy dentition that not only fulfills all functional and aesthetic requirements but lasts many years. Restoration of health, function, aesthetics, and longevity involves endodontic, orthodontic, periodontal, and prosthodontic considerations as well as the age, health, and desires of the patient. The financial impact of restoring the dentition to health, function, aesthetics, and longevity requires careful consideration and understanding by the patient. The intermediate goals may be quickly achieved or require treatments over months or even years, depending on the complexity of the case, the therapy involved, and the financial status of the patient.

The *long-term goal* is maintenance of health through prevention and professional supportive therapy. The long-term goal is set, and both the patient and the clinician work toward it from the very first visit. Once active disease has been controlled, all infectious and inflammatory processes have been eliminated, and health has been attained, health should be maintainable for the rest of the patient's life. Maintenance of health requires patient education on disease prevention and oral hygiene at the onset of treatment, meticulous daily home care by the patient, and patient adherence to professional recall maintenance.

The treatment plan is the blueprint for case management. It includes all procedures required for the establishment and maintenance of oral health and involves decisions regarding the following:

- Emergency treatment (pain, acute infections)
- Removal of nonfunctional and diseased teeth, and possibly strategic extraction of healthy teeth to facilitate the prosthetic reconstruction of the patient
- Treatment of periodontal diseases (surgical or nonsurgical, regenerative or resective)
- Endodontic therapy (necessary and intentional)
- Caries removal and placement of temporary and final restorations
- Occlusal adjustment and orthodontic therapy
- Replacement of missing teeth with removable or fixed dental prostheses or dental implants
- Aesthetic demands
- Sequence of therapy

Treatment decisions are made with the diagnosis and prognosis of the individual teeth and the overall dentition in mind. The prognosis is usually established based on the diagnosis. Treatment decisions are made based on the prognosis and to improve the prognosis. As such, *diagnosis and prognosis will change with treatment.*

Unforeseen developments during treatment may necessitate modification of the initial treatment plan. However, except for emergencies, no therapy should be initiated until a treatment plan has been established.

Overall Treatment Plan

The aim of the treatment plan is total treatment—that is, the coordination of all the immediate, intermediate, and long-term goals for the purpose of creating a well-functioning dentition in a healthy periodontal environment. The periodontal treatment encompasses different areas of therapeutic objectives for each patient according to his or her needs. It is based on the diagnosis, prognosis, disease severity, risk factors, and other factors outlined in previous chapters.

Extracting or Preserving a Tooth

Periodontal treatment requires long-range planning. Its value to the patient is measured in years of healthy functioning of the entire dentition and not by the number of teeth retained at the time of treatment. Treatment is directed to establishing and maintaining the health of the periodontium throughout the mouth rather than attempting spectacular efforts to "tighten loose teeth."

Implant replacement of missing teeth has become a predictable course of therapy. Therefore attempts to save questionable teeth may jeopardize adjacent teeth and may lead to the loss of bone needed for implant therapy. Teeth on the borderline of a hopeless prognosis do not contribute to the overall usefulness of the dentition. Such teeth become sources of recurrent problems for the patient and detract from the value of the greater service rendered by the establishment of periodontal health in the remainder of the oral cavity.

Removal, retention, or temporary (interim) retention of one or more teeth is an important part of the overall treatment plan. A tooth should be extracted under the following conditions:

- It is so mobile that function becomes painful.
- It can cause acute abscesses during therapy.
- There is no use for it in the overall treatment plan.

In some cases, a tooth can be retained temporarily, postponing the decision to extract until after treatment is completed. A tooth in this category can be retained under the following conditions:

- It maintains posterior stops; the tooth can be removed after treatment, when it can be replaced by an implant or another type of prosthesis.
- It maintains posterior stops and may be functional after implant placement in adjacent areas. When the implant is restored, these teeth can be extracted.
- In the anterior aesthetic zone, a tooth can be retained during periodontal therapy and removed when treatment is completed and a permanent restorative procedure can be performed. The retention of this tooth should not jeopardize the adjacent teeth. This approach avoids the need for temporary appliances during therapy.
- Extraction of hopeless teeth can also be performed during periodontal surgery of the adjacent teeth. This approach reduces the number of appointments needed for surgery in the same area.

In the formulation of the treatment plan, in addition to the proper function of the dentition, aesthetic considerations play an important role. Different patients value aesthetics differently, according to their age, gender, profession, and social status. The clinician should carefully evaluate and consider a final aesthetic outcome of treatment that will be acceptable to the patient without jeopardizing the basic need of attaining health.

With the predictable use of implants, questionable teeth should be carefully evaluated as to whether their removal and replacement with an implant may be a better and more satisfactory course of therapy.

In complex cases, interdisciplinary consultation with other specialty areas is necessary before a final plan can be made. The opinions of orthodontists and prosthodontists are especially important for the final decision in these patients.

Occlusal evaluation and therapy may be necessary during treatment, which may necessitate planning for occlusal adjustment (see Chapter 55), orthodontics see Chapter 56, and splinting. The correction of bruxism and other occlusal habits may also be necessary.

Systemic conditions should be carefully evaluated because they may require special precautions during the course of periodontal treatment. The tissue response to treatment procedures may be affected, or the preservation of periodontal health may be threatened after treatment is completed. The patient's physician should always be consulted when the patient presents with medical and systemic problems that may affect the periodontal therapy.

Supportive periodontal care is also of paramount importance for case maintenance. Such care entails all procedures for maintaining periodontal health after it has been attained. It consists of instruction in oral hygiene and recall therapy at regular intervals, according to the patient's needs.

Sequence of Therapy

The periodontal treatment sequence is presented in Box 36.1, and a nonsurgical periodontal treatment decision tree is presented in Fig. 36.1. Periodontal therapy is an inseparable part of dental therapy, and all treatments must be well coordinated.

Although the phases of treatment are numbered, the recommended sequence does not follow the numbers (Fig. 36.2). Phase I, or the *nonsurgical phase,* is directed to the elimination of the etiologic factors of dental, gingival, and periodontal diseases. When successfully performed, this phase stops the progression of dental and periodontal disease.

Immediately after completion of phase I therapy, the patient should be placed on the *maintenance phase* (phase IV) to preserve the results obtained and prevent any further deterioration and recurrence of disease. While on the maintenance phase, with its periodic evaluation, the patient enters into the *surgical phase* (phase II) and the *restorative phase* (phase III) of treatment (Fig. 36.3). These phases include periodontal surgery to treat and improve the condition of the periodontal and surrounding tissues. This may include regeneration of the gingiva and bone for function and aesthetics, placement of implants, and restorative therapy.

> **LEARNING BOX 36.3**
>
> Immediately after the completion of phase I therapy, the patient should be placed on the maintenance phase.

Explaining the Treatment Plan to the Patient

The following discussion includes suggestions for explaining the treatment plan to the patient.

Be specific. Tell your patient, "You have gingivitis" or "You have periodontitis," then explain exactly what the condition is.

Avoid vague statements. Do not use statements such as "You have trouble with your gums" or "Something should be done about your gums." The patient may not understand the significance of such statements and may disregard them.

Begin your discussion on a positive note. Talk about the teeth that can be retained and the long-term service they can be expected to render. Do not begin your discussion with the statement "The following teeth have to be extracted." This creates a negative impression, which adds to the erroneous attitude of hopelessness

---

BOX 36.1 Periodontal Treatment Sequence

Periodontal Evaluation

Comprehensive periodontal examination

Diagnosis and prognosis

Patient education
- Clinical findings and disease status
- Disease pathogenesis and prevention
- Personalized oral hygiene instruction

Reduction of systemic and environmental risk factors
- Physician consultation
- Smoking cessation

Periodontal treatment plan
- Oral hygiene assessment and education
- Nonsurgical therapy
- Periodontal reevaluation
- Periodontal supportive maintenance

Nonsurgical Therapy

Oral hygiene assessment and education*

Infection control
- Nonsurgical periodontal therapy
  - Supragingival and subgingival scaling and root planing
- Extraction of hopeless teeth

Reduction of local risk factors
- Removal or reshaping of overhangs and overcontoured restorations
- Restoration of carious lesions
- Restoration of open contacts

Periodontal Reevaluation

Inquiry of new concerns or problems

Inquiry of changes in patient's medical and oral health status

Oral hygiene assessment and education*

Comprehensive periodontal examination

Assessment of outcome of nonsurgical therapy

Determination of required additional nonsurgical and adjunctive therapy

Surgical Therapy

Adjunct to nonsurgical therapy

Should only occur once patient demonstrates proficient biofilm control

Objectives:
- Primary: Access for root instrumentation
- Secondary: Pocket reduction through soft tissue resection, osseous resection, or periodontal regeneration

Periodontal access surgery
- Resective
- Regenerative

Extraction of hopeless teeth

Periodontal plastic surgery
- Mucogingival surgery
- Aesthetic crown lengthening

Preprosthetic surgery
- Prosthetic crown lengthening
- Implant site preparation and implant placement

Periodontal Maintenance Therapy

Inquiry of new concerns or problems

Inquiry of changes in patient's medical and oral health status

Oral hygiene assessment and education*

Comprehensive periodontal examination

Professional maintenance care
- Supragingival and subgingival biofilm and calculus removal
- Selective scaling and root planing

Assessment of recall interval and plan for next visit

---

*Patient oral hygiene is critical to the overall short-term and long-term treatment outcome. Therefore oral hygiene must be repeatedly assessed and reinforced.

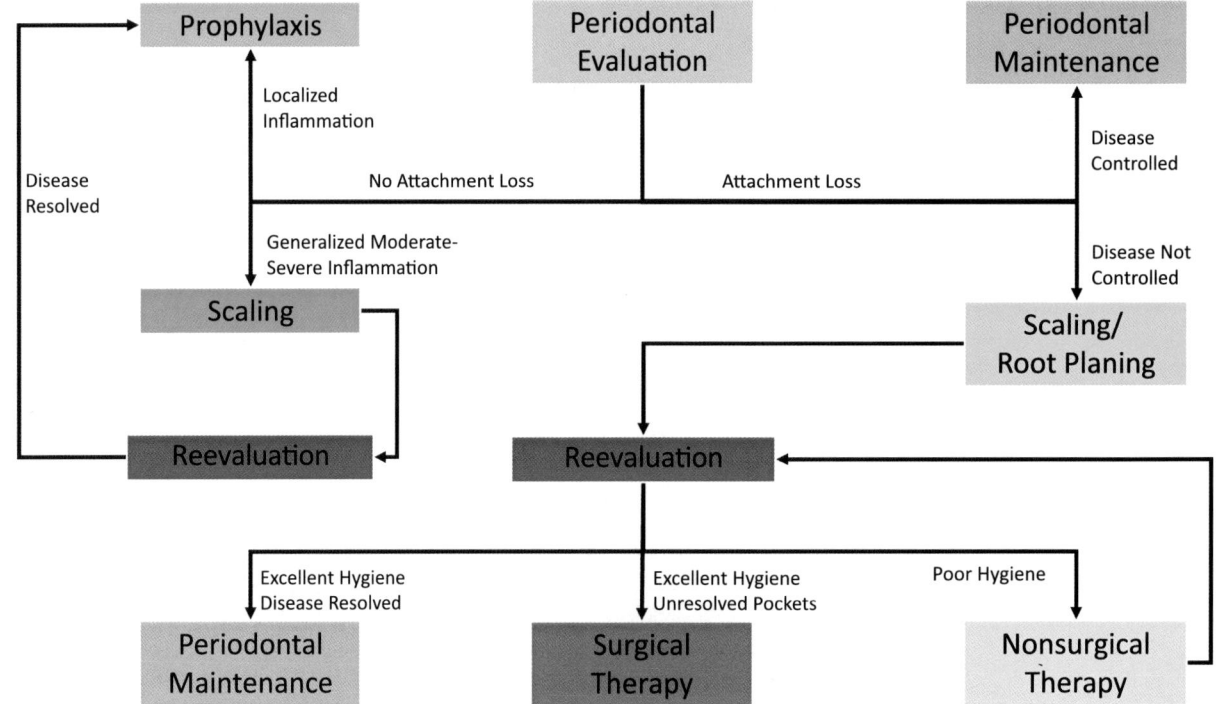

Fig. 36.1 Periodontal treatment decision tree.

the patient may already have regarding his or her mouth. Make it clear that every effort will be made to retain as many teeth as possible, but do not dwell on the patient's loose teeth. Emphasize that the important purpose of the treatment is to prevent the other teeth from becoming as severely diseased as the loose teeth.

Present the entire treatment plan as a unit. Avoid creating the impression that treatment consists of separate procedures, some or all of which may be selected by the patient. Make it clear that dental restorations and prostheses contribute as much to the health of the gingiva as the elimination of inflammation and periodontal pockets. Do not speak in terms of "having the gums treated and then taking care of the necessary restorations later" as if these were unrelated treatments.

Patients often seek guidance from the dentist with questions such as the following:
- "Are my teeth worth treating?"
- "Would you have them treated if you had my problem?"
- "Why don't I just go along the way I am until the teeth really bother me and then have them all extracted?"

Explain that "doing nothing" or holding onto hopelessly diseased teeth as long as possible is inadvisable for the following reasons:
1. Periodontal disease is a microbial infection, and research has clearly shown it to be an important risk factor for severe life-threatening diseases such as stroke, cardiovascular disease, pulmonary disease, and diabetes, as well as for premature low-birth-weight babies in women of childbearing age. Correcting the periodontal condition eliminates a serious potential risk of systemic disease, which in some cases ranks as high on the danger list as smoking.
2. It is not feasible to place restorations or fixed bridges on teeth with untreated periodontal disease because the usefulness of the restoration would be limited by the uncertain condition of the supporting structures.
3. Failure to eliminate periodontal disease not only results in the loss of teeth already severely involved, but also shortens the life span of other teeth. With proper treatment, these teeth can serve as the foundation for a healthy, functioning dentition.

Therefore the dentist should make it clear to the patient that if the periodontal condition is treatable, the best results are obtained by prompt treatment. If the condition is not treatable, the teeth should be extracted.

It is the dentist's responsibility to advise the patient of the importance of periodontal treatment. However, if treatment is to be successful, the patient must be sufficiently interested in retaining his or her natural teeth and to maintain the necessary oral hygiene. Individuals who are not particularly perturbed by the thought of losing their teeth are generally not good candidates for periodontal treatment.

Conclusion

The ultimate goal for every patient is to bring his or her mouth to a state of health and maintain it long term. This begins with educating the patient on the problems in his or her mouth and the

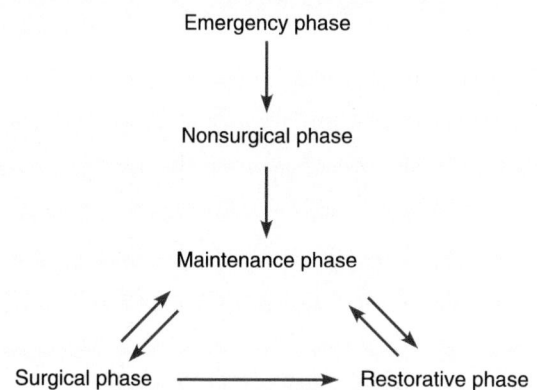

Fig. 36.2 Preferred sequence of therapy.

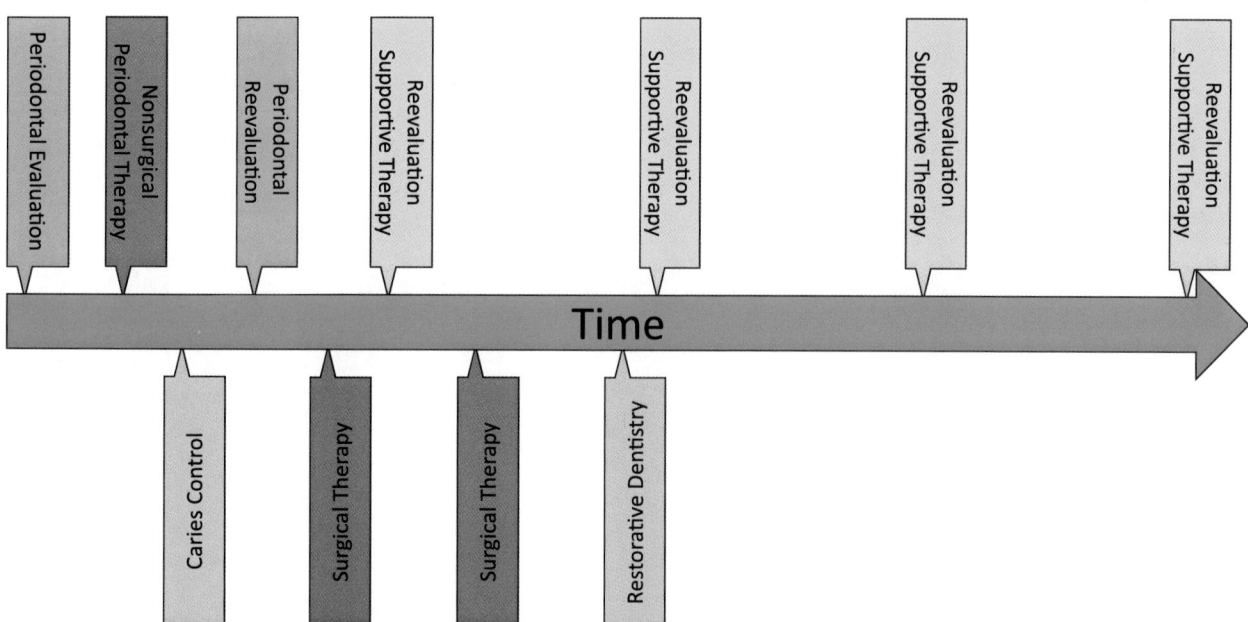

Fig. 36.3 Sample treatment timeline. Following nonsurgical periodontal therapy, the patient is placed on periodontal maintenance at regular intervals. Surgical and restorative treatments are scheduled between periodontal recalls.

etiologies, treatment, and prevention of these problems. A properly formulated treatment plan is paramount to achieving this goal. A treatment plan is a plan for therapy formulated only after a thorough examination has been completed, diagnosis and prognosis have been determined, and the needs and desires of the patient have been taken into consideration. It must be recognized that as diagnosis and prognosis will change with treatment, therapeutic needs may also change. As such, the treatment plan must be changed accordingly.

Examination → Diagnosis → Prognosis ↔ Treatment

- Diagnosis requires thorough and careful examination.
- Prognosis is based on accurate diagnosis.
- Treatment decisions are based on the the prognosis.
- Treatment decisions are made to improve the prognosis.
- Diagnosis and prognosis will change with treatment.

CHAPTER 38

Conscious Sedation

Robert L. Merin | Perry R. Klokkevold

CHAPTER OUTLINE

 For online-only content on mild sedation, anxiolysis, and moderate conscious sedation, please visit the companion website at www.expertconsult.com.

Periodontal and implant surgery should be performed painlessly and with minimal or no apprehension. The patient should be assured at the initial consultation. The most reliable means of providing painless surgery is effective administration of local anesthesia. However, patients who are apprehensive may require treatment under mild or moderate sedation. The use of sedation can help make patients more comfortable during periodontal and implant surgery, especially when the procedure is expected to continue for 2 hours or more. Routes of administration for sedation agents include inhalation, oral, intramuscular, and intravenous. The specific agents and modality of administration are based on the desired level of sedation, anticipated length of the procedure, overall condition of the patient, and training of the clinician and staff. This chapter reviews the rationale, definitions, techniques, and guidelines for the use of mild to moderate conscious sedation in the dental office for periodontal and implant surgical procedures.

Rationale for Sedation During Periodontal and Implant Surgical Procedures

Many patients delay or avoid having needed dental treatment because of fear and anxiety. This avoidance behavior often results in compromised health and quality of life. In a study of 174 patients referred for dental implant therapy, only 40.8% proceeded with therapy, and 24% listed dental fear as the reason for refusing to accept treatment.[33,41] Those who proceeded with therapy had low anxiety ratings as measured by the Modified Dental Anxiety Scale.[33]

Anxiety about dental therapy has not changed significantly during the past 50 years; publications report that about 30% to 50% of patients are at least somewhat fearful of dental procedures.[6,13-15,41,61,70] Evidence suggests that genetic variations are associated with anxiety related to dental care, which could help to explain the consistent avoidance patterns despite improved treatment methods.[7] According to a national survey of the Canadian population, more than 68% of patients would prefer to have sedation or general anesthesia for periodontal surgery[8] (Fig. 38.1). Anxiety reduction that includes moderate sedation is an important part of delivering advanced periodontal services.[1,53,65]

Because dental anxiety results in avoidance behavior and is associated with more dental and periodontal problems,[19,43,70] it is likely that disproportionate numbers of patients referred to periodontal specialists have dental anxiety. There appears to be a close relationship between anxiety and postoperative pain, and preoperative anxiety can be a predictor of postoperative pain.[22,25] High levels of anxiety (i.e., stress) can affect wound healing after periodontal treatment[37,40,68] (see Chapter 14). Sedation techniques have been effective in reducing physiologic markers of stress.[58] For these reasons, it is important for clinicians who provide advanced periodontal and implant therapy to be knowledgeable and skilled in providing sedation to reduce anxiety in their patients.

American Dental Association Policy Statement and Guidelines for Conscious Sedation

The American Dental Association (ADA) released three documents related to the use of sedation and general anesthesia in dentistry: the ADA Policy Statement on the Use of Sedation and General Anesthesia by Dentists,[2] the ADA Guidelines for the Use of Sedation and General Anesthesia by Dentists,[3] and the ADA Guidelines for Teaching Pain Control and Sedation to Dentists and Dental Students.[4] The policy statement and guidelines provide educational and practice standards for anxiety control in dental practice. The ADA Committee on Anesthesiology, consisting of representatives from dental organizations involved with sedation and anesthesia, produced these documents after reviewing the relevant scientific evidence, expert opinions, and comments by all communities of interest. The following sections describe the important elements of these documents as they relate to treating anxious periodontal patients.

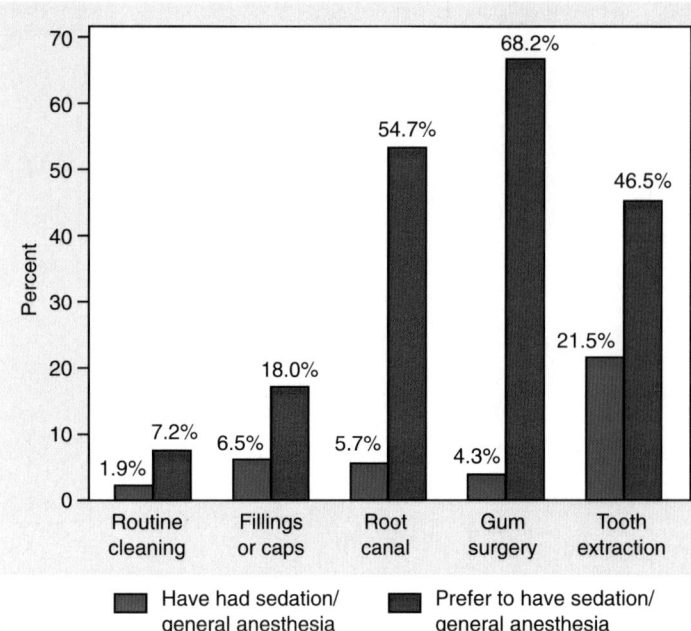

Fig. 38.1 Patient preferences for sedation or general anesthesia by dental procedure. *(From Chanpong B, Haas DA, Locker D: Need and demand for sedation or general anesthesia in dentistry: a national survey of the Canadian population,* Anesth Prog *52:3–11, 2005.)*

Use of Sedation and General Anesthesia by Dentists

The dental profession's continued ability to effectively control anxiety and pain depends on a strong educational foundation in the discipline. Training to competency in minimal and moderate sedation techniques may be acquired at the predoctoral, postgraduate, graduate, or continuing education level. Dentists who wish to use minimal or moderate sedation are expected to successfully complete formal training, which is structured in accordance with the ADA Guidelines for Teaching Pain Control and Sedation for Dentists and Dental Students.

The knowledge and skills required for administration of deep sedation and general anesthesia are beyond the scope of predoctoral and continuing education. Only dentists who have completed an advanced education program accredited by the Commission on Dental Accreditation (CODA) that provides training in deep sedation and general anesthesia are considered educationally qualified to use these modalities in practice.

Use of Sedation and General Anesthesia by Dentists

The 2016 ADA guidelines refer to the effects of sedation on the central nervous system and do not depend on the route of administration. The purpose of the guidelines is to assist dentists in the delivery of safe and effective sedation and anesthesia. The ADA adopted the American Society of Anesthesiologists (ASA) definitions for levels of sedation (Fig. 38.2) and expanded and commented on them as they relate to treating adult dental patients.[5]

For children, the ADA supports the use of the American Academy of Pediatric Dentistry (AAPD) series of Guidelines for Monitoring and Management of Pediatric Patients During and After Sedation for Diagnostic and Therapeutic Procedures.[11]

Definitions and Levels of Sedation
Pediatric Sedation

The definition of *child* is not discussed in the ADA guidelines but has been defined in other sources. The end of childhood can be defined by age, size, and development.[11,12,20,54] With normal size and development, an individual becomes an adolescent between the ages of 11 and 13 years.[20]

Sedation is often administered to children to control behavior, which often requires deeper levels of sedation. Children can become moderately sedated despite an intended level of minimal sedation. Except in extraordinary situations, the use of preoperative sedatives for children must be avoided because of the risk of unobserved respiratory obstruction during transport by untrained individuals. The management of conscious sedation in children is beyond the scope of this chapter but is addressed by the American Academy of Pediatrics/American Academy of Pediatric Dentists (APA/AAPD) Guidelines for Monitoring and Management of Pediatric Patients During and After Sedation for Diagnostic and Therapeutic Procedures.[11]

Adult Sedation
Minimal Sedation

Minimal sedation is defined as a minimally depressed level of consciousness produced by a pharmacologic method that retains the patient's ability to independently and continuously maintain an airway and respond normally to tactile stimulation and verbal commands. Although cognitive function and coordination can be modestly impaired, respiratory and cardiovascular functions are unaffected. Minimal sedation can be achieved by the administration of a drug (singly or in divided doses) by the enteral route to achieve the desired clinical effect, not to exceed the maximum recommended dose as printed in U.S. Food and Drug Administration (FDA)–approved labeling for unmonitored home use. The administration of enteral drugs exceeding the FDA-recommended dose during an appointment is considered moderate sedation, and the moderate sedation guidelines apply.

Inhalation sedation with nitrous oxide and oxygen (N_2O/O_2) can be used in combination with a single enteral drug for minimal sedation. When used in combination with one or more sedative agents, N_2O/O_2 can produce sedation that is minimal, moderate, or deep, and in some cases it can produce general anesthesia. If more than one enteral drug is administered to achieve the desired sedation effect, with or without the concomitant use of N_2O, the guidelines for moderate sedation apply.

CONTINUUM OF DEPTH OF SEDATION: DEFINITION OF GENERAL ANESTHESIA AND LEVELS OF SEDATION/ANALGESIA*
Committee of Origin: Quality Management and Departmental Administration (Approved by the ASA House of Delegates on October 13, 1999, and amended on October 27, 2004)

	Minimal Sedation/ Analgesia	Moderate Sedation/ "Conscious Sedation"	Deep Sedation/Anxiolysis	General Anesthesia/ Analgesia
Responsiveness	Normal response to verbal stimulation	Purposeful[†] response to verbal and tactile stimulation	Purposeful[†] response following repeated and painful stimulation	Unarousable even with painful stimulus
Airway	Unaffected	No intervention required	Intervention may be required	Intervention often required
Spontaneous ventilation	Unaffected	Adequate	May be inadequate	Frequently inadequate
Cardiovascular function	Unaffected	Usually maintained	Usually maintained	May be impaired

Minimal Sedation (Anxiolysis) is a drug-induced state during which patients respond normally to verbal commands. Although cognitive function and coordination may be impaired, ventilatory and cardiovascular functions are unaffected.

Moderate Sedation/Analgesia ("Conscious Sedation") is a drug-induced depression of consciousness during which patients respond purposefully[†] to verbal commands, either alone and accompanied by light tactile stimulation. No interventions are required to maintain a patent airway, and spontaneous ventilation is adequate. Cardiovascular function is usually maintained.

Deep Sedation/Analgesia is a drug-induced depression of consciousness during which patients cannot be easily aroused but respond purposefully[†] following repeated and painful stimulation. The ability to independently maintain ventilatory function may be impaired. Patients may require assistance in maintaining a patent airway, and spontaneous ventilation may be inadequate. Cardiovascular function is usually maintained.

General Anesthesia is a drug-induced loss of consciousness during which patients are not arousable, even by painful stimulation. The ability to independently maintain ventilatory function is often impaired. Patients often require assistance in maintaining a patent airway, and positive pressure ventilation may be required because of depressed spontaneous ventilation or drug-induced depression of neuromuscular function. Cardiovascular function may be impaired.

Because sedation is a continuum, it is not always possible to predict how an individual patient will respond. Hence, practitioners intending to produce a given level of sedation should be able to rescue[††] patients whose level of sedation becomes deeper than initially intended. Individuals administering Moderate Sedation/Analgesia ("Conscious Sedation") should be able to rescue[††] patients who enter a state of Deep Sedation/Analgesia, while those administering Deep Sedation/Analgesia should be able to rescue[††] patients who enter a state of General Anesthesia.

*Monitored anesthesia care does not describe the continuum of depth of sedation, rather it describes "a specific anesthesia service in which an anesthesiologist has been requested to participate in the care of a patient undergoing a diagnostic or therapeutic procedure."
[†]Reflex withdrawal from a painful stimulus is NOT considered a purposeful response.
[††]Rescue of a patient from a deeper level of sedation than intended is an intervention by a practitioner proficient in airway management and advanced life support. The qualified practitioner corrects adverse physiologic consequences of the deeper-than-intended level of sedation (such as hypoventilation, hypoxia, or hypotension) and returns the patient to the originally intended level of sedation.

Fig. 38.2 Continuum of depth of sedation: definitions of general anesthesia and levels of sedation or analgesia. The information was approved by the ASA House of Delegates on October 13, 1999, and it was last amended on October 15, 2014. *(From American Society of Anesthesiologists: Continuum of depth of sedation: definition of general anesthesia and levels of sedation/analgesia, 2014. http://www.asahq.org/quality-and-practice-management/standards-guidelines-and-related-resources/continuum-of-depth-of-sedation-definition-of-general-anesthesia-and-levels-of-sedation-analgesia.)*

Maximum Recommended Dose

The *maximum recommended dose* (MRD) is the maximum FDA-recommended dose of a drug as printed in FDA-approved labeling for unmonitored home use.

> **KEY FACT**
>
> Minimal sedation is a drug-induced minimally depressed level of consciousness. The ability to independently and continuously maintain an airway and respond to tactile stimulation and verbal commands is maintained. Respiratory and cardiovascular functions are unaffected.

Moderate Sedation

Moderate sedation is a drug-induced depression of consciousness during which patients respond purposefully to verbal commands, alone or accompanied by light tactile stimulation. No interventions are required to maintain a patent airway, and spontaneous ventilations are adequate. Cardiovascular function is usually maintained.

In accord with this definition, the drugs and techniques used should carry a margin of safety wide enough to render unintended loss of consciousness unlikely. Repeated dosing of an agent before the effects of previous dosing can be fully appreciated may result in greater alteration of the state of consciousness than intended by the dentist. A patient whose only response is reflex withdrawal from a painful stimulus is not considered to be in a state of moderate sedation.

Titration

Titration is the administration of incremental doses of an intravenous or inhalation drug until a desired effect is reached. Knowledge about each drug's time of onset, peak response, and duration of action is

TABLE 38.1   American Society of Anesthesiologists Physical Status Classification System

Class	Definition	Examples
ASA 1	A normal, healthy patient	No disease, nonsmoking, no or minimal alcohol use
ASA 2	A patient with mild systemic disease	Mild conditions or diseases without substantive functional limitations, such as current tobacco use, social drinking, pregnancy, obesity (BMI = 30–40), well-controlled DM or HTN, mild lung disease
ASA 3	A patient with severe systemic disease	Substantive functional limitations; one or more moderate to severe diseases, such as poorly controlled DM or HTN, COPD, morbid obesity (BMI ≥40), active hepatitis, alcohol dependence or abuse, implanted pacemaker, moderate reduction of ejection fraction, ESRD undergoing regularly scheduled dialysis, premature infant (PCA < 60 wk), history (>3 mo) of MI, CVA, TIA, or CAD/stents
ASA 4	A patient with severe systemic disease that is a constant threat to life	Recent (<3 mo) MI, CVA, TIA, or CAD/stents; ongoing cardiac ischemia or severe valve dysfunction; severe reduction of ejection fraction; sepsis, DIC, or ARD or ESRD not undergoing regularly scheduled dialysis
ASA 5	A moribund patient who is not expected to survive without the operation	Ruptured abdominal or thoracic aneurysm, massive trauma, intracranial bleed with mass effect, ischemic bowel in the setting of significant cardiac pathology or multiple organ or system dysfunction
ASA 6	A declared brain-dead patient whose organs are being removed for donation purposes	

ARD, Acute renal disease; *BMI*, body mass index; *CAD*, coronary artery disease; *COPD*, chronic obstructive pulmonary disease; *CVA*, cardiovascular accident; *DIC*, disseminated intravascular coagulation; *DM*, diabetes mellitus; *ESRD*, end-stage renal disease; *HTN*, hypertension; *MI*, myocardial infarction; *PCA*, postconceptional age; *TIA*, transient ischemic attack.
Modified from American Society of Anesthesiologists: ASA physical status classification system, 2014. https://www.asahq.org/resources/clinical-information/asa-physical-status-classification-system.

essential to avoid oversedation. The concept of titration to effect is critical for patient safety, and when the intent is moderate sedation, the clinician must know whether the previous dose has taken full effect before administering an additional drug increment.

 KEY FACT

Moderate sedation is a drug-induced depression of consciousness. Patients respond purposefully to verbal commands, possibly requiring light tactile stimulation. A patent airway is maintained, and spontaneous ventilation is adequate. Cardiovascular function is usually maintained.

Deep Sedation

Deep sedation is drug-induced depression of consciousness during which patients cannot be easily aroused but respond purposefully to repeated or painful stimulation. The ability to independently maintain respiratory function can be impaired. Patients may require assistance in maintaining a patent airway, and spontaneous ventilation may be inadequate. Cardiovascular function is usually maintained.

KEY FACT

Deep sedation is a drug-induced depression of consciousness. Patients may not be easily aroused but respond purposefully to repeated or painful stimulation. Respiratory function may be impaired, and assistance may be necessary to maintain a patent airway. Spontaneous ventilation may be inadequate. Cardiovascular function is usually maintained.

General Anesthesia

General anesthesia is drug-induced loss of consciousness during which patients are not aroused, even by painful stimulation. The ability to independently maintain respiratory function is often impaired.

Patients often require assistance in maintaining a patent airway, and positive-pressure ventilation may be required because of depressed spontaneous ventilation or drug-induced depression of neuromuscular function. Cardiovascular function can be impaired.

Clinical Guidelines for Minimal and Moderate Sedation

The following clinical guidelines apply to minimal and moderate sedation[3]: (1) patient evaluation, (2) preoperative preparation, (3) personnel and equipment, (4) monitoring and documentation, and (5) recovery and discharge. Differences between guidelines for minimal and moderate sedation are indicated.

Patient History and Evaluation

The patient's health status is assessed before any sedation procedure. Evaluation includes determination of the ASA physical status (ASA) (Table 38.1). For healthy or medically stable individuals (i.e., ASA 1 or 2), a review of the medical history and medication use may be adequate. For patients with significant medical considerations (i.e., ASA 3 or 4), a consultation with the primary care physician or consulting medical specialist is indicated. The evaluation must include a focused physical examination, including baseline vital signs and a focused examination of alertness, respiratory function, airway, and appearance, as well as a specific evaluation of identified medical conditions (Box 38.1 and Fig. 38.3). Assessment of body mass index (BMI) should be considered for patients undergoing moderate sedation.

Preoperative Preparation

The patient, or a parent, guardian, or caregiver if the patient is a minor, must be informed about the planned procedure that will occur while under sedation, including benefits, risks, and instructions for sedation (Fig. 38.4). Informed consent for the proposed procedure and sedation must be obtained.

Determination of an adequate oxygen supply and the equipment necessary to deliver oxygen under positive pressure must be completed. Baseline vital signs, including weight, height, blood pressure, pulse rate, and respiration rate, must be obtained. For moderate-sedation patients, blood oxygen saturation must be obtained by pulse oximetry.

BOX 38.1 Preoperative Physical Evaluation

1. Blood pressure and pulse
2. Oxygen saturation and respiration; ability to breathe deeply and cough
3. Mallampati airway classification and neck flexibility
4. Appearance and skin color
5. Alertness
6. Exercise tolerance and ambulation
7. Height, weight, body mass index

Body temperature should be measured when clinically indicated. Preoperative verbal or written instructions must be given to the patient, parent, escort, legal guardian, or caregiver. For moderate sedation, this includes preoperative fasting instructions based on the ASA summary of fasting and pharmacologic recommendations.

Preoperative dietary restrictions are based on the sedation technique prescribed (Boxes 38.2 and 38.3). For moderate sedation, NPO (nothing by mouth) status should be confirmed.

Personnel and Equipment

At least one person trained in basic life support (BLS) for health care providers must be present in addition to the dentist. Monitoring equipment includes a sphygmomanometer, positive-pressure oxygen delivery system, suction, and, if inhalation sedation is used, a fail-safe and scavenging system. In the case of moderate sedation, a pulse oximeter, equipment for monitoring end-tidal carbon dioxide (CO_2), a precordial or pretracheal stethoscope, equipment for intravenous

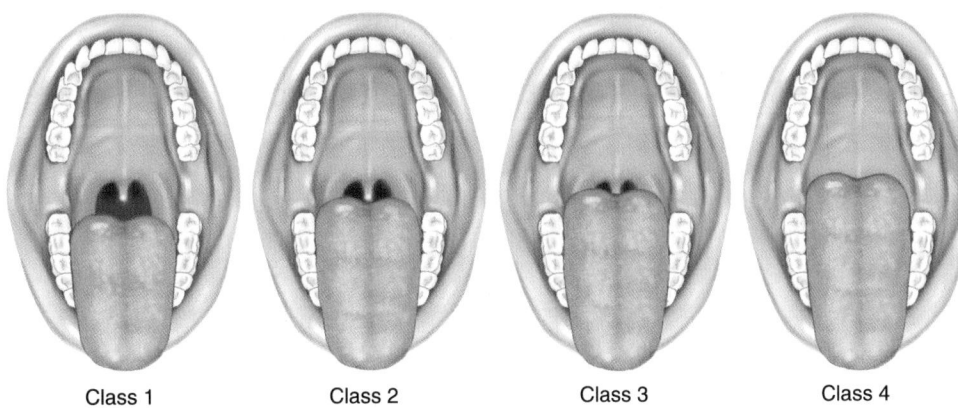

Class 1   Class 2   Class 3   Class 4

Class 1: soft palate, fauces, uvula, pillars
Class 2: soft palate, fauces, portion of uvula
Class 3: soft palate, base of uvula
Class 4: hard palate only

Fig. 38.3 Mallampati classifications used to predict difficult tracheal intubations. *(Modified from Mallampati SR, Gatt SP, Gugino LD, et al: A clinical sign to predict difficult tracheal intubation: a prospective study.* Can Anaesth Soc J *32:429–434, 1985.)*

An explanation of IV conscious sedation, its purpose, benefits, possible risks, and complications as well as alternative methods of anesthesia has been discussed with you at your consultation, and we obtained your verbal consent to undergo treatment planned for you. Please read this document, which repeats issues we discussed, and provide the appropriate signatures. Please ask us to clarify anything that you do not understand.

PRESEDATION INFORMATION

1. The premedication you will receive by vein is NOT sodium pentothal. Its purpose is not to put you to sleep but to relax and sedate you. In addition, local anesthetics will be administered in your mouth.
2. You must have a responsible adult bring you to the office and drive you home, and you must remain in the company of a responsible adult until you are fully alert. Make arrangements for the person driving you home to come to the waiting room.
3. You should not have any solid food for 6 hours before your appointment. You can have clear liquids up to 2 hours before your appointment. Examples of clear liquids are apple juice, lemonade, Jell-O, or decaffeinated coffee without cream or cream substitutes.
4. Please wear short sleeves or sleeves that may be raised above the elbows.
5. No alcoholic beverages for 12 hours before sedation.
6. Possible risks and side effects: I have been informed and understand that occasionally there are complications associated with IV conscious sedation including, but not limited to, pain, phlebitis (inflammation of the vein), infection, swelling, bleeding, numbness, discoloration, nausea, vomiting, allergic reaction, depressed breathing, and, in extremely rare instances, intraarterial injection with damage to the part of the body supplied by the artery.
7. I have read and understand the presedation instructions and have also read the enclosed postsedation instructions.

Patient's Signature   Date

Fig. 38.4 Consent form for and explanation of intravenous conscious sedation.

BOX 38.2 Mild Sedation: Protocol for the Use of Adult Oral Sedative Premedication for Anxious or Fearful Dental Patients

1. The dentist determines the extent of dental treatment, evaluates the patient's medical history, researches potential drug interactions, consults with the patient's physician if appropriate, and obtains informed consent.
2. The patient must have a responsible adult companion for travel to and from the dental office. The patient must be escorted by this companion to and from the parking lot to prevent stumbling.
3. The patient should take the prescribed medication according to directions and is instructed to have a light meal such as toast and a beverage without caffeine.
4. A patient who has received oral sedative is monitored visually and never left alone.
5. After treatment is complete, postoperative directions are given to the patient and a responsible adult, and the patient is released into the care of his or her companion for travel home. The companion is informed that the patient may have psychomotor and cognitive impairment for the rest of the day.

From Merin RL: Adult oral sedation in California: what can a dentist do without a special permit or certificate from the Dental Board of California? *J Calif Dent Assoc* 34:959–968, 2006.

BOX 38.3 Mild Sedation: Suggested Patient Pretreatment Instructions

1. The sedative _____ (name of medication) is being prescribed to help reduce your anxiety before and during your dental procedure.
2. The medication may make you sleepy and impair your thinking and coordination. You must have a responsible adult companion for travel to and from the dental office.
3. You must be escorted by this companion to and from the parking lot to prevent stumbling.
4. You should take the prescribed medication according to directions. You can have a light meal (no fat) such as toast without butter or margarine and a beverage without caffeine. No grapefruit juice is allowed.
5. After the treatment is complete, a responsible adult must escort you out of the office and take you home. Because the sedative effects may linger for the rest of the day, you should not plan to do anything, and it is advisable to have a responsible adult stay until you are able to take care of yourself.

From Merin RL: Adult oral sedation in California: what can a dentist do without a special permit or certificate from the Dental Board of California? *J Calif Dent Assoc* 34:959–968, 2006.

BOX 38.4 Safety Checklist for Office-Based Sedation

Check Before Patient Is Brought to the Procedure Room

1. Ensure functional monitors
   Pulse oximeter
   Capnograph
   Blood pressure monitor
   Printer
   Bluetooth pretracheal stethoscope
   Electrocardiograph if required
2. Oxygen source and delivery
3. Dinitrogen dioxide (N_2O) scavenger and fail-safe system
4. Suction functioning
5. Emergency equipment and medications
   Positive-pressure oxygen delivery system
   Airway adjuncts
   Laryngeal suction device
   Reversal agents
   Emergency medications
6. Fire hazard precautions with oxygen if laser, electrosurgery, flame sources, or burs and drills are used
7. Necessary instruments and devices for procedure

Preoperative Encounter With the Patient

1. Sedation record available
2. Correct patient chart
3. Recent radiographs
4. Correct procedure listed
5. Informed consent signed
6. Review of medical history, including allergies, adverse drug reactions, and changes in health
7. Medications taken
8. American Society of Anesthesiologists (ASA) score, Mallampati classification
9. NPO status (no oral intake)
10. Name of responsible adult escort
11. Preoperative vital signs

TABLE 38.2 Equipment Required for Mild or Moderate Sedation

Mild or Moderate Sedation	Moderate Sedation
Sphygmomanometer	Pulse oximeter
Positive-pressure oxygen delivery system	Equipment for establishing intravenous access
Suction equipment	Reversal agents for drugs used
Inhalation equipment with a fail-safe system and scavenging system	End-tidal CO_2 monitor (i.e., capnography)

---

or intraosseous access, and reversal agents for drugs used must be available (Table 38.2).

A positive-pressure oxygen delivery system suitable for the patient being treated must be immediately available. Documentation of compliance with the manufacturer's recommended maintenance of monitors, anesthesia delivery systems, and other anesthesia-related equipment should be maintained. A preprocedural check of equipment and a preoperative review of the patient's records and physical status are performed immediately before each administration of sedation (Box 38.4). When inhalation equipment is used, it must have a fail-safe system that is appropriately checked and calibrated. The equipment must also have a functioning device that prohibits the delivery of less than 30% oxygen or an appropriately calibrated and functioning in-line oxygen analyzer with an audible alarm. An appropriate scavenging system must be available if gases other than oxygen or air are used.

For moderate sedation, the equipment necessary to establish intravascular or intraosseous access should be available until the patient meets the discharge criteria. This includes a catheter or butterfly needle, an intravenous drip line, a solution bag (i.e., saline or dextrose), a tourniquet, and appropriate antiseptic or dermal disinfectant (Fig. 38.5). For moderate sedation, the equipment necessary for monitoring

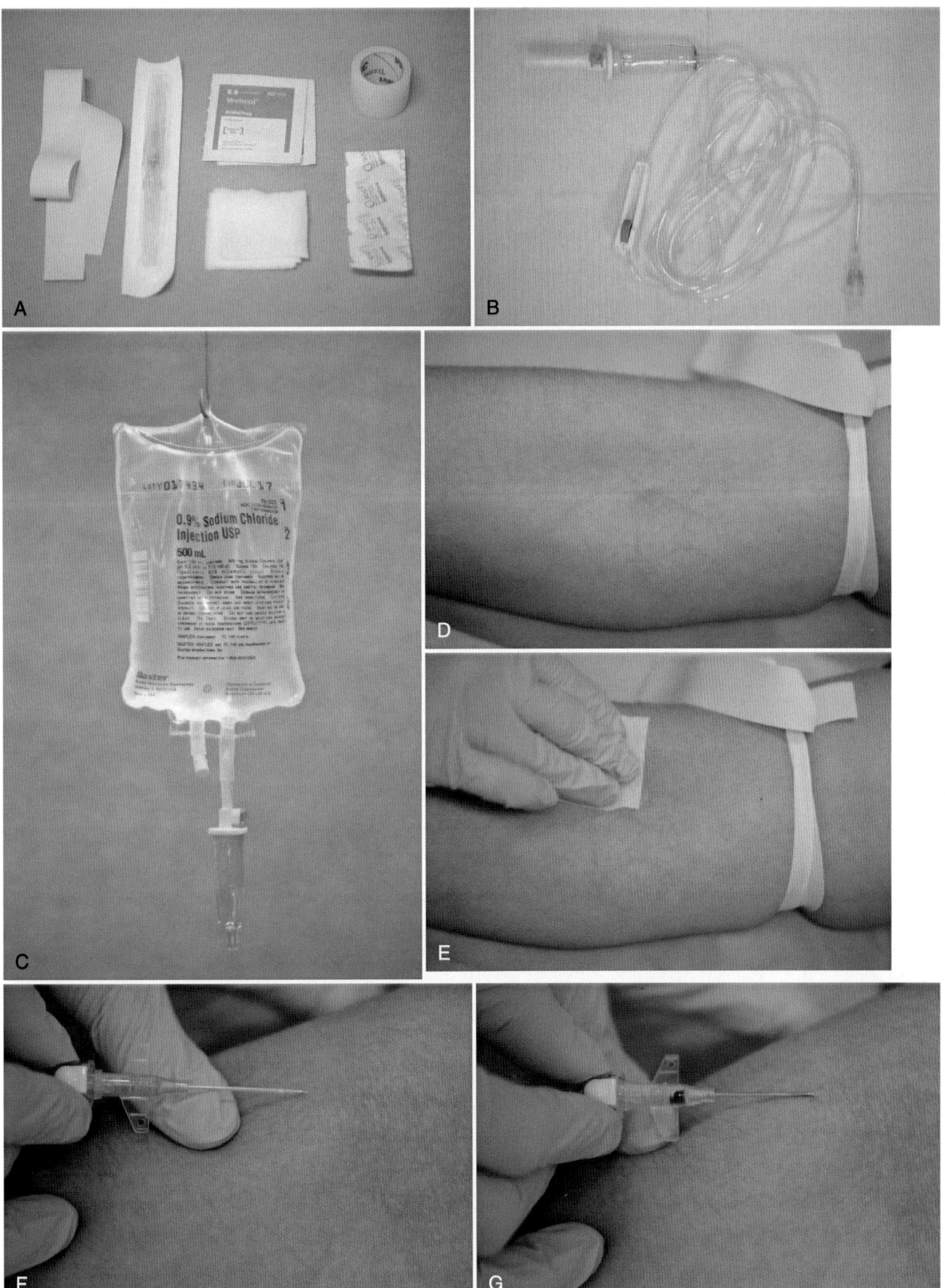

Fig. 38.5 Equipment and supplies needed for the administration of moderate intravenous (IV) sedation. (A) A tourniquet, indwelling catheter, appropriate antiseptic or dermal disinfectant wipes, tape, and adhesive bandage. (B) An IV line with drip chamber and administration ports. (C) Saline solution. (D) A tourniquet is placed proximal to the antecubital fossa, and veins are visualized and palpated. (E) The skin is prepared with an antiseptic wipe. (F) The indwelling catheter is directed toward a vein with the bevel of the needle facing up. (G) The needle with catheter is advanced into the vein (notice the blood flashback).   *Continued*

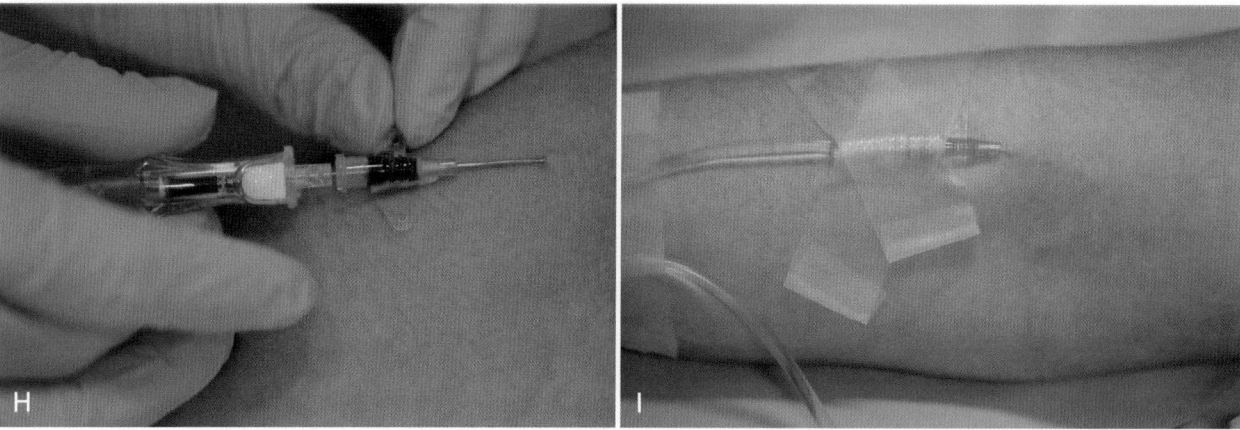

Fig. 38.5, cont'd (H) The catheter is advanced, and the needle is removed. (I) The IV line is connected, the tourniquet is removed, and the IV line is opened to check fluid flow and then secured with tape.

end-tidal CO_2 and auscultation of breath sounds must be immediately available.

Monitoring

For minimal sedation, a dentist or, at the dentist's direction, an appropriately trained individual must remain in the operating room during active dental treatment to monitor the patient continuously until he or she meets the criteria for discharge to the recovery area. The appropriately trained individual must be familiar with monitoring techniques and equipment.

In the case of moderate sedation, a dentist administering moderate sedation must remain in the room to monitor the patient continuously until he or she meets the criteria for recovery. When active treatment concludes and the patient recovers to a minimally sedated level, a qualified auxiliary may be directed by the dentist to remain with the patient and continue to monitor him or her as explained in the guidelines until discharged from the facility. The dentist must not leave the facility until the patient meets the criteria for discharge and is discharged to go home with a responsible adult (Box 38.5).

 KEY FACT

For moderate sedation, a dentist administering moderate sedation must remain in the operation room to monitor the patient continuously until he or she meets the criteria for recovery. When the patient recovers to a minimally sedated level, a qualified auxiliary person may be directed by the dentist to remain and monitor the patient until he or she meets the criteria for discharge. The dentist must not leave the facility until the patient meets the criteria for discharge and is discharged to home with a responsible adult.

Vital signs, level of sedation, and oxygen perfusion must be continuously monitored throughout the conscious sedation procedure. There are many methods of monitoring.

Circulation

For minimal sedation, blood pressure and heart rate should be evaluated preoperatively, postoperatively, and intraoperatively as necessary. For moderate sedation, the dentist must continually evaluate blood pressure and heart rate unless invalidated by the nature of the patient, procedure, or equipment, and this information is noted in the time-oriented anesthesia record. Continuous electrocardiographic monitoring

BOX 38.5 Discharge Criteria
Alertness: patient able to answer three simple questions
Who is driving you home?
Where are you?
What day is it?
Breathing
Normal oxygen saturation on room air
Able to breathe deeply and cough
Circulation
Systolic blood pressure within 20% of baseline
Ambulation
Able to walk with minimal assistance
Color
Normal skin color and appearance

should be considered for patients with significant cardiovascular disease. All-in-one monitors with printers can efficiently perform these functions.

Consciousness

The level of consciousness or sedation (e.g., responsiveness to verbal command) must be continually assessed. In 1990, Chernik and colleagues[8a] developed the Observer's Assessment of Alertness/Sedation Scale (Table 38.3), which has been used in many studies to evaluate the degree of alertness of patients undergoing sedation. The method developed by Dr. Katherine Wilson and coworkers in 2011 at the Newcastle University School of Dental Sciences is also an efficient method for assessing the level of sedation.[71]

Ventilation and Oxygenation

For minimal sedation, the dentist or appropriately trained individual must observe chest movements and verify respirations. Oxygen saturation by pulse oximetry may be clinically useful and should be considered. For moderate sedation, the dentist must observe chest movements continuously, and oxygen saturation must be evaluated continuously by pulse oximetry. Ventilation or breathing can also be assessed by monitoring end-tidal CO_2 (i.e., capnography). Ventilation should be monitored by continual observation of qualitative signs, including auscultation of breath sounds with a precordial or pretracheal stethoscope.

TABLE 38.3 Observer's Assessment of the Alertness/Sedation Scale

Category	Observation	Score[a]
Responsiveness	Responds readily to name spoken in normal tone	5
	Lethargic response to name spoken in normal tone	4
	Responds only after name is called loudly and/or repeatedly	3
	Responds only after mild prodding or shaking	2
	Does not respond to mild prodding or shaking	1
Speech	Normal	5
	Mild slowing or thickening	4
	Slurring or prominent slowing	3
	Few recognizable words	2
Facial expression	Normal	5
	Mild relaxation	4
	Marked relaxation (slack jaw)	3
Eyes	Clear, no ptosis	5
	Glazed or mild ptosis (less than half of the eye)	4
	Glazed and marked ptosis (half of the eye or more)	3

[a]This scored is used to evaluate the level of sedation.
Modified from Chernik DA, Gillings D, Laine H, et al: Validity and reliability of the Observer's Assessment of Alertness/Sedation Scale: study with intravenous midazolam, *J Clin Psychopharmacol* 10:244–251, 1990.

TABLE 38.4 Arterial Oxyhemoglobin Saturation and Oxygen Tension Values for Monitoring Tissue Oxygenation

Oximeter Arterial Oxyhemoglobin Saturation (SpO_2)	Arterial Oxygen Tension (PaO_2)	Interpretation
95%–99%	80–100 mm Hg	Normal oxygenation
90%	60 mm Hg	Alarm goes off; patient is hypoxemic
80%	45–50 mm Hg	Severe hypoxemia

The color of the mucosa, skin, or blood must be evaluated continuously to assess oxygenation. Oxygen saturation by pulse oximetry is clinically useful and should be considered for minimal sedation. For moderate sedation, oxygen saturation must be continuously evaluated by pulse oximetry. Approximately 98% to 99% of the total oxygen content in arterial blood is bound to hemoglobin in red blood cells. The pulse oximeter measures the degree to which hemoglobin is saturated with oxygen (SpO_2). The remaining 1% to 2% of oxygen is dissolved in plasma and produces a gas pressure referred to as arterial oxygen tension (PaO_2). The PaO_2 level is what determines how much oxygen is entering the body tissues and is referred to as *oxygenation*. Normally, the SpO_2 level is at 98% to 99% and sustains a PaO_2 level of about 95%. Normal oxygenation is defined as a PaO_2 of 80 to 100 mm Hg. There is a nonlinear relationship between SpO_2 and PaO_2. SpO_2 readings of 95% and higher maintain PaO_2 at or above 80 mm Hg and prevent hypoxemia (Table 38.4).

Capnography

Adequate ventilation and respiration can be monitored by assessing end-tidal CO_2 using capnography. This method monitors CO_2 concentrations in exhaled respiratory gases. A capnography monitor provides a graphic representation of the partial pressure of CO_2 and is more effective than other clinical assessments of ventilation.[62] A report of a randomized controlled clinical trial of patients undergoing moderate sedation demonstrated that capnography improved patient monitoring, with earlier detection of respiratory compromise prompting intervention to minimize hypoxemia compared with other care methods.[42]

> ### CLINICAL CORRELATION
>
> A capnography monitor provides a measure of exhaled CO_2 that is more effective than pulse oximetry. It provides an immediate alarm for life-threatening breathing problems during moderate sedation. Pulse oximeters, which have been the standard of care, take much longer to register respiratory distress because oxygen levels in the blood can remain normal for several minutes after a patient stops breathing. Capnography provides earlier detection.

Documentation

An appropriate, time-oriented anesthetic record (Fig. 38.6) must be maintained with the names of all administered drugs (including local anesthetics) along with dosages, times administered, and routes of administration. Physiologic parameters, including heart rate, respiratory rate, blood pressure, and level of consciousness, must be recorded. For moderate sedation, oxygen saturation (i.e., pulse oximetry) must be monitored and recorded continually. The anesthesia record should also include BMI, Mallampati classification, and capnography information.

Recovery and Discharge

Oxygen and suction equipment must be immediately available in the treatment room and the recovery room (if a separate recovery area is used). The qualified dentist or appropriately trained clinical staff must continually monitor the patient's blood pressure, heart rate, and respiration. In cases of moderate sedation, oxygen saturation and level of consciousness must be evaluated continuously. The qualified dentist must determine and document that the levels of consciousness, oxygenation, ventilation, and circulation are satisfactory before discharge (see Box 38.5). Postoperative verbal and written instruction must be given to the patient and a responsible adult (e.g., parent, escort, guardian, or caregiver).

If a reversal agent is administered before discharge criteria have been met, the patient must be monitored until recovery is ensured. A potential problem when using reversal agents is the possibility that the duration of action of the reversal agent can be shorter than the sedative agent used, and the patient can become sedated again. It is critical for the clinician to understand and appreciate the duration of action of all sedative and reversal agents used.

Sedation Failures

When performing outpatient mild or moderate sedation, the clinician must realize that sedation will not be 100% effective for all patients. A certain percentage of patients will not respond appropriately to minimal or moderate sedation protocols (Table 38.5). If a patient is not responding to the sedation procedure, it is extremely hazardous to go beyond dose limits or to attempt putting the patient into a

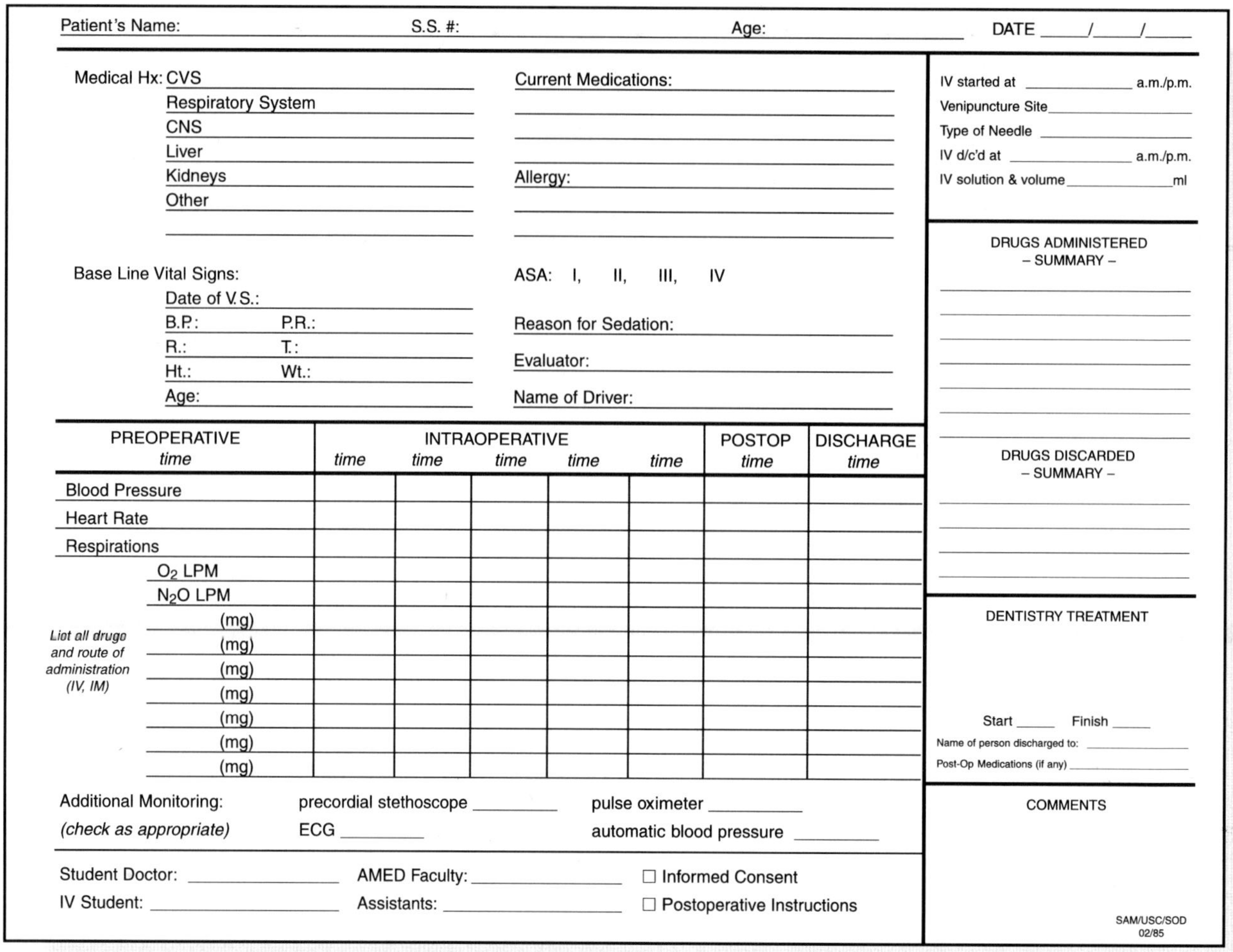

Patient's Name: S.S. #: Age: DATE ___/___/___

Medical Hx: CVS
Respiratory System
CNS
Liver
Kidneys
Other

Current Medications:

Allergy:

IV started at ______ a.m./p.m.
Venipuncture Site
Type of Needle
IV d/c'd at ______ a.m./p.m.
IV solution & volume ______ ml

DRUGS ADMINISTERED – SUMMARY –

Base Line Vital Signs:
Date of V.S.:
B.P.: P.R.:
R.: T.:
Ht.: Wt.:
Age:

ASA: I, II, III, IV

Reason for Sedation:

Evaluator:

Name of Driver:

PREOPERATIVE time	INTRAOPERATIVE time	time	time	time	time	POSTOP time	DISCHARGE time
Blood Pressure							
Heart Rate							
Respirations							
O_2 LPM							
N_2O LPM							
(mg)							
(mg)							
(mg)							
(mg)							
(mg)							
(mg)							
(mg)							

List all drugs and route of administration (IV, IM)

DRUGS DISCARDED – SUMMARY –

DENTISTRY TREATMENT

Start ____ Finish ____
Name of person discharged to:
Post-Op Medications (if any)

Additional Monitoring: precordial stethoscope ______ pulse oximeter ______
(check as appropriate) ECG ______ automatic blood pressure ______

COMMENTS

Student Doctor: AMED Faculty: ☐ Informed Consent
IV Student: Assistants: ☐ Postoperative Instructions

SAM/USC/SOD 02/85

Fig. 38.6 Example of a moderate sedation record. *(From Malamed SF:* Sedation: a guide to patient management, *5th ed, St. Louis, 2010, Elsevier.)*

TABLE 38.5 Sedation Failure in Dentistry by Route of Administration

Technique	Expected Failure Rate (%)
Oral (child, older)	40–50
Oral (child, younger)	50–65
Oral (adult)	20–50
Inhalation	15–20
Oral + inhalation	5–10
Intravenous	4.3–5
Oral + intravenous	2–3
Deep sedation/general anesthesia	1.6

Data from Malamed SF: Sedation and safety: 36 years of perspective *Alpha Omegan* 99:70–74, 2006; Senel FC, Buchanan JM Jr, Senel AC, et al: Evaluation of sedation failure in the outpatient oral and maxillofacial surgery clinic. *J Oral Maxillofac Surg* 65:645–650, 2007; Skehan SJ, Malone DE, Buckley N, et al: Sedation and analgesia in adult patients: evaluation of a staged-dose system based on body weight for use in abdominal interventional radiology. *Radiology* 216:653–659, 2000; Wilson KE, Thorpe RJ, McCabe JF, Girdler NM: Complications associated with intravenous midazolam sedation in anxious dental patients. *Primary Dental Care* 18:161–166, 2011.

deeper level of sedation. It is best to abort the procedure and reschedule the appointment for another day, with a different technique or with a dental anesthesiologist.

Emergency Preparedness

Because sedation and general anesthesia are on a continuum of drug-induced depression of consciousness to loss of consciousness, it is not always possible to predict how an individual patient will respond. Practitioners intending to produce a given level of sedation should be able to diagnose and manage the physiologic consequences for patients whose level of sedation becomes deeper than initially intended (i.e., rescue). For all levels of sedation, the practitioner must have the training, skills, drugs, and equipment to identify and manage such an occurrence until assistance arrives (i.e., emergency medical service) or the patient returns to the intended level of sedation without airway or cardiovascular complications. The qualified dentist is responsible for sedation management, adequacy of the facility, competence of the staff, diagnosis and treatment of emergencies related to the administration of sedation, and providing and maintaining the equipment and protocols for patient rescue.

If a patient enters a deeper level of sedation than the dentist is qualified to provide, the dentist must stop the procedure and focus attention on the patient until his or her condition returns to the intended level of sedation. This can involve monitoring the patient, providing airway management and support, administering reversal agents, or activating the emergency medical service. The qualified dentist is responsible for sedative management, adequacy of the facility and staff, diagnosis and treatment of emergencies related to the administration of minimal or moderate sedation, and providing the equipment, drugs, and protocol for patient rescue.

Conclusions

As periodontal procedures become more complex, there is an increased need for the use of conscious sedation techniques for patients with fear and anxiety. The ADA guidelines and policy are outlined in documents that need to be followed. Mild sedation with N_2O inhalation techniques must be used with appropriate patient monitoring. The doctor should have a minimum of 14 hours of instruction, including a clinical component.

After appropriate recovery, patients usually can be allowed to function normally and do not need another adult to monitor them. Mild sedation using oral agents, such as triazolam in one dose, should not exceed the MRD for home use, but after recovery, these patients cannot drive and need another adult to supervise them.

Moderate to deep sedation should be performed only by practitioners with appropriate postdoctoral training in an accredited advanced education program, which carries additional responsibilities for patient monitoring, restrictions on food and liquid intake, recovery, and additional trained support staff.

Patients with systemic problems should get preoperative evaluations from a physician, and elderly patients frequently need downward adjustments of normal dosage. Children require special care from trained doctors, and preoperative sedation in children younger than 12 years of age should be carried out by specialists in pediatric anesthesia. Patients with significant systemic problems are best treated in a hospital environment rather than in an outpatient surgical center.

 A Case Scenarios is found on the companion website www.expertconsult.com.

References

 References for this chapter are found on the companion website www.expertconsult.com.

CHAPTER 39

Periodontal Treatment of Medically Compromised Patients

Perry R. Klokkevold | Brian L. Mealey | Joan Otomo-Corgel

CHAPTER OUTLINE

Cardiovascular Diseases
Endocrine Disorders
Hemorrhagic Disorders
Renal Diseases *(e-only)*

Liver Diseases *(e-only)*
Pulmonary Diseases *(e-only)*
Medications and Cancer Therapies
Prosthetic Joint Replacement

Pregnancy *(e-only)*
Infectious Diseases *(e-only)*

 Content on thyroid and parathyroid disorders, adrenal insufficiency, thrombocytopenic purpuras, nonthrombocytopenic purpuras, blood dyscrasias, renal diseases, liver diseases, and pulmonary diseases can be accessed on the companion website at www.expertconsult.com.

Many patients seeking dental care have significant medical conditions that can alter the course of their oral disease and the therapy provided. Older periodontal patients are more likely to have underlying disease. The therapeutic responsibility of the clinician includes identification of the patient's medical problems to formulate a proper treatment plan. A thorough medical history is paramount.[81] If significant findings are unveiled, consultation with or referral of the patient to an appropriate physician is indicated. This ensures correct management and provides medicolegal coverage for the clinician.

This chapter covers common medical conditions and associated periodontal management. The review of each topic area can be supplemented by consulting other references for more detailed coverage of specific disorders. Understanding these conditions enables the clinician to treat the total patient, not merely the periodontal reflection of underlying disease.

Cardiovascular Diseases

Cardiovascular diseases are the most prevalent category of systemic disease in the United States and many other countries, and they are more common with increasing age.[113] Health histories should be closely scrutinized for cardiovascular problems, including hypertension, angina pectoris, myocardial infarction (MI), cardiac bypass surgery, cerebrovascular accident (CVA), congestive heart failure (CHF), infective endocarditis (IE), and implanted cardiac pacemakers or automatic cardioverter-defibrillators.

In most cases, the patient's physician should be consulted, especially if stressful or prolonged treatment is anticipated. Short appointments and a calm, relaxing environment help minimize stress and maintain hemodynamic stability.

Hypertension

Hypertension, the most common cardiovascular disease, affects more than 50 million American adults, many of whom are undiagnosed.[37]

In 2003, the National Heart, Lung, and Blood Institute issued revised guidelines for evaluation and management of hypertension.[18,38,47] The Seventh Report of the Joint National Committee on Prevention, Detection, Evaluation, and Treatment of High Blood Pressure (JNC-7 guidelines[18]) simplified the classification of blood pressure (Table 39.1).

Compared with previous classification schemes[43,44] that focused on diastolic blood pressure (BP), the JNC-7 guidelines[18] emphasize the importance of systolic BP. Systolic BP greater than 140 mm Hg is considered a greater risk factor for cardiovascular disease than elevated diastolic pressure. JNC-7 also introduced a category known as *prehypertension* to replace the more innocuous terms *high normal* and *borderline* hypertension. People with systolic BP between 120 and 139 mm Hg or diastolic BP between 80 and 89 mm Hg are classified as prehypertensive. It is not considered a disease category or diagnosis; it is instead a term used to describe a condition and identify individuals who are at high risk for hypertension.

The JNC-7 guidelines classify hypertension into two categories, versus the three under the previous classification schemes, for simplicity and because treatment for categories 2 and 3 was essentially the same. *Stage 1 hypertension* is defined as a systolic BP of 140 to 159 mm Hg or diastolic pressure of 90 to 99 mm Hg. *Stage 2 hypertension* is defined as a systolic pressure greater than 160 mm Hg or diastolic pressure greater than 100 mm Hg.

Hypertension is not diagnosed from a single elevated BP recording. Rather, classification is usually based on the average value of two or more BP readings taken at two or more appointments. The higher systolic or diastolic pressure determines the patient's classification. Patients with hypertension enter dental practices every day, and hypertension is particularly common among the older population seen in most periodontal practices. Evidence from the Framingham Heart Study revealed that people with normal BP at age 55 still have a 90% risk of becoming hypertensive later in life.[115]

Hypertension is divided into primary and secondary types. *Primary* (i.e., essential) *hypertension* occurs when no underlying pathologic

TABLE 39.1 Classification of Adult Blood Pressure

Classification	Systolic (mm Hg)	Diastolic (mm Hg)	Dental Treatment Modifications
Normal	<120	<80	No changes in dental treatment
Prehypertension	120–139	80–89	No changes in dental treatment Monitor BP at each appointment
Stage 1 hypertension	140–159	90–99	Inform patient of findings Medical consultation or referral Monitor BP at each appointment No changes in dental treatment; minimize stress
Stage 2 hypertension	≥160	≥100	Inform patient Medical consultation or referral Monitor BP at each appointment If systolic BP is <180 mm Hg and diastolic is <110 mm Hg, perform selective dental care (i.e., routine examination, prophylaxis, restorative nonsurgical endodontics and periodontics); minimize stress If systolic BP ≥180 mm Hg or diastolic ≥100 mm Hg, give immediate medical consultation or referral and perform emergency dental care only (to alleviate pain, bleeding, infection),[a] minimize stress Consider stress-reduction protocol

[a]Risk of providing emergency dental care must outweigh risk of possible hypertensive complications.[18,38,47]
BP, Blood pressure.

abnormality can be found to explain the disease. Approximately 95% of hypertensive patients have primary hypertension. The remaining 5% have *secondary hypertension,* in which an underlying cause can be found and is often treated. Conditions responsible for secondary hypertension include renal disease, endocrinologic changes, and neurogenic disorders.

In early hypertension, the patient may be asymptomatic. If not identified, diagnosed, and treated, hypertension can persist and increase in severity, leading eventually to coronary artery disease, angina, MI, CHF, CVA, or kidney failure.[55] The dental office can play a vital role in the detection of hypertension and maintenance care of the patient with hypertensive disease. The first dental office visit should include two BP readings spaced at least 10 minutes apart, which are averaged and used as a baseline. Before the clinician refers a patient to a physician because of elevated BP, readings should be taken at a minimum of two appointments, unless the measurements are extremely high (i.e., systolic pressure >180 mm Hg or diastolic pressure >100 mm Hg).

The periodontal recall system is an ideal method for hypertension detection and monitoring. Almost three of every four adult patients with hypertension in the United States do not control their BP well enough to attain the goal of systolic pressure less than 140 mm Hg and diastolic pressure less than 90 mm Hg.[14] Lack of compliance with antihypertensive therapy is the primary reason for this failure. Dentists can help achieve greater success in managing hypertension by taking BP readings at each periodontal recall visit.

Periodontal procedures should not be performed until accurate BP measurements and histories have been taken to identify patients with significant hypertensive disease. The time of day should be recorded because BP varies significantly throughout the day.[73] Table 39.1 outlines appropriate medical referral or consultation and dental treatment modifications, depending on the patient's stage of hypertension.

Dental treatment for hypertensive patients is safe as long as stress is minimized.[55,61] If a patient is receiving antihypertensive therapy, consultation with the physician may be warranted regarding the current medical status, medications, periodontal treatment plan, and

patient care. Many physicians are not knowledgeable about the specific details of dental or periodontal procedures. The dentist must inform the physician regarding the estimated degree of stress, length of the procedures, and complexity of the individualized treatment plan. Morning dental appointments were once suggested for hypertensive patients, but evidence indicates that BP usually increases around awakening and peaks at midmorning.[10,73,103] Because lower BP levels occur in the afternoon, afternoon dental appointments may be preferred.

No routine periodontal treatment should be given to a patient who is hypertensive and not under medical management. For patients with systolic BP greater than 180 mm Hg or diastolic BP greater than 110 mm Hg, treatment should be limited to emergency care until hypertension is controlled. Analgesics are prescribed for pain and antibiotics for infection. Acute infections may require surgical incision and drainage, although the surgical field should be limited because excessive bleeding can occur with elevated BP.

When treating hypertensive patients, the clinician should not use a local anesthetic containing an epinephrine concentration greater than 1:100,000 or a vasopressor to control local bleeding. Local anesthesia without epinephrine can be used for short procedures (<30 minutes). In a patient with hypertensive disease, however, it is important to minimize pain by providing profound local anesthesia to avoid an increase in endogenous epinephrine secretion.[55,61]

The benefits of the small doses of epinephrine used in dentistry far outweigh the potential for hemodynamic compromise. The smallest possible dose of epinephrine should be used, and aspiration before injection of local anesthetics is critical. Intraligamentary injection is usually contraindicated because hemodynamic changes are similar to intravascular injection.[102] If the hypertensive patient exhibits anxiety, use of conscious sedation in conjunction with periodontal procedures may be warranted[111] (see Chapter 38).

β-adrenergic receptor antagonists (i.e., β-blockers) are typically used to treat hypertension (Table 39.2). The β-blockers are *cardioselective,* blocking only β1 cardiac receptors (i.e., β1 receptors), or *nonselective,* blocking both β1 cardiac receptors and β2 peripheral

TABLE 39.2   Nonselective and Selective β-Adrenergic Receptor Antagonists

Generic Name	Trade Name
Nonselective β-Blockers	
Carvedilol	Coreg
Carteolol hydrochloride	Cartrol
Nadolol	Corgard
Penbutolol sulfate	Levatol
Pindolol	Visken
Propranolol hydrochloride	Inderal; Inderal LA
Timolol maleate	Blocadren
Selective β-Blockers	
Acebutolol hydrochloride	Sectral
Atenolol	Tenormin
Betaxolol hydrochloride	Kerlone
Bisoprolol fumarate	Zebeta
Metoprolol tartrate	Lopressor
Metoprolol succinate	Toprol-XL

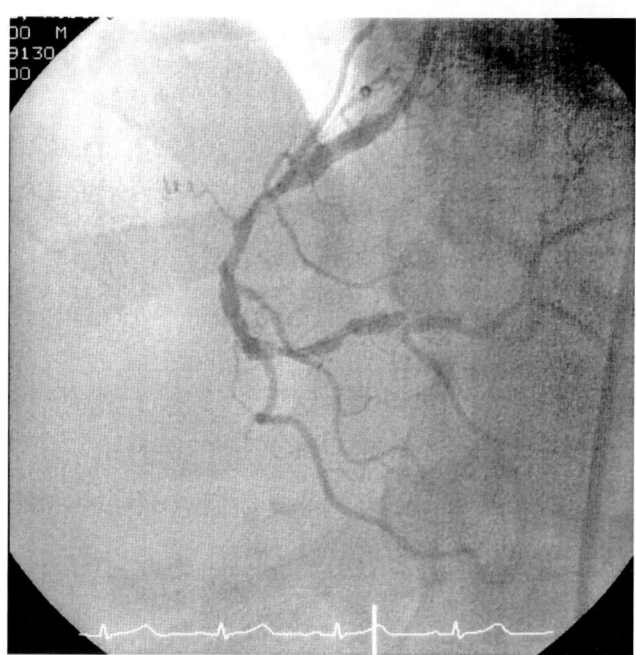

Fig. 39.1 As seen on a coronary angiogram, atherosclerosis can result in narrowing of the coronary arteries, producing signs and symptoms of ischemic heart disease.

receptors (i.e., β2 receptors). Epinephrine, an α-adrenergic and β-adrenergic agonist, increases heart rate through direct stimulation of cardiac β1 receptors. Epinephrine also stimulates α-adrenergic receptors, producing vasoconstriction of arteries, and β2 receptors, causing vasodilation of skeletal muscle arterioles.

Administration of local anesthetics containing epinephrine to patients taking nonselective β-blockers (e.g., propranolol, nadolol) can elevate BP.[127] Epinephrine-induced α-adrenergic stimulation results in vasoconstriction and increased BP. Because the patient's nonselective medication has blocked the β2 receptors, epinephrine cannot stimulate the normal compensatory β2 receptor–induced vasodilation. This can result in dramatically increased BP, followed by reflex bradycardia mediated by the vagus nerve and carotid baroreceptors. The end result is a patient with severe hypertension and bradycardia, producing a dangerous decrease in vascular perfusion and possibly causing death. Because of this potential complication, epinephrine-containing local anesthetics should be used cautiously and only in very small amounts in patients taking nonselective β-blockers, with careful monitoring of vital signs.[55,127]

The clinician should be aware of the many side effects of antihypertensive medications. *Postural hypotension* is common and can be minimized by slow positional changes in the dental chair.[55] *Depression* is a side effect of which many patients are unaware. Nausea, sedation, oral dryness, lichenoid drug reactions, and gingival overgrowth are associated with certain classes of antihypertensive agents.[61]

CLINICAL CORRELATION

Hypertension, the most common cardiovascular disease, affects more than 50 million American adults, many of whom are undiagnosed. Almost three of every four adults with hypertension do not control their blood pressure well enough. The dental office can play a vital role in the detection of undiagnosed hypertension and the compliance of patients being treated for hypertension. Blood pressure should be taken at the initial visit and at each recall visit.

Ischemic Heart Diseases

Ischemic heart disease (Fig. 39.1) includes disorders such as angina pectoris and MI. Angina pectoris occurs when myocardial oxygen demand exceeds supply, resulting in temporary myocardial ischemia.[38] Patients with a history of unstable angina pectoris (i.e., angina that occurs irregularly or on multiple occasions without predisposing factors) should be treated only for emergencies and then in consultation with their physician. Patients with stable angina (i.e., angina that occurs infrequently, is associated with exertion or stress, and is easily controlled with medication and rest) can undergo elective dental procedures. Because stress often induces an acute anginal attack, stress reduction is important. Profound local anesthesia is vital, and conscious sedation may be indicated for anxious patients[111] (see Chapter 38). Supplemental oxygen delivered by nasal cannula can help prevent intraoperative anginal attacks.

Patients who manage acute anginal attacks with nitroglycerin should be instructed to bring their medication to dental appointments. Nitroglycerin should also be kept in the office medical emergency kit. For particularly stressful procedures, the patient may take a nitroglycerin tablet preoperatively to prevent angina, although this usually is not necessary. The patient's nitroglycerin should be readily accessible on the dental tray in case it is needed during treatment. Because the shelf life of nitroglycerin is relatively short, the expiration date of the patient's nitroglycerin and that of the nitroglycerin in the office's medical emergency kit should be noted.

Patients with angina may be taking longer-acting forms of nitroglycerin (e.g., tablet, patch), β-blockers, or calcium channel blockers (also used for treating hypertension) for prevention of angina. Restrictions on the use of local anesthetics containing epinephrine are similar to those for the patient with hypertension. Intraosseous injection with epinephrine-containing local anesthetics using special systems (e.g., Stabident, Fairfax Dental) should be done cautiously in patients with ischemic heart disease because it results in transient increases in heart rate and myocardial oxygen demand.[78]

If the patient becomes fatigued or uncomfortable or has a sudden change in heart rhythm or rate during a periodontal procedure, the procedure should be discontinued as soon as possible. A patient who has an anginal episode in the dental chair should receive the following emergency medical treatment:

1. Discontinue the periodontal procedure.
2. Administer 1 tablet (0.3 to 0.6 mg) of nitroglycerin sublingually.
3. Reassure the patient, and loosen restrictive garments.
4. Administer oxygen with the patient in a reclined position.
5. If the signs and symptoms cease within 3 minutes, complete the periodontal procedure if possible, making sure that the patient is comfortable. Terminate the procedure at the earliest convenient time.
6. If the anginal signs and symptoms do not resolve with this treatment within 5 minutes, administer another dose of nitroglycerin, monitor the patient's vital signs, call the patient's physician, and be ready to accompany the patient to the emergency department.
7. A third nitroglycerin tablet can be given 5 minutes after the second. Chest pain that is not relieved by three tablets of nitroglycerin indicates likely MI. The patient should be transported to the nearest emergency medical facility immediately.

Nitroglycerin lingual spray formulations have been popular in hospital pharmacies because of the increased shelf life compared with nitroglycerin tablets.[72] The lingual spray can provide greater and more rapid vasodilation with a longer duration of action.[25,86] The convenience and advantages of a nitroglycerin lingual spray are appealing, but the accuracy of dose delivery has been questioned and warrants additional studies before the spray can be recommended to replace the known tablet regimen.[72]

MI is the other category of ischemic heart disease encountered in dental practice. Dental treatment is usually deferred for at least 6 months after MI because the peak mortality rate occurs during this time.[30] After 6 months, MI patients can usually be treated using techniques similar to those for stable angina patients.

Cardiac (aortocoronary) bypass, femoral artery bypass, angioplasty, and endarterectomy have become common surgical procedures in patients with ischemic heart disease. If one of these procedures was performed recently, the physician should be consulted before elective dental therapy to determine the degree of heart damage or arterial occlusive disease, the stability of the patient's condition, and the potential for infective endocarditis or graft rejection. Prophylactic antibiotics are not usually necessary for cardiac bypass patients unless recommended by the cardiologist.

Congestive Heart Failure

CHF is a condition in which the pump function of the heart is unable to supply sufficient amounts of oxygenated blood to meet the body's needs.[30] CHF usually begins with left ventricular failure caused by a disproportion between the hemodynamic load and the capacity to handle that load. CHF can be caused by a chronic increase in workload (as in hypertension or aortic, mitral, pulmonary, or tricuspid valvular disease), direct damage to the myocardium (as in MI or rheumatic fever), or an increase in the body's oxygen requirements (as in anemia, thyrotoxicosis, or pregnancy).

Patients with poorly controlled or untreated CHF are not candidates for elective dental procedures. These individuals are at risk for sudden death, usually from ventricular arrhythmias.[29] For patients with treated CHF, the clinician should consult with the physician regarding the severity of CHF, underlying cause, and current medical management. Medical management of CHF can include the use of calcium channel blockers, direct vasodilators, diuretics, angiotensin-converting enzyme (ACE) inhibitors, α-receptor blockers, or cardiotonic agents such as digoxin.[27,46] Each medication has potential side effects that can affect periodontal therapy. Because of orthopnea (i.e., inability to breathe unless in an upright position) in some CHF patients,

the dental chair should be adjusted to a comfortable level for the patient rather than placed in a supine position. Short appointments, stress reduction with profound local anesthesia and possibly conscious sedation, and use of supplemental oxygen should be considered.[30,55]

Cardiac Pacemakers and Implantable Cardioverter-Defibrillators

Cardiac arrhythmias are most often treated with medications, but some are also treated with implantable pacemakers or automatic cardioverter-defibrillators.[29,55,80] Pacemakers are usually implanted in the chest wall and enter the heart transvenously. Automatic cardioverter-defibrillators are more often implanted subcutaneously near the umbilicus and have electrodes passing into the heart transvenously or directly attached to the epicardium. Consultation with the patient's physician allows determination of the underlying cardiac status, the type of pacemaker or automatic cardioverter-defibrillator, and any precautionary measures to be taken.

Older pacemakers were unipolar and could be disrupted by dental equipment that generated electromagnetic fields, such as ultrasonic and electrocautery units. Newer units are bipolar and are usually not affected by dental equipment. Automatic cardioverter-defibrillators activate without warning when certain arrhythmias occur. This can endanger the patient during dental treatment because activation often causes sudden patient movement. Stabilization of the operating field during periodontal treatment with bite blocks or other devices can prevent unexpected trauma.

Infective Endocarditis

Infective endocarditis (IE) is a disease in which microorganisms colonize damaged endocardium or heart valves.[32] Although the incidence of IE is low, it is a serious disease with a poor prognosis despite modern therapy. The term *infective endocarditis* is preferred to the previous term *bacterial endocarditis* because the disease can also be caused by fungi and viruses. The organisms most often encountered in IE are α-hemolytic streptococci (e.g., *Streptococcus viridans*). However, nonstreptococcal organisms often found in the periodontal pocket have been increasingly implicated, including *Eikenella corrodens, Aggregatibacter actinomycetemcomitans, Capnocytophaga,* and *Lactobacillus* species.[8]

IE has been divided into acute and subacute forms. The acute form involves virulent organisms, usually nonhemolytic streptococci and strains of staphylococci, which invade normal cardiac tissue, produce septic emboli, and cause infections that run a rapid, usually fatal course. The subacute form results from colony formation on damaged endocardium or heart valves by low-grade pathogenic organisms. The classic example is rheumatic carditis from rheumatic fever.

Since the last American Heart Association (AHA) publication on prevention of IE in 1997,[22] many have questioned the efficacy of antimicrobial prophylaxis to prevent IE in patients who undergo dental or other procedures and have suggested that the AHA guidelines should be revised.[26,105] Members of the Rheumatic Fever, Endocarditis, and Kawasaki Disease Committee of the AHA Council on Cardiovascular Disease in the Young and a national and international group of experts on IE extensively reviewed data published on the prevention of IE. The committee concluded that only an extremely small number of IE cases might be prevented by antibiotic prophylaxis for dental procedures (even if such therapy were 100% effective). Consequently, the guidelines were changed and published in a 2008 report.[125] The new guidelines advise that IE prophylaxis should be recommended only for cardiac conditions with the highest risk of adverse outcome from IE (Box 39.1). For these patients, antibiotic prophylaxis is recommended for all dental procedures that involve manipulation of the gingival or periapical tissues, or perforation of the oral mucosa. Antibiotic prophylaxis is not indicated for individuals on the basis of an increased lifetime risk of contracting IE.

The practice of periodontics is intimately concerned with the prevention of IE. However, bacteremia may occur even in the absence of dental procedures, especially in individuals with poor oral hygiene and significant periodontal inflammation. IE is much more likely to result from frequent exposure to random bacteremias associated with daily activities than be caused by a dental procedure.[125] Prevention of periodontal inflammation is paramount. The AHA states that patients who are at risk for IE should "establish and maintain the best possible oral health to reduce potential sources of bacterial seeding." To provide adequate preventive measures for IE, the clinician's major concern should be to reduce the microbial population in the oral cavity to minimize soft tissue inflammation and bacteremia.

BOX 39.1 Cardiac Conditions Associated With the Highest Risk of Adverse Outcome From Infective Endocarditis for Which Prophylaxis With Dental Procedures Is Recommended[a]

Previous history of infective endocarditis
Prosthetic cardiac valves or prosthetic material used for cardiac valve repair
Congenital heart disease (CHD), with the following conditions:
- Unrepaired cyanotic CHD, including palliative shunts and conduits
- Completely repaired congenital heart defect with prosthetic material or device, whether placed by surgery or catheter intervention, during the first 6 months after the procedure
- Repaired CHD with residual defects at or adjacent to the site of a prosthetic patch or prosthetic device (which inhibits endothelialization)

Cardiac transplantation recipients who develop cardiac valvulopathy

[a]American Heart Association recommendations.[125]
From Wilson W, Taubert KA, Gewitz M, et al: Prevention of infective endocarditis: guidelines from the American Heart Association Rheumatic Fever, Endocarditis, and Kawasaki Disease Committee, Council on Cardiovascular Disease in the Young, and the Council on Clinical Cardiology, Council on Cardiovascular Surgery and Anesthesia, and the Quality of Care and Outcomes Research Interdisciplinary Working Group. *Circulation*, 116:1736–1754, 2007.

KEY FACT

The updated American Heart Association (AHA) guidelines on the prevention of infective endocarditis (IE) were published in a 2008 report. The guidelines recommend that prophylaxis should be provided only for cardiac conditions with the highest risk of adverse outcomes from IE (see Box 39.1).

Preventive measures to reduce the risk of IE consist of the following:

1. *Define the susceptible patient.* A careful medical history can disclose a susceptible patient. Health questioning should cover the history in all categories of risk. If any doubt exists, the patient's physician should be consulted.

2. *Provide oral hygiene instruction.* Oral hygiene should be practiced with methods that improve gingival health. In patients with significant gingival inflammation, oral hygiene should initially be limited to gentle procedures (i.e., oral rinses and gentle toothbrushing with a soft brush) to minimize bleeding. As gingival health improves, more aggressive oral hygiene can be initiated. Oral irrigators are usually not recommended because their use can induce bacteremia.[67] Susceptible patients should be encouraged to maintain the highest level of oral hygiene after soft tissue inflammation is controlled.

3. *Recommended antibiotic prophylactic regimens should be practiced with all high-risk patients during periodontal treatment* (Table 39.3). If any doubt regarding susceptibility exists, the patient's physician should be consulted. In patients who have been receiving continuous oral penicillin for secondary prevention of rheumatic fever, penicillin-resistant α-hemolytic streptococci are occasionally found in the oral cavity. An alternate regimen is recommended instead. If the periodontal patient is taking a systemic antibiotic as part of periodontal therapy, changes in the IE prophylaxis regimen may be indicated. For example, a patient taking a penicillin agent after regenerative therapy can be placed on azithromycin before the next periodontal procedure. Patients with early-onset forms of periodontitis often have high levels of *A. actinomycetemcomitans* in the subgingival plaque. This organism has been associated with IE and is often resistant to penicillins. In patients with aggressive periodontitis who should be given prophylaxis, Slots and colleagues[101] suggested using tetracycline (250 mg four times daily for 14 days) to eliminate or reduce *A. actinomycetemcomitans*, followed by the conventional prophylaxis protocol at the time of dental treatment.

TABLE 39.3 Recommended Antibiotic Prophylaxis Regimens for Periodontal Procedures in Adults at Risk for Infective Endocarditis

Regimen	Antibiotic	Dosage[a]
Standard oral regimen	Amoxicillin	2.0 g 30–60 min before procedure
Alternate regimen for patients allergic to amoxicillin or penicillin	Clindamycin	600 mg 30–60 min before procedure
	Azithromycin or clarithromycin	500 mg 30–60 min before procedure
	or	
	Cephalexin or cefadroxil[b]	2.0 g 30–60 min before procedure
Regimen for patients unable to take oral medications	Ampicillin	2.0 g intramuscularly or intravenously within 30 min before procedure
Regimen for patients unable to take oral medications and allergic to penicillin	Clindamycin	600 mg intravenously within 30 min before procedure (must be diluted and injected slowly)
	or	
	Cefazolin[b]	1.0 g intramuscularly or intravenously within 30 min before procedure

[a]Adult dosages are listed. Children's dosages are lower.
[b]Cephalosporins should not be used in patients with immediate-type hypersensitivity reactions to penicillins (e.g., urticaria, angioedema, anaphylaxis).

4. *Periodontal treatment should be designed for susceptible patients to accommodate their degree of periodontal involvement.* The nature of periodontal therapy enhances the problems related to the prophylaxis of subacute IE. Patients are faced with long-term therapy, healing periods that extend beyond a 1-day antibiotic regimen, multiple visits, and procedures that easily elicit gingival bleeding.

The following guidelines can aid in the development of periodontal treatment plans for patients susceptible to IE:

- Periodontal disease is an infection with potentially wide-ranging systemic effects. For patients at risk for IE, every effort should be made to eliminate this infection. Teeth with severe periodontitis and a poor prognosis may require extraction. Teeth with less severe involvement in a motivated patient should be retained, treated, and maintained closely.
- All periodontal treatment procedures (including probing) require antibiotic prophylaxis; gentle oral hygiene methods are excluded. Pretreatment chlorhexidine rinses are recommended before all procedures, including periodontal probing, because these oral rinses significantly reduce the bacteria on mucosal surfaces.[22]
- To reduce the number of visits required and thereby minimize the risk of developing resistant bacteria, numerous procedures can be accomplished at each appointment, depending on the patient's needs and ability to tolerate dental treatment.[55]
- When possible, allow at least 7 days between appointments (preferably 10 to 14 days). If this is not possible, select an alternative antibiotic regimen for appointments within a 7-day period.
- Evidence does not support or refute a need to place patients at risk for IE on extended antibiotic regimens after treatment.[55] Patients who have had periodontal surgery are not usually placed on antibiotics for the first week of healing unless there are specific indications to do so. If patients are placed on these regimens, the dosages are inadequate to prevent endocarditis during ensuing appointments. The standard prophylactic antibiotic dose is still needed. For example, if a patient was placed on 250 mg of amoxicillin three times a day for 10 days after periodontal surgery and was to return to the office for more treatment on the seventh day, the patient would require a full 2.0-g dose of amoxicillin before that treatment. Alternatively, clindamycin or azithromycin could be used at the second appointment.
- Regular recall appointments, with an emphasis on oral hygiene reinforcement and maintenance of periodontal health, are extremely important for patients susceptible to IE.

Cerebrovascular Accident

A CVA (i.e., stroke) results from ischemic changes (e.g., cerebral thrombosis caused by an embolus) or hemorrhagic phenomena. Hypertension and atherosclerosis are predisposing factors for CVA and should alert the clinician to evaluate the patient's medical history carefully for the possibility of early cerebrovascular insufficiency and to be aware of symptoms of the disease. A physician's referral should precede periodontal therapy if the signs and symptoms of early cerebrovascular insufficiency are evident.

To prevent a repeat stroke, active infections should be treated aggressively, because even a minor infection can alter blood coagulation and trigger thrombus formation and ensuing cerebral infarction. The clinician should counsel the patient about the importance of thorough oral hygiene.[82] Post-stroke weakness of the facial area or paralysis of extremities can make oral hygiene procedures extremely difficult.[66] The clinician may need to modify oral hygiene instruments for ease of use, perhaps in consultation with an occupational therapist. Long-term chlorhexidine rinses greatly aid in plaque control.

Dental clinicians should treat post-CVA patients with the following guidelines in mind:

1. No periodontal therapy (except for an emergency) should be performed for 6 months because of the high risk of recurrence during this period.
2. After 6 months, periodontal therapy can be performed during short appointments with an emphasis on minimizing stress. Profound local anesthesia should be obtained, using the minimal effective dose of local anesthetic agents. Concentrations of epinephrine greater than 1:100,000 are contraindicated.
3. Light conscious sedation (i.e., inhalation, oral, or parenteral) can be used for anxious patients. Supplemental oxygen is indicated to maintain thorough cerebral oxygenation.
4. Stroke patients are frequently placed on oral anticoagulants. Previously, it was thought that for procedures entailing significant bleeding, such as periodontal surgery or tooth extraction, the anticoagulant regimen might need adjustment, depending on the level of anticoagulation at which the patient is maintained. However, evidence regarding the risks of altering anticoagulation therapy suggests that it may be prudent to provide treatment without changing it (see Anticoagulant Medications). Any changes in anticoagulant therapy regimens for a stroke patient should be done in consultation with the patient's physician.
5. BP should be monitored carefully. Recurrence rates for CVAs are high, as are rates of associated functional deficits.

Endocrine Disorders

Diabetes

The diabetic patient requires special precautions before periodontal therapy. Type 1 diabetes was formerly known as insulin-dependent diabetes, and type 2 diabetes was referred to as non–insulin-dependent diabetes.[59] During the past decade, the medical management of diabetes has changed significantly in an effort to minimize the debilitating complications associated with this disease.[108,114] Blood glucose (i.e., glycemia) levels are more tightly managed through diet, oral agents, and insulin therapy.[56]

If the clinician detects intraoral signs of undiagnosed or poorly controlled diabetes, a thorough history is indicated.[77] The classic signs of diabetes include *polydipsia* (i.e., excessive thirst), *polyuria* (i.e., excessive urination), and *polyphagia* (i.e., excessive hunger, often with unexplained concurrent weight loss). If the patient has any of these signs or symptoms or the clinician suspects diabetes, further investigation with laboratory studies and physician consultation is indicated. Periodontal therapy has limited success in the setting of undiagnosed or poorly controlled diabetes.

If a patient is suspected of having undiagnosed diabetes, the following procedures should be performed:

1. Consult the patient's physician.
2. Analyze laboratory tests (Box 39.2), including fasting blood glucose and casual glucose test results.[5]
3. Rule out acute orofacial infection or severe dental infection; if present, provide emergency care immediately.
4. Establish the best possible oral health through nonsurgical debridement of plaque and calculus. Institute oral hygiene instruction. Limit more advanced care until the diagnosis has been established and good glycemic control obtained.

If a patient is known to have diabetes, it is critical that the level of glycemic control be established before initiating periodontal treatment. The fasting glucose and casual glucose tests provide snapshots of the blood glucose concentration at the time the blood was drawn; these tests reveal nothing about long-term glycemic control. The primary test used to assess glycemic control in a known

BOX 39.2   Diagnostic Criteria for Diabetes Mellitus

Diabetes mellitus can be diagnosed by any one of the following laboratory methods. Initial results using any method must be confirmed on a subsequent day.

1. Fasting plasma glucose level ≥126 mg/dL (≥7.0 mmol/L). *Fasting is defined as no caloric intake for at least 8 hours. The normal fasting glucose level is 70 to 100 mg/dL.*
2. Two-hour postprandial glucose level ≥200 mg/dL (≥11.1 mmol/L) during an oral glucose tolerance test. The test should be performed using a glucose load containing the equivalent of 75 g anhydrous glucose dissolved in water. The normal 2-hour postprandial glucose level is <140 mg/dL.
3. Glycated hemoglobin (HbA1c) value ≥6.5% (≥48 mmol/L). The test should be performed in a laboratory using a method that is certified by the National Glycohemoglobin Standardization Program (NGSP) and standardized according to the Diabetes Control and Complications Trial (DCCT) assay.[a]
4. Random plasma glucose level ≥200 mg/dL (≥11.1 mmol/L) for a patient with classic symptoms of hyperglycemia or hyperglycemic crisis, which include polyuria, polydipsia, and unexplained weight loss. Blood for casual glucose testing can be drawn without regard to the time since the last meal.

---

[a]In the absence of unequivocal hyperglycemia, results should be confirmed by repeat testing.
Data from American Diabetes Association: 2. Classification and diagnosis of diabetes. *Diabetes Care* 40(Suppl. 1):S11–S24, 2017.

BOX 39.3   Laboratory Evaluation of Diabetes Control by Glycated Hemoglobin (HbA1c) Assay Values

Normal	4%–6%
Good diabetes control	<7%
Moderate diabetes control	7%–8%
Action suggested to improve diabetes control	>8%

Data from American Diabetes Association: 2. Classification and diagnosis of diabetes. *Diabetes Care* 40(Suppl. 1):S11–S24, 2017.

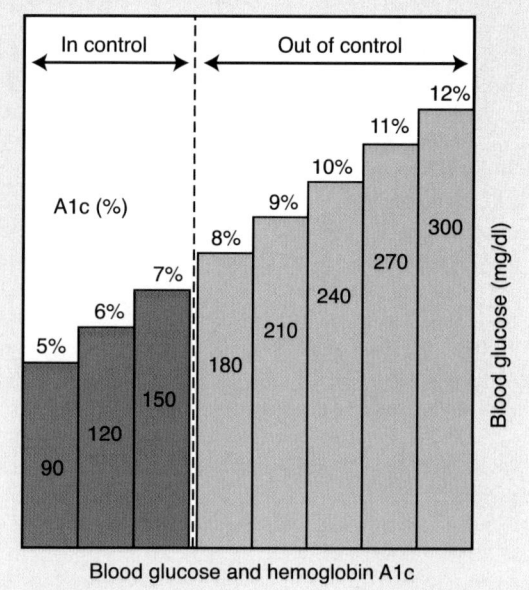

Fig. 39.2 Graphic representation of glycated hemoglobin (HbA1c) values that correspond to estimated average blood glucose levels.

diabetic individual is the glycated hemoglobin (Hb) assay (Box 39.3). Two tests are available, the HbA1 and HbA1c assays; the HbA1c is used more often.[56] This assay has been shown by a large international study to provide an accurate measure of the average blood glucose concentrations over the preceding 2 to 3 months.[64] Fig. 39.2 is a simplified graphic representation of the data from that study depicting the average blood glucose concentrations for HbA1c values.

The therapeutic goal for many patients is to achieve and maintain an HbA1c below 8%. Patients with relatively well-controlled diabetes (HbA1c <8%) usually respond to therapy in a manner similar to nondiabetic individuals.[19,107,124] Poorly controlled patients (HbA1c >10%) often have a poor response to treatment, with more postoperative complications and less favorable long-term results[59,107] (see Fig. 14.3 in Chapter 14). Improvements in HBA1c values after periodontal therapy may provide an indication of the potential response.

As discussed in Chapter 14, periodontal infection can worsen glycemic control and should be managed aggressively. Diabetic patients with periodontitis should receive oral hygiene instructions, mechanical debridement to remove local factors, and regular maintenance. When possible, an HbA1c of less than 10% should be established before surgical treatment is performed. Systemic antibiotics

are not needed routinely, although evidence indicates that tetracycline antibiotics in combination with scaling and root planing may positively influence glycemic control. If the patient has poor glycemic control and surgery is absolutely needed, prophylactic antibiotics can be given; penicillins are most often used for this purpose. Frequent reevaluation after active therapy is needed to assess treatment response and prevent recurrence of periodontitis.

Almost all diabetic patients use a glucometer for blood glucose self-monitoring. These devices use capillary blood from a fingerstick to provide blood glucose readings in seconds. Diabetic patients should be asked whether they have a glucometer and how often they use it. Because these devices provide instantaneous assessment of blood glucose, they are highly beneficial in the dental office environment. The following guidelines should be observed:

1. Patients should be asked to bring their glucometer to the dental office at each appointment.
2. Patients should check their blood glucose before any long procedure to obtain a baseline level. Patients with a blood glucose level at or below the lower end of normal before the procedure may become hypoglycemic intraoperatively. It is advisable to have the patient consume some carbohydrate before starting treatment. For example, if a 2-hour procedure is planned and the pretreatment glucose level is 70 mg/dL (i.e., lower end of normal range), providing 4 ounces of juice preoperatively may help prevent hypoglycemia during treatment. If the pretreatment glucose level is excessively high, the clinician should determine whether the patient's glycemic control has been poor recently. This can be done with thorough patient questioning and by determining the most recent HbA1c values. If glycemic control has been poor over the preceding few months, the procedure may need to be postponed until better glycemic control is established. If glycemic control has been good and the current high glucometer reading is a fairly isolated event, the surgical procedure may proceed.
3. If the procedure lasts several hours, it is often beneficial to check the glucose level during the procedure to ensure that the patient does not become hypoglycemic.
4. After the procedure, the blood glucose can be checked again to assess fluctuations over time.

5. Any time the patient feels the symptoms of hypoglycemia, the blood glucose level should be checked immediately. This may prevent the onset of severe hypoglycemia, a medical emergency.

The most common dental office complication seen in diabetic patients taking insulin is a symptomatic low blood glucose level (i.e., hypoglycemia) (Box 39.4). Hypoglycemia is also associated with the use of numerous oral agents (Table 39.4). In patients receiving conscious sedation, the warning signs of an impending hypoglycemic episode can be masked, making the patient's glucometer one of the best diagnostic aids. Hypoglycemia does not usually occur until the blood glucose level falls below 60 mg/dL. However, in patients with poor glycemic control who have prolonged hyperglycemia (i.e., high blood glucose levels), a rapid drop in glucose can precipitate signs and symptoms of hypoglycemia at levels well above 60 mg/dL.

As medical management of diabetes has intensified over the past decade, the incidence of severe hypoglycemia has risen.[109] The clinician should question diabetic patients about past episodes of hypoglycemia. Hypoglycemia is more common in patients with better glycemic control. When planning dental treatment, it is best to schedule appointments before or after periods of peak insulin

activity. This requires knowledge of the pharmacodynamics of the drugs being taken by the diabetic patient. Patients taking insulin are at greatest risk, followed by those taking sulfonylurea agents. Metformin and thiazolidinediones usually do not cause hypoglycemia (see Table 39.4).

Insulins are classified as rapid-acting, short-acting, intermediate-acting, or long-acting agents (Table 39.5). The categories vary in onset, peak, and duration of activity. It is important that the clinician establish exactly which insulin the diabetic patient takes, the amount, the number of times per day, and the time of the last dose. Periodontal treatment often can be timed to avoid peak insulin activity. Many diabetic patients take multiple injections each day, in which case it is difficult, if not impossible, to avoid peak insulin activity. Checking the pretreatment glucose with the patient's glucometer, checking again during a long procedure, and checking again at the end of the procedure provides a better understanding of the patient's insulin pharmacodynamics and can help prevent hypoglycemia.

If hypoglycemia occurs during dental treatment, therapy should be immediately terminated. If a glucometer is available, the blood glucose level should be checked. Treatment guidelines include the following[56]:

1. Provide approximately 15 g of oral carbohydrate to the patient
   - 4 to 6 ounces of juice or soda
   - 3 or 4 teaspoons of table sugar
   - Hard candy with 15 g of sugar
2. If the patient is unable to take food or drink by mouth or if the patient is sedated
   - Give 25 to 30 mL of 50% dextrose intravenously, which provides 12.5 to 15.0 g of dextrose, or

---

BOX 39.4   Signs and Symptoms of Hypoglycemia

Shakiness or tremors	Dizziness
Confusion	Feeling of impending doom
Agitation and anxiety	Unconsciousness
Sweating	Seizures
Tachycardia	

TABLE 39.4   Oral Agents Used for the Management of Diabetes

Agent	Action	Risk of Hypoglycemia[a]
Sulfonylureas (1st gen): Chlorpropamide Tolbutamide Tolazamide	Stimulate pancreatic insulin secretion	++
Sulfonylureas (2nd gen): Glyburide Glipizide	Stimulate pancreatic insulin secretion	+++
Sulfonylureas (3rd gen): Glimepiride	Stimulate pancreatic insulin secretion	+
Meglitinides: Repaglinide Nateglinide	Stimulate rapid pancreatic insulin secretion (different mechanism from sulfonylureas)	+
Biguanides: Metformin	Block production of glucose by liver; improve tissue sensitivity to insulin	−
Thiazolidinediones: Rosiglitazone Pioglitazone	Improve tissue sensitivity to insulin	−
α-Glucosidase inhibitors: Acarbose Miglitol	Slow absorption of some carbohydrates from gut, decreasing postprandial peaks in glycemia	−
Dipeptidyl peptidase-4 (DPP-4) inhibitors: Sitagliptin Saxagliptin	Inhibit the enzyme DPP-4; enable the pancreas to produce more insulin but only after food ingestion	−
Combination agents	Combine two different oral agents into single drug	Risk depends on which drugs are combined

[a]Hypoglycemia risk: +++, high; ++, moderate; +, low; −, none.

TABLE 39.5 Types of Insulin

Type	Classification	ACTIVITY		Duration
		Onset	**Peak**	
Lispro (Humalog), aspart (Novolog), glulisine (Apidra)	Rapid-acting	15 min	30–90 min	<5 hr
Regular R or Novolin R, Velosulin (used in insulin pump)	Short-acting	30–60 min	2–3 hr 1–2 hr	3–6 hr 2–3 hr
NPH (N), Humulin N, Novolin N	Intermediate-acting	2–4 hr	4–12 hr	14–18 hr
Insulin determir (Levemir)	Long-acting	1–2 hr	Relatively flat (fairly even over 24 hr)	up to 24 hr
Glargine (Lantus)	Long-acting	6–8 hr	There is no peak	20–24+ hr

- Give 1 mg of glucagon intravenously (i.e., glucagon results in rapid release of stored glucose from the liver), or
- Give 1 mg of glucagon intramuscularly or subcutaneously (if no intravenous access).

Emergencies resulting from hyperglycemia are rare in the dental office. They usually take days to weeks to develop. However, the glucometer may be used to rule out hyperglycemic emergencies such as diabetic ketoacidosis, a life-threatening event.

KEY FACT

The most common dental office complication seen in diabetic patients taking insulin is a symptomatic low blood glucose level, or hypoglycemia. It does not usually occur until blood glucose level falls below 60 mg/dL. However, in patients with poor glycemic control who have prolonged hyperglycemia, a rapid drop in glucose can precipitate signs and symptoms of hypoglycemia at higher levels. Clinicians must recognize the signs of hypoglycemia and be prepared to manage it. Hypoglycemia is more common in individuals with well-controlled glucose levels.

Because periodontal therapy can render the patient unable to eat for some time, adjustment in insulin or oral agent dosages may be required. It is critical that patients eat a normal meal before dental treatment. Taking insulin without eating is the primary cause of hypoglycemia. If the patient is restricted from eating before treatment (e.g., for conscious sedation), normal insulin doses need to be reduced. As a general guideline, *well-controlled diabetic patients having routine periodontal treatment may take their normal insulin doses as long as they also eat their normal meal.* If the procedure is going to be particularly long, the insulin dose before treatment may need to be reduced. Likewise, if the patient will have dietary restrictions after treatment, insulin or sulfonylurea dosages may need to be reduced.

Consultation with the patient's physician is prudent and allows both practitioners to review the proposed treatment plan and determine whether modifications are needed. When periodontal surgery is indicated, it is usually best to limit the size of the surgical field so that the patient will be comfortable enough to resume a normal diet immediately.

Hemorrhagic Disorders

Patients with a history of bleeding problems caused by disease or drugs should be managed to minimize the risks of hemorrhage. Identification of these patients through the health history, clinical examination, and clinical laboratory tests is paramount. Health questioning should cover (1) the history of bleeding after previous surgery or trauma, (2) past and current drug history, (3) history of bleeding problems among relatives, and (4) illnesses associated with potential bleeding problems.

Clinical examination can detect jaundice, ecchymosis, spider telangiectasia, hemarthrosis, petechiae, hemorrhagic vesicles, spontaneous gingival bleeding, and gingival hyperplasia. Laboratory tests include methods to measure the hemostatic, coagulation, or lytic phase of the clotting mechanism, depending on clues regarding which phase is involved (Table 39.6). These tests include bleeding time, tourniquet test, complete blood cell count, prothrombin time (PT), partial thromboplastin time (PTT), and coagulation time. Bleeding disorders are classified as coagulation disorders, thrombocytopenic purpuras, or nonthrombocytopenic purpuras.

Coagulation Disorders

The main inherited coagulation disorders include hemophilia A, hemophilia B, and von Willebrand disease[77,88] (Table 39.7). *Hemophilia A* results in a deficiency of coagulation factor VIII, and the clinical severity of the disorder depends on the level of factor VIII remaining.[68] Patients with severe hemophilia who have less than 1% of normal factor VIII levels can have severe bleeding on the slightest provocation, whereas those with more moderate hemophilia (i.e., 1% to 5% of factor VIII) have less frequent spontaneous hemorrhage but still bleed with minimal trauma.[55] Patients with mild hemophilia (i.e., 6% to 30% of factor VIII) rarely bleed spontaneously but may still hemorrhage after severe trauma or during surgical procedures.

The clinician should consult the patient's physician before dental treatment to determine the risk of bleeding and treatment modifications required. To prevent surgical hemorrhage, a factor VIII level of at least 30% is needed.[55,68] Parenteral 1-deamino-8-D-arginine vasopressin (DDAVP; desmopressin) can be used to raise factor VIII levels twofold to threefold in patients with mild or moderate hemophilia. DDAVP has the significant advantage of avoiding the risk of viral disease transmission from factor VIII infusion and is considered the drug of choice in responsive patients. Most patients with moderate or severe hemophilia require infusion of factor VIII concentrate before surgical procedures. Before 1985, the risk of viral disease transmission from these infusions was high. Since then, virally safe, highly purified monoclonal antibody or recombinant DNA factor VIII products have come into widespread use.

Hemophilia B (i.e., Christmas disease) results in a deficiency of factor IX. The severity of the disorder depends on the relative amount of existing factor IX. Surgical therapy requires a factor IX level of 30% to 50%, which is usually achieved by administration of purified prothrombin complex concentrate or factor IX concentrate.[68]

Von Willebrand disease results from a deficiency of von Willebrand factor, which mediates adhesion of platelets to the injured vessel walls and is required for primary hemostasis. Von Willebrand factor also carries the coagulant portion of factor VIII in the plasma. The disorder has three major subtypes, with a wide range of clinical

TABLE 39.6 Laboratory Tests for Bleeding Disorders

HEMOSTATIC TESTS			
Vascular	**Platelet**	**Coagulation**	**Lysis**

1. Tourniquet test
  N: 10 petechiae
  Abn: >10 petechiae
	1. Platelet count
	  N: 150,000-300,000/mm^3
	  Abn: Thrombocytopenia occurs at <100,000/mm^3; clinical bleeding occurs at <80,000/mm^3; spontaneous bleeding occurs at <20,000/mm^3
		1. PT measures extrinsic and common pathways: factors I, II, V, VII, and X.
		  N: 11–14 sec (depending on laboratory) measured against control
		  PT reported as international normalized ratio (INR):
		  N: INR = 1.0
		  Abn: INR >1.5
			1. Euglobin clot lysis time
			  N: <90 min
			  Abn: >90 min

2. Bleeding time
  N: 1–6 min
  Abn: >6 min
	2. Bleeding time
	3. Clot retraction
	4. Complete blood cell count
		2. PTT measures intrinsic and common pathways: factors III, IX, XI, and low levels of factors I, II, V, X, and XII.
		  N: 25–40 sec (depending on laboratory) measured against control
		  Abn: >1.5 times normal
		3. Clotting (coagulation) time
		  N: 30–40 min
		  Abn: >1 hr	

Clinical Disease Associations

Vascular (capillary) wall defect	Thrombocytopenia		Increase in fibrinolytic activity
Rule out:	*Rule out:*	*All three tests:*	
Thrombocytopenia Purpuras Telangiectasia Aspirin or NSAID therapy Leukemia Renal dialysis	Vascular wall defect Acute or chronic leukemia Aplastic anemia Liver disease Renal dialysis	Liver disease Warfarin therapy Aspirin or NSAID therapy Malabsorption syndrome or long-term antibiotic therapy (lack of vitamin K metabolism) PT: factor VII deficiency PTT: hemophilia Renal dialysis	

Abn, Abnormal; *N,* normal; *NSAID,* nonsteroidal antiinflammatory drug; *PT,* prothrombin time; *PTT,* partial thromboplastin time.

TABLE 39.7 Inherited Coagulation Disorders

Type	Prolonged	Normal	Treatment
Hemophilia A	PTT	PT Bleeding time	DDAVP factor VIII concentrate or cryoprecipitate Fresh frozen plasma Fresh whole blood ε-Aminocaproic acid (Amicar) Tranexamic acid
Hemophilia B	PTT	PT Bleeding time	Purified prothrombin complex concentrate Factor IX concentrates Fresh-frozen plasma
Von Willebrand disease	Bleeding time PTT Variable factor VIII deficiency	PT Platelet count	DDAVP factor VIII concentrate or cryoprecipitate

DDAVP, 1-deamino-8-D-arginine vasopressin (desmopressin); *PT,* prothrombin time; *PTT,* partial thromboplastin time.

severity. Many cases of von Willebrand disease go undiagnosed, and bleeding during dental treatment may be the first sign of the underlying disease. More severe forms require preoperative factor VIII concentrate or cryoprecipitate infusion. Patients with milder forms respond favorably to administration of DDAVP before periodontal surgery or tooth extraction.[68,69]

Periodontal treatment can be performed in patients with these coagulation disorders, provided that sufficient precautions are taken. Probing, scaling, and prophylaxis can usually be done without medical modification. More invasive treatment, such as local block anesthesia, root planing, or surgery, dictates prior physician consultation.

During treatment, local measures to ensure clot formation and stability are of major importance. Complete wound closure and application of pressure can reduce hemorrhage. Antihemostatic agents, such as oxidized cellulose or purified bovine collagen, can be placed over surgical sites or into extraction sockets. The antifibrinolytic agent *ε-aminocaproic acid* (Amicar), given orally or intravenously, is a potent inhibitor of initial clot dissolution.[42] *Tranexamic acid* is a more potent antifibrinolytic agent than Amicar and can prevent excessive oral hemorrhage after periodontal surgery and tooth extraction.[76] It is available as an oral rinse and may be used alone or in combination with systemic tranexamic acid for several days after surgery.[99]

Not all coagulation disorders are hereditary. Liver disease affects all phases of blood clotting because most coagulation factors are synthesized and removed by the liver. Long-term alcohol abusers or chronic hepatitis patients often demonstrate inadequate coagulation. Coagulation can be impaired by vitamin K deficiency, often caused by malabsorption syndromes, or by prolonged antibiotic administration, which alters the intestinal microflora that produces vitamin K. Dental treatment planning for patients with liver disease should include the following:

1. Physician consultation
2. Laboratory evaluations: PT, bleeding time, platelet count, and PTT (for patients in later stages of liver disease)
3. Conservative, nonsurgical periodontal therapy whenever possible
4. When surgery is required (may require hospitalization)
   - International normalized ratio (INR; PT) should be less than 2.0; for simple surgical procedures, an INR of less than 2.5 is usually safe.[39]
   - Platelet count should be more than 80,000/mm³.

KEY FACT

Periodontal treatment can be performed in patients with coagulation disorders, provided that sufficient precautions are taken. Probing, scaling, and prophylaxis usually can be done without medical modification. However, more invasive treatment, such as local block anesthesia, root planing, or surgery, should be considered only after consultation with a physician.

Anticoagulant Medications

The most common cause of abnormal coagulation may be drug therapy. Patients with a prosthetic heart valve or a history of MI, CVA, or thromboembolism are frequently placed on anticoagulant therapy using coumarin derivatives such as dicumarol and warfarin.[39,51] These drugs are vitamin K antagonists that decrease production of vitamin K–dependent coagulation factors II, VII, IX, and X. The effectiveness of anticoagulation therapy is monitored by a PT laboratory test. The recommended level of therapeutic anticoagulation for most patients is an INR of 2.0 to 3.0, with prosthetic heart valve patients usually in the 2.5 to 3.5 range.[39] Traditional recommendations for periodontal treatment are as follows:

1. Consult the patient's physician to determine the nature of the underlying medical problem and the degree of required anticoagulation.
2. The procedure to be done determines the acceptable INR. Infiltration anesthesia, scaling, and root planing can be done safely in patients with an INR of less than 3.0. Block anesthesia, minor periodontal surgery, and simple extractions usually require an INR of less than 2.0 to 2.5. Complex surgery or multiple extractions may require an INR of less than 1.5 to 2.0.
3. The physician must be consulted about any changes (i.e., discontinuing or reducing) in anticoagulant dosage until the desired INR is achieved. The dentist must inform the physician what degree of intraoperative and postoperative bleeding is usually expected with the planned procedure. If the INR is higher than the level at which significant bleeding is likely to accompany a particular procedure, the physician may elect to change anticoagulant therapy. Often, the anticoagulant is discontinued for 2 to 3 days before periodontal treatment (i.e., clearance half-life of warfarin is 36 to 42 hours), and the INR is checked on the day of therapy. If the INR is within the acceptable target range, the procedure is done and the anticoagulant resumed immediately after treatment.
4. Careful technique and complete wound closure are paramount. For all procedures, application of pressure can minimize hemorrhage. Use of oxidized cellulose, microfibrillar collagen, topical thrombin, and tranexamic acid should be considered for persistent bleeding.

Discontinuing anticoagulant therapy before dental surgery was common in the past. However, many clinicians no longer recommend discontinuing anticoagulation for many procedures because it poses significant risks for patient health.[41,90] Evidence related to the risks of altering anticoagulant therapy and the lack of evidence for bleeding complications suggest that treating patients without reducing or discontinuing medications may be more prudent. Details of anticoagulant or antiplatelet therapy are discussed in the next section.

Heparin typically is used for short-term anticoagulation and is given intravenously and usually in a hospital environment. It is a powerful anticoagulant with a duration of action of 4 to 8 hours. Periodontal treatment is rarely required while a patient is taking heparin.

Antiplatelet Medications

Aspirin interferes with normal platelet aggregation and can result in prolonged bleeding. Because it binds irreversibly to platelets, the effects of aspirin last at least 4 to 7 days. Aspirin typically is used in small doses of 325 mg or less per day, which usually does not alter bleeding time. Patients taking low doses of aspirin daily usually do not need to discontinue aspirin therapy before periodontal procedures.[90] However, higher doses can increase bleeding time and predispose the patient to postoperative bleeding.[55] For patients taking more than 325 mg of aspirin per day, it may need to be discontinued 7 to 10 days before surgical therapy that could result in significant bleeding; this should be done in consultation with the physician.

Nonsteroidal antiinflammatory drugs (NSAIDs) such as ibuprofen also inhibit platelet function. Because NSAIDs bind reversibly, the effect is transitory, lasting only a short time after the last drug dose. The bleeding time is used when questions arise about the potential effect of aspirin or NSAIDs. Aspirin should not be prescribed for patients who are receiving anticoagulation therapy or who have an illness related to bleeding tendency.

Leukemia

Altered periodontal treatment for patients with leukemia is based on their enhanced susceptibility to infections, bleeding tendency, and effects of chemotherapy.[55] The treatment plan for leukemia patients is as follows:

1. Refer the patient for medical evaluation and treatment. Close cooperation with the physician is required.
2. Before chemotherapy, a complete periodontal treatment plan should be developed with a physician (discussed in the previous discussion).
   - Monitor hematologic laboratory values daily: bleeding time, coagulation time, PT, and platelet count.
   - Administer antibiotic coverage before periodontal treatment because infection is a major concern.
   - If systemic conditions allow, extract all hopeless, nonmaintainable, or potentially infectious teeth at least 10 days before the initiation of chemotherapy.
   - Periodontal debridement (i.e., scaling and root planing) should be performed and thorough oral hygiene instructions given if the patient's condition allows. Twice-daily rinsing with 0.12% chlorhexidine gluconate is recommended after oral hygiene procedures. Recognize the potential for bleeding caused by thrombocytopenia. Use pressure and topical hemostatic agents as indicated.
3. During the acute phases of leukemia, patients should receive only emergency periodontal care. Any source of potential infection must be eliminated to prevent systemic dissemination. Antibiotic therapy is frequently the treatment of choice, combined with nonsurgical or surgical debridement as indicated.
4. Oral ulcerations and mucositis are treated palliatively with agents such as viscous lidocaine. Systemic antibiotics may be indicated to prevent secondary infection.
5. Oral candidiasis is common in leukemic patients and can be treated with nystatin suspension (400,000–600,000 U/mL four times daily) or clotrimazole vaginal suppositories (10 mg four or five times daily).[57]
6. For patients with chronic leukemia and those in remission, scaling and root planing can be performed without complication, but periodontal surgery should be avoided if possible. Platelet count and bleeding time should be measured on the day of the procedure. If either is low, postpone the appointment and refer the patient to a physician.

Agranulocytosis

Patients with agranulocytosis (i.e., cyclic neutropenia and granulocytopenia) have an increased susceptibility to infection. The total white blood cell count is reduced, and granular leukocytes (i.e., neutrophils, eosinophils, and basophils) are reduced in number or disappear. These disorders are often marked by early, severe periodontal destruction.[122] When possible, periodontal treatment should be done during periods of disease remission. At such times, treatment should be as conservative as possible while reducing potential sources of systemic infection. After physician consultation, severely affected teeth should be extracted. Oral hygiene instruction should include chlorhexidine rinses twice daily. Scaling and root planing should be performed carefully under antibiotic protection.

Medications and Cancer Therapies

Some medications prescribed to cure, manage, or prevent diseases have effects on periodontal tissues, wound healing, or the host immune response that sometimes require modification of treatment. Bisphosphonates, anticoagulation medications, antiplatelet medications, steroids, chemotherapy, and radiation therapy are briefly addressed in this chapter, and additional information and advice can be found in other sources.

Bisphosphonates

Bisphosphonate medications are primarily used to treat cancer (i.e., intravenous administration) and osteoporosis (i.e., oral administration). They act by inhibiting osteoclastic activity, which leads to less bone resorption, remodeling, and turnover.[83] Bisphosphonates are used in cancer treatment to prevent the often lethal imbalance of osteoclastic activity. In the treatment of osteoporosis, the goal is to harness osteoclastic activity to minimize or prevent bone loss. The major difference between these applications is the potency and route of administration. Potency is influenced by the chemical properties and pharmacokinetics of these agents in bone. Chapter 14 describes the chemical structure, activity, and role of bisphosphonates in the development of bisphosphonate-related osteonecrosis of the jaw (BRONJ).

Clinically, BRONJ manifests as exposed alveolar bone occurring spontaneously or after a dental procedure (see Figs. 14.20 and 14.21 in Chapter 14). Individuals treated with high-potency, nitrogen-containing bisphosphonates, especially those administered intravenously for cancer treatment (e.g., zoledronate), appear to be at greater risk for BRONJ than individuals taking oral bisphosphonates for prevention and treatment of osteoporosis. For patients treated for cancer, the incidence ranges from 2.5% to 5.4%.[121] Estimating the incidence for patients taking oral bisphosphonates for osteoporosis is more difficult but appears to range from 0.007% to 0.04%.[118] Even if this is an underestimation of the actual risk for individuals taking oral bisphosphonates, the incidence appears to be low. The risk for individuals treated with oral bisphosphonates for a period of less than 3 years appears to be minimal or zero.[52] Regular use of oral bisphosphonates for a period greater than 3 years suggests a risk profile that increases with time and length of use.[52]

As with many multifactorial diseases and conditions, it is likely that factors in addition to bisphosphonate therapy contribute to the individual risk of BRONJ. Potential risk factors include systemic corticosteroid therapy, smoking, alcohol, poor oral hygiene, chemotherapy, radiotherapy, diabetes, and hematologic disease.[25] Reported factors for BRONJ include extractions, root canal treatment, periodontal infections, periodontal surgery, and dental implant surgery.[54] Periodontal disease and treatment (especially surgery) poses a risk for patients treated with bisphosphonates. The bacteria-induced inflammatory process of periodontitis that causes bone resorption can lead to bone necrosis. Likewise, periodontal treatment can cause bone necrosis in the setting of bisphosphonates. Caution is warranted for all patients treated with bisphosphonates.

Health care providers need to evaluate patients carefully, communicate with other medical health care providers, inform patients, and consider treatment options and risks carefully. A careful intraoral examination is prudent for all patients treated with intravenous or oral bisphosphonate therapy to determine whether bone exposure exists and to assess local conditions that may predispose them to BRONJ. A thorough medical history should be reviewed, evaluated, and annotated with details about bisphosphonate treatment, including medication type, dose, route of administration, and duration. Comorbidities, such as previous and current medications, treatments, and existing disease or pathology, should be considered. Radiographs should be carefully evaluated for signs of bisphosphonate toxicity.

Marx suggested that a laboratory blood test for the serum C-terminal telopeptide fragment of type I collagen (CTX) could be used to assess an individual's risk of developing BRONJ.[52] Marx reported that lower CTX values were associated with greater risk (eTable 39.2). It is important to recognize that these values are based on retrospective evaluation of patients with osteonecrosis of the jaws and that prospective studies to validate these findings have not been done. The CTX laboratory test is a measure of the specific C-terminal fragment of type I collagen cleaved by osteoclasts and indicates bone resorption activity. However, its use as a measure of the risk for BRONJ is controversial and not confirmed by prospective studies.

Optimal periodontal and oral health should be achieved and maintained for all patients. For individuals treated with intravenous bisphosphonates, invasive treatment, such as extractions, periodontal surgery, implant surgery, and bone augmentation procedures, should be avoided. Risks must be considered before treatment of individuals with a history of taking oral bisphosphonates for longer than 3 years. This area of research will continue to evolve as the pathophysiology becomes better understood. Providers are encouraged to consult other sources for updates on this important topic.

KEY FACT

Bisphosphonate therapy and one or more comorbidity factors contribute to the individual risk of bisphosphonate-related osteonecrosis of the jaw (BRONJ). Potential risk factors include systemic corticosteroid therapy, smoking, alcohol, poor oral hygiene, chemotherapy, radiotherapy, diabetes, and hematologic disease.

Anticoagulant or Antiplatelet Therapy

Many patients with a variety of conditions are placed on anticoagulant or antiplatelet medications to prevent thrombosis (i.e., blood clotting) or thromboembolism. Patients at risk who may be on anticoagulant or antiplatelet therapy include those with heart valve replacements, heart rhythm disorders, congenital heart defects, or a history or risk of MI, stroke, or deep vein thrombosis. These medications, although effective in reducing the risk of thrombosis, may increase the risk for bleeding complications, especially in patients undergoing surgical procedures.

The traditional approach to patients on anticoagulant or antiplatelet therapy was to discontinue therapy about 3 to 5 days (antiplatelet therapy) or 7 to 10 days (anticoagulant therapy) before a planned surgical procedure. Evidence and theories about the care of patients on anticoagulant or antiplatelet therapy suggest that treating them (e.g., with periodontal surgery or extractions) without altering their anticoagulant or antiplatelet medications is safe and does not lead to intraoperative or postoperative bleeding complications. The increased risk of morbidity and mortality for those discontinuing the anticoagulant or antiplatelet therapy may be significant.

Controlled clinical studies have demonstrated that intraoperative bleeding is not likely to be a problem with simple extractions or periodontal surgery if antiplatelet therapy (e.g., aspirin) is continued.[6,50]

In these studies, there were no episodes of uncontrolled bleeding, all bleeding was controlled with local measures, and there were no cases of postoperative bleeding problems. Conversely, the risk of stopping antiplatelet therapy may be serious. In a retrospective evaluation of 52 patients undergoing cataract surgery, 1 in 10 whose antiplatelet therapy was stopped or reduced suffered a stroke.[85]

Clinical studies of patients on anticoagulant therapy undergoing extractions and other oral surgical procedures have demonstrated minimal bleeding problems when therapy is continued.[12,15,119,120,129] In a review of the literature, Wahl and colleagues[120] reported that only 12 (<1.3%) of 950 patients receiving continuous anticoagulant therapy required more than local measures to control hemorrhage after 2400 minor oral surgical procedures. Most of the 950 patients had anticoagulation levels that were well above currently recommended therapeutic levels. Only three patients (<0.31%) had anticoagulation levels within or below currently recommended therapeutic levels. In contrast, 5 (0.95%) of 526 patients who experienced 575 interruptions of continuous anticoagulant therapy suffered serious embolic complications; 4 patients died.

In a prospective study of 131 patients undergoing 511 extractions, those whose oral anticoagulant therapy was reduced 72 hours before surgery to achieve an INR of 1.5 to 2.0 (target, 1.8) had postoperative bleeding that warranted subsequent local intervention in 10 (15.1%) of 66 patients.[84] Postoperative bleeding occurred in only 6 (9.2%) of 65 patients in the group that continued the regular dosage of oral anticoagulant therapy (mean INR, 2.9).

These studies suggest that the risk of serious morbidity associated with discontinuing anticoagulant or antiplatelet therapy should be avoided and that the risk of bleeding while maintaining this therapy is minimal.

Corticosteroids

Approximately 5% of the adults in the United States habitually take corticosteroids for the treatment of various conditions, potentially putting them at risk for secondary adrenal insufficiency.[48] Patients who habitually use corticosteroids have an increased likelihood of developing hypertension, osteoporosis, and peptic ulcer disease. Care should be taken to minimize the risk of adverse outcomes in these patients. BP should be monitored, and medications that may exacerbate peptic ulceration (e.g., aspirin, NSAIDs) should be avoided.

Stressful events, such as trauma, illness, surgery, emotional upset, or athletic events, normally increase circulating endogenous cortisol levels through stimulation of the HPA axis. Pain appears to increase the requirement for cortisol release.[75] There is concern that the normal release of cortisol in response to a stressful event, such as a dental procedure may be impaired in patients exposed to habitual corticosteroid use. The concern is about whether these patients require perioperative supplementation for dental procedures. Historically, recommendations were based on the type, amount, and duration of corticosteroid use. However, current thinking about the need for perioperative corticosteroid supplementation has been adjusted.

Studies investigating the stress response to minor general and oral surgical procedures concluded that significant increases in cortisol were usually not seen until 1 to 5 hours after surgery and appeared to be associated more with postoperative pain and the loss of local anesthesia than with the preoperative and intraoperative stress of the procedure.[7,94,95] Administration of adequate analgesics in the postoperative period can diminish the release (requirement) of cortisol.[7]

Most individuals with adrenal insufficiency can receive routine dental treatment without the need for supplemental glucocorticosteroids.[13,48] Patients taking corticosteroids usually have enough exogenous and endogenous cortisol to handle routine dental procedures if the usual dose is taken within 2 hours of the planned procedure. For most patients, supplemental corticosteroid administration is not required when uncomplicated minor surgical procedures, including periodontal surgery, are performed with local anesthesia with or without sedation.[48] Topical corticosteroids usually have minimal HPA effect, and steroid supplementation is not required for these patients.

Individuals at risk for adrenal crisis who require supplementation include those undergoing lengthy major surgical procedures, those expected to have significant blood loss, and those who have extremely low adrenal function. Low adrenal function can be identified with an ACTH stimulation test. For these individuals, consultation with the physician and steroid supplementation are indicated.

Immunosuppression and Chemotherapy

Immunosuppressed patients have an impaired host defense as a result of an underlying immunodeficiency or use of drugs (primarily related to organ transplantation or cancer chemotherapy).[58,91] Because chemotherapy is often cytotoxic to bone marrow, destruction of platelets and red and white blood cells results in thrombocytopenia, anemia, and leukopenia. Immunosuppressed individuals are at greatly increased risk for infection, and even minor periodontal infections can become life-threatening if immunosuppression is severe.[74,77] Bacterial, viral, and fungal infections can manifest intraorally. Patients undergoing bone marrow transplantation require special attention because they receive extremely high-dose chemotherapy and are particularly susceptible to dissemination of oral infections.

Treatment should be directed toward prevention of oral complications that can be life-threatening. The greatest potential for infection occurs during periods of extreme immunosuppression; treatment should be conservative and palliative. It is always preferable to evaluate the patient before initiation of chemotherapy.[58,91] Teeth with a poor prognosis should be extracted, with thorough debridement of remaining teeth to minimize the microbial load. The clinician must teach and emphasize the importance of good oral hygiene. Antimicrobial rinses, such as chlorhexidine, are recommended, especially for patients with chemotherapy-induced mucositis, to prevent secondary infection.

Chemotherapy is usually performed in cycles, with each cycle lasting several days, followed by intervening periods of myelosuppression and recovery. If periodontal therapy is needed during chemotherapy, it is best done the day *before* chemotherapy is given, when white blood cell counts are relatively high. Coordination with the oncologist is critical. Dental treatment should be done when the white blood cell count is above 2000/mm³, with an absolute granulocyte count of 1000 to 1500/mm³.[55]

Radiation Therapy

The use of radiotherapy, alone or in conjunction with surgical resection, is common in the treatment of head and neck tumors. The side effects of ionizing radiation include dramatic perioral changes of significant concern to dental health personnel.[38,57,92] The extent and severity of mucositis, dermatitis, xerostomia, dysphagia, gustatory alteration, radiation caries (Fig. 39.3), vascular changes, trismus, temporomandibular joint degeneration, and periodontal changes depend on the type of radiation used, field of irradiation, number of ports, type of tissue in the field, and dosage.

Patients scheduled to receive head and neck radiation therapy require dental consultation *at the earliest possible time* to reduce the morbidity of known perioral side effects.[89] Preirradiation treatment depends on the patient's prognosis, compliance, and residual dentition in addition to the field, ports, dose, and immediacy of radiotherapy.

The initial visit should include panoramic and intraoral radiographs, a clinical dental examination, a periodontal evaluation, and a physician consultation. The physician should be asked about the amount of radiation to be administered, extent and location of the lesion, nature of surgical procedures already performed or to be performed, number of radiation ports, exact fields to be irradiated, mode of radiation therapy, and patient's prognosis (i.e., likelihood of metastasis). Preirradiation treatment should commence immediately after the physician consultation. The first decision should involve possible extractions because radiation can cause side effects that interfere with healing.

For head and neck squamous cell carcinomas, the radiation dose is usually 5000 to 7000 cGy (1 cGy = 1 rad) delivered in a fractionated method (150 to 200 cGy/day over a 6- to 7-week course).[11,57] This is considered full-course radiation treatment, and the degree of perioral side effects depends on which tissues are irradiated (i.e., radiation fields). If the radiation is administered to the salivary gland tissues, xerostomia will ensue. The parotid is the most radiosensitive of the salivary glands; saliva may become extremely viscous or nonexistent, depending on the dose delivered to the particular gland. Xerostomia causes a decrease in the normal salivary cleansing mechanisms, buffering capacity of saliva, and pH of oral fluids.[57] Oral bacterial populations shift to a preponderance of cariogenic forms (e.g., *Streptococcus mutans, Actinomyces* spp., *Lactobacillus* spp.). Radiation-induced caries may progress rapidly, and they primarily affect smooth tooth surfaces (see Fig. 39.3).

High-dose radiation therapy results in hypovascularity of irradiated tissues, with a reduction in wound-healing capacity.[66,116,117] Most severe among the resulting oral complications is osteoradionecrosis (ORN). Decreased vascularity renders the bone less capable of resolving trauma or infection. These events can cause severe destruction of bone. The risk of ORN continues for the remainder of the patient's life and does not decrease with time.[53]

Periodontal disease can be a precipitating factor in ORN.[16,31] Tooth extraction after radiation treatment involves a high risk of developing ORN, and surgical flap procedures are usually discouraged after radiation therapy. For these reasons, it is important that the clinician address the patient's periodontal disease *before* radiation begins, when possible. Teeth that are nonrestorable or severely periodontally diseased should be extracted, ideally at least 2 weeks before radiation therapy.[57] Extractions should be performed in a manner that allows primary closure. Mucoperiosteal flaps should be gently elevated; teeth should be extracted in segments; alveolectomy should be performed, allowing no rough bony spicules to remain; and primary closure should be provided without tension. It is not necessary to extract teeth that can be retained with conservative restorative, endodontic, or periodontal therapy. However, prudence dictates extraction of questionable teeth because periodontal treatment after irradiation may be limited to nonsurgical forms of therapy. Flap surgery or extraction of teeth after radiation can lead to ORN. Management of ORN is often difficult and costly, involving progressively more aggressive treatment if bone does not respond to conservative therapy. Costly hyperbaric oxygen therapy is frequently required for complete resolution.

During radiation therapy, patients should receive weekly prophylaxis, oral hygiene instruction, and professionally applied fluoride treatments, unless mucositis prevents treatment. Patients should be instructed to brush daily with a 0.4% stannous or 1.0% sodium fluoride gel. Custom gel trays allow optimal fluoride application.[116] All remaining teeth should receive thorough debridement (i.e., scaling and root planing).

Postirradiation follow-up consists of palliative treatment given as indicated. Viscous lidocaine can be prescribed for painful mucositis,

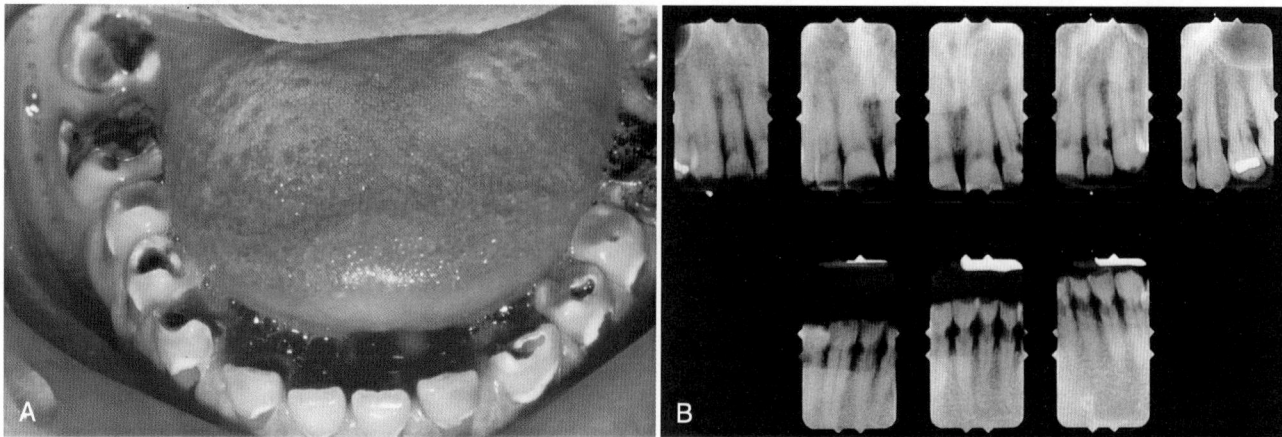

Fig. 39.3 (A) In a clinical view of a patient with radiation caries, notice how the caries primarily affected the smooth tooth surfaces, especially cervical areas and cusp tips. (B) Radiographs of anterior teeth of 52-year-old man with postradiation caries. The patient received a dose of 6000 cGy for radiation treatment of the posterior mandible and base of the tongue for squamous cell carcinoma. Radiation caries developed within 1 year after radiation treatment, affecting the cervical areas and incisal edges of the anterior teeth. *(A, courtesy Dr. Eric Sung, Hospital Dentistry, University of California Los Angeles.)*

and salivary substitutes can be given for xerostomia. Daily topical fluoride application and oral hygiene are the best means of preventing radiation caries over time. A long-term, 3-month recall interval is ideal.

Prosthetic Joint Replacement

The main treatment consideration for patients with prosthetic joint replacement is the potential need for antibiotic prophylaxis before periodontal therapy. No scientific evidence indicates that prophylactic antibiotics prevent late prosthetic joint infections, which can occur from transient bacteremia induced by dental treatment.[23,55,93] Although dental-induced bacteremia can theoretically cause prosthetic joint infection, scant reports demonstrate dental treatment as a source of joint infection, and none actually documents a cause-and-effect relationship.[19,81,112]

Reports of the American Dental Association (ADA), American Academy of Orthopedic Surgeons (AAOS), American Academy of Oral Medicine (AAOM), and British Society for Antimicrobial Chemotherapy (BSAC) agree that routine antibiotic prophylaxis before dental treatment is not indicated for most patients with prosthetic joint replacement.[2,3,21,28,110] However, antibiotic prophylaxis is indicated for almost all patients within the first 2 years after joint replacement and for high-risk patients, including those with previous prosthetic joint infections, immunosuppression, rheumatoid arthritis, systemic lupus erythematosus, type 1 diabetes, hemophilia, and malnourishment.[2] Many investigators consider patients with severe periodontal disease or other potential dental infections to be at high risk, and antibiotic prophylaxis may be indicated for them before dental treatment.[65,110]

Between 2009 and 2014, there was controversy and debate among experts, with a complete shift toward recommending prophylactic antibiotics before dental treatment for all patients with prosthetic joint replacement for life. After further review of the evidence and consensus among experts, new recommendations were published that did not recommend prophylactic antibiotics for dental procedures in patients with prosthetic joint replacement to prevent prosthetic joint infection. A historical description of the changes that were implemented from 2009 to 2012 can be found online (www.ada.org/en/member-center/oral-health-topics/antibiotic-prophylaxis).

Current advice for patients with orthopedic joint replacement stresses the importance of maintaining good dental health and hygiene and seeking prompt attention and treatment for oral infections when they occur. Dental procedures have not been associated with an increased risk of prosthetic joint infection, and the use of prophylactic antibiotics before dental procedures does not reduce the risk of infection.[9,100,128] Given the lack of evidence to support the need for prophylactic antibiotics, the AAOM, ADA, AAOS, and BSAC advise against universal use of antibiotic prophylaxis before dental procedures for the prevention of prosthetic joint infections.

In 2013, the ADA in conjunction with the AAOS published a joint guideline on the prevention of orthopedic implant infections in patients undergoing dental procedures. The publication stated that there was no convincing evidence to support the routine use of prophylactic antibiotics for patients with prosthetic joints.[123] In 2015, the ADA Council on Scientific Affairs published a clinical practice guideline to clearly state the findings of the 2013 ADA/AAOS joint guideline. The clinical practice guideline states that prophylactic antibiotics are not recommended before dental procedures for patients with prosthetic joint implants to prevent prosthetic joint infections.[104]

KEY FACT

In 2015, the American Dental Association (ADA) Council on Scientific Affairs published a clinical practice guideline to clearly state the findings published in the 2013 ADA and American Association of Orthopedic Surgeons (AAOS) joint guideline. The clinical practice guideline states that prophylactic antibiotics are *not* recommended before dental procedures for patients with prosthetic joint implants to prevent prosthetic joint infections.

 A Case Scenario is found on the companion website www.expertconsult.com.

References

 References for this chapter are found on the companion website www.expertconsult.com.

CHAPTER 40

Sleep-Disordered Breathing

Adrian K. Zacher | Michael J. McDevitt

CHAPTER OUTLINE

 Content on the diagnosis of obstructive sleep apnea, device design, and compliance with therapy can be accessed on the companion website at www.expertconsult.com.

New and Evolving Role of the Dentist

Everyone sleeps, and no one thinks much about sleep until something goes wrong. When sleep does go wrong—and it can in many ways—the effects can be more than just feeling a little tired in the morning. This chapter explores the exciting and evolving role of the dentist with an interest in sleep-disordered breathing (SDB) who helps patients to breathe, sleep, and ultimately function better each day.

Snoring and sleep apnea (i.e., cessation of breathing) are points along a spectrum that extends from benign or simple snoring with no sleep disturbance to obstructive sleep apnea (OSA) with excessive daytime sleepiness and the physiologic consequences of recurrent asphyxia.[21] Over the years, there have been many dubious claims made regarding snoring cures. However, knowledge has greatly improved,[13] and much can be done to manage OSA and its associated consequences. It is in the provision of oral devices for OSA that a key role for suitably trained dentists is developing.

Sleep apnea can be caused by the lack of a central drive to breathe. The central, mixed, and complex types of apnea are reviewed later in this chapter.

Professor Colin Sullivan invented the mainstay therapy for sleep apnea: positive airway pressure (PAP) therapy. He was also an internationally renowned key opinion leader, and he advocated[5] for dentists, as part of a multidisciplinary team, to play a critical role in four areas:

1. Treating adults with oral devices for snoring and mild to moderate OSA to slow the progression of the disease
2. Identifying at-risk children and adults by looking at their upper airway on a regular basis
3. Treating children with rapid maxillary expansion and avoiding deleterious orthodontic treatments
4. Recognizing the need for bimaxillary osteotomy in young adults requiring maxillofacial correction

Sleep-Related Breathing Disorders and the Periodontium

The prevalence of impaired breathing in patients who are also susceptible to periodontal disease and whose periodontitis experience may be affected by a sleep-related breathing disorder is sufficient to compel dentists and their teams to develop recognition strategies.

Whereas diagnosing OSA is the responsibility of a qualified physician, the dentist is capable of identifying and differentiating clinical signs of possible airway issues, often before the patient becomes suspicious of the health risk. Information shared by the patient regarding his or her overall health status should be reviewed and correlated with clinical observations of oral indicators of attempted compensation by the patient for a significant degree of airway obstruction or resistance.

The value of early recognition and intervention cannot be overstated. The deleterious effects of sleep-related breathing disorders and resultant periods of asphyxia on cardiovascular health, endocrine function, neurologic function, and masticatory system integrity add to the urgency for dentists to include recognition protocols during initial and recurring evaluations of their patients. A multidisciplinary team approach[25] that incorporates respect for each team member's professional role is essential to make an accurate diagnosis and facilitate provision of the most appropriate treatment.

The following sections discuss sleep, apnea, and the dentist's role in the provision of oral devices, which is one of the increasingly favored OSA treatment options.

Dental Identification of Signs and Symptoms

Review of Health Status and Systems

The frequency with which dentists see their patients places them in a unique position to recognize the symptoms of OSA. At the beginning of every dental appointment, the dentist or a member of the dental team should conduct an effective review and record the patient's health status. In addition to addressing specific items that might have been discussed previously, the inclusion of questions about breathing issues can alert the dentist to look for clinical indicators of sleep-related breathing disorders. Identification of clinical signs can reframe future discussions of the patient's overall health to prevent overlooking possible correlations with observations. For example, snoring or gasping reported to the patient by his or her bed partner may correlate with unexpected mobility of occluding anterior teeth. Important conditions or factors that may be reported by a patient include the following:

- Hypertension
- Gastroesophageal reflux disease
- Excessive daytime sleepiness
- Cardiovascular disease, including arrhythmias
- Type 2 diabetes
- Hypothyroidism
- Obesity
- Sudden onset of snoring
- Awareness of snoring or SDB
- Use of a snore appliance from a dentist or another source

Dental Signs and Symptoms of Obstructed Breathing

Neither the clinical indicators nor the health or breathing status reported by the patient can define the degree or implications of a sleep-related breathing disorder for the dentist. Developing a list of observations to discuss with the patient allows him or her to confirm the possibility of a breathing disorder and communicate the signs to the physician for further assessment and diagnosis.

Sleep Bruxism

Although patients commonly report SDB and sleep bruxism, there is only a suspected association because no evidence-based clinical trial has established a specific relationship. The bruxing patient's repeated patterns of mandibular movement are primarily mediated by the central nervous system. It has been hypothesized that the advancement of the mandible opens the oropharynx, relieving some of the consequences of SDB.[27,28]

Clinical Signs and Symptoms

- Wear patterns on opposing incisors can suggest that the patient positions the mandible anteriorly to open the airway.[42,43]
- The mobility of the anterior teeth may be in excess of that estimated on the basis of the patient's health and the support available from periodontal structures.
- In the periodontitis-susceptible patient, progressive bone loss may be located or exaggerated in sites of unusual wear or mobility. The possible role of occlusal trauma in the amplification of the consequences of periodontitis is described in the online version of Chapter 55 of this textbook (www.expertconsult.com).
- Tongue crenulations (i.e., scalloped borders) suggest that the patient is depressing the tongue forward against the mandibular teeth regularly to open the oral airway.
- Development of an anterior or lateral open-bite relationship of the opposing teeth may result from tongue posturing.
- Sleep bruxism may develop or increase.
- Dimpling of the cusps and lingual surfaces of the teeth can indicate related gastroesophageal reflux.
- The development of orofacial pain, temporomandibular joint (TMJ) dysfunction symptoms, masticatory muscle fatigue noticed on awakening, or morning headache can be related to the

positioning of the mandible to open the patient's airway. This topic is addressed in the online version of Chapter 26 of this textbook (www.expertconsult.com), where comprehensive diagnostic references can also be found.

- During evaluation of the oropharynx, prominent tonsils, a large uvula, or a narrow or tongue-obstructed airway may be seen. The patient's age can contribute to the loss of tone of the pharyngeal muscles.
- Mouth breathing while sleeping can manifest as drying of the surface of the gingiva.

Sleep, Breathing, and Apnea

A basic understanding of sleep physiology, normal sleep cycles, and the variety of sleep disorders can provide the dentist with the means for effective communication with patients and their physicians.

Sleep is classically defined as a cyclic, temporary, and physiologic loss of consciousness that is readily, promptly, and completely reversed with appropriate stimuli. Not being able to breathe would seem to qualify as an appropriate stimulus, but affected individuals are rarely aware of any difficulty. Normal sleep progresses through different stages that are typically depicted on a hypnogram (Fig. 40.1).

Snoring is a vibratory noise that is generated by the back of the relaxed tongue, pharynx, and soft palate. Further loss of tone or narrowing produces louder snoring and labored inspiration. Still further narrowing can cause complete collapse of the airway. This obstruction is known as an *apneic episode*.

There comes a point at which the increased inspiratory effort or oxygen desaturation that may accompany the apneic episode is sensed by the sleeping brain and a transient arousal is provoked. This is a brief awakening to breathe before the individual returns to sleep. These arousals can be seen in Fig. 40.2 as decreased-duration periods and increasingly frequent interruptions in the descent into deeper, more refreshing sleep. Disregarding complaints about the snoring

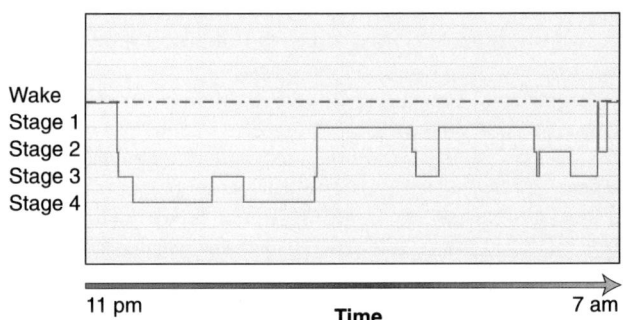

Fig. 40.1 Simplified hypnogram of a normal adult's sleep. *(Courtesy Adrian Zacher, 2013. Snorer.com.)*

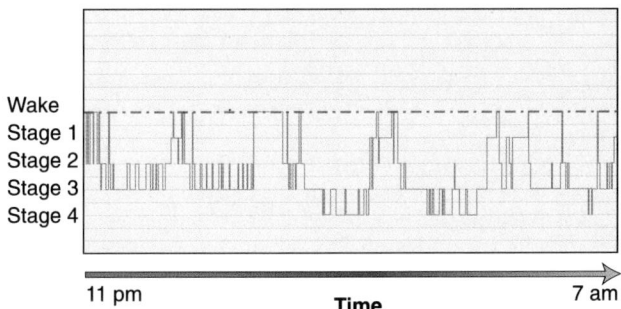

Fig. 40.2 Simplified hypnogram of an adult's fragmented sleep. *(Courtesy Adrian Zacher, 2013. Snorer.com.)*

noise, these repetitive arousals occur for the most part without the individual being aware, sometimes several hundred times a night.

Each apneic episode can last from a few seconds to approximately 2 minutes. The individual's descent into the deeper and more restorative slow-wave stages of sleep is interrupted because he or she has partially awakened to restore the airway. Sleep becomes highly fragmented, and the consequent daytime sleepiness known as *hypersomnolence* increases the individual's risk of accidents at home, at work, and on the road.[50]

OSA has a significant impact on an individual's quality of life.[10] If left untreated, it has neurologic and physiologic consequences,[37] including increased morbidity and mortality[35] and, particularly for men, impaired cardiovascular[51] and metabolic[18] function.

Prevalence of Obstructive Sleep Apnea

Sleep apnea affects a large number of people, but it continues to be largely unrecognized. Estimates suggest that 24% of men and 9% of women who are 30 to 60 years old with an average body mass index of 25 to 28 kg/m^2 are affected.[49] When considered in the context of the concurrent metabolic dysfunction epidemic (which is manifested in obesity, cardiovascular disease,[31,26] and type 2 diabetes in men[12,40,39]), the prevalence of sleep apnea becomes alarming. The International Diabetes Federation urges health care professionals to ensure that a person diagnosed with OSA is evaluated for type 2 diabetes and vice versa.[41]

Central, Mixed, and Complex Apnea

In contrast to OSA, central sleep apnea (CSA) occurs without physical obstruction of the airway. CSA is caused by disorders that are characterized by the intermittent loss of the respiratory drive. Fig. 40.3 shows the lack of chest wall movement in a patient with CSA. Cheyne–Stokes respirations as a form of CSA are most often seen in patients with heart failure. Mixed apnea is a combination of OSA and CSA. Complex apnea occurs when CSA events emerge in response to PAP therapy for OSA.[17]

This chapter is confined to OSA because it is by far the most common form of apnea, and it is in the provision of oral devices, also known as *mandibular repositioning devices* (MRDs), for OSA that the suitably trained dentist can play a role.[22]

Chronic Disease

The maintenance of a separate silo approach and viewing one aspect of an individual's symptomatology in isolation can be considered flawed thinking. OSA in isolation and as a potential component of metabolic syndrome (i.e., syndrome Z[47]) requires a multidisciplinary approach to chronic disease management. The World Health Organization[48] states that chronic diseases are projected to be the leading cause of disability; if they are not successfully prevented and managed by 2020, they will become the most expensive problems for health care systems.

Diagnosis of Obstructive Sleep Apnea

Snoring is a symptom of a partially impeded airway, the walls of which are vibrating as the air passes. How frequently the walls of the airway vibrate (i.e., snoring noise) or collapse (i.e., apnea events of varying duration) indicates the severity of OSA.

A multidisciplinary team approach is necessary for the diagnosis and treatment of OSA. Dentists are experts when it comes to the mouth and should be recognized as such. For OSA treatment, dentists need to build relationships with physicians so they can provide an appropriate dental solution for a medical condition. However, it is important to recognize that the diagnosis of OSA is not within the purview of dentistry.[7]

The closest thing to internationally accepted practice parameters, which are those issued by the American Academy of Sleep Medicine,[14] state that the "presence or absence and severity of OSA must be determined before initiating treatment." In practice, this means that a dentist must not initiate treatment with an oral device unless the patient has been assessed, medically diagnosed, and then referred to the dentist (Fig. 40.4).

If OSA is suspected, a referral is made for a sleep study. This can involve spending a night in a sleep laboratory or at home with an electronic monitoring device to wear while sleeping. A sleep laboratory is essentially a bedroom with monitoring equipment.

In a sleep laboratory, the patient undergoes *polysomnography* (PSG), during which multiple parameters are monitored while the patient is asleep. These parameters include, but are not limited to, sound, video, oxygen saturation, respiratory effort, electrocardiography, electroencephalography, and body position. Attended overnight PSG is an expensive assessment to perform, and availability and access vary based on geography.

Several screening protocols have been proposed over the years.[24,20] In January 2012, the California Dental Association[8] determined that it was appropriate for dentists to screen patients for the signs and

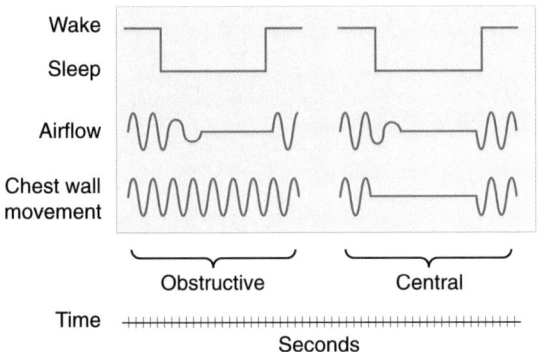

Fig. 40.3 Obstructive versus central apnea. *(Courtesy Learning Center, ResMed, San Diego, CA.)*

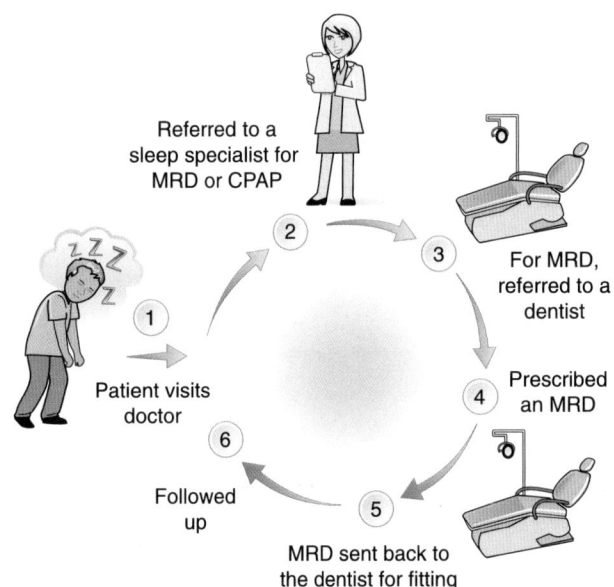

Fig. 40.4 Obstructive sleep apnea diagnosis and treatment route. *CPAP,* Continuous positive airway pressure; *MRD,* mandibular repositioning device. *(Courtesy ResMed, San Diego, CA, 2011.)*

symptoms of SDB and to work with physicians to diagnose and treat it. The association also stated that SDB is a medical condition and that its diagnosis is outside of the scope of the practice of dentistry.

Whether a PSG is essential to diagnose OSA is being questioned.[36] Since 2009 in the United Kingdom, a general dental practitioner working as part of a multidisciplinary team (including a sleep medicine specialist) can, in certain defined circumstances, screen, recognize the need for, and initiate treatment with an MRD without a prior medical diagnosis.[45] Currently in the United States, PSG and home study monitor results need to be interpreted by a physician.

The role of home sleep testing and who should interpret the data that it produces are points of contention that fuel the debate surrounding PSG. The need for mandatory PSG may be questioned in response to the following:

- Increasingly valid and competitively priced home sleep testing equipment
- Increase in the number of patients requiring assessment
- Perception that PSG is the point of contention in the treatment process
- Realization that oral devices are appropriate for milder forms of OSA and that dentists are uniquely positioned to provide them because they may see patients more frequently than sleep medicine specialists
- Realization that a trained dentist, as part of a multidisciplinary team, can filter referrals to the sleep medicine specialist

A sleep laboratory's main function is to diagnose OSA and then offer treatment to those who are likely to benefit from it. If the symptoms are fairly disabling and the diagnosis is confirmed by a sleep study, PAP therapy is routinely offered. Increasingly, around the world, oral devices are becoming a first-line treatment for mild to moderate OSA when they can be prescribed and monitored by a multidisciplinary team. Fig. 40.5 provides definitions and diagnostic criteria for SDB.[44]

Treatment Options for Obstructive Sleep Apnea

Otolaryngology or Oromaxillofacial Surgery

Surgical options for snoring and OSA are largely outside of the scope of this text. However, when physical obstructions to the airway (e.g., tonsils, deviated septum, nasal polyps) are present, surgical correction may improve breathing. For example, if adenotonsillar hypertrophy exists, childhood correction is considered advantageous.[30]

Apnea	Cessation of airflow > 10 seconds
Hypopnea	> 50% reduction in airflow for > 10 seconds
Apnea hypopnea index (AHI)	Number of apneas and hypopneas per hour of sleep
Severity	Normal: AHI < 5 Mild: AHI 5–15 Moderate: AHI 15–30 Severe: AHI > 30
Sleep apnea syndrome (SAS)	AHI > 5 with symptoms
Cheyne–Stokes respiration	> 3 consecutive cyclical crescendo-decrescendo changes in breathing apmplitude during 10 consecutive minutes and/or an AHI > 5

Fig. 40.5 Sleep-related disorders in adults: definitions and diagnostic criteria.

Limited evidence for adult palatal surgery, which is known as *uvulopalatopharyngoplasty,* exists; this surgery should be considered only after PAP therapy has failed.[6] Maxillary or bimaxillary orthognathic surgery is rarely considered, whereas tracheotomy is an effective option of last resort because it completely bypasses the affected area.

Positive Airway Pressure

PAP (Fig. 40.6) is considered the first-line treatment for OSA, and it is very effective in helping the patient to overcome daytime sleepiness symptoms. Individuals with severe sleep apnea do well with this therapy, despite the forbidding appearance. Possibly considered an arduous therapy, it involves wearing a mask over the nose (and sometimes the mouth and nose) at night while being connected to a quiet blower. It works by slightly pressurizing the upper airway, thereby pneumatically splinting it open and preventing it from collapsing. PAP is particularly useful when there is a need for rapid control of OSA.

The sleep laboratory may also suggest that oral device therapy is appropriate. This depends on the severity of the OSA and the existence of other comorbidities. Oral devices can be used to provide therapy for sleep apnea of any severity; however, effective results are considered less certain with increasing severity.[19] PAP and MRD therapies are complementary; in patients with moderate OSA, the two modalities in some circumstances can be considered equally appropriate. Fig. 40.7 illustrates this point in broad terms. Treatment of severe sleep apnea with an oral device necessitates careful patient

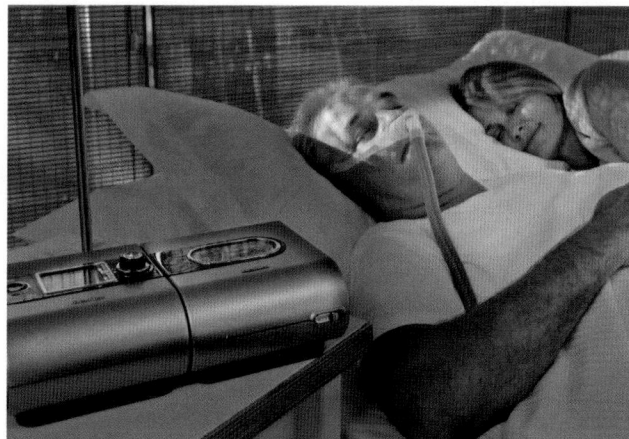

Fig. 40.6 Positive airway pressure therapy. *(Courtesy ResMed, San Diego, CA, 2011.)*

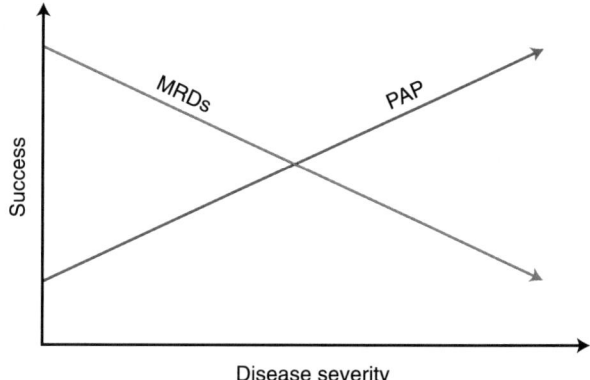

Fig. 40.7 Complementary therapies. *MRD,* Mandibular repositioning device; *PAP,* positive airway pressure. *(Courtesy Adrian Zacher, 2013, Snorer.com.)*

Normal airway   With apnea   With MRD

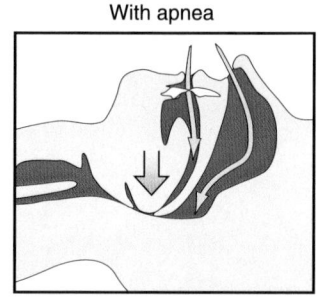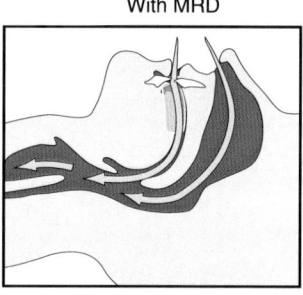

Fig. 40.8 Airway status: healthy and apneic, with a mandibular repositioning device (MRD). *(Courtesy ResMed, San Diego, CA, 2011.)*

monitoring, because things such as small weight changes can negate the effect.[34]

The technology of PAP and oral devices is fast developing, with particular focus on improving the patient's ability to tolerate their use and minimize their side effects. PAP development focuses on better mask design, the inclusion of air humidifiers, and the sensitive electronically controlled variation of air pressure in response to inspiration and expiration. Oral devices have become increasingly adjustable and thinner, and they can be designed to minimize some common side effects, such as hypersalivation and incisor sensitivity. Future developments in oral devices may focus on objective compliance monitoring and treatment efficacy.

Oral Devices for Mandibular Repositioning

The developing role of dentistry in the provision of oral devices for snoring and OSA has given rise to concerns about training and professional indemnity. Dentists may be asked to place antisnoring devices; consequently, state boards of dentistry (and insurance providers) are issuing position statements regarding whether the provision of these devices falls within the practice of dentistry. These statements will determine whether the devices are within the scope of the assistance normally provided.

Dentists should check with their state boards of dentistry and professional indemnity insurers to clarify the situation. Most insurers suggest that dentists are well placed to construct oral devices, provided that they have appropriate training to do so. However, the treatment of snoring and OSA does not routinely fall within the definition of the practice of dentistry and therefore would fall outside of the scope of assistance normally provided by the insurer.

Dentists should undergo a documented training course in the provision of antisnoring devices that includes training in appropriate screening for OSA. Candidates for oral devices should be properly assessed for the signs and symptoms of OSA in accordance with contemporary standards, and the assessment should be documented. If the patient exhibits signs or symptoms of OSA, there must be a referral for a medical assessment. Patients should be advised about the risks and benefits of antisnoring devices, including the potential impact on the occlusion, periodontium, and TMJs. Documentary evidence of the consent process must be retained. When OSA exists, an antisnoring device should be supplied only as part of an integrated treatment plan provided by a multidisciplinary team that includes the dentist.

Devices Pertinent to the Dentist

Oral devices for snoring and OSA aim to maintain the upper airway during sleep. Tongue-retaining devices and MRDs do this either directly, by acting on the tongue and holding it in a forward position, or indirectly, by forward repositioning of the mandible, which maintains upper airway patency (Fig. 40.8). MRDs are the most researched type of oral device for OSA, and they are the focus of this chapter.

Custom-made adjustable devices typically are associated with better treatment outcomes[46] compared with universal "boil and bite" MRDs. Adjustable MRDs are more likely to provide successful therapy in patients with moderate to severe OSA than nonadjustable MRDs.[29]

Predictor Devices

Sleep medicine specialists charged with caring for patients with OSA understandably desire certainty that the patient has been effectively treated. This has historically represented a legitimate concern when considering an MRD for a patient with OSA and has resulted in MRDs being confined to use for mild to moderate OSA. Predictor devices, which are sometimes known as *titration devices*,[11] are intended to do the following:
- Establish whether the patient can tolerate an intraoral device and whether it is subjectively effective
- Objectively determine whether mandibular repositioning delivers adequate therapy
- Provide a prescription jaw relationship for custom MRD manufacture if the outcome is positive

The use of predictor devices has been an area of MRD technologic innovation during recent years. In this role, it is important that predictor devices not be confused with thermoplastic universal treatment devices. Predictor devices are expressly designed for use for a limited number of nights; their use is self-limited, and they sacrifice patient convenience for functionality. Basic taxonomy for the oral devices of MRDs is shown in Fig. 40.9.

Characteristics of the Ideal Oral Device

From an individual wearer's perspective, any intraoral device feels foreign and invasive. The individual may seek treatment largely to please his or her partner and may perceive little or no personal benefit because hypersomnolence symptoms correlate poorly with OSA severity.[10] Affected individuals may have forgotten what it feels like to be fully awake.

Side effects of early devices included hypersalivation or dry mouth when worn, dental sensitivity, and perhaps a claustrophobic locking of the jaws in a protrusive position and a morning postwear TMJ ache. For these reasons, early oral devices required development. Some MRD manufacturers have reduced or eliminated these side effects, but there is no single perfect device.[2] Knowledge of a range of MRDs to suit different individuals is necessary. The characteristics of the ideal MRD vary for each patient, and some characteristics may preclude others. Table 40.1 presents several options.

Recognizing that a child may benefit from an SDB investigation is important. MRDs are *not* recommended for children unless they

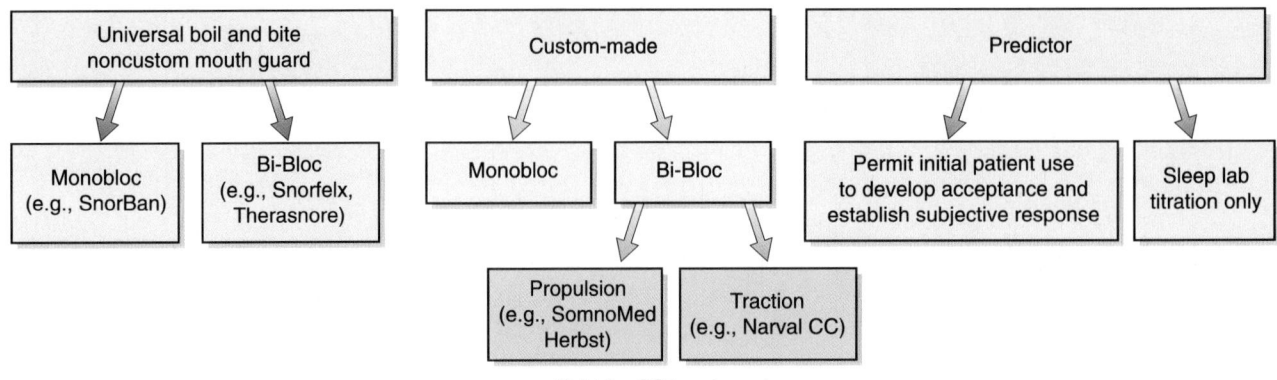

Monobloc: inherently not adjustable in protrusion
Bi-Bloc: varyingly adjustable in protrusion and sometimes vertical dimensions; may permit lateral movement for bruxism

Valid for OSA and snoring

Fig. 40.9 Mandibular repositioning device taxonomy. *(Courtesy Adrian Zacher, 2013, Snorer.com.)*

TABLE 40.1 Characteristics of the Ideal Mandibular Repositioning Device

Acceptance, Adherence, and Efficacy	Mitigation of Side Effects	Practical Considerations
Constructed of two separate pieces; to give the patient time to accept wearing the device, one half is worn alone before the complete device is worn	Metal-free; no parts that can fatigue, fracture, and then be inhaled or ingested to create a galvanic reaction with other dental restorations	Low cost
Enables titration anteroposteriorly for tolerability and effect	Minimal bulk for less impact on phonetic function and reduced hypersalivation	East to fit for the patient and dental practitioner
Enables starting titration from zero protrusion to improve comfort throughout the titration process	Does not dictate a protrusive path or final protruded position for the temporomandibular joints	Can be titrated in the sleep laboratory without waking the patient
Encourages the mouth to close and prevents the mouth from falling open at sleep onset	No unwanted orthodontic effects (e.g., incisor tilting)	Instant device; no impressions or laboratory work required
Permits lip seal and encourages nasal breathing		Minimal follow-up appointments
Enables titration of the vertical opening (i.e., <5 mm measured at the incisors) considered optimal for acceptance and adherence[38]		Easy to modify
Easy to clean		Does not necessitate a remake if a dental restoration is necessary
Permits lateral movement where there is evidence of parafunction		
Does not encroach on tongue space or impede forward movement of the tongue		
Includes compliance and efficacy monitoring		
Is it worn and does it work?		

From Adrian Zacher, 2013. https://snorer.com/snorer-training-for-dentists-who-want-to-help-snorers/.

are under the supervision of an orthodontist who is working as part of a multidisciplinary team.

Communication

Effective communication among the referring sleep laboratory, the patient, and the patient's general dental practitioner is essential and should begin before the patient is seen (Box 40.1).

Sleep Laboratory and Primary Care Physician Communication

The OSA diagnosis and the requirement for revaluation should be confirmed. Relevant medical history information should be exchanged. The existence of positional apnea (i.e., apnea that worsens when sleeping supine) should also be documented.

BOX 40.1 The Take-Home Message

1. Has the presence (and severity) or absence of obstructive sleep apnea been established?
2. Is the patient at least partially dentate? Does he or she have sufficient alveolar bone to withstand lateral loads?
3. Are you satisfied that there is no severe periodontal condition that the device would prejudice? Does the patient possess the competence to maintain his or her oral hygiene?
4. Are you satisfied there is no gross temporomandibular disorder?
5. Have you ensured that there is no pronounced gag reflex?
6. Does the patient have a competent nasal airway?
7. Does the patient comprehend the costs of therapy?
8. Have the patient's expectations of therapy been managed appropriately?

Patient Communication

Valid informed consent for treatment (including a risk-benefit analysis, information about side effects, and therapy limitations) and permission to obtain dental records from the general dental practitioner should be obtained.

General Dental Practitioner

With reference to the patient's existing dental records, a recent orthopantomogram may be valuable.

General Indications and Contraindications

When a patient who has been diagnosed with OSA is referred to a dentist, assessment to determine the suitability of MRD therapy is based on an individual analysis of indications and contraindications. It is essential to obtain valid informed consent and baseline records and to retain pre-MRD therapy casts. Uncontrolled epilepsy is an absolute contraindication.

All MRDs, which are also known as *mandibular advancement devices* (MADs) or *oral appliances,* protrude the mandible, but each MRD has a unique feature set. In 2010, Ahrens stated that "no [one] MAD design most effectively influences subjectively perceived treatment efficacy, but efficacy depends on many factors, including materials and method used for fabrication, type of MAD (monobloc or twin block [bi-bloc]), and the degree of protrusion."[1] Understanding the differences among these devices enables the dentist to prescribe appropriately, with knowledge of the indications, features, and design limitations, allowing him or her to maximize treatment efficacy and minimize unwanted side effects.

Temporomandibular Joint Dysfunction

Severe TMJ dysfunction, limited opening, and reports of jaw locking should be considered contraindications. A limited protrusive range (i.e., <5 mm) suggests a low likelihood of OSA treatment efficacy with an MRD.

Although basic assessment for TMJ dysfunction is essential, consideration of the validity of certain TMJ theories and diagnostic tools is necessary. Thorough record-keeping is advised. Referral to a dental practitioner who has advanced training in the diagnosis and management of TMJ dysfunction may be indicated if symptoms are identified at the initial evaluation or if they develop at any time during treatment. Reports of diffuse tenderness, ear canal stuffiness, clicks, significant deviation with opening or protruding, or pain associated with these movements necessitate referral to an expert.

Dentate State

The individual must have sound teeth. Edentulous patients are unable to use MRDs because they function by retaining the teeth, and retention is used to reposition the mandible anteriorly. The minimum number and distribution of teeth varies by device. Placement of the adjustment mechanism routinely needs to be on the teeth and not in an edentulous area. To avoid excessive lateral load, the 8 to 10 teeth distributed around the arch serve as a general guide. The shape and inclination of the teeth can affect retention of the MRD and the dentist's ability to provide effective MRD therapy; the presence of no teeth or grossly undercut teeth can be problematic. Difficulty taking impressions in the setting of a pronounced gag reflex suggests that the patient will have difficulty adhering to MRD therapy.

Periodontal Condition and Tooth Mobility

A healthy periodontium with evidence of adequate oral hygiene is essential before therapy with an MRD commences. Anything worn in the mouth can compromise oral hygiene if it is not kept clean.

Bruxism

Management of sleep bruxism is an important role for the dentist. Bruxism is not necessarily a contraindication to MRD therapy. An assessment for TMJ dysfunction is recommended. The bruxing individual should be advised that their parafunction will both limit their choice of MRD and negatively affect the life expectancy of the MRD.

Gastroesophageal Reflux Disease

Dentinal pooling that results from gastroesophageal reflux disease can be a symptom of OSA, and it is one that a dentist is ideally positioned to recognize.

Mandibular Repositioning Device Therapy

Long-term complications of MRD therapy are not well documented. Given the intricacies of determining which device is most likely to be successful, the role of titration, and the management of complications, the dentist should seek advanced training before supplying MRDs.

Complete periodontal assessment should precede the decision to fit a patient with an MRD. Management of inflammation can be more difficult with an MRD, which the patient must use consistently when sleeping. Bacterial biofilm formation and retention are likely to be encouraged on the tissues and the device, and additional instruction and encouragement regarding effective bacterial biofilm removal are often necessary. Careful and frequent monitoring of the periodontal status with ongoing use of the MRD is essential to confirm sustained health and tooth stability, to recognize negative changes, and to recommend intervention and consideration of an alternative treatment modality.

Conclusions

Around the world, the future of sleep medicine is being debated. In the United States, the American Academy of Sleep Medicine published a white paper on its website.[4] The aim of this publication was to devise "frameworks for health care delivery such as the patient-centered medical home (PCMH), patient registries, and new outcomes measures and tools for the diagnosis and treatment of sleep disorders." With the rise in awareness of how obesity, cardiology, diabetes, and OSA are interrelated, sleep laboratories may in the future evolve into metabolism centers.

In 1997, Loube and Strauss[32] concluded that "future efforts at enhancing cooperation between dentists and sleep disorders physicians in the treatment of OSA with oral appliances should be promoted as a means of standardizing treatment." Empowering appropriately trained team members to perform functions that they are well positioned to undertake seems logical and, in the face of an epidemic and a global financial crisis, necessary.

The role of dentistry in sleep medicine is developing to include increased emphasis on screening, and it may include patient evaluation (e.g., monitoring MRD compliance and objective efficacy). It may also include blood pressure and weight monitoring in an effort to recognize the best time to transition from an oral device to PAP.

The correlation of clinical indicators (e.g., incisal wear, tooth mobility) as signs of SDB with a patient's hypertension, for example, can help the physician develop a broad-based strategy of intervention. The roles of breathing obstruction in its various forms in the amplification of periodontal damage (see Chapter 55) and masticatory system disorders (see Chapter 26) are addressed in this textbook.

Perspective is essential and can be gained through working as part of a multidisciplinary team. Tooth movement that in isolation may appear to be significant can be considered relatively unimportant when placed in the context of breathing and sleeping.

 A Case Scenario is found on the companion website www.expertconsult.com.

References

 References for this chapter are found on the companion website www.expertconsult.com.

CHAPTER 41

Periodontal Therapy in the Female Patient

Joan Otomo-Corgel

CHAPTER OUTLINE

Puberty

Menses

Pregnancy

Oral Contraceptives

Menopause *(e-only)*

Conclusions

 Content on menopause can be accessed on the companion website at www.expertconsult.com.

Throughout a woman's life, hormonal influences affect therapeutic decision making in periodontics. Historically, therapies have been gender biased. Research has provided a keener appreciation of the unique systemic influences on oral, periodontal, and implant tissues. Oral health care professionals have greater awareness of and can better deal with hormonal influences associated with the reproductive process. Periodontal and oral tissue responses can be altered, creating diagnostic and therapeutic dilemmas. The clinician should recognize, customize, and appropriately alter periodontal therapy according to the individual woman's needs based on her stage of life.

Sex steroids exert profound biologic effects on immune function and bone metabolism.[137] Estrogen can significantly affect the periodontium, including maturation of gingival epithelium, osteoblastic differentiation of periodontal ligament cells, and bone formation.[136]

This chapter reviews phases of the female reproductive cycle from puberty through menopause. Periodontal manifestations, systemic effects, and clinical management are addressed.

Puberty

Puberty occurs, on average, between the ages of 11 to 14 in most girls. The production of sex hormones (i.e., estrogen and progesterone) increases and then remains relatively constant during the remainder of the reproductive phase. The prevalence of gingivitis increases without an increase in the amount of plaque. Gram-negative anaerobes, especially *Prevotella intermedia*, have been associated with puberty gingivitis. Kornman and Loesche[69] postulated that this anaerobic organism may use ovarian hormones as a substitute for vitamin K as a growth factor. Levels of black-pigmented *Bacteroides*, especially *P. intermedia* (formerly known as *Bacteroides intermedius*), are thought to increase with increased levels of gonadotropic hormones in puberty. *Capnocytophaga* species also increase in incidence and proportion. These organisms have been implicated in the increased bleeding tendency observed during puberty.

Studies of pubertal gingivitis indicate proportionately elevated numbers of motile rods, spirochetes, and *P. intermedia*.[47,96] Statistically significant increases in gingival inflammation and the proportions of *P. intermedia* and *Prevotella nigrescens* have been seen in pubertal gingivitis.[100] A study of 11- to 17-year-old adolescents found higher levels of *Actinobacillus actinomycetemcomitans* and *Fusobacterium nucleatum,* which were associated with bleeding indices, probing depth, and attachment loss.[83]

During puberty, periodontal tissues can have an exaggerated response to local factors. A hyperplastic reaction of the gingiva can occur in areas where food debris, materia alba, plaque, and calculus are deposited. The inflamed tissues become erythematous, lobulated, and retractable. Bleeding may occur easily with mechanical debridement of the gingival tissues. Histologically, the appearance is consistent with inflammatory hyperplasia.

During the reproductive years, women tend to have a more vigorous immune response, including higher immunoglobulin concentrations, stronger primary and secondary responses, increased resistance to the induction of immunologic tolerance, and a greater ability to reject tumors and homografts.[135] Allergy, sensitivity, and asthma occur more often in young men, but after puberty, women become more susceptible than their male counterparts.

KEY FACT

Sex steroids exert profound biologic effects on immune function and bone metabolism. Estrogen can have a significant impact on the periodontium, including maturation of gingival epithelium, osteoblastic differentiation of periodontal ligament cells, and bone formation. During puberty, periodontal tissues can have an exaggerated response to local factors. A hyperplastic reaction of the gingiva can occur. Inflamed tissues become erythematous, lobulated, retractable, and bleed easily. Histologically, the appearance is consistent with inflammatory hyperplasia.

Management

During puberty, education of the parent or caregiver is part of successful periodontal therapy. Preventive care, including a vigorous program of oral hygiene, is also vital.[5] Milder gingivitis cases respond well to scaling and root planing, with frequent oral hygiene reinforcement. Severe cases of gingivitis may require microbial culturing, antimicrobial mouthwashes and local site delivery, or antibiotic therapy. Periodontal maintenance appointments may need to be more frequent when periodontal instability is identified.

The clinician should recognize the periodontal manifestations and intraoral lesions associated with systemic diseases (e.g., diabetes).[23,106] Thorough review of the patient's medical history and medical referral should occur when deemed necessary. The clinician should be aware of the effects of chronic regurgitation of gastric contents on intraoral tissues; this age group is susceptible to eating disorders such as bulimia and anorexia nervosa.[15] *Perimolysis* (i.e., smooth erosion of enamel and dentin), typically on the lingual surfaces of maxillary anterior teeth, varies with the duration and frequency of the behavior.[17] Enlargement of the parotid glands (occasionally sublingual glands) has been estimated to occur in 10% to 50% of patients who binge and purge.[88] A diminished salivary flow rate may be identified, which can increase oral mucous membrane sensitivity, gingival erythema, and caries susceptibility.

Menses

Periodontal Manifestations

During the reproductive years, the ovarian cycle is controlled by the anterior pituitary gland. The gonadotropin follicle-stimulating hormone (FSH) and luteinizing hormone (LH) are produced by the anterior pituitary gland. The secretion of gonadotropins also depends on the hypothalamus. Ongoing changes in the concentration of the gonadotropins and ovarian hormones occur during the monthly menstrual cycle (Fig. 41.1). Under the influence of FSH and LH, estrogen and progesterone are steroid hormones produced by the ovaries during the menstrual cycle. During the reproductive cycle, the purpose of estrogen and progesterone is to prepare the uterus for implantation of an egg.

The monthly reproductive cycle has two phases. The first phase is referred to as the *follicular phase*. Levels of FSH are elevated, and estradiol (E2), the major form of estrogen, is synthesized by the developing follicle and peaks approximately 2 days before ovulation. Estrogen stimulates the egg to move down the fallopian tubes (i.e., ovulation) and stimulates proliferation of the stroma cells, blood vessels, and glands of the endometrium.

The second phase is called the *luteal phase*. The developing corpus luteum synthesizes estradiol and progesterone. Estrogen peaks at 0.2 ng/

mL and progesterone at 10.0 ng/mL to complete the rebuilding of the endometrium for implantation of a fertilized egg. If the egg is not fertilized, the corpus luteum involutes, ovarian hormone levels drop, and menstruation ensues. It has been postulated that ovarian hormones increase inflammation in gingival tissues and exaggerate the response to local irritants. Gingival inflammation seems to be aggravated by an imbalance or increase in sex hormones.[55,56] Menstrual cycle irregularity is a risk indicator for periodontal disease before menopause.[48] Numerous in vitro and in vivo studies have demonstrated that sex hormones affect and modify the actions of cells of the immune system.

Evidence suggests that the interaction between estrogen and cells of the immune system can have nonimmune regulatory effects.[7,22] Possible mechanisms have been suggested for the increase in hormonal gingival interaction in the menstrual cycle. Tumor necrosis factor alpha (TNF-α), which fluctuates during the menstrual cycle[13]; elevated prostaglandin E2 (PGE2) synthesis[93]; and angiogenetic factors, endothelial growth factors, and receptors may be modulated by progesterone and estrogen, contributing to increases in gingival inflammation during certain stages of the menstrual cycle.[65]

Progesterone has been associated with increased permeability of the microvasculature, altering the rate and pattern of collagen production in the gingiva,[84] increasing folate metabolism,[111,149] and altering the immune response. During menses, progesterone increases from the second week, peaks at approximately 10 days, and dramatically drops before menstruation (based on a 28-day cycle; individual cycles vary). Progesterone plays a role in stimulating the production of prostaglandins that mediate the body's response to inflammation. PGE2 is one of the major secretory products of monocytes, and the level is increased in inflamed gingiva. Miyagi and colleagues[92] found that the chemotaxis of polymorphonuclear leukocytes (PMNs) was enhanced by progesterone but reduced by estradiol. Testosterone did not have a measurable effect on PMN chemotaxis. The researchers suggested that the altered PMN chemotaxis associated with gingival inflammation might be caused by the effects of sex hormones. Physiologic, experimental, and clinical data confirm differences in immune responses between the two sexes.[158]

Gingival tissues have been reported to be more edematous during menses and erythematous before the onset of menses in some women.

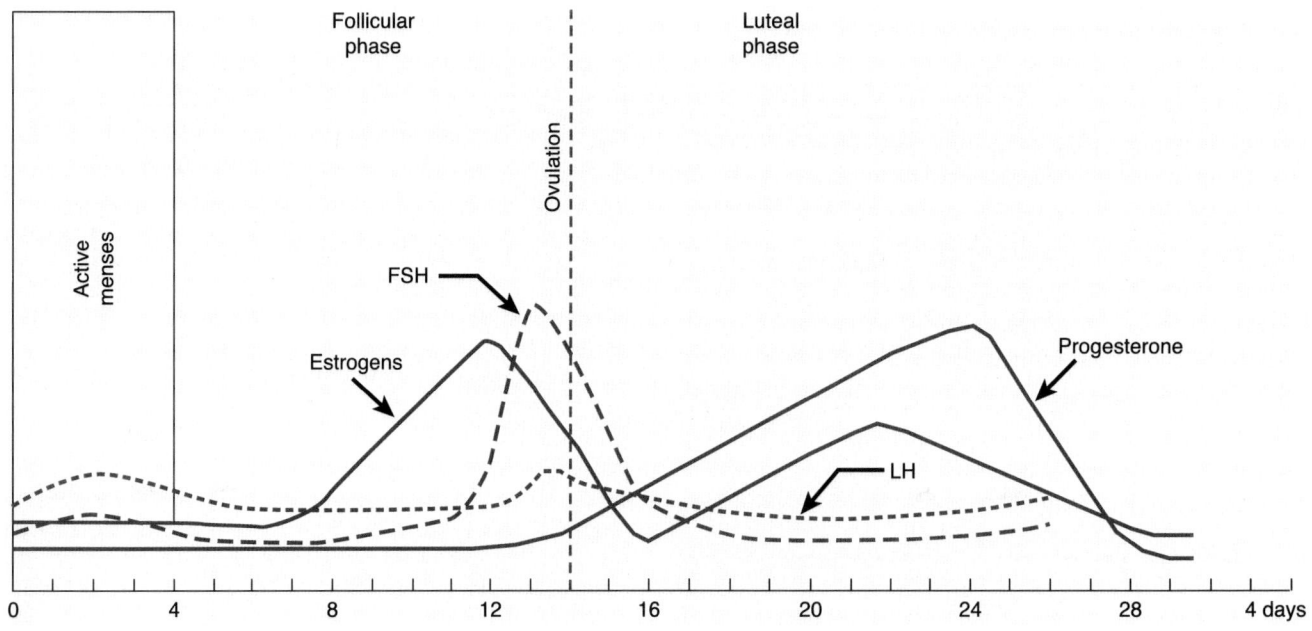

Fig. 41.1 Female menstrual cycle, showing the peak levels of progesterone and estrogen compared with follicle-stimulating hormone *(FSH)* and luteinizing hormone *(LH).*

One study reported higher gingival indices during ovulation and before menstruation despite reported increases in oral symptoms during menses.[85] An increase of gingival exudate has been observed during the menstrual period and is sometimes associated with a minor increase in tooth mobility.[43] The incidence of postextraction osteitis is also higher during initiation of menses. No significant hematologic laboratory findings accompany this, other than a slightly reduced platelet count and a slight increase in clotting time.

When the progesterone level is highest (during the luteal phase of the cycle), intraoral recurrent aphthous ulcers,[35] herpes labialis lesions, and candidal infections occur in some women in a cyclic pattern. Because the esophageal sphincter is relaxed by progesterone, women may be more susceptible to gastroesophageal reflux disease (GERD) during this time of the cycle. Symptoms of GERD include heartburn, regurgitation, and chest pain, and when reflux is severe, some patients develop unexplained coughing, hoarseness, sore throat, gingivitis, or asthma.[127]

Management

During the peak level of progesterone (about 7 to 10 days before menstruation), premenstrual syndrome (PMS) may also occur. There appears to be no significant difference in estrogen and progesterone levels between women with PMS and those without PMS. However, women with PMS seem to have lower levels of certain neurotransmitters such as enkephalins, endorphins, γ-aminobutyric acid (GABA), and serotonin. Depression, irritability, mood swings, and difficulty with memory and concentration are symptoms of neurotransmitter reduction. Patients are more sensitive and less tolerant of procedures, have a heightened gag reflex, and can have an exaggerated response to pain.

Increased gingival bleeding and tenderness associated with the menstrual cycle require closer periodontal monitoring. Periodontal maintenance should be titrated to the individual patient's need, and if problematic, 3- to 4-month intervals should be recommended. An antimicrobial oral rinse before cyclic inflammation may be indicated. Emphasis should be placed on oral hygiene. For the patient with a history of excessive postoperative hemorrhage or menstrual flow, scheduling surgical visits after cyclic menstruation is prudent. Anemia is common, and appropriate consultation with a physician and laboratory tests, when indicated, should be maintained.

During PMS, many women exhibit physical symptoms that include fatigue, sweet and salty food cravings, abdominal bloating, swollen hands or feet, headaches, breast tenderness, nausea, and gastrointestinal upset. GERD may make it more uncomfortable for the patient to lie fully supine, especially after a meal, and she may have a more sensitive gag reflex. The clinician should be aware that nonsteroidal antiinflammatory drugs (NSAIDs), infection, and acidic foods exacerbate GERD. Patients with GERD may take over-the-counter antacids, H_2-receptor antagonists (e.g., cimetidine, famotidine, nizatidine, ranitidine), prokinetic agents (e.g., cisapride, metoclopramide), or proton pump inhibitors (e.g., lansoprazole, omeprazole, pantoprazole, rabeprazole).[128] These medications interact with some antibiotics and antifungals, and a review of their pharmacology is necessary. Fluoride rinses and trays, frequent periodontal debridement, and avoidance of mouthwashes with high alcohol content can reduce the associated gingival and caries sequelae.

PMS is often treated with antidepressants. Selective serotonin reuptake inhibitors (SSRIs) usually are the first-line choice because they have fewer side effects than other antidepressants, do not require blood monitoring, and are safe if overdosed. Women with PMS taking the SSRI fluoxetine had a 70% response rate. Fluoxetine was ranked the fifth most dispensed prescription (i.e., new and refills) in the United States in 1998, but when the patent was lifted, sales

slowed. However, overall SSRIs ranked second in total dollar sales in the 2000s. Sertraline was ranked twelfth and is the drug of choice for treatment of PMS.[166]

The clinician should be aware that patients taking fluoxetine have increased side effects with highly protein-bound drugs (e.g., aspirin), and the half-life of diazepam and other central nervous system (CNS) depressants is increased. Other common SSRIs are fluvoxamine, paroxetine, and citalopram. Other prescribed antidepressants include selective serotonin-norepinephrine reuptake inhibitors (SNRIs), tricyclics, trazodone, mirtazapine, nefazodone, and maprotiline.

KEY FACT

Increased gingival bleeding and tenderness associated with the menstrual cycle require close periodontal monitoring. Periodontal maintenance should be adjusted to the individual patient's needs. If problematic, 3- to 4-month recall intervals should be recommended.

The PMS patient may be difficult to treat because of emotional and physiologic sensitivity. The dentist should treat the gingival and oral mucosal tissues gently. Gauze pads or cotton rolls should be moistened with a lubricant, chlorhexidine rinse, or water before placing them in the aphtha-prone patient. Careful retraction of the oral mucosa, cheeks, and lips is necessary in patients prone to aphthous or herpetic lesions. Because the hypoglycemic threshold is elevated, the clinician should advise the patient to have a light snack before her appointment. Of menstruating women, 70% have PMS symptoms, but only 5% meet the strict diagnostic criteria.

Pregnancy

Periodontal Manifestations

The link between pregnancy and periodontal inflammation has been known for many years. In 1778, Vermeeren discussed "toothpains" in pregnancy. In 1818, Pitcarin[118] described gingival hyperplasia in pregnancy. Despite awareness regarding pregnancy and its effect on periodontal disease, only recently has evidence indicated an inverse relationship with systemic health. Research confirms that periodontal disease alters the systemic health of the patient and adversely affects the well-being of the fetus by elevating the risk for preterm, low-birth-weight (PLBW) infants.

In 1877, Pinard[117] recorded the first case of pregnancy gingivitis. Only recently has periodontal research begun to focus on causative mechanisms. Pregnancy gingivitis is extremely common, occurring in 30% to 100% of pregnant women.[50,74,82,132] It is characterized by erythema, edema, hyperplasia, and increased bleeding. Histologically, the description is the same as for gingivitis. However, the etiologic factors are different despite clinical and histologic similarities. Cases range from mild to severe inflammation (Fig. 41.2), which can progress to severe hyperplasia, pain, and bleeding (Figs. 41.3 and 41.4).

Other growths that resemble pregnancy granulomas must be ruled out, such as central giant cell granulomas or underlying systemic diseases. Periodontal status before pregnancy may influence the progression or severity as the circulating hormones fluctuate. The anterior region of the mouth is affected more often, and interproximal sites tend to be most involved.[27] Increased tissue edema can lead to increased pocket depths and may be associated with transient tooth mobility.[120] Anterior site inflammation can be exacerbated by increased mouth breathing, primarily in the third trimester, from pregnancy rhinitis. The gingiva is the most common site involved (approximately 70% of cases), followed by the tongue and lips, buccal mucosa, and

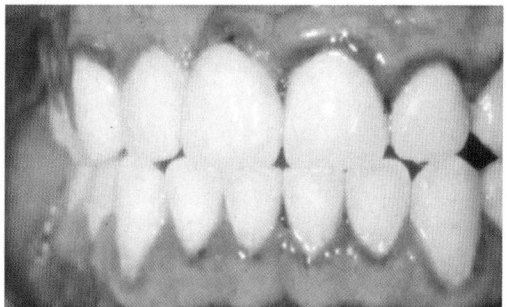

Fig. 41.2 Moderate form of pregnancy gingivitis.

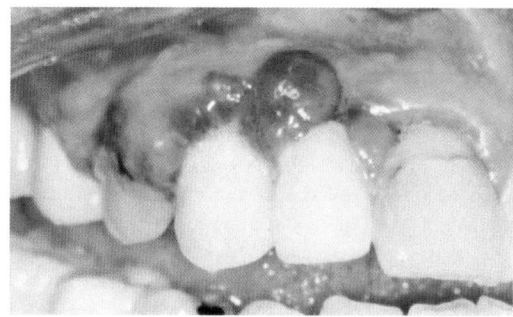

Fig. 41.3 Pyogenic granuloma of pregnancy (i.e., pregnancy tumor).

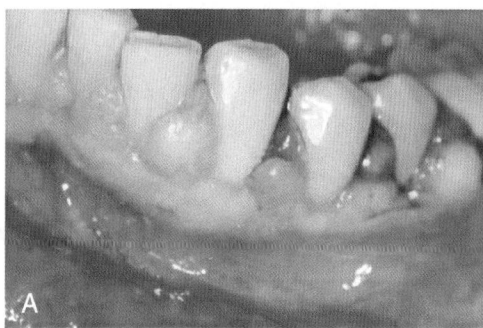

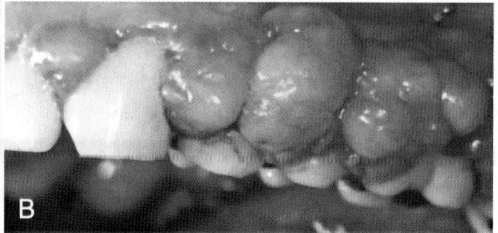

Fig. 41.4 Severe pregnancy gingivitis with hyperplasia can occur in patients with poorly controlled non–insulin-dependent diabetes mellitus. (A) Moderate gingival enlargement. (B) Severe gingival enlargement.

palate.[132] An increase in attachment loss can represent active periodontal infection accelerated by pregnancy.[75]

Pyogenic granulomas (i.e., pregnancy tumors or pregnancy epulis) occur in 0.2% to 9.6% of pregnancies. They are clinically and histologically indistinguishable from pyogenic granulomas occurring in nonpregnant women or in men. Pyogenic granulomas appear most often during the second or third month of pregnancy. Clinically, they bleed easily and become hyperplastic and nodular. When excised, the lesions usually do not leave a large defect. They may be sessile or pedunculated and ulcerated, ranging in color from purplish red to deep blue, depending on the vascularity of the lesion and degree of venous stasis.[10] The lesion classically occurs in an area of gingivitis and is associated with poor oral hygiene and calculus. Alveolar bone loss is usually not associated with pyogenic granulomas of pregnancy.

Role of Pregnancy Hormones
Subgingival Plaque Composition
Epidemiologic studies indicate a relationship between the level of home care and the severity of gingival inflammation. It appears that the association between signs of gingival inflammation and the amount of plaque is greater after parturition than during pregnancy. An alteration in the compositions of subgingival plaque occurs during pregnancy. Kornman and Loesche[70] found that during the second trimester, gingivitis and gingival bleeding increased without an increase in plaque levels. Bacterial anaerobic/aerobic ratios increased in addition to proportions of *Bacteroides melaninogenicus* and *P. intermedia* (2.2% to 10.1%). The study authors suggested that estradiol or progesterone could substitute for menadione (vitamin K) as an essential growth factor for *P. intermedia* but not *Porphyromonas gingivalis* or *Eikenella corrodens*. There was also an increase in *P. gingivalis* during the 21st through 27th weeks of gestation, but this was not statistically significant. The relative increase in the numbers of *P. intermedia* may be a more sensitive indicator of an

altered systemic hormonal situation than clinical parameters of gingivitis.[140]

One study concluded that subgingival levels of bacteria associated with periodontitis did not change. *P. gingivalis* and *Tannerella forsythia* counts were higher and associated with bleeding on probing at week 12.[2] Bacterial challenge to the gingival tissues, quantitatively (plaque scores) and qualitatively (*P. gingivalis*), appears to affect the level of gingival inflammation observed during pregnancy.[18]

Periodontal Disease and Preterm, Low-Birth-Weight Infants
Although most studies support a causal relationship regarding the hypothesis that periodontitis during pregnancy poses an increased risk of adverse pregnancy outcomes, there are conflicting results. Variations in study results may result from confounding factors, effect modifiers, populations studied, timing of intervention or evaluation, and severity of periodontal disease based on different definitions.

Several systematic reviews indicate that periodontal disease[134,153,161,162] adversely affects pregnancy outcomes. Intervention trials have shown a positive effect with periodontal therapy and reduction of adverse pregnancy outcomes,[60,80,81,105,147] but three large multicenter trials in the United States did not support these results.[90,102,141] Studies indicate that routine nonsurgical periodontal therapy after the first trimester is not associated with adverse pregnancy outcomes.[90]

Initially, Offenbacher and colleagues[104] provided evidence that untreated periodontal disease in pregnant women could be a significant risk factor for preterm (<37 weeks' gestation), low-birth-weight (<2500 g) infants. The relationship between genitourinary tract infection and PLBW infants is well documented in human and animal studies. Periodontal researchers, suspecting periodontal disease as another source of infection, found that otherwise low-risk mothers of PLBW infants had significantly more periodontal attachment loss than control mothers having normal-weight infants at birth.

Current opinion is that the correlation of periodontal disease with PLBW birth may result from infection and is mediated indirectly, principally by the translocation of bacterial products such as endotoxin (i.e., lipopolysaccharide [LPS]) and the action of maternally produced inflammatory mediators.[38] Jared and coworkers[58] found that fetal exposure to oral pathogens in utero increased the risk of neonatal intensive care unit admission and extended length of stay. Concentrations of biologically active molecules, such as PGE_2 and TNF-α, which usually are involved in normal parturition, are raised to artificially high levels by the infection process, which can foster premature labor.[3]

Gram-negative bacteria in periodontal diseases may permit their selective overgrowth or invasion within the genitourinary tract. Han and associates[49] documented hematogenous spread of oral bacteria to the amnion, and Madianos and colleagues[86] showed that oral bacteria crossed the placental barrier and triggered an immune response by the fetus.

Gingival crevicular fluid (GCF) levels of PGE_2 were positively associated with intraamniotic PGE_2 levels ($P = 0.018$), suggesting that gram-negative periodontal infection presents a systemic challenge sufficient to initiate the onset of premature labor as a source of LPS or through stimulation of secondary inflammatory mediators such as PGE_2 and interleukin-1 beta (IL-1β).[24] Offenbacher and coworkers[103] suggested a dose–response relationship for increasing GCF PGE_2 as a marker of current periodontal disease activity and decreasing birth weight.

Four organisms associated with mature plaque and progressing periodontitis—*T. forsythia, P. gingivalis, A. actinomycetemcomitans,* and *Treponema denticola*—were detected at higher levels in PLBW mothers compared with normal-birth-weight controls. Despite research supporting the association of periodontal disease and PLBW,[25,26] more studies with improved methodology are needed to assess the validity of the association.

KEY FACT

Current opinion suggests a possible association between periodontal disease and preterm, low-birth-weight (PLBW) infants. Adverse pregnancy events can result from an infection that is mediated by one of two major pathways: (1) directly by oral microorganisms or (2) indirectly, principally by the translocation of bacterial products such as endotoxin (i.e., lipopolysaccharide) and the action of maternally produced inflammatory mediators.

Preeclampsia

A systematic review of preeclampsia and periodontitis indicated an increased risk during pregnancy. Preeclampsia is a life-threatening condition in late pregnancy that is characterized by high blood pressure and excess protein in the urine. High C-reactive protein levels also are associated with preeclampsia in this population.[130,138,152]

Maternal Immunoresponse

The maternal immune system is thought to be suppressed during pregnancy. This response may allow the fetus to survive as an allograft. Documentation of immunosuppressive factors in the sera of pregnant women shows a marked increase of monocytes (which in large numbers inhibit in vitro proliferative responses to mitogens, allogenic cells, and soluble antigen),[151] and pregnancy-specific β1-glycoproteins contribute to diminished lymphocyte responsiveness to mitogens and antigens.[11] The ratio of peripheral helper T cells to suppressor T cells (CD4/CD8) decreases throughout pregnancy.[121]

The changes in maternal immunoresponsiveness suggest an increased susceptibility to developing gingival inflammation. In one study, the gingival index was higher, but percentages of T3 (CD3), T4 (CD4), and B cells appeared to decrease in peripheral blood and gingival tissues during pregnancy compared with a control group.[1] Other studies report decreased PMN (i.e., neutrophil) chemotaxis, depression of cell-mediated immunity, phagocytosis, and decreased T-cell response with elevated ovarian hormone levels, especially progesterone.[119] Decreased in vitro responses of peripheral blood lymphocytes to several mitogens and to a preparation of *P. intermedia* have been reported.[12,79,109] Evidence suggests a decrease in the absolute numbers of $CD4^+$ cells in peripheral blood during pregnancy compared with postpartum.[94,102]

Lapp and colleagues[73] suggested that high levels of progesterone during pregnancy affect the development of localized inflammation by downregulation of IL-6 production, rendering the gingiva less efficient at resisting the inflammatory challenges produced by bacteria. Another study indicated that live preterm birth was associated with decreased levels of immunoglobulin G (IgG) antibody to periodontal pathogens in women with periodontitis when assessed during the second trimester, but was not associated with birth outcomes.[29]

Ovarian hormone stimulates the production of prostaglandins, particularly PGE_1 and PGE_2, which are potent mediators of the inflammatory response. With the prostaglandin acting as an immunosuppressant, gingival inflammation can increase when the mediator level is high.[32,107] Kinnby and coworkers[66] found that high progesterone levels during pregnancy influenced plasminogen activator inhibitor type 2 (PAI-2) and disturbed the balance of the fibrinolytic system. Because PAI-2 is an important inhibitor of tissue proteolysis, this research implies that components of the fibrinolytic system may be involved in the development of pregnancy gingivitis.

During pregnancy, sex hormone levels rise dramatically (Box 41.1). Progesterone reaches levels of 100 ng/mL, 10 times the peak luteal phase of menses. Estradiol in the plasma may reach levels 30 times higher than during the reproductive cycle. In early pregnancy and during the normal ovarian cycle, the corpus luteum is the major source of estrogen and progesterone. During pregnancy, the placenta begins to produce estrogens and progesterone.

Estrogen regulates cellular proliferation, differentiation, and keratinization, whereas progesterone influences the permeability of the microvasculature,[76,77] alters the rate and pattern of collagen production, and increases the metabolic breakdown of folate (necessary for tissue maintenance).[164] High concentrations of sex hormones in gingival tissues, saliva, serum, and GCF also can exaggerate the response.

Regulation of most cellular processes by hormones occurs through the interaction of these products with intracellular receptors. The resulting effects depend on the concentration of unbound hormone diffused through the cell membrane. Vittek and associates[155] demonstrated specific estrogen and progesterone receptors in gingival tissues, providing direct biochemical evidence that this tissue functions as a target organ for sex hormones. Muramatsu and Takaesu[98] found increasing concentrations of sex hormones in saliva from the first month and peaking in the ninth month of gestation, along with increasing percentages of *P. intermedia*. Probing depth, number of gingival sites with bleeding, and redness increased until 1 month after delivery. Evidence indicates sex hormone concentration in GCF, providing a growth media for periodontal pathogens.

Other Oral Manifestations of Pregnancy

Perimolysis (i.e., acid erosion of teeth) can occur if morning sickness or esophageal reflux is severe and involves repeated vomiting of the gastric contents. Severe reflux can cause scarring of the esophageal sphincter, and the patient may become more susceptible to GERD later in life.

BOX 41.1 Causes of Gingival Responses to Elevated Estrogen and Progesterone During Pregnancy

Subgingival Plaque Composition
- Increase in anaerobic/aerobic ratio
- Higher concentrations of *Prevotella intermedia* (i.e., substitutes sex hormone for vitamin K growth factor)
- Higher concentrations of *Bacteroides melaninogenicus*
- Higher concentrations of *Porphyromonas gingivalis*

Maternal Immunoresponse
- Depression of cell-mediated immunity
- Decrease in neutrophil chemotaxis
- Depression of antibody and T-cell responses
- Decrease in ratio of peripheral helper T cells to suppressor-cytotoxic T cells (i.e., CD4/CD8 ratio)
- Cytotoxicity directed against macrophages and B cells can diminish immunoresponsiveness
- Decrease in absolute numbers of CD3$^+$, CD4$^+$, and CD19$^+$ cells in peripheral blood during pregnancy versus postpartum
- Stimulation of prostaglandin production

Sex Hormone Concentration
Estrogen
- Increases cellular proliferation in blood vessels (e.g., in the endometrium)
- Decreases keratinization while increasing epithelial glycogen
- Specific receptors are found in gingival tissues

Progesterone
- Increases vascular dilation and increases permeability, resulting in edema and accumulation of inflammatory cells
- Increases proliferation of newly formed capillaries in gingival tissues (i.e., increased bleeding tendency)
- Alters rate and pattern of collagen production
- Increases metabolic breakdown of folate (i.e., folate deficiency can inhibit tissue repair)
- Specific receptors are found in gingival tissues
- Decreases plasminogen activator inhibitor type 2, increasing tissue proteolysis

Estrogen and Progesterone
- Affect ground substance of connective tissue by increasing fluidity
- Concentrations increase in saliva and fluid, with increased concentrations in serum

Xerostomia is a frequent complaint among pregnant women. One study found this persistent dryness in 44% of pregnant participants.[30]

A rare finding in pregnancy is *ptyalism* (i.e., sialorrhea). Excessive secretion of saliva usually begins at 2 to 3 weeks' gestation and may abate at the end of the first trimester. The cause of ptyalism has not been identified, but it may result from the inability of a nauseated gravid woman to swallow normal amounts of saliva, rather than from a true increase in saliva production.[21]

Because pregnancy places the woman in an immunocompromised state, the clinician must be aware of her total health. Gestational diabetes, leukemia, and other medical conditions may appear during pregnancy.

Clinical Management

A thorough medical history is an imperative component of the periodontal examination, especially for the pregnant patient. Because of immunologic alterations, increased blood volume (i.e., ruling out mitral valve prolapse and heart murmurs), and fetal interactions, the clinician must diligently and consistently monitor the patient's medical and periodontal stability. Medical history discussion should include pregnancy complications, previous miscarriages, and recent history of cramping, spotting, or pernicious vomiting. The patient's obstetrician should be contacted to discuss her medical status, periodontal or dental needs, and the proposed treatment plan.

Establishing a healthy oral environment and maintaining optimal oral hygiene are primary objectives for the pregnant patient. A preventive periodontal program consisting of nutritional counseling and rigorous plaque control measures in the dental office and at home should be reinforced. Women of childbearing age, especially those trying to conceive, should be informed of the possible impact of inflammation on the unborn.

Plaque Control

The increased tendency for gingival inflammation during pregnancy should be clearly explained to the patient so that acceptable oral hygiene techniques may be taught, reinforced, and monitored throughout pregnancy. Scaling, polishing, and root planing can be performed whenever necessary during pregnancy. Some practitioners avoid the use of high-alcohol-content antimicrobial rinses for pregnant women and prefer to use non–alcohol-based oral rinses.

Prenatal Fluoride

Prescribing prenatal fluoride supplements has been an area of controversy. Although two studies have claimed beneficial results,[39,40] others suggest that the clinical efficacy of prenatal fluoride supplements is uncertain and the mechanism by which they might impart cariostasis is unclear.[139a] The American Dental Association (ADA) does not recommend the use of prenatal fluoride because its efficacy has not been demonstrated. The American Academy of Pediatric Dentistry also supports this position. The American Academy of Pediatrics has no stated position on prescribing prenatal fluorides.

Treatment
Elective Dental Treatment

Other than good plaque control, it is prudent to avoid elective dental care if possible during the first trimester and the last half of the third trimester. The first trimester is the period of organogenesis, when the fetus is highly susceptible to environmental influences. In the last half of the third trimester, a hazard of premature delivery exists because the uterus is very sensitive to external stimuli. Prolonged chair time may need to be avoided because the woman is most uncomfortable at this time.

Supine hypotensive syndrome may occur. In a semireclining or supine position, the great vessels, particularly the inferior vena cava, are compressed by the gravid uterus. By interfering with venous return, this compression causes maternal hypotension, decreased cardiac output, and eventual loss of consciousness. Supine hypotensive syndrome can usually be reversed by turning the patient on her left side, which removes pressure on the vena cava and allows blood to return from the lower extremities and pelvic area. A preventive 6-inch soft wedge (i.e., rolled towel) should be placed on the patient's right side when she is reclined for clinical treatment.

Early in the second trimester is the safest period for providing routine dental care. The emphasis at this time is on controlling active disease and eliminating potential problems that can arise in late pregnancy. Major elective oral or periodontal surgery may be postponed until after delivery. Pregnancy tumors that are painful, interfere with mastication, or continue to bleed or suppurate after mechanical debridement may require excision and biopsy before delivery.

It is hypothesized that when the inflammatory cascade is activated during pregnancy, interventions targeting this pathway may be ineffective in reducing the rate of preterm birth. Treatment during pregnancy may be too late; it is possible that treatment before pregnancy (in nulliparous women) or in the period between pregnancies (for multiparous women, especially those with a history of preterm birth) may yield more promising results.[41]

The American Academy of Periodontology (www.perio.org) developed a position statement regarding the need to provide proper periodontal therapy for pregnant patients (Fig. 41.5). Because of research indicating a possible impact on the fetus, acute infection, abscesses, or other potential disseminating sources of sepsis may warrant prompt intervention irrespective of the stage of pregnancy.[4] A consensus report of a Joint European Workshop of Periodontology and an American Academy of Periodontology Workshop stated that "although periodontal therapy has been shown to be safe and leads to improved periodontal conditions in pregnant women, case-related periodontal therapy, without systemic antibiotics does not reduce overall rates of preterm birth and low birth weight."[133]

CLINICAL CORRELATION

It is prudent to avoid elective dental care during the first trimester and the last half of the third trimester. The first trimester is the period of organogenesis, and the fetus is highly susceptible to environmental influences. During the last half of the third trimester, the fetus is vulnerable to premature delivery. The uterus is very sensitive to external stimuli. Early in the second trimester is the safest period for providing routine dental care.

Dental Radiographs

The safety of dental radiography during pregnancy has been well established, provided items such as high-speed film, filtration, collimation, and lead aprons are used. However, it is most desirable not to have any irradiation during pregnancy, especially during the first trimester, because the developing fetus is particularly susceptible to radiation damage.[78] When radiographs are needed for diagnosis, the most important aid for the patient is the protective lead apron. Studies have shown that when an apron is used during contemporary dental radiography, gonadal and fetal radiation is virtually unmeasurable.[9]

Even with the obvious safety of dental radiography, x-ray films should be taken selectively during pregnancy and only when necessary and appropriate to aid in diagnosis and treatment. In most cases, only bitewing, panoramic, or selected periapical films are indicated.

Medications

Drug therapy for the pregnant patient is controversial because drugs can affect the fetus by diffusion across the placenta. Prescriptions should be used only for the duration absolutely essential for the pregnant patient's well-being and only after careful consideration of potential side effects. The classification system established by the U.S. Food and Drug Administration (FDA) in 1979 to rate fetal risk levels associated with many prescription drugs provides safety guidelines (Box 41.2). The prudent practitioner should consult references, such as Briggs and colleagues' *Drugs in Pregnancy and Lactation*[16] and Olin's *Drug Facts and Comparisons*,[108] for information on the FDA pregnancy risk factors associated with prescription drugs.

Ideally, no drug should be administered during pregnancy, especially the first trimester.[78] However, it is sometimes impossible to adhere to this rule. Fortunately, most common drugs in dental practice can be given during pregnancy with relative safety, although there are a few important exceptions. Tables 41.1, 41.2, and 41.3

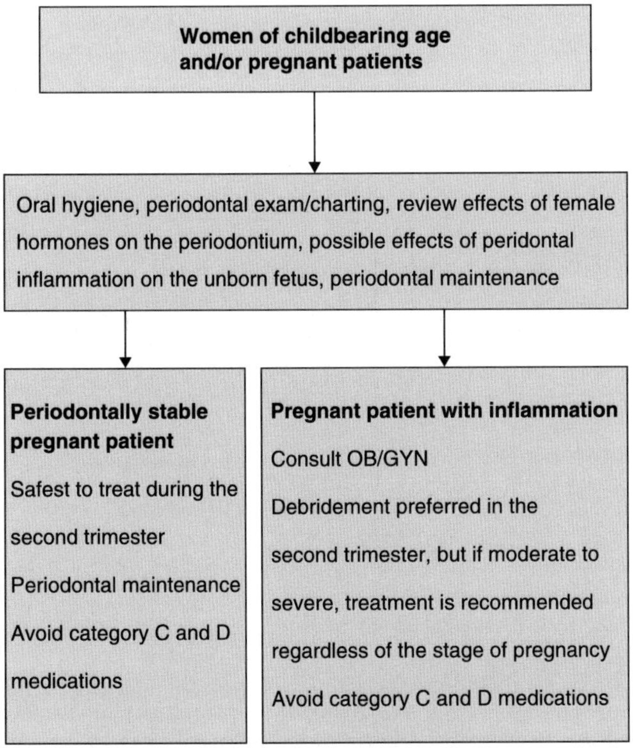

Fig. 41.5 Treatment algorithm for the pregnant patient.

BOX 41.2 FDA Drug Classification System Based on Potential to Cause Birth Defects

A: Controlled studies enrolling women fail to demonstrate a risk to the fetus in the first trimester (there is no evidence of risk in later trimesters), and the possibility of fetal harm appears remote.

B: Animal reproduction studies have not demonstrated a fetal risk, but there are no controlled studies in pregnant women; or animal reproduction studies have shown an adverse effect (other than decreased fertility) that was not confirmed in controlled studies in women in the first trimester (there is no evidence of risk in later trimesters).

C: Studies in animals have revealed adverse effects on the fetus (i.e., teratogenic, embryocidal, or other), and there are no controlled studies in women, or studies in women and animals are not available. Drugs should be given only if the potential benefit justifies the potential risk to the fetus.

D: There is positive evidence of human fetal risk, but the benefits of use in pregnant women may be acceptable despite the risk (e.g., the drug is needed in a life-threatening situation or for a serious disease for which safer drugs cannot be used or are ineffective).

X: Studies in animals or humans have demonstrated fetal abnormalities, or there is evidence of fetal risk based on human experience, or both, and the risk of using the drug in pregnant women clearly outweighs any possible benefit. The drug is contraindicated in women who are or may become pregnant.

TABLE 41.1 Local Anesthetic and Analgesic Administration During Pregnancy

Drug	FDA Category	During Pregnancy
Local Anesthetics[a]		
Lidocaine	B	Yes
Mepivacaine	C	Use with caution; consult physician
Prilocaine	B	Yes
Bupivacaine	C	Use with caution; consult physician
Etidocaine	B	Yes
Procaine	C	Use with caution; consult physician
Articaine	B	Yes; no blocks
Analgesics		
Aspirin	C/D, third trimester	Caution; avoid in third trimester
Acetaminophen	B	Yes
Ibuprofen	B/D, third trimester	Use with caution; avoid in third trimester
Codeine[b]	C	Use with caution; consult physician
Hydrocodone[b]	B	Use with caution; consult physician
Oxycodone[b]	B	Use with caution; consult physician
Propoxyphene	C	Use with caution; consult physician

[a]Can use vasoconstrictors if necessary.
[b]Avoid prolonged use.
FDA, U.S. Food and Drug Administration.

provide guidelines for anesthetic and analgesic, antibiotic, and sedative-hypnotic drugs, respectively.[122,150]

Antibiotics are often needed in periodontal therapy. The effect of a particular medication on the fetus depends on the type of antimicrobial, dosage, trimester, and duration of the course of therapy.[110] Research regarding subgingival irrigation and local site delivery in relation to the developing fetus is inadequate.

Breastfeeding

Usually, there is a risk that the drug can enter breast milk and be transferred to the nursing infant, on whom exposure could have adverse effects (Tables 41.4 and 41.5). Unfortunately, there is little conclusive information about drug dosage and effects through breast milk; however, retrospective clinical studies and empiric observations coupled with known pharmacologic pathways allow recommendations to be made.[78] The amount of drug excreted in breast milk is usually not more than 1% to 2% of the maternal dose; therefore it is highly unlikely that most drugs have any pharmacologic significance for the infant.[160]

The mother should take prescribed drugs just after breastfeeding and then avoid nursing for 4 hours or more if possible[78,142] to decrease the drug concentration in breast milk.

TABLE 41.3 Sedative-Hypnotic Drug Administration During Pregnancy

Drugs	FDA Category	During Pregnancy
Benzodiazepines	D	Avoid
Barbiturates	D	Avoid
Nitrous oxide	Not assigned	Avoid in first trimester; otherwise use with caution; consult physician

FDA, U.S. Food and Drug Administration.

TABLE 41.2 Antibiotic Administration During Pregnancy

Drugs	FDA Category	During Pregnancy	Risks
Penicillins	B	Yes	Diarrhea
Erythromycin	B	Yes; avoid estolate form	Intrahepatic jaundice in mother
Clindamycin	B	Yes, with caution	Drug concentrated in fetal bone, spleen, lung, and liver
Cephalosporins	B	Yes	Limited information
Tetracycline	D	Avoid	Depression of bone growth, enamel hypoplasia, gray-brown tooth discoloration
Ciprofloxacin	C	Avoid	Possible developing cartilage erosion
Metronidazole	B	Avoid; controversial	Theoretic carcinogenic data in animals
Gentamicin	C	Caution; consult physician	Limited information
Ototoxicity			
Vancomycin	C	Caution; consult physician	Limited information
Clarithromycin	D	Avoid; use only if potential benefit justifies risk to fetus	Limited information Adverse effects on pregnancy, outcome, and embryo and fetal development in animals

FDA, U.S. Food and Drug Administration.

TABLE 41.4 Local Anesthetic and Analgesic Administration During Breastfeeding

Drug	During Breastfeeding
Local Anesthetics	
Lidocaine	Yes
Mepivacaine	Yes
Prilocaine	Yes
Bupivacaine	Yes
Etidocaine	Yes
Procaine	Yes
Analgesics	
Aspirin	Avoid
Acetaminophen	Yes
Ibuprofen	Yes
Codeine	Yes
Hydrocodone	No data
Oxycodone	Yes
Propoxyphene	Yes

TABLE 41.5 Antibiotic and Sedative-Hypnotic Administration During Breastfeeding

Drugs	During Breastfeeding
Antibiotics[a]	
Penicillins	Yes
Erythromycin	Yes
Clindamycin	Yes, with caution
Cephalosporins	Yes
Tetracycline	Avoid
Ciprofloxacin	Avoid
Metronidazole	Avoid
Gentamicin	Avoid
Vancomycin	Avoid
Sedative-Hypnotics	
Benzodiazepines	Avoid
Barbiturates	Avoid
Nitrous oxide	Yes

[a]Antibiotics carry a risk of diarrhea and sensitization in the mother and infant.

Oral Contraceptives

Women may have responses to oral contraceptives (OCs) similar to those seen in pregnant patients. Mullally and associates found that current users of OCs had poorer periodontal health.[97] An exaggerated response to local irritants occurs in gingival tissues. Inflammation ranges from mild edema and erythema to severe inflammation with hemorrhagic or hyperplasic gingival tissues. It has been reported that more exudate is present in the inflamed gingival tissues of OC users than in those of pregnant women.[139,165]

Investigators have suggested several mechanisms for the heightened response in gingival tissues. Kalkwarf[63] reported that the response might be caused by an altered microvasculature, increased gingival permeability, and increased synthesis of prostaglandin. Levels of PGE, a potent mediator of inflammation,[33] appear to rise significantly with increasing levels of sex hormones. Jensen and colleagues[62] found dramatic microbial changes in pregnant and OC groups compared with a nonpregnant group. A 16-fold increase in *Bacteroides* species was seen in the OC group versus the nonpregnant group, despite no statistically significant clinical differences in gingival index or GCF flow. The study authors found that the increased female sex hormones substituting for the naphthoquinone requirement of certain *Bacteroides* species was most likely responsible for this increase.

OC-associated gingival inflammation may become chronic (versus the acute inflammation of pregnancy) because of the extended periods that women are exposed to elevated levels of estrogen and progesterone.[68,113] Some have reported that the inflammation increases with prolonged use of OCs. Kalkwarf[63] did not find that duration of use made a significant difference, but the brands used resulted in different responses. Further studies are needed to elucidate the effects of dosage, duration, and type of OC on the periodontium. The concentration of female sex hormones in current OCs is significantly less than that of the 1970s, while providing the same level of contraceptive efficacy.

Salivary composition changed notably in patients taking OCs in studies from the 1970s. Decreased concentrations of protein, sialic acid, hexosamine fucose, hydrogen ions, and total electrolytes have been reported. Salivary flow rates were increased in one report[87] and decreased in 30% of subjects in another report.[31]

The dental literature reports that women taking OCs experience a twofold to threefold increase in the incidence of localized osteitis after extraction of mandibular third molars.[144] The higher incidence of osteitis among these patients may be attributed to the effects of OCs (i.e., estrogens) on clotting factors. However, several studies refute these findings.[20] Evidence is inconclusive on osteitis after third molar extraction and OC use. A spotty melanotic pigmentation of the skin may occur with OC use. This suggests a relationship between the use of OCs and the occurrence of gingival melanosis,[52] especially in fair-skinned individuals.

Management

The medical history should include OCs along with other medications, and a discussion should include questions regarding OCs with women of childbearing age. The patient should be informed of the oral and periodontal side effects of OCs and the need for meticulous home care and compliance with periodontal maintenance. Treatment of gingival inflammation exaggerated by OCs should include establishing an oral hygiene program and eliminating local predisposing factors. Periodontal surgery may be indicated if resolution after initial therapy (i.e., scaling and root planing) is inadequate. It may be advisable to perform extraction of teeth (especially third molars) on nonestrogenic days of the OC cycle (i.e., days 23 to 28) to reduce the risk of a postoperative localized osteitis[36]; however, evidence of this association is inconclusive and warrants further investigation.

Although results from animal studies have demonstrated that antibiotic interference adversely affects contraceptive sex hormone levels, several human studies have failed to support such an interaction.[8,37,99,101] This issue is controversial, and antibiotics could render OCs ineffective in preventing pregnancy. In 1991, an ADA report stated that all women of childbearing age should be informed of possible reduced efficacy of steroid OCs during antibiotic therapy and advised women to use additional forms of contraception during short-term antibiotic therapy.[6] During long-term antibiotic therapy, women should consult their physician about using high-dose OC preparations. Although only research regarding oral manifestations attributed to OCs has been reported in the literature, the same effects presumably occur with the use of contraceptive implants. Similarly, the remote possibility of reduced efficacy of contraceptive implants with concurrent antibiotic use exists, and women can follow the same precautions as with OC use.

Conclusions

Clinical periodontal therapy includes an understanding of the clinician's role in the total health and well-being of female patients. Dentists do not treat localized infections without affecting other systems and the fetus or the breastfed infant. The periodontal and systemic difficulties of female patients can alter conventional therapy.

The cyclic nature of the female sex hormones often is reflected in the gingival tissues as initial signs and symptoms. Medical histories and discussions should include thoughtful investigation of the individual patient's problems and needs. Questioning should reflect hormonal stability and medications associated with regulation. Patients should be educated regarding the profound effects sex hormones have on periodontal and oral tissues and the consistent need for home and office removal of local irritants.

Research regarding female issues and medical/periodontal therapy is in process. In the near future, information about the specific management and causes of sex hormone–mediated infections will enhance dentists' ability to provide quality care to their patients.

 A Case Scenario is found on the companion website www.expertconsult.com.

References

 References for this chapter are found on the companion website www.expertconsult.com.

CHAPTER 42

Periodontal Treatment for Older Adults

Sue S. Spackman | Janet G. Bauer

CHAPTER OUTLINE

The Aging Periodontium
Demographics *(e-only)*
Dental and Medical Assessments
 (e-only)

Periodontal Diseases in Older
 Adults

Periodontal Treatment Planning
Conclusions

 Content on demographics, dental and medical assessment, and risk reduction can be accessed on the companion website at www.expertconsult.com.

Older adults are expected to comprise a larger proportion of the population than in the past. Population growth among long-lived older adults contributes to this increase worldwide. For dentistry, this means that older adults are retaining more of their natural dentition. Almost 70% of older adults in the United States have natural teeth.[30] However, retention of teeth may result in more teeth at risk for periodontal disease, and the prevalence of periodontal disease can be associated with aging. This association was addressed by Beck[23] at the 1996 World Workshop on Periodontics: "It may be that risk factors do change as people age or at least the relative importance of risk factors change." This chapter focuses on the associations between aging and oral health, with an emphasis on periodontal health.

The Aging Periodontium

Normal aging of the periodontium is a result of cellular aging, which is the basis for the intrinsic changes seen in oral tissues over time. The aging process does not affect every tissue in the same way. For example, muscle tissue and nerve tissue undergo minimal renewal, whereas epithelial tissue, which is one of the primary components of the periodontium, always renews itself.

Intrinsic Changes

In epithelium, a progenitor population of cells (i.e., stem cells) in the basal layer provides new cells. The cells of the basal layer are the least differentiated cells of the oral epithelium. A small subpopulation of these cells produces basal cells and retains the proliferative potential of the tissue. A larger subpopulation of these cells (i.e., amplifying cells) produces cells available for subsequent maturation. This maturing population of cells continually undergoes a process of differentiation or maturation.

By definition, the differentiated cell (i.e., epithelial cell) can no longer divide. Conversely, the basal cell remains as part of the progenitor population of cells ready to return to the mitotic cycle and again produce both types of cells. There is a constant source of renewal (Fig. 42.1).

In the aging process, cell renewal takes place at a slower rate and with fewer cells. The effect is to slow down the

regenerative processes. As the progenitor cells wear out and die, there are fewer and fewer of these cells to replace the dead ones. This effect is characteristic of the biologic changes that occur with aging.

 KEY FACT

With aging, stem cells undergo exhaustion that affects the regenerative potential of the organism. Reductions in the number of stem cells and in their response to stimuli in their local environment have been documented.

Through the action of gerontogenes or replicative senescence (i.e., Hayflick's limit and telomere shortening), the number of progenitor cells decreases. Hayflick, an American microbiologist, observed that fetal cells (i.e., fibroblasts) displayed a consistently greater growth potential (i.e., approximately 50 cumulative population doublings) than those derived from adult tissues (i.e., 20 to 30 cumulative population doublings). The decreased cellular component has a concomitant effect of decreasing both cellular reserves and protein synthesis. This causes the oral epithelial tissue to become thin, with reduced keratinization.

Stochastic Changes

Stochastic changes occurring in cells also affect tissue (e.g., glycosylation and cross-linking produce morphologic and physiologic changes). Structures become stiffer, with a loss of elasticity and increased mineralization (i.e., fossilization). With a loss of regenerative power, structures become less soluble and more thermally stable. Somatic mutations lead to decreased protein synthesis and structurally altered proteins. Free radicals contribute to the accumulation of waste in the cell.

All of these changes decrease the physiologic processes of tissue. Most changes are primarily a result of aging, although some result from physiologic deterioration. For example, loss of elasticity and increased resistance of the tissue can lead to decreased permeability, decreased nutrient flow, and accumulation of waste in the cell. Vascular

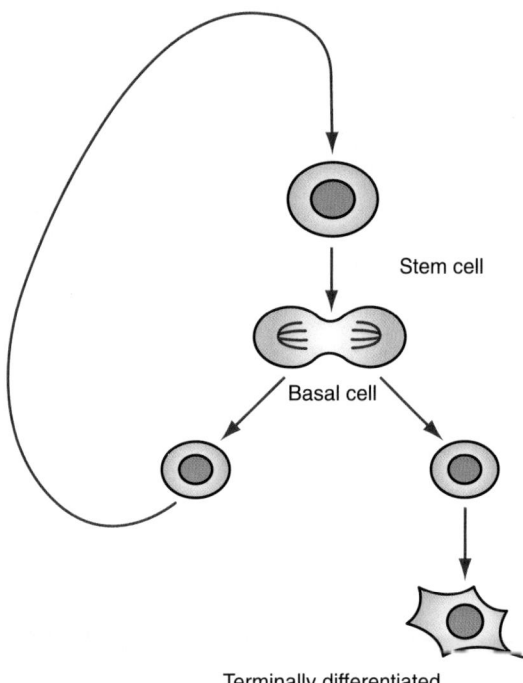

Fig. 42.1 Cell renewal cycle in which the basal cell produces an epithelial cell and returns to the progenitor cell population.

peripheral resistance (i.e., decreased blood supply) can decrease cellular function.

Physiologic Changes

In the periodontal ligament, a decrease in the number of collagen fibers leads to a reduction in or loss of tissue elasticity. Decreased vascularity reduces production of mucopolysaccharides.

All of these types of changes are seen in the alveolar bone. With aging, alveolar bone density decreases, bone resorption increases, and vascularity decreases. In contrast, cementum shows cemental thickening.

Functional Changes

With aging, the cells of the oral epithelium and periodontal ligament have reduced mitotic activity, and all cells experience a reduction in metabolic rate. These changes also affect the immune system and periodontium because of the reduced healing capacity and rate. Inflammation develops more rapidly and is more severe. Individuals are highly susceptible to viral and fungal infections because of abnormalities in T-cell function.

Clinical Changes

Compensatory changes that occur during aging or in response to disease manifest clinically as dental or periodontal conditions, such as gingival recession and reductions in bone height. Dental attrition, a type of tooth wear commonly seen as a normal part of aging, is a compensatory change that acts as a stabilizer between loss of bony support and excessive leveraging from occlusal forces imposed on the teeth.

A reduction in overjet of the teeth manifests as an increase in the edge-to-edge contact of the anterior teeth. Typically, this is related to the approximal wear of the posterior teeth. An increase is seen in the food table area, with loss of sluiceways, and in mesial migration.

Functional changes are associated with reduced efficiency of mastication. Although effectiveness of mastication may remain, efficiency is reduced because of missing teeth, loose teeth, poorly fitting prostheses, or noncompliance of the patient, who may refuse to wear prosthetic appliances.

KEY FACT

Key Periodontal Changes With Aging
- Thinning of oral epithelium and reduced keratinization
- Reduction or loss of periodontal ligament tissue elasticity
- Gingival recession
- Attachment and bone loss
- Thickening of cementum

Periodontal Diseases in Older Adults

Etiology

Periodontal disease in older adults is usually referred to as *chronic periodontitis*.[47,78] Because periodontitis is a chronic disease, much of the ravage of the disease detected in older adults accumulated over time. The advanced stages of periodontitis are less prevalent than the moderate stages in the older adult population.[27] One theory is that many sites of advanced periodontal disease have resulted in tooth loss earlier in life, suggesting that older age is not a risk factor for periodontal disease.[47,78]

Evidence is limited on whether the risk factors for periodontal disease fluctuate with age.[23] General health status, immune status, diabetes, nutrition, smoking, genetics, medications, mental health status, salivary flow, functional deficits, and finances can modify the relationship between periodontal disease and age.[23,95]

Some frequently prescribed medications for older adults can alter the gingival tissues. *Steroid-induced gingivitis* has been associated with postmenopausal women receiving steroid therapy. *Gingival overgrowth* can be induced by medications such as cyclosporine, calcium channel blockers, and anticonvulsants (e.g., nifedipine, phenytoin) in the setting of poor oral hygiene. Gingival overgrowth further decreases a person's ability to maintain good oral hygiene.[47]

Relation to Systemic Disease

Padilha and colleagues,[67] using data from the Baltimore Longitudinal Study of Aging, reached the conclusion that "the number of teeth is a significant risk indicator for mortality … and that improving oral health and preventing tooth decay may substantially improve the oral status of the population and increase longevity."

A review of the literature by Loesche and Lopatin[59] indicates that poor oral health has been associated with medical conditions such as aspiration pneumonia and cardiovascular disease. In particular, periodontal disease can be associated with coronary heart disease and cerebrovascular accident (CVA). The Surgeon General's Report on Oral Health emphasizes that animal- and population-based studies demonstrate an association between periodontal disease and diabetes, cardiovascular disease, and stroke.[82]

Investigations confirm these associations. For example, a periodontal examination can assist in cardiovascular risk assessment in hypertensive patients. Angeli and coworkers[11] reported an association between periodontal disease and left ventricular mass in untreated patients with essential hypertension. In another investigation, diabetes mellitus type 2 HbA1c levels declined with periodontal therapy in a large study by the U.S. Department of Veterans Affairs in South Carolina.[61]

Pneumonia is a common cause of morbidity and mortality in the older adult. Improvements in oral care have greatly reduced the incidence of pneumonia in elderly nursing home patients. Although the mechanism is under investigation, it is thought that the cough reflex can be improved by reducing the numbers of oropharyngeal microbial pathogens.[87] Expanding on these findings, studies have been conducted on the prevention of ventilator-associated pneumonia. Providing oral therapy for intensive care patients to reduce bacterial colonization in the mouth and teeth can reduce mortality and morbidity rates by 42%.[45]

The presence and extent of periodontal disease may be related to an increased risk of weight loss in older, well-functioning adults. This association is independent of smoking and diabetes mellitus. Changes in nutrient intake may be related to periodontal disease and a higher systemic burden of inflammation.[92]

Periodontal Treatment Planning

Periodontal disease in older adults usually is not a rapidly progressive disease but often manifests as long-standing chronic disease. Because periodontal disease has periods of exacerbation and remission, understanding and documenting periods of active disease compared with quiescent periods is essential to the formulation of the treatment plan and prognosis.[78]

Periodontal disease must be diagnosed regardless of age. The goal of periodontal treatment for young and old patients is to preserve function and eliminate or prevent the progression of inflammatory disease.[91]

The goal of clinically managing periodontal disease in older adults is based on specific, individualized care. The major consideration is improving or maintaining function, with an emphasis on quality-of-life issues. Emphasizing care over cure is the cornerstone of any proposed treatment plan. Prevention, comfort, function, aesthetics, and ease of maintenance are the criteria for successful care of an older adult, particularly a frail or functionally dependent older patient.

Several factors must be considered during treatment planning for older individuals.[78] It is important first to remember that periodontal healing and recurrence of disease are *not* influenced by age.[23] Factors to consider in the older patient are medical and mental health status, medications, functional status, and lifestyle behaviors that influence periodontal treatment, outcome, or progression of disease.[91] Periodontal disease severity, ability to perform oral hygiene procedures, and ability to tolerate treatment should be evaluated during treatment planning. The risks and benefits of surgical and nonsurgical therapy should be considered.[59] The amount of remaining periodontal support or past periodontal destruction, tooth type, number of occlusal contacts, and individual patient preferences are also important.[91]

Dental implants are reliable replacements for missing teeth in older adults[96]; age alone is not a contraindication for implant placement. Risk factors for the success of implants have been investigated. Although aging is a factor in decision making, most failures are associated with smoking, diabetes, head and neck irradiation, and postmenopausal estrogen therapy.[65]

For older adults, a nonsurgical approach is often the first treatment choice. Depending on the nature and extent of periodontal disease, surgical therapy may be indicated. Surgical technique should minimize the amount of additional root exposure. Individuals who respond best to surgical therapy are those who are able to maintain the surgical result. Age alone is not a contraindication to surgery. For individuals who are unable to comply with treatment, have poor oral hygiene, or are medically or mentally compromised or functionally impaired, palliative supportive periodontal care instead of surgical periodontal treatment is often the optimal approach.[59,76]

The U.S. Food and Drug Administration (FDA) approved silver diamine fluoride to reduce sensitivity, and its off-label use can arrest root caries and reduce bacteria on roots, where combined caries and periodontal infections is an issue and traditional dental treatment is not optimal or possible.[50]

A common goal for all older adults is to decrease bacteria through oral hygiene and mechanical debridement. Clinical trials enrolling older adults showed that the development or progression of periodontal disease could be prevented or arrested by controlling plaque. For certain patients, topical antibiotic therapy may complement repeated subgingival instrumentation during supportive care. Oral hygiene maintenance should also focus on root surfaces susceptible to caries.[91] Decision making for frail and functionally dependent older adults may be challenging for the general dentist. For this reason, dentists, other health care professionals, and other scientists are creating high-quality office-based methods to access evidence-based decision-making programs and accommodating websites to help with complicated oral health care issues.[4,77]

Disease Prevention and Maintenance of Periodontal Health in Older Adults

For younger and older people, the most important factors determining a successful outcome of periodontal treatment are plaque control and frequency of professional care. Advanced age does not decrease plaque control,[12] but older adults may have difficulty performing adequate oral hygiene because of compromised health, altered mental status, medications, or altered mobility and dexterity.[91] Older adults may change toothbrushing habits because of disabilities such as hemiplegia due to CVA, visual difficulties, dementia, or arthritis. The newer, lightweight electric-powered toothbrush may be more beneficial than a manual toothbrush for older adults with physical and sensory limitations.

The proportion of people who floss their teeth decreases after 40 years of age.[90] This may be partly caused by impairment of fine motor skills due to disease or injury. Interproximal brushes, shaped wooden toothpicks, and mechanical flossing devices often can be used in place of traditional flossing with satisfactory outcomes.

Multidisciplinary strategies are increasingly becoming part of periodontal health care promotion. Assessments of overall health, functional status, and patient education are fundamental to promoting and maintaining optimal periodontal health. Older adults, their families, and caregivers need to be informed and trained by dentists on the appropriate devices, chemotherapeutic agents, and techniques to provide oral self-care and maintain a healthy lifestyle.[40]

The outcomes are instrumental in achieving overall health, oral and periodontal health, self-esteem, nutrition, and quality of life. Barriers to achieving these benefits are access and cost. For older adults who are homebound or institutionalized, these barriers inhibit their achieving and maintaining optimal oral and periodontal health.

Chemotherapeutic Agents
Antiplaque Agents

Patients who are unable to remove plaque adequately due to disease or disability may benefit from antiplaque agents such as chlorhexidine, sub-antimicrobial tetracycline, or Listerine or its generic counterparts.[63,78,91]

Chlorhexidine is a cationic bisbiguanide that has been used as a broad-spectrum antiseptic in medicine since the 1950s. In Europe, a 0.2% concentration of chlorhexidine has been used for years as a preventive and therapeutic agent.[59,90] Chlorhexidine is bacteriostatic or bactericidal, depending on the dose. Adverse effects of chlorhexidine include an increase in calculus formation, dysgeusia (i.e., altered taste), and permanent staining of teeth.[8] Chlorhexidine is a prescription rinse for short-term use (<6 months); long-term use (>6 months) has not been extensively studied.[90]

The American Dental Association (ADA) Council on Dental Therapeutics[6] has approved chlorhexidine to help prevent and reduce supragingival plaque and gingivitis. Although chlorhexidine has not been studied in older adults, outcomes in younger persons, including those with disabilities, suggest that it is also effective in older adults. Chlorhexidine may be particularly useful for older adults who have difficulty with plaque removal and those who take phenytoin, calcium channel blockers, or cyclosporine and who are at risk for gingival hyperplasia.[78,90]

Sub-antimicrobial tetracycline (Periostat) is useful in treating moderate to severe chronic periodontitis. The active ingredient in Periostat is doxycycline hyclate. In concert with scaling and root planing, Mohammad and colleagues[63] showed this treatment to be effective in institutionalized older adults. Periostat is contraindicated for patients with an allergy to tetracycline.

Listerine antiseptic and its generic counterparts are approved by the ADA Council on Dental Therapeutics[8] to help prevent and reduce supragingival plaque and gingivitis. The active ingredients in Listerine are methyl salicylate and three essential oils (i.e., eucalyptol, thymol, and menthol). Listerine was effective in reducing plaque and gingivitis compared with placebo rinses in young healthy adults. Listerine may exacerbate xerostomia because of its high alcohol content, ranging from 21.6% to 26.9%. Listerine is generally contraindicated in patients under treatment for alcoholism who take disulfiram (Antabuse). Listerine may benefit patients who do not tolerate the taste or staining of chlorhexidine or who prefer OTC medicaments that are less expensive and easier to obtain.[78,90]

Antimicrobial photodynamic therapy (aPDT) is being investigated for the treatment of periodontitis. Using low-powered lasers and cells treated with a drug to make them susceptible to the light, it is possible to kill microorganisms specific to periodontal disease.[35]

Fluoride

Fluoride, nature's cavity fighter, is an effective caries-preventive agent (see Periodontal Treatment Planning). Fluoride's effects are as follows[78,90]:

1. Reduces enamel solubility
2. Promotes remineralization of early carious lesions
3. Is bactericidal for bacterial plaque

Topical fluorides are recommended for the prevention and treatment of dental caries. OTC fluorides include fluoride dentifrices, rinses, and gels that contain concentrations of 230 to 1500 parts per million (ppm) of fluoride ions. Prescription 1.1% neutral sodium fluoride gels are available with a fluoride concentration of 5000 ppm of fluoride ions. Professionally applied fluoride gel, foam, or varnish products have between 9050 and 22,600 ppm of fluoride ions.[8]

Saliva Substitutes

Saliva substitutes, which are intended to match the chemical and physical traits of saliva, are available to relieve the symptoms of dry mouth. Their composition varies, but they usually contain salt ions, a flavoring agent, paraben (a preservative), cellulose derivative or animal mucins, and fluoride. The ADA's seal of approval has been granted for some artificial saliva products (e.g., Saliva Substitute, Salivart).[8] Most saliva substitutes can be used as desired by patients and are dispensed in a spray bottle, rinse or swish bottle, or oral swab stick.[8,90] Products such as dry-mouth toothpastes and moisturizing gels are also available. Biotene products such as Oral Balance are marketed to relieve the symptoms of xerostomia.

Patients with dry mouth can benefit from stimulating saliva flow with sugarless candies and sugarless gum. Xylitol chewing gum has been shown to have anticariogenic properties in children. Medicated chewing gum with xylitol and chlorhexidine or xylitol alone has the added benefit of reducing oral plaque and gingivitis in elderly people who live in residential facilities.[9]

Salivary substitutes and stimulants are only effective in the short term. Under investigation is acupuncture-like transcutaneous nerve stimulation (Codetron), a method to treat radiation-induced xerostomia. Unlike traditional acupuncture therapy, Codetron does not use invasive needles to achieve stimulation. This method helps patients produce their own saliva and reduces symptoms of xerostomia for several months. Acupuncture therapy has demonstrated improvements lasting up to 3 years.[98]

Conclusions

Future oral health care trends will include increased numbers of older adults seeking periodontal therapy. Dental practitioners of the 21st century should be comfortable providing comprehensive periodontal care for this segment of the population. Aging dental patients have particular oral and general health conditions that dentists should be familiar with detecting, consulting on, and treating. Medical diseases and conditions that occur more often with age may require modification of periodontal preventive tools and the planning and treatment phases of periodontal care.

 A Case Scenario is found on the companion website www.expertconsult.com.

References

 References for this chapter are found on the companion website www.expertconsult.com.

CHAPTER 43

Treatment of Aggressive and Atypical Forms of Periodontitis

Perry R. Klokkevold

CHAPTER OUTLINE

Aggressive Periodontitis
Periodontitis Refractory to Treatment *(e-only)*
Necrotizing Ulcerative Periodontitis
Conclusions

 For online-only content on periodontitis refractory to treatment, please visit the companion website at www.expertconsult .com.

The majority of patients with common forms of periodontal disease respond predictably well to conventional therapy, including oral hygiene instruction, nonsurgical debridement, surgery, and supportive periodontal maintenance. However, patients diagnosed with aggressive periodontitis and some atypical forms of periodontal disease often do not respond as predictably or as favorably to conventional therapy. Fortunately, only a small percentage of patients with periodontal disease are diagnosed with aggressive periodontitis. Patients who are diagnosed with periodontal disease of any type that is *refractory* to treatment present in small numbers as well. Even fewer patients are diagnosed with necrotizing ulcerative periodontitis. Each of these atypical disease entities poses significant challenges for the clinician, not only because they are infrequently encountered but also because they may not respond favorably to conventional periodontal therapy.[24,40] Furthermore, the severe loss of periodontal support associated with these cases leaves the clinician faced with uncertainty about treatment outcomes and difficulty in making decisions about whether to save affected teeth or extract them.

Aggressive Periodontitis

Aggressive periodontitis, by definition, causes rapid destruction of the periodontal attachment apparatus and the supporting alveolar bone (see Chapter 28). The responsiveness of aggressive periodontitis to conventional periodontal treatment is unpredictable, and the overall prognosis for these patients is poorer than for patients with chronic periodontitis. Because these patients do not respond typically to conventional methods and their disease progresses unusually fast, the logical question is whether there are problems associated with an impaired host immune response that may contribute to such a *different* disease and result in a *limited* response to the usual therapeutic measures. There have been reports of defects in the function of polymorphonuclear leukocytes (i.e., neutrophils) in some patients with aggressive periodontitis.[30,31] Also, in a small number of cases, a systemic disease such as neutropenia can be identified that appears

to explain the unusual severity of the periodontal disease for that individual.[12,13] In most patients with aggressive periodontitis, however, these factors cannot be identified,[1] and in fact, these patients are typically quite healthy. Numerous attempts to examine immunologic profiles of patients with aggressive periodontitis have failed to identify any specific etiologic factors common to all patients.

The prognosis for patients with aggressive periodontitis depends on (1) whether the disease is generalized or localized, (2) the degree of destruction present at the time of diagnosis, and (3) the ability to control future progression. *Generalized* aggressive periodontitis rarely undergoes spontaneous remission, whereas *localized* forms of the disease have been known to arrest spontaneously.[29] This unexplained curtailment of disease progression has sometimes been referred to as a "burnout" of the disease. It appears that cases of localized aggressive periodontitis often have a limited period of rapid loss of periodontal attachment and alveolar bone, followed by a slower, more chronic phase of disease progression. Overall, patients with generalized aggressive periodontitis tend to have a poorer prognosis because they typically have more teeth affected by the disease and the disease is less likely to go into remission spontaneously compared with localized forms of aggressive periodontitis.

Therapeutic Modalities

Early detection is critically important in the treatment of aggressive periodontitis (generalized or localized) because prevention of further destruction is often more predictable than regeneration of lost supporting tissues. Therefore, at the initial diagnosis, it is helpful to obtain any previously taken radiographs to assess the rate of progression of the disease. Together with future radiographs, this documentation also facilitates the clinician's assessment of treatment success and control of the disease.

Treatment of aggressive periodontitis must be pursued with a logical and regimented approach. Several aspects of treatment must be considered. One of the most important aspects of treatment success is educating the patient about the disease, including the causes and risk factors, and stressing the importance of the patient's role in the success of treatment.[50] Essential therapeutic considerations for the clinician are controlling the infection, arresting disease progression, correcting anatomic defects, replacing missing teeth, and ultimately helping the patient maintain periodontal health with frequent periodontal maintenance care. Educating family members is another important factor because aggressive periodontitis is known to have familial aggregation. Family members, especially younger siblings of the patient diagnosed with aggressive periodontitis, should be examined for signs of disease, educated about preventive measures, and monitored closely. It cannot be stressed enough that early diagnosis, intervention, and, if possible, prevention of disease is more desirable than attempting to reverse the destruction that results from aggressive periodontitis.

Conventional Periodontal Therapy

Because aggressive periodontitis is primarily a bacterial infection, initial treatment is comparable to treatment rendered for chronic periodontitis. Conventional periodontal therapy for aggressive periodontitis consists of patient education, oral hygiene improvement, scaling and root planing, and regular (frequent) recall maintenance. It may or may not include periodontal flap surgery.[3] However, the response of aggressive periodontitis to conventional therapy alone may be limited and less predictable. Patients who are diagnosed with aggressive periodontitis at an early stage and are able to enter therapy may have a better outcome than those who are diagnosed at an advanced stage of destruction. In general, the earlier the disease is diagnosed, the more conservative the therapy and the more predictable the outcome.

Teeth with moderate to advanced periodontal attachment loss and bone loss often have a poor prognosis and pose the most difficult challenge. Depending on the condition of the remaining dentition, treatment of these teeth may offer a limited prospect of improvement and may even diminish the overall treatment success. Clearly, some of these teeth should be extracted; however, other teeth may be pivotal to the stability of the dentition, making it desirable to attempt treatment to maintain them. Treatment options for teeth with deep periodontal pockets and bone loss may be nonsurgical or surgical. Surgery may be purely resective, regenerative, or a combination of these approaches.

KEY FACT

Patients who are diagnosed with aggressive periodontitis at an early stage and who are able to enter therapy may have a better outcome than those who are diagnosed at an advanced stage of destruction. In general, the earlier the disease is diagnosed, the more conservative the therapy and the more predictable the outcome. Teeth with advanced periodontal attachment loss and bone destruction often have a poor prognosis and pose the biggest challenge for treatment.

Surgical Resective Therapy

Resective periodontal surgery can be effective in reducing or eliminating pocket depth in patients with aggressive periodontitis, but it may be difficult to accomplish if adjacent teeth are unaffected. If a significant height discrepancy exists between the periodontal support of the affected tooth and the adjacent unaffected tooth, the gingival transition (soft tissue following the bone) often results in deep probing pocket depth around the affected tooth that cannot be eliminated. A less-than-ideal outcome must be considered before deciding to treat increased pocket depth surgically.

It is important to realize the limitations of surgical therapy and to appreciate the possible risk that surgical therapy may further compromise teeth that are mobile due to extensive loss of periodontal support. For example, in a patient with severe horizontal bone loss, surgical resective therapy may result in increased tooth mobility that is difficult to manage, and a nonsurgical approach may be preferable. Careful evaluation of the risks versus the benefits of surgery must be performed on a case-by-case basis.

Regenerative Therapy

The concept and application of periodontal regeneration have been established in patients with chronic forms of periodontal disease (see Chapter 63). Regenerative materials, including bone grafts, barrier membranes, and wound-healing agents, are often employed, and their use is well documented. Intrabony defects, particularly vertical defects with multiple osseous walls, are often amenable to regeneration with these techniques. Most of the success and predictability of periodontal regeneration have been achieved in patients with chronic periodontitis; much less evidence is available regarding the use of periodontal regeneration for patients with aggressive periodontitis.

Periodontal regenerative procedures have been successfully demonstrated in patients with localized aggressive periodontitis in some clinical case reports. Dodson and colleagues[14] demonstrated the regenerative potential of a severe, localized osseous defect around a mandibular incisor in a healthy 19-year-old black man diagnosed with localized aggressive periodontitis. The patient presented with severe localized bone loss around one of the mandibular incisors. Using open flap surgical debridement, root surface conditioning (tetracycline solution), and an allogenic bone graft reconstituted with sterile saline and tetracycline powder, the surgeons reduced the probing pocket depth from 9–12 mm to 1–3 mm (3 mm of recession was noted); significant bone fill of the defect (about 80%) was reported (Fig. 43.1). This case illustrates the potential for healing of severe defects in patients with localized aggressive periodontitis, especially when local factors are controlled and sound surgical principles are followed. The authors cited several factors that likely contributed to the success of this case, including a probable transition of disease activity from aggressive to chronic, tooth stabilization before surgery, sound surgical management of hard and soft tissues, and good postoperative care.[14]

Although the potential for regeneration in patients with aggressive periodontitis appears to be good, expectations are limited for patients with severe bone loss. This is especially true if the bone loss is horizontal or has progressed to involve furcations.

 KEY FACT

Periodontal regeneration has been successfully demonstrated in patients with localized aggressive periodontitis, illustrating the potential for healing severe defects in these patients. As with periodontal regeneration in nonaggressive forms of periodontitis, it is important to control local factors and follow sound surgical principles.

Antimicrobial Therapy

Aggressive periodontitis is a disease with a bacterial etiology. The presence of periodontal pathogens, specifically *Aggregatibacter actinomycetemcomitans*, has been implicated as the reason that aggressive periodontitis does not respond to conventional therapy alone. These pathogens are known to remain in the tissues after therapy and to reinfect the pocket.[9,58] In the late 1970s and early

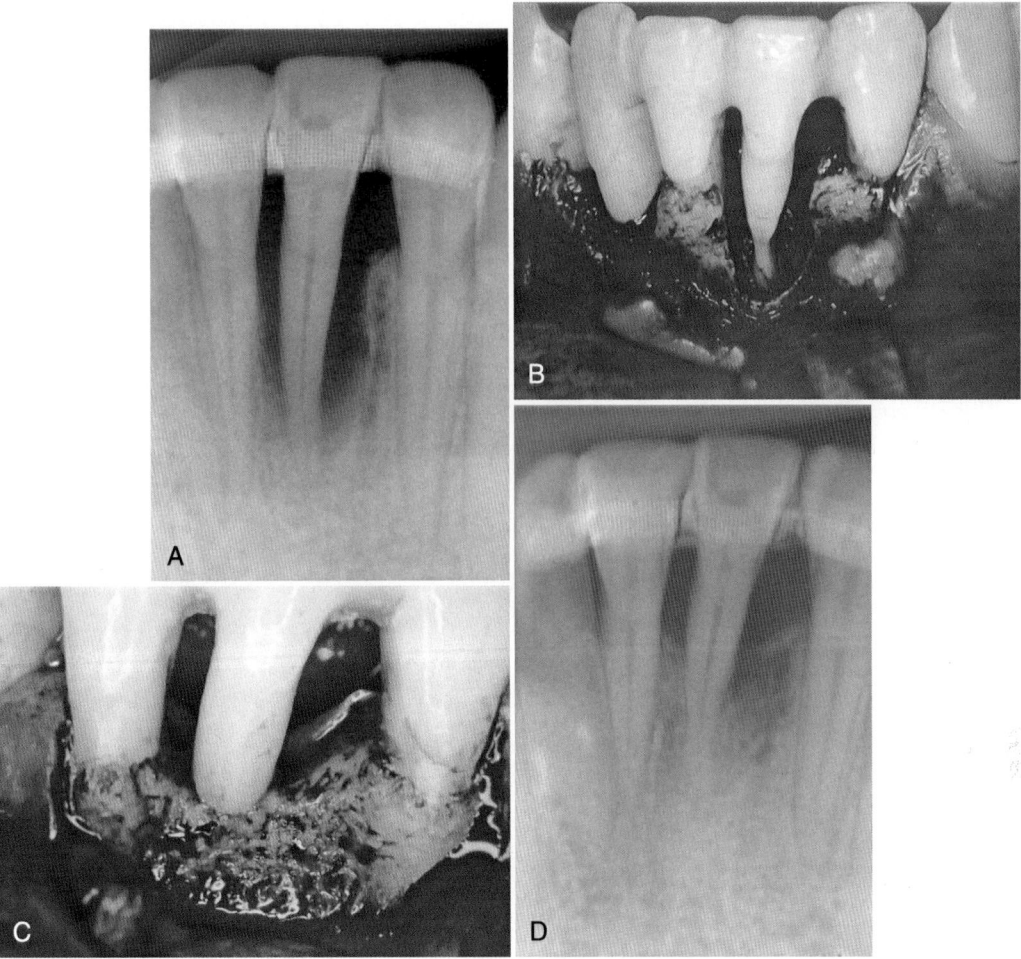

Fig. 43.1 Clinical photographs and periapical radiographs demonstrating regenerative success in a patient with localized aggressive periodontitis. (A) Periapical radiograph of the right lateral incisor at the initial diagnosis. Notice the severe vertical bone loss associated with the right lateral incisor. The tooth has been splinted to adjacent teeth for stability. (B) Facial view of the circumferential osseous defect around the lower right lateral incisor during open flap surgery. There is complete loss of buccal, lingual, mesial, and distal bone around the lateral incisor, with minimal bone support limited to the apical few millimeters. (C) Facial view of reentered surgical site 1 year after treatment. Bone fill around all surfaces demonstrates remarkable potential for regeneration of a large osseous defect in a young patient with localized aggressive periodontitis. (D) Periapical radiograph taken 1 year after regenerative therapy. Notice the increased radiopacity and bone fill. *(From Dodson SA, Takei HH, Carranza FA Jr: Clinical success in regeneration: report of a case.* Int J Periodont Restor Dent *16:455, 1996.)*

1980s, the identification of *A. actinomycetemcomitans* as a major culprit and the discovery that this organism penetrates the tissues offered another perspective on the pathogenesis of aggressive periodontitis and new hope for therapeutic success—namely, antibiotics.[9] The use of systemic antibiotics was thought to be necessary to eliminate pathogenic bacteria (especially *A. actinomycetemcomitans*) from the tissues. Indeed, several authors have reported success in the treatment of aggressive periodontitis using antibiotics as adjuncts to standard therapy.[33–35,71]

There is compelling evidence that adjunctive antibiotic treatment frequently results in a more favorable clinical response than mechanical therapy alone.[66] In a systematic review, Herrera and colleagues[23] found that systemic antimicrobials in conjunction with scaling and root planing offered benefits greater than scaling and planing alone in terms of clinical attachment level, probing pocket depth, and reduced risk of additional attachment loss. Patients with deeper, progressive pockets seemed to benefit the most from systemic administration of adjunctive antibiotics. Many different antibiotic types and regimens were reviewed, but because of limitations in

comparing data from different studies, definitive recommendations were not possible. In a meta-analysis of the literature (including six randomized clinical trials), Sgolastra and associates[60] found that the systemic use of combined amoxicillin and metronidazole as an adjunct to scaling and root planing for the treatment of generalized aggressive periodontitis resulted in significant clinical attachment gain ($P < 0.05$) and pocket reduction ($P < 0.05$) compared with scaling and root planing alone.

Fig. 43.2 shows the results of treatment in a case of aggressive periodontitis treated nonsurgically with scaling and root planing and adjunctive antibiotic therapy. The patient, a 34-year-old Asian man, presented with a complaint of loose teeth and bleeding gums. He requested treatment to save his teeth. Treatment consisted of patient education, including oral hygiene instructions, and nonsurgical therapy with adjunctive antibiotics. All teeth were thoroughly scaled and root planed under local anesthesia over two treatment appointments, and the patient was treated with systemic amoxicillin (500 mg, three times daily for 2 weeks) during the period of treatment. All areas responded favorably, with probing pocket depths decreasing from

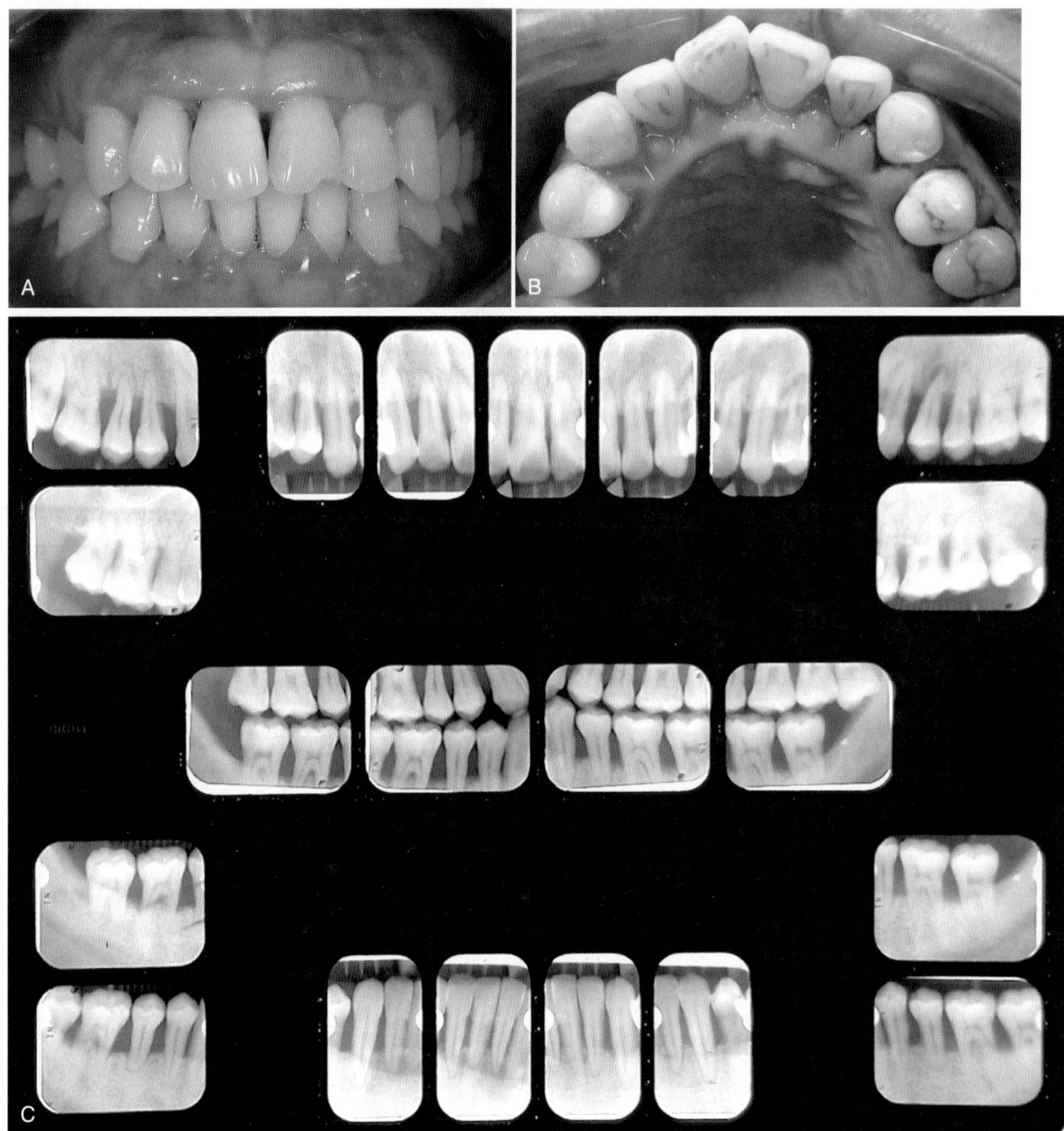

Fig. 43.2 Intraoral clinical photographs and full-mouth radiographs taken before and after treatment of aggressive periodontitis in a 34-year-old Asian man. (A and B) Intraoral clinical photographs of pretreatment periodontal condition. Notice the gingival edema, inflammation, and bleeding. Probing pocket depths ranged from 3 to 13 mm, with generalized bleeding on probing and purulent exudate. (C) Pretreatment full-mouth radiographs demonstrate generalized severe horizontal bone loss. Notice the periapical radiolucency at the apex of the upper left premolar, indicating pulpal disease.

3–13 mm to 2–5 mm. Bleeding on probing diminished from generalized to very few isolated areas. The patient continued on periodontal maintenance with good results for more than 5 years.

Genco and coworkers[18] treated localized aggressive periodontitis with scaling and root planing plus systemic administration of tetracycline (250 mg, four times daily for 14 days every 8 weeks). Measurements of vertical defects were made at intervals of up to 18 months after the initiation of therapy. Bone loss stopped, and

one-third of the defects demonstrated an increase in bone level, whereas in the control group, bone loss continued.

Liljenberg and Lindhe[33] treated localized aggressive periodontitis with systemic administration of tetracycline (250 mg, four times daily for 2 weeks), modified Widman flaps, and periodic recall visits (one visit every month for 6 months, then one visit every 3 months). The lesions healed more rapidly and more completely than similar lesions in control patients. These investigators reevaluated their results

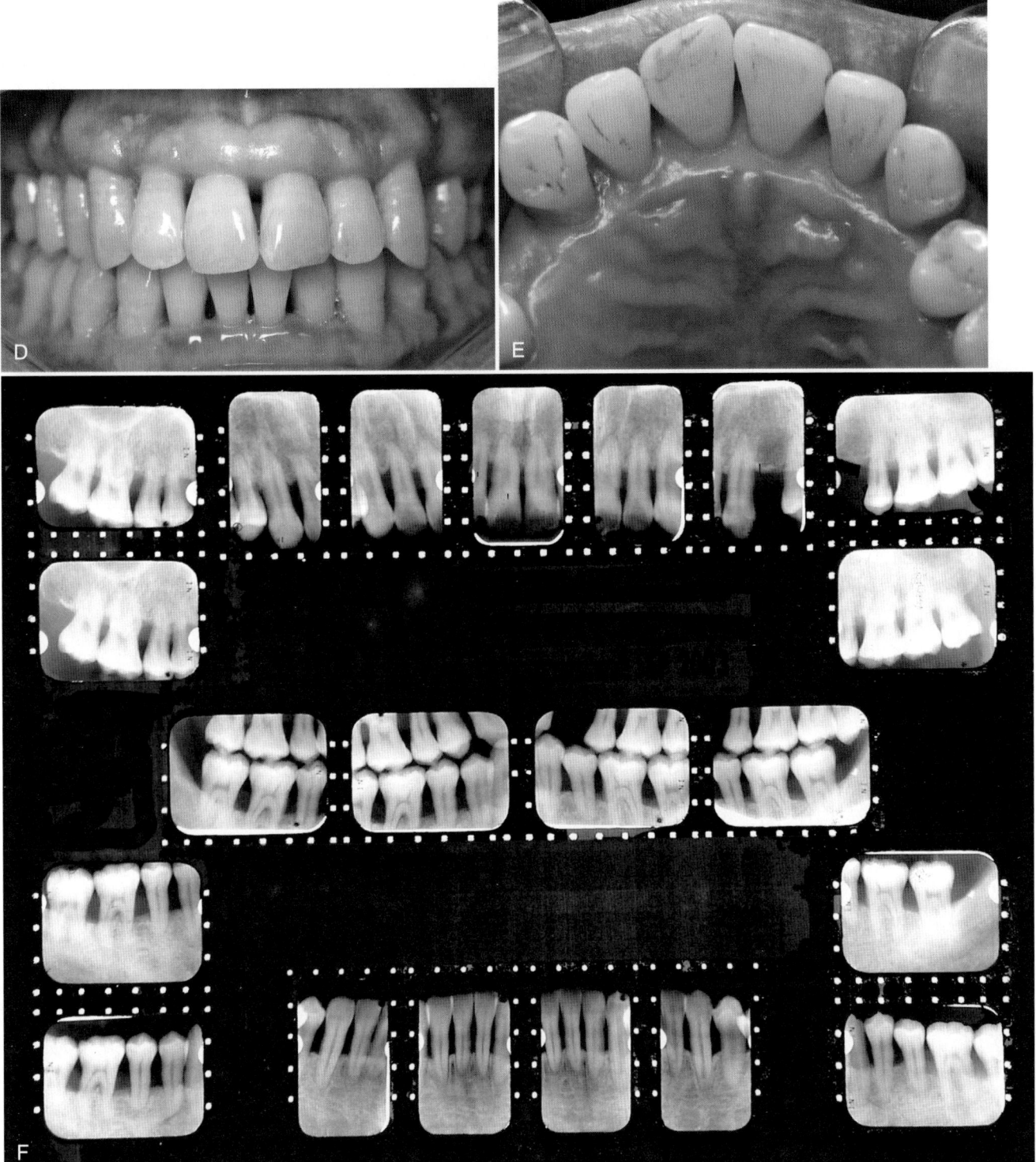

Fig. 43.2, cont'd (D and E) Intraoral clinical photographs of posttreatment results after 5 years. Treatment included nonsurgical scaling and root planing along with adjunctive systemic antibiotics (amoxicillin). Patient improved his oral hygiene and continued to be seen for professional maintenance every 3 months. Probing pocket depths have been maintained in the range of 2 to 5 mm, with only a few localized areas of bleeding on probing. (F) Full-mouth radiographs after 5 years demonstrate no additional bone loss. The endodontically involved maxillary premolar was extracted and replaced with a removable partial denture.

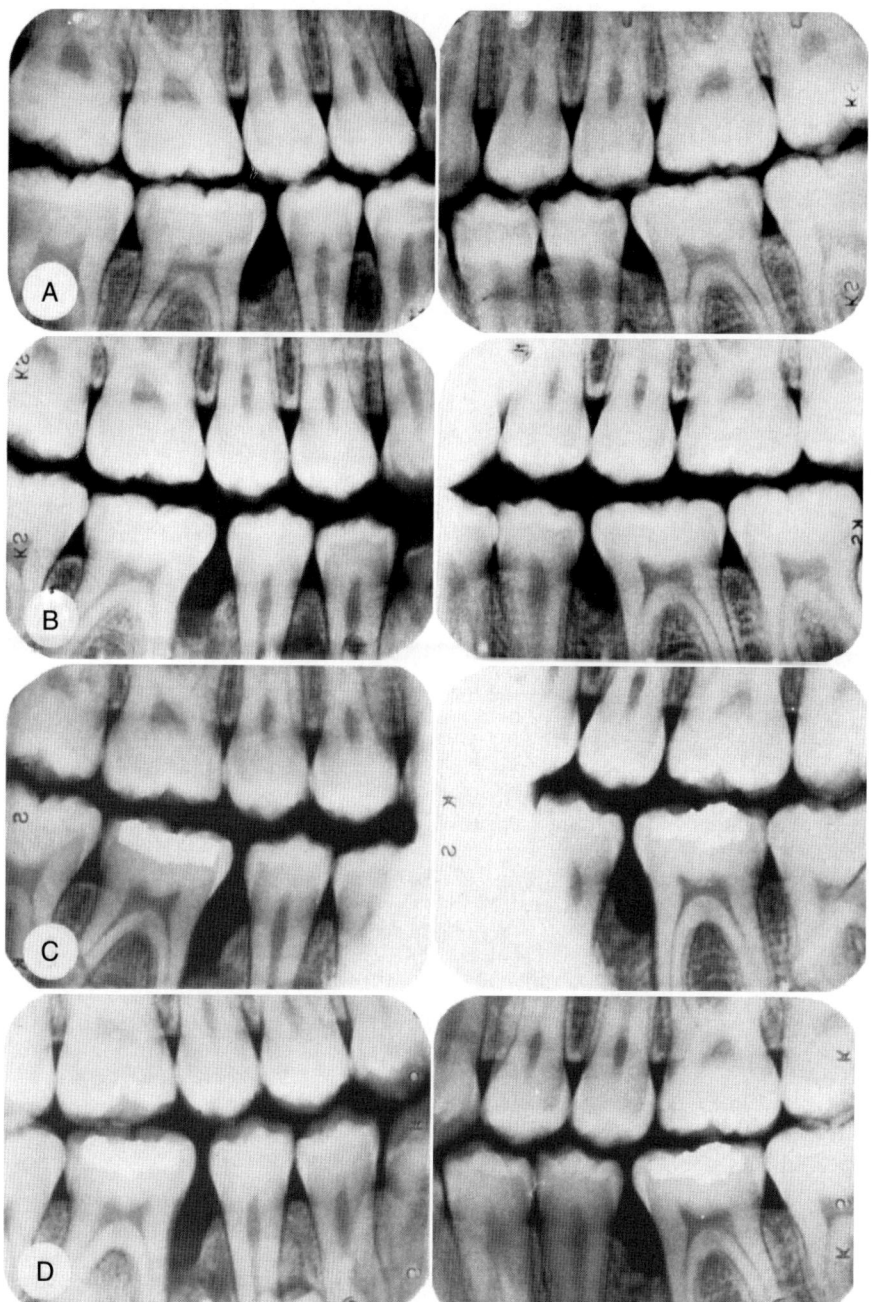

Fig. 43.3 Radiographs depicting progression of an osseous lesion in a patient with localized aggressive periodontitis (formerly "localized juvenile periodontitis"). (A) January 29, 1979; (B) August 16, 1979; (C) February 22, 1980; (D) May 15, 1981. Notice the progressive deterioration of the osseous level. *(From Barnett ML, Baker RL: The formation and healing of osseous lesions in a patient with localized juvenile periodontitis, case report.* J Periodontol *54:148, 1983.)*

after 5 years and found that the treatment group continued to demonstrate resolution of gingival inflammation, gain of clinical attachment, and refill of bone in angular defects.[34] Figs. 43.3 and 43.4 show radiographs of a case with similar treatment and results.[4]

Numerous studies support the use of adjunctive tetracycline along with mechanical debridement for the treatment of *A. actinomycetemcomitans*–associated aggressive periodontitis (Box 43.1). Given the possible emergence of tetracycline-resistant *A. actinomycetemcomitans,* there is concern that tetracycline may not be effective. In these cases, the combination of metronidazole and amoxicillin may be advantageous. The use of these two antibiotics

along with conventional periodontal therapy[21,22] provides better disease control and better clinical improvement in attachment levels in difficult-to-manage periodontitis than similar periodontal therapy without antibiotics. Similar effects have been seen for a variety of antibiotic types. However, a lack of sufficient sample sizes among studies makes it difficult to offer specific recommendations on which antibiotics are most effective.[23]

The criteria for selecting antibiotics are not clear. Good clinical and microbiologic responses have been reported with several individual antibiotics and antibiotic combinations (Table 43.1). The optimal antibiotic or combination for any particular infection probably

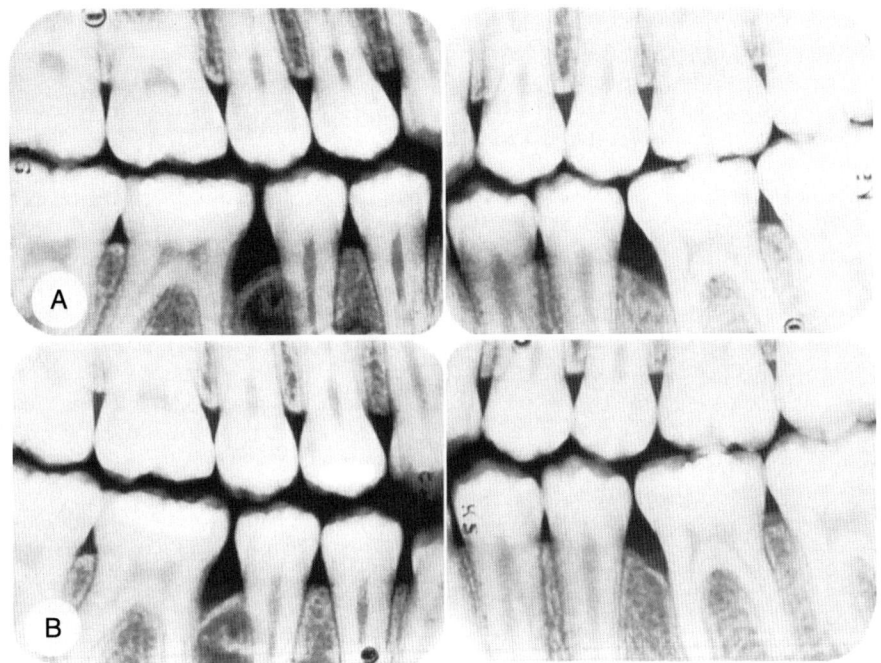

Fig. 43.4 Postoperative radiographs of the patient in Fig. 43.3. (A) November 6, 1981; (B) March 3, 1982. Treatment consisted of oral hygiene instruction, scaling and root planing concurrent with 1 g of tetracycline per day for 2 weeks, and modified Widman flaps. *(From Barnett ML, Baker RL: The formation and healing of osseous lesions in a patient with localized juvenile periodontitis, case report.* J Periodontol *54:148, 1983.)*

BOX 43.1   Systemic Tetracycline in the Treatment of Aggressive Periodontitis

Systemic tetracycline (250 mg of tetracycline hydrochloride four times daily for at least 1 week) should be given in conjunction with local mechanical therapy. If surgery is indicated, systemic tetracycline should be prescribed and the patient should be instructed to begin taking it approximately 1 hour before surgery. Doxycycline 100 mg/day may be used instead of tetracycline. Chlorhexidine rinses should be prescribed and continued for several weeks to enhance plaque control and facilitate healing.

TABLE 43.1   Antibiotic Therapy for Aggressive Periodontitis

Associated Microflora	Antibiotic of Choice
Gram-positive organisms	Amoxicillin–clavulanate potassium (Augmentin)[10,68]
Gram-negative organisms	Clindamycin[19,20,64,68]
Nonoral gram-negative facultative rods	Ciprofloxacin[36]
Pseudomonads, staphylococci	
Black-pigmented bacteria and spirochetes	Metronidazole[19,61]
Prevotella intermedia, Porphyromonas gingivalis	Tetracycline[51]
Aggregatibacter actinomycetemcomitans	Metronidazole-amoxicillin[19,61]
	Metronidazole-ciprofloxacin Tetracycline[48]
P. gingivalis	Azithromycin[49]

---

depends on the case. Choices must be made based on patient-related and disease-related factors.

CLINICAL CORRELATION

The use of amoxicillin and metronidazole as an adjunctive therapy to scaling and root planing for the treatment of aggressive periodontitis has been shown to significantly improve clinical attachment gain and pocket depth reduction when compared with scaling and root planing alone. Aggressive periodontitis is a disease with a bacterial etiology.

Microbial Testing

Some investigators and clinicians advocate microbial testing to identify the specific periodontal pathogens responsible for disease and selecting an appropriate antibiotic based on sensitivity and resistance. There may be specific cases in which bacterial identification and antibiotic-sensitivity testing is valuable. For example, in some cases of localized aggressive periodontitis, tetracycline-resistant *Actinobacillus* species have been suspected. If an antibiotic susceptibility test determines that tetracycline-resistant species exist in the lesion, the clinician may be advised to consider another antibiotic or an antibiotic combination, such as amoxicillin and metronidazole.[15,51,62]

In practice, antibiotics are often used empirically without microbial testing. One study evaluated and compared the results of microbial testing offered by two independent laboratories.[41,59] Two microbiologic cultures, sampled simultaneously from the same sites in 20 patients, were submitted separately to each of the two laboratories for bacterial identification and antibiotic-sensitivity testing. The reported presence of bacterial species varied between the two laboratories, as did their antimicrobial recommendations. The combination of amoxicillin and metronidazole yielded the highest level of agreement (80%), likely because of the effectiveness of this combination and a clinical predisposition to favor a known regimen. These findings suggested that the usefulness of microbial testing may be limited and led the authors to conclude that the empiric use of antibiotics, such as a combination of amoxicillin and metronidazole, may be more clinically sound and cost-effective than bacterial identification and antibiotic-sensitivity testing.[41,59]

Nonetheless, microbial testing should be considered whenever a case of aggressive periodontitis is not responding or if the destruction continues despite good therapeutic efforts.

Local Delivery

Local delivery for administration of antibiotics is a novel approach to the management of localized periodontal infections. The primary advantage of local therapy is that smaller total dosages of topical agents can be delivered inside the pocket, avoiding the side effects of systemic antibacterial agents while increasing the exposure of the target microorganisms to higher concentrations and therefore more therapeutic levels of the medication. Local delivery agents are available in many different forms, including solutions, gels, fibers, and chips[16,17,27] (see Chapter 53).

Full-Mouth Disinfection

Another approach to antimicrobial therapy in the control of infection associated with periodontitis is full-mouth disinfection. The concept, described by Quirynen and coworkers,[52] consists of full-mouth debridement (removal of all plaque and calculus) completed in two appointments within a 24-hour period. In addition to scaling and root planing, the tongue is brushed with chlorhexidine gel (1%) for 1 minute, the mouth is rinsed with chlorhexidine solution (0.2%) for 2 minutes, and periodontal pockets are irrigated with chlorhexidine solution (1%).

In a clinical and microbiologic study,[52] 10 patients with advanced chronic periodontitis were randomly assigned to a test or control group. Test patients were treated as just described, whereas control patients received scaling and root planing by quadrant at 2-week intervals along with oral hygiene instructions. At 1 and 2 months after treatment, the test group showed significantly higher reduction in probing pocket depth, especially for deeper pockets (7–8 mm). Patients in the test group also had significantly lower concentrations of pathogenic microorganisms after treatment compared with controls. Several follow-up studies by the same center demonstrated similar results for up to 6 months after therapy.[5,6,63] In another study, the same researchers included a test group who did *not* use chlorhexidine as part of the one-stage, full-mouth disinfection.[53] The results for both test groups (i.e., with and without chlorhexidine) were similar and were significantly better than for controls. The authors concluded that the beneficial effects of one-stage, full-mouth disinfection probably result from the full-mouth debridement within 24 hours rather than the adjunctive chlorhexidine treatment.

A few reports have included patients with aggressive (early-onset) periodontitis in their evaluation of the one-stage, full-mouth disinfection protocol.[11,45,54] As in patients with advanced chronic periodontitis, De Soete and colleagues[11] found a significant reduction in probing pocket depth and gain in clinical attachment in patients with aggressive periodontitis compared with controls up to 8 months after treatment (scaling and root planing by quadrant at 2-week intervals). They also found significant reductions in periodontal pathogens up to 8 months after therapy. *Porphyromonas gingivalis* and *Tannerella forsythia* were reduced to levels below detection.

Host Modulation

A novel approach in the treatment of aggressive periodontitis and difficult-to-control forms of periodontal disease is the administration of agents that modulate the host response. Several agents have been used or evaluated to modify the host response to disease (see Chapter 54).

Treatment Planning and Restorative Considerations

Successful management of aggressive periodontitis must include tooth replacement as part of the treatment plan. In some advanced cases, the overall treatment success for the patient may be enhanced if severely compromised teeth are extracted. The outcome of treatment for these teeth is limited, and, more important, the retention of severely diseased teeth over time may result in additional bone loss and teeth that are further compromised. The risk of further bone loss is an even greater concern now, with the current success and predictability of dental implants and the desire to preserve bone for implant placement. Any additional alveolar bone loss in an area that has already undergone severe bone loss may further compromise residual anatomy and impair the opportunity for tooth replacement with a dental implant. This is especially true for certain areas with poor bone quality or limited bone volume, such as the posterior maxilla. Fortunately, healing of extraction sites is typically uneventful in patients with aggressive periodontitis, and bone augmentation of defect sites is predictable.

In the patient with aggressive periodontitis, the approach to restorative treatment should be chosen based on a single premise: Extract severely compromised teeth early, and plan treatment to accommodate future tooth loss. The teeth with the best prognosis should be identified and considered when planning the restorative treatment. The lower cuspids and first premolars are typically more resistant to loss, probably because of the favorable anatomy (i.e., single roots, no furcations) and easier access for patient oral hygiene. As a rule, an extensive fixed prosthesis should be avoided, and removable partial dentures should be planned in such a way as to allow for the addition of teeth.

When hopeless teeth are extracted, they need to be replaced. The desire to replace missing teeth in a permanent manner without preparation of adjacent teeth for a fixed partial denture has motivated clinicians to attempt transplantation of teeth from one site to another. Transplantation of developing third molars to the sockets of hopeless first molars has been attempted with limited success.[7,32,39] Now, however, the success and predictability of dental implants have obviated the need to transplant teeth to edentulous sites.

Use of Dental Implants

Initially, the use of dental implants was suggested for and implemented in patients with aggressive periodontitis with much caution, because of an unfounded fear of bone and implant loss. However, evidence appears to support the use of dental implants in these patients.[37,43,44,46,70] Therefore, it is possible to consider the use of dental implants in the overall treatment plan for patients with aggressive periodontitis.

There is scant evidence to support the use of bone augmentation procedures in preparation for or in combination with implant placement in patients being treated for aggressive periodontitis. One case report with short-term follow-up suggested that it was successful.[25] A prospective study of 10 patients treated for generalized aggressive periodontitis who underwent guided bone regeneration followed by implant placement found that the implant survival rate was 100% after 3 years.[42] However, slightly greater attachment loss (0.65 mm) and bone loss (1.78 mm) were observed in the aggressive periodontitis group compared with 10 periodontally healthy controls who received implants without bone augmentation.

Periodontal Maintenance

When patients with aggressive periodontitis are transferred to maintenance care, their periodontal condition must be stable (i.e., no clinical signs of disease and no periodontal pathogens). Each maintenance visit should consist of a medical history review, an inquiry about any recent periodontal problems, an assessment of risk factors, a comprehensive periodontal and oral examination, thorough root debridement, and prophylaxis, followed by a review of oral hygiene instructions. If oral hygiene is not good, patients may benefit most from a review of oral hygiene instructions and visualization of plaque in their own mouth before debridement and prophylaxis.

Frequent maintenance visits appear to be one of the most important factors in the control of disease and the success of treatment in patients with aggressive periodontitis.[31,64] In a study of 25 individuals with aggressive (early-onset) periodontitis followed with maintenance every 3 to 6 months for 5 years, it was concluded that these patients can be effectively maintained with clinical and microbiologic improvements after active periodontal therapy.[26] High bacterial counts (particularly *P. gingivalis* and *Treponema denticola*), number of acute episodes, number of teeth lost, smoking, and stress appeared to be significant factors in the small percentage of sites that showed progressive bone loss. In a 5-year follow-up study of 13 patients with aggressive periodontitis treated with comprehensive mechanical, surgical, and antimicrobial therapy and supportive periodontal maintenance every 3 to 4 months, periodontal disease progression was arrested in 95% of the initially affected lesions. Only 2% to 5% experienced discrete episodes of loss of periodontal support.[8]

A supportive periodontal maintenance program aimed at early detection and treatment of sites that begin to lose attachment should be established. The interval between these recall visits is short during the first period after the patient's completion of therapy, usually no longer than 3 months. Acute episodes of gingival inflammation can be detected and managed earlier when the patient is on a frequent monitoring cycle. Monitoring as frequently as every 3 to 4 weeks may be necessary when the disease is thought to be active. If signs of disease activity and progression persist despite therapeutic efforts, frequent visits, and good patient compliance, microbial testing may be indicated. The rate of disease progression may be faster in younger individuals, and therefore the clinician should monitor such patients more frequently. Over time, the recall maintenance interval can be adjusted (more or less often) to suit the patient's level of oral hygiene and control of disease, as determined by each examination.

Close collaboration among members of the treatment team, including the periodontist, general dentist, dental hygienist, and patient's physician, is required for continuity of care and for patient motivation and encouragement. It is important to monitor and observe the patient's overall physical status as well, because weight loss, depression, and malaise have been reported in patients with generalized aggressive periodontitis. Finally, there is a constant need to reinforce patient education about disease etiology and preventive practices (i.e., oral hygiene and control of risk factors).

Necrotizing Ulcerative Periodontitis

Necrotizing ulcerative periodontitis (NUP) is a rare disease, especially in developed countries. Often, NUP is diagnosed in individuals with a compromised host immune response. The incidence of NUP in specific populations, such as patients who are positive for human immunodeficiency virus (HIV) infection or have acquired immunodeficiency syndrome (AIDS), has been reported to be between 0% and 6%. Most patients diagnosed with NUP have diseases or conditions that impair their host immune response. These patients often have an underlying predisposing systemic factor that renders them susceptible to NUP disease. For this reason, patients presenting with NUP should be treated in consultation with their physician.

A comprehensive medical evaluation and diagnosis of any condition that may be contributing to an altered host immune response should be completed. It is also important to rule out any hematologic disease (e.g., leukemia) before initiating treatment of any case that has a similar presentation to NUP (see Figs. 14.13 and 14.15 in Chapter 14).

Treatment can be initiated only after a thorough medical history and examination to identify the existence of any systemic diseases. Treatment for NUP includes local debridement of lesions with scaling and root planing, lavage, and instructions for good oral hygiene. It may be necessary to use local anesthesia during the debridement because lesions are frequently painful. The use of ultrasonic instrumentation with profuse irrigation may enhance debridement and flushing of deep lesions. Achieving good oral hygiene may also be challenging until the lesions and associated pain resolve.

Antimicrobial adjuncts, such as chlorhexidine, added to the oral hygiene regimen may contribute to the daily reduction of bacterial loads. Patients frequently complain of pain. Locally applied topical antimicrobials and systemic antibiotics, as well as systemic analgesics, should be used as indicated by signs and symptoms.

Patients with NUP often harbor bacteria, fungi, viruses, and other nonoral microorganisms, complicating the selection of antimicrobial therapy. Superinfection or overgrowth of fungi and viruses may be propagated by antibiotic therapy. Antifungal and/or antiviral agents may be considered against these infections prophylactically or after they are diagnosed. Because oral hygiene for these patients is complicated by the painful lesions, alternative methods should be encouraged. Irrigation with diluted cleansing and antibacterial agents can be of some benefit.

Ultimately, the successful treatment of NUP may depend on the resolution or treatment of the systemic condition (e.g., immune compromise) that predisposed the individual to the disease. Evaluation and treatment of patients with known systemic conditions, such as HIV infection, should be coordinated with the patient's physician.

Conclusions

Treatment of aggressive and atypical forms of periodontal disease is challenging for clinicians because these forms are infrequently encountered, can manifest with more severe bone loss, and do not respond as predictably or as favorably to conventional therapy. Fortunately, only a small percentage of patients are diagnosed with these forms of periodontitis. This chapter discussed therapies and rationales for management of these challenging cases.

 A Case Scenario is found on the companion website www.expertconsult.com.

References

 References for this chapter are found on the companion website www.expertconsult.com.

CHAPTER 44

Treatment of Acute Gingival Disease

Perry R. Klokkevold | Fermin A. Carranza

CHAPTER OUTLINE

Necrotizing Ulcerative Gingivitis
Primary Herpetic Gingivostomatitis
Pericoronitis
Conclusion

The treatment of acute gingival disease entails alleviation of the acute symptoms and elimination of all etiologic factors, including periodontal disease, both chronic and acute, throughout the oral cavity. Treatment is not complete if periodontal pathologic changes or predisposing factors capable of causing them remain. Systemic risk factors that increase susceptibility to these acute gingival diseases also need to be assessed and eliminated or modified if possible.

Necrotizing Ulcerative Gingivitis

Necrotizing ulcerative gingivitis (NUG) results from an impaired host response to a potentially pathogenic microflora. Depending on the degree of host compromise or immunosuppression, NUG may occur in a mouth essentially free of other gingival involvement or may be superimposed on underlying chronic gingival or periodontal disease. Treatment should include alleviation of the acute symptoms and correction of the underlying chronic gingival or periodontal disease. The former is the simpler part of the treatment; the latter often requires more comprehensive procedures, follow-up, and patient education.

The treatment of NUG consists of (1) alleviation of the acute inflammation by reduction of the microbial load and removal of necrotic tissue, (2) treatment of chronic disease either underlying the acute involvement or elsewhere in the oral cavity, (3) alleviation of generalized symptoms such as fever and malaise, and (4) correction of systemic conditions or factors that contribute to the initiation or progression of gingival changes. Chapter 30 provides further information on the management and treatment of NUG necrotizing ulcerative periodontitis (NUP) in patients with acquired immunodeficiency syndrome (AIDS).

Treatment of NUG should follow an orderly sequence, according to specific steps, at three clinical visits.

First Visit

At the first visit, the clinician should conduct a comprehensive evaluation of the patient, including a thorough medical history, with special attention to recent illness, living conditions, dietary background, cigarette smoking, type of employment, hours of rest, risk factors for human immunodeficiency virus (HIV) infection, and psychosocial parameters (e.g., stress, depression). The patient is questioned regarding the history of the acute disease, including its onset and duration, as follows:

- Is the disease recurrent?
- Are the recurrences associated with specific factors such as menstruation, particular foods, exhaustion, or mental stress?
- Has there been any previous treatment? When and for how long?

The clinician should also inquire as to the type of treatment received and the patient's impression regarding the effectiveness of previous treatment.

The initial physical examination should include an assessment of general appearance, presence of halitosis, presence of skin lesions, vital signs including temperature, and palpation for the presence of enlarged lymph nodes, especially submaxillary and submental nodes.

The oral cavity is examined for the characteristic NUG lesions (see Chapter 20), distribution, and the possible involvement of the oropharyngeal region. Oral hygiene is evaluated, with special attention to the presence of pericoronal flaps, periodontal pockets, and local risk factors (e.g., poorly contoured and ill-fitting restorations, presence and distribution of calculus). Periodontal probing of NUG lesions is likely to be very painful, will not aid in the primary diagnosis, and may need to be deferred until after the acute lesions are resolved.

> **KEY FACT**
>
> The goals of initial therapy for NUG are reduction of the microbial load and removal of necrotic tissue to facilitate the healing process of repair and regeneration so that normal tissue barriers can be reestablished.

The goals of initial therapy are reduction of the microbial load and removal of necrotic tissue to the degree that repair and regeneration of normal tissue barriers can be reestablished. Treatment during the initial visit is confined to the acutely involved areas, which are isolated with cotton rolls and dried. A topical anesthetic is applied, and after 2 or 3 minutes the areas are gently swabbed with a moistened cotton pellet to remove the pseudomembrane and nonattached surface debris. Bleeding may be profuse. Each cotton pellet is used in a small area, then discarded; sweeping motions over large areas with a single pellet are not recommended. After the area is cleansed with warm water, the superficial calculus is removed. Ultrasonic scalers are very useful for this purpose, because they do not elicit pain and the water jet and cavitation aid in lavage of the area.

Subgingival scaling and curettage are contraindicated at this time, because these procedures may extend the infection into the deeper tissues and may also cause bacteremia. *Unless an emergency exists, procedures such as extractions or periodontal surgery are postponed until the patient has been symptom free for 4 weeks, to minimize the likelihood of exacerbating the acute symptoms.*

Antibiotics are effective in the treatment of patients with NUG.[5] Patients with moderate or severe NUG and local lymphadenopathy or other systemic signs or symptoms are placed on an antibiotic regimen of amoxicillin 500 mg orally every 6 hours for 10 days. For amoxicillin-sensitive patients, other antibiotics are prescribed, such as erythromycin (500 mg every 6 hours) or metronidazole (500 mg twice daily for 7 days). Systemic complications should subside in 1 to 3 days. *Antibiotics are not recommended in NUG patients who do not have systemic complications.*

Instructions to the Patient

The patient is discharged with the following instructions:

1. Avoid tobacco, alcohol, and condiments.
2. Rinse with a glassful of an equal mixture of 3% hydrogen peroxide and warm water every 2 hours and/or 0.12% chlorhexidine solution twice daily.
3. Get adequate rest. Pursue usual activities, but avoid excessive physical exertion or prolonged exposure to the sun, as in golfing, playing tennis, swimming, or sunbathing.
4. Confine toothbrushing to removal of surface debris with either a bland dentifrice or just water and an ultrasoft brush; overzealous brushing and the use of dental floss or interdental cleaners will be painful. Chlorhexidine mouth rinses are also helpful in controlling biofilm throughout the mouth.
5. An analgesic, such as a nonsteroidal antiinflammatory drug (NSAID; e.g., ibuprofen), is appropriate for pain relief.
6. Patients who have systemic complications such as high fever, malaise, anorexia, or general debility are given antibiotics and instructed to get plenty of bed rest and drink lots of fluids.

Patients are asked to report back to the clinician in 1 to 2 days. They should be advised about the extent of total treatment required to resolve the condition and warned that treatment is not complete when pain stops. They should be informed of the presence of chronic gingival or periodontal disease, which must be eliminated to reduce the likelihood of recurrence of the acute symptoms.

A large variety of drugs have been used in the treatment of NUG.[3] Topical drug therapy, however, is only an adjunctive measure; no drug, when used alone, can be considered complete therapy. Systemic antibiotics, when used, also reduce the oral bacterial flora and alleviate the oral symptoms,[12,13] but they are only an adjunct to the complete local treatment that the disease requires. If patients are treated by drugs or systemic antibiotics alone, the acute painful symptoms often reoccur after treatment is discontinued.

Second Visit

At the second visit, 1 or 2 days after the first visit, the patient is evaluated for amelioration of signs and symptoms. The patient's condition is usually improved; the pain is diminished or is no longer present. The gingival margins of the involved areas are erythematous but without a superficial pseudomembrane.

Scaling is performed if it is necessary and sensitivity permits. Shrinkage of the gingiva may expose previously covered calculus, which is gently removed. Instructions to the patient are the same as those given previously.

Third Visit

At the next visit, approximately 5 days after the second visit, the patient is evaluated for resolution of symptoms, and a comprehensive plan for management of the patient's periodontal condition is formulated. The patient should be essentially symptom-free at this time. Some erythema may still be present in the involved areas, and the gingiva may be slightly painful on tactile stimulation (Fig. 44.1A and B). The patient is instructed in biofilm control procedures (see Chapter 48), which are essential for the success of the treatment and the maintenance of periodontal health. The patient is further counseled on nutrition, smoking cessation, and other conditions or habits associated with potential recurrence. The hydrogen peroxide rinses are discontinued, but chlorhexidine rinses may be maintained for an additional 2 or 3 weeks. Scaling and root planing is repeated if necessary. Unfortunately, patients often discontinue treatment because the acute condition has subsided; however, this is when comprehensive treatment of the chronic periodontal problem should begin. Patients need to be educated about the importance of comprehensive periodontal treatment and encouraged to complete it.

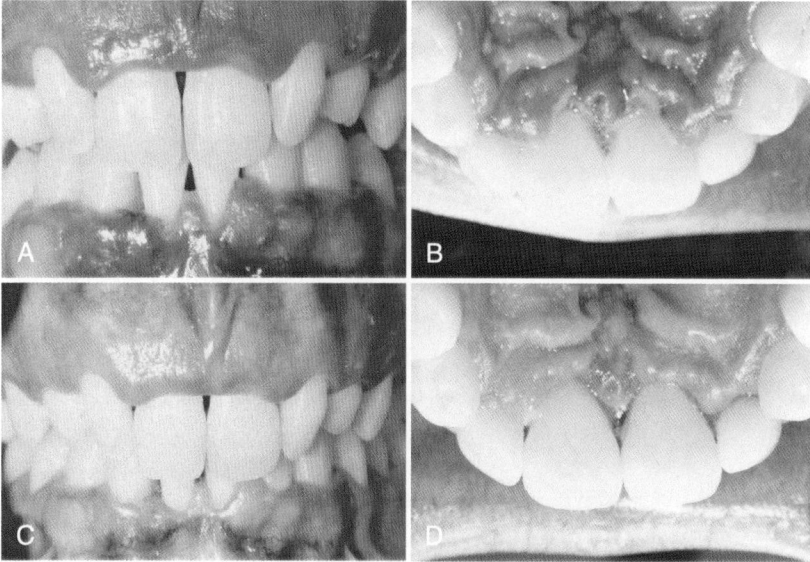

Fig. 44.1 (A) Initial view of the anterior gingival tissues in a 22-year-old white female smoker with acute necrotizing ulcerative gingivitis. (B) Palatal view of the same patient. (C) Facial view of the same patient, 2 days after initial scaling and cessation of smoking. (D) Palatal view of the same patient, 2 days after initial scaling and cessation of smoking. *(From Rose LF, Mealey BL, Genco RJ, Cohen DW: Periodontics: medicine, surgery, and implants, Mosby, St. Louis, 2005.)*

Appointments should be scheduled for treatment of chronic gingivitis, periodontal pockets, and pericoronal flaps, as well as for elimination of all forms of local risk factors (see Chapter 13). The patient should be reevaluated approximately 4 to 6 weeks after treatment to determine compliance with oral hygiene, health habits, psychosocial factors, the potential need for reconstructive or esthetic surgery, and the interval of subsequent recall visits.

Gingival Changes With Healing

The characteristic lesion of NUG undergoes the following changes during the course of healing in response to treatment:

1. Removal of the surface pseudomembrane exposes underlying red, hemorrhagic, craterlike depressions in the gingiva, indicating inflammation caused by necrosis and microbial infiltration of tissue that has lost the normal barrier function of the epithelium.
2. In the next stage, the bulk and redness of the crater margins are reduced, indicating a reduction in inflammation and reepithelialization, but the surface remains shiny (see Fig. 44.1C and D).
3. This is followed by the early signs of restoration of normal gingival contour and color, indicating reestablishment of the normal barrier function of the epithelium, including keratinization, and further reduction of inflammation.
4. In the final stage, the normal gingival color, consistency, surface texture, and contour may be restored. Portions of the root exposed by the acute disease may be covered by healthy gingiva (Fig. 44.2).

Additional Treatment Considerations
Contouring of Gingiva as an Adjunctive Procedure

Even in cases of severe gingival necrosis, healing often leads to restoration of the normal gingival contour, although normal architecture of the gingiva may be achieved only after several weeks or months. However, if there has been loss of interdental bone, if the teeth are irregularly aligned, or if the entire papilla is lost, healing sometimes results in the formation of a shelf-like gingival margin, which favors retention of biofilm and recurrence of gingival inflammation and is an esthetic problem. This can be corrected by an attempt to restore lost tissue through periodontal plastic procedures or by reshaping the gingiva surgically (Fig. 44.3). Effective biofilm control by the patient is particularly important to establish and maintain the normal gingival contour in areas of tooth irregularity.

Role of Drugs

A large variety of drugs have been used for topical treatment of NUG. Topical drug therapy is only an adjunctive measure. *No drug, when used alone, can be considered complete treatment.*

Escharotic drugs, such as phenol, silver nitrate, chromic acid, or potassium bichromate, should not be used. They are necrotizing agents that alleviate pain by destroying the nerve endings of the ulcerated gingiva but also destroy young cells that are needed for repair and delay healing. Repeated use of these agents results in loss of gingival tissue that is not restored when the disease subsides.[4]

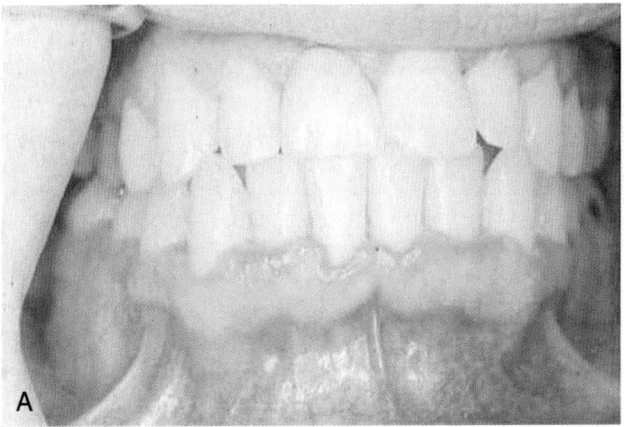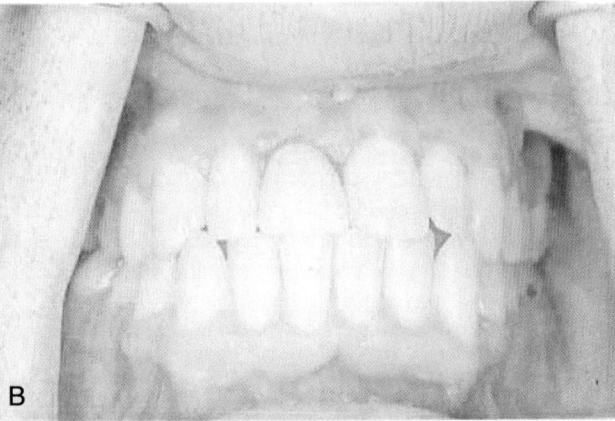

Fig. 44.2 Treatment of acute necrotizing ulcerative gingivitis. (A) Before treatment. Notice the characteristic interdental lesions. (B) After treatment, showing restoration of healthy gingival contour.

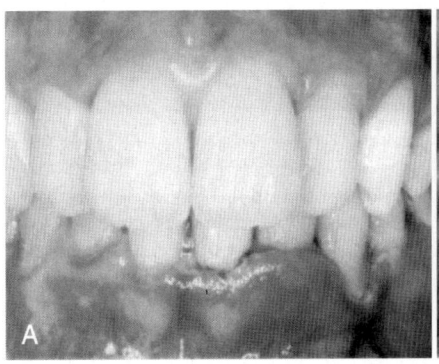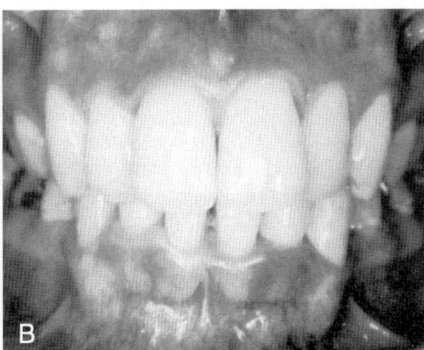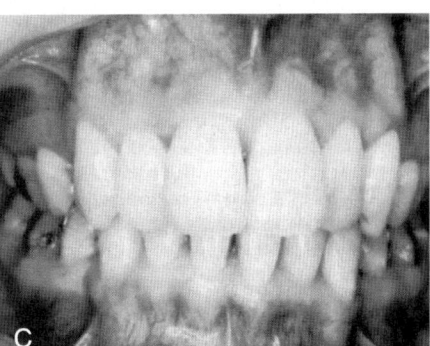

Fig. 44.3 Reshaping the gingiva in the treatment of acute necrotizing ulcerative gingivitis. (A) Before treatment. Bulbous gingiva and interdental necrosis are present in the mandibular anterior area. (B) After treatment. Gingival contours are still undesirable. (C) Final result. Physiologic contours are obtained by reshaping the gingiva.

Persistent or Recurrent Cases

Adequate local therapy with optimal home care will resolve most cases of NUG. If a case of NUG persists despite therapy or if it recurs, the patient should be reevaluated, with a focus on the following factors:

1. *Reassessment of differential diagnosis to rule out diseases that resemble NUG.* Several diseases and conditions (e.g., desquamative gingivitis) may initially manifest with an appearance similar to that of NUG. A renewed search for skin lesions and other signs or symptoms should be undertaken, with a biopsy if warranted (see Chapter 22).
2. *Underlying systemic disease causing immunosuppression.* In particular, HIV infection may frequently manifest with symptoms of NUG or necrotizing ulcerative periodontitis (NUP). The patient should be reassessed for risk factors and may need counseling about testing for HIV or other suspected underlying systemic diseases (e.g., lymphoproliferative disease). The patient will likely need referral to his or her physician for further evaluation.
3. *Inadequate local therapy.* Too often, treatment is discontinued when the symptoms have subsided, without elimination of the chronic gingival disease and periodontal pockets that remain after the superficial acute condition is relieved. Remaining calculus and other local factors that predispose to gingival inflammation may contribute to recurrence. Recurrent acute involvement in the mandibular anterior area can be associated with persistent pericoronal inflammation arising from partial eruption and pericoronal inflammation of third molars.[9] Anterior involvement is less likely to recur after the third molar situation is corrected.
4. *Inadequate compliance.* Poor biofilm control, heavy use of tobacco, ineffective stress management, and continued malnutrition can also contribute to persistence or recurrence of NUG. The clinician should evaluate the quality and consistency of biofilm control. Further assessment and counseling on tobacco use will also determine the role of tobacco. If the clinician perceives that unresolved psychosocial factors are complicating health, the patient should be referred to an appropriate professional. A reassessment of the patient's nutritional state, with dietary analysis or nutritional testing, may be required.[6,8]

Primary Herpetic Gingivostomatitis

Primary infection with herpes simplex virus in the oral cavity results in a condition known as acute herpetic gingivostomatitis, which is an oral infection that is often accompanied by systemic signs and symptoms (see Chapter 20). This infection typically occurs in children but can occur in adults as well. It runs a 7- to 10-day course and usually heals without scarring. A recurrent herpetic episode may be precipitated by dental treatment,[14] respiratory infection, sunlight exposure, fever, trauma, exposure to chemicals, or emotional stress in individuals with a history of herpesvirus infection.

Treatment consists of early diagnosis and immediate initiation of antiviral therapy. Historically, therapy for primary herpetic gingivostomatitis consisted of palliative care alone. However, since the development of antiviral therapy, the standard of care now includes the use of antiviral medications. In a randomized, double-blind, placebo-controlled study, Amir and colleagues[1] demonstrated that antiviral therapy with 15 mg/kg of an acyclovir suspension given five times daily for 7 days substantially changed the course of the disease without significant side effects. Acyclovir reduced the duration of symptoms, including fever, from 3 days to 1 day, decreased new extraoral lesions from 5.5 to 0 days, and reduced difficulty with eating from 7 to 4 days. Furthermore, viral shedding stopped at 1 day for the acyclovir group but persisted up to 5 days for the control group. Overall, oral lesions were present for only 4 days in the acyclovir group but persisted for 10 days in the control group. Although no clear clinical evidence indicates that this regimen will reduce recurrences, research data suggest that a greater number of latent virus copies incorporated into ganglia will increase the severity of recurrences.[1]

In summary, if primary herpetic gingivostomatitis is diagnosed within 3 days of onset, acyclovir suspension should be prescribed: 15 mg/kg 5 times daily for 7 days. If diagnosis occurs more than 3 days after onset in an immunocompetent patient, acyclovir therapy may have limited value. All patients, including those who present more than 3 days after disease onset, may receive palliative care, including removal of biofilm and food debris. An NSAID (e.g., ibuprofen) can be given systemically to reduce fever and pain. Patients may either take nutritional supplements or use topical anesthetics (e.g., viscous lidocaine) before eating to aid in proper nutrition during the early phases of acute herpetic gingivostomatitis. Periodontal therapy should be postponed until the acute symptoms subside to avoid the possibility of exacerbation (Fig. 44.4).

Local or systemic application of antibiotics is sometimes advised to prevent opportunistic bacterial or fungal infection of ulcerations, especially in the immunocompromised patient. If the condition does not resolve within 2 weeks, the patient should be referred to a physician for medical consultation.[7] The patient should be informed that herpetic gingivostomatitis is contagious at certain stages, such as when vesicles are present (highest viral titer). All individuals exposed to an infected patient should take precautions. Herpetic infection of a clinician's finger, referred to as *herpetic whitlow,* can occur if a seronegative clinician is exposed and becomes infected with herpesvirus from a patient's herpetic lesions.[10,11]

Pericoronitis

As described in Chapter 20, pericoronitis refers to inflammation of the excess flap of soft tissue that overlies the crown of an incompletely erupted tooth. It is most frequently associated with mandibular third molars (see Fig. 20.10 in Chapter 20). The treatment of pericoronitis depends on several factors, including position and quality of the

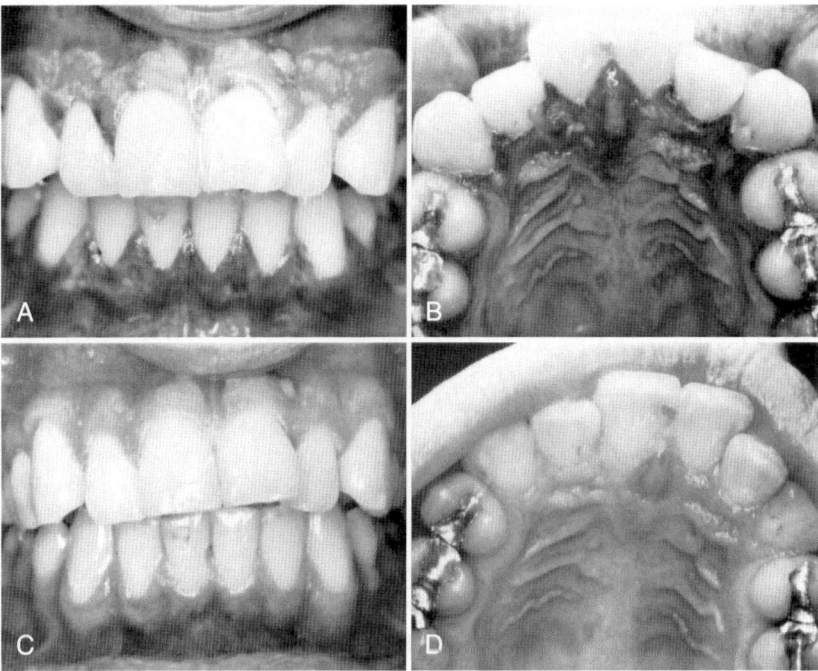

Fig. 44.4 Treatment of acute herpetic gingivostomatitis. (A) Before treatment. Note diffuse erythema and surface vesicles. (B) Before treatment, palatal view, showing gingival edema and ruptured vesicle on palate. (C) One month after treatment, showing restoration of normal gingival contour and stippling. (D) One month after treatment, palatal view.

surrounding tissues, severity of the inflammation, presence and/or risk of systemic complications, and advisability of retaining the involved tooth. All pericoronal flaps, even in the absence of symptoms, should be viewed with suspicion. Strong consideration should be given to removal of any pericoronal flaps that persist as a preventive measure against subsequent acute involvement.

The initial treatment of acute pericoronitis consists of (1) gently flushing the area with warm water to remove debris and exudate and (2) swabbing with antiseptic after the pericoronal flap has been lifted gently away from the tooth with an instrument. The underlying debris is removed, and the area is flushed with warm water. The occlusion is evaluated to determine whether an opposing tooth is contacting the pericoronal flap. It may be necessary to reduce soft tissue surgically and/or adjust the opposing tooth as a palliative measure to alleviate pain. Antibiotics can be prescribed in severe cases and for patients who have clinical evidence of diffuse microbial infiltration of the tissue. If the pericoronal flap is swollen and fluctuant, an incision and drainage procedure may be indicated to establish drainage and relieve pressure.

Once the acute symptoms have subsided, the prognosis of the tooth can be evaluated. The decision is governed by the likelihood that the tooth will continue erupting into a functional position or that impaction and the factors predisposing to pericoronitis will persist. Bone loss on the distal surface of the second molar is a concern when third molars are impacted along the distal surface (see Chapter 60).[2] The problem is significantly greater if the third molars are extracted after the roots are formed or when the patient is older (i.e., mid-twenties or later). To reduce the risk of bone loss around second molars, partially or completely impacted third molars should be extracted early in their development.

The quality of the soft tissues and the amount of space and vestibular depth are important factors to assess when deciding whether to retain or extract the tooth. If the decision is made to retain the tooth, the pericoronal flap is surgically reduced. It is necessary to reduce and reposition the tissue distal to the coronal aspect of the tooth, as well as remove the pericoronal flap on the occlusal surface. See Chapter 60 for a detailed description of distal surgical procedures and the proper management of tissues posterior to mandibular molars. Simply excising the occlusal portion of the pericoronal flap without managing the distal tissue leaves a deep periodontal pocket on the distal surface, which invites recurrence of acute pericoronal involvement. It is critical to leave the patient with a site that is cleansable and maintainable. As always, patient education and appropriate instruction in long-term maintenance of periodontal health is an essential part of successful therapy.

Conclusion

The treatment of acute gingival disease requires an accurate assessment and diagnosis of the problem that includes identification of risk factors. The objective of initial therapy is the alleviation of acute symptoms and elimination of all local and systemic contributing factors. Treatment is not complete if predisposing factors remain. Systemic risk factors that increase susceptibility to acute gingival disease should be eliminated or reduced.

 A Case Scenario is found on the companion website www.expertconsult.com.

References

 References for this chapter are found on the companion website www.expertconsult.com.

CHAPTER 45

Treatment of Periodontal Abscess

Philip R. Melnick | Henry H. Takei

Classification of Abscesses

The periodontal abscess is a localized purulent inflammation of the periodontal tissues.[6,15,18,19] It has been classified into three diagnostic groups: gingival abscess, periodontal abscess, and pericoronal abscess. The *gingival abscess* involves the marginal gingival and interdental tissues. The *periodontal abscess* is an infection located contiguous to the periodontal pocket and may result in destruction of the periodontal ligament and alveolar bone. The *pericoronal abscess* is associated with the crown of a partially erupted tooth.[15,18,25]

> ### LEARNING BOX 45.1
>
> Periodontal abscess has been classified into three categories: gingival abscess, periodontal abscess, and pericoronal abscess. Each category is classified according to the location and the tissue surrounding this localized lesion.

Periodontal Abscess

Periodontal abscesses are typically found in patients with untreated periodontitis and in association with moderate to deep periodontal pockets.[5,15,18,19,28] Periodontal abscesses often arise as acute exacerbations of preexisting pockets[6,15,18,19] (Fig. 45.1). Primarily related to incomplete calculus removal, periodontal abscesses have been linked to several clinical situations.[8,15–19,27] They have been identified in patients after periodontal surgery,[12] after preventive maintenance (Fig. 45.2),[7,10,20,24] after systemic antibiotic therapy,[29] and as the result of recurrent disease.[15–17] Conditions in which periodontal abscesses are not related to inflammatory periodontal disease include tooth perforation or fracture[1,27] (Fig. 45.3) and foreign body impaction.[2,26] Poorly controlled diabetes mellitus has been considered a predisposing factor for periodontal abscess formation[18,25] (Fig. 45.4). Formation of periodontal abscess has been reported as a major cause of tooth loss[12–14,16,17,20–24]; however, with proper treatment followed by consistent preventive periodontal maintenance, teeth with significant bone loss may be retained for many years[7] (see Fig. 45.10).

> ### LEARNING BOX 45.2
>
> Most periodontal abscesses are due to the incomplete removal of sub-gingival calculus in a periodontal pocket.

Gingival Abscess

The gingival abscess is a localized acute inflammatory lesion that may arise from a variety of sources, including microbial plaque infection, trauma, and foreign body impaction.[18,25] Clinical features include a red, smooth, sometimes painful, often fluctuant swelling (Fig. 45.5).[15]

Pericoronal Abscess

The pericoronal abscess results from inflammation of the soft tissue operculum, which covers a partially erupted tooth. This situation is most often observed around the mandibular third molars. As with the gingival abscess, the inflammatory lesion may be caused by the retention of microbial plaque biofilm, food impaction, or trauma.

Acute Versus Chronic Abscess

Abscesses are categorized as acute or chronic. The *acute abscess* is often an exacerbation of a chronic inflammatory periodontal lesion. Influencing factors include increased number and virulence of bacteria combined with lowered tissue resistance and lack of spontaneous drainage.[11,15,28] The drainage may have been prevented by deep, tortuous pocket morphology, debris, or closely adapted pocket epithelium blocking the pocket orifice. Acute abscesses are characterized by painful, red, edematous, smooth, and ovoid swelling of the gingival tissues.[16,17,28] Exudate may be expressed with gentle pressure; the tooth may be percussion sensitive and feel elevated in the socket (Fig. 45.6). Fever and regional lymphadenopathy are occasional findings.[25]

The *chronic abscess* forms after the spreading infection has been controlled by spontaneous drainage, host response, or therapy. Once homeostasis between the host and infection has been reached, the patient may have few or no symptoms.[9] However, dull pain may be associated with the clinical findings of a periodontal pocket, inflammation, and a fistulous tract.[25]

Box 45.1 compares the signs and symptoms of acute and chronic abscesses.

Periodontal Versus Pulpal Abscess

To determine the cause of an abscess and thus establish a proper treatment plan, it is often necessary to perform a differential diagnosis between periodontal abscess and pulpal abscess[4] (Box 45.2 and Figs. 45.7 and 45.8). Box 45.2 lists the differential diagnosis comparing the signs and symptoms of the two lesions. The correct diagnosis for these two lesions may overlap in some cases, but careful examination and patient questioning are important for an accurate diagnosis because the therapy for these two lesions is completely different.

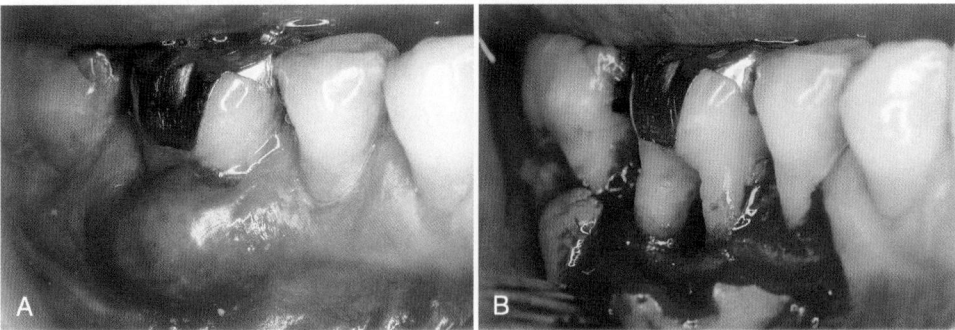

Fig. 45.1 (A) Deep furcation invasions are common locations for the periodontal abscess. (B) Furcation anatomy often prevents the definitive removal of calculus and microbial plaque.

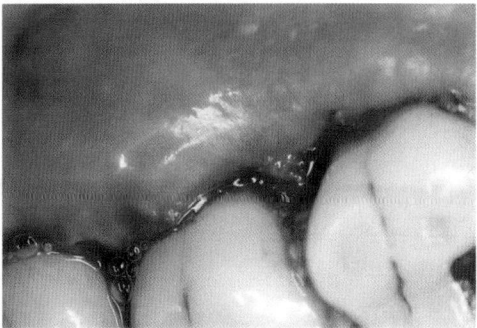

Fig. 45.2 Postprophylaxis periodontal abscess resulting from partial healing of a periodontal pocket over residual calculus.

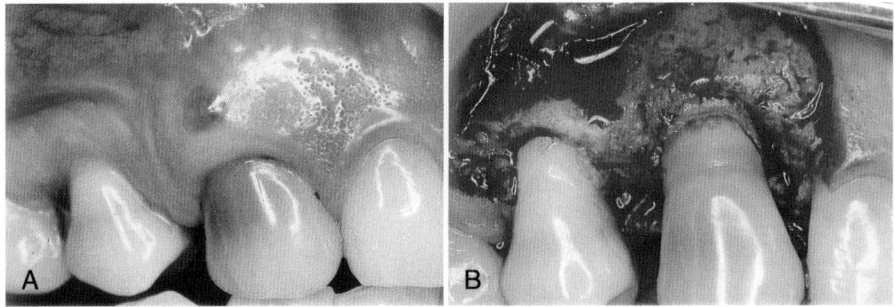

Fig. 45.3 (A) Fistula is observed in attached gingiva of a maxillary right canine. (B) Elevated flap shows the cause to be a root fracture.

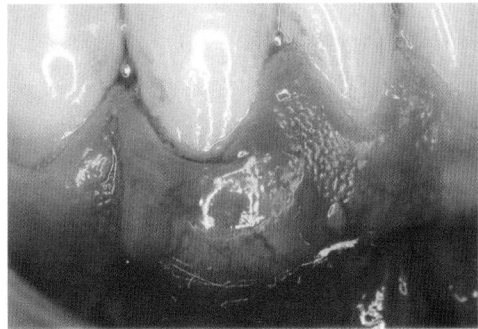

Fig. 45.4 Localized periodontal abscess of a mandibular right canine in a male adult with poorly controlled type 2 diabetes mellitus. For some patients, periodontal abscess formation may be the first sign of the disease.

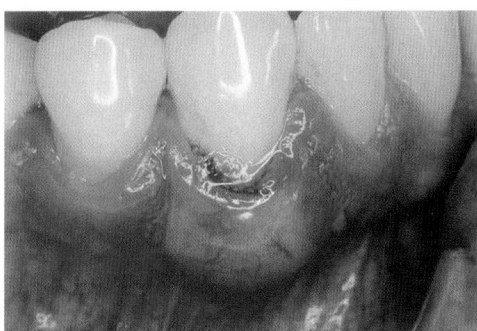

Fig. 45.5 Plaque-associated gingival abscess of a mandibular right canine.

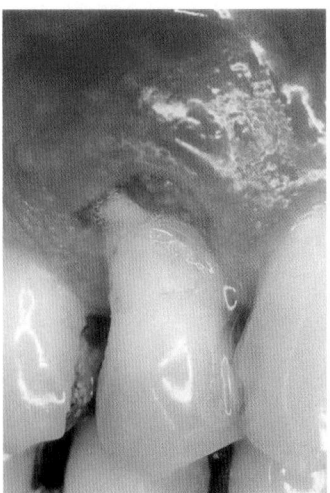

Fig. 45.6 Patient presenting with acute abscess complained of dull pain and a sensation of tooth elevation in the socket. Signs of tissue distention and exudation are evident.

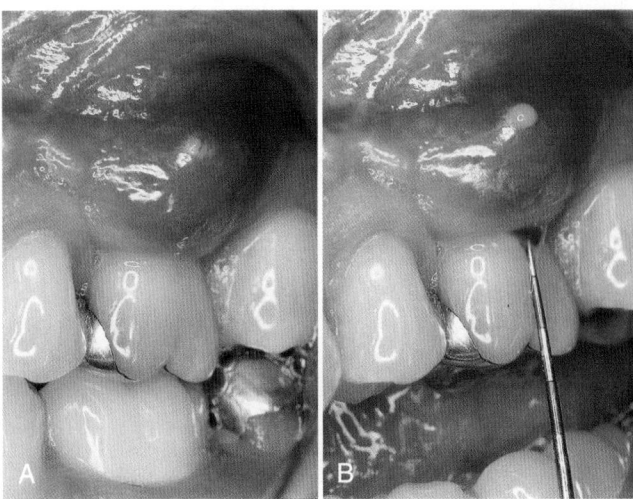

Fig. 45.8 (A) Periodontal abscess of maxillary left first molar. (B) Periodontal probe is used to retract the pocket wall gently.

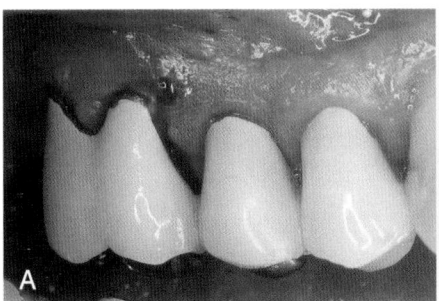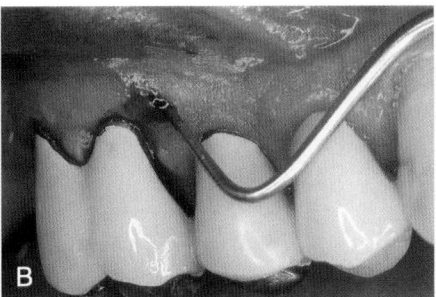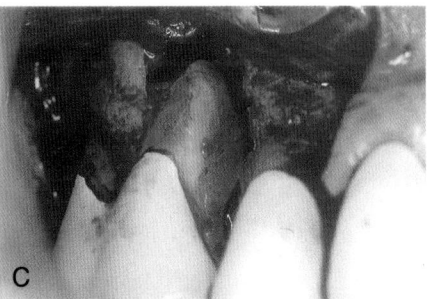

Fig. 45.7 (A) Maxillary right first molar with fistula on the attached gingiva. (B) With local anesthesia, periodontal probe is introduced through the fistula and angled toward the root end. (C) Surgical flap elevation demonstrates failed endodontic therapy and tooth fracture as causing the fistula.

BOX 45.1 Signs and Symptoms of Periodontal Abscess

Acute Abscess
Mild to severe discomfort
Localized red, ovoid swelling
Periodontal pocket
Mobility
Tooth elevation in socket
Tenderness to percussion or biting
Exudation
Elevated temperature[a]
Regional lymphadenopathy[a]

Chronic Abscess
No pain or dull pain
Localized inflammatory lesion
Slight tooth elevation
Intermittent exudation
Fistulous tract often associated with a deep pocket
Usually without systemic involvement

[a]May indicate the need for systemic antibiotics.
Data from Dahlen G: Microbiology and treatment of dental abscesses and periodontal-endodontic lesions. *Periodontol 2000* 28:206, 2002; Meng HX: Periodontal abscess. *Ann Periodontol* 4:79, 1999; and Sanz M, Herrera D, van Winkelhoff AJ: The periodontal abscess. In Lindhe J, editor: *Clinical periodontology*, Copenhagen, 2000, Munksgaard.

BOX 45.2 Differential Diagnosis of Periodontal and Pulpal Abscess

Periodontal Abscess
Associated with a preexisting periodontal pocket.
Radiographs show periodontal angular bone loss and furcation radiolucency.
Tests show vital pulp.
Swelling usually includes gingival tissue, with an occasional fistula.
Pain is usually dull and localized.
Sensitivity to percussion may or may not be present.

Pulpal Abscess
The offending tooth may have large restoration.
The tooth may have no periodontal pocket or, if present, it probes as a narrow defect.
Tests show nonvital pulp.
Swelling is often localized to the apex, with a fistulous tract.
Pain is often severe and difficult to localize.
Sensitivity to percussion is noted.

Modified from Corbet EF: Diagnosis of acute periodontal lesions. *Periodontol 2000* 34:204, 2004.

Specific Treatment Approaches

Treatment of the periodontal abscess includes two phases: resolving the acute lesion, then managing the resulting chronic condition[15,18,27] (Box 45.3).

Acute Abscess

The acute abscess is treated to alleviate symptoms, control the spread of infection, and establish drainage.[15,22] Before treatment, the patient's medical history, dental history, and systemic condition are reviewed and evaluated to assist in the diagnosis and determine the need for systemic antibiotics[3] (Boxes 45.4 and 45.5).

Drainage Through the Periodontal Pocket

The peripheral area around the abscess is anesthetized with sufficient topical and local anesthetic agents to ensure comfort. The pocket wall is gently retracted with a periodontal probe or curette in an attempt to initiate drainage through the pocket entrance (see Fig. 45.8). Gentle digital pressure and irrigation may be used to express the exudate and drain the pocket (Fig. 45.9). If the lesion is minimal and access is uncomplicated, debridement in the form of scaling and root planing may be undertaken at this appointment.

If the lesion is large and drainage cannot be established, root debridement by scaling and root planing or surgical access should be delayed until the major clinical signs have abated.[19,21] In these

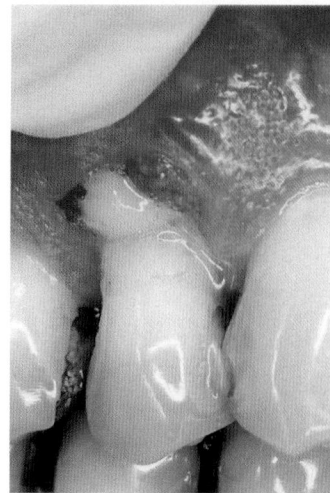

Fig. 45.9 Gentle digital pressure may be sufficient to express purulent discharge.

patients, use of adjunctive systemic antibiotics[13,14,16,17,19] with a short-term high-dose regimen is recommended[22] (see Box 45.5). Antibiotic therapy alone without subsequent drainage and subgingival scaling is contraindicated.[14]

Drainage Through an External Incision

To drain the abscess, the lesion is dried and isolated with gauze sponges. A topical anesthetic agent is applied, followed by a local anesthetic agent injected peripheral to the lesion. A vertical incision through the most fluctuant center of the abscess is made with a no. 15 surgical blade. The tissue lateral to the incision can be separated with a curette or periosteal elevator. The fluctuant matter is expressed, and the wound edges are approximated under light digital pressure with a moist gauze pad.

In abscesses manifesting with severe swelling and inflammation, aggressive mechanical instrumentation should be delayed in favor of antibiotic therapy to avoid damage to healthy contiguous periodontal tissues.[27]

Once bleeding and suppuration have ceased, the patient may be dismissed. For patients who do not need systemic antibiotics, post-treatment instructions include frequent rinsing with warm salt water (1 tbsp/8-oz glass) and periodic application of chlorhexidine gluconate 0.12% oral rinse either by rinsing or applied locally with a cotton-tipped applicator. Reduced physical exertion and increased fluid intake are often recommended for patients showing systemic involvement. Analgesics may be prescribed for comfort. By the following day, the signs and symptoms have usually subsided. If the problem continues and the patient is still uncomfortable, the previously recommended regimen is repeated for an additional 24 hours. This often results in satisfactory healing, and the lesion can be treated as a chronic abscess.[28]

Chronic Abscess

As with a periodontal pocket, the chronic abscess is usually treated with scaling and root planing and, if indicated, surgical therapy. Surgical treatment is suggested when deep vertical pocket or furcation defects are encountered that are beyond the therapeutic capabilities of nonsurgical instrumentation (Fig. 45.10). Access to subgingival calculus must be achieved in areas of deep pockets. The patient should be advised of the possible postoperative sequelae usually associated with periodontal nonsurgical and surgical procedures. As with the acute abscess, antibiotic therapy may be indicated.[15,19,28]

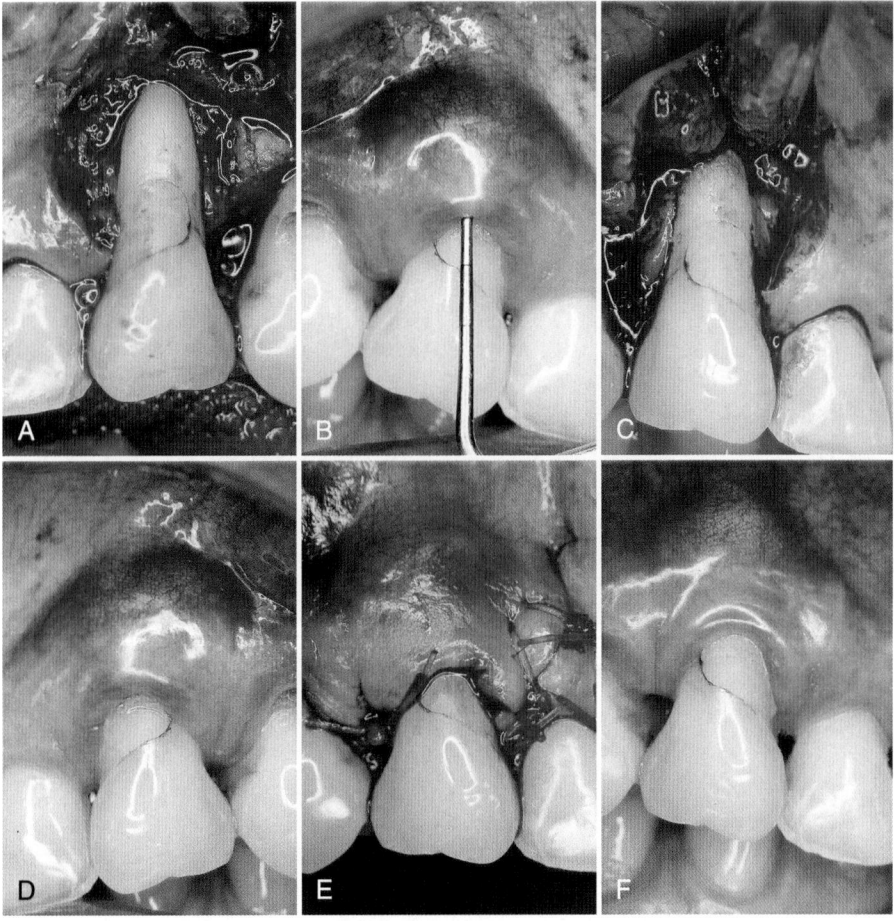

Fig. 45.10 (A) Chronic periodontal abscess of a maxillary right canine. (B) With local anesthesia, periodontal probe is inserted to determine severity of the lesion. (C) With mesial and distal vertical incisions, a full-thickness flap is elevated, exposing severe bone dehiscence, a subgingival restoration, and root calculus. (D) Root surface has been planed free of calculus, and the restoration has been smoothed. (E) Full-thickness flap has been replaced to its original position and sutured with absorbable sutures. (F) At 3 months, gingival tissues are pink, firm, and well adapted to the tooth, with minimal periodontal probing depth.

LEARNING BOX 45.3

Periodontal abscess due to a deep periodontal pocket often requires a surgical flap to access the subgingival calculus. This also allows the clinician to reduce the pocket at the same surgical appointment.

Gingival Abscess

Treatment of the gingival abscess is aimed at reversal of the acute phase and, when applicable, immediate removal of the cause. To ensure comfort, topical or local anesthesia by infiltration is administered. When possible, scaling and root planing are completed to establish drainage and remove microbial deposits. In more acute situations, the fluctuant area is incised with a no. 15 scalpel blade, and exudate may be expressed by gentle digital pressure. Any foreign material (e.g., dental floss, impression material) is removed. The area is irrigated with warm water and covered with moist gauze under light pressure.

Once bleeding has stopped, the patient is dismissed with instructions to rinse with warm salt water every 2 hours for the remainder of the day. After 24 hours, the area is reassessed, and if resolution is sufficient, scaling not previously completed is undertaken. If the residual lesion is large or poorly accessible, surgical access may be required.

Pericoronal Abscess

As with other abscesses of the periodontium, treatment of the pericoronal abscess is aimed at management of the acute phase, followed by resolution of the chronic condition. The acute pericoronal abscess is properly anesthetized for comfort, and drainage is established by gently lifting the soft tissue operculum with a curette. If the underlying debris is easily accessible, it may be removed, followed by gentle irrigation with sterile saline. If the patient has regional swelling, lymphadenopathy, or systemic signs, systemic antibiotics may be prescribed.

The patient is dismissed with instructions to rinse with warm salt water every 2 hours, and the area is reassessed after 24 hours. If discomfort was one of the original complaints, appropriate analgesics should be used. Once the acute phase has been controlled, the partially erupted tooth may be definitively treated with either surgical excision of the overlying tissue or removal of the offending tooth.

 A Case Scenario is found on the companion website www.expertconsult.com.

References

 References for this chapter are found on the companion website www.expertconsult.com.

CHAPTER 46

Endodontic-Periodontic Lesions: Pathogenesis, Diagnosis, and Treatment Considerations

Mo K. Kang | Kenneth C. Trabert | Shebli Mehrazarin

 CHAPTER OUTLINE

Factors Initiating Pulpal and Apical Diseases
Classification of Pulpal and Apical Diseases
Biologic Effects of Pulpal Infection on Periodontal Tissues
Biologic Effects of Periodontal Infection on the Dental Pulp

Effect of Endodontic Pathosis on Development of Retrograde Peri-Implantitis *(e-only)*
Interactions Between Extraradicular Infection and the Periodontium *(e-only)*

Differential Diagnosis of Pulpal and Periodontal Infection *(e-only)*
Treatment Considerations *(e-only)*
Summary

 For online-only content on perforations, tooth fractures (Video 46.1), sodium hypochlorite accident, resorptive defects, dental anomalies, and ultrasonic devices in the section on the effect on the periodontium of endodontic procedural complications and dental anomalies, as well as expanded discussions of the factors initiating pulpal and apical diseases and classification of pulpal and periradicular apical diseases, in addition to infections and diagnostic and treatment considerations, go to the companion website at www.expertconsult.com.

Periodontium and pulpal spaces represent the two primary sites of dental infection from oral bacteria. These two spaces are separated by hard shell of dentin, but they may communicate through various portals, such as root canal foramina, dentinal tubules, and even crack lines, through which bacteria and microbial irritants may trigger inflammatory responses in surrounding tissues. At the clinical level, compound dentoalveolar infections involving both periodontium and pulpal spaces are common and present challenges for diagnosis and treatment. Conversations occur daily among periodontists, endodontists, and general practitioners to try to ascertain whether a lesion surrounding one or more teeth is of periodontal or endodontic origin or is possibly a true combined lesion that affects both compartments and will require endodontic as well as subsequent periodontal treatment. In this chapter, we discuss the proper diagnosis of these various conditions and offer treatment modalities to ensure the retention of teeth that could otherwise be extracted.

Persistent infection in the pulp tissue leads to secondary infection and breakdown of tissues in the periodontium. Conversely, severe periodontal disease may initiate or exacerbate inflammatory changes in the pulp tissue. This mutuality of infection between pulp and periodontium is mediated through anatomic routes, allowing for communication between the two spaces. The main and obvious routes of communication are the apical foramina. Advanced pulpitis leads to pulp necrosis, which often is accompanied by inflammatory bone resorption at the root apex, as found in cases of apical periodontitis or an apical abscess (Fig. 46.1). This is also known as *retrograde periodontitis* because it represents periodontal tissue breakdown from an apical to a cervical direction and is the opposite of *orthograde*

periodontitis, which results from a sulcular infection. This condition is typically identified as a periapical radiolucency (Fig. 46.2). Retrograde periodontitis is the most common example of pulpal diseases leading to secondary periodontal breakdown. The presence of patent apical foramina may also lead to inflammatory changes in the pulp secondary to severe periodontitis in cases where the periodontal defect reaches the apical foramina.

Alternatively, lateral or accessory canals may comprise the route of periodontal and pulpal communication. The prevalence of accessory root canals in various human teeth and their contribution to the complexity of the root canal system have been well established. Accessory canals are found along the length of the root canals, albeit at varying frequencies depending on their location. By using the "clearing technique" for transparent root canal visualization, prior studies showed that 59.5% of maxillary second premolars possess lateral canals; 78.2% of those canals are located in the apical regions of the root canals.[105] Notably, accessory canals were also found in both midroot and cervical regions, albeit at reduced frequencies, at 16.2% and 4.0%, respectively. A subsequent study showed that 28.4% of permanent molars exhibit patent accessory canals in furcation regions,[27] a finding suggesting that these accessory canals allow a pulpal and periodontal communication to exist. Root canal therapies frequently fail in maxillary molars because of unidentified second mesiobuccal canals. These canals are found in a surprisingly high percentage (80.8%) of teeth.[40] Clearly, accessory canals can lead to asymptomatic apical periodontitis resulting from chronic pulpal diseases. This condition can be readily detected in periapical radiographs (Fig. 46.3), and the periodontal lesions usually heal after

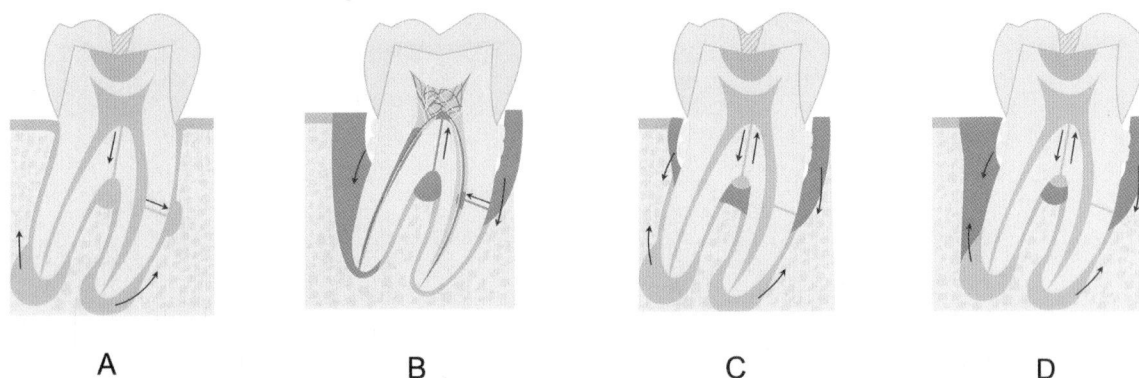

Fig. 46.1 Classification of endodontic-periodontic lesions. (A) Primary pulpal infection can lead to chronic periradicular periodontitis by which a periapical radiolucency can develop and migrate cervically. Mandibular molars can also have accessory canals in lateral orientation or in the furcation area. These accessory canals can allow migration of the primary pulpal infection and cause secondary breakdown of the periodontium at their respective loci. (B) Primary periodontal infection can lead to extensive breakdown of alveolar crest bone that migrates from the cervical area to the apex. In these lesions, one would find generalized bone loss around a single tooth or that often could involve multiple adjacent teeth. Because of the pulpal-periodontal continuum through main root canal foramina or through accessory canals, extensive periodontal infection can cause irritation in the pulp tissues. (C) Both primary pulpal infection and primary periodontal infection can occur simultaneously in an "independent" endo-perio lesion, exhibiting the characteristics of both. (D) Primary pulpal and primary periodontal infections can occur extensively in this "combined" endo-perio lesion.

Case 1

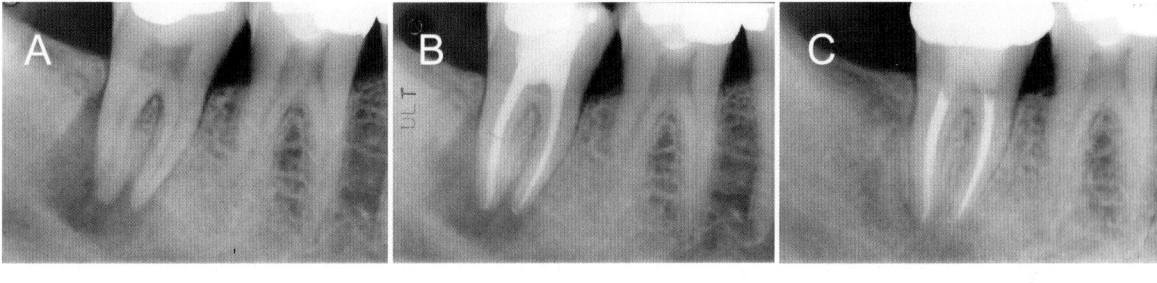

Case 2

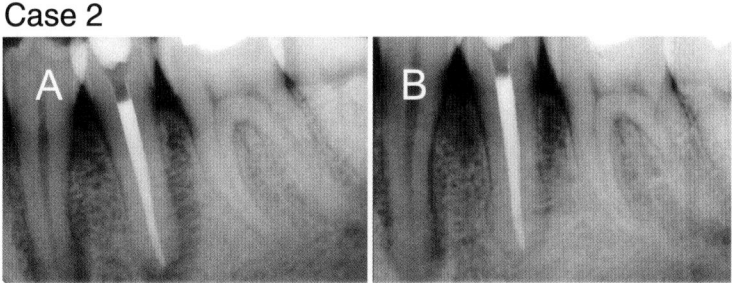

Fig. 46.2 Retrograde periodontitis. Case 1. (A) Large periapical lesion extending around the periapex of tooth #31. No visible fractures were detected on the mesial or distal marginal ridges. The tooth tested nonvital. A sinus tract was visible on the buccal gingiva. (B) Endodontic therapy was completed in two visits, and the canals were obturated. (C) Healing of the periradicular bone is evident at 6 months, and a crown providing complete coverage has been placed. Case 2. (A) Tooth #20 had a broad periradicular lesion extending from the apex to the distal root surface that resembled a J-shaped lesion. Conventional root canal therapy was completed. (B) Healing of periradicular bone lesion after 6-month recall. *(Case 1, Courtesy Dr. Thomas Rauth.)*

successful completion of endodontic therapy. Questions also arise about whether pulpitis develops from periodontal infections through accessory root canals. Kirkham[48] in 1975 reported that only 2% of teeth possessed accessory canals within the periodontal pockets among those teeth extracted for severe periodontal disease. Thus, the likelihood that primary periodontal infections will reach the dental pulp through accessory canals is highly remote.

The third route of communication between the periodontium and the pulp is through the dentinal tubules. Dentinal tubules maintain a tapered structure along the length from the pulpodentinal complex to the dentinoenamel junction with a diameter of 2.5 µm at the pulpodentinal complex and 0.9 µm at the dentinoenamel junction.[97] It is therefore conceivable that dentinal permeability changes at different locations along the root surface according to the size and

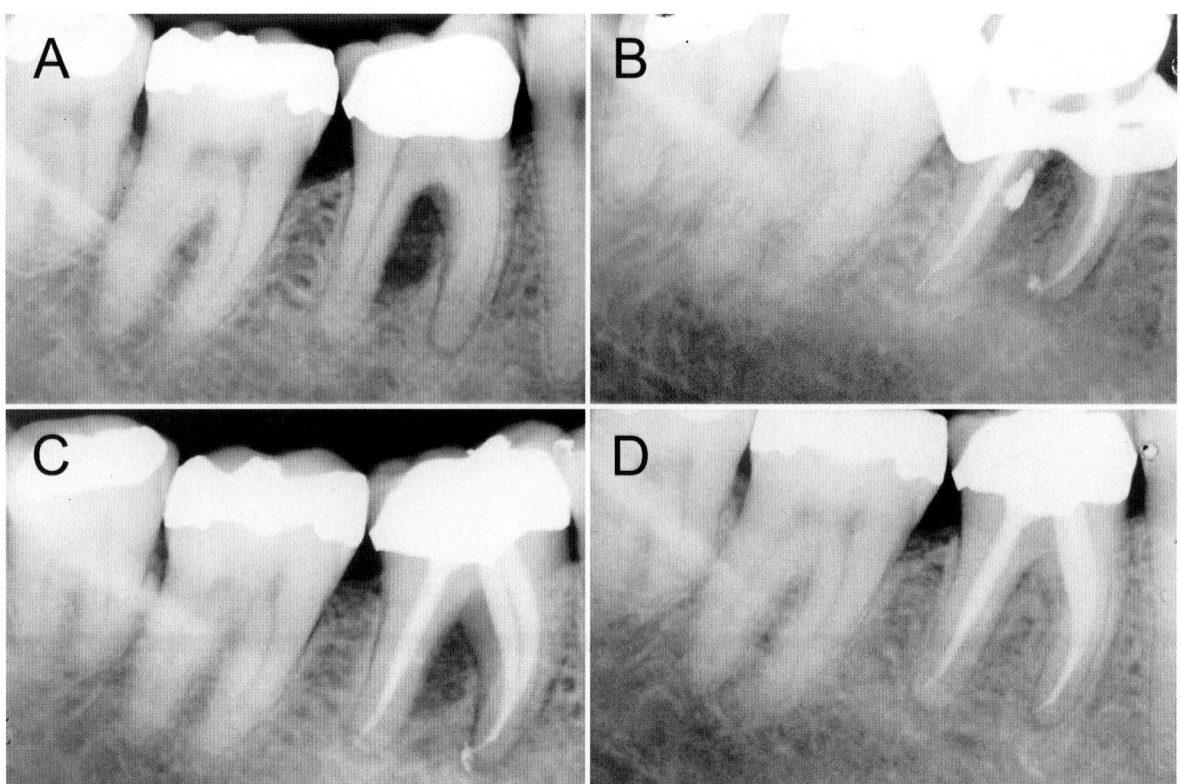

Fig. 46.3 Lateral canal-led periodontal defect from a primary endodontic infection. (A) Bone loss is present in the furcation with sinus tract present on the buccal mucosa. Tooth #30 tested nonvital. (B) During condensation, a large amount of sealer was expressed through a large lateral canal in the distal root. (C) Sealer was removed after obturation by curettage of the furcation and irrigation with anesthetic solution through the sinus tract. (D) Healing at 12 months demonstrates complete repair of periradicular bone. *(Courtesy Dr. Thomas Rauth.)*

density of the dentinal tubules. Bacterial colonization in the tubules from infected root canals has been well documented.[83] In addition, bacterial invasion into dentinal tubules from the periodontal pocket has been demonstrated,[23] suggesting that dentinal tubules may allow pulpal irritation from chronic periodontal infections. Periodontal pathogens penetrating into the dentinal tubules also may be the source of persistent periodontal infection.[23]

Dentin permeability through dentinal tubules is a clinically important issue. The permeability may be measured through hydraulic conductance, as described earlier.[71] Subsequently, investigators studied the effects of various agents and stresses on dentin permeability. Root planing as part of routine periodontal therapy, for example, is shown to decrease dentin permeability and result in the formation of a smear layer that is acid labile.[22] However, dentin permeability may increase on removal of the smear layer, thus resulting in tubular penetration of oral pathogens and subsequent pulpal irritation. Further study is necessary to delineate the role of dentinal tubules in causing secondary infection in pulpal or periodontal tissues. Clinicians need to be aware that patent dentinal tubules can provide effective irritant conduits between these two otherwise distinct tissues.

In addition to the foregoing routes of anatomic communication between pulpal and periodontal tissues, in some instances communication is established between the pulp and periodontium by iatrogenic defects such as vertical root fractures and tooth perforations. Both of these situations represent nonanatomic communication between the pulp and periodontium and result in the spread of infection from one compartment to the other.

Factors Initiating Pulpal and Apical Diseases

Pulpal and apical diseases are initiated by numerous external factors that may include microorganisms, trauma, excessive heat, restorative procedures, restorative agents, and malocclusion. These insults lead to inflammatory changes in the pulp, starting from reversible or irreversible pulpitis and ultimately progressing to pulpal necrosis and subsequent breakdown of the periodontium. Dental caries is a prominent cause of pulpal disease, and bacterial infection is the primary form of microbial insult to the pulp. A systematic review of literature from 1966 to 2000 showed causative effects of mutans streptococci and the lactobacilli for human dental caries, whereas other bacteria such as *Streptococcus sanguinis, Streptococcus salivarius*, and enterococci could not be associated with the disease.[94] More recent understanding of the caries process has emphasized the importance of homeostatic balance in biofilm, which describes the microbial ecosystem on tooth surfaces rather than the virulence of individual bacterial species.[93] Regardless, pulpal infection is polymicrobial and often starts from incipient caries causing localized pulpal inflammation or pulpitis.

Local invasion of the cariogenic bacteria or a shift in the bacterial content of biofilm can lead to inflammatory changes in the dental pulp. This frequently happens in the absence of caries extension into the pulp chamber. Bacterial byproducts relevant to pulpitis include lactic acid, ammonia, urea, lipopolysaccharide, and lipoteichoic acid. It is notable that the dental pulp is capable of managing numerous microbial insults because of its extensive intrapulpal lymphatic system. However, an overwhelming pulpal inflammatory response may be

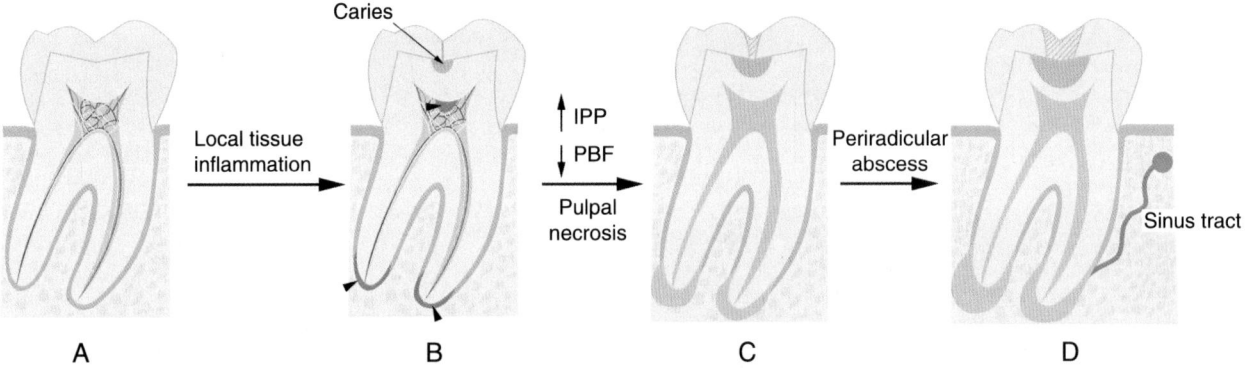

Fig. 46.4 Progression of the pulpal and periradicular pathosis. (A) Normal tooth without any pulpal pathosis is richly vascularized and innervated. (B) With microbial challenges such as caries, local tissue inflammation can occur in the pulp adjacent to the site of carious lesions, as well as in the apical regions *(arrowheads)*. (C) Pulpal inflammation can lead to reduction in pulpal blood flow *(PBF)* caused by an increase in intrapulpal pressure *(IPP)*, causing pulpal necrosis (shown in *gray*). (D) Pulpal necrosis, if left untreated, can cause chronic inflammation of periradicular tissues and abscess formation, leading to a draining sinus tract.

induced through various mechanisms and numerous microbial challenges. Lipopolysaccharide and lipoteichoic acid bind Toll-like receptors. These are present on the surface of some immune cells in the pulp and induce the release of inflammatory mediators such as prostaglandins, cytokines, and chemokines.[38] In particular, tumor necrosis factor alpha, interleukin-1 (IL-1), IL-8, IL-12, and chemokines CCL2 and CXCL2 are well described for their role in pulpitis.[28] IL-1 is known to be released from macrophages after stimulation with lipopolysaccharide and is responsible for bone resorption leading to apical periodontitis.[34] During acute pulpitis, the inflammatory mediators trigger vasodilation, a transient increase of pulpal blood flow, inflammatory cell infiltration, increased intrapulpal pressure, and finally ischemic necrosis of the pulp (Fig. 46.4).

In acute apical abscess, anaerobic bacteria are predominant over aerobic strains and anaerobes, and microaerophiles were predominant in 82% of the cases studied.[45] The most prevalent isolated bacteria are *Fusobacterium nucleatum, Parvimonas micra,* and *Porphyromonas endodontalis.*[86] Depending on the virulence of the organisms and host resistance, a lesion that has been chronic may exacerbate and become an acute apical abscess. The presence of spirochetes is also well documented in apical and periodontal abscesses and has been studied by various identification techniques.[16] Spirochetes most often isolated in root canal infections are *Treponema denticola* and *Treponema maltophilium.*[39,74] When comparing chronic and acute apical abscesses, Baumgartner and colleagues[6] found a significantly higher incidence of spirochetes in acute abscesses and cellulitis than in asymptomatic infected root canals. *Treponema socranskii* was the most frequently encountered species.[6]

Thermomechanical irritants can induce altered pulpal circulation and pulp tissue damage. Earlier studies demonstrated that thermal changes caused by dental procedures such as tooth preparation led to a marked diminution of pulpal blood flow and plasma extravasation, resulting in an inflammatory response.[47,70] Extreme heat caused by dry tooth preparation triggers vascular stasis and hemorrhage in the subodontoblastic vascular plexus.[60] Investigators noted that even a small increase in pulpal temperature (5° to 6° C) is capable of inducing necrotic changes in the pulp.[108] Pulpal necrosis eventually leads to apical periodontitis. Similarly, chemical irritants impose measurable changes in the pulp status. One study showed the cytotoxicity of dental resin material (2-hydroxyethyl methacrylate [HEMA]) on pulp stromal cells through induction of apoptotic cell death.[66] Etching the dentin surface with high phosphoric acid content causes deleterious

effects on dental pulp.[79] In addition, bonding resins used as pulp capping materials led to acute pulpitis and varying degrees of necrosis in human teeth.[1] Root canal overfills with gutta-percha and sealers invariably cause severe inflammatory reactions in the apical tissues, even though patients may be completely asymptomatic.[72] Thus, dental materials often contain chemical irritants that affect both the pulpal and periodontal tissues, and one must be aware of the potential iatrogenic endodontic pathosis associated with their misuse.

Classification of Pulpal and Apical Diseases

The diagnosis of endodontic lesions that may often have a periodontal component can be confusing. The diagnostic terminology used in various dental schools and textbooks further compounds the confusion for students and practitioners alike. In an attempt to simplify and unify a standardized diagnostic terminology, the American Association of Endodontists established new endodontic diagnosis terminology in 2009. The reader is referred to this revised terminology, published in the *Journal of Endodontics,* for a more complete discussion of this subject.[24] Throughout this chapter we refer to this new terminology, which is also summarized in Tables 46.1 and 46.2.

To make a proper endodontic diagnosis, the clinician must evaluate the symptoms of the patient, the radiographic and clinical findings, and the presence or absence and location of any swelling or drainage. Given all these variables, it is easy to understand why a lack of clarity exists and mistakes are made about whether the lesion is primarily endodontic or periodontal, or a true combined lesion.

The classification of diseases of the dental pulp depends on the extent of pulpal injury and its ability to repair. Many factors influence whether a tooth will be classified as normal, or whether it will develop reversible pulpitis or irreversible pulpitis, or will become necrotic.

Previous studies have found little correlation between the histologic features of pulpal disease and the symptoms that the patient experienced before treatment.[51,102] A review of the diagnosis of pulpal pain by Bender[7] in 2000 found that 80% of patients who gave a previous history of odontogenic pain manifested histopathologic evidence of pulpitis and partial necrosis in the dental pulp. Bender also concluded that a clinician can determine the degree of pulp histopathosis by asking the patient about his or her previous pain history and symptoms related to the involved tooth.[7] Controversy still remains, however, regarding the degree of correlation between pulpal symptoms and the histopathologic features of the pulpal tissues, and additional studies are needed to confirm the correlation between the two.

Apical pathoses of endodontic origin are inflammatory processes occurring in periradicular tissues surrounding root apices. They result from various microbial agents that originate from root canal infection and create a series of inflammatory and immunologic responses. These agents exit through the apical foramen, lateral canals, or dentinal tubules.[48,68] It is an infectious process caused by a large number of microbial species, unlike classic infectious diseases occurring elsewhere in the body that may be caused by only one or two specific organisms. These species reside in ecologically balanced communities discussed previously and constitute the *biofilm*.[65] The different characteristics of pulpal and periodontal lesions are summarized in Table 46.3.

Biologic Effects of Pulpal Infection on Periodontal Tissues

The effects of pulpal disease on the surrounding periodontal tissues are widely accepted by clinicians and researchers, and these effects have been studied since the 1960s. Early inflammatory changes in the pulp exert very little effect on the periodontium. Even a pulp that is significantly inflamed may have little or no effect on the surrounding periodontal tissues. Investigators believe that this initial pulpal inflammatory response is an attempt to prevent the spread of infection to the apical tissues.

When the pulp becomes necrotic, however, it produces a significant inflammatory response involving extremely complex inflammatory and immune reactions. This response can traverse the apical foramen, the furcation, lateral canals, dentinal tubules, and areas of trapped necrotic tissue along the surface of the root that extend past the periodontal ligament and into the surrounding apical tissues.[82] This initial inflammatory response of the pulp and subsequent necrosis that permeates the numerous spaces of the canal system include various bacterial strains, spirochetes, fungi, yeasts, and viruses.[61] The nature and extent of the periodontal destruction that follows depend on the virulence of the pathogens in the root canal system, the chronicity of the disease, and the defense mechanism of the host.[13]

In a classic study by Kakehashi and colleagues,[41] the infected pulp of germ-free rats remained vital, whereas the infected pulp of normal rats that were left open to the oral environment developed pulpal necrosis with subsequent inflammation and formation of periapical lesions. This was the first experimental evidence to demonstrate microbial infection as the etiology of pulpal and periapical pathoses. Similarly, bacterial infection plays a pivotal role in endodontic-periodontic lesions in the form of bacterial biofilm, which

TABLE 46.1 Classification of Pulpal Diseases[a]

Pulpal State	Symptom	Vitality	Response to Cold
Normal pulp	Asymptomatic	Vital	Within normal limits
Reversible pulpitis	Sensitive to pressure or temperature[b]	Vital	Hypersensitive to cold
Symptomatic irreversible pulpitis[c]	Spontaneous throbbing pain	Vital	Hypersensitive to cold and lingering response
Asymptomatic irreversible pulpitis[d]	None	Vital	Within normal limits
Pulp necrosis[e]	Asymptomatic[e]	Nonvital	No response
Previously treated	Variable	Nonvital	No response
Previously initiated therapy	Variable	Variable	Variable

[a]Different pulpal conditions cannot be discerned by periapical radiographs. Symptoms and responses to cold explained herein are the general findings, but there can be exceptions.
[b]Patients' response to pressure may be due to hyperocclusion in reversible pulpitis cases. In the absence of such factors, patients' complaints mainly revolve around thermal sensitivity.
[c]Symptomatic irreversible pulpitis may be symptomatic and painful as described or may be asymptomatic and nonpainful.
[d]Asymptomatic irreversible pulpitis is based on the presence of pulpal inflammation (e.g., extensive caries, hyperemia, or traumatic injury) in the absence of patients' subjective symptoms.
[e]Necrotic pulp may cause acute exacerbation of symptoms, including spontaneous throbbing pain. However, such sensitivity results from periradicular inflammation.
Diagnostic terminology based on the recommendations of the American Association of Endodontists consensus conference, as shown in Glickman GN: AAE consensus conference on diagnostic terminology: background and perspectives. *J Endod* 35:1634, 2009.

TABLE 46.2 Classification of Periradicular Diseases[a]

Periradicular State	Symptom	Pulpal Status	Percussion Response	Palpation Response	Periapical Radiolucency	Sinus Tract
Normal periapex	None	Varies[b]	None	None	Not present	Not present
Symptomatic apical periodontitis[c]	Painful	Inflamed	Painful	Varies[d]	Not present	Not present
Asymptomatic apical periodontitis	None	Nonvital	None	None	Present	Not present
Acute apical abscess[c]	Painful	Inflamed	Painful	Painful	Varies[e]	Not present
Chronic apical abscess	None	Nonvital	None	None	Present	Present
Condensing osteitis	None/pain	Inflamed	None	None	Radiopaque	Not present

[a]Symptom and other descriptions of the individual periradicular pathosis are the general findings, which can deviate.
[b]Normal periapex can be associated with normal, inflamed, or necrotic pulp.
[c]The difference between acute periradicular periodontitis and acute periradicular abscess is that the former is confined to the involved tooth and the latter is more generalized and frequently manifests with gross swelling of the affected periradicular tissues.
[d]Palpation in acute periradicular periodontitis may elicit tenderness after progression of the disease through the cortical plate.
[e]Periapical radiolucency may be present in advanced acute periradicular abscess.
Diagnostic terminology based on the recommendations of the American Association of Endodontists consensus conference, as shown in Glickman GN: AAE consensus conference on diagnostic terminology: background and perspectives. *J Endod* 35:1634, 2009.

TABLE 46.3   Different Characteristics of Pulpal and Periodontal Lesions[a]

	Primary Pulpal	Primary Periodontal	Independent Endodontic-Periodontic	Combined Endodontic-Periodontic
Patient symptom	Varies[b]	Mild discomfort	Varies[b]	Varies[b]
Coronal integrity	Compromised	Intact	Compromised	Compromised
Radiographic lesions	Periapical radiolucency	Crestal bone loss	Separate periapical radiolucency and crestal lesions	Continuous bony lesions from alveolar crest to apex
Vitality	Nonvital	Vital	Nonvital	Nonvital
Periodontal probing	Narrow probing to apex[c]	Generalized bone loss	Generalized bone loss	Generalized bone loss with narrow probing to apex

[a]These are generalized summaries, and there can be deviations.
[b]Patients' symptoms of pulpal lesions may vary, depending on the type of pathosis. Chronic lesions can be completely asymptomatic, whereas acute pain symptoms can be triggered without any radiographic lesions.
[c]Primary pulpal lesions may not manifest with any periodontal defect. Narrow probing in pulpal lesions may indicate a sinus tract through the sulcus.

is composed of a 15% cellular component and a matrix material that comprises the remaining 85%. The formation of biofilm communities is under the control of complex chemical signals that both regulate and guide the formation of the slime-enclosed colonies and water channels.[14] Proteolytic bacteria predominate in early root canal infections and then change over time to a flora that contains a greater number of anerobes.[21,90]

Several nonliving irritants have also been implicated in the inflammatory process. These include foreign bodies, epithelial rests, cholesterol crystals, Russell bodies, Rushton hyaline bodies, and Charcot-Leyden crystals. In addition, these irritants may also be responsible for the lack of healing of apical lesions in teeth that have received appropriate endodontic treatment.[75] If the growth of epithelial cells is stimulated by any of these living or nonliving pathogens, the integrity of the periodontal tissues also may be affected.

As the degree of pulpal inflammation becomes more extensive, a greater amount of destruction of the periodontal tissues ensues. Extension of the infection through the periodontal ligament space, tooth socket, and surrounding bone occurs, and the patient begins to experience a localized or diffuse swelling that may result in cellulitis that invades the various facial spaces. Most often, however, the infection erupts through the labial, buccal, or lingual mucosa and results in a draining sinus tract. In cases where the path of least resistance for the infectious process is along the attached gingiva, the infection may dissect the periodontal ligament space, resulting in the formation of a deep but narrow periodontal pocket. This pocket usually extends to the main site of the infection (e.g., root apex) when probed or traced with a gutta-percha point. Confusion often results among both general dentists and specialists about whether the probing defect is the result of an endodontic or periodontal problem or the result of vertical root crack. Generally, a narrow probing defect combined with a nonvital pulpal response indicates that the problem is usually of endodontic rather than periodontal origin. In addition, a probing defect associated with vertical root crack generally extends to the level of the crack, as opposed to the root apex. Vertical root crack is generally detected during access into the pulp chamber under high-power magnification or by using transillumination. If vertical root crack is not detected, it should be ruled out as a potential cause of the narrow probing defect.

In a few situations, adjacent teeth, their root surfaces, or furcation areas may also probe deeply. Care must be taken to test all maxillary and mandibular teeth thoroughly to assess correctly whether the problem is endodontic or periodontal. Once the correct diagnosis is

made, only then should the treatment plan be formulated and discussed with the patient. When endodontic therapy is the main cause of the swelling or breakdown of the periodontium, successful endodontic treatment usually results in healing of both the periapical and periodontal tissues. At times, however, trauma to the tooth, severe loss of adjacent periodontal tissues, continued tooth mobility, and occlusal trauma do not provide an environment that allows for apical healing to occur. In these cases, splinting is sometimes necessary to help stabilize the tooth and allow for potential repair of the apical tissues (Fig. 46.5).

If an endodontic infection is left untreated, the progression of periodontal disease continues. Untreated and unresolved infections of endodontic origin can sustain the growth of various endodontic pathogens that may lead to increased pocket formation, bone loss, calculus deposition, osteoclastic activity, and subsequent bone and tooth resorption. They may additionally impair wound healing and aggravate the development and progression of the periodontal disease state.[20]

The ability of the periodontium to regenerate and heal the lost attachment apparatus has been controversial. This is especially true when the teeth have been endodontically treated and the cement layer is no longer present.[44] A study by Sanders and associates[78] demonstrated a 60% osseous regeneration rate in teeth that had not undergone endodontic treatment compared with a regeneration rate of only 33% in teeth that had completed endodontic treatment. One study compared the loss of attached gingiva and found a 0.2-mm greater loss of attached tissue in the presence of teeth with root canal infection and periapical radiolucency.[36] These same investigators, in a later study, found a three times greater loss of marginal proximal bone when using radiographic measurements in teeth with endodontic infections compared with teeth without endodontic infections or subsiding endodontic involvement.[35] Other investigators, however, have reported that all periodontal tissues have the ability to regenerate, regardless of whether the tooth is vital, partially treated and medicated, or partially filled, or whether endodontic treatment has been successfully completed.[19] Additional studies need to be done to understand more clearly the relationship between the presence of endodontic infection and the increased loss of marginal bone and attached tissue in patients prone to periodontal disease.

It is evident that endodontium and periodontium are closely related from the structural, functional, and pathogenic perspective and that microorganisms and nonliving irritants play important roles in the disease progression of both structures. Proper diagnosis of

Case 1

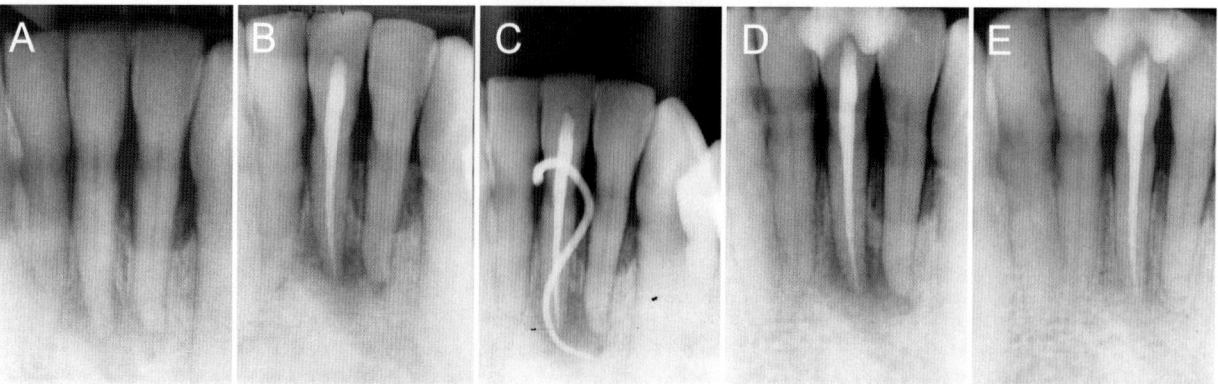

Case 2

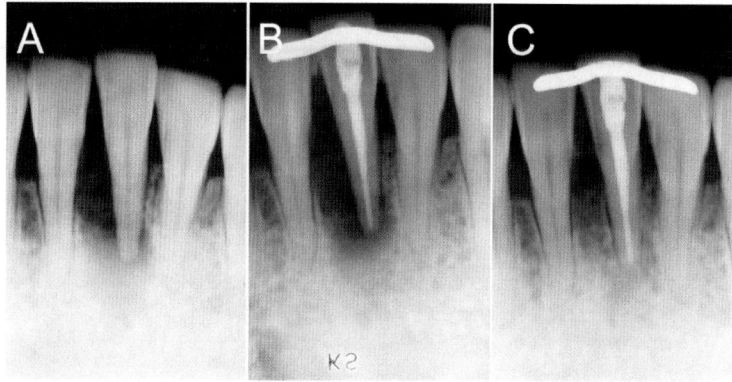

Fig. 46.5 Case 1. (A) Previous trauma of tooth #25 with complaints of pain on biting and chewing. The tooth tested nonvital, and tooth #26 probed 6 mm on the lingual surface. (B) Postoperative radiograph after obturation of the canal. Treatment was completed in two appointments with the interappointment placement of calcium hydroxide. (C) After 4 months, the tooth was mobile and a sinus tract was present. (D) The occlusion was adjusted, and composite resin was bonded to the mesial and distal surfaces to stabilize both teeth #25 and #26. (E) Healing of the periradicular lesion is apparent after 13 months, and tooth #26 probed only 4 mm. Case 2. (A) Previously traumatized tooth #25. The tooth was class III mobile and tested nonvital to both carbon dioxide and electric pulp testing. (B) After obturation of the tooth with gutta-percha, a cast gold splint was bonded to the lingual surface to stabilize it. (C) At 13-month recall, radiograph demonstrates repair of the periradicular bone and no mobility as a result of splint placement and stabilization. *(Case 1, Courtesy Dr. Thomas Rauth.)*

endodontic-periodontic lesions therefore is critically important and will dictate the appropriate course of treatment.

Biologic Effects of Periodontal Infection on the Dental Pulp

Effects of periodontal disease on the dental pulp appear to be more controversial compared with the effects of pulpal disease on the periodontium.[8,81] Not all studies agree about the effects of periodontal disease on the pulp. Even though inflammation and localized pulpal necrosis have been observed next to lateral canals exposed by periodontal diseases,[76,81,82] other studies have not confirmed a correlation between periodontal disease and changes within the pulp.[15,56,96] Langeland and colleagues[51] indicated that when pathologic changes do occur in the pulp as a result of advanced periodontal disease, the pulp does not usually undergo degenerative changes as long as the main canal has not been involved. If the vasculature of the pulp remains vital, no inflammatory reaction occurs and no symptoms of

pulpal pathosis develop. An animal study conducted by Bergenholtz and Lindhe[9] found that 70% of animal specimens showed no pathologic changes even when 30% to 40% of the periodontal attachment was lost. The remainder showed only minor inflammatory changes, formation of reparative dentin, or resorptive defects where the root had been exposed.

Researchers and clinicians, however, have observed the spread of advanced periodontal lesions that extend to the apical foramen and result in pulpal necrosis. This retrograde infection may proliferate through large accessory canals on the lateral surfaces of the tooth, canals positioned closer to the apical foramen, and the area where the main canal exits the tooth apex.[76] Kobayashi and associates[49] compared the microflora from root canals and periodontal pockets of caries-free teeth that were necrotic and tested nonvital with an electric pulp tester. The aerobic-to-anaerobic ratio in the periodontal pocket was 0.23 compared with 0.0022 in the root canal. Although far fewer bacteria were present in the root canal, both areas demonstrated similar bacterial strains. The similarity of strains in both

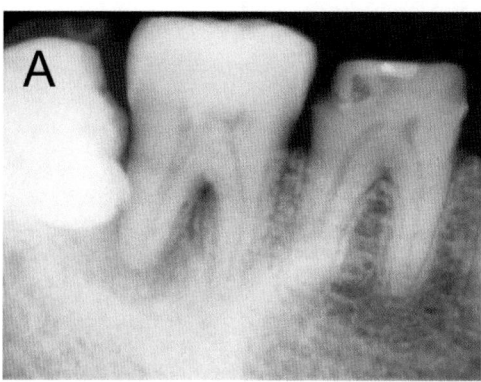
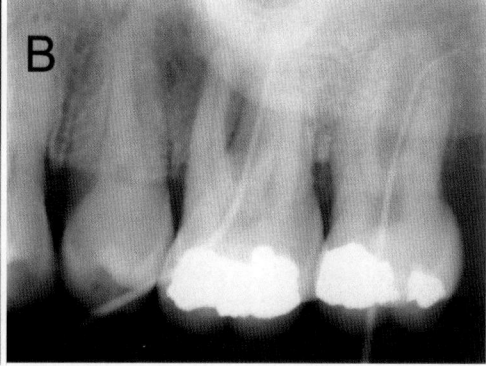

Fig. 46.6 Primary periodontal defects causing periradicular bony lesions and pulpal irritation. (A) Primary periodontal lesion is evident on the distal surface of tooth #31. The defect was probed to a depth of 7 mm, and the tooth tested vital to both thermal and electrical pulp testing. The defect was most likely the result of the impacted third molar and formation of a chronic periodontal abscess. (B) Primary periodontal lesions both probing 12 mm into the furcation. Teeth #14 and #15 tested vital to thermal and electrical testing. The patient's chief complaint was discomfort to cold, thus exemplifying pulpitis secondary to the primary periodontal infection. *(B, Courtesy Dr. Gregory Kolber.)*

areas suggested that the periodontal pocket may be the source of bacteria found in infections within the root canal system.

Protection and preservation of the cementum and dentin surrounding the tooth are also important in preserving the health of the pulp and preventing the ingress of periodontal pathogens. The presence of an intact layer of cementum is important in protecting the pulp from dental plaque and other periodontal pathogens that migrate along the root surface during the development of advanced periodontal disease. Excessive root planing and curettage that remove the cementum and dentin from the root surface encourage narrowing of the pulp canals. This process is thought to be reparative rather than inflammatory.[8,52] Several studies have also suggested that periodontal disease is degenerative to pulpal tissues and results in continued calcification, fibrosis, collagen resorption, and inflammation.[51,53]

Dentin thickness also contributes to the protection of the pulp. Stanley[89] stated that if a 2-mm thickness of dentin remains between the pulp and an irritating stimulus, little chance of pulpal damage exists. Weine[106] summarized the precautions that can be taken during the course of periodontal therapy: (1) avoid using irritating chemicals on the root surface, (2) minimize the use of ultrasonic scalers when less than 2 mm of dentin remains, and (3) allow minor pulpal irritations to subside before completing additional procedures. When these precautions are not followed and the microvasculature of the pulp is damaged during periodontal procedures that involve deep curettage or periodontal surgical efforts to save the tooth, necrosis may result.[107]

The healing success and failure rates after endodontic microsurgery were studied in teeth that had lesions of only endodontic origin compared with teeth that had lesions of combined endodontic-periodontal origin. Lesions of only endodontic origin had a success outcome of 95.2%, whereas teeth with combined lesions had a success outcome of only 77.5%. This finding suggests that bone healing and tissue healing are negatively affected after endodontic surgery for lesions of combined origin.[46]

It appears, therefore, that the pulp and periodontal compartments influence each other. Periodontal disease, however, seems to have less of an influence on the pulpal tissues compared with the influence of pulpal disease on the periodontium. Clearly, advanced periodontal disease has some biologic effects on the pulpal state (Fig. 46.6). Unless the microvasculature of the pulp is compromised during aggressive periodontal procedures or excessively deep curettage

severs the apical vessels, most periodontal interventions result in only a localized pulpal response and dentin hypersensitivity.[103]

Summary

Bacteria-induced inflammations of the pulpal and periodontal tissues often occur together. Endodontic lesions are more likely to spread to surrounding periodontal tissues, with subsequent bone and tissue destruction, compared with the less frequent involvement of periodontal infections in the pulpal tissues that result in retrograde pulpitis.

Understanding the etiology and making the diagnosis of dental abscess are based on the patient's history and clinical and radiographic findings. Pulpal pathosis often results in significant pain to thermal stimulus or tissue swelling, or it may be totally asymptomatic. Radiographic evaluation may demonstrate a circumscribed periapical lesion when the tooth tests necrotic and the origin of the lesion is pulpal. Vitality testing can detect changes of sensation caused by pulpal inflammation and necrosis. If evidence indicates pulpal disease and the possibility of associated periodontal bone loss, the endodontic treatment should be completed first, and then the patient should be reevaluated. In many cases, apparent periodontal disease, including bone loss, suppuration, and pocket depth, resolves if a pulpal lesion has been successfully treated endodontically.

Residual periodontal problems can be treated after completion of successful endodontic treatment, and in many cases, successful regeneration of periodontal defects is possible in endodontically treated teeth. Knowledge of these two disciplines is necessary for successful treatment outcomes.

Video 46.1 contains a slide show that discusses the treatment of fractured teeth.

A Case Scenario is found on the companion website www.expertconsult.com.

References

References for this chapter are found on the companion website www.expertconsult.com.

CHAPTER 47

Phase I Periodontal Therapy

Henry H. Takei

CHAPTER OUTLINE

Rationale

Treatment Sessions

Sequence of Procedures

Results

Healing

Decision to Refer for Specialist
   Treatment

Conclusion

Phase I therapy or cause-related therapy[10] is the first in the chronologic sequence of procedures that constitute periodontal treatment. The objective of phase I therapy is to alter or eliminate the microbial etiology and factors that contribute to gingival and periodontal diseases to the greatest extent possible, thereby halting the progression of disease and returning the dentition to a state of health and comfort.[5] Phase I therapy is referred to by a number of names, including *initial therapy*,[5,10] *nonsurgical periodontal therapy*,[18] and *cause-related therapy*.[10] All terms refer to the procedures performed to treat gingival and periodontal infections up to and including tissue reevaluation, which is the point at which the course of ongoing care is determined.

Rationale

Phase I therapy is defined by the evidence-based American Association of Periodontology practice guidelines[5] as the initiation of a comprehensive daily plaque or biofilm control regimen, management of periodontal-systemic interrelationships as needed, and thorough removal of supragingival and subgingival bacterial plaque or biofilm and calculus. Other problems that must be managed include the use of chemotherapeutic agents as necessary, and local factors[1-4,6] such as elimination of defective restorations and treatment of carious lesions.[7,9,15,16,20] These procedures are a required part of periodontal therapy, regardless of the extent of disease present. In many cases, only phase I therapy is required to restore periodontal health, or it constitutes the preparatory phase for surgical therapy. Figs. 47.1 and 47.2 show the results of phase I therapy in two patients with chronic periodontitis. Cause-related phase I periodontal therapy has been succinctly stated as the approach *aimed at removal of pathogenic biofilms, toxins, and calculus and the reestablishment of a biologically acceptable root surface.*[10]

Phase I therapy is a critical aspect of periodontal treatment. Data from clinical research indicate that the long-term success of periodontal surgical treatment is dependent on maintaining the plaque or biofilm control results achieved with phase I therapy. In fact, patients who do not have adequate plaque or biofilm control will continue to lose attachment regardless of what surgical procedures are performed.[12] In addition, phase I therapy provides an opportunity for the dentist to evaluate tissue response and provide reinforcement about home care, both of which are crucial to the overall success of treatment.

Based on the knowledge that microbial plaque or biofilm is the major etiologic agent in gingival inflammation, one specific aim of phase I therapy for every patient is *effective daily plaque or biofilm removal* at home. These home care procedures can be complex and time-consuming, and often require changing long-standing habits. Good oral hygiene is more easily accomplished if the tooth surfaces are free of calculus deposits and other irregularities so that they are easily accessible. Management of all contributing local factors is required in phase I therapy. The following list of elements makes up phase I therapy:

1. Patient education and oral hygiene instruction
2. Complete removal of supragingival calculus (see Chapters 50 and 51)
3. Correction or replacement of poorly fitting restorations and other prosthetic devices (see Chapter 70)
4. Restoration or temporization of carious lesions
5. Orthodontic tooth movement (see Chapter 56)
6. Treatment of food impaction areas
7. Treatment of occlusal trauma (see Chapter 55)
8. Extraction of hopeless teeth
9. Possible use of antimicrobial agents, including necessary plaque or biofilm sampling and sensitivity testing (see Chapters 8 and 52)

Treatment Sessions

After careful analysis and diagnosis of the specific periodontal condition present, the clinician must develop a treatment plan that includes all required procedures to treat the periodontal involvement and an estimate of the number of appointments necessary to complete phase I therapy. In most cases, patients require several treatment sessions for complete debridement of the tooth surfaces. All the following conditions must be considered when determining the phase I treatment plan[18]:

- General health and tolerance of treatment
- Number of teeth present
- Amount of subgingival calculus
- Probing pocket depths
- Attachment loss
- Furcation involvement
- Alignment of teeth
- Margins of restorations
- Developmental anomalies

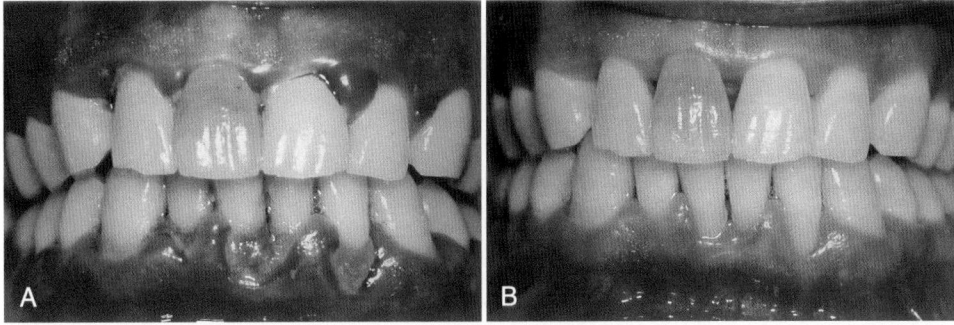

Fig. 47.1 Results of phase I therapy, severe chronic periodontitis. (A) A 45-year-old patient with deep probe depths, bone loss, severe swelling, and redness of the gingival tissues. (B) Results 3 weeks after the completion of phase I therapy. Note that the gingival tissue has returned to a normal contour, with redness and swelling dramatically reduced.

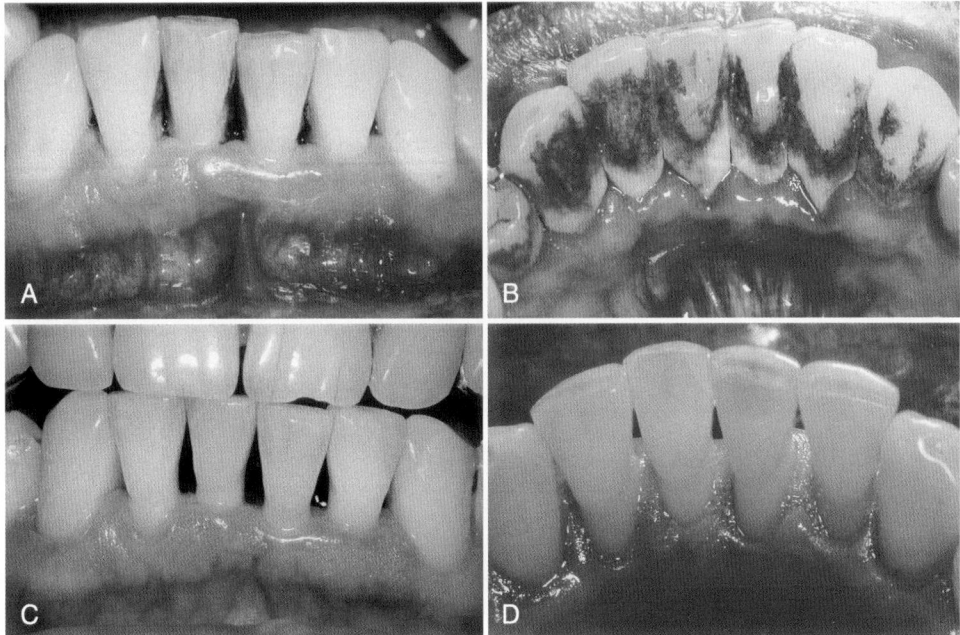

Fig. 47.2 Results of phase I therapy, moderate chronic periodontitis. (A) A 52-year-old patient with moderate attachment loss and probe depths in the 4- to 6-mm range. Note that the gingiva appears pink because it is fibrotic. Inflammation is present in the periodontal pockets but disguised by the fibrotic tissue. Bleeding occurs on probing. (B) Lingual view of the patient with more visible inflammation and heavy calculus deposits. (C) and (D) At 18 months after phase I therapy the same areas show significant improvement in gingival health. The patient returned for regular maintenance visits at 4-month intervals.

- Physical barriers to access the dentition (i.e., limited opening or tendency to gag)
- Patient cooperation and sensitivity to therapy (requiring use of anesthesia or analgesia)

Sequence of Procedures

Step 1: Plaque or Biofilm Control Instruction

Plaque or biofilm control is an essential component of successful periodontal therapy, and instruction should begin at the first treatment appointment. Before oral hygiene instruction, the patient must understand the reason that he or she must actively participate in therapy. The explanation of the etiology of the disease must be presented to the patient. Once the patient understands the nature of periodontal disease and the etiology, it will be easier to teach the hygiene that he or she must practice. The patient must be instructed on the correct technique to remove the plaque or biofilm; this means

focusing on applying the bristles at the gingival third of the clinical crowns, where the tooth meets the gingival margin. This technique is sometimes referred to as *targeted oral hygiene* (Takei H: Personal communication, 2009) and is synonymous with the Bass technique. Instructions are also initiated for interdental cleaning with dental floss and interdental brushes. The use of the multiple appointment approach to phase I therapy is favored by many clinicians because it permits the use of numerous appointments to evaluate, reinforce, and improve the patient's oral hygiene skills. (Chapter 48 details plaque and biofilm control options.)

Step 2: Removal of Supragingival and Subgingival Plaque or Biofilm and Calculus

Removal of calculus is accomplished using scalers, curettes, ultrasonic instrumentation, or combinations of these devices during one or more appointments. Evidence suggests that the treatment results for chronic periodontitis are similar for all instruments, which could be hand instrumentation or other mechanical instruments, such as ultrasonic scalers.[12,13] Most clinicians advocate the combination of hand instruments (scalers, curettes) and ultrasonic devices. In addition to calculus and plaque or biofilm removal, cementum exposed to the pocket environment should be removed. At one time it was thought that the removal of all cementum was necessary to attain a smooth, glassy, hard surface. The rationale was that cementum became necrotic from penetration of endotoxins from the microbial biofilm and would interfere with healing. Current studies have indicated that endotoxins do not penetrate into the cementum as deeply as once believed and complete removal of the cementum may not always be necessary, but removal of the plaque or biofilm and calculus is absolutely necessary. In a clinical situation, it is difficult to know whether the removal of some or all of the cementum is achieved.

Laser treatment has also been advocated for periodontal therapy by some clinicians.[8] However, some reviews suggest that further well-designed studies are needed to confirm the outcomes. In addition, gingival curettage, the systematic removal of the soft tissue lining of the pockets, has not been shown to improve the results of treatment. Thorough plaque or biofilm removal and excellent root therapy result in conversion of the soft, edematous, inflamed gingival tissue to a healthier state without removing this tissue by using intentional soft tissue curettage. Therefore curettage of the soft tissue pocket wall in phase I therapy is no longer advocated.

Photodynamic therapy has also been presented as an adjunct to scaling and root planing. This therapy uses lasers at specific wavelengths to "target microorganisms treated with a photosensitizer." Studies have not found this intervention to be useful as an alternative to scaling and root planing to improve treatment outcomes. Further research is necessary to ascertain the efficacy of this treatment.[12]

Another interesting approach to calculus removal and debridement is full-mouth disinfection. In this technique, full-mouth treatment is performed during one session or multiple sessions within a few days. Disinfectants are used after therapy, with the intention of preventing reinfection of treated sites from untreated sites.[14,17,19,22] This treatment approach is used during phase I therapy by some clinicians, but the results have not been shown to be superior to those of any other phase I therapy.[11,12,21]

Multiple approaches are used to plan and perform nonsurgical phase I therapy. Decisions on how to proceed should be discussed and agreed on by the patient and the dentist based on the amount of disease present and the patient's tolerance to the therapy.[11] Staged therapy has the advantage of evaluating and reinforcing the oral hygiene status of the patient, but the one- or two-appointment approach can be more efficient in reducing the number of office visits the patient is required to attend.

Step 3: Recontouring Defective Restorations and Crowns

Corrections of restorative defects, which are plaque or biofilm retentive areas, may be accomplished by smoothing the rough surfaces and removing overhangs from the faulty restorations with burs or hand instruments, or complete replacement of the failing restorations may be necessary. All these steps are important to remove the risk factors that perpetuate the inflammatory process. These procedures can be completed concurrently with other phase I procedures.

Step 4: Management of Carious Lesions

Removal of the carious lesions and placement of either temporary or permanent restorations are indicated in phase I therapy because of the infectious nature of the carious process. Healing of the periodontal tissues is maximized by removing the reservoir of bacteria in these lesions so that they cannot repopulate the microbial plaque.

Step 5: Tissue Reevaluation

After scaling, root planing, and other phase I procedures, the periodontal tissues require approximately 4 weeks to heal. This time allows the connective tissues to heal, and accurate probe depths can be measured. Patients will also have the opportunity to improve their home care skills to reduce gingival inflammation and adopt new habits that will ensure the success of treatment. At the reevaluation appointment, periodontal tissues are probed, and all related anatomic conditions are carefully evaluated to determine whether further treatment, including periodontal surgery, is indicated. Additional improvement from periodontal surgical procedures can be expected only if phase I therapy results in gingival tissues that are free of overt inflammation and the patient has adopted effective daily plaque or biofilm control procedures.

Results

Scaling and root planing therapy have been studied extensively to evaluate their effects on periodontal disease. Many studies have indicated that this treatment is both effective and reliable. Studies ranging from 1 month to 2 years in length demonstrated up to 80% reduction in bleeding on probing and mean probing depth reductions of 2 to 3 mm. Other studies demonstrated that the percentage of periodontal pockets of 4-mm or deeper was reduced by more than 50% and in many cases up to 80%.[9] Figs. 47.1 and 47.2 show examples of the effectiveness of phase I therapy.

In addition, deeper probing depths present the dentist with greatly increased instrumentation challenges due to the complexity of root anatomy and difficulty accessing the root surfaces. Badersten and colleagues[7] reported in the 1980s that residual calculus remained on 44% of the surfaces in deeper pockets. Other studies have confirmed these findings, including studies comparing the use of hand instruments with that of powered scaling instruments.[12]

Additional individual treatments, such as caries control and correction of poorly fitting restorations, clearly help the healing gained by good plaque or biofilm control and debridement by making tooth surfaces accessible to hygiene procedures. Fig. 47.3 demonstrates the effects of an overhanging amalgam restoration on gingival inflammation in an otherwise healthy periodontium. Maximal healing from phase I treatment is not possible when local conditions retain biofilm and provide reservoirs for repopulation of periodontal pathogens.

Healing

Healing of the gingival epithelium consists of the formation of a long junctional epithelium rather than new connective tissue attachment to the root surfaces. This long junctional epithelium occurs about 1 week after therapy. Gradual reductions in inflammatory cell population, crevicular fluid flow, and repair of connective tissue result in decreased clinical signs of inflammation, including less redness and swelling. One or two millimeters of recession is often apparent as the result of tissue shrinkage.[9] Connective tissue fibers are disrupted and lysed by the disease process and also by the inflammatory reaction to treatment. These tissues require 4 or more weeks to reorganize and heal, and many cases may require several weeks for complete healing.

Transient root sensitivity frequently accompanies the healing process. Although evidence suggests that relatively few teeth in a few patients become highly sensitive, this problem can be disconcerting to patients. The extent of the sensitivity can be diminished with good plaque or biofilm removal, but this may take several weeks to months.[23] Patients should also be warned and educated before the

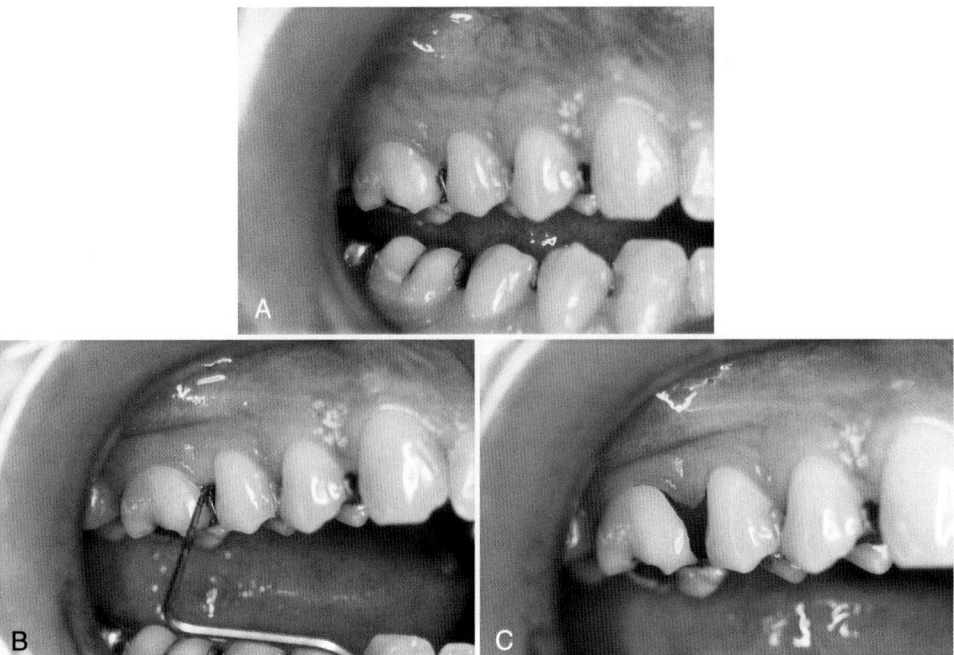

Fig. 47.3 Effects of overhanging amalgam margin on interproximal gingiva of maxillary first molar in otherwise healthy mouth. (A) Clinical appearance of rough, irregular, and overcontoured amalgam. (B) Gentle probing of interproximal pocket. (C) Extensive bleeding elicited by gentle probing indicating severe inflammation in the area.

therapy is undertaken regarding the potential outcomes of several changes, such as the teeth appearing longer due to shrinkage of the periodontal tissues and root sensitivity. Knowledge of these changes before therapy will prevent the possibility of the patient complaining if they should occur. Unexpected and possible uncomfortable consequences of treatment may result in the patient's distrust and loss of motivation to continue therapy.

Decision to Refer for Specialist Treatment

It is fortunate that many periodontally involved cases do not require any further therapy beyond phase I therapy. Therefore, these patients can be seen by general dentists for routine maintenance therapy. However, advanced or complicated cases benefit from specialist care. Heitz-Mayfield and Lang[12] demonstrated that surgical treatment in deep pockets, those >6 mm, gained 0.6 mm more probing depth reduction and 0.2 mm more clinical attachment gain than did deep pockets treated with scaling and root planing alone. This study also confirmed that in pockets of 4 to 6 mm probing depth, scaling and root planing resulted in 0.4 mm more attachment gain than surgical procedures, and shallow pockets of 1 to 3 mm had 0.5 mm less attachment loss compared with surgical results.[12] It is critical to be skilled in determining which patients would benefit from specialist care and deciding when a patient should be referred.

The concept of the *critical probing depth* of 5.4 mm has been advanced to assist in making the determination to proceed to surgical intervention. This is the measurement above which therapy will result in clinical attachment gain and below which it will result in clinical attachment loss. This determination was made based on statistical analysis of surgical outcomes data.[12] A similar *5-mm standard* has been commonly used as a guideline for identifying candidates for surgical referral based on the understanding that the typical root length is about 13 mm and the crest of the alveolar bone is at a level approximately 2 mm apical to the bottom of the pocket.

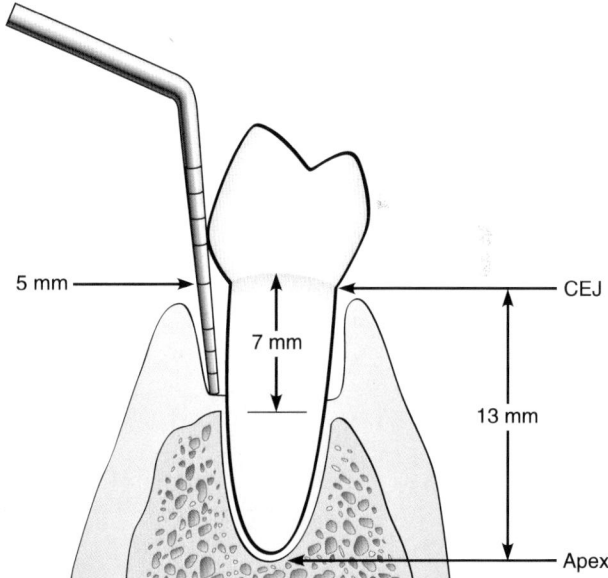

Fig. 47.4 The 5-mm standard for referral to a periodontist is based on root length, probing depth, and clinical attachment loss. The standard serves as a reasonable guideline to analyze the case for referral for specialist care. *CEJ,* Cementoenamel junction. *(Redrawn with permission from Armitage G, editor:* Periodontal maintenance therapy, *Berkeley, CA, 1974, Praxis.)*

When there is 5 mm of clinical attachment loss, the crest of bone is about 7 mm apical to the cementoenamel junction, and therefore only about half of the bony support for the tooth remains. Periodontal surgery can help improve support for teeth in these cases through pocket reduction, bone augmentation, and regeneration procedures. Fig. 47.4 depicts the relationship of clinical attachment loss to tooth support.

In addition to the 5-mm probing depth criterion, other factors must be considered in the decision to refer to a periodontal specialist:

1. *Extent of the disease and generalized or localized periodontal involvement.* The amount of bone loss, even in localized areas, suggests the need for specialized surgical techniques.
2. *Root length.* Short-rooted teeth are jeopardized to a greater extent by the 5-mm clinical attachment loss criterion than teeth with long roots.
3. *Hypermobility.* Excessive tooth mobility suggests that contributing factors may be responsible for the mobility. The extent of mobility could mean that the prognosis for the tooth may be guarded to poor.
4. *Difficulty of scaling and root planing.* The presence of deep pockets and furcations makes instrumentation difficult, but the results can often be improved with surgical access.
5. *Restorability and importance of particular teeth for reconstruction.* Long-term prognosis of each tooth is important when considering extensive restorative work.
6. *Age of the patient.* Younger patients with extensive attachment loss are more likely to have aggressive forms of disease that require advanced therapy.
7. *Lack of resolution of inflammation after thorough plaque or biofilm removal and excellent scaling and root planing.* If inflammation and progressive deepening of the pocket continue, further therapy will be necessary. Such cases require an understanding of the etiology to determine the best course of treatment.

Every patient is unique, and the decision process for each patient is complex and difficult. The considerations presented in this chapter should provide guidance for understanding the significance of phase I therapy and making referral decisions.

Conclusion

The major goal of phase I therapy is to control the factors responsible for periodontal inflammation; this involves educating the patient in the removal of bacterial plaque or biofilm. Phase I therapy also includes scaling, root planing, and other therapies such as caries control, replacement of defective restorations, occlusal therapy, orthodontic tooth movement, and cessation of confounding habits such as tobacco use. Comprehensive reevaluation after phase I therapy is essential to determine treatment options and establish a prognosis. Many patients can attain periodontal disease control with phase I therapy alone and do not require further surgical intervention. For patients who require surgical intervention, phase I therapy is an advantageous element of treatment in that it permits tissue healing, thus improving the surgical management and healing response of the tissues.

Periodontal surgical intervention should be considered for patients with deep pocket depths and those with 5 mm or more of attachment loss after phase I therapy. Periodontal specialists can best provide treatment to preserve the teeth for patients with advanced disease. Moreover, patients who do not demonstrate the ability to control plaque or biofilm on a daily basis effectively are poor candidates for surgery and should be closely monitored on a recall maintenance program unless conditions change.

References

 References for this chapter are found on the companion website www.expertconsult.com.

CHAPTER 48

Plaque Biofilm Control for the Periodontal Patient

Dorothy A. Perry | Henry H. Takei | Jonathan H. Do

CHAPTER OUTLINE

The Toothbrush
Powered Toothbrushes
Dentifrices
Toothbrushing Methods
Interdental Cleaning Aids
Gingival Massage

Oral Irrigation *(e-only)*
Caries Control *(e-only)*
Chemical Plaque Biofilm Control
 With Oral Rinses *(e-only)*
Disclosing Agents *(e-only)*

Frequency of Plaque Biofilm
 Removal *(e-only)*
Patient Motivation and Education
 (e-only)
Conclusion

 For online-only content on oral irrigation, caries control, chemical plaque biofilm control with oral rinses, disclosing agents, frequency of plaque biofilm removal, and patient motivation and education, please visit the companion website at www. expertconsult.com.

Microbial plaque biofilm control, also referred to as periodontal self-care,[32] is an effective way of treating and preventing gingivitis and is an essential part of all procedures involved in the treatment and prevention of periodontal diseases.[50] It is a critical element in the long-term success of all periodontal and dental treatment.[3] In 1965, Löe and colleagues[89] conducted the classic study demonstrating the relationship between microbial plaque biofilm accumulation and the development of experimental gingivitis in humans. Subjects in the study stopped brushing and other plaque biofilm control procedures, thus resulting in the development of gingivitis in every person within 7 to 21 days. The composition of the biofilm bacteria also shifted so that more virulent gram-negative organisms predominated, and these changes were shown to be reversible within 7 days. Good supragingival biofilm control has also been shown to affect the growth and composition of subgingival plaque biofilm so that it favors a healthier microflora and reduces calculus formation.[121] Carefully performed daily home plaque biofilm control, combined with frequent professionally delivered plaque biofilm and calculus removal, reduces the amount of supragingival biofilm, decreases the total number of microorganisms in moderately deep pockets, including furcation areas, and greatly reduces the quantity of periodontal pathogens.[29,61] Reviews of home care procedures in 2011 and 2013 confirmed the positive effects of daily plaque biofilm removal but cautioned that these gains appear to be small, and best results also require professional maintenance care.[32,107]

Microbial biofilm growth occurs within hours, and it must be completely removed at least once every 48 hours in the experimental setting with periodontally healthy subjects to prevent inflammation.[120] The American Dental Association (ADA) recommends that individuals should brush twice per day and use floss or other interdental cleaners once per day to effectively remove microbial plaque biofilms and prevent gingivitis.[3] The ADA recommends twice-daily brushing because most individuals do not adequately remove microbial biofilms at one brushing, and doing it a second time improves the results.

Periodontal lesions are predominantly found in interdental locations, so toothbrushing alone is not sufficient to control gingival and periodontal diseases.[75] It has been demonstrated in healthy subjects that plaque biofilm formation begins on the interproximal surfaces, where the toothbrush does not reach. Masses of biofilm first develop in the molar and premolar areas, followed by the proximal surfaces of the anterior teeth and the facial surfaces of the molars and premolars. Lingual surfaces accumulate the least amount of biofilm. Patients consistently leave more plaque biofilm on the posterior teeth than the anterior teeth, with interproximal surfaces retaining the highest amounts of biofilm. It is in these interproximal areas where periodontal infections and carious lesions begin.[120] In addition, periodontal patients tend to have increased susceptibility to disease[123] due to complex defects in gingival architecture and long exposed root surfaces to clean, which compounds the difficulty of practicing thorough hygiene.

CLINICAL CORRELATION

Daily plaque biofilm control practices result in improved periodontal and gingival health. Cessation of plaque control practices for 7 to 21 days results in:

- Accumulation of thick plaque on tooth surfaces
- Reddened gingiva that bleeds easily
- Shift to more virulent gram-negative flora
- Changes that are completely reversed in about 7 days when plaque control practices are resumed

Chemical inhibitors of plaque biofilm and calculus that are incorporated in mouthwashes or dentifrices also play an important role in controlling microbial biofilms.[32] Fluoride delivered through toothpastes and mouthrinses are essential for caries control.[38] Many products are available as adjunctive agents to mechanical techniques. These medicaments, as with any drug, should be recommended and prescribed according to the needs of the individual patient. Also note that the interest in supplementing oral hygiene procedures with natural products has increased in our society. However, the evidence base supporting the use of these products is currently lacking valid studies to determine their efficacy.[22]

Daily plaque biofilm control permits patients to assume responsibility for their own oral health every day. Without it, optimal oral health through periodontal treatment cannot be attained or preserved. Elements of biofilm control include mechanical cleaning and chemical adjuncts.

The Toothbrush

Toothbrushes vary in size and design, as well as in length, hardness, and arrangement of the bristles[115] (Fig. 48.1). Some toothbrush manufacturers claim superiority of design for such factors as minor modifications of bristle placement, length, and stiffness. These claims are primarily based on plaque biofilm removal shown to be significantly superior to other toothbrushes in short-term clinical studies. However, research does not indicate significant differences in gingivitis scores or bleeding indices, which are the more important measures of improved gingival health. In fact, at least one study compared four commercially available toothbrushes for total plaque biofilm removal at a single brushing. All four toothbrushes removed biofilm equally, and the investigators concluded that no one design was superior to the others.[25] In addition, systematic review of multiple studies did not identify a superior design.[32]

 FLASH BACK

Early toothbrushes were mostly made of hog bristles and were very stiff and hard. Hard-bristled toothbrushes have been shown to abrade tooth surfaces and scratch the gingiva. Few remain on the market, but in general, hard-bristled toothbrushes should be avoided.

When recommending a particular toothbrush, ease of use by the patient and the perception that the brush is effective are the important considerations. The effectiveness of and potential injury from different types of brushes depend to a great degree on how the brushes are used. Data from in vitro studies of abrasion by different manual toothbrushes suggest that brush designs that permit the bristles to carry a greater amount of toothpaste while brushing contribute to abrasion more than the bristles themselves.[33] However, it has been

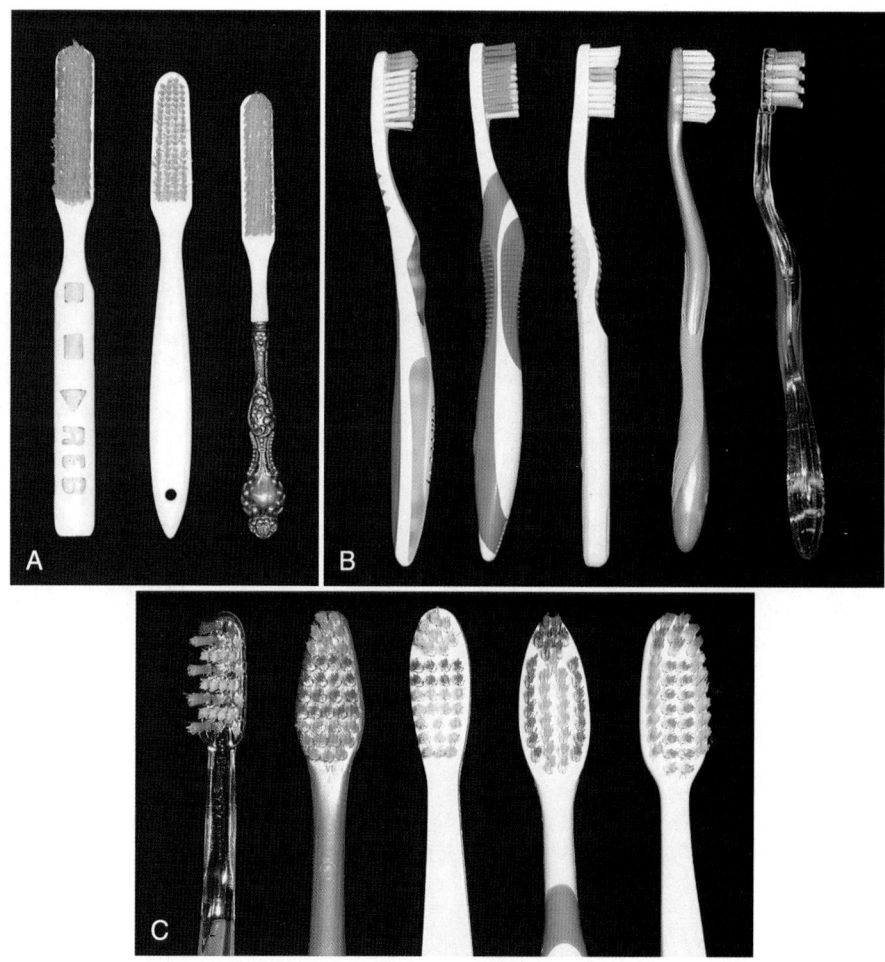

Fig. 48.1 Manual toothbrushes. (A) Toothbrushes from the 19th and 20th centuries, one with an ivory handle from about 1890 *(left),* one with a composition handle from the 1950s *(center),* and one with a sterling silver handle from the early 20th century *(right).* The ivory-handled brush belonged to a dental student who used the handle to practice cutting preparations and filling the "preps" with amalgam or gold foil. (B) Various types of toothbrushes are available; note the variations in brush head and handle design. (C) Brush heads, showing various bristle configurations. *(Antique brushes courtesy Dean John D.B. Featherstone, University of California, San Francisco School of Dentistry Historical Collection, San Francisco.)*

shown that several factors contribute to the problem of abrasion: (1) the use of hard toothbrushes, (2) vigorous horizontal brushing, and (3) the use of extremely abrasive dentifrices; all these factors may contribute to and lead to cervical abrasions of teeth and recession of the gingiva.[74]

Toothbrush Design

Toothbrush bristles are grouped in tufts that are usually arranged in three or four rows. Rounded bristle ends cause fewer scratches on the gingiva than flat-cut bristles with sharp ends[28,115] (see Fig. 48.1). Two types of bristle material are used in toothbrushes: natural bristles from hogs and artificial filaments made of nylon. Both remove microbial plaque biofilm, but nylon bristle brushes predominate in the market. Bristle hardness is proportional to the square of the diameter and inversely proportional to the square of the bristle length.[56] Diameters of common bristles range from 0.007 inch (0.2 mm) for soft brushes to 0.012 inch (0.3 mm) for medium brushes and 0.014 inch (0.4 mm) for hard brushes.[63] Soft-bristle brushes of the type described by Bass[11] have gained wide acceptance (Fig. 48.2). Handle design characteristics are entirely a matter of personal preference.

Softer bristles are more flexible, clean slightly below the gingival margin when used with a sulcular brushing technique,[12] and reach farther apically to the proximal surfaces[45] (see Fig. 48.2). As indicated earlier, the use of hard-bristled toothbrushes is associated with greater gingival recession.[74] However, the manner in which a brush is used and the abrasiveness of the dentifrice affect abrasion to a greater degree than the bristle hardness itself.[93] Bristle hardness does not significantly affect wear on enamel surfaces.[108]

The amount of force used to brush is not critical for effective plaque biofilm removal.[125] Vigorous brushing is not necessary and can lead to gingival recession, wedge-shaped defects in the cervical area of root surfaces,[109] and painful ulceration of the gingiva.[101]

Toothbrushes must also be replaced periodically, although the amount of visible bristle wear does not appear to affect plaque biofilm removal for up to 9 weeks.[27] Most clinicians recommend that toothbrushes be replaced every 3 to 4 months.

KEY FACTS

When recommending toothbrushes, keep these general recommendations in mind:

- Soft nylon bristle toothbrushes clean effectively when used properly and tend not to traumatize the gingiva or root surfaces.
- Toothbrushes become worn due to wear and should be replaced about every 3 to 4 months.
- If patients perceive a benefit from a particular design of toothbrush, they should use it as long as it is not too stiff and hard.

Powered Toothbrushes

Electrically powered toothbrushes designed to mimic back-and-forth brushing techniques were invented in 1939. Subsequent models featured circular or elliptical motions, and some had combinations of motions. Currently, powered toothbrushes have oscillating and rotating motions (Fig. 48.3), and some brushes use low-frequency acoustic energy to enhance cleaning ability. Powered toothbrushes rely primarily on mechanical contact between the bristles and the teeth to remove plaque biofilm. The addition of low-frequency acoustic energy generates dynamic fluid movement and provides cleaning slightly away from the bristle tips.[43] The vibrations have also been shown to interfere with bacterial adherence to oral surfaces. Neither the sonic vibration nor the mechanical motion of powered toothbrushes has been shown to affect bacterial cell viability.[91] Hydrodynamic shear forces created by these brushes disrupt biofilm a short distance

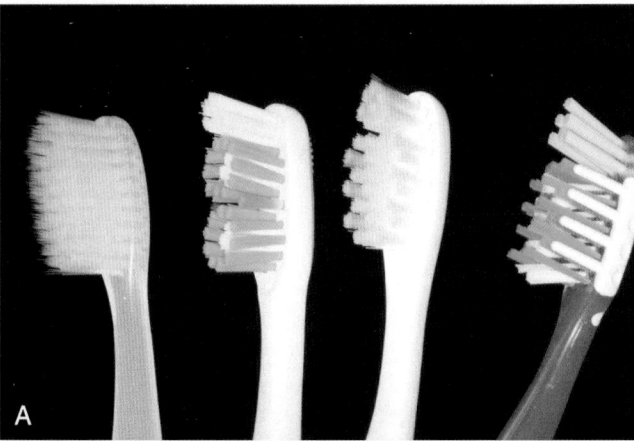
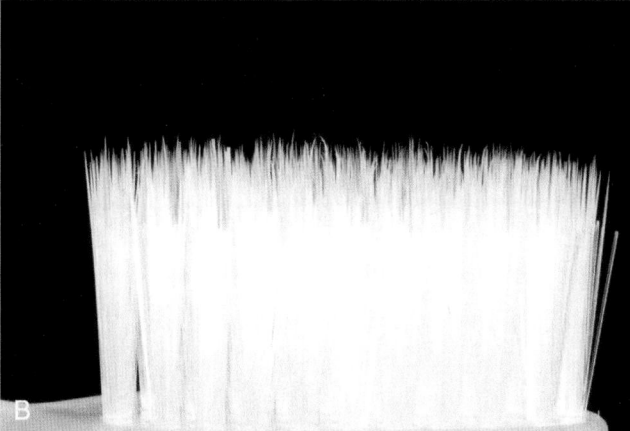

Fig. 48.2 (A) Toothbrushes of different bristle design and configuration. (B) The brush on the *far left* in (A) is the most appropriate of the four brushes displayed for biofilm removal.

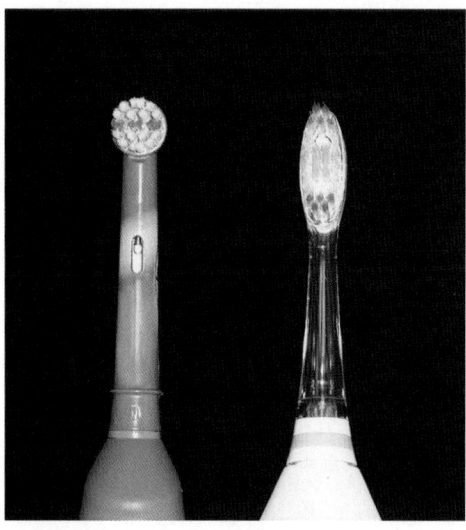

Fig. 48.3 Powered toothbrush designs offer options in head shape and size.

from the bristle tips, thus explaining the additional interproximal biofilm removal.[67]

Typically, comparison studies of powered toothbrushes, manual toothbrushes, and other powered devices demonstrate slightly improved plaque biofilm removal for the device of interest in short-term clinical trials.[95,106] A Cochrane review reported that mechanical brushes with oscillating and rotating motions reduced microbial plaque biofilm 11% better and demonstrated 6% greater reduction in gingival bleeding than manual brushing. These improvements were maintained over 3 months. Although long-term benefits have not been established, this particular style of mechanical brush resulted in better microbial plaque biofilm and gingivitis reduction in a number of well-controlled studies.[32,58]

Patients' acceptance of powered toothbrushes is favorable. One study reported that 88.9% of patients introduced to a powered toothbrush would continue to use it.[127] However, patients have been reported to discontinue the use of the powered toothbrushes after 5 or 6 months, presumably when the novelty has worn off. Powered toothbrushes have been shown to improve oral health for the following: (1) children and adolescents; (2) people with physical or mental disabilities; (3) hospitalized patients, including older adults who require the assistance of caregivers for hygiene; and (4) patients with fixed orthodontic appliances. Powered brushes have not been shown to provide benefits routinely for patients with rheumatoid arthritis, children who are motivated, or patients with chronic periodontitis.[60]

KEY FACTS

When recommending powered toothbrushes, keep in mind that:
- Powered toothbrushes with oscillating and rotating motions remove plaque biofilm and reduce gingival bleeding slightly better than manual toothbrushes.
- Patients who want to use powered toothbrushes should be encouraged to do so.
- Patients need to be instructed in the proper use of powered devices.
- Patients who are not dextrous, children, and caregivers may particularly benefit from using powered toothbrushes.

Dentifrices

Dentifrices aid in cleaning and polishing tooth surfaces. They are used mostly in the form of pastes, although powders and gels are also available. The contents of dentifrices are abrasives (e.g., silicon oxides, aluminum oxides, and granular polyvinyl chlorides), water, humectants, soap or detergent, flavoring and sweetening agents, therapeutic agents (e.g., fluoride, pyrophosphates), coloring agents, and preservatives.[57,119] Abrasives are insoluble inorganic salts that enhance the abrasive action of toothbrushing as much as 40 times and make up 20% to 40% of dentifrices.[93] Tooth powders are much more abrasive than pastes and contain about 95% abrasive materials. The abrasive quality of dentifrices affects enamel slightly and is a much greater concern for patients with exposed root surfaces. Dentin is abraded 25 times faster and cementum even faster, 35 times the rate of enamel. Therefore root surfaces with exposed dentin and cementum are easily abraded, leading to notching and tooth sensitivity.[119] It can be concluded that oral hygiene procedures that use abrasive toothpaste are the main cause of hard tissue damage, and it is possible that gingival lesions can also be produced[101,108] (Fig. 48.4). Dentifrices are very useful for delivering therapeutic

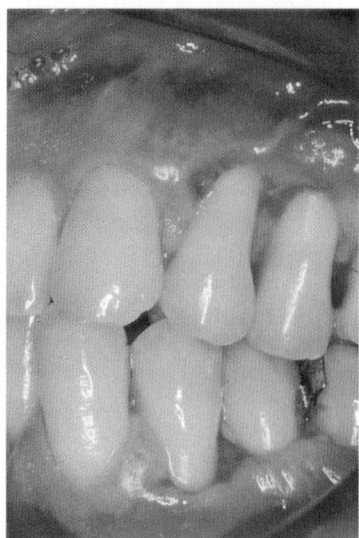

Fig. 48.4 Vigorous toothbrushing with an abrasive dentifrice can result in trauma to the gingiva and wearing away of the tooth surfaces, especially root surfaces, and can contribute to gingival recession.

agents to the teeth and gingiva. The successful caries-preventive effect of *fluoride* incorporated in dentifrices has been proven without question.[118] Fluoride ion must be available in the amount of 1000 to 1100 parts per million (ppm) to achieve caries-reduction effects. Toothpaste products that have been tested by the ADA and have fluoride ion available in the appropriate amount carry the ADA seal of approval to provide for caries control.[5]

"Calculus control" toothpastes, also referred to as "tartar control" toothpastes, contain *pyrophosphates* and have been shown to reduce the deposition of new calculus on teeth as it forms. These ingredients interfere with crystal formation in calculus but do not affect the fluoride ion in the paste or increase tooth sensitivity. Dentifrice with pyrophosphates has been shown to reduce the formation of new supragingival calculus by 30% or more.[70,92,131] Pyrophosphate-containing toothpastes do not affect subgingival calculus formation or gingival inflammation. The inhibitory effect reduces the deposition of new supragingival calculus but does not affect existing calculus deposits. To achieve the greatest effect from calculus control toothpaste, the teeth must be cleaned and completely free of supragingival calculus when adding these products to the daily home care regimen.

KEY FACTS

Considering dentifrices, keep in mind that:
- Dentifrices increase the effectiveness of brushing.
- Products containing fluoride and antimicrobial agents provide additional benefits for controlling caries and gingivitis.
- Patients who form significant amounts of supragingival calculus benefit from the use of a calculus control dentifrice, but remember that calculus formation is directly related to plaque biofilm accumulation.

Toothbrushing Methods

Many methods for brushing the teeth have been described and promoted as being efficient and effective. These methods can be

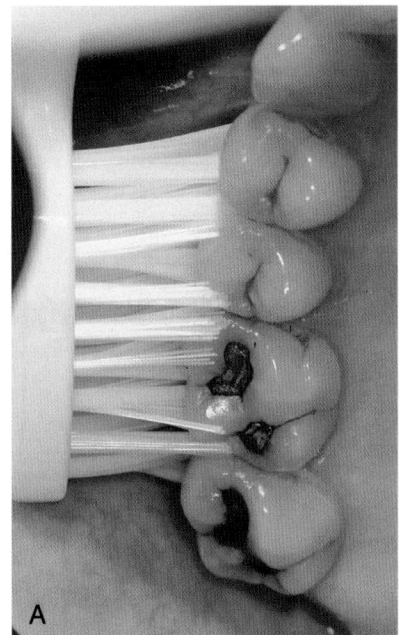
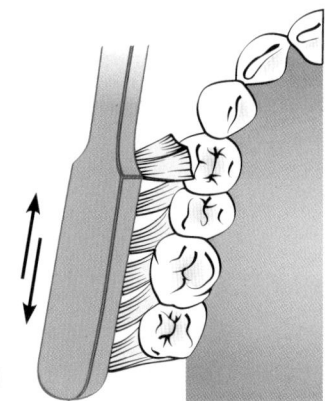

Fig. 48.5 Bass method. (A) Place the toothbrush so that the bristles are angled approximately 45 degrees from the tooth surfaces. (B) Start at the most distal tooth in the arch, and use a vibrating back-and-forth motion to brush.

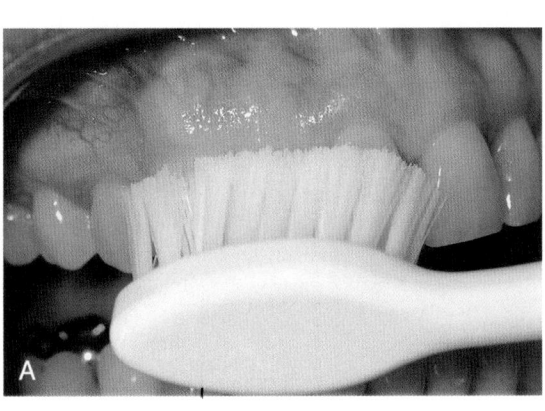
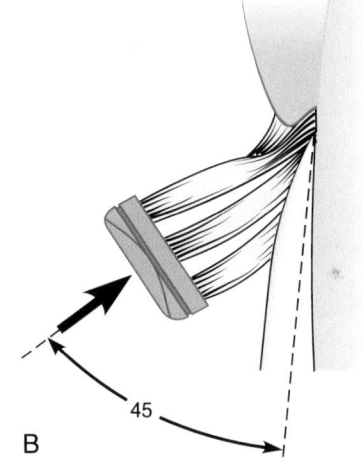

Fig. 48.6 Bass method. (A) Proper positioning of the brush in the mouth aims the bristle tips toward the gingival margin. (B) Diagram shows the ideal placement, which permits slight subgingival penetration of the bristle tips.

categorized primarily according to the pattern of motion when brushing and are primarily of historic interest, as follows[68]:

Roll: Roll[2] or modified Stillman technique[64]
Vibratory: Stillman,[117] Charters,[21] and Bass[12] techniques
Circular: Fones technique[42]
Vertical: Leonard technique[82]
Horizontal: Scrub technique[103]

Patients with periodontal disease are most frequently taught a sulcular brushing technique using a vibratory motion to improve access to the gingival margin areas. It is important for patients to understand that plaque biofilm removal at the dentogingival junction is necessary to prevent caries as well as periodontal disease. This emphasis to clean the area of the dentogingival junction is referred to as *target hygiene* (Takei H: Personal communication, 2009). The method most often recommended is the *Bass technique* because it emphasizes the placement of the bristles at this most important area. Sulcular placement of the bristles and adapting the bristle tips to the gingival margin to reach the supragingival plaque biofilm and accessing some of the subgingival biofilm may be the most important aspects of target hygiene. A controlled vibrating motion is used to dislodge microbial plaque biofilm and avoid trauma. The brush is systematically placed on all the teeth in both arches. Figs. 48.5 and 48.6 illustrate this brushing technique. Almost everybody brushes their teeth, but some individuals may have both carious and periodontal problems. Patients must understand why, where, and how to practice meaningful plaque biofilm removal properly at the target area to prevent oral diseases.

Bass Technique

1. Place the head of a soft brush parallel to the occlusal plane, with the brush head covering three to four teeth. This hygiene procedure begins at the most distal tooth in the arch and systematically proceeds mesially.[11]

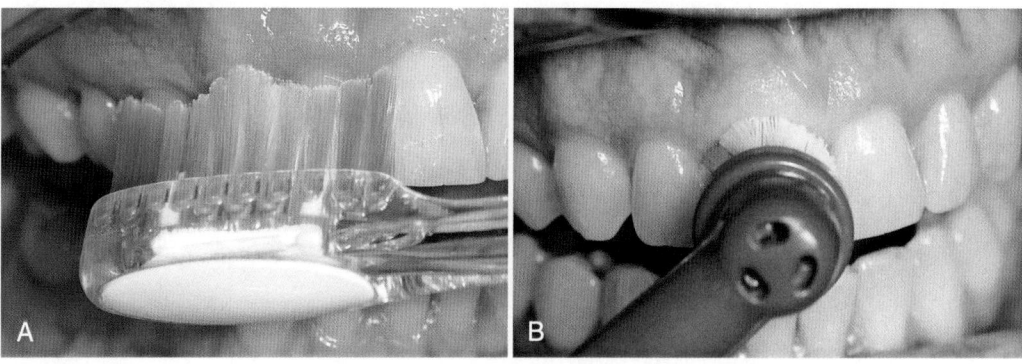

Fig. 48.7 Positioning the powered toothbrush head and bristle tips so that they reach the gingival margin is critical to achieving the most effective cleaning results. (A) Straight-head placement. (B) Round-head placement.

2. Place the bristles at the gingival margin, pointing at a 45-degree angle to the long axis of the teeth.
3. Exert gentle vibratory pressure using short, back-and-forth motions without dislodging the tips of the bristles. This motion forces the bristle ends into the gingival sulcus area (see Fig. 48.5), as well as partly into the interproximal embrasures. The pressure should be firm enough to blanch the gingiva

Brushing With Powered Toothbrushes

The various mechanical motions built into powered toothbrushes means they do not require special techniques. The patient should place the brush head next to the teeth at the gingival margin, similar to the position with the manual brush. This is the target hygiene area, and it proceeds systematically around the arch.[124] As indicated earlier, it is the routine brushing method described for manual brushing, except it is with the powered toothbrush (Fig. 48.7).

KEY FACTS

When recommending toothbrushing techniques, remember what research has taught us:
• Targeted hygiene[121] focuses brushing efforts on the critical cervical and interproximal areas of teeth.
• Brushing with either a manual or powered toothbrush requires a systematic routine to be effective.[95]
• Patients will modify any technique to their needs, so emphasize brushing all the surfaces of the teeth effectively.

Interdental Cleaning Aids

Any toothbrush, regardless of the brushing method used, does not completely remove interdental plaque biofilms. This is true for all patients, even for periodontal patients with wide-open embrasures.[47,111] Daily interdental plaque biofilm removal is crucial to augment the effects of toothbrushing because most dental and periodontal diseases originate in interproximal areas.[1]

Tissue destruction associated with periodontal disease often leaves large, open spaces between teeth and exposed root surfaces with anatomic concavities and furcations. These defects also occur after resective periodontal surgery. The best example of an anatomic root concavity is the mesial root surface of the maxillary first bicuspid. With attachment loss, the concavity located on this mesial surface is exposed where plaque biofilm will accumulate. These areas shelter plaque biofilm and are difficult for patients to clean with the toothbrush alone.[75] In addition, dental floss does not reach these concave surfaces

(see Fig. 48.16). Patients should understand that the purpose of interdental cleaning is to remove microbial plaque biofilm, not just food that has wedged between two approximating teeth. Many instruments are available for interproximal cleaning, and they should be recommended based on the size of the interdental spaces, the presence of furcations, root surface concavities, tooth alignment, and the presence of orthodontic appliances or other fixed prostheses. Moreover, ease of use and patient cooperation are important considerations. Common aids for interdental hygiene are dental floss, interdental brushes, rubber tips, and wooden or plastic tips.

Dental Floss

Dental floss is the most widely recommended tool for removing biofilm from proximal tooth surfaces.[46] Floss is made from nylon filaments or plastic monofilaments, and it comes in waxed, unwaxed, thick, thin, and flavored varieties. Some prefer monofilament floss made of nonstick material because they are slick and do not fray. Clinical research has demonstrated no significant differences in the ability of the various types of floss to remove dental plaque biofilm; they all work equally well.[40,62,72,73] Waxed dental floss was thought to leave a waxy film on proximal surfaces, thus contributing to biofilm accumulation and gingivitis. It has been shown, however, that wax is not deposited on tooth surfaces,[102] and improvement in gingival health is unrelated to the type of floss used.[40] Factors influencing the choice of dental floss include the tightness of tooth contacts, the roughness of proximal surfaces, and the patient's manual dexterity, not the superiority of any one product. Therefore, recommendations about type of floss should be based on ease of use and personal preference. As indicated previously, the limitations of dental floss must also be explained to the patient, and alternative methods must be demonstrated.

FLASH BACK

Recommended by Bass in the 1930s, and popularized in the 1960s, unwaxed floss is still recommended as being superior to waxed versions. The rationale is that it does not leave a waxy film that would cause more plaque deposition on the interproximal surfaces of the teeth. No evidence supports this. Given that waxed floss is easier for most people to use, patients should floss with whatever type they like. The important thing is that they adopt the flossing habit!

Technique for the Use of Dental Floss

The floss must contact the proximal surface from line angle to line angle to clean effectively. It must also clean the entire proximal

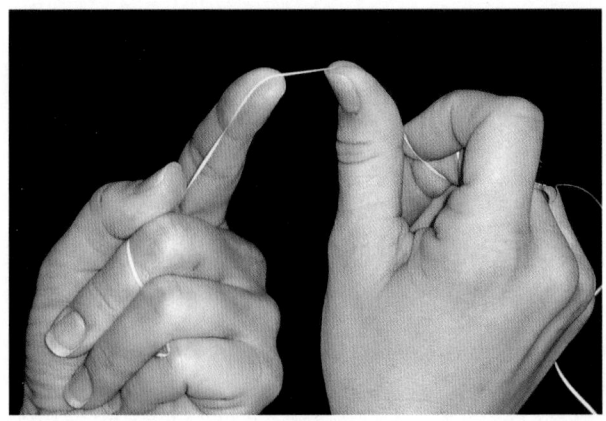

Fig. 48.8 Dental floss should be held securely in the fingers or tied in a loop.

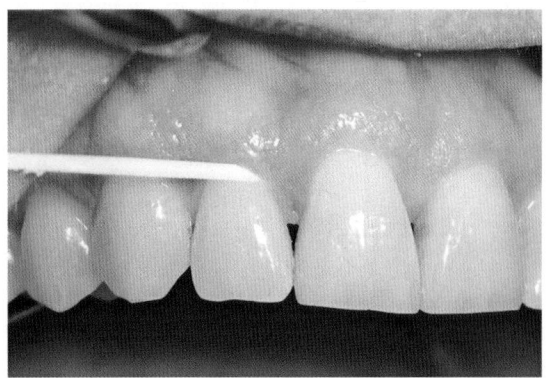

Fig. 48.9 Dental floss technique. The floss is slipped between the contact areas of the teeth (in this case, teeth #7 and #8) and wrapped around the proximal surface, and removes plaque by using several up-and-down strokes. The process must be repeated for the distal surface of tooth #8.

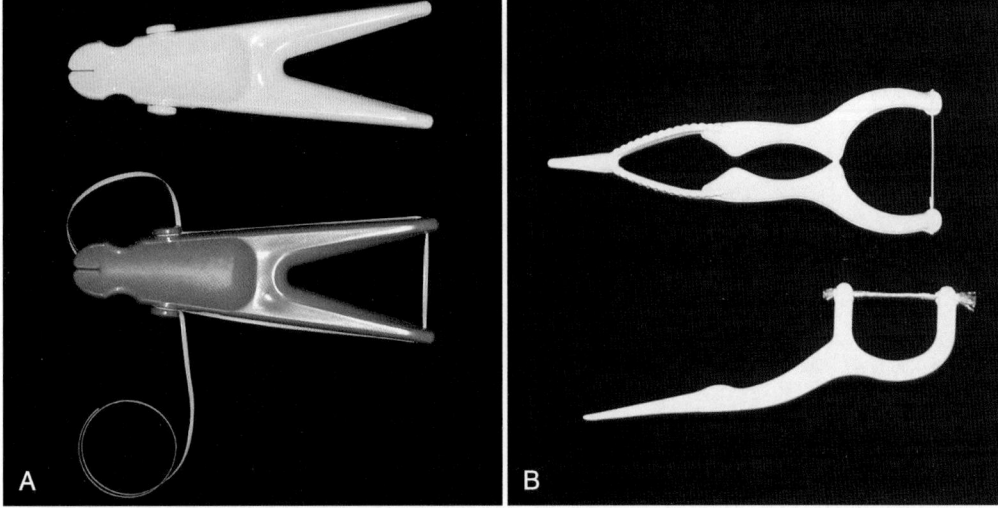

Fig. 48.10 Floss holders can simplify the manipulation of dental floss. (A) Reusable floss tools require stringing the floss around a series of knobs and grooves to secure it. (B) Disposable floss tools have prestrung floss and are easy to use, but the floss may shred and break, requiring several tools to complete flossing the teeth.

surface, including accessible subgingival areas. Flossing technique requires the following:

1. Start with a piece of floss long enough to grasp securely; 12 to 18 inches is usually sufficient. It may be wrapped around the fingers, or the ends may be tied together in a loop.
2. Stretch the floss tightly between the thumb and forefinger (Fig. 48.8) or between both forefingers, and pass it gently through each contact area with a firm back-and-forth motion. Do not snap the floss past the contact area, because this may injure the interdental gingiva. In fact, zealous snapping of floss through contact areas creates proximal grooves in the gingiva.
3. Once the floss is apical to the contact area between the teeth, wrap the floss around the proximal surface of one tooth and slip it under the marginal gingiva. Move the floss firmly along the tooth up to the contact area and gently down into the sulcus again, repeating this up-and-down stroke two or three times (Fig. 48.9). Then move the floss across the interdental gingiva, and repeat the procedure on the proximal surface of the adjacent tooth.
4. Continue through the whole dentition, including the distal surface of the last tooth in each quadrant. When the working portion of the floss shreds or becomes contaminated, move the floss to a fresh portion.

Flossing can be facilitated by using a *floss holder* (Fig. 48.10A). Floss holders are helpful for patients lacking manual dexterity and for caregivers assisting patients in cleaning their teeth. A floss holder should be rigid enough to keep the floss taut when penetrating tight contact areas, and it should be simple to string the floss onto the holder. The disadvantage of these floss holders is that using them tends to be time-consuming because they must be rethreaded frequently when the floss shreds.

Disposable single-use floss holders with prethreaded floss are also available. Short-term clinical studies suggested that plaque biofilm reduction and improvement in gingivitis scores are similar for patients using disposable floss devices and patients who hold the floss with their fingers[19,116] (Fig. 48.10B).

Powered flossing devices are also available (Fig. 48.11). These devices have been shown to be safe and effective, but they are no better at plaque biofilm removal than holding the floss with the fingers.[26,51]

Establishing a lifelong habit of flossing the teeth is difficult to achieve for both patients and dentists, regardless of whether one uses a tool or flosses with fingers. In fact, it is thought that the daily use of dental floss by patients is inconsistent. Investigators reported that only about 8% of young teenagers in Great Britain flossed daily,[90] with similar percentages reported for other countries.[75]

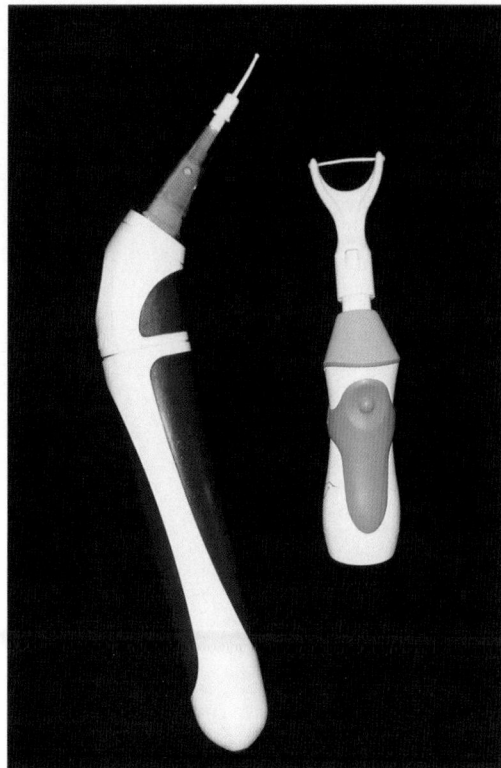

Fig. 48.11 Powered flossing devices can be easier for some patients to use than handheld floss. The tip is inserted into the proximal space, and a bristle or wand comes out of the tip and moves in a circular motion when the device is turned on *(left)*. Alternately, the device moves the prestrung floss in short motions to provide interproximal cleaning *(right)*.

It has been suggested that motivational interviewing and instructional techniques are helpful in encouraging this habit.[44] No information is available regarding long-term flossing habits comparing the various instruments used to floss with flossing with one's fingers. However, these instruments may be useful to help individuals begin flossing or to make flossing possible for patients who have limited dexterity.

 KEY FACTS

The benefits to gingival health of interproximal cleaning are undisputed.
- Dental floss is a simple and readily available tool to clean where the toothbrush cannot reach. The thorough removal of plaque biofilm from the interdental tooth surfaces is the most important hygiene step in the treatment of periodontal disease.
- Flossing tools work as well as flossing using one's fingers.
- The flossing habit is difficult to establish and requires positive reinforcement during dental visits.

Interdental Brushes

Probably the most effective plaque biofilm removal method for interdental areas, where the papilla does not completely fill the space, is the use of interdental brushes. As indicated earlier, the concave root surfaces, such as the mesial aspect of the maxillary first bicuspid and furcation areas, are usually not cleaned efficiently with dental floss. A comparison study of dental floss and interdental brushes used by patients with moderate to severe periodontal disease indicated

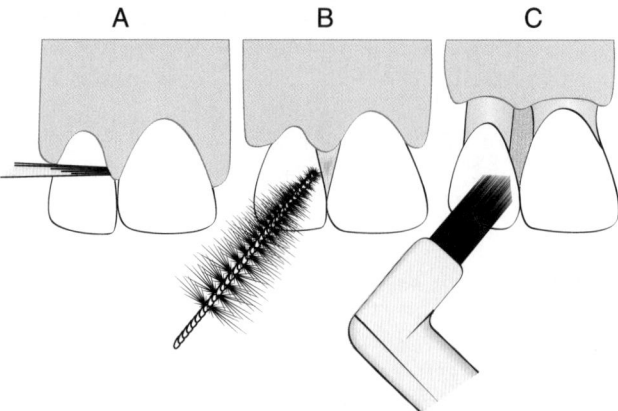

Fig. 48.12 Interproximal embrasure spaces vary greatly in patients with periodontal disease. (A) In general, embrasures with no gingival recession are adequately cleaned using dental floss. (B) Larger spaces with exposed root surfaces require the use of an interproximal brush. (C) Single-tufted brushes clean efficiently in interproximal spaces with no papillae.

that the interproximal brushes removed a greater amount of interproximal plaque biofilm and that the subjects found it easier to use these brushes than dental floss. However, no difference was found when probe depth reductions or bleeding indices were compared.[23] Therefore, interproximal cleaning aids such as dental floss and interdental brushes are excellent for proximal cleaning of teeth when interdental spaces permit their access.[75]

Embrasure spaces vary greatly in size and shape. Fig. 48.12 provides a representation of the size and anatomy of three types of embrasures and the interdental cleaning instrument most often recommended for each. As a general rule, the larger the spaces, the larger the instruments needed to clean them properly.

Technique

An interdental brush of any style is inserted through the interproximal spaces and moved back and forth between the teeth with short strokes. The diameter of the brush should be slightly larger than the gingival embrasures to be cleaned. This size permits the bristles to exert pressure on both proximal tooth surfaces by working their way into concavities on the roots. The brush bristles must also reach the interdental gingival margin.

Single-tufted brushes provide access to furcation areas, or isolated areas of deep recession, and are effective on the lingual surfaces of mandibular molars and premolars. These areas are often missed when using a toothbrush and floss.

Other Interdental Cleaning Devices: Rubber Tips, Wooden Toothpicks, and Tufted Brushes

Other interdental cleaning devices are available for removing microbial plaque biofilm from between the teeth (Fig. 48.13). Rubber tips with angled shanks, tapered wooden toothpicks that are round or triangular in cross-section, and single-tufted brushes are all helpful in attaining interdental hygiene. Many interdental devices have handles and contoured shanks for convenient manipulation around the teeth and in posterior areas. Clinical research has indicated that these devices are all effective for both lingual and facial tooth surfaces, as well as for proximal surfaces.[75,111]

Wooden toothpicks are used either with or without a handle (see Fig. 48.13A and B). Access is easier from the buccal surfaces for tips without handles but is limited primarily to the anterior and bicuspid areas. Wooden toothpicks on handles improve access to all areas and have been shown to be as effective as dental floss in reducing plaque biofilm and bleeding scores in subjects with gingivitis.[84] Triangular wooden tips are also available; this design is most useful in the anterior areas when used from the buccal surfaces of the teeth.

Rubber tips are conical and are mounted on handles or the ends of toothbrushes. They are reusable and can be easily adapted to all proximal surfaces in the mouth. The rubber tips that are mounted on handles with a curved shank, as in curettes, are excellent not only for cleaning the interdental spaces but also for demonstrating to the patient the location of the plaque biofilm during oral hygiene instruction. For hygiene purposes, the rubber tip should be placed into the embrasure space, resting on the gingiva, and used in a circular motion. It can be applied to interproximal spaces and other defects throughout the mouth and is easily adaptable to lingual surfaces. Plastic tips that resemble wooden or rubber tips are also available and are used in the same way.

Technique

Toothpicks are common devices and readily available in most homes. They can be used around all surfaces of the teeth when attached to commercially available handles (see Fig. 48.13B). Once mounted on the handle, the toothpick is broken off so that it is only 5 or 6 mm long. The tip of the toothpick is used to trace along the gingival margin and into the proximal areas from both the facial and lingual surface of each tooth (Fig. 48.14). Toothpicks mounted on handles are efficient for cleaning along the gingival margin,[46] can penetrate periodontal pockets and furcations, and permit patients to target their hygiene efforts at the gingival margin (Takei H: Personal communication, 2009).

Soft triangular wooden picks or plastic picks are placed in the interdental space with the base of the triangle resting on the gingiva and the sides in contact with the proximal tooth surfaces (Fig. 48.15). The pick is then moved in and out of the embrasure several times to remove the biofilm. The disadvantage of triangular wooden or plastic tips is that they do not reach into the posterior areas or on the lingual surfaces.

KEY FACTS

Periodontal patients often have to clean large interdental spaces, so it is extremely important to find an interdental device that is easy to manipulate and that the patient will use regularly.

- Patients may need to try several of the many devices available before finding one that satisfies their needs.
- In general, the largest brush or device that fits into a space will clean most efficiently (Fig. 48.16).

Gingival Massage

Massaging the gingiva with a toothbrush or an interdental cleaning device produces epithelial thickening, increased keratinization, and

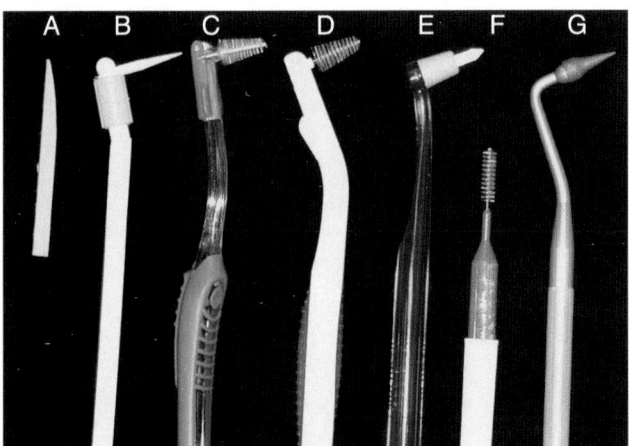

Fig. 48.13 (A) and (B) Interproximal cleaning devices include wooden tips, (C to F) interproximal brushes, and (G) rubber-tip stimulators.

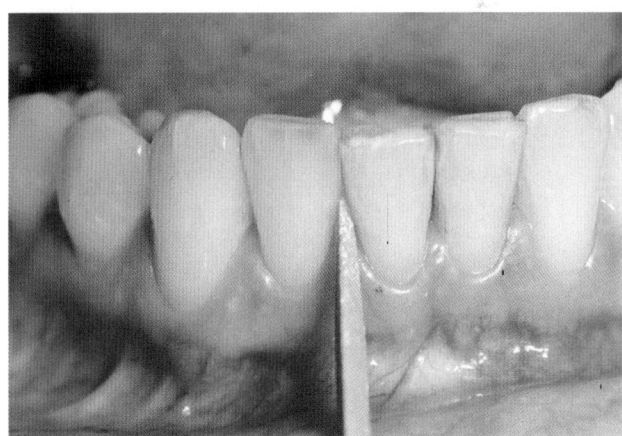

Fig. 48.15 Triangular wooden tips are also popular with patients. The tip is inserted between the teeth, with the triangular portion resting on the gingival papilla. The tip is moved in and out to remove plaque; however, it is very difficult to use on posterior teeth and from the lingual aspect of all teeth.

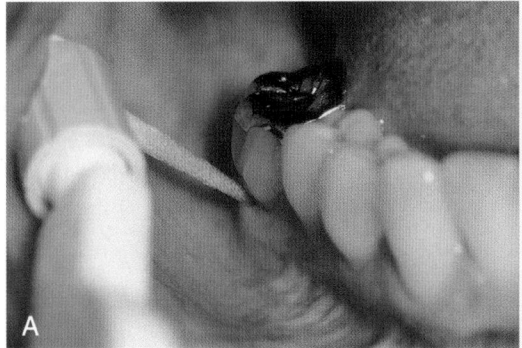

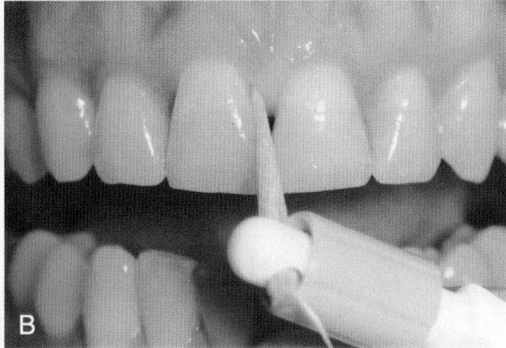

Fig. 48.14 Wooden toothpick. (A) The tip is a common wooden toothpick held in a handle and broken off. It is used to clean subgingivally and reach into periodontal pockets. (B) The tip can also be used to clean along the gingival margins of the teeth and reach under the gingiva.

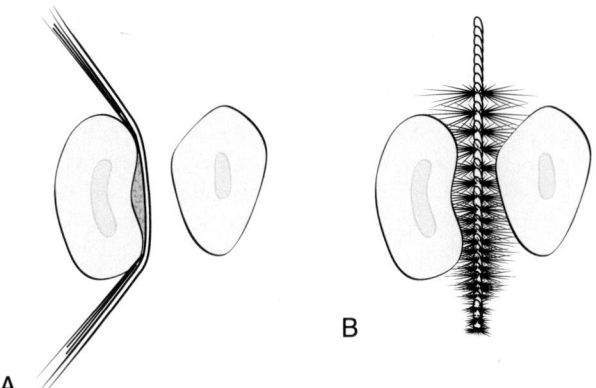

A

B

Fig. 48.16 Cleaning of concave or irregular proximal tooth surfaces. (A) Dental floss may be less effective than (B) an interdental brush on long root surfaces with concavities.

increased mitotic activity in the epithelium and connective tissue.[17,20,49] The increased keratinization occurs only on the gingiva facing the oral cavity (oral epithelium), but not on the areas more vulnerable to microbial attack, which are the sulcular epithelium and the interdental areas where the gingival col is present. Epithelial thickening, increased keratinization, and blood circulation have not been shown to be beneficial for restoring gingival health.[48] Improved gingival health associated with interdental stimulation is the result of inadvertent microbial plaque biofilm removal rather than the effects of gingival massage. No clinical evidence indicates that massaging the gingiva is essential or necessary to attain gingival health.

Conclusion

- After thorough patient education regarding the disease and the etiology, the hygiene technique is initiated by demonstrating the procedure in the patient's own mouth. The rubber tip is an excellent instrument to demonstrate plaque biofilm. All patients require regular use of a toothbrush, either manual or electric, at least once per day. The brushing method should emphasize access to the gingival margins (dentogingival junction) of all accessible tooth surfaces. Emphasize the importance of *targeted hygiene* and extending as far onto the proximal surfaces as possible.
- Dental floss should be used in all interdental spaces that are filled with gingiva.

- Interdental aids such as interproximal brushes, rubber tips, wooden tips, or toothpicks should be used in all areas where the toothbrush and floss techniques cannot adequately remove the plaque biofilm. This includes large embrasure spaces and furcation areas, as well as the mesial surface of the maxillary first bicuspid, which presents a concavity on the root surface near the cementoenamel junction.
- Daily at-home subgingival irrigation and lavage are useful for reduction of inflammation and maintenance for patients with residual deep pockets and those who struggle with mechanical interproximal cleaning devices. The effectiveness of irrigation and lavage is enhanced by the addition of a chlorhexidine or essential oil rinse as an irrigant.
- Caries control requires the daily use of a dentifrice with low-concentration fluoride. Topical oral rinses and gels with higher concentrations of fluoride should be used for patients with a high risk for caries.
- Chemical antimicrobial agents, such as chlorhexidine and essential oils, can be used to disinfect the patient's mouth and control infection. These oral rinses may be continued indefinitely. Staining of teeth and taste alteration are side effects that may limit the patient's acceptance of these products.
- Reinforcement of daily plaque biofilm control practices and routine visits to the dental office for maintenance care are essential for successful microbial plaque biofilm control and the long-term success of therapy.

Successful prevention, treatment, and maintenance in periodontal therapy are based on scientific knowledge of the etiology, risk factors, and host resistance involved in periodontal disease. The importance of the patient's understanding of the etiology and active participation in partnership with the therapist to prevent and treat periodontal disease is well understood in the current understanding of periodontal therapy.

A Case Scenario is found on the companion website www.expertconsult.com.

References

References for this chapter are found on the companion website www.expertconsult.com.

CHAPTER 49

Breath Malodor

Marc Quirynen | Isabelle Laleman | Sophie De Geest | Charlotte De Hous | Christel Dekeyser | Wim Teughels

CHAPTER OUTLINE

 For online-only content on extraoral causes of breath malodor and the portable volatile sulfur monitor, as well as expanded discussions on epidemiology and etiology of malodor, fundamentals of malodor detection, diagnosis of malodor including organoleptic rating and gas chromatography, and chlorhexidine use in treating malodor, please go to the companion website www.expertconsult.com.

Semantics and Classification

Breath odor can be defined as the subjective perception after smelling someone's breath. It can be pleasant, unpleasant, or even disturbing, if not repulsive. If unpleasant, the terms *breath malodor, halitosis, bad breath,* or *fetor ex ore* can be applied. Breath malodor is a common complaint in the general population. One in four persons has bad breath at a given time in his/her life. It has a significant socioeconomic impact but unfortunately has been neglected until recently by scientists and clinicians, and it is still hardly covered in the medical curricula. Halitosis can lead to personal discomfort and social embarrassment, and it remains one of the biggest taboos of society.

The three main categories of halitosis are genuine halitosis, pseudo-halitosis, and halitophobia. *Genuine halitosis* is the term that is used when the breath malodor really exists and can be diagnosed organoleptically or by measurement of the responsible compounds. A distinction should be made between physiologic and pathologic halitosis (Fig. 49.1).

Transient disturbing odors caused by food intake (e.g., garlic, onions, and certain spices), smoking, or medications (e.g., metronidazole) do not reveal a health problem and are common examples of physiologic halitosis. The same is true for "morning" bad breath, as habitually experienced on awakening. This malodor is caused by decreased salivary flow and increased putrefaction during the night, and it spontaneously disappears after breakfast or after oral hygiene measures. A persistent breath malodor, by definition, does reflect some pathology (pathologic halitosis). The causes of this condition are discussed later in the chapter. When the origin of pathologic halitosis can be found in the oral cavity, one speaks of *oral malodor.* When an obvious breath malodor cannot be perceived but the patient is convinced that he or she suffers from it, this is called *pseudo-halitosis.* If the patient still believes that bad breath is present after treatment of genuine halitosis or diagnosis of pseudo-halitosis, one considers halitophobia, which is a recognized psychiatric condition.[167]

Important Terms for the Diagnosis of Bad Breath

Genuine halitosis	Malodor that can be verified objectively
Physiologic halitosis	Malodor that is transient and caused by physiologic factors, such as food intake or smoking
Oral malodor or intraoral halitosis	Obvious malodor originating from the oral cavity
Extraoral halitosis	Bad breath originating from pathologic conditions outside the oral cavity
Pseudo-halitosis	Malodor that cannot be perceived objectively even though the patient complains of its existence. This condition can be improved by oral hygiene instruction and counseling.
Halitophobia	No malodor that can be perceived objectively after treatment of halitosis or pseudo-halitosis even though the patient persists in believing that halitosis exists

Etiology

In most patients, breath malodor originates from the oral cavity. Tongue coating is the predominant cause of oral malodor. Furthermore, periodontal diseases (gingivitis and periodontitis) are the second most important causative factors.[27,97,98,107,168,169]

A large-scale study including 2000 patients with halitosis complaints showed that for those patients whose bad breath could be objectively detected, the cause was mostly found within the oral cavity (90%). Tongue coating (51%), gingivitis or periodontitis

(13%), or a combination (22%) accounted for the majority of the cases.[107] Because a large part of the population has tongue coating or gingivitis/periodontitis, the risk always exists that an intraoral condition is too easily considered as the cause, whereas more important pathologic conditions are overlooked. Indeed, for a minority of patients (4% in the same study), extraoral causes could be identified, including ear, nose, and throat (ENT) disorders, systemic diseases (e.g., diabetes), metabolic or hormonal changes, hepatic or renal insufficiency, bronchial and pulmonary diseases, or gastroenterologic disorders.[27,86,102,107,152]

Intraoral Causes

Tongue coating, poor oral hygiene, gingivitis, and periodontitis are the predominant causative factors.[107,130] In these cases the term *oral malodor* applies. It is the result of the degradation of organic substrates by anaerobic bacteria. During the process of bacterial putrefaction, peptides and proteins present in saliva, food debris, gingival crevicular fluid, interdental plaque, shed epithelial cells, postnasal drip, and blood are hydrolyzed to sulfide-containing and non–sulfide-containing amino acids, which can be further metabolized. The proteolytic degradation of sulfur-containing amino acids (cysteine, cystine and methionine) by gram-negative bacteria produces sulfur-containing gases such as hydrogen sulfide (H_2S) and methylmercaptan (CH_3SH).[162]

The most commonly involved bacteria are *Porphyromonas gingivalis, Prevotella intermedia, Prevotella nigrescens, Aggregatibacter actinomycetemcomitans, Campylobacter rectus, Fusobacterium nucleatum, Peptostreptococcus micros, Tannerella forsythia, Eubacterium* spp., and spirochetes. A study by Niles and Gaffar[88] made clear that these gram-negative species in particular cause an unpleasant smell by the production of sulfur compounds. However, because of the large microbial diversity found in patients with halitosis, it is suggested that breath malodor is the result of complex interactions among several bacterial species. One study indicated that some gram-positive microorganisms, such as *Streptococcus salivarius,* also contribute to oral malodor production by deglycosylating salivary glycoproteins, thus exposing their protein core to further degradation

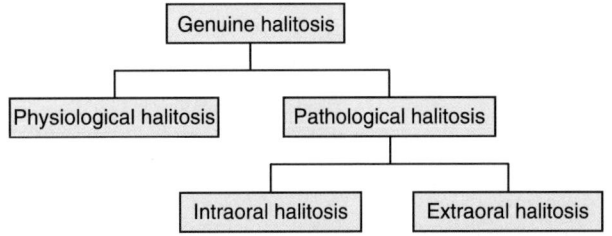

```
                    Genuine halitosis
                          │
            ┌─────────────┴─────────────┐
  Physiological halitosis       Pathological halitosis
                          │
            ┌─────────────┴─────────────┐
    Intraoral halitosis         Extraoral halitosis
```

Fig. 49.1 Genuine halitosis: classification.

by gram-negative microorganisms.[139] More recently, the presence of *Solobacterium moorei,* a gram-positive bacterium, has also been linked to oral malodor.[49,50,58]

Thus, for oral malodor, the unpleasant smell of the breath mainly originates from volatile sulfur compounds (VSCs), especially hydrogen sulfide, methylmercaptan, and (less significantly) dimethyl sulfide $((CH_3)_2S)$, as first discovered by Tonzetich.[149] Other compounds, such as the diamines indole and skatole, the polyamines putrescine and cadaverine, and the carboxylic acids acetic, butyric, and propionic acid, are also formed by proteolytic degradation of non–sulfur-containing amino acids by oral microorganisms.[42]

Tongue and Tongue Coating

The dorsal tongue mucosa, with an area of 25 cm^3, has a very irregular surface topography.[19,129] The innumerable depressions in the tongue surface are ideal niches for bacterial adhesion and growth, sheltered from cleaning actions.[25,168] Moreover, desquamated cells and food remnants also remain trapped in these retention sites and consequently can be putrefied by the bacteria.[8] A fissured tongue (deep fissures on the dorsum, also called *scrotal tongue* or *lingua plicata*) and a hairy tongue (*lingua villosa*) have an even rougher surface (Fig. 49.2).

Accumulated food remnants intermingled with exfoliated cells and bacteria form a coating on the tongue dorsum. The latter cannot be easily removed because of retention by the irregular surface of the tongue dorsum (see Fig. 49.2). As such, the two factors essential for putrefaction (bacteria and their nutrients) are united. Several investigators have identified the dorsal posterior surface of the tongue as the primary source of oral malodor.[8,18,25,118] Indeed, high correlations have been reported between tongue coating and odor formation.[8,21,78,168]

In both healthy individuals and patients with periodontitis with or without complaints of oral halitosis, a significant positive correlation was found between the presence or amount of tongue coating and levels of VSCs[78,108] and/or organoleptic scores of the mouth odor.[25] In a group of 2000 patients visiting a multidisciplinary halitosis clinic,[107,159] significant correlations were found between organoleptic scores and tongue coating ($R = 0.52$; $P < 0.001$). In another study,[92] it was also observed that the amount of tongue coating was significantly greater in the halitosis-positive group compared with the halitosis-negative group. Morita and Wang[80] found that the volume of tongue coating and the percentage of sites with bleeding on probing were significantly associated with oral malodor.[80] In 1992, Yaegaki and Sanada[168,169] demonstrated that even in patients with periodontal disease, 60% of the VSCs were produced from the tongue surface.[168,169]

Research has showed that the strongest determinant of the presence of tongue coating is suboptimal oral hygiene. Other influencing factors were periodontal status, presence of a denture, smoking, and dietary habits.[158]

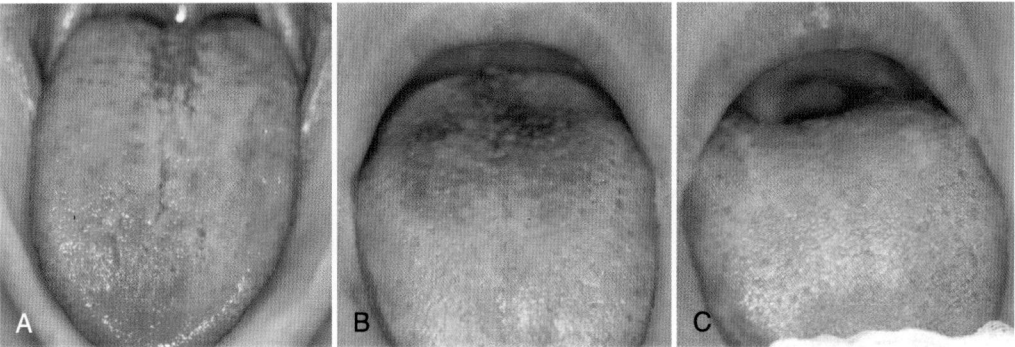

Fig. 49.2 (A) to (C) Clinical pictures of heavily coated tongues.

Periodontal Infections

A relationship between periodontitis and oral malodor has been shown. However, periodontally healthy patients can suffer from halitosis, not all patients with gingivitis and/or periodontitis complain about bad breath, and some disagreement exists in the literature over to what extent oral malodor and periodontal disease are related.[8,119,136] Bacteria associated with gingivitis and periodontitis are indeed able to produce VSCs.[61,84,88,97,98,149]

Several studies have shown that VSC levels in the mouth correlate positively with the depth of periodontal pockets (the deeper the pocket, the more bacteria, particularly anaerobic species) and that the amount of VSCs in the breath increases with the number, depth, and bleeding tendency of the periodontal pockets.[18,96,107,169] VSCs aggravate the periodontitis process by increasing the permeability of the pocket and mucosal epithelium, therefore exposing the underlying connective tissues of the periodontium to bacterial metabolites. Methylmercaptan enhances interstitial collagenase production, interleukin-1 production by mononuclear cells, and cathepsin B production, thus further mediating connective tissue breakdown.[70,112] It was shown that human gingival fibroblasts developed an affected cytoskeleton when exposed to methylmercaptan.[10,112] Furthermore, the reaction of hydrogen sulfide with collagen can alter the protein structure, thereby rendering the periodontal ligament and bone collagen more susceptible to destruction by proteases.[87] Investigators have shown, in cases of gingivitis and periodontitis, a decrease in the content of acid-soluble and total collagen in the affected tissues.[128] These findings suggest that increased production of VSCs may accelerate the progression of periodontal disease. Toxic VSCs are able to damage the periodontal tissues and create even more loss of attachment. A mutual reinforcement of the loss of periodontal attachment and production of VSCs occurs, resulting in a vicious cycle.

Some studies, however, have shown that when the presence of tongue coating is taken into account, the correlation between periodontitis and oral malodor is much lower, thus indicating that tongue coating remains a key factor for halitosis. The prevalence of tongue coating is six times higher in patients with periodontitis, and the same bacterial species associated with periodontal disease can also be found in large numbers on the dorsum of the tongue, particularly when tongue coating is present.[168] The reported association between periodontitis and oral malodor may thus primarily be due to the effects of periodontal disease on tongue coating. It may also explain why other articles did not find a correlation.[8,136]

Other relevant malodorous pathologic manifestations of the periodontium are pericoronitis (the soft tissue "cap" being retentive for microorganisms and debris), major recurrent oral ulcerations, herpetic gingivitis, and necrotizing gingivitis/periodontitis. Microbiologic observations indicate that ulcers infected with gram-negative anaerobes (i.e., *Prevotella* and *Porphyromonas* species) are significantly more malodorous than noninfected ulcers.[9]

CLINICIAN'S CORNER

What is the influence of bad breath in patients with periodontitis?

The increased production of volatile sulfur compounds in people with bad breath may accelerate the progression of periodontal disease. For example, it is known that methylmercaptan and hydrogen sulfide can adversely affect collagen structure and gingival fibroblasts.

Dental Disorders

Possible causes within the dentition are deep carious lesions with food impaction and putrefaction, extraction wounds filled with blood clots, and purulent discharge leading to important putrefaction. Other causes include interdental food impaction in large interdental areas and crowding of teeth favoring food entrapment and accumulation of debris. Acrylic dentures, especially when kept continuously in the mouth at night or not regularly cleaned, can lead to infections (e.g. candidiasis), which produce a typical smell. The denture surface facing the gingiva is porous and retentive for bacteria, yeasts, and debris, which are compounds needed for putrefaction.

Dry Mouth

Saliva has an important cleaning function in the oral cavity. Patients with xerostomia often present with large amounts of plaque on teeth and extensive tongue coating. The increased microbial load and the escape of VSCs when salivary flow is reduced explain the strong breath malodor.[61] Several studies link stress with VSC levels, but it is not clear whether this can simply be explained by a reduction of salivary flow.[67,104] Other causes of xerostomia are medication,[79] alcohol abuse,[36] Sjögren syndrome (a common autoimmune rheumatic disease),[74] and diabetes.[160]

Extraoral Causes

For a minority of patients, extraoral causes can be identified, including ENT disorders, systemic disease (e.g., diabetes or kidney disease), metabolic or hormonal changes, hepatic or renal insufficiency, bronchial and pulmonary diseases, or gastroenterologic disorders.[4,5] Moreover, multiple causes may be present at the same time, and over the course of time the etiology may shift.

Extraoral halitosis can be subdivided into two types: non–blood-borne halitosis and blood-borne halitosis.[147] Non–blood-borne halitosis is uncommon, and most information about it comes from case reports. Non–blood-borne halitosis encompasses, for example, throat infections, nasal infections, infections of the respiratory system, lung diseases, and stomach disorders.

Blood-borne halitosis is the result of bad-smelling metabolites that can be formed or absorbed at any place in the body (e.g., the liver, the gut) and transported by the bloodstream to the lungs. Exhalation of these volatiles in the alveolar air then causes halitosis, at least when the concentrations of the bad-smelling metabolites are sufficiently high. The crevicular fluid reflects the circulating molecules in the blood and can thus also play a relevant role, but due to the small amount, probably not a very dominant one.

The extraoral causes are much more difficult to detect, although they can sometimes be recognized by a typical odor. Uncontrolled diabetes mellitus can be associated with a sweet odor of ketones, liver disease can be revealed by a sulfur odor, and kidney failure can be characterized by a fishy odor because of the presence of dimethylamine and trimethylamine.[102]

CLINICIAN'S CORNER

What is the most important cause of halitosis?

Tongue coating is the most important cause of halitosis. The innumerable depressions in the tongue surface are ideal niches for bacterial adhesion and growth; additionally, desquamated cells and food remnants also remain trapped in these retention sites. The degradation of organic substrates by anaerobic bacteria results in the production of a range of unpleasant-smelling volatile compounds.

Pseudo-halitosis or Halitophobia

If a patient presents with complaints but no objective halitosis can be detected, one speaks of pseudo-halitosis or *imaginary breath odor,* which can lead to *halitophobia.*[94] The latter is the case when, even after repeated diagnosis of an absence of bad breath, the patient cannot accept the absence of halitosis. This condition has been associated with obsessive-compulsive disorder and hypochondria. Well-established personality disorder questionnaires (e.g., Symptom Checklist 90) allow the clinician to assess the patient's tendency for illusional breath malodor.[28,29,31] Having a psychologist or psychiatrist at the malodor consultation can be especially helpful for such patients. Because of the complexity of this disorder, a malodor consultation is thus preferably multidisciplinary, combining the knowledge of a periodontologist or dentist, an ENT specialist, an internist (if necessary), and a psychologist or psychiatrist. In a study of 2000 patients, 16% were diagnosed with pseudo-halitosis or halitophobia.[107]

KEY FACT

Only in a few cases is the cause of bad breath found outside the oral cavity. Thus, dentists play an important role in the diagnosis and treatment of halitosis.

Diagnosis of Malodor
Preconsultation Approach

A proper diagnostic approach starts with providing the right information to the patient before the appointment. It is recommended that the patient does not eat garlic, onions, or spices for 2 days before the consultation because they can cause bad breath and body odor that can last from several hours to 2 days.[48] To remove confounding odors, the patient is also instructed to refrain from alcohol, coffee, and smoking during the 12-hour period before the consultation. For the same reason, it is advisable not to use chewing gum, mints, drops, or mouthrinses during the 8 hours preceding the appointment, both for the patient and for the oral malodor judge. The day of the consultation, the use of fragranced shampoo, body lotion, and perfume should also be avoided, so as not to disturb the organoleptic ratings. In most halitosis consultations, the patient is asked not to eat or drink on the morning of the examination. However, if breakfast is consumed, morning bad breath can be excluded.

Course of a Halitosis Consultation
Preconsultation patient information
Anamnesis
Organoleptic examination
Examination of the breath with portable sulfur monitor
Oropharyngeal examination
Explanation of halitosis and instructions for oral hygiene
If necessary, explanation of additional therapy

The patient should be encouraged to bring a confidant to the consultations who can identify whether the perceived odor is the one previously noticed. Some of these guidelines are crucial not only for the organoleptic evaluation, but also for a correct interpretation of the results obtained with certain breath analyzers (see later).

Anamnesis

Each consultation should start with thorough questioning about the breath malodor, eating habits, and medical and dental history. This can be done with a questionnaire that the patient fills out in the waiting room and/or verbally at the beginning of the consultation, depending on the preference of the examiner and the practical

possibilities. To start with, the patient should be asked about the frequency of the halitosis (e.g., constantly, every day), the time of appearance during the day (e.g., after meals can indicate a stomach hernia), when the problem first appeared, and whether others have identified the problem (to exclude imaginary breath odor). In addition, the medical history has to be recorded, with an emphasis on medications and systemic diseases of the lungs, liver, kidneys, stomach, and pancreas. Concerning the ENT history, attention should be paid to the presence of nasal obstruction, mouth breathing, postnasal drip, allergy, tonsillitis, dysphagia, and previous ENT encounters. The dental history includes questions assessing the frequency of dental visits, the use of mouthrinses, the presence and maintenance of a dental prosthesis, and the frequency of and instruments used for toothbrushing, interdental cleaning, and tongue brushing and scraping. Finally, the patient is asked about smoking, drinking, and dietary habits.

Examinations

After obtaining a thorough anamnesis, the clinician checks whether an unpleasant odor can be perceived and inspects the mouth to detect possible causes of bad breath. Different ways exist to examine the breath. The easiest and least expensive way is to smell the breath. However, several devices are on the market that mainly detect VSCs.

Organoleptic Rating

Even though devices are available, organoleptic assessment by a judge is still the gold standard in the examination of breath malodor. It is the easiest and most often used method because it gives a reflection of the everyday situation when halitosis is noticed. Moreover, the human nose can smell 10,000 different odors, many more than any device on the market.[48,51] In an organoleptic evaluation, a trained and preferably calibrated "judge" sniffs the expired air and assesses whether it is unpleasant by using an intensity rating.[124] Scoring is normally done according to the intensity scale of Rosenberg, where 0 represents the absence of odor, 1 is barely noticeable odor, 2 is slight malodor, 3 is moderate malodor, 4 is strong malodor, and 5 is severe malodor.[124] In this six-point system, 0 indicates a concentration of odorant below a threshold, 1 to 4 are increasing occupancy of receptor binding sites, and 5 is assumed to be close to saturation.[43,44] To avoid bias, it is advisable that the organoleptic assessment precedes all other measurements.

In an organoleptic assessment, the judge smells a series of air samples (Fig. 49.3), as follows:

1. *Nasal breath odor:* The subject expires through the nose while keeping the mouth closed. When the nasal expiration is malodorous yet the air expired through the mouth is not, an ENT problem can be suspected.
2. *Oral cavity odor:* The subject opens the mouth and refrains from breathing while the judge places his or her nose close to the mouth opening (approximately 10 cm from the patient's mouth).
3. *Oral cavity odor:* The patient counts from 1 to 10. This reveals the same as described earlier, but favors oral malodor because of drying of the palatal and tongue mucosa.
4. *Tongue coating:* The judge smells a tongue scraping from the posterior part of the tongue, obtained with an odorless plastic spoon or tongue scraper, at a distance of approximately 5 cm from his or her nose. This odor resembles that emanating from the tongue dorsum.

Although the organoleptic assessment is still the gold standard for diagnosis of halitosis, the method also has some important drawbacks. The assessment can, for example, be influenced by several aspects, such as the position of the head, hunger, and the experience of the judge. Odor judges are also supposed to rest their nose for several

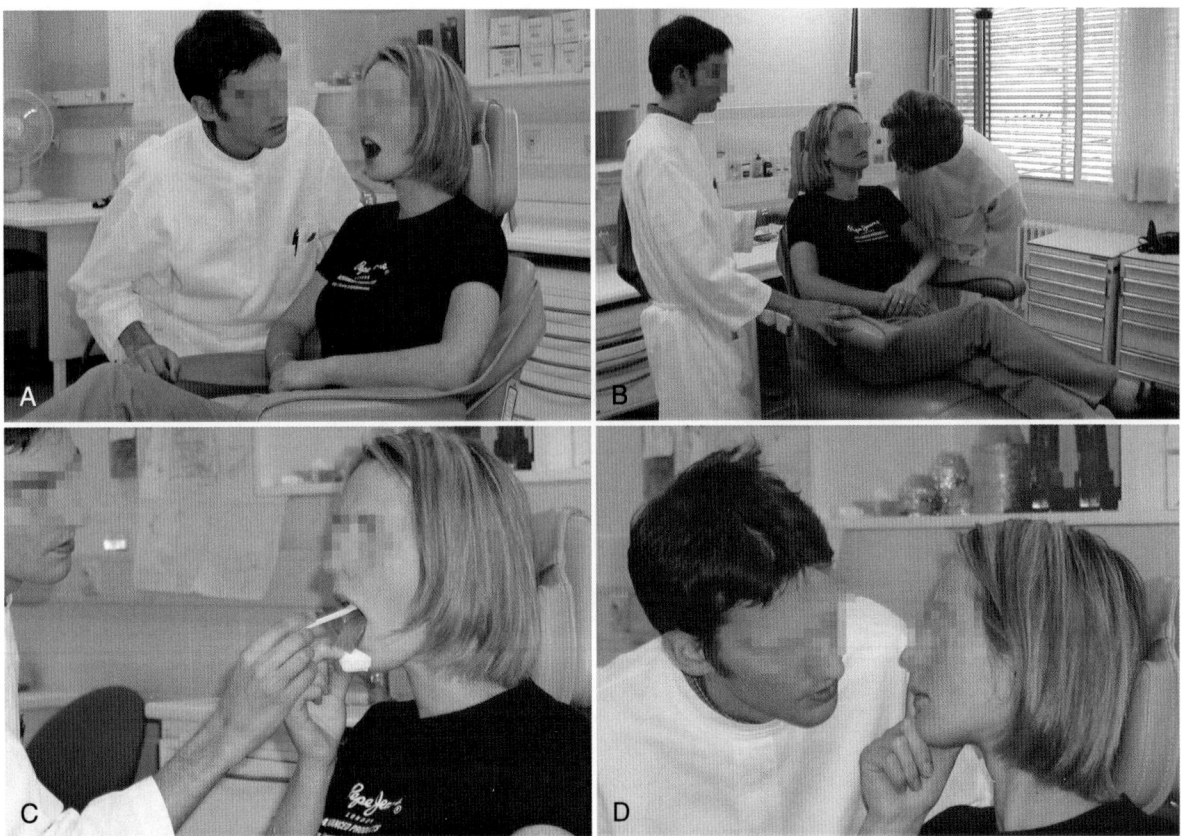

Fig. 49.3 (A) Organoleptic assessement of the oral cavity odor while the patients refrains from breathing. (B) assessment of the oral cavity odor when the patient counts out loud from 1 to 10. (C) A sample of the tongue coating is taken to smell afterward. (D) The nasal odor is rated.

minutes between tests to avoid habituation. The most important disadvantage of the method, however, is that it clearly has a degree of subjectivity. Researchers are trying to improve the reliability and reproducibility of the organoleptic method.[44] When using a panel of odor judges instead of one judge, the reliability is already considered to increase.[167] Furthermore, the agreement among judges may be improved by standardization of the sense of smell using an odor solution kit for measuring the olfactory response.[173] Training is also considered to reduce odor judges' errors.[82]

Portable Volatile Sulfur Monitor

The Halimeter (Interscan, Chatsworth, CA) is an electronic device that detects the presence of VSCs such as hydrogen sulfide and methylmercaptan in breath. The instrument cannot discriminate among the different sulfur compounds. The sensitivity for methylmercaptan is five times lower than for hydrogen sulfide, and the device is almost insensitive to dimethyl sulfide.[37] Moreover, ethanol and other compounds can disturb the measurements.

To allow an increase in concentration of VSCs, the patient has to keep his or her mouth closed for 2 to 3 minutes before sampling. The mouth air is aspirated by inserting a drinking straw fixed on the flexible tube of the instrument (Fig. 49.4). The straw is kept inside the mouth, preferably above the posterior part of the tongue dorsum, not touching the oral mucosa or the tongue, while the subject keeps the mouth slightly open and breathes through the nose. The sulfur meter uses a voltametric sensor that generates a signal when exposed to sulfur-containing gases. Using a recorder or specific software, a graphic presentation can be obtained, called a *haligram* (Fig. 49.5), which gives the response as a function of time. For the most optimal results, the manufacturer recommends performing three

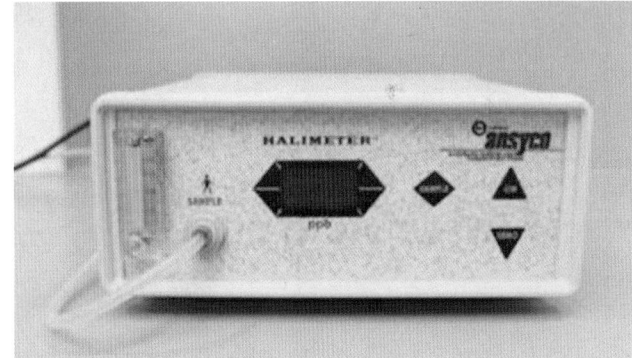

Fig. 49.4 Halimeter.

measurements and using the average value. Between measurements, it is important to allow the meter to restabilize before repeating. The monitor needs regular calibration and replacement of the sensor biannually.

The Halimeter is easy to use as a chair-side test and is relatively inexpensive. Patients are usually less embarrassed by this examination than by organoleptic assessment. Moreover the absence of odor in cases of halitophobia can be more convincingly proven than by an organoleptic assessment. Several studies have shown good correlations between the organoleptic measurement and the Halimeter.[122,125] An important drawback of the device is that it detects only sulfur compounds and thus is useful only for intraoral causes of halitosis. The absence of VSCs does not prove that no breath odor is present.

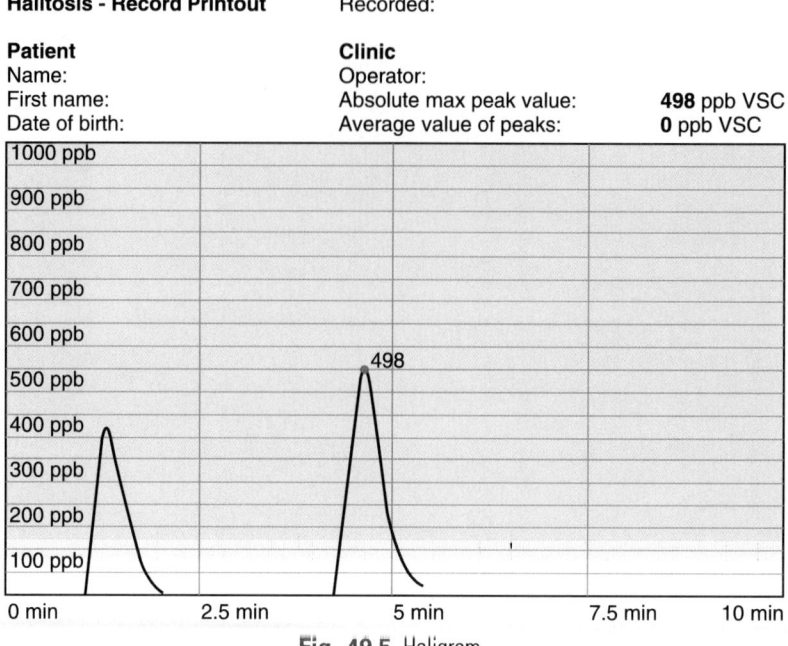

Halitosis - Record Printout   Recorded:

Patient   **Clinic**
Name: Operator:
First name: Absolute max peak value: **498** ppb VSC
Date of birth: Average value of peaks: **0** ppb VSC

Fig. **49.5** Haligram.

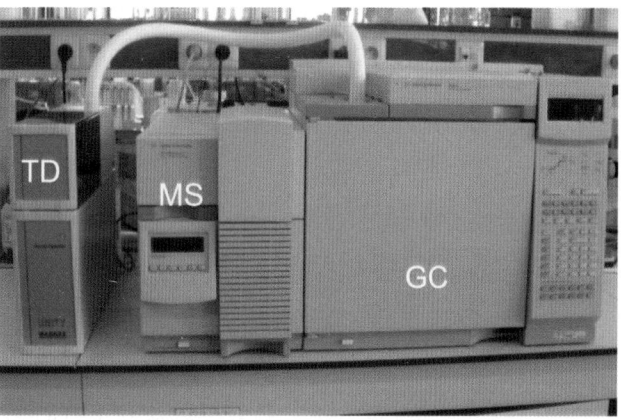

Fig. **49.6** Gas chromatography machinery, including thermal desorber (TD) to release molecules trapped in special collectors, gas chromatograph (GC) for separation of molecules, and mass spectrometer (MS) for identification of molecules.

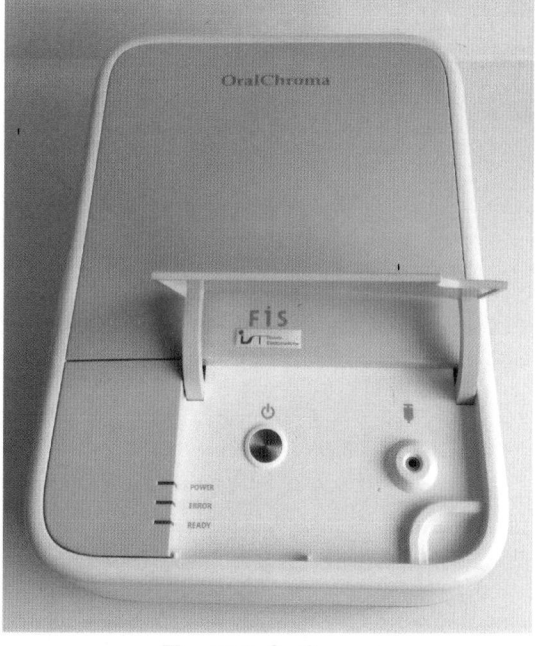

Fig. **49.7** OralChroma.

A wide range of threshold limits for halitosis has been proposed. Yaegaki and Sanade[168] recommended a value of 75 ppb as the limit for social acceptance, whereas the Halimeter's manufacturer proposes 150 ppb. Following this recommendation, the sensitivity and specificity of the device for the organoleptic score have been calculated to be 63% and 98%, respectively. Previous studies from our group showed that a reduction in this threshold to 120 ppb improves the sensitivity of the device without detriment to specificity.[159] In patients with oral malodor, VSC concentrations can easily reach 300 to 400 ppb.

Gas Chromatography

A gas chromatograph can analyze air, saliva, or crevicular fluid (Fig. 49.6). About 100 compounds have been isolated from the headspace of saliva and tongue coating, including ketones, alkanes, sulfur-containing compounds, and phenyl compounds.[17] In the expired air of a person, at least 150 compounds can be found.[100,155-157] The most important advantage of the technique is that when coupled with mass spectrometry, it can detect virtually any compound when using

adequate materials and conditions. Moreover, it has very high sensitivity and specificity.

Elaborate gas chromatography is available only in specialized centers but is especially useful for identifying nonoral causes.[54,99,142,154] It is expensive and requires trained personnel.

A small, portable "gas chromatograph" (OralChroma, Nissha FIS, Inc., Japan) has been introduced, which makes this technique available for periodontal clinics (Fig. 49.7). More recently, the second generation of this portable gas chromatograph was introduced: the OralChroma CHM-2. The CHM-2 is a little bit smaller than the first-generation OralChroma, the measurements only take half the time, and it comes with optimized software. Sample collection is done by use of a disposable syringe, which is inserted two-thirds of the way into the oral cavity. The patient must close the mouth for 30 seconds before sample collection, and afterward the sample is injected into the gas chromatograph.

The analysis starts automatically. A software packet, OralChroma Data Manager, collects the data from the OralChroma and graphically displays the sensor responses on a computer screen. After 4 minutes for the OralChroma CHM-2, the process is completed, and the concentrations of the three gases are displayed in either ng/10 mL or ppb (nmol/mol) (Fig. 49.8). The accompanying software packet gives a clear overview of the VSC measurement. However, with the OralChroma CHM-1, sometimes these graphics are not correct because the place of the VSCs is incorrectly assigned in the chromatogram. The latter can be corrected by analyzing the chromatograph.[146,148]

The OralChroma has the capacity to measure the concentration of the three key sulfur compounds (hydrogen sulfide, methylmercaptan, and dimethyl sulfide) separately. This can be helpful for a differential diagnosis. A high concentration of methylmercaptan compared with hydrogen sulfide indicates, for example, periodontitis.[169] If only hydrogen sulfide is increased, a problem with oral hygiene may exist. Dimethyl sulfide can indicate an extraoral cause.[145] Just like the Halimeter, the OralChroma cannot detect compounds other than sulfur compounds, and some intraoral and extraoral causes can thus be overlooked. The apparatus needs calibration and the sensor and column need to be replaced every 2 years.[159]

Halimeter Versus OralChroma

Halimeter	OralChroma
Easy to handle	Easy to handle
Affordable	More expensive
Displays results immediately	Takes 4 min (CHM-2) or 8 min (CHM-1) before measurements are shown
Cannot discriminate among different gases	Can discriminate among hydrogen sulfide, methylmercaptan, and dimethyl sulfide
Maintenance needed	Maintenance needed

Dark-Field or Phase-Contrast Microscopy

Oral malodor is typically associated with a higher incidence of motile organisms and spirochetes, so shifts in their proportions allow monitoring of therapeutic progress. Another advantage of direct microscopy is that the patient becomes aware of bacteria present in plaque, tongue coating, and saliva. Too often, patients confuse plaque with food remnants.

Oropharyngeal Examination

The oropharyngeal examination includes inspection of deep carious lesions, interdental food impaction, wounds, bleeding of the gums, periodontal pockets, tongue coating, dry mouth, and the tonsils and pharynx (for tonsillitis and pharyngitis).

The tongue coating can be scored with regard to thickness and surface. Several methods have been proposed for thickness; Gross and coworkers in 1975[47] proposed an index ranging from 0 (no coating) to 3 (severe coating). Miyazaki[78] (Fig. 49.9A) assessed tongue-coating status according to area: 0 = none visible, 1 = less than one-third of the tongue dorsum covered, 2 = less than two-thirds, and 3 = more than two-thirds.

Winkel and coworkers[165] considered both the extension and the thickness of the tongue coating. The dorsum of the tongue is divided into six areas, three in the posterior and three in the anterior of the tongue (see Fig. 49.9B). The tongue coating in each sextant is scored as follows: 0 = no coating, 1 = light coating, and 2 = severe coating. A score of 1 is given when the pink color underneath the coating is still visible; when this is not the case, 2 is given.

Attention should be paid to the morphology of the tongue. For example, the clinician should note whether the tongue looks normal or rough or has a deep sulcus or large papillae vallatae.[165]

Self-Examination

Smelling one's own breath by expiring into the hands in front of the mouth is not relevant because the nose becomes used to the odor,[141] and the smell of the skin and soap used for handwashing may interfere. Moreover, studies have shown that self-assessment of oral malodor is notoriously unreliable, and one should be careful with such information obtained from the patient.[6,30]

CLINICIAN'S CORNER

When one of your patients complains of bad breath and he or she is periodontally healthy but has a thick tongue coating, what can you do?

You give the patient oral hygiene instruction and stress the importance of using a tongue scraper. Optionally, a mouthrinse can be advised, with active ingredients of proven efficacy such as chlorhexidine, cetylpyridinium chloride, or a zinc formulation.

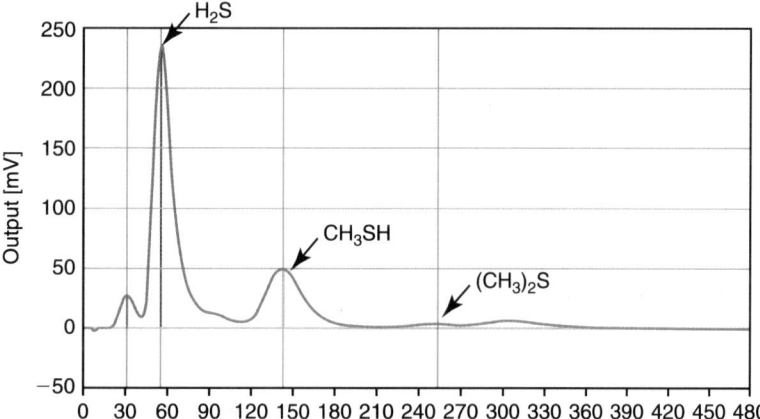

Fig. 49.8 Graphic from the OralChroma. The first peak indicates the level of hydrogen sulfide *(HS)*, the second the level of methylmercaptan *(CHSH)*, and the third the level of dimethyl sulfide *([CH]S). 2332*

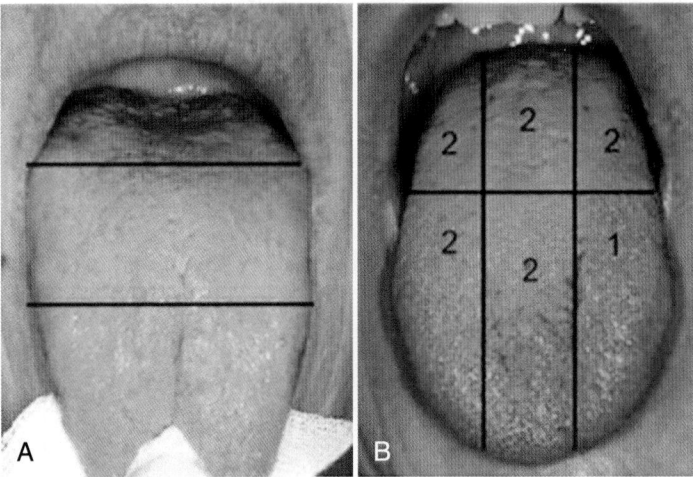

Fig. 49.9 (A) Miyazaki tongue coating index. Score 0 = none visible, score 1 = less than one-third of the tongue dorsum covered, score 2 = less than two-thirds, and score 3 = more than two-thirds; here score 2 applies because less than two-thirds of the tongue dorsum is covered. (B) Winkel tongue coating index. Divide the dorsum of the tongue into six areas, (i.e., three in the posterior and three in the anterior part of the tongue). The tongue coating in each sextant is scored as 0 = no coating, 1 = light coating, and 2 = severe coating.

Treatment of Oral Malodor

The treatment of oral malodor (with an intraoral origin) should preferably be cause related. Because oral malodor is caused by the metabolic degradation of available proteins to malodorous gases by certain oral microorganisms, the following general treatment strategies can be applied:

- Mechanical reduction of intraoral nutrients (substrates) and microorganisms
- Chemical reduction of oral microbial load
- Rendering malodorous gases nonvolatile
- Masking the malodor

Treatment should be centered on reducing the bacterial load and micronutrients by effective mechanical oral hygiene procedures, including tongue scraping. Periodontal disease should be treated and controlled, and as an auxiliary aid, oral rinses containing chlorhexidine and other ingredients may further reduce the oral malodor. If breath malodor persists after these approaches, other sources of the malodor, such as the tonsils, lung disease, gastrointestinal disease, or metabolic abnormalities (e.g., diabetes), should be investigated.

Mechanical Reduction of Intraoral Nutrients and Microorganisms

Because of the extensive accumulation of bacteria on the dorsum of the tongue, tongue cleaning should be emphasized.[15,126,168] Previous investigations demonstrated that tongue cleaning reduces both the amount of coating (and thus bacterial nutrients) and the number of bacteria and thereby improves oral malodor effectively.[25,40,41,47,111] Other reports indicated that the reduction of the microbial load on the tongue after cleaning is negligible and that the reduced malodor probably results from the reduction of bacterial nutrients.[76,106]

Cleaning of the tongue can be done with a normal toothbrush, but preferably with a tongue scraper if a coating is established.[93,95] Tongue cleaning using a tongue scraper reduces halitosis levels by 75% after 1 week.[95] This should be gentle cleaning to prevent soft tissue damage. It is best to clean as far backward as possible; the posterior portion of the tongue has the most coating.[123] Tongue cleaning should be repeated until almost no coating material can be removed.[16] The gagging reflex is often elicited, especially when using brushes[106];

practice helps to prevent this.[14] It can also be helpful to pull the tongue out with a gauze pad. Tongue cleaning has the additional benefit of improving taste sensation.[106,166]

Interdental cleaning and toothbrushing are essential mechanical means of dental plaque control. Both remove residual food particles and organisms that cause putrefaction. Clinical studies have shown that the mechanical action of toothbrushing alone has no appreciable influence on the concentration of VSCs.[143] In a short-term study, Tonzetich[150] showed a short-term effect on bad breath after brushing with a sodium monofluorophosphate toothpaste. However, the effect was half of what was observed when combined with tongue brushing (73% and 30% reduction in VSCs, respectively).[150]

When chronic oral malodor arises as a consequence of periodontitis, professional periodontal therapy is needed.[8,18,96,169] A one-stage full-mouth disinfection, combining scaling and root planing with the application of chlorhexidine, reduced organoleptic malodor levels up to 90% in one study.[108] In another study by the same investigators, initial periodontal therapy had only a weak impact on VSC levels, except when combined with a mouthrinse containing chlorhexidine.[109]

Chewing gum may control bad breath temporarily because it can stimulate salivary flow.[114] The salivary flow itself also has a mechanical cleaning capability. Not surprisingly, therefore, subjects with extremely low salivary flow rate have higher VSC ratings and tongue coating scores than those with normal saliva production.[64] Waler[161] showed that chewing gum without any active ingredient can reduce halitosis modestly.

Chemical Reduction of Oral Microbial Load

Together with toothbrushing, mouth rinsing has become a common oral hygiene practice.[38] Formulations have been modified to carry antimicrobial and oxidizing agents, impacting the process of oral malodor formation. The active ingredients usually include antimicrobial agents such as chlorhexidine, cetylpyridinium chloride (CPC), essential oils, chlorine dioxide, triclosan, amine fluoride and stannous fluoride, hydrogen peroxide, and baking soda. Some of these agents have only a temporary effect on the total number of microorganisms in the oral cavity.

Chlorhexidine

Chlorhexidine is considered the most effective antiplaque and antigingivitis agent.[1-3,5,56] Its antibacterial action can be explained by disruption of the bacterial cell membrane by the chlorhexidine molecules, thus increasing its permeability and resulting in cell lysis and death.[56,68] Because of its strong antibacterial effects and superior substantivity in the oral cavity, chlorhexidine rinsing provides significant reductions in VSC levels and organoleptic ratings.[12,120,122,153,171]

Unfortunately, as mentioned in some trials, chlorhexidine at a concentration of 0.2% or greater also has some disadvantages, such as increased tooth and tongue staining, unpleasant taste, and some temporary reduction in taste sensation.[32]

Essential Oils

Previous studies evaluated the short-term effect (3 hours) of a Listerine rinse (which contains essential oils) compared with a placebo rinse.[101] Listerine was found to be only moderately effective against oral malodor (±25% reduction vs. 10% for placebo of VSCs after 30 minutes) and caused a sustained reduction in the levels of odorigenic bacteria. Similar VSC reductions were found after rinsing for 4 days.[12]

Chlorine Dioxide

Chlorine dioxide (ClO_2) is a powerful oxidizing agent that can eliminate bad breath by oxidation of hydrogen sulfide, methylmercaptan, and the amino acids methionine and cysteine. Studies demonstrated that a single use of a chlorine dioxide–containing oral rinse slightly reduced mouth odor.[34,35]

Two-Phase Oil-Water Rinse

Rosenberg and colleagues[120] designed a two-phase oil-water rinse containing CPC. The efficacy of oil-water-CPC formulations is thought to result from the adhesion of a high proportion of oral microorganisms to the oil droplets that is further enhanced by the CPC. A twice-daily rinse with this product (before bedtime and in the morning) showed reductions in both VSC levels and organoleptic ratings. These reductions were superior to those seen with Listerine and were significantly superior to placebo.[65,120]

Triclosan

Triclosan, a broad-spectrum antibacterial agent, has been found to be effective against most oral bacteria and has good compatibility with other compounds used for oral home care. A pilot study demonstrated that an experimental mouthrinse containing 0.15% triclosan and 0.84% zinc (Zn^{++}) produced a stronger and more prolonged reduction in mouth odor than Listerine rinse.[113] The anti-VSC effect of triclosan, however, seems strongly dependent on the solubilizing agents.[170] Flavoring oils or anionic detergents and copolymers are added to increase the oral retention and decrease the rate of release in toothpaste formulations containing triclosan. The effects of these formulations in oral malodor have been illustrated in several studies.[53,89,90,132,133] Significant reduction of breath scores were observed after a single use as well as after a week (28% and >50%, respectively), with a similar effect on VSC levels (57% reduction after 1 week of using the paste).

Amine Fluoride or Stannous Fluoride

The association of amine fluoride with stannous fluoride resulted in encouraging reductions of morning breath odor, even when oral hygiene was insufficient.[105] More recent evidence supporting the use of this rinse has become available. The formulation showed not only short-term but also long-term effects on malodor indicators in patients with obvious malodor.[22]

Stannous fluoride has also been shown to be effective in the management of oral malodor as a component of a dentifrice, reducing both organoleptic scores and VSC levels.[39] A superior short-term and overnight benefit of a stannous-containing dentifrice versus a control dentifrice on morning bad breath was demonstrated in a meta-analysis.[33]

Hydrogen Peroxide

Suarez and colleagues[143] reported that rinsing with 3% hydrogen peroxide (H_2O_2) produced impressive reductions (±90%) in sulfur gases that persisted for 8 hours.

Oxidizing Lozenges

Greenstein and associates[46] reported that sucking a lozenge with oxidizing properties reduced tongue dorsum malodor for 3 hours. This antimalodor effect may be caused by the activity of dehydro-ascorbic acid, which is generated by peroxide-mediated oxidation of ascorbate in the lozenges.

Baking Soda

Baking soda dentifrices have been shown to confer a significant odor-reducing benefit for up to 3 hours.[11,88] The mechanism by which baking soda produces its inhibition of oral malodor is related to its bactericidal effects.[103]

Conversion of Volatile Sulfur Compounds
Metal Salt Solutions

Metal ions with an affinity for sulfur are efficient in capturing the sulfur-containing gases. Zinc is an ion with two positive charges (Zn^{++}), which will bind to the twice-negatively loaded sulfur radicals and thus reduce the expression of VSCs. The same applies for other metal ions such as stannous, mercury, and copper. Clinically, the VSC inhibitory effect was copper chloride > stannous fluoride > zinc chloride ($CuCl_2 > SnF_2 > ZnCl_2$). In vitro, the inhibitory effect was mercury chloride = copper chloride = cadmium chloride > zinc chloride > stannous fluoride > tin chloride > lead chloride ($HgCl_2 = CuCl_2 = CdCl_2 > ZnCl_2 > SnF_2 > SnCl_2 > PbCl_2$).[172]

Compared with other metal ions, Zn^{++} is relatively nontoxic and noncumulative and gives no visible discoloration. Thus, Zn^{++} has been one of the most-studied ingredients for the control of oral malodor.[161,172] Schmidt and Tarbet[127] reported that a rinse containing zinc chloride was remarkably more effective than a saline rinse (or no treatment) in reducing the levels of both VSCs (±80% reduction) and organoleptic scores (±40% reduction) for 3 hours.

As mentioned, Halita, a rinse containing 0.05% chlorhexidine, 0.05% CPC, and 0.14% zinc lactate, has been even more efficient than a 0.2% chlorhexidine formulation in reducing VSC levels and organoleptic ratings.[110,153] The special effect of Halita may result from the VSC conversion ability of Zn^{++}, besides its antimicrobial action. The combination of Zn^{++} and chlorhexidine seems to act synergistically.[171]

Similar observations have been reported for a chlorhexidine-free mouthrinse. The addition of zinc ions to a basic formulation containing amino fluoride and stannous fluoride caused short- and long-term reduction of oral malodor indicators in volunteers with morning bad breath[163,164] as well as in volunteers with obvious halitosis.[22]

In a study by Hoshi and van Steenberghe,[52] a zinc citrate/triclosan toothpaste applied to the tongue dorsum appeared to control morning breath malodor for 4 hours. If the flavor oil was removed, however, the antimalodor efficacy of the active ingredients decreased. Another clinical study reported up to a 41% reduction in VSC levels after 7 days' use of a dentifrice containing triclosan and a copolymer, but the benefit compared with a placebo was relatively small (17%

reduction).[90] Similar reductions were also found in two other more recent studies.[53,89]

Chewing gum can be formulated with antibacterial agents, such as fluoride or chlorhexidine, helping to reduce oral malodor through both mechanical and chemical approaches. Tsunoda and associates[151] investigated the beneficial effect of chewing gum containing tea extracts for its deodorizing mechanism. *Epigallocatechin* is the main deodorizing agent among the tea catechins. The chemical reaction between epigallocatechin and methylmercaptan results in a nonvolatile product. Waler[161] compared different concentrations of Zn^{++} in a chewing gum and found that a 2-mg Zn^{++} acetate–containing chewing gum that remained in the mouth for 5 minutes resulted in an immediate reduction in VSC levels of up to 45%, but the long-term effect was not mentioned.

Masking the Malodor

Treatment with rinses, mouth sprays, or lozenges containing volatiles with a pleasant odor has only a short-term effect.[114,115] Typical examples are mint-containing lozenges and the aroma of rinses without antibacterial components.[22]

Another pathway is to increase the solubility of malodorous compounds in the saliva by increasing the secretion of saliva; a larger volume allows the retention of larger volumes of soluble VSCs.[62] The latter can also be achieved by ensuring proper liquid intake or using chewing gum; chewing triggers the periodontal-parotid reflex, at least when the lower (pre)molars are still present.

Conclusion

Breath malodor has important socioeconomic consequences and can reveal important diseases. A proper diagnosis and determination of the etiology allow initiation of the proper etiologic treatment. Although tongue coating and (less frequently) periodontitis and gingivitis are by far the most common causes of malodor, a clinician cannot take the risk of overlooking other, more challenging diseases. This can be done with a multidisciplinary consultation or, if this is not feasible, a trial therapy to deal quickly with intraoral causes (e.g., full-mouth one-stage disinfection, including the use of proper mouthrinses, tongue scrapers, and toothpastes). For more detailed information, the reader is encouraged to consult review articles.[45,69,131]

 A Case Scenario is found on the companion website www.expertconsult.com.

References

 References for this chapter are found on the companion website www.expertconsult.com.

CHAPTER 50

Scaling and Root Planing*

Anna M. Pattison | Gordon L. Pattison

CHAPTER OUTLINE

Classification of Periodontal Instruments
General Principles of Instrumentation *(e-only)*
Principles of Scaling and Root Planing *(e-only)*
Instrument Sharpening *(e-only)*

 For online-only content on general principles of instrumentation, principles of scaling and root planing, and instrument sharpening, please visit the companion website at www.expertconsult.com.

Periodontal instruments are designed for specific purposes, such as calculus removal, biofilm removal, and root planing. On first investigation, the variety of instruments available for similar purposes appears confusing. With experience, however, clinicians select a relatively small set that fulfills all requirements.

Classification of Periodontal Instruments

Periodontal instruments are classified according to the purposes they serve, as follows:

1. *Periodontal probes* are used to locate, measure, and mark pockets, as well as determine their course on individual tooth surfaces.
2. *Explorers* are used to locate calculus deposits and caries.
3. *Scaling, root-planing, and curettage instruments* are used for removal of biofilm and calcified deposits from the crown and root of a tooth, removal of altered cementum from the subgingival root surface, and debridement of the soft tissue lining the pocket. Scaling and curettage instruments are classified as follows:
   - *Sickle scalers* are heavy instruments used to remove supragingival calculus.
   - *Curettes* are fine instruments used for subgingival scaling, root planing, and removal of the soft tissue lining the pocket.
   - *Hoe, chisel, and file scalers* are used to remove tenacious subgingival calculus and altered cementum. Their use is limited compared with that of curettes.
   - *Implant instruments* are plastic or titanium scalers and curettes designed for use on implants and implant restorations.
   - *Ultrasonic and sonic instruments* are used for scaling and cleansing tooth surfaces and curetting the soft tissue wall of the periodontal pocket.[42,43,66]
4. *Periodontal endoscopes* are used for deep visualization into subgingival pockets and furcations, thereby allowing the detection of deposits.
5. *Cleansing and polishing instruments,* such as rubber cups, brushes, and dental tape, are used to clean and polish tooth surfaces.

Air-powder abrasive systems are also available for supragingival and subgingival cleaning and polishing of tooth, root, and implant surfaces.

The wearing and cutting qualities of some types of steel used in periodontal instruments have been tested,[88,89,157] but specifications vary among manufacturers.[157] Stainless steel is used most often in instrument manufacture. High–carbon content steel instruments are available and are considered by some clinicians to be superior. Newer advanced proprietary manufacturing processes for heat treating and cryogenically tempering stainless steel are producing blades that are sharper and longer lasting than ever before. In addition, other processes produce stainless steel instruments with titanium nitride or other surface coatings that are not embedded or diffused into the base material. Their cutting edges are sharp when new, but these coatings wear down during normal use and cannot be resharpened. Each group of instruments has characteristic features; individual therapists often develop variations with which they operate most effectively. Small instruments are recommended to fit into periodontal pockets without injuring the soft tissues.[116,118,119,174]

The parts of each instrument are referred to as the working end, shank, and handle (Fig. 50.1).

Periodontal Probes

Periodontal probes are used to measure the depth of pockets and to determine their configuration. The typical probe is a tapered, rodlike instrument calibrated in millimeters, with a blunt, rounded tip (Fig. 50.2). Several other designs with various millimeter calibrations are available (Fig. 50.3). The World Health Organization probe has millimeter markings and a small, round ball at the tip (Fig. 50.3E). Ideally, these probes are thin, and the shank is angled to allow easy insertion into the pocket. Furcation areas can best be evaluated with the curved, blunt Nabers probe (Fig. 50.4).

LEARNING BOX 50.1

Periodontal probes are used to measure the depth of pockets and to determine their configuration.

---

*Material in this chapter was derived from Pattison A, Pattison G, Matsuda S: *Periodontal instrumentation,* ed 3, New York, 2018, Pearson Education.

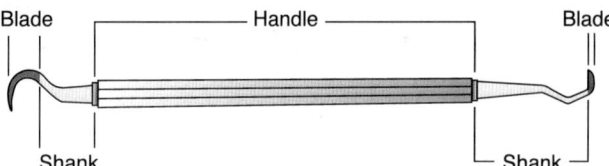

Fig. 50.1 Parts of a typical periodontal instrument.

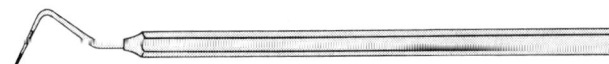

Fig. 50.2 Periodontal probe is composed of the handle, shank, and calibrated working end.

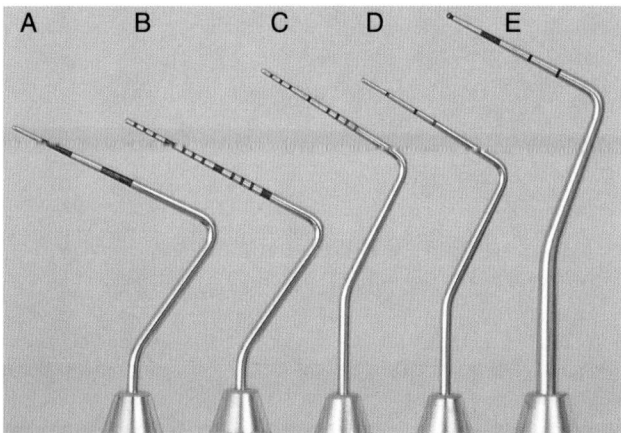

Fig. 50.3 Types of periodontal probes. *A,* Marquis color-coded probe. Calibrations are in 3-mm sections. *B,* University of North Carolina 15 probe, a 15-mm long probe marked at each millimeter and color coded at the 5th, 10th, and 15th millimeters. *C,* University of Michigan "O" probe, with Williams markings (at 1, 2, 3, 5, 7, 8, 9, and 10 mm). *D,* Michigan "O" probe with markings at 3, 6, and 8 mm. *E,* World Health Organization probe, which has a 0.5-mm ball at the tip and markings at 3.5, 8.5, and 11.5 mm and color coding from 3.5 to 5.5 mm.

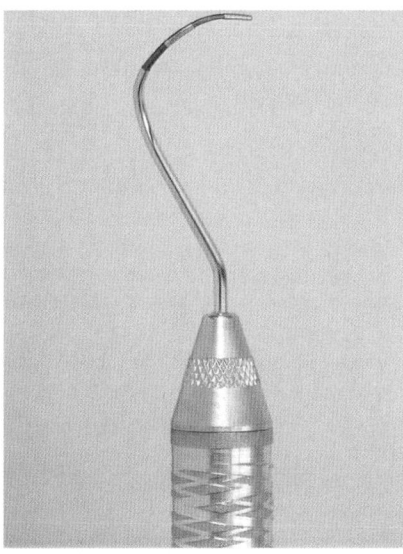

Fig. 50.4 Curved #2 Nabers probe for detection of furcation areas, with color-coded markings at 3, 6, 9, and 12 mm.

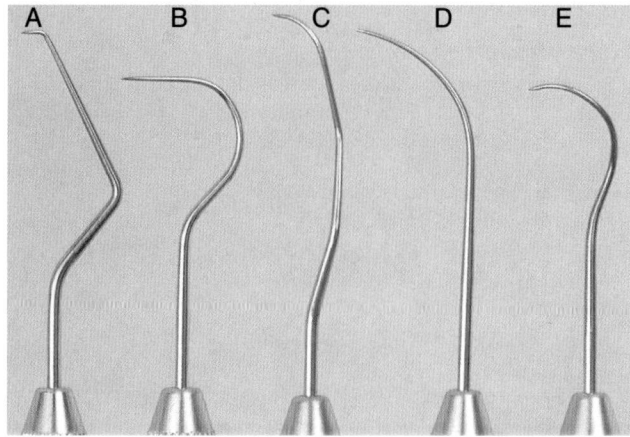

Fig. 50.5 Five typical explorers. *A,* #17; *B,* #23; *C,* EXD 11-12; *D,* #3; *E,* #3CH pigtail.

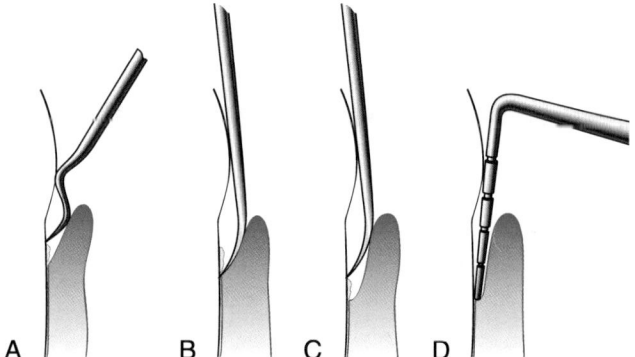

Fig. 50.6 Insertion of two types of explorers and a periodontal probe in a pocket for calculus detection. (A) The limitations of the pigtail explorer in a deep pocket. (B) Insertion of the #3 explorer. (C) Limitations of the #3 explorer. (D) Insertion of the periodontal probe.

When measuring a pocket, the probe is inserted with firm, gentle pressure to the bottom of the pocket. The shank should be aligned with the long axis of the tooth surface to be probed. Several measurements are made to determine the level of attachment along the surface of the tooth.

Explorers

Explorers are used to locate subgingival deposits and carious areas and to check the smoothness of the root surfaces after root planing. Explorers are designed with different shapes and angles, with various uses (Fig. 50.5), as well as limitations (Fig. 50.6). The periodontal probe can also be useful in the detection of subgingival deposits (Fig. 50.6D).

Scaling and Curettage Instruments

Scaling and curettage instruments are illustrated in Fig. 50.7.

Sickle Scalers

Sickle scalers have a flat surface and two cutting edges that converge in a sharply pointed tip. The shape of the instrument makes the tip strong so that it will not break off during use (Fig. 50.8). The sickle

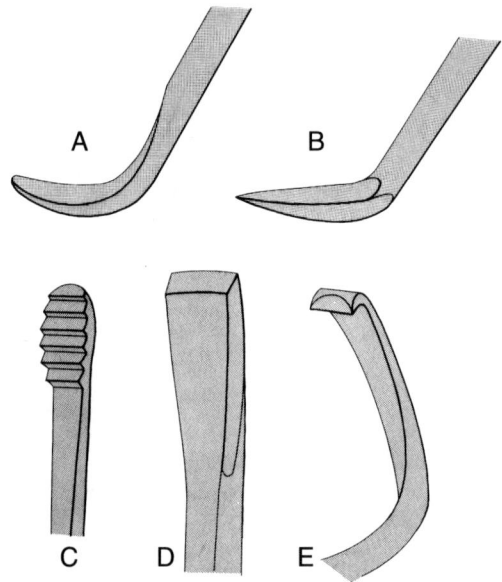

Fig. 50.7 The five basic scaling instruments. (A) Curette; (B) sickle; (C) file; (D) chisel; (E) hoe.

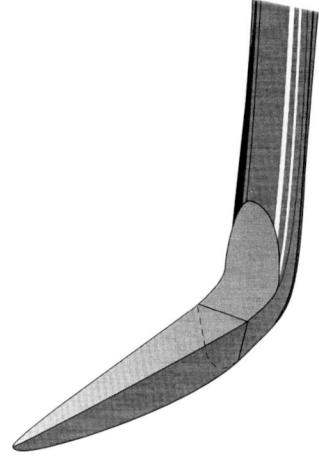

Fig. 50.8 Basic characteristics of a sickle scaler: triangular shape, double-cutting edge, and pointed tip.

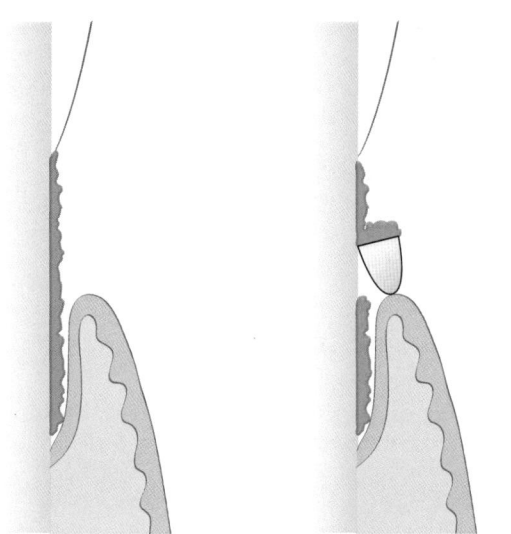

Fig. 50.9 Use of a sickle scaler for removal of supragingival calculus.

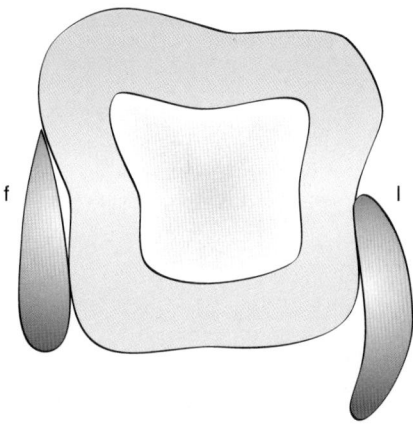

Fig. 50.10 Subgingival adaptation around the root is better with the curette than with the sickle. *f*, Facial; *l*, lingual.

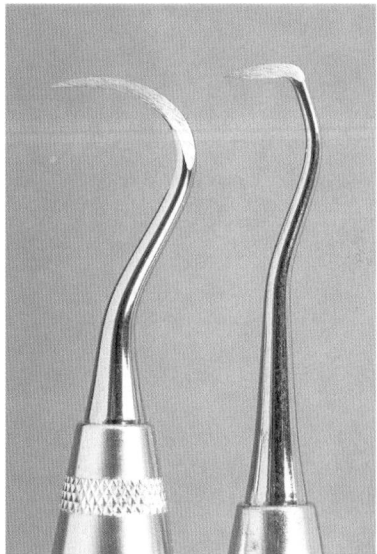

Fig. 50.11 Both ends of a U15/30 scaler.

scaler is used primarily to remove supragingival calculus (Fig. 50.9). Because of the design of this instrument, it is difficult to insert a large sickle blade under the gingiva without damaging the surrounding gingival tissues (Fig. 50.10). Small, curved sickle scaler blades such as the 204SD can be inserted under ledges of calculus several millimeters below the gingiva. Sickle scalers are used with a pull stroke.

Sickle scalers of the same basic design can be obtained with different blade sizes and shank types to adapt to specific uses. The U15/30 (Fig. 50.11), Ball, and Indiana University sickle scalers are large. Jaquette sickle scalers #1, #2, and #3 have medium-size blades. Curved 204 posterior sickle scalers are available with large, medium, or small blades (Fig. 50.12). The Montana Jack sickle scaler and the Nevi 2, Nevi 3, and Nevi 4 curved posterior sickle scalers are all thin enough to be inserted several millimeters subgingivally for removal of light to moderate ledges of calculus. The selection of these instruments should be based on the area to be scaled. Sickle scalers with straight shanks are designed for use on anterior teeth and premolars. Sickle scalers with contra-angled shanks adapt to posterior teeth.

Curettes

The curette is the instrument of choice for removing deep subgingival calculus, root planing altered cementum, and removing the soft tissue lining the periodontal pocket (Fig. 50.13). Each working end has a

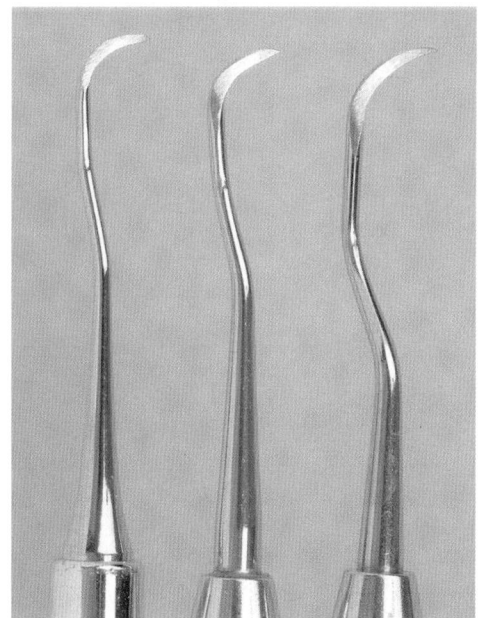

Fig. 50.12 Three different sizes of 204 sickle scalers.

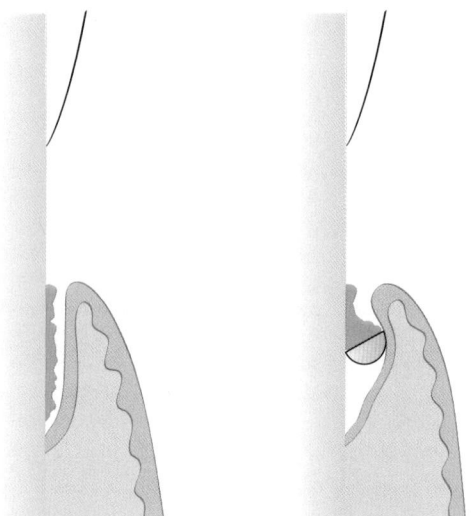

Fig. 50.13 The curette is the instrument of choice for subgingival scaling and root planing.

cutting edge on both sides of the blade and a rounded toe. Curettes are finer than sickle scalers and do not have any sharp points or corners other than the cutting edges of the blade (Fig. 50.14). Therefore curettes can be adapted for and provide good access to deep pockets, with minimal soft tissue trauma (see Fig. 50.10). In cross section, the blade appears semicircular with a convex base. The lateral border of the convex base forms a cutting edge with the face of the semi-circular blade. Cutting edges are present on both sides of the blade. Both single- and double-end curettes may be obtained, depending on the preference of the operator.

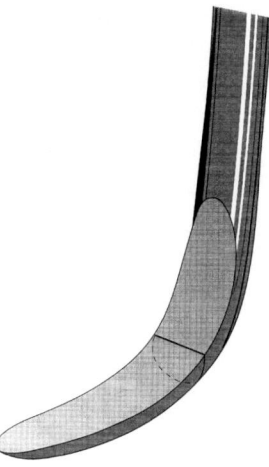

Fig. 50.14 Basic characteristics of a curette: spoon-shaped blade and rounded tip.

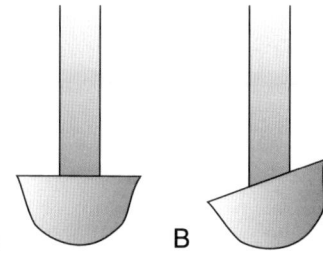

Fig. 50.15 Principal types of curettes as seen from the toe of the instrument. (A) Universal curette. (B) Gracey curette. Note the offset blade angulation of the Gracey curette.

As shown in Fig. 50.10, the curved blade and rounded toe of the curette allow the blade to adapt better to the root surface, unlike the straight design and pointed end of a sickle scaler, which can cause tissue laceration and trauma. The two basic types of curettes are universal and area specific.

Universal Curettes

Universal curettes have cutting edges that may be inserted in most areas of the dentition by altering and adapting the finger rest, fulcrum, and hand position of the operator. The blade size and the angle and length of the shank may vary, but the face of the blade of every universal curette is at a 90-degree angle (perpendicular) to the lower shank when seen in cross section from the tip (Fig. 50.15A). The blade of the universal curette is curved in one direction from the head of the blade toward the toe. Barnhart curettes #1-2 and #5-6 and Columbia curettes #13-14, #2R-2L, and #4R-4L (Figs. 50.16 and 50.17A) are examples of universal curettes. Other popular universal curettes are Younger-Good #7-8, McCall's #17-18, and Indiana University #17-18 (Fig. 50.17B).

Area-Specific Curettes

Gracey Curettes. Gracey curettes are representative of the area-specific curettes, a set of several instruments designed and angled

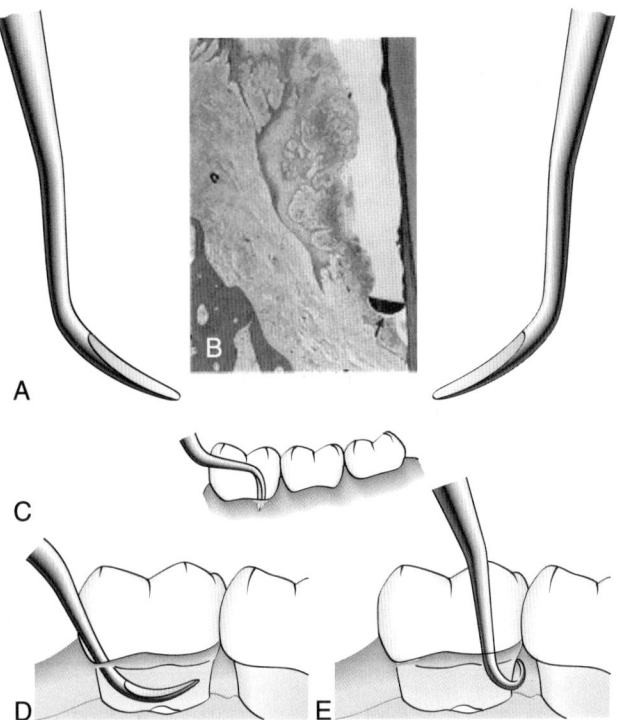

Fig. 50.16 (A) Double-ended curette for the removal of subgingival calculus. (B) Cross section of the curette blade *(arrow)* against the cemental wall of a deep periodontal pocket. (C) Curette inserted in a pocket with the tip directed apically. (D) Curette in position at the base of a periodontal pocket on the facial surface of a mandibular molar. (E) Curette in position at the base of a pocket on the distal surface of the mandibular molar.

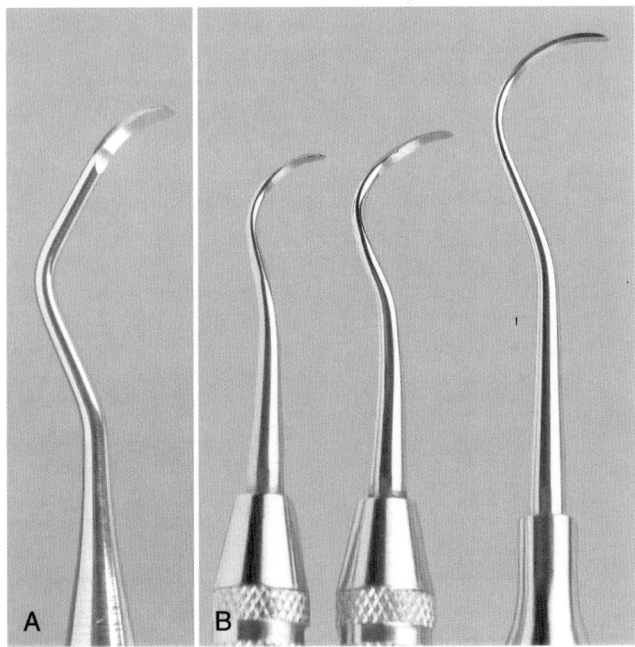

Fig. 50.17 (A) Columbia #4R-4L universal curette. (B) Younger-Good #7-8, McCall's #17-18, and Indiana University #17-18 universal curettes.

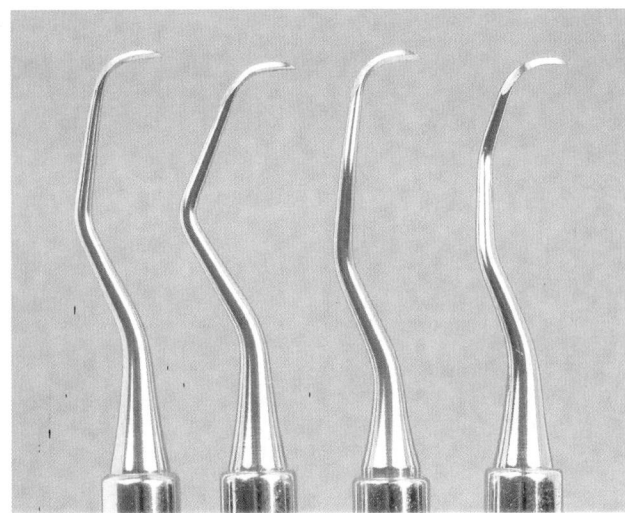

Fig. 50.18 Reduced set of Gracey curettes. *Left to right,* #5-6, #7-8, #11-12, and #13-14.

to adapt to specific anatomic areas of the dentition (Fig. 50.18). These curettes and their modifications are probably the best instruments for subgingival scaling and root planing because they provide the best adaptation to complex root anatomy.

LEARNING BOX 50.5

Gracey curettes are representative of the area-specific curettes, a set of several instruments designed and angled to adapt to specific anatomic areas of the dentition.

Double-ended Gracey curettes are paired in the following manner:
Gracey #1-2 and #3-4: Anterior teeth
Gracey #5-6: Anterior teeth and premolars
Gracey #7-8 and #9-10: Posterior teeth, facial and lingual
Gracey #11-12: Posterior teeth, mesial (Fig. 50.19)
Gracey #13-14: Posterior teeth, distal (Fig. 50.20)

Single-ended Gracey curettes can also be obtained; a set comprises 14 instruments. Although these curettes are designed to be used in specific areas, an experienced operator can adapt each instrument for use in several different areas by altering the position of his or her hand and the position of the patient.

Gracey curettes also differ from universal curettes in that the blade is not at a 90-degree angle to the lower shank. The term *offset blade* is used to describe Gracey curettes because they are angled approximately 70 degrees from the lower shank (see Fig. 50.15B). This unique angulation allows the blade to be inserted in the precise position necessary for subgingival scaling and root planing, provided the lower shank is parallel to the long axis of the tooth surface being scaled.

LEARNING BOX 50.6

Gracey curettes also differ from universal curettes in that the blade is not at a 90-degree angle to the lower shank.

Area-specific curettes also have curved blades. Whereas the blade of the universal curette is curved in one direction (Fig. 50.21A), the Gracey blade is curved from shank to toe and also appears to be curved along the side of the cutting edge (Fig. 50.21B).

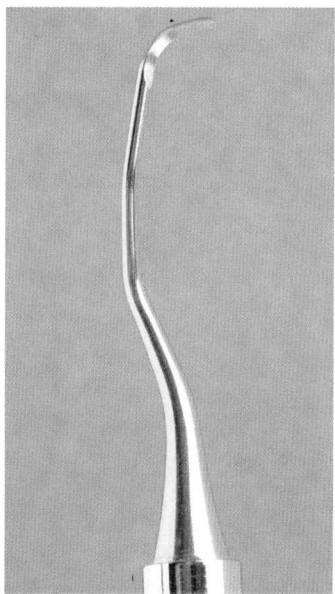

Fig. 50.19 Gracey #11-12 curette. For mesial surfaces.

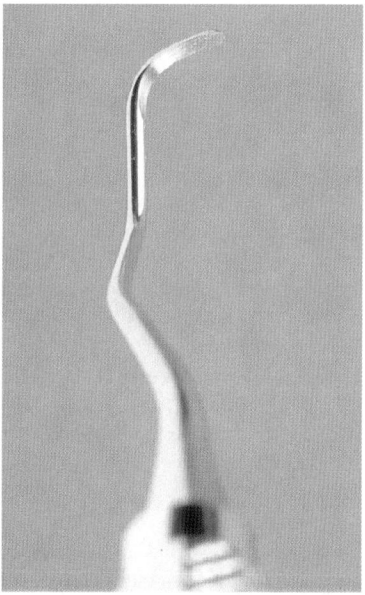

Fig. 50.20 Gracey #13-14 curette. For distal surfaces.

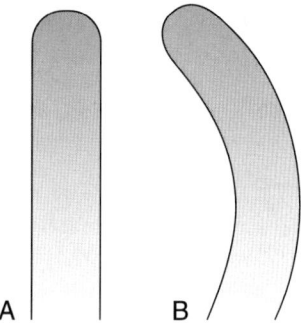

Fig. 50.21 (A) Universal curette as seen with the face of the blade parallel to the floor. Note that the blade is straight. (B) Gracey curette as seen with the face of the blade parallel to the floor. Only the outer convex cutting edge is used.

TABLE 50.1 Comparison of Area-Specific (Gracey) and Universal Curettes

	Gracey Curette	Universal Curette
Area of use	Set of many curettes designed for specific areas and surfaces	One curette designed for all areas and surfaces
Cutting Edge		
Use	One cutting edge used; work with outer edge only	Both cutting edges used; work with either outer or inner edge
Curvature	Blade curves from the shank toward the toe and also appears to curve to the side	Blade curves only from the shank toward the toe, not to the side
Blade angle	Offset blade; face of blade beveled at 60 degrees to shank	Blade not offset; face of blade beveled at 90 degrees to shank

Modified from Pattison G, Pattison A: *Periodontal instrumentation*, ed 2, Norwalk, CT, 1992, Appleton & Lange.

Table 50.1 lists some of the major differences between Gracey (area-specific) curettes and universal curettes.

Gracey curettes are available with either a "rigid" or "finishing" type of shank. The rigid Gracey has a larger, stronger, and less flexible shank and blade than the standard finishing Gracey. The rigid shank allows the removal of moderate to heavy calculus without using a separate set of heavy scalers, such as sickles and hoes. Although some clinicians prefer the enhanced tactile sensitivity that the flexible shank of the finishing Gracey provides, both types of Gracey curettes are suitable for root planing.

More recent additions to the Gracey curette set have been #15-16 and #17-18. The Gracey #15-16 is a modification of the standard #11-12 and is designed for the mesial surfaces of posterior teeth (Fig. 50.22). It consists of a Gracey #11-12 blade combined with the more acutely angled #13-14 shank. When the clinician is using an intraoral finger rest, it is often difficult to position the lower shank of the Gracey #11-12 so that it is parallel to the mesial surfaces of the posterior teeth, especially on the mandibular molars. The newer shank angulation of the Gracey #15-16 allows better adaptation to posterior mesial surfaces from a front position with intraoral rests. If alternative fulcrums, such as extraoral or opposite-arch rests, are used, the Gracey #11-12 works well and the #15-16 is not essential. The Gracey #17-18 is a modification of the #13-14. It has a terminal shank elongated by 3 mm and a more accentuated angulation of the shank to provide complete occlusal clearance and better access to all posterior distal surfaces. The horizontal handle position minimizes interference from opposing arches and allows a more relaxed hand position when scaling distal surfaces. In addition, the blade is 1 mm shorter to allow better adaptation of the blade to distal tooth surfaces.

Extended-Shank Curettes. Extended-shank curettes, such as *After Five* curettes (Hu-Friedy, Chicago, IL), are modifications of the standard Gracey curette design. The terminal shank is 3 mm longer, allowing extension into deeper periodontal pockets of 5 mm or more (Figs. 50.23 and 50.24). Other features of After Five curettes include a thinned blade for smoother subgingival insertion and reduced tissue distention and a large-diameter, tapered shank. All standard Gracey numbers except for the #9-10 (i.e., #1-2, #3-4, #5-6, #7-8, #11-12, or #13-14) are available in the After Five series.

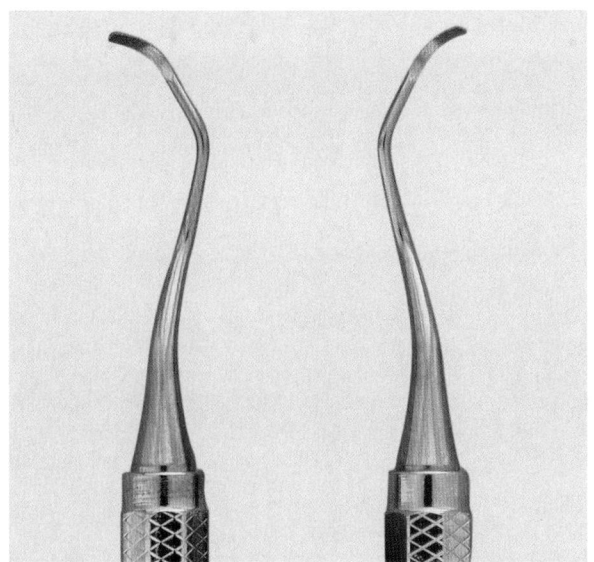

Fig. 50.22 Gracey #15-16. New Gracey curette, designed for mesioposterior surfaces, combines a Gracey #11-12 blade with a Gracey #13-14 shank. (Copyright A. Pattison.)

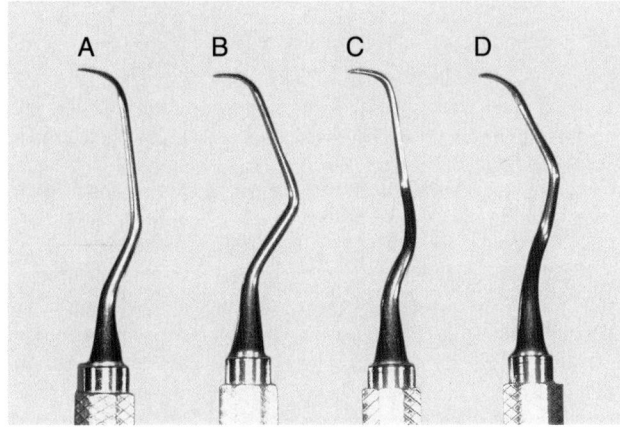

Fig. 50.23 After Five curettes. Note the extra 3 mm in the terminal shank of After Five curettes compared with standard Gracey curettes. *A*, #5-6; *B*, #7-8; *C*, #11-12; *D*, #13-14. (Copyright A. Pattison.)

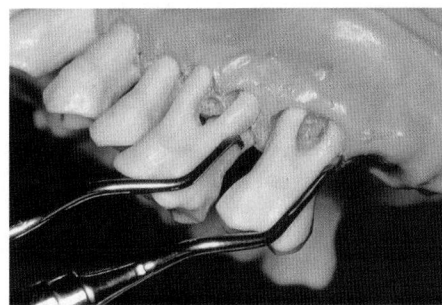

Fig. 50.24 Comparison of After Five curette with standard Gracey curette. Rigid Gracey #13-14 adapted to the distal surface of the first molar and rigid After Five #13-14 adapted to the distal surface of the second molar. Notice the extralong shank of the After Five curette, which allows deeper insertion and better access. (Copyright A. Pattison.)

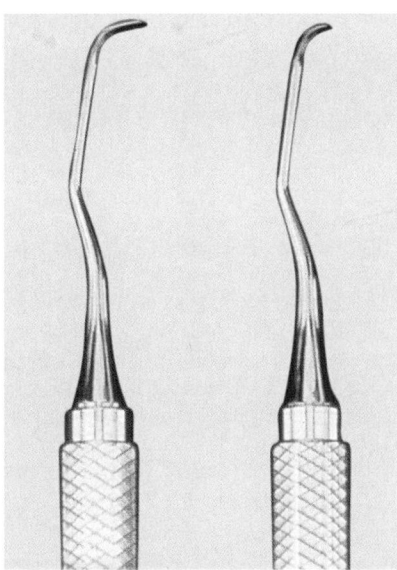

Fig. 50.25 Comparison of After Five curette and Mini Five curette. The shorter Mini Five blade (half the length) allows increased access and reduced tissue trauma.

After Five curettes are available in finishing or rigid designs. For heavy or tenacious calculus removal, rigid After Five curettes should be used. For light scaling or deplaquing in a periodontal maintenance patient, the thinner finishing After Five curettes will insert subgingivally more easily.

LEARNING BOX 50.7

Extended-shank curettes, such as After Five curettes (Hu-Friedy, Chicago, IL), are modifications of the standard Gracey curette design.

Mini-Bladed Curettes. Mini-bladed curettes, such as Hu-Friedy *Mini Five* curettes, are modifications of the After Five curettes. Mini Five curettes feature blades that are half the length of After Five or standard Gracey curettes (Fig. 50.25). The shorter blade allows easier insertion and adaptation in deep, narrow pockets; furcations; developmental grooves; line angles; and deep, tight facial, lingual, or palatal pockets. In any area where root morphology or tight tissue prevents full insertion of the standard Gracey or After Five blade, Mini Five curettes can be used with vertical strokes, with reduced tissue distention and no tissue trauma (Fig. 50.26).

LEARNING BOX 50.8

Mini Five curettes (Hu-Friedy, Chicago, IL) feature blades that are half the length of After Five or standard Gracey curettes. The shorter blade allows easier insertion and adaptation in deep, narrow pockets; furcations; developmental grooves; line angles; and deep, tight facial, lingual, or palatal pockets.

In the past the only solution in most of these areas of difficult access was to use Gracey curettes with a toe-down horizontal stroke. Mini Five curettes, along with other short-bladed instruments recently introduced, opened a new chapter in the history of root instrumentation by allowing access to areas that previously were extremely difficult or impossible to reach with standard instruments. Mini Five curettes are available in both finishing and rigid designs. Rigid Mini Five curettes are recommended for calculus removal.

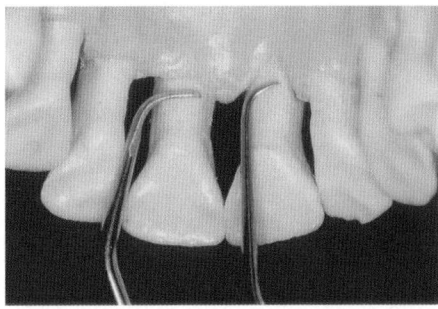

Fig. 50.26 Comparison of standard rigid Gracey #5-6 with rigid Mini Five #5-6 on the palatal surfaces of the maxillary central incisors. Mini Five curette can be inserted to the base of these tight anterior pockets and used with a straight vertical stroke. The standard Gracey or After Five curette usually cannot be inserted vertically in this area because the blade is too long. (Copyright A. Pattison.)

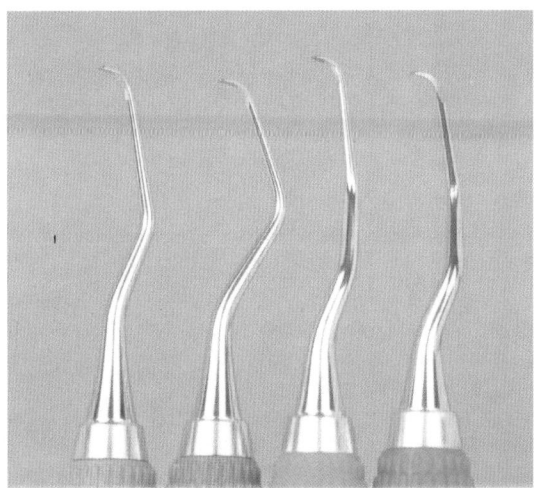

Fig. 50.27 Micro Mini Five Gracey curettes. *Left to right,* #1-2, #7-8, #11-12, #13-14. (Copyright A. Pattison.)

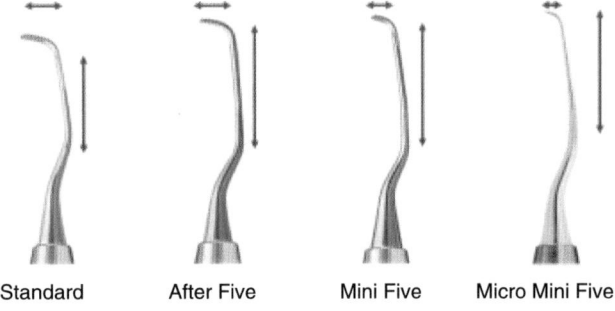

Standard   After Five   Mini Five   Micro Mini Five

Fig. 50.28 Comparison of Gracey curette designs. *Left to right,* Standard #1-2, After Five #1-2, Mini Five #1-2, Micro Mini Five #1-2. (Courtesy Hu-Friedy, Chicago, IL.)

The more flexible shanked finishing Mini Five curettes are appropriate for light scaling and deplaquing in periodontal maintenance patients with tight pockets. As with the After Five series, Mini Five curettes are available in all standard Gracey numbers, except the #9-10.

The recently introduced *Micro Mini Five* Gracey curettes (Hu-Friedy) have blades that are 20% thinner and smaller than the Mini Five curettes (Figs. 50.27 and 50.28). These are the smallest of all curettes, and they provide exceptional access and adaptation to tight, deep, or narrow pockets; narrow furcations; developmental

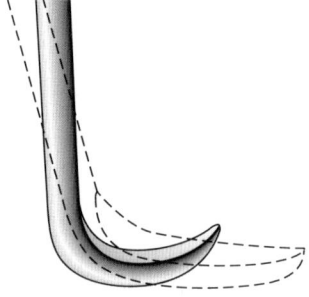

Fig. 50.29 Gracey Curvette blade. This diagram shows the 50% shorter blade of the Gracey Curvette superimposed on the standard Gracey curette blade *(dotted lines)*. Notice the upward curvature of the Curvette blade and blade tip. *(Redrawn from Pattison G, Pattison A: Periodontal instrumentation, ed 2, Norwalk, CT, 1992, Appleton & Lange.)*

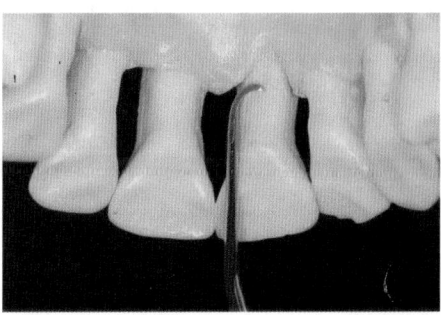

Fig. 50.30 Gracey Curvette Sub-0 on the palatal surface of a maxillary central incisor. The long shank and short, curved, blunted tip make this a superior instrument for deep anterior pockets. This curette provides excellent blade adaptation to the narrow root curvatures of the maxillary and mandibular anterior teeth. *(Copyright A. Pattison.)*

depressions; line angles; and deep pockets on facial, lingual, or palatal surfaces. In areas where root morphology or tight, thin tissue prevents easy insertion of other mini-bladed curettes, Micro Mini Five curettes can be used with vertical strokes without causing tissue distention or tissue trauma.

Gracey Curvettes comprise another set of four mini-bladed curettes; the Sub-0 and #1-2 are used for anterior teeth and premolars, the #11-12 is used for posterior mesial surfaces, and the #13-14 is used for posterior distal surfaces. The blade length of these instruments is 50% shorter than that of the conventional Gracey curette, and the blade is curved slightly upward (Fig. 50.29). This curvature allows Gracey Curvettes to adapt more closely to the tooth surface than any other curettes, especially on the anterior teeth and on line angles (Fig. 50.30). However, this curvature also carries the risk of gouging or "grooving" into the root surfaces on the proximal surfaces of the posterior teeth when #11-12 or #13-14 is used. Additional features that represent improvements on the standard Gracey curettes are a precision-balanced blade tip in direct alignment with the handle, a

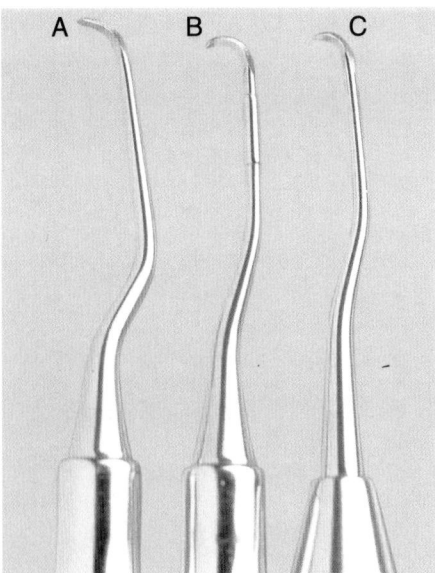

Fig. 50.31 Comparison of three different mini-bladed instruments designed for use on the maxillary and mandibular anterior teeth. *A,* Hu-Friedy Mini Five #5-6; *B,* Hu-Friedy Curvette Sub-0; *C,* Hartzell Sub-0. (Copyright A. Pattison.)

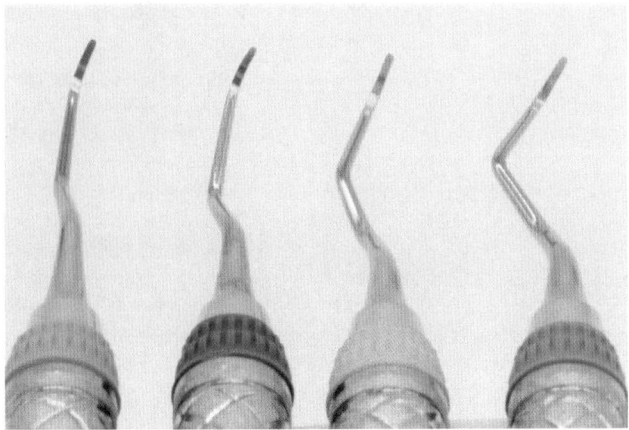

Fig. 50.32 Periodontal maintenance Gracey curettes (Hu-Friedy) Shorter, thinner three-quarter–sized Gracey curettes with modified rigid shanks. *Left to right,* Pattison Gracey Lite #1-2, Pattison Gracey Lite #7-8, Pattison Gracey Lite #11-12, Pattison Gracey Lite #13-14. (Copyright A. Pattison.)

blade tip perpendicular to the handle, and a shank closer to parallel with the handle.

For many years, the *Morse scaler,* a miniature sickle, was the only mini-bladed instrument available. However, mini-bladed curettes have largely replaced this instrument (Fig. 50.31).

Periodontal Maintenance Curettes. The most recent Gracey curette innovation is a category called periodontal maintenance Gracey curettes, introduced in November 2015. These instruments are specifically designed for patients with tight tissue, recession, and residual pocket depth following initial periodontal therapy or periodontal surgery. They can also be used on maintenance patients with healthier tight tissue without attachment loss or recession. In both cases, patients require a small, thin blade to allow subgingival insertion with ease (Fig. 50.32).

The most recent Gracey curette innovation is a category called periodontal maintenance Gracey curettes, introduced in November 2015. These instruments are specifically designed for patients with tight tissue, recession, and residual pocket depth following initial periodontal therapy or periodontal surgery.

This newer blade is 1 mm shorter and 20% thinner, and the face of the blade is offset from the terminal shank at 60 degrees as opposed to all other Gracey designs, which are offset at 70 degrees. This slight modification to the blade-to-shank angle and the thinner, narrow blade allow easier insertion and better access to root surfaces with tight tissue and loss of attachment. Working angulation can be achieved without as much tissue distention, thus increasing patient comfort. The three-quarter blade length of this new type of Gracey curette is between the blade lengths of the standard and mini-bladed Gracey curettes. The shorter blade adapts more easily to root anatomy and furcation areas and helps to prevent spanning across root depressions.

The shank length is 2 mm longer than that of the standard Gracey curette, but 1 mm shorter than that of the extended shank Gracey curette. This length enables better access to molar areas with attachment loss but still allows ease of use in the anterior areas where a very long shank is not necessary. The shank angle of the new Gracey #11-12 is between the regular Gracey #11-12 and the Gracey #15-16, and the shank angle of the new Gracey #13-14 is between the regular Gracey #13-14 and the Gracey #17-18. These shank angle modifications were developed to enhance access to the mesial and distal surfaces of the posterior teeth.

The shanks of these newer instruments are rigid so they can withstand firm pressure when removal of residual burnished calculus is necessary. However, they are not designed for moderate or heavy calculus removal. The clinician must be mindful that the instrument blade is at a slightly more closed angle than the traditional Gracey curette, so if more substantial or tenacious calculus is encountered, the clinician must slightly open the blade angulation, or switch to a rigid standard Gracey curette, or use a different manual or ultrasonic instrument.

Langer and Mini-Langer Curettes. Langer and Mini Langer curettes comprise a set of three curettes combining the shank design of standard Gracey #5-6, #11-12, and #13-14 curettes with a universal blade honed at 90 degrees rather than the offset blade of the Gracey curette. This marriage of the Gracey and universal curette designs allows the advantages of the area-specific shank to be combined with the versatility of the universal curette blade. The Langer #5-6 curette adapts to the mesial and distal surfaces of anterior teeth; the Langer #1-2 curette (Gracey #11-12 shank) adapts to the mesial and distal surfaces of mandibular posterior teeth; and the Langer #3-4 curette (Gracey #13-14 shank) adapts to the mesial and distal surfaces of maxillary posterior teeth (Fig. 50.33). These instruments can be adapted to both mesial and distal tooth surfaces without changing instruments. The standard Langer curette shanks are heavier than a finishing Gracey but less rigid than the rigid Gracey. Langer curettes are also available with either rigid or finishing shanks and can be obtained in extended-shank (After Five) and mini-bladed (Mini Five) versions.

Schwartz Periotrievers

Schwartz Periotrievers comprise a set of two double-ended, highly magnetized instruments designed for retrieval of a broken instrument

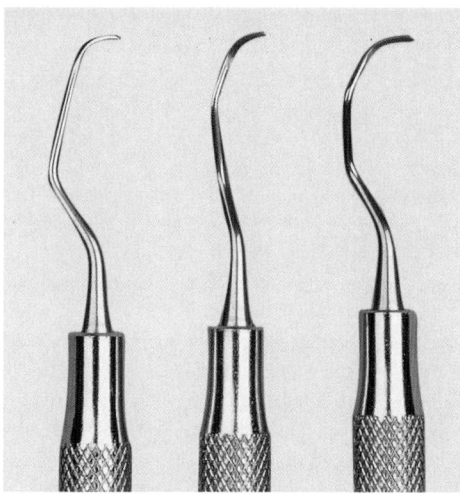

Fig. 50.33 Langer curettes combine Gracey-type shanks with universal curette blades. *Left to right, #5-6, #1-2, and #3-4. (Copyright A. Pattison.)*

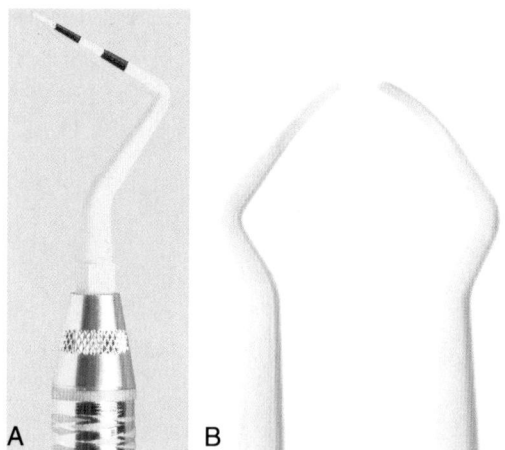

Fig. 50.35 (A) Plastic probe: Colorvue. (B) New Implacare II Barnhart #5-6 cone socket plastic curette tips that screw into an autoclavable stainless steel handle. *(Courtesy Hu-Friedy, Chicago, IL.)*

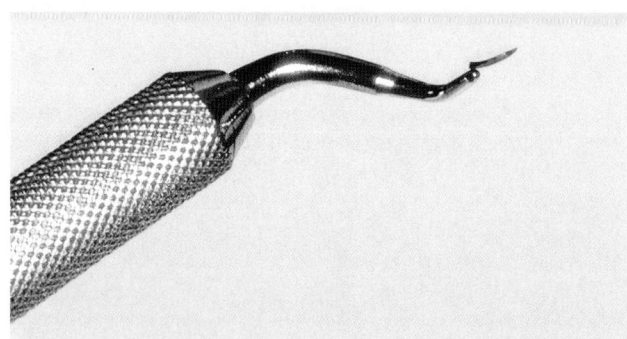

Fig. 50.34 Broken instrument tip attached to the magnetic tip of a Schwartz Periotriever (Daness Dental Distributors, Nyack, N.Y.). *(From Pattison G, Pattison A: Periodontal instrumentation, ed 2, Norwalk, CT, 1992, Appleton & Lange.)*

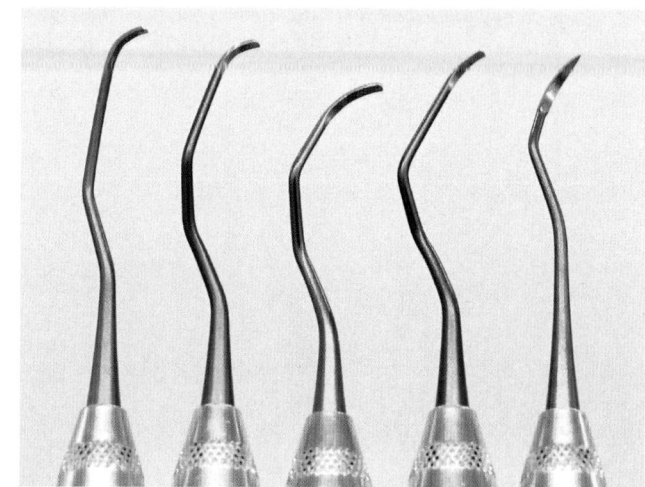

Fig. 50.36 New Mini titanium implant scalers (Hu-Friedy, Chicago). *Left to right,* Mini Five Gracey #1-2, Mini Five Gracey #11-12, Langer #1-2, Mini Five Gracey #13-14, 204SD Sickle Scaler.

tip from the periodontal pocket (Fig. 50.34). They are indispensable when the clinician has broken a curette tip in a furcation or deep pocket.[148]

Plastic and Titanium Instruments for Implants

Several companies are manufacturing plastic and titanium instruments for use on titanium and other implant abutment materials. It is important that plastic or titanium instruments be used to avoid scarring and permanent damage to implants[a] (Figs. 50.35 through 50.37).

Mini-bladed titanium implant instruments are now available in both universal and Gracey curette designs (Fig. 50.37B). Although most standard titanium implant instrument blades are large, the newer mini-bladed titanium curettes insert more easily under tight tissue and adapt more easily around implants and implant restorations. They may be used for implant maintenance with careful, light-pressured strokes for biofilm and light calculus removal. Moderate- or heavy-pressured strokes should be avoided to prevent scratching or roughening of implant surfaces. These instruments are not intended for removal of heavy calculus or cement. Such deposits are often found in cases of peri-implantitis with moderate to advanced bone

loss and exposure of implant threads. Removal of tenacious deposits requires other forms of instrumentation and surgical treatment of the implant. (See Chapter 85 for information on treatment of peri-implantitis.)

Hoe Scalers

Hoe scalers are used for scaling of ledges or rings of calculus (Fig. 50.38). The blade is bent at a 99-degree angle, and the cutting edge is formed by the junction of the flattened terminal surface with the inner aspect of the blade. The cutting edge is beveled at 45 degrees. The blade is slightly bowed so that it can maintain contact at two points on a convex surface. The back of the blade is rounded, and the blade has been reduced to minimal thickness

---

[a]References 23, 39, 43, 48, 57, 96, 142.

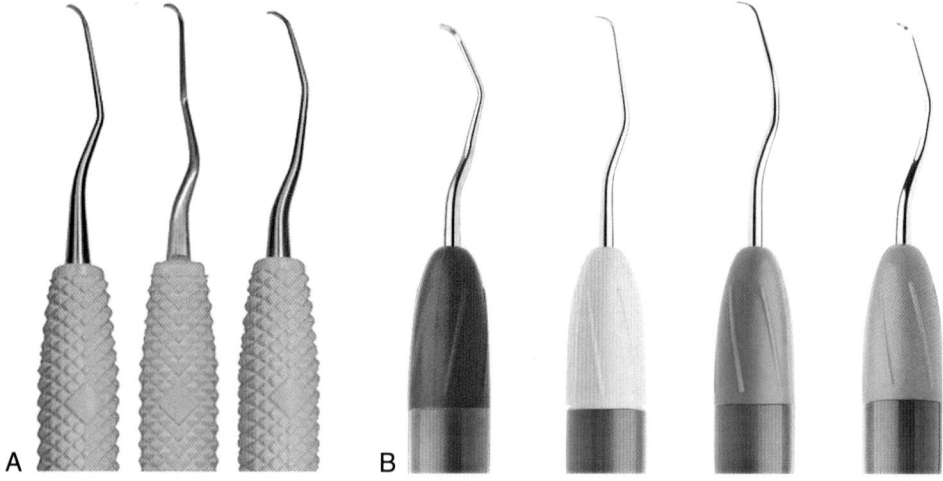

Fig. 50.37 (A) Micro Mini titanium implant curettes (Paradise Dental Technologies, Missoula, MT). *Left to right,* Gracey #1-2 Micro Mini, Gracey #11-12 Micro Mini, Gracey #13-14 Micro Mini. (B) Mini-bladed titanium implant curettes (LM Instruments, Parainen, Finland) : Mini universal curette, Mini Gracey #1-2, Mini Gracey #13-14, Mini Gracey #11-12.

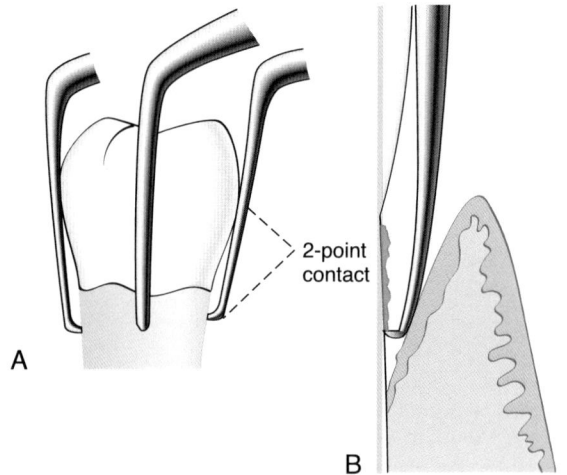

Fig. 50.38 (A) Hoe scalers designed for different tooth surfaces, showing "two-point" contact. (B) Hoe scaler in a periodontal pocket. The back of the blade is rounded for easier access. The instrument contacts the tooth at two points for stability.

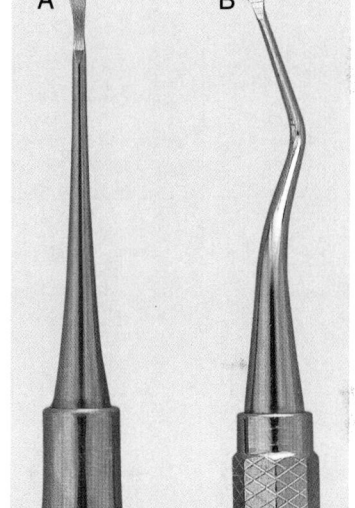

Fig. 50.39 (A) Chisel scaler and (B) file scaler.

to permit access to the roots without interference from the adjacent tissues.

Hoe scalers are used in the following manner:
1. The blade is inserted into the base of the periodontal pocket so that it makes two-point contact with the tooth (see Fig. 50.38). This stabilizes the instrument and prevents nicking of the root.
2. The instrument is activated with a firm pull stroke toward the crown, with every effort made to preserve the two-point contact with the tooth.

McCall's #3, #4, #5, #6, #7, and #8 comprise a set of six hoe scalers designed to provide access to all tooth surfaces. Each instrument has a different angle between the shank and the handle.

Files

Files have a series of blades on a base (Fig. 50.39). Their primary function is to fracture or crush large deposits of tenacious calculus or burnished sheets of calculus. Files can easily gouge and roughen

root surfaces when they are used improperly. Therefore they are not suitable for fine scaling and root planing. Mini-bladed curettes are currently preferred for fine scaling in areas where files were once used. Files are sometimes used for removing overhanging margins of dental restorations.

> **LEARNING BOX 50.12**
>
> Files have a series of blades on a base. Their primary function is to fracture or crush large deposits of tenacious calculus or burnished sheets of calculus.

Chisel Scalers

The chisel scaler, designed for the proximal surfaces of teeth too closely spaced to permit the use of other scalers, is usually used in the anterior part of the mouth. It is a double-ended instrument with a curved shank at one end and a straight shank at the other (see

Fig. 50.39); the blades are slightly curved and have a straight cutting edge beveled at 45 degrees.

The chisel is inserted from the facial surface. The slight curve of the blade makes it possible to stabilize it against the proximal surface, while the cutting edge engages the calculus without nicking the tooth. The instrument is activated with a push motion while the side of the blade is held firmly against the root.

Quétin Furcation Curettes

Quétin furcation curettes are actually hoes with a shallow, half-moon radius that fits into the roof or floor of the furcation. The curvature of the tip also fits into developmental depressions on the inner aspect of the roots. The shanks are slightly curved for better access, and the tips are available in two widths (Fig. 50.40). The BL1 *(buccal-lingual)* and MD1 *(mesial-distal)* instruments are small and fine, with a 0.9-mm blade width. The BL2 and MD2 instruments are larger and wider, with a 1.3-mm blade width.

These instruments remove burnished calculus from recessed areas of the furcation where curettes, even mini-bladed curettes, are often too large to gain access. Using mini-bladed Gracey curettes and Gracey Curvettes on the ceiling or floor of the furcation may unintentionally create gouges and grooves. The Quétin instruments,

however, are well suited for this area and lessen the likelihood of root damage.

Diamond-Coated Files

Diamond-coated files are unique instruments used for final finishing of root surfaces. These files do not have cutting edges; instead, they are coated with very fine-grit diamond (Fig. 50.41). The most useful diamond files are the buccal-lingual instruments, which are used in furcations and also adapt well to many other root surfaces.

New diamond files are sharply abrasive and should be used with light, even pressure against the root surface to avoid gouging or grooving. When viewing the root surface with the dental endoscope after all tactilely detectable deposits are gone, one can observe small embedded remnants of calculus in the root surface. Diamond files are used similar to an emery board to remove these minute remnants of calculus from the root, to create a surface that is free of all visible accretions. Diamond files can produce a smooth, even, clean, and highly polished root surface.

Diamond files must be used carefully because they can cause overinstrumentation of the root surface. They will remove too much root structure if they are used with excessive force, are poorly adapted to root morphology, or are used too long in one place.

Diamond files are particularly effective when used with the dental endoscope, which reveals residual deposits and directs the clinician to the exact area for instrumentation.

Ultrasonic and Sonic Instruments

Ultrasonic instruments may be used for removing biofilm, scaling, curetting, and removing stain (see Chapter 51).

Dental Endoscope

A dental endoscope has been introduced for use subgingivally in the diagnosis and treatment of periodontal disease (Fig. 50.42). The *Perioscopy* system (Perioscopy, Inc., Oakland, CA) consists of a 0.99-mm-diameter reusable fiberoptic endoscope over which is fitted a disposable sterile sheath. The fiberoptic endoscope fits onto periodontal probes and ultrasonic instruments that have been designed to accept it (Fig. 50.43). The sheath delivers water irrigation that flushes the pocket while the endoscope is being used, thereby keeping the field clear. The fiberoptic endoscope attaches to a medical-grade charge-coupled device (CCD) video camera and light source that produces an image on a flat-panel monitor for viewing during

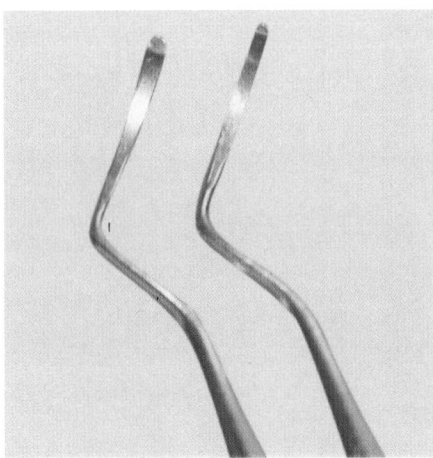

Fig. 50.40 Quétin furcation curettes: BL2 (larger) and BL1 (smaller). *(Copyright A. Pattison.)*

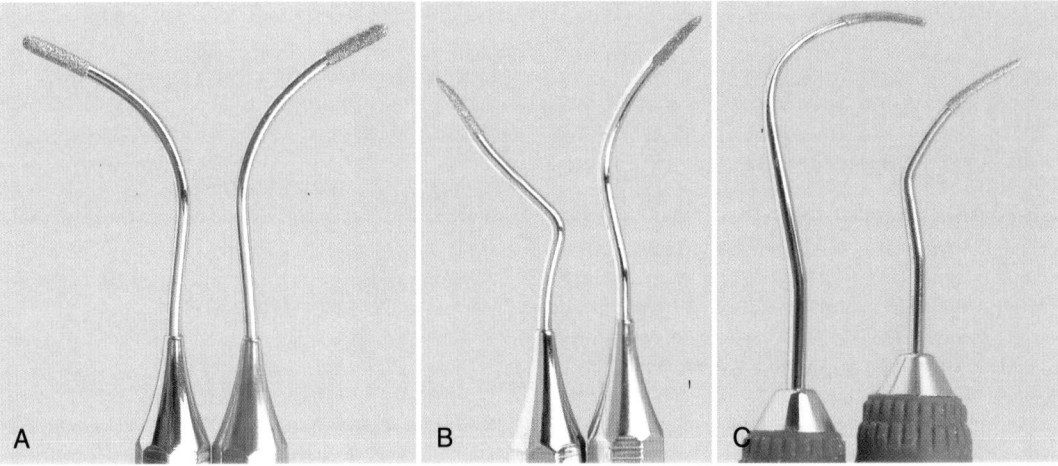

Fig. 50.41 Diamond files. (A) #1, #2 and (B) #3, #4. (Brasseler, Savannah, GA.) (C) SDCN 7, SDCM/D 7. (Hu-Friedy, Chicago.) (Copyright A. Pattison.)

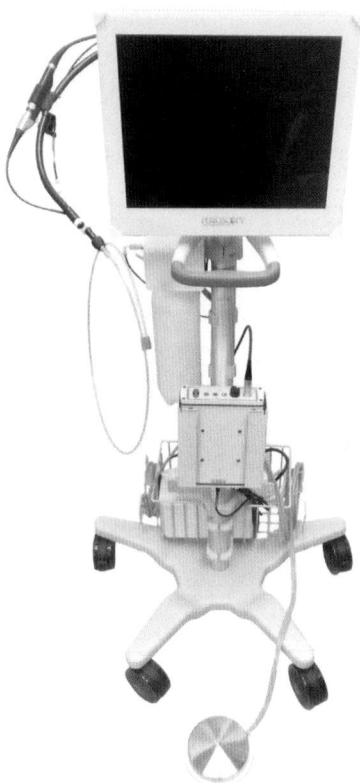

Fig. 50.42 **Perioscopy system, dental endoscope.** *(Courtesy Perioscopy, Inc., Oakland, CA.)*

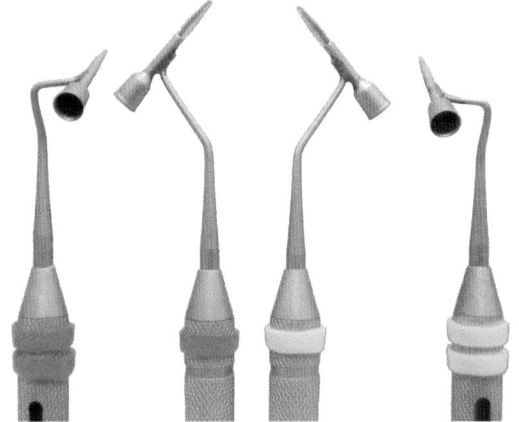

Fig. 50.43 **Viewing periodontal explorers (left/right/full viewing) for the Perioscopy system.** *(Courtesy Perioscopy, Inc., Oakland, CA.)*

subgingival exploration and instrumentation. This device allows clear visualization deep into subgingival pockets and furcations (Fig. 50.44). It permits operators to detect the presence and location of subgingival deposits and guides them in the thorough removal of these deposits. Magnification ranges from 24 to 48 times, enabling visualization of even minute deposits of plaque and calculus. Using this device, operators can achieve levels of root debridement and cleanliness that are much more difficult or impossible to produce without it.[160,161,179,180] The Perioscopy system can also be used to evaluate subgingival areas for caries, defective restorations, root fractures, and resorption.

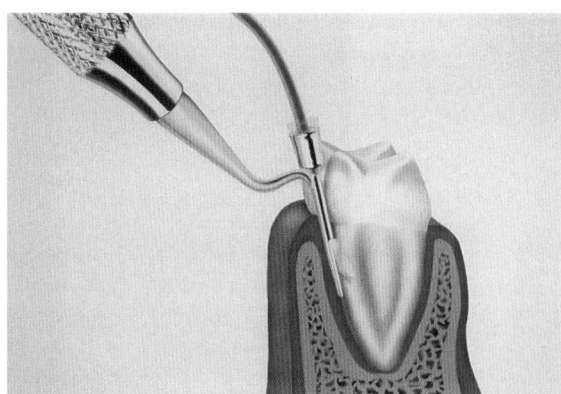

Fig. 50.44 **Perioscopic instrumentation permits deep subgingival visualization in pockets and furcations.** *(Courtesy Perioscopy, Inc., Oakland, CA.)*

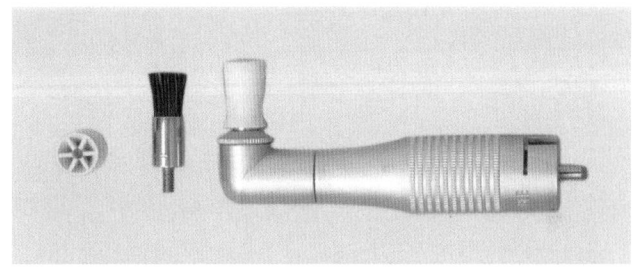

Fig. 50.45 **Metal prophylaxis angle with rubber cup and brush.**

LEARNING BOX 50.13

Using this device, operators can achieve levels of root debridement and cleanliness that are much more difficult or impossible to produce without it. The Perioscopy system (Perioscopy, Inc., Oakland, CA) can also be used to evaluate subgingival areas for caries, defective restorations, root fractures, and resorption.

Cleansing and Polishing Instruments
Rubber Cups

Rubber cups consist of a rubber shell with or without webbed configurations in the hollow interior (Fig. 50.45). They are used in the handpiece with a special prophylaxis angle. The handpiece, prophylaxis angle, and rubber cup must be sterilized after each patient use, or a disposable plastic prophylaxis angle and rubber cup may be used and then discarded (Fig. 50.46). A good cleansing and polishing paste that contains fluoride should be used and kept moist to minimize frictional heat as the cup revolves. Polishing pastes are available in fine, medium, or coarse grit and are packaged in small, convenient, single-use containers. Aggressive use of the rubber cup with any abrasive may remove the layer of cementum, which is thin in the cervical area.

Bristle Brushes

Bristle brushes are available in wheel and cup shapes (see Fig. 50.45). The brush is used in the prophylaxis angle with a polishing paste. Because the bristles are stiff, use of the brush should be confined to the crown to avoid injuring the cementum and the gingiva.

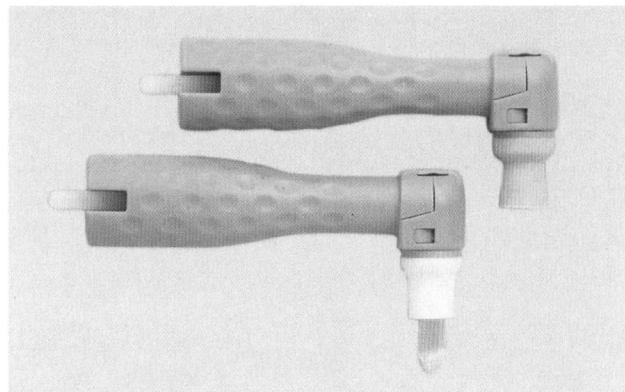

Fig. 50.46 Disposable plastic prophylaxis angle with rubber cup and with brush.

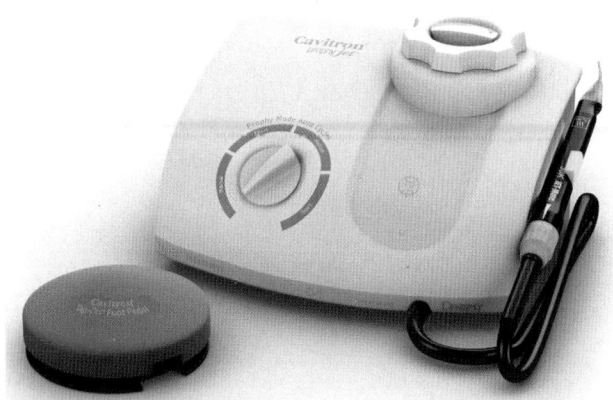

Fig. 50.47 Cavitron ProphyJet air-powder polishing device. *(Courtesy Dentsply International, York, PA.)*

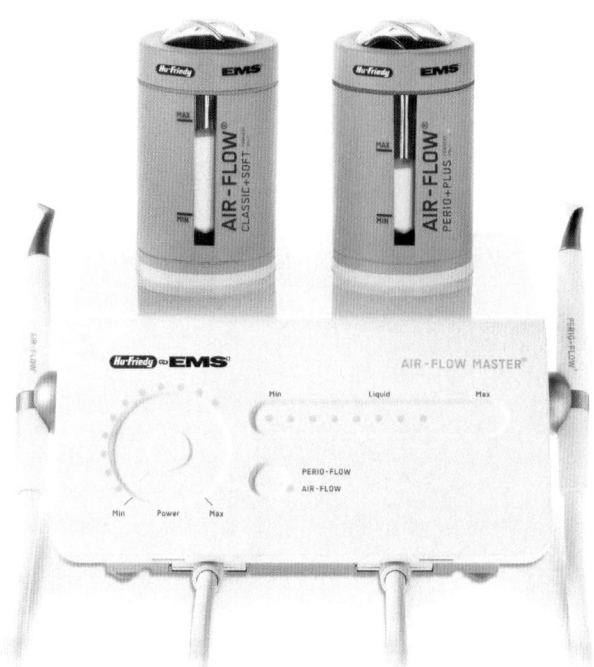

Fig. 50.48 Hu-Friedy EMS Air Flow Master air polishing device with perio and standard handpieces and tips for both supragingival and subgingival air polishing. *Courtesy Hu-Friedy, Chicago, IL.)*

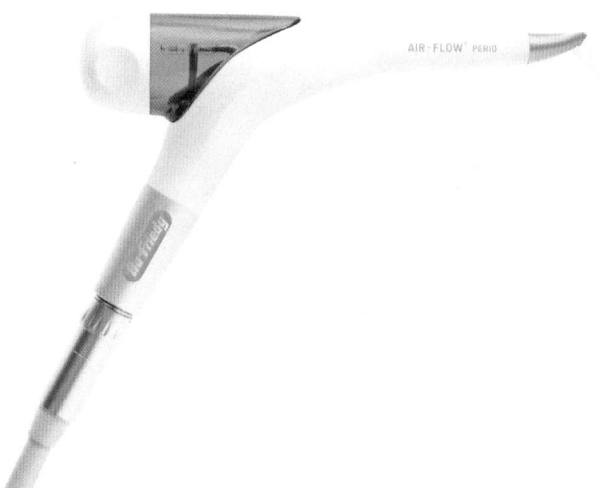

Fig. 50.49 Hu-Friedy EMS Air Flow Perio Handy smaller air polishing device with subgingival air polishing tip for glycine or erythritol powder polishing. *(Courtesy Hu-Friedy, Chicago, IL.)*

Dental Tape

Dental tape with polishing paste is used for polishing proximal surfaces that are inaccessible to other polishing instruments. The tape is passed interproximally while being kept at a right angle to the long axis of the tooth and is activated with a firm labiolingual motion. Particular care is taken to avoid injury to the gingiva. The area should be cleansed with warm water to remove all remnants of paste.

Air-Powder Polishing

The first specially designed handpiece to deliver an air-powered slurry of warm water and sodium bicarbonate for polishing was introduced in the early 1980s. This device, called the *Prophy-Jet* (Dentsply International, York, PA), is very effective for removing extrinsic stains and soft deposits (Fig. 50.47). The slurry removes stains rapidly and efficiently by mechanical abrasion and provides warm water for rinsing and lavage. The flow rate of the abrasive cleansing power can be adjusted to increase the amount of powder for heavier stain removal. Currently, many manufacturers produce air-powder polishing systems that use various powder formulas (Fig. 50.48).

The results of studies on the abrasive effect of the air-powder polishing devices using sodium bicarbonate and aluminum trihydroxide on cementum and dentin show that significant tooth substance can be lost.[2,20,117,125] Damage to gingival tissue is transient and insignificant clinically, but amalgam restorations, composite resins, cements, and other nonmetallic materials can be roughened.[13,44,72,94,172] Polishing powders containing glycine or erythritol rather than sodium

bicarbonate are commonly used in Europe for subgingival biofilm removal from root surfaces.[103,124]

Both supragingival and subgingival air polishing with glycine or erythritol powder are safe and very effective for removal of biofilm from titanium implant surfaces and restorative materials[79,96,136] (Fig. 50.49).

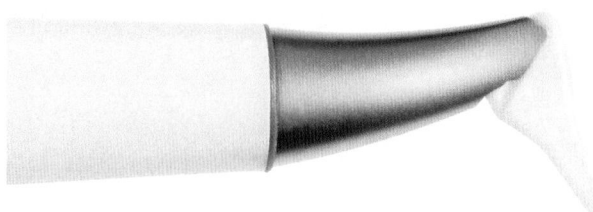

Fig. 50.50 Hu-Friedy EMS Perio Flow Tip disposable plastic tip with millimeter markings for subgingival air polishing of implants or deep pockets with glycine or erythritol powder. *(Courtesy Hu-Friedy, Chicago IL.)*

No soft tissue abrasion occurs, and at probing depths of 1 mm to greater than 5 mm, the use of glycine or erythritol powder in an air-polishing device with a subgingival nozzle (Fig. 50.50) is more effective for subgingival biofilm removal than the use of either manual or ultrasonic instruments.[b]

LEARNING BOX 50.15

The use of glycine or erythritol powder in an air-polishing device with a subgingival nozzle is more effective for subgingival biofilm removal than the use of either manual or ultrasonic instruments.

Patients with a medical history of respiratory illness or hemodialysis are not candidates for the use of the air-powder polishing device.[156,177] Powder containing sodium bicarbonate should not be used on patients with a history of hypertension, sodium-restricted diet, or medication use affecting electrolyte balance.[135] Patients with infectious diseases should not be treated with this device because of the large quantity of aerosol created. A preprocedural rinse with 0.12% chlorhexidine gluconate should be used to minimize the microbial content of the aerosol.[18] High-speed evacuation should also be performed to eliminate as much of the aerosol as possible.[61]

Summary

Various periodontal instruments and devices are specifically designed for examination of the periodontium, removal of calculus and biofilm from tooth and implant surfaces, and root planing.

 Important information on techniques for use and sharpening of these instruments is described in detail in the online continuation of this chapter.

 A Case Scenario is found on the companion website www.expertconsult.com

References

 References for this chapter are found on the companion website www.expertconsult.com.

[b]References 14, 46, 47, 63, 64, 102, 109, 126, 128, 129, 149, 175.

CHAPTER 51

Sonic and Ultrasonic Instrumentation and Irrigation

Carol A. Jahn

CHAPTER OUTLINE

Scaling and root planing are considered the initial nonsurgical treatments of choice for chronic periodontitis.[60] Practitioners often try to enhance and prolong the outcomes from scaling and root planing. In the office setting, technologic advances and new designs of ultrasonic and sonic power scalers have transformed the role of power-driven oscillating instruments in periodontal therapy. At home, the pulsating oral irrigator has been clinically proven to help patients maintain periodontal health by removing biofilm supragingivally and subgingivally and reducing inflammation.

Power-Driven Instruments: Overview

Power-driven instruments are everyday mainstays in periodontal therapy and maintenance. They may be used alone or combination with hand instruments. Evidence indicates that power-driven instruments provide clinical outcomes similar to those derived from hand instruments.[49,50,64,68] Power instrumentation has the potential to make scaling less demanding and more time efficient.[11,64] Potential hazards from using power-driven devices include rough root surfaces, production of bioaerosols, and interference with cardiac pacemakers.[40,63]

⚠ CLINICAL CORRELATION

Power instruments are useful tools that can be used alone or in combination with hand instruments. Evidence indicates that power and hand instruments have similar clinical outcomes. Although power instruments can make scaling less demanding, thorough debridement takes time regardless of the type of instrument used.

Mechanism of Action of Power Scalers

Various physical factors play a role in the mechanism of action of power scalers. These factors include frequency, stroke, and water flow. In addition to rate of flow, the physiologic effects of water may contribute to the efficacy of power instruments.

Water contributes to three physiologic effects that play a role in the efficacy. These are acoustic streaming, acoustic turbulence, and cavitation. Acoustic steaming is unidirectional fluid flow caused by ultrasound waves. Acoustic turbulence is created when the movement of the tip causes the coolant to accelerate, producing an intensified swirling effect. This turbulence continues until cavitation occurs. Cavitation is the formation of bubbles in water caused by the high turbulence. The bubbles implode and produce shock waves in the liquid, thus creating further shock waves throughout the water.[40,66] In vitro, the combination of acoustic streaming, acoustic turbulence, and cavitation has been shown to disrupt biofilm.[36,67]

Type and Benefit of Power Instruments

Sonic units work at a frequency of 2000 to 6500 cycles per second and use a high- or low-speed air source from the dental unit. Water is delivered via the same tubing used to deliver water to a dental handpiece. Sonic scaler tips are large in diameter and universal in design. A sonic scaler tip travels in an elliptical or orbital stroke pattern. This stroke pattern allows the instrument to be adapted to all tooth surfaces. Box 51.1 outlines the advantages and disadvantages of mechanized instruments compared with manual instruments.

Magnetostrictive ultrasonic devices work in a frequency range of 18,000 to 50,000 cycles per second (Figs. 51.1 and 51.2). Metal stacks that change dimension when electrical energy is applied power the magnetostrictive technology. Vibrations travel from the metal stack to a connecting body that causes the vibration of the working tip. Tips move in an elliptical or orbital stroke pattern. This gives the tip four active working surfaces (Fig. 51.3).

Piezoelectric ultrasonic units work in a frequency range of 18,000 to 50,000 cycles per second (Fig. 51.4). Ceramic disks located in the handpiece power the piezoelectric technology and change in dimension as electric energy is applied. Piezoelectric tips move primarily in a linear pattern, giving the tip two active surfaces (Fig. 51.5). Various insert tip designs and shapes are available for use.

BOX 51.1   Advantages and Disadvantages of Mechanized Instruments Compared With Manual Instruments

Advantages

Increased efficiency

    Multiple surfaces of tip are capable of removing deposits

    No need to sharpen

    Less chance for repetitive stress injuries

    Large handpiece size

    Reduced lateral pressure

    Less tissue distention

    Water

    Lavage

    Irrigation

    Acoustic microstreaming

Disadvantages

More precautions and limitations

    Client comfort (water spraying)

    Aerosol production

    Temporary hearing shifts

    Noise

    Less tactile sensation

    Reduced visibility

From Darby ML, Walsh MM: *Dental hygiene*, ed 3, St. Louis, 2010, Saunders.

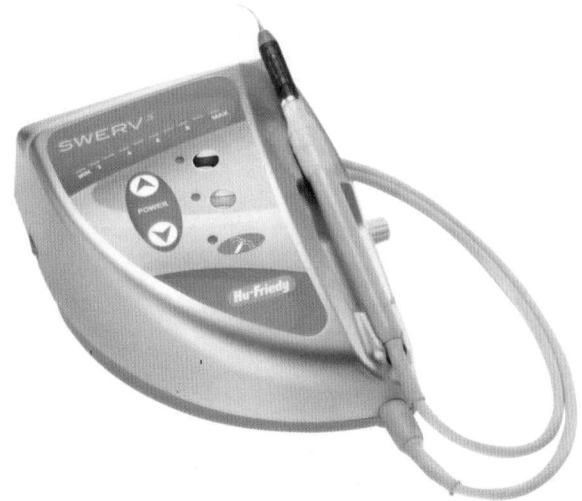

Fig. 51.2 A magnetostrictive ultrasonic device. *(Courtesy Hu-Friedy, Chicago, IL.)*

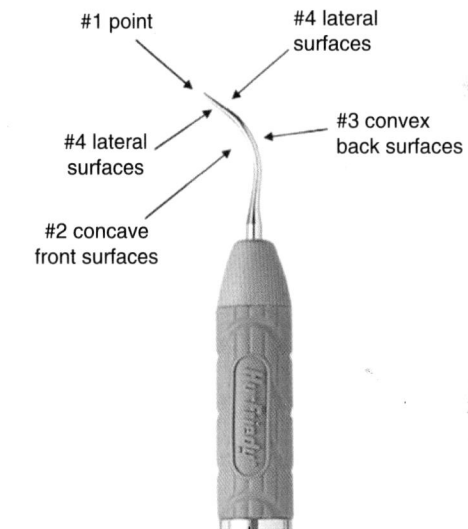

Fig. 51.3 Working sides of a magnetostrictive tip. *(Courtesy Hu-Friedy, Chicago, IL.)*

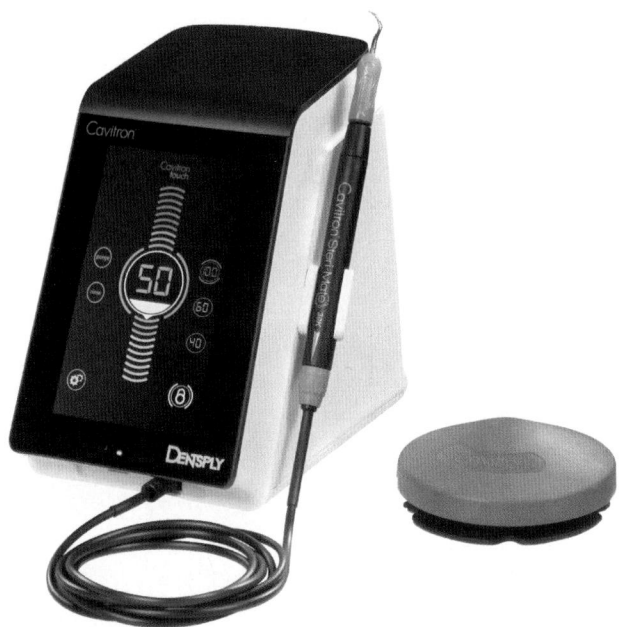

Fig. 51.1 Magnetostrictive ultrasonic device. *(Courtesy Dentsply Sirona, York, PA.)*

Efficiency

Modified tip designs allow for improved access in many areas, including furcations. Newer, slimmer designs operate effectively at lower power settings, thus improving patients' comfort. Flat-edged tips (rectangular in cross section) or bladed designs seem to engage deposits and remove them more efficiently than conical (in cross section) tips.

Tip Designs

Some tips are designed to remove heavy supragingival calculus or debride periodontal pockets definitively. Large-diameter tips are created with a universal design and are indicated for the removal of large, tenacious deposits. A medium to medium-high power setting is generally recommended. Thinner-diameter tips may be site specific in design. The straight-tip design is ideal for use in treating patients with gingivitis and deplaquing maintenance patients[51] (Fig. 51.6). The right and left contra-angled instruments allow for greater access and adaptation to root morphology. These inserts are designed to work on a low-power setting. A deactivated tip can be used for exploration. The amount of water delivered for lavage can be controlled through the selection of either traditional flow or focused-tip delivery flow. Contra-angled designs and larger ergonomic grips enhance comfort and ergonomics (Figs. 51.7 and 51.8).

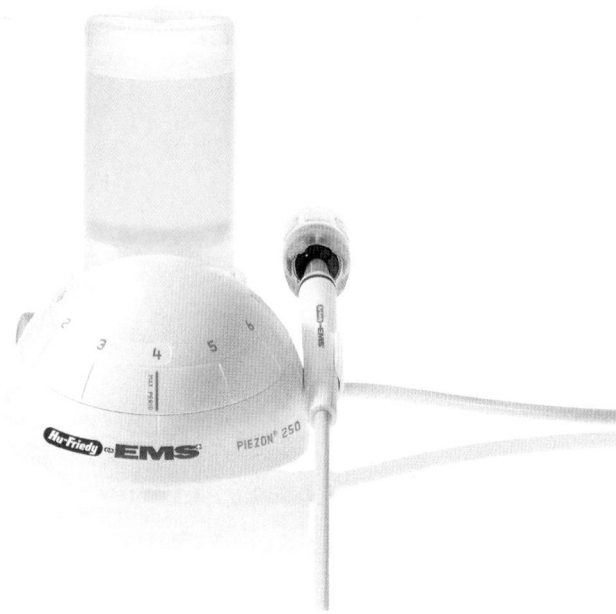

Fig. 51.4 A piezoelectric ultrasonic device. *(Courtesy Hu-Friedy, Chicago, IL.)*

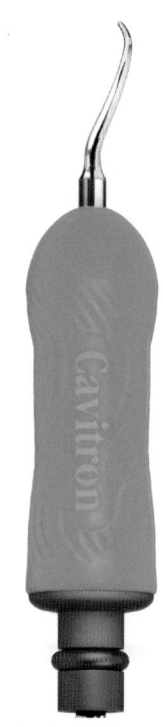

Fig. 51.8 Site-specific designed insert. *(Courtesy Dentsply Sirona, York, PA.)*

Clinical Outcomes of Power-Driven Instruments

Numerous clinical outcomes have been evaluated from the use of power-driven instruments. Reviews of the literature have found the effectiveness of subgingival debridement using ultrasonic or sonic scalers to be similar to that achieved with hand instruments.[2,50,64,68]

It is well established that power-driven instruments remove bacterial biofilm and calculus through mechanical action.[26,32,39,58,62] With the advent of newer designs and thinner tips, deplaquing of root surfaces may be effectively accomplished by power scalers.[51] Power-driven instruments have been shown to be effective in removing calculus, similar to hand instrumentation.[39,58] Ultrasonic instruments, through high-speed action, produce cavitational activity and acoustic microstreaming that some believe may help enhance the disruption of bacteria in subgingival biofilm.

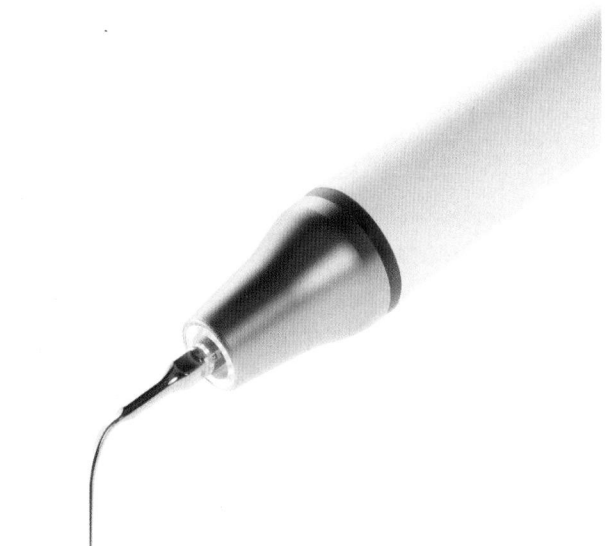

Fig. 51.5 Working sides of a piezoelectric tip. *(Courtesy Hu-Friedy, Chicago, IL.)*

KEY FACT

Power-driven instruments are not just for heavy calculus removal. Depending on tip design and size, they are beneficial for supragingival calculus removal, subgingival debridement, and general deplaquing.

The primary expected clinical outcomes from scaling and root planing are reductions in bleeding and probing depth and a gain in clinical attachment.[60] Comparing power scalers with hand instruments, both types demonstrate similar outcomes for reductions in bleeding on probing and probing depth and gains in clinical attachment.[16,43,49] Because the opening of a furcation is narrower than with conventional hand instruments, power scalers may be recommended as a means to improve access when scaling this type of defect.[3]

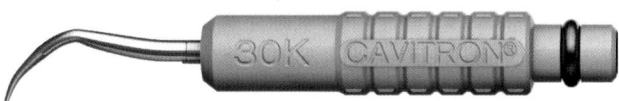

Fig. 51.6 An ultrasonic insert with universal design. *(Courtesy Dentsply Sirona, York, PA.)*

Special Considerations

Power-driven instruments must be used with some caution. Roots may be rougher post scaling than with hand instruments. Due to

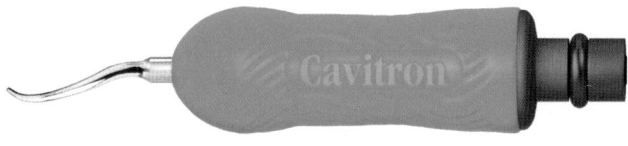

Fig. 51.7 Site-specific designed insert. *(Courtesy Dentsply Sirona, York, PA.)*

aerosol production, proper infection control procedures need to be implemented. Power-driven instruments may be contraindicated for people with pacemakers.

Root Surface Roughness

The data are mixed on whether power-driven instruments cause more root surface roughness than hand instruments.[38,40,41,59] Although it could be assumed that using the device at a higher power may cause more roughness, this is not been proven.[39] It is also not known how much root surface roughness affects the healing process.[40] Power-driven instruments may increase the roughness of resin or glass ionomer restorative materials; therefore, repolishing post scaling is recommended.[20]

Aerosol Production

Power-driven devices produce bioaerosols and splatter, which can contaminate the operator and remain in the air for up to 30 minutes.[65] Good infection control practices can minimize the hazard. Data have shown that preprocedural rinsing with 0.12% chlorhexidine and high-speed evacuation are the most efficient ways to reduce bioaerosols.[46]

KEY FACT

Bioaerosols from power-driven devices can remain in the air for up to 30 minutes. If the operator's face mask becomes damp during the procedure, it should be changed. A face shield may be required. To help minimize bioaerosols, preprocedural rinsing and high-speed evacuation have been shown to be effective.

Cardiac Pacemakers

The use of ultrasonics on patients with cardiac pacemakers is somewhat controversial.[63] Newer models of pacemakers often have bipolar titanium insulation that is believed to make ultrasonic and sonic instruments generally safe for use. An in vivo study supports this; 12 patients underwent continuous electrocardiogram monitoring during piezoelectric ultrasonic scaling and had no abnormal pacemaker functions.[45] Conversely, an in vitro study found that ultrasonic scalers interfered with the activity of dual-system pacemakers.[52] If in doubt, consult with the physician regarding any precautions or warnings from the manufacturer of the product. Box 51.2 outlines the indications, precautions, and contraindications of using mechanized instrumentation.

Principles of Instrumentation

Ultrasonic technique is different from instrumentation with hand scalers. A pen grasp is used with an ultrasonic scaler, along with an extraoral fulcrum (Fig. 51.9). The purpose of the extraoral fulcrum is to allow the operator to maintain a light grasp and have easier access physically and visually to the oral cavity. Alternate cross-arch or opposite-arch fulcrums are acceptable alternatives.

CLINICAL CORRELATION

Instrumentation with the ultrasonic device is different from hand instrumentation. A pen grasp with light pressure is preferred, as is using an extraoral fulcrum. Deposits are removed coronally to apically. For deposits in the embrasure area, a horizontal or transverse stroke is recommended.

BOX 51.2   Indications, Precautions, and Contraindications for Use of Mechanized Instruments

Indications
- Supragingival debridement of dental calculus and extrinsic stains
- Subgingival debridement of calculus, oral biofilm, root surface constituents, and periodontal pathogens
- Removal of orthodontic cement
- Gingival and periodontal conditions and diseases
- Surgical interventions
- Margination (reduces amalgam overhangs)

Precautions
- Unshielded pacemakers
- Infectious diseases: human immunodeficiency virus, hepatitis, tuberculosis (active stages)
- Demineralized tooth surface
- Exposed dentin (especially associated with sensitivity)
- Restorative materials (porcelain, amalgam, gold, composite)
- Titanium implant abutments unless using special insert (e.g., Quixonic SofTip Prophy Tips)
- Children (primary teeth)
- Immunosuppression from disease or chemotherapy
- Uncontrolled diabetes mellitus

Contraindications
- Chronic pulmonary disease: asthma, emphysema, cystic fibrosis, pneumonia
- Cardiovascular disease with secondary pulmonary disease
- Swallowing difficulty (dysphagia)

From Darby ML, Walsh MM: *Dental hygiene*, ed 3, St. Louis, 2010, Saunders.

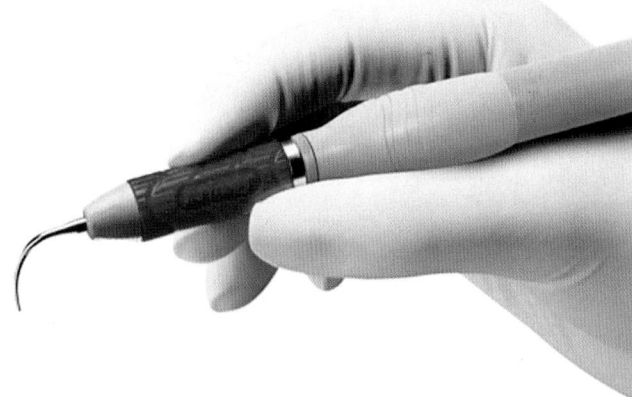

Fig. 51.9 Pen grasp of tip. *(Courtesy Hu-Friedy, Chicago, IL.)*

Light pressure is needed with a power instrument. The tip is traveling at a set frequency in a set stroke pattern. Increased clinician pressure on the tip causes decreased clinical efficacy.

Sonic or ultrasonic instrumentation requires removal from the coronal to the apical portion of the deposit. This stroke pattern allows the insert to work at its optimal stroke pattern and frequency for quick, effective deposit removal. For coronal deposits located in the embrasure area, a horizontal or transverse tip orientation is recommended. A deplaquing stroke should be used when the focus is removal of biofilm and soft debris for the resolution of gingival inflammation. This stroke entails accessing every square millimeter

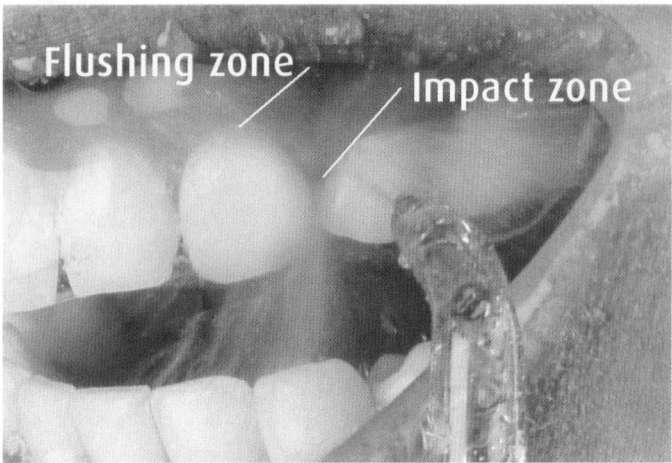

Fig. 51.10 Pulsation creates two zones of hydrokinetic activity: the impact zone and the flushing zone. *(Courtesy Water Pik, Inc., Fort Collins, CO.)*

of the tooth surface during ultrasonic deplaquing as a result of the limited lateral dispersion of the lavage subgingivally (Videos 51.1 and 51.2).

Home and Self-Applied Irrigation

The oral irrigator (also called a dental water jet or water flosser) was introduced in 1962. Contrary to myth and misunderstanding, the body of evidence on this device has consistently shown that it safely and effectively improves periodontal health.[33,35] Emerging evidence indicates that the oral irrigator effectively removes biofilm[28,29] and is as effective as dental floss when added to toothbrushing.[4,44,54,57]

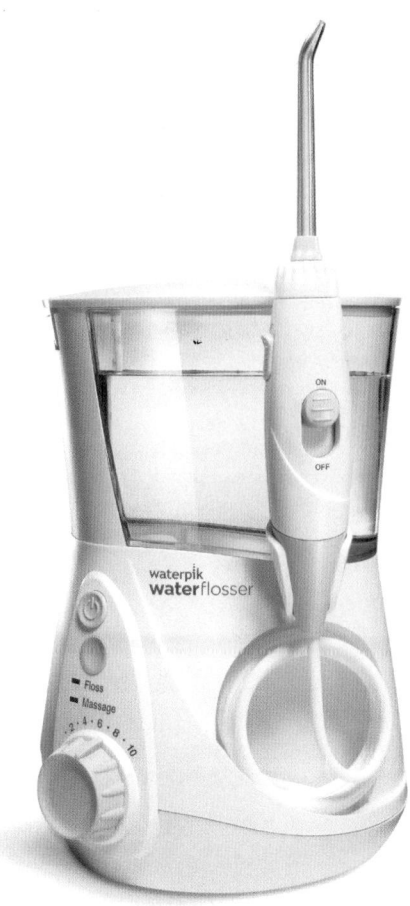

Fig. 51.11 A dental water jet with 1200 ppm and a pressure setting that ranges from 20 to 90 psi. *(Courtesy Water Pik, Inc., Fort Collins, CO.)*

FLASH BACK

The oral irrigator has had many different names throughout the years. It has been referred to as a water jet or dental water jet. Today, the more common name is water flosser. The term is supported by clinical evidence and has been shown to be useful in helping patients understand the benefit of the device.

Mechanism of Action of Irrigation

The mechanism of action of irrigation is through pulsation and pressure.[5,7,55] Pulsation creates a decompression phase that allows the water or solution to penetrate subgingivally. It is followed by a compression phase that expels bacteria and debris from the pocket (Fig. 51.10). Physiologically, pulsation, along with pressure and water velocity, creates shear hydraulic forces that are capable of removing bacterial biofilm from treated areas.[28] Clinical efficacy of home irrigation has been found for units that pulsate from 1200 to 1400 pulses per minute set at a minimum of 60 psi.[33] The oral irrigator is safe to use at higher pressure settings.[5,7,55] Many types of oral irrigators are commercially available, but as with other self-care products, research available from one product brand should not be extrapolated to other brands, because they may have used different pressure settings and pulsation rates (Figs. 51.11 and 51.12).

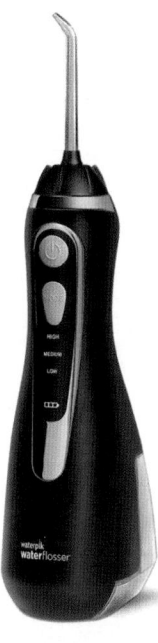

Fig. 51.12 A cordless dental water jet, which also has 1200 ppm. *(Courtesy Water Pik, Inc., Fort Collins, CO.)*

A variety of tips can be used with an oral irrigator. One type of tip is placed supragingivally at a 90-degree angle, and the other is placed slightly subgingivally. Tips placed above the gingival margin result in a pocket penetration of 50% on average[19] (Fig. 51.13). The soft, site-specific subgingival tip (Pik Pocket subgingival irrigation tip, Water Pik, Inc., Fort Collins, CO) (Fig. 51.14) penetrates to about 90% of the depth of pockets that are 6 mm or less and 64% of pockets that are 7 mm or greater[8] (Videos 51.3 and 51.4).

Tips that are placed supragingivally are recommended for full-mouth irrigation or cleansing. These tips include a traditional jet tip along with jet tips of this configuration that have been enhanced with bristles or filaments to assist in biofilm removal[54,57] (Figs. 51.15 and 51.16). The subgingival tip is generally used after full-mouth cleaning for localized irrigation of a specific site that is difficult to access, such as a deep pocket, a furcation, an implant, or a crown and bridge (Fig. 51.17).

Safety

Oral irrigation is supported by a large body of scientific evidence and has been used by people since the 1960s.[35] Clinical studies on oral irrigation evaluate for adverse events, and none have been reported. Despite the scientific evidence, myths about trauma to soft

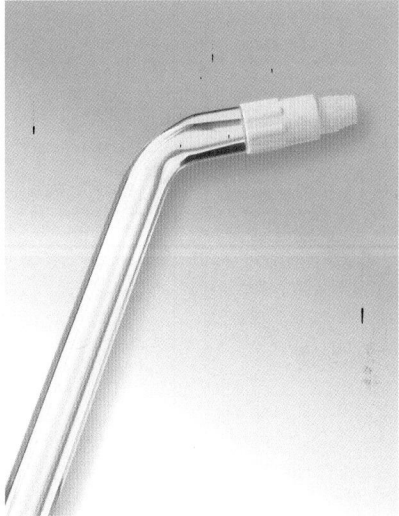
Fig. 51.15 Tip with soft tapered bristles. *(Courtesy Water Pik, Inc., Fort Collins, CO.)*

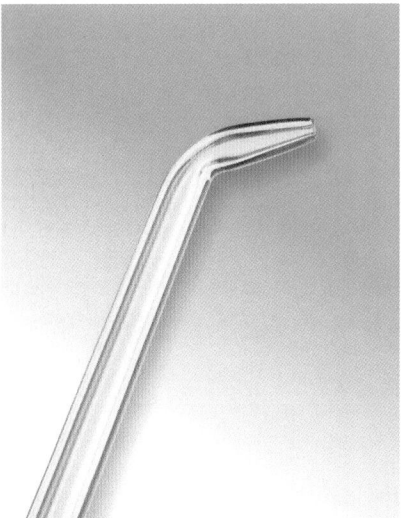
Fig. 51.13 Jet tip. *(Courtesy Water Pik, Inc., Fort Collins, CO.)*

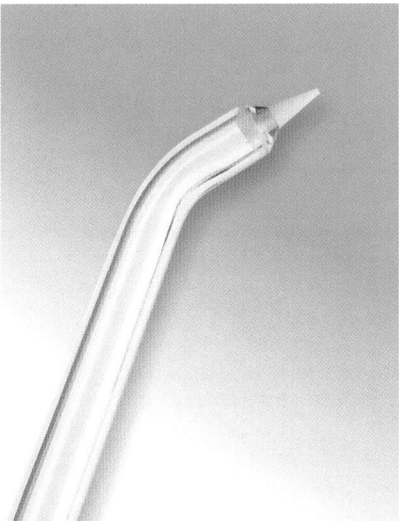
Fig. 51.14 Site-specific tip. *(Courtesy Water Pik, Inc., Fort Collins, CO.)*

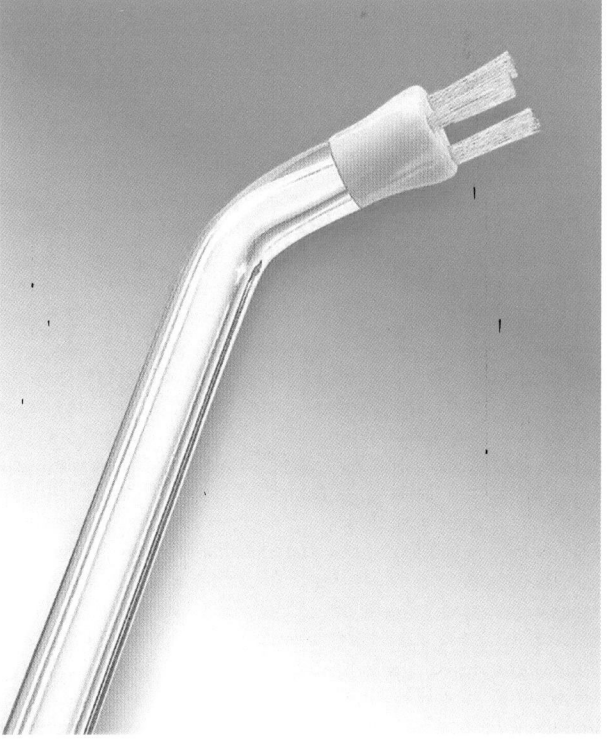
Fig. 51.16 Tip with soft filaments. *(Courtesy Water Pik, Inc., Fort Collins, CO.)*

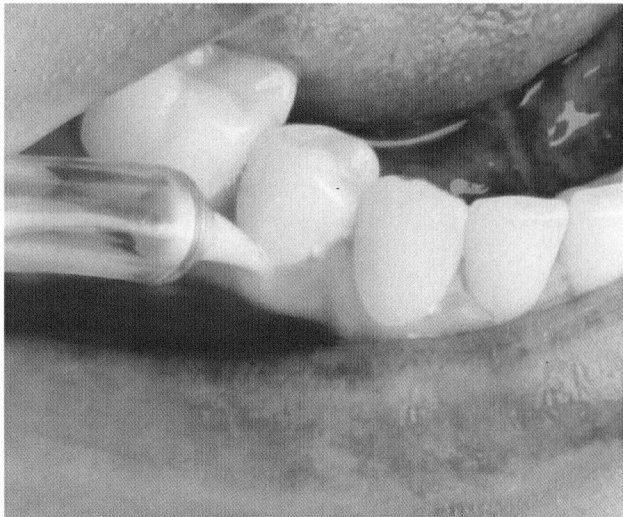

Fig. 51.17 The Pik Pocket tip is gently placed slightly subgingivally. *(Courtesy Water Pik, Inc., Fort Collins, CO.)*

tissue, penetration of bacteria into the pocket, increased pocket depth, and rates of bacteremia still exist.

KEY FACT

Using an oral irrigation is both safe and effective. "Stories" about trauma to soft tissue, penetration of bacteria into the pocket, and increased pocket depth are not supported by clinical evidence. The device has been recommended by dental professionals and used by the general population since the 1960s.

Trauma to tissue and penetration of bacteria were evaluated in a study that used scanning electron microscopy to assess the differences between irrigated and nonirrigated untreated chronic periodontal pockets. Examination with scanning electron microscopy showed no observable differences between the irrigated and nonirrigated pocket tissue with regard to physical features and appearance of the epithelium. The investigators also found that irrigated pockets had significantly fewer bacteria up to 6 mm, compared with nonirrigated pockets.[15] These findings are supported by other investigations. Histologic studies have shown that irrigated tissue has less inflammation.[12,37] Researchers who have looked at the reduction of bacteria agree that irrigation reduces pathogens and that irrigation for a period of 3 to 6 months results in reduced periodontal bacteria.[13,23,48]

Probing pocket depth has been evaluated in several studies.[a] None have found that the use of an oral irrigator increases pocket depth. The findings consistently show small improvements in probing depth.[b]

One long-held assumption is that using an oral irrigator will result in a higher incidence of bacteremia compared with flossing. However, the data show that the incidence of bacteremia can range from 7% in people with gingivitis[53] to 50% in those with periodontitis.[21] Other investigators have found similar results, with one study finding no incidence of bacteremia[61] post irrigation and another study noting a rate of 27%.[6] In comparison, the incidence of bacteremia from string flossing has been shown to be 40% in people with periodontitis and 41% in periodontally healthy individuals.[17]

Clinical Outcomes of Irrigation

Table 51.1 highlights the body of evidence on the oral irrigator. Evaluated outcomes include removal of plaque biofilm and reductions in calculus, gingivitis, bleeding on probing, probing depth, periodontal pathogens, and inflammatory mediators.[c] Home irrigation has been studied and found safe and effective for those with gingivitis,[d] implants,[22,44] crown and bridge,[37] orthodontics,[10,57] and diabetes,[1] as well as in periodontal maintenance.[18,23,24,27,35,47]

Emerging evidence indicates that using an oral irrigator can lead to oral health improvements over what has been traditionally seen with string floss.[4,29,44,54,57] When an oral irrigator was added to either manual or power toothbrushing and compared with manual brushing and flossing, subjects who added the oral irrigator, regardless of toothbrush type, had significantly better reductions in both bleeding and gingivitis.[4] This finding is supported by other studies that have found the oral irrigator to be more effective than string floss in reducing bleeding.[44,54,57]

CLINICAL CORRELATION

Nearly 70 studies have been conducted on the oral irrigator. Consistent clinical outcomes demonstrate reductions in biofilm, periodontal pathogens, bleeding on probing, gingivitis, and probing depth. The device has been tested on people in periodontal maintenance and in those with gingivitis, orthodontic appliances, implants, crowns, bridges, and diabetes.

As early as the 1960s, it was shown that oral irrigation with water added to toothbrushing reduced gingivitis by 52% compared with a 30% reduction for toothbrushing alone.[42] Throughout the years, other researchers have found concurring results with the use of plain water.[e] The use of an antimicrobial agent, such as diluted chlorhexidine (Table 51.2), or an essential oil generally enhances reductions in gingivitis and bleeding.[9,13,14,22-25,35]

The oral irrigator has been demonstrated to remove biofilm.[f] The combination of pulsation, pressure, and water velocity creates shear hydraulic forces that can significantly remove biofilm. Researchers who assessed the action of the oral irrigator with scanning electron microscopy found that a 3-second application at medium pressure removed 99.9% of biofilm from treated areas[28] (Figs. 51.18 and 51.19).

Individuals With Special Considerations

Some clinical trials have focused on groups with special oral or medical health needs. Both children and adults undergoing orthodontic therapy have shown significant benefits from using a dental water jet.[10,57] A newer small brush tip that cleans and irrigates simultaneously has been shown to remove 3.76 times more plaque than brushing and flossing with a floss threader.[57] For individuals with implants, a modified jet tip with filaments has been found to be both safe and effective. Patients who used the oral irrigator at 60 psi with warm water had twice the reduction in bleeding around implants compared with patients who used floss. No adverse events were reported.[44] The site-specific subgingival tip has also been shown to be safe and effective for use on implants.[22] The oral irrigator has also been found

---

[a]References 1, 10, 14, 18, 24, 25, 27, 34, 47.
[b]References 1, 10, 14, 18, 24, 25, 27, 34, 47.

[c]References 1, 4, 9, 10, 13, 14, 18, 22, 23, 25, 27, 30, 31, 34, 37, 42, 44, 47, 54, 56, 57.
[d]References 4, 9, 13, 14, 25, 30, 31, 42, 54, 57.
[e]References 1, 4, 13, 18, 25, 27, 30, 31, 42, 44, 47, 54, 56, 57.
[f]References 1, 4, 18, 28-31, 54, 56, 57.

TABLE 51.1 Reduction of Inflammation and Plaque Biofilm

Study	Duration	N	Agent Used	Bleeding Reduction (%)	Gingivitis Reduction (%)	Plaque Biofilm Reduction (%)
Al-Mubarak et al[1]	3 months	50	Water	43.8	66.9	64.9
Barnes et al[4]	4 weeks	105	Water	36.2–59.2	10.8–15.1	8.8–17.3
Brownstein et al[9]	8 weeks	44	CHX (0.06%) Water	52–59 NR	25.4–31.1[a]	14.3–19[a] NR
Burch et al[10]	2 months	47	Water	57.1–76.6	NR	52–55.7
Chaves et al[13]	6 months	105	CHX (0.04%) Water	54 50	26 26	35 16
Ciancio et al[14]	6 weeks	61	Essential oils[b] Water and alcohol 5%	27.6 13.6–31.2	54–55.7 59.8–61.9	23–24 9/6–13.3
Cutler et al[18]	2 weeks	52	Water	56	50	40
Flemmig et al[25]	6 months	175	CHX (0.06%) Water	35.4 24	42.5 23.1	53.2 0.1
Flemmig et al[24]	6 months	60	Acetylsalicylic acid 3% Water	50	8.9 29.2	55.6 0
Felo et al[22]	3 months	24	CHX (0.06%)	62	45	29
Fine et al[23]	6 weeks	50	Essential oils[b] Water	14.8–21.7 7.5–10.6	NR NR	36.8–37.7 15.5–18.4
Genovesi et al[27]	30 days	30	Water Minocycline hydrochloride, 1 mg per pocket in-office/1 time	81% 75%	NR NR	45% 61%
Jolkovsky et al[35]	3 months	58	CHX (0.4%) Water	NR NR	33.1 18.6	51.6 25.6
Lobene et al[42]	5 months	155	Water	NR	52.9	7.9
Magnuson et al[44]	30 days	44 implants	Water	82%	NR	NR
Newman et al[47]	6 months	155	Water Water and zinc sulfate (0.57%)	22.8 8.8	17.8 6.5	6.1 9.2
Rosema et al[54]	30 days	104	Water	17%	NR	?
Sharma et al[57]	4 weeks	128	Water	84.5	NR	38.9

[a]Percentages were reported for differences between CHX and water irrigation groups.
[b]Reported the range for prophy and nonprophy groups.
CHX, Chlorhexidine; *NR*, not reported.

TABLE 51.2 Chlorhexidine Dilutions (Based on 0.12% Concentration) Shown Effective in Clinical Trials

Concentrations	Amount of Water	Amount of Chlorhexidine
0.04%[13,35]	3 parts	1 part
0.06%[9,22,25,48]	1 part	1 part

to improve periodontal health in people with type 1 or 2 diabetes.[1] For patients who prefer natural products, subjects who used the oral irrigator for 30 days post scaling and root planing effectively reduced the clinical parameters of periodontitis and periodontal bacteria similar to scaling and root planing followed by the placement of 1 mg of minocycline hydrochloride. Any differences between the two therapies was not statistically significant (Videos 51.5 and 51.6).[27]

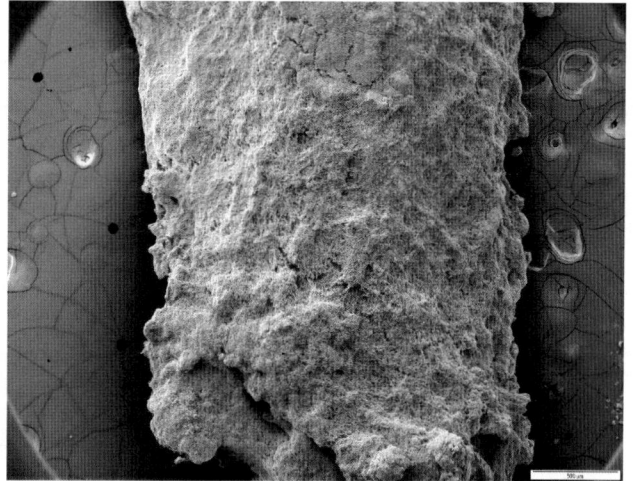

Fig. 51.18 Control tooth with no irrigation. *(Courtesy Water Pik, Inc., Fort Collins, CO.)*

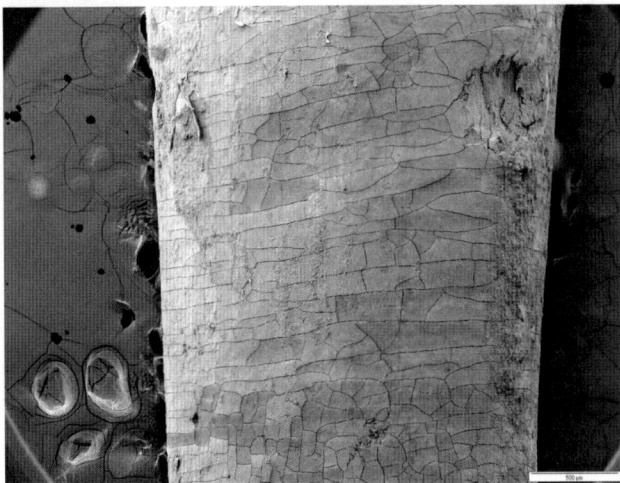

Fig. 51.19 Tooth after a 3-second pulsating lavage with a jet tip at medium pressure. *(Courtesy Water Pik, Inc., Fort Collins, CO.)*

Action of a Tip With Filaments Cleaning Around an Implant

Video 51.7 shows the action of the site-specific tip in a periodontal pocket.

Conclusion

Power scalers have emerged from being adjuncts for removing heavy supragingival calculus to a tool that may be used for all aspects of scaling: deplaquing, supragingival scaling, and subgingival scaling. The clinical outcomes achieved are similar to those seen with hand instrumentation. The advantages gained from using power instruments are potentially greater access subgingivally and in furcation areas and increased efficiency in time needed for scaling.

Home irrigation is safe and effective for a wide variety of patients, including those in periodontal maintenance; those with calculus buildup, gingivitis, orthodontic appliances, maxillary fixation, crown and bridge, implants, or diabetes; and those who are noncompliant with floss. Clinical outcomes include reductions of plaque, calculus, gingivitis, bleeding on probing, probing depth, periodontal pathogens, and inflammatory mediators.

 A Case Scenario is found on the companion website www.expertconsult.com

References

 References for this chapter are found on the companion website www.expertconsult.com.

CHAPTER 52

Systemic Anti-infective Therapy for Periodontal Diseases

Sebastian G. Ciancio | Angelo J. Mariotti

CHAPTER OUTLINE

Definitions
Systemic Administration of Antibiotics
Serial and Combination Antibiotic Therapy
Conclusion

Learning Objectives
- Evaluate the rationale for use of anti-infective agents as adjuncts to periodontal therapy.
- List the clinical indications for use of anti-infective agents.
- Evaluate the pharmacology of anti-infective agents indicated as adjuncts to periodontal therapy.

It has been well established that the various periodontal diseases are caused by bacterial infection. Bacteria begin reattaching to tooth surfaces soon after the teeth have been cleaned and start to form a *biofilm*. Over time, this supragingival plaque biofilm becomes more complex, which leads to a succession of bacteria that are more pathogenic. Bacteria grow in an apical direction and become subgingival. Eventually, as bone is destroyed, a periodontal pocket is formed. In a periodontal pocket, the bacteria form a highly structured and complex biofilm. As this process continues, the bacterial biofilm extends so far subgingivally that the patient cannot reach it during oral hygiene efforts. In addition, this complex biofilm may now offer some protection from the host's immunologic mechanisms in the periodontal pocket as well as from antibiotics used for treatment. It has been suggested that an antibiotic strength that is 500 times greater than the usual therapeutic dose may be needed to be effective against bacteria that have become arranged in biofilms.[26]

Systemic Administration of Antibiotics
Tetracyclines
Metronidazole
Penicillins
Cephalosporins
Clindamycin
Ciprofloxacin
Macrolides

It is therefore logical to treat periodontal pockets by mechanically removing local factors (including the calculus that harbors bacteria) and by disrupting the subgingival plaque biofilm itself. Mechanical removal includes manual instrumentation (e.g., scaling and root planing) and machine-driven instrumentation (e.g., ultrasonic scalers), and these procedures can be considered "anti-infective therapy." Many chemotherapeutic agents are now available to clinicians who treat periodontal diseases. *Systemic* anti-infective therapy (oral antibiotics) and *local* anti-infective therapy (placing anti-infective agents directly into the periodontal pocket) can reduce the bacterial challenge to the periodontium. It is also possible that systemically administered nonsteroidal antiinflammatory agents may play a role in future adjunctive therapy.[42,58]

Bacteria and their toxic products may cause a loss of attachment and a loss of bone. Ultimately, however, the host's own immunologic response to this bacterial infection can cause even more bone destruction (i.e., indirect bone loss) than that caused by pathogenic bacteria and their by products. This immunologic response can be influenced by environmental (e.g., tobacco use), acquired (e.g., systemic disease), or genetic risk factors.[49] Chemotherapeutic agents can modulate the host's immune response to bacteria and reduce the host's self-destructive immunologic response to bacterial pathogens, thereby reducing bone loss.[45-47] It is also incumbent on health care providers to counsel patients about the detrimental effects of systemic factors, including medications, stress, and tobacco use.[26]

This chapter reviews the indications and protocols for optimizing the use of systemically administered anti-infective agents during the treatment of periodontal diseases. It is important to note that there has been significant work with the use of a systematic *evidence-based approach* to evaluate the various anti-infective and host modulation therapies.[64] A meta-analysis of similar research studies has given power to statistical analysis to evaluate anti-infective chemotherapeutic agents for the treatment of periodontal disease. Unfortunately, a standardized research protocol has not yet been implemented. As a result, some studies, although relevant, have not been used in the evidence-based approach because of their study design. Further evidence-based and similar research is needed to define protocols

TABLE 52.1 Antibiotics Used to Treat Periodontal Diseases

Category	Agent	Major Features
Penicillin[a]	Amoxicillin	Extended spectrum of antimicrobial activity; excellent oral absorption; used systemically
	Augmentin[b]	Effective against penicillinase-producing microorganisms; used systemically
Tetracyclines	Minocycline	Effective against a broad spectrum of microorganisms; used systemically and applied locally (subgingivally)
	Doxycycline	
	Tetracycline	Effective against a broad spectrum of microorganisms; used systemically and applied locally (subgingivally)
		Chemotherapeutically used in subantimicrobial doses for host modulation (Periostat)
		Effective against a broad spectrum of microorganisms
Quinolone	Ciprofloxacin	Effective against gram-negative rods; promotes health-associated microflora
Macrolide	Azithromycin	Concentrates at sites of inflammation; used systemically
Lincomycin derivative	Clindamycin	Used in penicillin-allergic patients; effective against anaerobic bacteria; used systemically
Nitroimidazole[c]	Metronidazole	Effective against anaerobic bacteria; used systemically and applied locally (subgingivally) as gel

[a]Indications: localized aggressive periodontitis, generalized aggressive periodontitis, medically related periodontitis, and refractory periodontitis.
[b]Amoxicillin and clavulanate potassium.
[c]Indications: localized aggressive periodontitis, generalized aggressive periodontitis, medically related periodontitis, refractory periodontitis, and necrotizing ulcerative periodontitis.

more precisely for the use of anti-infective agents to treat various periodontal diseases.

KEY FACT

Bacteriostatic Versus Bactericidal Antibiotics

Pharmacologic agents that prevent the growth of bacteria are bacteriostatic antibiotics, whereas pharmacologic agents that actually kill the bacteria are bactericidal antibiotics. Examples of bacteriostatic antibiotics include tetracycline and clindamycin, and penicillin and metronidazole are good examples of bactericidal antibiotics.

Definitions

An anti-infective agent is a *chemotherapeutic agent* that acts by reducing the number of bacteria present. An antibiotic is a naturally occurring, semisynthetic, or synthetic type of anti-infective agent that destroys or inhibits the growth of select microorganisms, generally at low concentrations. An antiseptic is a chemical antimicrobial agent that can be applied topically or subgingivally to mucous membranes, wounds, or intact dermal surfaces to destroy microorganisms and inhibit their reproduction or metabolism. In dentistry, antiseptics are widely used as the active ingredient in antiplaque and antigingivitis oral rinses and dentifrices. Disinfectants (a subcategory of antiseptics) are antimicrobial agents that are generally applied to inanimate surfaces to destroy microorganisms.[13]

When anti-infective agents are administered orally, many of these agents can be found in the gingival crevicular fluid (GCF). The purpose of a *systemic administration* of antibiotics is to reduce the number of bacteria present in the diseased periodontal pocket; this is often a necessary adjunct for controlling bacterial infection, because bacteria can invade periodontal tissues, thereby making mechanical therapy alone sometimes ineffective.[2,11,12,21,48]

A single chemotherapeutic agent can also have a dual mechanism of action. For example, tetracyclines (especially doxycycline) are chemotherapeutic agents that can reduce collagen and bone destruction via their ability to inhibit the enzyme collagenase. As antibiotic agents, they can also reduce periodontal pathogens in periodontal tissues.[12]

Systemic Administration of Antibiotics

Background and Rationale

The treatment of periodontal diseases is based on their infectious nature (Table 52.1). Ideally, the causative microorganisms should be identified, and the most effective agent should be selected with the use of antibiotic-sensitivity testing. Although this appears simple, the difficulty lies primarily in identifying the specific etiologic microorganisms rather than the microorganisms that are simply associated with various periodontal disorders.[12]

An ideal antibiotic for use in the prevention and treatment of periodontal disease should be specific for periodontal pathogens, allogenic, nontoxic, substantive, not in general use for the treatment of other diseases, and inexpensive.[22] Currently, however, an ideal antibiotic for the treatment of periodontal disease does not exist.[32] Although oral bacteria are susceptible to many antibiotics, no single antibiotic at the concentrations achieved in body fluids inhibits all putative periodontal pathogens.[61] Indeed, a combination of antibiotics may be necessary to eliminate all putative pathogens from some periodontal pockets[43] (Table 52.2).

As always, the clinician, in concert with the patient, must make the final decision regarding any treatment. Thus the treatment of an individual patient must be based on the patient's clinical status, the nature of the colonizing bacteria, the ability of the agent to reach the site of infection, and the risks and benefits associated with the proposed treatment plan. The clinician is responsible for choosing the correct antimicrobial agent. Some adverse reactions include allergic or anaphylactic reactions, superinfections of opportunistic bacteria, development of resistant bacteria, interactions with other medications, upset stomach, nausea, and vomiting.[3] Most adverse reactions take the form of gastrointestinal upset.[32] Other concerns include the cost of the medication and the patient's willingness and ability to comply with the proposed therapy.

No consensus exists regarding the magnitude of risk for the development of bacterial resistance. The common and indiscriminate use of antibiotics worldwide has contributed to increasing numbers of resistant bacterial strains since the late 1990s, and this trend is likely to continue given the widespread use of antibiotics.[10,18,62] The overuse, misuse, and widespread prophylactic application of anti-infective drugs are some of the factors that have led to the emergence of resistant microorganisms. Increasing levels of resistance of subgingival microflora to antibiotics have been correlated with the increased use of antibiotics in individual countries.[10,57] However, researchers have noted that the subgingival microflora tends to revert to similar proportions of antibiotic-resistant isolates 3 months after therapy.[20,28]

Tetracyclines

Tetracyclines have been widely used for the treatment of periodontal diseases. They have been frequently used to treat refractory periodontitis, including *localized aggressive periodontitis* (LAP)[31,63] (see Table 52.1). Tetracyclines have the ability to concentrate in the periodontal tissues and inhibit the growth of *Aggregatibacter actinomycetemcomitans*. In addition, tetracyclines exert an anticollagenase effect that can inhibit tissue destruction and may help with bone regeneration.[9,37,60]

TABLE 52.2 Common Antibiotic Regimens Used to Treat Periodontal Diseases[a]

	Regimen	Dosage/Duration
Single Agent		
Amoxicillin	500 mg	Three times daily for 8 days
Azithromycin	500 mg	Once daily for 4 to 7 days
Ciprofloxacin	500 mg	Twice daily for 8 days
Clindamycin	300 mg	Three times daily 10 days
Doxycycline or minocycline	100 mg to 200 mg	Once daily for 21 days
Metronidazole	500 mg	Three times daily for 8 days
Combination Therapy		
Metronidazole + amoxicillin	250 mg of each	Three times daily for 8 days
Metronidazole + ciprofloxacin	500 mg of each	Twice daily for 8 days

[a]These regimens are prescribed after a review of the patient's medical history, periodontal diagnosis, and antimicrobial testing. Clinicians must consult pharmacology references such as *Mosby's GenRx*[41] or the manufacturer's guidelines for warnings, contraindications, and precautions.
Data from Jorgensen MG, Slots J: Practical antimicrobial periodontal therapy. *Compend Contin Educ Dent* 21:111, 2000.

Pharmacology

The tetracyclines are a group of antibiotics that are produced naturally from certain species of *Streptomyces* or derived semisynthetically. These antibiotics are bacteriostatic and are effective against rapidly multiplying bacteria. They generally are more effective against gram-positive bacteria than against gram-negative bacteria. Tetracyclines are effective for the treatment of periodontal diseases in part because their concentration in the gingival crevice is 2 to 10 times that found in serum.[1,4,24] This allows a high drug concentration to be delivered into the periodontal pockets. In addition, several studies have demonstrated that tetracyclines at a low GCF concentration (i.e., 2 μg/ml to 4 μg/ml) are very effective against many periodontal pathogens.[5,6]

Clinical Use

Tetracyclines have been investigated as adjuncts for the treatment of LAP.[31,51] *A. actinomycetemcomitans* is a microorganism that is frequently associated with LAP, and it invades tissue. Therefore the mechanical removal of calculus and plaque from root surfaces may not eliminate this bacterium from the periodontal tissues. Systemic tetracycline can eliminate tissue bacteria and has been shown to arrest bone loss and suppress *A. actinomycetemcomitans* levels in conjunction with scaling and root planing.[50] This combination therapy allows for the mechanical removal of root surface deposits and the elimination of pathogenic bacteria from within the tissues.[53] Increased posttreatment bone levels have been noted with the use of this method (Figs. 52.1 to 52.4).

As a result of increased resistance to tetracyclines, metronidazole or amoxicillin with metronidazole has been found to be more effective for the treatment of aggressive periodontitis in children and young adults. Some investigators think that metronidazole in combination with amoxicillin–clavulanic acid is the preferable antibiotic.[59]

Long-term use of low antibacterial doses of tetracyclines has been advocated in the past. One long-term study of patients taking low doses of tetracycline (i.e., 250 mg/day for 2 to 7 years) demonstrated the persistence of deep pockets that did not bleed after probing. These sites contained high proportions of tetracycline-resistant gram-negative rods *(Fusobacterium nucleatum)*. After the antibiotic was discontinued, the flora was characteristic of sites with disease.[32] Therefore it is not advisable to prescribe a long-term regimen of tetracyclines because of the possible development of resistant

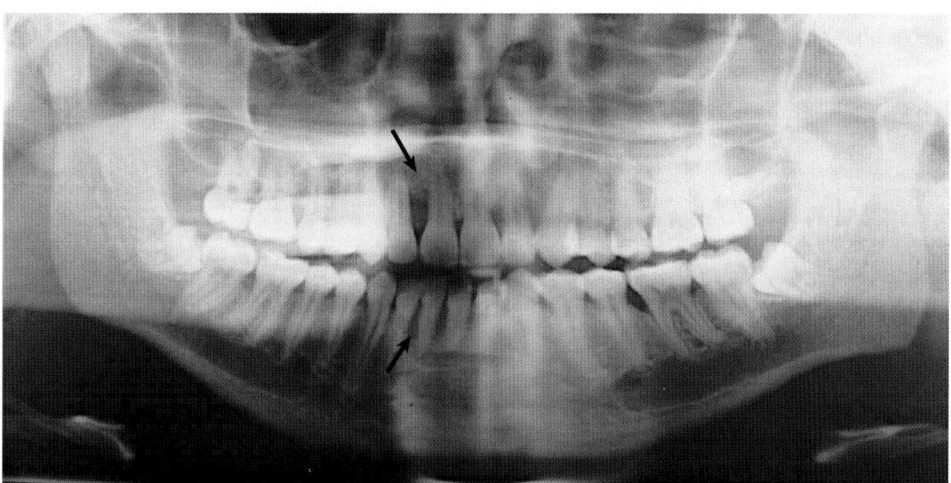

Fig. 52.1 Panoramic image of 17-year-old African American male exhibiting signs of localized aggressive periodontitis. *(Photo courtesy Dr. Sasi Sunkari.)*

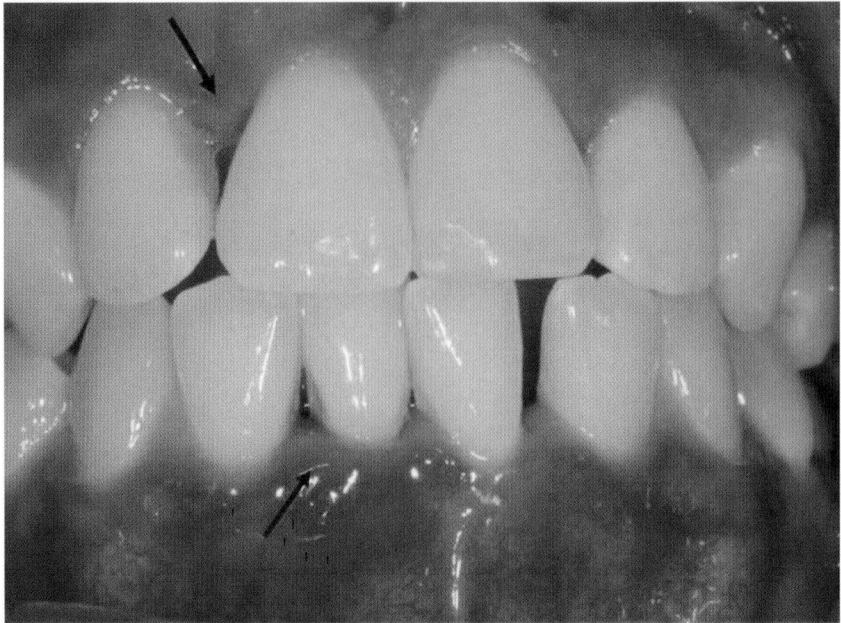

Fig. 52.2 Image of anterior dentition in 17-year-old African American male with localized aggressive periodontitis. *(Photo courtesy Dr. Sasi Sunkari.)*

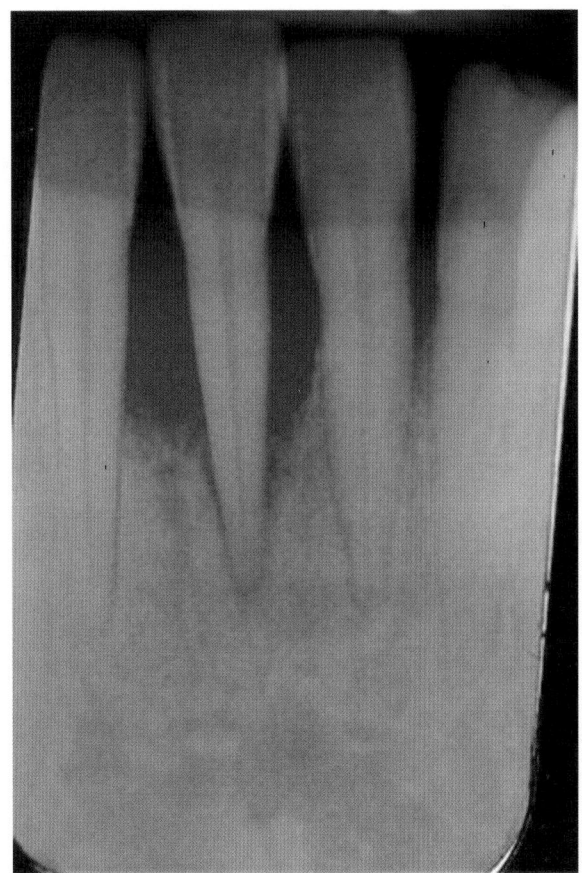

Fig. 52.3 Preoperative radiograph of anterior mandible in localized aggressive periodontitis patient. *(Photo courtesy Dr. Sasi Sunkari.)*

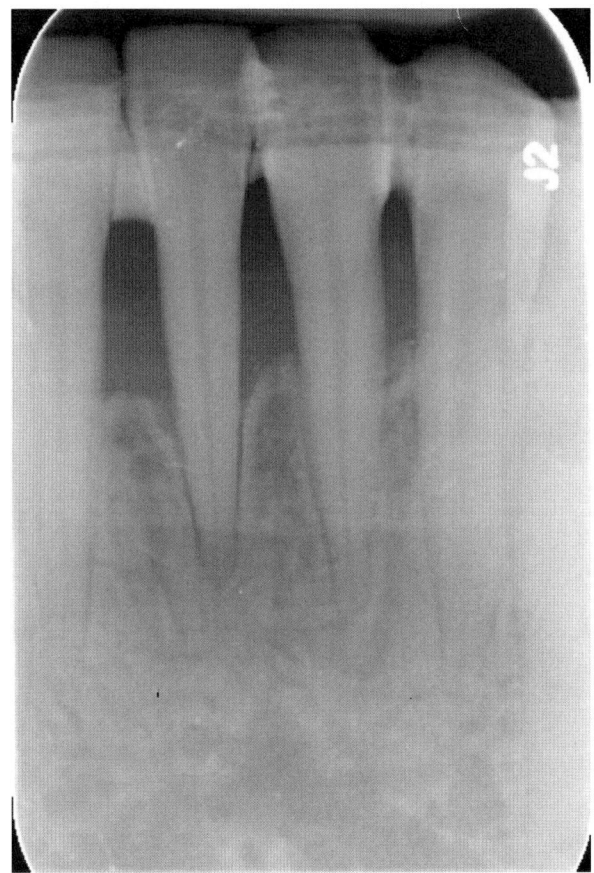

Fig. 52.4 Postoperative radiograph of anterior mandible in localized aggressive periodontitis patient treated with a combination of antibiotic therapy, scaling and root planing, and surgical intervention. *(Photo courtesy Dr. Sasi Sunkari.)*

bacterial strains.[34] Although tetracyclines were often used in the past as anti-infective agents, especially for LAP and other types of aggressive periodontitis, they are now frequently replaced by more effective combination antibiotics.[32]

Specific Agents

Tetracycline, minocycline, and doxycycline are semisynthetic members of the tetracycline group that have been used in periodontal therapy.

Tetracycline

Treatment with tetracycline hydrochloride requires the administration of 250 mg four times daily. It is inexpensive, but compliance may be reduced by the need to take the medication so frequently. Side effects include gastrointestinal disturbances, photosensitivity, hypersensitivity, increased blood urea nitrogen levels, blood dyscrasias, dizziness, and headache. In addition, tooth discoloration occurs when this drug is administered to children who are 12 years old or younger.

KEY FACT

Tetracycline and Tooth Discoloration
Tetracycline has the ability to chelate with calcium and therefore gets deposited in mineralized tissues such as bone or teeth during the mineralization process, resulting in yellow to brown discoloration of teeth.

Minocycline

Minocycline is effective against a broad spectrum of microorganisms. In patients with adult periodontitis, it suppresses spirochetes and motile rods as effectively as scaling and root planing, with suppression evident up to 3 months after therapy. Minocycline can be given twice daily, thereby facilitating compliance as compared with tetracycline. Although it is associated with less phototoxicity and renal toxicity than tetracycline, minocycline may cause reversible vertigo. Minocycline administered at a dose of 200 mg/day for 1 week results in a reduction of total bacterial counts, complete elimination of spirochetes for up to 2 months, and improvement of all clinical parameters.[13,14]

Side effects are similar to those of tetracycline; however, there is an increased incidence of vertigo. It is the only tetracycline that can permanently discolor erupted teeth and gingival tissue when administered orally.

Doxycycline

Doxycycline has the same spectrum of activity as minocycline and can be equally effective.[12] Because doxycycline can be given only once daily, patients may be more compliant. Compliance is also improved because its absorption from the gastrointestinal tract is only slightly altered by calcium, metal ions, or antacids, as is absorption of other tetracyclines. Side effects are similar to those of tetracycline hydrochloride; however, it is the most photosensitizing agent in the tetracycline category.

The recommended dosage when doxycycline is used as an anti-infective agent is 100 mg twice daily the first day, which is then reduced to 100 mg daily. To reduce gastrointestinal upset, 50 mg can be taken twice daily after the initial dose. When given as a sub-antimicrobial dose (to inhibit collagenase), 20 mg of doxycycline twice daily is recommended.[9,16]

Metronidazole
Pharmacology

Metronidazole is a nitroimidazole compound that was developed in France to treat protozoal infections. It is bactericidal to anaerobic

organisms and is thought to disrupt bacterial DNA synthesis in conditions with a low reduction potential. Metronidazole is not the drug of choice for treating *A. actinomycetemcomitans* infections. However, metronidazole is effective against *A. actinomycetemcomitans* when used in combination with other antibiotics.[43,44] Metronidazole is also effective against anaerobes such as *Porphyromonas gingivalis* and *Prevotella intermedia*.[25]

Clinical Use

Metronidazole has been used clinically to treat acute necrotizing ulcerative gingivitis, chronic periodontitis, and aggressive periodontitis. It has been used as monotherapy and also in combination with root planing and surgery or with other antibiotics. Metronidazole has been used successfully to treat necrotizing ulcerative gingivitis.[39]

Studies in humans have demonstrated the efficacy of metronidazole for the treatment of periodontitis.[38] A single dose of metronidazole (250 mg orally) appears in both serum and GCF in sufficient quantities to inhibit a wide range of suspected periodontal pathogens. When it is administered systemically (i.e., 750 mg/day to 1000 mg/day for 2 weeks), metronidazole reduces the growth of anaerobic flora, including spirochetes, and it decreases the clinical and histopathologic signs of periodontitis.[38] The most common regimen is 250 mg 3 times daily for 7 days.[39] Currently, the critical level of spirochetes that is needed to diagnose an anaerobic infection, the appropriate time to give metronidazole, and the ideal dosage or duration of therapy are unknown.[25] As monotherapy (i.e., with no concurrent root planing), metronidazole is inferior and at best only equivalent to root planing. Therefore if it is used, metronidazole should not be administered as monotherapy.

Soder and colleagues[52] demonstrated that metronidazole was more effective than placebo for the management of sites that were unresponsive to root planing. Nevertheless, many patients still had sites that bled with probing, despite metronidazole therapy. The existence of refractory periodontitis as a diagnostic consideration indicates that some patients do not respond to conventional therapy, which may include root planing, surgery, or both.

Studies have suggested that when it is combined with amoxicillin or amoxicillin–clavulanate potassium (Augmentin), metronidazole may be of value for the management of patients with LAP or refractory periodontitis. This is discussed in more detail later in this chapter.

Side Effects

Metronidazole has an Antabuse effect when alcohol is ingested. The response is generally proportional to the amount ingested and can result in severe cramps, nausea, and vomiting. Products that contain alcohol should be avoided during therapy and for at least 1 day after therapy is discontinued. Metronidazole also inhibits warfarin metabolism. Patients who are undergoing anticoagulant therapy should avoid metronidazole, because it prolongs prothrombin time.[39] It also should be avoided in patients who are taking lithium. This drug produces a metallic taste in the mouth, which may affect compliance.

Penicillins
Pharmacology

Penicillins are the drugs of choice for the treatment of many serious infections in humans and are the most widely used antibiotics. Penicillins are natural and semisynthetic derivatives of broth cultures of the *Penicillium* mold. They inhibit bacterial cell wall production and therefore are bactericidal.

Clinical Use

Penicillins other than amoxicillin and amoxicillin–clavulanate potassium (Augmentin) have not been shown to increase periodontal attachment levels, and their use in periodontal therapy does not appear to be justified.

Side Effects

Penicillins may induce allergic reactions and bacterial resistance.

KEY FACT

Penicillin Allergy

Up to 10% of patients may be allergic to penicillin. Reactions to ingestion of penicillin or its derivatives, such as amoxicillin, in allergic patients can range from skin rash to life-threatening anaphylaxis.

Amoxicillin

Amoxicillin is a semisynthetic penicillin with an extended anti-infective spectrum that includes gram-positive and gram-negative bacteria. It demonstrates excellent absorption after oral administration. Amoxicillin is susceptible to penicillinase, which is a β-lactamase produced by certain bacteria that breaks the penicillin ring structure and thus renders penicillins ineffective.

Amoxicillin may be useful for the management of patients with aggressive periodontitis in both localized and generalized forms. The recommended dosage is 500 mg 3 times daily for 8 days.[32,33]

Amoxicillin–Clavulanate Potassium

The combination of amoxicillin with clavulanate potassium makes this anti-infective agent resistant to penicillinase enzymes produced by some bacteria. Amoxicillin with clavulanate (Augmentin) may be useful for the management of patients with LAP or refractory periodontitis.[42] Bueno and colleagues[8] reported that Augmentin arrested alveolar bone loss in patients with periodontal disease that was refractory to treatment with other antibiotics, including tetracycline, metronidazole, and clindamycin.

Cephalosporins

Pharmacology

The family of β-lactams known as cephalosporins is similar in action and structure to the penicillins. These drugs are frequently used in medicine, and they are resistant to a number of β-lactamases that are normally active against penicillin.

Clinical Use

Cephalosporins are generally not used to treat dental-related infections. The penicillins are superior to cephalosporins with regard to their range of action against periodontal pathogenic bacteria.

Side Effects

Patients who are allergic to penicillins must be considered to be allergic to all β-lactam products. More specifically, up to 10% of patients who have an allergy to penicillin may also have an adverse reaction to cephalosporins. Rashes, urticaria, fever, and gastrointestinal upset have all been associated with cephalosporins.[62]

Clindamycin

Pharmacology

Clindamycin is effective against anaerobic bacteria and has a strong affinity for osseous tissue.[56] It is effective for situations in which the patient is allergic to penicillin.

Clinical Use

Clindamycin has demonstrated efficacy in patients with periodontitis that is refractory to tetracycline therapy. Walker and colleagues[62] showed that clindamycin helped stabilize refractory patients; the dosage used was 150 mg 4 times daily for 10 days. Jorgensen and Slots[33] recommend a regimen of 300 mg twice daily for 8 days.

Side Effects

Clindamycin has been associated with pseudomembranous colitis, but the incidence is higher with cephalosporins and ampicillin. When needed, however, clindamycin can be used with caution, but it is not indicated for patients with a history of colitis. Diarrhea or cramping that develops during clindamycin therapy may be indicative of colitis, and it should be discontinued. If symptoms persist, the patient should be referred to an internist.

Ciprofloxacin

Pharmacology

Ciprofloxacin is a quinolone that is active against gram-negative rods, including all facultative and some anaerobic putative periodontal pathogens.[41]

Clinical Use

Because it demonstrates a minimal effect on *Streptococcus* species, which are associated with periodontal health, ciprofloxacin therapy may facilitate the establishment of a microflora that is associated with periodontal health. At present, ciprofloxacin is the only antibiotic in periodontal therapy to which all strains of *A. actinomycetemcomitans* are susceptible. It has also been used in combination with metronidazole.[43]

Side Effects

Nausea, headache, metallic taste in the mouth, and abdominal discomfort have been associated with ciprofloxacin. Quinolones inhibit the metabolism of theophylline, and caffeine and concurrent administration can produce toxicity. Quinolones have also been reported to enhance the effects of warfarin and other anticoagulants.[62]

Macrolides

Pharmacology

Macrolide antibiotics contain a many-membered lactone ring to which one or more deoxy sugars are attached. They inhibit protein synthesis by binding to the 50S ribosomal subunits of sensitive microorganisms. Macrolides can be bacteriostatic or bactericidal, depending on the concentration of the drug and the nature of the microorganism. The macrolide antibiotics used for periodontal treatment include erythromycin, spiramycin, and azithromycin.

Clinical Use

Erythromycin does not concentrate in GCF and is not effective against most putative periodontal pathogens. For these reasons, erythromycin is not recommended as an adjunct to periodontal therapy.

Spiramycin is active against gram-positive organisms; it is excreted in high concentrations in saliva. It is used as an adjunct to periodontal treatment in Canada and Europe but is not available in the United States. Spiramycin has a minimal effect on attachment levels.

Azithromycin is a member of the azalide class of macrolides. It is effective against anaerobes and gram-negative bacilli. After an oral dosage of 500 mg 4 times daily for 3 days, significant levels of azithromycin can be detected in most tissues for 7 to 10 days.[7,30] The concentration of azithromycin in tissue specimens from periodontal lesions is significantly higher than that of normal gingiva.[40] It has been proposed that azithromycin penetrates fibroblasts and phagocytes in concentrations that are 100 to 200 times greater than that of the extracellular compartment. Azithromycin is actively transported to sites of inflammation by phagocytes, where it is released directly into the sites of inflammation as the phagocytes rupture during phagocytosis.[23] Therapeutic use requires a single dose of 250 mg/day for 5 days after an initial loading dose of 500 mg.[62]

Data have suggested that azithromycin may be an effective adjunctive therapy for increasing attachment levels in patients with aggressive periodontitis[27] as well as for reducing the degree of gingival enlargement.[15] These data must be carefully considered, because they were derived from small subject populations. Currently, the literature presents conflicting reports regarding the efficacy of this antibiotic as an adjunct to periodontal therapy. One study concluded that adjunctive azithromycin provides no additional benefit over nonsurgical periodontal treatment for the parameters investigated in patients with severe generalized chronic periodontitis. Furthermore, an additional study reported that there was an increase in cardiovascular deaths among patients who received azithromycin; this increase was most pronounced among patients with a high baseline risk of cardiovascular disease. As a result of this study, the US Food and Drug Administration issued a warning that the drug can alter the electrical activity of the heart, which may lead to a potentially fatal heart rhythm known as *prolonged QT interval*. This rhythm causes the timing of the heart's contractions to become irregular. The warning stated that physicians should use caution when giving the antibiotic to patients who are known to have this condition or who are at risk for cardiovascular problems.

To ascertain the efficacy of azithromycin for the management of periodontal diseases, future studies will need to increase the number of subjects, improve diagnostic methods and tools, and determine the appropriate dose, duration, and frequency of azithromycin therapy.

Serial and Combination Antibiotic Therapy
Rationale
Because periodontal infections may contain a wide variety of bacteria, no single antibiotic is effective against all putative pathogens. Indeed, differences exist in the microbial flora associated with the various periodontal disease syndromes.[63] These "mixed" infections can include a variety of aerobic, microaerophilic, and anaerobic bacteria, which may be both gram negative and gram positive. In these cases, it may be necessary to use more than one antibiotic, either serially or in combination.[44] Before combinations of antibiotics are used, however, the periodontal pathogens being treated should be identified and antibiotic-susceptibility testing performed.[65]

Clinical Use
Antibiotics that are bacteriostatic (e.g., tetracycline) generally require rapidly dividing microorganisms to be effective. They do not function well if a bactericidal antibiotic (e.g., amoxicillin) is given concurrently. *When both types of drugs are required, they are best given serially rather than in combination.*

Rams and Slots[44] reviewed combination therapy involving the use of systemic metronidazole along with amoxicillin, amoxicillin–clavulanate (Augmentin), or ciprofloxacin. The metronidazole–amoxicillin and metronidazole–Augmentin combinations provided excellent elimination of many organisms in adults with LAP who had been treated unsuccessfully with tetracyclines and mechanical debridement. These drugs have an additive effect that involves the suppression of A. actinomycetemcomitans. Tinoco and colleagues[55] found metronidazole and amoxicillin to be clinically effective for the treatment of LAP, although 50% of patients who were treated with this regimen harbored A. actinomycetemcomitans 1 year later. The metronidazole–ciprofloxacin combination is effective against A. actinomycetemcomitans; metronidazole targets obligate anaerobes,

and ciprofloxacin targets facultative anaerobes. This is a powerful combination against mixed infections. Studies of this drug combination for the treatment of refractory periodontitis have documented marked clinical improvement. This combination may provide a therapeutic benefit by reducing or eliminating pathogenic organisms and a prophylactic benefit by giving rise to a predominantly streptococcal microflora.[43]

Systemic antibiotic therapy in combination with mechanical therapy appears to be valuable for the treatment of recalcitrant periodontal infections and LAP infections that involve A. actinomycetemcomitans. Antibiotic treatment should be reserved for specific subsets of periodontal patients who do not respond to conventional therapy. The selection of specific agents should be guided by the results of cultures and sensitivity tests for subgingival plaque microorganisms.

Pharmacologic Implications
Principles of antibiotic therapy for the proper selection of an antibiotic minimally require identification of the causative organism, determination of the antibiotic sensitivity, and an effective method of administration.[29] The use of antibiotics to treat gingival diseases is contraindicated, because this is a local infection that can be easily treated with scaling and appropriate home care by the patient.[54] With regard to destructive periodontal diseases, there are limited data to support the use of systemic antibiotic treatment. Although bacterial infections of the periodontium are considered to be important to initiation of the disease, currently no one microbe or group of microbes has been demonstrated to be the cause of these diseases. It is therefore not surprising that systemic antibiotics have had only a modest effect on the management of periodontal diseases. At this time, systemic antibiotics for the treatment of periodontal diseases have been indicated primarily for adjunctive use in the treatment of aggressive periodontal diseases[26,28] (Table 52.3).

Guidelines for the use of antibiotics in periodontal therapy include the following:
1. The clinical diagnosis and situation dictate the need for possible antibiotic therapy as an adjunct for controlling active periodontal disease (Fig. 52.5). The patient's diagnosis can change over time. For example, a patient who presents with generalized mild chronic periodontitis can return to a diagnosis of periodontal health after initial therapy. However, if the patient has been treated and continues to have active disease, the diagnosis may change to generalized severe chronic periodontitis.
2. Disease activity as measured by continuing attachment loss, purulent exudate, and bleeding on probing[35,36] may be an indication for periodontal intervention and possible microbial analysis through plaque sampling.
3. When they are used to treat periodontal disease, antibiotics are selected on the basis of the patient's medical and dental status and current medications,[32] and the results of microbial analysis, if it is performed.
4. Microbiologic plaque sampling may be performed according to the instructions of the reference laboratory. The samples are usually taken at the beginning of an appointment, before instrumentation of the pocket. Supragingival plaque is removed, and an endodontic paper point is inserted subgingivally into the deepest pockets to absorb bacteria in the loosely associated plaque. This endodontic point is placed in reduced transfer fluid or a sterile transfer tube and sent to the laboratory. The laboratory will then send the referring dentist a report that includes the pathogens that are present and any appropriate antibiotic regimen. At this time, there are scant data to suggest that microbial identification from a

TABLE 52.3 Therapeutic Uses of Systemic Antimicrobial Agents for Various Periodontal Diseases

Disease	Systemic Antimicrobial Agents	Adjunct or Stand-Alone Therapy
Gingival diseases	Antibiotic use not recommended	Not applicable
Necrotizing ulcerative gingivitis	Antibiotic use not recommended unless there are systemic complications (e.g., fever, swollen lymph nodes)	As an adjunct when necessary
Chronic periodontitis	Limited benefit; antibiotic use not recommended	Not applicable
Aggressive periodontitis	Antibiotic use recommended; for greatest benefit, therapeutic levels of antibiotics should be achieved by the time scaling and root planing are completed (all debridement should be completed within a week); the optimal antibiotic type, dose, frequency, and duration have not been identified	As an adjunct
Necrotizing ulcerative periodontitis	Antibiotic use dependent on the systemic condition of the patient	As an adjunct when necessary
Periodontitis as a manifestation of systemic disease	Antibiotic use dependent on the systemic condition of the patient	As an adjunct when necessary
Periodontal abscess	Antibiotic use not recommended	Not applicable

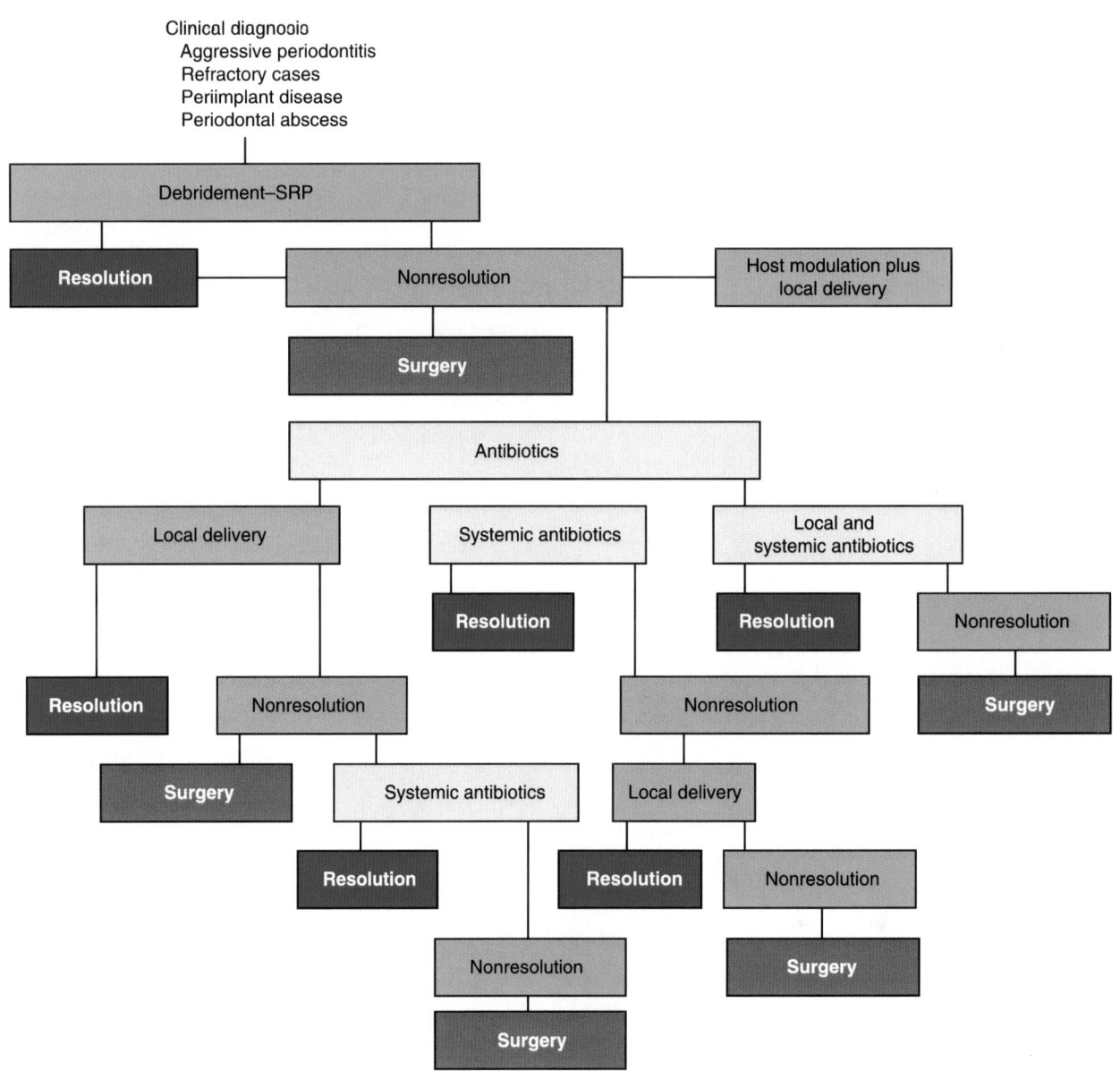

Fig. 52.5 A decision tree for the selection of antibiotic therapy.

plaque sample can be used to clinically improve the periodontal condition of the patient.

5. Meta-analyses of randomized clinical trials and quasi-experimental studies have shown that systemic antibiotics can improve attachment levels when they are used as adjuncts to scaling and root planing. The same benefits could not be demonstrated when antibiotics were used as a stand-alone therapy.[28]

6. When systemic antibiotics were used as adjuncts to scaling and root planing, improvements were observed in the attachment levels of patients with chronic and aggressive periodontitis, although patients with aggressive periodontitis experienced greater benefits.[28] The mean attachment level change depended on the antibiotic used and ranged from 0.09 mm to 1.10 mm.[28]

7. The identification of which antibiotics were most effective for the treatment of destructive periodontal diseases was limited by the insufficient sizes of the samples found in the randomized clinical trials used as part of a systematic review.[28] A meta-analysis evaluating eight different antibiotics or antibiotic combinations showed that only tetracycline and metronidazole significantly improved attachment levels when they were used as adjuncts to scaling and root planing for patients with destructive periodontal diseases.[28]

8. Debridement of root surfaces, optimal oral hygiene, and frequent periodontal maintenance therapy are important parts of comprehensive periodontal therapy. As mentioned previously, an antibiotic strength that is 500 times greater than the systemic therapeutic dose may be required to be effective against bacteria that have been arranged into biofilm. It is therefore important to disrupt the biofilm physically so that the antibiotic agents can have access to the periodontal pathogens.[26]

9. Although there are adequate data to suggest that systemic antibiotics can be of benefit for the treatment of destructive periodontal diseases, there are limited data available to identify which antibiotics are suitable for which infection; the optimum dosage, frequency, and duration of antibiotic therapy; when the regimen should be introduced during the treatment schedule; the long-term outcomes of antibiotic use; the potential hazards of these agents (e.g., antibiotic resistance, changes in oral microflora)[28]; and the economic ramifications of this type of pharmacologic intervention.

The selection of an antibiotic must be made on the basis of factors other than the empirical decisions made by the clinician. Unfortunately, there is no one best choice of antibiotic at present (i.e., there is no "silver bullet"). Therefore the clinician must integrate the history of the patient's disease, the clinical signs and symptoms, and the results of radiographic examinations and possibly microbiologic sampling to determine the course of periodontal therapy. The clinician must obtain a thorough medical history, including current medications and the possible adverse effects of combining these medicines, before prescribing any antibiotic therapy. The clinician must make the final decision with the patient. Risks and benefits concerning antibiotics as adjuncts to periodontal therapy should be discussed with the patient before antibiotics are used.

Conclusion

Scaling and root planing alone are effective for reducing pocket depths, gaining increases in periodontal attachment levels, and decreasing inflammation levels (i.e., bleeding with probing). When systemic antibiotics are used as adjuncts to scaling and root planing, the evidence indicates that some systemic antibiotics (e.g., metronidazole, tetracycline) provide additional improvements in attachment levels (0.35 mm for metronidazole; 0.40 mm for tetracycline) when used as adjuncts to scaling and root planing.[28] The use of anti-infective chemotherapeutic treatment adjuncts does not result in significant adverse effects for patients.

The decision regarding when to use systemic antimicrobials should be made on the basis of the clinician's consideration of the clinical findings, the patient's medical and dental history,[17,19] the patient's preferences, and the potential benefits of adjunctive therapy with these agents.

CHAPTER HIGHLIGHTS

- The *systemic administration* of antibiotics may be a necessary adjunct for controlling bacterial infection, because bacteria can invade periodontal tissues, thereby making mechanical therapy alone sometimes ineffective.
- Although oral bacteria are susceptible to many antibiotics, no single antibiotic at the concentrations achieved in body fluids inhibits all putative periodontal pathogens.
- The protocol for use of anti-infective agents depends on the mechanism of action, the patient's health status and history, and the clinical presentation.

 A Case Scenario is found on the companion website www.expertconsult.com.

References

 References for this chapter are found on the companion website www.expertconsult.com.

Host Modulation

Maria Emanuel Ryan | *Ying Gu*

Content on emerging host modulatory therapies, bacteria–host interactions, host modulation factors in systemic disorders such as diabetes and cardiovascular disease, management of periodontal and other inflammatory diseases, and the clinical efficacy and safety of sub-antimicrobial–dose doxycycline can be accessed on the companion website at www.expertconsult .com.

Introduction

The term *host modulation* has been incorporated in dental jargon, but it has not been well defined. *Host* can be defined as the organism from which a parasite obtains its nourishment or, in the transplantation of tissue, the individual who receives the graft. *Modulation* is the alteration of function or status of something in response to a stimulus or an altered chemical or physical environment.

In diseases of the periodontium that are initiated by bacteria, the host is the individual who harbors the pathogens, but it was not clear for many years whether it was possible to modulate the host response to the pathogens and other stimuli that led to breakdown of the attachment apparatus. Host modulation with chemotherapeutic agents or drugs is the latest adjunctive therapeutic option for the management of periodontal diseases.

The concept of host modulation is fairly new to the field of dentistry but is universally understood by most physicians who routinely apply the principles of host modulation to the management of chronic progressive disorders such as arthritis and osteoporosis. The concept of host modulation was introduced to dentistry by Williams[113] and Golub and colleagues[42] and then expanded on by many other scholars in the dental profession. In 1990, Williams concluded that "there are compelling data from studies in animals and human trials indicating that pharmacologic agents that modulate the host responses believed to be involved in the pathogenesis of periodontal destruction may be efficacious in slowing the progression of periodontitis."[113] In 1992, Golub and colleagues discussed host modulation with tetracyclines and their chemically modified analogues.[42] The future that these investigators described has arrived, and to better understand this new era in disease management, we first consider the pathogenesis of periodontitis.

Many clinicians previously thought that periodontal disease was an inevitable consequence of aging and was uniformly distributed in the population. They thought that disease severity was directly correlated with plaque levels (i.e., the worse the oral hygiene, the

worse the periodontal disease) and that disease progression occurred in a continuous, linear manner throughout life. As a result of better epidemiologic data, there has been a paradigm shift in how clinicians and scientists view the prevalence and progression of this common disease. It has been established that periodontal disease is not a natural consequence of aging and disease severity is not necessarily correlated with plaque levels. Theories about the pathogenesis of periodontitis have evolved from a purely plaque-associated disease to the hypotheses that place considerable emphasis on the host's response to the bacteria.[13]

The Surgeon General's report on *Oral Health in America*, published in 2000, recognized the importance of dental health in the overall general health and well-being of a patient.[104] Research findings indicate possible associations between chronic oral infections, such as periodontitis, and systemic disorders, such as diabetes, cardiovascular and lung diseases, stroke, osteoporosis, and rheumatoid arthritis. The Surgeon General's report assesses these emerging associations and explores factors that may underlie oral-systemic disease connections. Along with these findings and the emergence of the discipline of periodontal medicine, there have been many developments in therapeutic approaches to the management of periodontitis. Development of the chemotherapeutic approach known as *host modulation* required a thorough understanding of the host response and the impact of a variety of risk factors.

Anecdotally, many dentists have identified patients with abundant plaque and calculus deposits that manifest as gingivitis with shallow pocketing. In contrast, other patients, despite maintaining a high standard of plaque control, succumb to aggressive forms of periodontitis, with deep pocketing, tooth mobility, and early tooth loss. The former group of patients is *periodontal disease resistant,* whereas the latter group is *periodontal disease susceptible.* The response of the periodontal tissues to plaque is different in these two types of patients, and certain patients undergo advanced periodontal breakdown even though they achieve a high standard of oral hygiene.

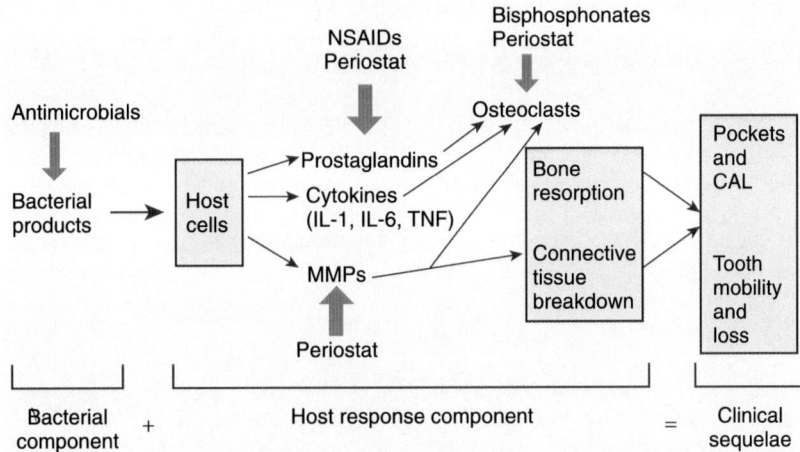

Fig. 54.1 Potential adjunctive therapeutic approaches and points of intervention in the treatment of periodontitis are shown in the context of the pathologic cascade of events. *CAL,* clinical attachment loss; *IL,* interleukin; *MMPs,* matrix metalloproteinases; *NSAIDs,* nonsteroidal antiinflammatory drugs; *TNF,* tumor necrosis factor.

These observations led researchers to realize that the *host response* to the bacterial challenge of subgingival plaque is the most important determinant of disease severity, progression, and response to therapy. Although plaque bacteria are capable of causing direct damage to the periodontal tissues (e.g., by release of hydrogen sulfide, butyric acid, and other enzymes and mediators), most destructive events occurring in the periodontal tissues result from activation of destructive processes that occur as part of the host immune-inflammatory response to plaque bacteria. The host response is essentially protective but paradoxically can also result in significant tissue damage, including breakdown of connective tissue fibers in the periodontal ligament and resorption of alveolar bone.

HMT is a *means of treating the host side of the host–bacteria interaction.* The host response is responsible for most of the tissue breakdown that occurs and leads to the clinical signs of periodontitis (i.e., loss of connective tissue attachment and bone). HMTs offer the opportunity for modulating or reducing this destruction by treating aspects of the chronic inflammatory response. HMTs do not block normal defense mechanisms or inflammation; instead, they ameliorate excessive or pathologically elevated inflammatory processes to enhance the opportunities for wound healing and periodontal stability.

HMT can be used to reduce excessive levels of enzymes, cytokines, and prostanoids and should not reduce levels below constitutive levels. HMTs can also modulate osteoclast and osteoblast function (Fig. 54.1) but should not affect normal tissue turnover. HMT is key to addressing many of the risk factors that have adverse effects on the host response that are not easily managed (e.g., smoking, diabetes) or cannot be changed (e.g., genetic susceptibility). Host modulatory agents can be used to increase the levels of a person's protective or antiinflammatory mediators. Use of systemic HMTs for treatment of a patient's periodontal condition may also provide benefits for other inflammatory disorders, such as arthritis, cardiovascular disease, dermatologic conditions, diabetes, rheumatoid arthritis, and osteoporosis. Patients who are currently taking host modulatory agents, such as nonsteroidal antiinflammatory drugs (NSAIDs), bisphosphonates, or tetracyclines, and newer agents targeting specific cytokines for the management of medical conditions, may experience periodontal benefits from the systemic medications prescribed for the management of other chronic inflammatory conditions.

Systemically Administered Agents

A variety of drug classes have been evaluated as host modulation agents, including NSAIDs, bisphosphonates, tetracyclines, enamel matrix proteins, growth factors, and bone morphogenetic proteins. Chemotherapeutic agents have been researched as adjunct treatments for periodontitis in clinical practice, and HMTs are still evolving.

Nonsteroidal Antiinflammatory Drugs

NSAIDs inhibit the formation of prostaglandins, including PGE_2, which is produced by neutrophils, macrophages, fibroblasts, and gingival epithelial cells in response to LPS, a component of the cell wall of gram-negative bacteria. PGE_2 has been extensively studied in periodontal disease because it up-regulates bone resorption by osteoclasts.[44,55,79] Levels of PGE_2 are elevated in patients with periodontal disease compared with healthy patients.[45,79] PGE_2 also inhibits fibroblast function and has inhibitory and modulatory effects on the immune response.[46]

NSAIDs inhibit prostaglandin synthesis and therefore reduce tissue inflammation. They are used to treat pain, acute inflammation, and a variety of chronic inflammatory conditions. NSAIDs include the salicylates (e.g., aspirin), indomethacin, and propionic acid derivatives (e.g., ibuprofen, flurbiprofen, naproxen). The ability of NSAIDs to block PGE_2 production, thereby reducing inflammation and inhibiting osteoclast activity in the periodontal tissues, has been investigated in patients with periodontitis. Short-term administration of NSAIDs reduced gingival crevicular fluid (GCF) MMP-8 levels, but no statistically significant differences were observed in clinical attachment levels (CALs).[11] Studies also suggested that low-dose aspirin as an adjunct periodontal therapy was beneficial in reducing periodontal attachment loss.[27,29]

Studies have shown that systemic NSAIDs, such as indomethacin,[114] flurbiprofen,[115] and naproxen,[54] administered daily for up to 3 years significantly slowed the rate of alveolar bone loss compared with placebo. However, NSAIDs have some serious disadvantages when considered as an HMT for periodontitis. Daily administration for extended periods is necessary for periodontal benefits to become apparent, and NSAIDs are associated with significant side effects, including gastrointestinal problems, hemorrhage (from decreased platelet aggregation), and renal and hepatic impairment. Research shows that the periodontal benefits of taking long-term NSAIDs are lost when patients stop taking the drugs, with a return to or an acceleration of the rate of bone loss seen before NSAID therapy, often referred to as a *rebound effect*.[116] For these reasons, the long-term use of NSAIDs as an adjunctive treatment for periodontitis has never developed beyond research studies.

Selective cyclooxygenase-2 (COX-2) inhibitors may offer promise as adjunctive treatments for periodontitis. The enzyme cyclooxygenase, which converts arachidonic acid to prostaglandins, exists in two functionally distinct isoforms: COX-1 and COX-2. COX-1 is constitutively expressed and has antithrombogenic and cytoprotective functions. Inhibition of COX-1 by nonselective NSAIDs therefore causes side effects such as gastrointestinal ulceration and impaired hemostasis.

COX-2 is induced after stimulation by various cytokines, growth factors, and LPS, resulting in the production of elevated quantities of prostaglandins. Inhibition of COX-2 by selective COX-2 inhibitors reduces inflammation. Researchers thought that the use of selective COX-2 inhibitors could reduce periodontal inflammation without the side effects typically observed after long-term (nonselective) NSAID therapy, and preliminary studies found that selective COX-2 inhibitors slowed alveolar bone loss in animal models[5,53] and modified prostaglandin production in human periodontal tissues.[107] However, the selective COX-2 inhibitors were later associated with significant and life-threatening adverse effects (e.g., myocardial infarction), resulting in some drugs being withdrawn from the market. NSAIDs, including selective COX-2 inhibitors, are not indicated as adjunctive HMTs for the treatment of periodontal disease.

Bisphosphonates

Bisphosphonates are bone-seeking agents that inhibit bone resorption by disrupting osteoclast activity. Their precise mechanism of action is unclear, but research has shown that bisphosphonates interfere with osteoblast metabolism and secretion of lysosomal enzymes.[112] Evidence suggests that bisphosphonates also possess anticollagenase properties.[74]

The ability of bisphosphonates to modulate osteoclast activity may be useful in the treatment of periodontitis. Research has demonstrated that in naturally occurring periodontitis in beagle dogs, treatment with the bisphosphonate alendronate significantly increased bone density compared with placebo.[90] In animal models of experimentally induced periodontitis, bisphosphonates reduced alveolar bone resorption.[98,112] In human studies, these agents resulted in enhanced alveolar bone status and density.[7,21,92]

Some bisphosphonates have the unwanted effects of inhibiting bone calcification and altering white blood cell counts. Reports of avascular necrosis of the jaws after bisphosphonate therapy highlight the risk of bone necrosis after dental extractions.[14] Reports of bisphosphonate-related osteonecrosis of the jaw (BRON/ONJ), although primarily associated with intravenous administration of bisphosphonates rather than oral administration, has impeded the development of bisphosphonates as an HMT to manage periodontitis. As with NSAIDs, no bisphosphonate drugs are approved and indicated for the treatment of periodontal disease.

◀◀   **FLASH BACK**

Down-regulation of the destructive elements of the host immune response can add to treatment choices in the future. However, agents such as systemic nonsteroidal antiinflammatory drugs (e.g., ibuprofen) can cause significant side effects with long-term use and are not advised. Antiosteoporotic agents (e.g., bisphosphonates) have a minimal effect on periodontal bone loss but carry risks such as localized bone necrosis.

Sub-antimicrobial–Dose Doxycycline

Sub-antimicrobial–dose doxycycline (SDD) is a 20-mg dose of doxycycline (Periostat) that is approved and indicated as an adjunct to SRP in the treatment of chronic periodontitis (see Fig. 54.4). It is taken twice daily for 3 months, up to a maximum of 9 months of continuous dosing. The 20-mg dose exerts its therapeutic effect by enzyme, cytokine, and osteoclast inhibition rather than by any antibiotic effect. Research studies have found no detectable antimicrobial effect on the oral flora or the bacterial flora in other regions of the body and have identified clinical benefit when used as an adjunct to SRP.

SDD (Periostat) is the only systemically administered HMT specifically indicated for the treatment of chronic periodontitis that is approved by the U.S. Food and Drug Administration (FDA) and accepted by the American Dental Association (ADA). Studies conducted by Preshaw and colleagues[89] comparing this same modified-release SDD with placebo in 266 subjects with periodontitis as an adjunct to SRP resulted in significantly greater clinical benefits than SRP alone. A review paper on the nonsurgical treatment of chronic periodontitis by means of SRP with or without adjuncts showed that clinical improvements with SRP alone resulted in a mean gain of 0.5 mm in CALs, whereas adjunctive therapy with SDD resulted in an additional 0.35 mm gain in CALs beyond that seen with mechanical therapy alone, representing a 70% improvement in CALs.[99]

A modified-release SDD (i.e., Oracea) was approved by the FDA for the treatment of the common skin disorder rosacea, and it is routinely prescribed within the dermatology community. It will be interesting to see what the long-term benefits to oral health will be in rosacea patients prescribed the time-release formulation of SDD. There has been considerable off-label use of this drug for the treatment of periodontal disease based on the understanding that once-daily administration can increase the level of compliance compared with twice-daily oral administration. Preshaw and coworkers demonstrated that this modified-release SDD resulted in significantly improved clinical benefits in the treatment of periodontitis.[89]

◢ !   **CLINICAL CORRELATION**

- Host modulatory therapy (HMT) is an emerging option for the management of periodontitis.
- A promising form of HMT is the use of chemically modified tetracyclines.
- An FDA-approved agent for host modulation treatment of periodontal disease is sub-antimicrobial–dose doxycycline (SDD) at 20 mg, taken twice daily.
- SDD is the only systemically administered HMT approved, and it is indicated as an adjunct to scaling and root planing (SRP) for treating periodontitis.
- Clinical trials have demonstrated a clear benefit for SDD compared with SRP alone.

Locally Administered Agents
Nonsteroidal Antiinflammatory Drugs

Topical NSAIDs have shown benefit in the treatment of periodontitis. One study of 55 patients with chronic periodontitis who received topical ketorolac mouthrinse reported that GCF levels of PGE_2 were reduced by approximately one-half over 6 months and that bone loss was halted.[57] Locally administered ketoprofen also has been investigated. Topically administered NSAIDs have not been approved as local HMTs for the management of periodontitis.

Enamel Matrix Proteins, Growth Factors, and Bone Morphogenetic Proteins

Several local HMTs have been investigated for use as adjuncts to surgical procedures to improve wound healing and stimulate regeneration of lost bone, periodontal ligament, and cementum, restoring the complete periodontal attachment apparatus. They include enamel matrix proteins, bone morphogenetic proteins (e.g., BMP-2, BMP-7), growth factors (e.g., platelet-derived growth factor, insulin-like growth factor), and tetracyclines. The locally applied HMTs approved by the FDA for adjunctive use during surgery are enamel matrix proteins (Emdogain), recombinant human platelet-derived growth factor-BB (GEM 21S), and BMP-2 (rhBMP-2 [Infuse]), which are covered more extensively in Chapter 63.

The initial local host modulatory agent approved by the FDA for adjunctive use during surgery to assist with clinical attachment gain and wound healing was Emdogain. It was followed by platelet-derived growth factor combined with a resorbable synthetic bone matrix (GEM 21S) to assist in regenerative procedures approved by the FDA and by rhBMP-2 (Infuse) soaked onto an absorbable collagen sponge to assist with ridge and sinus augmentation. The technology behind GEM 21 also has been approved and marketed for use in wound healing, particularly in patients with diabetes, and Infuse has been used for some time for healing fractures by the orthopedic community. However, adverse events associated with the administration of BMPs have been reported, including osteolysis, seroma or hematoma, infection, arachnoiditis, dysphagia, increased neurologic deficits, and cancer.[26] The remainder of this chapter focuses on the clinical utility of host modulation for nonsurgical procedures in clinical practice and the use of SDD (Periostat) in clinical practice.

Host Modulation and Comprehensive Periodontal Management

The term *periodontal management* suggests a much broader concept of periodontal care than the term *periodontal treatment*. This concept is extremely important considering the chronic nature of the disease. Management includes thorough medical and dental history and examination (i.e., clinical charting and radiographs), assessment of risk factors, diagnosis, development of a treatment strategy, initial and definitive treatment planning, review of treatment outcomes and reevaluation, long-term supportive periodontal therapy (i.e., maintenance care), and assessment of prognosis.

As new data continue to emerge regarding biochemical assessments of disease activity (i.e., measuring levels of proinflammatory mediators, bone and connective tissue breakdown products in the GCF, saliva, and tissues of the oral cavity), new diagnostic and prognostic tests may become part of established protocols for comprehensive periodontal disease management in the future. However, controlling the bacteria that cause periodontal infections remains a central focus of effective periodontal treatment. Understanding the importance of the host response and the impact of risk factors allows clinicians to provide complementary treatment strategies simultaneously for their patients (Fig. 54.2).

Patients most likely to require the use of HMT include those with risk factors that are nonmodifiable or not easily modified. If the decision is made to use HMT, it must be discussed with the patient and the rationale for treatment thoroughly explained. This takes time at chairside, but it is time well spent; patients become increasingly interested in their periodontal status and are more likely to develop ownership of their management, enhancing compliance with all aspects of care, including plaque control, risk reduction,

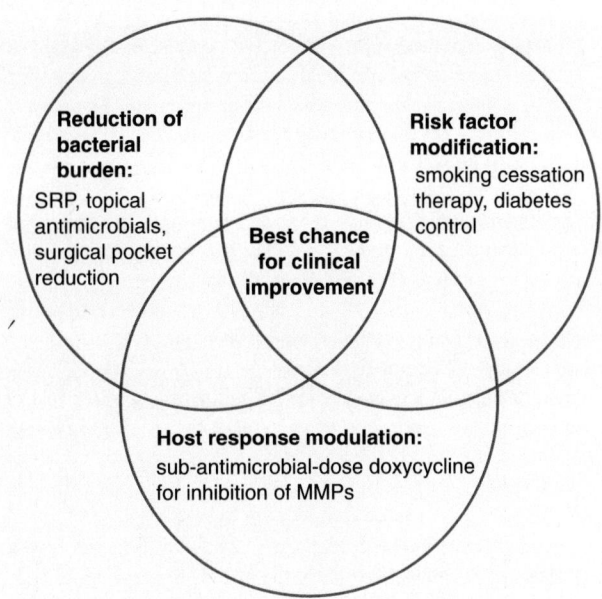

Fig. 54.2 The best chance for clinical improvement may come from implementing complementary treatment strategies for periodontitis that target different aspects of the periodontal balance. Reduction of the bacterial burden by scaling and root planing *(SRP)* is the cornerstone of treatment, and it can be augmented by the use of topical antimicrobials and surgical pocket therapy. In addition to antibacterial treatment, the host response can be treated with host modulatory therapy, such as sub-antimicrobial–dose doxycycline, for the inhibition of matrix metalloproteinases *(MMPs)*. Risk factor assessment and modification, including smoking cessation counseling, must form a key part of the periodontal treatment strategy. These different treatment strategies can be used together as part of a comprehensive management approach.

and treatment protocols. Compliance with HMT is greatly facilitated if the rationale for prescribing is clearly explained.

The need for compliance with the prescribed drug regimen is important because with SDD, for example, a tablet must be taken twice daily (i.e., once in the morning and once in the evening) and should not be taken with calcium supplements. Compliance may be improved by administration of a modified-release SDD capsule taken only once daily. It should be emphasized to the patient that the use of HMT is not a substitute for excellent plaque control (just as it is not a substitute for excellent debridement and root surface instrumentation by the treating clinician). To achieve the best results, patients must be interested and well informed about their condition so that compliance is maximized. Patients must also be convinced that comprehensive and frequent recall appointments are necessary in the maintenance phase of this chronic and often progressive disease, which can be very well controlled with adequate follow-up.

In addition to patient motivation, oral hygiene instruction, and SRP to reduce the bacterial challenge, a key treatment strategy when managing periodontitis is *risk factor modification*. The harmful effects of smoking on the periodontal tissues are well documented,[60] and successful smoking cessation therapy can be a major benefit to patients with periodontitis. Smoking cessation counseling can be undertaken in the dental office (if staff are appropriately trained) or through collaboration with the patient's physician or specialized clinics. Given the evidence that smokers have worse periodontal disease than nonsmokers[100,117] and that the magnitude and predictability of clinical improvements after treatment are significantly reduced in smokers,[1,85] smoking cessation counseling should form a major part of treatment for smokers with periodontitis.

Patients with poorly controlled diabetes are also at increased risk for periodontitis,[69] and periodontal therapy can have an impact on diabetic control.[46] Collaboration with medical colleagues when treating patients with diabetes and periodontitis is warranted to ascertain the degree of diabetic control.[31]

Other possible risks for periodontitis include nonmodifiable factors such as genetics, gender, and race. As the relevance of different risk factors is established through epidemiologic research, clinicians must remain aware of their responsibilities for informing and attempting to change patients' behaviors in relation to modifiable risks. The management of patients with periodontitis can involve the following complementary treatment strategies:

- Patient education and motivation, including oral hygiene instruction; use of powered toothbrushes, antiseptics in rinses, toothpastes, and irrigation; and explanation of the rationale for any adjunctive treatments
- Reduction of the bacterial burden by high-quality SRP
- Site-specific antibacterial treatment with local delivery systems or systemic antimicrobial therapy in selected cases
- Host response modulation by HMT
- Risk factor modification and risk reduction strategies
- Periodontal surgery with or without HMT

It is the responsibility of the dentist to customize the treatment plan for each patient by selecting and providing appropriate treatments after discussion and informed decision making by the patient. Good communication and showing an interest in the patient's condition are essential to maximize compliance and modify risk factors. The best chance for clinical improvement may come from a combination of targeted treatment approaches for each patient (see Fig. 54.2). Novak and colleagues published striking improvements in probing depth reductions and CAL gains in a 6-month, randomized, multicenter, examiner-blinded, placebo-controlled study, which showed that combination therapy of HMT (i.e., SDD) plus a locally delivered antimicrobial (i.e., doxycycline hyclate gel) and SRP provided optimal improvements in clinical parameters compared with SRP alone in the treatment of moderate to severe periodontitis.[76]

Sub-antimicrobial–Dose Doxycycline

SDD is the only FDA-approved, systemically administered HMT indicated specifically for the treatment of periodontitis. SDD is used as an adjunct to SRP and must not be used as a stand-alone therapy (i.e., monotherapy). Because SDD, previously called low-dose doxycycline (LDD) and currently marketed as Periostat, is based on a sub-antimicrobial dosage of doxycycline, a member of the tetracycline family of compounds, the use of tetracyclines for the management of periodontal diseases must be put in perspective.

No class of drugs has made more of an impact on periodontal therapy than the tetracyclines. They have been used in conjunction with SRP, the gold standard of nonsurgical therapy, and with resective and regenerative surgical procedures. The tetracyclines have been used locally and systemically as antimicrobial agents and as host modulation agents (i.e., SDD). Tetracyclines have been prescribed to address chronic periodontitis and to manage specific and often more aggressive types of periodontitis.

Tetracyclines have been advocated for treatment of patients with systemic diseases such as diabetes, rheumatoid arthritis, and rosacea (i.e., treated with Oracea). Doxycycline has led to improvements in the periodontal health of compromised diabetic patients and long-term markers of glycemic control (i.e., glycated hemoglobin).[47] As an adjunct to mechanical therapies, the goal of tetracycline therapy has

been to enhance reattachment or stimulate new attachment of the supporting apparatus and osseous formation. The following sections concentrate on the use of pleiotropic compounds for modulation of the host response in the treatment of periodontitis.

Mechanisms of Action

In addition to its antibiotic properties, doxycycline (and other members of the tetracycline family) has the ability to down-regulate MMPs, a family of zinc-dependent enzymes that can degrade extracellular matrix molecules, including collagen.[8,95] MMPs are secreted by the major cell types in the periodontal tissues (e.g., fibroblasts, keratinocytes, macrophages, PMNs, endothelial cells) and play a key role in periodontitis. Excessive quantities of MMPs are released in inflamed periodontal tissues, resulting in breakdown of the connective tissue matrix. The predominant MMPs in periodontitis, particularly MMP-8 and MMP-9, are derived from PMNs[41] and are extremely effective in degrading type I collagen, the most abundant collagen type in gingiva and periodontal ligament.[67] Levels of PMN-type MMPs increase with the severity of periodontal disease and decrease after therapy.[34,41] The release of large quantities of MMPs in the periodontium leads to significant anatomic disruption and breakdown of the connective tissues, contributing to the clinical signs of periodontitis.

The rationale for using SDD as an HMT in the treatment of periodontitis is that doxycycline down-regulates the activity of MMPs by a variety of synergistic mechanisms, including reductions in cytokine levels, and stimulates osteoblastic activity and new bone formation by up-regulating collagen production (Fig. 54.3).

Clinical Research Data on Distinct Patient Populations

Tetracyclines work well as host modulation agents because of their pleiotropic effects on multiple components of the host response (see Fig. 54.1). The only enzyme (MMP) inhibitors that have been approved for clinical use and tested for the treatment of periodontitis are members of the tetracycline family of compounds. In early studies investigating the use of commercially available tetracyclines, Golub and colleagues[43] reported that the semisynthetic compound doxycycline was more effective than the parent compound tetracycline in reducing excessive collagenase activity in the GCF of chronic periodontitis patients. Because doxycycline was a more effective inhibitor of collagenase than minocycline or tetracycline[11,35] and because of its safety profile, pharmacokinetic properties, and ready systemic absorption, clinical trials have focused on this compound.

In an effort to eliminate the side effects of long-term tetracycline therapy, especially the emergence of tetracycline-resistant organisms, SDD capsules were prepared and tested.[41] Each capsule contained 20 mg of doxycycline, compared with the commercially available 50-mg and 100-mg, antimicrobially effective capsules or tablets. Multiple clinical studies using sub-antimicrobial doses of doxycycline have shown no difference in the composition or resistance level of the oral flora.[102,111] Later studies demonstrated no appreciable differences in fecal or vaginal microflora samples.[109] These studies have shown no overgrowth of opportunistic pathogens, such as *Candida,* in the oral cavity, gastrointestinal system, or genitourinary system.

In a study of MMP inhibition, Golub and coworkers[34] reported that a 2-week regimen of SDD reduced collagenase in GCF and in the adjacent gingival tissues surgically excised for therapeutic purposes. Subsequent studies using SDD therapy adjunctive to routine scaling and prophylaxis indicated continued reductions in the excessive levels of collagenase in the GCF after 1 month of treatment. After cessation of SDD administration, however, there was a rapid rebound

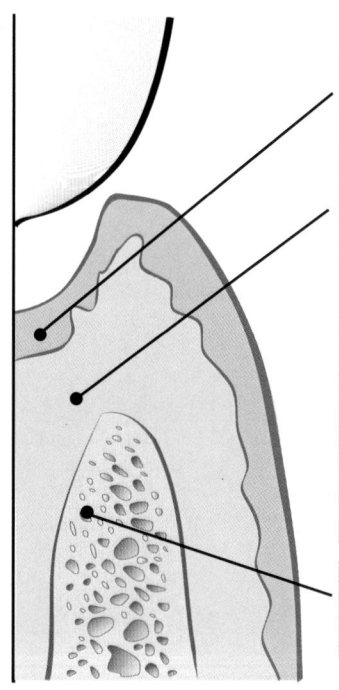

• Inhibition of production of epithelial-derived MMPs by inhibiting cellular expression and synthesis

• Direct inhibition of active MMPs by cation chelation (dependent on Ca^{2+} and Zn^{2+} binding properties)
• Inhibition of oxidative activation of latent MMPs (independent of cation-binding properties)
• Downregulates expression of key inflammatory cytokines including IL-1, IL-6, and TNF-α as well as PGE_2
• Scavenges and inhibits production of reactive oxygen species (ROS) produced by PMNs (e.g., HOCl, which activates latent MMPs)
• Inhibition of MMPs and ROS protects α_1 proteinase inhibitor (α_1-PI), thereby indirectly reducing tissue proteinase activity
• Stimulates fibroblast collagen production

• Reduces osteoclast activity and bone resorption
• Blocks osteoclast MMPs
• Stimulates osteoblast activity and bone formation

Fig. 54.3 Schematic drawing of a periodontal pocket shows the pleiotropic mechanisms by which doxycycline inhibits connective tissue breakdown. Down-regulation of destructive events in periodontal tissues by doxycycline results from modulation of a variety of proinflammatory pathways. *IL,* Interleukin; *MMPs,* matrix metalloproteinases; *PGE₂,* prostaglandin E_2; *PMNs,* polymorphonuclear leukocytes; *TNF,* tumor necrosis factor. *(From Golub LM, Lee HM, Ryan ME, et al: Tetracyclines inhibit connective tissue breakdown by multiple non-antimicrobial mechanisms.* Adv Dent Res *12:12, 1998.)*

of collagenase activity to placebo levels, suggesting that a 1-month treatment regimen with this host modulation agent was insufficient to produce a long-term benefit.[3] During the same study, a 3-month regimen produced a prolonged drug effect without a rebound in collagenase levels to baseline during the no-treatment phase of the study. The mean levels of GCF collagenase were significantly reduced (i.e., 47.3% from baseline levels) in the SDD group compared with the placebo group of patients, who received scaling and prophylaxis alone (i.e., 29.1% reduction from baseline levels). Accompanying the reductions in collagenase levels were gains in the relative attachment levels in the SDD group.[3,40]

A review paper reported that adjunctive therapy with SRP and SDD resulted in a 70% improvement in CAL.[99] Continuous drug therapy over several months appears to be necessary for maintaining collagenase levels near normal over prolonged periods. It is reasonable to speculate that levels of MMPs will eventually increase again in more susceptible patients after drug cessation and that individuals having the most risk factors and the greatest microbial challenge will require more frequent HMT than other patients.

General Patient Populations

Data from clinical trials of SDD are summarized in Table 54.1. A series of double-blind, placebo-controlled studies of 3, 6, and 9 months' duration showed clinical efficacy based on reductions in probing depth, gains in clinical attachment, and biochemical efficacy based on the inhibition of collagenase activity and protection of serum α_1-antitrypsin (a naturally occurring protective mediator) from collagenase attack in the periodontal pocket.[18,35,62] Golub and associates[37] showed that a 2-month regimen of SDD significantly decreased the level of bone-type collagen breakdown products (i.e., carboxy-terminal telopeptide of type I collagen [ICTP], a pyridinoline-containing, cross-linked peptide of type I collagen) and MMP-8 and

MMP-13 enzyme levels (i.e., neutrophil and bone-type collagenase) in chronic periodontitis subjects (Fig. 54.4).

High-Risk Patients: Smokers

The harmful effects of cigarette smoking and the reduced response to periodontal treatment in smokers compared with nonsmokers are well established.[60] A meta-analysis of randomized clinical trials of SDD used as an adjunct to SRP revealed a benefit when using SDD in smokers with periodontitis[75,87] (see Table 54.1). A hierarchical treatment response was observed; nonsmokers who received SDD demonstrated the best clinical improvements and smokers who received placebo had the poorest treatment response. The responses of the smokers who received SDD and the nonsmokers who received placebo were intermediate to the two extremes and were broadly identical. This suggests that even patients traditionally considered resistant to periodontal treatment (i.e., smokers) can benefit from SDD, with a treatment response similar to that expected when treating a nonsmoker by SRP alone.

Special Patient Populations

More recent phase IV (i.e., after licensing) clinical studies have revealed success using SDD in particular populations of susceptible individuals. Much interest has focused on genetic susceptibility to periodontal disease, particularly whether a specific variation in the genes that regulate the cytokine IL-1 confers increased susceptibility to disease. This polymorphism is known as the *periodontitis-associated genotype* (PAG), which can be characterized using the PST Genetic Test (Interleukin Genetics, Waltham, MA). Investigation of patients who possess these polymorphisms (i.e., two single nucleotide polymorphisms in the *IL-1A* promoter region and *IL-1B* gene) has been driven by the assumption that local phenotypic differences exist in chronic periodontitis associated with this genotype (e.g.,

TABLE 54.1 Summary of Data From Clinical Trials of Sub-antimicrobial–Dose Doxycycline[86]

Study (Year)	Duration	Study Groups (n)	MEAN CAL CHANGE (mm) 4–6 mm Pockets	7+ mm Pockets	MEAN PD REDUCTION (mm) 4–6 mm Pockets	7+ mm Pockets	% SITES WITH CAL GAIN[a] ≥2 mm	≥3 mm	% SITES WITH PD REDUCTION[b] ≥2 mm	≥3 mm
Caton et al. (2000)[15]	Study: 9 mo (drug: 9 mo)	SRP + SDD (90)	1.03[c]	1.55[c]	0.95[b]	1.68[b]	46	22	47[c]	22[c]
		SRP + placebo (93)	0.86	1.17	0.69	1.20	38	16	35	13
Novak et al. (2002)[77]	Study: 9 mo (drug: 6 mo)	SRP + SDD (10)	1.00	1.78	1.20	3.02	29	15	48	26
		SRP + placebo (10)	0.56	1.24	0.97	1.42	21	11	21	6
Emingil et al. (2004)[23]	Study: 12 mo (drug: 3 mo)	SRP + SDD (10)	0.21 (all sites)	1.59[c] (all sites)	—	—	—	—	—	—
		SRP + placebo (10)	0.05 (all sites)	1.32 (all sites)	—	—	—	—	—	—
Preshaw et al. (2004)[88]	Study: 9 mo (drug: 9 mo)	SRP + SDD (107)	1.27[b]	2.09[c]	1.29[b]	2.31[b]	58[c]	33[b]	62[b]	37[b]
		SRP + placebo (102)	0.94	1.60	0.96	1.77	44	20	45	21
Lee et al. (2004)[63]	Study: 9 mo (drug: 9 mo)	SRP + SDD (240)	1.56[c] (all sites)	1.63[c] (all sites)	—	—	—	—	—	—
		SRP + placebo (17)	0.80 (all sites)	1.19 (all sites)	—	—	—	—	—	—
Choi et al. (2004)[16]	Study: 4 mo (drug: 4 mo)	SRP + SDD (15)	2.2[c] (test sites)	1.6[c] (test sites)	—	—	—	—	—	—
		SRP + placebo (17)	0.6 (test sites)	1.1 (test sites)	—	—	—	—	—	—
Gurkan et al. (2005)[51]	Study: 6 mo (drug: 3 mo)	SRP + SDD (13)	1.12	2.15	1.80	3.38	—	—	—	—
		SRP + placebo (13)	0.78	1.76	1.46	2.57	—	—	—	—
Preshaw et al. (2005)[87,e]	Study: 9 mo (drug: 9 mo)	SRP + SDD[#] (116)	1.23[c]	1.89[b]	1.22[c]	2.16[c]	59[b]	33[b]	63[d]	37
		SRP + placebo[#] (135)	0.96	1.43	0.88	1.53	43	19	44	18
		SRP + SDD[##] (81)	1.03	1.71	1.01	1.80	44	21	45[b]	20
		SRP + placebo[##] (60)	0.85	1.58	0.80	1.62	37	15	31	13
Mohammad et al. (2005)[73]	Study: 9 mo (drug: 9 mo)	SRP + SDD (12)	2.14[d]	3.18[c]	1.57[d]	3.22[d]	—	—	—	—
		SRP + placebo (12)	0.02	0.25	0.63	0.98	—	—	—	—
Górska and Nedzi-Góra (2006)[33]	Study: 3 mo (drug: 3 mo)	SRP + SDD (33)	0.33[c] (all sites)	0.29[c] (all sites)	—	—	—	—	—	—
		SRP + placebo (33)	0.04 (all sites)	0.08 (all sites)	—	—	—	—	—	—
Needleman et al. (2007)[75]	Study: 6 mo (drug: 3 mo)	SRP + SDD[##] (18)	0.65 (all sites)	1.40 (all sites)	—	—	—	—	—	—
		SRP + placebo[##] (16)	0.40 (all sites)	0.98 (all sites)	—	—	—	—	—	—

[a]Percentage of sites with CAL gain and PD reduction of ≥2 mm and ≥3 mm, respectively, calculated for all sites that had 6+ mm probing depths at baseline.
[b]$P < .01$ compared with placebo.
[c]$P < .05$ compared with placebo.
[d]$P < .001$ compared with placebo.
[e]Same study population as in Preshaw et al (2004),[88] which was stratified by smoking status: nonsmokers (#) and smokers (##).
CAL, Clinical attachment level (CAL gain or CAL loss); n, number of subjects; PD, probing depth; SDD, sub-antimicrobial–dose doxycycline; SRP, scaling and root planing.
Summary data from Preshaw PM: Host response modulation in periodontics, Periodontol 2000 48:92, 2008.

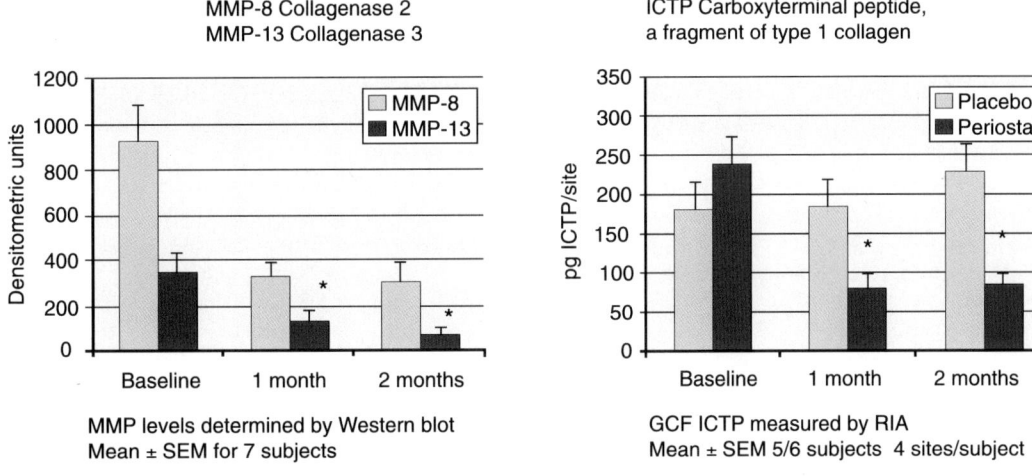

Fig. 54.4 Effects are shown for sub-antimicrobial–dose doxycycline (SDD) on gingival crevicular fluid *(GCF)*, collagenase (e.g., MMP-8, MMP-13), and carboxy-terminal telopeptide of type I collagen *(ICTP)*. A 2-month regimen of SDD significantly decreased levels of matrix metalloproteinases (i.e., neutrophil type [*MMP-8*] and bone-type [*MMP-13*]) and ICTP compared with placebo in GCF samples from adult periodontitis patients. Decreased levels of GCF bone-type collagen breakdown products (i.e., ICTP, a pyridinoline-containing cross-linked peptide of type I collagen) in the SDD group versus placebo provides biochemical evidence of a reduction in bone resorption. *MMPs,* Matrix metalloproteinases; *RIA,* radioimmunoassay. *(From Golub LM, Lee HM, Greenwald RA, et al: A matrix metalloproteinase inhibitor reduces bone-type collagen degradation fragments and specific collagenases in gingival crevicular fluid during adult periodontitis.* Inflamm Res *46:310, 1997.)*

that PAG-positive patients produce more IL-1 cytokines for a given bacterial challenge, resulting in increased tissue damage and more extensive periodontal disease). IL-1β levels in shallow periodontal pockets are higher in patients with this genotype than those without.[25]

Studies that have investigated associations between PAG and periodontal disease status have generated conflicting data.[101] A reasonable assumption is that there are genetic associations between polymorphisms in the *IL-1* gene cluster and periodontal disease but that unambiguous results are not apparent because of the heterogeneity of the disease or the various study designs. Cullinan and colleagues concluded that the IL-1 genotype is a contributory but nonessential risk factor for periodontal disease progression.[19] Despite the controversy surrounding the acceptance of this genotype as a risk factor, insurance companies are using testing as a determinant of covered treatment.[9]

A 5-month preliminary investigation by Ryan and coworkers[94] was designed to evaluate the impact of treatment on IL-1β and MMP levels in PST-positive (i.e., PAG) patients who had elevated levels of these biochemical markers in the GCF. They were initially treated with SRP, resulting in no change in the levels of these biochemical markers after 1 month. Al-Shammari and colleagues[2] reported similar findings, with no changes in GCF levels of IL-1β and ICTP before and after SRP in patients who had not been genotyped. When the genotype-positive patients received SDD and the biochemical markers were monitored at 2 and 4 months, a significant decrease (50% to 61%) in the IL-1β and MMP-9 levels was found after treatment with SDD. Gains in clinical attachment and reduced probing depths were also observed. The study concluded that a sub-antimicrobial dose of doxycycline could provide PST-positive patients with a therapeutic strategy that specifically addresses their exaggerated host response.

Another study enrolling susceptible patients with severe generalized periodontitis looked at host modulation (i.e., SDD) as an adjunct to repeated subgingival debridement.[77] Seventy percent of the patients who completed the 9-month, double-blind, placebo-controlled study were smokers. SDD as an adjunct to mechanical therapy compared with mechanical therapy alone resulted in significantly greater mean probing depth reductions in pockets of 7 mm or greater at baseline as early as 1 month after therapy (2.52 mm vs. 1.25 mm). Improvements in the SDD group compared with those in the group receiving mechanical therapy were maintained during the 5.25 months of therapy (2.85 mm vs. 1.48 mm) and even at 3 months after stopping drug therapy (3.02 mm vs. 1.41 mm), demonstrating that no rebound effect occurred. Because of the beneficial effects of HMT in susceptible patients, multicenter studies are using SDD in other susceptible populations, including diabetic, osteoporotic, and institutionalized geriatric patients and smokers.

Suggested Uses and Other Considerations

Until recently, treatment options for periodontal disease have focused solely on reducing the bacterial challenge by nonsurgical therapy, surgery, and systemic or local antimicrobial therapy. Development of SDD as an HMT, driven by research into the pathogenesis of periodontal disease, is a great example of how translational research can lead to new treatments. By better understanding the biochemical processes that are important in periodontal disease, a pharmacologic principle (i.e., doxycycline down-regulates MMP activity) has been used in the development of a new drug treatment. Data from research studies show the clinical benefits of adjunctive SDD, and the science behind SDD has been transferred into clinical practice. Dentists have the opportunity to use SDD for patient care, with the aim of enhancing the treatment response to conventional therapy.

Candidate Patients

When deciding whether to use SDD as an adjunct to SRP, the dentist should first consider the patient's motivation for periodontal care, the medical history, and the patient's willingness to take a systemic drug treatment. SDD is contraindicated in any patient with a history of allergy or hypersensitivity to tetracyclines. It should not be given to pregnant or lactating women or to children younger than 12 years of age because of the potential for discoloration of the developing dentition. Because doxycycline can reduce the efficacy of oral contraceptives, alternative forms of birth control should be discussed if necessary. There is a risk of increased sensitivity to sunlight (manifested by an exaggerated sunburn) seen with higher doses of doxycycline, although this has not been reported in the clinical trials using the sub-antimicrobial dose.

The rationale for using SDD must be clearly explained to the patient. By discussing the cause of periodontal disease, the available treatment options, and the anticipated outcomes, patients become more interested in periodontal management, are more likely to comply with treatment, and take more responsibility for managing their disease. The anticipated compliance and likely commitment to treatment must also be gauged when considering SDD therapy. Patients who show little enthusiasm for complying with the treatment plan or with oral hygiene practices are less likely to be good candidates for systemic drug therapy.

Treatable Periodontal Conditions

SDD is indicated in the management of chronic periodontitis, and studies have focused on chronic and aggressive forms of periodontitis.[15,23,77,88] SDD should not be used in conditions such as gingivitis and periodontal abscess or when an antibiotic is indicated. SDD can be used in patients with aggressive periodontitis who are being treated nonsurgically. Studies have supported efficacy of SDD as an adjunct to periodontal surgery.[28] SDD may also be of benefit in cases that are refractory to treatment and in patients with risk factors such as smoking, diabetes, osteoporosis or osteopenia, and genetic susceptibility and those in whom the treatment response is limited.

Side Effects

Doxycycline at antibiotic doses ($\geq$100 mg) is associated with adverse effects, including photosensitivity, hypersensitivity reactions, nausea, vomiting, and esophageal irritation. However, in the clinical trials of SDD using a 20-mg dose, the drug was well tolerated, and the profile of unwanted effects was virtually identical in the SDD and placebo groups.[15,23,77,88] The types of adverse events were not significantly different between treatment groups, and the typical side effects of the tetracycline class of drugs were not observed, indicating that adverse events are dose related.[15,88] There was no evidence of adverse events that could be attributed to antimicrobial effects of treatment and no evidence of developing antibiotic resistance of the microflora after 2 years of continuous use.[15,102,103,110,111] The drug appears to be well tolerated, with a very low incidence of adverse effects.

Sequencing Prescription With Periodontal Treatment

SDD is indicated as an adjunct to mechanical periodontal therapy and should not be used as a stand-alone treatment or monotherapy. SDD should be prescribed to coincide with the first round of SRP and is prescribed for 3 months, up to a maximum of 9 to 24 months of continuous dosing depending on the patient's risk. Modification of any risk factors, such as smoking, nutrition, stress, contributing medications, faulty restorations, poor oral hygiene, and poor diabetic control, should also be addressed at this time. A patient's refusal or inability to modify contributing risk factors is an important consideration for treatment planning and evaluation of therapeutic responses.

Combining With Periodontal Surgery or Local Delivery Systems

Most clinical research has focused on using SDD as an adjunct to nonsurgical periodontal treatment. However, data from studies in which SDD was used as an adjunct to access flap surgery in 24 patients revealed better probing depth reductions in surgically treated sites greater than 6 mm compared with surgically treated sites in patients given placebo.[28] The SDD group demonstrated greater reductions in ICTP, a breakdown product of collagen, than the placebo group, indicating that collagenolytic activity was reduced in the patients taking SDD.

SDD treatment can also be combined with the local delivery of antibiotics into the periodontal pocket through sustained-delivery systems. The two treatment approaches target different aspects of the pathogenic process. Local delivery systems deliver antimicrobial concentrations of an antibacterial agent directly into the site of the pocket, whereas SDD is a systemic host response modulator. Combining these two complementary treatment strategies is another example of how antibacterial therapy (i.e., SRP plus local antibiotics) can be combined with HMT (i.e., SDD) to maximize the clinical benefit for patients. Preliminary results from a 6-month, 180-patient clinical trial designed to evaluate the safety and efficacy of SDD combined with a locally applied antimicrobial (Atridox) and SRP compared with SRP alone demonstrated that patients receiving the combined treatments had more than a 2-mm improvement in mean attachment gains and probing depth reductions ($P < .0001$) compared with SRP alone.[76]

Monitoring Benefits of Therapy

To improve the ability of dentists to make appropriate treatment decisions for patients undergoing periodontal therapy, they need access to the types of diagnostic tests available to their medical colleagues. The tests could be used, for example, to distinguish between active and inactive lesions. Studies have shown that SRP alone, although effective for improving clinical parameters such as probing depths, may not be sufficient to reduce excessive levels of many underlying destructive mediators, particularly in more susceptible patients.

It would be valuable to monitor the levels of inflammatory mediators as treatment progresses. SDD results in down-regulation of MMP activity in inflamed periodontal tissues.[34,37] In theory, MMP levels could be monitored before, during, and after SRP plus SDD treatment. Published data support a concomitant reduction in MMP levels in GCF[16,23] and improvements in clinical parameters when combining SDD and SRP.[23] Although chairside tests for MMPs have been developed,[66] they are not in widespread use because of concerns about their specificity and sensitivity.

In the absence of new chairside tests or a centralized diagnostic facility for monitoring the inflammatory status of the tissues, dentists must rely on clinical periodontal monitoring to assess the outcomes of treatment. In addition to the reductions in probing depths and gains in attachment that may be observed after SRP plus SDD, the quality of the periodontal tissues tends to improve after treatment with SDD with significant reductions in gingival indices and bleeding on probing. More sensitive radiographic techniques, assessments of bone density, and bone height changes used solely in clinical trials in the past may be possible in clinical practice in the future. Until such diagnostic techniques are made widely available, clinicians must rely on clinical judgment to determine the most appropriate course of therapy.

Summary

Periodontal pathogens and destructive host responses are involved in the initiation and progression of periodontitis. Successful long-term management can require an integrated treatment strategy that addresses both etiologic components. Evidence for the role of MMPs, cytokines, and other mediators in the pathogenesis of periodontal disease distinguishes them as targets for a chemotherapeutic approach. The introduction of novel, adjunctive therapies such as host modulation to enhance the efficacy of mechanical procedures can contribute favorably to an integrated approach for the long-term clinical management of periodontitis.

HMTs are an emerging treatment concept in the management of periodontitis. The use of HMT as an adjunct can be particularly useful in susceptible, high-risk patients in whom a prolonged and excessive host response to bacteria promotes the activity of MMPs and osteoclasts.

SDD is the only systemically administered HMT currently approved and indicated as an adjunct to SRP for treating periodontitis. Clinical trials have demonstrated a clear benefit for using SDD compared with SRP alone. SDD should be used as part of a comprehensive treatment strategy that includes antibacterial treatments (i.e., SRP, plaque control, oral hygiene instruction, local antimicrobials, and periodontal surgery), host response modulation (i.e., SDD), and assessment and management of periodontal risk factors.

In the future, a range of HMTs targeting different aspects of the destructive cascade of breakdown events in periodontal tissues are likely to be developed as adjunctive treatments for periodontitis. Development of these agents will permit dentists to treat specific aspects of the underlying biochemistry of periodontal disease. The goal is to maximize and make more predictable the treatment response by reducing inflammation and inhibiting destructive processes in the tissues, resulting in enhanced periodontal stability after conventional periodontal treatments such as SRP and surgery. The dentist is now in the exciting position of being able to combine established treatment strategies with new systemic and local drug treatments for this common, chronic disease.

The use of HMT to better manage chronic periodontal disease may have applications to other chronic systemic diseases such as arthritis, diabetes, osteoporosis, and CVD. Studies using locally applied antimicrobials as part of an intensive periodontal therapy (IPT) regimen have shown promising results. Future studies may demonstrate that in addition to current standard therapies, IPT with adjunctive antibiotics and host modulation for the management of periodontal disease can have profound positive effects on the overall health status of high-risk patients. The proper management of local infection and inflammation (i.e., periodontitis) will have a significant impact on the general overall health of the population.

KEY FACT

Host modulatory therapies directed at various aspects of the destructive cascade of breakdown events in periodontal tissues are being developed as adjunctive treatments for periodontitis. These agents target specific aspects of the underlying biochemistry of periodontal disease. The goal is to enhance response to therapy and achieve periodontal stability.

References

References for this chapter are found on the companion website www.expertconsult.com.

CHAPTER 55

Occlusal Evaluation and Therapy

Michael J. McDevitt

CHAPTER OUTLINE

Pathogenesis
Evidence-Based Decision Making
Terminology

Occlusal Function and Dysfunction
Parafunction
Clinical Examination

Occlusal Therapy
Conclusions

Among the numerous local and systemic factors with the potential to influence the progression of periodontitis, the patient's occlusion remains a variable that requires an exact diagnosis. All of the disciplines of dentistry include the comprehensive analysis of occlusal relationships for determination of appropriate care.

The functional demands of the occlusion may fall within or substantially exceed the tolerances and the adaptability of the patient's periodontium and masticatory system. The full range of knowledge and skill needed to analyze all aspects of occlusal anatomy and function is beyond the scope of this chapter, which does present practical guidelines for the assessment and management of the occlusion specific to a patient's unique susceptibility to periodontitis.

Pathogenesis

The host-driven inflammatory response of each patient to a pathogenic bacterial biofilm[39] is so specific that the patient is his or her only reference for the interpretation of possible contributing factors to the progressive loss of supporting bone. Destructive events can be episodic and are site specific.

A dentist's diagnostic responsibility includes careful measurement of periodontal structures in the entire circumference of each tooth, accurate documentation, and timely reassessment. Periodontal deterioration that occurs rapidly or that is excessive for a person's age should prompt the clinician to investigate all variables that can amplify his or her periodontitis. If a local factor such as an occlusal relationship can influence the course of the disease, its analysis must be as precise as any other aspect of the periodontal examination.

Evidence-Based Decision Making

In a perfect world, all diagnostic and therapeutic decisions would reflect evidence from multiple prospective clinical trials that have been subject to systematic review. Prospective human investigations of occlusal trauma are considered unethical, and periodontics has conscientiously struggled to reach discipline-wide consensus regarding the interaction of a patient's occlusion with his or her periodontal status.[15] To be clinically applicable, the investigation's methodology must parallel the clinical diagnosis and treatment of an individual with periodontitis.[17]

Historically, data management and statistical credibility and methodology within retrospective studies limited the ability of dedicated researchers to interpret the role of occlusion in an individual's periodontitis experience.[19,38,44] The grouping of data points, especially for large study populations, departs from the site specificity that periodontal diagnosis requires. If occlusal trauma is affecting a tooth, the effect on the periodontium is site specific for only that tooth. Treatment for a patient with periodontitis would never be based on an average of diagnostic references, but rather on his or her unique susceptibility, anatomy, occlusion, and history.

In 2001, Nunn and Harrell[34] reported the retrospective findings for a group of patients with periodontitis. The analysis was based on measurement of the loss of attachment of each tooth and the presence or absence of occlusal interferences. This study and a similar investigation[4] confirmed that trauma from occlusion amplified the loss of attachment. Harrell and Nunn[18] also reported that eliminating occlusal interferences had a positive influence on the outcome of treatment when trauma from occlusion was found to be a contributing local factor. The positive influence of occlusal adjustment on the outcome of surgical and nonsurgical periodontal therapies was also reported by Burgett.[6] Evidence supports the possibility that trauma from occlusion can amplify damage to an inflamed periodontium.

Although animal studies do not carry the evidence-based hierarchic weight of ideally structured clinical trials, several newer studies seem to support the potential for excessive occlusal forces to amplify damage from inflammatory periodontitis. In two studies using a periodontitis-induced rat model, occlusal trauma resulted in readily identifiable changes in the periodontal ligament of the experimental group compared with the controls. Greater numbers of osteoclasts, perhaps related to increased receptor activator of nuclear factor kappa-B ligand (RANKL) expression, supported the observation of greater alveolar bone loss in the inflammation plus trauma group. That group also demonstrated increased numbers of immune complexes, which may be a product of the damaged periodontal ligament collagen fibers' greater permeability.[31,49] An in vitro study of human periodontal ligament fibroblasts from healthy individuals and chronic periodontitis patients also supported the observation of significant differences in healthy and diseased periodontal ligament fibroblasts when subjected to compression. Several matrix metalloproteins, interleukin-l6 and -21, and other inflammation-associated proteins were expressed by the diseased, compressed fibroblasts compared with healthy fibroblasts, suggesting the diseased fibroblasts could produce additional damage to the periodontium of patients with chronic periodontitis.[12]

Interest in occlusion in the discipline of periodontics appears to be increasing, especially with the rapid growth of the replacement of missing teeth with implants. Despite some conflicting reports in the literature, common ground for consensus exists, as shown in Fig. 55.1.

Occlusal force has an effect on the periodontium (see Chapters 24 and 25) and that susceptibility to periodontitis is unique to each patient. Occlusal forces occur across a broad spectrum. No or minimal occlusal contact on a tooth results in disuse atrophy of the periodontium, which can result in instability of that tooth. Harmonious occlusal force on a tooth stimulates the physiologic arrangement of the periodontal attachment fibers and osseous architecture and encourages stability. Forces that exceed the tolerance of the periodontium result in resorption of the bone and disruption of the attachment.[21,30,33] In the healthy person, the periodontium around teeth that are subject to excessive occlusal force experiences adaptation and repair or remodeling with no loss of attachment, which often occurs with orthodontics.

For the patient who is losing bone as a result of periodontitis, coupling the ongoing inflammatory disease with excessive occlusal force can amplify destruction and damage to the periodontium of affected teeth.[34] If this conclusion is valid, the clinician has the responsibility to correlate the periodontal status of each tooth with its occlusal responsibilities and possible occlusal excesses.

Terminology

The following is a list of key descriptive terms, as used in this chapter, and their common synonyms:

Centric relation: Position of the mandible when both condyle–disc assemblies are in their most superior positions in their respective glenoid fossae and against the slope of the articular eminences of each respective temporal bone.

Disclusion: Separation of certain teeth caused by the guidance provided by other teeth during an excursion. When anterior guidance provides separation of posterior teeth during an excursion, posterior disclusion is achieved.

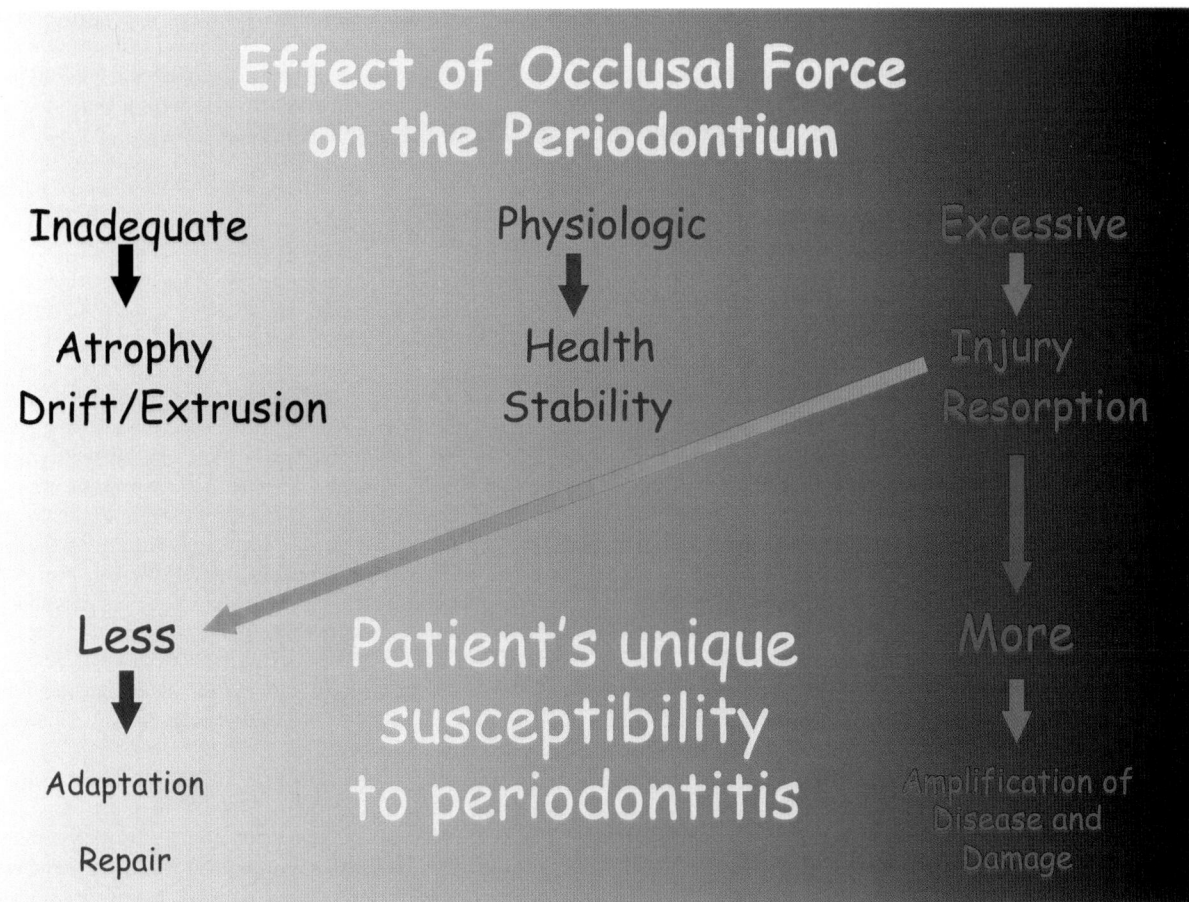

Fig. 55.1 The degree of occlusal force is depicted as a spectrum of white to black, representing none to excessive force.

Excursive movement: Any movement of the mandible away from maximum intercuspation.

Guidance: The pattern of opposing tooth contact during excursive movements of the mandible.

Initial contact in centric relation: The first occlusal contact in the centric relation closure arc.

Interference: Any occlusal contact in the centric relation closure arc or in any excursion that prevents the remaining occlusal surfaces from achieving stable contact or functioning harmoniously or that encourages masticatory system disharmony; also called an *occlusal discrepancy.*

Lateral excursion: Movement of the mandible laterally to the right or to left from maximal intercuspation.

Maximal intercuspation: Position of the mandible when there is maximal interdigitation and occlusal contact between the maxillary and mandibular teeth; also called *centric occlusion* and *intercuspal position.*

Nonworking side: The side of either arch that corresponds with the side of the mandible moving toward the midline during a lateral excursion; also called the *balancing side.*

Protrusion: Movement of the mandible anteriorly from maximal intercuspation.

Retrusion: Movement of the mandible posteriorly relative to a more anterior position.

Working side: The side of either dental arch that corresponds with the side of the mandible moving away from the midline during a lateral excursion.

Occlusal Function and Dysfunction

Excellent sources for a comprehensive understanding of dental anatomy and function include textbooks by Ash and Nelson,[3] McNeill,[28] and Dawson.[9,10] Trauma from occlusion is determined by whether the composite of all occlusal forces on a specific tooth exceeds the tolerance or adaptability of its periodontium. Identification of masticatory system disharmonies begins with an appreciation of physiologic norms; this allows the clinician to recognize dysfunctional relationships, which can influence the accuracy of the diagnosis.[10,33,35]

Centric relation is a term used to describe the position of both condyles when they are fully seated in the fossae of their respective temporomandibular joints (TMJs). Rotation of the mandible around an axis through both condyles is called the *centric relation closure arc* (see Chapter 26). This is strictly a skeletal relationship until tooth contact occurs. Maximal intercuspation occurs when opposing teeth make contact, with optimal interdigitation, at the most stable endpoint of mandibular closure. Stability is enhanced by the simultaneous bilateral contact of multiple posterior teeth with occlusal forces in the long axis of most posterior teeth. If the initial tooth contact in the centric relation arc of closure occurs simultaneously with maximal intercuspation, the teeth do not displace the condyles. Conversely, if the teeth are firm and any contact occurs before maximal intercuspation, incline relationships of opposing occlusal surfaces guide the mandible into intercuspal position, thereby requiring one or both condyles to become dislocated from their fossa.[10,34] If the teeth are mobile and contact first in the centric relation closure arc, then *they may move away from opposing teeth rather than cause condylar displacement.*

Cusp–fossa or cusp–marginal ridge relationships of the posterior teeth provide resistance to vertical loading and functional stability for the patient's dentition. When occlusal forces load teeth in their long axis, the periodontium is the most resistant and supportive.[9,10] The anterior teeth can be stable with little occlusal loading in centric occlusion if they are favorably influenced by the oral musculature. If the anterior teeth are in contact in maximal intercuspation, they are coupled.

Movement of the mandible from centric occlusion is called an *excursion.* Movement forward is called a *protrusive excursion,* and movement to either side is called a *lateral excursion.* If the mandible can move posteriorly, it is called *retrusion.* There is evidence that the contact of posterior teeth in excursions can overload those teeth, which results in negative dental, periodontal, muscular, and TMJ consequences.[1,7,10,35,50–52] The ideal relationship may be a light coupling of the anterior teeth in centric occlusion with immediate separation (i.e., disclusion) of all posterior teeth in all excursions.[51]

During a lateral excursion, posterior teeth that make contact on the same side as the direction of mandibular movement are described as having a working contact. Posterior teeth that make contact on the side opposite the direction of the lateral excursion are described as having a nonworking contact. Although nonworking contacts are classically associated with negative consequences,[52] the analysis of working contacts and the function of anterior teeth are critically important. Contacts that are disruptive to mandibular movement or stressful to individual teeth are called *occlusal interferences* or *discrepancies.* Dentists' ability to analyze the occlusion to identify contacts that can amplify a patient's periodontitis, thereby affecting certain teeth, is strategic to making the correct diagnosis.

Inflammation disrupts the integrity of the attachment apparatus, which results in less resistance to force from opposing teeth. When bone loss has occurred, less root surface area is supported,[2,20] and there are fewer sensory fibers in the periodontal ligament, which limits the protective muscle modulation of the occlusal forces.[41] The clinician must differentiate among inflammation-caused intolerance to occlusal forces, normal forces on teeth with reduced periodontal support, excessive occlusal forces, and well-tolerated forces on teeth affected by periodontitis.

Parafunction

Bruxism can cause occlusal forces on teeth that are susceptible to periodontitis to be increased in intensity or frequency, thereby magnifying the potential amplification of damage.[8,23,24,47] Daytime or awake occlusal parafunction is commonly limited to clenching the teeth during incidents that require a person's focused effort or mental concentration. Patients can be engaged in identification of daytime teeth clenching, as was the case in a study of sleep bruxism and myofascial pain. Awake clenching was reported by 58 of the 60 participants.[42] Selection criteria for a study must be very exacting because self-reports of sleep bruxism by patients is usually unreliable.[40] Patients' identification of their parafunction can help them to understand its importance, and it supports the clinical experience that daytime clenching can be a frequent contributor to a patient's increased susceptibility to bone loss in sites of inflammatory periodontitis.

Nighttime or sleep bruxing of the teeth can take the form of grinding the teeth during various excursions or clenching the teeth. Sleep bruxism is probably an extension of the rhythmic masticatory muscle activity that is also observed in nonbruxers. Why nuclei in the brain stem allow bruxing to occur in some individuals while others are spared is unclear.[8,23,24] Bruxing is associated with the greater frequency and persistence of TMJ dysfunction, orofacial pain, and possibly periodontal attachment loss.[47] The sensory input of teeth that are subject to bruxism is probably dampened, which may interfere with the diagnosis and treatment.[37] There seems to be limited influence on bruxing tendencies from occlusal interferences.[25] An exception was discovered in a clinical study of 30 bruxers and 30 nonbruxers; there was a significant difference in nonworking interferences in the bruxing population compared with their absence in the nonbruxing group.[43] When these findings are viewed along with those reported by Youdelis and Mann decades ago, the correlation of bruxing and site-specific inflammatory bone damage appears meaningful.[52]

Gerber and Lynd studied selective serotonin reuptake inhibitor–induced movement disorders.[14] They found that selective serotonin reuptake inhibitors such as Prozac encouraged bruxism.

Evidence is emerging that sleep-disordered breathing can influence or be associated with inflammatory diseases such as periodontitis.[5,11,16] Although a causal relationship between obstructive sleep apnea and sleep bruxism has not been firmly established, the reported data and observations support a definite association.[36,45,46] A patient with periodontitis with clinical evidence of occlusal trauma may be experiencing the consequences of sleep-disordered breathing. Chapter 40 provides an overview of sleep-disordered breathing, offering a reference for the dentist who is seeking to develop skill in the recognition of oral signs of sleep-disordered breathing to complement his or her diagnostic skills in evaluation of a patient's occlusion. If an occlusal appliance is being considered to address the periodontal implications of excessive occlusal force experienced by a periodontitis-susceptible patient, compliance may be problematic for a person with sleep-disordered breathing because the appliance can contribute to airway obstruction.[13]

Clinical Examination

Before clinical evaluation, a conversation with the patient can help to provide a more complete diagnosis. With minimal symptoms, a patient may not associate loose teeth or significant dental wear with TMJ dysfunction or orofacial pain with occlusal function or parafunction. The list of questions in Chapter 26 and inquiries specific to the condition of the patient's teeth can help the clinician to open the lines of communication and set the tone for patient education during the clinical examination. Comprehensive evaluation of occlusal anatomy and relationships is accomplished by the analysis of many factors in the clinical setting and by mounted diagnostic casts.

Clinical evaluation of the occlusion is sequenced to support the patient's learning. It should always include a clinical assessment of masticatory system function and identification of disharmonies.

Temporomandibular Disorders Screening and Evaluation

Complete assessment of the masticatory system and identification of temporomandibular disorders are described in Chapter 26 and should be part of a patient's initial comprehensive examination. The temporomandibular disorder screening and clinical evaluation then become part of subsequent examinations.

The patient's range of motion is observed, maximal opening and the lateral and protrusive excursions are measured, and any deviation from the midline during opening and closing is defined. Light finger pressure applied over each TMJ can detect deflection of the tissue while the patient opens and closes the mouth; deflection suggests condyle–disc discoordination. Tenderness on palpation can indicate TMJ capsulitis. Listening to the joint with a stethoscope or a Doppler instrument during opening and closing can detect sounds that are consistent with uncoordinated condyle–disc relationships, arthritic changes, and other diagnostic sounds.[10]

Palpation of the muscles of mastication and the related head and neck musculature can reveal muscle tension or spasm related to

BOX 55.1 Temporomandibular Disorder Screening Evaluation
1. Maximal interincisal opening (range, 40 to 50 mm)
2. Opening or closing pathway
3. Range of lateral and protrusive excursions (7 to 9 mm)
4. Auscultation for temporomandibular joint sounds
5. Palpation for temporomandibular joint tenderness or tissue displacement
6. Palpation for muscle tenderness
7. Load testing of the patient's temporomandibular joints

compensation for occlusal or TMJ disharmonies.[10,35] Load testing of the TMJ is described in Chapter 26. Significant discoveries revealed during the screening examination summarized in Box 55.1 should lead the clinician to complete the comprehensive evaluation.

Testing for the Mobility of Teeth

Two basic methods are used to assess the firmness or looseness of a tooth. Classically, a dental instrument is used to exert pressure in the facial or lingual direction, and the dentist places his or her finger on the opposite side of the tooth to feel and see movement if it occurs (see Chapter 32). Recording a numeric value (range, 0 to 3) for the degree of mobility allows the clinician to track changes that may occur in response to therapy.

The other method is to test for the movement of teeth that are subject to pressure generated by the patient. Fremitus, vibration, or micromovement of a tooth can be felt when patients tap their teeth together. When the patient mimics clenching the teeth and then attempts to move the mandible in excursions, tooth movement can be observed. The patient placing a finger where the clinician felt tooth movement helps the patient to appreciate the looseness of his or her teeth (Fig. 55.2).

If the mobility of the teeth exceeds what is expected on the basis of the loss of support or the level of inflammation observed, trauma from occlusion is included in the diagnosis. The assimilation of all of the occlusal and periodontal diagnostic references can lead the clinician to conclude that even without mobility, there may be evidence of amplified periodontal damage as a result of unfavorable occlusal forces.

LEARNING BOX 55.3
An inflamed periodontium often contributes to the mobility of a tooth.

Centric Relation Assessment

Bimanual manipulation of the mandible in the axis of rotation of the condyles in their respective glenoid fossae has become a standard method of assessing centric relation.[3,9,10,35] This method is illustrated in Fig. 55.3, and it involves gentle guidance rather than the forced positioning of the mandible. This technique is essential for load testing of the TMJs, and it is effective for generating centric relation records for mounting diagnostic casts. Telling the patient that he or she will feel modest lifting pressure on the inferior borders of the mandible and a light depressing force in the mental region often allows for relatively free and comfortable hinging of the mandible.[9,10] If hinging is uncomfortable or not repeatable, muscle deprogramming (see Chapter 26) may be beneficial. Other methods for guiding the condyles toward a seated position (e.g., leaf gauges, anterior bite stops) can be effective.[10]

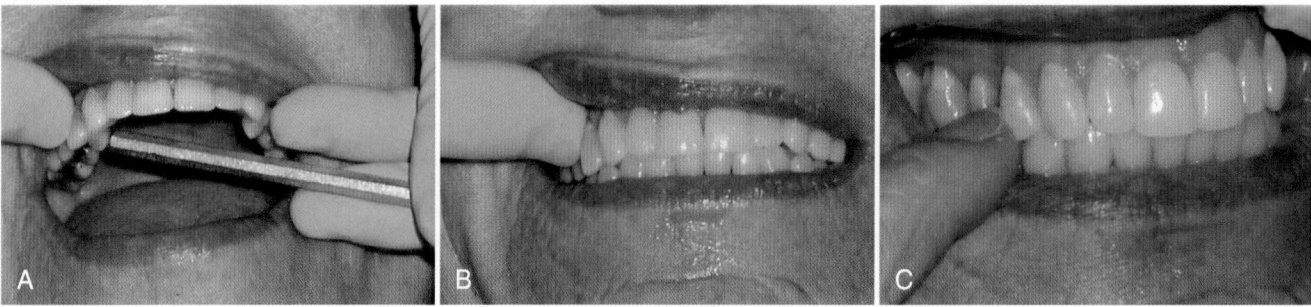

Fig. 55.2 (A) Tactile and visual testing for mobility is done with a dental instrument by the dentist. (B) Tactile and visual testing for mobility is done with the patient clenching and while beginning right lateral excursion by the dentist. (C) The patient feels movement of her tooth when lateral excursion is attempted while the teeth are clenched.

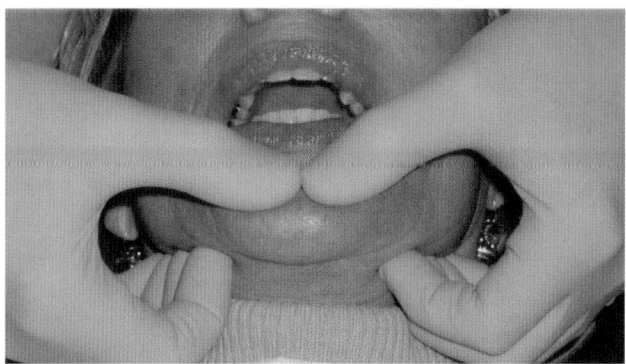

Fig. 55.3 Bimanual manipulation is used to hinge the mandible in centric relation and to load test the temporomandibular joints.

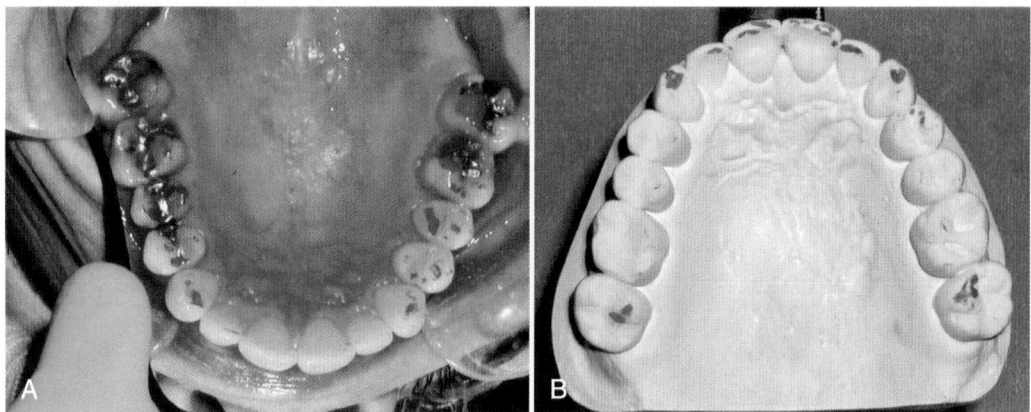

Fig. 55.4 (A) Teeth are marked clinically in maximal intercuspation and in excursions while clenching. (B) Teeth are marked in centric relation and maximal intercuspation on a diagnostic cast mounted in centric relation. Marks only on the second molars indicate that they were mobile and that they moved to permit the contact of other teeth.

Asking the patient to identify the first tooth to touch in the centric relation arc of closure may indicate that interferences to closure into maximal intercuspation exist. Asking the patient to close further may demonstrate a slide from centric relation to centric occlusion because teeth are firm enough to dislocate one or both condyles.[35] Drying the occlusal surfaces, positioning marking paper, and then guiding the patient to the initial contact in centric relation allows marking of occlusal contact points, thereby identifying any interference. Asking the patient to then close into maximal intercuspation marks the points or surfaces that contact during the slide. An early occlusal contact in centric relation before closure to centric occlusion is obtained that does not cause a slide may indicate the early contact that occurs on teeth that are mobile enough to move, allowing maximal intercuspation to be gained without condylar accommodation (Fig. 55.4). Confirmation of permissive intercuspation is a product of marking the teeth clinically and comparing the marks with the ones on mounted diagnostic casts, which demonstrates that mobile teeth can move out of the way to allow others to contact.

Evaluation of Excursions

Marking the teeth in all excursions reveals the pathways of contact of opposing occlusal or incisal surfaces during function, and it may identify interferences to harmonious function.[3,10,28] Movement of any teeth during marking may lessen the intensity of the marks and the assessed severity of the forces experienced by the affected teeth.

Vectors of force and steepness of the opposing inclines are studied to determine whether the force is excessive. Interpreting contacts on a tooth-by-tooth basis can suggest or deny occlusal trauma as a contributing factor to the loss of attachment of each affected tooth. When patients are engaged in the evaluation of their occlusion, they can be given suggestions to observe certain habits, such as clenching their teeth during the day or sleeping with pressure on their mandible. As they contribute to their own diagnosis, patients become better prepared to make informed choices about treatment options.

Articulated Diagnostic Casts

When the maxillary diagnostic cast is mounted on an articulator with a facebow transfer technique, the occlusal surfaces become oriented to the axis of rotation of the patient's condyles. The centric relation transfer record orients the mandibular teeth to the maxillary teeth in centric relation.[9,10] Study of the accurately mounted diagnostic casts can reveal occlusal discrepancies between initial contact in the centric relation closure arc and maximal intercuspation and occlusal disharmonies in excursions. Mobile teeth may produce a mark on a solid model but little or no mark in that patient's mouth during clinical assessment. Accuracy of the observations made on the models should be confirmed clinically to whatever degree possible.

Occlusal Therapy

Effective nonsurgical therapy usually reduces inflammation within the periodontium and results in some healing of attachment,[32] which often results in mobile teeth becoming more stable. If the clinician concludes that inflammation has been optimally controlled and that occlusal forces on individual teeth still exceed the tolerance of the periodontium, the basis for intervention is established.

The harmonious function of both TMJs and their associated muscles is required for occlusal stability. When there is sufficient evidence of excessive occlusal forces on the patient's teeth or when masticatory system disharmony exists and the patient desires a more stable occlusion, an occlusal appliance is prescribed.

Chapter 26 reviews TMJ anatomy, This can provide a better understanding of the therapy.

LEARNING BOX 55.4

Optimal resolution of inflammation is necessary to accurately interpret tooth mobility.

Occlusal Appliance Therapy

A well-designed and accurately fitted appliance can benefit masticatory system function while encouraging loose teeth in both arches to tighten as the supporting periodontium heals. The bilateral simultaneous contact of all opposing posterior teeth in centric relation, shallow anterior guidance, and the immediate disclusion of all posterior teeth in every excursion are essential elements of maxillary and mandibular occlusal appliances (Figs. 55.5 and 55.6).

Teeth that are opposing an appliance should be loaded as close as possible to their long axis. Maxillary appliances engage a portion of the hard palate, which provides substantial bracing of teeth and resistance to vertical and lateral forces. A horseshoe-shaped maxillary appliance relies on other, possibly compromised teeth to attempt to protect the most mobile teeth. Soft or partial coverage appliances are contraindicated for long-term protection and stabilization.[32] The protective role of occlusal appliances was addressed in the 8-year study by McGuire.[27] Occlusal appliances are not expected to cure bruxism,[26] but they are often prescribed for patients with habitual parafunction as a compensating or protective intervention to limit masticatory system disharmony, damage to the teeth, and overstressing of implants.[22]

Occlusal Adjustment

As teeth tighten from consistent use of the appliance, occlusal interferences may become more evident, and greater discrepancy between the initial dental contact and maximal intercuspation may be observed. Interferences with harmonious excursive movement of the mandible may also become more obvious. When the clinician confirms that the interferences correlate with a greater than expected loss of attachment, direct intervention in the patient's occlusion is considered. With the patient's full understanding and consent, occlusal adjustment or selective reshaping of the occluding surfaces of the teeth can reduce the magnitude of occlusal interferences or direct the forces to be more compatible with the long axes of the affected teeth.

Clinical analysis of the occlusion should be combined with a detailed analysis of diagnostic casts mounted in centric relation on an adjustable articulator. Accurately mounted duplicate models can be used to accomplish a trial occlusal adjustment to determine safety and efficacy for a patient.[10,28] Scheduling patients so that they leave their appliances on overnight and in place until they are seated in the dental chair allows assessment of their teeth at maximal firmness, when interferences are most readily identifiable. Teeth usually progressively tighten with continued compliance with the appliance and repeated careful occlusal adjustment.

Other methods that can be employed to alter occlusal relationships include orthodontics and restorative dentistry. Provisional restoration of teeth is another method of improving occlusal contacts and stability, and it often simplifies the process of occlusal adjustment and final restoration.

Occlusal Stability for Restorative Dentistry

A stable occlusion is considered a prerequisite for any restorative therapy (Box 55.2). Implants to replace the teeth of a partially dentate patient add to the occlusal considerations. Osseointegration of implants eliminates micromovement, which can allow teeth to accommodate occlusal forces. The extent and timing of occlusal loading and the

---

BOX 55.2 Requirements for Occlusal Stability

1. Forces on an individual tooth that do not exceed the support and resistance of the tooth's periodontium and that are vertically oriented to the long axis of each tooth as much as possible
2. Even and simultaneous contact of all posterior teeth in the centric relation closure or in maximal intercuspation, with minimal difference between the two
3. Little or no contact of the anterior teeth in centric occlusion, although such contact is readily available to provide guidance in excursion and to produce posterior disclusion
4. Harmonious excursive movement of the mandible within the patient's envelope of function and with complete absence of occlusal interference

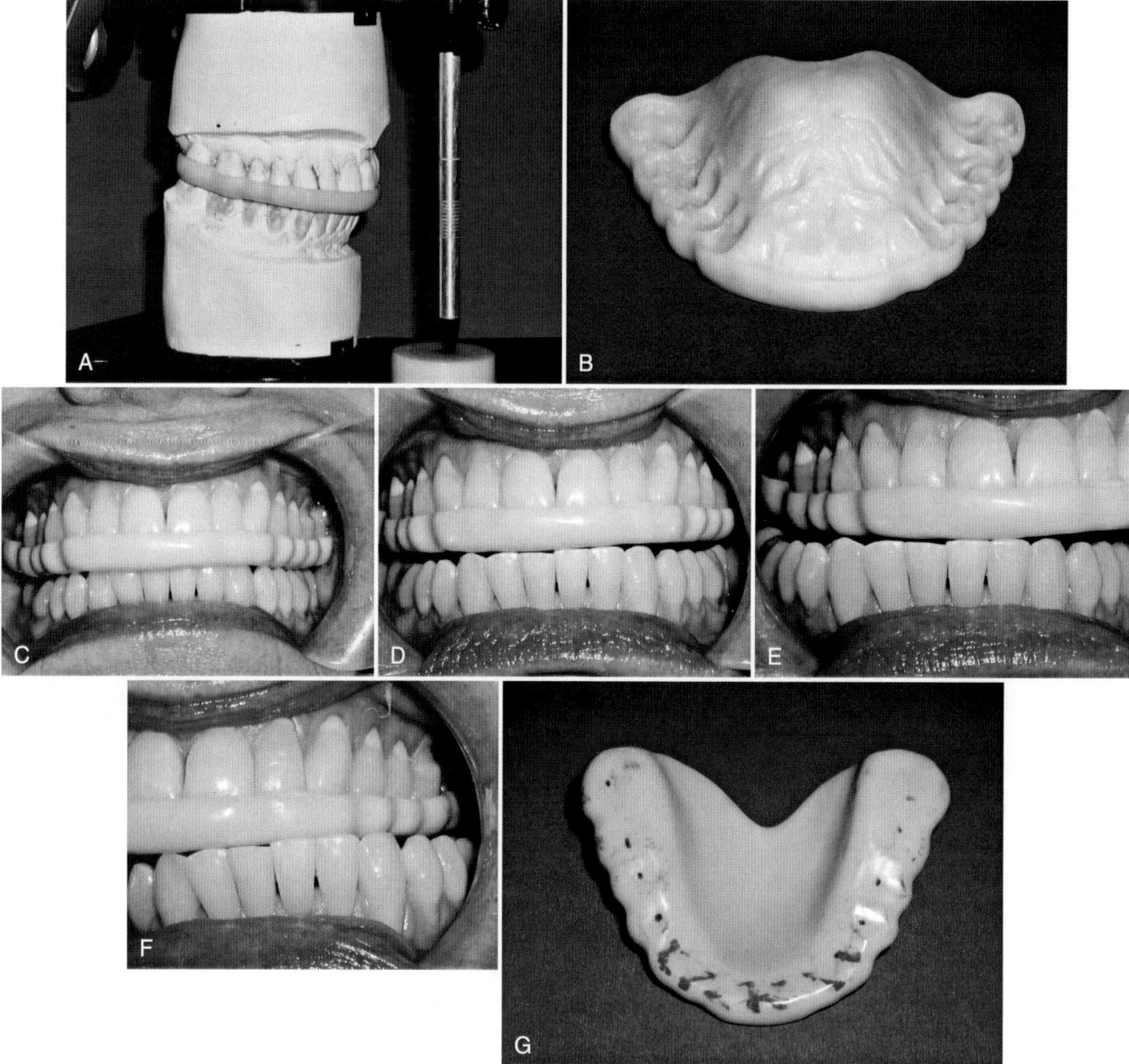

Fig. 55.5 (A) An occlusal appliance is fabricated on accurately mounted diagnostic casts. (B) The entire dental and palatal surface has been carefully relined to promote an optimal stabilizing influence on mobile teeth. (C) There is bilateral, simultaneous contact of the cuspids and all posterior teeth in centric relation, fabricated to enhance axial loading of opposing mandibular teeth. (D) There is smooth, relatively flat anterior guidance with immediate and sustained disclusion of all posterior teeth in protrusion. (E) There is smooth, relatively flat anterior guidance with immediate and sustained disclusion of all posterior teeth in right lateral excursions. (F) There is extreme left lateral excursion with smooth, harmonious transitions across the anterior teeth to maintain the disclusion of all posterior teeth. (G) Marks created by the opposing dentition demonstrate bilateral, simultaneous contact in centric relation and the immediate disclusion of the opposing posterior teeth in all excursions.

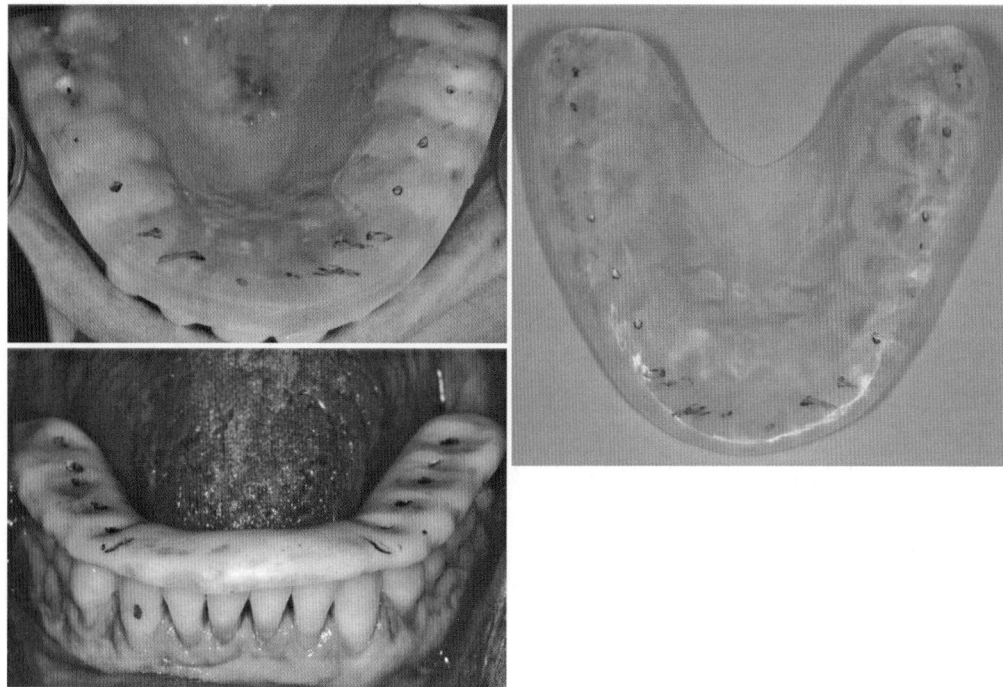

Fig. 55.6 A mandibular occlusal appliance is fabricated after surgery to provide a stabilizing influence for the incisors in particular and to demonstrate occlusal attributes similar to those of the maxillary appliance.

guidance requirement for each tooth and for each implant must be carefully harmonized (see Chapter 74). This is especially critical if any of the teeth are mobile or the patient bruxes to a significant degree.[48] If bruxism is suspected or the functional forces are considered to be excessive, the occlusal appliance as described may be a valuable application.[22,29]

Conclusions

Confirmation of the appropriateness of occlusal therapy is the product of a thorough evaluation of the patient's occlusion and his or her masticatory system. The sequence of occlusal treatment begins with antiinflammatory therapy and progresses through reversible appliance therapy before any irreversible options are considered. This provides the clinician with the most careful approach to assessing and treating the occlusion of a patient with periodontitis.

 A Case Scenario is found on the companion website www.expertconsult.com.

References

 References for this chapter are found on the companion website www.expertconsult.com.

CHAPTER 56

Orthodontics: Interdisciplinary Periodontal and Implant Therapy

CHAPTER 56A

Adjunctive Role of Orthodontic Therapy

†*Vincent G. Kokich*

CHAPTER OUTLINE

Benefits of Orthodontic Therapy
Preorthodontic Osseous Surgery *(e-only)*
Orthodontic Treatment of Osseous Defects *(e-only)*

Orthodontic Treatment of Gingival Discrepancies
 (e-only)
Conclusion

 For discussions of preorthodontic osseous surgery, orthodontic treatment of osseous defects, the orthodontic treatment of gingival discrepancies, and implant interactions in orthodontics, please go to the companion website at www.expertconsult.com.

Orthodontic tooth movement may be of substantial benefit to the adult periorestorative patient. Many adults who seek routine restorative dentistry have problems with tooth malposition, which compromises their ability to clean and maintain their dentition. If these individuals also are susceptible to periodontal disease, tooth malposition may be an exacerbating factor that could cause premature loss of specific teeth.

Orthodontic appliances have become smaller, less noticeable, and easier to maintain during orthodontic therapy. Many adults are taking advantage of the opportunity to have their teeth aligned to improve the aesthetics of their smile. Underlying gingival or osseous periodontal defects often can be improved during orthodontic therapy if the orthodontist is aware of the situation and designs the appropriate tooth movement. In addition, implants have become a major part of the treatment plan for many adults with missing teeth. If adjacent teeth have drifted into edentulous spaces, orthodontic therapy is often helpful to provide the ideal amount of space for implants and subsequent restorations. This chapter shows the ways in which adjunctive orthodontic therapy can enhance the periodontal health and restorability of teeth and presents the role of implant dentistry in both periodontics and orthodontics.

Benefits of Orthodontic Therapy

Orthodontic therapy can provide several benefits to adult periodontal patients. The following seven factors should be considered:
1. Aligning crowded or malpositioned maxillary or mandibular anterior teeth permits adult patients better access to clean all

surfaces of their teeth. This could be a tremendous advantage for patients who are susceptible to periodontal disease or do not have the dexterity to maintain oral hygiene.
2. Vertical orthodontic tooth repositioning can improve certain types of osseous defects in periodontal patients. Often, moving the tooth eliminates the need for resective osseous surgery.
3. Orthodontic treatment can improve the aesthetic relationship of the maxillary gingival margins before restorative dentistry. Aligning the gingival margins orthodontically avoids gingival recontouring, which could also entail bone removal and exposure of the roots of the teeth (eFig. 56A.1).
4. Orthodontic therapy also benefits the patient with a severe fracture of a maxillary anterior tooth that requires forced eruption to permit adequate restoration of the root. Erupting the root allows the crown preparation to have sufficient resistance form and retention for the final restoration.
5. Orthodontic treatment allows open gingival embrasures to be corrected to regain lost papillae. If open gingival embrasures are located in the maxillary anterior region, this can present an aesthetic problem. In most patients, these areas can be corrected with a combination of orthodontic root movement, tooth reshaping, and restoration.
6. Orthodontic treatment could improve adjacent tooth positioning before implant placement or tooth replacement. This is especially true for the patient who has been missing teeth for several years and has drifting and tipping of the adjacent dentition.
7. A common tooth malalignment problem that results in periodontal pockets is the mesially tipped molar. Orthodontic

†Deceased.

uprighting of tipped molars corrects the deep gingival contours and eliminates or reduces the mesial periodontal pocket (eFig. 56A.2).

Conclusion

There are many benefits to integrating orthodontics and periodontics in the management of adult patients with underlying periodontal defects. The key to treating these patients is communication and proper diagnosis before orthodontic therapy, as well as continued dialog during treatment. Not all periodontal problems are treated in the same way. This chapter provides a framework for the integration of orthodontics to solve periodontal problems.

 Case Scenarios are found on the companion website www.expertconsult.com.

References

 References can be found on the companion Expert Consult website at www.expertconsult.com.

Orthodontics, Implants, and Periodontal Interactions

Frank Celenza

CHAPTER OUTLINE

Introduction
Implant Interactions in Orthodontics *(e-only)*
Conclusion

 ## Introduction

Whereas the interrelationships between the disciplines of orthodontics and implantology might not seem close to the casual observer, in fact they are quite intimate. In addition, the integration of periodontics with orthodontics and implants presents an even more interesting and important combination. Although the conventional orthodontic patient might be quite different in nature from the periodontal patient, there are many useful and interesting interactions between the disciplines that can and should be harnessed for the best treatment outcomes. This is especially true in current treatment planning in which implants are used as anchors to move teeth.

The conventional orthodontic patient might be characterized as an adolescent or young adult, usually with a healthy, although not always complete, dentition. This patient most often does not present with a significant medical or dental history. Conversely, the periodontal patient often does present with a significant and contributory medical history and a long list of dental problems, which often includes restorative considerations. Further, the periodontium will be compromised and in need of treatment, usually preparatory to orthodontic intervention. Also, there will often be tooth replacement considerations to be sequenced into the therapy. It is in this situation that implant therapy may be part of the treatment scenario. How, then, are these two divergent patient types to be managed by combining treatment modalities from these three disciplines?

This section delineates some of the interrelationships that can be utilized for better therapeutic outcomes. When the clinician gains an appreciation for the periodontal apparatus that supports a tooth and applies an understanding of the physiology of tooth movement,

one can utilize the body's reparative and remodeling capacities to effect periodontal alterations as a result of tooth movement. Further, as implant modalities are called upon, a greater demand for accurate tooth position arises. Moreover, as more adult patients are seeking orthodontic and implant treatment, an understanding of the need for and methods of ensuring periodontal health before and during orthodontic and implant care becomes paramount. Consequently, the intimate relationships among these three distinct dental disciplines become apparent in both the treatment planning and treatment execution phases of therapy. We can truly address this topic as *interdisciplinary dentistry*.

Conclusion

Significant and fascinating interplays exist between the practices of orthodontics and periodontics, which also includes implantology. Reciprocal relationships can be harnessed through proper sequencing of treatments to enhance outcomes. Utilization of various implants can facilitate orthodontic mechanotherapy, streamline treatment, eliminate compliance dependency, improve predictability and even introduce new treatment options. Conversely, orthodontic preparation prior to implant placement can yield a more favorable environment through orthodontically induced site development in which both hard and soft tissue can be augmented and remodeled. Further, spatial management of implant sites and neighboring tooth positions is often essential to ideal implant location.

Periodontal treatment preparatory to orthodontic treatment is often required to eliminate inflammation and bolster the investing tooth structures, thereby permitting successful tooth movement without further loss of attachment. Likewise, orthodontic modalities can be employed to remodel the hard and soft tissues of the periodontium to benefit various situations, such as defect eradication.

Consequently, there are many instances in which interdisciplinary interactions can facilitate treatment, and these interactions can be considered bidirectional. Thus implant utilization can sometimes enhance orthodontic outcomes, while other times orthodontic treatment should be employed to enhance implant outcomes. Just as applicable are the bidirectional possibilities between orthodontics and periodontics. This chapter has illustrated these concepts and has stressed the importance of proper sequencing of therapy to maximize these possibilities.

 Case Scenarios are found on the companion website www.expertconsult.com.

References

 References can be found on the companion Expert Consult website at www.expertconsult.com.

CHAPTER 57

Phase II Periodontal Therapy

Henry H. Takei

CHAPTER OUTLINE

Objectives of the Surgical Phase
Pocket Elimination Versus Pocket Maintenance

Reevaluation After Phase I Therapy
Critical Zones in Pocket Surgery
Indications for Periodontal Surgery

Methods of Pocket Therapy
Conclusions

Therapy for periodontal disease, which encompasses many techniques and procedures, depends on the disease status and objective of the final outcome. Early problems can be corrected with successful phase I therapy, consisting of biofilm removal by the patient on a daily basis, scaling, and root planing when necessary.

Many moderate to advanced cases cannot be resolved without surgically gaining access to the root surface for root planing and reducing or eliminating pocket depth to allow the patient to remove biofilm. The surgical phase of therapy is also referred to as phase II therapy. This chapter describes the surgical techniques used for the following purposes:

- Controlling or eliminating periodontal disease
- Correcting anatomic conditions that favor periodontal disease, impair aesthetics, or impede placement of prosthetic appliances
- Placing implants to replace lost teeth and improving the environment for their placement and function

Many cases are successfully treated and maintained by phase I therapy. The chapters in Section V discuss the techniques and concepts used to treat periodontal diseases that require a surgical approach to reduce or eliminate pockets and obtain access to the root surface to remove accretions.

Objectives of the Surgical Phase

The surgical phase of periodontal therapy has the following objectives:
1. To improve the prognosis for teeth and their replacements
2. To improve aesthetics

Surgical techniques are used for pocket therapy and for correction of related morphologic problems (i.e., mucogingival defects). In many cases, therapies are combined to provide one surgical intervention that fulfills both objectives.

Surgical techniques (1) increase access to the root surface, allowing the clinician to remove all irritants; (2) reduce or eliminate pocket depth, making it possible for the patient to maintain the root surfaces free of biofilm; and (3) reshape soft and hard tissues to attain a harmonious topography. Resective or regenerative surgery, or both, is used to reduce pocket depth (Box 57.1) (see Chapters 60 to 61).

The second objective of phase II therapy is to correct anatomic defects that favor plaque or biofilm accumulation and pocket recurrence or impair aesthetics. The aim of correcting anatomic problems is to alter defects of the gingival and mucosal tissues that predispose

these areas to disease. Three types of techniques are performed on noninflamed tissues and in the absence of periodontal pockets (see Box 57.1):

- *Plastic surgery techniques* are used to create or widen the attached keratinized gingiva by placing grafts of various types.
- *Aesthetic surgery techniques* are used to cover denuded root surfaces resulting from recession and to recreate lost papillae.
- *Pre-prosthetic techniques* are used to modify the periodontal and neighboring tissues to receive prosthetic replacements. They include crown lengthening, ridge augmentation, and vestibular deepening.

Fig. 57.1 provides a three-tiered classification of the surgical procedures used in periodontics: pocket reduction surgery, periodontal plastic surgery, and pre-prosthetic surgery. Pocket reduction surgery consists of resective and regenerative procedures, and periodontal plastic surgery includes aesthetic and gingival augmentation (anatomic) procedures. Crown lengthening, ridge augmentation, and implant procedures are listed under pre-prosthetic surgery. Plastic and aesthetic surgery techniques are explored in Chapter 65, and pre-prosthetic techniques are discussed in Chapter 69.

Periodontal surgical procedures also are available for the placement of dental implants. They include implant placement techniques and a variety of surgical procedures to modify neighboring tissues for the placement of implants. Bone augmentation of the sinus floor or for a narrow edentulous ridge is an example (see Box 57.1). These topics are discussed in Chapters 79 and 80.

Surgical Pocket Therapy

Surgical pocket therapy can be used to gain access to the diseased root surface to ensure the removal of calculus located subgingivally before surgery and to eliminate or reduce the depth of the periodontal pocket.

Successful periodontal therapy completely eliminates calculus, plaque or biofilm, and diseased cementum from the tooth surface. Numerous investigations have shown that the difficulty of this task increases as the pocket becomes deeper.[2,5] The irregularities and concavities on the root surface also increase, which adds to the difficulty of instrumenting the root surfaces.[11,15] Furcations also create problems for scaling and root planing in these areas[4] (see Chapter 50). Most of these problems can be remedied by resecting or displacing the soft tissue wall of the pocket, which increases the visibility

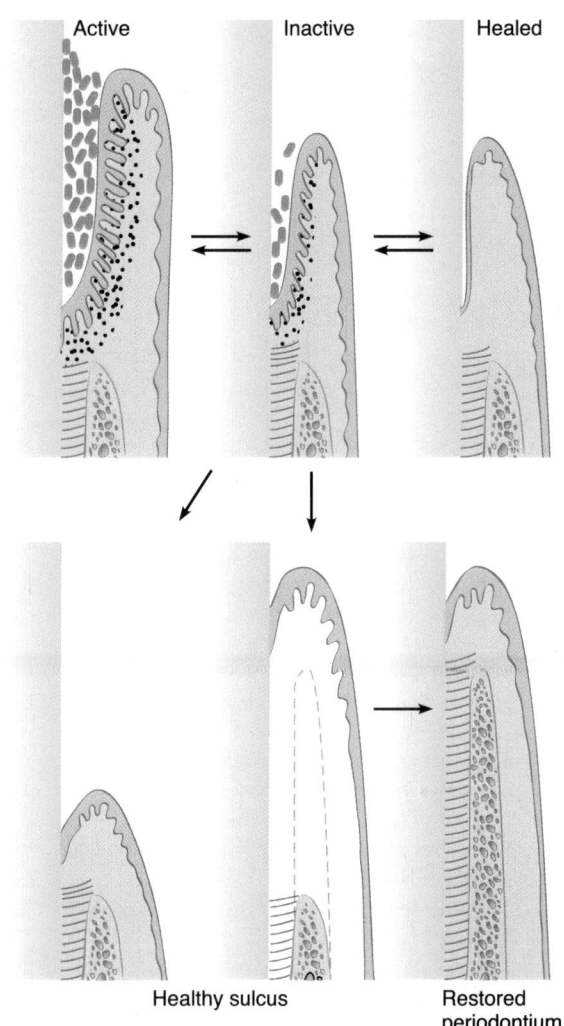

BOX 57.1 Periodontal Surgery

Pocket Reduction Surgery
- Resective (e.g., gingivectomy, apically displaced flap, undisplaced flap with or without osseous resection)
- Regenerative (e.g., flaps with grafts, membranes)

Correction of Anatomic or Morphologic Defects
- Plastic surgery techniques used to widen attached gingiva (e.g., free gingival grafts)
- Esthetic surgery (e.g., root coverage, recreation of gingival papillae)
- Pre-prosthetic techniques (e.g., crown lengthening, ridge augmentation, vestibular deepening)
- Placement of dental implants, including techniques for site development for implants (e.g., guided bone regeneration, sinus grafts)

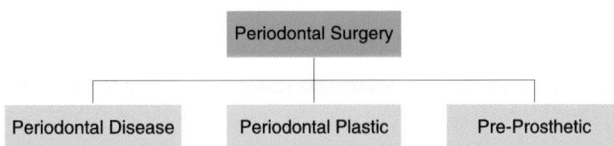

Fig. 57.1 Classification of periodontal surgery. The surgical procedures accomplished in periodontics are organized as pocket reduction surgery, periodontal plastic surgery, and pre-prosthetic surgery.

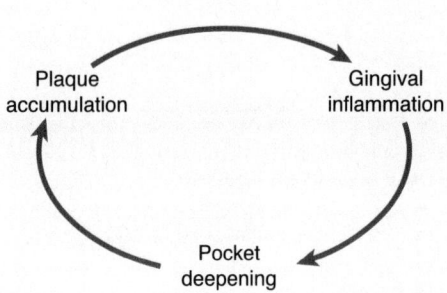

Fig. 57.2 Accumulation of plaque leads to gingival inflammation and pocket deepening, which increases the area of plaque accumulation.

Fig. 57.3 Possible results of pocket therapy are shown. An active pocket can become inactive and heal by means of a long junctional epithelium. Surgical pocket therapy can result in a healthy sulcus, with or without gain of attachment. Improved gingival attachment promotes restoration of bone height, with re-formation of periodontal ligament fibers and layers of cementum.

and accessibility of the root surface.[3] The surgical flap technique allows the clinician to overcome these problems of access to the root surface.

Pocket elimination is another important consideration. It consists of reducing the depth of the periodontal pocket to that of a physiologic sulcus to enable cleaning by the patient. By proper case selection, resective and regenerative techniques can be used to accomplish this goal. A pocket makes it impossible for the patient to remove biofilm, which is part of the vicious cycle depicted in Fig. 57.2.

Results of Pocket Therapy

A periodontal pocket can be in an active state or a period of inactivity or quiescence. In an active pocket, underlying bone is being lost (Fig. 57.3, *top left*). It often is diagnosed clinically by bleeding that occurs spontaneously or in response to probing. After phase I therapy, the inflammatory changes in the pocket wall subside, rendering the pocket inactive and reducing its depth (see Fig. 57.3, *top center*). The extent of this reduction depends on the depth before treatment

and the degree to which the depth is the result of the edematous and inflammatory component of the pocket wall (i.e., pseudopocket).

Whether the pocket remains inactive depends on the depth, the individual characteristics of the plaque or biofilm components, and the host response. Recurrence of the initial activity is likely.

Inactive pockets sometimes heal with a long junctional epithelium (see Fig. 57.3, *top right*). This condition can be unstable, and the chance of recurrence and re-formation of the original pocket remains because the epithelial union with the tooth is weak. However, one study in monkeys showed that the long junctional epithelial union could be as resistant to biofilm infection as a true connective tissue attachment.[9]

Several studies reported that inactive pockets could be maintained for long periods with little loss of attachment by means of frequent therapy[6,10,12] and by excellent plaque or biofilm removal by the patient on a daily basis. A more reliable and stable result is obtained by transforming the pocket into a healthy sulcus. The bottom of the healthy sulcus can be located where the bottom of the pocket was localized or coronal to it. In the first case (see Fig. 57.3, *bottom left*), there is no gain of attachment, and the area of the root that was previously the tooth wall of the pocket becomes exposed. Rather than causing recession, periodontal treatment uncovers the recession previously caused by disease.

The healthy sulcus can be located coronal to the bottom of the preexisting pocket (see Fig. 57.3, *bottom center* and *right*). This is conducive to a restored marginal periodontium; the result is a sulcus of normal depth with a gain of attachment. The creation of a healthy sulcus and a restored periodontium entails total restoration of the status that existed before periodontal disease began, which is the ideal result of treatment. The bone regeneration diagram in Fig. 57.3 (*bottom center* and *right)* is for illustrative purpose only because bone regeneration without an osseous wall is seldom achieved (see Chapter 24).

Pocket Elimination Versus Pocket Maintenance

Pocket elimination (i.e., depth reduction to gingival sulcus levels) has traditionally been considered a type of periodontal therapy. It was considered vital because of the need to improve access to root surfaces for the therapist during treatment and for the patient after healing. Prevailing opinion considers deep pockets after therapy to represent a greater risk of disease progression than shallow sites. Individual probing depths are not good predictors of future clinical attachment loss. Conversely, the absence of deep pockets in treated patients is an excellent predictor of a stable periodontium.[5]

Longitudinal studies of different therapeutic modalities over the past 30 years have produced conflicting results,[7,16] probably because of problems created by the split-mouth design. After surgical therapy, pockets that rebound to a shallow or moderate depth can be maintained in a healthy state and without radiographic evidence of advancing bone loss by maintenance visits consisting of scaling and root planing, with oral hygiene reinforcement performed at regular intervals of 3 months or less. In these patients, the residual pocket can be examined with a thin periodontal probe without pain, exudate, or bleeding. This indicates that biofilm has not formed on the subgingival root surfaces.

These findings do not alter the indications and need for periodontal surgery because the results are based on surgical exposure of the root surfaces for thorough elimination of irritants. However, the findings also emphasize the importance of the maintenance phase and close monitoring of the level of attachment and pocket depth along with the other clinical variables (e.g., bleeding, exudation, tooth mobility). *Transformation of the initial deep, active pocket into a shallower, inactive, maintainable pocket requires some form of definitive pocket therapy and constant supervision thereafter.*

Pocket depth is an extremely useful and widely employed clinical determination, but it must be evaluated together with the level of attachment and degree of bleeding, exudation, and pain. The most important variable for evaluating whether a pocket is progressing is the *level of attachment,* which is measured in millimeters from the cementum–enamel junction. Apical displacement of the level of attachment places the tooth in jeopardy, not the increase in pocket depth, which may be caused by coronal displacement of the gingival margin.

Pocket depth remains an important clinical variable in making decisions about treatment. Lindhe and colleagues[8] compared the effect of root planing alone or using a modified Widman flap with the resultant level of attachment and in relation to initial pocket depth. They reported that scaling and root planing procedures induced loss of attachment if performed in pockets shallower than 2.9 mm, whereas gain of attachment occurred in deeper pockets. The modified

Widman flap induced loss of attachment if performed in pockets shallower than 4.2 mm but resulted in a greater gain of attachment than root planing in pockets deeper than 4.2 mm. The loss is a true loss of connective tissue attachment, whereas the gain can be considered a false gain because of reduced penetrability of connective tissues apical to the bottom of the pocket after treatment.[9,17]

Probing depths established about 6 months after active therapy and healing can be maintained, remain unchanged, or be reduced even further during a maintenance period involving careful reevaluation, plaque or biofilm removal, and root therapy as necessary every 3 months.[8]

Ramfjord[12] and Rosling[13] and their colleagues reported that a certain pocket depth recurs regardless of the surgical technique used for pocket therapy. *Maintaining this depth without any further loss of attachment becomes the goal.*

Reevaluation After Phase I Therapy

Longitudinal studies found that all patients should be treated initially with scaling, root planing, and plaque or biofilm control and that a final decision on the need for periodontal surgery should be made only after a thorough evaluation of the effects of phase I therapy.[5] Assessment typically is made no less than 1 to 3 months and sometimes as much as 9 months after the completion of phase I therapy.[1] Reevaluation of the periodontal condition includes repeat probing of the entire mouth. Calculus, root caries, defective restorations, and signs of persistent inflammation should also be evaluated.

Critical Zones in Pocket Surgery

Criteria for the selection of a surgical technique for pocket therapy are based on clinical findings in the soft tissue pocket wall, tooth surface, underlying bone, and attached gingiva.

Zone 1: Soft Tissue Pocket Wall

The clinician should determine the morphologic features, thickness, and topography of the soft tissue pocket wall and persistence of inflammatory changes in the wall.

Zone 2: Tooth Surface

The clinician should identify the deposits on and alterations of the cementum surface and determine the accessibility of the root surface to instrumentation. Phase I therapy should have solved many or all of the problems on the tooth surface. Evaluation of the results of phase I therapy can determine the need for further therapy and the method to be used.

Zone 3: Underlying Bone

The clinician should establish the shape and height of the alveolar bone next to the pocket wall through careful probing and clinical and radiographic examinations. The number of osseous walls—one, two, or three—helps to determine whether resective or regenerative therapy can be used (see Chapter 24). Bony craters, horizontal or angular bone losses, and other bone deformities also are important criteria in selection of the treatment technique.

Zone 4: Attached Gingiva

The clinician should consider the presence or absence of an adequate band of keratinized, attached gingiva when selecting the pocket treatment method. Diagnostic techniques for mucogingival problems are described in Chapter 65. An inadequate attached gingiva can be caused by a high frenum attachment, marked gingival recession, or a deep pocket that reaches the level of the mucogingival junction.

All of these conditions should be explored and their influence on pocket therapy considered.

Indications for Periodontal Surgery

The following findings can indicate the need for a surgical phase of therapy:

1. Areas with irregular bony contours, deep craters, and other defects usually require a surgical approach.
2. Pockets around teeth where access to the root surface for complete removal of root irritants is not clinically possible are an indication for surgery. This occurs frequently around molars and premolars.
3. Furcation involvement of grade II or III may require a surgical approach to ensure the removal of irritants around root surfaces. If root resection or hemisection is necessary, surgical intervention will be needed.
4. Intrabony pockets distal to the last molars, which in many cases are complicated by mucogingival problems, often require surgery.
5. Persistent inflammation in areas after past procedures that have moderate to deep pockets may require a surgical approach. These are usually areas where all of the subgingival calculus could not be removed. Cases with shallow pockets and good hygiene but bleeding on probing can be caused by mucogingival problems in areas where there is no keratinized tissue. Trauma to these areas can cause bleeding.

Methods of Pocket Therapy

The methods for pocket therapy can be classified as follows:

1. *New attachment techniques* offer the ideal result because they eliminate pocket depth by reuniting the gingiva with the tooth at a position coronal to the bottom of the preexisting pocket. New attachment involves regeneration of bone, connective tissue, periodontal ligament, and cementum.
2. *Removal of the pocket wall* is the most common method. The wall of the pocket consists of soft tissue and can include bone in the case of intrabony pockets. It can be removed by the following methods:
   - Retraction or shrinkage, where plaque or biofilm removal by the patient and scaling and root planing resolve the inflammatory process, can occur. The gingival tissue shrinks, reducing the pocket depth.
   - Surgical removal of the pocket is done by gingivectomy or the undisplaced flap technique.
   - Apical displacement of the flap is performed with an apically displaced flap.
3. *Removal of the tooth side of the pocket*, which is accomplished by tooth extraction or by partial tooth extraction in the case of furcation involvement (i.e., hemisection or root resection).

The techniques, what they accomplish, and the factors governing their selection are discussed in Chapters 60 through 63.

Criteria for Selection of the Method of Surgical Therapy

Scientific criteria to establish indications for the use of each technique are difficult to determine. Criteria are based on longitudinal studies that follow a significant number of cases over a number of years, standardization of multiple factors, and long-term clinical experience. Selection of a technique for treating a particular periodontal lesion is based on the following considerations:

1. Characteristics of the pocket: depth, relation to bone, and configuration

2. Accessibility to instrumentation, including furcation involvement
3. Existence of mucogingival problems
4. Response to phase I therapy
5. Patient cooperation, including the ability to perform effective oral hygiene and stop smoking
6. Age and general health of the patient
7. Overall diagnosis of the case: various types of gingival enlargement and types of periodontitis (e.g., chronic marginal periodontitis, localized aggressive periodontitis, generalized aggressive periodontitis)
8. Aesthetic considerations
9. Previous periodontal treatments

Each variable is analyzed in relation to the pocket therapy techniques available. A specific technique is then selected. The one most likely to successfully solve the problem with the fewest undesirable effects should be selected. Clinicians who adhere to one technique to solve all problems do not take advantage of the wide repertoire of techniques that are at their disposal.

Approaches to Specific Pocket Problems

Therapy for Gingival Pockets

Gingival pockets do not have an osseous component (i.e., no attachment loss) and usually have edematous or fibrotic gingival tissue. Two factors are taken into consideration: the character of the pocket wall and the accessibility of the pocket.

The pocket wall can be edematous or fibrotic. *Edematous tissue* shrinks after the elimination of local factors, reducing or totally eliminating pocket depth. Scaling and root planing is the technique of choice for these cases.

Pockets with a *fibrotic wall* are not appreciably reduced in depth after scaling and root planing. These pockets are eliminated or reduced by surgical therapy. In the past, gingivectomy was frequently used to reduce these pockets. This solved the problem, but in cases of marked gingival enlargement (e.g., severe phenytoin-related enlargement), treatment could leave a large, open wound, and the patient had to endure a painful and prolonged healing process. Currently, a modified flap technique is used, and fewer postoperative problems are associated with primary closure of the wound (see Chapter 61). Some clinicians have advocated the use of laser therapy to manage gingival enlargement (see Chapter 68),

Therapy for Incipient Periodontitis

In patients with slight or incipient periodontitis with minimal attachment and bone loss, the pocket depths are shallow or a moderate depth. In these patients, the conservative approach of good oral hygiene, scaling, and root planing when necessary usually suffices to control the disease. Incipient periodontitis that recurs in previously treated sites with good hygiene may require a thorough analysis of the recurrence, which may be caused by remnants of calculus that were missed during previous treatment or other factors such as open margins of a restoration located subgingivally. Occasionally, a surgical approach may be required to correct these problems.

Therapy for Moderate to Severe Periodontitis in the Anterior Sector

Because the maxillary anterior teeth are important aesthetically, techniques that cause the least amount of visual root exposure should be considered. However, each patient has different expectations regarding the final result of therapy. The clinician must explain that the therapy may be a compromise between complete pocket elimination and achieving an aesthetic result that is acceptable to the patient. The patient must be educated before therapy that the result may be some degree of gingival recession and some loss of the interdental papilla (see Chapter 65).

The anterior dentition has two advantages for using a conservative (nonsurgical) approach: (1) the teeth are all single rooted and easily accessible for subgingival scaling and root planing, and (2) patient compliance and thoroughness in plaque or biofilm control may be easier to attain. *Nonsurgical therapy is therefore the technique of choice for the maxillary anterior dentition.*

In some situations, surgical therapy may be necessary to improve accessibility for root planing, or regenerative therapy may be possible. Chapters 59, 60, and 63 discuss the surgical aspects in detail. The papilla preservation flap or modified papilla preservation flap can be used for both purposes and offers a better postoperative result with less recession and reduced soft tissue crater formation interproximally.[14]

When the interdental space is minimal, papilla preservation techniques may not be feasible. Instead, a technique that splits the papilla and retains as much of the papilla as possible is the appropriate surgical technique.

When the aesthetic outcome is not the primary consideration and a flap procedure is necessary for root surface access, the *modified Widman flap* can be selected. This technique uses an internal bevel incision about 1 to 2 mm from the gingival margin without thinning the flap. This procedure may result in minor recession of the surrounding gingival tissue.

In cases with advanced osseous involvement, bone contouring may be needed despite the resultant root exposure. The technique of choice is the *apically displaced flap with osseous bone contouring.* The clinician must educate the patient before therapy about the possibility of aesthetic difficulties due to the expected recession of gingival tissue.

Therapy for Moderate to Severe Periodontitis in Posterior Areas

Treatment for the maxillary and mandibular premolars and molars does not entail aesthetic problems but frequently involves difficult access for root therapy. Bone defects occur more often in the posterior area than the anterior, with many areas having deep infrabony lesions and anatomic root problems with concavities, such as the mesial surface of the maxillary first premolar. A difficult problem encountered in the posterior area is the furcation lesion. Because this area can pose insurmountable problems for instrumentation unless a flap is reflected, surgery is frequently indicated.

Surgery is used in the posterior area for enhanced access to the root surface or for definitive pocket reduction requiring osseous surgery. Access can be obtained by an undisplaced or apically displaced flap (see Chapter 60).

Most patients with moderate to severe periodontitis have developed osseous defects that require some degree of bone remodeling or reconstruction. For osseous defects amenable to reconstruction, the *papilla preservation flap* or *modified papilla preservation flap* is the technique of choice because it better protects the interproximal areas where defects frequently occur. Second and third choices are the *sulcular flap* and *modified Widman flap,* maintaining as much of the papilla as possible.

For osseous defects with no possibility of reconstructive therapy, such as interdental craters, the technique of choice is an undisplaced or apically displaced flap with osseous contouring. All surgical flap procedures are discussed in Chapters 57, 59, and 60.

Surgical Techniques for Correction of Morphologic Defects

The rationales and objectives for techniques performed to correct morphologic defects (i.e., mucogingival, aesthetic, and pre-prosthetic) are described in Chapters 60 and 62.

Surgical Techniques for Implant Placement and Related Problems

The rationales and objectives for techniques performed for implant placement and related problems are described in Chapters 78 through 80.

Conclusions

Many steps are required to achieve and maintain a healthy periodontal status. After completion of phase I therapy, which consists of patient education, biofilm control, and thorough root therapy, the involved periodontal areas are reevaluated. The necessity of phase II therapy, which is the surgical phase of treatment, depends on the success of the initial phase and the severity of the periodontal condition. Periodontal surgery, which includes plastic, aesthetic, resective, and regenerative procedures, becomes necessary when access for root therapy is required or correction of anatomic or morphologic defects is necessary. Placement of dental implants can be part of this therapy.

References

 References for this chapter are found on the companion website www.expertconsult.com.

CHAPTER 58

Periodontal and Peri-Implant Surgical Anatomy

Perry R. Klokkevold | *Fermin A. Carranza*

CHAPTER OUTLINE

Mandible

Maxilla

Exostoses

Muscles

Anatomic Spaces

Conclusion

A sound knowledge of the anatomy of the periodontium and the surrounding hard and soft tissue structures is essential to determine the scope and possibilities of periodontal and implant surgical procedures and to minimize their risks. The spatial relationship of bones, muscles, blood vessels, and nerves, as well as the anatomic spaces located in the vicinity of the periodontal or implant surgical field, are particularly important. Only those features of periodontal and implant surgery relevance are mentioned in this chapter; the reader is referred to books about oral anatomy for a more comprehensive description of these structures.[4,6]

Mandible

The mandible is a horseshoe-shaped bone connected to the skull by the temporomandibular joints. It presents several landmarks of great surgical importance for both periodontal and implant surgical procedures.

The *mandibular canal,* which is occupied by the inferior alveolar nerve and vessels, begins at the mandibular foramen on the medial surface of the mandibular ramus and curves downward and forward until it becomes horizontal below the apices of the molars (Fig. 58.1). The distance from the canal to the apices of the teeth is shortest in the third molar area. A small percentage (1%) of mandibular canals bifurcates in the body of the mandible, thereby resulting in two canals and two mental foramina.[5,10] In the premolar area, the mandibular canal divides in two branches, with one exiting the mandible and the other continuing anteriorly: the *incisive canal,* which continues horizontally to the midline, and the *mental canal,* which turns upward and opens in the mental foramen.

The *mental foramen,* from which the mental nerve and vessels emerge, is located on the buccal surface of the mandible below the apices of the premolars, sometimes closer to the second premolar and usually halfway between the lower border of the mandible and the alveolar margin (Fig. 58.2). It is often but not always visible on conventional radiographs. The opening of the mental foramen, which may be oval or round, typically faces upward and distally, with its posterior-superior border slanting gradually to the bone surface. An "anterior loop" of the mental foramen has been described, with the use of cadaver dissection, as a reverse turn and looping back of the mental nerve within the body of the mandible before its exit out of the mental foramen; the estimated length of the anterior loop ranges from 0.5 to 5.0 mm.[10] A more recent evaluation of the anterior loop of the mental nerve involving the use of cone beam scans and cadaveric

dissection reported this loop extension to range from 0.0 to 9.0 mm.[22,23] The anterior loop of the mental nerve has a high prevalence (88%), symmetric occurrence, and a mean length of 4.13 ± 1.08 mm.[18] As it emerges, the *mental nerve* divides into three branches. One branch of the nerve turns forward and downward to supply the skin of the chin. The other two branches course anteriorly and upward to supply the skin and mucous membrane of the lower lip and the mucosa of the labial alveolar surface.

Surgical trauma (e.g., pressure, manipulation, postsurgical swelling) to the mental nerve can produce paresthesia of the lip, which recovers slowly. Partial or complete cutting of the nerve can result in permanent paresthesia, dysesthesia, or both. Familiarity with the location and appearance of the mental nerve reduces the likelihood of injury (Fig. 58.3).

KEY FACT

Surgical trauma, including pressure, manipulation, or postsurgical swelling of the mental nerve tissues, may result in transient paresthesia of the lip. Partial or complete nerve cutting of the mental nerve may result in permanent paresthesia, dysesthesia, or both.

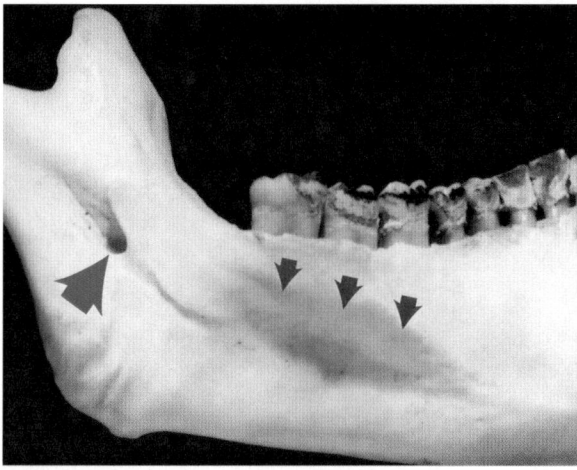

Fig. 58.1 Mandible, lingual surface view. Note the lingual or mandibular foramen *(blue arrow),* where the inferior alveolar nerve enters the mandibular canal, and the mylohyoid ridge *(red arrows).*

In partially or totally edentulous jaws, the disappearance of the alveolar portion of the mandible brings the mandibular canal and mental foramen closer to the superior border (Figs. 58.4 and 58.5). When these patients are evaluated for the placement of implants, the distance between the canal and the superior surface of the bone, as well as the location of the mental foramen, must be carefully determined to avoid surgical injury to the nerve (see Chapter 76).

The anterior extension of the inferior alveolar nerve or incisive nerve has been measured with the use of conventional radiographs, computed tomography (CT) scans, cadaver dissections, and cone beam scans.[3,10,22,23] This nerve, which is less evident on conventional radiographs and often unnoticed, extends beyond the anterior loop of the mental foramen in a horizontal direction toward the midline. The length of the incisive canal has been reported to be up to 21.45 mm from the mesial aspect of the mental foramen and to terminate just 4 mm from the midline.[3]

The *lingual nerve,* along with the inferior alveolar nerve, is a branch of the posterior division of the mandibular nerve. It descends along the mandibular ramus medial to and in front of the inferior alveolar nerve. The lingual nerve lies close to the surface of the oral mucosa in the third molar area and goes deeper as it travels forward (Fig. 58.6). It can be damaged during anesthetic injections and during oral surgery procedures (e.g., third molar extractions).[14] Less often, the lingual nerve may be injured when a periodontal partial-thickness flap is raised in the third molar region or when releasing incisions are made in the area.

The *alveolar process,* which provides the supporting bone to the teeth, has a narrower distal curvature than the body of the mandible (Fig. 58.7), thus creating a flat surface in the posterior area between the teeth and the anterior border of the ramus. This results in the formation of the *external oblique ridge,* which runs downward and forward to the region of the second or first molar (Fig. 58.8) to create a shelflike bony area. Resective osseous therapy may be difficult or impossible in this area because of the amount of bone that must be removed distally toward the ramus to achieve resection of a periodontal osseous defect on the distal aspect of the mandibular second or third molar.

Distal to the third molar, the external oblique ridge circumscribes the *retromolar triangle* (see Fig. 58.8). This region is occupied by glandular and adipose tissue and covered by unattached, nonkeratinized mucosa. If sufficient space exists distal to the last molar, a band of attached gingiva may be present; only in such a case can a distal flap procedure be performed effectively (see Chapter 60).

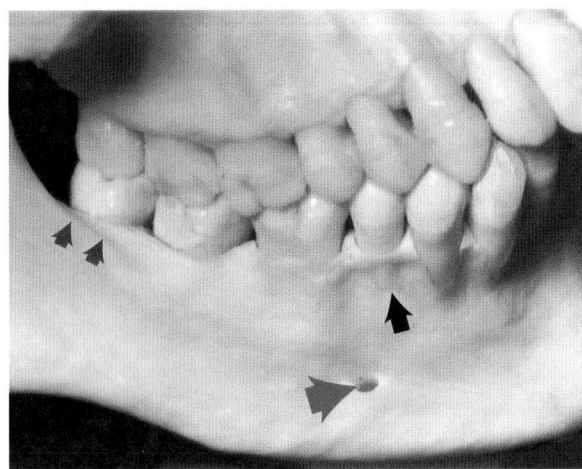

Fig. 58.2 Mandible, facial surface view. Note the location of the mental foramen *(blue arrow),* which is slightly distal and apical to the apex of the second premolar, and the shelflike area in the region of the molars *(red arrows)* that is created by the external oblique ridge. Note also the fenestration that is present in the second premolar *(black arrow).*

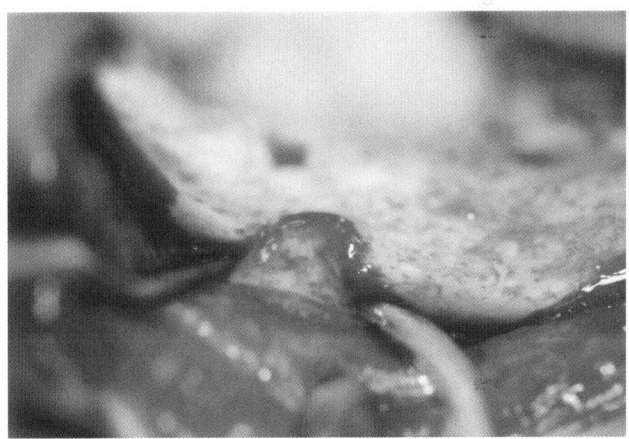

Fig. 58.3 Mental nerve emerging from the foramen in the premolar area.

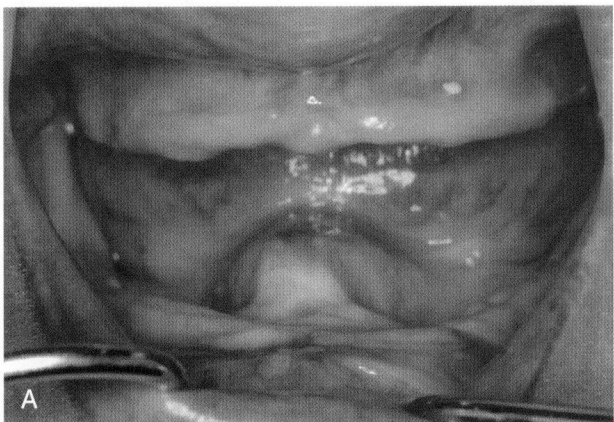
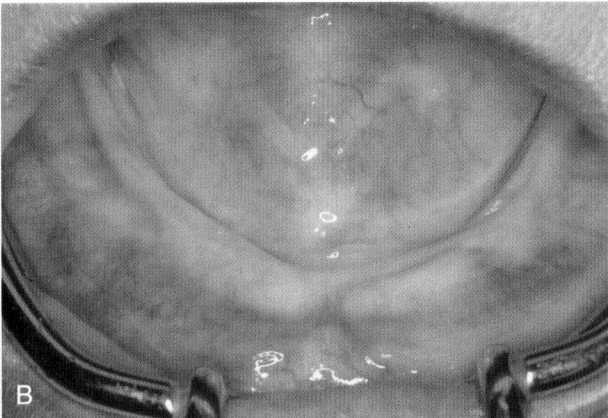

Fig. 58.4 Loss of the alveolar ridge in an edentulous patient brings the mental foramen and the inferior alveolar nerve canal closer to the surface, which may lead to discomfort for the patient. (A) Anterior view demonstrating a severe loss of vertical alveolar ridge height. (B) Occlusal view of the same patient demonstrating a loss of vestibular depth with alveolar bone loss.

The medial side of the body of the mandible is traversed obliquely by the *mylohyoid ridge,* which starts close to the alveolar margin in the third molar area and continues anteriorly in an apical direction, thereby increasing its distance from the osseous margin as it travels forward (Fig. 58.9). The *mylohyoid muscle* inserts along this ridge and separates the *sublingual space,* which is located above or more anteriorly and superiorly, from the submandibular space, which is located below or more posteriorly and inferiorly.

Maxilla

The maxilla is a paired bone that is hollowed out by the maxillary sinus and the nasal cavity. The maxilla has the following four processes:

*   The *alveolar process* contains the sockets for and supports the maxillary teeth.

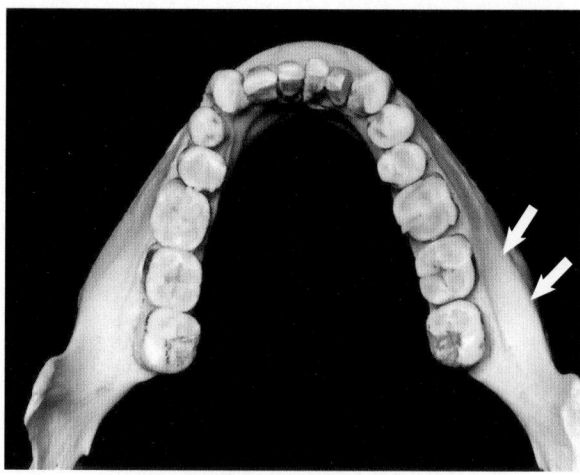

Fig. 58.7 Occlusal view of the mandible. Note the shelf that is created in the facial molar areas by the external oblique ridge. *Arrows* show the attachment of the buccinator muscle.

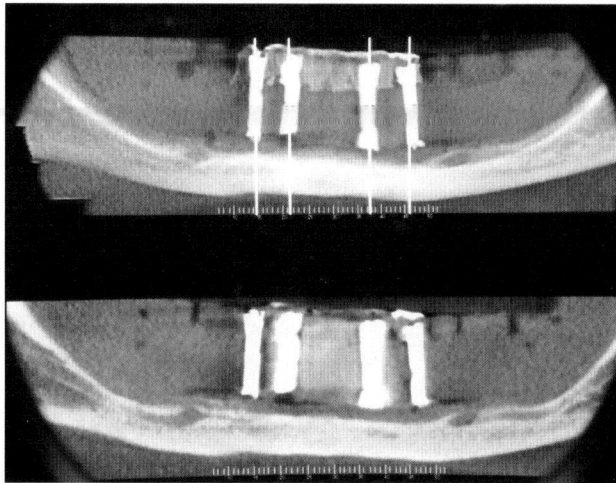

Fig. 58.5 Panoramic radiograph of an edentulous patient with a loss of alveolar bone height. This results in the mental foramen exiting the jaw at the superior aspect of the remaining bone (ridge crest), which is the denture-bearing surface. Pressure from the complete removable denture over this area causes pain.

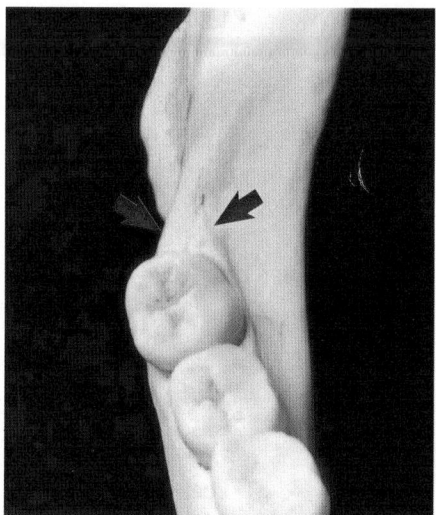

Fig. 58.8 Mandible; occlusal view of the ramus and molars. Note the retromolar triangle area distal to the third molar *(arrows).*

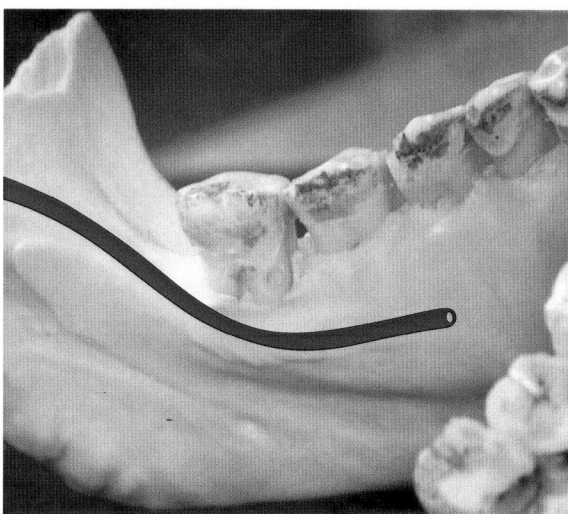

Fig. 58.6 Lingual view of the mandible showing the pathway of the lingual nerve *(red),* which goes near the gingiva in the third molar area and then continues forward, going deeper and medially.

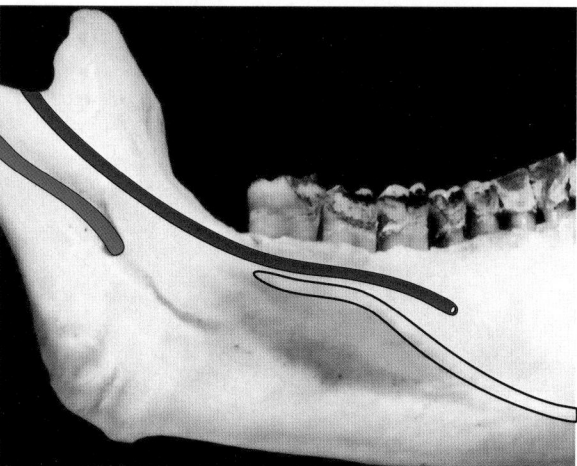

Fig. 58.9 Lingual view of the mandible showing, The inferior alveolar nerve entering the mandibular canal *(blue),* the lingual nerve traversing near the lingual surface of the third molar *(red),* and the attachment of the mylohyoid muscle inferiorly *(outline).*

- The *palatine process* extends horizontally from the alveolar process to meet its counterpart from the opposite maxilla at the midline intermaxillary suture, and it extends posteriorly with the horizontal plate of the palatine bone to form the hard palate.
- The *zygomatic process* extends laterally from the area above the first molar and determines the depth of the vestibular fornix on the lateral aspect of the maxilla.
- The *frontal process* extends in an ascending direction and articulates with the frontal bone at the frontomaxillary suture.

The terminal branches of the nasopalatine nerve and vessels pass through the incisive canal, which opens in the midline anterior area of the palate (Fig. 58.10). The mucosa overlying the incisive canal presents a slight protuberance called the *incisive papilla.* Vessels that emerge through the incisive canal are of small caliber, and their surgical interference is of little consequence.

The *greater palatine foramen* opens 3 to 4 mm anterior to the posterior border of the hard palate (Fig. 58.11). The greater palatine nerve and vessels emerge through this foramen and run anteriorly

in the submucosa of the palate, between the palatal and alveolar processes (Fig. 58.12). Palatal flaps and donor sites for gingival and connective tissue grafts should be carefully performed and selected to avoid invading these areas because profuse hemorrhage may ensue, particularly if vessels are damaged at the greater palatine foramen. Vertical incisions in the molar region should be avoided.

The mucous membrane that covers the hard palate is firmly attached to the underlying bone. The submucous layer of the palate posterior to the first molars contains the *palatal glands,* which are more compact in the soft palate and extend anteriorly, thereby filling the gap between the mucosal connective tissue and the periosteum and protecting the underlying vessels and nerve (see Fig. 58.22, later).

The area distal to the last molar, called the *maxillary tuberosity,* consists of the posterior-inferior angle of the infratemporal surface of the maxilla. Medially it articulates with the pyramidal process of the palatine bone. It is covered by dense, fibrous connective tissue, and it contains the terminal branches of the middle and posterior palatine nerves. Excision of the area for distal flap surgery may reach medially to the tensor palati muscle. The tensor palati muscle comes from the greater wing of the sphenoid bone and ends in a tendon that forms the palatine aponeurosis, which expands, fanlike, to attach to the posterior border of the hard palate.

The body of the maxilla is occupied by the *maxillary sinus,* which is the largest of the paranasal sinuses. It is an air-filled cavity located in the posterior maxilla superior to the teeth. The lateral wall of the nasal cavity borders the sinus medially; it is bordered superiorly by the floor of the orbit and laterally by the lateral wall of the maxilla, the alveolar process, and the zygomatic arch (Fig. 58.13). It is pyramidal, with its apex in the zygomatic arch and its base at the lateral wall of the nasal cavity. The size of the maxillary sinus varies from one individual to another (depending on the individual and his or her age) and from very small and narrow to quite large and expansive.

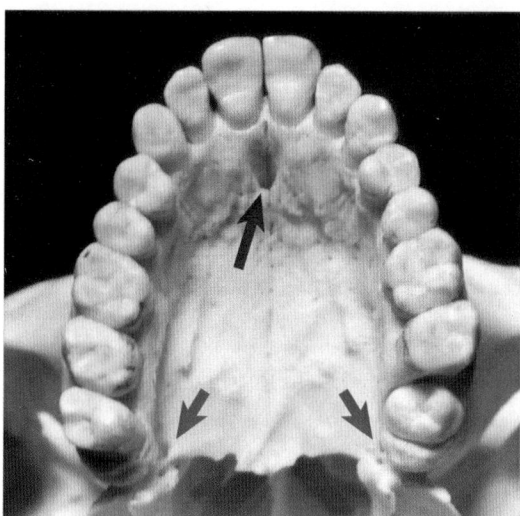

Fig. 58.10 Occlusal view of the maxilla and the palatine bone. Note the opening of the incisive canal or the anterior palatine foramen *(red arrow)* and the greater palatine foramen *(blue arrows).*

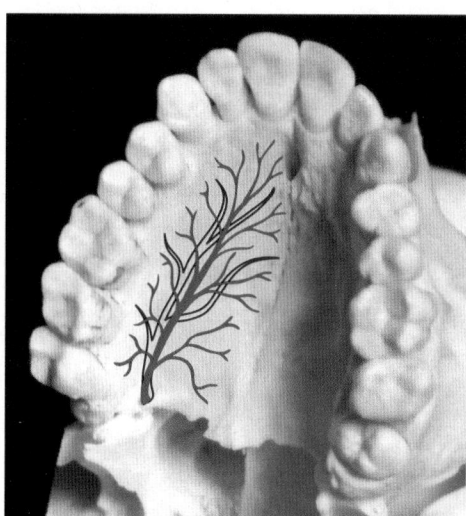

Fig. 58.11 Occlusolateral view of the palate showing nerves *(red)* and vessels *(blue)* emerging from the greater palatine foramen and continuing anteriorly on the palate.

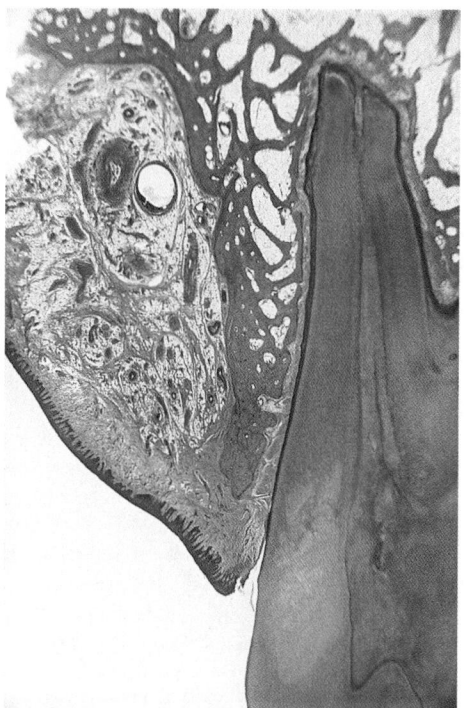

Fig. 58.12 Histologic frontal section of a human palate at the level of the first molar showing the location of the vessels and the nerve surrounded by adipose and glandular tissue.

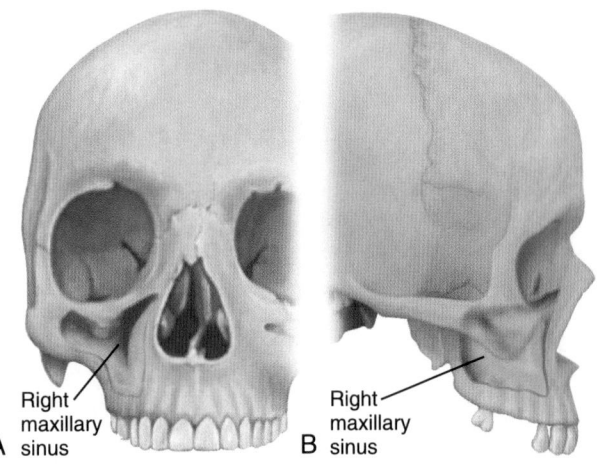

Fig. 58.13 Location and anatomy of the maxillary sinus. (A) Frontal view. (B) Lateral view.

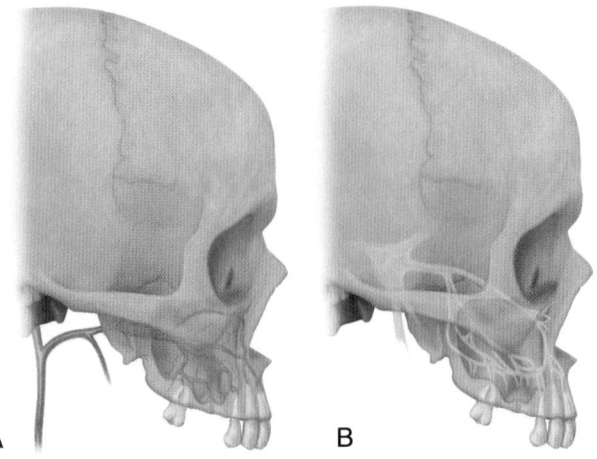

Fig. 58.14 Blood supply and innervation of the maxillary sinus. (A) Arterial blood supply. (B) Innervation of the maxillary sinus.

The maxillary sinus is frequently subdivided (incompletely) into recesses by one or more septa. Maxillary sinus septa vary in size and location. Clinical and radiographic examinations suggest that septa are frequently present (≤39% of sinuses).[8,13,25] CT scanning is the preferred method for detecting septa because panoramic radiographs are not reliable (i.e., 26.5% false diagnosis of the presence or absence of septa).[13,15] Septa are found in the anterior (24%), middle (41%), and posterior (35%) aspects of the maxillary sinus, with the most common location being between the second premolar and the first molar.[12,25] The height of septa varies as well, ranging from 0 to 20.6 mm.[25] Only 0.5% of septa form a complete separation of the sinus spaces into separate chambers.[16]

The entire maxillary sinus is lined with a thin mucosal membrane called the *schneiderian membrane*. This specialized structure of the respiratory mucous membrane, with its motile cilia and rich blood supply, is well adapted to purifying, moistening, and warming air to protect the lungs. The entrance to the maxillary sinus, through the orifice or maxillary duct, is located at the superior medial aspect of the cavity. The orifice is relatively small, measuring only 3 to 6 mm in length and diameter. An accessory opening is occasionally found inferior and posterior to the main opening. The maxillary sinus drains into the middle meatus of the nasal cavity through the maxillary duct, which passes secretions medially to the semilunar hiatus. Normal amounts of secretion are moved from the sinus by the spiral pattern of the beating cilia that surround the orifice. If the maxillary sinus becomes infected or chronically inflamed, swelling of the mucosa around the orifice impairs drainage. The floor of the maxillary sinus extends down below the level of the nasal cavity into the alveolar process.

The roots of the maxillary first and second molars are often close to the floor of the sinus. Less frequently, the roots of the premolars and third molars may protrude into the floor of the sinus. With increasing age, the maxillary sinus expands. It becomes more and more pneumatized down around the roots of the maxillary teeth, sometimes resulting in exposure of the roots through the bony floor into the sinus, with only the thin mucosal membrane covering the root surface. The ability to perform periodontal osseous surgery in the posterior maxilla may be limited when the sinuses are severely pneumatized. Extraction of teeth with roots exposed into the maxillary sinus (i.e., without bone to maintain integrity of the maxillary sinus floor) can result in an oroantral communication.

Blood supply to the maxillary sinus arises from the superior alveolar (anterior, middle, and posterior) branches of the maxillary

artery (Fig. 58.14A).[24] The maxillary artery, which is a large terminal branch of the external carotid artery, gives off many branches to supply the maxillary sinus, including the infraorbital artery, which travels superiorly and anteriorly and gives off the anterior superior alveolar artery.[9] Branches of the greater palatine artery contribute to a lesser extent. Venous blood drains via the pterygoid plexus. Much of the vasculature travels through channels in the bony walls of the maxillary sinus, with many branches anastomosing with the highly vascularized schneiderian membrane. Innervation of the maxillary sinus is supplied by the superior alveolar (anterior, middle, and posterior) nerves and the branches of the maxillary nerve (Fig. 58.14B).

Knowledge of the arterial blood supply is particularly important when considering a lateral window approach to sinus floor elevation and bone augmentation. Solar and colleagues[19] found an intraosseous branch of the posterior superior alveolar artery anastomosing with the infraorbital artery in 100% of their human cadaver specimens (134 sinuses, all in male cadavers). On average, the vessel was located 18.9 mm from the alveolar crest. By studying 50 CT scans from 625 patients (both male and female) who were undergoing sinus bone augmentation, Elian and colleagues[7] found that the vessel was radiographically evident in 52.9% of sinuses. The vessel was located an average of 16.4 mm from the alveolar crest, a slightly shorter distance but consistent with the previous study. Human cadaver dissection and CT scan evaluations of the vessels running through the lateral wall of the maxillary sinus have revealed that intraosseous vessels are present in the lower two-thirds of the anterolateral wall in approximately 10.5% of cases (Fig. 58.15).[9] In 57.1% of those cases (about 6% of all sinuses), the vessel diameter ranged in size from 1 to 2.5 mm. The location of the artery in relation to the position of the lateral window for sinus augmentation presents a risk for bleeding complications in 10% to 20% of cases.[7,9]

The inferior wall of the maxillary sinus is frequently separated from the apices and roots of the maxillary posterior teeth by a thin, bony plate (Fig. 58.16). In edentulous posterior areas, the maxillary sinus bony wall may be only a thin plate that is in intimate contact with the alveolar mucosa (Fig. 58.17). Adequate determination of the extension of the maxillary sinus into the surgical site is important to avoid creating an oroantral communication, particularly in relation to osseous reduction in periodontal surgery or surgical procedures for bone augmentation or the placement of implants in edentulous areas. Determining the amount of available bone in the anterior area, below the floor of the nasal cavity, is also critical for the placement of implants (see Chapter 76).

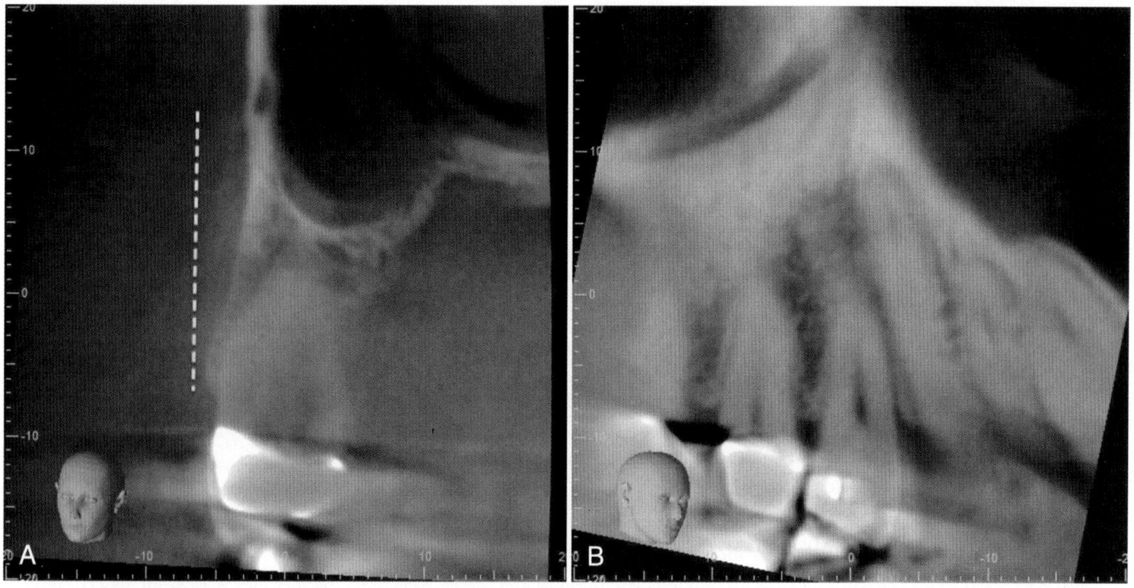

Fig. 58.15 (A) Cross-sectional image from a cone beam computed tomography scan of the maxillary sinus demonstrating the presence of an intraosseous vessel in the lateral wall approximately 20 mm from the alveolar crest. (B) Sagittal section through the maxillary sinus in the same patient demonstrating an intraosseous vessel extending along the maxillary sinus. The diameter of the intraosseous canal is 2 mm.

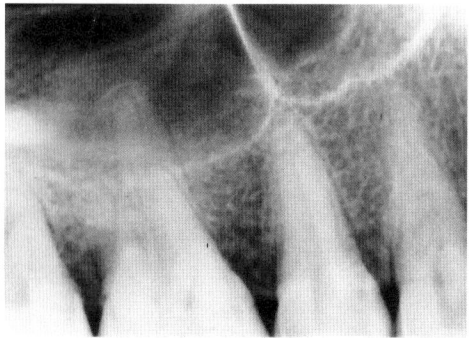

Fig. 58.16 Radiograph of the maxillary molars and premolars, with the maxillary sinus apparently near the apices.

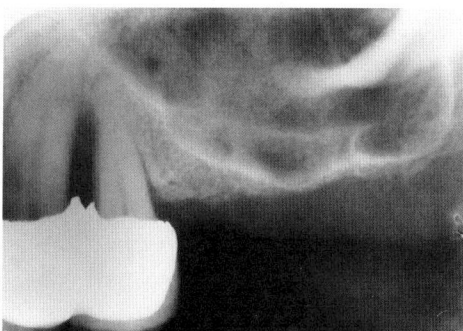

Fig. 58.17 Radiograph of an edentulous molar maxillary area demonstrating severe pneumatization of the maxillary sinus. Only a thin layer of cortical bone separates the sinus from the oral cavity.

Exostoses

Both the maxilla and the mandible may have exostoses or tori, which are considered to be within the normal range of anatomic variation. Sometimes these structures may hinder the removal of plaque by the patient and may have to be removed to improve the prognosis

of neighboring teeth. Additional indications for the removal of exostoses include the inability to wear removable prostheses comfortably over these areas. The most common location of a mandibular torus is in the lingual area of the canines and the premolars, above the mylohyoid muscle (Fig. 58.18). Mandibular tori can also be found on the buccal and labial surfaces of the mandibular teeth. Maxillary tori are usually located in the midline of the hard palate (Fig. 58.19). Smaller tori may be seen over the palatal roots of the maxillary molars, in the area above the greater palatine foramen (see Fig. 58.19), or on the buccal and labial surfaces of the maxillary teeth (Fig. 58.20).

Muscles

Several muscles may be encountered when performing periodontal and implant flap surgery, particularly during mucogingival surgery and bone augmentation procedures. These are the mentalis, the incisivus labii inferioris, the depressor labii inferioris, the depressor anguli oris (triangularis), the incisivus labii superioris, and the buccinator muscles. Their bony attachments are shown in Fig. 58.21. These muscles provide mobility to the lips and cheeks.

Anatomic Spaces

Several anatomic spaces or *compartments* are found close to the operative field of periodontal and implant surgery sites. These spaces contain loose connective tissue, but they can be easily distended by hemorrhage, inflammatory fluid, and infection.

Surgical invasion of these areas may result in dangerous hemorrhage (intraoperative) or infections (postoperative) and should be carefully avoided. Some of these spaces are briefly described in the following paragraphs. For more information, the reader is referred to other sources.[2,11,20,21]

The *canine fossa* contains varying amounts of connective tissue and fat. It is bounded superiorly by the quadratus labii superioris muscle, anteriorly by the orbicularis oris, and posteriorly by the buccinator. Infection of this area results in swelling of the upper lip,

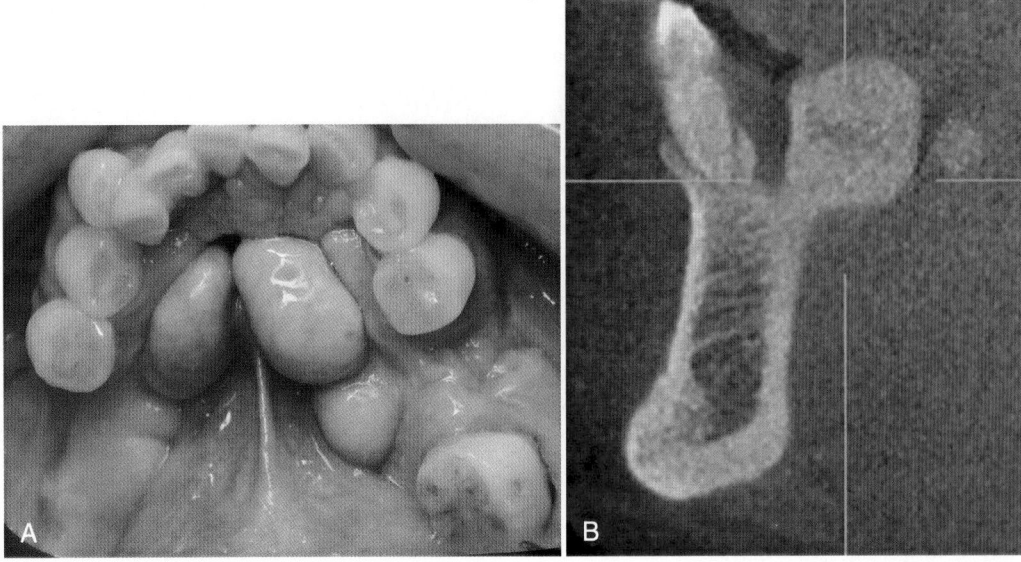

Fig. 58.18 (A) Clinical photograph of large mandibular tori on the lingual aspect of both the right and left mandible. (B) Cross-sectional image of a mandibular torus in the premolar area in the same patient.

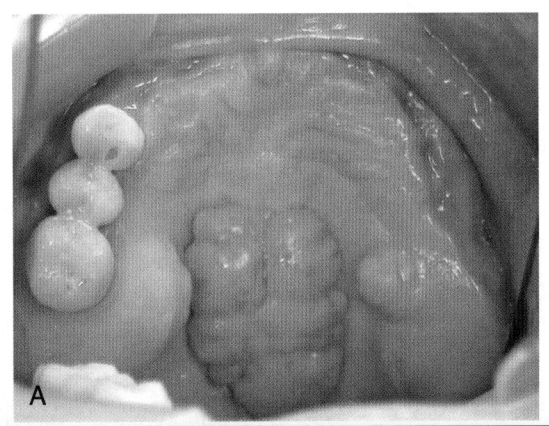

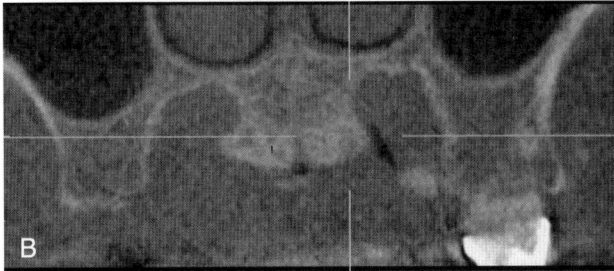

Fig. 58.19 (A) Clinical photograph of a large palatal torus located in the midline of the palate. Notice also the large tori on the palatal aspects of the maxillary alveolar ridge. (B) Cross-sectional image of the maxillary midline torus in the same patient. Notice also the torus located on the palatal aspect of the alveolar ridge.

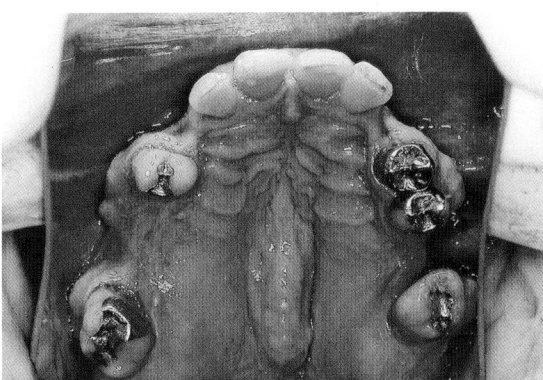

Fig. 58.20 Clinical photograph of large buccal exostosis in the maxillary arch. The patient also has a large midline palatal torus.

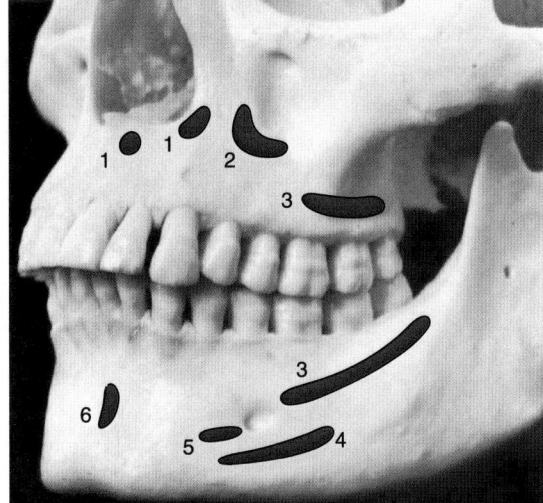

Fig. 58.21 Muscle attachments that may be encountered in mucogingival surgery. *1,* Nasalis; *2,* levator anguli oris; *3,* buccinator; *4,* depressor anguli oris; *5,* depressor labii inferioris; *6,* mentalis.

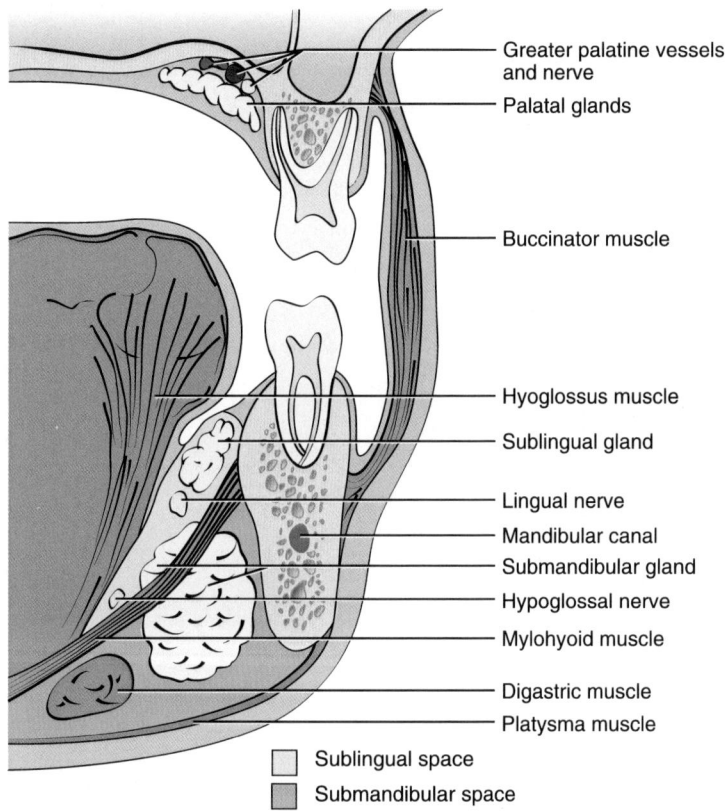

Greater palatine vessels
and nerve

Palatal glands

Buccinator muscle

Hyoglossus muscle

Sublingual gland

Lingual nerve

Mandibular canal

Submandibular gland

Hypoglossal nerve

Mylohyoid muscle

Digastric muscle

Platysma muscle

□ Sublingual space

■ Submandibular space

Fig. 58.22 Diagram of a frontal section of the human head at the level of the first molars depicting the most important structures in relation to periodontal surgery. Note the location of the sublingual space, the submandibular space, and the greater palatine nerve and vessels.

which obliterates the nasolabial fold, and of the upper and lower eyelids, which closes the eye.

The *buccal space* is located between the buccinator and the masseter muscles. Infection of this area results in swelling of the cheek that may extend to the temporal space or the submandibular space, with which the buccal space communicates.

The *mental* or *mentalis space* is located in the region of the mental symphysis, where the mental muscle, the depressor muscle of the lower lip, and the depressor muscle of the corner of the mouth are attached. Infection of this area results in large swelling of the chin that extends downward.

The *masticator space* contains the masseter muscle, the pterygoid muscles, the tendon of insertion of the temporalis muscle, the mandibular ramus, and the posterior part of the body of the mandible. Infection of this area results in swelling of the face and severe trismus and pain. If the abscess occupies the deepest part of this compartment, facial swelling may not be obvious, but the patient may complain of pain and trismus. Patients may also have difficulty and discomfort when moving the tongue and swallowing.

The *sublingual space* is located below the oral mucosa in the anterior part of the floor of the mouth. It contains the sublingual gland and its excretory duct, the submandibular or Wharton duct; it is traversed by the lingual nerve and vessels and by the hypoglossal nerve (Fig. 58.22). Its boundaries are the geniohyoid and genioglossus muscles medially, the lingual surface of the mandible below, and the mylohyoid muscle laterally and anteriorly (Fig. 58.23). Infection of this area raises the floor of the mouth and displaces the tongue, which results in pain and difficulty swallowing but little facial swelling.

The *submental space* is found between the mylohyoid muscle superiorly and the platysma inferiorly. It is bounded laterally by the

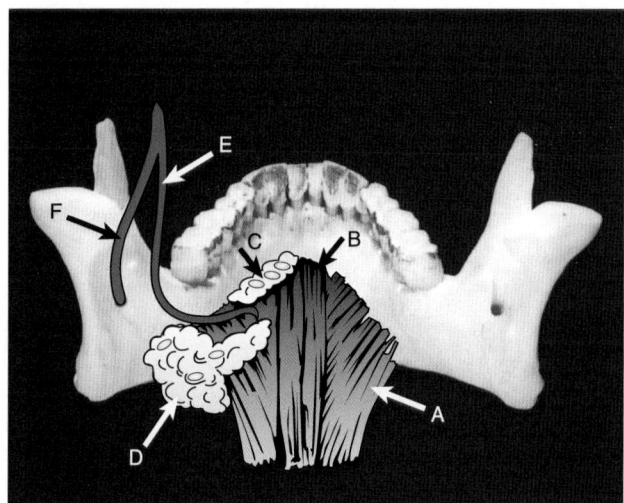

Fig. 58.23 Posterior view of the mandible showing, *A,* the attachment of the mylohyoid muscles; *B,* the geniohyoid muscles; *C,* the sublingual gland; *D,* the submandibular gland, which extends below and also to some extent above the mylohyoid muscle; *E,* the sublingual nerve; and *F,* the inferior alveolar nerve.

mandible and posteriorly by the hyoid bone. It is traversed by the anterior belly of the digastric muscle. Infections of this area arise from the region of the mandibular anterior teeth and result in swelling of the submental region; infections become more dangerous as they proceed posteriorly.

The *submandibular space* is found external to the sublingual space, below the mylohyoid and hyoglossus muscles (see Figs. 58.22

and 58.23). This space contains the submandibular gland, which extends partially above the mylohyoid muscle, thereby communicating with the sublingual space and numerous lymph nodes. Infections of this area originate in the molar or premolar area and result in swelling that obliterates the submandibular line and in pain with swallowing. Ludwig angina is a severe form of infection of the submandibular space that may extend to the sublingual and submental spaces. It results in the hardening of the floor of the mouth, and it may lead to asphyxiation from edema of the neck and glottis. Although the bacteriology of these infections has not been completely determined, they are presumed to be mixed infections with an important anaerobic component.[1,17]

≪ FLASH BACK

Ludwig angina is a life-threatening fascial space infection involving the submandibular, sublingual, and submental spaces. It is characterized by extraoral swelling and edema of the lower face and neck with intraoral swelling that raises the floor of the mouth and tongue. If not treated urgently, it can lead to airway obstruction requiring tracheostomy. Infection can spread to other fascial spaces of the head and neck including the retrosternal space.

Conclusion

Having a thorough understanding of the anatomic structures of the periodontium and the surrounding hard and soft tissues is essential for periodontal and implant surgical procedures. Knowledge of anatomy and function is important for proper execution of surgical procedures, as well as to minimize the risk of injury and complications. The spatial relationship of bones, muscles, blood vessels, and nerves, as well as the anatomic spaces located in the vicinity of the periodontal or implant surgical field, are particularly important. This chapter describes anatomic features that are significant to clinicians performing periodontal and implant surgical therapy.

 Case Scenarios are found on the companion website www.expertconsult.com.

References

 References for this chapter are found on the companion website www.expertconsult.com.

CHAPTER 59

General Principles of Periodontal Surgery

Perry R. Klokkevold | Henry H. Takei | Fermin A. Carranza

 CHAPTER OUTLINE

Outpatient Surgery
Hospital Periodontal Surgery
Surgical Instruments
Conclusion

> For online-only content on the treatment of root sensitivity and hospital periodontal surgery, please visit the companion website at www.expertconsult.com.

All surgical procedures must be carefully planned. The patient should be adequately prepared medically, psychologically, and practically for all aspects of the intervention. This chapter covers the preparation of the patient and the general considerations that are common to all periodontal surgical techniques. Complications that may occur during or after surgery are also discussed.

Although periodontal surgical procedures are usually performed in the dental office, an online section of this chapter briefly discusses situations that may require hospitalization and treatment using general anesthesia in the operating room. This chapter is concluded with a review of common surgical instruments.

Outpatient Surgery

Patient Preparation

Reevaluation After Phase I Therapy

Almost every patient undergoes the so-called initial or preparatory phase of therapy, which basically consists of thorough scaling and root planing and the removing of all irritants responsible for the periodontal inflammation. When these procedures are executed well and are combined with patient education, the results will: (1) eliminate some lesions entirely; (2) render the tissues firm and consistent, thereby allowing for accurate and minimally invasive surgery; and (3) acquaint the patient with the office, the clinician, and the assistants, thereby reducing the patient's apprehension and fear.

> **LEARNING BOX 59.1**
>
> Phase I therapy and reevaluation are important to minimize the necessity for periodontal surgery. When excellent biofilm removal by the patient and scaling and root planing are accomplished, numerous cases may not require surgical therapy, or if it is necessary, the surgical therapy may be minimal.

The reevaluation phase consists of reprobing and reexamining all of the pertinent findings that previously indicated the need for

the surgical procedure. The persistence of these findings confirms the indication for surgery. The number of surgical procedures, the expected outcome, and the postoperative care necessary are all determined before therapy and are explained to the patient. After all of the important information regarding the surgery is discussed, a final decision is made that incorporates any necessary adjustments to the original plan.

Premedication

For patients who are not medically compromised, the value of administering antibiotics routinely for periodontal surgery has not been clearly demonstrated.[29] However, some studies have reported reduced postoperative complications, including reduced pain and swelling, when antibiotics are given before periodontal surgery and continued for 4 to 7 days after surgery.[4,12,21,32]

The prophylactic use of antibiotics in patients who are otherwise healthy has been advocated for bone-grafting procedures and purported to enhance the chances of new attachment. Although the rationale for such use appears logical, no research evidence is available to support it. In any case, the risks inherent in the administration of antibiotics should be evaluated together with the potential benefits. Additional presurgical medications that may be administered include a nonsteroidal antiinflammatory drug such as ibuprofen (e.g., Motrin) 1 hour before the procedure and an antimicrobial mouthrinse such as 0.12% chlorhexidine gluconate (e.g., Peridex or PerioGard).[38]

Precautions to be taken with medically compromised patients are discussed in Chapter 39.

Smoking

The deleterious effect of smoking on the healing of periodontal wounds has been amply documented[20,33,43] (see Chapter 12). Patients should be clearly informed of this fact and asked to quit smoking completely or to stop smoking for a minimum of 3 to 4 weeks after the procedure. For patients who are unwilling to follow this advice, an alternate treatment plan that does not include complicated techniques (e.g., regenerative, mucogingival, aesthetic) should be considered.

Informed Consent

The patient should be informed at the initial visit regarding the diagnosis, prognosis, and recommended treatment options including explanations about expected outcomes. The pros and cons of each approach should be discussed, and the patient should be encouraged to ask questions. At the time of surgery, the patient should again be informed both verbally and in writing of the procedure to be performed, including the risks and expected outcomes. Patients should be given the opportunity to ask any additional questions, and, once their questions are answered, they should indicate their agreement to undergo the procedure by signing the informed consent form.

Emergency Equipment

The clinician, all assistants, and office personnel should be trained to handle all possible emergencies that may arise. Drugs and equipment for emergency use should be readily available at all times.

The most common emergency is syncope, which is a transient loss of consciousness caused by a reduction in cerebral blood flow. The most common causes of syncope are fear and anxiety. Syncope is usually preceded by a feeling of weakness, and then the patient experiences pallor, sweating, coldness of the extremities, dizziness, and a slowing of the pulse. The patient should be placed in a supine position with the legs elevated; tight clothes should be loosened, and a wide-open airway should be ensured. The administration of oxygen should be started. Unconsciousness may persist for a few minutes. A previous history of syncope during dental appointments should be explored before the treatment is started. If the patient has had other experiences with syncope, every effort should be made to minimize the patient's fear and anxiety, as well as considering the use of oral sedatives. The reader is referred to Chapter 38 and other texts for a complete analysis of this important topic.[3]

Measures to Prevent Transmission of Infection

The danger of transmitting infections to the dental team or to other patients is an important precaution that must be a part of every appointment in the dental office, especially with the threat of acquired immunodeficiency syndrome and hepatitis B virus infection. Universal precautions (e.g., protective attire) and barrier techniques must be incorporated into the surgical protocol of every procedure. These include the use of disposable sterile gloves, surgical masks, and protective eyewear. All surfaces that may be contaminated with blood or saliva and cannot be sterilized (e.g., light handles, unit syringes) must be covered with sterile aluminum foil or plastic wrap. Aerosol-producing devices (e.g., ultrasonic scalers) should not be used on patients with suspected infections, and their use should be kept to a minimum in all other patients. Special care should be taken when using and disposing of sharp items such as needles and scalpel blades.

Sedation and Anesthesia

Pain control in periodontal surgery is important. Most procedures should either be painless or minimally painful. The patient should be assured of this at the beginning and throughout the procedure. The most reliable means of providing painless surgery is the effective administration of local anesthesia. The area to be treated should be thoroughly anesthetized by means of regional block and local infiltration. Injections directly into the interdental papillae may also be helpful.

Apprehensive and neurotic patients may require special management with antianxiety or sedative–hypnotic agents. Modalities for the administration of these agents include inhalation, oral, intramuscular, and intravenous routes. The specific agents and the modality of administration are based on the desired level of sedation, the anticipated length of the procedure, and the overall condition of the patient. Specifically, the patient's medical history and physical and emotional status should be considered when determining the need for sedation, as well as the specific agents and techniques to be used. The reader is referred to Chapter 38 for a detailed description of conscious sedation methods.

Hospital Periodontal Surgery

For most patients, periodontal surgical procedures are managed well in the dental office with local anesthesia only or with some form of sedation and are performed in quadrants or sextants, usually at biweekly or longer intervals. However, certain patients and procedures warrant treatment in the hospital operating room with general anesthesia. These include patients who are not well enough to undergo treatment in a dental office and procedures that are more extensive and difficult for patients to endure. Readers are referred to the online material for a discussion of indications and procedures in a hospital setting.

Tissue Management

1. *Operate gently and carefully.* In addition to being most considerate to the patient, this is also the most effective way to operate. Tissue manipulation should be precise, deliberate, and gentle. It is essential to be thorough, but traumatic instrumentation must be avoided because it produces excessive tissue injury, causes postoperative discomfort, and delays healing.
2. *Observe the patient at all times.* It is essential to pay careful attention to the patient's reactions. Facial expressions, pallor, and perspiration are distinct signs that may indicate when a patient is experiencing pain, anxiety, or fear. The clinician's responsiveness to these signs can be the difference between success and failure.
3. *Be certain that the instruments are sharp.* Instruments must be sharp to be effective; successful treatment is not possible without sharp instruments. Dull instruments inflict unnecessary trauma as a result of poor cutting and excessive force applied to compensate for their ineffectiveness. A sterile sharpening stone should be available on the operating table at all times.

Scaling and Root Planing

Although scaling and root planing have been performed previously as part of phase I therapy, all exposed root surfaces should be carefully explored and planed as needed during the surgical procedure. In particular, areas of difficult access (e.g., furcations, deep infrabony pockets) often have rough areas or even calculus that was undetected during the preparatory sessions. The assistant who is retracting the tissues and using the aspirator should also check for the presence of calculus and the smoothness of each surface from a different angle.

LEARNING BOX 59.2

The most important objective of periodontal pocket reduction surgery is to gain access to the root surface for scaling and root planing. The exposure obtained to the subgingival root surfaces when the flap is reflected allows not only access for root therapy but also the opportunity to alter the osseous defects that may exist.

Hemostasis

Hemostasis is an important aspect of periodontal surgery because good intraoperative control of bleeding permits accurate visualization of the extent of disease, the pattern of bone destruction, and the anatomy and condition of the root surfaces. It provides the operator with a clear view of the surgical site, which is essential for wound debridement and scaling and root planing. In addition, good hemostasis also prevents excessive loss of blood into the mouth, oropharynx, and stomach.

Periodontal surgery can produce profuse bleeding, especially during the initial incisions and flap reflection. After flap reflection and the removal of granulation tissue, bleeding stops or is considerably reduced. Typically, the control of intraoperative bleeding can be managed with aspiration. Continuous suctioning of the surgical site with an aspirator is indispensable when performing periodontal surgery. The application of pressure to the surgical wound with moist gauze can be a helpful adjunct to control site-specific bleeding. Intraoperative bleeding that is not controlled with these simple methods may indicate a more serious problem and require additional control measures.

Excessive hemorrhaging after initial incisions and flap reflection may be caused by the laceration of venules, arterioles, or larger vessels. Fortunately, the laceration of medium or large vessels is rare because incisions near highly vascular anatomic areas (e.g., the posterior mandible [the lingual and inferior alveolar arteries], the posterior midpalatal regions [the greater palatine arteries]) are avoided by incision and flap procedures. Proper design of the flaps that takes these areas into consideration will help avoid these accidents (see Chapter 58). However, even when all anatomic precautions are taken, it is possible to cause bleeding from medium or large vessels due to anatomic variations that occur and may result in inadvertent laceration. If a medium or large vessel is lacerated, a suture around the bleeding end may be necessary to control the hemorrhage. Pressure should be applied through the tissue to determine the location that will stop blood flow in the severed vessel. A suture can then be passed through the tissue and tied to restrict blood flow. Excessive bleeding from a surgical wound may also result from incisions across a capillary plexus. Minor areas of persistent bleeding from capillaries can be stopped by applying cold pressure to the site with moist gauze for several minutes.

The use of a local anesthetic with a vasoconstrictor (epinephrine) may also be useful for controlling minor bleeding from the periodontal flap. Both of these methods act through vasoconstriction, thereby reducing the flow of blood through incised small vessels and capillaries. This action is relatively short lived, and it should not be relied on for long-term hemostasis. It is important to avoid the use of vasoconstrictors to control bleeding before sending a patient home. If a more serious bleeding problem exists or if a firm blood clot is not established, bleeding is likely to recur when the vasoconstrictor has metabolized and the patient is no longer in the office.

For a slow, constant blood flow and for oozing, hemostasis may be achieved with hemostatic agents. Absorbable gelatin sponge (Gelfoam), oxidized cellulose (Oxycel), oxidized regenerated cellulose (Surgicel Absorbable Hemostat), and microfibrillar collagen hemostat (Avitene, CollaCote, CollaTape, CollaPlug) are useful hemostatic agents for the control of bleeding in capillaries, small blood vessels, and deep wounds (Table 59.1).

Absorbable gelatin sponge is a porous matrix prepared from pork skin that helps to stabilize a normal blood clot. The sponge can be cut to the desired dimensions and either sutured in place or positioned within the wound (e.g., an extraction socket). It is absorbed in 4 to 6 weeks.

Oxidized cellulose is a chemically modified form of surgical gauze that forms an artificial clot. The material is friable, and it can be difficult to keep it in place. It is absorbed in 1 to 6 weeks.

TABLE 59.1 Absorbable Hemostatic Agents

Generic (Brand)	Directions	Adverse Effects	Precautions
Absorbable gelatin sponge (Gelfoam)	May be cut into various sizes and applied to bleeding surfaces	May form nidus for infection or abscess	Should not be overpacked into extraction site or wound—may interfere with healing
Oxidized cellulose (Oxycel)	Most effective when applied to wound dry as opposed to moistened	May cause foreign-body reaction	Extremely friable and difficult to place; should not be used adjacent to bone—impairs bone regeneration; should not be used as a surface dressing—inhibits epithelialization
Oxidized regenerated cellulose (Surgicel Absorbable Hemostat)	May be cut to various shapes and positioned over bleeding sites; thick or excessive amounts should not be used	Encapsulation, cyst formation, and foreign-body reaction possible	Should not be placed in deep wounds—may physically interfere with wound healing and bone formation
Microfibrillar collagen hemostat (Avitene, CollaCote, CollaTape, CollaPlug)	May be cut to shape and applied to bleeding surface	May potentiate abscess formation, hematoma, and wound dehiscence; possible allergic reaction or foreign-body reaction	May interfere with wound healing; placement in extraction sockets has been associated with increased pain
Thrombin (Thrombostat)	May be applied topically to bleeding surface	Allergic reaction can occur in patients with known sensitivity to bovine materials	Must not be injected into tissues or vasculature—can cause severe (and possibly fatal) clotting

Oxidized regenerated cellulose is prepared from cellulose via a reaction with alkali to form a chemically pure and uniform structure than oxidized cellulose. The material is prepared in a cloth or thin gauze form that can be cut to the desired size and sutured or layered on the bleeding surface. It can be used as a surface dressing because it does not impair epithelialization, and it is bactericidal against many gram-negative and gram-positive microorganisms that are both aerobic and anaerobic. Caution should be used when wounds are infected or have an increased potential to becoming infected (e.g., immunocompromised patients) because the absorbable hemostatic agents can serve as a nidus for infection.

Microfibrillar collagen hemostat is type I collagen derived from bovine skin. It is commonly dispensed in a flour form but also comes in a nonwoven sponge form. It binds tightly to blood surfaces and causes the aggregation of platelets, thus working even when the field is not dry. In addition to its blood binding properties as a collagen product, it also activates platelets.

Thrombin is a drug that is capable of hastening the process of blood clotting. It is intended for topical use only, and it is applied as a liquid or powder. Thrombin should never be injected into tissues because it can cause serious or even fatal intravascular coagulation. In addition, because thrombin is a bovine-derived material, caution should be used for any patient with a known allergic reaction to bovine products.

Finally, it is imperative to recognize that excessive bleeding may be caused by systemic disorders, including (but not limited to) platelet deficiencies, coagulation defects, medications, and hypertension. As a precaution, all surgical patients should be asked about any current medications that may contribute to bleeding, any family history of bleeding disorders, and hypertension. All patients, regardless of health history, should have their blood pressure evaluated before surgery, and anyone who is diagnosed with hypertension must be advised to see a physician before surgery. Patients with known or suspected bleeding deficiencies or disorders must be carefully evaluated before any surgical procedure. A consultation with the patient's physician is recommended, and laboratory tests should be performed to assess the risk of bleeding. It may be necessary to refer the patient to a hematologist for a comprehensive workup.

LEARNING BOX 59.4

Thrombin is a very effective drug to help coagulate blood and is applied topically. This drug should never be injected into tissues because it can cause serious or even fatal intravascular coagulation. In addition, thrombin is a bovine-derived drug, so caution should be used for patients with a known allergy to bovine products.

Periodontal Dressings (Periodontal Packs)

At completion of the periodontal surgical procedure, clinicians may elect to cover the area with a surgical dressing. In general, dressings have no curative properties but assist healing by protecting the tissue rather than providing "healing factors." The dressing minimizes the likelihood of postoperative infection, facilitates healing by preventing surface trauma during mastication, and protects the patient from pain induced by contact of the wound with food or with the tongue during mastication. (For a complete literature review on this subject, see the article by Sachs and colleagues.[37])

Zinc Oxide–Eugenol Dressing

Dressings that are based on the reaction of zinc oxide and eugenol include the Wonder Pak, which was developed by Ward[46] in 1923, and several other dressings that use modified forms of Ward's original

formula. The addition of accelerators such as zinc acetate gives the dressing a better working time.

Zinc oxide–eugenol dressings are supplied as a liquid and a powder that are mixed before use. Eugenol in this type of dressing may induce an allergic reaction that produces reddening of the area and burning pain in some patients.

Noneugenol Dressing

The reaction between a metallic oxide and fatty acids is the basis for the Coe-Pak, which is the most widely used dressing in the United States. This is supplied in two tubes, the contents of which are mixed immediately before use until a uniform color is obtained. One tube contains zinc oxide, an oil (for plasticity), a gum (for cohesiveness), and lorothidol (a fungicide).

The other tube contains liquid coconut fatty acids that have been thickened with colophony resin (or rosin) and chlorothymol (a bacteriostatic agent).[37,40] This dressing does not contain asbestos or eugenol, thereby avoiding the problems associated with these substances.

Other noneugenol dressings include cyanoacrylates[6,19,24] and tissue conditioners (methacrylate gels).[2] However, these products are not in common use.

Retention of Dressing

Periodontal dressings are usually kept in place mechanically by interlocking the dressing in interdental spaces and joining the lingual and facial portions of the dressing. In isolated teeth or when several teeth in an arch are missing, retention of the dressing may be difficult. Numerous reinforcements and splints and stents for this purpose have been described.[17,18,47] The placement of dental floss tied loosely around the teeth enhances retention of the dressing.

Antibacterial Properties of Dressing

Improved healing and patient comfort with less odor and taste[6] have been obtained by incorporating antibiotics into the dressing. Bacitracin,[5] oxytetracycline (Terramycin),[13] neomycin, and nitrofurazone have been used. Care must be taken when any antibiotic products are used because they may produce hypersensitivity reactions. The emergence of resistant organisms and opportunistic infections has been reported.[35] The incorporation of tetracycline powder into the Coe-Pak is generally recommended, particularly when long and traumatic surgical procedures are performed.

Allergy

Contact allergies to eugenol and rosin have been reported.[34]

Preparation and Application of Dressing

Zinc oxide dressings are mixed with eugenol or noneugenol liquids on a wax paper pad with a spatula or a wooden tongue depressor. The powder is gradually incorporated with the liquid until a thick paste is formed.

The Coe-Pak is prepared by mixing equal lengths of paste from tubes that contain the accelerator and the base until the resulting paste is a uniform color (Fig. 59.1A to C). A capsule of tetracycline powder can be added at this time. The dressing is then placed in a cup of water at room temperature (Fig. 59.1D). After 2 to 3 minutes, the paste loses its tackiness, and it can be handled and molded. The mixed dressing remains workable for 15 to 20 minutes. The working time can be shortened by adding a small amount of zinc oxide to the accelerator (pink paste) before spatulating.

The dressing is then rolled into two strips that are approximately the length of the treated area. The end of one strip is bent into a hook shape and fitted around the distal surface of the last tooth to

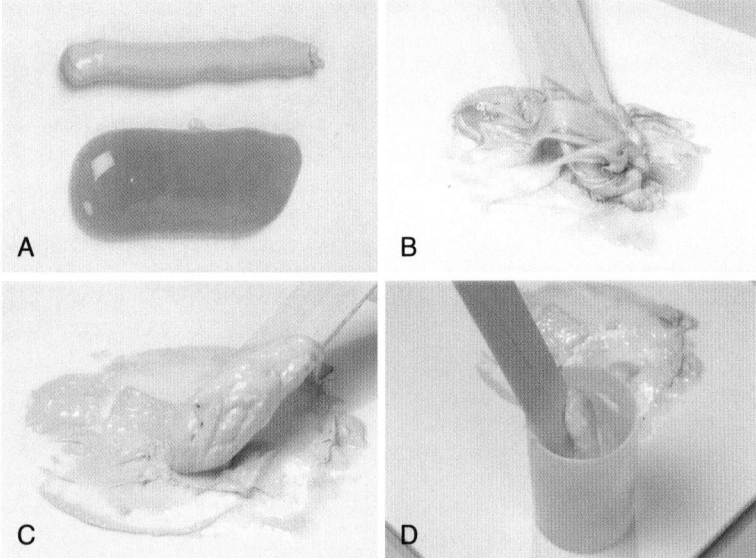

Fig. 59.1 Preparing the surgical pack (Coe-Pak). (A) Equal lengths of the two pastes are placed on a paper pad. (B) The pastes are mixed with a wooden tongue depressor for 2 or 3 minutes until (C) the paste loses its tackiness. (D) The mixed paste is placed in a paper cup of water at room temperature. With lubricated fingers, it is then rolled into cylinders and placed on the surgical wound.

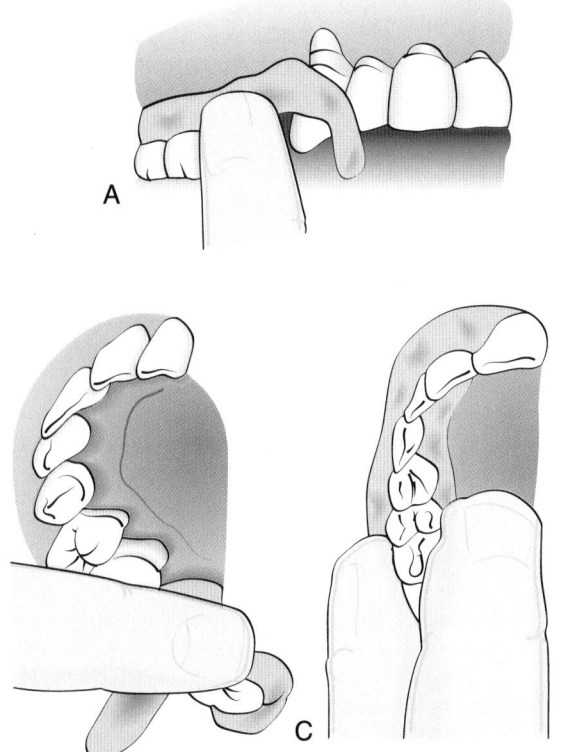

Fig. 59.2 Inserting the periodontal pack. (A) A strip of pack is hooked around the last molar and pressed into place anteriorly. (B) The lingual pack is joined to the facial strip at the distal surface of the last molar and fitted into place anteriorly. (C) Gentle pressure on the facial and lingual surfaces joins the pack interproximally.

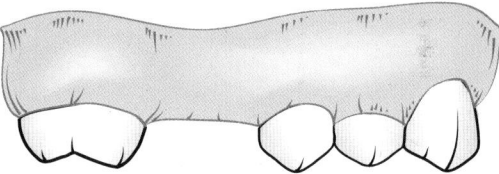

Fig. 59.3 Continuous pack covers the edentulous space.

approach that tooth from the distal surface (Fig. 59.2A). The remainder of the strip is brought forward along the facial surface to the midline and gently pressed into place along the gingival margin and interproximally. The second strip is applied from the lingual surface. It is joined to the dressing at the distal surface of the last tooth and then brought forward along the gingival margin to the midline (Fig. 59.2B). The strips are joined interproximally by applying gentle pressure on the facial and lingual surfaces of the dressing (Fig. 59.2C). For isolated teeth separated by edentulous spaces, the dressing should be made continuous from tooth to tooth to cover the edentulous areas (Fig. 59.3).

When split-thickness flaps have been performed, the area should be covered with a sterile tinfoil to protect the sutures before the dressing is placed.

The dressing should cover the gingiva, but overextension onto uninvolved mucosa should be avoided. *Excess dressing irritates the mucobuccal fold and the floor of the mouth, and it interferes with the tongue.* Overextension also jeopardizes the remainder of the dressing because the excess tends to break off and loosens the dressing from the operated area. *Dressing that interferes with the occlusion should be removed before the patient is dismissed* (Fig. 59.4). Failure to do this causes discomfort and jeopardizes the retention of the dressing.

The operator should ask the patient to move the tongue forcibly out and to each side, and the cheek and lips should be displaced in all directions to mold the dressing while it is still soft. After the dressing has set, it should be trimmed to eliminate all excess.

As a general rule, the dressing is kept on for 1 week after surgery. This guideline is based on the usual timetable of healing and clinical experience. It is not a rigid requirement; the period may be extended, or the area may be redressed for an additional week.

Portions of the dressing may not remain during the week, but this should not present a problem. If the dressing is lost from the operated area and the patient is uncomfortable, it is usually best to

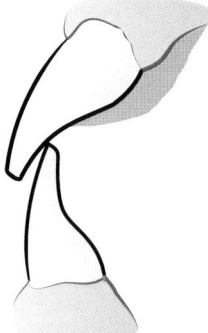

Fig. 59.4 Periodontal pack should not interfere with the occlusion.

redress the area. The clinician should remove the remaining dressing, irrigate the area with warm water, and apply a topical anesthetic before replacing the dressing, which is then retained for another week. The excess dressing should be trimmed away with care taken to ensure that the new margin is not rough before the patient is dismissed.

Postoperative Instructions

After the dressing is placed, oral and printed postoperative instructions are given before the patient is dismissed from the chair (eBox 59.1, online).

First Postoperative Week

When the therapy is properly performed, periodontal surgery should present minimal postoperative problems. Patients should be instructed to rinse with 0.12% chlorhexidine gluconate (Peridex, PerioGard) immediately after the surgical procedure and twice daily thereafter until normal biofilm control can be resumed.[30,38,45] The following complications may arise during the first postoperative week, although they are the exception rather than the rule:

1. *Persistent bleeding after surgery.* The dressing is removed, and local anesthesia may be needed before the bleeding areas are located. The bleeding is stopped with pressure, or if necessary the area may have to be anesthetized and resutured. After the bleeding has been stopped, the area is again redressed.
2. *Sensitivity to percussion.* Extension of inflammation into the periodontal ligament may cause sensitivity to percussion. The patient should be questioned regarding the progress of the symptoms. Gradual diminishing discomfort is a favorable sign. The dressing should be removed and the surgical area checked for localized areas of infection or irritation. The area should be irrigated or incised to provide drainage if areas of localized exudate are present. Particles of calculus that may have been overlooked should be removed. Relieving the occlusion can be helpful. Sensitivity to percussion may also be caused by excess dressing, which interferes with the occlusion. Removal of the excess usually corrects the condition.
3. *Swelling.* During the first 2 postoperative days, some patients may report a soft, painless swelling of the cheek in the surgical area. Lymph node enlargement may occur, and the temperature may be slightly elevated. The area of operation itself is usually symptom free. This type of involvement results from a localized inflammatory reaction to the surgical procedure. It generally subsides by the fourth postoperative day without necessitating the removal of the dressing. If swelling persists, enlarges, or is associated with increased pain, amoxicillin (500 mg) should be taken every 8 hours for 1 week. The patient should

also be instructed to apply moist heat intermittently over the area.

4. *Feeling of weakness.* Occasionally, patients report having experienced a "washed-out," weakened feeling for about 24 hours after surgery. This represents a systemic reaction to transient bacteremia induced by the procedure. This reaction can be prevented by premedication with amoxicillin (500 mg) every 8 hours. This protocol should be started 24 hours before the next procedure and continued for 5 days postoperatively.

Removal of the Dressing and Return Visit

When the patient returns in 1 week, the periodontal dressing is removed by inserting a curette along the margin and exerting gentle lateral pressure. Pieces of the dressing retained interproximally and particles adhering to the tooth surfaces are also removed with curettes. Particles of dressing and debris may be enmeshed in the surgical surfaces and should be carefully removed with cotton pliers. The entire area is irrigated with peroxide to remove the superficial debris.

Findings at the Time of Dressing Removal

The following are usual findings when the dressing is removed:
- If *gingivectomy* has been performed, the incised surface is covered with a friable meshwork of new epithelium. This tissue should not be disturbed. If calculus has not been completely removed, red, beadlike protuberances of granulation tissue will persist. The granulation tissue must be removed with a curette to expose the calculus so the root can be planed. Granulation tissue will recur if the residual calculus is not completely removed.
- After a *flap operation*, the areas that correspond to the incisions are epithelialized, but they may bleed readily if irritated. These areas should not be disturbed nor probed.
- The facial and lingual mucosa may be covered with a grayish-yellow or white granular layer of debris that has entered under the dressing. This is easily removed with a moist cotton pellet. The root surfaces may be sensitive to touch or to thermal change. The patient should be assured that these changes will disappear with time (4 to 6 weeks). The dentition that was beneath the dressing may be stained in a brownish-yellow color that can be removed by polishing at a later date.
- *Fragments of calculus delay healing.* Each root surface should be carefully rechecked visually to be certain that no calculus was missed during surgery. The grooves on the proximal root surfaces and the furcations are areas where calculus is likely to be overlooked.

Redressing

After the dressing is removed, it is usually not necessary to replace it. However, redressing for an additional week is advised for the following types of patients: (1) those with a low pain threshold who are particularly uncomfortable when the dressing is removed; (2) those with unusually sensitive root surfaces postsurgically; or (3) those with an open wound where the flap edges have necrosed. Clinical judgment helps when deciding whether to redress the area or to leave the initial dressing for a longer period.

Tooth Mobility

Tooth mobility usually increases immediately after surgery.[8] This results from edema in the periodontal ligament space from the inflammation that occurs postsurgically. The mobility diminishes to the pretreatment level by the fourth week.[25] The patient should be reassured before surgery that the mobility is temporary.

Mouth Care Between Procedures

Care of the mouth by the patient between the treatments as well as after the surgery is completed is extremely important.[48] These measures should begin after the dressing is removed from the first surgical procedure. The patient has had instructions on oral hygiene before surgical therapy but must be instructed again after surgical therapy. Plaque or biofilm removal post surgery is different from that of presurgical hygiene because the areas are still healing and uncomfortable.

Vigorous brushing is not feasible during the first week after the dressing is removed. However, the patient is informed that biofilm and food accumulation impair healing and is advised to try to keep the area as clean as possible with the gentle use of a soft toothbrush and light water irrigation. Rinsing with a chlorhexidine mouthwash or applying such a rinse topically with cotton-tipped applicators is indicated for the first few postoperative weeks. Brushing is introduced when the healing of the tissues permits, and the overall hygiene regimen is increased as healing progresses. Patients should be told that (1) some gingival bleeding will occur when the wounded areas are gently cleaned; (2) this bleeding is normal and will subside as healing progresses; and (3) the bleeding should not deter them from following their oral hygiene regimen.

Management of Postoperative Pain

Periodontal surgery that follows the basic principles outlined here should produce only minimal pain and discomfort.[41] A study of 304 consecutive periodontal surgical interventions revealed that 51.3% of the patients reported minimal or no postoperative pain, and only 4.6% reported severe pain. Of these, only 20.1% took five or more doses of analgesic.[11] The same study indicated that mucogingival procedures result in six times more discomfort and that osseous surgery is three and a half times more uncomfortable than plastic gingival surgery. For the few patients who may have severe pain, the control of pain becomes an important part of patient management.[29]

As indicated earlier, a common source of postoperative pain is overextension of the periodontal dressing onto the soft tissue apical to the mucogingival junction or onto the frena. Overextended dressings cause localized areas of edema that are usually noticed 1 to 2 days after surgery. The removal of excess dressing is followed by resolution in about 24 hours. Extensive and excessively prolonged exposure of bone with poor irrigation during surgery induces greater pain. For most healthy patients, a preoperative dose of ibuprofen (600 to 800 mg) followed by one tablet every 8 hours for 24 to 48 hours is very effective for reducing discomfort after periodontal surgery. Patients are advised to continue taking ibuprofen or acetaminophen thereafter, if needed. If pain persists, acetaminophen plus codeine (Tylenol #3) can be prescribed. Caution should be used when prescribing or dispensing ibuprofen to patients with hypertension that is controlled by medications because it can interfere with the effectiveness of the medication. Patients experiencing severe postoperative pain should be seen on an emergency basis. The area should be anesthetized by infiltration, and the dressing should be removed to allow for the examination of the area in

pain. Postoperative pain related to infection is accompanied by localized lymphadenopathy and a slight elevation in temperature.[31] This type of pain should be treated with systemic antibiotics and analgesics.

Dentin (Root) Hypersensitivity

Dentin or root hypersensitivity is a relatively common problem in periodontal practice. It may occur spontaneously when the root becomes exposed as a result of gingival recession or pocket formation, or it may appear after scaling and root planing and other periodontal surgical procedures. The reader is referred to the online discussion for a detailed discussion of root sensitivity and its management.

Surgical Instruments

Periodontal surgery is accomplished with numerous instruments; Fig. 59.5 shows a typical surgical cassette. Periodontal surgical instruments are classified as follows:
1. Excisional and incisional instruments
2. Surgical curettes and sickles
3. Periosteal elevators
4. Surgical chisels
5. Surgical files
6. Scissors
7. Hemostats and tissue forceps

Excisional and Incisional Instruments

Periodontal Knives (Gingivectomy Knives)

The Kirkland knife is representative of the knives that are typically used for gingivectomy. These knives can be obtained as either double-ended or single-ended instruments. The entire periphery of these kidney-shaped knives is the cutting edge (Fig. 59.6A).

Interdental Knives

The Orban knife (#1 and #2; Fig. 59.6B) and the Merrifield knife (#1 through #4) are examples of knives that can be used for interdental areas. These spear-shaped knives have cutting edges on both sides of the blade, and they are designed with either double-ended or single-ended blades.

Surgical Blades

Scalpel blades of different shapes and sizes are used in periodontal surgery. The most common blades are #12D, #15, and #15C (Fig. 59.7). The #12D blade is a beak-shaped blade with cutting edges on both sides that allow the operator to engage narrow, restricted areas with both pushing and pulling cutting motions. The #15 blade is used for thinning the flaps and is also used for general purposes. The #15C blade, which is a narrower version of the #15 blade, is useful for making the initial, scalloping-type incision. The slim design of this blade allows for incising into the narrow interdental portion of the flap. All of these blades are discarded after one use.

Electrosurgery (Radiosurgery) Techniques and Instrumentation

The terms *electrosurgery* and *radiosurgery*[39] are currently used to identify surgical techniques performed on soft tissue with the use of controlled, high-frequency electrical (radio) currents in the range of 1.5 to 7.5 million cycles per second (megahertz). Three classes of active electrodes are available: single-wire electrodes for incising or excising; loop electrodes for planing tissue; and heavier, bulkier electrodes for coagulation procedures.[16,28]

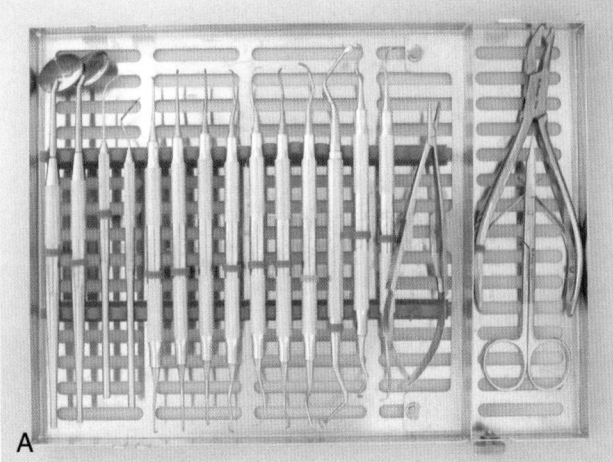
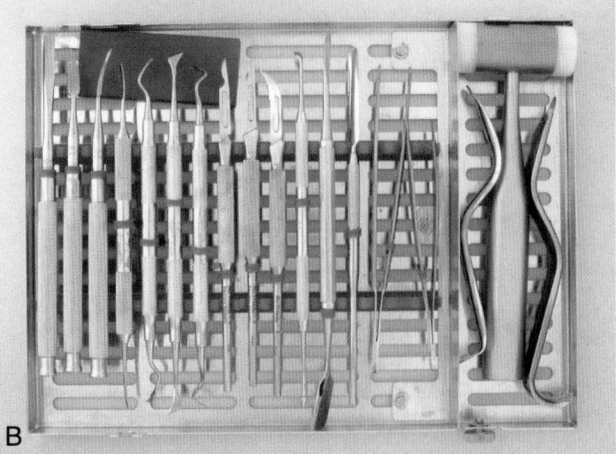

Fig. 59.5 A typical series of periodontal surgical instruments, divided into two cassettes. (A) *From left,* Mirrors, explorer, probe, series of curettes, needleholder, rongeurs, and scissors. (B) *From left,* Series of chisels, Kirkland knife, Orban knife, scalpel handles with surgical blades (#15C, #15, and #12D), periosteal elevators, spatula, tissue forceps, cheek retractors, and mallet; also shown is a sharpening stone. *(A, Courtesy Hu-Friedy, Chicago, IL. B, Courtesy G. Hartzell & Son, Concord, CA.)*

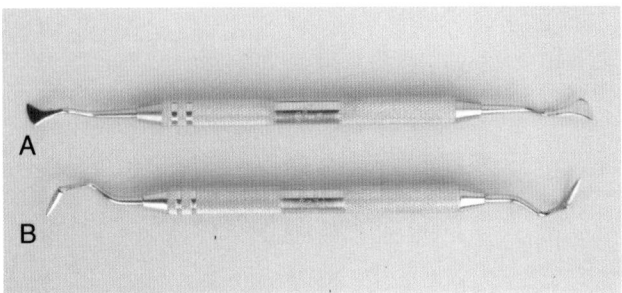

Fig. 59.6 Gingivectomy knives. (A) Kirkland knife. (B) Orban interdental knife.

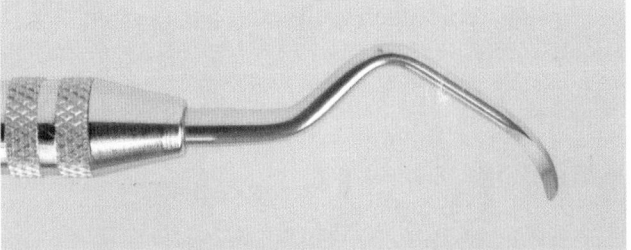

Fig. 59.8 A Prichard surgical curette. The curettes that are used in surgery have wider blades than those that are used for conventional scaling and root planing.

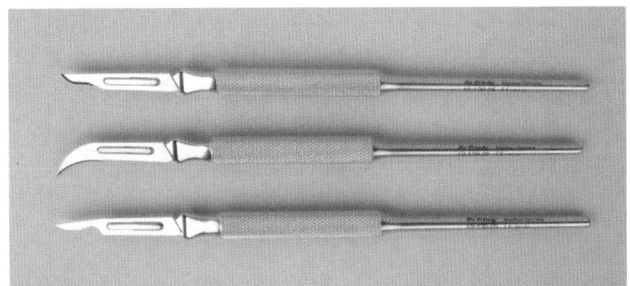

Fig. 59.7 Surgical blades. *Top to bottom,* #15, #12D, and #15C. These blades are disposable.

The four basic types of electrosurgical techniques are electrosection, electrocoagulation, electrofulguration, and electrodesiccation.

Electrosection, which is also referred to as *electrotomy* or *acusection,* is used for incisions, excisions, and tissue planing. Incisions and excisions are performed with single-wire active electrodes that can be bent or adapted to accomplish any type of cutting procedure.

Electrocoagulation provides a wide range of coagulation and hemorrhage control by using the electrocoagulation current. Electrocoagulation can prevent bleeding or hemorrhage at the initial entry into soft tissue, but it cannot stop bleeding after the blood is present. All forms of hemorrhage must be stopped first by some form of direct pressure (e.g., air, compress, hemostat). After bleeding has momentarily stopped, the final sealing of the capillaries or large vessels can be accomplished with a short application of the electrocoagulation current. The active electrodes that are used for coagulation are much bulkier than the fine tungsten wire used for electrosection. Electrosection and electrocoagulation are the procedures that are most often used in all areas of dentistry. The two monoterminal techniques, electrofulguration and electrodesiccation, are not in general use in dentistry.

The most important basic rule of the use of electrosurgery is *always keep the tip moving.* The prolonged or repeated application of current to tissue induces heat accumulation and undesired tissue destruction, whereas interrupted application at intervals adequate for tissue cooling (5 to 10 seconds) reduces or eliminates heat buildup. Electrosurgery is not intended to destroy tissue; it is a controllable means of sculpturing or modifying oral soft tissue with little discomfort and hemorrhage for the patient. Electrosurgery is contraindicated for patients who have incompatible or poorly shielded cardiac pacemakers.

Surgical Curettes and Sickles

Larger and heavier curettes and sickles are often needed during surgery for the removal of granulation tissue, fibrous interdental

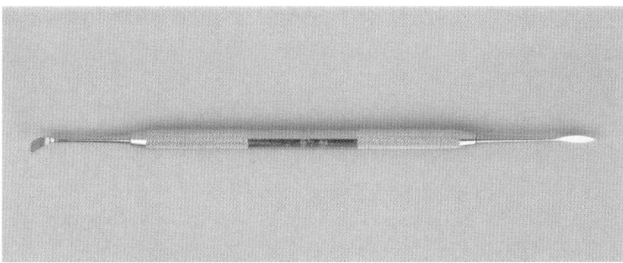

Fig. 59.9　Woodson periosteal elevator.

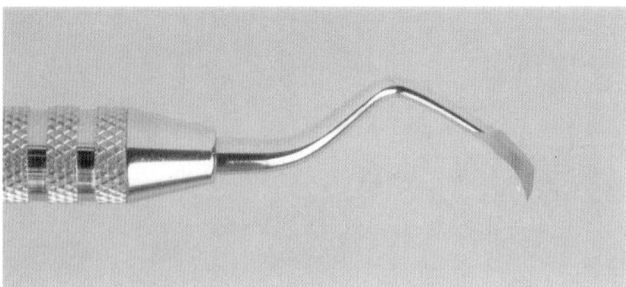

Fig. 59.10　Back-action chisel.

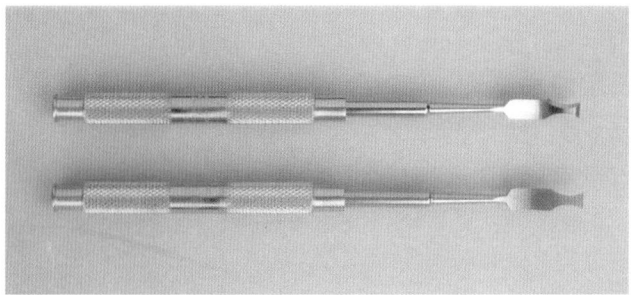

Fig. 59.11 Ochsenbein chisels are paired, with their cutting edges in opposite directions.

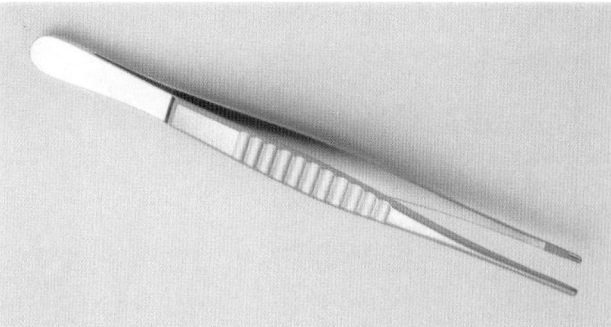

Fig. 59.12　DeBakey tissue forceps.

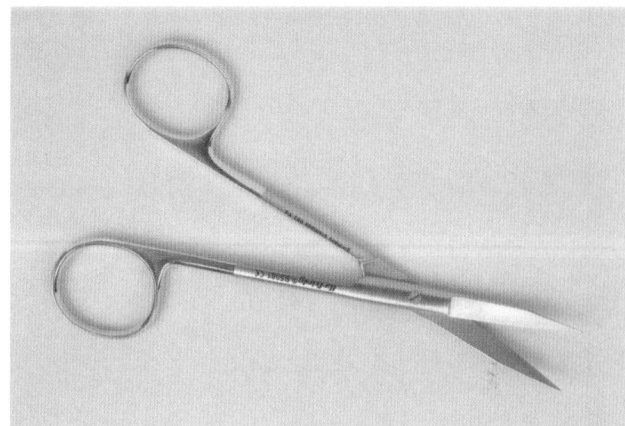

Fig. 59.13　Goldman–Fox scissors.

tissues, and tenacious subgingival deposits. The Prichard curette (Fig. 59.8) and the Kirkland surgical instruments are heavy curettes, whereas the Ball scaler (#B2 and #B3) is a popular heavy sickle. The wider, heavier blades of these instruments are suitable for surgical procedures that require the removal of tenacious tissues and calculus.

Periosteal Elevators

The periosteal elevators are needed to reflect and move the flap after the incision has been made for flap surgery. The Woodson and Prichard elevators are well-designed periosteal instruments (Fig. 59.9).

Surgical Chisels

The back-action chisel is used with a pull motion (Fig. 59.10), whereas the straight chisel (e.g., Wedelstaedt, Ochsenbein [#1 and #2]) are used with a push motion (Fig. 59.11). The Ochsenbein chisel is a useful chisel with a semicircular indentation on both sides of the shank that allows the instrument to engage around the tooth and into the interdental area. The Rhodes chisel is another popular back-action chisel.

Tissue Forceps

The tissue forceps are used to hold the flap during suturing. This instrument is also used to position and displace the flap after the

flap has been reflected. The DeBakey forceps are efficient instruments for this purpose (Fig. 59.12).

Scissors and Nippers

Scissors and nippers are used in periodontal surgery to remove tabs of tissue during gingivectomy, to trim the margins of flaps, to enlarge incisions in periodontal abscesses, and to remove muscle attachments in mucogingival surgery. Many types are available, and individual preference determines the choice. Goldman–Fox #16 scissors have a curved, beveled blade with serrations (Fig. 59.13).

Needleholders

Needleholders are used to suture the flap at the desired position after the surgical procedure has been completed. In addition to the regular types of needleholders (Fig. 59.14A), the Castroviejo needleholder is used for delicate, precise techniques that require quick and easy grasp and release of the suture (Fig. 59.14B).

Conclusion

The majority of periodontal surgical procedures can be carried out with the thorough application of local anesthesia. Clinicians have the obligation to ensure a patient-centered approach that includes oral, intravenous, and inhalational sedation in their spectrum of available services for their patients.

The efficient, precise, and minimally traumatic management of tissues is necessary to achieve the most predicable and comfortable result and outcome for the patient. Most patients need oral analgesic support, and they should be given the necessary pain-relieving medications so that an effective level of analgesia is present during

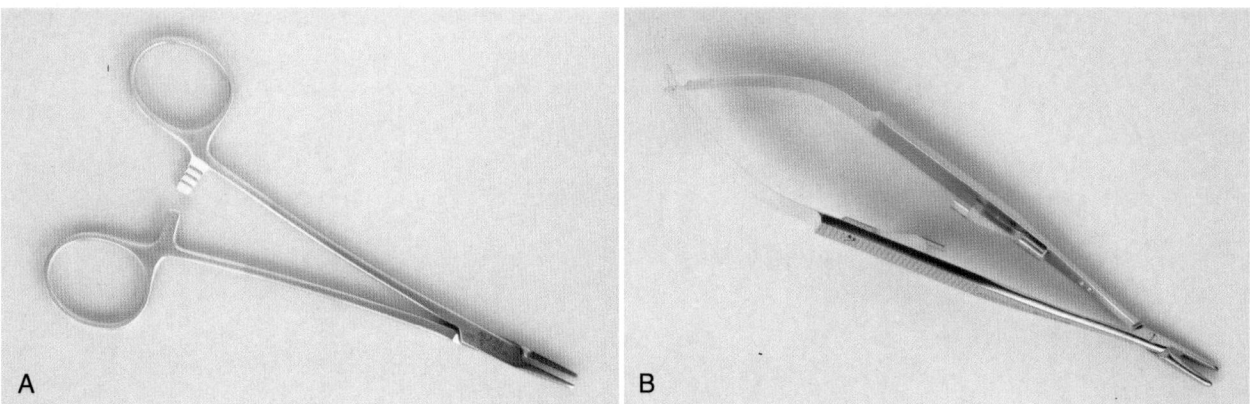

Fig. 59.14 (A) Conventional needleholder. (B) Castroviejo needleholder.

the immediate postsurgical period. The use of longer-acting local anesthetic agents (e.g., bupivacaine) and protective periodontal dressings also helps to reduce postsurgical pain.

During the immediate postsurgical weeks, biofilm control and healing are enhanced by the use of antimicrobial mouthrinses such as chlorhexidine. Postsurgical root sensitivity is well controlled by ensuring that biofilm control is optimal, and occasionally desensitizing agents will be needed.

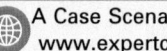
A Case Scenario is found on the companion website www.expertconsult.com.

References

References for this chapter are found on the companion website www.expertconsult.com.

CHAPTER 60

Periodontal Surgical Therapy

Jonathan H. Do | Henry H. Takei | Michael Whang | Kitetsu Shin

CHAPTER OUTLINE

Rationale for Periodontal Access Surgery
Fundamentals of Periodontal Surgery
Periodontal Surgical Techniques
Conclusion

 For online-only content on periodontal surgery fundamentals and specific techniques, please visit the companion website at www.expertconsult.com.

Rationale for Periodontal Access Surgery

In moderate to advanced cases, and in cases with furcation invasion and infrabony defects, it may be difficult and even impossible to resolve periodontal inflammation completely with nonsurgical therapy alone. Adjunctive periodontal access surgery is necessary in many of these cases to treat the periodontal disease definitively, create anatomies that are maintainable long-term by both the patient and the clinician, and, when feasible, reconstruct lost periodontal structures. Periodontal access surgery enhances access for root instrumentation and allows for reduction of periodontal pockets and correction of osseous defects. However, periodontal access surgery frequently results in gingival recession and loss of interdental papillae.

In the anterior maxilla, where aesthetics is of high priority, recession and loss of interdental papillae can present major aesthetic problems that are both difficult and unpredictable to treat. As such, in the anterior aesthetic area, periodontal disease is treated first and foremost nonsurgically, and periodontal access surgery is reserved for instances where surgical access is absolutely necessary. Fortunately, the anterior location of these teeth and their single-rooted and convex root surface anatomies facilitate nonsurgical root instrumentation. When specialized instruments such as mini Gracey curettes and Vision Curvettes are used in conjunction with illumination and magnification, access to these periodontal pockets are enhanced, and nonsurgical periodontal therapy can be very efficacious.

In the posterior sextants, access for definitive root instrumentation is much more restricted due to multiple anatomic factors, especially around multirooted teeth. Wide proximal surfaces, root grooves and concavities, furcations, angulation and proximity of roots, depth of the periodontal pocket, the cheek, the tongue, and the opposing dentition can all contribute to hinder the removal of subgingival biofilm and calculus on these teeth. Fortunately, gingival recession and loss of interdental papillae generally do not present aesthetic problems for most patients. Many patients and clinicians are willing to accept recession and the associated transient root sensitivity and food impaction in exchange for periodontal health. As such, periodontal access surgery is a treatment modality that is essential and

frequently used in the treatment of periodontal disease in the nonaesthetic area.

Periodontal access surgery is an adjunct to nonsurgical periodontal therapy and should occur only once the patient has demonstrated effective biofilm control. The *primary* objective of periodontal access surgery is to obtain access for root instrumentation to remove bacterial biofilm and calculus accretion on the root surfaces thoroughly. The *secondary* objective of periodontal access surgery is pocket reduction via soft and hard tissue resection or periodontal regeneration to facilitate home care and long-term professional supportive maintenance. These objectives are achieved by two main modalities of periodontal access surgery, gingivectomy and periodontal flap surgery. Both gingivectomy and flap surgery provide access for root instrumentation. Pocket reduction is achieved only by resection of the suprabony soft tissue pocket in gingivectomy, whereas with periodontal flap surgery pocket reduction is achieved via soft tissue resection, osseous resection, or periodontal regeneration.

LEARNING BOX 60.1

The primary objective of periodontal access surgery is access for root instrumentation. The secondary objective of periodontal access surgery is pocket reduction via soft and hard tissue resection or periodontal regeneration.

Fundamentals of Periodontal Surgery
Incisions

Periodontal surgery involves the use of horizontal (mesial-distal) and vertical (occlusal-apical) incisions. The #15 or #15C surgical blade is used most often to make these incisions.

Horizontal Incisions

Horizontal incisions are directed along the gingiva in a mesial or distal direction. Flaps can be reflected with the use of only horizontal incision if sufficient access can be obtained in this way and if apical,

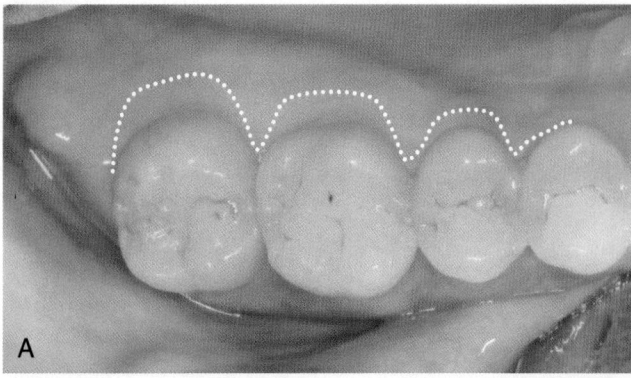

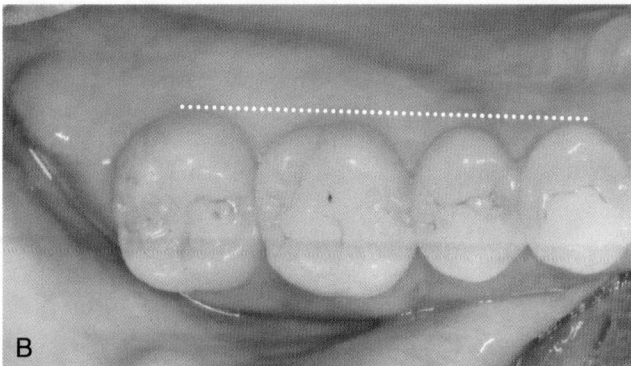

Fig. 60.1 (A) Scalloped incision. (B) Straight incision.

lateral, or coronal displacement of the flap is not anticipated. If vertical incisions are not made, the flap is called an *envelope flap*.

Straight and Scalloped Incisions

A horizontal incision that follows the scalloped morphology of the gingival architecture is called a scalloped incision, as opposed to a straight incision, which follows a straight line (Fig. 60.1). The scalloped incision is advantageous in preserving the interdental architecture in gingivectomy and in creating surgical papillae and preserving soft tissue over the interdental areas to allow coverage of the interdental bone in flap surgery. Historically, the horizontal incisions were used in both gingivectomy and flap surgery to eliminate the interdental tissue, where periodontal disease and periodontal pockets frequently occur. The *interdental denudation procedure* used horizontal internal bevel incisions to remove the gingival papillae and to denude the interdental spaces.[3,4,25,29] This technique completely eliminates the inflamed interdental tissue. Healing is by secondary intention and results in excellent gingival contour and shallow probing depths. However, the initial healing is slow and uncomfortable due to exposure and necrosis of interdental bone. For this reason, the interdental denudation procedure has very limited clinical application. The use of scalloped incisions in flap surgery allows the interdental bone to be covered once the flap is coapted. This enhances patients' comfort and allows for faster closure of the wound.

When scalloping the incision, the scallop is from the mesial line angle to the distal line angle to maximize the width of the surgical papillae and to allow tight adaptation of the flap to the roots once the flap is coapted. In the interdental areas, the incision is maintained close to or in the sulcus to maximize coverage of the interdental bone. The scallop incision should take into account root anatomy to optimize primary closure. For example, the mesial-distal palatal dimension of a maxillary molar decreases from the cementoenamel junction down to the palatal root as the tooth transitions from a root

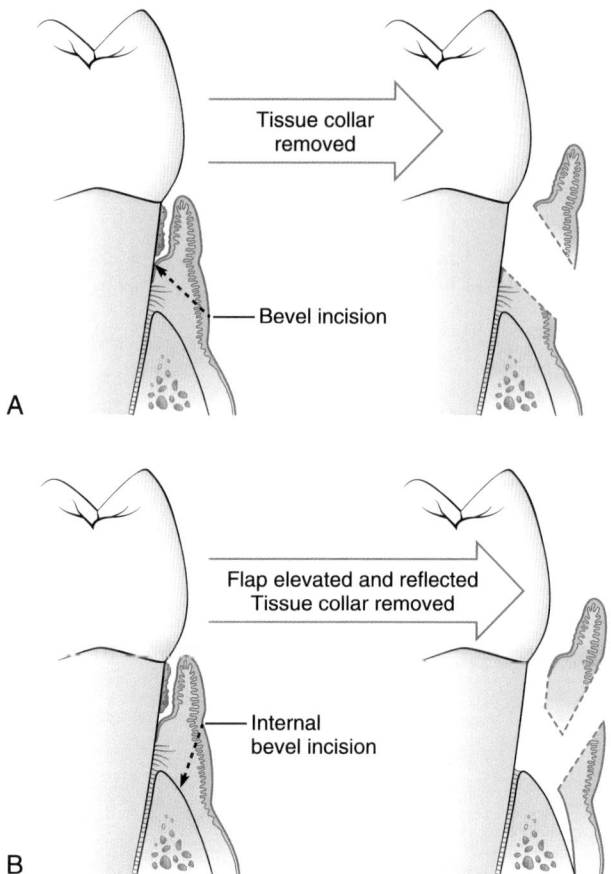

Fig. 60.2 (A) Bevel incision. (B) Internal bevel incision.

trunk to a single root. An aggressive scallop may leave bone around the palatal root of a maxillary molar exposed.

External Bevel and Internal Bevel Incisions

The external bevel incision starts at the surface of the gingiva apical to the periodontal pocket and is directed coronally toward the tooth apical to the bottom of the periodontal pocket. The external bevel incision, or simply bevel incision, is used primarily in gingivectomy, and it can be made with a scalpel or a knife. The internal bevel incision, also called the reverse bevel incision and inverse bevel incision, is the opposite of the external bevel incision (Fig. 60.2). The internal bevel incision[28] starts at the surface of the gingiva and is directed apically to the bone crest. It is the incision from which the flap is reflected to expose the underlying bone and root. The internal bevel incision accomplishes three important objectives: (1) it removes the pocket lining; (2) it conserves the relatively uninvolved outer surface of the gingiva, which, if apically positioned, becomes attached gingiva; and (3) it produces a sharp, thin flap margin for adaptation to the bone–tooth junction. The internal bevel incision is basic to most periodontal flap procedures. Both bevel and internal bevel incisions can be straight or scalloped.

Crevicular, Crestal, and Submarginal Incisions

The crevicular incision is also called intercrevicular incision, intracrevicular incision, sulcular incision, intrasulcular incision, and intersulcular incision. It starts in the gingival crevice and is directed apically through the junctional epithelium and connective tissue attachment and down to the bone (Fig. 60.3). The crestal incision is also called the marginal incision. It starts at the surface of the gingiva at the gingival margin and is directed apically down through

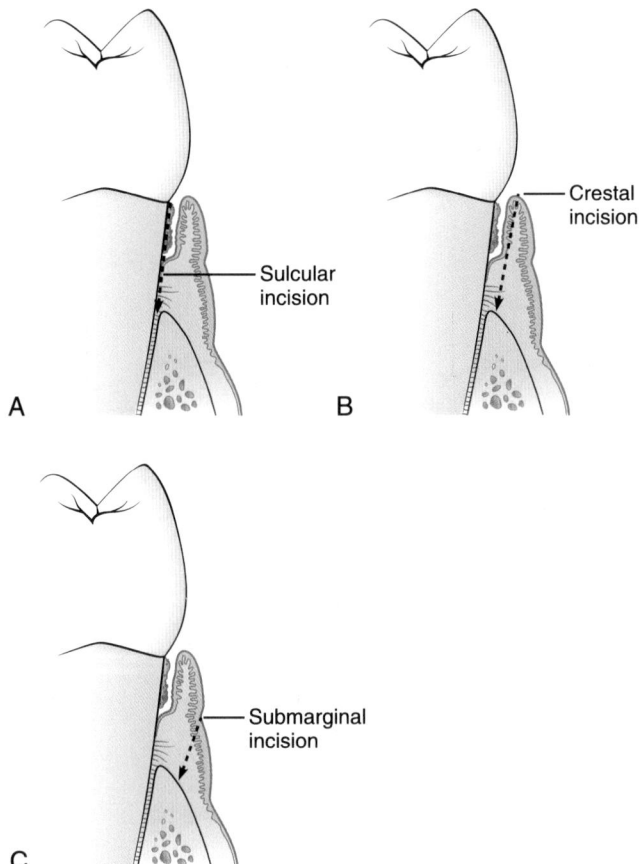

A   B

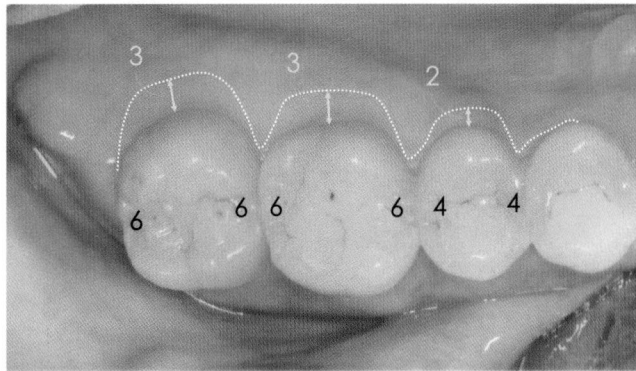

Fig. 60.4 The submarginal scalloped incision is placed a distance of one-half to two-thirds the transgingival interdental probing depth away from the tooth surface.

C

Fig. 60.3 (A) Sulcular incision. (B) Crestal incision. (C) Submarginal incision.

Placement of the submarginal scalloped incision depends on (1) the transgingival interdental probing depth, (2) the mucogingival junction, and (3) the depth of the palatal vault.

the epithelium and connective tissue to the bone. Both the crevicular and crestal incisions are internal bevel incisions. The submarginal incision starts at the surface of the gingiva apical to the gingival margin and can be external bevel or internal bevel. In flap surgery, the submarginal incision is an internal bevel incision, whereas in gingivectomy, it is an external bevel incision.

The use of a crevicular, marginal, or submarginal internal bevel incision in periodontal flap surgery depends on the objectives of the surgery and the anatomy of the area. The crevicular incision is frequently used in regenerative periodontal surgery to retain all gingival tissue to maximize blood supply and to obtain primary wound closure. The crevicular incision is also the incision of choice when recession is not desired. The anterior maxilla is an area where recession and loss of interdental papillae can compromise aesthetics. When flap surgery is required in the anterior maxilla, the crevicular incision is recommended. In resective periodontal surgery, the marginal and submarginal scalloped incisions are frequently used to create flaps with thin margins and to leave a collar of tissue around the tooth that contains the epithelium of the pocket lining and the adjacent granulomatous tissue. This collar of tissue is discarded after flap elevation. The marginal incision maximizes the remaining keratinized tissue, whereas the submarginal scalloped incision allows for more aggressive soft tissue resection and reduction of the periodontal pocket.

When the submarginal scalloped incision is used, *how submarginal should be incision be?* The placement of the submarginal incision always depends on two of three factors, depending on the location: (1) the transgingival interdental probing depth, (2) the mucogingival junction, and (3) the depth of the palatal vault.

The transgingival interdental probing depth is used to provide a guide for the placement of the submarginal scalloped incision. The transgingival probing depth is the distance from the gingival margin down to the bone. It is measured by inserting the probe into the gingival crevice through the attachment apparatus and down to the bone. Transgingival probing is also called *bone sounding*. The submarginal scalloped incision is placed a distance of one-half to two-thirds the transgingival interdental probing depth away from the tooth surface (Fig. 60.4). For example, if the mesial and distal interdental probing depths are 6 mm, then the submarginal scalloped incision will be placed 3 mm apical to the gingival margin at the midbuccal and midlingual surface of the tooth. *Why is the transgingival interdental probing depth used as a guide for the placement of the submarginal scalloped incision in resective periodontal surgery?* Periodontal disease occurs most commonly in the interdental areas due to inadequate biofilm removal below the interdental proximal contact. Interdental attachment and bone loss result in reverse/negative bony architecture. To reestablish positive architecture, the radicular bone is resected apical to the interdental bone, whereas the interdental bone is maintained. Therefore, the transgingival interdental probing depth is used as the guide for submarginal incision placement.

Although the presence of keratinized tissue is not required for periodontal health, its presence facilitates oral hygiene. Therefore, the submarginal scalloped incision will be placed depending on the mucogingival junction to preserve ≥3 mm of keratinized tissue. If the width of keratinized tissue is narrow, the submarginal scalloped incision will be placed closer to the gingival margin. A marginal incision would be used in lieu of a submarginal incision if the width of the keratinized tissue is <3 mm. If the width of the keratinized tissue is broad, then the submarginal scalloped incision will be placed based on the transgingival interdental probing depth (Fig. 60.5).

On the *palatal maxilla*, where the lack of keratinized tissue is not a concern, placement of the submarginal scalloped incision must take into consideration the depth of the palatal vault (Fig. 60.6). A high palatal vault will allow the submarginal incision to be placed based on one-half to two-thirds the transgingival interdental probing depth. In shallow palates, the more submarginal an incision, the closer it will be to the midline and the farther away it will be from the tooth surface. A submarginal incision placed in a shallow palatal

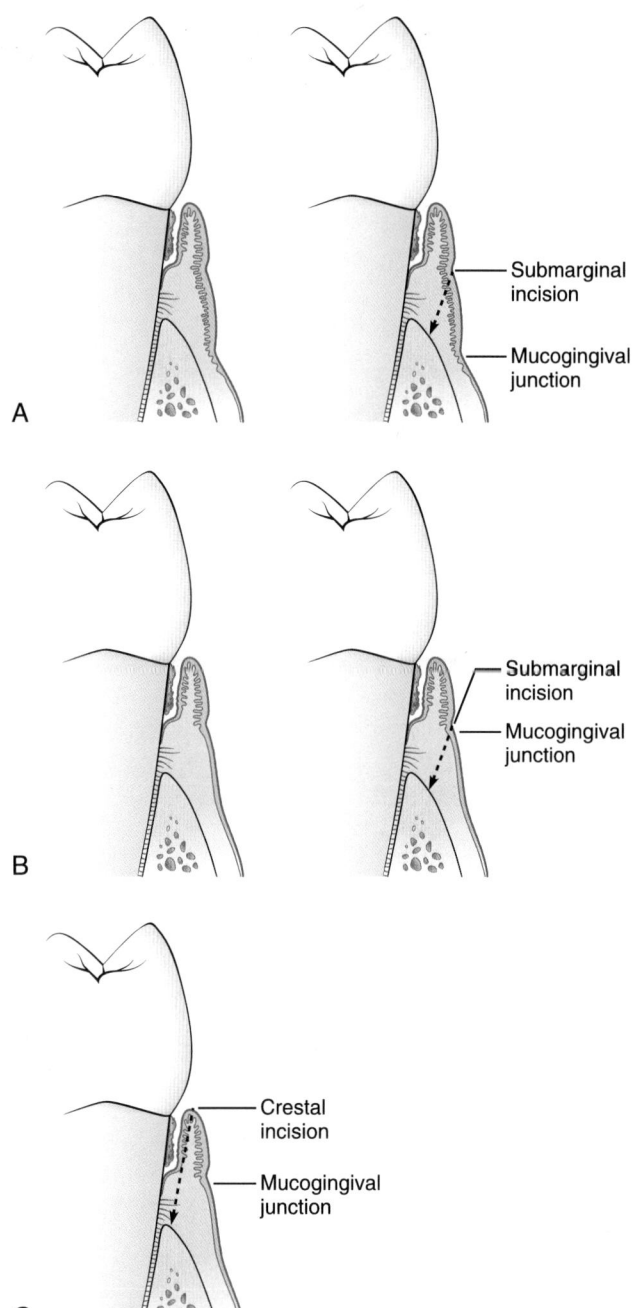

Fig. 60.5 (A) When keratinized tissue is abundant, a submarginal incision may be used. (B) When keratinized tissue is limited, a submarginal incision eliminates keratinized tissue that must be retained. (C) A crestal incision maximizes the retained keratinized tissue.

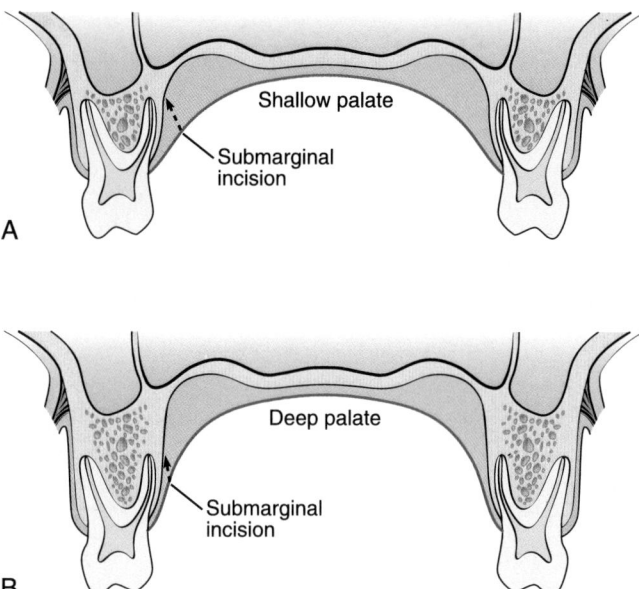

Fig. 60.6 (A) In a shallow palate, the more submarginal an incision, the closer it will be to the midline and the farther away it will be from the tooth surface. (B) In a high palate, a submarginal incision remains close to the tooth and allows for primary closure of the flap.

the flap margin to the level of the alveolar crest. The only area in the mouth where the submarginal incision must be used to reduce soft tissue height is the palate, where it is not possible to reposition the soft tissue apically due to the absence of a mucogingival junction.

LEARNING BOX 60.3

Reduction of soft tissue height may be achieved with the use of the submarginal scalloped incision or a combination of a marginal scalloped incision and an apically displaced flap.

Vertical Incisions

Vertical or oblique releasing incisions can be used on one or both ends of the horizontal incision, depending on the design and purpose of the flap. Vertical incisions at both ends may be necessary if the flap is to be apically displaced. Vertical incisions must extend beyond the mucogingival junction to reach the alveolar mucosa; this allows for the release of the flap to be displaced.

In general, vertical incisions in the lingual and palatal areas are avoided. Facial vertical incisions should not be made in the center of an interdental papilla or over the radicular surface of a tooth. Incisions should be made at the line angles of a tooth either to include the papilla in the flap or to avoid it completely. The vertical incision should also be designed to avoid long (coronal-apical) and narrow (mesial-distal) flaps, and flaps with the base narrower than the margin, because this could jeopardize the blood supply to the flap (Fig. 60.7).

Papilla Management

The papilla may be thinned, preserved, or split beneath the contact point. Management of the papilla depends on the dimension of the interdental space, aesthetics, and the secondary objective of the surgery, which could be resective or regenerative. In resective surgery, the scalloped incision creates surgical papillae to cover the interdental bone. The surgical papilla may or may not include the original papilla, depending on submarginal placement of the scalloped incision. The

vault based on the transgingival probing depth may result in a palatal flap that is too short to provide complete coverage of the alveolar bone and primary closure once it is coapted. Therefore, the flatter the palatal vault, the closer the submarginal incision must be to the gingival margin. If the palatal flap is too long when it is coapted, it can always be trimmed and rescalloped.

In areas where a mucogingival junction is present, such as the buccal or facial maxilla and the buccal or facial and lingual mandible, resection of soft tissue with the submarginal scalloped internal bevel incision is not the only way to obtain pocket reduction. A marginal incision can be used to maximize remaining keratinized tissue, and reduction of soft tissue height can be achieved by apically repositioning

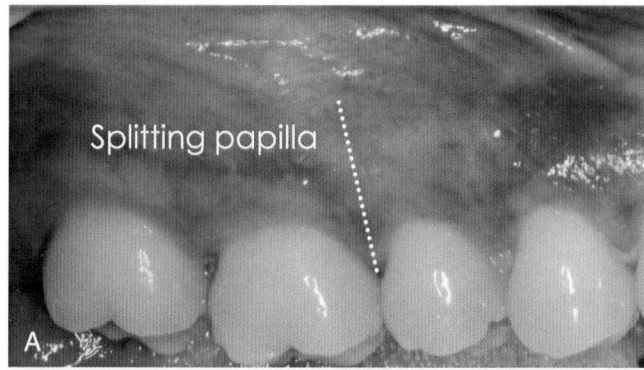

Splitting papilla

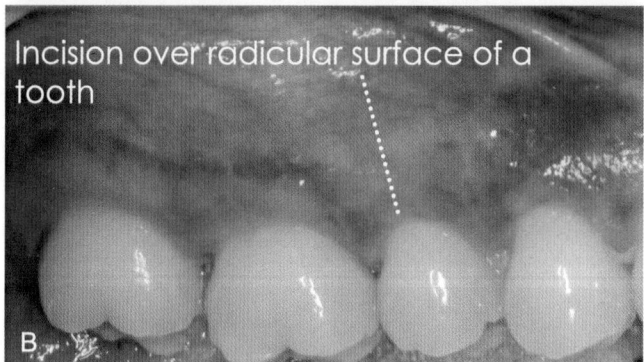

Incision over radicular surface of a tooth

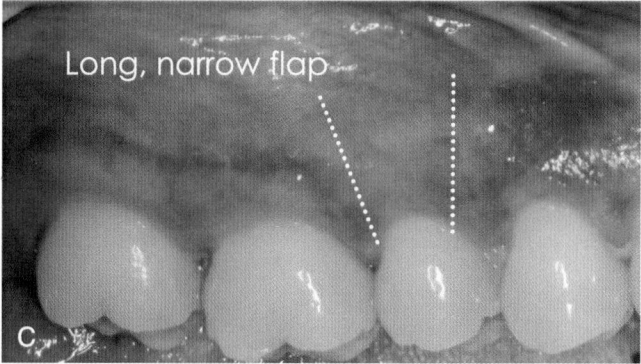

Long, narrow flap

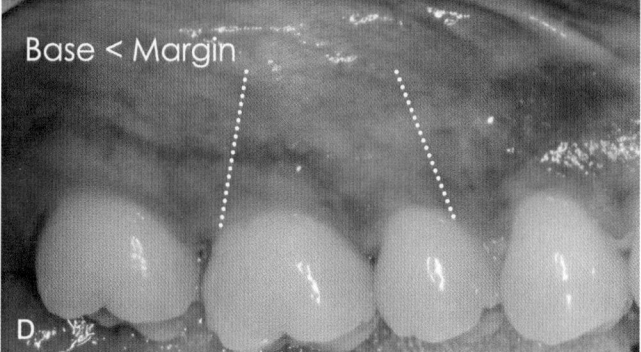

Base < Margin

Fig. 60.7 Vertical incisions should not (A) split a papilla or (B) be placed over a root prominence. When two vertical incision are used, (C) the length of the flap should not be longer than the width of the flap, and (D) the base of the flap should not be narrower than the margin of the flap.

surgical papilla is thinned to create the same thickness as the remainder of the flap to allow intimate adaptation of the papilla and the flap with the bone once the flap is coapted. In regenerative therapy and in aesthetic cases, the *papilla preservation technique*[35] (Fig. 60.8), which retains the entire papilla, is favored when the interdental space is adequate to allow the intact papilla to be reflected with the facial

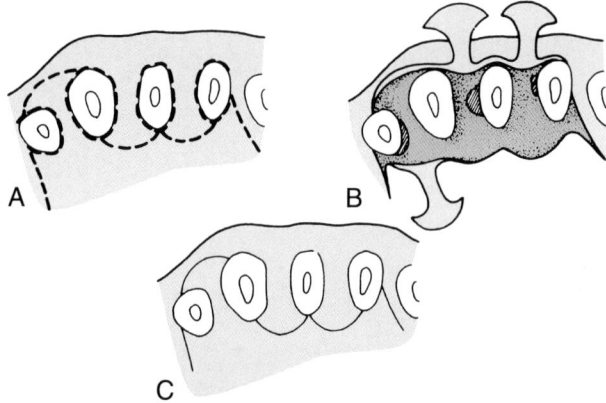

Fig. 60.8 Flap design for a papilla preservation flap. (A) Incisions for this type of flap are depicted by interrupted lines. The preserved papilla can be incorporated into the facial or the lingual–palatal flap. (B) The reflected flap exposes the underlying bone. Several osseous defects are seen. (C) The flap has been returned to its original position, where it covers all of the interdental spaces.

or lingual-palatal flap. When the interdental space is narrow and reflection of an intact papilla is not possible, the interdental papilla is split beneath the contact point of the two approximating teeth to allow for the reflection of the buccal and lingual flaps. The papilla is not thinned in these cases to minimize tissue shrinkage.

Flap Elevation

A periodontal flap may be elevated in full thickness or partial thickness (Fig. 60.9).

In a *full-thickness flap,* all of the soft tissue, including the periosteum, is reflected to expose the underlying bone. This complete exposure of and access to the underlying bone are indicated when resective or regenerative osseous surgery is contemplated. This type of flap is also called the mucoperiosteal flap. Elevation of a full-thickness flap requires the internal bevel incision to penetrate the periosteum, the last tissue overlying the bone. Once the periosteum has been completely incised along the length of the flap, a full-thickness flap is reflected by elevating the periosteum off the bone via blunt dissection. A periosteal elevator or curette is used to separate the periosteum from the bone by moving it mesially, distally, and apically on the bone until the desired reflection is accomplished, usually a millimeter apical to the mucogingival junction. Elevation of the periosteum off the bone should be performed with ease, and it can even be done with gauze. Difficulty in elevating a full-thickness flap is usually due to incomplete and noncontiguous incision of connective tissue and periosteum along the length of the flap.

The *partial-thickness flap* includes only the epithelium and a layer of the underlying connective tissue. The bone remains covered by a layer of connective tissue that includes the periosteum. This type of flap is also called the *split-thickness flap.* The partial-thickness flap is indicated when the flap is to be positioned apically or when exposure of bone is not desired. Elevation of a partial-thickness flap is completed by sharp dissection with a surgical scalpel (#15). When the tissue is thin, a flap may be elevated at full thickness slightly past the mucogingival junction and at partial thickness apical to the mucogingival junction. The combination of full-thickness and partial-thickness flaps reduces the risk of flap perforation at the mucogingival junction, where the tissue is often the thinnest. This also allows for access to bone around the teeth and preserves tissue over the bone apical to the mucogingival junction, which can be used to help stabilize the flap should it be apically displaced.

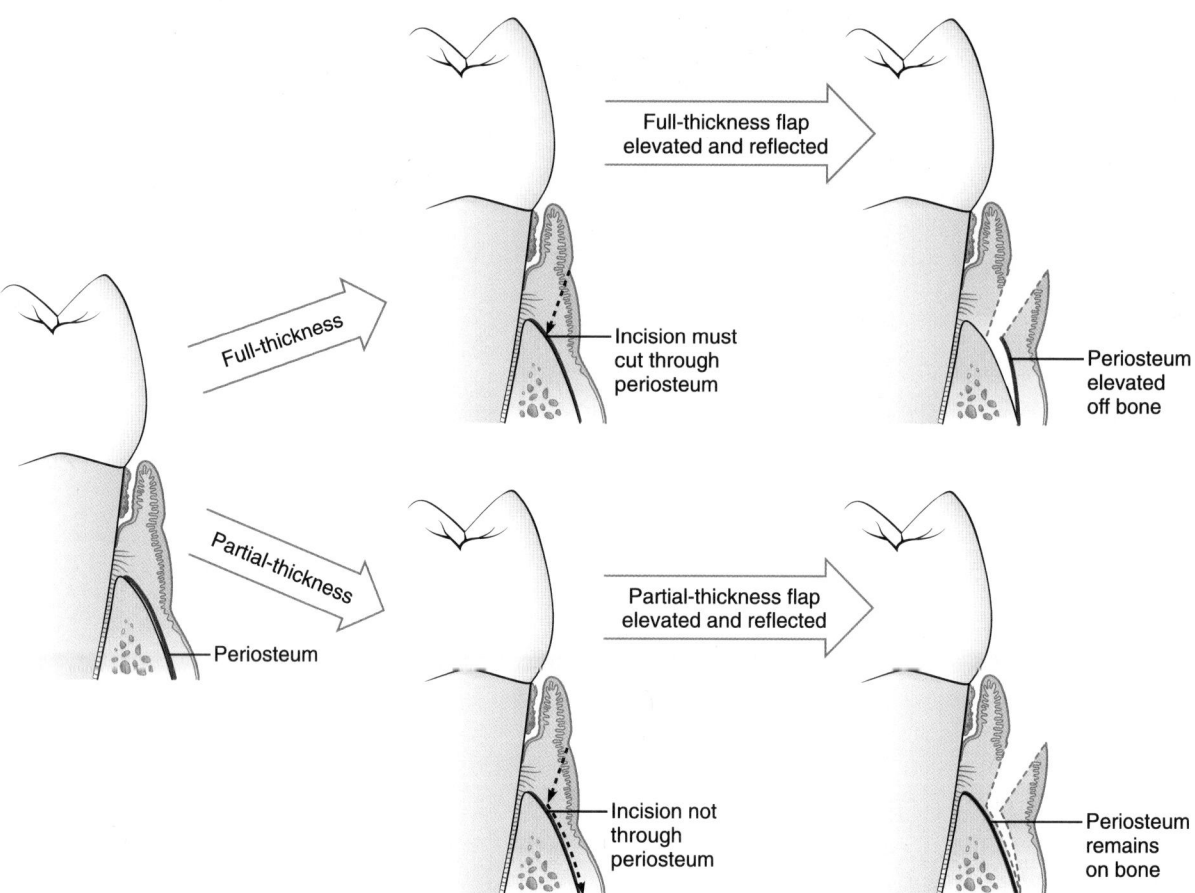

Fig. 60.9 In full-thickness flap elevation, the periosteum is elevated off the bone by blunt dissection. In partial-thickness flap elevation, the flap is split by sharp dissection to leave the periosteum and connective tissue intact over the bone.

Conflicting data surround the advisability of uncovering the bone when this is not actually needed. When bone is stripped of its periosteum, a loss of marginal bone occurs, and this loss is prevented when the periosteum is left on the bone.[7] Although this is usually clinically insignificant,[14] the difference may be significant in some cases. The partial-thickness flap may be necessary when the crestal bone margin is thin or when dehiscences or fenestrations are present. An apically displaced flap may be stabilized by suturing it to the intact periosteum.

Flap Coaptation

For flap coaptation after surgery, flaps are classified as either (1) *nondisplaced flaps,* when the flap is placed and sutured in its original position, or (2) *displaced flaps,* which are placed apically, coronally, or laterally to their original position (Fig. 60.10). Both full-thickness and partial-thickness flaps can be displaced. For a full-thickness flap to be displaced, the attached gingiva must be completely separated from the underlying bone and the flap must be elevated apical to the mucogingival junction, thereby enabling mobility of the flap. Flap mobility may also require the use of vertical incisions and the release of the periosteum, especially for full-thickness flaps. Although the periosteum is only a few cells thick, it is not elastic. The periosteum may be folded over itself to allow apical displacement of the flap. However, it does not stretch, and coronal flap displacement requires the periosteum to be incised along the length of the flap. Palatal flaps cannot be displaced due to absence of a mucogingival junction and mobile elastic tissue.

Apically displaced flaps have the important advantage of preserving the outer portion of the pocket wall and transforming it into attached gingiva. Therefore, these flaps accomplish the double objective of eliminating the pocket and increasing the width of the attached gingiva. The apically displaced flap also allows for pocket reduction in instances where keratinized tissue is limited and the internal bevel incision must be made close to or at the gingival margin.

At locations where keratinized tissue is abundant, and pocket reduction is desired, such as the palate, a nondisplaced flap is created with a submarginal scalloped incision to eliminate marginal tissue.

Periodontal Surgical Techniques

Periodontal surgery limited to the gingival tissues only without the use of periodontal flaps can be classified as *gingival curettage* and *gingivectomy.* The current understanding of disease etiology and therapy limits the use of both techniques, but their place in surgical therapy is essential.

Periodontal flap surgery is one of the most frequently employed procedures, particularly for moderate and deep pockets in the posterior areas. Periodontal flap surgery provides access for root instrumentation and pocket reduction via gingival resection, osseous resection, and periodontal regeneration.

Non-displaced flap

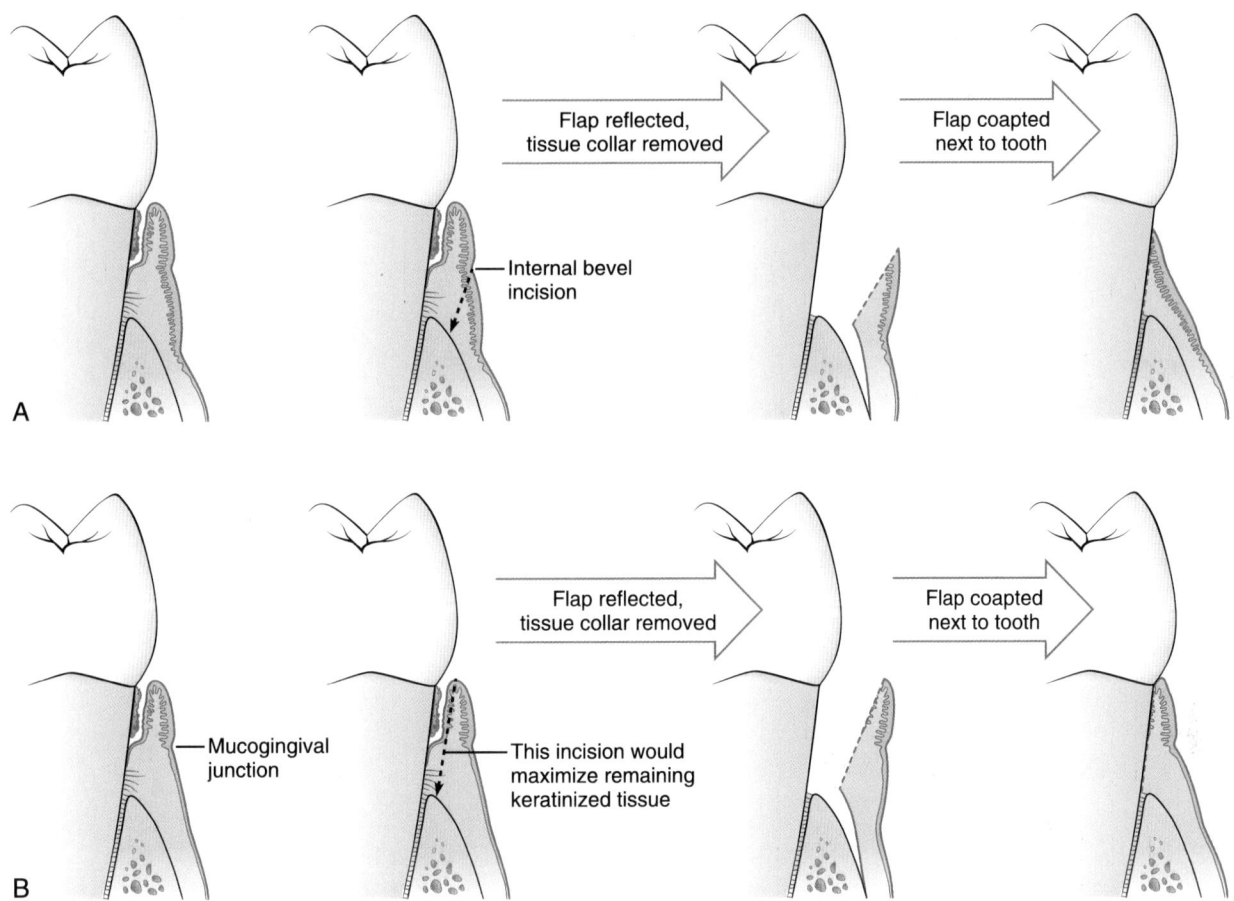

Fig. 60.10 (A) In the presence of abundant keratinized tissue, reduction in soft tissue height is obtained with a submarginal scalloped incision. (B) A marginal incision is used to maximize remaining keratinized tissue. A nondisplaced flap results in thick soft tissue height. This is desirable in an aesthetic area where recession needs to be minimized.

Continued

Gingival Surgery

Gingivectomy

The word *gingivectomy* means "excision of the gingiva." By removing the pocket wall, gingivectomy provides visibility and accessibility for complete calculus removal and thorough root planing. This creates a favorable environment for gingival healing and restoration of a physiologic gingival contour.

Although gingivectomy was widely performed in the past, improved understanding of healing and the development of sophisticated flap techniques have relegated it to a lesser role in periodontal surgery. However, it remains an effective form of treatment when indicated (Fig. 60.11).

Gingivectomy may be performed for the following indications[11]:
1. Elimination of suprabony pockets if the pocket wall is fibrous and firm
2. Elimination of gingival enlargements

Contraindications to gingivectomy include the following:
1. Access to bone required
2. Narrow zone of keratinized tissue
3. Aesthetics
4. Patients with high postoperative risk of bleeding

The step-by-step technique for gingivectomy is as follows:

Step 1: The periodontal pocket is mapped out on the external gingival surface by inserting a probe to the bottom of the pocket and puncturing the external surface of the gingiva at the depth of probe penetration (see Figs. 60.11C and D; Figs. 60.12 and 60.13).

Step 2: Periodontal knives (e.g., Kirkland) are used for incisions on the facial and lingual surfaces. Orban periodontal knives are used for interdental incisions (see Fig. 60.11E to G). Bard–Parker blades (#12 and #15), and scissors are used as auxiliary instruments.

The external bevel incision is started apical to the points marking the course of the pockets,[30,36] and it is directed coronally to a point between the base of the pocket and the crest of the bone. It should be as close as possible to the bone without exposing it to remove the soft tissue coronal to the bone. Exposure of bone is undesirable. If this occurs, healing usually presents minimal complications if the area is adequately covered by the surgical dressing.

Either interrupted or continuous incisions may be used. The incision should be beveled at approximately 45 degrees to the tooth surface, and it should re-create the normal festooned pattern of the gingiva. Failure to bevel the incision will leave a broad, fibrous plateau that will delay development of a physiologic contour.

Step 3: Remove the excised pocket wall, irrigate the area, and examine the root surface.

Step 4: Scale and root plane.

Step 5: Cover the area with a surgical dressing (see Fig. 60.11I and Chapter 59).

Apically displaced flap

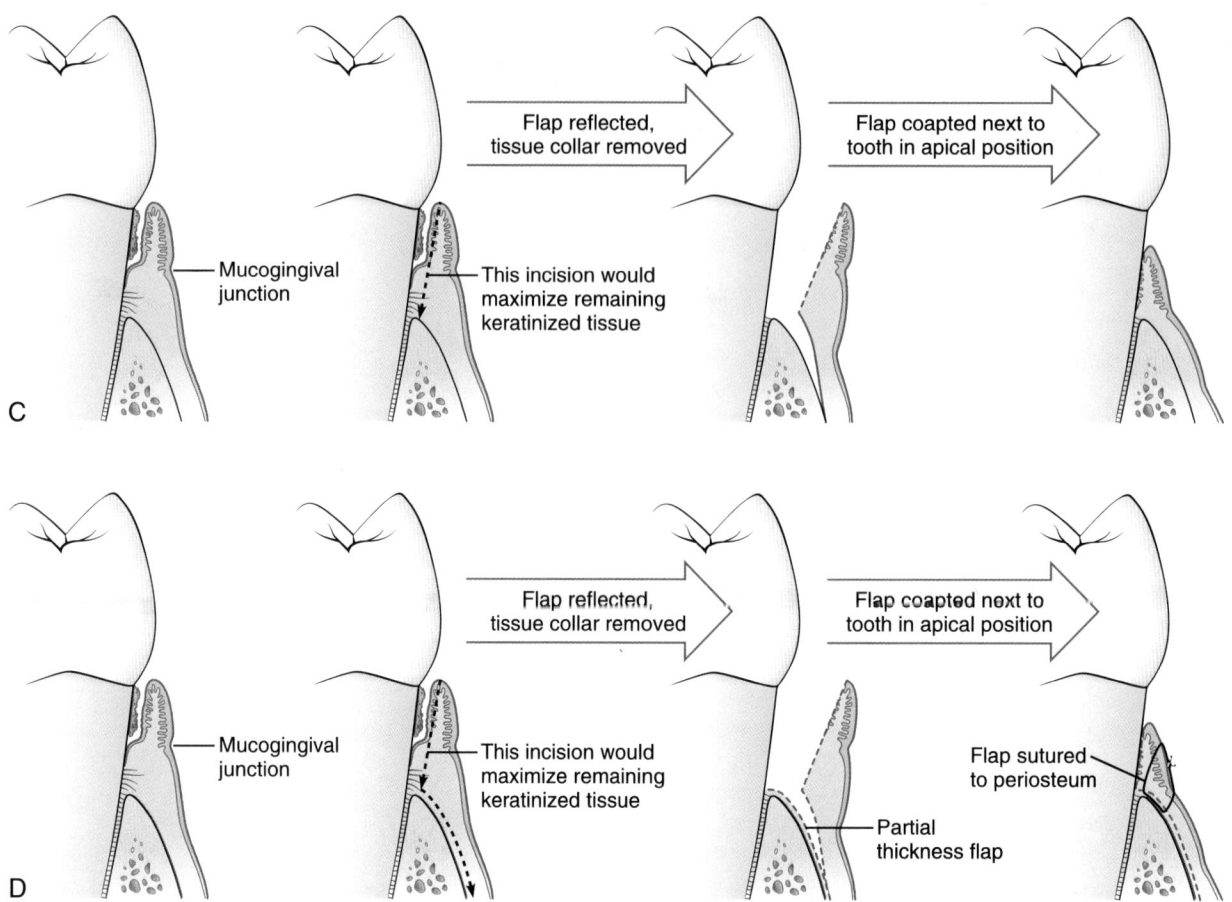

Fig. 60.10, cont'd (C) A marginal incision, to maximize keratinized tissue, is combined with an apically displaced flap to reduce soft tissue height. (D) A partial-thickness flap is used to allow stabilization of an apically positioned flap with a periosteal suture.

Gingivoplasty

Gingivoplasty is *recontouring the gingiva* in the absence of pockets.[12] It may be accomplished with a periodontal knife, a scalpel, or rotary coarse diamond stones.[24]

Healing After Gingivectomy

The *initial response* after gingivectomy is the formation of a protective surface blood clot. The underlying tissue becomes acutely inflamed with necrosis. The clot is then replaced by granulation tissue. In 24 hours, an increase occurs in new connective tissue cells, which are mainly angioblasts beneath the surface layer of inflammation and necrotic tissue. By the third day, numerous young fibroblasts are located in the area.[27] The highly vascular granulation tissue grows coronally and creates a new free gingival margin and sulcus.[23] Capillaries derived from the blood vessels of the periodontal ligament migrate into the granulation tissue, and within 2 weeks they connect with the gingival vessels.[37]

After 12 to 24 hours, epithelial cells at the margins of the wound begin to migrate over the granulation tissue, thereby separating it from the contaminated surface layer of the clot. Epithelial activity at the margins reaches a peak after 24 to 36 hours.[10]

The new epithelial cells arise from the basal and deeper spinous layers of the epithelial wound edge and migrate over the wound over a fibrin layer that is later resorbed and replaced by a connective tissue bed.[15] The epithelial cells advance by a tumbling action, with the cells becoming fixed to the substrate by hemidesmosomes and a new basement lamina.[13,16]

After 5 to 14 days, surface epithelialization is generally complete (see Fig. 60.11J). During the first 4 weeks after gingivectomy, keratinization is less than it was before surgery. Complete epithelial repair takes about 1 month.[34] Vasodilation and vascularity begin to decrease after the fourth day of healing, and they appear to be almost normal by the 16th day.[21] Complete repair of the connective tissue takes about 7 weeks.[34]

The flow of gingival fluid in humans is initially increased after gingivectomy, and it diminishes as healing progresses.[2,32] Maximal flow is reached after 1 week, which coincides with the time of maximal inflammation.

Although the tissue changes that occur during postgingivectomy healing are the same in all individuals, the time required for complete healing varies considerably among sites and individuals. In patients with physiologic gingival melanosis, the pigmentation is diminished in the healed gingiva.

Flap Surgery

Periodontal flaps are used in surgical periodontal therapy to accomplish the following:

1. Access for root instrumentation
2. Gingival resection

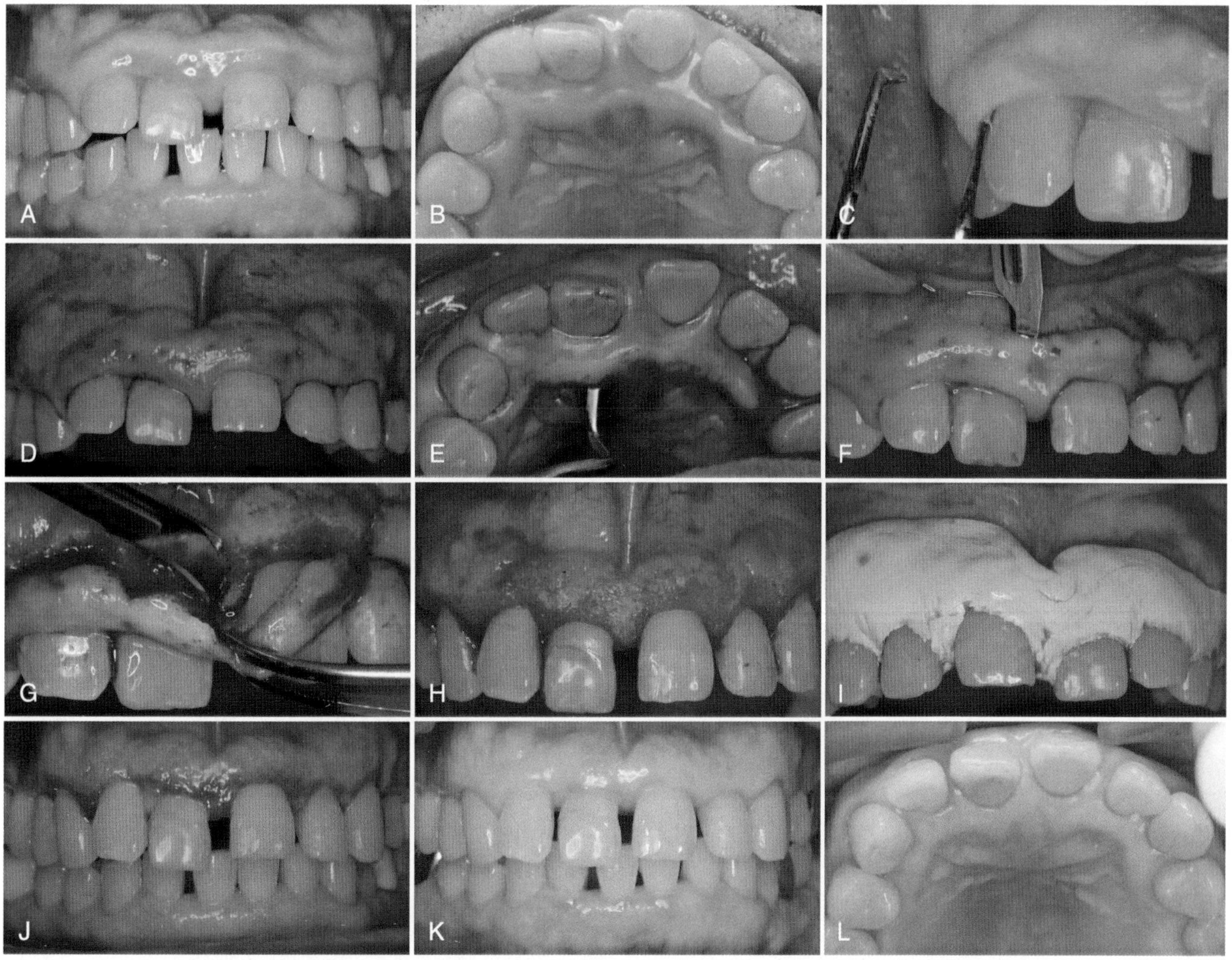

Fig. 60.11 Results obtained by treating a suprabony pocket with gingivectomy. (A) and (B) Preoperative facial and palatal views. (C) Marking of the depth of the suprabony pocket. (D) The bottoms of the pockets are indicated by pinpoint markings. (E) A beveled palatal incision with an Orban knife. (F) A facial beveled incision with a Bard–Parker #15 blade extends apical to the perforations made by the pocket marker. Note that the beveled incision can also be made with a Kirkland knife. (G) The interdental incision and excision of the pocket wall with a Bard–Parker #12 blade. (H) A completed gingivectomy. (I) The surgical site covered with periodontal dressing. (J) One week after healing. (K) and (L) Results 22 months after the operation. *(Courtesy Dr. Kitetsu Shin, Saitama, Japan.)*

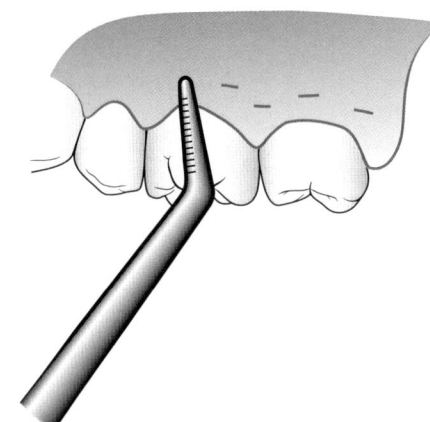

Fig. 60.12 The pocket marker makes pinpoint perforations that indicate pocket depth.

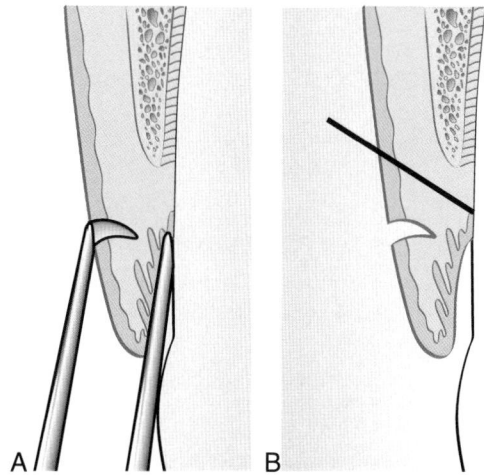

Fig. 60.13 Marking the depth of a suprabony pocket. (A) A pocket marker in position. (B) The beveled incision extends apical to the perforation made by the pocket marker.

3. Osseous resection
4. Periodontal regeneration

To fulfill these purposes, five different flap techniques are used: (1) the modified Widman flap,[28] (2) the undisplaced flap, (3) the apically displaced flap, (4) the papilla preservation flap,[8,35] (5) and the distal terminal molar flap.

The modified Widman flap facilitates root instrumentation. It does not attempt to reduce the pocket depth, but it does eliminate the pocket lining. The objectives of the undisplaced and apically displaced flaps include root surface access and the reduction of probing depth. The choice of which procedure to use depends on two important anatomic landmarks: the transgingival probing depth and the location of the mucogingival junction. These landmarks establish the presence and width of the attached gingiva, which are the basis for the decision.

The papilla preservation flap is used when possible in regenerative and aesthetic cases to minimize recession and loss of interdental papillae. The distal terminal molar flap is used for treating pockets and osseous defects on the distal surface of the terminal maxillary and mandibular molars.

Modified Widman Flap

The original Widman[38] flap used two vertical releasing incisions connected by a submarginal scalloped internal bevel incision to demarcate the area of surgery. A full-thickness flap was reflected and the marginal collar of tissue was removed to provide access for root instrumentation and osseous recontouring. In 1974, Ramfjord and Nissle[28] published the "modified Widman flap" (Fig. 60.14), which used only horizontal incisions. This technique offers the

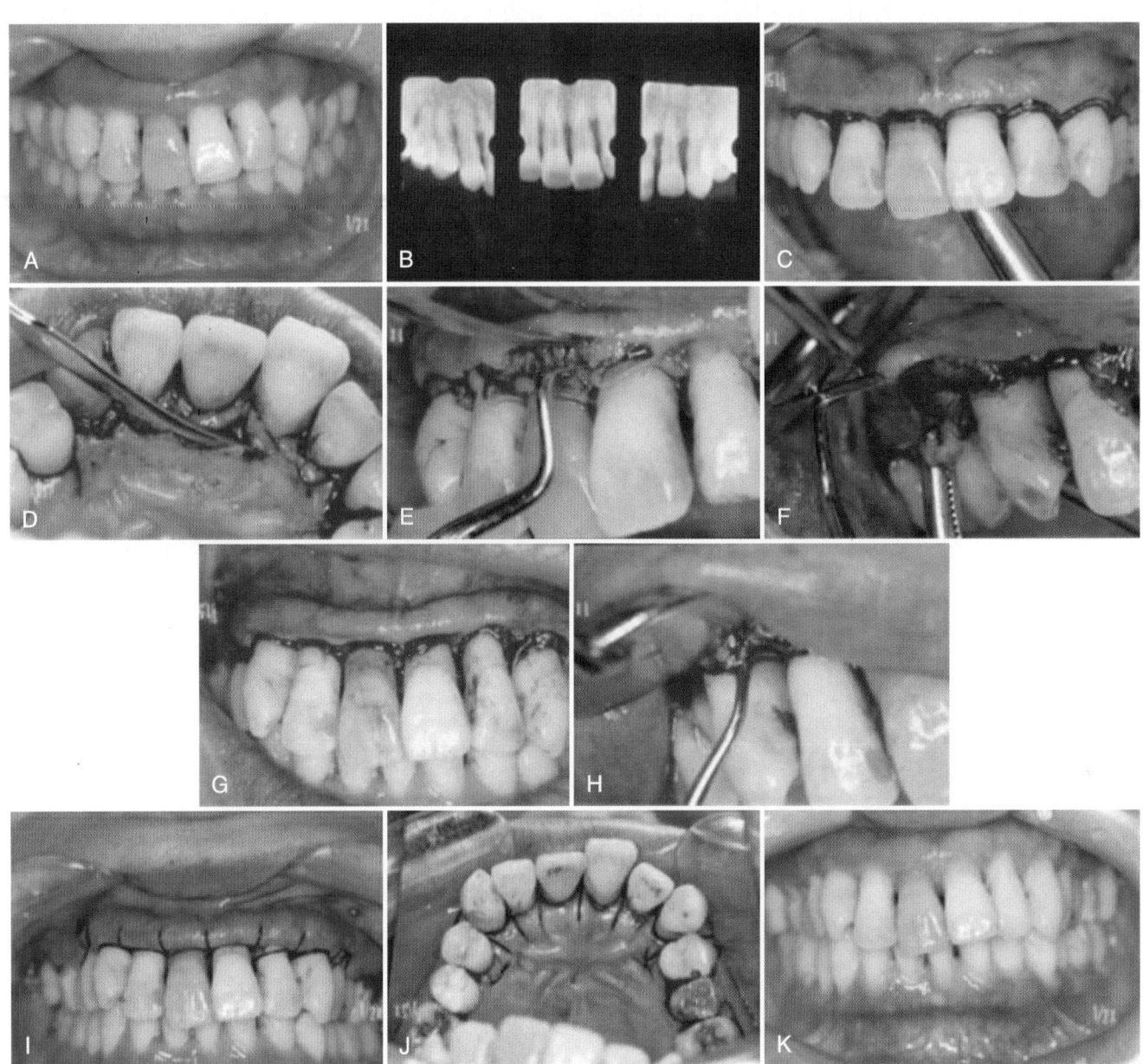

Fig. 60.14 Modified Widman flap technique. (A) Facial view before surgery. The probing of pockets revealed interproximal depths that ranged from 4 to 8 mm and facial and palatal depths of 2 to 5 mm. (B) Radiographic survey of the area. Note the generalized horizontal bone loss. (C) Facial internal bevel incision. (D) Palatal incision. (E) Elevation of the flap, which left a wedge of tissue attached to its base. (F) Removal of tissue. (G) Tissue removed and ready for scaling and root planing. (H) Scaling and root planing of exposed root surfaces. (I) Continuous, independent sling suture of facial portion of surgery. (J) Continuous, independent sling suture of palatal portion of surgery. (K) Postsurgical result. *(Courtesy Dr. Kitetsu Shin, Saitama, Japan.)*

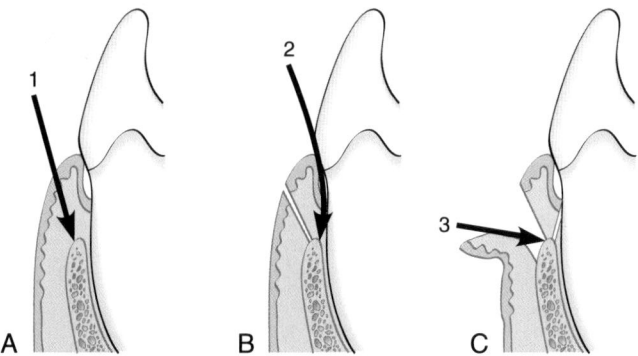

Fig. 60.15 The three incisions necessary for flap surgery. (A) First (internal bevel) incision; (B) second (crevicular) incision; and (C) third (interdental) incision.

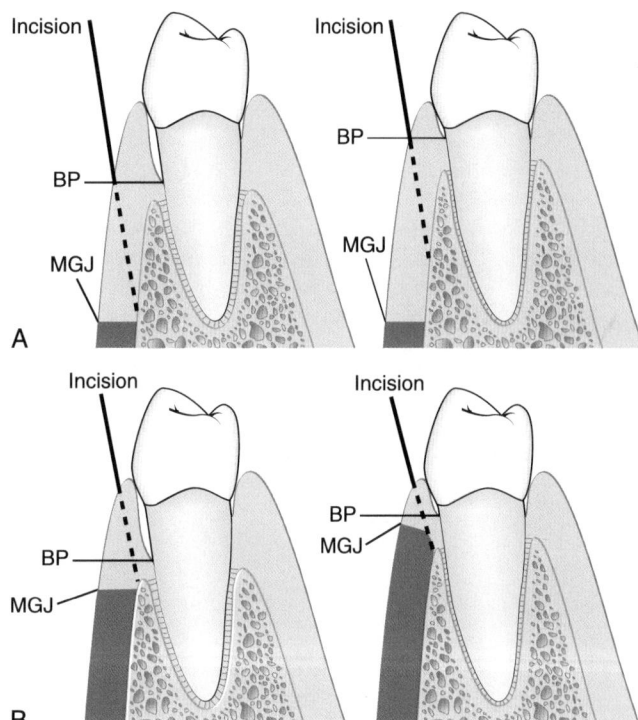

Fig. 60.16 (A) and (B) The location of two different areas where the internal bevel incision is made in an undisplaced flap. The incision is made at the level of the pocket to discard the tissue coronal to the pocket if remaining attached gingiva is sufficient. *BP,* Bottom of pocket; *MCJ,* mucogingival junction.

possibility of establishing an intimate postoperative adaptation of healthy collagenous connective tissue to tooth surfaces,[5,18,26,28] and it provides access for adequate instrumentation of the root surfaces and immediate closure of the area.

The step-by-step technique for the modified Widman flap is as follows:

Step 1: The first incision (Fig. 60.15A) parallel to the long-axis of the tooth is a scalloped internal bevel incision to the alveolar crest starting 0.5 to 1 mm away from the gingival margin (see Fig. 60.14C). The papillae are dissected and thinned to have a thickness similar to that of the remaining flaps.

Step 2: Full-thickness flaps are reflected 2 to 3 mm away from the alveolar crest (see Fig. 60.14D).

Step 3: The second, crevicular incision (Fig. 60.15B) is made in the gingival crevice to detach the attachment apparatus from the root.

Step 4: The interdental tissue and the gingival collar are detached from the bone with a third incision (Fig. 60.15C; see Fig. 60.14E and F).

Step 5: The gingival collar and granulation tissue are removed with curettes. The root surfaces are scaled and planed (see Fig. 60.14G and H). Residual periodontal fibers attached to the tooth surface should not be disturbed.

Step 6: Bone architecture is not corrected unless it prevents intimate flap adaptation. Every effort is made to adapt the facial and lingual interdental tissue in such a way that no interdental bone remains exposed at the time of suturing. The flaps may be thinned to allow for close adaptation of the gingiva around the entire circumference of the tooth.

Step 7: The flaps are stabilized with sutures (see Fig. 60.14I and J) and covered with a surgical dressing.

Ramfjord[26] performed an extensive longitudinal study that compared the modified Widman procedure with the curettage technique and the pocket elimination (gingivectomy and osseous surgery) methods. Patients were assigned randomly to one of the techniques, and results were analyzed yearly for up to 7 years after therapy. The researchers reported similar results for each of the three methods tested. Pocket depth was initially similar for all methods, but it was maintained at shallower levels with the modified Widman flap; the attachment level remained higher with the modified Widman flap.

Undisplaced Flap

Currently, the undisplaced flap may be the most frequently performed type of periodontal surgery. For the undisplaced flap, the submarginal scalloped internal bevel incision is initiated at a distance from the tooth that is roughly one-half to two-thirds the interdental transgingival probing depth. This incision can be accomplished only if sufficient

attached gingiva remains apical to the incision. Therefore, the two anatomic landmarks, the transgingival interdental probing depth and the mucogingival junction, must be considered to evaluate the amount of attached gingiva that will remain after surgery. The internal bevel incision should be scalloped to create surgical papillae, which are essential to covering the interdental bone (see Fig. 60.4). If the tissue is too thick, the flap margin should be thinned with the initial incision. Proper placement of the flap margin at the alveolar crest during closure is important to prevent either recurrence of the pocket or exposure of bone.

The step-by-step technique for the undisplaced flap is as follows:

Step 1: The periodontal probe is inserted into the gingival crevice and penetrates the junctional epithelium and connective tissue down to bone.

Step 2: The mucogingival junction is assessed to determine the amount of keratinized tissue.

Step 3: The initial placement of the submarginal scalloped internal bevel incision is based on the transgingival interdental probing depth and the mucogingival junction (Fig. 60.16). The incision is made parallel to the long axis of the tooth and directed down to the alveolar bone. The angulation of the incision may be altered depending on the thickness of the gingiva, as well as the initial placement of the submarginal scalloped incision, to produce a thin flap margin. The thicker the tissue, the more apically the incision will end (see Fig. 60.16). A short mesial vertical incision may be employed to allow flap release on the palate or to avoid extension of the horizontal incision into the aesthetic area.

Step 4: Full-thickness flaps are reflected 1 mm apical to the mucogingival junction.

Step 5: The crevicular is made in the gingival crevice to detach the attachment apparatus from the root.

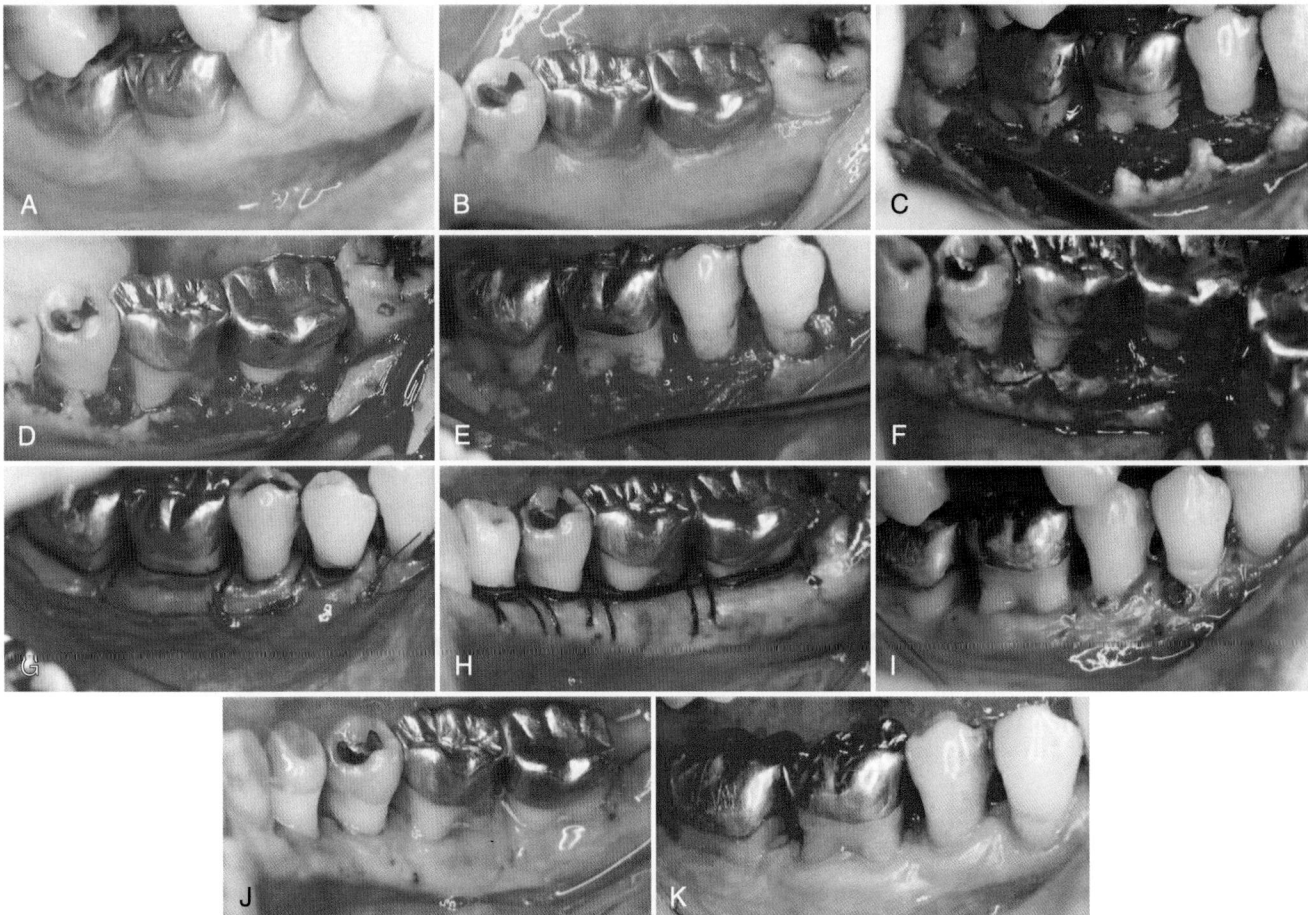

Fig. 60.17 An apically displaced flap. (A) and (B) Facial and lingual preoperative views. (C) and (D) The facial and lingual flaps have been elevated. (E) and (F) After debridement of the areas. (G) and (H) The sutures are in place. (I) and (J) Healing after 1 week. (K) Healing after 2 months. Note the preservation of attached gingiva displaced to a more apical position. *(Courtesy Dr. Thomas Han, Los Angeles, CA.)*

Step 6: The gingival collar and granulation tissue are removed with curettes. The root surfaces are scaled and planed.

Step 7: Osseous recontouring is performed to eliminate defects and reestablish positive architecture.

Step 8: The flaps are coapted on the alveolar crest with the flap margin well adapted to the roots. The flaps may be trimmed and rescalloped if necessary.

Step 9: The flaps are stabilized with sutures and covered with a surgical dressing.

Apically Displaced Flap

The apically displaced flap is selected for cases that present with a minimal amount (<3 mm) of attached gingiva. For this reason, the internal bevel incision should be made as close to the tooth as possible (i.e., 0.5 to 1.0 mm). No need exists to determine where the bottom of the pocket is in relation to the incision for the apically displaced flap as one would for the undisplaced flap. The flap is placed at the tooth–bone junction by apically displacing the flap. Its final position is not determined by the placement of the first incision.

With some variants, the apically displaced flap can be used for pocket eradication, widening the zone of attached gingiva, or both. Depending on the purpose, the apically displaced flap can be a full-thickness flap or a split-thickness flap. The split-thickness flap requires more precision and finesse, as well as a gingiva that is thick enough to split. The split-thickness flap can be more precisely

positioned and sutured in an apical position with the use of a periosteal suturing technique.

The step-by-step technique for the apically displaced flap is as follows:

Step 1: A marginal scalloped internal bevel incision parallel to the long axis of the tooth is made down to the crest of bone (Fig. 60.17).

Step 2: If used, vertical incisions are made extending beyond the mucogingival junction. It is important that the vertical incisions—and therefore the flap elevation—reach past the mucogingival junction to provide adequate mobility to the flap for its apical displacement.

Step 3: The flap is reflected in full thickness or partial thickness, depending on the thickness of the gingiva and the objective of the surgery.

Step 4: Crevicular and interdental incisions are made, and the marginal collar of tissue is removed.

Step 5: After degranulation, scaling and root planing, and osseous surgery if needed, the flap is displaced apically.

Step 6: If a full-thickness flap was reflected, an independent sling suture positions the flap margin at the alveolar crest, and a surgical dressing can prevent its coronal movement. If a partial-thickness flap was reflected, it can be apically displaced with an independent sling suture, and further stabilized with periosteal sutures. A periodontal dressing can prevent its coronal movement.

After 1 week, dressings and sutures are removed. The area is usually repacked for another week, after which the patient is to brush gently along the gingival margin with a soft brush and interdentally with interdental brushes.

Distal Terminal Molar Flap

The treatment of periodontal pockets on the distal surface of terminal molars is often complicated by the presence of bulbous fibrous tissue over the maxillary tuberosity or prominent retromolar pads in the mandible. Some of these osseous lesions may result from incomplete repair after the extraction of impacted third molars (Fig. 60.18).

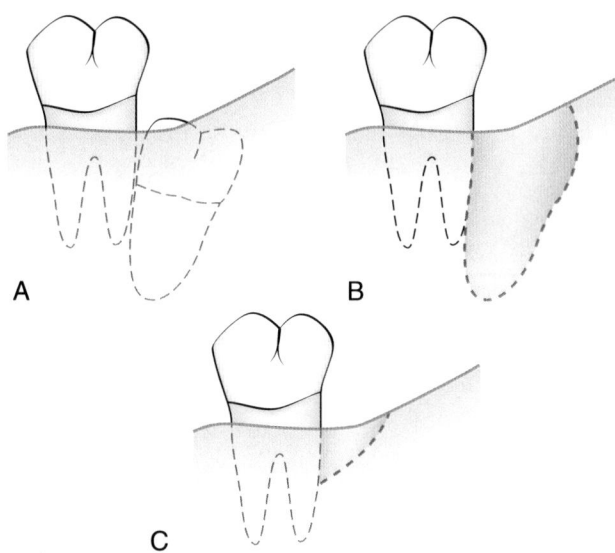

Fig. 60.18 (A) Impaction of a third molar distal to a second molar with little or no interdental bone between the two teeth. (B) Removal of the third molar creates a pocket with little or no bone distal to the second molar. (C) This often leads to a vertical osseous defect distal to the second molar.

Access to these distal areas may be obtained by a single horizontal incision, two converging horizontal incisions, or two parallel incisions extending distally from the distal surface of the terminal molar to the mucogingival junction distal to the tuberosity or the retromolar pad. The distal horizontal incision is connected with the crevicular incision on the distal surface of the terminal molar, which merges mesially with the buccal and lingual or palatal scalloped incisions. If the secondary objective of surgery is regenerative or the buccolingual width of the distal keratinized tissue is limited, a single horizontal incision in keratinized tissue is used. If the secondary objective of surgery is resective and adequate keratinized tissue is present buccolingually, two distal horizontal incisions are placed in keratinized tissue. The two horizontal incisions technique were described by Robinson[31] and Braden[5] and modified by several other investigators. These techniques are called the *distal wedge* and the *modified distal wedge*.

The distal wedge technique employs two horizontal incisions that begin at the distal surface of the terminal molar and *converge* distally at the mucogingival junction distal to the tuberosity or the retromolar pad. The modified distal wedge technique employs two *parallel* horizontal incisions that extend distally from the distal surface of the terminal molar and are connected by a transverse incision distal to the mucogingival junction distal to the tuberosity or retromolar pad. The buccolingual distance between the two horizontal incisions in both techniques depends on the transgingival probing depth and the amount of fibrous tissue involved. When the flaps are thinned and the tissue between the two incisions is removed, the two flap edges must approximate each other at a new apical position without overlapping (Fig. 60.19). Generally, the distance between the two parallel incisions is roughly one-half to two-thirds the distal transgingival probing depth and should never be farther apart than the distance between the buccal and lingual line angles of the tooth.

To ensure primary closure of the distal flaps, especially in the tuberosity, it is advantageous to use one horizontal incision or two horizontal incisions that are closer together rather than farther apart.

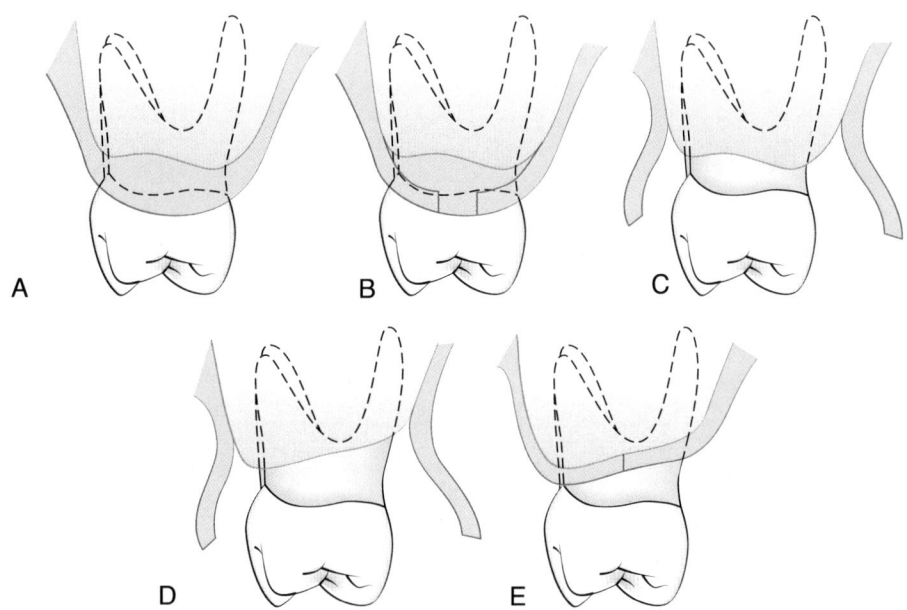

Fig. 60.19 (A) Coronal view from behind a maxillary second molar with an osseous defect. (B) Distal terminal flap surgery employing two horizontal incisions; both buccal and lingual flaps are thinned. (C) Buccal and lingual flaps are elevated, and the "wedge" of tissue is removed. (D) The bone is sloped to the palatal side to eliminate the osseous defect. (E) The flaps are coapted on the bone in the apical position.

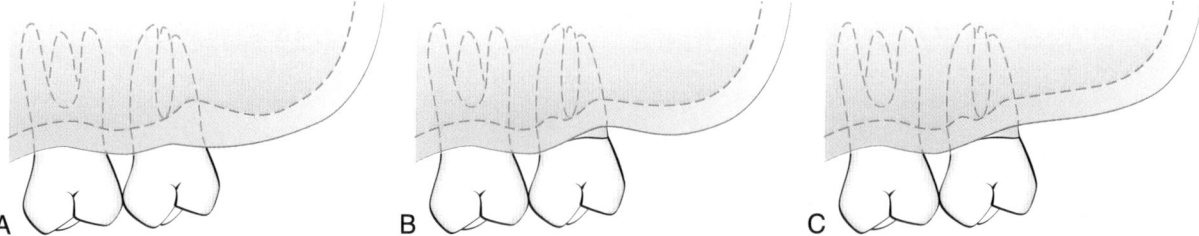

Fig. 60.20 (A) Sagittal view of a distal defect on a maxillary second molar. (B) Treatment with a distal wedge results in an acute angle between the tuberosity and the distal surface of the second molar. (C) Treatment with a modified distal wedge results in a wider angle between the tuberosity and the distal surface of the second molar that is more accessible for hygiene.

Flaps that overlap when they are coapted can be easily trimmed by placing one flap over the other, grabbing the superficial flap with a hemostat, and cutting away the overlapped tissue with a sharp scalpel or scissors.

In regenerative therapy, the distal flaps are not thinned; they are reflected in full thickness. Whereas in resective therapy, before the flaps are completely reflected, they are undermined and thinned with a #15 blade. It is easier to thin the flap before it is completely reflected and mobile. The flaps are then reflected in full thickness.

Maxillary Molars

The treatment of distal pockets in the maxilla is usually less challenging than that in the mandible. The tuberosity presents a greater amount of fibrous attached gingiva than does the retromolar pad. The use of the distal wedge with two converging incisions causes the tissue next to the tooth to be displaced more apically than the tissue away from the tooth. Consequently, healing of a distal wedge in the maxilla results in an acute angle between the distal tooth surface and the tuberosity that is biofilm retentive and difficult to clean (Fig. 60.20B). In contrast, the use of the modified distal wedge with two parallel distal incisions allows the soft tissue along the whole length of the distal flap to be evenly displaced apically (Fig. 60.20C). This is advantageous in the maxilla in maintaining a wide angle between the tooth and the tuberosity that is much easier to clean. Therefore, the modified distal wedge is preferred in the maxilla. The two parallel incisions are usually made at the midline of the tuberosity where the tissue is the thickest or slightly to the palatal side to maximize buccal keratinized tissue and to provide easier access for flap closure (Fig. 60.21).

LEARNING BOX 60.5

The two parallel distal horizontal incisions in the maxillary tuberosity are advantageous in allowing the soft tissue along the whole length of the distal flap to be evenly displaced. This results in a wide angle between the tooth and the tuberosity that is much easier to clean.

Mandibular Molars

Incisions in the distal mandible differ from those in the tuberosity due to differences in the anatomy of the area. The retromolar pad usually has limited attached gingiva and vestibular depth. The attached gingiva, if present, may not be found directly distal to the molar. The greatest amount may be distolingual or distobuccal, and it may not be over the bony crest. The ascending ramus of the mandible may also create a short or completely eliminate the horizontal area distal to the terminal molar (Fig. 60.22). The shorter this area, the more difficult it is to treat any deep distal lesion around the terminal

molar. The anatomy of the posterior mandible is further discussed in Chapter 58.

The mandibular retromolar tissue ascends distally to merge with the ascending ramus. This anatomy favors the distal wedge technique in the mandible, although the parallel distal incisions and the single horizontal incision may be used. The two distal incisions should follow the area with the greatest amount of attached gingiva and must be made over bone (Fig. 60.23). Therefore, the incisions could be directed distally or distobuccally, depending on which area has more attached gingiva. Incisions directing distolingually should be avoided due to the potential presence of the lingual nerve.

Papilla Preservation Flap

In current regenerative therapy, bone grafts, membranes, or a combination of these are used with or without other biologics (see Chapter 63). The flap design should maximize the amount of gingival tissue and papilla retained to cover the material placed in the osseous defect. In the aesthetic area, when surgery is necessary, flap design must minimize recession and loss of interdental papillae. As such, the crevicular incision is the incision of choice for the anterior aesthetic area and regenerative therapy. The interdental papilla is retained with the papilla preservation technique when the interdental space is adequate for reflection of the intact papilla; otherwise, it is split beneath the contact point of the two approximating teeth. The flap is elevated in full thickness without thinning of the flap or the papilla.

The step-by-step technique for the papilla preservation flap (see Fig. 60.8; Fig. 60.24) is as follows:

Step 1: A crevicular incision is made around each tooth, with no incisions across the interdental papilla.

Step 2: The preserved papilla can be incorporated into the facial-buccal flap (original papilla preservation technique[35]) or lingual-palatal flap (modified papilla preservation technique[8]). If the preserved papilla is reflected with the facial-buccal flap, the semilunar incision at the base of the papilla is on the lingual-palatal side of the interdental space. If the preserved papilla is reflected with the lingual-palatal flap, the semilunar incision at the base of the papilla is on the facial-buccal side of the interdental space. This semilunar incision dips apically from the line angles of the tooth so that the incision is at least 5 mm from the crest of the papilla.

Step 3: The papilla is then elevated with an Orban knife or curettes and is reflected intact with the flap.

Step 4: The flap is reflected without thinning the tissue.

Healing After Flap Surgery

Immediately after suturing (≤24 hours), a connection between the flap and the tooth or bone surface is established by a blood clot,

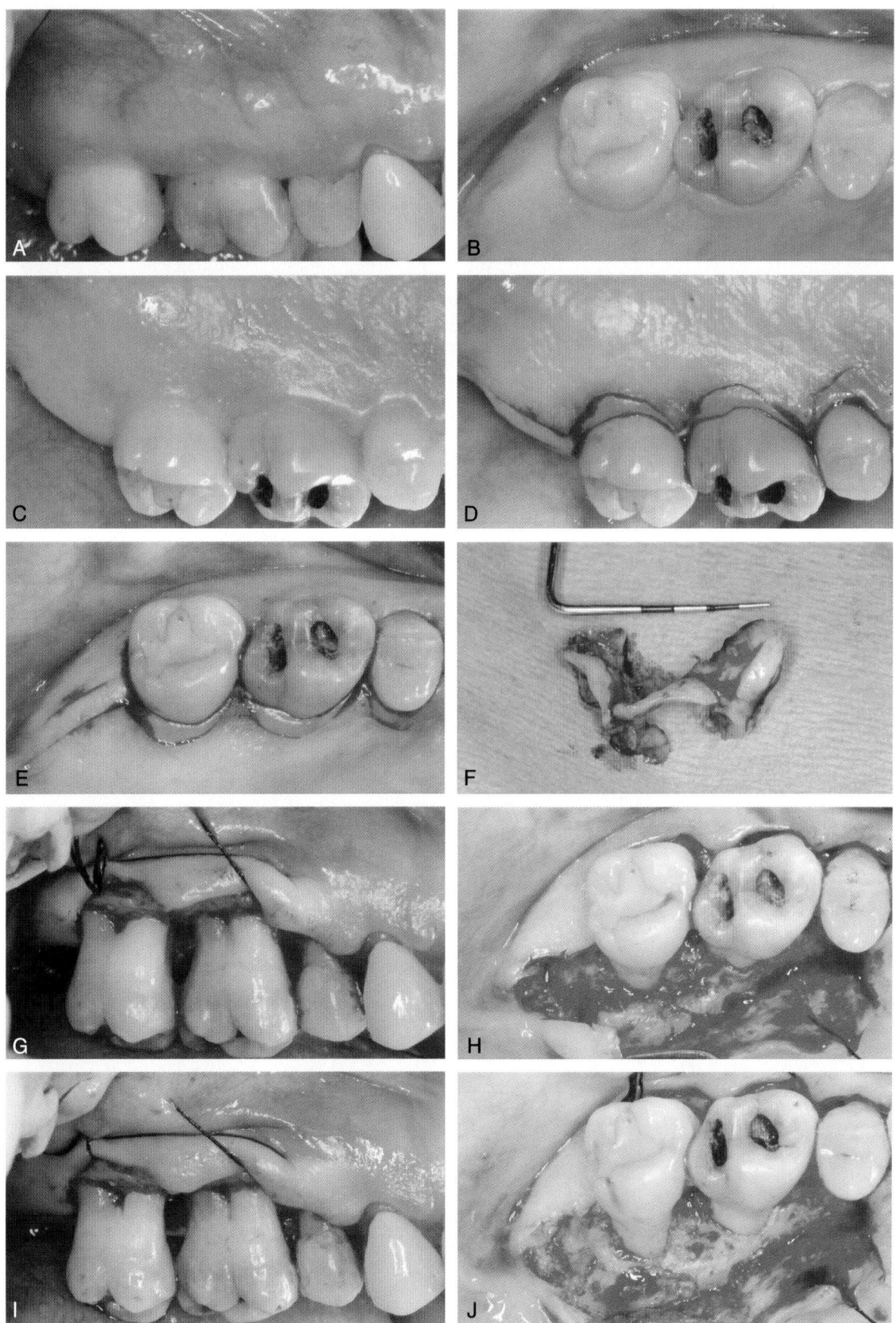

Fig. 60.21 (A) to (C) Presurgical views. (D) and (E) Palatal submarginal scalloped incision and parallel distal horizontal incisions. (F) Distal "wedge" of tissue removed. (G) Buccal and (H) palatal bone before osseous recontouring. (I) Buccal and (J) palatal bone after osseous recontouring.   *Continued*

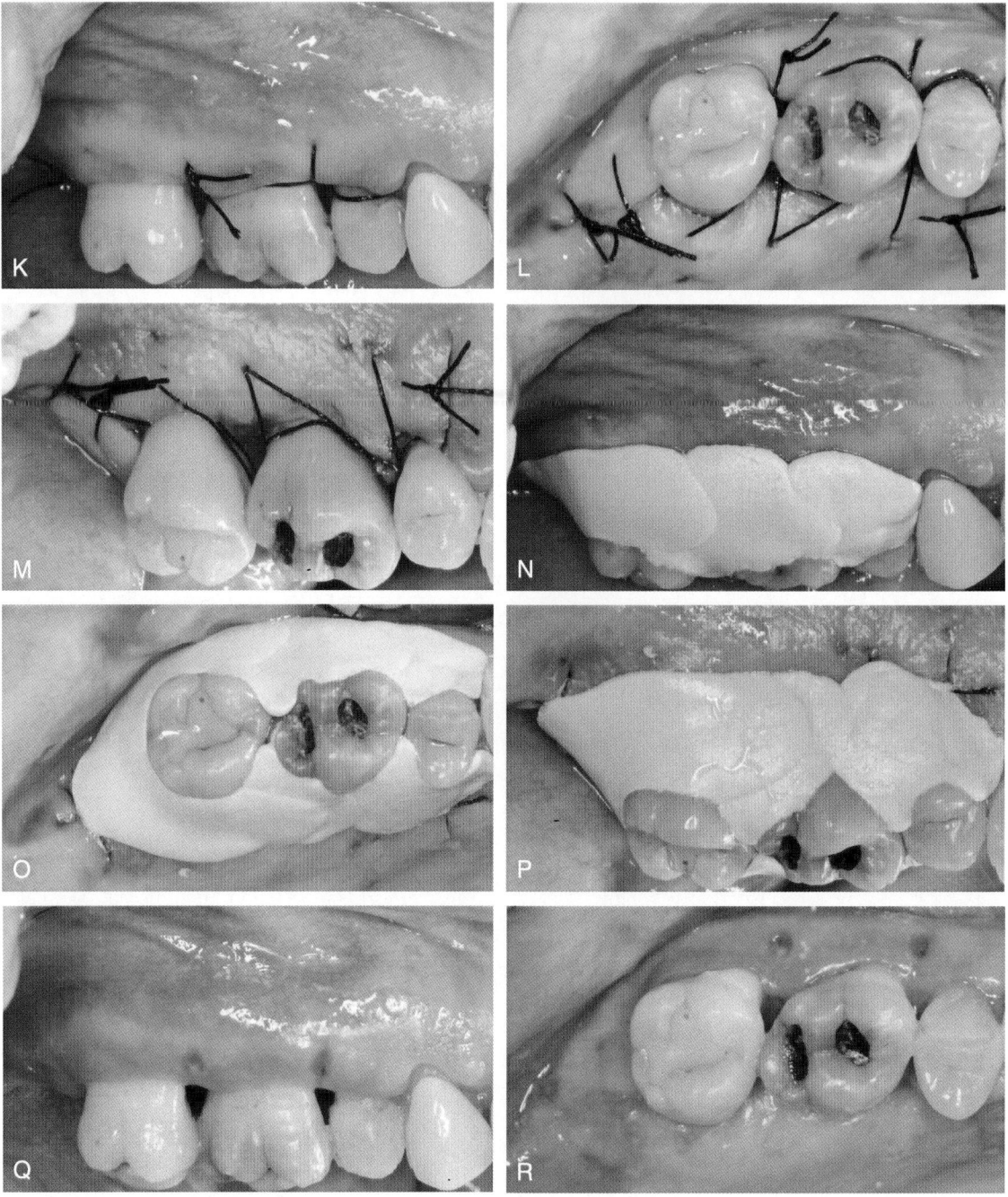

Fig. 60.21, cont'd (K) to (M) Primary closure of flaps with 4-0 silk sutures. (N) to (P) Placement of surgical dressing. (Q) to (S) Postoperative healing at 2 weeks.

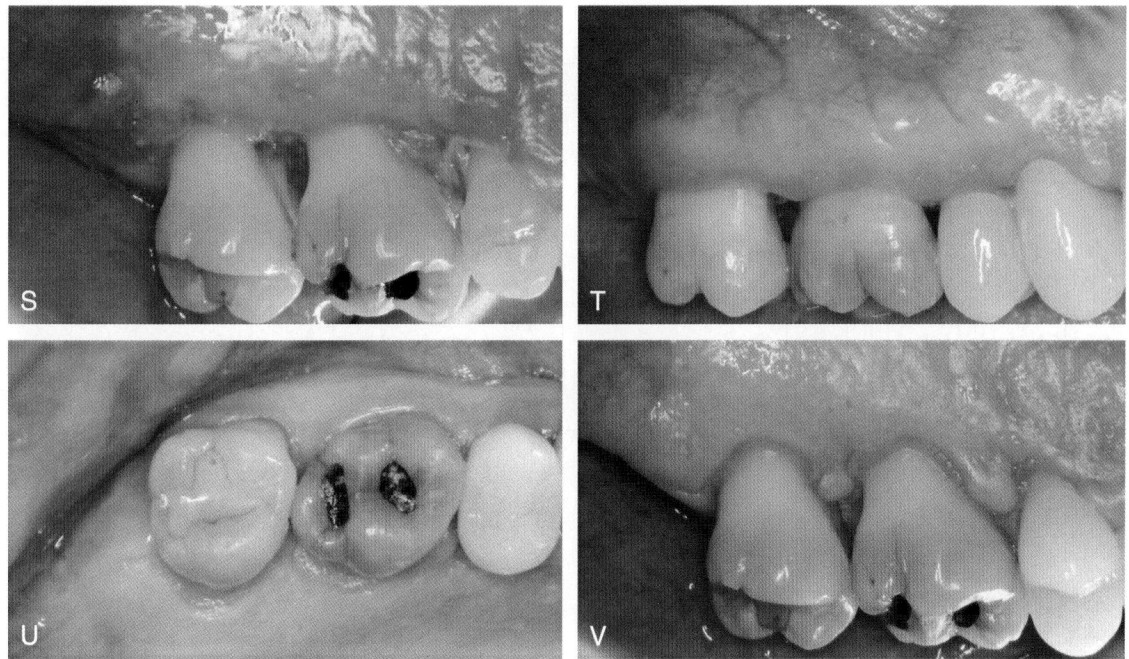

Fig. 60.21, cont'd (T) to (V) Postoperative healing at 8 months. (Copyright Jonathan H. Do, DDS. All rights reserved.)

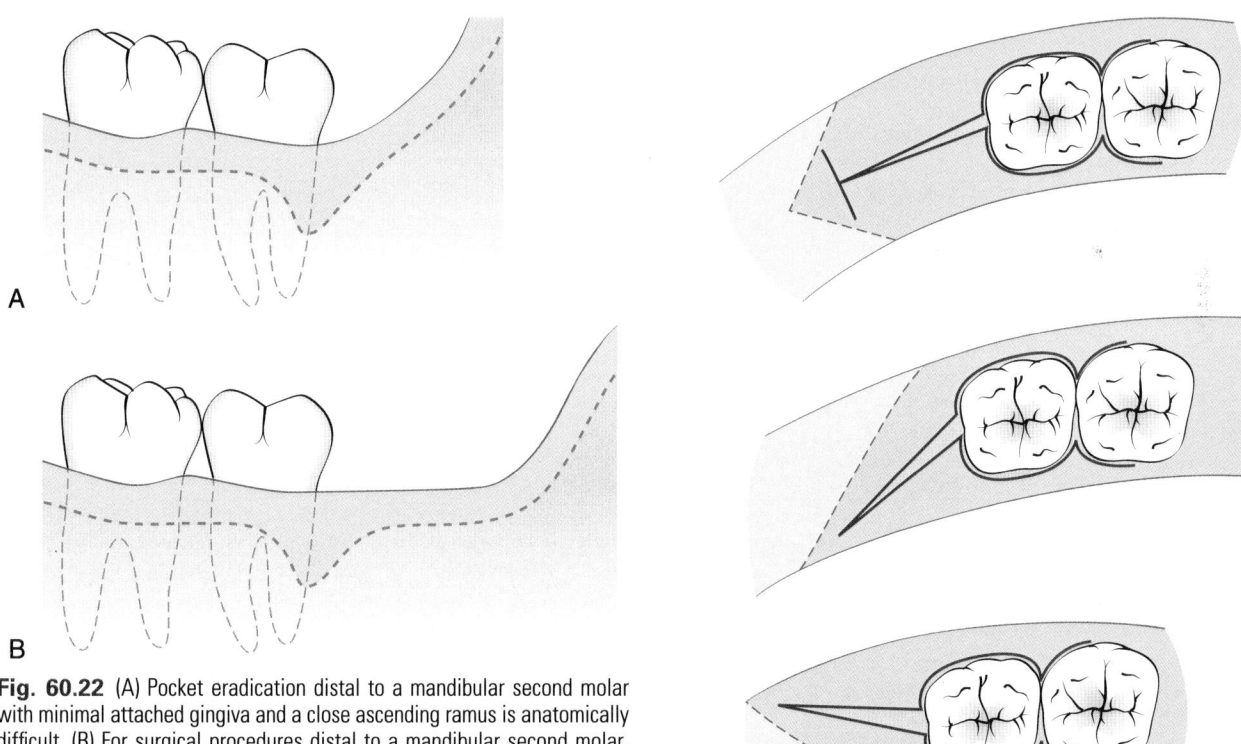

Fig. 60.22 (A) Pocket eradication distal to a mandibular second molar with minimal attached gingiva and a close ascending ramus is anatomically difficult. (B) For surgical procedures distal to a mandibular second molar, abundant attached gingiva and distal space are ideal.

Fig. 60.23 Incision designs for surgical procedures distal to the mandibular second molar. The incision should follow the areas of greatest attached gingiva and underlying bone.

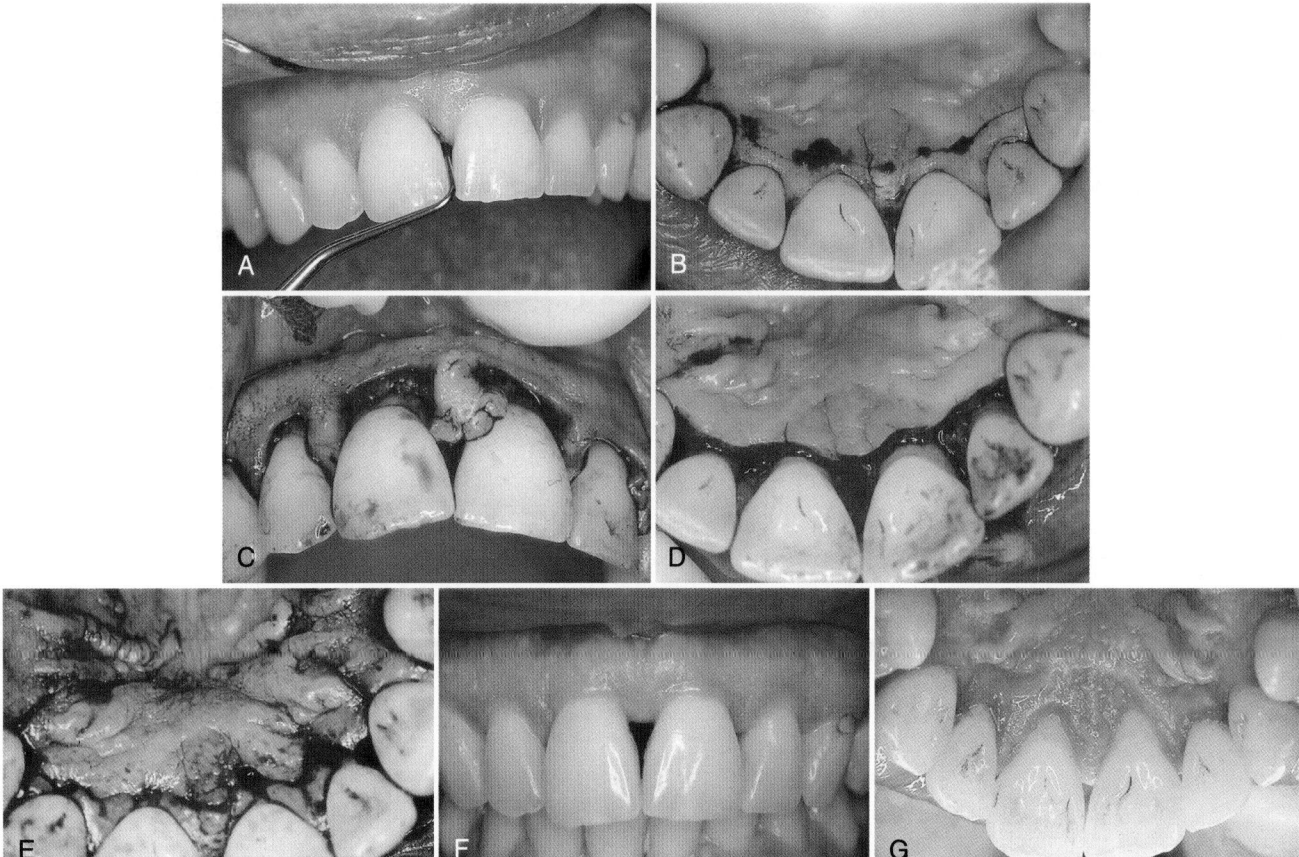

Fig. 60.24 Papilla preservation flap. (A) Facial view after sulcular incisions have been made. (B) Straight-line incision in the palatal area about 3 mm from the gingival margins. This incision is then connected to the margins with vertical incisions at the midpart of each tooth. (C) Papillae are reflected with the facial flap. (D) Lingual view after the reflection of the flap. (E) Lingual view after the flap is brought back to its original position. It is then sutured with independent sutures. (F) Facial view after healing. (G) Palatal view after healing. *(Courtesy Dr. Thomas Han, Los Angeles, CA.)*

which consists of a fibrin reticulum with many polymorphonuclear leukocytes, erythrocytes, debris of injured cells, and capillaries at the edge of the wound.[6] Bacteria and an exudate or transudate also result from tissue injury.

One to 3 days after flap surgery, the space between the flap and the tooth or bone is thinner. Epithelial cells migrate over the border of the flap, and they usually contact the tooth at this time. When the flap is closely adapted to the alveolar process, the inflammatory response is minimal.[6]

One week after surgery, an epithelial attachment to the root has been established by means of hemidesmosomes and a basal lamina. The blood clot is replaced by granulation tissue derived from the gingival connective tissue, the bone marrow, and the periodontal ligament.

Two weeks after surgery, collagen fibers begin to appear parallel to the tooth surface.[6] Union of the flap to the tooth is still weak because of the presence of immature collagen fibers, although the clinical aspect may be almost normal.

One month after surgery, a fully epithelialized gingival crevice with a well-defined epithelial attachment is present. A functional arrangement of the supracrestal fibers is beginning.

Full-thickness flaps, which denude the bone, result in superficial bone necrosis after 1 to 3 days. Osteoclastic resorption follows and reaches a peak at 4 to 6 days and then declines thereafter.[33] This

results in a loss of bone of about 1 mm^3; the bone loss is greater if the bone is thin.[39,40]

Osteoplasty with the use of diamond burs results in areas of bone necrosis with a reduction in bone height, which is later remodeled by new bone formation. The final shape of the crest is determined more by osseous remodeling than by surgical reshaping.[17] Therefore, osseous surgery around the crestal areas must be carefully managed.

This may not be the case when osseous remodeling does not include excessive thinning of the radicular bone.[19] Bone repair reaches its peak after 3 to 4 weeks.[40]

A loss of bone occurs during the initial healing stages both in the radicular bone and in the interdental bone areas. However, in the interdental areas, which have cancellous bone, the subsequent repair stage results in total restitution without any loss of bone; in radicular bone (particularly if it is thin and unsupported by cancellous bone), bone repair results in the loss of marginal bone.[40]

Conclusion

Periodontal access surgery is an adjunct to nonsurgical periodontal therapy, and should occur only once the patient has demonstrated effective biofilm control. The primary objective of periodontal access surgery is access for root instrumentations. The secondary objective of periodontal access surgery is pocket reduction through soft tissue resection, osseous resection, or periodontal regeneration. The clinician must also take aesthetics into consideration; in some areas, such as the anterior maxilla, periodontal disease should be treated nonsurgically, and periodontal access surgery is rendered only when absolutely necessary.

Periodontal surgical therapy has a long history and evolution. It started with subgingival curettage and pocket elimination with gingivectomy. Understanding of healing, development of sophisticated periodontal flap techniques, and aesthetic demands have made gingival curettage obsolete and have relegated gingivectomy to limited cases of gingival enlargement or instances where flap surgery is not possible.

Periodontal flap surgery is the most widely used surgical procedure for periodontal pocket therapy. Periodontal flaps are advantageous and versatile in providing not only access for root instrumentation but also access for osseous surgery and periodontal regeneration. Flap surgery also allows for primary closure, which enhances wound healing and minimizes patients' discomfort. Papilla preservation techniques are useful in regenerative therapy, as well as minimizing recession and loss of interdental papilla in the aesthetic area.

Although the submarginal scalloped incision is useful in reducing periodontal pockets, it must be used with caution. Placement of a submarginal scalloped incision without regard for the mucogingival junction and the width of keratinized tissue may result in a mucogingival problem. The only area in the mouth where the submarginal scalloped incision is necessary is the palatal maxilla. In places where a mucogingival junction is present, marginal incisions and apically displaced flaps may be used in lieu of submarginal scalloped incisions

to maximize remaining keratinized tissue and reduce soft tissue height. The palatal maxilla is unique in that all the tissue is keratinized, attached, and immobile. Pocket reduction must be obtained by tissue resection. The precise placement of the submarginal scalloped incision on the palatal maxilla is essential for intimate adaptation of the flap and primary closure.

Although the "distal wedge" procedure is popular and widely practiced, it is perhaps one of the most difficult procedures to execute well due to the location of the surgical site, as well as the challenges presented by the anatomy of the mandibular retromolar pad and the maxillary tuberosity. The distal wedge procedure is not simply removing a "wedge of tissue" distal to the terminal molar to reduce or eliminate a pocket. Well-executed distal terminal molar flap surgery requires the flaps to approximate intimately to allow for primary closure and in an apical position to achieve pocket reduction. Execution of distal terminal molar flap surgery requires understanding of the anatomy and behavior of the tissue, as well as surgical finesse.

Short-term and long-term success of periodontal access surgery is dependent on biofilm control and long-term maintenance. The patient must understand the etiology of the periodontal disease and its prevention. Surgery in the absence of effective biofilm control and maintenance will result in failure and recurrence of disease.

References

 References for this chapter are found on the companion website www.expertconsult.com.

CHAPTER 61

Treatment of Gingival Enlargement

Paulo M. Camargo | Flavia Q. Pirih | Henry H. Takei | Fermin A. Carranza

CHAPTER OUTLINE

Chronic Inflammatory Enlargement
Periodontal and Gingival Abscesses
Drug-Induced Gingival Enlargement

Leukemic Gingival Enlargement
Gingival Enlargement During
Pregnancy

Gingival Enlargement During
Puberty

The treatment of gingival enlargement is based on an understanding of the cause and underlying pathologic changes of this condition (see Chapter 19). Gingival enlargements are of special concern to the patient and the dentist because they pose problems that include biofilm control, impaired function (mastication, tooth eruption, and speech), and aesthetics. Because gingival enlargements differ with regard to etiology, the treatment of each type is best considered individually.

Chronic Inflammatory Enlargement

Chronic inflammatory enlargements, which are characterized by gingival tissues that are soft and have an altered gingival color, are usually caused by edema and cellular infiltration. Typical therapy consists of scaling and root planing, provided the size of the enlargement does not interfere with the complete removal of deposits from the involved tooth surfaces.

When chronic inflammatory gingival enlargements include a significant fibrotic component that does not undergo shrinkage after scaling and root planning, or if the extent of the gingival enlargement is so severe that access to the deposits on the tooth surface is impossible, surgical removal is the treatment of choice. Two techniques exist for this purpose: gingivectomy and the flap operation. Before instituting surgical therapy, biofilm control, scaling, and root planing should always be completed, and sufficient time should be allowed to heal before reevaluating the periodontal status. It is important that the decision to implement surgical therapy should be made after this reevaluation.

Once the decision is made that surgical therapy is necessary, the selection of the appropriate surgical technique will depend on the extent of the enlargement and the status of the gingival tissues. When the enlarged gingiva remains soft and friable even after scaling and root planing, the gingivectomy technique may be preferable because management of the periodontal flap may be technically difficult on the friable tissues. If the gingival tissue is firm and fibrotic, preference is given to the flap operation, which is always the favorable choice because the healing is by primary intention and the keratinized tissue is better preserved. Therefore, conservation of the keratinized, attached gingiva must be considered along with removal of the excessive gingival tissue.

Tumor-like, localized, and severe inflammatory enlargements (Fig. 61.1) can be treated by gingivectomy as follows. With the patient under local anesthesia, the tooth surfaces beneath the mass are scaled to remove calculus and other debris. The lesion is separated from the mucosa at its base by using a surgical blade. If the lesion extends interproximally, the interdental gingiva is included in the incision to ensure the exposure of deposits. After the enlarged tissues are removed and access is sufficient, the root surfaces are scaled and planed, and the area is irrigated with saline solution. A periodontal dressing is applied and removed after a week, but in some cases, depending on the extent of the surgery, the postoperative appointment may have to be scheduled in 2 weeks to allow for further healing. It is important at this time that proper biofilm control is instituted.

For more information regarding the surgical techniques, see Chapters 59 and 60.

Periodontal and Gingival Abscesses

Periodontal and gingival abscesses result in areas of gingival enlargement. However, the enlargement due to abscesses is usually localized around the area of the lesion, and the content of the enlarged area is purulent material, which must be drained and the area curetted.

The reader is referred to Chapter 45 for a complete discussion of abscess treatment.

Drug-Induced Gingival Enlargement

Gingival enlargement has primarily been associated with the administration of three different types of drugs: anticonvulsants, calcium channel blockers, and the immunosuppressant cyclosporine. Chapter 16 provides a comprehensive review of the clinical and microscopic features and the pathogenesis of gingival enlargement induced by these drugs. Although the clinical presentation of the gingival enlargement induced by the three drug categories listed here may be similar, evidence suggests that their cellular and molecular mechanisms may differ.[29] Limited evidence indicates that other drugs may also induce gingival enlargement, albeit at a lower prevalence and with a lesser severity.[5]

The examination of cases of drug-induced gingival enlargement reveals the overgrown tissues to have two components: fibrotic, which is the result of the action of the drug on the physiologic gingival collagen turnover; and inflammatory, which is induced by the bacterial biofilm. Although the fibrotic and inflammatory components present in the enlarged gingiva are the result of distinct pathologic processes, they almost always are observed as gingival enlargement induced by the combination of drugs and biofilm. The role of bacterial biofilm in

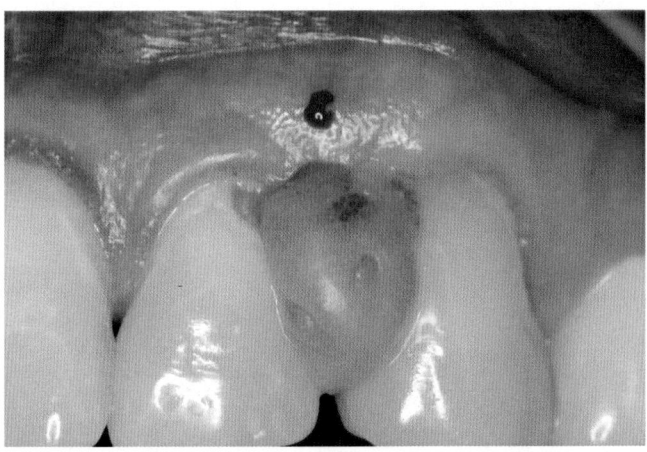

Fig. 61.1 Localized, fibrotic, tumor-like gingival enlargement on a female young adult. This lesion may be treated via gingivectomy.

the overall pathogenesis of drug-induced gingival enlargement is not clear. Some studies indicate that biofilm is a prerequisite for gingival enlargement,[13] whereas others suggest that the presence of biofilm is a consequence of biofilm accumulation caused by the enlarged gingiva. In patients taking calcium channel blockers, termination and/or substitution of the drug with another class of medication resulted in significant decreases in gingival enlargement, with no differences observed between patients with poor or good oral hygiene.[11] These studies suggest that the gingival enlargement process is independent of biofilm-related inflammation.

> **LEARNING BOX 61.1**
>
> The inflammatory components present in the enlarged gingiva are the result of plaque biofilm accumulating beneath the enlarged gingiva, and the fibrotic portion may be drug induced. The enlarged gingiva is almost always the result of the combination of both the biofilm and the drug.

Treatment Options

The treatment of drug-induced gingival enlargement should be based on the medication used and the clinical features of the case.

First, consideration should be given to the possibility of discontinuing the drug[10,14] or changing the medication. These possibilities should be examined in consultation with the patient's physician. Simple discontinuation of the offending drug is often not practical, but substitution of the drug with another medication may be an option. If any drug substitution is attempted, it is important to allow a 6- to 12-month period to elapse between discontinuation of the offending drug and substitution with an alternative drug. The changes instituted with the drug should always be in combination with oral hygiene instructions, scaling, and root planing. Reevaluation of the gingival enlargement after the alteration of drug therapy is necessary before any surgical treatment is planned.

Alternative medications to the anticonvulsant phenytoin include carbamazepine[2,9] and valproic acid, both of which have been reported to induce gingival enlargement to a lesser degree. A murine study suggested that lovastatin may attenuate the onset of gingival enlargement induced by phenytoin.[2] Further research is necessary to confirm the therapeutic value of lovastatin.

For patients who are taking nifedipine, which has a reported prevalence of gingival enlargement of up to 86%, other calcium channel blockers such as diltiazem or verapamil may be viable alternatives. The reported prevalence of inducing gingival enlargement is 20% for diltiazem and 4% for verapamil.[4,12,19] In addition, consideration should be given to the use of another class of antihypertensive medications rather than calcium channel blockers. None of these drugs are known to induce gingival enlargement.

Drug substitutions for cyclosporine are more limited. Tacrolimus is another immunosuppressant that is used in organ transplant recipients.[26] The incidence of gingival enlargement in patients receiving tacrolimus therapy is approximately 65% lower than that in individuals who are receiving cyclosporine.[1] Clinical trials have also shown that the substitution of cyclosporine with tacrolimus results in a significant decrease in the severity of gingival enlargement as compared with patients who continue cyclosporine therapy.[15,24,30] In another study,[17] the same drug substitution resulted in a strong decrease or complete resolution of gingival enlargement in more than 70% of the patients who initially presented with cyclosporine-induced gingival enlargement. Therefore, the dental practitioner should consult with the treating physician to investigate the possibility of a change in immunosuppressant therapy as one of the steps in the treatment of cyclosporine-induced gingival enlargement. Patients who take cyclosporine in combination with a calcium channel blocker tend to have an overall lower prevalence of and less severe gingival enlargement if the antihypertensive drug is amlodipine as compared with nifedipine.[16]

> **LEARNING BOX 61.2**
>
> The prescribing of a substitute drug can help reduce gingival enlargement. The drug tacrolimus, which is another drug used as an immunosuppressant, if used as a substitute for cyclosporine can reduce the amount of gingival enlargement by almost 65%.

The administration of the antibiotic azithromycin has been shown to decrease the severity of gingival enlargement induced by cyclosporine. A 3-day course of systemic azithromycin significantly decreased gingival enlargement, and the effect was observed as early as 7 to 30 days after the initiation of antibiotic therapy.[28] The use of azithromycin to decrease cyclosporine-induced gingival enlargement resulted in significantly greater changes than those observed with an improvement in oral hygiene.[22] The topical administration of azithromycin in the form of a toothpaste also decreased the severity of cyclosporine-induced gingival enlargement.[1]

> **LEARNING BOX 61.3**
>
> The decrease in gingival enlargement with the administration of antibiotics indicates the association of plaque biofilm (bacteria) as one cause of gingival enlargement, along with medications such as cyclosporine.

Second, the clinician should emphasize biofilm control as the first step in the treatment of drug-induced gingival enlargement. Although the exact role played by bacterial biofilm is not fully understood, evidence suggests that good oral hygiene, chemotherapeutic agents,[25] and the frequent professional removal of biofilm decrease the degree of gingival enlargement and improve overall gingival health.[10,13,27] The presence of drug-induced enlargement is associated with pseudo-pocket formation, frequently with abundant biofilm accumulation, which may lead to the development of periodontitis. Therefore, meticulous biofilm control helps to maintain attachment levels. In addition, adequate biofilm control may help to prevent the recurrence of gingival enlargement in surgically treated cases.

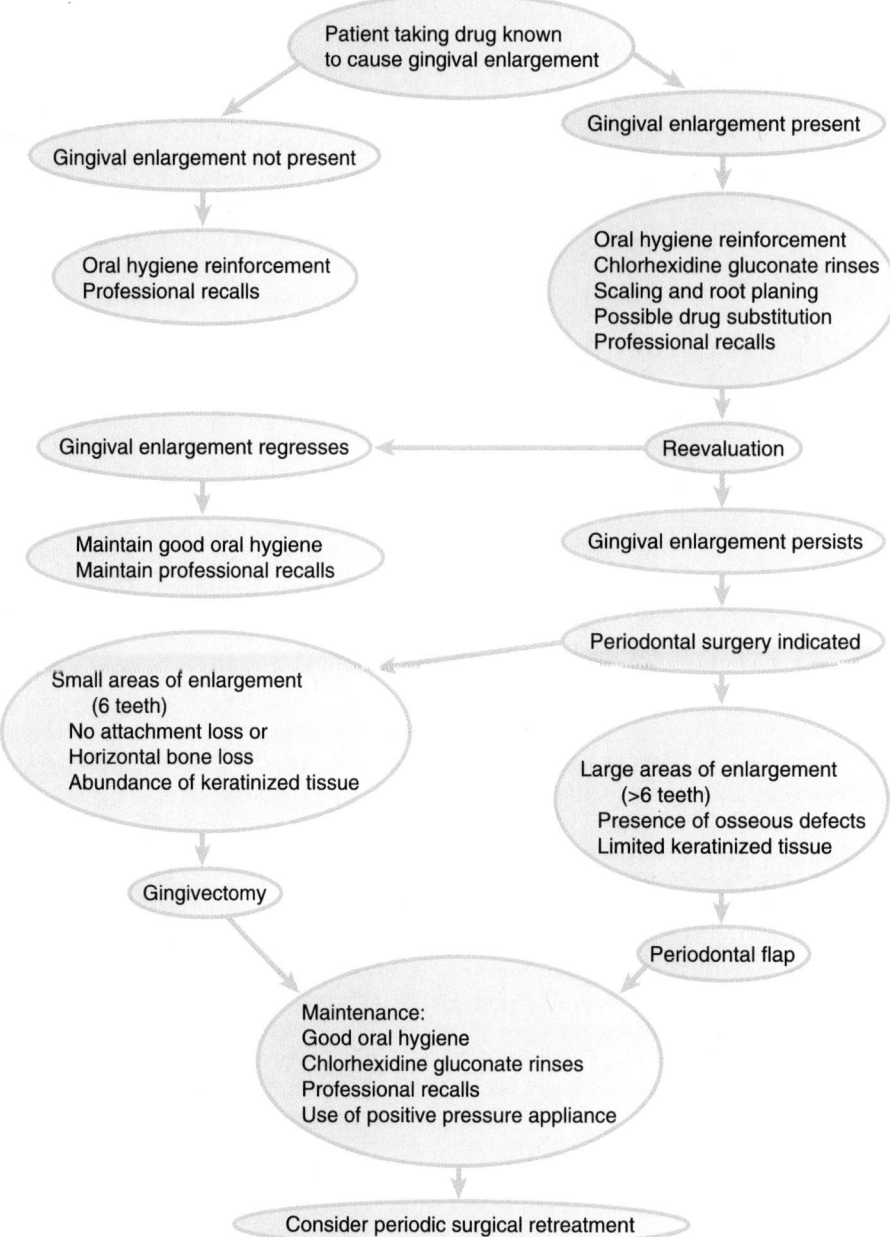

Fig. 61.2 Decision tree for treatment of drug-induced gingival enlargements.

Third, in many patients, gingival enlargement persists after careful consideration of the previous two approaches. With these patients, surgical removal of the enlarged gingiva must be considered.

Fig. 61.2 is a decision tree that outlines the sequence of events and options for the treatment of drug-induced gingival enlargement.

Gingivectomy

The advantages of gingivectomy are the ease and simplicity of the procedure, but it has the disadvantages of more postoperative discomfort and an increased chance of postoperative bleeding. It also sacrifices keratinized tissue and does not allow for osseous recontouring. The flap operation, in contrast, is more technically demanding, but it tends to create less postoperative discomfort and bleeding, besides preserving keratinized tissue. The clinician's decision between the two surgical techniques available should include the extent of the area to be operated on, the severity of the enlargement, the presence of periodontitis and osseous defects, and the

location of the base of the pockets in relation to the mucogingival junction.

In general, small areas (i.e., up to six teeth) of drug-induced gingival enlargement with no evidence of clinical attachment loss (and therefore no anticipated need for osseous surgery) can be effectively treated with the gingivectomy technique. An important consideration is the amount of keratinized tissue present. The removal of excessive amount of keratinized gingiva will create a mucogingival problem.

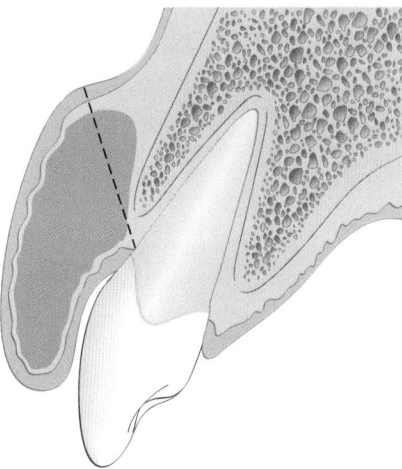

Fig. 61.3 Gingivectomy technique as used to treat patients with drug-induced gingival enlargement. The *dashed line* represents the external bevel incision, and the *shaded area* corresponds to the tissue to be excised. The gingivectomy incision may not remove the entire hyperplastic tissue *(shaded area).* This may leave a wide wound of exposed connective tissue.

Chapters 59 and 60 describes the gingivectomy technique in detail. Fig. 61.3 depicts the procedure diagrammatically, and Fig. 61.4 illustrates a case of cyclosporine-induced gingival enlargement treated with the gingivectomy technique.

Gingivectomy or gingivoplasty can also be performed with electrosurgery or via a laser device[8] (see Chapter 60). Some evidence indicates that recurrence of drug-induced gingival enlargement is reduced in patients treated via laser as compared with conventional gingivectomy or flap surgery.[18]

Flap Operation

For larger areas of gingival enlargement (i.e., more than six teeth), and where attachment loss and osseous defects are present, flap surgery is recommended.

The periodontal flap technique used for the treatment of gingival enlargements is a simple variation of the one used to treat periodontitis, as described in Chapters 59 and 60. Fig. 61.5 shows the basic surgical steps in the use of the flap technique.

The flap surgical technique is as follows:

1. After anesthetizing the area, sounding of the underlying alveolar bone is performed with a periodontal probe to determine the presence and extent of the osseous defects.
2. On the buccal and lingual aspects, with a #15 surgical blade, the initial scalloped internal bevel incision is made at least 3 mm coronal to the mucogingival junction, which includes the creation of new surgical interdental papillae in each interproximal space.
3. The same blade is used to thin the gingival tissues in the buccolingual direction to the mucogingival junction. At this point, the blade establishes contact with the alveolar bone, and a full-thickness or split-thickness flap is elevated.
4. On the palatal aspect, a scalloped internal bevel incision is made at the level of the intended postoperative gingival margin level, which is usually the cementoenamel or more apical in cases where periodontitis is combined with gingival enlargement. The whole extent of the palatal flap is thinned as needed in the apical direction. The base of the flap is then scored to bone and elevated.
5. With the use of an Orban knife, the base of each papilla that connects the facial and the lingual incisions is released.

6. Intrasulcular incisions are made on buccal, lingual, and palatal areas that are being treated to release the tissue collar.
7. The marginal and interdental tissues are removed with curettes.
8. After all tissue tags are removed, the roots are thoroughly scaled and planed, and the bone is recontoured as needed.
9. The flap is replaced or apically displaced and, if necessary, retrimmed to reach the bone–tooth junction exactly (palatal flaps). The flaps are then sutured with an interrupted or a continuous mattress technique, and the area is protected with periodontal dressing.

Sutures and periodontal dressing are removed after 1 to 2 weeks, depending on the extent of the surgery. The patient is instructed to begin biofilm control practices. Usually it is convenient for the patient to use chlorhexidine oral rinses once or twice daily for 2 to 4 weeks.

Fig. 61.6 shows a kidney transplant recipient who was receiving cyclosporine and nifedipine therapy and was treated with the flap technique. Fig. 61.7 depicts the treatment of a 9-year-old kidney transplant recipient whose upper anterior teeth could not break through the enlarged gingival tissues because of their overgrowth, which was induced by cyclosporine therapy; treatment via flap operation allowed for exposure of the anatomic crowns and for the maintenance of keratinized tissue, which could have been completely eliminated if the case had been treated with gingivectomy.

The recurrence of drug-induced gingival enlargement is a reality in surgically treated cases.[23] The major cause of the recurrence of gingival enlargement is the difficulty with postsurgical oral hygiene. Meticulous home care,[7,20] with a soft, postsurgical brush and chlorhexidine gluconate rinses,[27] is indicated. Frequent professional cleanings can also help reduce the degree of recurrence. A hard, rubber, custom-fitted occlusal guard worn at night may also be helpful to control recurrence.[3,31]

Although the periodontal flap approach may be technically more difficult than the gingivectomy procedure, as indicated previously, the postsurgical healing of the flap technique causes less discomfort and decreases the chances of postoperative bleeding. The primary closure of the surgical site with the flap procedure is a great advantage over the secondary open wound that results from the gingivectomy technique. In addition, postsurgical home care can be instituted earlier with the periodontal flap.[6]

Recurrence may occur as early as 3 to 6 months after surgical treatment. In general, surgical results with minimal recurrence are possible for at least 12 months. In one study, healing of flap surgery was compared with that of gingivectomy after a 6-month postsurgical examination. This comparative study of the recurrence of cyclosporine-induced gingival enlargement after periodontal flap surgery compared with that of the gingivectomy technique indicated that the return of the pocket depth took longer with flap surgery.[21]

LEARNING BOX 61.5

The use of flap surgery to reduce gingival enlargement is favored over the gingivectomy technique. By using flap surgery, recurrence of gingival tissue is minimized both in amount of tissue and in time to recurrence.

Leukemic Gingival Enlargement

Leukemic enlargement occurs with acute or subacute leukemia (Fig. 61.8), and it is uncommon among patients in the chronic leukemic state. The patient's bleeding and clotting times and platelet count should be checked before treatment, and the hematologist should be consulted before periodontal treatment is instituted (see Chapters 19 and 39). Gingival bleeding, sometimes spontaneous, is often associated with leukemic gingival enlargement.

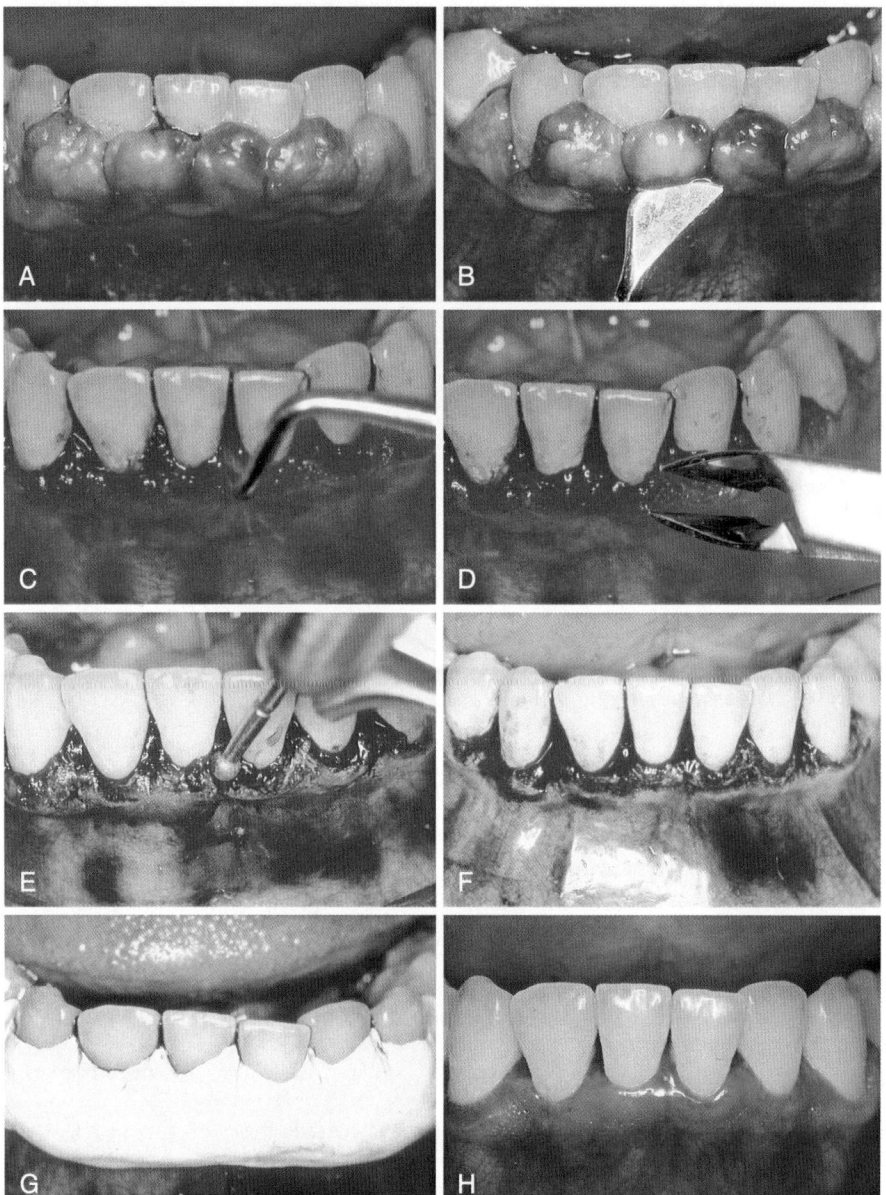

Fig. 61.4 Surgical treatment of cyclosporine-induced gingival enlargement with the use of the gingivectomy technique on a 16-year-old girl who had received a kidney allograft 2 years earlier. (A) Enlarged gingival tissues and pseudo-pocket formation. No attachment loss or radiographic evidence of bone loss existed. (B) Initial external bevel incision performed with a Kirkland knife. (C) Interproximal tissue release achieved with an Orban knife. (D) and (E) Gingivoplasty performed with tissue nippers and a round diamond at high speed with abundant cooling. (F) Aspect of the surgical wound at conclusion of the surgical procedure. (G) Placement of noneugenol periodontal dressing. (H) The surgical area 3 months postoperatively. Note the successful elimination of the enlarged gingival tissue, the restoration of a physiologic gingival contour, and the maintenance of an adequate band of keratinized tissue.

The treatment of periodontal conditions in patients with leukemia is described in Chapters 19 and 30. After acute symptoms subside, attention is directed to correction of the gingival enlargement. The rationale is to remove the local irritating factors to control the inflammatory component of the enlargement, and this is achieved by scaling and root planing. The initial treatment steps consist of gently removing all loose debris with cotton pellets, performing superficial scaling, and instructing the patient in oral hygiene for biofilm control. This hygiene should include, at least initially, the daily use of chlorhexidine mouthrinses. Oral hygiene procedures are extremely important for these patients and, if necessary, may require the assistance of a nurse.

Definitive scaling and root planing are carried out at subsequent visits using local anesthesia. Treatment sessions are confined to a small area of the mouth if hemostasis poses a challenge. Antibiotics are administered systemically the evening before and for a week after each treatment to reduce the risk of infection.

Gingival Enlargement During Pregnancy

Treatment requires the elimination of all local irritants that may be responsible for precipitating the gingival changes that occur during pregnancy. The elimination of local irritants early in pregnancy is

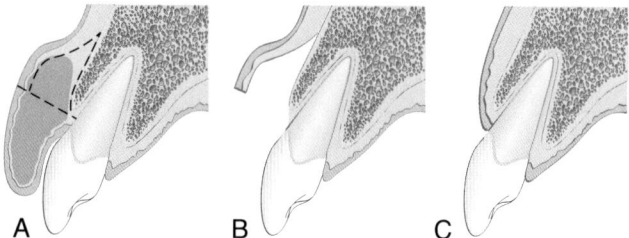

Fig. 61.5 Periodontal flap treatment for drug-induced gingival enlargement. (A) Initial reverse bevel incision followed by thinning of the enlarged gingival tissue; *dotted lines* represent incisions, and the *shaded area* represents the tissue portion to be excised. (B) After flap elevation, the enlarged portion of the gingival tissue is removed. (C) The flap is placed on top of the alveolar bone and sutured.

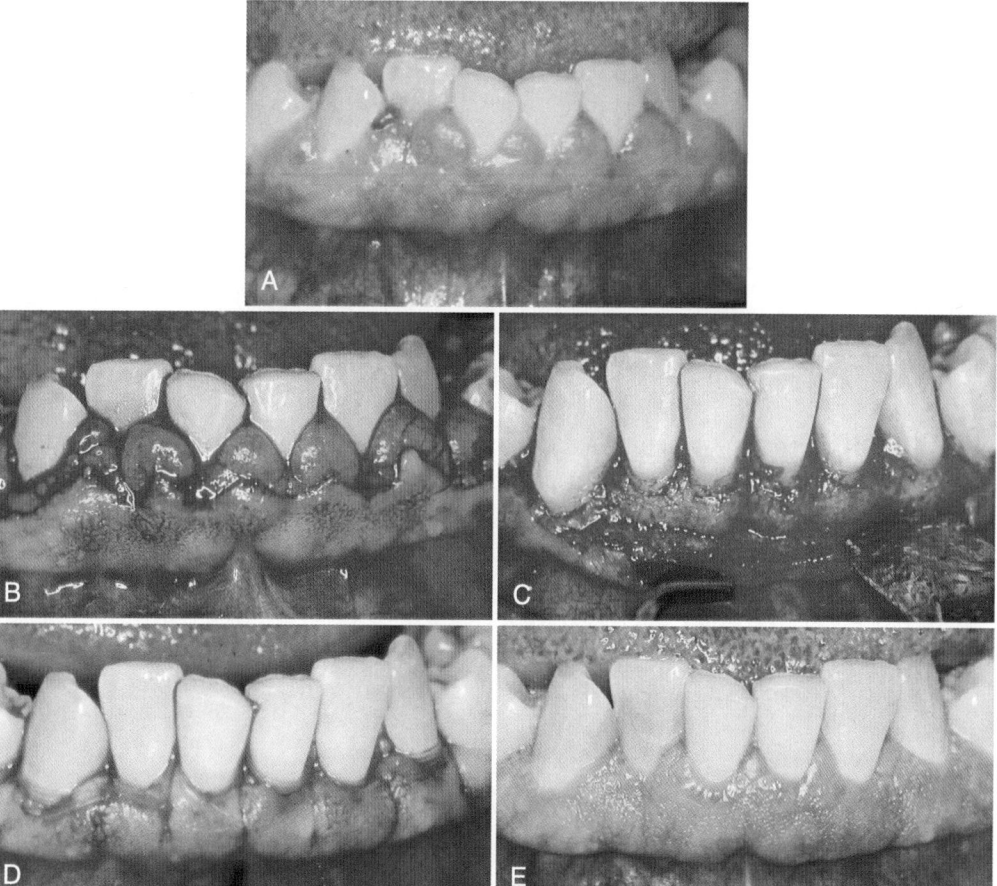

Fig. 61.6 Treatment of combined cyclosporine and nifedipine–induced gingival enlargement with a periodontal flap on a 35-year-old female patient who had received a kidney allograft 3 years earlier. (A) Presurgical clinical aspect of the lower anterior teeth, showing severe gingival enlargement. (B) Initial scalloped reverse bevel incision, including maintenance of keratinized tissue and creation of surgical papillae. (C) Elevation of a full-thickness flap and removal of the inner portion of the previously thinned gingival tissue. After scaling and root planing, osseous recontouring can be performed if necessary. (D) The flap is positioned on top of the alveolar crest. (E) Postsurgical aspect of the treated area at 12 months. Note the reduction of enlarged tissue volume and acceptable gingival health.

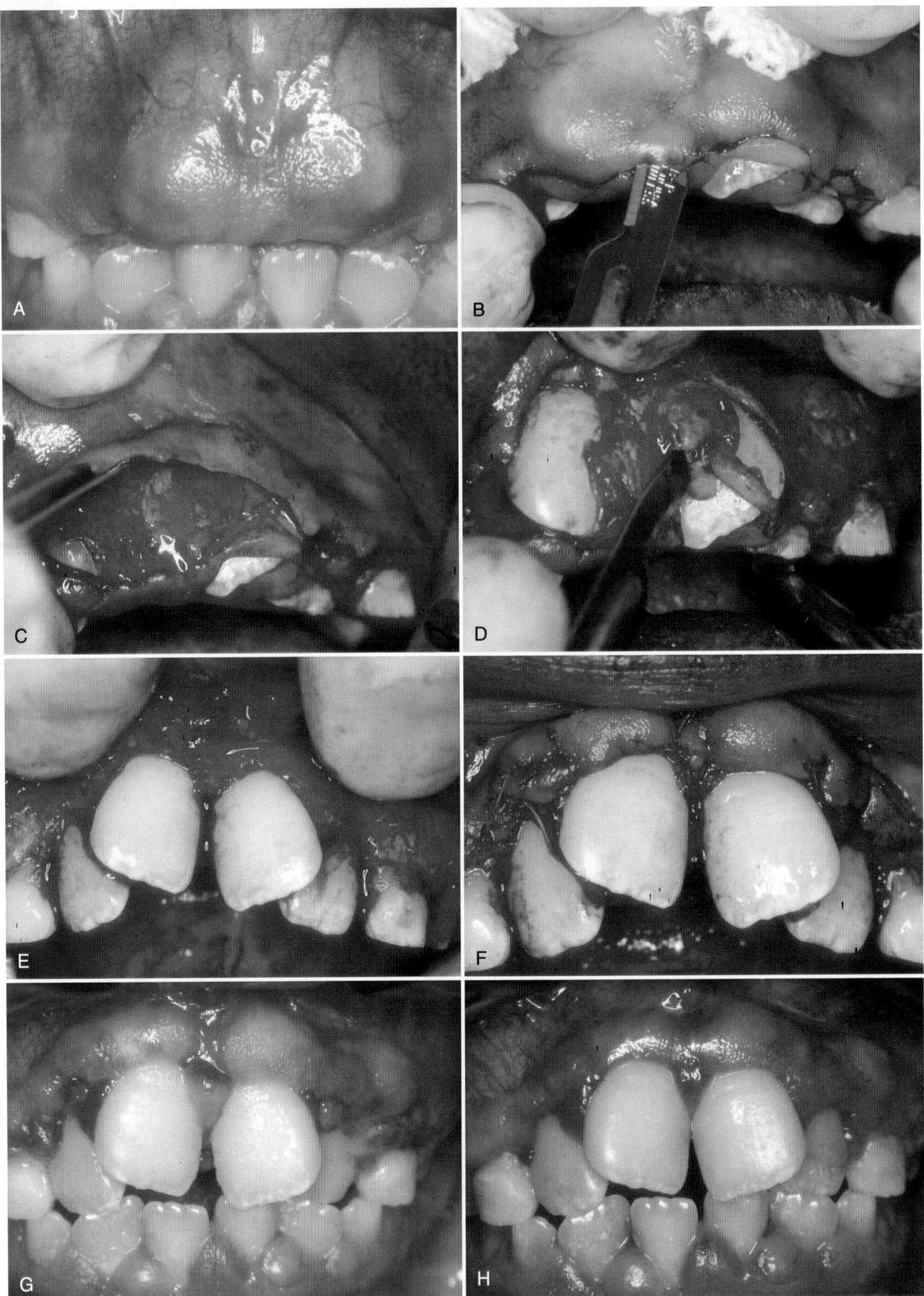

Fig. 61.7 Treatment of a 9-year old recipient of an allogeneic kidney transplant who had been receiving Cyclosporin A and nifedipine therapy for $2\frac{1}{2}$ years. Surgical treatment was with an apically positioned flap. (A) Upper incisors were in an occluding position, but they did not erupt through the drug-enlarged gingival tissues. (B) Crestal reversed bevel incision maintaining most of the buccal keratinized tissue. (C) Flap thinning via split-thickness dissection. (D) Removal of excess gingival connective tissue on the buccal surfaces of the anterior teeth and interproximal spaces. (E) Clinical crowns fully exposed; periosteum preserved over alveolar bone. (F) Flap was apically positioned and sutured to periosteum with 5-0 plain gut. (G) Healing at 14 days after surgery. (H) Healing at 3 months postoperatively with acceptable gingival health and presence of adequate buccal keratinized tissue.

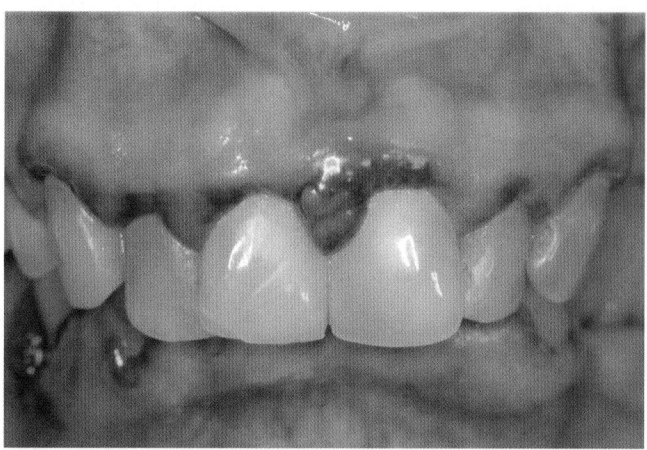

Fig. 61.8 A 74-year-old patient with acute leukemia. Gingival enlargement is observed in combination with a hemorrhagic appearance, which sometimes causes spontaneous bleeding.

a preventive measure against gingival disease, and prevention is preferable to treatment of gingival enlargement after it occurs. Marginal and interdental gingival inflammation and enlargement are treated by scaling and root planing (see Chapters 48, 50, and 51). Treatment of tumor-like gingival enlargements consists of surgical excision, as well as the scaling and planing of the tooth surfaces adjacent to the lesion. The enlargement may recur unless all irritants are removed. Food impaction is frequently an inciting factor.

Gingival lesions during pregnancy should be treated as soon as they are detected, although not necessarily by surgical means. Scaling and root planing procedures and adequate oral hygiene measures may reduce the extent of the enlargement. Gingival enlargements do shrink after pregnancy, but they usually do not disappear. After pregnancy, the entire periodontal status of the patient should be reevaluated, and comprehensive treatment should be undertaken.

Lesions should be removed surgically during pregnancy if they interfere with mastication or produce an aesthetic disfigurement that bothers the patient.

During pregnancy, the emphasis should be on (1) preventing gingival disease before it occurs and (2) treating existing gingival disease before it worsens. All patients should be seen as early as possible after becoming pregnant. Patients without gingival disease should be examined for potential sources of local irritation and should be instructed on meticulous oral hygiene procedures. In addition, patients who already have signs and symptoms of periodontal disease should be treated promptly, before the effect of pregnancy on the gingiva becomes manifest. Chapter 41 presents the necessary precautions for the periodontal treatment of pregnant women.

Every pregnant patient should be scheduled for periodic maintenance visits. The importance of such visits in the prevention of serious periodontal disturbances should be stressed.

Gingival Enlargement During Puberty

Gingival enlargement during puberty is treated by performing scaling and root planing, removing all sources of irritation, and controlling biofilm. Surgical removal may be required in severe cases. The most important problem in these young patients is recurrence, for which close maintenance therapy is recommended.

 A Case Scenario is found on the companion website www.expertconsult.com.

References

 References for this chapter are found on the companion website www.expertconsult.com.

CHAPTER 62

Resective Osseous Surgery

Thomas N. Sims | Henry H. Takei

 For online-only content on osseous resection technique, flap placement and closure, postoperative maintenance, and specific osseous reshaping situations, please visit the companion website at www.expertconsult.com.

The damage resulting from periodontal disease manifests in variable destruction of the tooth-supporting bone. Generally, bony deformities are not uniform; they are not indicative of the alveolar housing of the tooth before the disease process and do not reflect the overlying gingival architecture. Bone loss has been classified as either "horizontal" or "vertical," but in fact, bone loss is most often a combination of horizontal and vertical loss. Horizontal bone loss generally results in a relative thickening of the marginal alveolar bone because bone tapers as it approaches its most coronal margin.

The effects of this thickening and the development of vertical defects leave the alveolar bone with countless combinations of bony shapes. If these various topographic changes are to be altered to provide a more physiologic bone pattern, a method for osseous recontouring must be followed.

Osseous surgery may be defined as the procedure by which changes in the alveolar bone can be accomplished to rid it of deformities induced by the periodontal disease process or other related factors such as exostosis and tooth supraeruption.

Osseous surgery can be either additive or subtractive. *Additive osseous surgery* includes procedures directed at restoring the alveolar bone to its original level, whereas *subtractive osseous surgery* is designed to restore the form of preexisting alveolar bone to the level present at the time of surgery or slightly more apical to this level (Fig. 62.1).

Additive osseous surgery brings about the ideal result of periodontal therapy; it implies regeneration of lost bone and reestablishment of the periodontal ligament, gingival fibers, and junctional epithelium at a more coronal level. This type of osseous surgery is discussed in Chapter 63.

Subtractive osseous surgery procedures provide an alternative to additive methods and should be used when additive procedures are not feasible.[4] These subtractive procedures are discussed in this chapter.

Selection of Treatment Technique

The morphology of the osseous defect largely determines the treatment technique to be used. *One-wall angular defects* usually need to be recontoured surgically. *Three-wall defects,* particularly if they are narrow and deep, can be successfully treated with techniques that strive for new attachment and bone reconstruction. *Two-wall angular defects* can be treated with either method, depending on their depth, width, and general configuration. Therefore, except for one-wall defects and wide, shallow two-wall defects, and interdental craters, osseous defects are treated with the objective of obtaining optimal repair by natural healing processes.

Rationale

Osseous resective surgery necessitates following a series of strict guidelines for proper contouring of alveolar bone and subsequent management of the overlying gingival soft tissues. The specifics of these techniques are discussed later in this chapter. The techniques discussed here for osseous resective surgery have limited applicability in deep intrabony or hemiseptal defects, which could be treated with a different surgical approach (see Chapter 63). Osseous surgery provides the purest and surest method for reducing pockets with bony discrepancies that are not overly vertical and also remains one of the principal periodontal modalities because of its long-term success and predictability.

Osseous resective surgery is the most predictable pocket reduction technique.[10–12] However, more than any other surgical technique, osseous resective surgery is performed at the expense of bony tissue and attachment level.[1,2,8] Thus its value as a surgical approach is limited by the presence, quantity, and shape of the bony tissues and by the amount of attachment loss that is acceptable.

The major rationale for osseous resective surgery is based on the tenet that discrepancies in level and shapes of the bone and gingiva

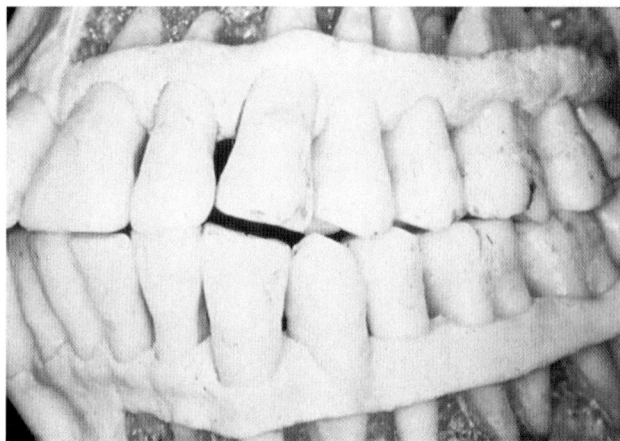

Fig. 62.2 Photograph of a healthy bony periodontium in a skull. Although a slight amount of attachment may have been lost, this skull demonstrates the characteristics of normal form.

Fig. 62.1

Fig. 62.1 Additive and subtractive osseous surgery. (A) Before and (B) immediately after subtractive osseous surgery; the osseous wall of the two adjoining infrabony pockets has been removed. (C) Before and (D) 1 year after additive osseous surgery; the area has been flapped and thoroughly instrumented, resulting in reconstruction of the interdental and periapical bone. *(Courtesy Drs. E.A. Albano and B.O. Barletta, Buenos Aires, Argentina.)*

predispose patients to the recurrence of pocket depth postsurgically.[6] Although this concept is not universally accepted,[3,5] and the procedure induces loss of radicular bone in the healing phase, recontouring of bone is the only logical treatment choice in some cases. The goal of osseous resective therapy is to reshape the marginal bone to resemble that of the alveolar process undamaged by periodontal disease. The technique is performed in combination with apically positioned flaps, and the procedure eliminates periodontal pocket depth and improves tissue contour to provide a more easily maintainable environment.[4] The relative merits of pocket reduction procedures are discussed in Chapter 60; this chapter discusses the osseous resective technique and how and where it may be accomplished.

 KEY FACT

Bone dictates the form of the gingiva and determines much of the residual pocket depth.

It is proposed that the conversion of the periodontal pocket to a shallow gingival sulcus enhances the patient's ability to remove plaque and oral debris from the dentition. Similarly, the ability of dental professionals to maintain the periodontium in a state free of gingivitis and periodontitis is more predictable in the presence of shallow sulci. The more effective the periodontal maintenance

therapy, the greater is the longitudinal stability of the surgical result. The efficacy of osseous surgery therefore depends on its ability to affect pocket depth and to promote periodontal maintenance.[11,22,23] The merits of resection versus other treatment procedures are discussed in Chapter 63.

Normal Alveolar Bone Morphology

Knowledge of the morphology of the bony periodontium in a state of health is required to perform resective osseous surgery correctly (Fig. 62.2). The characteristics of a normal bony form are as follows:
1. The interproximal bone is more coronal in position than the labial or lingual-palatal bone and pyramidal in form.
2. The form of the interdental bone is a function of the tooth form and the embrasure width. The more tapered the tooth, the more pyramidal is the bony form. The wider the embrasure, the more flattened is the interdental bone mesiodistally and buccolingually.
3. The position of the bony margin mimics the contours of the cementoenamel junction. The distance from the facial bony margin of the tooth to the interproximal bony crest is flatter in the posterior than the anterior areas. This "scalloping" of the bone on the facial surfaces and lingual-palatal surfaces is related to tooth and root form, as well as tooth position within the alveolus. Teeth with prominent roots or those displaced to the facial or lingual side may also have fenestrations or dehiscences (Fig. 62.3). The molar teeth have less scalloping and a flatter profile than bicuspids and incisors.

Although these general observations apply to all patients, the bony architecture may vary from patient to patient in the extent of contour, configuration, and thickness. These variations may be both normal and healthy.

Terminology

Numerous terms have been developed to describe the topography of the alveolar housing, the procedure for its removal, and the resulting correction. These terms should be clearly defined.

Procedures used to correct osseous defects have been classified in two groups: osteoplasty and ostectomy.[7] *Osteoplasty* refers to reshaping the bone without removing tooth-supporting bone. *Ostectomy,* or *osteoectomy,* includes the removal of tooth-supporting bone. One or both of these procedures may be necessary to produce the desired result.

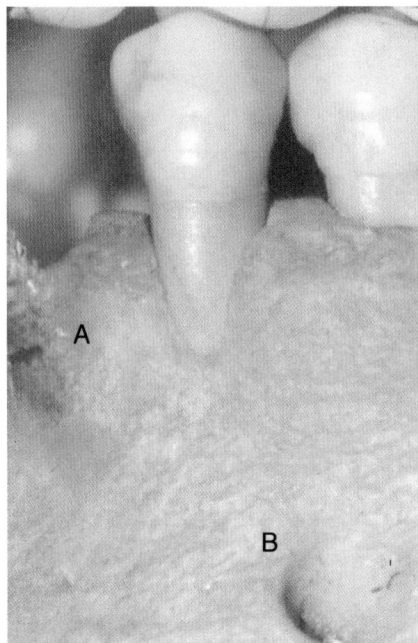

Fig. 62.3 Effects of tooth position on facial bony contours. Bony dehiscence *(A)* and bony fenestration *(B)*. These deformities can and should be detected by palpation, probing, and sounding before flap surgery.

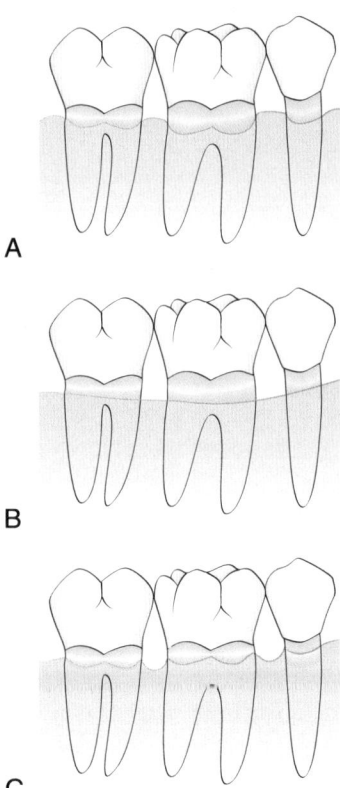

Fig. 62.4 Diagram of types of bony architecture. (A) Positive bony architecture. (B) Flat bony architecture. (C) Reversed, or negative, bony form.

Terms that describe the bone form after reshaping can refer to morphologic features or to the thoroughness of the reshaping performed. Examples of morphologically descriptive terms include *negative, positive, flat,* and *ideal*. These terms all relate to a preconceived standard of ideal osseous form.

Positive architecture and *negative architecture* refer to the relative position of interdental bone to radicular bone (Fig. 62.4). The architecture is "positive" if the radicular bone is apical to the interdental bone. The bone has "negative" architecture if the interdental bone is more apical than the radicular bone. *Flat architecture* is the reduction of the interdental bone to the same height as the radicular bone.

Osseous form is considered to be "ideal" when the bone is consistently more coronal on the interproximal surfaces than on the facial and lingual surfaces. The ideal form of the marginal bone has similar interdental height, with gradual, curved slopes between interdental peaks (Fig. 62.5).

Terms that relate to the thoroughness of the osseous reshaping techniques include "definitive" and "compromise." *Definitive osseous reshaping* implies that further osseous reshaping would not improve the overall result. *Compromise osseous reshaping* indicates a bone pattern that cannot be improved without significant osseous removal that would be detrimental to the overall result. References to compromise and definitive osseous architecture can be useful to the clinician, not as description of a morphologic feature, but as terms that express the expected therapeutic result.

Factors in Selection of Resective Osseous Surgery

The relationship between the depth and configuration of the bony lesion or lesions with root morphology and the adjacent teeth determines the extent that bone and attachment are removed during resection. Bony lesions have been classified according to their configuration and number of bony walls.[9] The technique of ostectomy is best applied to patients with early to moderate bone loss (2 to

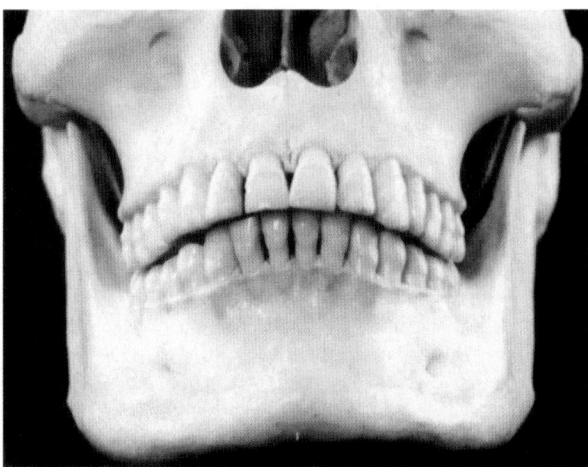

Fig. 62.5 Skull photograph of healthy periodontium. Note the shape of the alveolar bone housing. This bone is considered to have ideal form. It is more coronal in the interproximal areas, with a gradual slope around and away from the tooth.

3 mm) with moderate-length root trunks[18] that have bony defects with one or two walls. These shallow to moderate bony defects can be effectively managed by osteoplasty and ostectomy. Patients with advanced attachment loss and deep intrabony defects are not candidates for resection to produce a positive contour. To simulate a normal architectural form, so much bone would have to be removed that the survival of the teeth could be compromised.

Two-walled defects, or craters, occur at the expense of the interseptal bone. As a result, they have buccal and lingual or palatal walls that extend from one tooth to the adjacent tooth. The interdental loss of bone exposes the proximal aspects of both adjacent teeth.

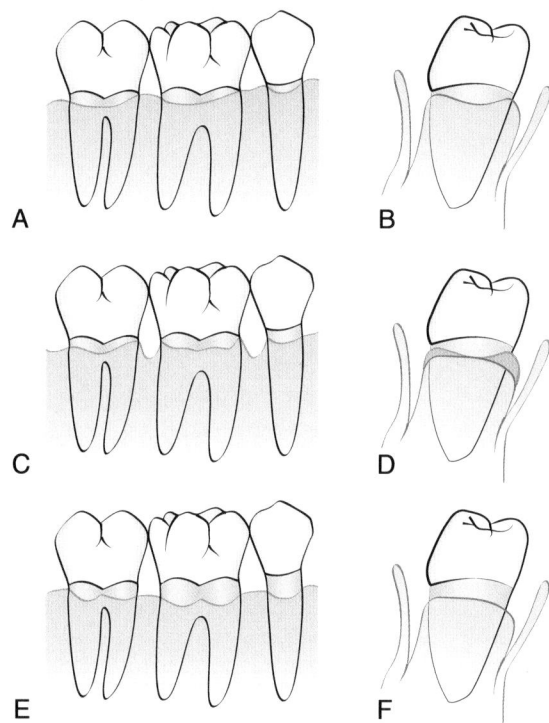

A

B

C

D

E

F

Fig. 62.6 Effect of correction of craters. (A) and (B) Facial and interproximal bony contours after flap reflection. Note the loss of some interproximal bone and cratering. (C) and (D) Line angles; this is only osteoplasty and has resulted in a reversed architecture. (E) and (F) Ostectomy on the facial and lingual bone and the removal of the residual widow's peaks to produce a positive bony architecture.

The buccal-lingual interproximal contour that results is opposite to the contour of the cementoenamel junction of the teeth (Fig. 62.6A and B). *Two-walled defects* (*craters*) *are the most common bony defects found in patients with periodontitis.*[14,20] If the facial and lingual plates of this bone are resected, the resultant interproximal contour would become more flattened or ovate (Fig. 62.6C and D). However, confining resection only to ledges and the interproximal lesion results in a facial and lingual bone form in which the interproximal bone is located more apically than the bone on the facial or lingual aspects of the tooth. This resulting anatomic form is reversed, or negative, architecture[17,18,22] (see Fig. 62.6C and D).

Although the production of a reversed architecture minimizes the amount of ostectomy that is performed, it is not without consequences.[5] Peaks of bone typically remain at the facial and lingual-palatal line angles of the teeth (*widow's peaks*). During healing, the soft tissue tends to bridge the embrasure from the most coronal height of the bone on one tooth to the most coronal heights on the adjacent teeth. The result is therefore the tendency to replicate the attachment contour on the tooth. The interproximal soft tissues invest these peaks of bone, which may subsequently resorb with a tendency to rebound without gain in attachment over time. Interproximal pocket depth can recur.[22,24]

Ostectomy to a positive architecture requires the removal of the line–angle inconsistencies (widow's peaks), as well as some of the facial, lingual, and palatal and interproximal bone. The result is a loss of some attachment on the facial and lingual root surfaces but a topography that more closely resembles normal bone form before disease (see Fig. 62.6E and F). Proponents of osseous resection to create a positive contour believe that this architecture, devoid of sharp angles and spines, is conducive to the formation of a more uniform and reduced soft tissue dimension postoperatively.[17,21] The

therapeutic results are less pocket depth and increased ease of periodontal maintenance by the patient, dental hygienist, or dentist.

The amount of attachment lost from the use of ostectomy varies with the depth and configuration of the treated osseous defects. Osseous resection applied to two-wall intrabony defects (craters), the most common osseous defects, results in attachment loss at the proximal line angles and the facial and lingual aspects of the affected teeth without affecting the base of the pocket. The extent of attachment loss during resection to a positive architecture has been measured. When the technique is properly applied to appropriate patients, the mean reduction in attachment circumferentially around the tooth has been determined to be 0.6 mm at six probing sites.[22] In practical terms, this means that the technique is best applied to interproximal lesions 1 to 3 mm deep in patients with moderate to long root trunks.[17] Patients with deep, multiwalled defects are not candidates for resective osseous surgery. They are better treated with regenerative therapies or by combining osteoplasty to reduce bony ledges and to facilitate flap closure with new attachment and regeneration procedures.

KEY FACT

Osseous resective surgery should never compromise the prognosis of the tooth.

Examination and Treatment Planning

The potential for the use of resective osseous surgery is usually identified during a comprehensive periodontal examination. Suitable patients display the signs and symptoms of periodontitis (see Chapter 32). The gingiva may be inflamed, and deposits of plaque, calculus, and oral debris may be present. An increased flow of crevicular fluid may be detected, and bleeding on probing and exudation are often observed.

Periodontal probing and exploration are key aspects of the examination. Careful probing reveals the presence of (1) pocket depth greater than that of a normal gingival sulcus, (2) the location of the base of the pocket relative to the mucogingival junction and attachment level on adjacent teeth, (3) the number of bony walls, and (4) the presence of furcation defects. Transgingival probing, or sounding, using local anesthesia confirms the extent and configuration of the intrabony component of the pocket and of furcation defects.[6,16]

Routine dental radiographs do not identify the presence of periodontitis and do not accurately document the extent of bony defects. Radiographs cannot accurately document the number of bony walls and the presence or extent of bony lesions on the facial-buccal or lingual-palatal walls. Well-made radiographs provide useful information about the extent of interproximal bone loss, the presence of angular bone loss, caries, root trunk length, and root morphology. Films also facilitate the identification of other dental pathoses that require treatment. In addition, a radiographic survey serves as a means of evaluating the success of therapy and documenting the patient's longitudinal stability.[19]

Treatment planning should provide solutions for active periodontal diseases and correction of deformities that result from periodontitis. Planning should also facilitate the performance of other dental procedures included in a comprehensive dental treatment plan. The extent of periodontal involvement can vary significantly from tooth to tooth in the same patient. The response to therapy from patient to patient may also vary, as may the treatment objectives for the patients. Therefore a treatment plan may encompass a number of steps and combinations of procedures in the same surgical area.

After oral hygiene instruction, scaling and root planing, and other disease control procedures, the response of the patient to these treatment procedures is evaluated by reexamination and recording the changes in the periodontium. Because the extent of periodontal involvement can vary significantly from tooth to tooth in the same patient, the local response to therapy is also variable. The resolution of inflammation and decrease in edema and swelling may have resulted in a return to normal depth and configuration of some pockets, and additional therapy beyond periodic maintenance may not be required.

The patient with moderate to advanced periodontitis and bony defects may display a persistence of pocket depth bleeding on probing and suppuration, although the overt signs of periodontitis may be reduced. These signs may indicate the presence of residual plaque and calculus, attributable to the difficulty of achieving instrumentation in these deep pockets or the patient's inability or unwillingness to perform adequate oral hygiene in these sites. Patients with inadequate oral hygiene are not good candidates for periodontal surgery. If the supragingival plaque or biofilm control is good and the residual pocket depths are 5 mm or more, patients with such areas may be candidates for periodontal surgery.[13]

Resective osseous surgery is also used to facilitate certain restorative and prosthetic dental procedures. Dental caries can be exposed for restoration; fractured roots of abutment teeth can be exposed for removal; and bony exostoses and ridge deformities can be altered in contour to improve the performance of removable or fixed prostheses (Fig. 62.7). Severely decayed teeth or teeth with short anatomic crowns can be lengthened by resection or by a combination of orthodontic tooth extrusion and osseous resection. Such procedures allow the therapist to expose more tooth for restoration, prevent an invasion of the biologic width of attachment, and create a periodontal attachment of normal dimension.[8,15] Resection can also provide a means of producing optimal crown length for cosmetic purposes.

Methods of Resective Osseous Surgery

The reshaping process is fundamentally an attempt to gradualize the bone sufficiently to allow soft tissue structures to follow the contour of the bone. The soft tissue predictably attaches to the bone within certain specific dimensions. The length and quality of connective tissue and junctional epithelium that reform in the surgical site depend on numerous factors, including the health of the tissue, condition and topography of the root surface, and proximity of the bone surrounding the tooth. Each of these factors must be controlled to the best of the clinician's ability to obtain the optimal result, making osseous resective surgery an extremely precise technique.

It is assumed in this chapter that the gingival tissue has been reflected by the apically positioned flap described in Chapter 60. Reshaping of the bone may necessitate selective changes in gingival height. These changes must be calculated and accounted for in the initial flap design. For this reason, it is important for the clinician to know about the underlying bone tissue before flap reflection. The clinician must gain as much indirect knowledge as possible from soft tissue palpation, radiographic assessment, and transgingival probing (sounding).

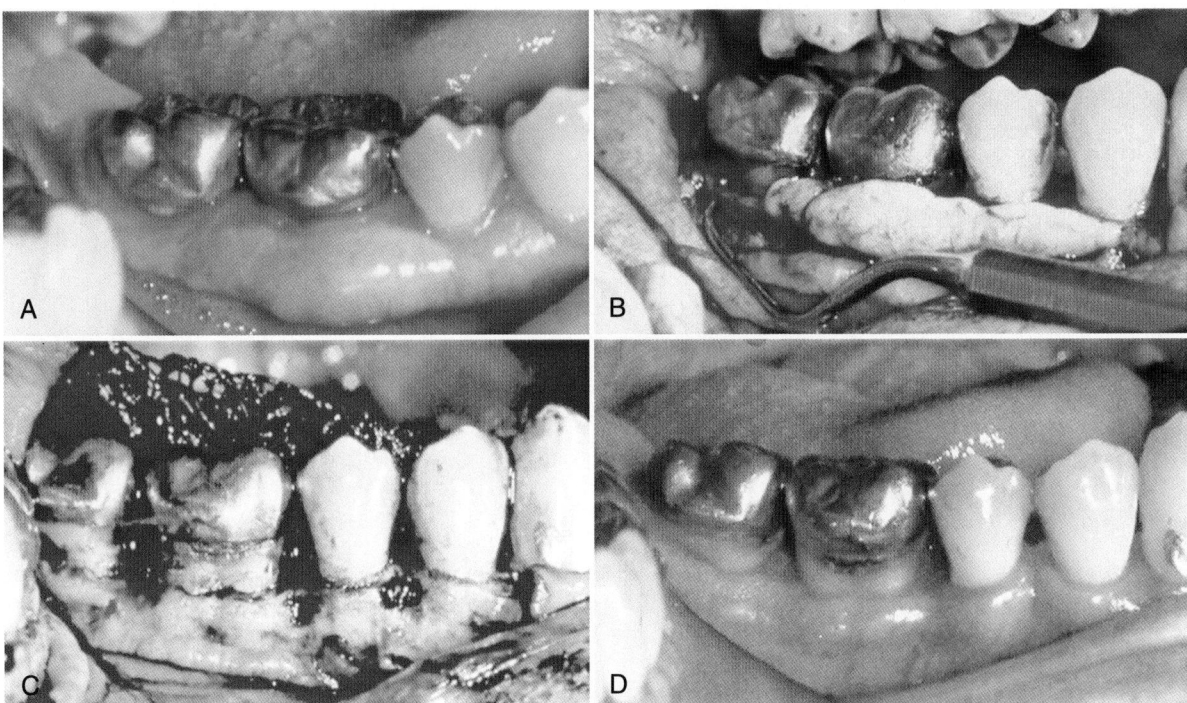

Fig. 62.7 Reduction of bony ledges and exposure of caries by osteoplasty. (A) Buccal preoperative photograph showing two crowns, exostoses, and caries. (B) Flap reflected to reveal caries on both molars at the restoration margins, interdental cratering, and a facial exostosis. (C) After osseous surgery; the bulk of the bony removal was by osteoplasty, with minor ostectomy between the two molars. The caries is now exposed, and the crowns are lengthened for restoration. (D) Postoperative photograph at 6 weeks. Plaque control is deficient, but the teeth should be readily restorable at this time. *(Courtesy Dr. Joseph Schwartz, Portland, OR.)*

Radiographic examination can reveal the existence of angular bone loss in the interdental spaces; these areas usually coincide with intrabony pockets. The radiograph does not show the number of bony walls of the defect or document with any accuracy the presence of angular cone defects on facial or lingual surfaces. Clinical examination and probing are used to determine the presence and depth of periodontal pockets on any surface of any tooth and can also provide a general sense of the bony topography, although intrabony pockets can go undetected by probing. Both clinical and radiographic examinations can indicate the presence of intrabony pockets when the clinician finds (1) angular bone loss, (2) irregular bone loss, or (3) pockets of irregular depth in adjacent areas of the same tooth or adjacent teeth.

The experienced clinician can use transgingival probing to predict many features of the underlying bony topography. The information thus obtained can change the treatment plan. For example, an area that had been selected for osseous resective surgery may be found to have a narrow defect that was unnoticed in the initial probing and radiographic assessment and is ideal for augmentation procedures. Such findings can and do change the flap design, osseous procedure, and results expected from the surgical intervention. Transgingival probing is extremely useful just before flap reflection. It is necessary to anesthetize the tissue locally before inserting the probe. The probe should be "walked" along the tissue–tooth interface so that the operator can feel the bony topography. The probe may also be passed horizontally through the tissue to provide three-dimensional information regarding bony contours (i.e., thickness, height, and shape of the underlying base). However, this information is still "blind," and although it is undoubtedly better than probing alone, it has significant limitations. Nevertheless, this step is recommended immediately before the surgical intervention.

The situations that can be encountered after periodontal flap reflection vary greatly. When all soft tissue is removed around the teeth, there may be larger exostoses, ledges, troughs, craters, vertical defects, or combinations of these defects. Therefore, each osseous situation presents uniquely challenging problems, especially if reshaping to the optimal level is contemplated.

Conclusion

Although osseous surgical techniques cannot be applied to every bony abnormality or topographic modification, it has been clearly demonstrated that properly used osseous surgery can eliminate and modify defects, as well as gradualize excessive bony ledges, irregular alveolar bone, early furcation involvement, excessive bony exostosis, and circumferential defects. When properly performed, resective osseous surgery achieves a physiologic architecture of marginal alveolar bone conducive to gingival flap adaptation with minimal probing depth. The advantages of this surgical modality include a predictable amount of pocket reduction that can enhance oral hygiene and periodic maintenance. It also preserves the width of the attached tissue while removing granulomatous tissue and providing access for debridement of the radicular surfaces. In addition, the osseous resection technique permits recontouring of bony abnormalities, including hemiseptal defects, tori, and ledges. Its substantial benefits include proper assessment for restorative procedures (e.g., crown lengthening) and assessment of restorative overhangs and tooth abnormalities (e.g., enamel projections, enamel pearls, perforations, fractures). Consequently, resective osseous surgery can be an important technique in the armamentarium necessary to provide a maintainable periodontium for periodontal patients.

 A Case Scenario is found on the companion website www.expertconsult.com.

References

 References for this chapter are found on the companion website www.expertconsult.com.

CHAPTER 63

Periodontal Regeneration and Reconstructive Surgery

Richard T. Kao | Henry H. Takei | David L. Cochran

 For online-only content on non–graft-associated reconstructive procedures of historical interest, as well as expanded discussions on assessment of periodontal wound healing, guided tissue regeneration, graft-associated reconstructive procedures of historical interest, factors that influence therapeutic success, and future directions for periodontal regeneration, please visit the companion website at www.expertconsult.com.

Intrabony and furcation defects are sequelae of periodontal disease. Ideally, these defects are managed in a timely fashion through periodontal regeneration. In the past, the results of regenerative therapy were inconsistent and unpredictable. The current status of regenerative therapy has dramatically changed and improved due to research and a better understanding of the biology of the tissues that comprise the periodontal attachment. The various surgical approaches including bone replacement grafts, guided tissue regeneration (GTR), and a better understanding of biologic mediators and tissue engineering have improved the predictability of regeneration as another choice for therapy. This chapter reviews the current strategies and clinical decision making for optimizing regenerative success.

When the periodontium is damaged by inflammation or as a result of surgical treatment, the defect heals either through periodontal regeneration or repair.* In periodontal regeneration, healing occurs through the reconstitution of a new periodontium, which involves the formation of alveolar bone, functionally aligned periodontal ligament, and new cementum. Alternatively, repair due to healing by replacement with epithelial and/or connective tissue that matures into various nonfunctional types of scar tissue is termed *new attachment*. Histologically, patterns of repair include long junctional epithelium, ankylosis, and/or new attachment (see Chapter 3). Although the stability of periodontal repair is not clear, the ideal goal of periodontal surgical therapy is periodontal regeneration.

Today, several highly reproducible regenerative approaches are used, as evidenced by clinical attachment gain, decreased pocket probing depth, radiographic evidence consistent with bone fill, and overall improvements in periodontal health. These clinical improvements can be maintained over long periods (>10 years).[2,9,136,243]

Assessment of Periodontal Wound Healing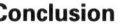

It is sometimes difficult in clinical and experimental situations to determine whether regeneration or new attachment has occurred and the extent to which it has occurred. Although various types of evidence of reconstruction exist, the *proof of principle* for the type of healing is determined by histologic studies. Once defined, the evidence found subsequently by clinical, radiographic, and surgical reentry findings is implied.[36,37,168] All these methods have advantages and shortcomings that should be well understood and considered in individual cases and when critically evaluating the literature. A comparative analysis of regenerative approaches is detailed in Table 63.1.

LEARNING BOX 63.1

It is difficult to obtain *proof of principle* for periodontal regeneration with today's bioethics because of the *human* histologic requirements for the regeneration of new bone, cementum, and periodontal ligament. A need exists for redefining periodontal regeneration with a broader basis for acceptance of *proof of principle*. This may include proofs through animal models.

Reconstructive Surgical Techniques

Reconstructive techniques can be subdivided into three major therapeutic approaches: non–bone graft–associated, graft-associated, and biologic mediator–associated new attachment and regeneration. In clinical practice, it is common for clinicians to combine these various approaches.†

---

*References 66, 84, 176, 195, 202, 217, 232, 242.

†References 9, 84, 104, 136, 164, 242, 243.

TABLE 63.1 Comparative Analysis of Regenerative Approaches

Graft Material	CAL Gain (mm)	Defect Fill (% or mm)	Histologic Assessment	Comments
Autologous				
Extraoral (iliac crest)	3.3–4.2[259] • 2.60 mm in 0-wall • 3.75 mm in 1-wall • 4.16 mm in 2-wall	—	33 of 39 defects showed evidence of regeneration[49]	Only evidence of regeneration in 0-wall and (2.5 mm) supracrestal regeneration
Intraoral autologous	2.88–3.44 mm[36,73,79,117]	73%[47]	0.7 mm of regeneration[49,55]	Only one controlled study with 2.98 mm of bone gain vs. 0.66 mm with debridement[47] No significant difference in one study[54]
Allograft (vital)				
Human vital	3.6 mm mean[259] • 3.6 mm in 1-, 2-, and 3-wall • 2.1 mm in 0-wall	—	Evidence of regeneration[49]	Potential risk of disease transmission
Allograft (Nonvital)				
FDBA	2.0 mm mean[174,180,256,277]	60%–68% of 1401 defects had ≥50% fill[61–64]	None available	Only controlled study using paired defects shows no difference between FDBA vs. debridement[65] No histologic study of healing pattern The addition of autologous osseous coagulum enhances healing
Comparative Studies				
FDBA vs. FDBA + autologous graft	—	63%–67% had ≥50% fill 78%–80% had ≥50% fill[62]		
Allograft (Nonvital)				
DFDBA vs. debridement	2.3–2.9 mm vs. 0.3–1.3 mm[177,217]	65% vs. 11%[72,73,78]	1.21 mm of periodontal regeneration[70,71]	
Comparative Studies				
DFDBA vs. FDBA	1.7 vs. 2.4 mm[252]	59% vs. 66%[79]		
Ceramics				
HA vs. debridement	1.3–2.8 mm vs. 0.5–0.9 mm[171,329,330]	67% vs. 10%[92]	No new periodontal attachment, osteogenesis, or centogenesis[98]	
PHA vs. debridement	3.6 mm vs. 1.2 mm[139]	55%-60% vs. 23% had ≥ 50% fill[91,93,94]	Bone formation in the implant pores and periphery. No new attachment. Pocket reduction by long JE[104–106]	
TCP	2.3–2.7 mm[33,141,288]	24 mm vs. 9 mm[100] 58 mm vs. 22 mm[101] 67%[107]	Fibrous encapsulation followed by rapid resorption. No evidence of new attachment. Healing by long JE[112]	
Calcium Carbonates				
NCS vs. debridement	2.3 mm vs. 0.7 mm	67% vs. 26%[121]		NCS is superior to debridement
GTR				
ePTFE	2.0–5.3 mm[47,93,314]		0.5–1.7 mm of new attachment	
Resorbable barrier polyglactin-910 vs. ePTFE	4.0 mm vs. 3.5 mm[42,43]	77.5% vs. 70.7%[165,169]		

Continued

TABLE 63.1 Comparative Analysis of Regenerative Approaches—cont'd

Graft Material	CAL Gain (mm)	Defect Fill (% or mm)	Histologic Assessment	Comments
Comparative Studies				
ePTFE + DFDBA + citric acid root conditioning	4.7 mm[263]			Clinical series suggest improved results with DFDBA + citric acid root conditioning
ePTFE vs. ePTFE + HA-collagen graft vs. HA-collagen graft vs. debridement	3.70 mm[140] 3.80 mm 2.60 mm 2.1 mm	1.50 mm[140] 1.55 mm 0.85 mm 0.60 mm		ePTFE membranes ± HA-collagen was better than HA-collagen or debridement
EMDs				
EMD vs. placebo control or debridement	2.2 mm vs. 1.7 mm[113] 4.28 mm vs. 2.65 mm[75]	— 74.0% vs. 22.7%[196]	Histologic analysis of 2 cases. Both cases had new cementum and attachment but only one had new bone[191,192]	Suggests EMD can stimulate new attachment
Comparative Studies				
EMD vs. GTR (evaluate after 24 and 48 months)	3.0 mm vs. 2.9 mm[266] 2.9 mm vs. 3.1 mm[225]	—		Both techniques improve CAL; comparable results and appear to be stable over 4 years
EMD vs. DFDBA	3.2 mm vs. 3.0 mm[97]	—		Improved results over published debridement results but no difference between treatment modality
EMD + anorganic bone vs. EMD + fibrin glue	2.89 mm vs. 2.83 mm[161]			
rhPDGF + β-TCP				
rhPDGF+ β-TCP vs. placebo (pivotal trail 6-month data)	3.8 mm vs. 3.3 mm[204]	57% vs. 18% LBF: 2.6 mm vs. 0.9 mm		
rhPDGF + β-TCP vs. placebo (pivotal trail 36-month data)	4.3 mm vs. 3.2 mm[203]	60.5% vs. 32.6% LBF 2.88 mm vs. 1.42 mm		Maximum regeneration seen with 0.3 mg/mL rhPDGF was at the 1-year mark and the results were stable

CAL, Clinical attachment level; *DFDBA*, demineralized freeze-dried bone allograft; *EMD*, enamel matrix derivative; *ePTFE*, expanded polytetrafluoroethylene; *FDBA*, freeze-dried bone allograft; *GTR*, guided tissue regeneration; *HA*, hydroxyapatite; *JE*, junctional epithelium; *LBF*, linear bone fill; *NCS*, calcium carbonates; *PHA*, porous hydroxyapatite; *rhPDGF*, recombinant human platelet-derived growth factor; *TCP*, tricalcium phosphate.

All recommended techniques include careful case selection and complete removal of all irritants on the root surface. Although this can be done in some cases as a closed procedure, in most cases it should be done after exposure of the area with a flap.[5,6] Flap design and incisions should follow the description given in Chapter 60 for flaps used in reconstructive surgery. Trauma from occlusion, as well as other factors, may impair posttreatment healing of the supporting periodontal tissues, thus reducing the likelihood of new attachment. Occlusal adjustment or splinting, if needed, is therefore indicated.

Systemic antibiotics are generally used after reconstructive periodontal therapy, although definitive information on the advisability of this measure is still lacking. Case reports have shown extensive reconstruction of periodontal lesions after scaling, root planing, and curettage, with systemic and local treatment using penicillin or tetracycline, in combination with other forms of therapy.[32,197]

Non–Graft-Associated Reconstructive Procedures

The following sections discuss the rationale and techniques that must be considered for a successful outcome in achieving new attachment or periodontal bone regeneration in response to non–graft-associated reconstructive surgical therapy. This approach is used in Europe and Asia where human bone graft is not available due to regulatory restraints. Of these procedures, GTR is the main procedure used in clinical practice. More recent evidence suggests that the laser-assisted new attachment procedure (LANAP) may also result in new attachment and regeneration, but further clinical trials are needed to test its efficacy and parameters for success. Additionally, several procedures are of historical interest: (1) the removal of the junctional and pocket epithelium; (2) the prevention of their migration into the healing area after therapy; (3) clot stabilization, wound protection, and space creation; and (4) biomodification of the root surfaces. Although these procedures are not used individually as reconstructive approaches, some of these strategies are currently incorporated into reconstructive surgery as adjuncts.

Guided Tissue Regeneration

GTR is used for the prevention of epithelial migration along the cemental wall of the pocket and for maintaining space for clot stabilization. Derived from the classic studies of Nyman, Lindhe, Karring, and Gottlow, this method is based on the assumption that periodontal ligament and perivascular cells have the potential for regeneration of the attachment apparatus of the tooth.[‡] GTR consists of placing barriers of different types (membranes) to cover the bone and periodontal ligament, thus temporarily separating them from the gingival epithelium and connective tissue. Excluding the epithelium and the gingival connective tissue from the root surface during the postsurgical healing phase not only prevents epithelial migration into the wound but also favors repopulation of the area by cells from the periodontal ligament and the bone[38] (see also Chapter 3). In the United States, GTR is often performed with some type of bone graft as a scaffolding agent, so it is a combined therapy. As indicated earlier, in Europe and in other parts of the world, because of regulatory and religious constraints, human graft materials are not available, so it is performed as a traditional GTR procedure and may be occasionally used in conjunction with other graft materials as combined therapy.

Initial animal experiments using Millipore filters (Millipore Sigma, Burlington, MA) and Teflon membranes resulted in regeneration of cementum and alveolar bone and a functional periodontal ligament.[32,33,38,129] Clinical case reports indicate that GTR results in a gain in attachment level.[15,16] Histologic studies in humans provided evidence of periodontal reconstruction in most cases, even with horizontal bone loss.[93,294,296]

The use of polytetrafluoroethylene (PTFE) membranes has been tested in controlled clinical studies in mandibular molar furcations and has shown statistically significant decreases in pocket depths and improvement in attachment levels after 6 months, but bone level measurements have been inconclusive.[162,227] A study of maxillary molar furcations did not result in significant gain in attachment or bone levels.[186]

With the regenerative success associated with the use of nonresorbable membrane, the advantages and disadvantages of this approach became apparent. Notably, problems such as membrane exposure, which resulted in no or limited regeneration and the need for a secondary procedure for surgical removal, resulted in the development of biodegradable membranes.[277] Today in clinical practice, most GTR procedures use biodegradable membranes, whereas the nonresorbable membranes, especially those with titanium reinforcement struts, are used for regeneration of large intrabony defects and implant site development. Nevertheless, the historical research using nonresorbable membranes and the development of various types of biodegradable membranes are valuable.

Laser-Assisted New Attachment Procedure

The role of laser in periodontal therapy remains controversial (see Chapter 68). Nevertheless, the use of neodymium:yttrium-aluminum-garnet (Nd:YAG) to perform surgical LANAPs has been reported for the management of chronic periodontitis,[139,191] and it can potentially result in new attachment and periodontal regeneration (see Chapter 68).[210,334]

Many questions remain about LANAP. The first refers to the exact mechanism and parameter by which healing by new attachment versus regeneration occurs with LANAP therapy. The frequency, consistency, and extent of regeneration have not been defined, nor has this approach been compared with other established regenerative therapies. This comparison, along with other randomized controlled trials, will be needed for meta-analysis to determine whether LANAP is equivalent or superior to other conventional therapy. As with all periodontal therapy, the long-term stability of the regeneration also needs to be explored.

Graft Materials and Procedures

Numerous therapeutic grafting modalities for restoring periodontal osseous defects have been investigated. Periodontal reconstruction can be attained without the use of bone grafts in meticulously treated three-wall defects (intrabony defects) and in periodontal and endodontic abscesses.[32,117,138,232] New attachment is more likely to occur when the destructive process has occurred rapidly, such as after treatment of pockets complicated by acute periodontal abscesses and after treatment of acute necrotizing ulcerative lesions.[204] The use of graft materials at one time was to provide regenerative inductive effect, but it should be viewed primarily as providing a scaffold for healing.

The following classifications of bone graft material are important. Grafts are categorized either by their origins or function during healing. Categorizations by origin include the following: (1) *autografts* are bone obtained from the same individual; (2) *allografts* are bone obtained from a different individual of the same species; and (3) *xenografts* are bone from a different species. Bone graft materials are also evaluated based on their osteogenic, osteoinductive, or osteoconductive potential. *Osteogenesis* refers to the formation or development of new bone by cells contained in the graft. *Osteoinduction* is a chemical process by which molecules contained in the graft (e.g., bone morphogenetic proteins) convert the neighboring cells into osteoblasts, which in turn form bone. *Osteoconduction* is a physical effect by which the matrix of the graft forms a scaffold that favors outside cells to penetrate the graft and form new bone.

Periodontal defects as sites for transplantation differ from osseous cavities surrounded by bony walls. Saliva and bacteria may easily penetrate along the root surface, and epithelial cells may proliferate into the defect, thus resulting in contamination and possible exfoliation of the grafts. Therefore the principles established to govern transplantation of bone or other materials into closed osseous cavities are not fully applicable to transplantation of bone into periodontal defects.[64]

Schallhorn[263] defined the considerations that govern the selection of a material as follows: biologic acceptability, predictability, clinical feasibility, minimal operative hazards, minimal postoperative sequelae, and patients' acceptance. It is difficult to find a material with all these characteristics, and to date, no ideal material or technique exists.

Graft materials have been developed and tried in many forms. To familiarize the reader with various types of graft material, as defined by either the technique or the material used, a brief discussion of each is provided.

All grafting techniques require presurgical scaling, occlusal adjustment as needed, and exposure of the defect with a full-thickness flap. The flap technique best suited for grafting purposes is the *papilla preservation flap* because it provides complete coverage of the interdental area after suturing (see Chapter 60). The use of antibiotics after the procedure is generally recommended.

Autogenous Bone Grafts

Historically, extraoral sites for bone harvesting have been from the iliac crest, but this approach is seldom performed due to medical and legal concerns. Intraoral sites can be effective, especially when

---

[‡]References 47, 64, 92–94, 187, 213, 214, 294.

donor sites adjacent to the defects are available. Despite the popularity of using allograft, this should always be a consideration, especially as one reviews the historical development of the use of autografts from intraoral sites.

Bone Allografts

Obtaining donor material for autograft purposes necessitates inflicting surgical trauma on another part of the patient's body. Obviously, it would be to the patient's and therapist's advantage if a suitable substitute could be used for grafting purposes that would offer similar potential for repair and not require the additional surgical removal of donor material from the patient. However, both allografts and xenografts are foreign to the patient and therefore have the potential to provoke an immune response. Attempts have been made to suppress the antigenic potential of allografts and xenografts by radiation, freezing, and chemical treatment.[24]

Bone allografts are commercially available from tissue banks. They are obtained from cortical bone within 12 hours of the death of the donor, defatted, cut in pieces, washed in absolute alcohol, and deep-frozen. The material may then be demineralized, subsequently ground and sieved to a particle size of 250 to 750 μm, and freeze-dried. Finally, it is vacuum-sealed in glass vials.

Numerous steps are also taken to eliminate viral infectivity. These include exclusion of donors from known high-risk groups and various tests on the cadaver tissues to exclude individuals with any type of infection or malignant disease. The material is then treated with chemical agents or strong acids to inactivate the virus, if still present. The risk of human immunodeficiency virus (HIV) infection has been calculated as 1 in 1 to 8 million and is therefore characterized as highly remote.[184]

Freeze-Dried Bone Allograft

Several clinical studies by Mellonig, Bowers, and coworkers reported bone fill exceeding 50% in 67% of the defects grafted with freeze-dried bone allograft (FDBA) and in 78% of the defects grafted with FDBA in combination with autogenous bone.[21,182,203,257,278] FDBA, however, is considered an osteoconductive material, whereas demineralized FDBA (DFDBA) is considered an osteoinductive graft. Laboratory studies have found that DFDBA has a higher osteogenic potential than FDBA and is therefore preferred.[178,180,181]

Demineralized Freeze-Dried Bone Allograft

Experiments by Urist[312–315] established the osteogenic potential of DFDBA. Demineralization in cold, diluted hydrochloric acid exposes the components of bone matrix, which are closely associated with collagen fibrils and have been termed *bone morphogenetic proteins* (BMPs).[40,315]

In 1975, Libin and colleagues[163] reported three patients with 4 to 10 mm of bone regeneration in periodontal osseous defects. Subsequent clinical studies were made with cancellous DFDBA and cortical DFDBA.[221,230,233] DFDBA resulted in more desirable results (2.4 mm vs. 1.38 mm of bone fill).

Bowers and associates,[22] in a histologic study in humans, showed new attachment and periodontal regeneration in defects grafted with DFDBA. Mellonig and colleagues[180,181,183] tested DFDBA against autogenous materials in the calvaria of guinea pigs and showed it to have similar osteogenic potential.

These studies provided strong evidence that DFDBA in periodontal defects results in significant probing depth reduction, attachment level gain, and osseous regeneration. The combination of DFDBA and GTR has also proved to be very successful[264]; however, limitations of the use of DFDBA include the possible, although remote, potential of disease transfer from the cadaver.

A bone-inductive protein isolated from the extracellular matrix of human bones, termed *osteogenin* or *BMP-3,* has been tested in human periodontal defects and seems to enhance osseous regeneration.[23] This bone-inductive protein is discussed later in this chapter.

Xenografts

Bone products from other species have a long history of use in periodontal therapy. A few of these xenograft products are mentioned here for historical purposes but are no longer used today. Bovine-derived bone (Bio-Oss, Geistlich Pharma, Princeton, NJ) is used in combination with GTR for periodontal regeneration. This material is also used in combination with autologous bone for ridge augmentation.

Calf bone (Boplant), treated by detergent extraction, sterilized, and freeze-dried, has been used for the treatment of osseous defects.[8,259] Kiel bone is calf or ox bone denatured with 20% hydrogen peroxide, dried with acetone, and sterilized with ethylene oxide. Anorganic bone is ox bone from which the organic material has been extracted by means of ethylenediamine; it is then sterilized by autoclaving.[177] These materials have been tried and discarded for various reasons.

Currently, an anorganic, bovine-derived bone marketed under the brand name Bio-Oss (Geistlick Pharma) has been successfully used both for periodontal defects and in implant surgery. It is an osteoconductive, porous bone mineral matrix from bovine cancellous or cortical bone. The organic components of the bone are removed, but the trabecular architecture and porosity are retained.[30,176] The physical features permit clot stabilization and revascularization to allow for migration of osteoblasts, leading to osteogenesis. Bio-Oss is biocompatible with the adjacent tissues, and it elicits no systemic immune response.

LEARNING BOX 63.2

Due to the osteoconductive nature and slow resorption rate of anorganic, bovine-derived bone graft, it acts as a bioexclusive graft material in that it excludes epithelial mesenchymal cell migration into the regeneration site. The slow resorption rate is also advantageous for grafting in implant surgical sites in that it may be corrective for soft tissue defects and remain fairly stable. However, the use of this material in implant placement sites must be cautioned because overcompaction of this material may result in such low volume of native bone that it will not provide an adequate level of osseointegration for implant stability.

Several studies have reported successful bone regeneration and new attachment with Bio-Oss in periodontal defects,[30,179] as well as regeneration around implants and sinus grafting (see Chapter 80).

Periodontally, Bio-Oss has been used as a graft material covered with a resorbable membrane (Geistlich Bio-Gide, Geistlich Pharma). The membrane prevents the migration of fibroblasts and connective tissues into the pores and between the granules of the graft. Histologic studies of this technique have shown significant osseous regeneration and cementum formation.

Yukna and associates[336] have used Bio-Oss in combination with a cell-binding polypeptide (P-15) that is a synthetic analogue of a 15-amino acid sequence of type I collagen marketed as PepGen P-15 (Dentsply Sirona, York, PA); this combination seems to enhance the bone regenerative results of the matrix alone in periodontal defects.

Graft-Associated Reconstructive Procedures of Historical Interest

In addition to bone graft materials, many nonbone graft materials have been used in an attempt to restore the periodontium. These

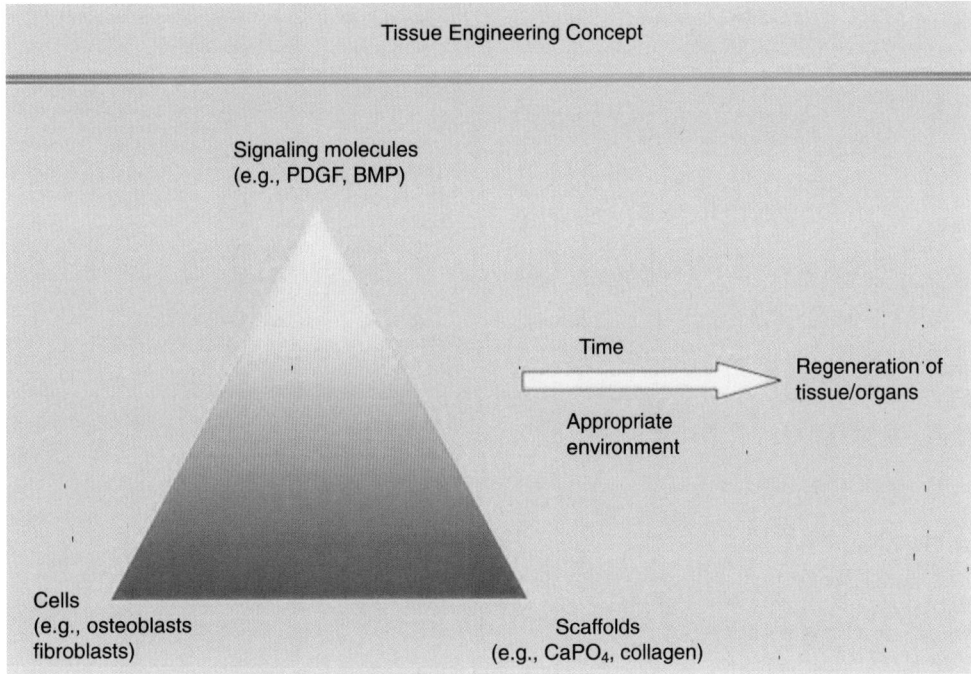

Fig. 63.1 Tissue engineering is the manipulation of one or more of the three elements: signaling molecules, scaffolds, or cells. *BMP,* Bone morphogenetic protein; *CaPO₄,* calcium phosphate; *PDGF,* platelet-derived growth factor. *(Courtesy Dr. Samuel Lynch.)*

include sclera, dura, cartilage, cementum, dentin, plaster of Paris, plastic materials, ceramics, and coral-derived materials.[26,158,159] None offers a reliable substitute for bone graft materials; some of these materials are briefly presented here to offer a complete picture of the many attempts that have been made to solve the critical problem of periodontal regeneration.

Tissue Engineering With Biologic Mediators

In wound healing, the natural healing process usually results in tissue scarring or repair. By using tissue engineering, the wound healing process is manipulated so that tissue regeneration occurs.[95] This manipulation usually involves one or more of the three key elements: the signaling molecules, scaffold or supporting matrices, and cells (Fig. 63.1). The use of tissue engineering for periodontal regeneration and dental implant site preparation has been reviewed.[86,135,137]

Early clinical examples involving tissue engineering principles include the use of bone allografts and autologous platelet-rich plasma (PRP). Investigations indicated that the success rates with these materials were inconsistent. With the development of recombinant growth factors and morphogens, and the use of synthetic scaffolds, the level of success has improved. Once considered experimental, tissue engineering is now clinically applicable with two commercially available tissue engineering systems for periodontal regeneration that involve the use of enamel matrix derivative (EMD) and platelet-derived growth factor-BB (PDGF-BB)–beta-TCP (β-TCP).[136] The ability of BMP type I collagen sponge to enhance periodontal regeneration has been studied, but the mixed results and the concern for ankylosis have relegated this differentiation factor to be used primarily for implant site development. The development of a fourth promising system using basic fibroblast growth factor (FGF-2) is completing multicenter clinical trials.

Because tissue engineering approaches are likely to improve clinical results, clinicians need to understand the biology and clinical parameters and limitations of these techniques. In the following sections, each of the three key elements of tissue engineering and how they are applied to the spectrum of periodontal and other orofacial surgery procedures are reviewed.

Enamel Matrix Derivative for Periodontal Regeneration

EMD has been effective in the treatment of infrabony defects (Fig. 63.2). The histologic evidence of EMD-induced periodontal regeneration has been confirmed in a clinical case report.[114,115] A mandibular lateral incisor destined for orthodontic extraction was treated with acid etching and EMD. After 4 months, the tooth was extracted and examined histologically. Regenerated cementum covered 73% of the defect, and regenerated alveolar bone covered 65%. This histologic finding was later confirmed in other case reports,[268,338] whereas new connective tissue attachment was reported in another case series where EMD was used in combination with a bone-derived xenograft.[275]

EMD has been shown to be safe for clinical use.[110,339] Evidence of clinical efficacy was first reported in a multicenter study consisting of 33 patients with at least 2 defects, which were treated in a split-mouth design. The experimental site was treated with acid etching and EMD, whereas the control site was treated with a placebo.[114] Patients were examined at 8, 16, and 36 months after surgery. Increased bone fill of the osseous defect was observed over time for 25 of the 27 (93%) EMD-treated teeth, but no bone fill was detected in the controls. The mean radiographic bone fill was greater for the EMD-treated defects compared with the control sites treated with open flap debridement (2.7 mm vs. 0.7 mm, respectively). Statistically significant improvements were also observed for EMD-treated sites over control sites in mean pocket reduction (3.1 mm vs. 2.3 mm, respectively) and mean attachment level gain (2.2 mm vs. 1.7 mm, respectively). These clinical findings have been supported by additional studies.¶ However, one randomized, double-masked, placebo-controlled

---

¶References 75, 80, 81, 99, 112, 214, 216, 228, 274, 304, 342, 343.

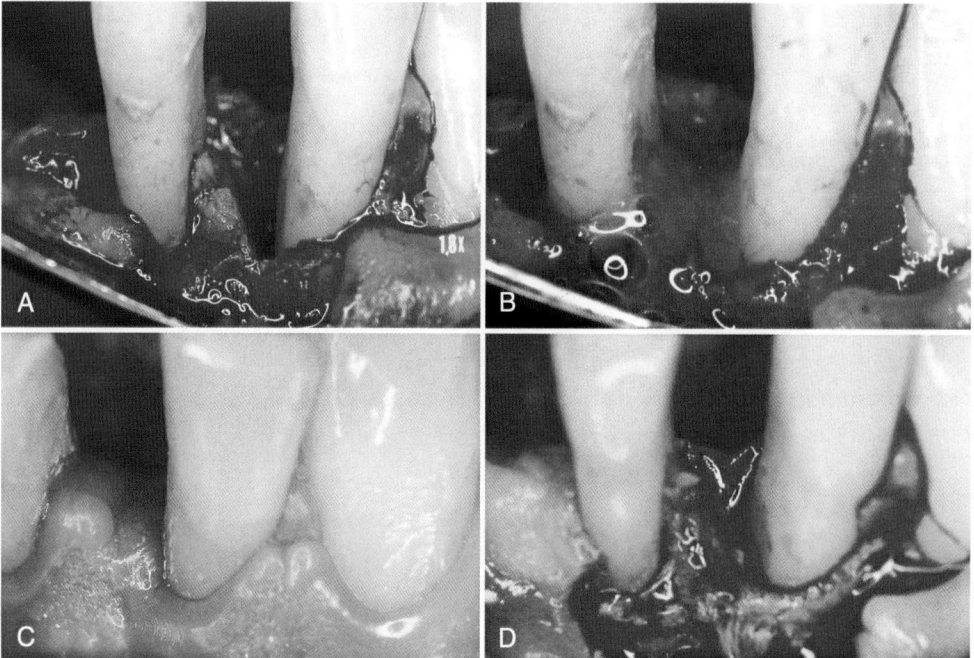

Fig. 63.2 (A) Deep vertical bone loss distal to the lower left central incisor. (B) Area flapped, root prepared, and defect filled with enamel matrix protein (Emdogain, Straumann, Andover, Mass.). (C) Postoperative photograph 6 months later. (D) Reentry surgery showing extensive bone fill. *(Courtesy Dr. Marco Orsini, Aquila, Italy.)*

clinical trial failed to show significant differences in clinical and radiographic measure between EMD and control.[251] Long-term stability of EMD regenerative therapy was reported in a case series that followed 106 EMD-treated defects in 90 patients.[112] The data suggest that radiographic bone level, clinical attachment level gain, and reduced pocket depth reached near-maximal response after 1 year, and the results remained stable over 5 years. Other long-term studies have confirmed these findings.[72,237,270,271]

Several studies have compared the use of EMD alone or in conjunction with other regenerative approaches. When EMD treatment was compared with GTR using bioresorbable membranes, the clinical results were comparable and stable over as much as a 10-year period.[59,179,270,271,273,284,287] In a study comparing EMD, GTR, or EMD in combination with GTR with open flap debridement, all three had results superior to those of open flap surgery, with no additional improvement when EMD was used in conjunction with GTR.[274] Other investigators have confirmed this finding.[188,269,287]

The use of EMD in combination with other graft materials is controversial. When EMD is used in conjunction with autogenous bone, DFDBA, xenograft, and bioactive glass, additional improvements in clinical parameters were observed as compared with the use of either EMD or DFDBA alone.[#] However, others studies failed to demonstrate clinical improvement when EMD was used in conjunction with TCP or bioactive glass.[20,127,159]

EMD remains a very intriguing biologic mediator.[136,205] As we better understand the mechanism of action of the potpourri of proteins and growth factors, this may strengthen the biologic rationale for clinical use of this material. The concern remains whether commercial batches of EMD will be consistent and provide comparable clinical results in all cases. Perhaps the message is that the achievement of maximum regenerative response will require

a mixture of biologic mediators. With further characterization of EMD, we may better develop a synergistic blend that will provide an optimal result.

Recombinant Human Platelet-Derived Growth Factor for Periodontal Regeneration

PDGF is one of the earliest growth factors studied for its effect on wound healing because it is a potent mitogenic and chemotactic factor for mesenchymal cells in cell culture. Histologic evidence of periodontal regeneration was first reported in experimental defects in beagle dog.[163,167] During the development of PDGF for clinical use, recombinant human PDGF (rhPDGF) was used in conjunction with allogenic bone to correct class II furcations and interproximal intrabony defects on hopeless teeth.[29,207] Histologic evidence of successful periodontal regeneration in the furcation lesion with excellent fill has been noted.

A human clinical trial was conducted using rhPDGF and recombinant human insulin-like growth factor 1 (rhIGF-1).[121] Using a split-mouth design, defects were treated with either a low dose (50 µg/mL) or high dose (150 µg/mL) of rhPDGF–rhIGF-1. After 9 months, the high-dose rhPDGF–rhIGF-1 induced 2.08 mm of new bone and 43.2% defect fill, compared with 0.75 mm vertical bone height and 18.5% bone fill in controls. Low-dose rhPDGF–rhIGF-1 results were statistically similar to those of the controls. Additionally, this study demonstrated that no adverse immunologic or clinical reaction resulted from use of these agents. A primate study examined the regenerative effects of PDGF–IGF-1 individually and in combination.[166] PDGF alone was found to be as effective as the PDGF–IGF-1 combination in producing new attachment after 3 months. No significant effect was found when IGF was used alone. This study suggests that IGF may not be important at the dose level tested.

Subsequently, the effectiveness of 0.3 mg/mL of rhPDGF in combination with β-TCP to improve attachment level gain, bone level, and bone volume significantly compared with β-TCP alone

---

[#]References 99, 100, 136, 154, 272, 318, 330.

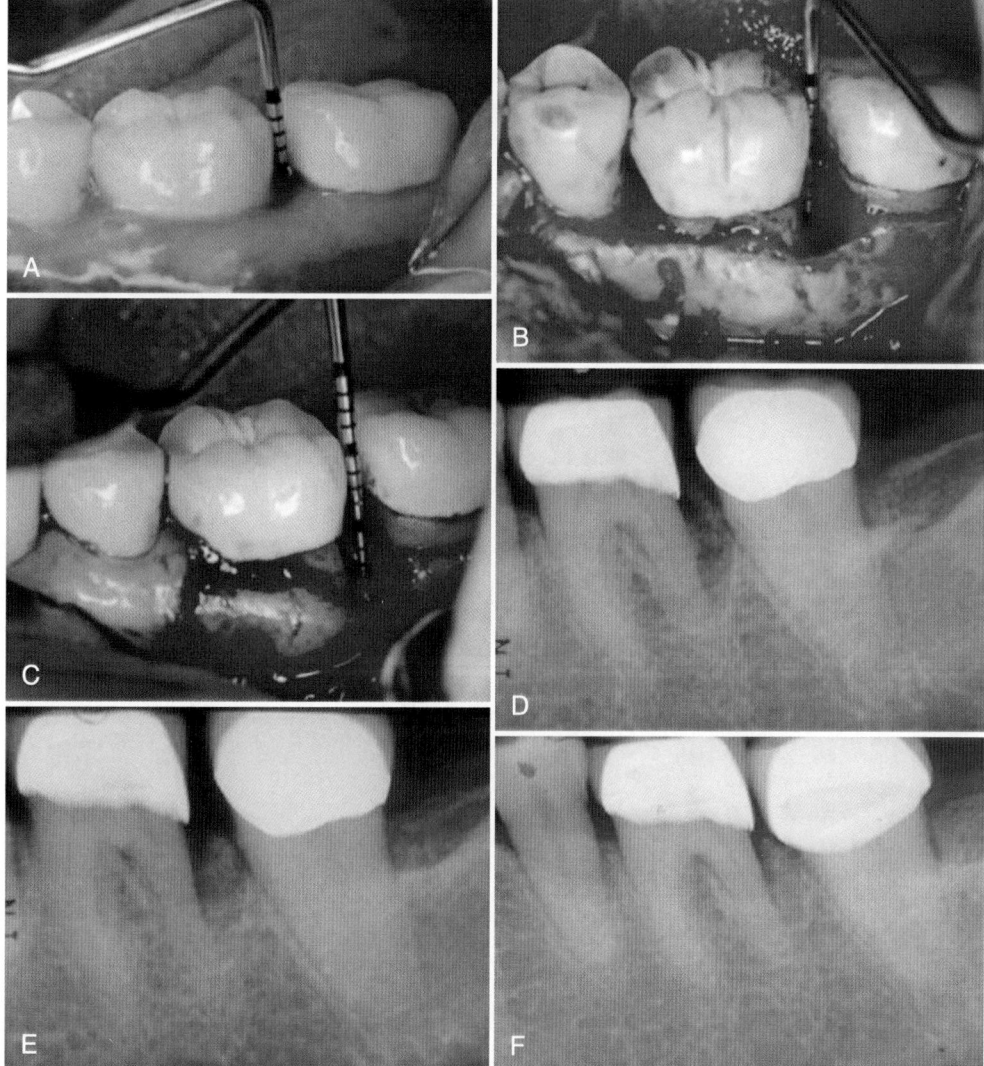

Fig. 63.3 A sample case of a patient treated in the pivotal trial. (A) to (C) The pretreatment situation preoperatively, at surgical debridement, and at postsurgical reentry. (D) to (F) The radiographic appearance after 12, 24, and 60 months. Surgical reentry after 12 months indicates good bone fill of the circumferential intrabony defect (C). The clinical pocket depth was 3 mm after 5 years.

was demonstrated after 6 months in a multicenter clinical trial.[208] A subset of these patients was followed for 24 months, and a representative case series was reported to be stable, with increases in radiographic bone fill compared with the end results after 6 months (Fig. 63.3).[174] A review of these cases indicates that the results were stable after 3 and 5 years.[134,209] Another case series suggested that rhPDGF with freeze-dried bone allograft can be combined to achieve excellent results in severe periodontal intrabony defects.[29] These findings were confirmed by another randomized control trial.[126]

The combination of rhPDGF with a β-TCP carrier is now commercially available (GEM 21S, Osteohealth, Shirley, NY). These preliminary studies using rhPDGF-TCP suggest that it is easy to use, requires no barrier membranes, and has results comparable or superior to those of other regenerative graft materials. The potential for using rhPDGF for regeneration of furcation defects and implant site preparation still needs to be evaluated. Additionally, considerable clinical interest has been expressed in combining rhPDGF-BB with other bone replacement grafts, particularly bone allografts and xenografts.

LEARNING BOX 63.3

Note that the use of biologic agents such as enamel matrix derivative and platelet-derived growth factor is a relatively recent concept for periodontal regeneration. The process can proceed even with the short biologic half-life of these materials; this means that it is often not present in the later stages of development. Readers should appreciate that these stimulated cells can somehow organize themselves to differentiate and in a timely fashion become three histologic structures: new bone, cementum, and periodontal ligament. In addition, it is amazing that these three histologic structures "intertwine" with each other and stimulate regeneration using a different mechanism from the bioexclusion principle, as demonstrated with the use of guided tissue regeneration membranes. Finally, randomized controlled studies indicate that the addition of guided tissue regeneration membranes confers no advantage. All these factors indicate that the use of biologic agents can stimulate stem cells to be recruited to the intrabony or furcation defect site, proliferate, and differentiate into a newly regenerated periodontal apparatus. It is also interesting that this occurs in very rapid fashion, faster than the migration of epithelial and mesenchymal cells.

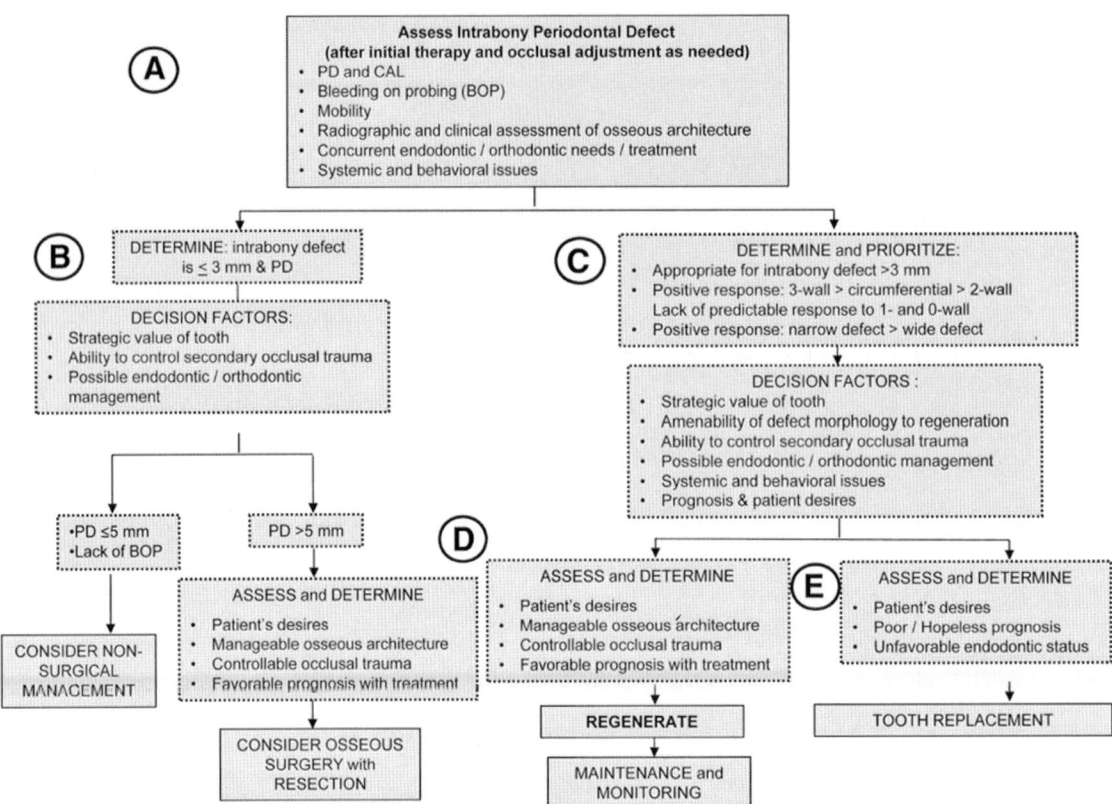

Fig. 63.4 Clinical decision tree for the management of advanced periodontal defects. *A* to *E* are explained in the text in the section titled "Clinical Guidelines to Guide Clinicians in Their Patient Management." *CAL,* Clinical attachment level; *PD,* periodontal defect. *(From American Academy of Periodontology: J Periodontol 86[Suppl]:S77, 2015.)*

Combined Techniques

Periodontal new attachment and bone reconstruction have been challenges for clinicians throughout the history of periodontal therapy. To take advantage of the different bone graft materials and biologic mediators, clinicians have combined these graft materials with the use of membranes in an attempt to find a predictable technique to regenerate bone.

Several clinicians have proposed a combination of the techniques previously described in an attempt to enhance their results.[11,104,160,177] A classic paper published by Schallhorn and McClain[264] in 1988 described a combination technique using graft material, root conditioning with citric acid, and coverage with a nonresorbable membrane (the only available one at the time). More recently, with the advent of osteopromotive agents, such as the EMD (Emdogain, Straumann, Andover, MA) and osteoconductive bovine-derived anorganic bone (Bio-Oss) graft materials, other combination techniques have been advocated.[158] The combined use of these products, along with autogenous bone with resorbable membrane coverage, has resulted in an increased percentage of cases with successful new attachment and periodontal reconstruction. Many of these combination techniques were reviewed in previous sections of this chapter. Whereas the use of combination technique may be appealing, it is important for clinicians to remember that these added materials often escalate the cost of the procedure and should be balanced with the quality and the long-term stability of the clinical results.

Factors That Influence Therapeutic Success

Factors that adversely affect periodontal regeneration were reviewed at the 1996 World Workshop in Periodontics and the 1997 Proceedings of the Second European Workshop on Periodontology.[217,232] Some of the therapeutic factors that have been implicated or shown to influence periodontal regenerative therapy adversely include (1) the selection of the appropriate surgical technique, accurate assessment of the periodontal defect, and the clinician's clinical experience (Fig. 63.4); (2) the importance of the tooth in the overall restorative treatment plan; and (3) the patient's selection of the regenerative options.

Clinical Guidelines to Guide Clinicians in Their Patient Management

Clinical guidelines for the management of patients with periodontal disease are depicted in Fig. 63.4.[136] The ideal management of periodontal defects consists of the early diagnosis and appropriate addressing of the defect (Fig. 63.4, *A*). When defects are detected early, before the formation of intrabony and furcation lesions, a predictable outcome can be obtained with scaling, root planing, and conventional osseous surgery (Fig. 63.4, *B*). Even early narrow intrabony (<3 mm) and furcation defects can be blended in with the adjacent osseous contour. When the intrabony and furcation defects are >3 mm, periodontal regeneration should be considered (Fig. 63.4, *C*). Assessment of defect morphology and the patient's clinical and systemic-behavioral determinants is critical for regenerative success. Consideration of these issues, in addition to the patient's desires, will define the selection of the regenerative approach to be used (Fig. 63.4, *D*). Long-term stability is possible, but the individual outcome is influenced by patient-related considerations such as smoking and compliance with periodontal maintenance and monitoring. Should patient-related or clinical determinants be unfavorable for periodontal regeneration, appropriate therapy must be selected

TABLE 63.2   In Vitro Effects of Growth Factors on Periodontal Ligament Cells and Osteoblasts

	PDGF	FGF-2	BMP	EMD	TGF-α	IGF-1 and IGF-2
PDL Cells						
Cell proliferation	++	+++	++	++	−	+
Chemotaxis	++	+++	+	++	0	++
Collagen synthesis	+	−	+	+	+	+
Protein synthesis	+	+	+	+	+	+
Matrix gene expression	++	++/−	?	+	+	+
Cementoblasts						
Cell proliferation	+++	?	−	++	++	++
Chemotaxis	++	?	?	?	?	?
Collagen synthesis	+	?	++	++	+	+
Protein synthesis	+	?	++	++	+	+
Matrix gene expression	±	?	++	++/−	±	±
Osteoblasts						
Cell proliferation	++	+++	0	++	+++	++
Chemotaxis	+++	+++	+	++	+++	+
Collagen synthesis	0	++	0	+	+	+
Protein synthesis	0	+	ND	+	±	0
Matrix gene expression	±	++/−	++	++/−	++	++
Alkaline phosphatase synthesis	0	−	++	++	±	0

(−) Inhibition; (0) no effect; (+) effect; (?) unknown effect; *BMP*, bone morphogenetic protein; *EMD*, enamel matrix derivative; *FGF*, fibroblast growth factor; *IGF*, insulin-like growth factor; *PDGF*, platelet-derived growth factor; *PDL*, periodontal ligament; *TGF-α*, transforming growth factor alpha.
Adapted and updated from Kao RT, Murakami S, Beirne OR: The use of biologic mediators and tissue engineering in dentistry. *Periodontol 2000* 20:127, 2009.

in place of regeneration that may consist of long-term maintenance or the removal of the tooth and replacement with a prosthesis such as a dental implant or another form of prosthesis.(Fig. 63.4, *E*).[133]

Before regenerative therapy, it is important to perform an endodontic assessment. This is to eliminate the possibility that the defect is the result of an endodontic-periodontal lesion. Should this be case, endodontic treatment may resolve that portion of the defect due to the endodontic lesion. If a residual defect still persists, periodontal therapy should be initiated.

A common misconception is that regenerative therapy ends with a postoperative assessment a few months after treatment. Most therapeutic approaches have maximal healing results after 12 months. As such, postoperative monitoring should occur at least 12 months later. Additionally, these regenerated areas should be monitored at every recall visit because poor hygiene, uncorrectable tooth anatomy, and undiagnosed endodontic problems will cause these areas to relapse. Should failures due to these causes be determined, it may be prudent to consider strategic extraction.[133]

The endpoint for active periodontal therapy should comprise a stable periodontal attachment level, absence of inflammation or bleeding, and a periodontal anatomic environment that is conducive for the patient and the clinician to maintain excellent oral hygiene. A successful long-term periodontal outcome is also dependent on a patient who will be compliant with the maintenance visits.

 Future Directions for Periodontal Regeneration

In wound healing, the natural healing process usually results in tissue scarring or repair. By using tissue engineering, the wound healing process is manipulated so that tissue regeneration occurs.[87,165] This manipulation usually involves one or more of the three key elements: (1) the signaling molecules, (2) scaffold or supporting matrices, and (3) cells (see Fig. 63.1). The cellular responses to these biologic mediators in vitro have been studied and are summarized in Table 63.2. Some of these biologic mediators are commercially available (recombinant human bone morphogenetic protein [rhBMP], rhPDGF, EMD). The potential of tissue engineering in periodontal regeneration has been reviewed.[164,246]

Conclusion

Since the 1980s, the periodontal literature has been filled with numerous reports related to periodontal regeneration. This therapeutic goal, although ideal, is difficult to achieve. Various graft materials and regenerative strategies are now available; however, they all have limitations. The surgical procedure can be technically demanding, and when success is achieved, maintenance of positive results is highly dependent on patients' oral hygiene habits and compliance with periodontal maintenance. Despite all these difficulties, periodontal regeneration is a clinical possibility that can be offered to patients. The clinician must carefully evaluate the various regenerative and reparative approaches and decide which technique may result in the best clinical outcome. With the advent of new regenerative approaches, such as biologic modifiers such as EMD and growth factors, we must critically evaluate how they may improve our ability to regenerate periodontal defects.

Treatment planning in periodontics also has changed dramatically because of the acceptance of dental implants as viable long-term options for replacing missing teeth. With the increased predictability of implants, questions arise regarding when to treat severe periodontal defects with regenerative procedures and when to perform strategic extraction in preparation for implant placement. Sometimes the best management of a periodontal defect may be extraction in lieu of periodontal regeneration or when regenerative efforts have been unsuccessful. Extraction would minimize further bone loss and provide the maximum volume of bone at the future implant healing site. This paradigm shift has complicated our views about regeneration. With dental implants as viable alternatives, we need to redefine periodontal prognosis and consider strategic extraction more often. Conversely, heroic regenerative procedures would be contraindicated.

Periodontal regeneration continues to be one of the primary therapeutic approaches toward the management of periodontal defects. Although evidence suggests that present regenerative techniques can lead to periodontal regeneration, the use of GTR and biologic modifiers can enhance these results. The crucial challenge for the clinician is to assess critically whether a periodontal defect can be corrected with a regenerative approach, or whether it would be better managed with osseous resection for a slight periodontal defect and with strategic extraction for an advanced diseased state. In this assessment, the clinician should attempt to differentiate between techniques that have been studied in depth and with acceptable results and those that are still experimental and promising. Research articles must be critically evaluated for adequacy of controls, selection of cases, methods of evaluation, and long-term postoperative results. In addition, the clinician should remember that we treat patients on the basis of "clinical" success and not "statistical" success. A resulting clinical attachment gain of half a millimeter may be a "statistical" success, but it is meaningless for the patients we treat and manage over the long term.

 Case Scenarios are found on the companion website www.expertconsult.com.

References

 References for this chapter are found on the companion website www.expertconsult.com.

CHAPTER 64

Furcation: Involvement and Treatment

Thomas N. Sims | Henry H. Takei

For online-only content on root resection, hemisection, and root resection or hemisection procedure in the surgical therapy section, please visit the companion website at www.expertconsult.com.

Editors' note: An animation (slide show) has been added by the editors as a supplement to the chapter. It was produced by My Dental Hub as a patient education tool and covers the basic elements in a conceptual manner. It is not intended to be a procedural guide for dental professionals.

Inflammatory periodontal disease, if unabated, ultimately progresses to attachment loss sufficient to affect the bifurcation or trifurcation of multirooted teeth. The furcation is an area of complex anatomic morphology[5,6,11] that may be difficult or impossible to debride by routine periodontal instrumentation.[29,36] Routine home care methods may not keep the furcation area free of plaque[17,23] (Video 64.1).

The presence of furcation involvement is a clinical finding that can lead to a diagnosis of advanced periodontitis and potentially to a less favorable prognosis for the affected tooth or teeth. Thus furcation involvement presents both diagnostic and therapeutic dilemmas.

Etiologic Factors

The primary etiologic factor in the development of furcation defects is *bacterial plaque* and the inflammatory consequences that result from its long-term presence. The extent of attachment loss required to produce a furcation defect is variable and related to local anatomic factors (e.g., root trunk length, root morphology)[13,27] and local developmental anomalies (e.g., cervical enamel projections [CEPs]).[22,27] Local factors may affect the rate of plaque deposition or complicate the performance of oral hygiene procedures, thereby contributing to the development of periodontitis and attachment loss. Studies indicate that prevalence and severity of furcation involvement increase with age.[21,22,36] Dental caries and pulpal death may also affect a tooth with furcation involvement or even the area of the furcation. All of these factors should be considered during the diagnosis, treatment planning, and therapy of the patient with furcation defects.

Diagnosis and Classification of Furcation Defects

A thorough clinical examination is the key to diagnosis and treatment planning. Careful probing is required to determine the presence and extent of furcation involvement, the position of the attachment relative to the furca, and the extent and configuration of the furcation defect.[38] The Nabors probe may be helpful to enter and measure difficult to access furcal areas (Fig. 64.1). Transgingival sounding may further define the anatomy of the furcation defect.[29] The goals of this examination are to identify and classify the extent of furcation involvement and to identify factors that may have contributed to the development of the furcation defect or that could affect treatment outcome. These factors include (1) the morphology of the affected tooth, (2) the position of the tooth relative to adjacent teeth, (3) the local anatomy of the alveolar bone, (4) the configuration of any bony defects, and (5) the presence and extent of other dental diseases (e.g., caries, pulpal necrosis).

The dimension of the furcation entrance is variable but usually quite small; 81% of furcations have an orifice of 1 mm or less, and 58% are 0.75 mm or less.[5,6] The clinician should consider these dimensions, and the local anatomy of the furcation area,[11–13] when selecting instruments for probing. A probe of small cross-sectional dimension is required if the clinician is to detect early furcation involvement.

Local Anatomic Factors

Clinical examination of the patient should allow the therapist to identify not only furcation defects but also many of the local anatomic factors that may affect the result of therapy (prognosis). Well-made dental radiographs, although not allowing a definitive classification of furcation involvement, provide additional information vital for treatment planning (Fig. 64.2). Important local factors include anatomic features of the affected teeth, as described next.

Root Trunk Length

A key factor in both the development and the treatment of furcation involvement is the root trunk length. The distance from the cementoenamel junction to the entrance of the furcation can vary extensively. Teeth may have very short root trunks, moderate root trunk length, or roots that may be fused to a point near the apex (Fig. 64.3). The combination of root trunk length with the number and configuration of the roots affects the ease and success of therapy. The shorter the root trunk, the less attachment needs to be lost before the furcation is involved. Once the furcation is exposed, teeth with short root trunks may be more accessible to maintenance procedures, and the short root trunks may facilitate some surgical procedures. Alternatively, teeth with unusually long root trunks or fused roots may not be appropriate candidates for treatment once the furcation has been affected.

Root Length

Root length is directly related to the quantity of attachment supporting the tooth. Teeth with long root trunks and short roots may have lost a majority of their support by the time that the furcation becomes affected.[12,20] Teeth with long roots and short to moderate root trunk length are more readily treated because sufficient attachment remains to meet functional demands.

Root Form

The mesial root of most mandibular first and second molars and the mesiofacial root of the maxillary first molar are typically curved to the distal side in the apical third. In addition, the distal aspect of this root is usually heavily fluted. The curvature and fluting may increase the potential for root perforation during endodontic therapy or complicate post placement during restoration.[1,25] These anatomic features may also result in an increased incidence of vertical root fracture. The size of the mesial radicular pulp may result in removal of most of this portion of the tooth during preparation.

Interradicular Dimension

The degree of separation of the roots is also an important factor in treatment planning. Closely approximated or fused roots can preclude adequate instrumentation during scaling, root planing, and surgery. Teeth with widely separated roots present more treatment options and are more readily treated.

Anatomy of Furcation

The anatomy of the furcation is complex. The presence of bifurcational ridges, a concavity in the dome,[11] and possible accessory canals[16] complicates not only scaling, root planing, and surgical therapy,[28] but also periodontal maintenance. Odontoplasty to reduce or eliminate these ridges may be required during surgical therapy for an optimal result.

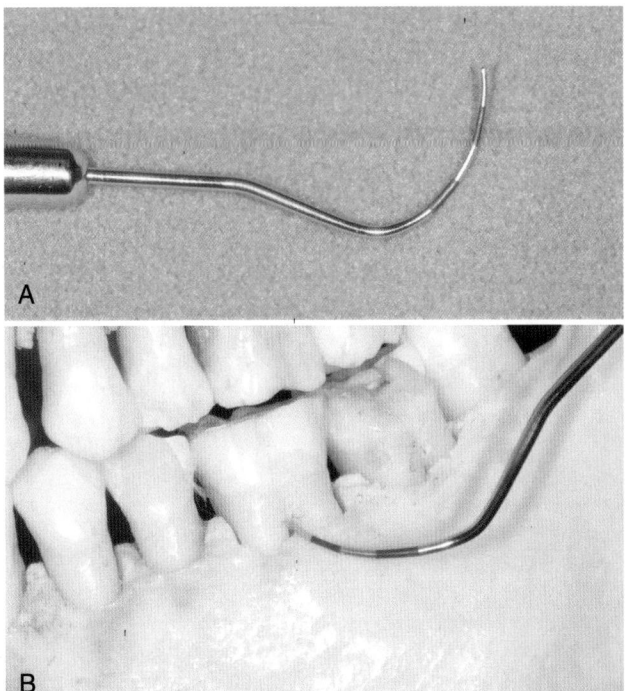

Fig. 64.1 (A) The Nabors probe is designed to probe into the furcation. (B) The probe placed into a class II furcation of a dried skull.

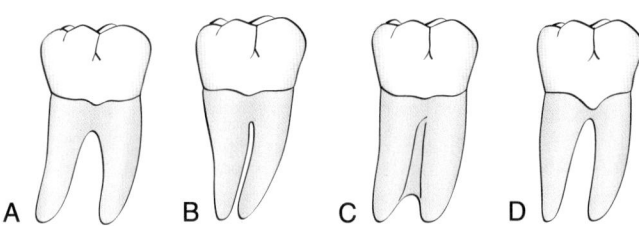

Fig. 64.3 Different anatomic features that may be important in prognosis and treatment of furcation involvement. (A) Widely separated roots. (B) Roots are separated but close. (C) Fused roots separated only in their apical portion. (D) Presence of enamel projection that may be conducive to early furcation involvement.

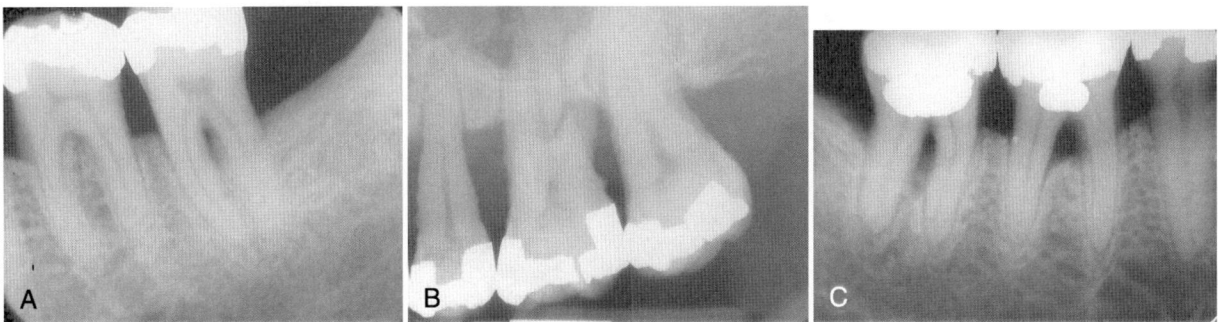

Fig. 64.2 Different degrees of furcation involvement in radiographs. (A) Grade I furcation on the mandibular first molar and a grade III furcation on the mandibular second molar. The root approximation on the second molar may be sufficient to impede accurate probing of this defect. (B) Multiple furcation defects on a maxillary first molar. Grade I buccal furcation involvement and grade II mesiopalatal and distopalatal furcations are present. Deep developmental grooves on the maxillary second molar simulate furcation involvement in this molar with fused roots. (C) Grades III and IV furcations on mandibular molars.

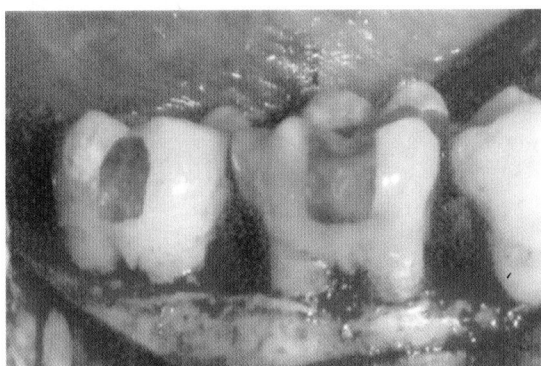

Fig. 64.4 Furcation involvement by grade III cervical enamel projections.

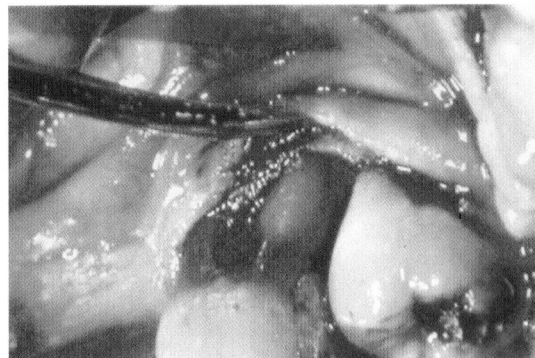

Fig. 64.5 Advanced bone loss, furcation involvement, and root approximation. Note the buccal furcation, which communicates with the distal furcation of a maxillary first molar that also displays advanced attachment loss on the distal root and approximation with the mesial root of the maxillary second molar. The patient with such teeth may benefit from root resection of the distobuccal root of the first molar or extraction of the molar.

BOX 64.1   Classification of Cervical Enamel Projections

Grade I: The enamel projection extends from the cementoenamel junction of the tooth toward the furcation entrance.

Grade II: The enamel projection approaches the entrance to the furcation. It does not enter the furcation, and therefore no horizontal component is present.

Grade III: The enamel projection extends horizontally into the furcation.

From Masters DH, Hoskins SW: Projection of cervical enamel into molar furcations. *J Periodontol* 35:49, 1964.

Cervical Enamel Projections

Cervical enamel projections (CEPs) are reported to occur on 8.6% to 28.6% of molars.[26,27,35] The prevalence is highest for mandibular and maxillary second molars. The extent of CEPs was classified by Masters and Hoskins[27] in 1964 (Box 64.1). Fig. 64.4 provides an example of a grade III CEP. These projections can affect plaque removal, can complicate scaling and root planing, and may be a local factor in the development of gingivitis and periodontitis. CEPs should be removed to facilitate maintenance.

Anatomy of the Bony Lesions
Pattern of Attachment Loss

The form of the bony lesions associated with the furcation can vary significantly. Horizontal bone loss can expose the furcation as thin facial or lingual plates of bone that may be totally lost during resorption. Alternatively, areas with thickened bony ledges may persist and predispose to the development of furcations with deep vertical components. The pattern of bone loss on other surfaces of the affected tooth and adjacent teeth must also be considered during treatment planning. The treatment response in deep, multiwalled bony defects is different from that in areas of horizontal bone loss. Complex multiwalled defects with deep, interradicular vertical components may be candidates for regenerative therapies. Alternatively, molars with advanced attachment loss on only one root may be treated by resective procedures.

Other Dental Findings

The dental and periodontal condition of the adjacent teeth must be considered during treatment planning for furcation involvement. The combination of furcation involvement and root approximation with an adjacent tooth represents the same problem that exists in furcations without adequate root separation. Such a finding may dictate the removal of the most severely affected tooth or the removal of a root or roots (Fig. 64.5).

The presence of an adequate band of gingiva and a moderate to deep vestibule will facilitate the performance of a surgical procedure, if indicated.

Indices of Furcation Involvement

The extent and configuration of the furcation defect are factors in both diagnosis and treatment planning. This has led to the development of a number of indices to record furcation involvement. These indices are based on the horizontal measurement of attachment loss in the furcation,[14,17] on a combination of horizontal and vertical measurements,[37] or a combination of these findings with the localized configuration of the bony deformity.[10] Glickman[14] classified furcation involvement into four grades (Fig. 64.6).

Grade I

A grade I furcation involvement is the incipient or early stage of furcation involvement (see Fig. 64.6A). The pocket is suprabony and primarily affects the soft tissues. Early bone loss may have occurred with an increase in probing depth, but radiographic changes are not usually found.

Grade II

A grade II furcation can affect one or more of the furcations of the same tooth. The furcation lesion is essentially a cul-de-sac (see Fig. 64.6B) with a definite horizontal component. If multiple defects are present, they do not communicate with each other because a portion of the alveolar bone remains attached to the tooth. The extent of the horizontal probing of the furcation determines whether the defect is early or advanced. Vertical bone loss may be present and represents a therapeutic complication. Radiographs may or may not depict the furcation involvement, particularly with maxillary molars because of the radiographic overlap of the roots. In some views, however, the presence of furcation "arrows" indicates possible furcation involvement (see Chapter 33).

Grade III

In grade III furcations, the bone is not attached to the dome of the furcation. In early grade III involvement, the opening may be filled

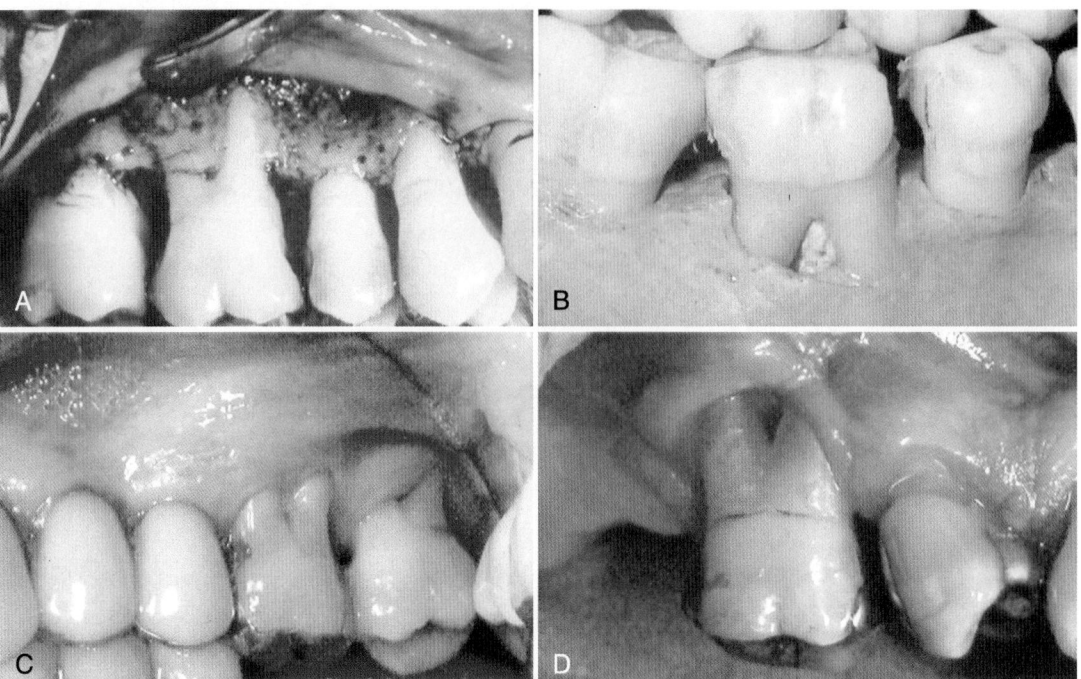

Fig. 64.6 Glickman's classification of furcation involvement. (A) Grade I furcation involvement. Although a space is visible at the entrance to the furcation, no horizontal component of the furcation is evident on probing. (B) Grade II furcation in a dried skull. Note both the horizontal and the vertical components of this cul-de-sac. (C) Grade III furcations on maxillary molars. Probing confirms that the buccal furcation connects with the distal furcation of both these molars, yet the furcation is filled with soft tissue. (D) Grade IV furcation. The soft tissues have receded sufficiently to allow direct vision into the furcation of this maxillary molar.

with soft tissue and may not be visible. The clinician may not even be able to pass a periodontal probe completely through the furcation because of interference with the bifurcational ridges or facial-lingual bony margins. However, if the clinician adds the buccal and lingual probing dimensions and obtains a cumulative probing measurement that is equal to or greater than the buccal-lingual dimension of the tooth at the furcation orifice, the clinician must conclude that a grade III furcation exists (see Fig. 64.6C). Properly exposed and angled radiographs of early class III furcations display the defect as a radiolucent area in the crotch of the tooth (see Chapter 33).

Grade IV

In grade IV furcations, the interdental bone is destroyed, and the soft tissues have receded apically so that the furcation opening is clinically visible. A tunnel therefore exists between the roots of such an affected tooth. Thus the periodontal probe passes readily from one aspect of the tooth to another (see Fig. 64.6D).

 KEY FACT

Despite the valuable information found in the clinical examination, radiographs are essential for a complete and thorough diagnosis of furcation involvement.

Other Classification Indices

Hamp and associates[17] modified a three-stage classification system by attaching a millimeter measurement to separate the extent of horizontal involvement. Easley and Drennan[10] and Tarnow and Fletcher[37] have described classification systems that consider both horizontal and vertical attachment loss in classifying the extent of furcation involvement. The Tarnow and Fletcher article uses a

subclassification that measures the probeable vertical depth from the roof of the furca apically. The subclasses being proposed are: A, B, and C. "A" indicates a probeable vertical depth of 1 to 3 mm, "B" indicates 4 to 6 mm, and "C" indicates 7 or more mm of probeable depth from the roof of the furca apically. Furcations would thus be classified as IA, IB, and IC; IIA, IIB, and IIC; and IIIA, IIIB, and IIIC.

Consideration of defect configuration and the vertical component of the defect provides additional information that is useful in planning therapy.

 KEY FACT

The functions of classification systems are to assist in communication among therapists and to provide a framework for treatment.

Treatment

The objectives of furcation therapy are to (1) facilitate maintenance, (2) prevent further attachment loss, and (3) obliterate the furcation defects as a periodontal maintenance problem. The selection of therapeutic mode varies with the class of furcation involvement, the extent and configuration of bone loss, and other anatomic factors.

Therapeutic Classes of Furcation Defects
Class I: Early Defects

Incipient or early furcation defects (class I) are amenable to conservative periodontal therapy.[15] Because the pocket is suprabony and has not entered the furcation, oral hygiene, scaling, and root planing are effective.[16] Any thick overhanging margins of restorations, facial grooves, or CEPs should be eliminated by odontoplasty, recontouring,

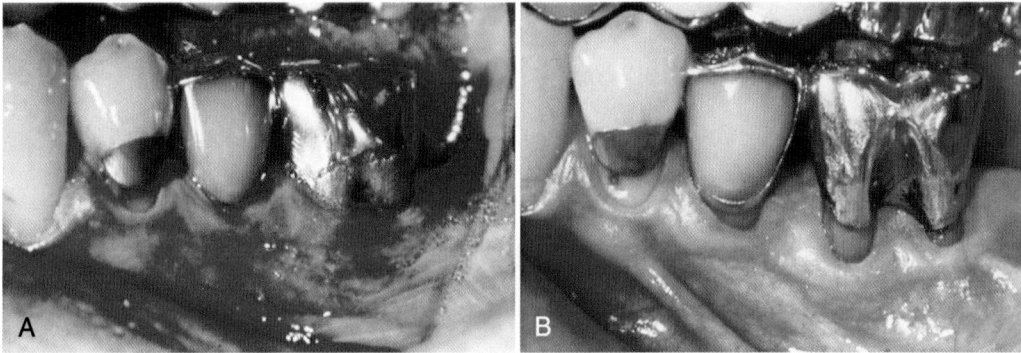

Fig. 64.7 Treatment of a grade II furcation by osteoplasty and odontoplasty. (A) This mandibular first molar has been treated endodontically and an area of caries in the furcation has been repaired. A class II furcation is present. (B) Results of flap debridement, osteoplasty, and severe odontoplasty 5 years postoperatively. Note the adaptation of the gingiva into the furcation area. *(Courtesy Dr. Ronald Rott, Sacramento, CA.)*

or replacement. The resolution of inflammation and subsequent repair of the periodontal ligament and bone are usually sufficient to restore periodontal health.

Class II

Once a horizontal component to the furcation has developed (class II), therapy becomes more complicated. Shallow horizontal involvement without significant vertical bone loss usually responds favorably to localized flap procedures with odontoplasty, osteoplasty, and ostectomy. Isolated deep class II furcations may respond to flap procedures with osteoplasty and odontoplasty (Fig. 64.7). This treatment reduces the dome of the furcation and alters gingival contours to facilitate the patient's plaque removal.

Classes II to IV: Advanced Defects

The development of a significant horizontal component to one or more furcations of a multirooted tooth (late class II, class III, or class IV[12]) or the development of a deep vertical component to the furca poses additional problems. Nonsurgical treatment is usually ineffective because the ability to instrument the tooth surfaces adequately is compromised.[31,40] Periodontal surgery, endodontic therapy, and restoration of the tooth may be required to retain the tooth.

Nonsurgical Therapy

Oral Hygiene Procedures

Furcal management is difficult at best. Therapeutic modalities for the treatment and maintenance of furcations have long been a dilemma for periodontists and restorative dentists. Nonsurgical therapy is a very effective way of producing a satisfactory stable result. Ideal results with furcations are impossible to obtain. Once furcation breakdown has begun, the clinical result is always somewhat compromised. Both surgical and nonsurgical therapies have been shown to work effectively over time. Nonsurgical therapy, a combination of oral hygiene instruction and scaling and root planing, has provided excellent results in some patients. The earlier the furcation is detected and treated, the more likely it will be that a good long-term result can be obtained. Nonetheless, even advanced furcation lesions can have successful long-term treatment.[34] Several oral hygiene procedures have been used over time. All include access to the furcation. Obtaining access to the furcation requires a

combination of the awareness of the furcation by the patient and an oral hygiene tool that facilitates that access. Many tools, including rubber tips, periodontal aids, both specific and general toothbrushes, and other aids have been used over time for access to the patient (Fig. 64.8).

Scaling and Root Planing

Nonsurgical maintenance by the clinician has also improved over time as instrumentation has improved. In recent decades, instruments beyond simple curettes have been used to instrument the furcation. The frustration of instrumenting the furcation was illustrated beautifully by Bower in 1979 in his articles[5,6] showing that only 58% of furcations could be entered by typically using curettes (see Chapter 35). Subsequently, other instrumentation has evolved, including DeMarco curettes, diamond files, Quétin furcation curettes, and Mini Five Gracey Curettes. See Chapter 50 for a detailed discussion on this subject.

Svärdström and Wennström[34] illustrated that in the long term, furcations could be maintained using nonaggressive techniques over a 10-year period in patients who were participants in consistent maintenance. Other studies also illustrate that maintenance therapy is useful for patients to facilitate furcation cleanliness. Chemotherapy has proven disappointing. Ribeiro and colleagues[32] found that nonsurgical therapy can effectively treat class II furcation involvements, but using povidone-iodine did not provide additional benefits to subgingival instrumentation.

KEY FACT

The maintenance of a furcation-involved tooth is difficult and requires special attention and care. This is especially true for Class III and IV cases.

The area most critical in furcation management is maintaining a relatively plaque-free status to the furcation. Attaining access is a problem in this regard, but with the previously mentioned instruments and an effective nonsurgical approach, much can be accomplished. The most critical component of multirooted tooth maintenance is always the successful reduction or elimination of plaque retention areas from the furcation area; meticulous oral hygiene by the patient and effective nonsurgical therapy can play a major role in attaining this goal.[21,33]

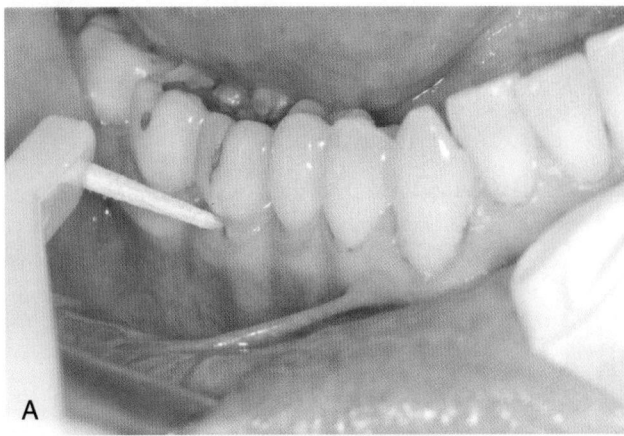

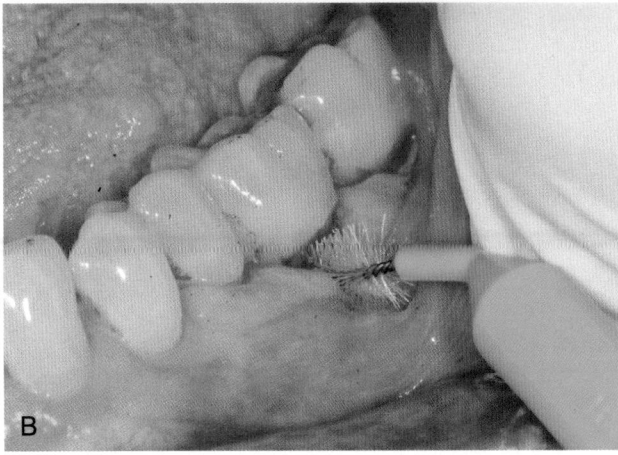

Fig. 64.8 (A) The utilization of a Perio-Aid into the furcation for plaque removal. (B) Proxy brush is used for plaque removal into the furcation lesion. *(Courtesy Karen DeYoung, RDH, and Janet Shigekawa, RDH.)*

 ## Surgical Therapy
Osseous Resection

Osseous surgical therapy can be divided into resective and regenerative therapy. This also applies to the furcation areas when surgical therapy is contemplated. For many years, osteoplasty and ostectomy have been used to make the furcation areas cleansable. In advanced cases, techniques were used to open the furcation into a class IV from a severe class II or III case. This would allow easier hygiene into the furcation area for the patient. These techniques have limited usefulness today, but in the compromised individual whose teeth cannot be extracted or in whom conservative therapy has failed, these surgical techniques have been used. The immediate goal with these surgical approaches is to create access for the patient to maintain good hygiene.

Regeneration

In furcal lesions, bone regeneration is often thought to be relatively futile. The periodontal literature has well-documented therapeutic efforts designed to induce new attachment and reconstruction on molars with furcation defects. Many surgical procedures using a variety of grafting materials have been tested on teeth with different classes of furcation involvement. Some investigators have reported clinical success,[24] whereas others have suggested that the use of these materials in class II, III, or IV furcations offers little advantage compared with surgical controls.[3,9,30]

Furcation defects with deep two-walled or three-walled components may be suitable for reconstruction procedures. These vertical bony deformities respond favorably to a variety of surgical procedures, including debridement with or without membranes and bone grafts. Chapter 63 addresses therapies designed to induce new attachment or reattachment.

Tsao and associates[39] have shown that the furcation defect is a graftable lesion. They found that lesions that were grafted had greater vertical fill than areas treated with open flap debridement alone. Bowers and colleagues[7] have shown that furcation bone grafting using various membranes can improve the clinical status of these lesions. Nonetheless, bone grafting remains an elusive goal with variable results in furcation lesions.

Another area of interest has been barrier membrane technology. Analysis of published studies demonstrated a great variability in the clinical outcomes in mandibular grade II furcations treated with different types of nonbioabsorbable and bioabsorbable barrier membranes. Although many barrier membrane studies show a slight clinical improvement after treatment in both maxillary and mandibular furcations, the results are generally inconsistent.

Extraction

The extraction of teeth with through-and-through furcation defects (classes III and IV) and advanced attachment loss may be the most appropriate therapy for some patients. This is particularly true for individuals who cannot or will not perform adequate plaque control, who have a high level of caries activity, who will not commit to a suitable maintenance program, or who have socioeconomic factors that may preclude more complex therapies. Some patients are reluctant to accept periodontal surgery or even allow the removal of a tooth with advanced furcation involvement, even though the long-term prognosis is poor. The patient may elect to forego therapy, opt to treat the area with scaling and root planing or site-specific antibacterial therapies, and delay extraction until the tooth becomes symptomatic. Although additional attachment loss may occur, such teeth may survive a significant number of years.[21,33]

Dental Implants

The advent of osseointegrated dental implants as an alternative abutment source has had a major impact on the retention of teeth with advanced furcation problems. The high level of predictability of osseointegration may motivate the therapist and patient to consider removal of teeth with a guarded or poor prognosis and to seek an implant-supported prosthetic treatment plan. Therefore careful evaluation of the long-term periodontal, endodontic, and restorative prognosis must be considered before invasive surgical therapy is undertaken to save a tooth with an advanced furcated lesion (Fig. 64.9).

Prognosis

For many years the presence of significant furcation involvement meant a hopeless long-term prognosis for the tooth. Clinical research, however, has indicated that furcation problems are not as severe a complication as originally suspected if one can prevent the development of caries in the furcation. Relatively simple periodontal therapy is sufficient to maintain these teeth in function for long periods.[21,33] Other investigators have defined the reasons for clinical failure of root-resected or hemisected teeth.[2,25] Their data indicate that recurrent periodontal disease is not a major cause of the failure of these teeth. Investigations of root-resected or hemisected teeth have shown that such teeth can function successfully for long periods.[2,8,25]

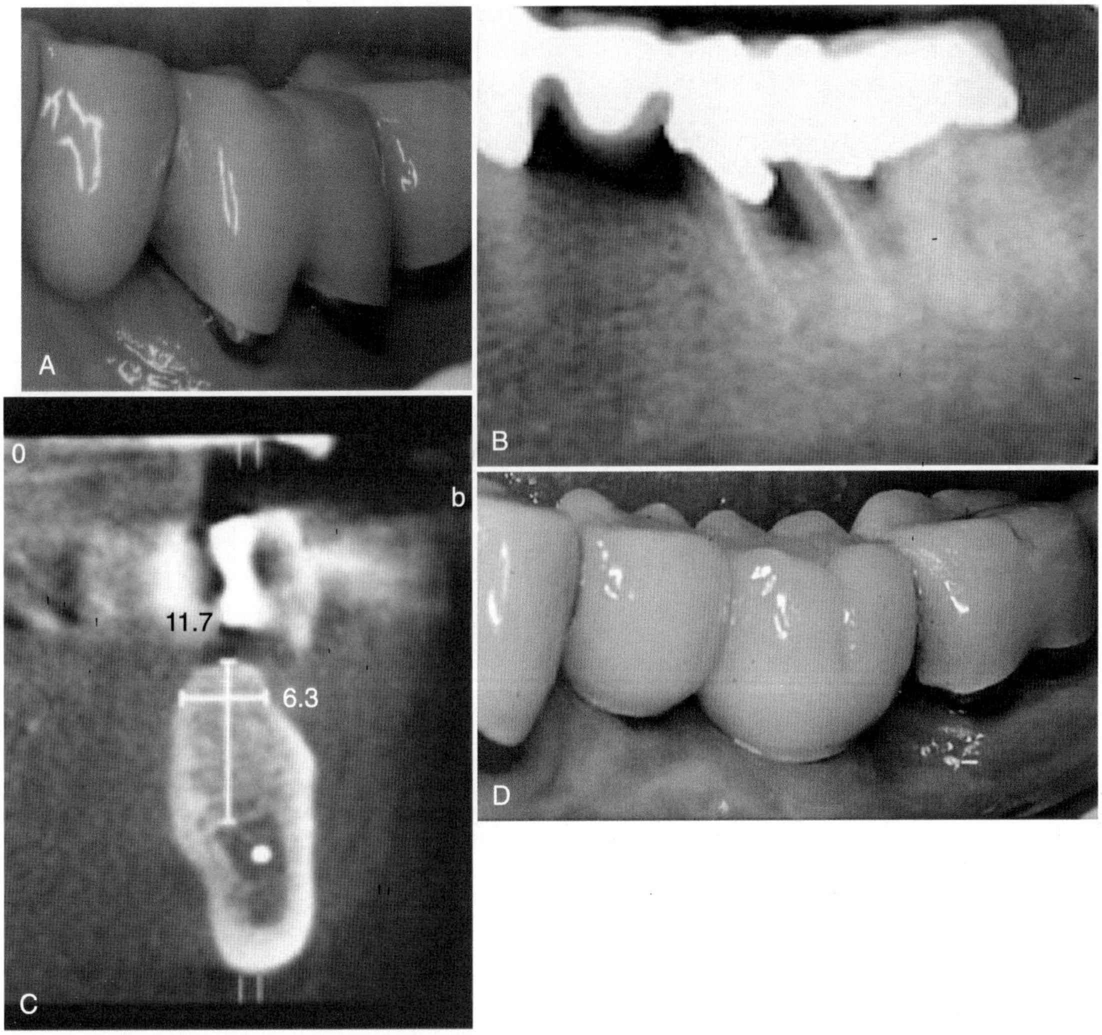

Fig. 64.9 (A) Clinical picture of a class III furcation involvement. (B) Radiographic appearance is far more grave than the clinical appearance. (C) After the tooth is removed, a computed tomography image is taken to plan treatment for implant replacement. (D) The implant restored. *(Courtesy Dr. Sarvenaz Angha, Los Angeles, CA.)*

The keys to long-term success appear to be (1) thorough diagnosis, (2) selection of patients with good oral hygiene, (3) excellence in nonsurgical therapy, and (4) careful surgical and restorative management.

 A Case Scenario is found on the companion website www.expertconsult.com.

References

 References for this chapter are found on the companion website www.expertconsult.com.

CHAPTER 65

Periodontal Plastic and Aesthetic Surgery

Henry H. Takei | E. Todd Scheyer | Robert R. Azzi | Edward P. Allen | Thomas J. Han

CHAPTER OUTLINE

Terminology
Objectives
Cause of Marginal Tissue
 Recession
Factors That Affect Surgical
 Outcome

Techniques to Increase Attached
 Gingiva *(e-only)*
Techniques to Deepen the Vestibule
 (e-only)
Techniques to Remove the Frenum
 (e-only)

Techniques to Improve Aesthetics
 (e-only)
Tissue Engineering *(e-only)*
Criteria for Selection of Techniques
Conclusions

> Content on techniques to increase attached gingiva, gingival augmentation coronal to recession, tissue engineering, and techniques used to deepen the vestibule, remove the frenum, and improve aesthetics can be accessed on the companion website at www.expertconsult.com.

Terminology

The term *mucogingival surgery* was initially introduced in the literature by Friedman[38] to describe surgical procedures for the correction of relationships between the gingiva and the oral mucous membrane, with special reference to three problem areas: attached gingiva, shallow vestibules, and a frenum interfering with the marginal gingiva. With the advancement of periodontal surgical techniques, the scope of nonpocket surgical procedures has increased and now encompasses a multitude of areas that were not addressed in the past. Recognizing this, the 1996 World Workshop in Clinical Periodontics renamed mucogingival surgery as *periodontal plastic surgery*,[4] a term originally proposed by Miller in 1993 and broadened to include the following areas[3,4]:

- Periodontal-prosthetic corrections
- Crown lengthening
- Ridge augmentation
- Aesthetic surgical corrections
- Coverage of the denuded root surface
- Reconstruction of papillae
- Aesthetic surgical correction around implants
- Surgical exposure of unerupted teeth for orthodontics

Periodontal plastic surgery is defined as the surgical procedures performed to correct or eliminate anatomic, developmental, or traumatic deformities of the gingiva or alveolar mucosa.[3,4] Muco-gingival therapy is a broader term that includes non-surgical procedures such as papilla reconstruction by means of orthodontic or restorative therapy. Periodontal plastic surgery includes only the surgical pro-cedures of mucogingival therapy (Video 65.1).

The periodontal plastic surgical techniques included in the traditional definition of mucogingival surgery are (1) widening of attached gingiva, (2) deepening of shallow vestibules, and (3) resection of the aberrant frena. Aesthetic surgical therapy for natural dentition and tissue engineering (i.e., biologic mediators) also are addressed in this chapter. Other aspects of periodontal plastic surgery, such as periodontal-prosthetic surgery, aesthetic surgery around implants, and surgical exposure of teeth for orthodontic therapy, are covered in Chapters 56, 69, and 81.

A classification system for periodontal surgery is shown in Fig. 65.1. It indicates the category of periodontal plastic surgery in surgical procedures that are used in periodontal therapy.

Objectives

Five objectives of periodontal plastic surgery are addressed in this chapter:

1. Problems associated with attached gingiva
2. Problems associated with a shallow vestibule
3. Problems associated with an aberrant frenum
4. Aesthetic surgical therapy
5. Tissue engineering

Problems Associated With Attached Gingiva

The ultimate goal of mucogingival surgical procedures is the creation or widening of attached gingiva around teeth and implants.[4] The width of the attached gingiva varies in different individuals and on different teeth of the same individual (see Chapter 3). Attached gingiva is not synonymous with keratinized gingiva because the latter also includes the free gingival margin. The width of the attached gingiva is determined by subtracting the depth of the sulcus or pocket from the distance between the crest of the gingival margin and the mucogingival junction.

The original rationale for mucogingival surgery was predicated on the assumption that a minimal width of attached gingiva was required to maintain optimal gingival health. However, several studies have challenged the view that a wide, attached gingiva is more protective against the accumulation of biofilm than a narrow or a nonexistent zone. No minimal width of attached gingiva has been established as a standard necessary for gingival health. People who practice good, atraumatic oral hygiene can maintain excellent gingival health with almost no attached gingiva.

However, individuals whose oral hygiene practices are less than optimal can be helped by the presence of keratinized gingiva and vestibular depth. Vestibular depth provides space for easier placement of the toothbrush and prevents brushing on mucosal tissue. To improve

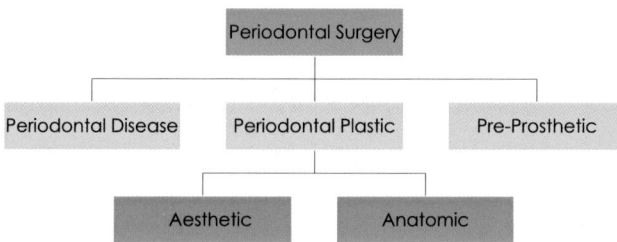

Fig. 65.1 Classification of periodontal surgery.

aesthetics, the objective is the coverage of the denuded root surface. The maxillary anterior area, especially the facial aspect of the canine, often has extensive gingival recession. In these cases, the covering of the denuded root surface widens the zone of attached gingiva and creates an improved aesthetic result. Recession and the resultant denuded root surface have special aesthetic concerns for individuals with a high smile line. A wider zone of attached gingiva is also needed around teeth that serve as abutments for fixed or removable partial dentures and in the ridge areas bearing a denture. Teeth with subgingival restorations and narrow zones of keratinized gingiva have higher gingival inflammation scores than teeth with similar restorations and wide zones of attached gingiva.[96,97] In these cases, techniques for widening the attached gingiva are considered preprosthetic periodontal surgical procedures. Chapter 69 discusses this subject in detail.

Widening the attached gingiva accomplishes four objectives:
1. Enhances plaque removal around the gingival margin
2. Improves aesthetics
3. Reduces inflammation around restored teeth
4. Allows gingival margin to bind better around teeth and implants with attached gingiva

Problems Associated With a Shallow Vestibule

Another objective of periodontal plastic surgery is the creation of vestibular depth when it is lacking. Gingival recession displaces the gingival margin apically, reducing vestibular depth, which is measured from the gingival margin to the bottom of the vestibule. With minimal vestibular depth, proper hygiene procedures are jeopardized. The sulcular brushing technique (i.e., Bass technique) requires placement of the toothbrush at the gingival margin, which may not be possible with reduced vestibular depth.

Minimal attached gingiva with adequate vestibular depth may not require surgical correction if proper atraumatic hygiene is practiced with a soft brush. Minimal amounts of keratinized attached gingiva with no vestibular depth benefit from mucogingival correction. Adequate vestibular depth is also necessary for the proper placement of removable prostheses.

Problems Associated With an Aberrant Frenum

An important objective of periodontal plastic surgery is correction of frenal or muscle attachments that may extend coronal to the mucogingival junction. If adequate keratinized, attached gingiva exists coronal to the frenum, it may not be necessary to remove the frenum. A frenum that encroaches on the margin of the gingiva can interfere with biofilm removal, and the tension on the frenum tends to open the sulcus. In these cases, surgical removal of the frenum is indicated.

Aesthetic Surgical Therapy

Recession of the facial gingival margin alters the proper gingival symmetry and results in an aesthetic problem. The interdental papilla is also important to satisfy the aesthetic goals of the patient. A missing papilla creates a space that many call a *black hole*. Regeneration of the lost or reduced papilla is one of the most difficult goals in aesthetic periodontal plastic surgery.

Another area of concern is an excessive amount of gingiva in the visible area. This condition is often called as a *gummy smile,* and it can be corrected surgically by crown lengthening. Correction of these anatomic defects has become an important part of periodontal plastic surgery.

Tissue Engineering

The future of periodontal plastic surgery will encompass the use of tissue-engineered products at the recipient site to reduce donor site morbidity. Results of numerous experimental and clinical studies support the clinician's use of a minimally invasive approach to periodontal plastic surgery.

Cause of Marginal Tissue Recession

The most common cause of gingival recession and the loss of attached gingiva is abrasive and traumatic toothbrushing habits. The bone and soft tissue anatomy of the facial, radicular surface of the dentition is usually thin, especially around the anterior area. Teeth positioned facially may have an even thinner bone and gingiva. In many instances, the areas have a complete absence of bone beneath the thin overlying gingival tissue. This defect in the bone is called a *dehiscence*. This anatomic status combined with external trauma from overzealous brushing can lead to the loss of gingival tissue. Recession of the gingival tissue and bone exposes the cemental surface of the root, which results in abrasion and ditching of the cemental surface apical to the cementoenamel junction (CEJ). The cementum is softer than enamel and is destroyed before the enamel surface of the crown.

Another cause of gingival recession is periodontal disease and chronic marginal inflammation. The loss of attachment caused by the inflammation is followed by the loss of bone and gingiva. Advanced periodontal involvement in areas of minimally attached gingiva results in the base of the pocket extending close to or apical to the mucogingival junction. Periodontal therapy for these areas results in gingival recession caused by the loss of gingiva and bone.

Frenal and muscle attachments that encroach on the marginal gingiva can distend the gingival sulcus, which creates an environment for biofilm accumulation. This condition increases the rate of periodontal recession and contributes to the recurrence of recession, even after treatment (Fig. 65.2). These problems are more common on facial surfaces, but they may also occur on the lingual surface.[11]

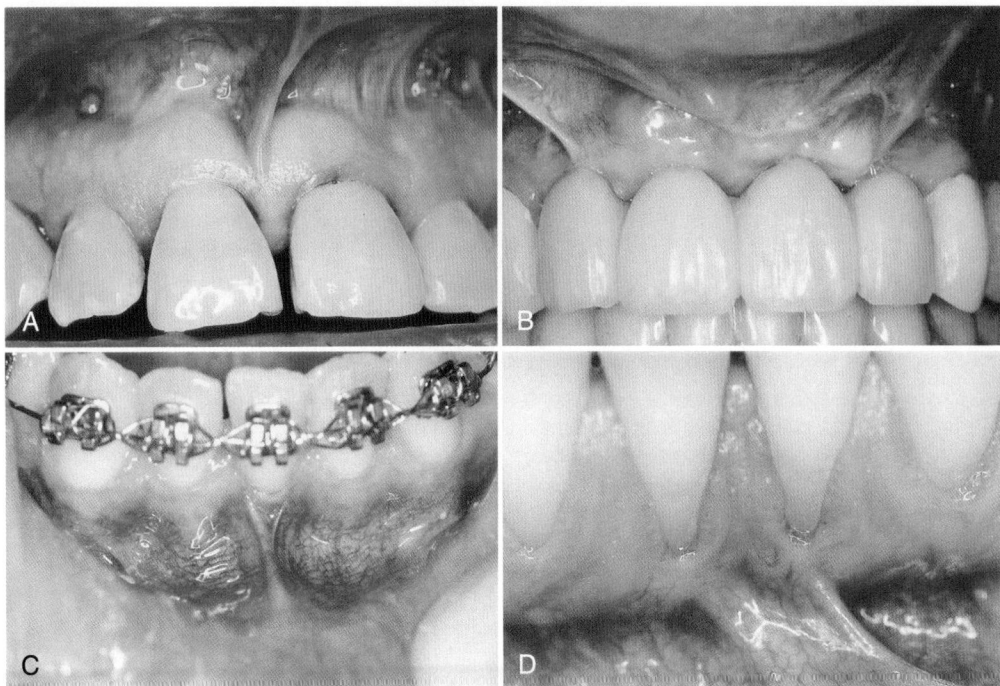

Fig. 65.2 High frenum attachments. (A) Frenum between the maxillary central incisors. (B) Frenum attached to the facial surface of the maxillary lateral incisors. (C) Frenum attached to the facial surface of a mandibular incisor. (D) Frenum attached to the facial surface of an incisor.

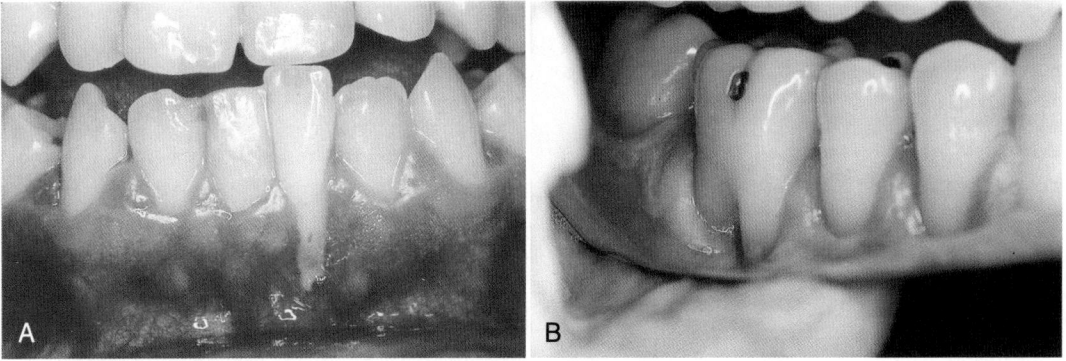

Fig. 65.3 (A) Gingival recession and extreme inflammation around a lower central incisor. (B) Advanced recession of the mesial root of a first lower molar.

Orthodontic tooth movement through a thin buccal osseous plate may lead to a dehiscence beneath a thin gingiva. This situation can also lead to the recession of the gingival margin[46,117] (Fig. 65.3).

Factors That Affect Surgical Outcome

Irregularity of Teeth

Abnormal tooth alignment is an important cause of gingival deformities that require corrective surgery and an important factor in determining the outcome of treatment. Location of the gingival margin, width of the attached gingiva, and alveolar bone height and thickness are affected by tooth alignment. On teeth that are tilted or rotated labially, the labial bony plate is thinner and located further apically than on the adjacent teeth. The gingival margin is recessed apically to follow the bone, which leads to the exposure of the root.[117] On the lingual surface of these teeth, the gingiva is bulbous, and the bone margins are closer to the CEJ. The level of gingival attachment on the root surfaces and the width of the attached gingiva after

mucogingival surgery are affected as much by tooth alignment as by variations in treatment procedures.

Orthodontic correction is indicated when mucogingival surgery is performed on malposed teeth in an attempt to widen the attached gingiva or to restore the gingiva over denuded roots. If orthodontic treatment is not feasible, the prominent tooth should be reduced to within the borders of the alveolar bone, with special care taken to avoid pulp injury.

Roots covered with thin bony plates pose a hazard in mucogingival surgery. Even the most minimally invasive flap, such as the partial-thickness flap, creates the risk of bone resorption on the periosteal surface.[49] Resorption in amounts that ordinarily are not significant may cause loss of bone height when the bone plate is thin or tapered at the crest.

Mucogingival Line

Normally, the mucogingival line (i.e., junction) in the incisor and canine areas is located approximately 3 mm apical to the crest of the alveolar bone on the radicular surfaces and 5 mm interdentally.[98] In periodontal disease and on malposed, disease-free teeth, the bone margin is located further apically and may extend beyond the mucogingival line. The distance between the mucogingival line and the CEJ before and after periodontal surgery is not necessarily constant. After inflammation is eliminated, the tissue tends to contract and draw the mucogingival line in the direction of the crown.[31]

Criteria for Selection of Techniques

Numerous techniques are used for solving the mucogingival problems outlined in this chapter. Proper selection of a technique must be based on the predictability of success, which is based on specific criteria.

The following criteria are used for selection of mucogingival techniques:
1. Surgical site free of biofilm, calculus, and inflammation
2. Adequate blood supply to the donor tissue
3. Anatomy of the recipient and donor sites
4. Stability of the grafted tissue to the recipient site
5. Minimal trauma to the surgical site

Surgical Site Free of Biofilm, Calculus, and Inflammation

Periodontal plastic surgical procedures should be undertaken in a biofilm-free and inflammation-free environment to enable the clinician to manage gingival tissue that is firm. Meticulous, precise incisions and flap reflection cannot be achieved when tissue is inflamed and edematous. Thorough scaling and root planing and meticulous biofilm removal by the patient must be accomplished before any surgical procedure.

Adequate Blood Supply

To obtain the maximal amount of blood supply to the donor tissue, gingival augmentation apical to the area of recession provides a better blood supply than coronal augmentation because the recipient site is entirely periosteal tissue. Root coverage procedures involve a portion of the recipient site (i.e., denuded root surface) without blood supply. If aesthetics is not a factor, gingival augmentation apical to the recession may be more predictable. A pedicle-displaced flap has a better blood supply than a free graft, with the base of the flap intact. If the anatomy is favorable, the pedicle flap or any of its variants may be the best procedure for root coverage.

The Langer subepithelial connective tissue graft (SECTG) procedure and the pouch and tunnel techniques use a split flap with the connective tissue sandwiched between the flaps. This flap design maximizes the blood supply to the donor tissue. If large areas require root coverage, these sandwich-type recipient sites provide the best flap design for blood supply.

Anatomy of the Recipient and Donor Sites

The presence or absence of vestibular depth is an important anatomic criterion at the recipient site for gingival augmentation. If gingival augmentation is indicated apical to the area of recession, there must be adequate vestibular depth apical to the recessed gingival margin to provide space for a free or pedicle graft. If a vestibule is necessary, only a free graft can accomplish this objective apical to the recession.

Mucogingival techniques, such as free gingival grafts and free connective tissue grafts, can be used to create vestibular depth and widen the zone of attached gingiva. Other techniques require vestibular depth to exist before the surgery, including pedicle grafts (i.e., lateral and coronal), the Langer SECTG, and pouch and tunnel procedures.

Availability of donor tissue is another anatomic factor that must be considered. Pedicle displacement of tissue necessitates an adjacent donor site that has gingival thickness and width. Palatal tissue thickness is also necessary for the connective tissue donor autograft. Gingival thickness is required at the recipient site for techniques using a split-thickness, sandwich-type flap or the pouch and tunnel techniques.

Stability of the Grafted Tissue to the Recipient Site

Good communication of the blood vessels from the grafted donor tissue to the recipient site requires a stable environment. This necessitates sutures that stabilize the donor tissue firmly against the recipient site. The least amount of sutures and maximal stability should be achieved.

Minimal Trauma to the Surgical Site

As with all surgical procedures, periodontal plastic surgery is based on the meticulous, delicate, and precise management of oral tissues. Unnecessary tissue trauma caused by poor incisions, flap perforations, tears, or traumatic and excessive placement of sutures can lead to tissue necrosis. The proper selection of instruments, needles, and sutures is mandatory to minimize tissue trauma. Sharp contoured blades (see eFig. 65.16), smaller-diameter needles, and resorbable monofilament sutures are important factors in achieving atraumatic surgery.

Conclusions

Periodontal plastic surgery refers to soft tissue relationships and manipulations. In all of these procedures, blood supply is the most significant concern and must be the underlying issue for all decisions regarding the individual surgical procedure. A major complicating factor is the avascular root surface, and many modifications to existing techniques are used to overcome this. Diffusion of fluids is short term and of limited benefit as tissue size increases. The formation of a circulation through anastomosis and angiogenesis is crucial to the survival of these therapeutic procedures.

Formation of vascularity is based on growth molecules, such as vascular endothelial growth factor (VEGF), and on cellular migration, proliferation, and differentiation. As tissue-engineering techniques improve, the success and predictability of mucogingival surgery should dramatically increase. However, all advancements must have adequate circulation and blood supply as their basis.

New techniques are being developed and are slowly being incorporated into periodontal practice. The practitioner should be aware that new methods sometimes are published without adequate clinical research to ensure the predictability of the results and the extent to which the techniques may benefit the patient. Critical analysis of recently presented techniques should guide the evolution toward better clinical methods.

 A Case Scenario is found on the companion website www.expertconsult.com.

References

 References for this chapter are found on the companion website www.expertconsult.com.

CHAPTER 66

Leukocyte- and Platelet-Rich Fibrin: Biologic Properties and Applications

Nelson R. Pinto | Andy Temmerman | Ana B. Castro | Simone Cortellini | Wim Teughels | Marc Quirynen

CHAPTER OUTLINE

 Content on the use of L-PRF for extraoral applications, sinus floor elevation, implant surgery, and medication-related osteonecrosis of the jawbone, as well as initial observations on the PRF-Block, can be accessed on the companion website at www.expertconsult.com.

Introduction

Wound healing has been and remains an important topic in dentistry and other medical fields. Biomaterials proved to be beneficial in the process of wound healing.[10] They can be derived from nature or synthesized in the laboratory using a variety of chemical approaches. Countless efforts have been made to find new and specific bioactive additives that promote and accelerate healing, regulate inflammation, and improve regeneration. The impact of platelet concentrates to achieve these goals has been explored in sports medicine and orthopedics.[26] By facilitating recruitment, proliferation, and maturation of cells participating in regeneration, platelet concentrates clearly improve wound healing.[14]

Tissue adhesives (fibrin glues) were the precursors of platelet concentrates. Afterward, different types of platelet concentrates were developed. Based on the leukocyte content and fibrin structure, platelet concentrates can be classified into four main categories[26]:

- Pure platelet-rich plasma (P-PRP) without leukocytes and with a low-density fibrin network after activation
- Leukocyte- and platelet-rich plasma (L-PRP) with leukocytes and with a low-density fibrin network after activation
- Pure platelet-rich fibrin (P-PRF) without leukocytes and with a high-density fibrin network
- Leukocyte- and platelet-rich fibrin (L-PRF) with leukocytes and a high-density fibrin network

The literature is at times contradictory on the benefits of these platelet concentrates, and the data is often difficult to interpret. This chapter focuses on the use of L-PRF as a platelet concentrate for tissue regeneration.

From Fibrin Sealers to Platelet Concentrates

Fibrin sealers were one of the first biologic adjuvants in surgery. They were used in the 1970s to stimulate wound healing in rats.[65] It was the derivatives of human plasma that mimicked the last steps in the process of blood coagulation by the formation of a fibrin clot. Fibrin sealers are divided into two groups:

- Homologous fibrin sealers: products made from a combination of fibronectin, fibrinogen, factor VIII, and a thrombin concentrate in calcium chloride
- Autologous fibrin sealers: products of plasma in which the fibrin polymerization is started by the addition of thrombin of animal origin

The main action of these fibrin sealers is to stimulate local angiogenesis, minimize edema or hematoma formation, and reduce postoperative pain. The fibrin matrix is the main component of fibrin sealers. The properties of this matrix are determined by interactions among circulating fibrinogen, platelet aggregation, and molecules produced by the platelets.

Further research led to an upgraded version of the sealers, called platelet-derived wound healing factor (PDWHF). This group of sealers contains a significant concentration of platelets to strengthen the fibrin gel and simultaneously promote healing capacities. The addition of more components from blood forms a more natural product. The results in general surgery, neurosurgery, and ophthalmology are encouraging.

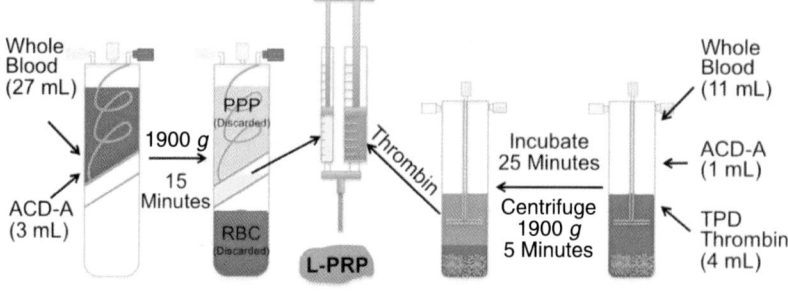

Fig. 66.1 Centrifugation protocol for L-PRP (leucocyte- and platelet rich plasma) according to the manufacturer's protocol (Biomet Inc., Dietikon, Switzerland). *ACD-A*, Adenosine-citrate-dextrose acid anticoagulant; *PPP*, plasma-poor platelets; *RBC*, red blood cells; *TPD*, thrombin processing device (Thermogenesis Corp., Rancho Cordova, CA). *(From Schär MO, Diaz-Romero J, Kohl S, Zumstein MA, Nesic D: Platelet-rich concentrates differentially release growth factors and induce cell migration in vitro.* Clin Orthop Relat Res *473:1635–1643, 2015.)*

The First Generation of Platelet Concentrates: Platelet-Rich Plasma

Whitman, Berry, and Green in 1997[90] and Marx and colleagues in 1998[63] were the first to promote the use of PRP in oral and maxillofacial surgery. In essence, PRP is an increased concentration of autologous platelets in a small amount of plasma that is obtained after centrifugation. The preparation is quite complex (Fig. 66.1). Briefly, 27 mL of blood is collected in a 30-mL syringe containing 3 mL of adenosine-citrate-dextrose acid (ACD-A) anticoagulant. The content of the syringe is transferred to the 30-mL separation tube and centrifuged at a relative centrifugal force (RCF) of 1900g for 15 min at room temperature. After removal of the plasma, the buffy coat is resuspended in the leftover plasma by shaking the tube for 30 seconds. A second syringe containing 1 mL of ACD-A is used to collect an additional 11 mL of blood, which is transferred into a Clotalyst disposable tube (Biomet Inc., Dietikon, Switzerland) containing 4 mL thrombin. After gentle mixing, the tube is placed into a Clotalyst disposable tube heater for 25 min. Subsequently, the mix is centrifuged for 5 min at 1900g. Coagulation is performed with the use of a double syringe (spray applicator) that allows uniform mixing of the two components, resulting in the formation of a clot. The time between centrifugation and clinical use is approximately 45 min.

The benefits of using PRP in medicine have been studied extensively. Most reviews are found within the field of orthopedics and sports medicine. According to a meta-analysis,[16] the intra-articular injection of PRP in patients with osteoarthritis of the knee is beneficial. However, results are not conclusive.[55] In oral and maxillofacial surgery, PRP is particularly used after extraction of third molars,[9] in the treatment of periodontal intrabony defects,[34,71] in sinus elevation techniques,[53] and for hard and soft tissue augmentation.[69] The purpose of using PRP in these types of surgeries was to accelerate the vascularization of the graft, improve soft tissue healing and bone regeneration, and reduce postoperative morbidity. However, results remained inconclusive.

To improve its efficacy, the preparation protocol for this platelet concentrate has been changed and adapted several times over the years. A well-known example is platelet-rich growth factor (PRGF), which was first described by Anitua and coworkers.[4] PRGF differs from other platelet concentrates in its versatility. Depending on the degree of coagulation and activation of the blood, four different types of preparations with different therapeutic potentials were obtained (e.g., PRGF structure as a liquid substance or a dense elastic fibrin). Research showed that PRGF may be used as a treatment modality for osteoarthritis, treatment of ulcers, tissue engineering, and oral surgery applications. However, the results should be interpreted with some caution.[5] Overall, we can say that there is a shortage of critical scientific data on the positive effects of PRP in clinical procedures. There is great variability in study designs (e.g., small groups of patients, no control groups) and also in preparation protocols (e.g., without clear classification), which makes comparisons

Table 66.1   Major Differences Between Platelet-Rich Plasma (PRP) and Leukocyte- and Platelet-Rich Fibrin (L-PRF)

Blood Products	PRF (2004)	PRP (1998)
Protocol	Easy	Very complex
Speed	Fast	Slow
Reproducibility	No bias	Possible bias
Use of anticoagulants	No	Yes
Amount obtainable	Good	Enough
Cost of the protocol	Low	Moderate
Amount of fibrin obtainable	High	Low
Speed of fibrin formation	Physiological	High
Fibrin morphology	Trimolecular	Tetramolecular
Leukocyte amount	65%	0–50%
Immunomodulatoy properties	Yes	Poor
Neoangiogenic potential	+++++	+
Osteoconductive potential (scaffolding)	High	Poor
Mechanical properties (sol-gel membrane)	Good	Enough
Presence of MSCs	Yes	Yes

MSCs, Mesenchymal stem cells.
From Giannini S, Cielo A, Bonanome L, et al: Comparison between PRP, PRGF and PRF: lights and shadows in three similar but different protocols. *Eur Rev Med Pharmacol Sci* 19:927–930, 2015.

difficult. Furthermore, the use of PRP has a number of significant disadvantages: the preparation protocol is expensive, complicated, and very operator dependent, and the need for animal thrombin as a coagulant raises legal issues in some countries.[51]

The Second Generation of Platelet Concentrates: Platelet-Rich Fibrin

New techniques were investigated to overcome the disadvantages of PRP (Table 66.1). This resulted in the introduction of PRF by Choukroun and coworkers in 2001.[22] PRF can be seen as an autologous biomaterial made of a fibrin matrix that contains the following[41]:

- The highest concentration of platelets
- The highest concentration of growth factors, including platelet-derived growth factor (PDGF), vascular endothelial growth factor (VEGF), and transforming growth factor (TGF)
- A representative concentration of fibrin, fibronectin, vitronectin, and thrombospondin
- An approximately 65% concentration of leukocytes

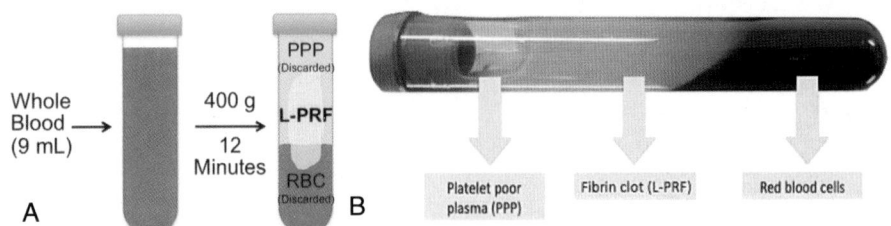

Fig. 66.2 (A) L-PRF tube after centrifugation, with its three compartments. (B) Photograph of a tube after the preparation of L-PRF. *PPP*, platelet-poor plasma; *RBC*, red blood cells. (A, *from Schär MO, Diaz-Romero J, Kohl S, Zumstein MA, Nesic D: Platelet-rich concentrates differentially release growth factors and induce cell migration in vitro.* Clin Orthop Relat Res *473:1635–1643, 2015.)*

Nowadays, PRF can be regarded as the least expensive and most streamlined way to produce platelet concentrate. PRF is classified according to its leukocyte content as either L-PRF or P-PRF. L-PRF contains up to 90% of the platelets and at least 75% of the leukocytes present in the patient's blood. This chapter deals only with L-PRF.

Preparation of L-PRF

Blood samples (9–10 mL) are collected in sterile glass or plastic-coated tubes. The tubes are placed in pairs and centrifuged at 400*g* RCF for 12 min using the Intraspin centrifuge (Intra-Lock International, Boca Raton, FL); 400*g* RCF is equivalent to 2700 rpm. The Intraspin centrifuge is approved by the U.S. Food and Drug Administration and has a level 2 CE certificate. It is very important that the collection of blood and placement of the tubes in the centrifuge happen as rapidly as possible, before the spontaneous coagulation process occurs. Ideally, the tubes should be centrifuging within 60 seconds after the start of the venipuncture. This often requires loading the centrifuge with tubes two by two or one by one. In the latter case, a tube filled with the same amount of glycerine or saline should be considered to balance the centrifugation.

There is no manipulation of the blood; no anticoagulants are used in the tubes, and hence there is no need for animal thrombin and calcium chloride for fibrin polymerization. Plastic tubes are coated with silica and silicon to activate the coagulation. The absence of anticoagulants allows the activation of platelets in contact with the inner walls of the tube. After a few minutes, a coagulation cascade is initiated. Initially, the fibrinogen is positioned in the upper part of the tube. However, after centrifugation, due to the activation of autologous thrombin, it is converted to fibrin and a fibrin clot is created. After centrifugation, three distinct layers can be seen in the tube (Fig. 66.2): red blood cells (RBCs) at the bottom of the tube, platelet-poor plasma (PPP) at the top of the tube, and the fibrin clot (containing most leukocytes and platelets) in the middle of the tube.

The L-PRF clot can be removed from the tube with surgical tweezers. With an instrument similar to a spatula, the RBC fraction can be gently separated from the fibrin clot. The clot by itself contains a great amount of exudate, which is rich in growth factors. This exudate can be expressed by gentle compression of the clot (about 5 min) in order to obtain stronger L-PRF membranes. For this compression, one can utilize a specially engineered box. The box contains a weighted press plate that is designed to express serum from the L-PRF clot in a controlled manner. It forms standard 1-mm-thick L-PRF membranes (Box 66.1 and Fig. 66.3). The membranes remain stable at room temperature for several hours.

These autologous membranes, which have a dense fibrin network, are strong (one membrane can withstand a load of approximately 400 g before rupture) and have excellent biologic properties (rich in platelets, growth factors, and cytokines), opening many new clinical avenues. L-PRF provides a scaffold consisting of fibrin that promotes cellular migration, a fundamental aspect in the process of regeneration.[62] L-PRF membranes remain solid and intact in vitro and continuously release large quantities of growth factors for 7 to 14 days.

> ### KEY FACT
>
> The blood tubes have to be in the centrifuge within 60 seconds after the start of the venipuncture and centrifuged at 400*g* RCF for at least 12 minutes.

BOX 66.1   Step-by-Step Approach for the Preparation of L-PRF (Simple Chair-Side Procedure)

Protocol for Preparation of L-PRF Clots:

- Venipuncture: collect between four and eight 9-mL tubes of blood (see Fig. 66.3A,B).
- Tubes have to be in the centrifuge within 60 seconds. *(Often, the centrifuge is loaded step-wise with two tubes at a time; centrifugation is performed between collections of new tubes.)*
- Centrifuge at 400*g* RCF (2700 rpm) using the IntraSpin centrifuge (Intra-Lock International, Boca Raton, FL) for at least 12 min (see Fig. 66.3C). *(Start timing after the centrifuge has been loaded with the last two tubes.)*
- After at least 12 min of centrifugation (for patients taking anticoagulant medication, 15–18 min is recommended), the L-PRF clots are ready (see Fig. 66.3D).
- Take the clots out of the tubes and separate them from the red blood cells (see Fig. 66.3E,F).

Protocol for Preparation of L-PRF Membranes:

- Place clots in Xpression kit (Intra-Lock) for gentle compression by gravity (e.g., with light metal plate) (see Fig. 66.3G,H).
- Five minutes later, the L-PRF membranes are ready for use (see Fig. 66.3I).
- Membranes can be used during at least the next 2 hours but should be prevented from drying out.

Protocol for Preparation of L-PRF Plugs:

- Place clots in the small cylinder of the metal Xpression box.
- Use the piston to carefully compress the clot.
- Plugs can be used during at least the next 2 hours, but prevent them from drying out.

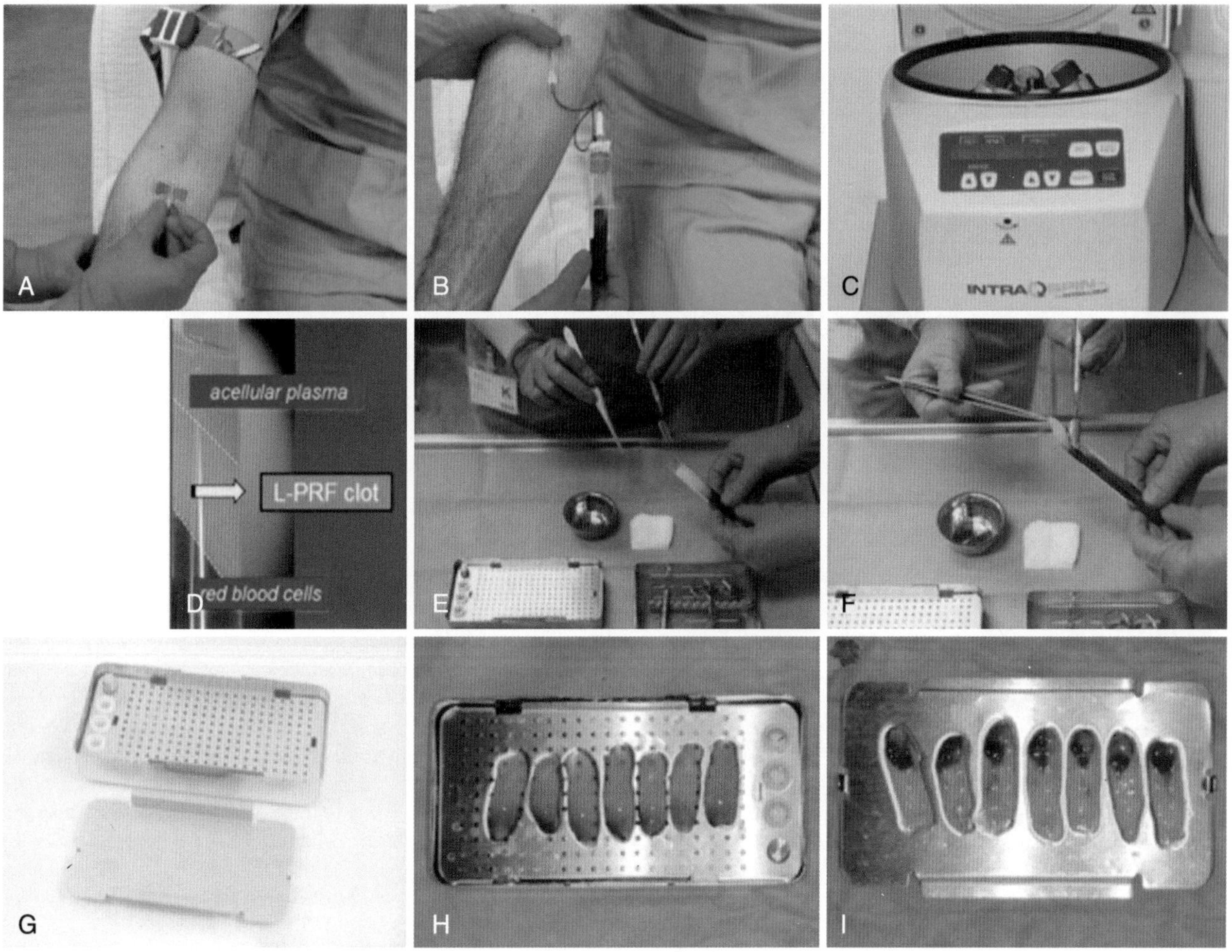

Fig. 66.3 Process of preparing L-PRF clots and membranes. (A and B) Venipuncture and blood collection. (C) Centrifugation at 400*g* RCF (2700 rpm) with the IntraSpin centrifuge (Intra-Lock International, Boca Raton, FL). (D) L-PRF clot in tube, showing clear separation: red blood cells (RBCs) at the bottom, PPP (platelet-poor plasma) on the top, and L-PRF fibrin clot in the middle. (E and F) Removal of clot from tube and separation of clot from RBCs. (G) A specially designed kit (Xpression box; Intra-Lock International) is used to compress L-PRF clots into L-PRF membranes with a consistent thickness of 1 mm. A piston and cylinder assembly *(left side of kit)* can be used for the creation of L-PRF plugs, which are suitable for filling extraction sockets. (H) L-PRF clots before compression. (I) L-PRF membranes after gentle compression; the red area of the membrane represents the face side, where most leukocytes and platelets are concentrated.

General Characteristics of L-PRF Membranes

Platelets in L-PRF

After centrifugation, at least 90% of the platelets derived from the blood sample are present in the fibrin clot. The platelets are mainly present in the lower portion of the clot, at the border between the RBCs and the clot itself. As a result, the lower portion of the clot, also called the *face*, is considered to be the most biologically active. The platelet cytoplasm contains several granules. The content is released at the time of activation. These granules contain many cytokines and many active substances such as serotonin, von Willebrand factor, factor V, osteonectin, and antimicrobial proteins. When platelets come in contact with the collagen of a damaged blood vessel, they get activated. This activation is necessary for platelet aggregation and thus starts and maintains hemostasis. Activation of the platelets involves degranulation and the sequential release of various cytokines. They stimulate cell migration and proliferation into the fibrin matrix. The principal role of the platelets is the maintenance of homeostasis; however, they are capable of binding, aggregating, and internalizing

microorganisms, which enhances the clearance of pathogens from the bloodstream. Platelets participate in antibody-dependent cell cytotoxicity functions to kill protozoal pathogens and to release an array of potent antimicrobial peptides.[12,83]

KEY FACT

After centrifugation, at least 90% of the platelets derived from the blood sample are present in the fibrin clot. The platelets are mainly present in the lower portion of the clot, at the border between the red blood cells and the clot itself. As a result, the lower portion of the clot, also called the face, is considered to be the most biologically active.

Leukocytes in L-PRF

Dohan and associates[32] analyzed the cellular content of L-PRF membranes and concluded that more than 50% of the leukocytes are concentrated in the fibrin matrix. A cell count performed at the KU Leuven (Periodontology and Oral Microbiology Laboratory) shows that more than 75% of the leukocytes remain within the L-PRF membrane (Table 66.2), whereas the concentration in the L-PRF exudate is very low. The latter, however, contains a high concentration of growth factors.

TABLE 66.2 Cellular Content of the L-PRF Membrane or L-PRF Exudate Based on the Analysis of 15 Patients

Cells	L-PRF Exudate (%)	L-PRF Membrane (%)
Red blood cells	1.1 ± 0.9	42.8 ± 17.7
Platelets	1.0 ± 0.8	96.9 ± 2.0
White blood cells (leukocytes)	3.5 ± 2.3	74.3 ± 8.9
Neutrophils	1.5 ± 2.2	62.9 ± 13.1
Lymphocytes	4.9 ± 3.9	82.1 ± 21.9
Monocytes	1.9 ± 2.5	93.3 ± 4.5
Eosinophils	1.6 ± 1.7	36.0 ± 29.9
Basophils	1.9 ± 2.8	84.4 ± 10.6

L-PRF, Leukocyte- and platelet-rich fibrin.
Adapted from Castro AB, Meschi N, Temmerman A, et al: Regenerative potential of leucocyte- and platelet-rich fibrin (L-PRF) Part B: sinus floor elevation, alveolar ridge preservation, and implant therapy. A systematic review. *J Clin Periodontol* 44:225–234, 2017b.

The presence of leukocytes in platelet concentrates is of great importance. Leukocytes have potential antibacterial characteristics but can also regulate cell proliferation and cell differentiation. In addition, they are the basic cells responsible for the wound healing process and the first cells to start neoangiogenesis. In fact, they contain VEGF, which acts as a potent vascular growth factor. The leukocytes are also a source of production of the aforementioned growth factors.

Neutrophils are recruited to the site of injury within minutes after trauma and are the hallmark of acute inflammation. They migrate toward the damaged site and get embedded in the fibrin network, forming a dense barrier against pathogens and preventing infection. Their main function is the production of inflammatory cytokines and growth factors.[4]

Monocytes are the largest type of leukocyte and can differentiate into macrophages, playing a central role in healing. They have immunologic functions as antigen-presenting cells and phagocytes.

Macrophages have been implicated in inflammation processes. However, they also play an essential role in bone repair. The role of monocytes and macrophages in bone repair has become an area of increased interest. Macrophages apparently direct osteogenic cell signals and promote mineralization during in vitro studies.[20] During bone injury, monocytes and macrophages modulate the acute inflammatory response, produce growth factors such as bone morphogenetic protein 2 (BMP-2) and PDGF-BB, and induce osteogenesis in mesenchymal stem cells.[19,91,92,93] Macrophages secrete collagenase, which promotes the cleaning of the wound. Additionally, they are a source of growth factors such as TGF, which stimulates the keratinocytes, and PDGF, which plays an important role in angiogenesis. Granulocytes and macrophages promote the production of inflammatory mediators such as leukotriene B4 and platelet-activating factor, which stimulate the expansion and increased permeability of blood vessels as well as the production of inflammatory cytokines and protolithic enzymes. These factors also act on the endothelial cells of blood vessels, stimulating the adhesion of neutrophils and lymphocytes and their migration out of blood vessels.[4]

Despite the release of activated oxygen species (free radicals) from leukocytes during phagocytosis activity and the ischemia reperfusion process, it seems that the inclusion of leukocytes in blood derivatives such as L-PRF may play a beneficial role.[38]

KEY FACT

More than 75% of the leukocytes remain within the L-PRF membrane. The presence of leukocytes in platelet concentrates is important. They can regulate cell proliferation and cell differentiation. Leukocytes are the basic cells responsible for wound healing and the first cells to start neoangiogenesis. They contain vascular endothelial growth factor (VEGF), which acts as a potent vascular growth factor.

Growth Factors in L-PRF

Platelets have an important function in the release of growth factors. The alpha-granules in platelets contain PDGF, insulin-like growth factor-1 (IGF-1), epidermal growth factor (EGF), VEGF, and TGF-β, which initiate wound healing by attracting and activating macrophages, fibroblasts, and endothelial cells. L-PRF membranes continuously release (≥7 days) a large quantity of growth factors. A significant amount of them are produced by the platelets (Fig. 66.4). These growth factors are also present in PRP gel. However, their release occurs specifically in the first hours, and they are completely dissolved in the medium after 3 days due to the chemical activation of the platelet content. This difference can be explained by the differences in fibrin architecture between the PRF families. PRF has a natural polymerization with intrinsic growth factor enmeshment, whereas PRP gel families have an artificial provoked polymerization with extrinsic growth factor enmeshment, leading to their immediate release and use or destruction.[28,74]

Fibrin in L-PRF

Fibrin is an insoluble clotting protein that plays a major role in platelet aggregation during hemostasis and wound healing. Fibrinogen, the precursor of fibrin, is converted by thrombin into fibrin, which forms long, nonsoluble strands that bind to platelets. Present in physiologic concentrations, thrombin allows the formation of a fibrin matrix in a slow and physiologic manner. The fibrin wires tend to polymerize and form a biochemical structure with trimolecular or equilateral junctions, providing a fine and flexible fibrin network that favors the entrapment of cytokines and cell migration (Fig. 66.5). This three-dimensional network has an important function as a matrix, promoting the invasion of various types of inflammatory, endothelial, and other cells. This matrix is also able to capture glycosaminoglycans (originating from the blood platelets). These glycosaminoglycans have a high affinity for circulating peptides (e.g., cytokines) and a large capacity to support cell migration and healing processes.[28]

Stem Cells in L-PRF

Dohan and colleagues[33] showed a significant stimulation of human bone mesenchymal stem cells when in contact with L-PRF. This effect was dose-dependent during the first weeks in normal conditions and during the whole experiment in differentiation conditions. The cultures without L-PRF in differentiation conditions did not rise above the degree of differentiation of the cultures in normal conditions with L-PRF up to the 14th and 28th day, respectively. The scanning electron microscopy (SEM) culture analysis at day 14 showed mineralization nodules more numerous and more structured in the groups with L-PRF compared to the control groups.

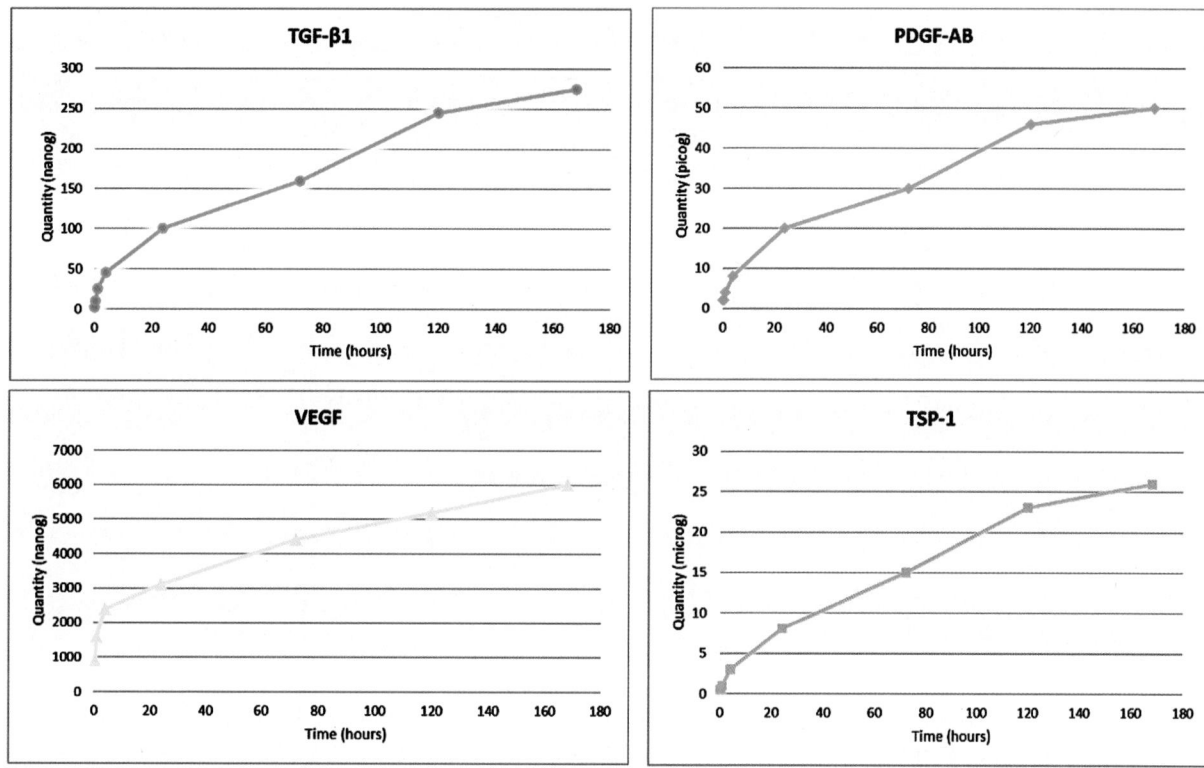

Fig. 66.4 Slow release of TGF-β1, PDGF-AB, VEGF, and thrombospondin-1 from an L-PRF membrane over 7 days. Values are expressed as the cumulative mean quantity of molecules at 20 min, 1h, 4h, 24h, 72h (3 days), 120h (5 days), and 168h (7 days). *PDGF,* Platelet-derived growth factor; *TGF,* transforming growth factor; *TSP,* thrombospondin; *VEGF,* vascular endothelial growth factor. *(From Dohan DM, de Peppo GM, Doglioli P, Sammartino G: Slow release of growth factors and thrombospondin-1 in Choukroun's platelet-rich fibrin (PRF): a gold standard to achieve for all surgical platelet concentrates technologies.* Growth Factors *27:63–69, 2009.)*

L-PRF in the Treatment of Periodontal Bony Defects

The use of L-PRF in the treatment of periodontal or bone defects can be described as natural tissue regeneration and natural bone regeneration, analogous to guided tissue regeneration and guided bone regeneration.[23] The defect is filled with L-PRF (optionally combined with a biomaterial to prevent collapse) and sealed with L-PRF membranes.

These membranes have a protective function (induction of the periosteum) and serve as a competitive barrier (Fig. 66.6 and Box 66.2). Epithelium and connective tissues are kept away from the intrabony crater, so that the cells from the periodontal ligament or periosteum have time to regenerate cementum, bone, and ligament. These cells can also migrate through the membranes, which results in fast neo-angiogenesis. L-PRF also promotes the proliferation and differentiation of osteoblasts and bone marrow stromal cells in vitro.[31] This stimulation appears to be dose dependent, with leukocytes playing a key role.

FLASH BACK

Guided tissue regeneration uses a barrier membrane to separate tissues. This allows slower-moving cells from the periodontal ligament and periosteum to occupy the wound, facilitating periodontal regeneration, while delaying the faster-moving cells of epithelium and connective tissue from entering the site.

A series of clinical studies evaluated the benefits of applying L-PRF alone during open flap debridement (Table 66.3). A systematic review and meta-analysis on the use of L-PRF in regenerative procedures reported an adjunctive improvement, when L-PRF was

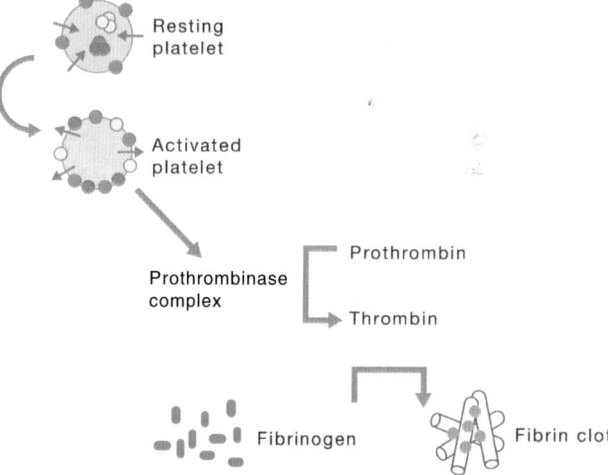

Fig. 66.5 Interaction between release of granules by activated platelets and conversion of prothrombin to thrombin, which by itself regulates the conversion of fibrinogen into a fibrin clot. This principle is also used in the preparation of an L-PRF block. The activation of the platelets occurs during centrifugation.

used, on parameters such as probing pocket depth reduction (1.1 ± 0.5 mm extra reduction), clinical attachment level (1.2 ± 0.6 mm extra gain), and bone defect fill (1.5 ± 0.3 mm or 46% ± 12.8% extra bone fill).[17] In some studies, L-PRF was combined with a bone substitute, and even here an additional benefit could be observed. When L-PRF was compared to enamel matrix derivative, similar improvements were reported (see Table 66.3).

L-PRF for Ridge Preservation

After tooth extraction and loss of the bundle bone, the alveolar ridge undergoes a remodeling process in both vertical and horizontal directions. This process often complicates the placement of implants in an ideal position. Many surgical techniques have been developed to prevent, or at least minimize, this bone resorption. Different bone grafts or bone substitutes have been developed to be used in extraction sockets, with or without the addition of a soft tissue graft or soft tissue

substitute to seal the alveolus. However, a systematic review[89] concluded that today there is no clear guideline on which technique to use for this purpose. Another approach suggests keeping the vestibular part of the tooth root in the extraction socket, with the implant inserted behind this dentine shield.[47] The use of L-PRF in an extraction socket could be a less costly, more simplified, and more effective treatment alternative (Fig. 66.7 and Box 66.3), but standardization of the protocol is required to obtain reproducible results. The use of enough L-PRF clots or membranes seems to be crucial to obtain an optimal effect.[18]

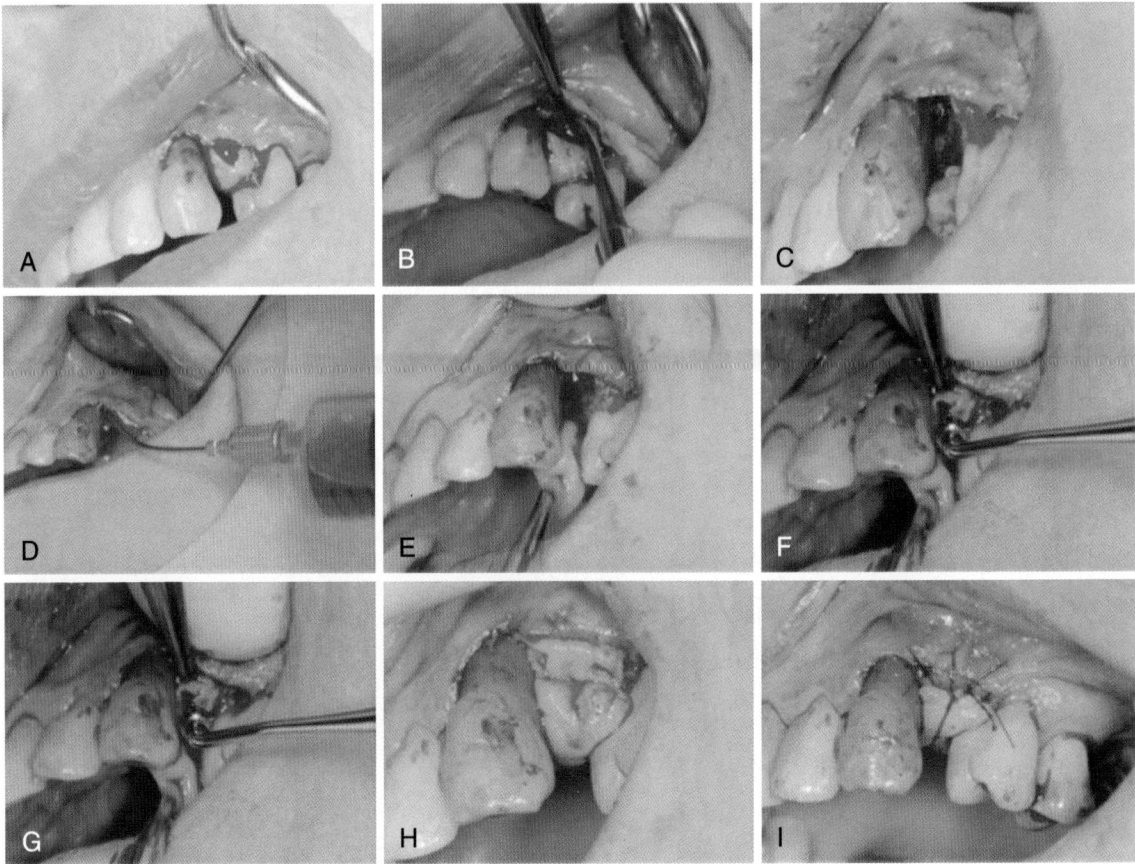

Fig. 66.6 Regenerative treatment of intrabony defects with L-PRF. (A) Intrasulcular incision with papilla preservation. (B) Minimal flap elevation (palatally pediculated). (C) Defect after root planing. (D) Rinsing of the intrabony defect with L-PRF exudate. (E and F) Application of chopped L-PRF membrane in the defect (preferably face side). (G and H) Coverage of bony defect with at least two layers of L-PRF membranes. (I) Flap suturing, preferably with primary closure of the interdental papilla, in the absence of tension.

BOX 66.2 Step-by-Step Approach for the Use of L-PRF During Open Flap Debridement

Protocol for L-PRF as Sole Biomaterial for Intrabony Defect Regeneration During Open Flap Debridement (Fig. 66.9):
- Intrasulcular incision with maximal preservation of gingival complex (see Fig. 66.6A).
- Minimal flap elevation and degranulation of intrabony defects (see Fig. 66.6B).
- Optimal root planing (see Fig. 66.6C).
- Rinse defect with L-PRF fluid (see Fig. 66.6D). *(The fluid is collected at the bottom of the Xpression kit [Intra-Lock International, Boca Raton, FL] after compression of the clots.)*
- Apply L-PRF membrane (or part of it) in the defect (preferably with the face part of the membrane toward bone) (see Fig. 66.6E,F).
- Cover bony defect with at least two layers of L-PRF membranes, running at least 2 mm over the bony borders underneath the periosteum, in order to seal the socket and to force the soft tissues to grow over instead of underneath the membranes (see Fig. 66.6G,H).
- Suture flap and try to provide primary closure of the interdental papilla in the absence of tension (see Fig. 66.6I).

Postoperative Care:
- Soft food intake; no biting in treated area; no mechanical cleaning of the treated area.
- Use of 0.12% chlorhexidine mouthwash twice daily for 1 min for at least 3 weeks.
- Painkillers.

TABLE 66.3 Most Important and Most Relevant RCTs and CCTs on the Use of L-PRF in Periodontal Defects

Article	Type	Subjects	Groups	Conclusions
Thorat et al. 2011[86]	RCT	32 defects	test: L-PRF + OFD control: OFD	OFD + L-PRF: -More PPD reduction, CAL gain, and defect fill
Sharma & Pradeep, 2011b[77]	RCT	56 defects	test: L-PRF + OFD control: OFD	OFD + L-PRF: -More PPD reduction, CAL gain, and defect fill
Sharma & Pradeep, 2011a[76]	RCT split-mouth	36 furcation class 2 mandible	test: L-PRF + OFD control: OFD	OFD + L-PRF: -Significantly better clinical and radiologic parameters
Lekovic et al. 2012[57]	CCT split-mouth	17	test: L-PRF + DBBM control: L-PRF	L-PRF improved the clinical parameters L-PRF + DBBM: greater filling of the defect and greater PPD reduction
Pradeep et al. 2012[70]	RCT	57	test 1: L-PRF + OFD test 2: L-PRF + HA + OFD control: OFD	Both test conditions resulted in greater reduction of PPD, greater gain in CAL, and greater filling of the intrabony defects.
Rosamma Joseph et al. 2012[72]	RCT split-mouth	15	test: OFD + L-PRF control: OFD	OFD + L-PRF: -More effective than OFD alone in the treatment of intrabony periodontal defects
Bansal & Bharti, 2013[8]	RCT split-mouth	10	test: L-PRF + DFDBA control: DFDBA	OFD + L-PRF: -More PPD reduction and CAL gain
Gupta et al. 2014[44]	RCT	44 defects	test: L-PRF control: EMD	Similar results in both groups; EMD was superior in filling defects.
Rosamma Joseph et al. 2014[73]	CCT split-mouth	15	t1: L-PRF gel + OFD t2: L-PRF + OFD control: OFD	L-PRF in any form was more effective in PPD reduction and CAL gain than OFD alone.
Agarwal et al. 2015[1]	RCT split-mouth	30	test: L-PRF + DFDBA control: DFDBA	DFDBA in combination with L-PRF gave significant advantages in PPD reduction and CAL gain and an increase in bone density.
Ajwani et al. 2015[2]	RCT split-mouth	20	test: L-PRF + OFD control: OFD	OFD + L-PRF: -More filling of the defect
Elgendy & Abo Shady, 2015[35]	RCT split-mouth	20	test: L-PRF + HA control: HA	HA in combination with L-PRF gave more PPD reduction and CAL gain and an increase in bone density.
Mathur et al. 2015[64]	RCT	38	test: OFD + L-PRF control: OFD + ABG	Both groups resulted in a reduction of PPD and gain in CAL and were effective in the treatment of intrabony defects.
Shah et al. 2015[75]	RCT split-mouth	20	test: L-PRF + OFD control: OFD + DFDBA	Similar results in both groups

ABG, Autologous bone graft; *CAL*, clinical attachment level; *CCT*, controlled clinical trial; *DBBM*, deproteinized bovine bone mineral; *DFDBA*, demineralized freeze-dried bone allograft; *EMD*, enamel matrix derivative; *HA*, hydroxyapatite; *L-PRF*, leukocyte- and platelet-rich fibrin; *OFD*, open flap debridement; *PPD*, probing pocket depth; *RCT*, randomized controlled trial.

Hauser and coworkers[46] carried out a randomized controlled trial with a so-called split-mouth design in order to ascertain preservation of the alveolar ridge after tooth extraction. They concluded that L-PRF application resulted in better preservation of the width of the alveolar ridge and better intrinsic bone quality (measured by bone biopsies with micro-computed tomography). A split-mouth comparison[84] between natural healing of extraction sockets and sockets filled with L-PRF (comprising 22 patients) confirmed the above-mentioned benefits with significantly less horizontal and vertical resorption, more socket fill, higher bone quality, and faster soft tissue and bone healing. This was reported even at sites with bone dehiscences. The observed reduction in bone resorption was comparable to the best-performing clinical procedures using bone substitutes in combination with connective tissue grafting and/or the placement of a membrane, similar to what was observed by Anwandter and coworkers.[6] These studies do, however, contradict a paper by Suttapreyasri and Leepong,[80] who did not record such significant differences (Table 66.4).

Several papers on third molar extractions indicated that L-PRF as a filling material has a beneficial effect on postoperative pain and soft tissue healing.[37,59]

The L-PRF clot enables fast neoangiogenesis and compensates for the bone trauma caused by the extraction with bone regeneration stimulated by growth factors.

L-PRF for Periodontal Mucogingival Surgery

Several procedures have been introduced to successfully cover an exposed root surface. These procedures resolve the hypersensitivity and aesthetic problems but biologically lead to an important clinical attachment level, an increase in the amount of keratinized mucosa, and an increase in gingival thickness. One can divide the treatment options into the following: a free gingival graft, a coronally advanced flap (CAF), a modified CAF, a coronally advanced tunnel technique, and combinations of these techniques using an autologous graft (often

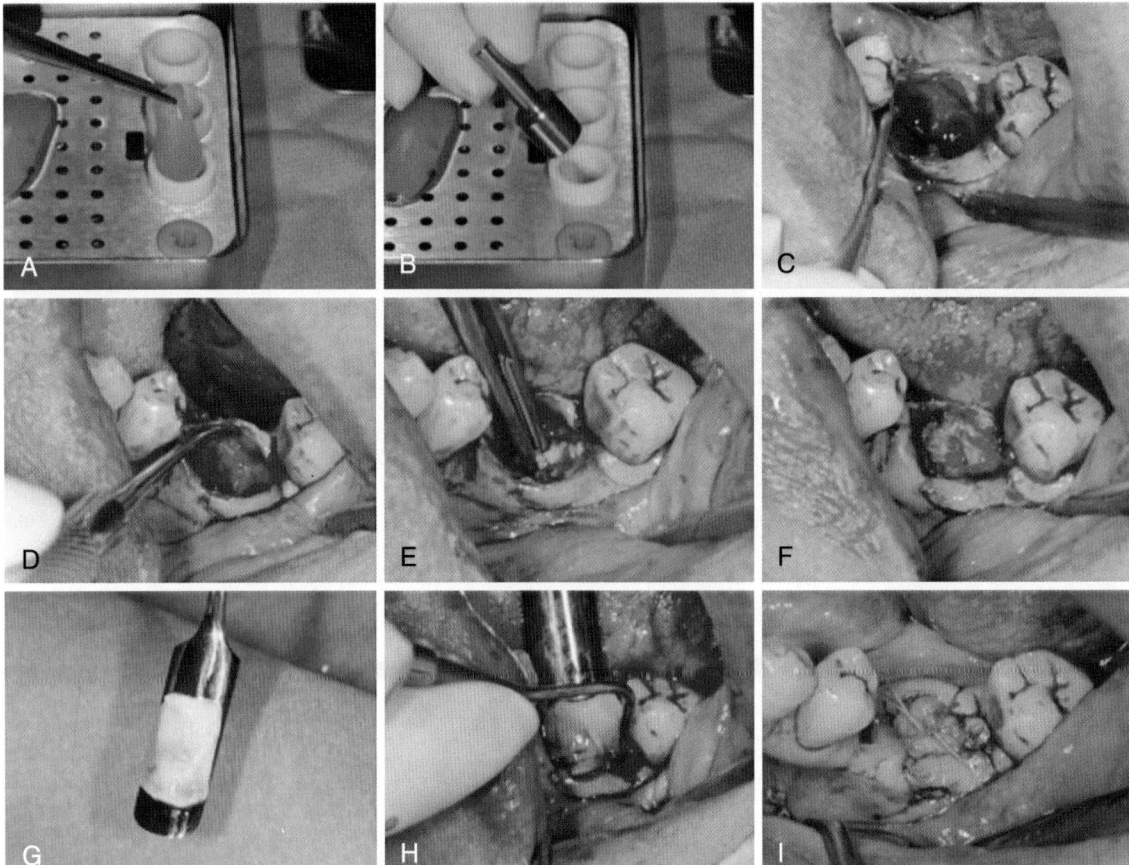

Fig. 66.7 The use of L-PRF as a filling material for a tooth socket, with the aim of maintaining the alveolar bone dimensions. (A and B) Preparation of L-PRF plugs with the Xpression kit (Intra-Lock International, Boca Raton, FL). (C) Accurate removal of all inflammation and granulation tissue. (D) Preparation of envelope (approximately 2 mm in width) between the bony borders of the socket and surrounding soft tissues; this is needed to slide in the L-PRF membranes at the end, in order to prevent the fast ingrowth of connective tissue and to force the epithelium to grow over the membranes. (E and F) Placement, one by one, of three to five L-PRF plugs in the socket and vigorous compression. (G and H) Coverage of socket with at least a double layer of L-PRF membranes, sliding the borders of the membranes into the prepared envelope. (I) Tension-free suturing with, for example, a modified internal mattress or external mattress technique; primary closure is not necessary.

BOX 66.3 Step-by-Step Approach for Ridge Preservation With L-PRF

Protocol for Ridge Preservation With L-PRF (Fig. 66.10):

- Atraumatic tooth extraction with maximal preservation of alveolar bone.
- Accurate removal of inflammation and granulation tissue (with bur, if needed) (see Fig. 66.7C).
- Preparation of envelope (approximately 2 mm in width) between the bony borders of the socket and surrounding soft tissues. This allows insertion of part of the L-PRF membranes between the periosteum and the flap, in order to seal the socket and force the soft tissues to grow over, instead of underneath, the membranes (see Fig. 66.7D).
- If applicable, use L-PRF exudate (aspirated in syringe), obtained after compression of clots, to irrigate and clean the socket.
- Place three to five L-PRF plugs, one by one, into the socket, compressing them vigorously with amalgam condenser and absorbing superfluous serum with gauze (see Fig. 66.7E,F).
- Cover the socket with at least a double layer of L-PRF membranes, and slide their margins between soft and hard tissues around the socket (envelope) to seal the socket and to prevent epithelial infiltration (see Fig. 66.7G,H).
- Suture with, for example, a modified internal mattress or external mattress technique, not with the intention to close the wound, but to keep the membranes in place without traction (see Fig. 66.7I).

Postoperative Care:

- No use of chlorhexidine during first 2 days, in order to not disturb initial soft tissue healing.

TABLE 66.4   Most Relevant RCTs and CCTs on the Use of L-PRF for Ridge Preservation

Article	Design	Subjects	Socket Fill	Conclusion
Hauser et al. 2013[46]	RCT	23 subjects	control: blood clot (8) test 1: L-PRF (9) test 2: L-PRF + flap (6)	L-PRF alone: -Improved bone healing with improved microarchitecture and quality -Better preservation of the alveolar bone L-PRF + flap: -Flap preparation negatively influenced benefits of L-PRF
Suttapreyasri & Leepong 2013[80]	RCT split-mouth	8 subjects	control: blood clot (10) test: L-PRF (10)	L-PRF: -Better preservation of the alveolar ridge -Less vestibular/lingual bone loss -No enhanced bone formation
Marenzi et al. 2015[59]	RCT split-mouth	26 subjects	2–8 sockets/patient control: blood clot test: L-PRF	L-PRF (up to 21 days): -Reduced postoperative pain -Improved healing of the soft tissues
Eshghpour et al. 2014[37]	RCT split-mouth	78 subjects	control: blood clot (78) test: L-PRF (7)8	L-PRF: -Decreased risk of alveolar osteitis after extraction of mandibular third molar
Anwandter et al. 2016[6]	prospective cohort	18 subjects	1 socket/patient test: L-PRF (18)	L-PRF: - Mean horizontal resorption of 1.2 ± 2.4 mm at the crest, 1.2 ± 2 mm and 0.8 ± 2.0 mm at 2 and 4 mm apically
Temmerman et al. 2016[84]	RCT split-mouth	22 subjects	2 sockets/patient control: blood clot (22) test: L-PRF (22)	L-PRF: -Less buccal bone resorption -Better preservation of the alveolar bone

CCT, Controlled clinical trial; L-PRF, leukocyte- and platelet-rich fibrin; RCT, randomized controlled trial.

a connective tissue graft) or nonautologous graft between flap and root surface. Optionally, even enamel matrix derivative can be used.

L-PRF can be helpful in mucogingival surgery because of its strong three-dimensional fibrin network, which provides the possibility of its use as a membrane but also as a soft tissue graft. It slowly releases growth factors and matrix proteins that stimulate healing for more than 7 days. This release promotes two biologic mechanisms:

- *Impregnation:* The root surface is impregnated with blood proteins, which are the first biologic link between the surface and the new attachment.
- *Induction:* The release of growth factors lasts long enough to trigger cell induction—the growth factors stimulate periosteal cell proliferation, new blood vessels develop within the fibrin matrix, gingival fibroblasts migrate within the fibrin matrix and provide slow remodeling, and the membrane surface induces epithelialization.

These processes allow rapid wound closure and healing and, in the longer term, could result in more stable recession coverage and thicker gingiva. The potential advantages of this technique triggered research (Table 66.5) in which L-PRF was added during periodontal plastic surgery or L-PRF membranes were used to replace connective tissue grafts (Fig. 66.8 and Box 66.4). To date, most studies have examined the use of L-PRF in combination with a CAF technique.

In general, one can conclude that L-PRF might successfully replace connective tissue graft, with, of course, less morbidity for patients owing to the absence of a donor site (see Table 66.5). However, long-term studies are needed to verify the stability of the outcomes. When CAF is applied with the use of L-PRF, additional advantages have been reported, compared to CAF without L-PRF.[17]

One study examined the benefits of L-PRF in the coverage of the donor site after harvesting of a free gingival graft.[39] The results were faster healing at the donor site and less postoperative pain with the use of L-PRF compared to spontaneous healing.

 CLINICAL CORRELATION

L-PRF can be helpful in mucogingival surgery because of its strong three-dimensional fibrin network, which provides the possibility of its use as a membrane but allows its use (alone) as a soft tissue graft. It slowly releases growth factors and matrix proteins that stimulate healing for more than 7 days.

Conclusions

The benefits of using the first-generation platelet concentrates were very controversial; however, the second-generation platelet concentrate (L-PRF) seems to produce more consistent and predictable results. The advantages of using L-PRF are its autologous nature, simple collection, ease of chair-side preparation, and simple clinical application without the risks associated with allogeneic products. Therefore, it seems suitable to be used in either a specialized or general practice. The special texture of L-PRF allows its clinical use in the amorphous form (clot) but mainly in the membranous form (obtained after slight compression). The membranes can be used to cover and protect wounds like a tissue graft. The biologic properties of L-PRF clearly show interesting surgical versatility and all the characteristics that can support faster tissue regeneration and high-quality clinical outcomes. L-PRF is able to stimulate osteogenesis in addition to angiogenesis, and it provides a scaffold that allows cellular migration. These are certainly the fundamental aspects of the process of bone regeneration. All of these features support the conclusion that L-PRF

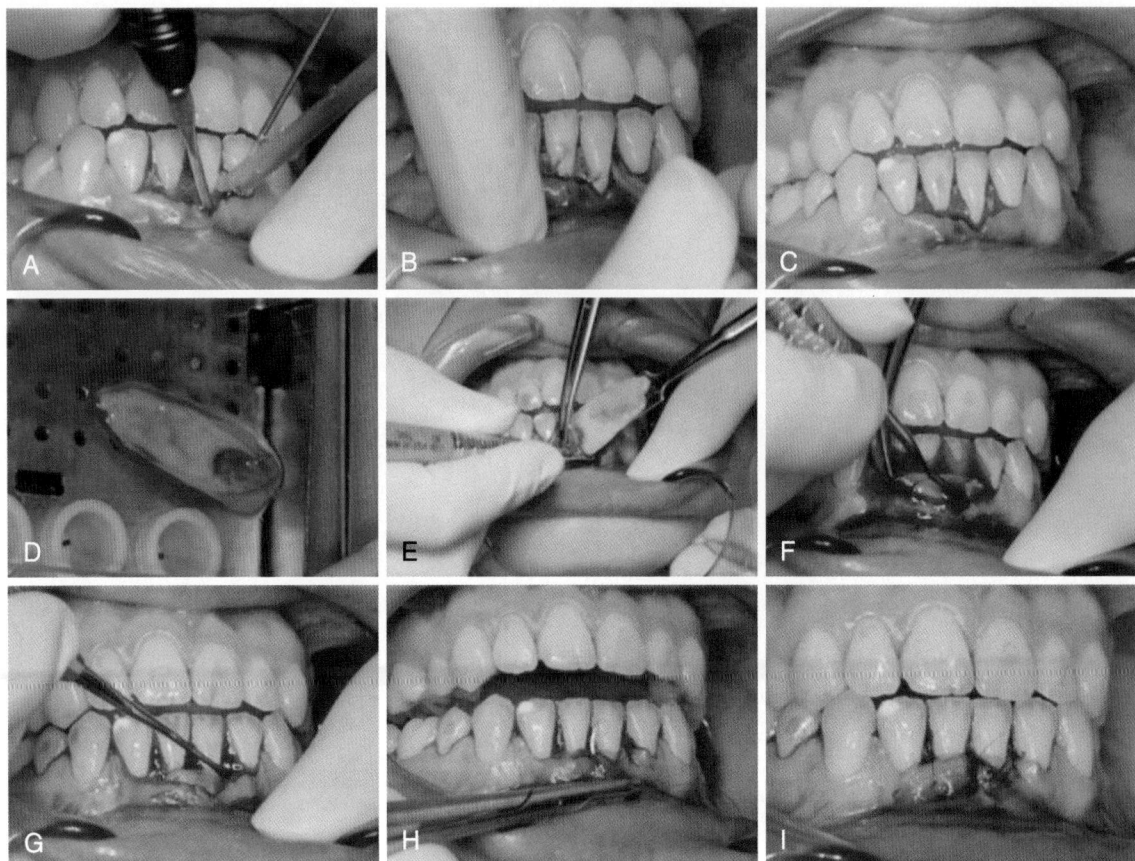

Fig. 66.8 Gingival recession coverage with the coronally advanced flap (CAF) procedure and L-PRF membranes. (A) Split-thickness preparation of receptor site. (B and C) Deepithelialization of papillae. (D) Fix (glue together) three or more L-PRF membranes with dimensions of receptor bed. (E through G) Place L-PRF graft on exposed connective tissue (receptor bed) and over the recession. (H and I) Suture with a coronal advancement of the flap for coverage of the graft.

TABLE 66.5   Most Relevant RCTs and CCTs on the Use of L-PRF in Mucogingival Surgery

Article	Design	Subjects	Groups	Conclusion
Aroca et al. 2009[7]	CCT	20	test: CAF + L-PRF control: CAF	CAF + L-PRF: -More GTH after 6 mo
Aleksic et al. 2010[3]	RCT split-mouth	19	test: CAF + L-PRF control: CAF + CTG	No difference between groups Better healing and less postoperative pain in CAF + L-PRF group
Jankovic et al. 2010[48]	RCT split-mouth	20	test: CAF + L-PRF control: CAF + EMD	No difference between groups More GTH with CAF + L-PRF
Jankovic et al. 2012[49]	RCT	15	test: CAF + L-PRF control: CAF + CTG	Greater KM width with CAF + CTG Improved wound healing in the CAF + L-PRF group
Eren & Atilla 2014[36]	RCT split-mouth	22	test: CAF + L-PRF control: CAF + CTG	No difference in % coverage, GTH, or KM between groups L-PRF is easier and requires no donor site
Gupta et al. 2015[43]	RCT	23	test: CAF + L-PRF control: CAF	No difference between groups GTH greater in CAF + L-PRF group
Keceli et al. 2015[52]	RCT	40	test: CAF + CTG + L-PRF control: CAF + CTG	No difference between groups; more GTH with CAF + L-PRF
Thamaraiselvan et al. 2015[85]	RCT	20	test: CAF + L-PRF control: CAF	No difference between groups More GTH in CAF + L-PRF group
Tunali et al. 2015[88]	RCT	44 recessions	test: CAF + L-PRF control: CAF + CTG	No difference between groups after 12 months

CAF, Coronally advanced flap; CAL, clinical attachment level; CCT, controlled clinical trial; CTG, connective tissue graft; GTH, gingival thickness; KM, keratinized mucosa; L-PRF, leukocyte- and platelet-rich fibrin; RCT, randomized controlled trial.

BOX 66.4   Step-by-Step Approach for Gingival Recession Coverage

Protocol for Gingival Recession Coverage With Coronally Advanced Flap (CAF) Procedure Using L-PRF as Graft Material (Fig. 66.11)

- Create incision (following surgical technique protocol) and prepare full-split, full-thickness receptor bed (see Fig. 66.8A).
- Perform de-epithelialization of papilla (see Fig. 66.8B,C).
- Fix at least three L-PRF membranes (with correct dimensions) together with resorbable 6-0 sutures (see Fig. 66.8D).
- Place L-PRF graft on exposed connective tissue (receptor bed) and over the recession, and fix it to the periosteum (see Fig. 66.8E,F,G).

- Suture with a coronal advancement of the flap for coverage of the graft (see Fig. 66.8H,I).

Postoperative Care

- No pressure or applied forces on the graft site for at least 6 months.
- Soft food intake; no biting in treated area. No mechanical cleaning of the treated area. Moderate use of the mouth.
- Chlorhexidine 0.12% (from day 3) three times per day for 1 min for at least 3 weeks.
- Prescribe sufficient painkillers.

---

has numerous advantages compared with other similar blood products, and L-PRF has demonstrated the capability to enhance the natural healing of soft and hard tissue.

The use of L-PRF has already been investigated in many periodontal treatments, including the placement of implants. However, some areas are still unexplored, and well-designed clinical studies are needed. Clearly, the arrival of L-PRF does not mean that the whole way of thinking and acting in oral surgery should be changed. Nonetheless, for many indications, L-PRF can replace bone substitutes or membranes. Also very relevant is the fact that its autogenous origin makes it 100% safe.

 A Case Scenario is found on the companion website www.expertconsult.com.

References

 References for this chapter are found on the companion website www.expertconsult.com.

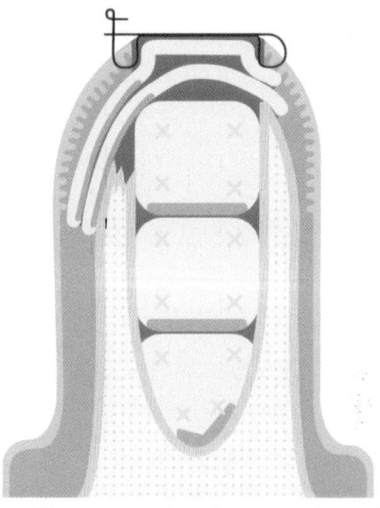

Fig. 66.10 Graphic representation of an extraction socket filled with L-PRF. Several L-PRF plugs or membranes (≥3) are condensed at the bottom (face toward bone), and the socket is sealed with at least two layers of L-PRF membranes. These membranes are slid under the periosteum at the bony socket borders (in the created envelope between the periosteum and the bony borders; 2 mm coverage is sufficient). Suturing is done without any attempt to close the wound (healing by secondary intention).

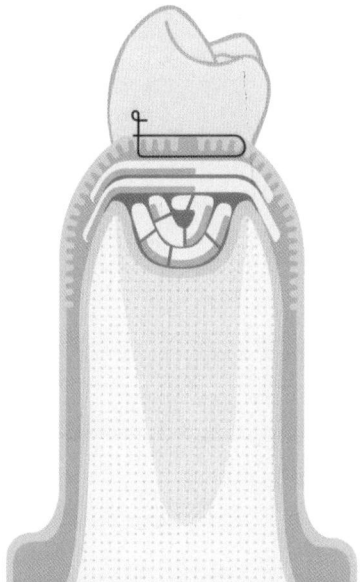

Fig. 66.9 Graphic representation of an intrabony defect filled with chopped L-PRF membrane parts (preferably the face part) and covered with L-PRF membranes (at least two layers with face side toward bony defect and running over the buccal and lingual bony borders). Primary closure is not mandatory.

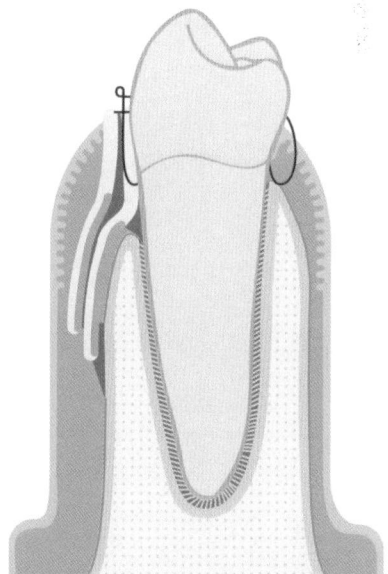

Fig. 66.11 Graphic representation of the final situation after gingival recession coverage with a coronally advanced flap (CAF) and L-PRF membranes. Several L-PRF membranes (≥3) are placed on the receptor bed and over the recession. Suturing is done to advance the flap coronally over the recession. (The periosteum [blue line] has been cut to enable coronal advancement of the flap.)

CHAPTER 67

Periodontal Microsurgery

Dennis A. Shanelec | Leonard S. Tibbetts | Adriana McGregor | J. David Cross*

CHAPTER OUTLINE

Philosophy of Periodontal
  Microsurgery
Advantages of Microsurgery
Magnification Systems

Microsurgical Sutures
Aesthetic Periodontal Microsurgery
  (e-only)

Microsurgical Knots *(e-only)*
Conclusions

 Content on aesthetic periodontal microsurgery and microsurgical knots can be accessed on the companion website at www.expertconsult.com.

Microsurgery is surgery performed under a magnification of ×10 or more, which is possible only by using a surgical microscope.[5] The hallmarks of microsurgery are increased visual acuity and improved manual dexterity.[17] When visibility is increased 10-fold, motor movement precision is increased 1 mm to 10 µm.[3] This is the approximate size of an epithelial cell.[12] Large incisions for visibility are therefore unnecessary.

Small surgical instruments are used to advantage in the reduced surgical field (Fig. 67.1). This minimally invasive philosophy results in less injury, diminished morbidity, and rapid healing.[9,12] Sharp microsurgical blades are used to create incisions at a virtually cellular level (Fig. 67.2). These incisions are closed with meticulous apposition to eliminate wound edge gaps and dislocations, allowing healing by primary intention to begin within hours of microsurgical closure. This circumvents the need for an extensive secondary mitotic stage of wound healing to bridge wound gaps and fill surgical voids.

---

*Bryan S. Pearson, Scott O. Kissel, Leslie Broline, and Robert Henshaw also contributed to this chapter.

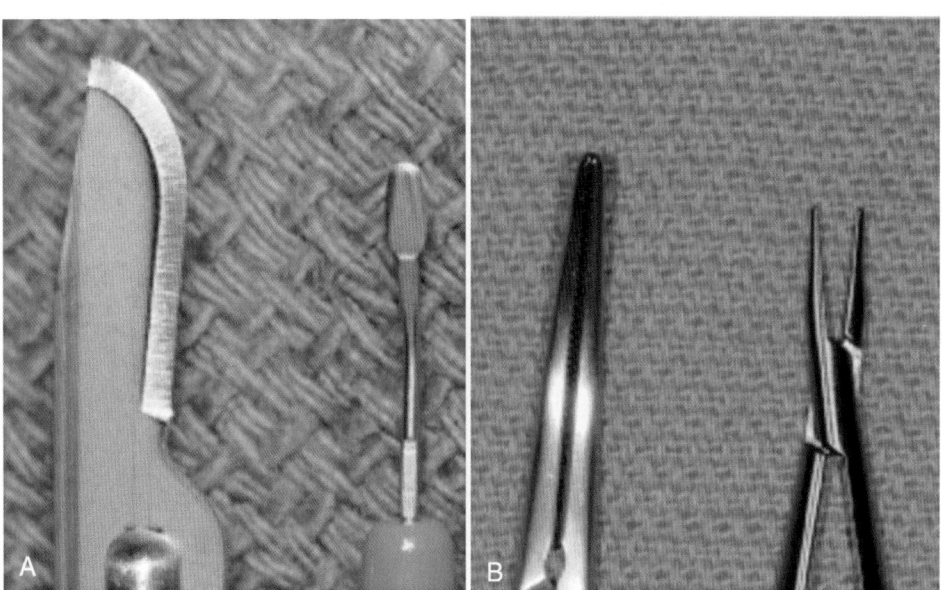

Fig. 67.1 Side-by-side dimensional comparison of commonly used conventional versus microsurgical instruments. (A) A #15 blade versus an ophthalmic blade. (B) Working tip of a conventional needle holder versus a McGregor microsuturing forceps.

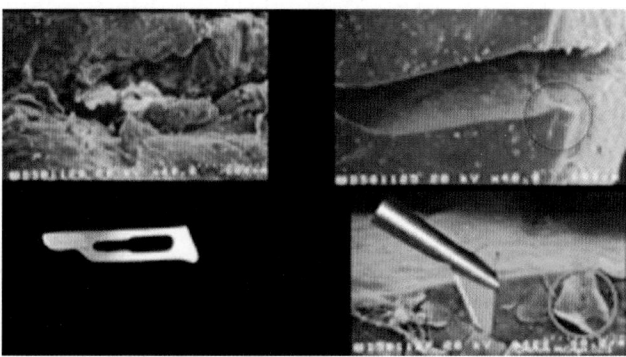

Fig. 67.2 Scanning electron microscopy (SEM) comparison of the incisions made with a #15 blade *(upper left)* and an ophthalmic microsurgical "feather" blade *(upper right and lower right)*. The *red circle* in the upper right image shows the area magnified in the lower right image. The *green circle* shows the disruption of only one epithelial cell. (SEM photographs courtesy Masana Susuki, DDS, Tokyo, Japan.)

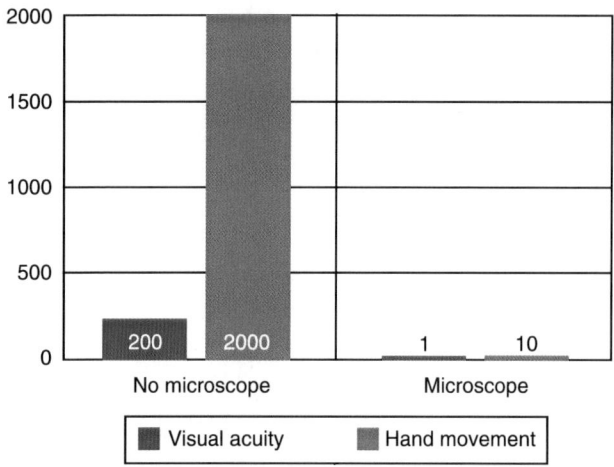

Fig. 67.3 Chart shows the correlation between enhanced visual acuity through magnification and a dramatic reduction in minimal hand movement. *(From Shanelec DA: Periodontal microsurgery.* Esthet Restor Dent *15:402–407, 2003.)*

Philosophy of Periodontal Microsurgery

The philosophy of microsurgery embraces three core values. The first is enhanced motor skill for better surgical performance. This is accomplished through improved visual acuity and the use of a precise hand grip to increase accuracy and reduce tremor (Fig. 67.3). The second is minimal tissue trauma, which is accomplished through smaller incisions and reduced surgical fields (Fig. 67.4). The third value is primary passive wound closure.[18] This is accomplished by microsuturing to eliminate gaps and dead spaces at the wound edge (Fig. 67.5).

Advanced periodontics has an increasing need for clinical procedures that require intricate surgical skills. Regenerative procedures, periodontal plastic surgery, and dental implants are a few of the surgical procedures that demand clinical performance that frequently challenge the skills of periodontal surgeons beyond the range of possibility with ordinary vision. Microsurgery establishes a minimally invasive surgical approach to periodontics exemplified by fewer vertical incisions and smaller surgical sites. Every field of microsurgery has recognized the extent to which reduced incision size and less retraction directly correlates with reduced postoperative morbidity and rapid healing[2] (Fig. 67.6).

In addition to the use of magnification and reliance on atraumatic technique, microsurgery requires specially constructed instruments designed specifically to minimize trauma. An important characteristic of microsurgical instruments is their ability to create clean incisions that prepare wounds for healing by primary intention. Microsurgical

incisions are established at a 90-degree angle to the surface using ophthalmic microsurgical scalpels (Fig. 67.7).

Microscopy permits easy identification of ragged wound edges for trimming and freshening. For primary wound closure, microsutures in the range of 6-0 to 9-0 are needed to approximate the wound edges accurately (Fig. 67.8). Microsurgical wound apposition minimizes gaps or voids at the wound edges and encourages rapid healing with less postoperative inflammation and less pain. Figs. 67.9 and 67.10 illustrate periodontal surgery cases using microsurgical techniques.

Advantages of Microsurgery

Periodontal microsurgery raises the treatment bar in many ways. Surgical decision making is enhanced because the quality and quantity of visual data reaching the cerebral cortex is increased by a square of the magnification level. Ergonomic and body posture advantages also occur when using the surgical microscope[1] (Fig. 67.11). Issues such as neuromuscular fatigue and occupational skeletal pathology are reduced. Sitting comfort, good body posture, arm support, and controlled breathing are inherent to proper microscope use. Motor skills are enhanced through instruments designed for a precision grip of the hand. Titanium instruments are used for strength and lightness and are made with round handles to permit precise rotation (Fig. 67.12). This reduces hand fatigue and tremor for precise surgical movement. Ergonomic benefit is a significant aspect of microscope use in periodontics.

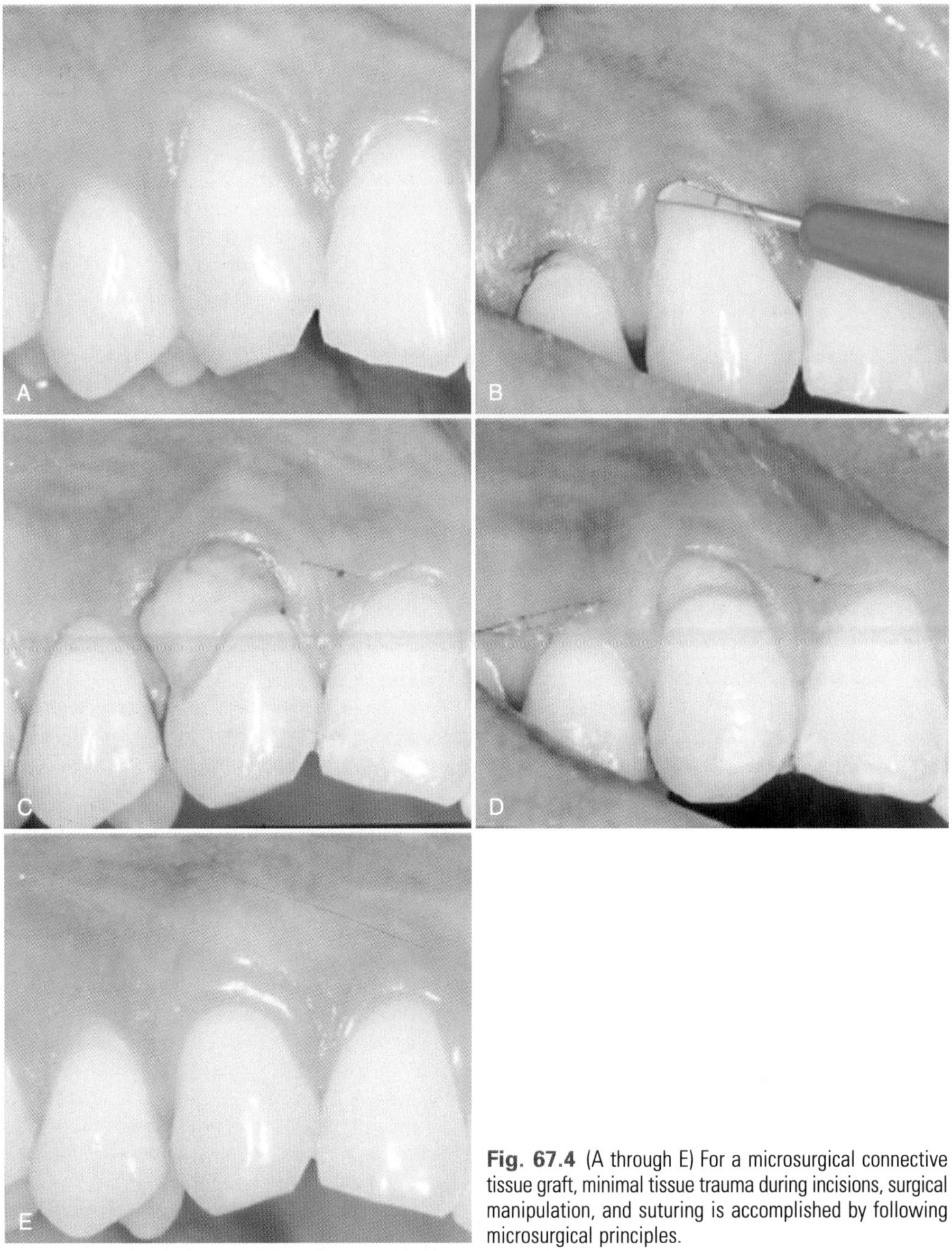

Fig. 67.4 (A through E) For a microsurgical connective tissue graft, minimal tissue trauma during incisions, surgical manipulation, and suturing is accomplished by following microsurgical principles.

Fig. 67.5 (A through C) Primary wound closure is achieved using microsurgical principles.

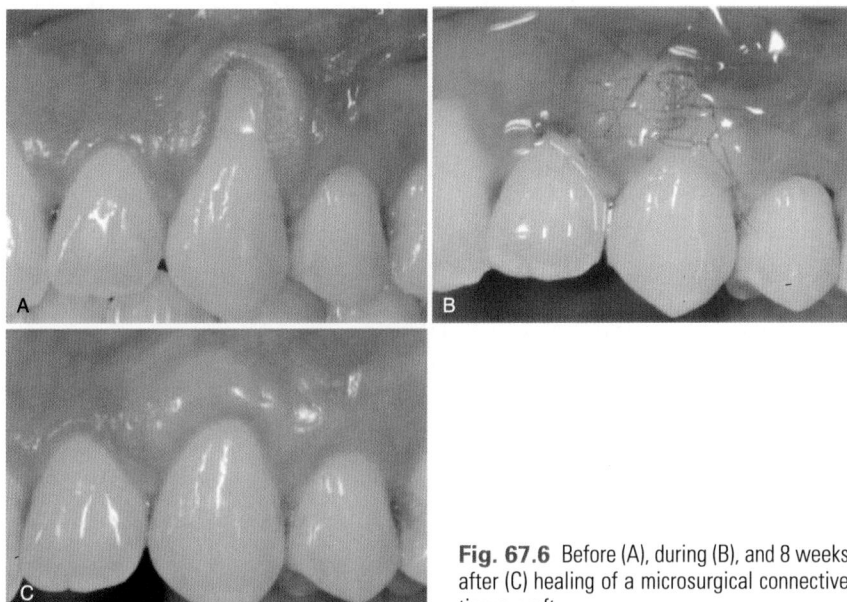

Fig. 67.6 Before (A), during (B), and 8 weeks after (C) healing of a microsurgical connective tissue graft.

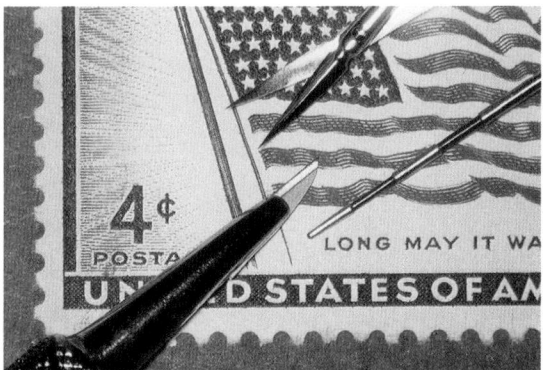

Fig. 67.7 Castroviejo microsurgical scalpel.

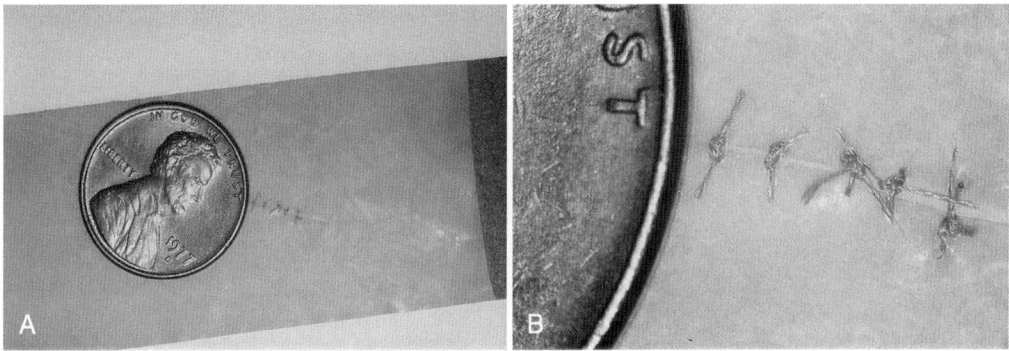

Fig. 67.8 (A and B) Microsurgical suturing.

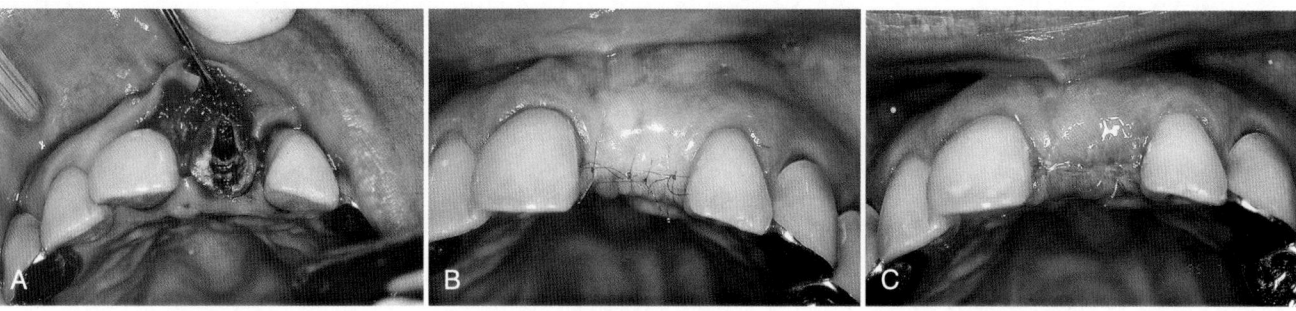

Fig. 67.9 Microsurgical extraction. (A) Before surgery. (B) Microsurgical view. (C) One week after surgery.

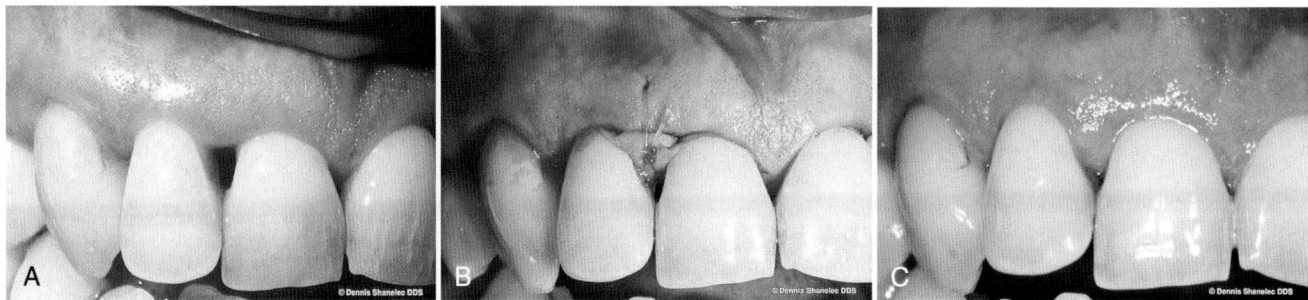

Fig. 67.10 Papilla reconstruction. (A) Before surgery. (B) Microsurgical view. (C) After surgery.

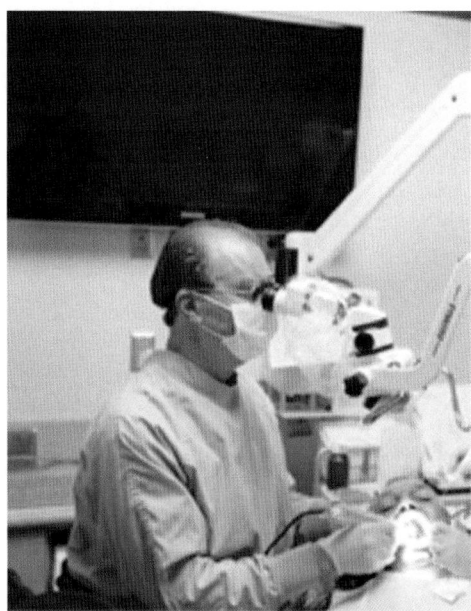

Fig. 67.11 Muscle strain and potential career-ending injuries can be prevented through a more ergonomic position facilitated by the proper use of a microscope.

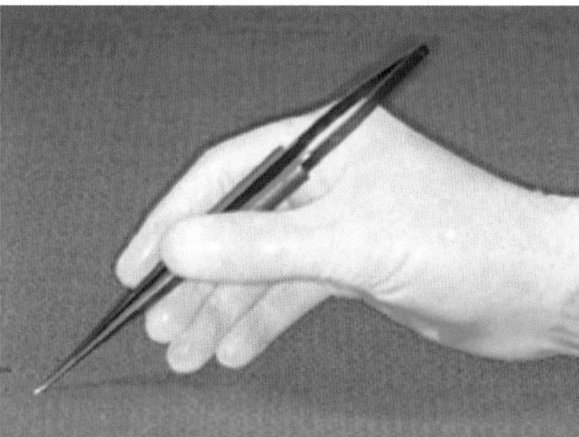

Fig. 67.12 Rounded, titanium microsurgical instruments, ideally 9 mm in diameter, reduce muscle fatigue and facilitate precise, rotational hand movements.

An important aspect of periodontal microsurgery is technical improvement in surgical performance. Higher skill levels have been shown in many surgical disciplines and can be fully appreciated when a surgeon tries his or her hand under the microscope. Viewing surgery under the microscope impresses a surgeon with the coarseness of conventional surgical manipulation (Fig. 67.13). What appears to the unaided eye as gentle surgery is revealed under the microscope as gross crushing and tearing of delicate tissues. Periodontics has long advocated atraumatic surgery, but the limits of normal vision have made this goal unattainable.

Proprioceptive guidance is of little value at the microsurgical level. Visual guidance is used for midcourse correction of scalpels and instruments to achieve the finest degrees of skill and dexterity.[4,9] Incisions can be accurately mapped, flaps elevated with minimal damage, and wounds closed accurately without tension (Fig. 67.14). Periodontal microsurgery is a natural progression from conventional surgical principles to a surgical ethic in which the surgical microscope

is employed for the most accurate and atraumatic handling of tissue (Fig. 67.15).

The resulting appearance of microsurgery is superior to that of conventional surgery. The difference is often startling (Figs. 67.16 to 67.18). As much as judgment and knowledge play a role in surgery, in the end, surgery is a craft. Surgeons appreciate this, especially when microsurgery raises their work to levels of artistic expression. Personal gratification in performing better surgery leads to acceptance of periodontal microsurgery by surgeons motivated to improve the quality of their work.

Microsurgery offers another advantage in the area of root preparation. The importance of root debridement is recognized universally as an essential component of periodontal therapy.[10,17] Research in clinical dentistry has shown that microscope-enhanced vision more readily accomplishes the established clinical goals of endodontic and restorative dentistry. In periodontics, studies demonstrated that root debridement performed without magnification was incomplete. When debrided roots were examined with the aid of a microscope, substantial deposits remained. Even in the absence of clinical studies, it may be inferred that microscope-enhanced vision in periodontics permits more definitive root debridement.

The primary goals of periodontal surgery include visual access to the root surface for plaque and calculus removal and for removing pathologically altered tooth structures. Magnification greatly improves the surgeon's ability to create a clean, smooth root surface (Fig. 67.19). The root surface represents one opposing edge of the periodontal wound. Root planing is therefore analogous to establishing a clean soft tissue incision. Magnification permits preparation of hard and soft tissue wound surfaces so that they can be joined together according to the accepted microsurgical principle of butt-joint wound approximation. This encourages primary wound healing and enhanced periodontal reconstruction. Studies of wound healing show epithelial anastomosis of microsurgically joined surgical wounds in animals within 48 hours.[4,16] With training, the average periodontal microsurgeon can consistently produce better-crafted work than the most talented conventional surgeon (Fig. 67.20).

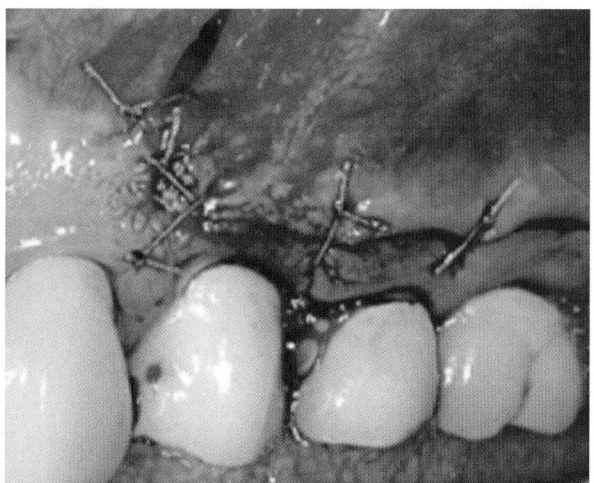

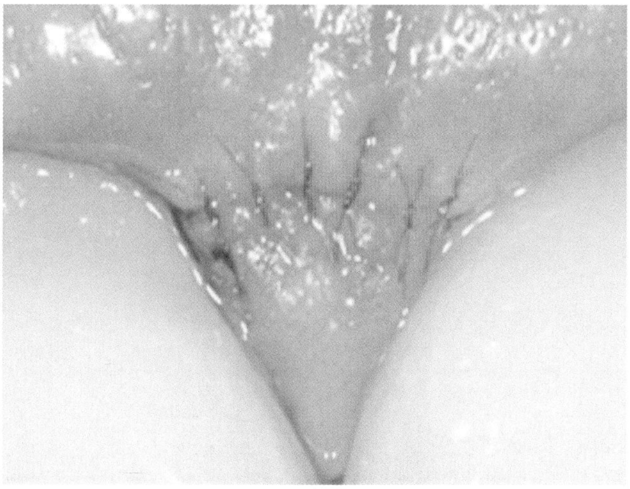

Fig. 67.13 The coarseness of conventional periodontal surgery is readily apparent under microscopic magnification.

Fig. 67.14 Tension-free wound closure is one of the goals of a microsurgical approach.

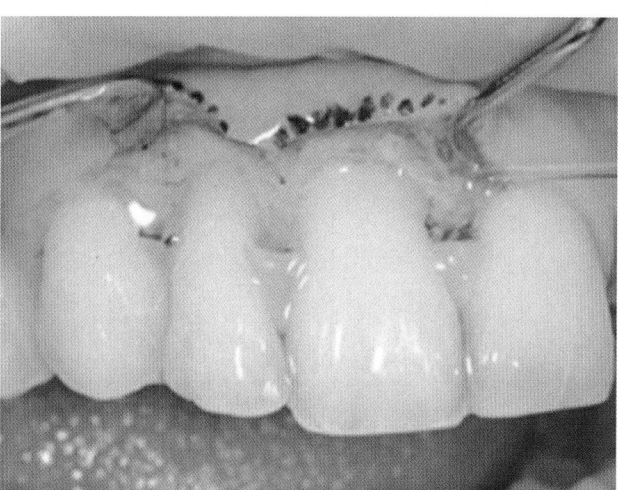

Fig. 67.15 Atraumatic microsurgical tissue manipulation during a microsurgical crown-lengthening procedure.

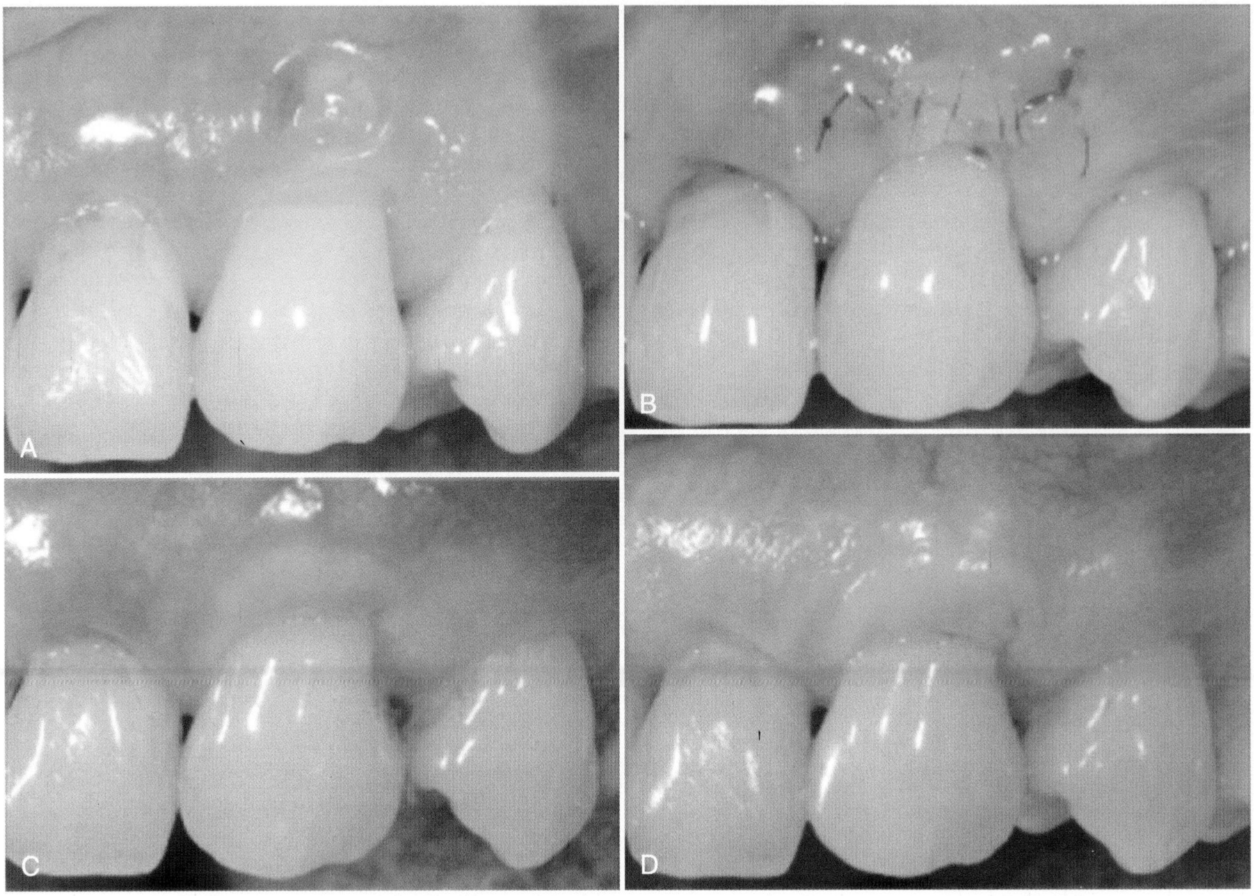

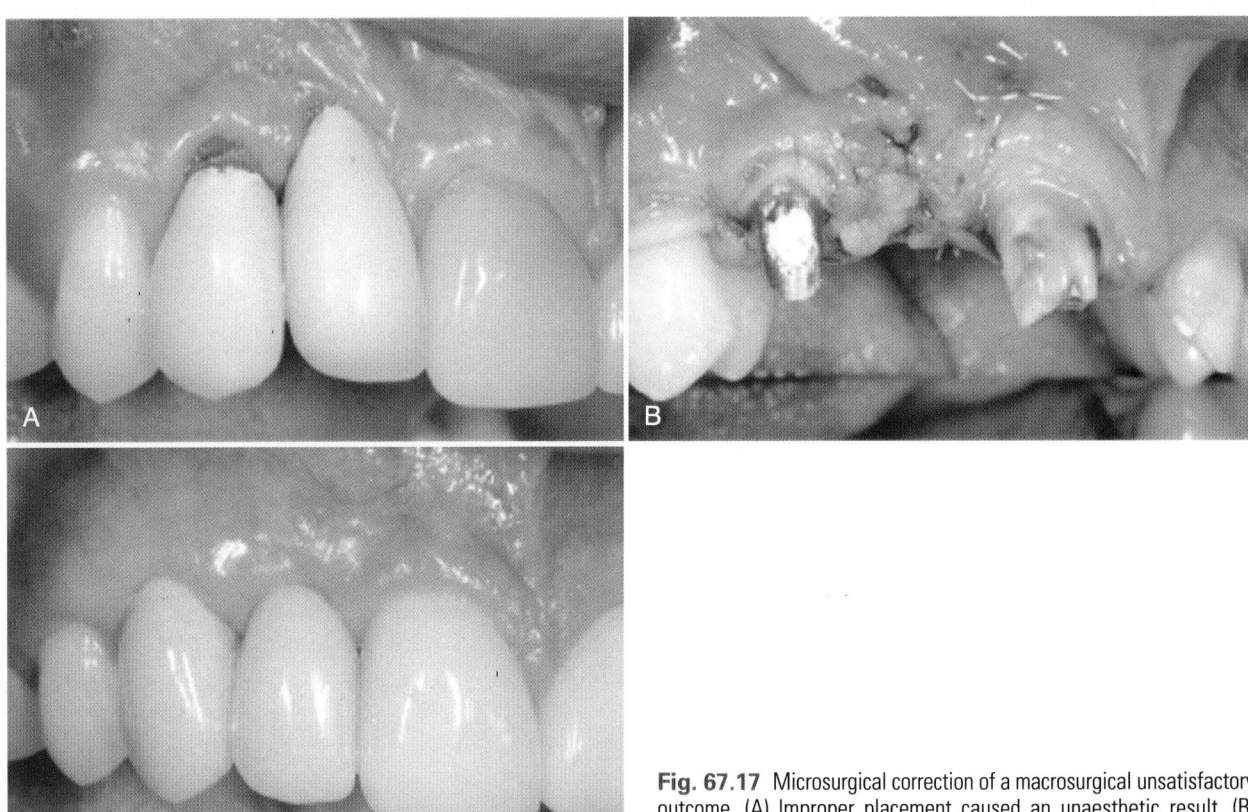

Fig. 67.16 (A) Suppurating gingival fenestration. (B) After careful root planing, a connective tissue graft (CTG) was carefully sutured under the envelope flap. (C) Postoperative healing at 3 weeks. (D) Postoperative follow-up at 1 year.

Fig. 67.17 Microsurgical correction of a macrosurgical unsatisfactory outcome. (A) Improper placement caused an unaesthetic result. (B) Microsurgical grafting procedure. (C) Final surgical result after fabrication of new crowns.

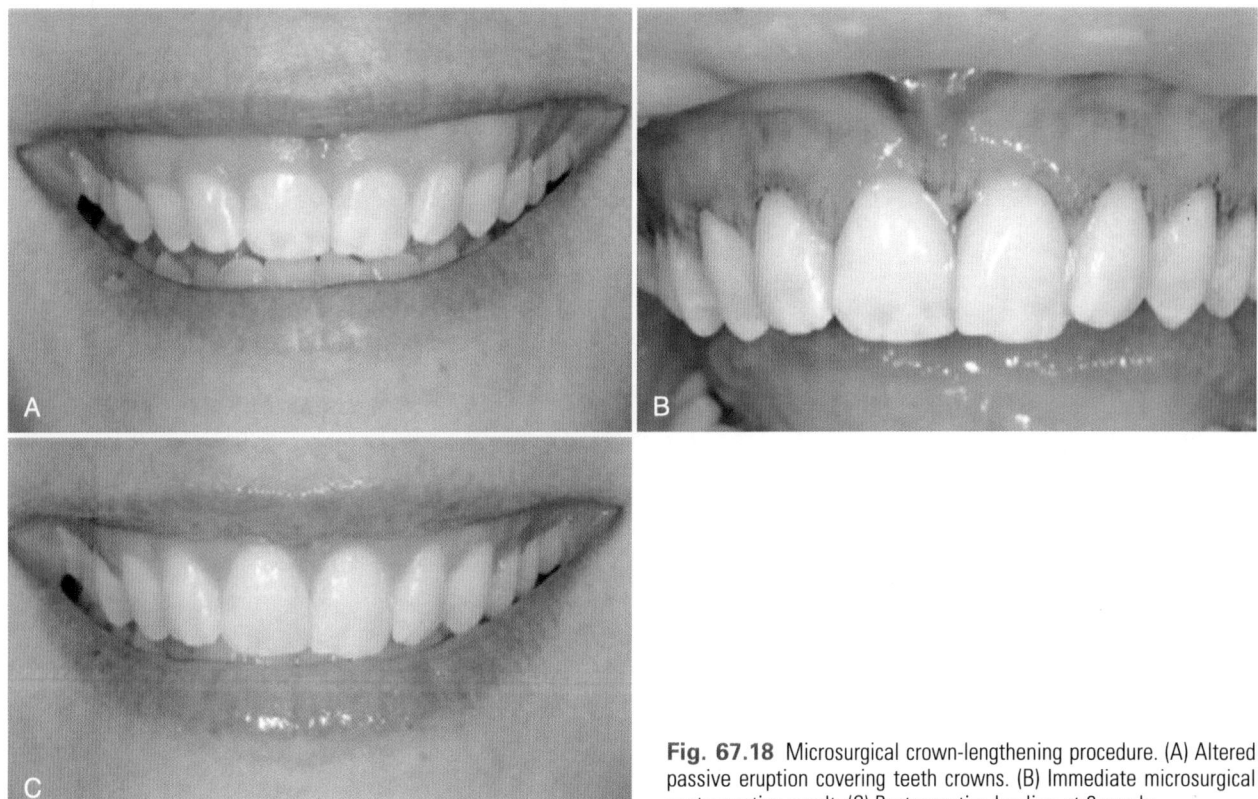

Fig. 67.18 Microsurgical crown-lengthening procedure. (A) Altered passive eruption covering teeth crowns. (B) Immediate microsurgical postoperative result. (C) Postoperative healing at 3 weeks.

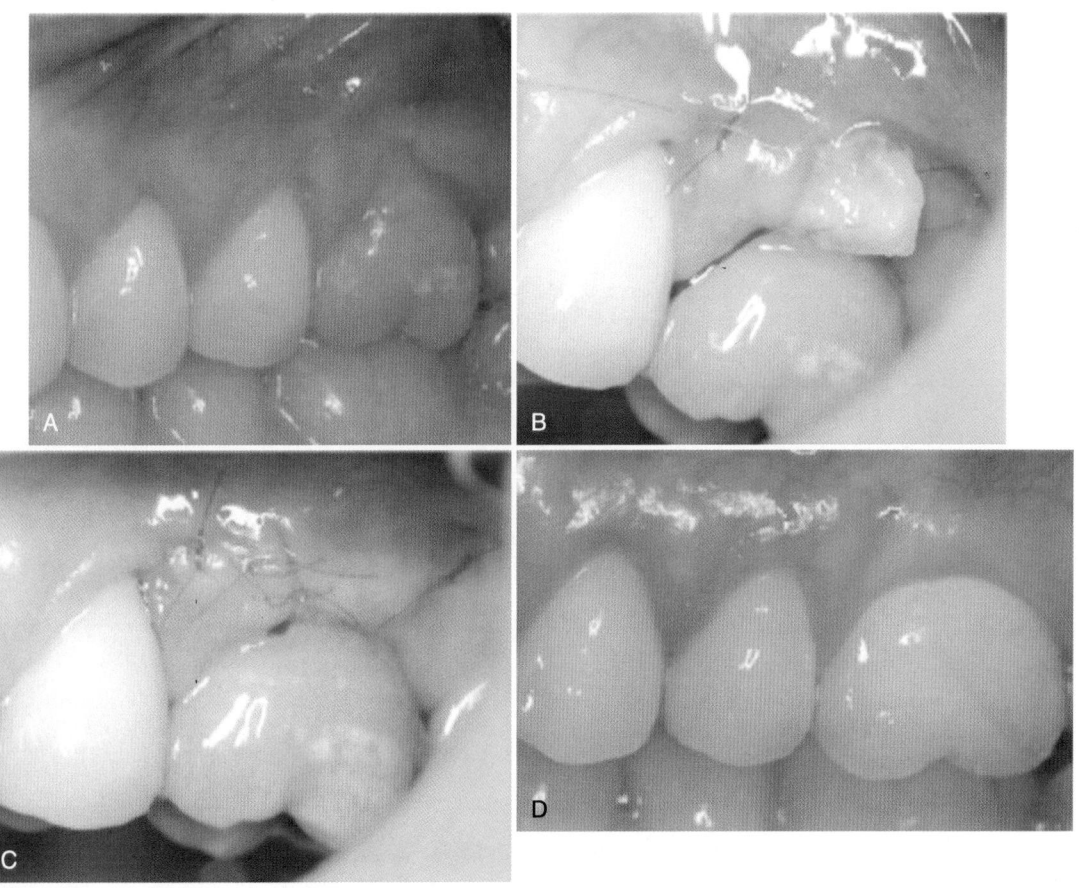

Fig. 67.19 Magnified root planing.

Magnification Systems

Simple and complex magnification systems are available to dentists. They range from simple loupes to prism telescopic loupes and surgical microscopes. Each magnification system has specific advantages and limitations. Although magnification improves the accuracy of clinical and diagnostic skills, it requires an understanding of optical principles that govern all magnification systems. The assumption that "more magnification is better" must always be weighed against the decrease in field of view and depth of focus that can occur as magnification increases, which is a problem more common with dental loupes than operating microscopes.

Magnifying Loupes

Dental loupes are the most common system of optical magnification used in periodontics. Loupes are fundamentally dual monocular telescopes with side-by-side lenses convergent to focus on the operative field. The magnified image formed has stereoscopic properties by virtue of their convergence. A convergent lens optical system is called a *Keplerian optical system.*

Although dental loupes are widely used, they have disadvantages compared with the microscope. The clinician's eyes must converge to view the operative field. This can result in eyestrain, fatigue, and pathologic vision changes, especially after prolonged use.

Three types of Keplerian loupes are typically used in periodontics: simple or single-element loupes, compound loupes, and prism telescopic loupes. Each type can differ widely in optical sophistication and individual design.

Simple Loupes

Simple loupes consist of a pair of single meniscus lenses (Fig. 67.21). Simple loupes are primitive magnifiers with limited capabilities. Each lens is limited to only two refracting surfaces. Their magnification can increase only by increasing lens diameter and thickness. Size and weight constraints make simple loupes impractical for magnification beyond ×1.5. Another disadvantage of simple loupes is that they are greatly affected by spherical and chromatic aberration. This distorts the image shape and color of objects being viewed.

Compound Loupes

Compound loupes use multielement lenses with intervening air spaces to gain additional refracting surfaces (Fig. 67.22). This allows increased magnification with more favorable working distance and depth of field. Magnification of compound loupes can be increased by lengthening the distance between lenses, thereby avoiding excessive size and weight.

In addition to offering improved optical performance, compound lenses can be *achromatic,* which is an optical feature that clinicians should always choose when selecting magnifying loupes. Achromatic lenses consist of two glass lenses joined together with clear resin. The specific density of each lens counteracts the chromatic aberration of its paired lens to produce a color-correct image. However, multielement compound loupes become optically inefficient at magnifications above ×3.

Prism Telescopic Loupes

The most advanced loupe optical magnification currently available is the prism telescopic loupe. These loupes employ Schmidt or rooftop prisms to lengthen the light path through a series of switchback mirrors between the lenses. This arrangement folds the light so that the barrel of the loupes can be shortened. Prism loupes produce better magnification, wider depths of field, longer working distances, and larger fields of view than other types of loupes. The barrels of prism loupes are short enough to be mounted on eyeglass frames (Fig. 67.23) or headbands. However, increased weight of prism telescopic loupes with magnification above ×4 makes headband mounting more

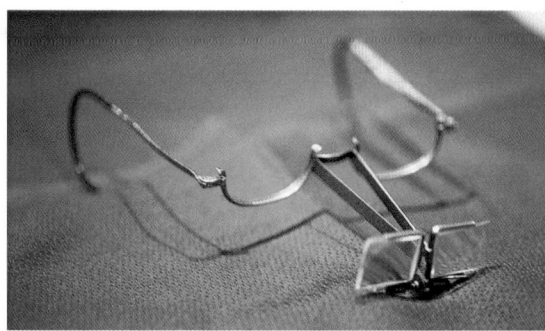

Fig. 67.21 Simple loupes.

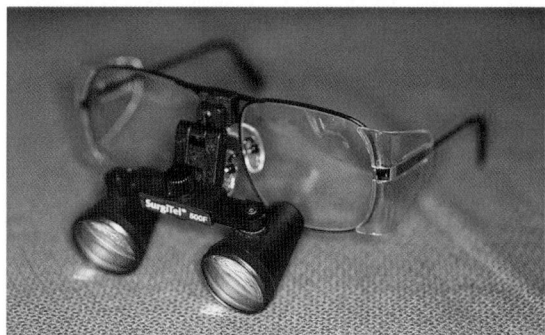

Fig. 67.22 Compound loupes.

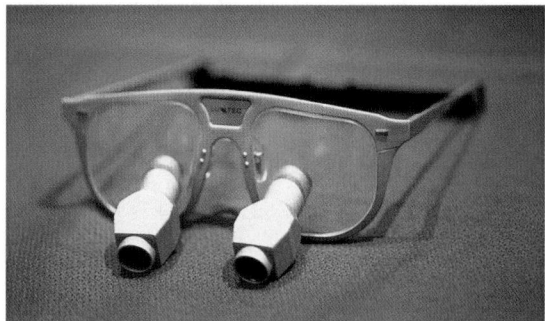

Fig. 67.23 Eyeglass-mounted prism loupes.

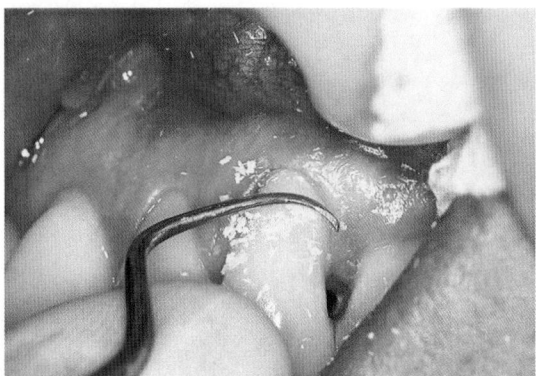

Fig. 67.20 Procedure accessibility is enhanced through microsurgery. (A) Connective tissue graft (CTG) on a maxillary molar. (B) Before surgery. (C) During surgery. (D) Seven weeks postoperatively.

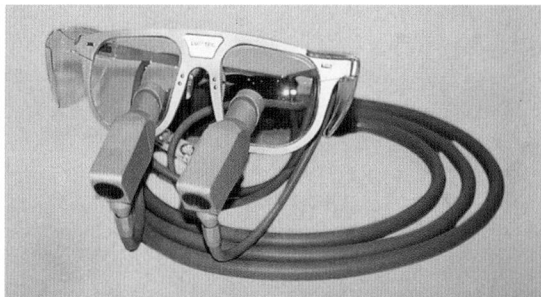

Fig. 67.24 Coaxial lighted prism loupes.

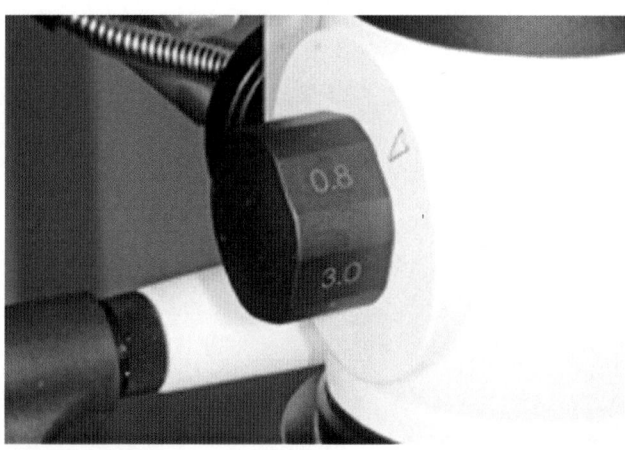

Fig. 67.26 Rotating magnification element with a field of view ranging from the full mouth to approximately 3 cm when using a 250-mm objective lens.

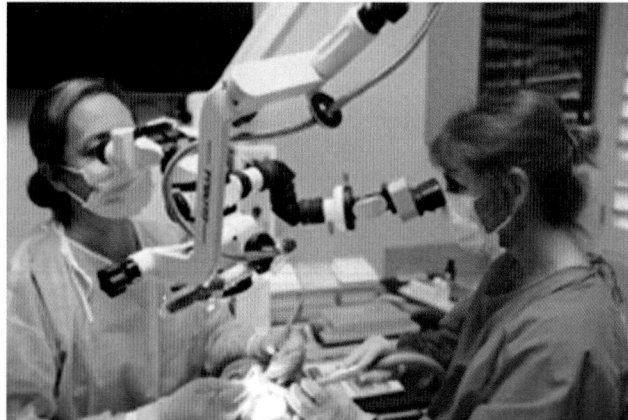

Fig. 67.25 Accessory binocular module allows the assistant to better support the operator during the procedure.

comfortable and stable than eyeglass frame mounting. Innovations in prism telescopic loupes include coaxial fiberoptic lighting incorporated in the lens elements to improve illumination (Fig. 67.24).

Magnification Range of Surgical Loupes

Dental loupes provide a limited range of magnification (×1.5 to ×6). Loupes delivering magnification of less than ×3 are usually inadequate for the visual acuity necessary for clinical periodontics. Surgical loupes providing magnification of more than ×4 are impractical because of their small field of view, shallow depth of focus, and excessive weight. Excessively heavy loupes can make it difficult to maintain a stable visual field.

For some periodontal procedures, prism telescopic loupes with magnification of ×4 provide an adequate combination of magnification, field of view, and depth of focus. However, the surgical microscope offers much higher magnification and superior optics compared with any of the loupe optical systems mentioned.

The Surgical Microscope

The surgical microscope offers greater versatility than dental loupes by providing a range of magnification with superior optical performance. A surgical microscope can last an entire career, making its long-term expense practical. Proficient use of the microscope requires training and practice. Surgical microscopes designed for dentistry employ galilean optics, which have binocular eyepieces joined by offset prisms to establish a parallel optical axis and permit stereoscopic vision without eye convergence or eyestrain. An additional binocular eyepiece can aid the microsurgical assistant (Fig. 67.25).

Surgical microscopes have coated achromatic lenses, high optical resolution, and a rotating magnification element that allows the

microsurgeon to easily change magnification to a value appropriate for the surgical task at hand (Fig. 67.26). Because the optical elements of surgical microscopes are more advanced than those in loupes, depth-of-focus and field-of-view characteristics are greatly enhanced. Surgical microscopes have objective lenses with various working distances. A useful range in dentistry is 250 to 350 mm.

For practical use, a surgical microscope must have maneuverability and stability. Mountings are available for the ceiling, wall, or floor. Adjustable inclining eyepieces enhance postural flexibility for various procedures (Fig. 67.27). This maneuverability provides visual access to every area of the mouth and is an important factor in choosing to use a surgical microscope.

Illumination of the microsurgical field is also an important consideration. Dentists are accustomed to working with lateral illumination from side-mounted dental lights or headlamps. Fiberoptic coaxial illumination is a major advantage because it focuses light parallel to the microscope's optical axis, which eliminates shadows. Surgeons can visualize the deepest reaches of the oral cavity, including subgingival pockets and angular bony defects. Definitive visualization of root surface to detect deposits and irregularities is possible. Surgeons can view anatomy to make clinical decisions based on accurate assessment of pathology rather than blind, educated guesses.

Documentation is important for patient and professional education and for dental-legal reasons. The surgical operating microscope is an ideal platform for documenting periodontal pathology and clinical procedures. Digital images can be captured using a beam splitter and camera attachment. A foot-controlled switch permits a surgeon to record as the procedure unfolds without interrupting surgery. These images represent the surgical field exactly as the surgeon sees it, as opposed to a camera view over the surgeon's shoulder. High-definition video cameras capture still and video images simultaneously to permit documentation of periodontal procedures for educational purposes (Fig. 67.28).

Microsurgical Sutures

To achieve ideal microsurgical wound closure, a surgeon depends on how the incisions were planned and executed, how the surgery was performed, and the suturing technique. Selection of proper suture needles and materials is essential for successful microsurgical wound closure. The choice of suture and needle size is critical for atraumatic tissue passage. Suture material must maintain wound closure until healing is sufficiently advanced to withstand functional stress.

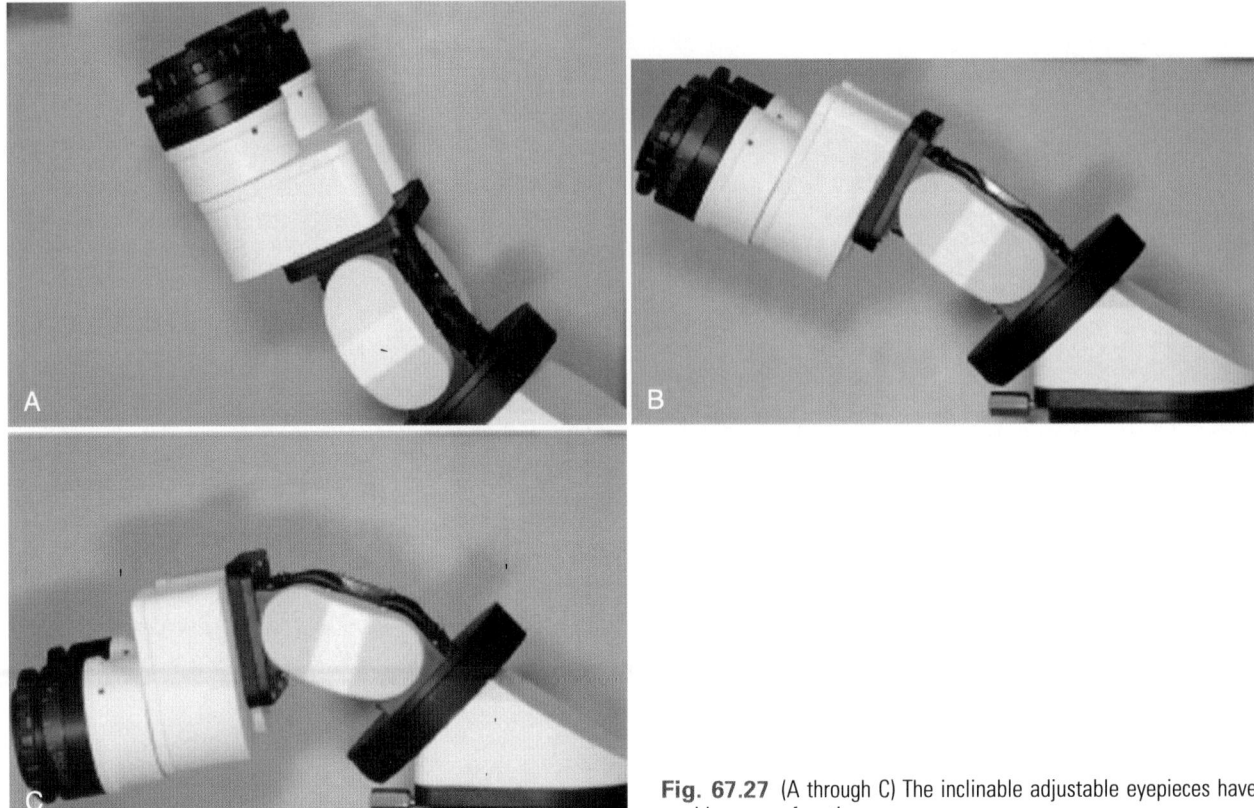

Fig. 67.27 (A through C) The inclinable adjustable eyepieces have a wide range of motion.

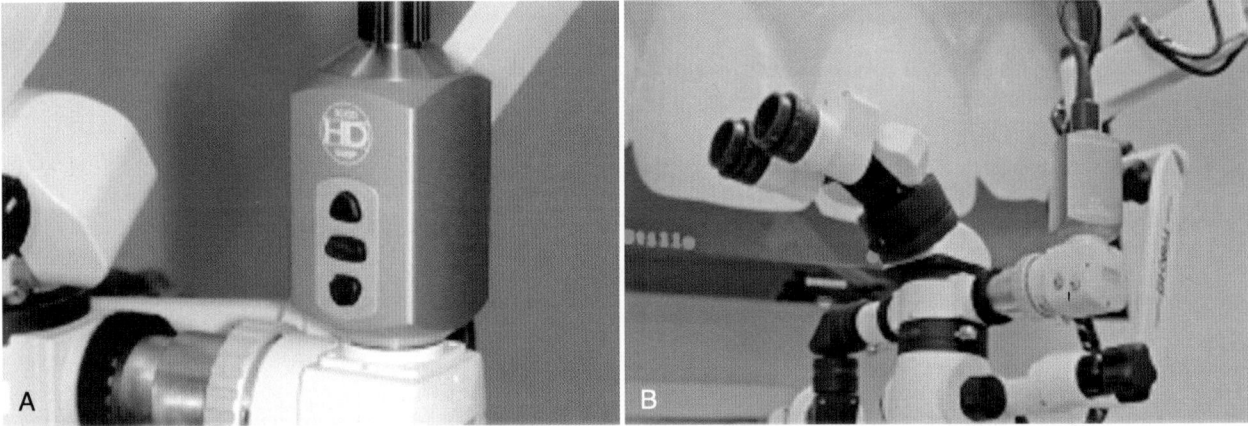

Fig. 67.28 (A) High-definition (HD) video and still capture camera mounts conveniently fit into the microscope and (B) can be viewed in real time on an HD monitor. *(Courtesy Optronics Microcast HD Studio, Optronics Medical Grade HD Microimaging Systems, Goleta, CA.)*

Sutures are classified according to structure as monofilament or braided, according to surface as coated or uncoated, and according to biologic properties as absorbable or nonabsorbable.[2] The suture of choice in microsurgery is a monofilament suture material such as polypropylene or polydioxanone. These materials are bacteriostatic and noninflammatory, hold a knot extremely well, and are easily removed. The purpose of sutures is to provide initial wound support. They are chosen to appropriate wounds based on the fragility of the tissue. The smallest suture capable of supporting the wound produces the least tissue trauma and the least interruption of the blood supply.

In periodontal microsurgery, the suture size ranges from 6-0 (i.e., diameter of a human hair) to 9-0 (Fig. 67.29). The size and shape of the needle used is essential for the atraumatic passage of the suture. The needle diameter is ideally slightly larger than the suture size. Sutures used in microsurgery are swaged, making the needle and the suture continuous[1] (Fig. 67.30). Penetration and passage of the needle depends on the angle of entry of the needle point. Cutting needles pass through gingival tissue easily but can tear tissue. Tapered needles are less traumatic and less likely to tear tissue.

An important component of needle design is the chord distance (see Fig. 67.30). The chord of a needle is the length of a line drawn between the cutting point and the swaged end.[1] The radius of a needle is the arc of its circumference. A half-round needle has an

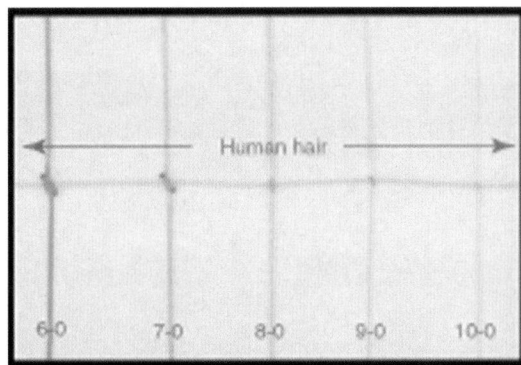

Fig. 67.29 Size comparison of microsutures in relation to the dimension of a human hair.

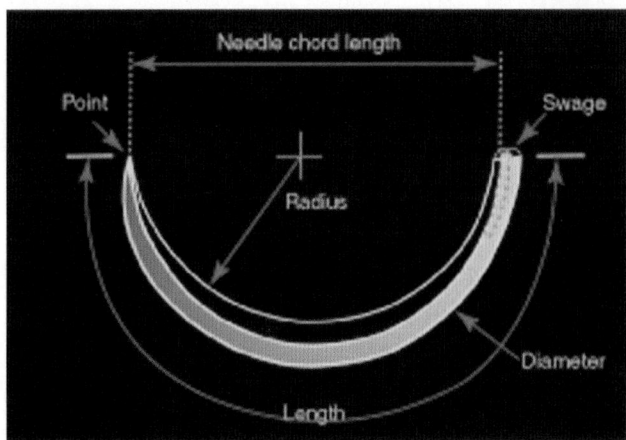

Fig. 67.30 Anatomy of a needle. Microsutures are hand-inserted into the laser-drilled swaged end of the needle, forming a seamless, contiguous unit.

arc of 180 degrees. The chord determines the ease in passing a suture between adjacent teeth. The arc determines the bite size and angle of entry taken by the needle. These needle dimensions are important when selecting sutures for periodontal microsurgery.[4]

Conclusions

As medicine and dentistry continue the pursuit of minimally invasive treatment, periodontal microsurgery and its principles will emerge as the methodology to meet professional and public demand.[14] The microscope provides a tremendous platform from which the microsurgical clinician can gather and observe detailed and precise amounts of information for the diagnosis and treatment of patients with skill and accuracy.[6] Microsurgery leads to improved aesthetics, rapid healing, reduced morbidity, and enhanced patient acceptance.[3,15,16]

References

References for this chapter are found on the companion website www.expertconsult.com.

CHAPTER 68

Lasers in Periodontal and Peri-implant Therapy

Perry R. Klokkevold | Bobby Butler | Richard T. Kao

CHAPTER OUTLINE

Laser Physics and Biologic
  Interactions
Laser Applications in
  Periodontics

Lasers in the Management of
  Periodontitis *(e-only)*
Lasers in the Management of
  Peri-implantitis *(e-only)*

Complications and Risks of Laser
  Therapy
Conclusion

 For online-only content on specific laser types (diode, Nd:YAG, Er:YAG, Er,Cr:YSGG, and CO_2) and lasers in the management of periodontitis and peri-implantitis, go to the companion website www.expertconsult.com. Some figures may be out of numeric order in this printed chapter.

The first working laser was made in 1960 by Theodore H. Maiman at Hughes Research Laboratories, a subdivision of Hughes Aircraft in Malibu, California.[68] Maiman created the laser by pumping very high energy from a flashtube into a solid state ruby medium, which emitted a monochromatic beam of deep red visible light with a wavelength of 694.3 nm. Almost immediately thereafter researchers began investigating the use of lasers for dental applications.[47,76,94,115] Early uses focused on removal of hard tissues and caries, but these lasers offered little benefit over standard rotary instruments. Consequently, interest in the use of lasers for dentistry faded. Laser activity for dental applications remained nominal until the 1990s when advances in new wavelengths, delivery units, and power maximums refocused the use of lasers for soft tissue as well as hard tissue procedures (Table 68.1).[39,66] More recently, there has been an increased interest in the use of lasers for periodontal therapy including both surgical and nonsurgical applications. In addition to their application as a cutting device, lasers have been advocated in antimicrobial photodynamic therapy mode for biofilm disruption to reduce or eliminate pathogens from the periodontal pocket. Yet another potential laser application in periodontics is the use of low-level laser therapy (LLLT) to stimulate cellular activity for enhanced wound healing and tissue regeneration.

As with the introduction of most new technologies, advocates of laser therapy for periodontics hope it will be able to replace or enhance traditional therapies. It is important to recognize that making the determination of whether a new technology should be incorporated into practice requires evidence from clinical studies to demonstrate equivalence or superiority to accepted therapies. The sample size required to statistically test superiority versus equivalence is generally much larger than what has been tested in clinical trials evaluating lasers to date. Hence, the only reasonable conclusions will state that lasers are equivalent, at best, as compared with conventional therapies. The limited number of longitudinal clinical trials and cohort studies for each laser type along with the fact that different exposure settings and various protocols are used in these studies make justification to implement this new technology for periodontal applications difficult. Published studies to date are too small and heterogeneous to make

definitive conclusions. Nonetheless, if a new therapy is found to be equivalent, albeit not superior to a conventional therapy, there may be other reasons such as safety, cost, or ease of use that warrant utilization of the new technology.[48] Systematic reviews and meta-analyses of available reports have attempted to define whether lasers provide additional benefits for periodontal applications.[111–113,115] Unfortunately, there is a lack of well-designed randomized controlled clinical trials (RCTs), which is the optimal type of study needed for meta-analyses, and those studies that exist are often heterogeneous with regard to laser type, settings, and exposure. As such, the conclusions should be interpreted with caution. This chapter describes some of the clinical applications of lasers for periodontal therapy and discusses the currently available literature.

⚠ CLINICAL CORRELATION

Laser energy delivered to target tissues will vary depending on laser type (wavelength), settings (power), and exposure (time). It is difficult to compare the results of multiple studies unless the same laser is used with identical settings and exposure time.

Laser Physics and Biologic Interactions

Laser is an acronym for "*L*ight *A*mplification by *S*timulated *E*mission of *R*adiation." Lasers function by stimulating the emission of light energy from a given medium in a collimated, focused monochromatic ray of light. The energy beam reacts with a target tissue by being absorbed, reflected, or scattered depending on wavelength and absorption characteristics (Fig. 68.1). Some lasers (e.g., Nd:YAG lasers) may be transmitted through surface tissues to interact with deeper tissues. When the laser is well absorbed, the energy explodes the target tissue cells and extracellular matrix in a process called *ablation*.[93] The efficiency of ablation is related to the wavelength and the affinity of the laser beam for the target tissue. Laser beams may also be reflected or bounced off the target (e.g., reflected off a metal surface) without interaction. This is typically an undesirable

TABLE 68.1   Types of Lasers Currently Used in Dentistry

Laser Medium	Wavelength (nm)	Dental Uses
Argon	488–514	Tooth bleaching and advanced curing lights
Diode	655–980	Gingivectomy/gingivoplasty, oral medicine uses (aphthous ulcer therapy, biopsies, dentinal desensitizing), second-stage implant exposure, periodontal curettage (advocated but not evidence based)
Neodymium:yttrium-aluminum-garnet (Nd:YAG)	1064	Gingivectomy/gingivoplasty, oral medicine uses (aphthous ulcer therapy, biopsies, dentinal desensitizing), second-stage implant exposure, periodontal curettage (advocated but not evidence based)
Erbium, chromium:yttrium-scandium-gallium-garnet (Er,Cr:YSGG)	2780	Gingivectomy/gingivoplasty, oral medicine uses (aphthous ulcer therapy, biopsies, dentinal desensitizing), second-stage implant exposure, periodontal curettage (advocated but not evidence based), hard tissue cutting (dentin and osseous)
Erbium:yttrium-aluminum-garnet (Er:YAG)	2940	Gingivectomy/gingivoplasty, oral medicine uses (aphthous ulcer therapy, biopsies, dentinal desensitizing), second-stage implant exposure, periodontal curettage (advocated but not evidence based), hard tissue cutting (dentin and osseous)
Carbon dioxide (CO_2)	10,600	Gingivectomy/gingivoplasty, second-stage implant exposure, periodontal curettage (advocated but not evidence based)

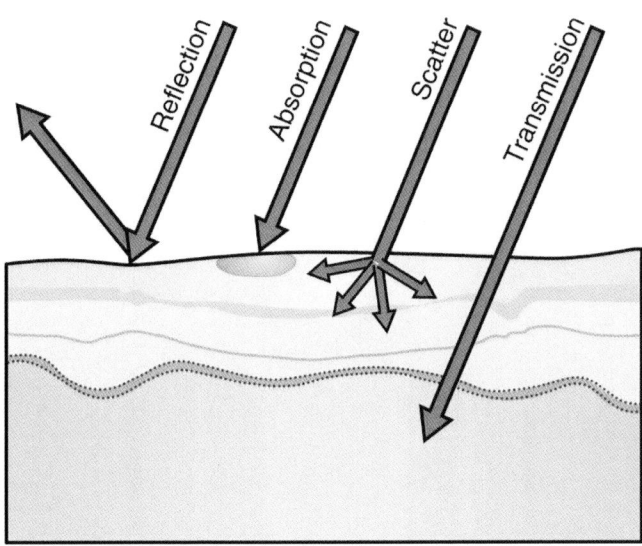

Fig. 68.1 Four potential laser-tissue interactions. The laser beam may be reflected, absorbed, scattered or transmitted. *(From Convissar RA: Principles and practice of laser dentistry, ed 2, St. Louis, 2016, Mosby.)*

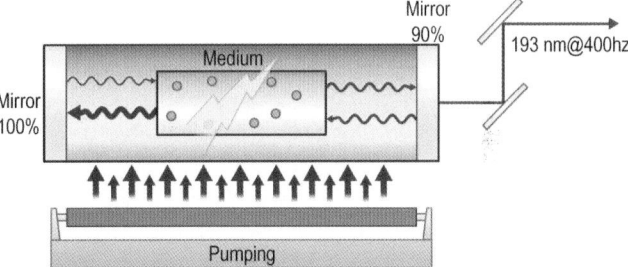

Fig. 68.2 Diagrammatic presentation of the main components of a laser device. Lasers require a medium, an optical chamber or laser tube, and an externally applied energy source to create an emitted monochromatic energy beam. *(From Spaeth GL, Danesh-Meyer H, Goldberg I, et al: Ophthalmic surgery: principles and practice, ed 4, Edinburgh, 2012, Saunders.)*

effect because there is no effect on the target tissue and the reflected beam can interact with unintended targets. If the wavelength is not well absorbed, there can be scattering and a thermal reaction in the adjacent tissues with carbonization, charring, and melting. Clinicians must understand and appreciate not only how this energy is affecting the target tissues but also how it affects the adjacent tissues as well.

Production of a laser requires a medium, an optical chamber or laser tube, and an externally applied energy source to create an emitted monochromatic energy beam (Fig. 68.2). When energy is applied to the medium, electrons are "excited" to a higher energy orbit. When they return to the normal orbit, a photon (particle of light) is emitted. Because the photons are all the same wavelength, the laser beam is "coherent." The medium, which can be a gas, a solid, or a semiconductor, determines the laser wavelength. Lasers are named in relationship to the active element(s) that, when stimulated, generates the energy beam. Typical lasers used in dentistry include argon, GaAs (diode), Nd:YAG, Er:YAG, Er,Cr:YSGG, and

CO_2 lasers. Wavelengths are delivered either in a continuous, pulsed (gated) or in a running pulse waveform.[27] Argon lasers have wavelengths in the ultraviolet and visible light range with primary dental applications in composite resin placement, enamel and dentin bonding, preventive therapies, and endodontic procedures.[57] Reported periodontal applications for the other lasers include soft tissue incision, ablation, depigmentation, subgingival curettage, scaling of root surfaces, calculus removal, bacterial killing, osteoplasty, and ostectomy.

KEY FACT

Lasers function by stimulating the emission of light energy from a given medium in a collimated, focused monochromatic ray of light. The energy beam reacts with a target tissue by being absorbed, reflected, or scattered depending on wavelength and absorption characteristics.

Each laser has a unique wavelength spectrum resulting in specific absorption characteristics that must be understood and appreciated for the desired purpose (Figs. 68.3 and 68.4). When applied to the various periodontal tissues such as the gingiva, periodontal ligament, cementum, dentin, and bone, the biologic interactions will be unique

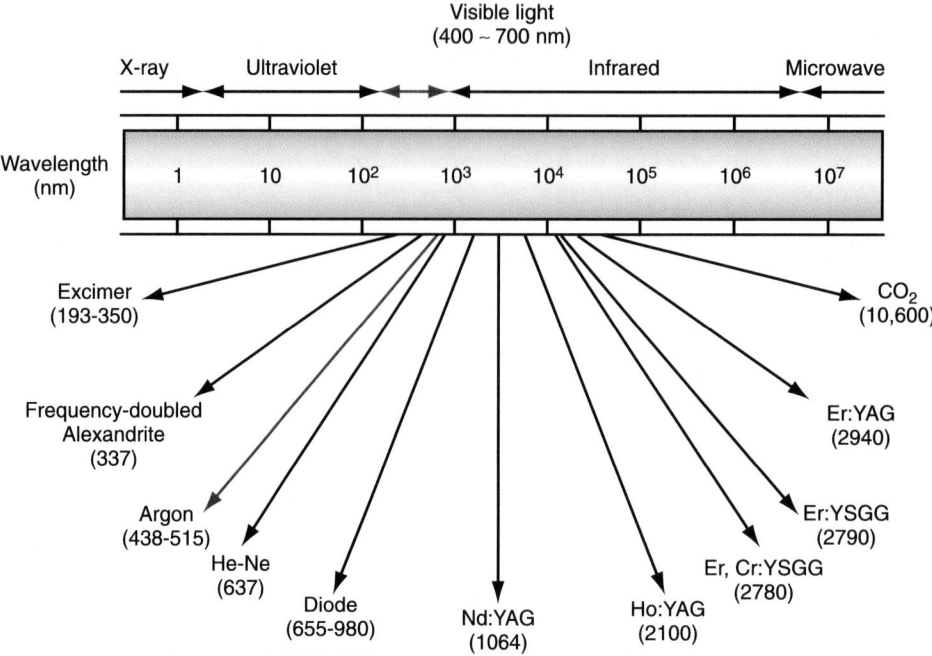

Fig. 68.3 Laser wavelengths. Each laser has a unique wavelength spectrum resulting in specific absorption characteristics. The wavelength of most of the lasers used in dentistry/periodontics is in the red and near-infrared spectrum.

DEPTH OF OPTICAL PENETRATION BY VARIOUS LASERS

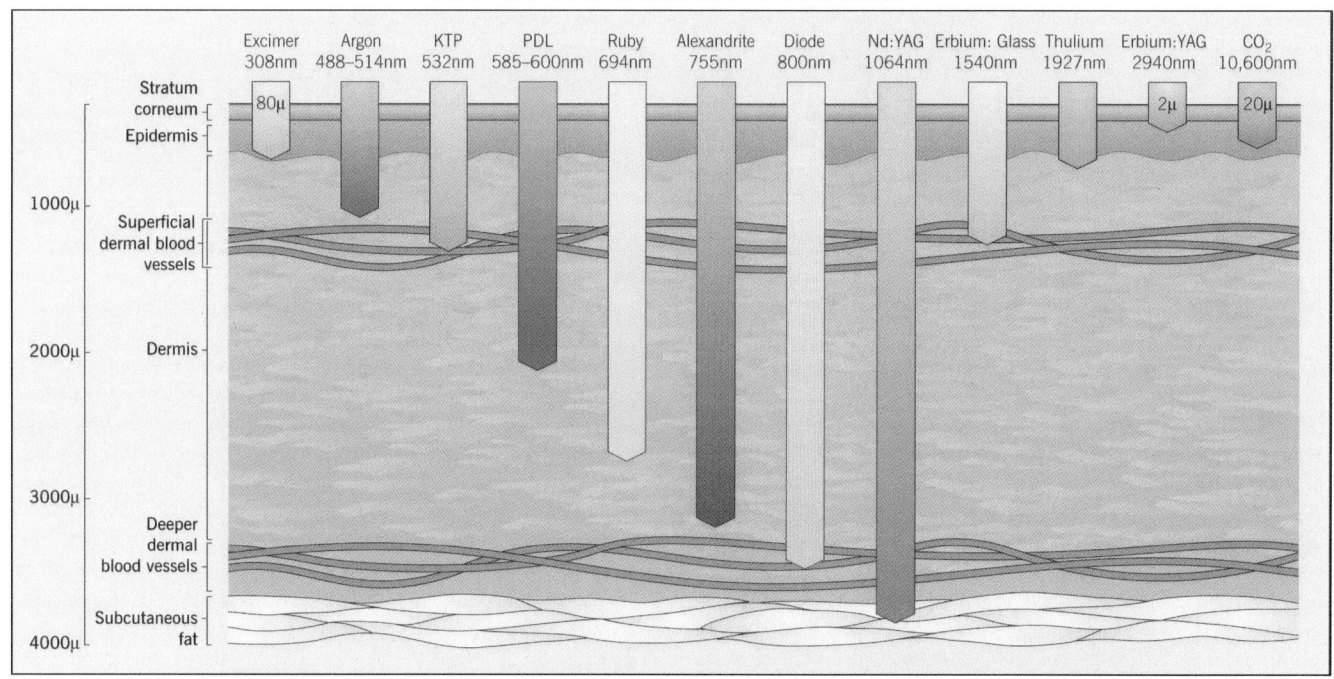

Fig. 68.4 Depth of optical penetration by various lasers. Tissue penetration is a function of laser wavelength and absorption characteristics. It should be noted that the treatment depth can greatly exceed the optical penetration depth for ablative lasers. On the face, the fat can be present at depth of 2 to 3 mm. For example, the depth of optical penetration for CO_2 lasers is only ~20 microns, but fractional CO_2 lasers can vaporize nearly full-thickness microchannels through the dermis. KTP, potassium titanyl phosphate; Nd, neodymium; PDL, pulsed dye laser; YAG, yttrium aluminum garnet. *(From Bolognia JL, Jorizzo JL, Schaffer JV: Dermatology, two-volume set, ed 3, Philadelphia, 2012, Saunders.)*

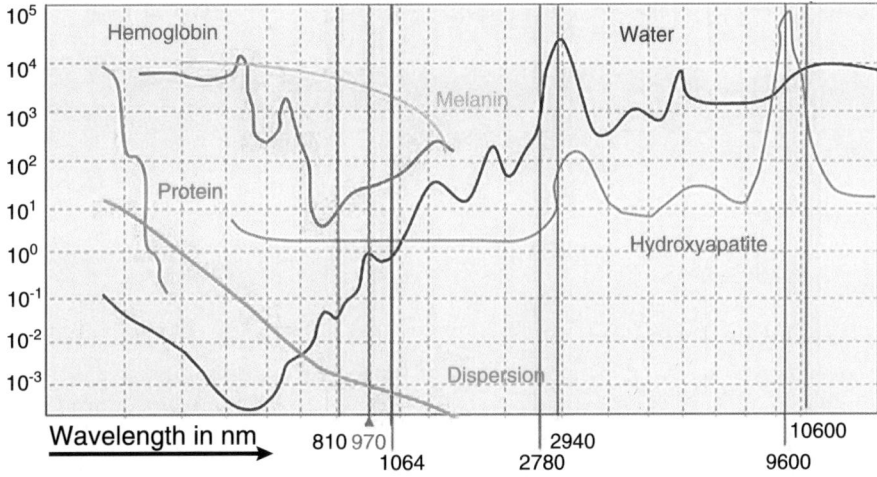

Fig. 68.5 Laser absorption coefficient of various tissue constituents as a function of wavelength.

for that wavelength. Tissues are composite structures of inorganic and organic elements with various constituents. Gingiva is composed of fibrous connective tissue, extracellular matrix components (including melanin pigmentation), and 70% water. Bone is composed of 67% inorganic minerals (calcium hydroxyapatite) and 33% organic elements (collagen, noncollagenous proteins, and water). Other factors to consider are the textures, compositions, and densities of these structures. For example, the varying percentages of mineralized structures, blood vessels, and fluid found in cortical bone versus cancellous bone will result in the laser energy beam encountering differing fluctuations in absorption and scattering, regardless of the wavelength, due to these differences. Blood contains 55% plasma (water) and 45% cells including red blood cells with hemoglobin, white blood cells, and platelets. Thus, when considering the use of lasers for a given clinical application, it is important to appreciate not only the type of laser being used and the target tissue but also the composition of that tissue.

The affinity of a laser wavelength for the target tissue (absorption coefficient) is critical to its effectiveness for the procedure (Fig. 68.5). The relatively short wavelengths of the diode (655 to 980 nm) and Nd:YAG (1064 nm) are well absorbed by pigment and are better suited for soft tissue procedures than for hard tissue procedures. The CO_2 laser, which has a very long wavelength (10,600 nm), has an affinity for water and is best suited for soft tissue procedures. Diode and Nd:YAG wavelengths are not absorbed by hydroxyapatite and thus are not effective for hard tissues such as cementum, dentin, and bone. The wavelengths of Er:YAG (2940 nm) and Er,Cr:YSGG (2780 nm) lasers have a positive affinity for both water and hydroxyapatite. The specificity for hydroxyapatite allows erbium lasers to cut hard tissues including bone, dentin, and enamel.[14,15,18–20] The selective absorption by water also makes erbium lasers effective for soft tissue procedures.

Selection of the laser type is ultimately based on the amount of energy transmitted to the tissue during a procedure. Photothermal energy is measured in watts (W = joules/second) and hertz (Hz = cycles/second). The energy beam can be delivered in a continuous or pulsed manner. A continuous laser transmits more energy than a pulsed laser, as there are momentary breaks or cooling periods in the latter. When comparing outcomes of different laser therapies, it is imperative to consider the type of laser, the wavelength, *and* the amount of energy delivered to tissues including watts, hertz, and total time of exposure.

Care must be taken to avoid the transmission of excessive thermal energy to target and adjacent tissues. The amount of energy delivered

to target tissues is critical to the desired outcome. Although the optimal energy delivered to tissues can be advantageous, excessive energy may completely negate the potential benefits. Consider a study that compared wound healing of incisions made with a scalpel versus Nd:YAG laser with two different power settings. Healing was best following the incision with the laser applied with settings of 1.75 W, 20 Hz. However, healing was delayed when the energy was increased to 3 W, 20 Hz. Healing of the scalpel incision was better than that for the laser incision at the higher energy setting.[97] The study demonstrates that differences in energy level delivered to tissues from the same laser can have significantly different results. It also shows the dilemma faced when attempting to compare the results of one study to another unless both studies use the same laser with the same energy settings and the same quantity of energy delivered. Unfortunately, the literature is inundated with reports of various applications using different lasers, varied settings, and a wide range of protocols.

 KEY FACT

It is important for clinicians to recognize not only the type of tissue (e.g., hard vs. soft tissue) but also the quality of target tissue makeup when applying laser therapy. For example, the varying percentages of mineralized structures, blood vessels, and fluid found in cortical bone versus cancellous bone will result in the laser energy beam encountering differing fluctuations in absorption and scattering, regardless of the wavelength.

Laser Applications in Periodontics

Currently, lasers are used in periodontal therapy for (1) aesthetic surgical procedures such as gingivectomy, osseous crown lengthening, and depigmentation; (2) nonsurgical therapy; (3) decontamination and antimicrobial therapy; and (4) biomodulation.

Aesthetic and Pre-Prosthetic Surgical Applications

Several types of laser wavelengths have been used for soft tissue surgical procedures.[11,72,73] Appropriate use of lasers for procedures such as frenectomy, gingivectomy/gingivoplasty, reshaping of drug-induced gingival overgrowth, exposure of short crowns associated with altered passive/delayed eruption, and management of excess mucosal tissue such as pericoronitis situations distal of mandibular second molars have been well documented.[7,13,44,56] Some of the positive aspects of laser therapy are good visibility during the surgical procedure as a result of coagulation, hemostasis, and minimal tissue damage

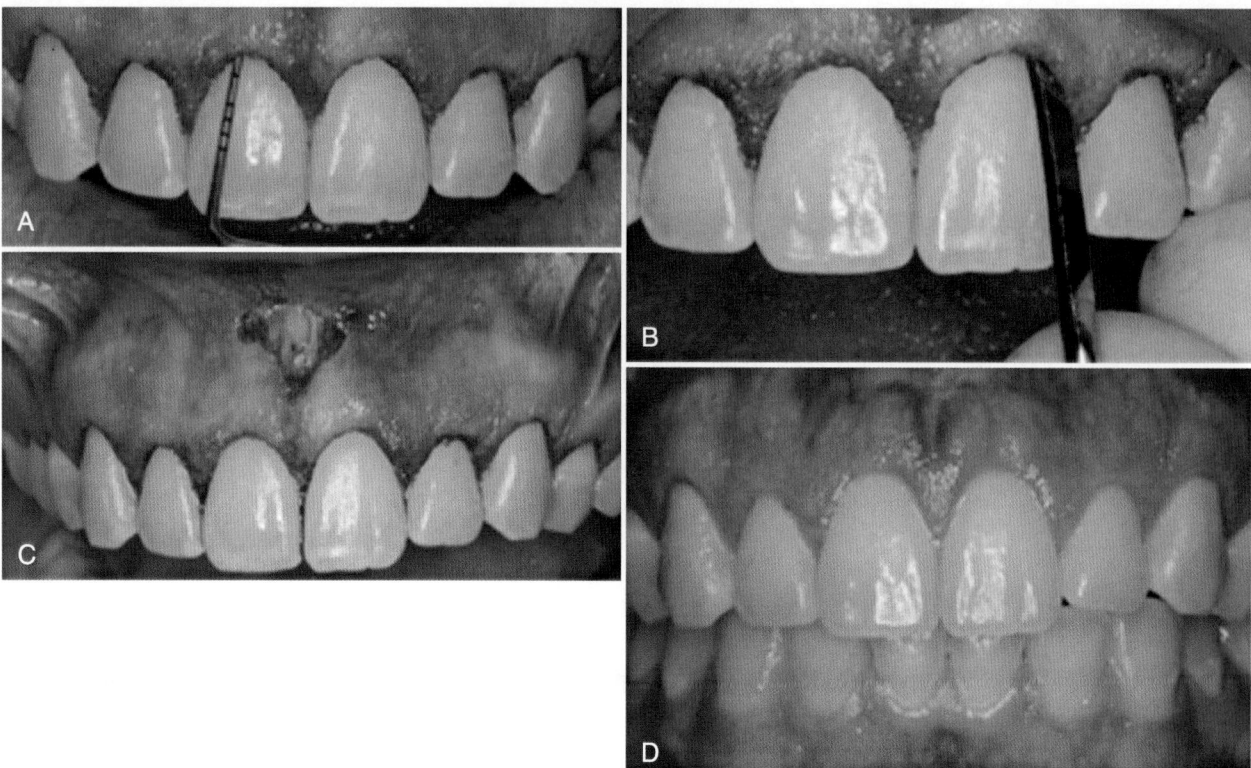

Fig. 68.6 Crown-lengthening procedure performed using a closed approach with a laser. (A) Periodontal sounding after the initial gingivectomy, which indicated the need for osseous contouring to achieve biologic width. (B) The osseous contouring was done via intrasulcular access. Sounding confirms 3 mm from the gingival to osseous crest. Final small fragments of bone are checked and removed with a small chisel. (C) Final surgical photograph shows minimal bleeding with no need for sutures. A frenectomy was also completed at the time of surgery. (D) Smile at 3 months postsurgery. *(Case courtesy Dr. Bobby Butler, Seattle, Washington.)*

adjacent to the laser wound. Additionally, laser therapy can offer extreme precision and may be easier than using a scalpel.

Aesthetic applications for gingivectomy and gingivoplasty procedures allow delicate tissue reshaping. The laser is effective for the removal of pigmentation from the gingival tissues, which can significantly improve the aesthetics of highly pigmented areas. The CO_2, diode, Nd:YAG, Er:YAG, and Er,Cr:YSGG lasers have been used for depigmentation.[8,34,40,45,63,79]

Some clinicians advocate the use of lasers for crown-lengthening procedures. Whereas crown lengthening involving only soft tissue can be effectively performed with a wide variety of lasers, only lasers with wavelengths that have an affinity for hydroxyapatite are effective for crown-lengthening procedures that require osseous resection. Erbium lasers (e.g., Er:YAG and Er,Cr:YSGG), which have an affinity for water and hydroxyapatite, have been advocated for clinical crown lengthening without gingival flap reflection.[42,43,59,118,126–129] The Er,Cr:YSGG laser can safely cut bone without burning or altering the calcium-to-phosphate ratio of the irradiated bone.[59,127] This approach has been described in case reports and case series, but there are no controlled longitudinal or cohort studies supporting the use of lasers for clinical crown lengthening using the closed-flap technique. The use of lasers for flapless crown lengthening with osseous contouring remains controversial.

Decision making for the use of lasers in crown lengthening in an open or closed approach is based on osseous biotypes.[60] In the closed approach, the Er,Cr:YSGG or Er:YAG laser is only feasible in medium biotype cases with an osseous crest that is approximately 1 mm in thickness and may be limited to situations where only 1 to 2 mm of osseous removal is required. In this technique, bone sounding

with a probe is used after the external gingivectomy to determine the thickness of the osseous biotype and to determine the amount of bone removal required. The laser tip is aligned parallel to the root surface in contact with the bone and fired for 1 to 2 seconds. The tip is moved slowly around the tooth, firing intermittently while in contact with the bone until the desired osseous reduction is achieved. The osseous removal is verified by sounding, and detailing is performed with a small chisel (Fig. 68.6). This technique can be surgically conservative and result in symmetric gingival levels in the aesthetic zone.[11,65,72]

Case selection based on osseous biotypes is critical for the success of this closed approach for crown lengthening. In a thick biotype, the laser will likely create a "trough" or an intrabony defect. Because inadequate bone removal is performed, the soft tissue will often rebound soon after the procedure. An open-flap approach with direct vision of bone is indicated for cases with a thick osseous biotype so definitive osseous contouring can be performed. Closed or flapless laser crown lengthening should absolutely be avoided in all cases of thin biotype. Using laser therapy in an ablative mode for osseous removal in thin biotype cases poses a high risk for overheating tissues and adversely affecting the healing response, leading to unfavorable or possibly disastrous clinical outcomes.

Further issues of concern include the limited ability to assess the appropriateness of osseous recontouring and the inability to avoid or detect damage to root surfaces.[27] These concerns and the possible need for retreatment because of tissue rebound or poor healing suggest that this is not a superior or equivalent technique as compared with traditional functional crown lengthening that requires osseous contouring.

1. Do the in vivo studies demonstrate a reduction in pathogenic bacteria as compared with conventional therapy (e.g., scaling and root planing [SRP])?
2. Are positive microbial changes sustained, or do the periodontal pathogens return and recolonize the sites?
3. Are there any differences in clinical parameters following laser-assisted versus conventional therapy SRP? When evaluating nonsurgical periodontal therapy, gain in clinical attachment level (CAL) represents the gold standard. Pocket depth (PD) and levels of subgingival microbes are important because they correlate with changes in CAL.[26,99]
4. Are there changes in root surface condition based on in vitro or in vivo studies?

Nonsurgical Periodontal Therapy

One of the more prevalent applications of lasers in periodontics is the nonsurgical treatment of moderate to advanced chronic periodontitis. Lasers have been used as a monotherapy or as an adjunct to scaling and root planing. The purported benefits of lasers for nonsurgical periodontal therapy include subgingival curettage, minimally invasive access for scaling and root planning, and calculus removal, as well as detoxification and killing of subgingival periodontal pathogens.[49,102,114,131]

In the clinical situation, periodontal pathogenic bacteria exist within a protective biofilm in a periodontal pocket. Consequently, it is difficult for conventional periodontal therapies to completely eliminate them. Laser therapy is proposed to improve access to areas that are difficult for instruments to reach and to facilitate killing bacteria. Indeed, lasers with various wavelengths have been shown to effectively kill periodontal pathogens.[20,50] See the Photodynamic Therapy section.

When assessing the effectiveness of any particular laser type used for nonsurgical periodontal therapy, several questions need to be considered, as listed in Box 68.1.

 CLINICAL CORRELATION

Laser therapy used to treat moderate to advanced chronic periodontitis is one of the more prevalent applications of this technology. The purported benefits of lasers for nonsurgical periodontal therapy include minimally invasive access for scaling and root planing, calculus removal, and the detoxification and killing of subgingival periodontal pathogens. Laser therapy may reach difficult-to-access areas more effectively than conventional therapy.

Photodynamic Therapy

Photodynamic therapy (PDT) involves the use of a photosensitizer (photoactive dye) that is activated by exposure to a specific wavelength of light in the presence of oxygen. The activated photosensitizer transitions to an excited state and subsequently reacts with oxygen to create singlet oxygen and free radicals, which are damaging to proteins, lipids, nucleic acids, and other vital elements causing destruction of the target tissues. In the case of biofilm and periodontal pathogens, antimicrobial photodynamic therapy (aPDT) may *appear* to offer a magic bullet effect of target killing bacteria. PDT may be an effective means of disrupting the biofilm.[96] Most studies evaluating photodynamic therapy have been conducted in Europe. The US Food and Drug Administration does not yet approve PDT.

The use of lasers for photodynamic therapy has been reviewed.[30,88,119] Antimicrobial PDT for periodontitis uses a photosensitizer dye that specifically targets microorganisms and is activated by low-level laser light. Photosensitizer activation can be achieved with low-level energy exposure from various laser light sources including but not limited to argon, Nd:YAG, and diode. The introduction of a photosensitizer can greatly increase the bactericidal ability of a laser.[19,20,22,29,92,117] This is supported by an in vitro study using methylene blue with a diode laser to destroy black-pigmented bacteria (*P. gingivalis* and *P. intermedia*)[117]; 99% to 100% of bacteria were eliminated. However, it is important to recognize that pathogenic bacteria within the protective biofilm that exists in vivo may not be killed to the same degree observed during in vitro studies. Laboratory analysis of laser bactericidal properties is not clinically relevant in that these bacteria do not exist as a suspension or monolayer in vivo.

 KEY FACT

Antimicrobial photodynamic therapy uses a photosensitizer (nontoxic dye), which specifically targets microorganisms and is activated by low-level laser light. The introduction of a photosensitizer can greatly increase the bactericidal ability of a laser.

To date, the results of clinical studies evaluating the effectiveness of aPDT are mixed and not convincing.[116] A systematic review including 17 clinical studies found that 4 studies demonstrated significantly reduced bacteria with laser photodynamic therapy, whereas 13 studies showed equivalent effectiveness as compared with conventional scaling root planing (SRP) alone.[2] The authors concluded that the bactericidal efficacy of aPDT as an adjunct to SRP against periodontal pathogens remains debatable. The incomplete elimination of periodontal pathogens and the protective nature of the biofilm environment may be responsible for the observed persistence and recolonization of microbial pathogens in this microniche. Several individual clinical studies have been published on the use of aPDT as adjunct to SRP. A majority of these studies reported significant clinical and microbiologic improvements in the PDT + SRP combination as compared with SRP alone.[4,18,19,20,22,23,128] One study found the results to be comparable.[30] A clinical and microbiologic evaluation of the effectiveness of PDT in the nonsurgical treatment of aggressive periodontitis, using a split-mouth design (PDT + SRP versus SRP only), found no additional benefits from PDT as compared with SRP alone.[21] A meta-analysis evaluating the effectiveness of aPDT as an adjunct to nonsurgical periodontal therapy in patients with diabetes included four RCTs reporting clinical and metabolic parameters.[1] Although aPDT with SRP was shown to be effective in treating chronic periodontitis, no difference was observed between the test (aPDT + SRP) and control (SRP only) groups. The authors concluded that aPDT has no additional benefit. More clinical trials are required prior to clinical implementation.

Low-Level Laser Therapy

The use of low-level laser therapy (LLLT) for photobiomodulation is prevalent in medicine. Soon after the discovery of lasers in the 1960s, it was recognized that laser "light" therapy had the potential to reduce pain, inflammation, and swelling and to improve wound healing.[24,70,71] The term *low-level laser therapy* refers to the therapeutic application of light to tissues with the goal of reducing pain or stimulating healing. The wavelengths of light used for LLLT are in the red to near-infrared range (600–1070 nm). It is referred to as "low level" because the density of light energy is low compared with other lasers, which are used for ablation, cutting, and thermally heating tissue. The power of low-level light (energy) is typically in the range of 1 to 1000 mW.[24] LLLT is thought to promote wound healing by reducing inflammation, increasing the formation of granulation tissue, enhancing epithelialization, fibroblast proliferation, and matrix synthesis, as well as neovascularization.[28,124,125]

Although LLLT is widely used in medicine, it continues to be controversial because the biologic mechanism(s) are not understood and the parameters of use (i.e., wavelength, power, pulse, and timing or exposure duration) are not defined. As with other laser investigations, there is heterogeneity of experimental protocols, parameters used, and results reported. Some published reports are positive, whereas others are negative. In the case of LLLT, perhaps more than other forms of laser therapy, the therapeutic effectiveness greatly depends on the optimal parameters being applied, and those details have yet to be defined.

Low-level laser therapy has been shown to reduce inflammation and enhance nonsurgical periodontal treatment in healthy subjects as well as subjects with diabetes.[9,82] In a meta-analysis of eight publications (seven RCTs) evaluating the effectiveness of LLLT as an adjunct to nonsurgical periodontal therapy, short-term (1–2 months) improvements in probing pocket depth and crevicular fluid levels of IL-1ß were shown.[95] However, LLLT failed to show significant intermediate-term (3–6 months) effects in terms of clinical parameters.

Case reports and case controlled series have suggested that LLLT *may* improve the effects of periodontal regenerative procedures.[17,35,36]

One clinical study evaluated the effectiveness of enamel matrix derivative (EMD, Emdogain) with or without the application of a low-level laser (diode) to treat intrabony defects in 22 periodontitis patients.[83] The EMD + LLLT sites healed with less gingival recession, less swelling, and less visual analog scale pain scores as compared with the EMD-only sites. More research, preferably well-designed, randomized controlled clinical trials, is needed to assess the effectiveness of LLLT on periodontal therapy.

Complications and Risks of Laser Therapy

The primary disadvantage of laser therapy is the potential for unintended tissue damage, as lasers can easily generate excessive temperatures. The exposure of bone to temperatures ≥47°C (116.6°F) can induce cellular damage and osseous resorption.[39] Extreme temperature levels of ≥60°C (140°F) result in tissue necrosis.[66]

Overexposure of laser energy has been the basis for complications, reports of tissue damage, and destruction of the periodontium. New, inexperienced operators as well as more seasoned, "cutting-edge" clinicians may encounter disastrous results from their initial treatments (Fig. 68.7). To avoid these negative outcomes, knowledge of the laser mechanics and technique is essential to minimize tissue damage.

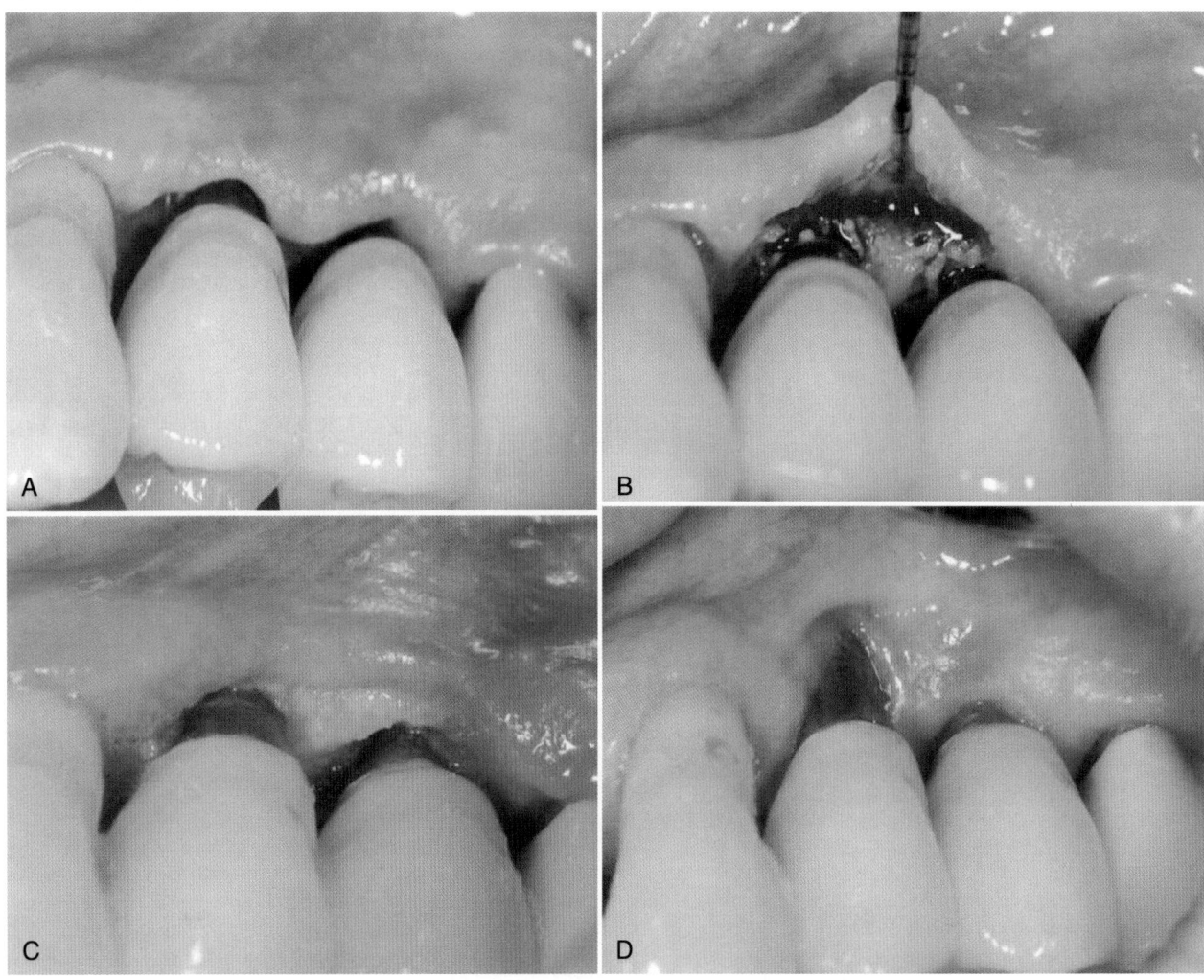

Fig. 68.7 Interproximal soft tissue cratering with underlying bone necrosis around two dental implants following laser treatment of peri-implantitis using inappropriate energy density and duration of exposure. Photos in sequence: (A–B) One-month post laser treatment. (C) Sequestration of necrotic interproximal and facial bone at 2 months post treatment. (D) Healing at 3 months post treatment. *(Courtesy Dr. Charles Cobb, University of Missouri, Kansas City.)*

Once mastery of the information has been achieved, it is critical to identify the desired laser application and the fashion in which it will be used.

Conclusion

There are many potential advantages to using laser therapy, including better visualization of cutting, patient acceptance, wound detoxification, less invasive surgical access, and minimal wound contraction with less scarring.[11,54,72] Although these laser applications hold promise, many require more well-designed, controlled research to validate their effectiveness.[55]

The literature has numerous positive findings for the use of lasers in the management of periodontal and peri-implant disease. The quality of the literature is largely dominated by case reports and case series. There are limited well-designed randomized controlled clinical trials. Further clouding the issue is the number of different lasers in use and the variety of settings and protocols being tested for each laser. The lack of consistency from one study to another has left the profession with no lasers that have been researched extensively enough to provide predictable parameters of use. Therefore laser use for the treatment of periodontal or peri-implant disease continues to have numerous unknowns.

As in all professions, technology is constantly advancing with new research to provide the clinician with better equipment, drugs, and techniques to improve the therapy rendered to patients. Lasers may become an integral part of periodontal therapy, but at the present time, further research as to the parameters for clinical efficacy and the biologic basis for laser therapy is required. Clinicians considering incorporating laser therapy should be familiar with what is known, understand the appropriate parameter for use, and receive adequate training to master the laser of interest.

 A Case Scenario is found on the companion website www.expertconsult.com.

References

 References for this chapter are found on the companion website www.expertconsult.com.

CHAPTER 69

Preparation of the Periodontium for Restorative Dentistry

Philip R. Melnick | Henry H. Takei

CHAPTER OUTLINE

Rationale for Therapy
Sequence of Treatment

Control of Active Disease
Preprosthetic Surgery *(e-only)*

Conclusion

 For online only content on preprosthetic surgery, please visit the companion website at www.expertconsult.com.

Editors' note: An animation (slide show) has been added by the editors as a supplement to the chapter. It was produced by My Dental Hub as a patient education tool and covers the basic elements in a conceptual manner. It is not intended to be a procedural guide for dental professionals.

Periodontal health is the *sine qua non*, a prerequisite, of successful comprehensive dentistry.[25] To achieve the long-term therapeutic targets of comfort, good function, treatment predictability, longevity, and ease of restorative and maintenance care, active periodontal infection must be treated and controlled before the initiation of restorative, aesthetic, and implant dentistry. In addition, the residual effects of periodontal disease or anatomic aberrations inconsistent with realizing and maintaining long-term stability must be addressed. This phase of treatment includes techniques performed in anticipation of aesthetic or implant dentistry, such as clinical crown lengthening, covering denuded roots, alveolar ridge retention or augmentation, and implant

 site development (Video 69.1: Effects of Single Tooth Loss).

Rationale for Therapy

The many reasons for establishing periodontal health before performing restorative dentistry include the following[52]:

1. Periodontal treatment is undertaken to ensure the establishment of stable gingival margins before tooth preparation. Noninflamed, healthy tissues are less likely to change (e.g., shrink) as a result of subgingival restorative treatment or postrestoration periodontal care.[28,29] In addition, tissues that do not bleed during restorative manipulation allow for a more predictable restorative and aesthetic result.[22,23]

2. Certain periodontal procedures are designed to provide for adequate tooth length for retention, access for tooth preparation, impression making, tooth preparation, and finishing of restorative margins in anticipation of restorative dentistry.[22,47] Failure to complete

these procedures before restorative care can add to the complexity of treatment and introduce unnecessary risk for failure.[22]

3. Periodontal therapy should antecede restorative care because the resolution of inflammation may result in the repositioning of teeth[46] or in soft tissue and mucosal changes.[20,48] Failure to anticipate these changes may interfere with prosthetic designs planned or constructed before periodontal treatment.

4. Traumatic forces placed on teeth with ongoing periodontitis may increase tooth mobility, discomfort, and possibly the rate of attachment loss.[9] Restorations constructed on teeth free of periodontal inflammation, synchronous with a functionally appropriate occlusion, are more compatible with long-term periodontal stability and comfort (see Chapters 18 and 55).

5. Quality, quantity, and topography of the periodontium may play important roles as structural defense factors in maintaining periodontal health. Orthodontic tooth movement and restorations completed without the benefit of periodontal treatment designed for this purpose may be subject to negative changes that complicate construction and future maintenance.[55]

6. Successful aesthetic and implant procedures may be difficult or impossible without the specialized periodontal procedures developed for this purpose.

LEARNING BOX 69.1

Periodontal treatment is undertaken to ensure the establishment of stable gingival margins before tooth preparation. Noninflamed, healthy tissues are less likely to change (e.g., shrink) as a result of subgingival restorative treatment or postrestoration periodontal care. In addition, tissues that do not bleed during restorative manipulation allow for a more predictable restorative and aesthetic result.

Sequence of Treatment

Treatment sequencing should be based on logical and evidence-based methodologies, taking into account not only the disease state

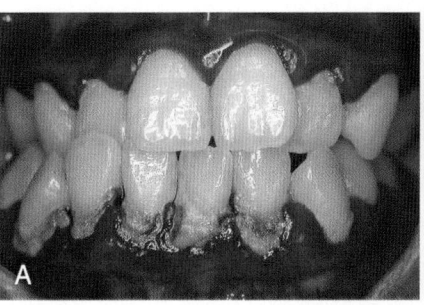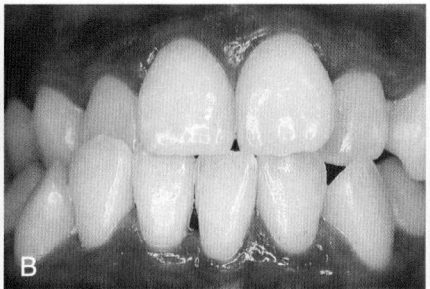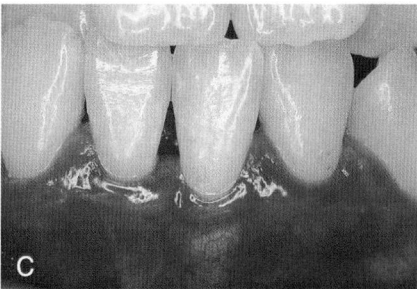

Fig. 69.1 Root planing has resolved the gingival inflammation of this patient.

BOX 69.1   Sequence of Treatment in Preparing Periodontium for Restorative Dentistry

Control of Active Disease
Emergency treatment
Extraction of hopeless teeth
Oral hygiene instructions
Scaling and root planing
Reevaluation
Periodontal surgery
Adjunctive orthodontic therapy

Preprosthetic Surgery
Management of mucogingival problems
Preservation of ridge morphology after tooth extraction
Crown-lengthening procedures
Alveolar ridge reconstruction

---

encountered but also the psychological and aesthetic concerns of the patient. Because periodontal and restorative therapy is situational and specific to each patient, a plan must be adaptable to change depending on the variables encountered during the course of treatment. For example, teeth initially determined to be salvageable may be judged "hopeless," thus altering the established treatment scheme.[20,48]

Generally, the preparation of the periodontium for restorative dentistry can be divided into two phases: (1) control of periodontal inflammation with nonsurgical and surgical approaches and (2) preprosthetic periodontal surgery (Box 69.1).

Control of Active Disease

When the clinician is presented with a patient with different stages of periodontal involvement, this condition must be treated before one can contemplate any restorative dentistry. This step is the most important part of preparing the periodontium for restorative dentistry. The inflammatory state of the supporting tissues must be eliminated or controlled with biofilm removal, scaling, root planing, and, if necessary, periodontal surgery.

The periodontal therapy is intended to control the active disease (see Chapters 47 to 57). In addition to the removal of biofilm and root surface accretions that are the primary etiologic agents, secondary local factors, such as plaque-retentive overhanging margins and untreated caries, must be addressed.[14,19]

Emergency Treatment

Emergency treatment is undertaken to alleviate symptoms and stabilize acute infection. This includes endodontic as well as periodontal conditions (see Chapters 45 and 46). To the patient, the control of

acute pain, especially endodontic, is the most important reason for seeking dental therapy. Therefore this aspect of therapy must be properly addressed before any other therapy is instituted.

Extraction of Hopeless Teeth

Extraction of hopeless teeth is followed by provisionalization with fixed or removable prosthetics. Retention of hopeless teeth without periodontal treatment may result in bone loss around the adjacent teeth.[32] It is also important to consider the extraction of teeth with a poor prognosis when implant replacement has become a predictable alternative to keeping and attempting periodontal therapy.

Oral Hygiene Measures

As indicated earlier, oral hygiene measures, when properly applied, will reduce plaque biofilm scores and gingival inflammation[30,51] (see Chapter 48). However, in patients with deep periodontal pockets (>5 mm), plaque biofilm control measures alone are insufficient for resolving subgingival infection and inflammation.[5,30] Hygiene alone does not allow the brush to reach into the deep pocket area to remove nor disturb the plaque biofilm.

Scaling and Root Planing

Scaling and root planing combined with oral hygiene measures have been demonstrated to significantly reduce gingival inflammation and the rate of the progression of periodontitis[3,4,31] (see Chapter 50). This applies even to patients with deep periodontal pockets[5,15] (Fig. 69.1).

LEARNING BOX 69.2

When the clinician is presented with a patient with any stage of periodontal involvement, this condition must be treated before one can contemplate any restorative dentistry.

Reevaluation

After 4 weeks the gingival tissues are evaluated to determine oral hygiene adequacy, soft tissue response, and pocket depth (see Chapter 47). This permits sufficient time for healing, reduction in inflammation and pocket depths, and gain in clinical attachment levels. However, in deeper pockets (>5 mm), plaque biofilm and calculus removal are often incomplete[2,54] with risk of future breakdown[8,49] (Fig. 69.2). As a result, periodontal surgery to access the root surfaces for instrumentation and to reduce periodontal pocket depths must be considered before restorative care proceeds.

Periodontal Surgery

Periodontal surgery may be required for some patients (see Chapters 60, 62, and 63). This should be undertaken with future restorative and implant dentistry in mind. Some procedures are intended to treat active periodontal disease successfully,[12,37] and others are

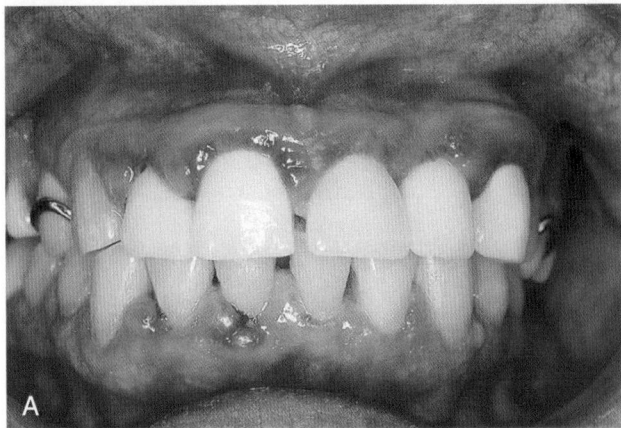

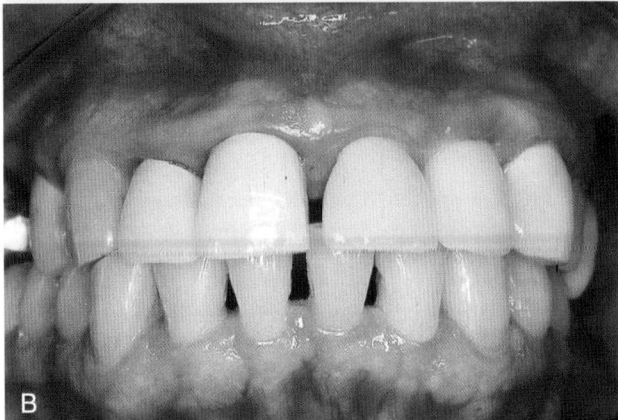

Fig. 69.2 (A) Before treatment. (B) After 4 weeks, oral hygiene instructions and scaling and root planing have improved this patient's periodontal status. However, inflammation associated with pockets deeper than 5 mm suggests a need for periodontal surgery.

aimed at preparing the mouth for restorative or prosthetic care.[55] Crown lengthening is an example of such surgery. Both types of surgery are for preparing the periodontium for restorative dentistry.

Adjunctive Orthodontic Therapy

Orthodontic treatment has been shown to be a useful adjunct to periodontal therapy[6,17,18,24,34] (see Chapter 56). It should be undertaken only after active periodontal disease has been controlled. If nonsurgical treatment is sufficient, definitive periodontal pocket therapy may be postponed until after the completion of orthodontic tooth movement. This allows for the advantage of the positive bone changes that orthodontic therapy can provide. However, deep pockets and furcation invasions may require surgical access for root instrumentation in advance of orthodontic tooth movement. Failure to control active periodontitis can result in acute exacerbations and bone loss during tooth movement.[10] As long as the periodontium is periodontally healthy, teeth with preexisting bone loss may be moved orthodontically without incurring additional attachment loss.[39,40]

If teeth that are to be orthdontically moved lack keratinized attached gingiva, soft tissue–grafting procedures are often indicated in anticipation of orthodontic therapy. The procedure is necessary to increase the dimension of attached tissue to prevent the possibility of gingival margin recession.[34,55]

LEARNING BOX 69.3

Periodontal surgery is performed for the treatment of active periodontal disease as well as for the preprosthetic preparation of the periodontium. Some procedures are intended to treat active disease successfully, and others are aimed at preparing the mouth for restorative or prosthetic care.

Conclusion

As described in this and other sections of this textbook, the therapeutic goals of patient comfort, function, aesthetics, predictability, longevity, and ease of restorative and maintenance care are attainable only by a carefully constructed interdisciplinary approach with accurate diagnosis and comprehensive treatment planning serving as the cornerstones. The complex interaction between periodontal therapy and successful restorative dentistry only serves to underscore this premise.

 Case Scenarios are found on the companion website www.expertconsult.com.

References

 References for this chapter are found on the companion website www.expertconsult.com.

CHAPTER 70

Restorative Interrelationships

Frank M. Spear | Todd R. Schoenbaum | Joseph P. Cooney

CHAPTER OUTLINE

Biologic Considerations
Aesthetic Tissue Management
Occlusal Considerations in Restorative Therapy
Special Restorative Considerations *(e-only)*

 For expanded discussions on margin placement, biologic width, and aesthetic tissue management as well as online-only content on special restorative considerations, please visit the companion website at www.expertconsult.com.

Editors' note: An animation (slide show) has been added by the editors as a supplement to the chapter. It was produced by My Dental Hub as a patient education tool and covers the basic elements in a conceptual manner. It is not intended to be a procedural guide for dental professionals.

The relationship between periodontal health and the restoration of teeth is intimate and inseparable. For restorations to survive long term, the periodontium must remain healthy so that the teeth are maintained. For the periodontium to remain healthy, restorations must be critically managed in several areas so that they are in harmony with their surrounding periodontal tissues. To maintain or enhance the patient's aesthetic appearance, the tooth–tissue interface must present a healthy natural appearance, with gingival tissues framing the restored teeth in a harmonious manner. This chapter reviews the key areas of restorative management necessary to optimize periodontal health, with a focus on the aesthetics and function of restorations.

Biologic Considerations
Margin Placement and Biologic Width

One of the most important aspects of understanding the periodontal–restorative relationship is the location of the restorative margin to the adjacent gingival tissue. Restorative clinicians must understand the role of biologic width in preserving healthy gingival tissues and controlling the gingival form around restorations. They must also apply this information in the positioning of restoration margins, especially in the aesthetic zone, where a primary treatment goal is to mask the junction of the margin with the tooth.

A clinician is presented with three options for margin placement: supragingival, equigingival (even with the tissue), and subgingival.[69] The *supragingival margin* has the least impact on the periodontium. Classically, this margin location has been applied in unaesthetic areas because of the marked contrast in color and opacity of traditional restorative materials against the tooth. With the advent of more translucent restorative materials, adhesive dentistry, and resin cements, the ability to place supragingival margins in aesthetic areas is now a reality (Figs. 70.1 and 70.2). Therefore whenever possible, these

restorations should be chosen not only for their aesthetic advantages but also for their favorable periodontal impact.

The use of *equigingival margins* traditionally was not desirable because they were thought to retain more plaque than supragingival or subgingival margins and therefore resulted in greater gingival inflammation. There was also the concern that any minor gingival recession would create an unsightly margin display. These concerns are not valid today, not only because the restoration margins can be aesthetically blended with the tooth, but also because restorations can be finished easily to provide a smooth, polished interface at the gingival margin. From a periodontal viewpoint, both supragingival and equigingival margins are well tolerated.

The greatest biologic risk occurs when placing *subgingival margins*.[42] These margins are not as accessible as supragingival or equigingival margins for finishing procedures. In addition, if the margin is placed too far below the gingival tissue crest, it violates the gingival attachment apparatus.

As described in Chapter 3, the dimension of space that the healthy gingival tissues occupy between the base of the sulcus and the underlying alveolar bone is composed of the junctional epithelial attachment and the connective tissue attachment. The combined attachment width is now identified as the *biologic width*. Most authors credit Gargiulo, Wentz, and Orban's 1961 study[18] on cadavers with the initial research establishing the dimensions of space required by the gingival tissues. They found that, in the average human, the connective tissue attachment occupies 1.07 mm of space above the crest of the alveolar bone and that the junctional epithelial attachment below the base of the gingival sulcus occupies another 0.97 mm of space above the connective tissue attachment. The combination of these two measurements, averaging approximately 1 mm each, constitutes the biologic width (Fig. 70.3). Clinically, this information is applied to diagnose biologic width violations when the restoration margin is placed 2 mm or less away from the alveolar bone and the gingival tissues are inflamed with no other etiologic factors evident.

Restorative considerations frequently dictate the placement of restoration margins beneath the gingival tissue crest. Restorations may need to be extended gingivally (1) to create adequate resistance and retentive form in the preparation, (2) to make significant contour alterations because of caries or other tooth deficiencies, (3) to mask

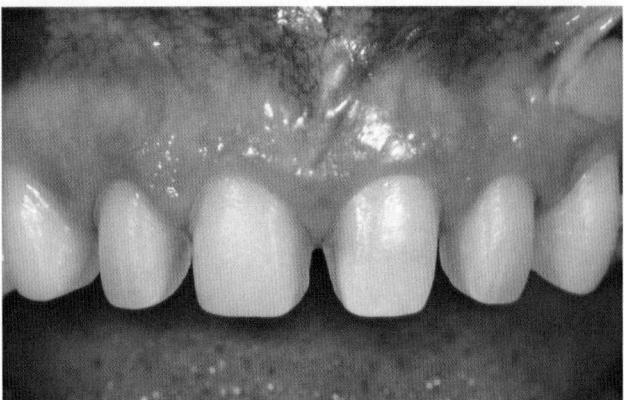

Fig. 70.1 With the advent of adhesive dentistry and ultrathin ceramic veneers, it now is possible to prepare restorations equigingival without visible margins. The preparations for six porcelain veneers with the margins placed at the level of tissue are shown.

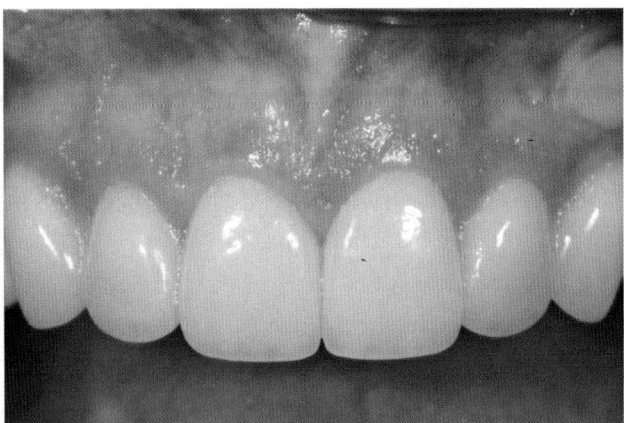

Fig. 70.2 The completed veneers from Fig. 70.1. Note the invisible gingival finish line, even though the margin has not been carried below tissue.

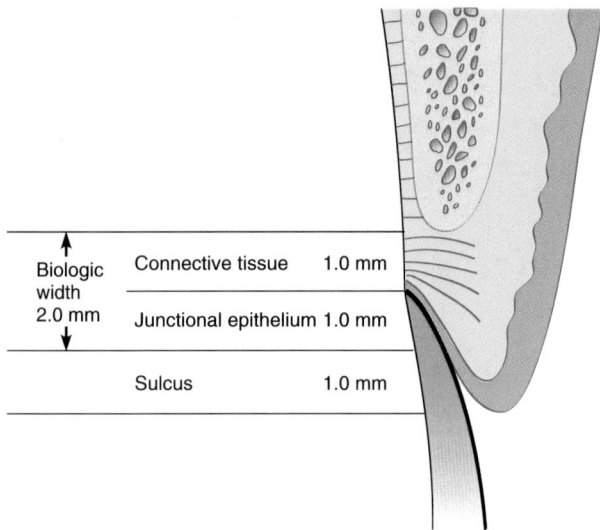

Fig. 70.3 Average human biologic width: connective tissue attachment 1 mm in height; junctional epithelial attachment 1 mm in height; sulcus depth of approximately 1 mm. The combined connective tissue attachment and junctional epithelial attachment, or biologic width, equals 2 mm.

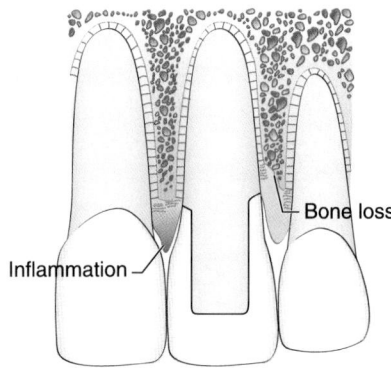

Fig. 70.4 Ramifications of a biologic width violation if a restorative margin is placed within the zone of the attachment. On the mesial surface of the left central incisor, bone has not been lost, but gingival inflammation occurs. On the distal surface of the left central incisor, bone loss has occurred, and a normal biologic width has been reestablished.

the tooth–restoration interface by locating it subgingivally, or (4) to lengthen the tooth for aesthetic reasons. When the restoration margin is placed too far below the gingival tissue crest, it impinges on the gingival attachment apparatus and creates a violation of biologic width.[49] Two different responses can be observed from the involved gingival tissues (Fig. 70.4).

One possibility is that bone loss of an unpredictable nature and gingival tissue recession occurs as the body attempts to re-create room between the alveolar bone and the margin to allow space for tissue reattachment. This is more likely to occur in areas in which the alveolar bone surrounding the tooth is very thin in width. Trauma from restorative procedures can play a major role in causing this fragile tissue to recede. Other factors that may impact the likelihood of recession include (1) whether the gingiva is thick and fibrotic or thin and fragile and (2) whether the periodontium is highly scalloped or flat in its gingival form. It has been found that highly scalloped, thin gingiva is more prone to recession than a flat periodontium with thick fibrous tissue.[47]

KEY FACT

Thin gingiva and highly scalloped papilla are more highly prone to recession after normal restorative procedures.

The more common finding with deep margin placement is that the bone level appears to remain unchanged, but gingival inflammation develops and persists. To restore gingival tissue health, it is necessary to establish space clinically between the alveolar bone and the margin. This can be accomplished either by surgery to alter the bone level or by orthodontic extrusion to move the restoration margin farther away from the bone level.

Biologic Width Evaluation

Radiographic interpretation can identify interproximal violations of biologic width. However, with the more common locations on the mesiofacial and distofacial line angles of teeth, radiographs are not diagnostic because of tooth superimposition. If a patient experiences tissue discomfort when the restoration margin levels are being assessed with a periodontal probe, it is a good indication that the margin extends into the attachment and that a biologic width violation has occurred.

A more positive assessment can be made clinically by measuring the distance between the bone and the restoration margin using a

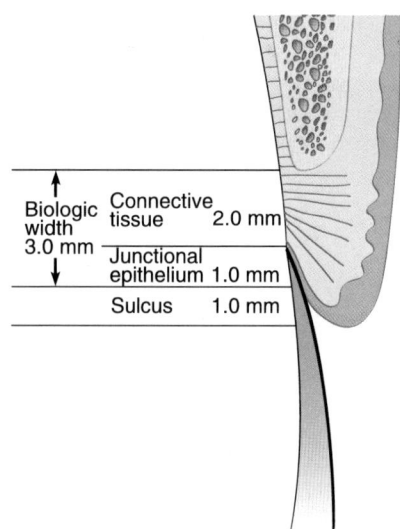

Fig. 70.5 Possible variations exist in biologic width. Connective tissue attachments and junctional epithelial attachments may be variable. In this example, the connective tissue attachment is 2 mm in height, the junctional epithelial attachment 1 mm in height, and the sulcus depth 1 mm, for a combined total tissue height above bone of 4 mm. However, the biologic width is 3 mm. This is just one variation that can occur from the average depicted in Fig. 70.3.

sterile periodontal probe. The probe is pushed through the anesthetized attachment tissues from the sulcus to the underlying bone. If this distance is less than 2 mm at one or more locations, a diagnosis of biologic width violation can be confirmed. This assessment is completed circumferentially around the tooth to evaluate the extent of the problem. However, biologic width violations can occur in some patients in whom the margins are located more than 2 mm above the alveolar bone level.[22] In 1994 Vacek and colleagues[70] also investigated the biologic width phenomenon. Although their average width finding of 2 mm was the same as that previously presented by Gargiulo and associates,[18] they also reported a range of different biologic widths that were patient specific. They reported biologic widths as narrow as 0.75 mm in some individuals, whereas others had biologic widths as tall as 4.3 mm (Fig. 70.5).

This information dictates that specific biologic width assessment should be performed for each patient to determine if the patient needs additional biologic width, in excess of 2 mm, for restorations to be in harmony with the gingival tissues. The biologic, or attachment, width can be identified for the individual patient by probing to the bone level (referred to as "sounding to bone") and subtracting the sulcus depth from the resulting measurement. This measurement must be done on teeth with healthy gingival tissues and should be repeated on more than one tooth to ensure an accurate assessment. The technique allows the variations in sulcus depths found in individual patients to be assessed and factored into the diagnostic evaluation. The information obtained is then used for definitive diagnosis of biologic width violations, the extent of correction needed, and the parameters for placement of future restorations.

Margin Placement Guidelines

When determining where to place restorative margins relative to the periodontal attachment, it is recommended that the patient's existing sulcular depth be used as a guideline in assessing the biologic width requirement for that patient. The base of the sulcus can be viewed as the top of the attachment, and therefore the clinician accounts for variations in attachment height by ensuring that the margin is placed in the sulcus and not in the attachment.[4,36,37,56] The variations in

sulcular probing depth are then used to predict how deep the margin can safely be placed below the gingival crest. With shallow probing depths (1 to 1.5 mm), extending the preparation more than 0.5 mm subgingivally risks violating the attachment. This assumes that the periodontal probe will penetrate into the junctional epithelial attachment in healthy gingiva an average of 0.5 mm. With shallow probing depths, future recession is unlikely because the free gingival margin is located close to the top of the attachment. Deeper sulcular probing depths provide more freedom in locating restoration margins farther below the gingival crest. In most circumstances, however, the deeper the gingival sulcus, the greater is the risk of gingival recession. Locating the restorative margin deep subgingivally should be avoided, as it increases the difficulty in making an accurate impression, finishing the restoration margins, and increases the likelihood of inflammation and recession.

Provisional Restorations

Three critical areas must be effectively managed to produce a favorable biologic response to provisional restorations.[3,74] The marginal fit, crown contour, and surface finish of the interim restorations must be appropriate to maintain the health and position of the gingival tissues during the interval until the final restorations are delivered. Provisional restorations that are poorly adapted at the margins, that are overcontoured or undercontoured, and that have rough or porous surfaces can cause inflammation, overgrowth, or recession of gingival tissues. The outcome can be unpredictable, and unfavorable changes in the tissue architecture can compromise the success of the final restoration.

Marginal Fit

Marginal fit has clearly been implicated in producing an inflammatory response in the periodontium. It has been shown that the level of gingival inflammation can increase corresponding with the level of marginal opening.[15] Margins that are significantly open (several tenths of a millimeter) are capable of harboring large numbers of bacteria and may be responsible for the inflammatory response seen. However, the quality of marginal finish and the margin location relative to the attachment are much more critical to the periodontium than the difference between a 20-μm fit and a 100-μm fit.[42,46,59]

Crown Contour

Restoration contour has been described as extremely important to the maintenance of periodontal health.[26,75] Ideal contour provides access for hygiene, has the fullness to create the desired gingival form, and has a pleasing visual tooth contour in aesthetic areas. Evidence from human and animal studies clearly demonstrates a relationship between overcontouring and gingival inflammation, whereas undercontouring produces no adverse periodontal effect.[48,51] The most frequent cause of overcontoured restorations is inadequate tooth preparation by the dentist, which forces the technician to produce a bulky restoration to provide room for the restorative material. In areas of the mouth in which aesthetic considerations are not critical, a flatter contour is always acceptable.

Subgingival Debris

Leaving debris below the tissue during restorative procedures can create an adverse periodontal response. The cause can be retraction cord, impression material, provisional material, or either temporary or permanent cement.[55] The diagnosis of debris as the cause of gingival inflammation can be confirmed by examining the sulcus surrounding the restoration with an explorer, removing any foreign bodies, and then monitoring the tissue response. It may be necessary to provide tissue anesthesia for patient comfort during the procedure.

Hypersensitivity to Dental Materials

Inflammatory gingival responses have been reported related to the use of nonprecious alloys in dental restorations.[52] Typically, the responses have occurred to alloys containing nickel, although the frequency of these occurrences is controversial.[50] Hypersensitivity responses to precious alloys are extremely rare, and these alloys provide an easy solution to the problems encountered with the nonprecious alloys. Importantly, tissues respond more to the differences in surface roughness of the material than they do to the composition of the material.[1,66] The rougher the surface of the restoration subgingivally, the greater are the plaque accumulation and gingival inflammation. In clinical research, porcelain, highly polished gold, and highly polished resin all show similar plaque accumulation. Regardless of the restorative material selected, a smooth surface is essential on all materials subgingivally.

 ## Aesthetic Tissue Management

Managing Interproximal Embrasures

Current restorative and periodontal therapy must consider a good aesthetic result, especially in the "aesthetic zone." As discussed in Chapters 58 and 65, the interproximal papilla is an important part in creating this aesthetic result. The interproximal embrasure created by restorations and the form of the interdental papilla have a unique and intimate relationship.[61,62] The ideal interproximal embrasure should house the gingival papilla without impinging on it and should also extend the interproximal tooth contact to the top of the papilla so that no excess space exists to trap food and to be aesthetically displeasing.

Papillary height is established by the level of the bone, the biologic width, and the form of the gingival embrasure. Changes in the shape of the embrasure can impact the height and form of the papilla. The tip of the papilla behaves differently than the free gingival margin on the facial aspect of the tooth. Whereas the free gingival margin averages 3 mm above the underlying facial bone, the tip of the papilla averages 4.5 to 5 mm above the interproximal bone (Fig. 70.6). This means that if the papilla is farther above the bone than the facial tissue but has the same biologic width, the interproximal area will have a sulcus 1 to 1.5 mm deeper than that found on the facial surface.

 CLINICAL CORRELATION

If you create restorations with no more than 5 mm from the contact to the bone, open gingival embrasures can be avoided. The downside to this approach is that the teeth will look square and blocky. However, some patients can support a 7-mm papilla. Well-made provisional restorations allow accurate determination of actual papilla length.

Van der Veldon[72] completely removed healthy papillae to the bone level and found that they routinely regenerated 4 to 4.5 mm of total tissue above bone, with an average sulcus depth of 2 to 2.5 mm. The height above bone that the papilla strives to maintain was indirectly confirmed by Tarnow and coworkers,[67] who studied the relationship of the papilla between the interproximal contact and the underlying bone. When the distance from the interproximal bone to the interproximal contact of the teeth measured 5 mm or less, 98% of these sites had complete papilla fill. When the distance was 6 mm, only 56% of the sites had complete papilla fill. When the distance was 7 mm, only 27% of the sites had complete papilla fill (Fig. 70.7).

Because there is individual variability to the required biologic width, this information relative to the papilla is applied by locating the lowest point of the interproximal contact in relation to the top of the epithelial attachment. The ideal contact should be 2 to 3 mm coronal to the attachment, which coincides with the depth of the average interproximal sulcus. In assessing the soft tissues to determine margin location, it is imperative that they be healthy and mature. Performing the analysis on inflamed or immature tissues will result in supragingival margins when the tissues heal. If the papillary sulcus measures greater than 3 mm, there is some risk of recession with restorative procedures. Critical adjustments to margin and soft tissue positions should be ultimately diagnosed with the use of well-designed and adapted provisional restorations. This will allow for treatment to be accurately designed based on the individual's unique biologic width.

The clinician most frequently confronts a normal or shallow sulcus with a papilla that appears too short rather than a tall papilla with a deep sulcus. Management of this situation is best approached by viewing the papilla as a balloon of a certain volume that sits on the

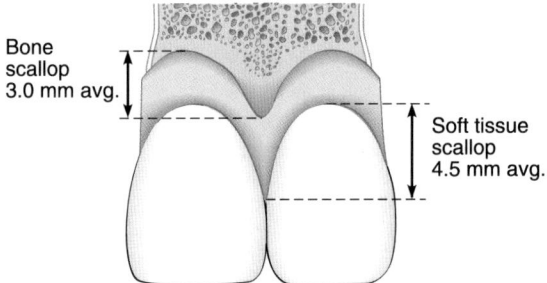

Fig. 70.6 Comparison of the behavior of the interproximal papilla relative to bone and the free gingival margin relative to bone in the average human. There is a 3-mm scallop from the facial bone to the interproximal bone. However, on average, a 4.5- to 5-mm gingival scallop exists between the facial tissue height and the interproximal papilla height. This extra scallop of 1.5 to 2 mm of gingiva compared with bone is the result of the extra soft-tissue height above the attachment interproximally.

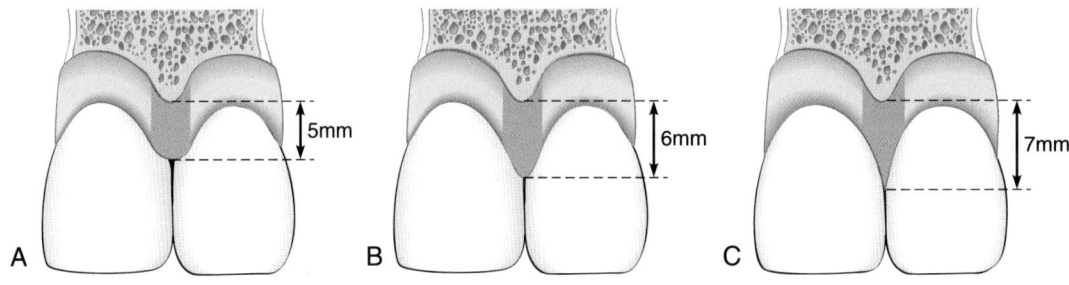

Fig. 70.7 The probability of complete fill of gingival embrasure by papilla. (A) With 5 mm from crest of bone to the apical contact point, there is a 98% chance of complete fill of the space. (B) At 6 mm from crest to contact, the chance of filled embrasure drops to 56%. (C) At 7 mm from crest to contact, the chance of complete fill drops to 27%.

attachment. This balloon of tissue has a form and height dictated by the gingival embrasure of the teeth. With an embrasure that is too wide, the balloon flattens out, assumes a blunted shape, and has a shallow sulcus (Fig. 70.8).

If the embrasure is the ideal width, the papilla assumes a pointed form, has a sulcus of 2.5 to 3 mm, and is healthy. If the embrasure is too narrow, the papilla may grow out to the facial and lingual, form a col, and become inflamed. This information is applied when evaluating an individual papilla with an open embrasure. The papilla in question is compared with the adjacent papillae. If the papillae are all on the same level, and if the other areas do not have open embrasures, the problem is one of gingival embrasure form. If the papilla in the area of concern is apical to the adjacent papillae, however, the clinician should evaluate the interproximal bone levels. If the bone under that papilla is apical to the adjacent bone levels, the problem is caused by bone loss. If the bone is at the same level, the open embrasure is caused by the embrasure form of the teeth and not a periodontal problem with the papilla. The papillae in the anterior maxilla average 4 mm long and are the same heights at the mesial and distal sides of the tooth. Ultimately, deficient papillae and open gingival embrasures are most predictably corrected with restorations to close the space.

Pontic Design

Classically, there are four options to consider in evaluating pontic design: hygienic, ridge lap, modified ridge lap, and ovate designs (Fig. 70.9). Regardless of design, the pontic should provide an occlusal surface that stabilizes the opposing teeth, allows for normal mastication, and does not overload the abutment teeth. The area of the pontic interfacing with the gingiva can be porcelain, metal, zirconia, lithium disilicate, or some other material with no variation in the biologic response of the tissue provided it has a smooth surface finish.[25,53,63]

The key differences between the four pontic designs relate to the aesthetics and access for hygiene procedures. The primary method for cleaning the undersurface of pontics is to draw dental floss mesiodistally along the undersurface. The shape of this undersurface determines the ease with which plaque and food debris can be removed in the process. The hygienic and ovate pontics have convex undersurfaces, which makes them easiest to clean. The ridge lap and modified ridge-lap designs have concave surfaces, which are more difficult to access with the dental floss. Although the hygienic pontic design provides the easiest access for hygiene procedures, it is much less aesthetic and objectionable by some patients.

The ovate pontic is the ideal pontic form, particularly in areas of aesthetic concern.[61] It is created by forming a receptor site in the edentulous ridge with a diamond bur, electrosurgery, pressure, or wound healing. The site is shaped to create either a flat or a concave contour so that when the pontic is created to adapt to the site, it will have a flat or convex outline. The depth of the receptor site depends on the aesthetic requirements of the pontic. In highly aesthetic areas such as the maxillary anterior region, it is necessary to create a receptor area that is 1 to 1.5 mm below the tissue on the facial aspect. This creates the appearance of a free gingival margin and produces optimal aesthetics (Fig. 70.10). This site can then be tapered to the height of the palatal tissue to facilitate hygiene access from the palatal side. In the posterior areas, a deep receptor site can complicate hygiene access. In these situations, the ideal site has the facial portion of the pontic at the same level as the ridge, and then the site is created as a straight line to the lingual side of the pontic. This removes the convexity of the ridge and produces a flat, easily cleanable tissue surface on the pontic (Fig. 70.11).

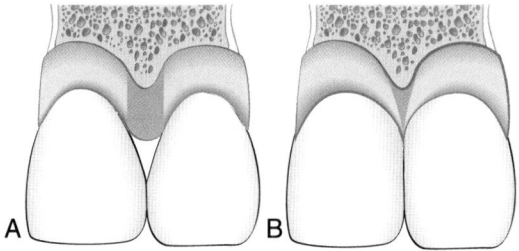

Fig. 70.8 Relationship between gingival embrasure volume and papillary form. (A) Gingival embrasure of the teeth is excessively large as the result of a tapered tooth form. Because of the large embrasure form, the volume of tissue sitting on top of the attachment is not molded to the shape of a normal papilla but rather has a blunted form and a shallower sulcus. (B) Ideal tooth form in which the same volume of tissue sits on top of the attachment as in part A. Because of the more closed embrasure form from the teeth in part B, however, the papilla completely fills the embrasure and has a deeper sulcus, averaging 2.5 to 3 mm. Note that the ideal contact position is 3 mm coronal to the attachment.

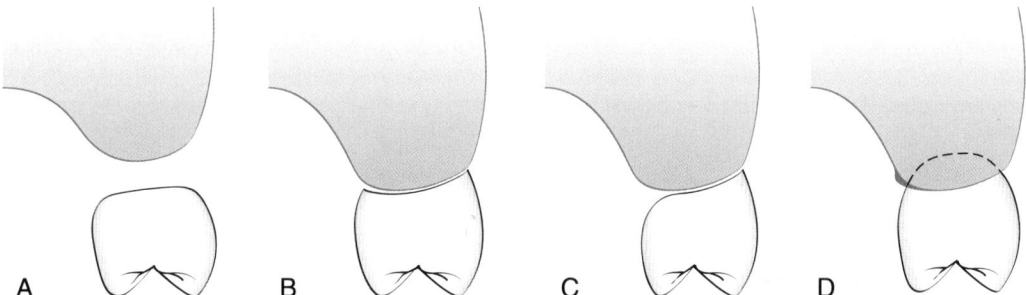

Fig. 70.9 Four options to designing the shape of a pontic. (A) Hygienic pontic. Tissue surface of the pontic is 3 mm from the underlying ridge. (B) Ridge-lap pontic. Tissue surface of the pontic straddles the ridge in saddle-like fashion. The entire tissue surface of the ridge-lap pontic is convex and very difficult to clean. (C) Modified ridge-lap pontic. Tissue surface on the facial is concave, following the ridge. However, the lingual saddle has been removed to allow access for oral hygiene. (D) Ovate pontic. The pontic form fits into a receptor site within the ridge. This allows the tissue surface of the pontic to be convex and also optimizes aesthetics.

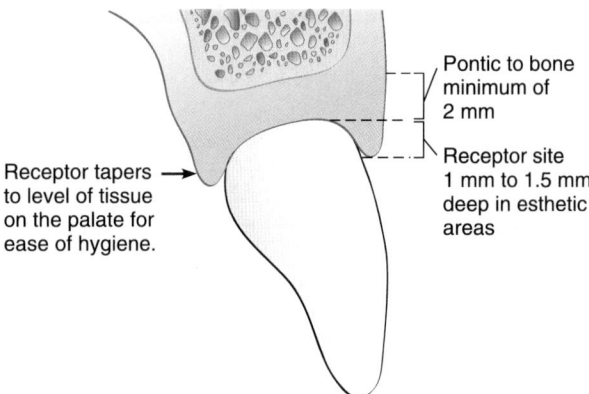

Fig. 70.10 Ideal shape and form of an ovate pontic in the aesthetic area. The receptor site has been created 1 to 1.5 mm apical to the free gingival margin on the facial aspect. This creates the illusion of the pontic erupting from the tissue. On the palatal side, the pontic is tapered so that the receptor site is not extended below tissue; this allows easier access for oral hygiene. Note that when the receptor site is created, the bone must be a minimum of 2 mm from the most apical portion of the pontic.

Pontic to bone minimum of 2 mm

Receptor site 1 mm to 1.5 mm deep in esthetic areas

Receptor tapers to level of tissue on the palate for ease of hygiene.

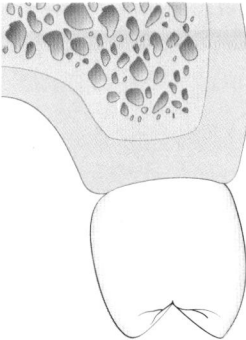

Fig. 70.11 Option for creating an ovate pontic receptor site in less aesthetic areas of the mouth. Rather than creating the receptor site so that the pontic extends into the ridge, it is possible to create a flattened receptor site in which the pontic sits flush with the ridge. This facilitates oral hygiene.

Occlusal Considerations in Restorative Therapy

 KEY FACT

A mutually protective occlusion is created when all the teeth touch at the same time in a normal closing arc, but when the mandible moves, all contacts are on the anterior teeth.

Chapter 55 presents details on the biology of occlusion and related clinical evaluation procedures. The importance of occlusal trauma as a factor in periodontal disease and its role in orofacial pain have been deemphasized in numerous papers.[8,14,34,35,44,45,54,65,71] However, the role that occlusion plays in restorative dentistry has been reemphasized. The increased use of dental implants and nonmetallic restorations has resulted in increased concern over force management. Some of these materials are more sensitive to occlusal trauma, and resulting fracture, than are metal restorations. Consequently, for the clinician who wants a high degree of predictability, understanding occlusion is critical. The clinician must know how to create an occlusion, with the following guidelines as a goal:

1. There should be even, simultaneous contacts on all teeth in maximal intercuspal position (MIP). This distributes the force of closure over all the teeth instead of the few teeth that may touch first.

2. When the mandible moves from maximum intercuspal position (MIP), some form of canine or anterior guidance is desirable, with no posterior tooth contacts. This mutually protective occlusion reduces the ability and force of the muscles of mastication, while it more evenly distributes the forces. It has been shown that, as a result of the class III lever action, the anterior teeth receive approximately one-ninth the force of a second molar.[24,60]

3. The anterior guidance needs to be in harmony with the patient's envelope of function. The harmony of this relationship is demonstrated by a lack of fremitus and mobility on the anterior teeth, by the ability of the patient to speak clearly and comfortably, and by the patient's general sense of comfort with the overbite, overjet, and guidance created during chewing and when holding the head upright.

4. The occlusion should be created at a occlusal vertical dimension (OVD) that is stable for the patient. It is generally accepted that the patient's existing vertical dimension is at equilibrium between the eruptive forces of the teeth and the repetitive contracted length of the elevator muscles. It has been demonstrated that vertical dimension can be altered with no sense of pain from muscles and joints.[8,10,21,29] However, if this alteration lengthens the pterygomasseteric sling beyond its ability to adapt, the patient will not maintain the vertical change and will close the occlusal vertical dimension back down by intruding the teeth.[11,33,39-41]

5. When managing a pathologic occlusion or when restoring a complete occlusion, the clinician needs to work with a repeatable condylar reference position. Centric relation, defined as the most superior condylar position, provides such a starting point.[20] Centric relation has been shown to be reproducible over multiple appointments, allowing the clinician to create the occlusion indirectly on an articulator and return it to the same reference position in the mouth.[13,38,43,73] It is the only position that has been shown to shut off lateral pterygoid muscle contraction.[19] Because it is a border position, any mandibular movement will result in the condyle moving inferiorly. Therefore centric relation is the most predictable position from which an interference-free occlusion can be created.

To manage the occlusion as previously described, the clinician must be able to make accurate casts, use a facebow, and create centric relation records so that the information can be transferred to a suitable articulator. Although the details of these procedures are beyond the scope of this chapter, they are a routine part of any restorative treatment plan and must be mastered for the clinician to achieve predictable, long-term restorative success. The reader is referred to Chapter 55 for a more comprehensive overview of occlusal evaluation and therapy.

 Case Scenarios are found on the companion website www.expertconsult.com.

References

 References for this chapter are found on the companion website www.expertconsult.com.

CHAPTER 71

Multidisciplinary Versus Interdisciplinary Approaches to Dental and Periodontal Problems

Dennis P. Tarnow | Mitchell J. Bloom

CHAPTER OUTLINE

Educational Trends Toward Multidisciplinary Specialist Education in Implant Treatment
The Future

Traditionally, periodontal treatment has been delivered using an *interdisciplinary* model of therapy, with general dentists and specialists each providing their respective aspects of care to the same patients according to a comprehensive plan of therapy (Figs. 71.1 to 71.22). Conversely, a *multidisciplinary* approach is centered on a single provider delivering care across a range of dentistry disciplines. This practitioner can be a general dentist or a specialist, as traditional modes of practice have evolved and in some aspects look quite different from the classic model. The interdisciplinary system has worked well because the patient benefits from the best mix of talent from a "team" of dentists. Regardless of whether an interdisciplinary or multidisciplinary approach is utilized, it is critical for primary providers to have a thorough understanding of the signs, symptoms, local and systemic risk factors, and pathophysiology of disease processes as they relate to periodontal and dental implant therapy. Additionally, they must possess a strong working knowledge of the range of treatment options available along with their respective indications, contraindications, benefits, and liabilities to effectively formulate a proper treatment plan. At this point the dentist can then decide whether he or she has the requisite knowledge, expertise, and experience to meet the patient's needs to proceed in a multidisciplinary fashion or should refer the patient to a specialist for care at a more advanced level.

Many of the early innovators in the field of implant dentistry were general practitioners. Subsequently, their early accomplishments were built on using rigid and narrowly defined surgical and prosthetic protocols whose effectiveness and predictability were supported by well-documented long-term research studies put forth by Dr. P.I. Brånemark. His namesake implant design, when used precisely as directed with respect to case type and patient selection, strict surgical protocols, specialized armamentarium, and a narrow range of treatment options, made it possible for clinicians to achieve highly predictable treatment outcomes. The initial offering of training in the Brånemark method was limited only to specialist prosthodontists and oral surgeons, the former group focusing on the restorative aspect of care and the latter group on the surgical phase of therapy. However, as implant dentistry continued to evolve, periodontists became increasingly more active in the field, ultimately sharing the same role and stature as their oral surgeon colleagues in this arena. The same was true for many general practitioners with respect to their prosthodontist colleagues in terms of delivering implant restorative care.

The range of indications for the use of dental implants expanded beyond the limited mandibular full arch case type Brånemark initially taught to include partial edentulism, single teeth, and even orthodontic and maxillofacial applications. Regenerative techniques have been developed as well to address hard- and soft-tissue deficiencies that, for many patients, had previously deemed them unsuitable candidates for dental implant therapy. Autogenous intraoral block grafting, guided bone regeneration, maxillary sinus grafting, transposition of the inferior alveolar nerve, ridge splitting, distraction osteogenesis, and biologics are among the many strategies that have emerged to overcome limitations for less-than-optimal sites.

Early implant designs and materials were subject to limitations and even prone to problems. Those with machined surfaces suffered from a significantly higher failure rate in sites with poor-quality bone, whereas those with rough surfaces, coupled with other design flaws, were prone to late failure resulting from inflammatory peri-implant disease or prosthetic complications. With all of these variables in play and emerging so rapidly during the formative years, implant dentistry was relegated largely to the specialty care arena. Through innovative implant designs, advances in material science, opportunities for simplified surgical techniques, digital planning and manufacturing

Text continued on p. 711

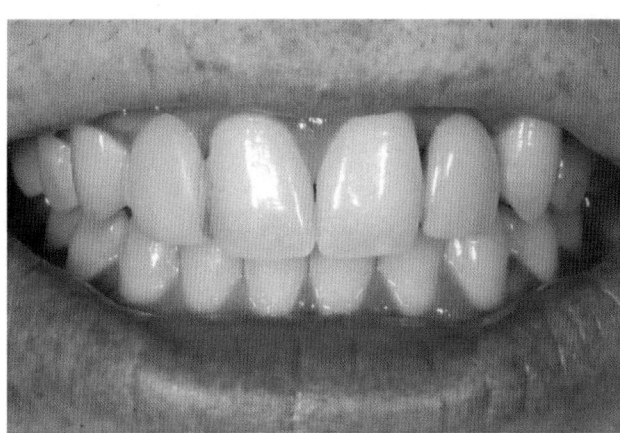

Fig. 71.1 Complex interdisciplinary implant care scenario. Extraoral preoperative condition. Aesthetic compromise is evident in this challenging treatment scenario where there is significant gingival display.

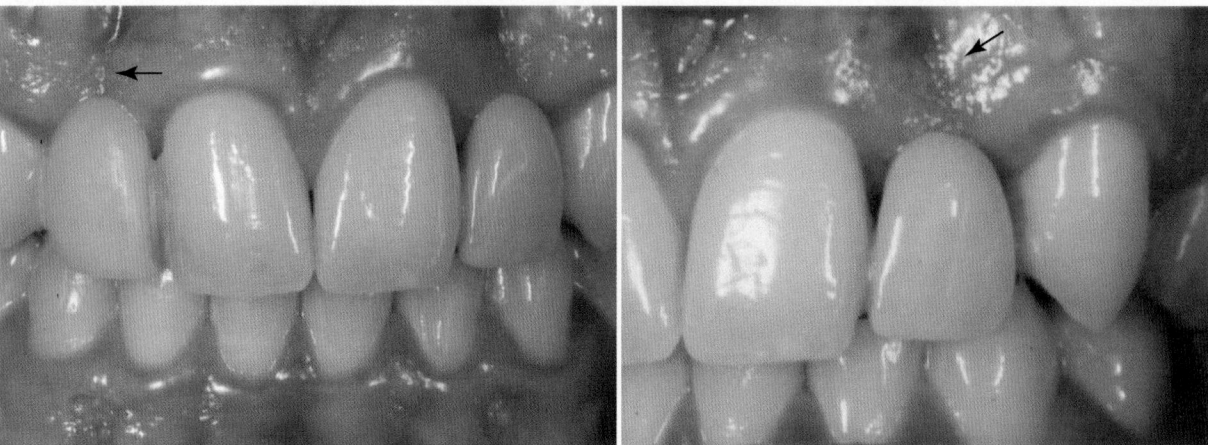

Fig. 71.2 Intraoral preoperative condition. A concave soft-tissue profile that contributes to a dark shadow and aesthetic compromise is evident bilaterally *(arrows)*.

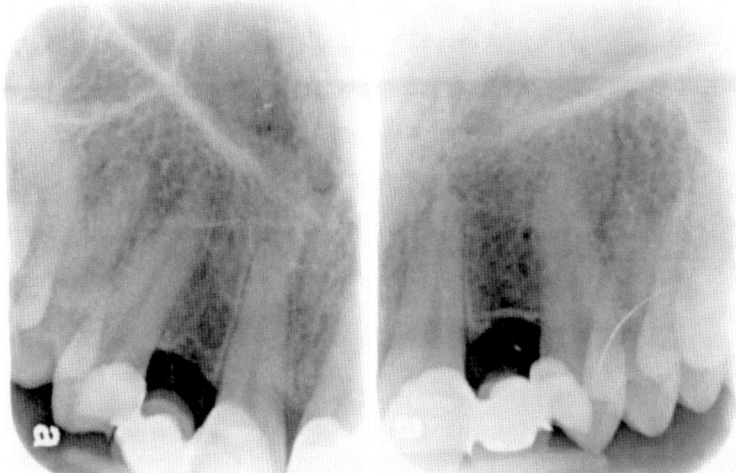

Fig. 71.3 Preoperative radiographs. The roots of adjacent teeth do not converge to interfere with proper orientation of the positions of the planned dental implants. However, there is limited space between the adjacent tooth roots.

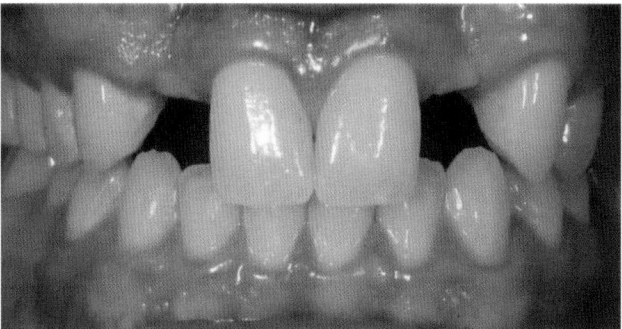

Fig. 71.4 Intraoral preoperative clinical view. Soft-tissue contours as seen with the existing restorations removed.

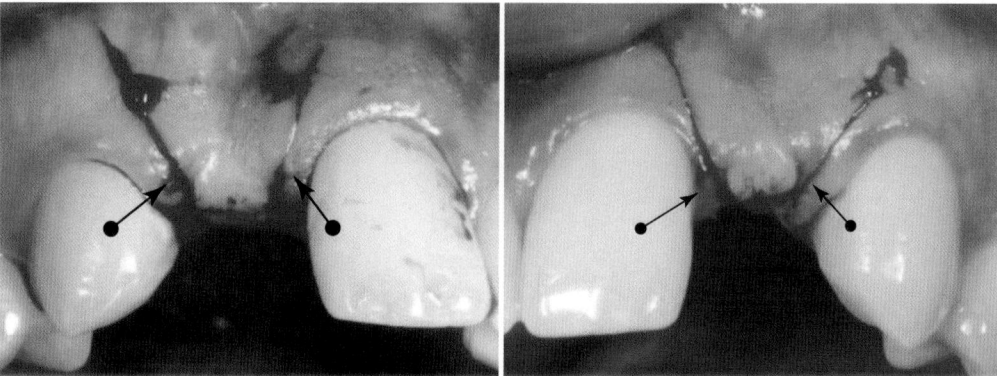

Fig. 71.5 Implant surgery. Initial incisions using a papilla-sparing technique to minimize disturbing the healthy supracrestal attachment on the surfaces of the adjacent teeth.

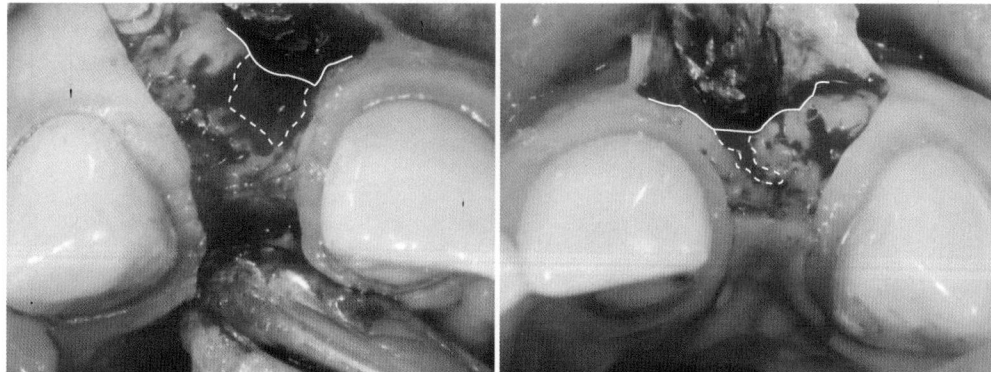

Fig. 71.6 Intraoperative clinical view. Edentulous right and left treatment areas both show concave bony defects labially.

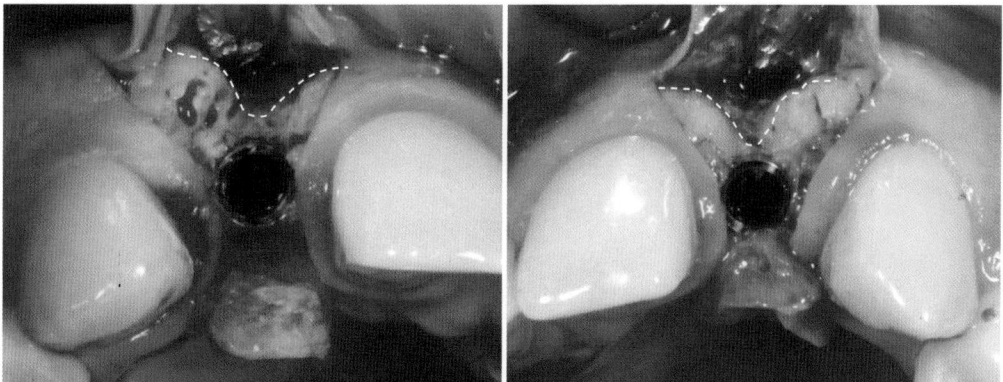

Fig. 71.7 Intraoperative clinical view. Implants placed in a prosthetically guided orientation that is palatal to the buccal depression.

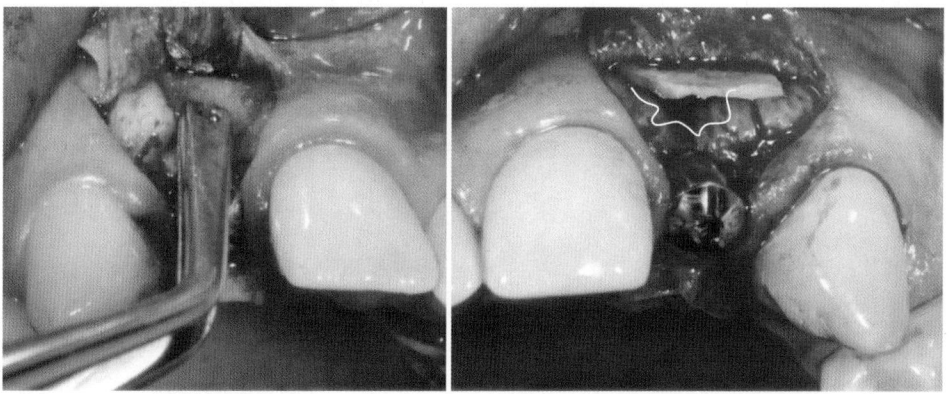

Fig. 71.8 Intraoperative clinical view. Correction of bony defects using guided bone regeneration technique. Resorbable barrier membranes are shown in position after being trimmed to a suitable shape and fitted in place.

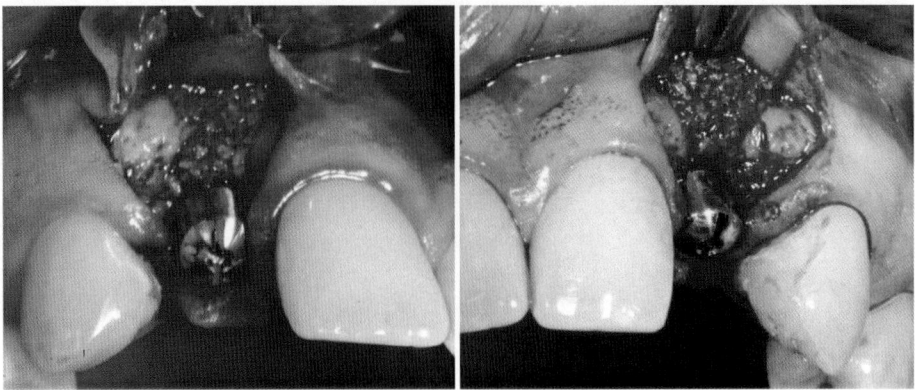

Fig. 71.9 Intraoperative clinical view. A particulate bone graft material is placed and shaped to fill the bony depression under the previously fitted membrane.

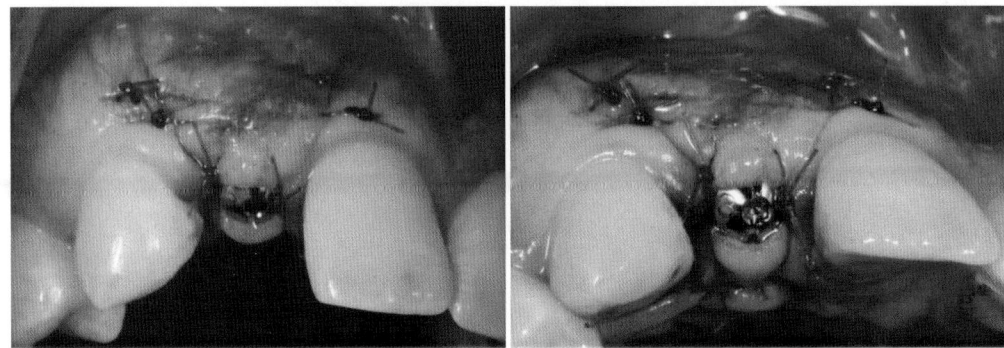

Fig. 71.10 Implant healing abutments, which act to facilitate coronal and labial positioning of the soft-tissue flap, were previously placed. This will work in conjunction with the augmentation procedure to correct the preoperative soft-tissue concavity.

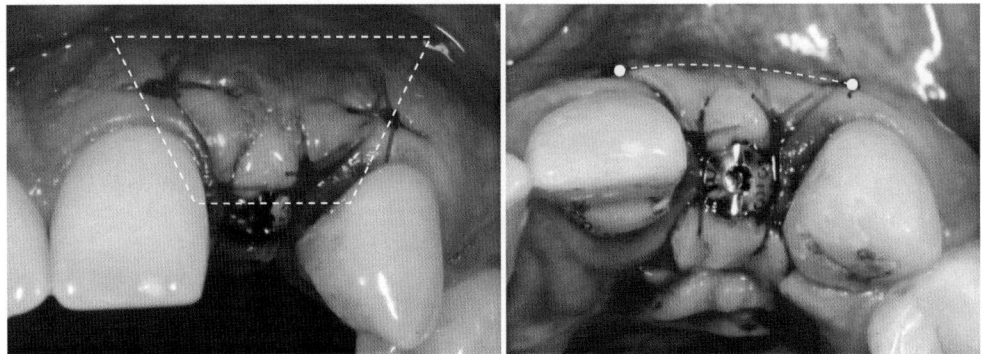

Fig. 71.11 Convex ridge shape after augmentation is shown after completion of the surgical procedure.

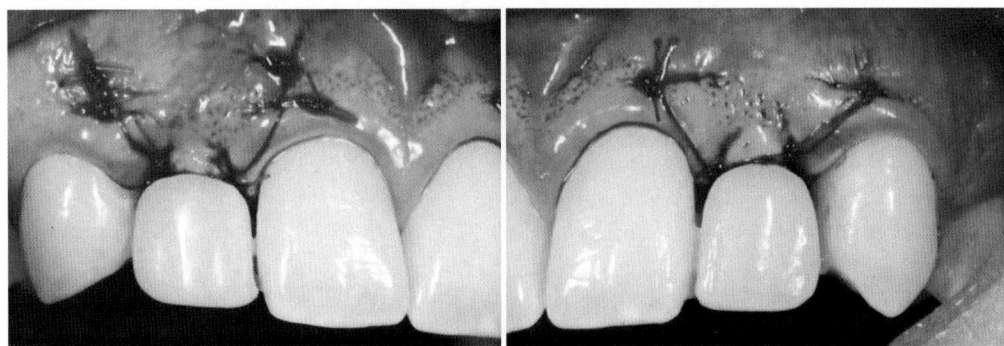

Fig. 71.12 The gingival third of the provisional restoration has been reduced so it does not impinge on the surgical site. The vertical position of the soft-tissue height on completion of the surgery is favorable as compared with that of the adjacent natural teeth.

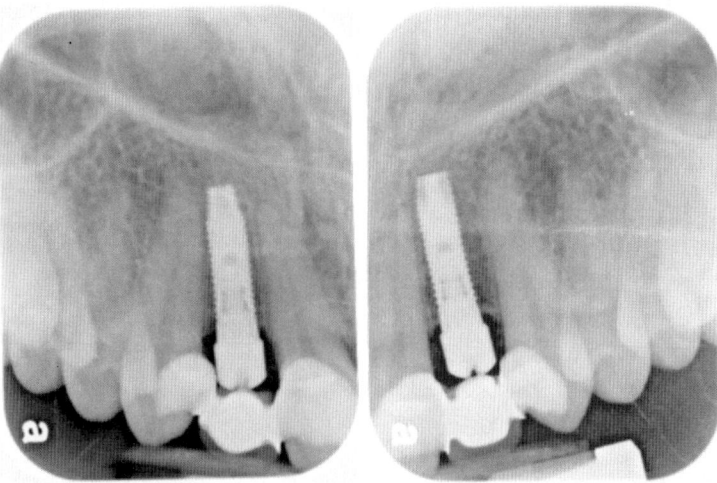

Fig. 71.13 Postoperative radiograph. The dental implants are in good position. Given the amount of available space between the adjacent tooth roots, a narrow-diameter implant was selected as part of the treatment plan to yield a biologically and prosthetically favorable result.

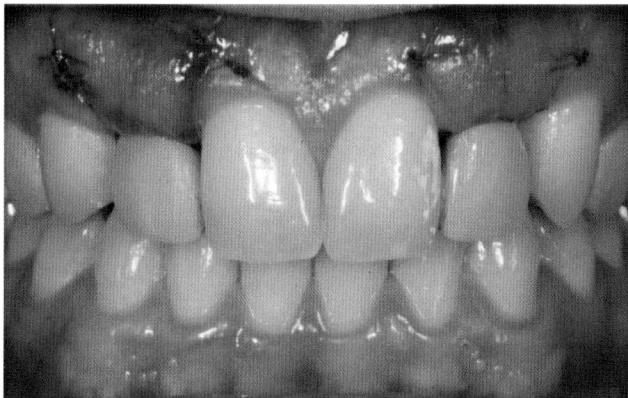

Fig. 71.14 Postoperative clinical view at 1 week after surgery. The soft tissue is healing well. Note the favorable soft-tissue response where the papillae were not disturbed using a conservative incision design.

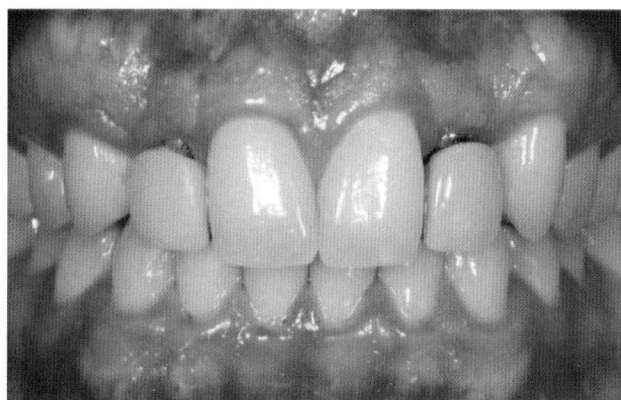

Fig. 71.15 Postoperative clinical view 3 months after surgery. The soft tissues have healed favorably with maintenance of the free gingival margin position situated to yield a prosthetic clinical crown of appropriate length.

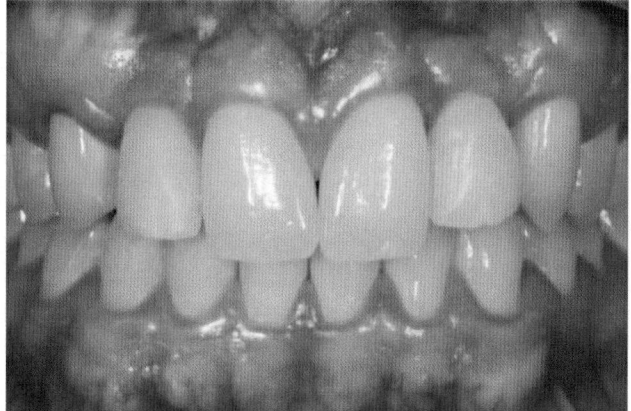

Fig. 71.16 Screw-retained single provisional crowns inserted and connected to the dental implants to begin nonsurgical sculpting of the peri-implant soft tissue.

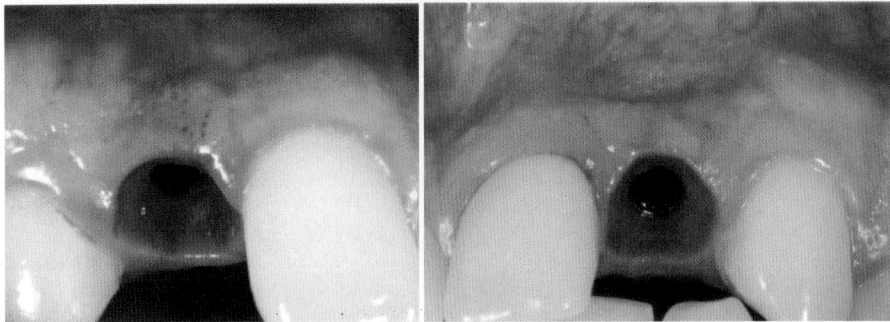

Fig. 71.17 The peri-implant soft tissue is sculpted three-dimensionally to represent the cross section of the natural tooth being replaced to create a more natural appearance in the final restoration than possible with prefabricated round healing abutments.

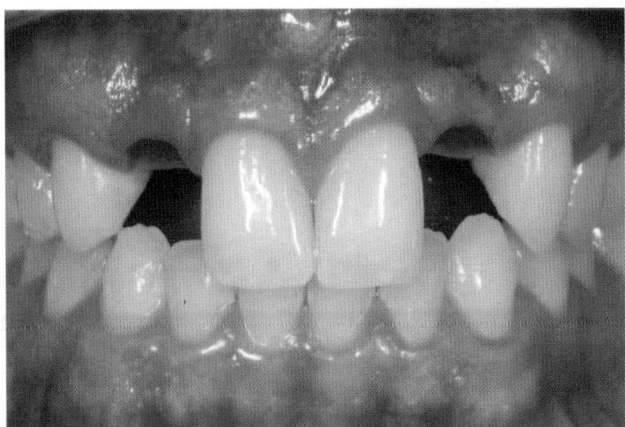

Fig. 71.18 Peri-implant soft tissue after nonsurgical sculpting. Notice the early stages of papillae reforming in the spaces between the natural teeth and dental implants.

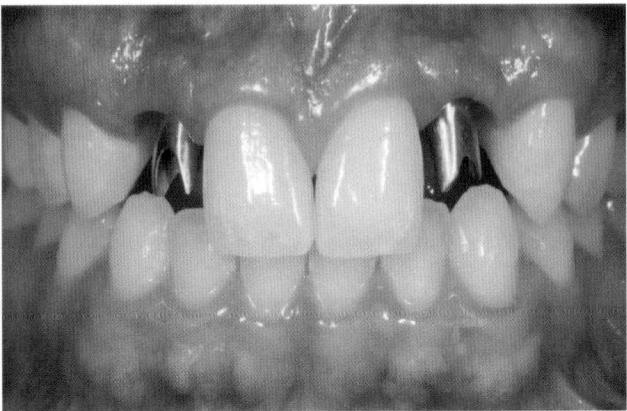

Fig. 71.19 Custom abutments in place on the dental implants. Gold plating of the custom abutments was done to impart a hue to the peri-implant sulcus and soft tissue to optimize the aesthetic outcome.

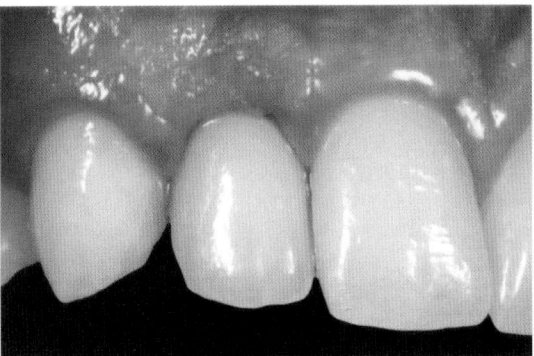

Fig. 71.20 Final crowns are seen here on the date of insertion. The crown contours dictate the gingival contours.

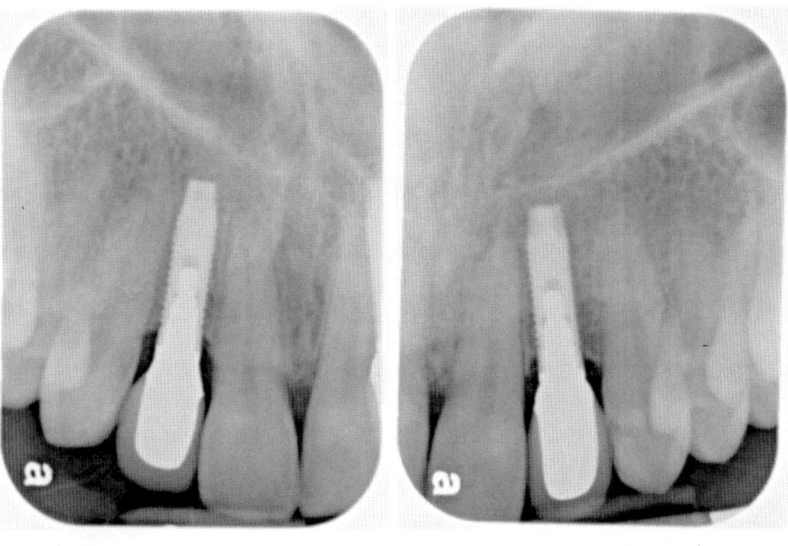

Fig. 71.21 Radiograph following final crown insertion. Note the customized emergence profile of the prosthetic components on the dental implants.

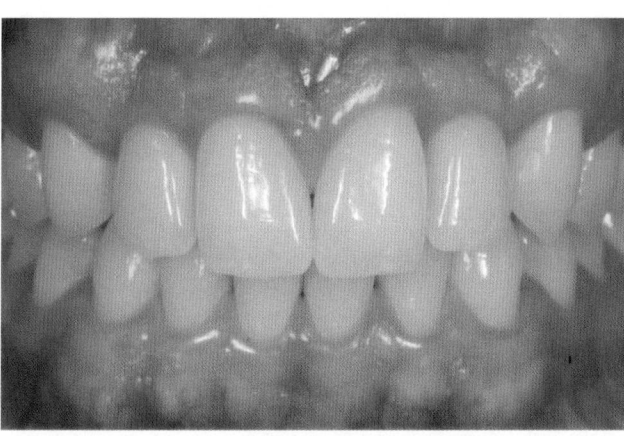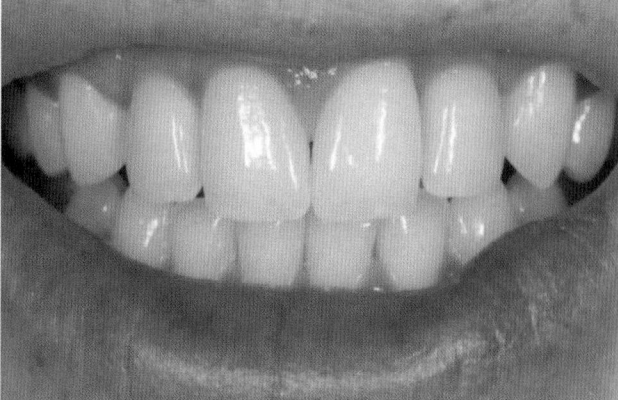

Fig. 71.22 Final aesthetic outcome from both an intraoral and extraoral perspective.

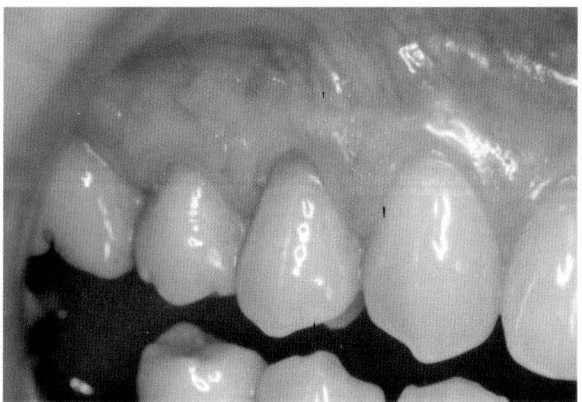

Fig. 71.23 Multidisciplinary simple implant care scenario: favorable soft-tissue parameters combined with a low smile line. Preoperative view of the maxillary right first premolar. With the exception of a small degree of gingival recession, all other aspects of the surrounding periodontium are intact.

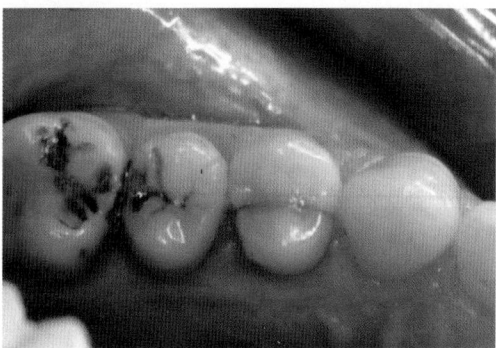

Fig. 71.24 A fracture extending in a mesiodistal orientation is evident on the occlusal surface of the maxillary first premolar.

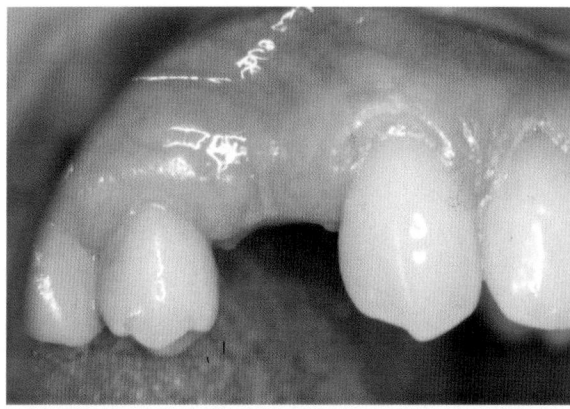

Fig. 71.25 Healed ridge 3 months after tooth extraction. Note the wide zone of keratinized tissue present and favorable maintenance of the height of the adjacent interdental papillae.

technologies, systematic treatment protocols, and better data to appreciate success and risk factors, predictable outcomes have become readily achievable. The widespread emergence and acceptance of implant dentistry and the fact that it is both a surgical and prosthetic modality puts it at the center of many of the trends transforming traditional practice models.

Periodontology, like other specialties, has evolved to embrace a more global view of patient care. It is suggested that in addition to learning all of the standard periodontal procedures of the past, the contemporary periodontist should also be able to *restore* simple implant cases such as those located outside of the aesthetic zone (Figs. 71.23 to 71.32). Periodontists will continue to be trained to manage hard and soft tissues and perform all of the latest periodontal plastic surgical procedures to preserve and reconstruct pleasing gingival architecture in the aesthetic zone to the highest level of sophistication and complexity. However, as the definition of what is deemed a successful outcome continues to evolve and the bar for the definition is raised, the surgeon must remain acutely aware of the restorative aspects of care and abreast of related advances. In other words, it has become essential that periodontists not limit their knowledge and care to the treatment of periodontal disease alone.

Surgical specialists (i.e., periodontists) who are trained according to a multidisciplinary approach will provide even greater benefit to their patients from this evolved philosophy. Consider the case for immediate dental implant placement along with simultaneous fabrication and insertion of a provisional restoration at the time of tooth

extraction. This treatment is a series of steps that integrates both surgical and restorative areas of dentistry. As such, suitable depth of knowledge in all phases is needed to allow for proper diagnosis, case selection, and clinical delivery of care for predictable outcomes and to yield the wide range of benefits this treatment offers to both the patient and the doctor. Even when the role of implant surgeons is limited to the surgical phase of therapy, achieving the best and most predictable outcomes requires that they possess a thorough understanding of the realities and intricacies related to the fabrication and delivery of the planned prosthesis. This "restorative" knowledge and experience will help them to place implants in as close to ideal

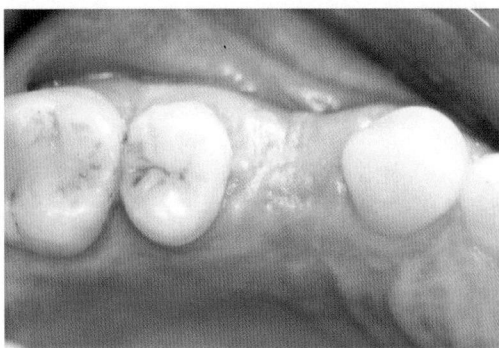

Fig. 71.26 The healed ridge demonstrates favorable buccolingual dimension and soft-tissue quality. Based on preoperative clinical and radiographic evaluation, placement of a dental implant in an uncomplicated fashion can be expected.

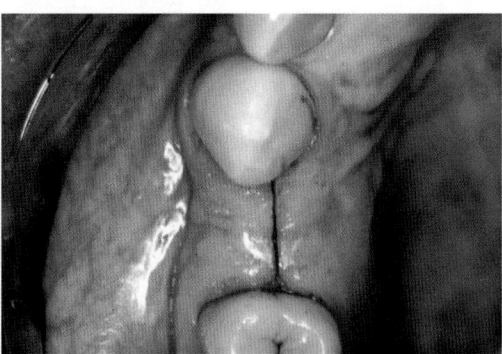

Fig. 71.27 Surgical access for placement of the dental implant using a horizontal incision that extends intrasulcularly to the nearest buccal and palatal line angles of the adjacent teeth.

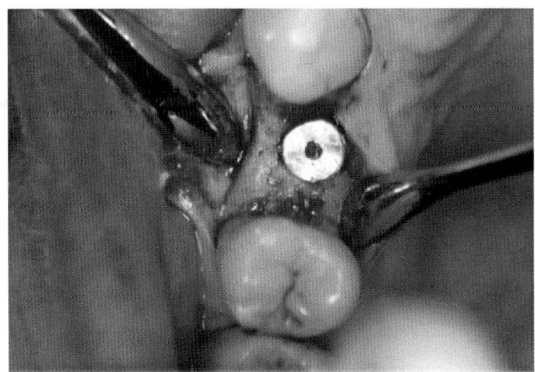

Fig. 71.28 The endosseous implant is properly positioned to facilitate an optimal prosthetic outcome in the final restoration.

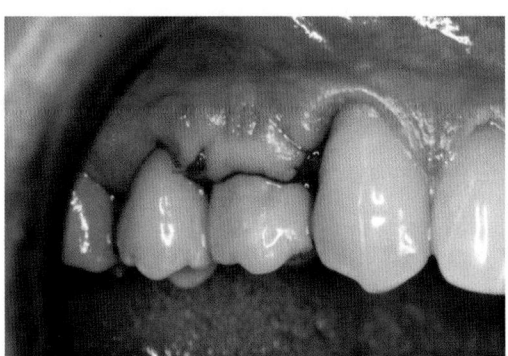

Fig. 71.29 After a period of healing during which the implant was submerged, stage II surgery to expose it was accomplished. In this scenario, a fixed provisional restoration was secured to the implant to serve as a matrix and begin sculpting the resultant soft-tissue profile in lieu of using a conventional nonanatomic round healing abutment. Note the position of the flap margin on the prosthetic crown. It is located occlusal to the expected cementoenamel junction (CEJ) location to compensate for expected soft-tissue healing and remodeling and yield a favorable aesthetic outcome.

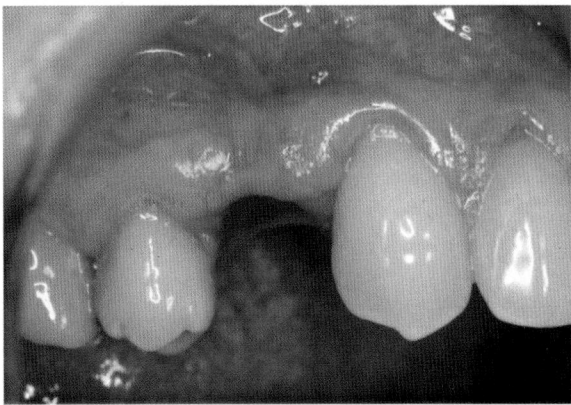

Fig. 71.30 The healed peri-implant sulcus demonstrates the three-dimensionally generated result achieved using a provisional crown for soft-tissue sculpting. Note the recreation of the interdental papilla, the result of a favorable relationship between the interproximal bone height of the adjacent teeth and reestablishment of contact areas between the natural teeth and the provisional restoration.

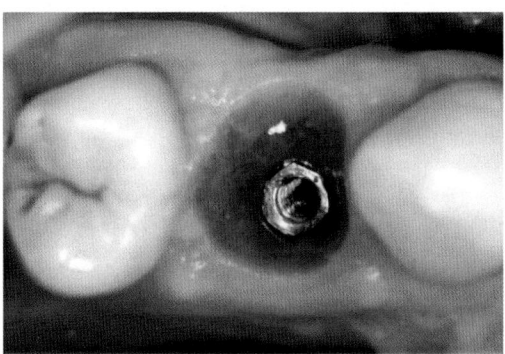

Fig. 71.31 Occlusal view of the anatomic peri-implant sulcus formed by the contours of the provisional restoration subgingivally.

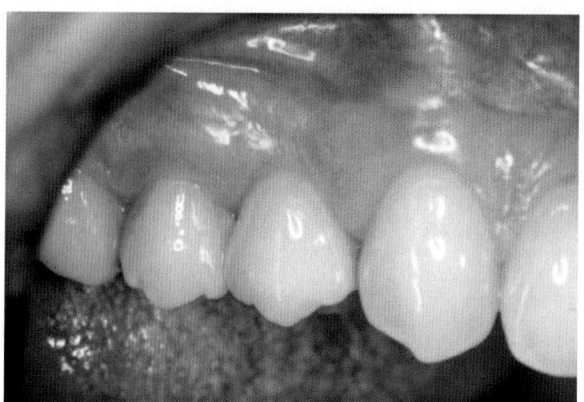

Fig. 71.32 Final implant-supported restoration in place.

orientation in all three spatial dimensions and to avoid such common errors as excessive implant angulation by understanding the restorative challenges that may otherwise result. Additionally, the well-versed periodontist will be better able to communicate effectively with restorative colleagues and may even serve as a resource to guide and educate those who might have less familiarity with the subject matter when an interdisciplinary approach is utilized.

Educational Trends Toward Multidisciplinary Specialist Education in Implant Treatment

For the multidisciplinary model of practice to be able to deliver care at the level presently available through the interdisciplinary model, the provider (general practitioner or specialist) needs to be comprehensively trained with a broader scope and depth of expertise than typical contemporary norms often deliver. This is reflected in the many changes and opportunities in continuing and postgraduate training, particularly those centered on the surgical aspects of dental implant therapy.

Continuing education offerings span a broad range. Some are limited to didactic teaching with laboratory simulation, whereas others take the form of clinical fellowship-style programs that encompass a patient care component lasting a year or longer. As such, some general practitioners and traditionally trained prosthodontists who have sought out advanced postgraduate training might add some aspects of surgical care (commensurate with the scope and level of their respective training) to the range of services they personally provide. Conversely, members of the surgical specialties (e.g., periodontists and oral surgeons) would have received a level of training that would enable them to recommend, guide, and, if necessary, provide a range of restorative treatments. Indeed, rigidly defined accreditation standards for some postgraduate specialties have already been revised and reflect this trend toward encouraging multidisciplinary training. Traditional nonsurgical restorative training programs now include basic implant surgical training in their curricula. Advanced education specialty programs in prosthodontics, among other topics, now include an increased allocation of time in their didactic and clinical curricula in the area of diagnosis, as well as training to the level of competency with respect to simple single-tooth implants in healed ridges of favorable dimension and in sites outside the aesthetic zone.

The Future

It has already become the accepted norm that not all surgery will be done by a periodontist or oral surgeon, nor is it likely that all restorative work will be done by a general dentist or prosthodontist. Instead, simple cases that require surgery and restoration will probably be performed entirely by either a well-trained general dentist or a specialist. In fact, many periodontists have already begun working with their restorative colleagues by making the final impression or index of the implant at the time of surgery and forwarding it to them. In such a scenario, the restorative dentist may now only need to insert the final restoration when it comes back from the laboratory, thus expediting treatment and enhancing the experience for both the patient and the doctor. Although it is conceivable that simple implant cases will more likely be treated in a multidisciplinary fashion, an interdisciplinary approach will still exist and be utilized for patients who require advanced treatments, particularly when there is a deficiency of soft and/or hard tissues.

Periodontists of the future will have a multidisciplinary approach to patient care. They will continue to provide all of the specialty services that "classically" trained periodontists have done for decades, but they will also be well suited to better support their restorative colleagues.

CHAPTER 72

Supportive Periodontal Treatment

Robert L. Merin

CHAPTER OUTLINE

Rationale for Supportive Periodontal
Treatment
Maintenance Program

Classification of Posttreatment
Patients and Risk Assessment
Referral of Patients to the
Periodontist

Tests for Disease Activity
Conclusion

Preservation of the periodontal health of the treated patient requires a supportive program that is just as important as the therapy used to treat the periodontal disease. After phase I therapy has be4en completed, patients are placed on a schedule of periodic recall visits for maintenance care to prevent the recurrence of the disease (Figs. 72.1 and 72.2).

LEARNING BOX 72.1

The long-term preservation of the dentition is closely associated with the frequency and quality of recall maintenance.

Transfer of the patient from active treatment status to a maintenance program is a definitive step in total patient care that requires time and effort on the part of the dentist and staff. Patients must understand the purpose of the maintenance program, and the dentist must emphasize that preservation of the teeth depends on maintenance therapy.[5] Patients who are not maintained in a supervised recall program subsequent to active treatment show obvious signs of recurrent periodontitis (e.g., increased pocket depth, bone loss, or tooth loss).[6,7,11,12,16,17,37] The more often patients present for recommended supportive periodontal treatment (SPT), the less likely they are to lose teeth.[17,28,34,37,40,54,61] One study indicated that treated patients who do not return for regular recall have a 5.6 times greater risk for tooth loss than compliant patients.[12] Another study showed that patients with inadequate SPT after successful regenerative therapy have a 50-fold increase in risk of probing attachment loss compared with those who have regular recall visits.[15]

LEARNING BOX 72.2

Patients who do not return for SPT lose five to six times more teeth than compliant patients,

Motivational techniques and reinforcement of the importance of the maintenance phase of treatment should be considered before performing definitive periodontal surgery.[7] Studies show that few patients display complete compliance with recommended maintenance schedules[1,33,34,38,39,59,61] (Fig. 72.3). *It is meaningless simply to inform*

patients that they are to return for periodic recall visits without clearly explaining the significance of these visits and describing what is expected of patients between visits.

The maintenance phase of periodontal treatment starts immediately after the completion of phase I therapy (see Figs. 72.1 and 72.2). While the patient is in the maintenance phase, the necessary surgical and restorative procedures are performed. This ensures that all areas of the mouth retain the degree of health attained after phase I therapy.

Rationale for Supportive Periodontal Treatment

Studies indicate that even with appropriate periodontal therapy, some progression of disease is possible.[23,25,41,44,46,53,62] One likely explanation for the recurrence of periodontal disease is incomplete subgingival plaque/biofilm and calculus removal.[56,62] If subgingival biofilm is left behind during scaling, it regrows within the pocket. The regrowth of subgingival biofilm is a slow process compared with that of supragingival biofilm. During this period (perhaps months), the subgingival biofilm may not induce inflammatory reactions that can be discerned at the gingival margin. The clinical diagnosis may be further confused by the introduction of adequate supragingival biofilm control because the inflammatory reactions caused by the biofilm in the soft-tissue wall of the pocket are not likely to manifest clinically as gingival erythema and edema.[18] Thus inadequate subgingival biofilm control can lead to continued loss of attachment, even without the presence of clinical gingival inflammation. Scaling and root planing are generally not effective at sites with probing depths of 6 mm or greater.[5]

Bacteria are present in the gingival tissues in chronic and aggressive periodontitis cases.[9,14,19,43] Eradication of intragingival microorganisms may be necessary for a stable periodontal result.[19] Scaling, root planing, and even flap surgery may not eliminate intragingival bacteria in some areas.[9] These bacteria may recolonize the pocket and cause recurrent disease.

Bacteria associated with periodontitis can be transmitted between spouses and other family members.[2,55] Patients who appear to be successfully treated can become infected or reinfected with potential pathogens. This is especially likely in patients with remaining pockets.

Another possible explanation for the recurrence of periodontal disease is the microscopic nature of the dentogingival unit healing

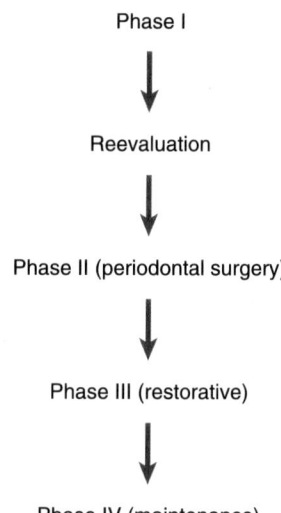

Fig. 72.1 Incorrect sequence of periodontal treatment phases. Maintenance phase should be started immediately after the reevaluation of phase I therapy.

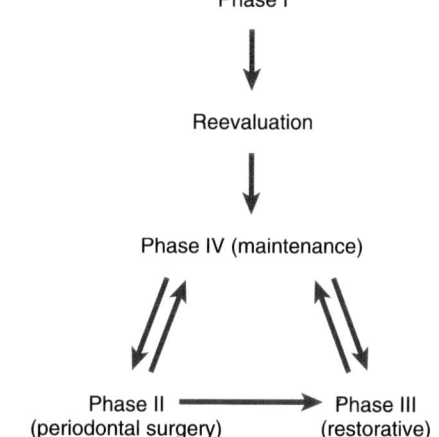

Fig. 72.2 Correct sequence of periodontal treatment phases.

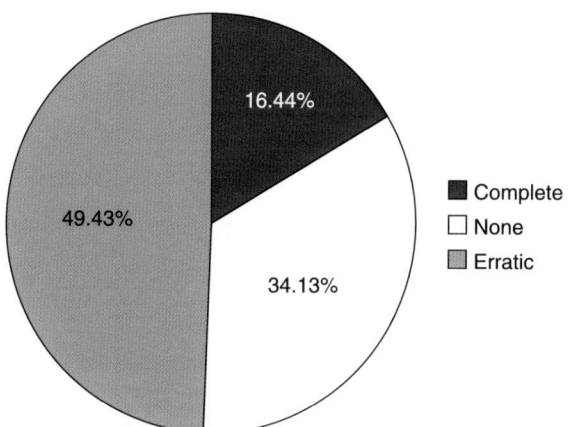

Fig. 72.3 Compliance with maintenance therapy in 961 patients studied for 1 to 8 years. *(Modified from Wilson TG Jr, Glover ME, Schoen J, et al: Compliance with maintenance therapy in a private periodontal practice. J Periodontol 55:468, 1984.)*

after periodontal treatment. Histologic studies have indicated that after periodontal procedures, tissues usually heal by the formation a long junctional epithelium instead of new connective tissue attachment to root surfaces.[10,49,50] It has been speculated that this type of dentogingival unit may be weaker and that inflammation may rapidly separate the long junctional epithelium from the tooth. Thus treated periodontal patients may be predisposed to recurrent pocket formation if maintenance care is not optimal.

Subgingival scaling alters the microflora of periodontal pockets.[35,42,47] In one study, a single session of scaling and root planing in patients with chronic periodontitis resulted in significant changes in subgingival microflora.[35] Reported alterations included a decrease in the proportion of motile rods for 1 week, a marked elevation in the proportion of coccoid cells for 21 days, and a marked reduction in the proportion of spirochetes for 7 weeks.

Although pocket debridement suppresses components of the subgingival microflora associated with periodontitis, periodontal pathogens may return to baseline levels within days or months.[3,46] The return of pathogens to pretreatment levels generally occurs in approximately 9 to 11 weeks but can vary dramatically among patients.[3]

LEARNING BOX 72.3

Scaling and root planing are generally not effective at sites with probing depths of 6 mm or greater.

Both the mechanical debridement performed by the therapist and the motivational environment provided by the appointment seem to be necessary for good maintenance results. Patients tend to reduce their oral hygiene efforts between appointments.[4,61] Knowing that their hygiene will be evaluated motivates them to perform better oral hygiene in anticipation of the appointment.

In one study, the proportion of spirochetes obtained in baseline samples of subgingival flora was highly correlated with clinical periodontal deterioration over 1 year.[31] However, subsequent reports in the same longitudinal study concluded that the arbitrary assignment of treated periodontitis patients to 3-month maintenance intervals appears to be as effective in preventing recurrences of periodontitis as assignment of recall intervals based on microscopic monitoring of the subgingival flora.[30,31] Microscopic monitoring was found not to be a reliable predictor of future periodontal destruction in patients on 3-month recall programs, presumably because of the alteration of subgingival flora produced by subgingival instrumentation.

In conclusion, there is a sound scientific basis for recall maintenance because subgingival scaling alters the pocket microflora for variable but relatively long periods.

Maintenance Program

Periodic recall visits form the foundation of a meaningful long-term prevention program. The interval between visits is initially set at 3 months but may vary according to the patient's needs.[5,20,26,27]

Periodontal care at each recall visit comprises three parts (Box 72.1). The first part involves examination and evaluation of the patient's current oral health. The second part includes the necessary maintenance treatment and oral hygiene reinforcement. The third part involves scheduling the patient for the next recall appointment, additional periodontal treatment, or restorative dental procedures. The time required for a recall visit for patients with multiple teeth in both arches is approximately 1 hour.[45]

BOX 72.1   Maintenance Recall Procedures

Part I: Examination

(Approximate time: 14 minutes)
Patient greeting
Medical history changes
Oral pathologic examination
Oral hygiene status
Gingival changes
Pocket depth changes
Mobility changes
Occlusal changes
Dental caries
Restorative, prosthetic, and implant status

Part II: Treatment

(Approximate time: 36 minutes)
Oral hygiene reinforcement
Scaling
Polishing
Chemical irrigation or site-specific antimicrobial placement

Part III: Report, Cleanup, and Scheduling

(Approximate time: 10 minutes)
Write report in chart.
Discuss report with patient.
Clean and disinfect operatory.
Schedule next recall visit.
Schedule further periodontal treatment.
Schedule or refer for restorative or prosthetic treatment.

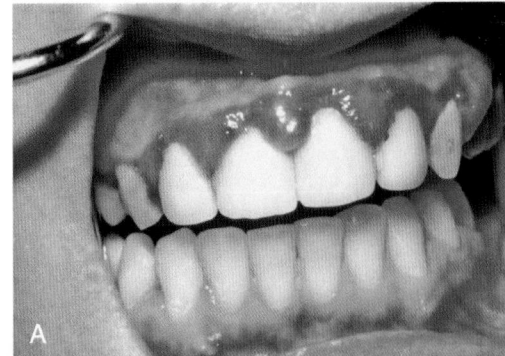
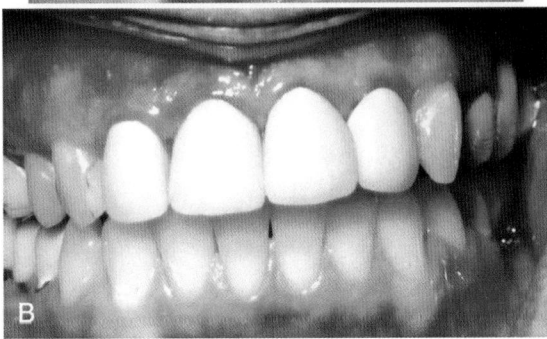

Fig. 72.4 (A) Hyperplastic gingivitis related to crown margins and plaque accumulation in a 27-year-old woman. (B) Four months after treatment, there is significant improvement. However, some inflammation around crown margins still exists, which cannot be resolved without replacing the crowns.

LEARNING BOX 72.4

There are three parts to an SPT appointment: (1) examination; (2) treatment; and (3) report, cleanup, and scheduling.

Examination and Evaluation

The recall examination is similar to the initial evaluation of the patient (see Chapter 32). However, because the patient is not new to the office, the dentist or hygienist primarily looks for changes that have occurred since the last evaluation. Analysis of the current oral hygiene status of the patient is essential. Updating of changes in the medical history and evaluation of restorations, caries, prostheses, occlusion, tooth mobility, gingival status, and periodontal and periimplant probing depths are important parts of the recall appointment. The oral mucosa should be carefully inspected for pathologic conditions (Figs. 72.4 to 72.9).

Radiographic examination must be individualized,[22] depending on the initial severity of the case and the findings during the recall visit (Table 72.1). These are compared with findings on previous radiographs to check the bone height and look for repair of osseous defects, signs of trauma from occlusion, periapical pathologic changes, and caries.

Checking of Plaque/Biofilm Control

To assess the effectiveness of their plaque control, patients should perform their hygiene regimen immediately before the recall appointment. Plaque/biofilm control must be reviewed and corrected until the patient demonstrates the necessary proficiency, even if additional instruction sessions are required. A motivational interviewing

TABLE 72.1   Radiographic Examination of Recall Patients for Supportive Periodontal Treatment

Patient Condition/Situation	Type of Examination
Clinical caries or high-risk factors for caries	Posterior bitewing examination at 6- to 18-month intervals
No clinical caries and no high-risk factors for caries	Posterior bitewing examination at 24- to 36-month intervals
Periodontal disease not under good control	Periapical or vertical bitewing radiographs of problem areas every 12 to 24 months
History of periodontal treatment with disease under good control	Bitewing examination every 24 to 36 months
Root form dental implants	Periapical or vertical bitewing radiographs after prosthetic placement and at 12 and 24 months, then every 24 to 36 months unless clinical problems arise
Transfer of periodontal or implant maintenance patients	Full-mouth series if a current set not available; if full-mouth series has been taken within 24 months, radiographs of implants and periodontal problem areas should be taken

Radiographs should be taken when they are likely to affect diagnosis and patient treatment. The recommendations in this table are subject to clinical judgment and may not apply to every patient.
Adapted from Guide to Patient Selection and Limiting Radiation Exposure. American Dental Association website, http://ada.org/2760/aspx, 2013.

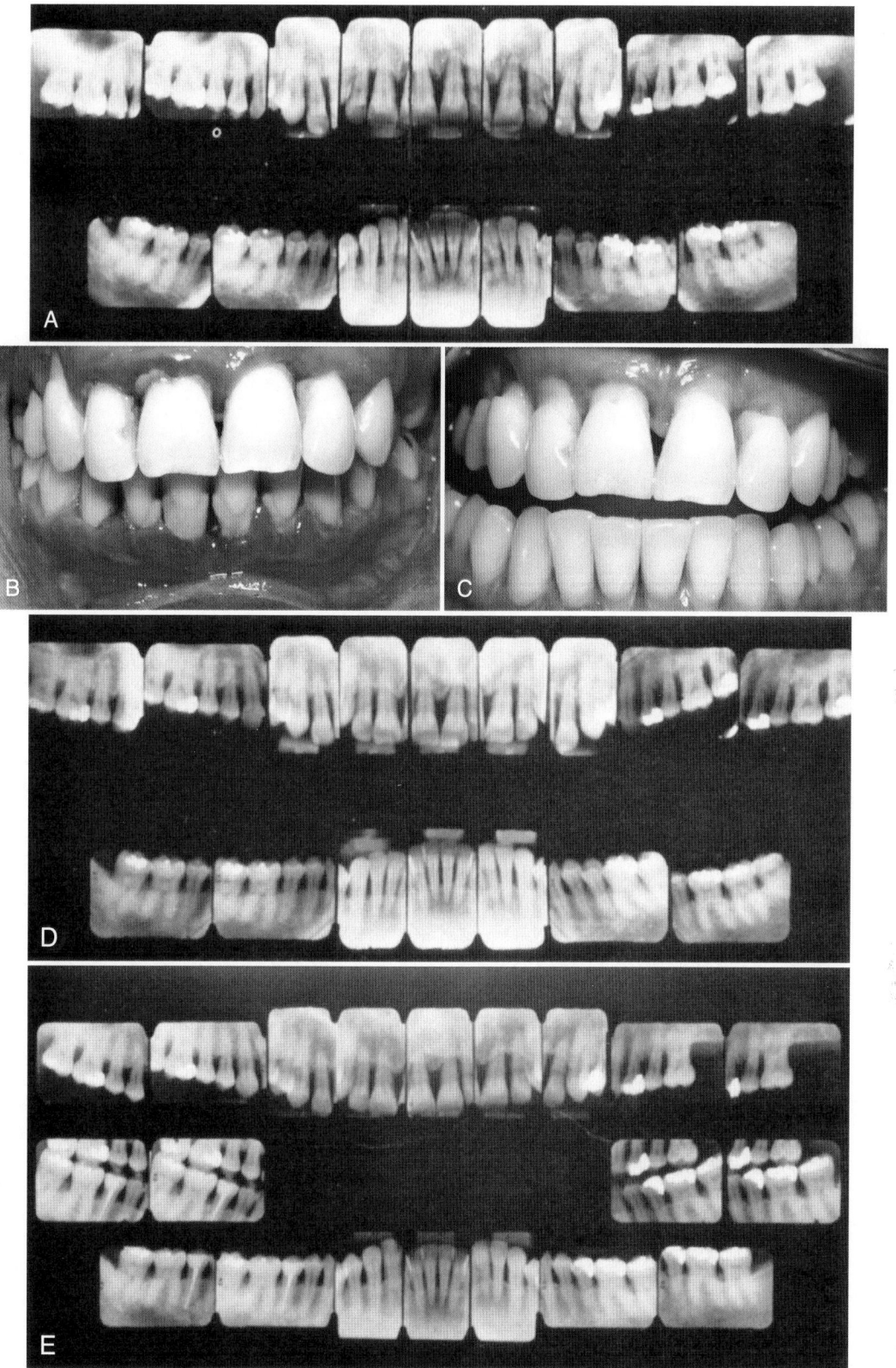

Fig. 72.5 (A) Patient was 38 years old when these original radiographs were taken and was treated with a combination of surgical and nonsurgical therapy. This individual is a classic class C maintenance patient. (B) Pretreatment photograph. Note the inflammation and heavy calculus deposits. (C) Photograph taken 10 years after treatment. (D) Radiographs taken 5 years after treatment. (E) Radiographs taken 10 years after treatment. The radiographic appearance is as good as can be expected in such a severe case. Teeth #15 and #17 were extracted 8 years after treatment.

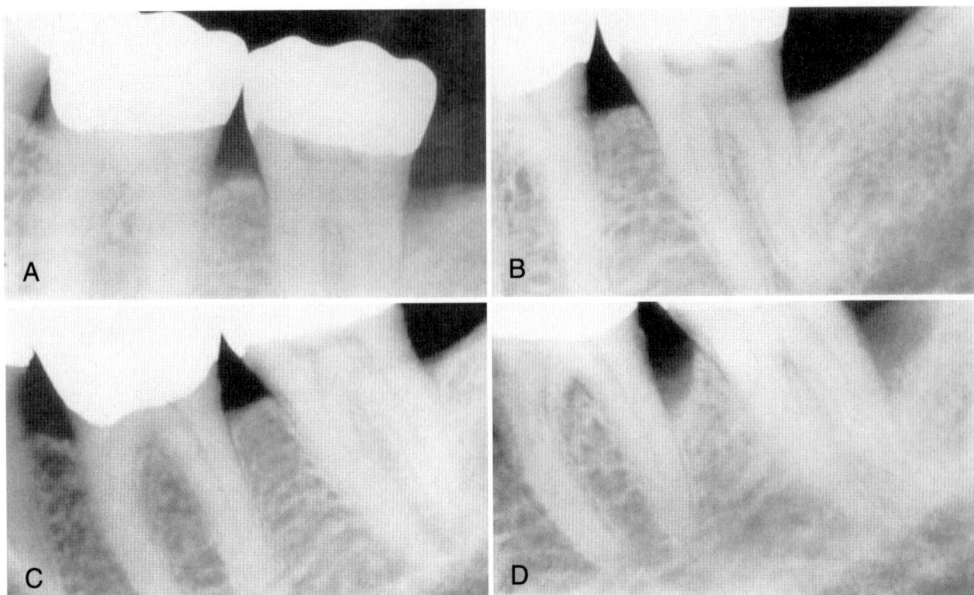

Fig. 72.6 This series of radiographs clearly shows the importance of maintenance therapy. (A) Original radiograph of a 58-year-old male. Note the deep distal bone loss on tooth #18 and the moderate distal lesion of tooth #19. Surgical treatment included osseous grafting. (B) Radiograph 14 months after surgical therapy. The patient had recall maintenance performed every 3 to 4 months. (C) Appearance 3 years after surgery, with regular recalls every 3 to 4 months. (D) Appearance after 2 years without recalls (7 years after surgery). Note the progression of the disease on the distal surfaces of teeth #18 and #19.

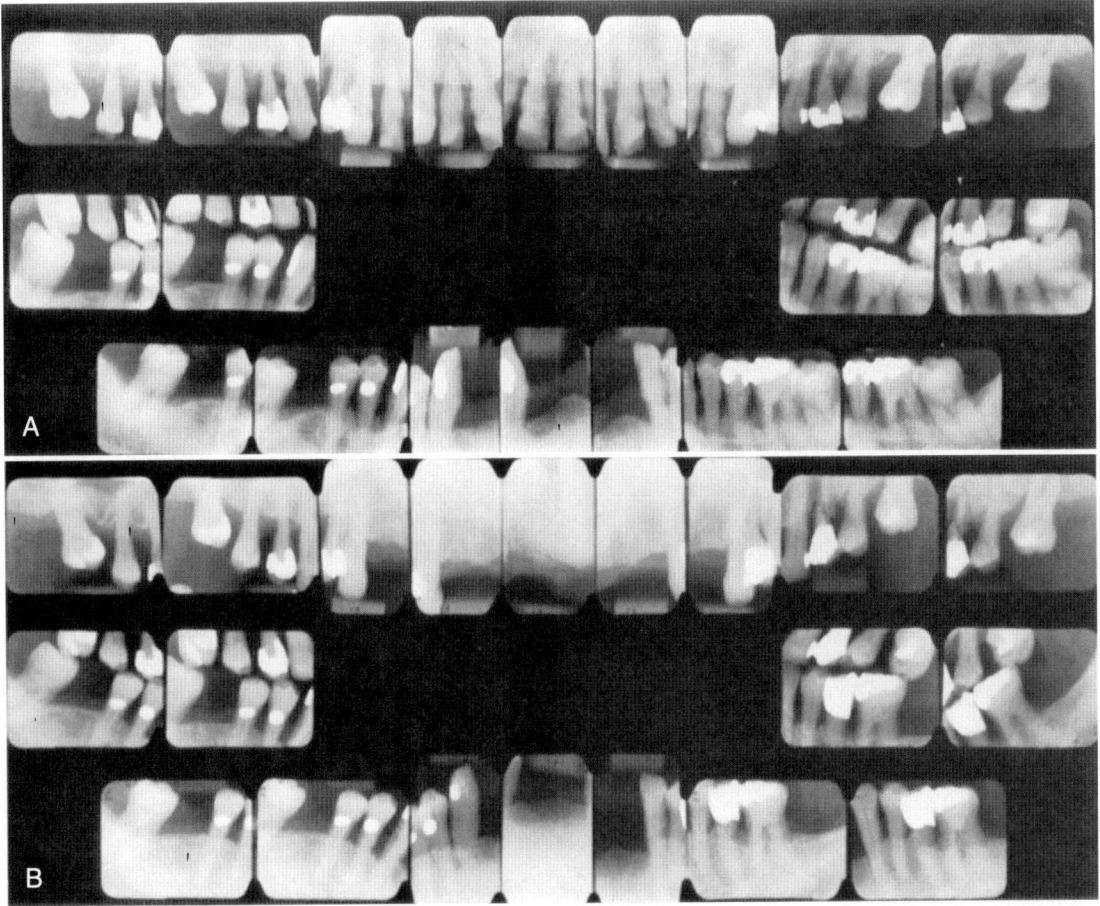

Fig. 72.7 Advanced cases sometimes do better than expected when the patient complies with maintenance therapy. (A) Initial radiographs showing an advanced case. The maxillary arch had extractions and nonsurgical treatment. A plastic partial denture was placed and was expected to grow into a full denture within a few years. The mandibular arch was treated with periodontal surgery, and a permanent, metal and plastic, removable partial denture was placed. (B) Radiographs taken 8 years later. The patient performed good oral hygiene and had 3-month recalls. Teeth #12 and #15 required extraction.

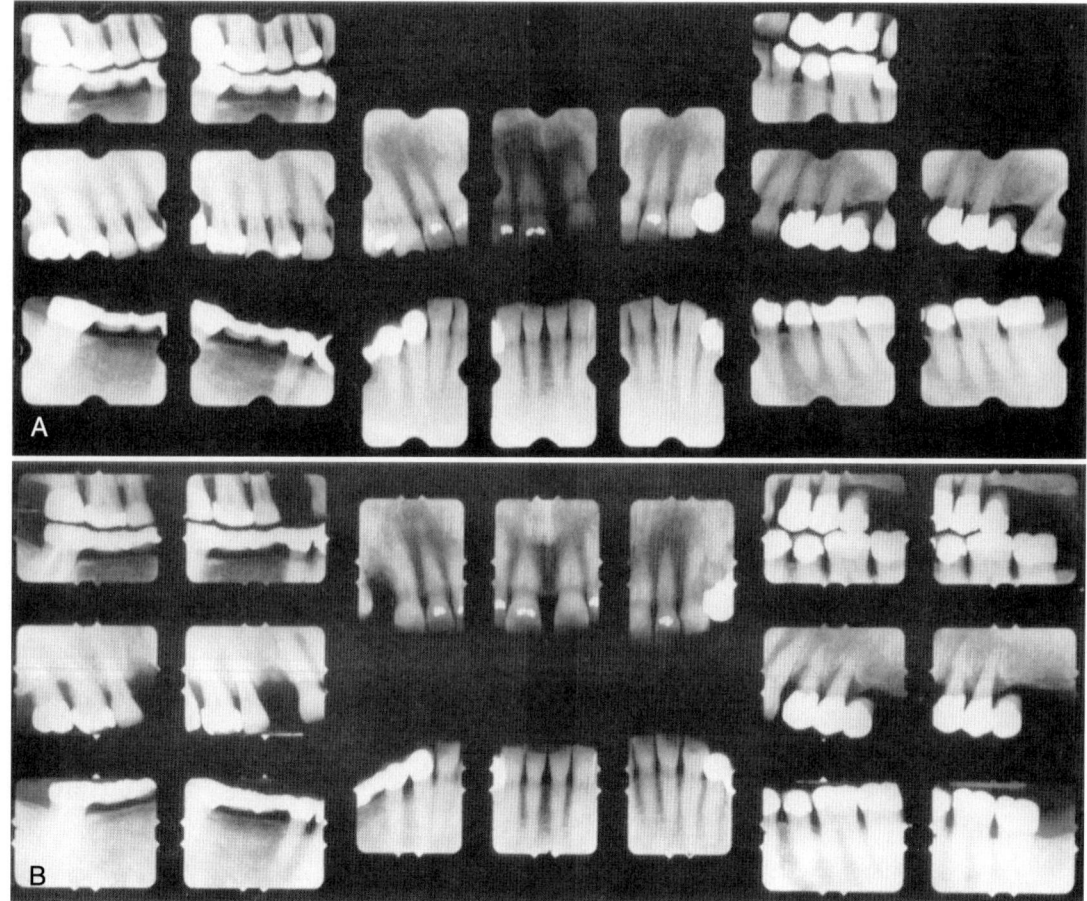

Fig. 72.8 (A) Initial radiographs. The patient was advised to have localized areas of periodontal surgery and periodontal recall every 3 months. However, the patient did not comply and only had dental cleanings once or twice yearly. (B) Radiographs 4 years later. Note the loss of teeth #5 and #15 and the increased bone loss of several premolars and molars.

technique of teaching may help to produce positive results.[57] Patients instructed in plaque/biofilm control have less biofilm and gingivitis than uninstructed patients,[6,51,52] and because the amount of supragingival plaque/biofilm is less, there is a decrease in the number of subgingival anaerobic organisms.[10,48]

Treatment

Following consultation, examination, consultation, and oral hygiene instruction, the required scaling and root planing are performed (see Chapter 50). Care must be taken not to instrument healthy sites with shallow sulci (1 to 3 mm deep) and an absence of gingival inflammation because studies have indicated that repeated subgingival scaling and root planing of sites not periodontally involved result in significant loss of attachment and gingival recession, which will affect aesthetics.[29] Irrigation with antimicrobial agents or placement of site-specific antimicrobial devices may be performed in maintenance patients with remaining pockets.[3,24,32]

Recurrence of Periodontal Disease

Occasionally, lesions may recur, which is often due to inadequate plaque/biofilm control on the part of the patient or failure to comply with recommended SPT schedules. It should be understood, however, that it is the responsibility of the dentist to educate and motivate patients to improve their oral hygiene techniques. Surgery should not be undertaken unless the patient participates in disease prevention and demonstrates proficiency in plaque/biofilm control.[7,53,60]

Other causes for recurrence include the following:

1. Inadequate or insufficient treatment that has failed to remove all of the potential factors favoring biofilm accumulation (see Fig. 72.4). Incomplete calculus removal in areas of difficult access is a common source of problems.
2. Inadequate restorations placed after the periodontal treatment was completed.
3. Failure of the patient to return for periodic maintenance care (see Fig. 72.6). This may be a result of the patient's conscious or unconscious decision not to continue treatment or the failure of the dentist and staff to emphasize the need for periodic supportive therapy.
4. Presence of some systemic diseases that may affect host resistance to previously acceptable levels of biofilm.

A failing case can be recognized by the following:

1. Recurring inflammation revealed by gingival changes and bleeding of the sulcus on probing.
2. Increasing depth of sulci, leading to the recurrence of pocket formation.
3. Gradual increases in bone loss, as determined by radiographs.
4. Gradual increases in tooth mobility, as ascertained by clinical examination.

The decision to retreat a periodontal patient should not be made at the preventive maintenance appointment but should be postponed for 1 to 2 weeks.[11] Often, the mouth appears improved at that time because of the resolution of edema and the resulting improved tone of the gingiva. Table 72.2 summarizes the symptoms of the recurrence of periodontal disease and their probable causes.

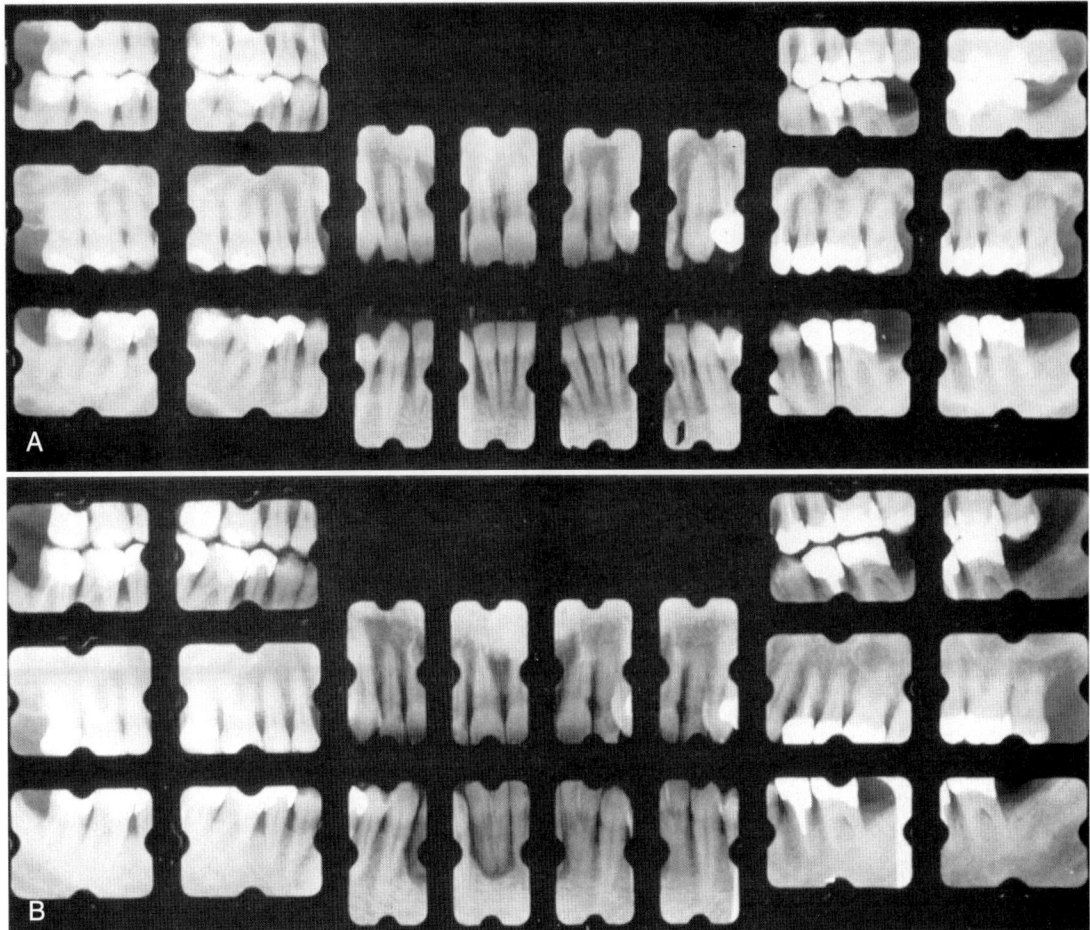

Fig. 72.9 (A) Initial radiographs. The patient was advised to have localized areas of periodontal surgery and periodontal recall every 3 months. However, the patient did not comply and had no treatment other than emergency care and occasional dental cleanings. (B) Radiographs 7 years later. Note the advanced bone loss and caries on many teeth.

TABLE 72.2   Symptoms and Causes of Recurrence of Disease

Symptom	Possible Causes	Symptom	Possible Causes
Increased mobility	Increased inflammation Poor oral hygiene Subgingival calculus Inadequate restorations Deteriorating or poorly designed prostheses Systemic disease modifying host response to plaque	Increased pocket depth with no radiographic change	Poor oral hygiene Infrequent recall visits Subgingival calculus Poorly fitting partial denture Mesial inclination into edentulous space Failure of new attachment surgery Cracked teeth Grooves in teeth New periodontal disease Gingival overgrowth caused by medication
Recession	Toothbrush abrasion Inadequate keratinized gingiva Frenum pull Orthodontic therapy	Increased pocket depth with increased radiographic bone loss	Poor oral hygiene Subgingival calculus Infrequent recall visits Inadequate or deteriorating restorations Poorly designed prostheses Inadequate surgery Systemic disease modifying host response to plaque Cracked teeth Grooves in teeth New periodontal disease
Increased mobility with no change in pocket depth and no radiographic change	Occlusal trauma caused by lateral occlusal interference, bruxism, high restoration Poorly designed or worn-out prosthesis Poor crown-to-root ratio		

Classification of Posttreatment Patients and Risk Assessment

The first year after periodontal therapy is important in terms of indoctrinating the patient in a recall pattern and reinforcing oral hygiene techniques. In addition, it may take several months to evaluate accurately the results of some periodontal surgical procedures. Consequently, some areas may have to be retreated because the results may not be optimal. Furthermore, the first-year patient often has etiologic factors that may have been overlooked and may be amenable to treatment at this early stage. For these reasons, the recall interval for first-year patients should not be longer than 3 months.

Patients who are on a periodontal recall schedule are a varied group. Table 72.3 lists several categories of maintenance patients and a suggested recall interval for each group. Patients can improve or may relapse to a different classification, with a reduction in or exacerbation of periodontal disease. When one dental arch is more involved than the other, the patient's periodontal disease is classified by the arch with the worse condition.

Table 72.3 is a traditional method of assigning the risk of a recurrence of periodontal destruction. A practitioner uses the listed risk factors and his or her own diagnostic and prognostic gestalt to assign a risk category and maintenance schedule. New risk factor assessment tools for the prevention of periodontal destruction have been developed.[21,26,27,36] The Periodontal Risk Assessment (PRA) (Fig. 72.10) and the Periodontal Risk Calculator (PRC) have the most studies documenting their ability to predict the progression of periodontitis and tooth loss.[26] The PRC is marketed by the PreViser Corporation and offers a web-based system for periodontal risk analysis and prognosis.[21] The PRA is offered free of charge by the Clinical Research Foundation and the University of Bern at http://www.perio-tools.com/PRA/en/index.asp. Patient data are entered into the online form, and the program automatically calculates whether the patient is at low risk, moderate risk, or high risk; an appropriate recall interval is then suggested. Fig. 72.9A is a sample assessment from the PRA website. Because the different assessment tools use

TABLE 72.3 Recall Intervals for Various Classes of Recall Patients

Merin Classification	Characteristics	Recall Interval
First year	First-year patient: routine therapy and uneventful healing.	3 months
	First-year patient: difficult case with complicated prosthesis, furcation involvement, poor crown-to-root ratios, or questionable patient cooperation	1–2 months
Class A	Excellent results well maintained for 1 year or longer	6 months to 1 year
	Patient displays good oral hygiene, minimal calculus, no occlusal problems, no complicated prostheses, no remaining pockets, and no teeth with less than 50% of alveolar bone remaining	
Class B	Generally good results maintained reasonably well for 1 year or more, but patient displays some of the following factors: 1. Inconsistent or poor oral hygiene 2. Heavy calculus formation 3. Systemic disease that predisposes to periodontal breakdown 4. Some remaining pockets 5. Occlusal problems 6. Complicated prostheses 7. Ongoing orthodontic therapy 8. Recurrent dental caries 9. Some teeth with less than 50% of alveolar bone support 10. Smoking 11. Positive family history or genetic test 12. More than 20% of pockets bleed on probing	3–4 months (decide on a recall interval based on the number and severity of negative factors)
Class C	Generally poor results after periodontal therapy or several negative factors from the following list: 1. Inconsistent or poor oral hygiene 2. Heavy calculus formation 3. Systemic disease that predisposes to periodontal breakdown 4. Many remaining pockets 5. Occlusal problems 6. Complicated prostheses 7. Recurrent dental caries 8. Periodontal surgery indicated but not performed for medical, psychological, or financial reasons 9. Many teeth with less than 50% of alveolar bone support 10. Condition too far advanced to be improved by periodontal surgery 11. Smoking 12. Positive family history or genetic test 13. More than 20% of pockets bleed on probing	1–3 months (decide on a recall interval based on the number and severity of negative factors; consider retreating some areas or extracting severely involved teeth)

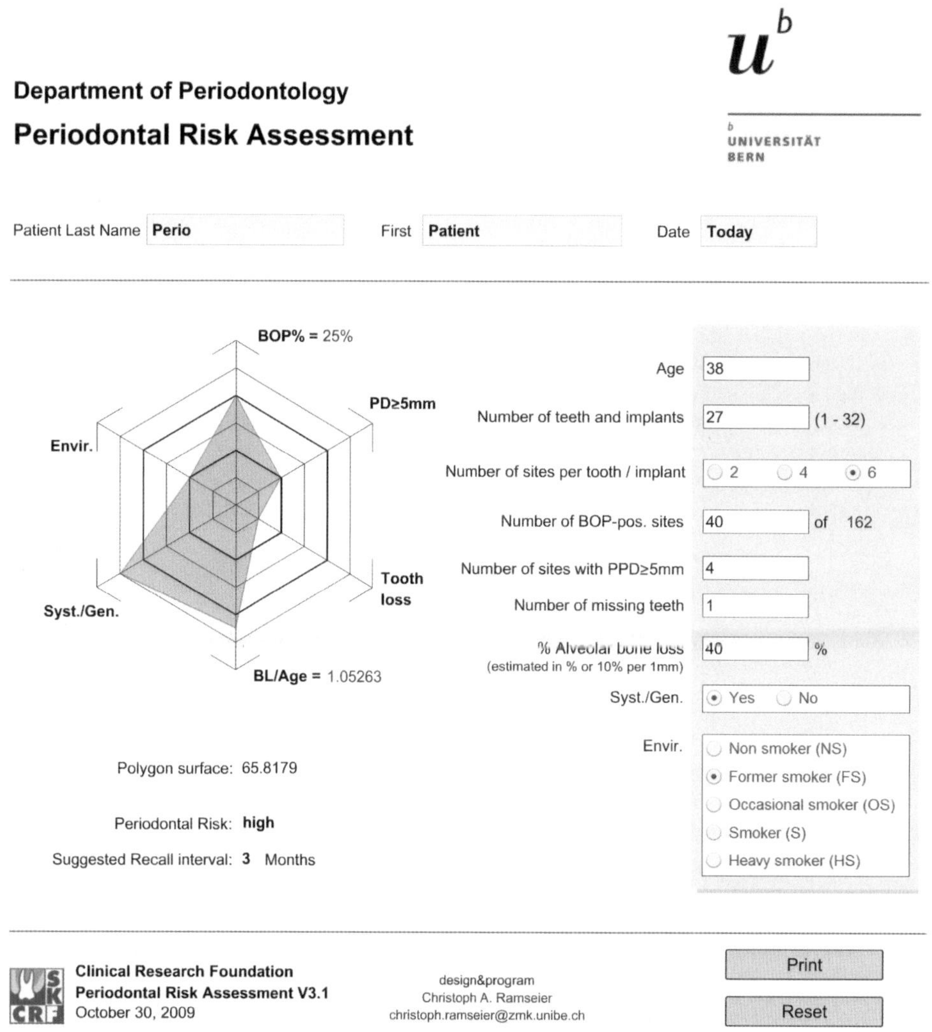

Department of Periodontology

Periodontal Risk Assessment

u^b

b
UNIVERSITÄT
BERN

Patient Last Name **Perio**   First **Patient**   Date **Today**

BOP% = 25%

PD≥5mm

Envir.

Tooth loss

Syst./Gen.

BL/Age = 1.05263

Polygon surface: 65.8179

Periodontal Risk: **high**

Suggested Recall interval: **3** Months

Age [38]

Number of teeth and implants [27] (1 - 32)

Number of sites per tooth / implant ○ 2 ○ 4 ◉ 6

Number of BOP-pos. sites [40] of 162

Number of sites with PPD≥5mm [4]

Number of missing teeth [1]

% Alveolar bone loss [40] %
(estimated in % or 10% per 1mm)

Syst./Gen. ◉ Yes ○ No

Envir. ○ Non smoker (NS)
◉ Former smoker (FS)
○ Occasional smoker (OS)
○ Smoker (S)
○ Heavy smoker (HS)

[Print]

[Reset]

Clinical Research Foundation
Periodontal Risk Assessment V3.1
October 30, 2009

design&program
Christoph A. Ramseier
christoph.ramseier@zmk.unibe.ch

Fig. 72.10 Sample Periodontal Risk Assessment(PRA) report completed and downloaded from http://www.perio-tools.com/PRA/en/index.asp.

different risk factors and algorithms, they will not be in complete agreement. In one study, 57 patients were assessed with the PRC and PRA.[36] The PRC classified 14 as low risk, 17 as medium risk, and 26 as high risk, whereas the PRA classified 8 as low risk, 28 as medium risk, and 21 as high risk.[36]

Currently, there is no universally accepted objective method of predicting periodontitis progression, and there has been little research to determine if the risk calculators are more accurate than good clinical judgment.[21] In summary, maintenance care is a critical phase of therapy. The long-term preservation of the dentition is closely associated with the frequency and quality of recall maintenance.

Referral of Patients to the Periodontist

A general dentist can properly manage many periodontal patients, as a greater number of people retain their teeth throughout their lifetime. Another important fact to consider is that as the proportion of older people in the population increases, more teeth will be at risk for periodontal disease. Numerous studies indicate possible links between periodontal disease and systemic diseases, such as heart disease, stroke, diabetes, and adverse pregnancy outcomes. Therefore the prevalence of patients requiring SPT is likely to increase in the future.

This expected increase in the number of periodontal patients will necessitate a greater understanding of periodontal problems and an increased level of expertise for the solution of such problems on the part of the general practitioner. General dentists must know when co-management with a periodontist is indicated. Specialists are needed to treat difficult periodontal cases, patients with systemic health problems, dental implant patients, and those with a complex prosthetic construction that requires predictable results.

The criteria for cases to be treated in the general dental office and cases to be referred to a specialist vary for different practitioners and patients. The American Academy of Periodontology has issued guidelines to help the general practitioner decide when co-management with a periodontist is indicated.[4] The diagnosis will indicate the type of periodontal treatment required. If periodontal destruction necessitates surgery on the distal surfaces of second molars, extensive osseous surgery, or complex regenerative procedures, the patient is usually best treated by a specialist. Patients who require localized nonsurgical therapy or minor flap surgery can usually be managed by the general practitioner. General dentists have a primary responsibility to do what is best in the interest of the patient. According to Christensen, quality dentistry for a complex case requires a team effort partnering with a periodontal specialist to provide optimal care for the patient.[13]

The decision to have the general practitioner treat a patient's periodontal disease should be guided by consideration of the risk that the patient will lose a tooth or teeth due to periodontal involvement or the periodontal disease negatively affecting the patient's systemic health.

The most important factors in the decision to refer a patient to a periodontist are the severity and location of the periodontal disease. Teeth with pockets of 5 mm or more, as measured from the cementoenamel junction, may have a questionable prognosis, as do teeth with furcation invasions even when more than 50% of bone support remains. Therefore patients with strategically important teeth that have moderate to severe attachment loss or furcation invasions are usually best treated by specialists.

An important question remains: Should the maintenance phase of therapy be performed by the general practitioner or the specialist? This should be determined by the extent and severity of periodontal disease present. Class A recall patients should be maintained by the general dentist, whereas class C patients should be maintained by the specialist (see Table 72.3). Class B patients can alternate recall visits between the general practitioner and the specialist (Fig. 72.11). The suggested rule to decide who should maintain the recall therapy is determined by the initial category of the patient's disease and the result of the therapy. Patients with moderate to severe initial bone loss, advanced grades 2 or 3 furcation invasions, or pockets that could not be completely eradicated are those who should be seen by the periodontist. The specialist and the general dentist must work together, respect the other's knowledge and skills, and decide on a maintenance schedule that is in the best interest of the patient.

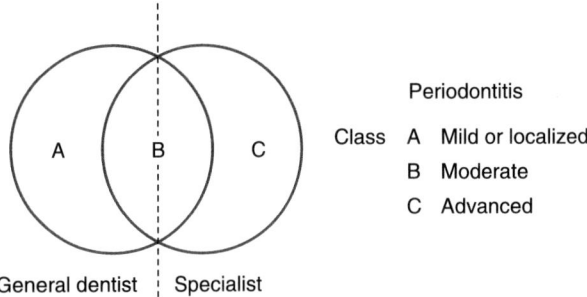

Fig. 72.11 Scheme for determining which practitioner should perform periodontal maintenance in patients with different degrees of periodontitis.

Periodontitis

Class A Mild or localized

B Moderate

C Advanced

General dentist   Specialist

of sequential probing measurements, which may be facilitated by a dental practice management software, gives the most accurate indication of the rate of loss of attachment. A number of other clinical and laboratory variables have been correlated with disease activity.

No accurate method exists to predict disease activity, and clinicians rely on the information obtained from evaluating multiple risk factors.[21,25,30,58] Patients whose disease is clearly refractory are candidates for bacterial culturing and antibiotic therapy in conjunction with additional mechanical therapy.

New methods will undoubtedly be developed in the future to help predict disease activity.[3] The clinician must be able to interpret whether a test may be useful in determining disease activity and future loss of attachment.[8] Tests should be adopted only when they are based on research that includes a critical analysis of the sensitivity, specificity, disease incidence, and predictive value of the proposed test.[21]

Conclusion

The long-term preservation of the dentition is closely associated with the frequency and quality of recall maintenance. The therapist should use risk assessment and educate the patient on the need for periodontal maintenance. Supportive periodontal therapy is a lifetime effort to prevent the disease from recurring. Patients who do not return for supportive periodontal therapy lose more teeth than compliant patients.

> A Case Scenario is found on the companion website www.expertconsult.com.

LEARNING BOX 72.6

Quality dentistry for a complex case requires a team effort partnering with a periodontal specialist to provide optimal care for the patient.[13]

Tests for Disease Activity

Periodontal patients, even though they have received effective periodontal therapy, are at risk of disease recurrence for the remainder of their lives.[23,24] In addition, pockets in and around the furcation areas are difficult to eliminate even with surgical therapy. These areas with pockets may continue to lose attachment.[3] Comparison

References

> References for this chapter are found on the companion website www.expertconsult.com.

CHAPTER 73

Results of Periodontal Treatment

Robert L. Merin

The prevalence of periodontal disease, the resulting high rate of tooth mortality, and the potential for multiple systemic health complications aggravated by chronic periodontitis raise an important question: Is periodontal treatment effective in preventing and controlling the chronic infection and progressive destruction of periodontal disease? Current concepts of evaluating health care require a scientific basis for treatment, referred to as *evidence-based therapy*. Evidence is now overwhelming that periodontal therapy is effective in preventing periodontal disease, slowing the destruction of the periodontium, and reducing tooth loss.

Prevention and Treatment of Gingivitis

> **LEARNING BOX 73.1**
>
> Gingivitis is reversible.

For many years, the belief that good oral hygiene is necessary for the successful prevention and treatment of gingivitis has been widespread among periodontists. In addition, worldwide epidemiologic studies have confirmed a close relationship between the incidence of gingivitis and the lack of oral hygiene.[8,9]

Löe and coworkers[20,38] provided conclusive evidence on the association between oral hygiene and gingivitis. After 9 to 21 days without performing oral hygiene measures, healthy dental students with previously excellent oral hygiene and healthy gingiva developed heavy accumulations of biofilm and generalized mild gingivitis. When oral hygiene techniques were reinstituted, the biofilm in most areas disappeared in 1 or 2 days, and gingival inflammation in these areas disappeared approximately 1 week after the biofilm was removed. Thus gingivitis is reversible and can be resolved by daily, effective biofilm removal.

A number of long-term studies have shown that gingival health can be maintained by a combination of effective oral hygiene maintenance and scaling procedures.[1,2,11,13–15,22,24,36,37] A 3-year study was conducted on 1248 General Telephone workers in California to determine whether progression of gingival inflammation is reduced in an oral environment in which high levels of hygiene are maintained.[36,37] Experimental and control groups were computer matched based on periodontal and oral hygiene status, past caries experience, age, and gender. During the study period, several procedures were instituted to ensure that the oral hygiene status of the experimental group was maintained at a high level. Subjects were given a series of frequent oral prophylaxis treatments combined with oral hygiene instruction. Subjects in the control group received no attention from the study team except for annual examinations. They were advised to continue their usual daily practices and accustomed visits for professional care. After 3 years, the increase in biofilm and debris in the control group was four times as great as that in the experimental group. Similarly, gingivitis scores were much higher in control subjects than in the matching experimental group. Therefore chronic marginal gingivitis can be controlled with good oral hygiene and dental prophylaxis.

> **LEARNING BOX 73.2**
>
> A number of long-term studies have shown that gingival health can be maintained by a combination of effective oral hygiene maintenance and scaling procedures.[1,2,11,13–15,22,24,36,37]

Prevention and Treatment of Loss of Attachment

Although periodontal therapy has been used for more than 100 years, it is only since the mid-1970s that a number of studies have been conducted to determine the effect of treatment on reducing the progressive loss of periodontal support for the natural dentition.

Prevention of Loss of Attachment

Löe and coworkers[19,20] conducted a longitudinal investigation to study the natural development and progression of periodontal disease. The first study group, established in Oslo, Norway, in 1969, consisted of 565 healthy male nondental students and academicians between 17 and 40 years of age. Oslo was selected mainly because this city had an ongoing preschool, school, and postschool dental program offering systematic preventive, restorative, endodontic, orthodontic, and surgical therapy on an annual recall basis for all children and adolescents, complete with a documented attendance record, for the previous 40 years. Members of the study population had experienced maximum exposure to conventional dental care throughout their lives. A second study group, established in Sri Lanka in 1970, consisted of 480 male tea laborers between 15 and 40 years of age. They were

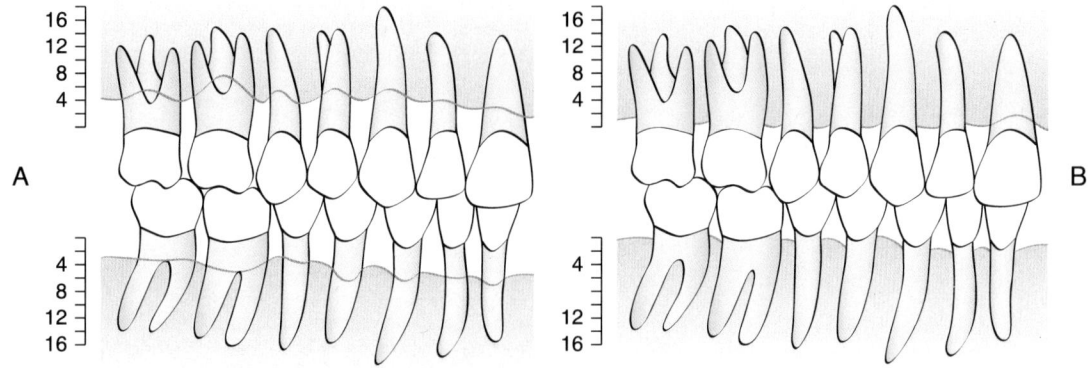

Fig. 73.1 (A) Mean periodontal support of teeth of Sri Lankan tea laborers at approximately 40 years of age. (B) Mean periodontal support of teeth of Norwegian academicians at approximately 40 years of age. *(From Löe H, Anerud A, Boysen H, et al: The natural history of periodontal disease in man: the rate of periodontal destruction before 40 years of age.* J Periodontol *49:607, 1978.)*

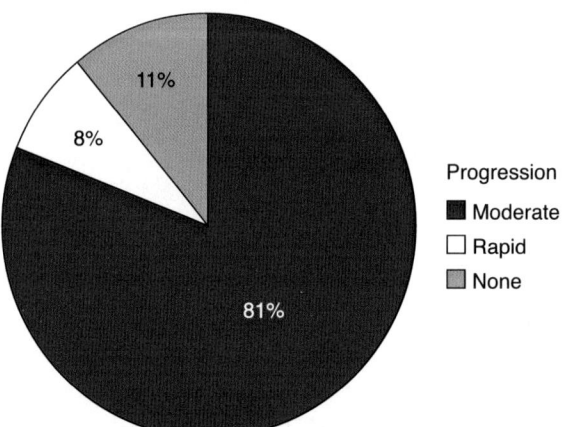

Classification of 480 Sri Lankan Laborers
According to Progression of Periodontal Disease

Progression
■ Moderate
□ Rapid
■ None

Fig. 73.2 Progression of periodontal disease in an untreated population. *(Data from Löe H, Anerud A, Boysen H, et al: Natural history of periodontal disease in man: rapid, moderate and no loss of attachment in Sri Lankan laborers 14 to 46 years of age.* J Clin Periodontol *13:431, 1986.)*

Mean Loss of Attachment at Various Ages (mm)

Age	Progression Group	
	Rapid	**Moderate**
35	9	4
45	13	7

Fig. 73.3 Loss of attachment in untreated Sri Lankan laborers. *(Data from Löe H, Anerud A, Boysen H, et al: Natural history of periodontal disease in man: rapid, moderate and no loss of attachment in Sri Lankan laborers 14 to 46 years of age.* J Clin Periodontol *13:431, 1986.)*

healthy and in excellent physical condition by local standards, and their nutritional condition was clinically fair. The workers had never been exposed to any programs relative to the prevention or treatment of dental diseases. Oral care was unknown, and dental caries was virtually nonexistent.

The results of this study are interesting. As the members of the Norwegian group approached 40 years of age, the mean individual loss of attachment was slightly above 1.5 mm and the mean annual rate of attachment loss was 0.08 mm for interproximal surfaces and 0.1 mm for buccal surfaces. As the Sri Lankans approached 40 years of age, the mean individual loss of attachment was 4.5 mm, and the mean annual rate of progression of the lesion was 0.3 mm for interproximal surfaces and 0.2 mm for buccal surfaces. Fig. 73.1 shows a graphic interpretation of the difference between the two groups. This study suggests that without oral care, periodontal lesions progress continually and at a relatively even pace.

Further analysis of the Sri Lankan laborers showed that they were not all losing attachment at the same rate (Figs. 73.2 and 73.3).[20] Virtually all gingival areas showed inflammation, but attachment loss varied tremendously. Based on interproximal loss of attachment

and tooth mortality, three subpopulations were identified as individuals with "rapid progression" (RP) of periodontal disease (8%), individuals with "moderate progression" (MP) (81%), and individuals who exhibited "no progression" (NP) of periodontal disease beyond gingivitis (11%). At age 35, the mean loss of attachment in the RP group was 9 mm; in the MP group, 4 mm; and in the NP group, less than 1 mm. At the age of 45, the mean loss of attachment in the RP group was 13 mm and in the MP group it was 7 mm. Therefore under natural conditions and in the absence of therapy, 89% of the Sri Lankan laborers had severe periodontitis that progressed at a much greater rate than that observed in the Norwegian group.

In the previously discussed study of General Telephone workers in California, loss of attachment was measured clinically and alveolar bone loss was measured radiographically.[36,37] After 3 years, the control group showed loss of attachment at a rate more than three times that of the matching experimental group during the same period (Fig. 73.4). In addition, subjects who received frequent oral prophylaxis and were instructed in good oral hygiene practices showed less bone loss radiographically after 3 years than did control subjects. It is clear that loss of attachment can be reduced by good oral hygiene and frequent dental prophylaxis.

Treatment of Loss of Attachment

A longitudinal study of patients with moderate-to-advanced periodontal disease conducted at the University of Michigan indicated that the progression of periodontal disease can be terminated for 3 years postoperatively regardless of the modality of treatment.[29-32] With long-term observations, the average loss of attachment was only

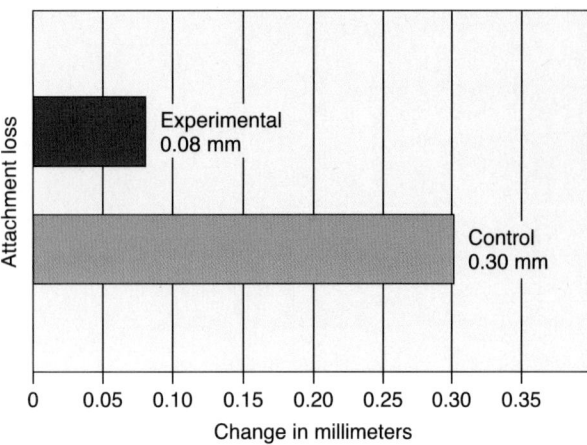

Fig. 73.4 Change in mean attachment level from baseline to third-year examination for experimental and control groups. *(From Suomi JD, Greene JC, Vermillion JR, et al: The effect of controlled oral hygiene procedures on the progression of periodontal disease in adults: results after third and final year.* J Periodontol *42:152, 1971.)*

0.3 mm over 7 years.[30] These results indicated a more favorable prognosis for treatment of advanced periodontal lesions than previously assumed.

LEARNING BOX 73.3

Patient compliance for regular, thorough biofilm removal by the patient with periodic maintenance therapy can predictably stop ongoing attachment loss.

Another study was conducted in 75 patients with advanced periodontal disease to determine the effect of biofilm control and surgical pocket elimination on the establishment and maintenance of periodontal health.[16] This study indicated that no further alveolar bone loss occurred during the 5-year observation period. The meticulous biofilm control practiced by the patients in this study was considered a major factor in the excellent results produced. After 14 years, results for 61 of the initial 75 individuals were reported.[14] Repeated examinations demonstrated that treatment of advanced forms of periodontal disease resulted in clinically healthy periodontal conditions and that this state of health was maintained in most patients and sites during the 14-year period. A more detailed analysis of the data, however, revealed that a small number of sites in a few patients lost a substantial amount of attachment. Approximately 43 surfaces in 15 different patients were exposed to recurrent periodontal disease of significant magnitude. The frequency of sites that lost more than 2 mm of attachment during the 14 years of maintenance was 0.8% to 0.1% per year.

Neither of these studies used a control group because failing to treat advanced periodontal patients cannot be justified for ethical reasons. However, in a study in a private practice, an effort was made to find and evaluate patients with diagnosed moderate-to-advanced periodontitis who had not followed through with recommended periodontal therapy.[3] Thirty patients ranging in age from 25 to 71 years were evaluated after periods ranging from 18 to 115 months. All of these untreated patients had progressive increases in pocket depth and radiographic evidence of progressive bone resorption.

In a study of the progression of periodontal disease in the absence of therapy, two different populations were monitored.[18] One group

TABLE 73.1 Average Loss of Teeth During a 5-Year Period Compared With Normal Loss of Teeth in 1428 Men and Women Ages 20 Through 59

	GRADE OF ORAL HYGIENE		
	Good	Fairly Good	Not Good
"Normal" loss of teeth[a]	1.1	1.4	1.8
Actual loss of teeth during 5-year period	0.4	0.6	0.9

[a]Estimate based on data recorded at initiation of study period.
From Lovdal A, Arno A, Schei O, et al: Combined effect of subgingival scaling and controlled oral hygiene on the incidence of gingivitis. *Acta Odontol Scand* 19:537, 1961.

of 64 Swedish adults with mild-to-moderate periodontal disease and one group of 36 American adults with advanced destructive disease were monitored but not treated for 6 years and 1 year, respectively. During the course of 6 years, 11.6% of all sites in the Swedish population (1.9% per year) showed attachment loss of greater than 2 mm, and the corresponding figure for the American population was 3.2% per year. Thus the frequency of sites with disease progression was 20 to 30 times higher in untreated groups of patients than in the treated and well-maintained groups described in the preceding discussion.[18] Thus treatment is effective in reducing loss of attachment.

Tooth Mortality

The ultimate test for the effectiveness of periodontal treatment is whether the loss of teeth can be prevented. Sufficient studies from both private practice and research institutions are now available to document that therapy reduces or prevents loss of teeth.

The combined effect of subgingival scaling every 3 to 6 months and controlled oral hygiene was evaluated over a 5-year period in 1428 factory workers in Oslo.[22] Tooth loss was significantly reduced in all patients. This study showed that frequent subgingival scaling reduces tooth loss even when oral hygiene is "not good" (Table 73.1).

The previously mentioned longitudinal study conducted at the University of Michigan included 104 patients with a total of 2604 teeth.[29-32] After 1 to 7 years of treatment, 53 teeth were lost for various reasons (Table 73.2). Approximately 32 teeth were lost during the first and second years after the initiation of treatment. The remaining 21 teeth were lost in a random pattern over the next 6 years. Therefore the loss of teeth caused by advanced periodontal disease after treatment was minimal (1.15%).

Another study was undertaken to test the effect of periodontal therapy in cases of advanced disease.[16-17] The subjects were 75 patients who had lost 50% or more of their periodontal support (Fig. 73.5). Treatment consisted of oral hygiene measures, scaling procedures, extraction of untreatable teeth, periodontal surgery, and prosthetic therapy if indicated. After completion of periodontal treatment, none of the patients showed further loss of periodontal support for the next 5 years. None of the teeth were extracted in the 5-year post-treatment period. Patients in this study were selected because of their capacity to meet the high requirements of biofilm control after repeated instruction in oral hygiene techniques. This fact does not detract from the validity of the study but tends to indicate the etiologic importance of bacterial biofilm. The results indicate that periodontal surgery coupled with a detailed biofilm control program not only temporarily cures the disease but also reduces further progression

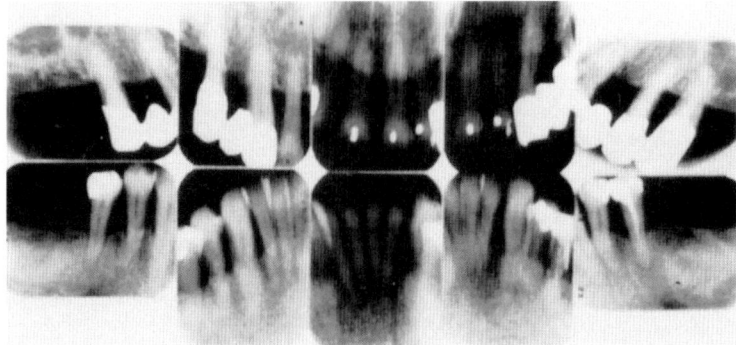

Fig. 73.5 Radiographs taken 5 years after typical periodontal treatment. Note the advanced bone loss, despite the teeth retained in a healthy condition for the duration of the study. *(From Lindhe J, Nyman S: The effect of plaque control and surgical pocket elimination on the establishment and maintenance of periodontal health: a longitudinal study of periodontal therapy in cases of advanced disease. J Clin Periodontol 2:67, 1975.)*

TABLE 73.2   Tooth Mortality After Treatment of Advanced Periodontitis in 104 Patients With 2604 Teeth Treated Over a 10-Year Period

Teeth Lost[a]	Reason
2	Pulpal disease
3	Accidents
4	Prosthetic considerations
14	Various reasons; for example, one patient wanted a maxillary denture for cosmetic reasons
30	Periodontal
53	All reasons

[a]Two percent of the teeth were lost during the study period. Note that US health surveys conducted in the 1960s indicated that an average of 4.3 teeth were lost after age 35 in the general population.[9]
Data from Ramfjord SP, Knowles JW, Nissle RR, et al: Longitudinal study of periodontal therapy. *J Periodontol* 44:66, 1973.

Cumulative Tooth Loss after 10-14 Years of Therapy in 61 Patients

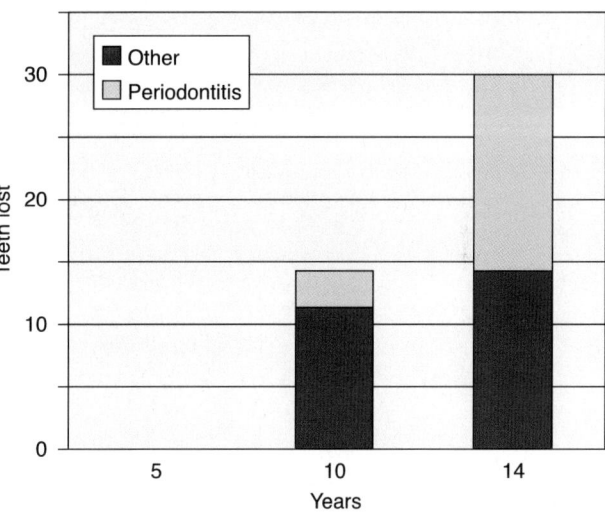

Fig. 73.6 Tooth loss in treated patients with very advanced periodontal disease. *(Data from Lindhe J, Nyman S: Long-term maintenance of patients treated for advanced periodontal disease. J Clin Periodontol 11:504, 1984.)*

of periodontal breakdown, even in patients with severely reduced periodontal support.

After 14 years, 61 of the original patients were still in the study.[17] Recurrence of destructive periodontal disease in isolated sites of the dentition resulted in loss of a certain number of teeth during the observation period (Fig. 73.6). In the 6 to 10 years after active therapy, one tooth in each of three different patients was lost, and during the final observation period (11 to 14 years), three teeth in one patient, two teeth in each of three patients, and one tooth in each of four patients had to be extracted because of recurrent periodontal disease. In addition, three teeth in each of three different patients and one tooth in each of five patients were extracted because of the development of extensive caries, periapical lesions, or other endodontic complications. Throughout the course of the study, the total loss was 30 teeth (for all reasons) from the total of 1330 teeth. Therefore the tooth mortality rate was 2.3%.

University-based studies on the treatment of moderate to severe periodontitis continue to show minimal tooth loss in patients who comply with periodontal maintenance therapy. [5,26]

Several studies in private practice have attempted to measure the frequency of tooth loss after periodontal therapy. In one study, 180 patients who had been treated for chronic destructive periodontal disease were evaluated.[33] The average age of the patients before treatment was 43.7 years. A total of 141 teeth were lost. From the

beginning of treatment to the time of the survey, the majority of patients did not lose any teeth (Fig. 73.7). Three of 180 patients (1.7%) lost 35 teeth; approximately 25% of the teeth were lost. Twelve additional patients lost 46 teeth, or 32.6% of the teeth were lost. Many patients in the study had advanced alveolar bone loss, including extensive furcation involvements. However, only a relatively small number (141) of the teeth were lost in the study group of 180 patients between the beginning of periodontal treatment and the time of the study.

The teeth were lost for several reasons, including periodontal disease, caries, and other nonperiodontal causes. The length of time after treatment varied from 2 to 20 years, with an average of 8.6 years. Of considerable significance is the large number of teeth (81 teeth, or 57.5%) lost by a few patients (15 patients, or 8.4%). Even when this group is considered with the remaining 165 patients, the periodontal care helped to retain most teeth because the average loss was slightly less than one tooth (0.9) over the 10 years after treatment.

In a follow-up study, the long-term results of periodontal therapy were evaluated after 15 to 34 years (average of 22.2 years).[7] The average tooth loss at this time was 1.6 teeth per 10 years. Patients

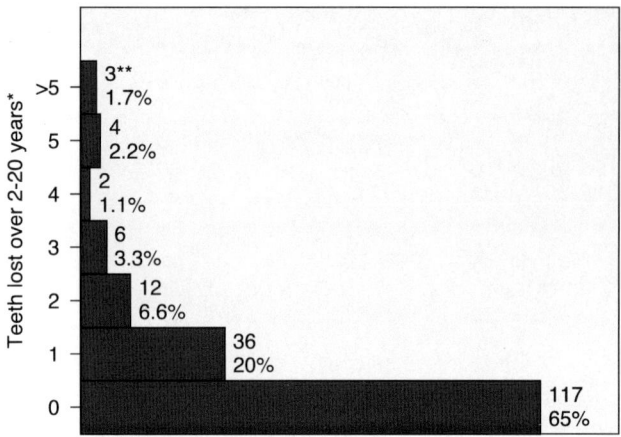

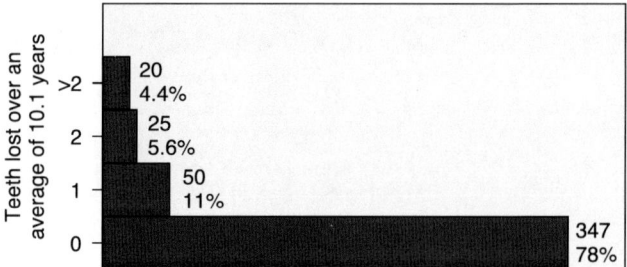

Fig. 73.9 Tooth mortality in 442 periodontal patients treated over 10 years. *(Courtesy Dr. R.C. Oliver, Rio Verde, AZ.)*

*Average of 8.6 years.
**3 patients lost 35 teeth.

The average tooth loss per patient was 0.9 per 10 years.

Fig. 73.7   Tooth mortality. Average tooth loss per patient was 0.9 per 10 years. *(Modified from Ross IF, Thompson RH, Galdi M: The results of treatment: a long term study of one hundred and eighty patients.* Parodontologie *25:125, 1971.)*

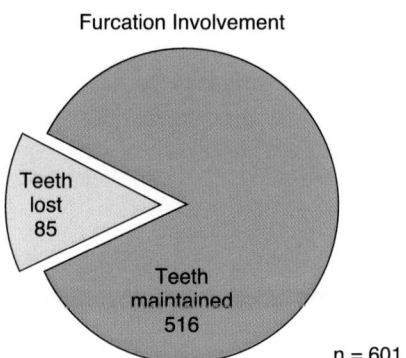

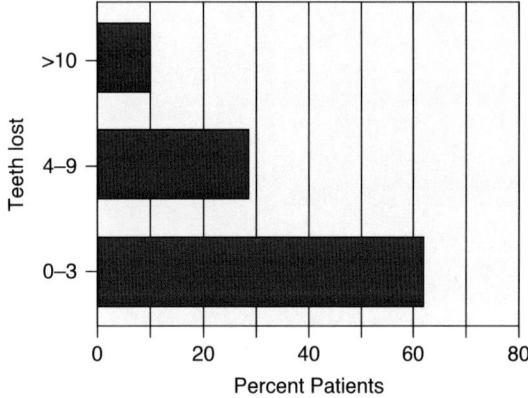

Fig. 73.8   Tooth mortality 15 to 34 years after initiation of therapy (average of 22.2 years). Average tooth loss per patient was 1.6 teeth per 10 years. Compare with the same study population in Fig. 73.7. As the treated population ages, the rate of bone loss appears to increase. *(Modified from Goldman MJ, Ross IF, Goteiner D: Effect of periodontal therapy on patients maintained for 15 years or longer: a retrospective study.* J Periodontol *57:347, 1986.)*

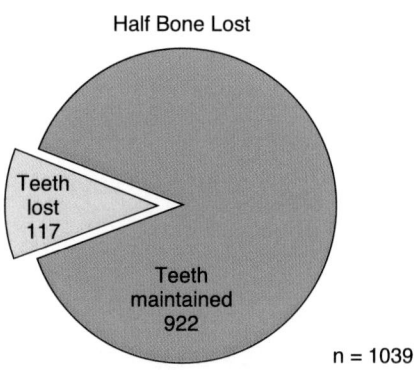

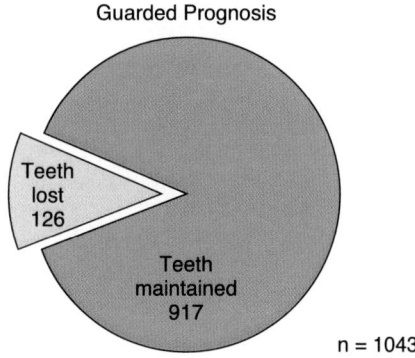

Fig. 73.10   Loss of teeth with advanced periodontal disease over 10 years. *(Courtesy Dr. R.C. Oliver, Rio Verde, AZ.)*

were classified into three groups according to tooth loss. Approximately 62% had an average tooth loss of 0.45 per 10 years and were considered "well maintained"; 28% lost an average of 2.6 teeth per 10 years and were considered "downhill"; and 10% lost an average of 6.4 teeth per 10 years and were considered "extreme downhill" (Fig. 73.8).

Another study included all patients in a practice who had been treated 5 or more years previously and had received regular preventive periodontal care since that time.[28] The 442 patients had an average of 10.1 years since treatment. Two-thirds of the patients were older than 40 years of age at the time of treatment. These patients had been seen every 4.6 months, on average, for their preventive periodontal care, which consisted of oral hygiene instruction and prophylaxis (Figs. 73.9 and 73.10).

The total tooth loss resulting from periodontal disease was 178 of more than 11,000 teeth available for treatment. More important, 78% of the patients did not lose a single tooth after periodontal therapy, and 11% lost only one tooth. Considering that more than 600 teeth had furcation involvements at the time of the original treatment and that far more than 1000 teeth had less than half the alveolar bone support remaining, there was minimal tooth loss. During the same average 10-year period after periodontal therapy, only 45 teeth were lost through caries or pulpal involvement. Even more surprising are the statistics over an average 10-year period for teeth with a poor prognosis. Only 85 (14%) of a total of 601 teeth with furcation involvement were lost, and 117 (11%) of 1039 teeth with half or less of the bone remaining were lost. Of the 1043 teeth listed as having a "guarded prognosis" by the clinician performing the initial examination, only 126 (12%) were lost over this 10-year period. The average tooth mortality rate was 0.72 tooth lost per patient per 10 years.

In a third study in a private practice, 600 patients were followed for 15 to 53 years after periodontal therapy (Figs. 73.11 and 73.12).[10] The majority (76.5%) had advanced periodontal disease at the start of treatment. There were 15,666 teeth present, for an average of 26 teeth per patient. During the follow-up period (an average of 22 years), a total of 1312 teeth were lost from all causes. Of this number, 1110 were lost for periodontal reasons. The average tooth mortality rate per patient was 2.2 teeth, and when this is converted to a 10-year rate, an average of one tooth was lost per 10 years in each patient. During this period of observation, 666 teeth with a questionable prognosis were lost out of a total of 2141. This means that 31% of the teeth with a questionable prognosis were lost over 22 years of treatment. A total of 1464 teeth with furcation involvement were

treated, and 31.6% were lost during the period of study. Approximately 83% of the patients lost fewer than three teeth over the 22-year average treatment period and were classified as "well maintained." The remaining 17% of the patients were divided into two groups: "downhill" (4 to 9 teeth lost) or "extreme downhill" (10 to 23 teeth lost). Thus 17% of the patients studied accounted for 69% of the teeth lost from periodontal causes. This study also indicated that relatively few teeth are lost after periodontal therapy. In addition, few teeth with a guarded prognosis, including those with furcation involvement, are lost, and a small percentage of patients lose most of the teeth.

Clinical studies have also indicated a relatively low rate of tooth loss in patients who are involved in a supportive periodontal maintenance program. One study showed that 0.9% of teeth were lost over 7.8 years, whereas another showed 1.5% were lost over a 9.8-year period after the initiation of active periodontal treatment.[4,6] Another study showed that questionable teeth in patients with aggressive periodontitis can be maintained for longer than 15 years if the patient is compliant.[41]

A study at the University of Bern looked at the outcome of multirooted teeth treated for longer than 11.5 years.[42] The study found that grade 1 furcation status was not a risk factor for tooth loss compared with no furcation bone loss in patients treated for periodontal disease. Risk factors for the loss of multirooted teeth included furcation involvements grades 2 and 3, smoking, and lack of compliance with regular maintenance therapy (Fig. 73.13).

Three studies give insight into tooth mortality in untreated patients. The studies of Löe and coworkers[20,21] in Sri Lankan laborers showed that after age 35, an average of 5 and 16 teeth were lost per 10 years in the "moderate progression" and "rapid progression" groups, respectively (Fig. 73.14). In a previously discussed study in private practice,[3] an effort was made to find and evaluate patients with diagnosed moderate-to-advanced periodontitis who did not follow through with recommended periodontal therapy. Patients with untreated periodontal disease were losing teeth at a rate greater than 0.61 per year (6.1 teeth per 10 years). A total of 83 teeth were lost in 30 patients, but the investigators excluded one patient who had lost 25 teeth. Including this patient would have increased the tooth loss in untreated patients to an even higher rate. In another study, reporting on patients with moderate-to-advanced periodontitis examined at the Department of Periodontology at the University of Kiel in Germany, Kocher and associates[12] found a marked increase in tooth loss in the untreated patients compared with the treated patients when they were examined after 7 years.

When Tables 73.3 and 73.4 are compared, it is obvious that tooth mortality is much greater in untreated groups.

Conclusion

The prevalence of periodontal disease and the resulting high rate of tooth mortality have increased the need for effective treatment. Strong evidence now indicates that periodontal disease can contribute to numerous health problems, including pregnancy complications, heart disease, stroke, and diabetes.[25,27,34,35] For patients with periodontitis, treatment effectively prevents periodontal disease and stops the

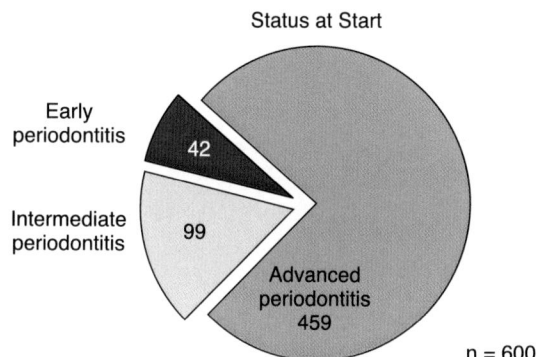

Fig. 73.11 Status at the start of a study of 600 patients. *(Data from Hirschfeld L, Wasserman B: A long-term survey of tooth loss in 600 treated periodontal patients.* J Periodontol *49:225, 1978.)*

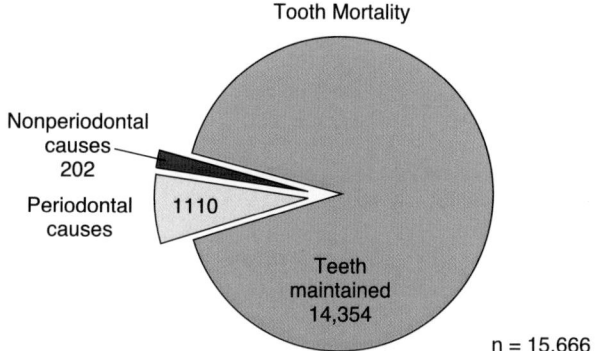

Fig. 73.12 Loss of teeth in 600 patients over 15 to 53 years from nonperiodontal and periodontal causes. *(Data from Hirschfeld L, Wasserman B: A long-term survey of tooth loss in 600 treated periodontal patients.* J Periodontol *49:225, 1978.)*

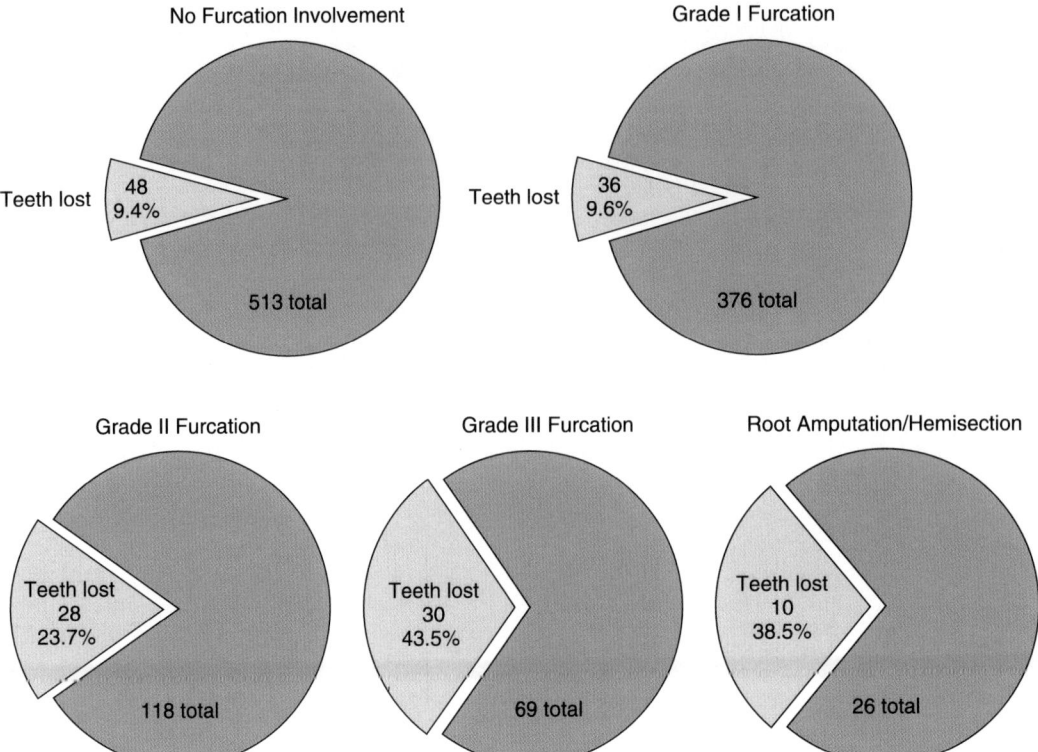

Fig. 73.13 Loss of multirooted teeth during 11.5 years of supportive periodontal therapy. *(Data from Salvi GE, Mischler DC, Schmidlin K, et al: Risk factors associated with longevity of multi-rooted teeth: long-term outcomes after active supportive periodontal therapy. J Clin Periodontol 41:701–707, 2014.)*

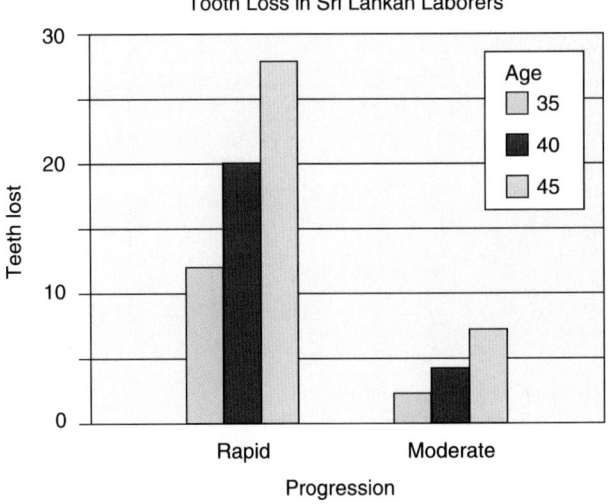

Fig. 73.14 Tooth loss in a population with untreated periodontal disease. *(Data from Löe H, Anerud A, Boysen H, et al: Natural history of periodontal disease in man: rapid, moderate and no loss of attachment in Sri Lankan laborers 14 to 46 years of age. J Clin Periodontol 13:431, 1986.)*

TABLE 73.3 Tooth Mortality in Treated Periodontitis Patients

Study	Average Number of Teeth Lost per 10 Years With Periodontal Treatment[a]
Hirschfeld and Wasserman[10]	1.0
Kocher et al.[12]	1.6
McFall[23]	1.4
Oliver[28]	0.7
Ross et al.[33]	0.9
Goldman et al.[7]	1.6
McLeod et al.[24]	1.5
Tsami et al.[39] (nonsmokers)	1.7
Tsami et al.[39] (smokers)	3.7
Ng et al.[26] (compliant with maintenance)	0.8
Ng et al.[26] (noncompliant with maintenance)	2.8
Costa et al.[40] (compliant with maintenance)	1.2
Costa et al.[40] (noncompliant with maintenance)	3.6
Graetz et al.[41] (aggressive periodontitis)	1.4
Graetz et al.[41] (chronic periodontitis)	1.6

[a]Tooth mortality adjusted to 10 years by chapter author.

TABLE 73.4 Tooth Mortality in Untreated Periodontitis Patients

Study	Average Number of Teeth Lost per 10 Years Without Periodontal Treatment[a]
Becker et al[3]	6
Kocher et al[12]	5
Löe et al[20] (moderate progression)	5
Löe et al[20] (rapid progression)	16

[a]Tooth mortality adjusted to 10 years by chapter author.

progression of the disease. In addition, overwhelming evidence suggests that periodontal therapy greatly reduces tooth mortality. Every dental practitioner should be familiar with the philosophy, recognition, and techniques for periodontal therapy. Failure to diagnose and treat periodontal disease or not to make periodontal treatment available to patients causes unnecessary dental problems and tooth loss and places the patient at risk for other systemic health problems.

 A Case Scenario is found on the companion website www.expertconsult.com.

References

 References for this chapter are found on the companion website *www.expertconsult.com*.

CHAPTER 74

Peri-implant Anatomy, Biology, and Function

Joseph Fiorellini | Keisuke Wada | Hector Leonardo Sarmiento | Perry R. Klokkevold

CHAPTER OUTLINE

Implant Geometry (Macrodesign)
Implant Surface Characteristics (Microdesign) *(e-only)*

Hard Tissue Interface
Soft Tissue Interface

Clinical Comparison of Teeth and Implants
Conclusion

 For online-only content on endosseous implants, root form (cylindrical) implants, transmandibular implants, subperiosteal implants, and implant surface characteristics (microdesign), go to the companion website at www.expertconsult.com. Some figures may be out of numeric order in this printed chapter.

The history of modern implant dentistry began with the introduction of titanium implants.[41] In the 1950s, Per-Ingvar Brånemark, a Swedish professor of anatomy, had a serendipitous finding while studying blood circulation in bone that became a historical breakthrough in medicine. He discovered an intimate bone-to-implant apposition with titanium that offered sufficient strength to cope with load transfer. He called the phenomenon *osseointegration* and developed an implant system with a specific protocol to predictably achieve it. The implants were used to anchor prosthetic replacement teeth in the edentulous jaw,[27] and the first patient was successfully treated in 1965.[30,72] Subsequent clinical studies proved that commercially pure (CP) titanium implants, placed with a strict protocol, including an unloaded healing period, could predictably achieve osseointegration and retain a full-arch prosthesis in function with long-term success (15 years).[8]

FLASH BACK

The history of modern implant dentistry began with the introduction of titanium implants. In the 1950s, Per-Ingvar Brånemark, a Swedish professor of anatomy, had a serendipitous finding while studying blood circulation in bone that became a historical breakthrough in medicine. He coined the phenomenon *osseointegration* and developed an implant system with a specific protocol to achieve it predictably.

Today, implant designs, surgical placement techniques, healing times, and restorative protocols continue to evolve with the goal of improving outcomes. It is important for clinicians to know peri-implant anatomy, to understand the biology, and to appreciate the functional capacity of osseointegrated implants. This chapter reviews implant geometry and surface characteristics, as well as the anatomic and biologic relationships of peri-implant tissues.

Implant Geometry (Macrodesign)

Numerous implant systems with various geometric (macrodesign) designs have been developed and used before the current implant systems in use today. Previous implant designs included blade vents (narrow, flat shape; tapped into bony trough prepared with rotary burs),[69] press-fit cylindrical (bullet shape; pressed or tapped into prepared hole),[102] subperiosteal (custom-made framework; adapted to the surface of jawbone),[37] and transmandibular (long rods or posts; placed through the anterior mandible).[107] Some of these implant systems were initially stable and appeared to be successful over short-term periods (e.g., 5 years) but failed to remain stable, became symptomatic or loose, and failed over longer periods.[100,124] Lacking predictability, these implant systems are no longer used.

Since the time of the Brånemark studies, millions of patients have been treated worldwide using variations of these techniques with implants of different geometries and surface characteristics. Similar research including that of André Schroeder in Switzerland in the mid-1970s contributed to the success of endosseous dental implants. The serendipitous finding of Brånemark was that when a hole is prepared into bone without overheating or otherwise traumatizing the tissues, an inserted biocompatible implantable device would predictably achieve an intimate bone apposition, as long as micromovements at the interface were prevented during the early healing period. The history of the research endeavors in Sweden provides a better understanding of the relevant biologic parameters involved.[72]

The macroscopic configuration of implants has varied widely; the most common types are listed in Box 74.1. Currently, most endosseous implants have a cylindrical or tapered, screw-shaped/threaded design. The disastrous results with other implant configurations were largely responsible for the evolution toward the current popular designs.[13] See online for a detailed description of the various implant designs including blades, pins, disks, root form, transmandibular, and subperiosteal implants.

Hard Tissue Interface

The primary goal of implant installation is to achieve and maintain a stable bone-to-implant connection (i.e., osseointegration).[29,30] Histologically, osseointegration is defined as the direct structural and functional connection between ordered, living bone and the surface of a load-bearing implant without intervening soft tissues (Fig. 74.1).[27,28] Clinically, osseointegration is the asymptomatic rigid fixation of an alloplastic material (implant) in bone with the ability to withstand occlusal forces.[12,126] The hard tissue interface is a fundamental requirement for and an essential component of implant success.

> ### KEY FACT
>
> Histologically, osseointegration is defined as the direct structural and functional connection between ordered, living bone and the surface of a load-bearing implant without intervening soft tissues. Clinically, osseointegration is the rigid fixation of an alloplastic material (implant) in bone with the ability to withstand occlusal forces.

Initial Bone Healing

The osseointegration process observed after implant insertion can be compared with bone fracture healing. Implant site osteotomy preparation (bone wounding) initiates a sequence of events, including an inflammatory reaction, bone resorption, release of growth factors, and attraction by chemotaxis of osteoprogenitor cells to the site. Differentiation of osteoprogenitor cells into osteoblasts leads to bone formation at the implant surface. Extracellular matrix proteins, such as osteocalcin, modulate apatite crystal growth.[123] Specific conditions, optimal for bone formation, must be maintained at the healing site to achieve osseointegration.

Immobility of the implant relative to the bone must be maintained for bone formation at the surface. A mild inflammatory response enhances the bone healing, but moderate inflammation or movement above a certain threshold is detrimental.[6] When micromovements at the interface exceed 150 μm, the movement will impair differentiation of osteoblasts and fibrous scar tissue will form between the bone and implant surface.[91] Therefore it is important to avoid excessive forces, such as occlusal loading, during the early healing period.

BOX 74.1 Implant Geometry (Macrodesign)

1. Endosseous implants
   - Blade like
   - Pins
   - Root form, cylindrical (hollow and full)
   - Disk like
   - Screw shaped
   - Tapered and screw shaped
2. Subperiosteal (custom frame) implants
3. Transmandibular implants

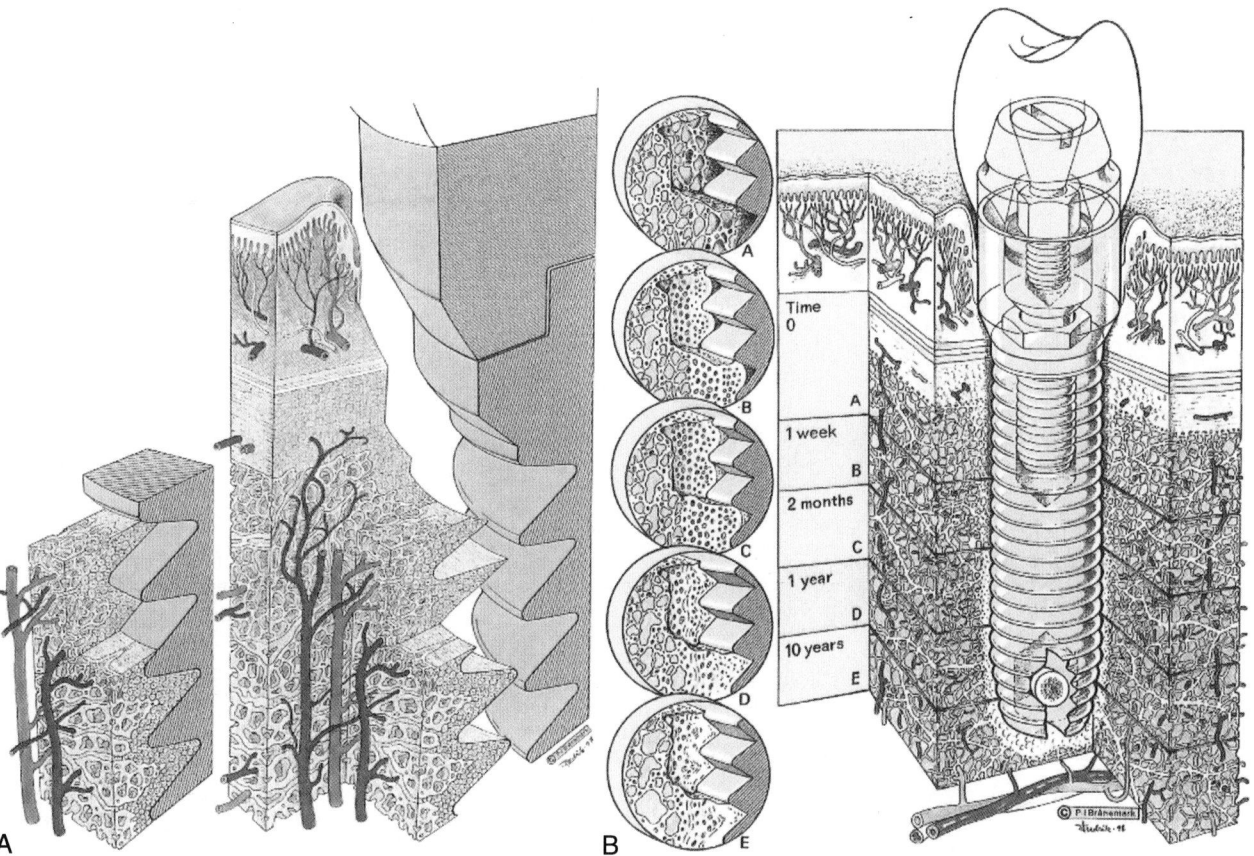

Fig. 74.1 (A) Three-dimensional diagram of the tissue and titanium interrelationship showing an overall view of the intact interfacial zone around the osseointegrated implant. (B) Physiologic evolution of the biology of the interface over time.

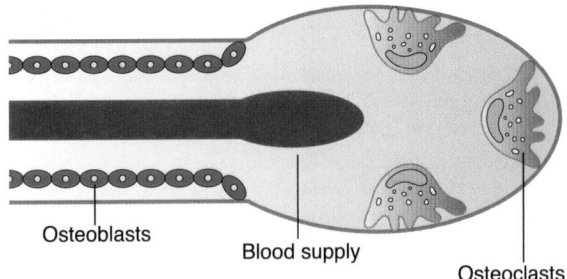

Osteoblasts

Blood supply

Osteoclasts

Fig. 74.2 The basic multicellular unit is the basic remodeling process for bone renewal. Osteoclasts are imported by the vascular supply, and the resorption lacunae are soon filled by the lining osteoblasts.

Bone tissue damage and debris created by the osteotomy site preparation must be cleared up by osteoclasts for normal bone healing. These multinuclear cells, originating from the blood, can resorb bone at a pace of 50 to 100 μm per day. There is a coupling between bone apposition and bone resorption (Fig. 74.2). Preosteoblasts, derived from primary mesenchymal cells, depend on a favorable oxidation-reduction (redox) potential of the environment. Thus a proper vascular supply and oxygen tension are needed. If oxygen tension is poor, the primary stem cells may differentiate into fibroblasts, form scar tissue, and lead to implant failure (nonintegration).

If bone is overheated or crushed during preparation, it will become necrotic and may lead to nonmineralized (soft tissue) scar formation or be sequestered. The critical temperature for bone cells that should not be exceeded is 47°C (116.6°F) at an exposure time of 1 minute.[6] Thus preparation of implant osteotomy sites requires profuse irrigation (cooling) along with gentle, intermittent, moderate-speed drilling using sharp drills. Another complicating factor, well recognized from open wound fractures, is that microbial contamination jeopardizes the normal bone healing. Accordingly, strict aseptic techniques should be maintained.

KEY FACT

Immobility of the implant must be maintained during the early postinsertion healing for bone formation at the surface. Moderate inflammation or movement above a certain threshold is detrimental and may lead to implant failure. If micromovements exceed 150 μm, the movement will impair the differentiation of osteoblasts, and fibrous scar tissue will form between the bone and implant surface.

New bone formation follows a specific sequence of events. Woven bone is quickly formed in the gap between the implant and the bone; it grows fast, up to 100 μm per day, and in all directions. Characterized by a random orientation of its collagen fibrils, high cellularity, and limited degree of mineralization, the biomechanical capacity of woven bone is poor (Fig. 74.3A). Thus any occlusal load should be well controlled or avoided in the early phase of healing. After several months, woven bone is progressively replaced by lamellar bone with organized, parallel layers of collagen fibrils and dense mineralization. Contrary to the fast-growing woven bone, lamellar bone formation occurs at a slow pace (only a few microns per day). Ultimately, after 18 months of healing, a steady state is reached where lamellar bone is continuously resorbed and replaced (Fig. 74.3B).[27] At the light microscopic level, an intimate bone-to-implant contact has been extensively reported (Fig. 74.4).[98] Once the bone-to-implant interface has reached a steady state, it can maintain itself over decades, as

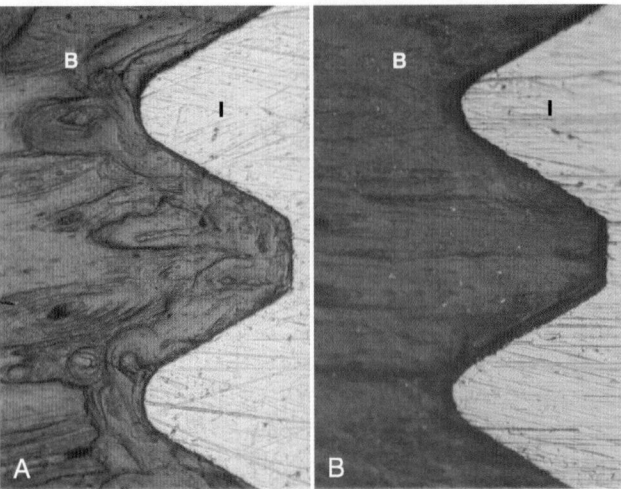

Fig. 74.3 (A) After initial healing, woven bone, as characterized by its irregular pattern, is laid down. (B) After weeks or months, progressively a lamellar bone is laid down, with regular concentric lamellae. *B,* Bone; *I,* implant. *(Courtesy Professor T. Albrektsson, Gothenburg, Sweden.)*

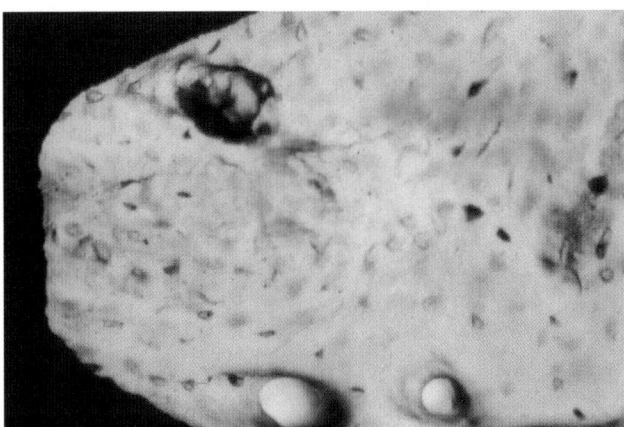

Fig. 74.4 Once a steady state has been achieved at the bone-to-implant interface, an intimate contact can be observed, with some marrow spaces seen in between at the light microscopic level.

ascertained by human histology from implants retrieved because of hardware fractures.[10]

FLASH BACK

The biomechanical capacity of woven bone is poor. New bone formation adjacent to an implant follows a specific sequence of events with woven bone forming quickly in the gap; it grows fast (100 μm per day) and in all directions. It is characterized by a random orientation of its collagen fibrils, high cellularity, and a limited degree of mineralization.

Bone Remodeling and Function

Clinically, both primary stability and secondary stability of an implant are critical to success. Primary stability, achieved at the time of surgical placement, depends on the implant geometry (macrodesign), as well as the quality and quantity of bone available for implant anchorage at a specific site. Studies using resonance frequency analysis (RFA) have reported decreased implant stability in the early weeks of postinsertion healing.[18,44,56,93] Secondary stability, achieved over time with healing, depends on the implant surface (microdesign), as well as the quality and quantity of adjacent bone, which will determine the percentage of contacts between the implant and bone.[18,48,96,113] For example, areas such as the anterior mandible have dense cortical bone and provide rigid primary stabilization and good support throughout the healing process. Conversely, areas such as the posterior maxilla have thin cortical bone, and large marrow spaces provide less primary stability. For this reason, the posterior maxilla has been associated with lower success rates compared with other sites with greater bone density and support.[17,60] Interestingly, a new implant with unique knife-edge wide threads (macrodesign) has been shown, in completely healed sites, to maintain stability without the typical drop in the implant stability quotient (ISQ) through the early bone remodeling phase.[73]

Once osseointegration is achieved, implants can resist and function under the forces of occlusion for many years. Longitudinal biomechanical assessments seem to indicate that during the first weeks after placement of one-stage implants, decreased rigidity is observed.[46] This may be indicative of bone resorption during the initial phase of healing. Subsequently, rigidity increases and continues to increase for years.[112] Thus when a prosthesis is installed immediately (in 1 day) or early (in 1 to 2 weeks), care must be taken to control against overload. It is important to recognize that sites with limited primary stability or less bone-to-implant contact (e.g., posterior maxilla) will likely go through a period of even less bone support in the early stages of bone healing due to the initial phase of bone resorption.

Soft Tissue Interface

Not surprisingly, for two decades, research and clinical interest focused on the bone-to-implant interface of osseointegrated implants, and the overlying soft tissues were largely ignored. Except for a few descriptive sentences, the classic handbook by Brånemark and colleagues[27] presented no data or information about the soft tissue interface. This may be due in part to the fact that most patients were fully edentulous and the Brånemark system implants had turned (machined) surfaces, which are less likely to be associated with soft tissue inflammatory problems.[5] Today, there is greater interest in and appreciation for peri-implant soft tissues and the soft tissue-to-implant interface as a function of aesthetics and maintenance of a seal or barrier against microbial invasion.

Peri-implant soft tissues are similar in appearance and structure to periodontal soft tissues (see Chapter 3).[5] Clearly, both implants and teeth emerge through the soft tissues on the alveolar ridge. The soft tissues consist of connective tissue covered by epithelium. There is a gingival/mucosal sulcus, a long junctional epithelial attachment, and a zone of connective tissue above the supporting bone (Fig. 74.5). Despite the apparent similarities in soft tissues around teeth and implants, the presence of a periodontal ligament around teeth and not around implants is an important, distinct difference. Whereas natural teeth have a periodontal ligament with connective tissue fibers inserting into the cementum and suspending them in the alveolar bone, osseointegrated implants do not. There are no inserting collagen fibers anywhere along the interface of osseointegrated implants. Bone is in direct contact with the implant surface without intervening soft tissues.

 FLASH BACK

Sharpey's fibers are bundles of collagenous fibers that pass into the outer circumferential lamellae of alveolar bone and the cementum of teeth.

Clinically, the thickness of the peri-implant soft tissues varies from 2 to several millimeters (Fig. 74.6). An animal study determined the total height of the peri-implant "biologic width" to be approximately 3 to 4 mm, where about 2 mm is the epithelial attachment and about 1 to 2 mm is the supracrestal connective tissue zone.[19] Consistent with this finding, a human histologic study determined the height of the peri-implant "biologic width," consisting of an epithelial attachment and supracrestal connective tissue, to be about 4 to 4.5 mm[47] (Fig. 74.7).

Epithelium

As in the natural dentition, the oral epithelium around implants is continuous with a sulcular epithelium that lines the inner surface of the gingival sulcus; the apical part of the gingival sulcus is lined with long junctional epithelium.[71] Ultrastructural examination of the long junctional epithelial attachment adjacent to dental implants has demonstrated that epithelial cells attach with a basal lamina and hemidesmosomes[2,4,49,62,115] (Fig. 74.8). Histologic studies indicate that these epithelial structures and the surrounding lamina propria cannot be distinguished from those structures around teeth.[33] In health, the dimension of the sulcular epithelium is about 0.5 mm,[95] and the dimension of the epithelial attachment is about 2 mm,[19] which is higher than that of the periodontal epithelial attachment.

The apical edge of the epithelial attachment is about 1.5 to 2 mm above the bone margin.[89] In healthy peri-implant tissues, progressive epithelial downgrowth does not occur, indicating that factors other than inserted collagen fiber bundles (i.e., Sharpey's fibers in natural dentition) prevent it.

Connective Tissue

Peri-implant connective tissue morphology closely resembles that of the natural dentition except that it lacks a periodontal ligament, cementum, and inserting fibers (Fig. 74.9). No significant differences were found at the biochemical level between the peri-implant and the periodontal soft tissues,[34] whereas the dimension of the peri-implant connective tissue is 1 to 2 mm, which is higher than that of the average periodontal connective tissue.[19,89]

The zone of supracrestal connective tissue has an important function in the maintenance of a stable soft tissue–implant interface and as a seal or barrier to the "outside" oral environment. The orientation of connective tissue fibers adjacent to an implant differs from that of periodontal connective tissue fibers. In the absence of cementum and inserting connective tissue fibers (i.e., as in a natural tooth), most peri-implant connective tissue fibers run in a direction more or less parallel to the implant surface. Even when the fiber bundles are oriented perpendicularly, which occurs more often in the gingiva than in the mucosa surrounding implants, the bundles are never embedded in the implant surface.

The fiber bundles can also have a cufflike circular orientation.[20,93] The role of these fibers remains unknown, but it appears that their presence helps to create a soft tissue "seal" around the implant. The adaptation of the connective tissue to an implant surface may also be affected by the mobility of the soft tissue around the implant. The connective tissue in direct contact with the implant surface is characterized by an absence of blood vessels and an abundance of fibroblasts interposed between collagen fibers.[68] Several animal and human studies have shown that the alignments of connective fibers were circular and horizontal around the implants[1,15,35,48,51,52,99] (Fig. 74.10).

More recent studies have shown histologic evidence of connective tissue attachment perpendicular to the microgrooved implant surface on both animal and human studies.[78-80] These laser-microtextured grooves (Fig. 74.11) have been shown to be able to stop the epithelial

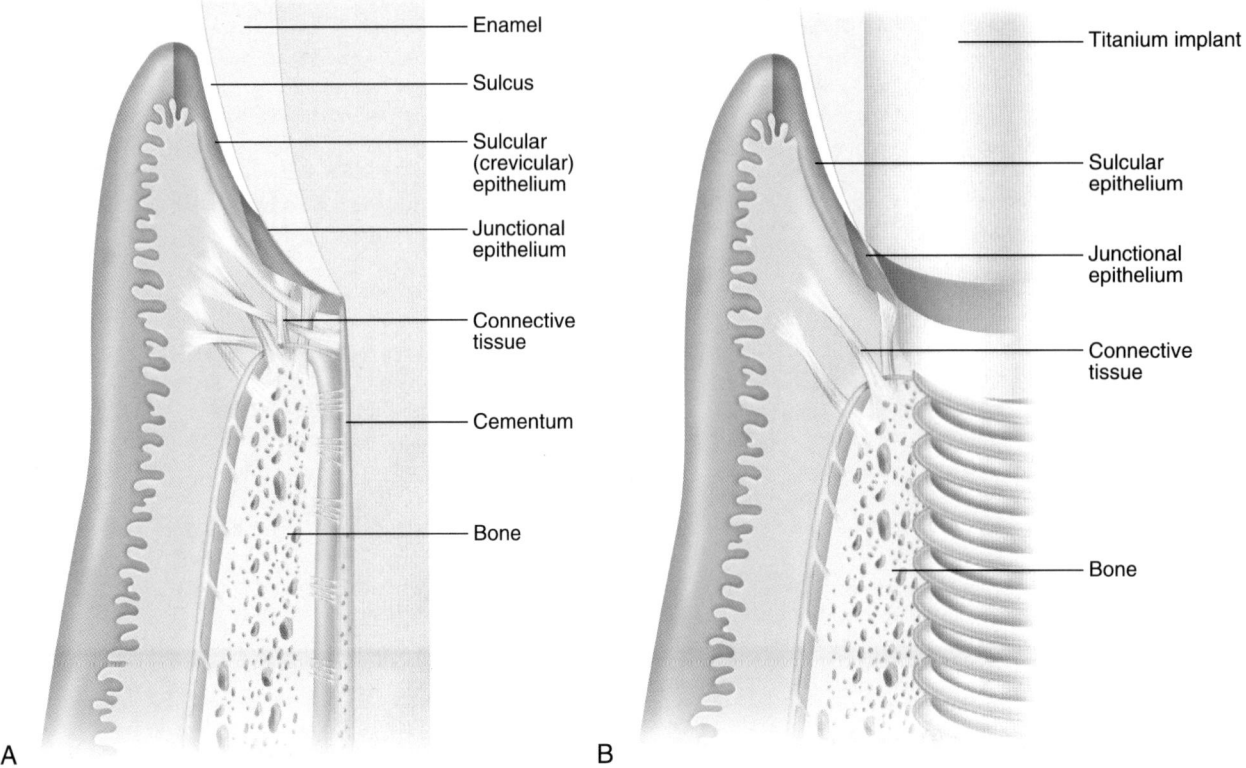

Fig. 74.5 Schematic illustration of hard and soft tissue around a tooth and an implant. (A) Hard and soft tissue anatomy around a natural tooth demonstrates bone support with a periodontal ligament, a connective tissue zone above the crest of bone with connective tissue fibers (Sharpey's) inserting into dentin, a long junctional epithelial attachment, a gingival sulcus lined with sulcular epithelium, and oral gingival epithelium (outer surface of gingiva). (B) Hard and soft tissue anatomy around an implant demonstrates some similarities and some distinct differences. There is supporting bone in direct approximation to the implant surface without any intervening soft tissues (i.e., no periodontal ligament). A connective tissue zone is present above the level of bone with fibers running parallel to the implant surface and no inserting fibers. There is a long junctional epithelial attachment, a gingival/mucosal sulcus lined with sulcular epithelium, and oral gingival/mucosal epithelium (outer surface of soft tissue). *(From Rose LF, Mealey BL:* Periodontics: medicine, surgery, and implants, *St. Louis, 2004, Mosby.)*

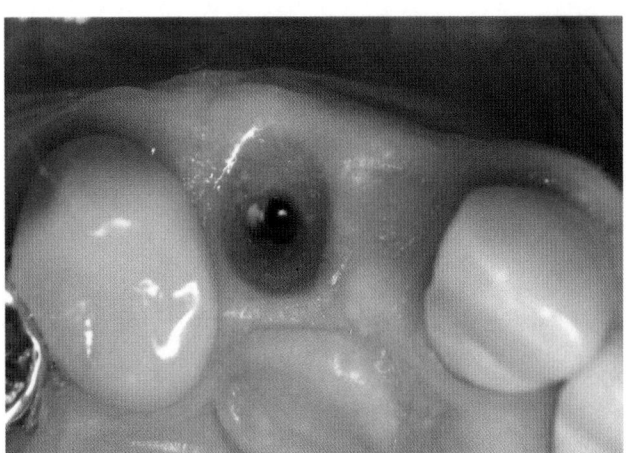

Fig. 74.6 Clinical appearance of normal, healthy peri-implant tissue with implant restoration removed. Soft tissue thickness varies from site to site, depending on quantity and quality of tissue, as well as the anatomy of the surrounding area (e.g., adjacent to natural teeth with healthy periodontal attachment versus adjacent to a space). Note that the intrasulcular tissue appears more erythematous as the result of the thin, nonkeratinized layer of epithelium overlying the connective tissue.

downgrowth and establish connective tissue insertion right at the most coronal part of the laser microgrooved area. (Fig. 74.12). A prospective controlled clinical study showed that laser-grooved surface resulted in shallower probing depth and less peri-implant crestal bone loss than that seen around implants with machined collars.[25,85]

This connective tissue interface has been examined by probing attachment level measurements in patients. Probing attachment levels were consistently found coronal to the alveolar crest in patients with peri-implant tissue health, indicating the presence of a zone of direct connective tissue contact to the implant surface. This means that the probing depth measurement performed with a periodontal probe may be about 1.5 mm higher above the bone level in healthy tissues. At inflamed sites, the probe may penetrate to the bone, with the probing depth measurement reflecting the total soft tissue thickness above bone. In cases with inflammatory peri-implant tissue disease, increasing probing depth and reduced attachment levels have been reported.[3,40,86,117]

Keratinized Tissue

Questions emerged decades ago, as it did for the natural dentition, about the need for keratinized tissue to surround implants. Prospective and cross-sectional studies, evaluating screw-shaped implants with a machined surface, suggest that the presence or absence of keratinized gingiva is not a prerequisite for long-term stability.[101] However, it has been suggested that implants surrounded by mucosa only (i.e.,

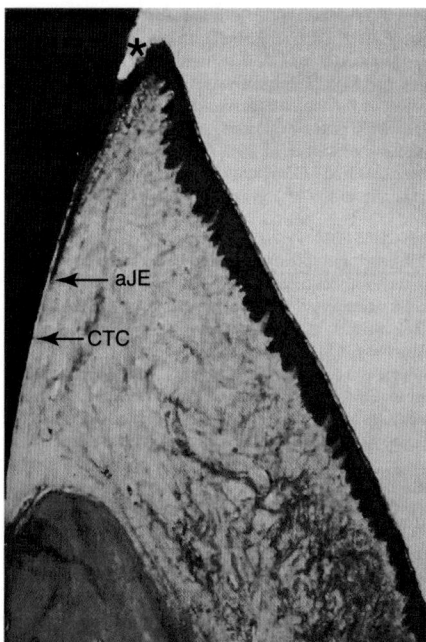

Fig. 74.7 Buccolingual section (basic fuchsin stain; original magnification, ×12.5; one-part SLA implant, 3 months unloaded) showing the gingiva and the most coronal part of alveolar bone. Rete peg formation is only apparent in the area of the keratinized oral gingival epithelium. The oral sulcular epithelium exhibits no keratinization. In the area of the most coronal point of the junctional epithelium (cJE), the soft tissues are slightly torn away (artifact) because of nondecalcified histologic processing. The most apical point of the junctional epithelium is indicated *(aJE)*. No rete peg formation is evident adjacent to the basal cell layer of the junctional epithelium (JE), all showing healthy and physiologic soft tissue structures. In addition, the area of connective tissue contact *(CTC)* adjacent to the machined titanium surface is marked. A slight round cell infiltrate in the connective tissue indicates a mild inflammation. Note bone remodeling/new bone formation in the crestal bone region indicated by saturated, dark red stained areas.

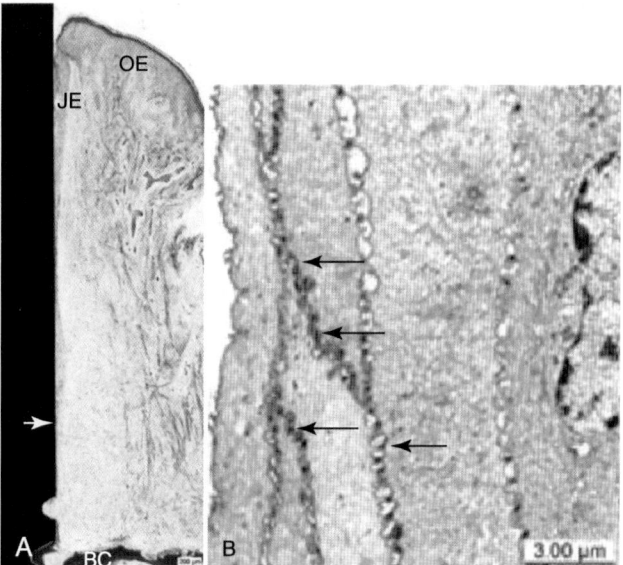

Fig. 74.8 (A) Overview of ground section showing peri-implant tissues covered with keratinizing oral epithelium *(OE)*. Junctional epithelium *(JE)* is interposed between connective tissue and alveolar bone crest *(BC)*. Apical end of junctional epithelium *(arrow)*. Toluidine blue stain. (Bar = 200 μm.) (B) Transmission electron microscopic view of sulcular epithelium showing tightly sealed intercellular spaces by numerous spot desmosomes *(arrows)*, contributing to low permeability of this portion of peri-implant mucosa. Bar = 3 μm.[14]

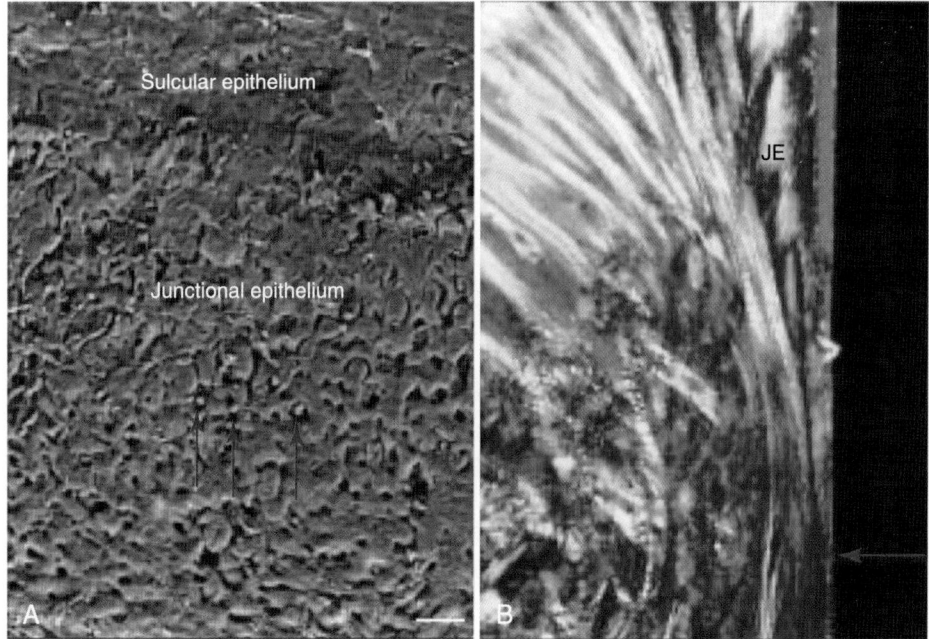

Fig. 74.9 (A) Scanning electron microscope (SEM) image of the junctional epithelium. Note the neutrophils located between the cells *(red arrows)*. Bar = 40 μm. (B) Higher magnification of Fig. 74.8 with polarized light showing the apical extent *(red arrow)* of the junctional epithelium *(JE)*. Note the dense collagen fibers running apicocoronal (i.e., parallel to the implant surface).

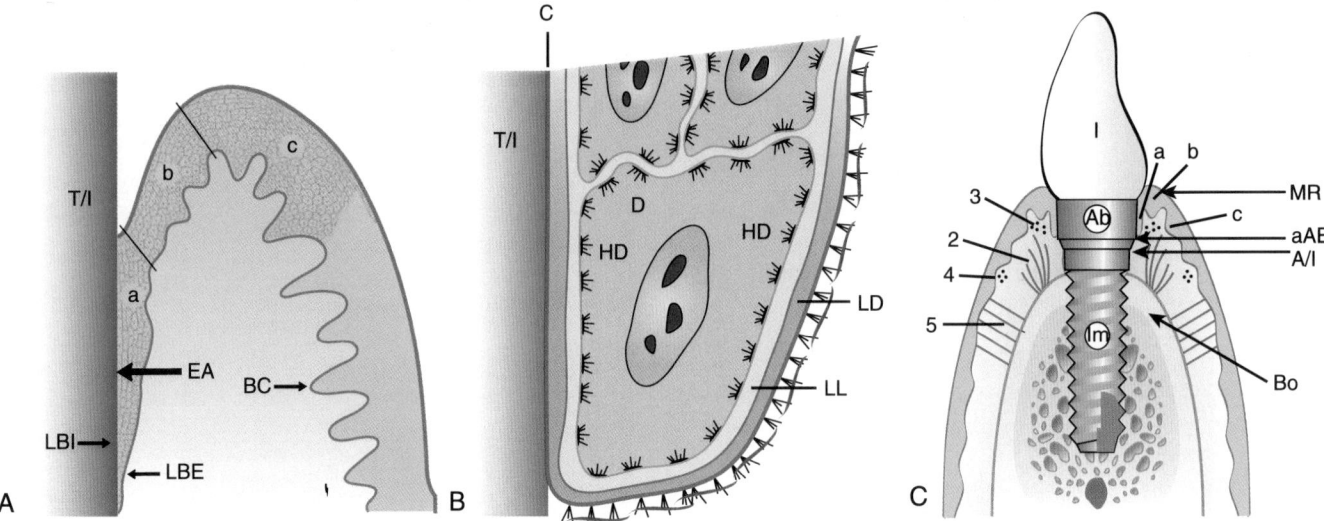

Fig. 74.10 (A) Histologic scheme of epithelial attachment *(EA)* (identical for tooth and implant). *T/I*, Titanium implant; *BC*, basal complex; *LBI*, lamina basalis interna; *LBE*, lamina basalis externa (only location where cell divisions occur); *a*, long junctional epithelial attachment zone; *b*, sulcular epithelial zone; *c*, oral epithelial zone. (B) At the electron microscopic level, basal complex at the epithelial attachment (three most apical cells) and connection with stroma. *HD*, Hemidesmosomes; *D*, desmosome; *LL*, lamina lucida; *LD*, lamina densa; *C*, cuticle. (C) Implant, abutment *(Ab)*, and crown within alveolar bone and soft tissues. *Im*, Endosseous part of implant; *MR*, margin of gingiva/alveolar mucosa; *Bo*, marginal bone level; *1*, implant crown; *2*, vertical alveolar-gingival connective tissue fibers; *3*, circular gingival connective tissue fibers; *4*, circular gingival connective tissue fibers; *5*, periosteal-gingival connective tissue fibers; *a*, junctional epithelium; *b*, sulcular epithelium; *c*, oral epithelium; *A/I*, abutment/implant junction; *aAE*, apical (point) of attached epithelium.

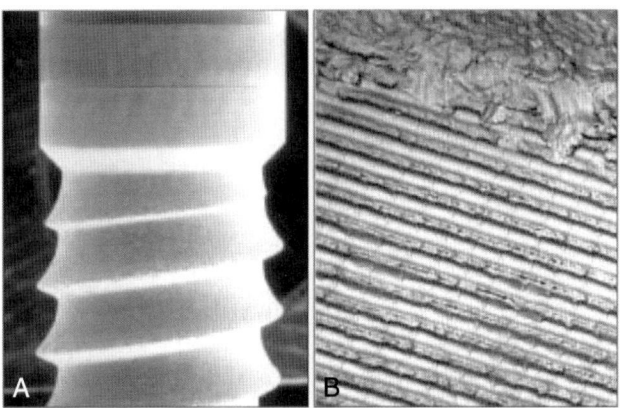

Fig. 74.11 (A) Laser-microtextured surface. (B) Machined collar, original magnification, ×500. *(Botos S, Yousef H, Zweig B, et al: The effects of laser microtexturing of the dental implant collar on crestal bone levels and peri-implant health.* Int J Oral Maxillofac Implants *26:492–498, 2011. With the permission of Dr. Spyros Botos.)*

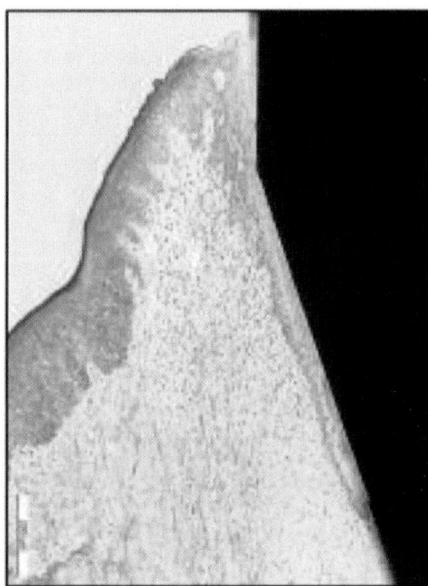

Fig. 74.12 Laser-ablated surface: epithelial downgrowth was stopped right at the coronal-most microgrooved area *(arrow)*. Apical to the junctional epithelium, healthy connective tissue fibers attached perpendicularly to the laser-ablated channels. *(Courtesy Dr. Myron Nevins.)*

nonkeratinized) are more susceptible to peri-implant problems. An animal study observed that ligature-induced peri-implantitis occurs more frequently when alveolar mucosa surrounds the implant as compared with when keratinized mucosa surrounds the implant.[116]

Keratinized mucosa tends to be more firmly anchored by collagen fibers to the underlying periosteum than nonkeratinized mucosa, which has more elastic fibers and tends to be movable relative to the underlying bone. In clinical studies evaluating intraoral implants, with or without peri-implant keratinized mucosa, no clinically significant difference in implant success was reported.[66,121] However, when there is a lack of keratinized tissue, patients tend to complain about pain and discomfort while performing oral hygiene procedures or other functions in the area. The symptoms are alleviated by increasing the amount of keratinized (firmly bound) tissue around

the implant(s) via soft tissue grafting (see online Fig. 65.5, A–L).[9,66,121] Finally, although it may not be comparable to intraoral implants, mobility of soft tissues surrounding extraoral implants is associated with a higher incidence of implant failure.[9]

Vascular Supply and Inflammation

The vascular supply of the peri-implant gingival or alveolar mucosa may be limited, as compared with periodontal gingiva, due to the lack of a periodontal ligament (Fig. 74.13).[21] This is especially true in the tissue immediately adjacent to the implant surface. However, capillary loops in the connective tissue under the junctional and sulcular epithelium around implants appear to be anatomically similar to those found in the normal periodontium (Fig. 74.14).[114]

Emerging knowledge indicates that the peri-implant gingival or alveolar mucosa has the same morphology as the corresponding tissues around teeth. These soft tissues also react the same way to plaque accumulation. Studies investigating the histology (light microscopic and ultrastructural) of healthy and inflamed tissues surrounding implants in humans have indicated that the inflammatory response to plaque is similar to that observed in periodontal tissues.[95] Polymorphonuclear cells and mononuclear cells transmigrate normally through the peri-implant sulcular epithelium (Fig. 74.15).[95]

Clinical Comparison of Teeth and Implants

Although the soft tissue-to-implant (abutment) interface offers striking similarities with tissue surrounding the natural dentition, some differences should be considered. At the bone level, the lack of a periodontal ligament is the most striking difference. The following discussion elaborates on the clinical perspectives of these similarities and differences.

At the bone level, the absence of the periodontal ligament surrounding an implant has important clinical consequences. This means that no resilient connection exists between implants and supporting bone. Implants cannot intrude or migrate to compensate for the presence of a premature occlusal contact (as teeth can). Implants and the rigidly attached implant restorations do not move. Thus any occlusal disharmony will have repercussions at either the restoration-to-implant connection, the bone-to-implant interface, or both.

Proprioception in the natural dentition comes from the periodontal ligament. The absence of a periodontal ligament around implants reduces tactile sensitivity[58] and reflex function.[23] This can become even more challenging when osseointegrated, implant-supported, fixed prostheses are present in both jaws.

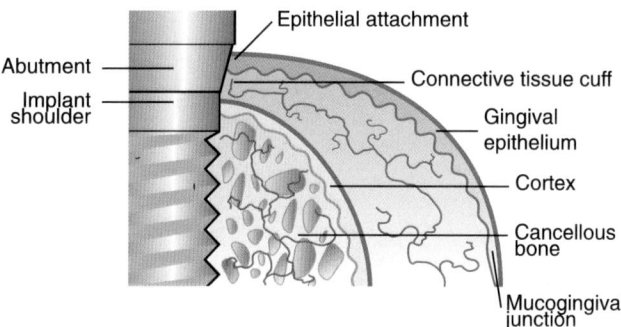

Fig. 74.13 Schematic illustration of the blood supply in the connective tissue cuff surrounding the implant/abutment, which is scarcer than in the gingival complex around teeth because none originates from a periodontal ligament.

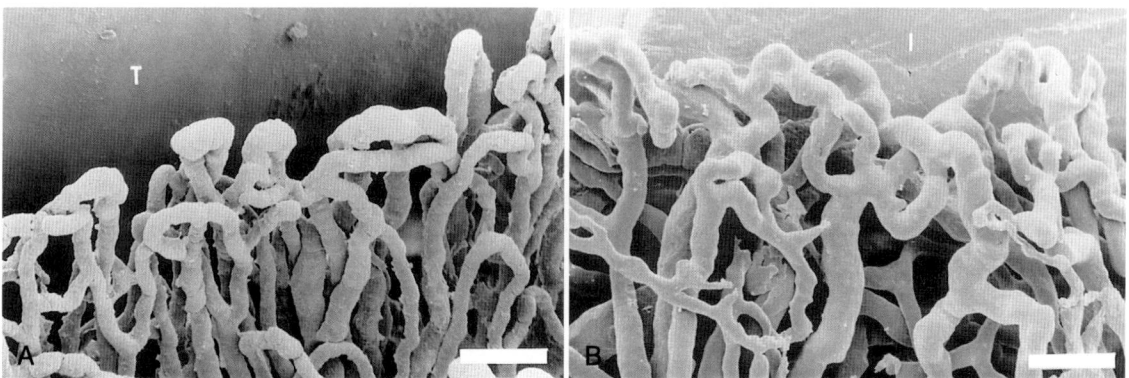

Fig. 74.14 (A) Microvascular topography surrounding a tooth. (B) Microvascular topography surrounding an implant. Bar = 5 µm.[105] *(Courtesy Drs. N. Selliseth and K. Selvig, Bergen, Norway.)*

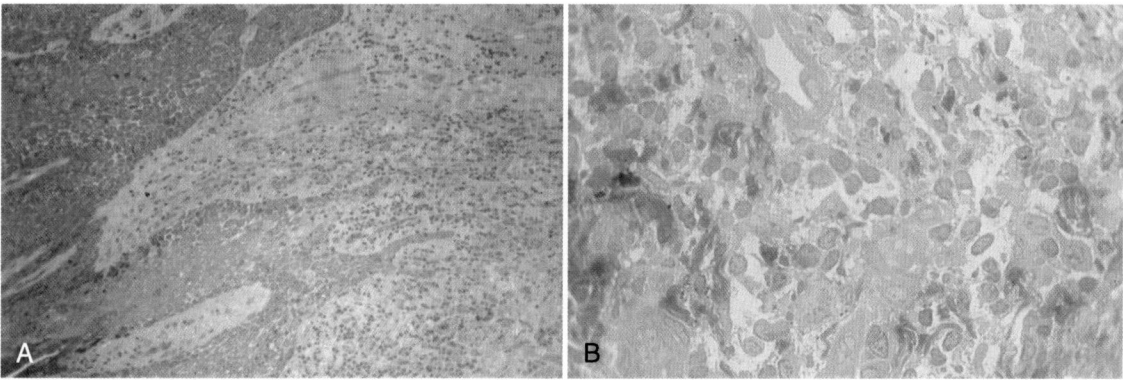

Fig. 74.15 (A) Histologic slide from healthy gingiva surrounding a well-functioning implant in a human patient. No morphologic characteristics differentiate tissue around implant from that around teeth. (B) When gingivitis occurs, a profuse migration of inflammatory cells through the pocket epithelium can be observed. *(Courtesy Professor Mariano Sanz, Madrid, Spain.)*

The lack of a periodontal ligament and the inability of implants to move contraindicates their use in growing individuals. Natural teeth continue to erupt and migrate during growth, whereas implants do not. Implants placed in individuals prior to the completion of growth can lead to occlusal disharmonies with implants.[83] Likewise, it may be problematic to place one or more implants in a location adjacent to teeth that are very mobile from the loss of periodontal support because, as the teeth move in response to or away from the occlusal forces, the implant(s) will bear the entire load.

Overload, because of improper superstructure design, parafunctional habits, or excessive occlusal load, may cause microstrains and microfractures in the bone, which will lead to bone loss and a fibrous inflammatory tissue at the implant interface.[114]

Conclusion

A thorough understanding of bone biology is essential for clinicians to fully appreciate the phenomenon and limitations of osseointegration. Many factors can interfere with the predictable establishment and maintenance of a long-term rigid connection between the implant surface and the surrounding bone that is able to sustain occlusal loads. The bone-to-implant interface and its rigidity are a predominant biomechanical aspect of coping with the time and intensity of loading. The quality of the soft tissue-to-implant interface also plays an important role in the long-term maintenance of stable marginal bone levels around implants. Clinicians must familiarize themselves with the underlying molecular and cellular events to evaluate the future evolution of implant design and implant protocols, including surgical placement, restoration, and maintenance.

 A Case Scenario is found on the companion website www.expertconsult.com.

References

 References for this chapter are found on the companion website www.expertconsult.com.

CHAPTER 75

Clinical Evaluation of the Implant Patient

Perry R. Klokkevold | David L. Cochran

CHAPTER OUTLINE

Case Types and Indications
Risk Factors and Contraindications
Posttreatment Evaluation
Conclusion

Over the past several decades, following the landmark research and development of osseointegrated dental implants by Brånemark and colleagues,[15-17] treatment options and treatment planning in dentistry have evolved tremendously. Initially, prosthetic reconstructions with osseointegrated implants were limited to use in the edentulous patient, with many reports documenting excellent long-term success.[1,2,25]

Shortly thereafter, the original implant treatment protocols were adapted for use in partially edentulous patients. There were some transitional challenges associated with the early use of dental implants being adapted to the partially edentulous patient, but ultimately successes were achieved for this population as well. Modifications in implant design, procedural techniques, and treatment planning greatly improved implant therapy for the partially edentulous patient. Currently, the long-term success of dental implants used to replace single and multiple missing teeth in the partially edentulous patient is very good[29,40,42,48,52] (see Chapter 87). The implementation of bone augmentation procedures further increased the option for patients with inadequate bone volume to be successfully restored with implant-retained prostheses.[27,34,53] Virtually any patient with an edentulous space could be a candidate for endosseous implants, and studies suggest that success rates of 90% to 95% can be expected in healthy patients with good bone and normal healing capacity.[24]

The ultimate goal of dental implant therapy is to satisfy the patient's desire to replace one or more missing teeth in an aesthetic, secure, functional, and long-lasting manner. To achieve this goal, clinicians must accurately diagnose the dentoalveolar condition, as well as the overall mental and physical well-being of the patient. It is necessary to determine whether implant therapy is possible, practical, and, perhaps most important, whether it is indicated for the particular patient who is seeking implants. Local evaluation of potential jaw sites for implant placement (e.g., measuring available alveolar bone height, width, and spatial relationship) and prosthetic restorability are essential considerations in determining whether an implant(s) is possible. However, making as assessment of the patient and determining whether that patient is a good candidate for implants is an equally important part of the evaluation process. The patient evaluation includes identifying factors that might increase the risk of failure or the possibility of complications, as well as determining whether the patient's expectations are reasonable.

This chapter presents an overview of the clinical aspects of dental implant therapy, including an assessment of possible risk factors and contraindications. It also provides guidelines for the pretreatment evaluation of potential implant patients and the posttreatment evaluation of patients with implants.

Case Types and Indications

Edentulous Patients

The patients who seem to benefit most from dental implants are those with fully edentulous arches. These patients can be effectively restored, both aesthetically and functionally, with an implant-assisted removable prosthesis, an implant-supported removable prosthesis, or an implant-supported fixed prosthesis.

The original design for the edentulous arch was a fixed-bone–anchored bridge that used five to six implants in the anterior area of the mandible or the maxilla to support a fixed, hybrid prosthesis. The design is a denture-like complete arch of teeth attached to a substructure (metal framework), which in turn is attached to the implants with cylindrical titanium abutments (Fig. 75.1). The prosthesis is fabricated without flange extensions and does not rely on any soft tissue support. It is entirely implant supported. Usually, the prosthesis includes bilateral distal cantilevers, which extend to replace posterior teeth (back to premolars or first molars).

Another implant-supported design used to restore an edentulous arch is the ceramic-metal fixed bridge (Fig. 75.2). Some patients prefer this design because the ceramic restoration emerges directly from the gingival tissues in a manner that makes its appearance similar to that of natural teeth.

One limitation of both hybrid and ceramometal implant-supported fixed prostheses is that they provide very little lip support and thus may not be indicated for patients who have lost significant alveolar dimension. This is often more problematic for maxillary reconstructions because lip support is more critical in the upper arch. Furthermore, for some patients, the lack of a complete seal (i.e., spaces under the framework) allows air to escape during speech, thus creating phonetic problems.

Depending on the volume of existing bone, the jaw relationship, the amount of lip support, and phonetics, some patients may not be able to be rehabilitated with an implant-supported fixed prosthesis.

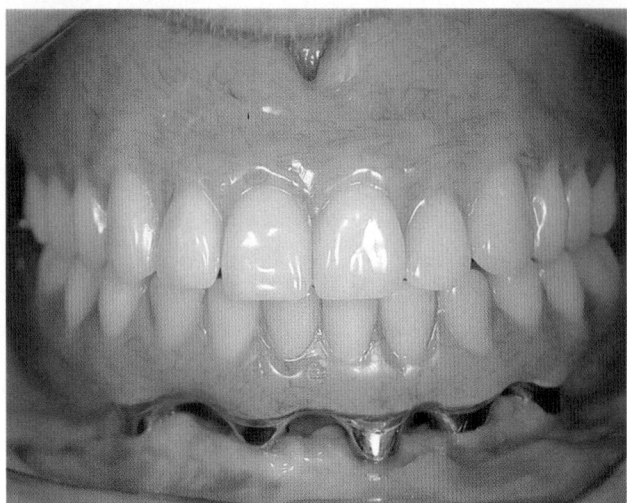

Fig. 75.1 Clinical photograph of patient with a complete maxillary denture opposing a full-arch implant-supported fixed prosthesis in the mandibular arch.

For these patients, a removable, complete-denture type of prosthesis is a better choice because it provides a flange extension that can be adjusted and contoured to support the lip, and there are no spaces for unwanted air escape during speech. This type of prosthesis can be retained and stabilized by two or more implants placed in the anterior region of the maxilla or mandible. Methods used to secure the denture to the implants vary from separate attachments on each individual implant to clips or other attachments that connect to a bar, which splints the implants together (Fig. 75.3). It is also possible to design a removable prosthesis to intimately and securely attach to a precision-fit substructure (e.g., milled bar), making it an implant-supported removable prosthesis.

Although the stability of the implant-retained overdenture does not compare with the rigidly attached, implant-supported fixed prosthesis, the increased retention and stability over conventional complete dentures is an important advantage for denture wearers.[55] Additionally, implant-assisted and implant-supported prostheses are thought to lessen the amount of alveolar bone loss associated with long-term use of removable prostheses that bear directly on the alveolar ridges.

Partially Edentulous Patients

Multiple Teeth

Partially edentulous patients with multiple missing teeth represent another viable treatment population for osseointegrated implants, but the remaining natural dentition (occlusal schemes, periodontal health status, spatial relationships, and aesthetics) introduces additional challenges for successful rehabilitation.[41] The juxtaposition of implants with natural teeth in the partially edentulous patient presents the clinician with challenges not encountered with implants in the edentulous patient. As a result of distinct differences in the biology and function of implants compared with natural teeth, clinicians must educate themselves and use a prescribed approach to the evaluation and treatment planning of implants for partially edentulous patients (see Chapter 77). In general, endosseous dental implants can support a freestanding fixed partial denture. Adjacent natural teeth are not necessary for support, but their close proximity requires special attention and planning.[11] The major advantage of an implant-supported restoration in the partially edentulous patient is that it replaces missing teeth without invasion or alteration of adjacent

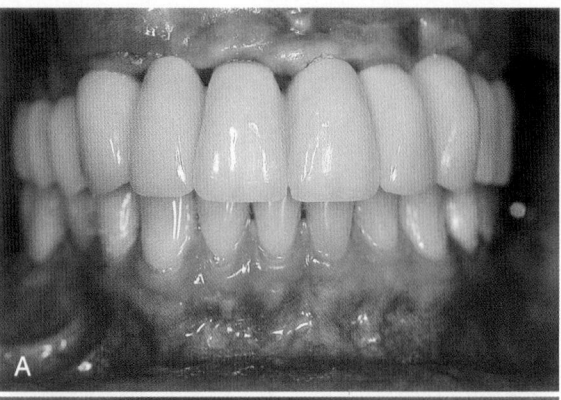
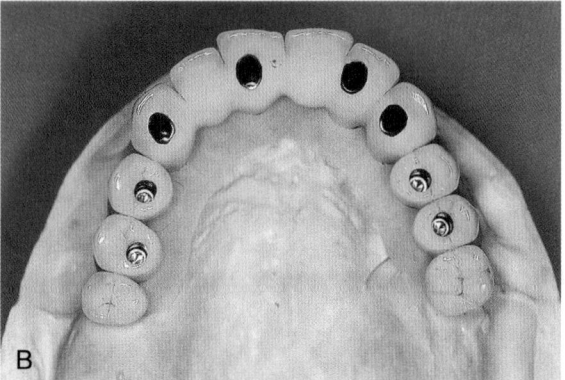
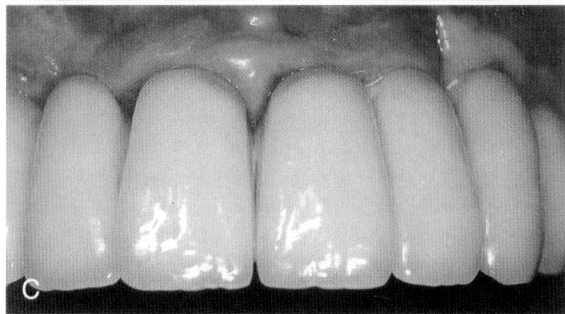

Fig. 75.2 (A) Clinical photograph of acrylic provisional fixed full-arch prosthesis in the maxilla. (B) Clinical photograph of the final ceramometal restoration, anterior view. (C) Occlusal view of final restoration on master cast. *(Courtesy Dr. Russell Nishimura, Westlake Village, California.)*

teeth. Preparation of natural teeth becomes unnecessary, and larger edentulous spans can be restored with implant-supported fixed bridges.[49] Moreover, patients who previously did not have a fixed option, such as those with Kennedy class I and II partially edentulous situations, can be restored with an implant-supported fixed restoration (Fig. 75.4).

Early attempts to use endosseous implants to replace missing teeth in the partially edentulous patient were a challenge partly because the implants and armamentarium were designed for the edentulous patient and did not have much flexibility for adaptation and use in the partially edentulous patient. Today, clinicians have many choices in terms of implant length, diameter, and abutment connection to choose for the optimal replacement of any missing tooth, large or small (Fig. 75.5).

The primary challenge with partially edentulous cases is an underestimation of the importance of treatment planning for implant-retained restorations with an adequate number of implants to withstand occlusal loads. For example, one problem that required correction was the misconception that two implants could be used to support

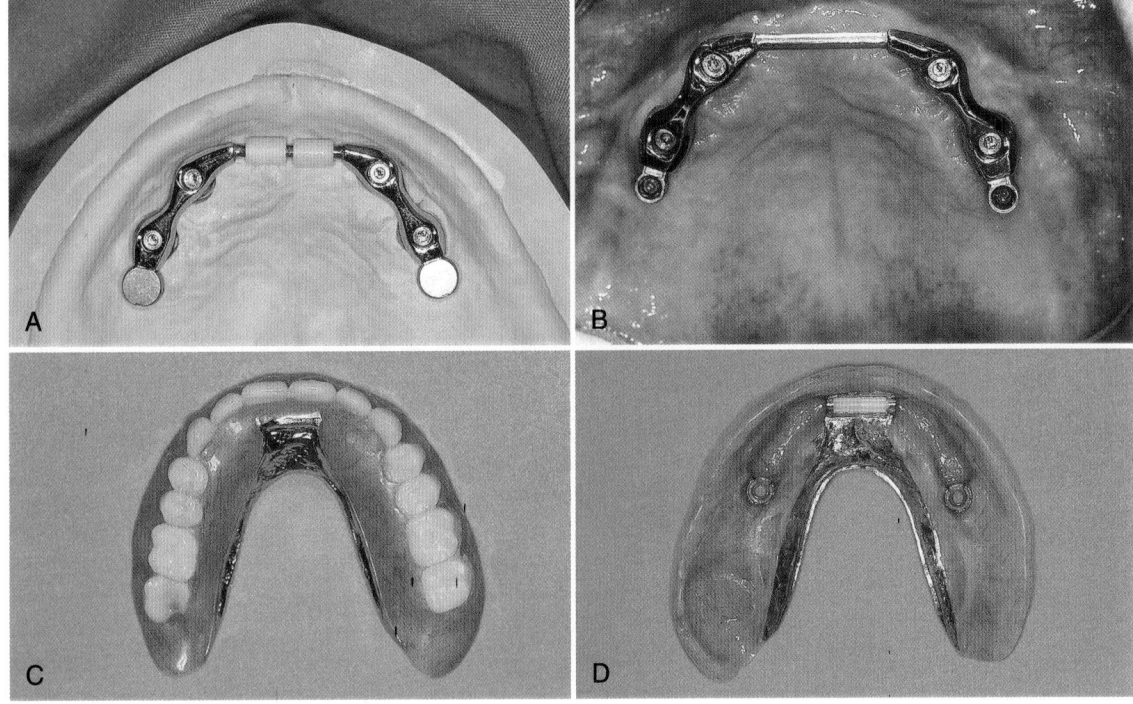

Fig. 75.3 (A) Maxillary overdenture bar attached to four implants with anterior clips and posterior extracoronal resilient attachments (ERAs). (B) Clinical view of maxillary overdenture bar. (C) Palateless maxillary complete overdenture. (D) Tissue surface of the same maxillary implant-assisted overdenture showing clips and ERAs. *(Courtesy Dr. John Beumer, University of California, Los Angeles, Maxillofacial Prosthodontics.)*

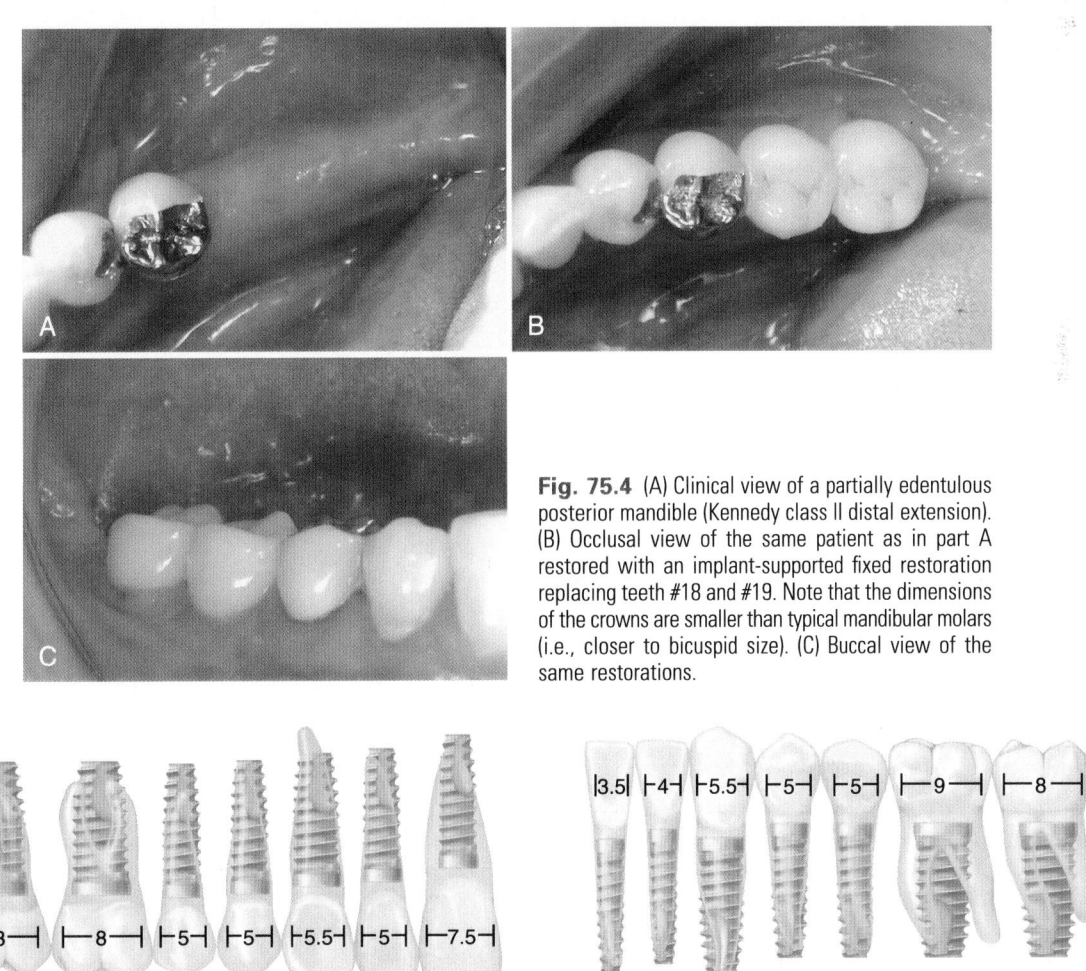

Fig. 75.4 (A) Clinical view of a partially edentulous posterior mandible (Kennedy class II distal extension). (B) Occlusal view of the same patient as in part A restored with an implant-supported fixed restoration replacing teeth #18 and #19. Note that the dimensions of the crowns are smaller than typical mandibular molars (i.e., closer to bicuspid size). (C) Buccal view of the same restorations.

Fig. 75.5 Diagram representing the use of wide-, narrow-, and standard-diameter implants for molars, mandibular incisors, and other teeth (different-sized implants superimposed over various teeth). (A) Maxillary teeth. (B) Mandibular teeth.

a long-span, multiunit fixed bridge in the posterior area. Multiunit fixed restorations in the posterior jaw are more likely to experience complications or failures (mechanical or biologic) when they are inadequately supported in terms of the number of implants, quality of bone, or strength of the implant material (see Chapter 77). Better treatment planning with the use of an adequate number and size of implants, particularly in areas of poor-quality bone, has solved many of these problems.

≪ FLASH BACK

The Kennedy Classification refers to a system developed by Dr. Edward Kennedy for the classification of an edentulous jaw and partial dentures. It is based on the distribution of edentulous spaces. Kennedy class I is a bilateral free-end posterior edentulous area. Kennedy class II is a unilateral free-end posterior edentulous area. Kennedy class III is a single bounded edentulous area that does not cross the midline (unilateral). Kennedy class IV is a single anterior bounded edentulous area that crosses the midline (bilateral).

Single Tooth

Patients with a missing single tooth (anterior or posterior) represent another type of patient who benefits greatly from the success and predictability of endosseous dental implants (Video 75.1). Replacement of a single missing tooth with an implant-supported crown is a much more conservative approach than preparing two adjacent teeth for the fabrication of a tooth-supported fixed partial denture. It is no longer necessary to "cut" healthy or minimally restored adjacent teeth to replace a missing tooth with a nonremovable prosthetic replacement (Fig. 75.6). Reported success rates for single-tooth implants are excellent.[23]

Replacement of an individual missing posterior tooth with an implant-supported restoration has been successful as well. The greatest challenges to overcome with the single-tooth implant restorations were screw loosening and implant or component fracture. Because of the increased potential to generate forces in the posterior area, the implants, components, and screws often failed. Both of these problems have been addressed with the use of wider-diameter implants and internal fixation of components (Fig. 75.7). Wide-diameter implants often have a wider platform (restorative interface) that resists tipping forces and thus reduces screw loosening. The wide-diameter implant also provides greater strength and resistance to fracture as a result of increased wall thickness (i.e., the thickness of the implant between the inner screw thread and the outer screw thread). Implants with an internal connection are inherently more resistant to screw loosening and thus have an added advantage for single-tooth applications.

Aesthetic Considerations

Anterior single-tooth implants present some of the same challenges as the single posterior tooth supported by an implant, but they also are an aesthetic concern for patients. Some cases are more aesthetically challenging than others because of the nature of each individual's smile and display of teeth. The prominence and occlusal relationship of existing teeth, the thickness and health of periodontal tissues, and the patient's own psychological perception of aesthetics all play a role in the aesthetic challenge of the case. Cases with good bone volume, bone height, and tissue thickness can be predictable in terms of achieving satisfactory aesthetic results (see Fig. 75.6). However, achieving aesthetic results for ipatients with less-than-ideal tissue qualities poses difficult challenges for the restorative and surgical team.[12] Replacing a single tooth with an implant-supported crown

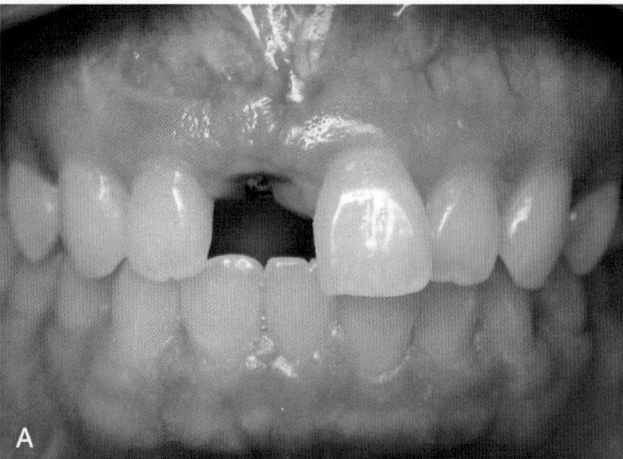

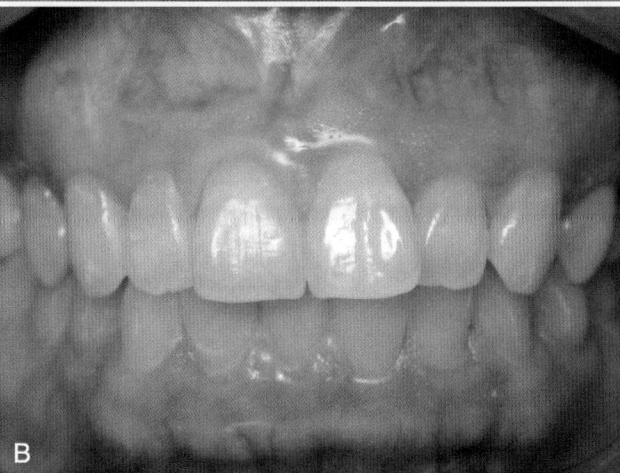

Fig. 75.6 Single-tooth replacement. (A) Implant in place. (B) Metalloceramic crown.

in a patient with a high smile line, compromised or thin periodontium, inadequate hard or soft tissues, and high expectations is probably one of the most difficult challenges in implant dentistry and should not be attempted by novice clinicians.

Pretreatment Evaluation

A comprehensive evaluation is indicated for any patient who is being considered for dental implant therapy. The evaluation should assess all aspects of the patient's current health status, including a review the patient's past medical history, medications, and medical treatments. Patients should be questioned about parafunctional habits, such as clenching or grinding teeth, as well as any substance use or abuse, including tobacco, alcohol, and drugs. The assessment should also include an evaluation of the patient's motivations, level of understanding, compliance, and overall behavior. For most patients, this involves simply observing their demeanor and listening to their comments for an impression of their overall sensibility and coherence with other patient norms.

An intraoral and radiographic examination must be done to determine whether it is possible to place implant(s) in the desired location(s). Properly mounted diagnostic study models and intraoral clinical photographs are useful parts of the clinical examination and treatment-planning process to aid in the assessment of spatial and occlusal relationships. Once the data collection is completed, the

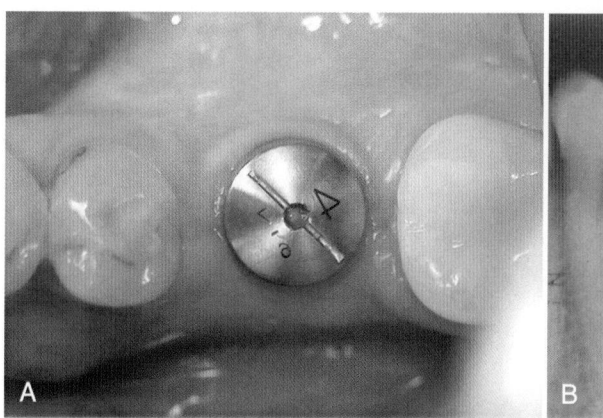
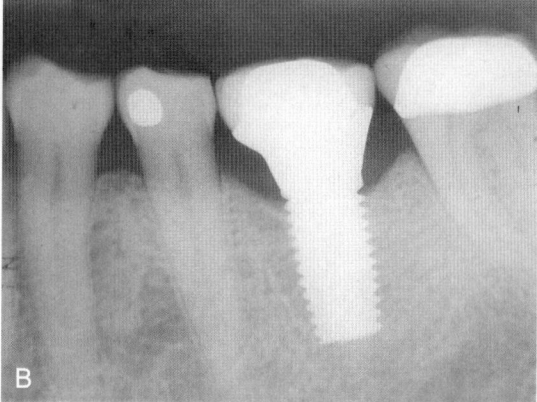

Fig. 75.7 (A) Occlusal view of healing abutment, which is attached to a wide-diameter implant used to replace a single missing molar. (B) Radiograph of the same patient depicted in part A, showing the wide-diameter implant supporting the final restoration (molar replaced with a single-tooth implant-supported crown).

clinician will be able to determine whether implant therapy is possible, practical, and indicated for the patient.

Conducting an organized, systematic history and examination is essential to obtaining an accurate diagnosis and creating a treatment plan that is appropriate for the patient. Each treatment plan should be comprehensive and provide several treatment options for the patient, including periodontal and restorative therapies. Then, in consultation, the clinician can agree on the final treatment plan with the patient. Information gathered throughout the process will help the clinician's decision making and determination of whether a patient is a good candidate for dental implants. A thoughtful and well-executed evaluation can also reveal deficiencies and indicate what additional surgical procedures may be necessary to accomplish the desired goals of therapy (e.g., localized ridge augmentation, sinus bone augmentation). Each part of the pretreatment evaluation is briefly discussed here.

 KEY FACT

Every treatment plan should be comprehensive. It should provide multiple treatment options, including periodontal and restorative therapies. Then, once presented with good information, the patient can ask questions and make an informed decision about the final treatment plan. Information gathered throughout the process will help the clinician's decision making and determination of whether a patient is a good candidate for dental implants.

Chief Complaint

What is the problem or concern in the patient's own words? What is the patient's goal of treatment? How realistic are the patient's expectations? The patient's chief concern, desires for treatment, and vision of the successful outcome must be taken into consideration. The patient will measure implant success according to his or her personal criteria. The overall comfort and function of the implant restoration are often the most important factors, but satisfaction with the appearance of the final restoration will also influence the patient's perception of success. Furthermore, patient satisfaction may be influenced simply by the impact that the treatment has on the patient's perceived quality of life. Patients will evaluate for themselves whether the treatment helped them to eat better, look better, or feel better about themselves.

The clinician could consider an implant and the retained prosthesis a success using standard criteria of symptom-free implant function,

implant stability, and lack of peri-implant infection or bone loss. At the same time, however, the patient who does not like the aesthetic result or does not think the condition has improved could consider the treatment a failure. Therefore it is critical to inquire, as specifically as possible, about the patient's expectations before initiating implant therapy and to appreciate the patient's desires and values. With this goal in mind, it is often helpful and advisable to invite patients to bring their spouses or family members to the consultation and treatment-planning visits to add an independent "trusted" observer to the discussion of treatment options. Ultimately, it is the clinician's responsibility to determine if the patient has realistic expectations for the outcome of therapy and to educate the patient about realistic outcomes for each treatment option.

CLINICAL CORRELATION

It is essential to listen to a patient's chief concerns. The patient will ultimately decide whether the implant is successful based on his or her personal criteria. The overall comfort and function of the implant restoration are often the most important factors, but satisfaction with the appearance will also influence the patient's perception of success. Patient satisfaction will be influenced by the impact of treatment on their perceived quality of life. Patients will evaluate for themselves whether the implant treatment helped them to eat better, look better, or feel better.

Medical History

A thorough medical history is required for any patient in need of dental treatment, regardless of whether implants are part of the plan. This history should be documented in writing by the patient's completion of a standard health history form and verbally through an interview with the treating clinician. The patient's health history should be reviewed for any condition that might put the patient at risk for adverse reactions or complications.

Patients must be in reasonably good health to undergo surgical therapy for the placement of dental implants. Any disorder that may impair the normal wound-healing process, especially as it relates to bone metabolism, should be carefully considered as a possible risk factor or contraindication to implant therapy (discussed later).

A thorough physical examination is warranted if any questions arise about the patient's health status.[15] Appropriate laboratory tests (e.g., coagulation tests for a patient receiving anticoagulant therapy) should be requested to evaluate further any conditions that may affect the patient's ability to undergo the planned surgical and restorative procedures safely and effectively. If any questions remain about the patient's health status, a medical clearance for surgery should be obtained from the patient's treating physician.

Dental History

A review of a patient's past dental experiences can be a valuable part of the overall evaluation. Does the patient report a history of recurrent or frequent abscesses, which may indicate a susceptibility to infections or diabetes? Does the patient have many restorations? How compliant has the patient been with previous dental recommendations? What are the patient's current oral hygiene practices?

The individual's previous experiences with surgery and prosthetics should be discussed. If a patient reports numerous problems and difficulties with past dental care, including a history of dissatisfaction with past treatment, the patient may have similar difficulties with implant therapy. It is essential to identify past problems and to elucidate any contributing factors. The clinician must also assess the patient's dental knowledge and understanding of the proposed treatment, as well as the patient's attitude and motivation toward implants.

Intraoral Examination

The oral examination is performed to assess the current health and condition of existing teeth, as well as to evaluate the condition of the oral hard and soft tissues. It is imperative that no pathologic conditions are present in any of the hard or soft tissues in the maxillofacial region. All oral lesions, especially infections, should be diagnosed and appropriately treated before implant therapy. Additional criteria to consider include the patient's habits, level of oral hygiene, overall dental and periodontal health, occlusion, jaw relationship, temporomandibular joint condition, and ability to open wide.

After a thorough intraoral examination, the clinician can evaluate potential implant sites. All sites should be clinically evaluated to measure the available space in the bone for the placement of implants and in the dental space for prosthetic tooth replacement (Box 75.1). The mesial-distal and buccal-lingual dimensions of edentulous spaces can be approximated with a periodontal probe or other measuring instrument. The orientation or tilt of adjacent teeth and their roots should be noted as well. There may be enough space in the coronal area for the restoration but not enough space in the apical region for the implant if roots are directed into the area of interest (Fig. 75.8). Conversely, there may be adequate space between roots, but the coronal aspects of the teeth may be too close for emergence and restoration of the implant. If either of these conditions is discovered, orthodontic tooth movement may be indicated. Ultimately, edentulous areas need to be precisely measured using diagnostic study models and imaging techniques to determine whether space is available and whether adequate bone volume exists to replace missing teeth with implants and implant restorations. Fig. 75.9 diagrams the minimal space requirements for standard-, wide-, and narrow-diameter implants placed between natural teeth, and the minimal interocclusal space needed to restore implants.

Diagnostic Study Models

Mounted study models are an excellent means of assessing potential sites for dental implants. Properly articulated models with diagnostic wax-up of the proposed restorations allow the clinician to evaluate the available space and to determine potential limitations of the planned treatment (eFig. 75.1). This is particularly useful when multiple teeth are to be replaced with implants or when a malocclusion is present.

> **BOX 75.1** How Much Space Is Required for Placement of One or More Implants?[a]
>
> **Alveolar Bone**
> Assuming an implant is 4 mm in diameter and 10 mm long, the minimal width of the jawbone needs to be 6 to 7 mm, and the minimal height should be 10 mm (minimum of 12 mm in the posterior mandible, where an additional margin of safety is required over the mandibular nerve). This dimension is desired to maintain at least 1 to 1.5 mm of bone around all surfaces of the implant after preparation and placement.
>
> **Interdental Space**
> Edentulous spaces need to be measured to determine whether enough space exists for the placement and restoration with one or more implant crowns. The minimal space requirements for the placement of one, two, or more implants are illustrated diagrammatically in Fig. 75.9. The minimal mesial-distal space for an implant placed between two teeth is 7 mm. The minimal mesial-distal space required for the placement of two standard-diameter implants (4-mm diameter) between teeth is 14 mm. The required minimal dimensions for wide-diameter or narrow-diameter implants will increase or decrease incrementally according to the size of the implant. For example, the minimal space needed for the placement of an implant 6 mm in diameter is 9 mm (7 mm + 2 mm). Whenever the available space between teeth is greater than 7 mm and less than 14 mm, only one implant, such as placement of a wide-diameter implant, should be considered. Two narrow-diameter implants could be positioned in a space that is 12 mm. However, the smaller implant may be more vulnerable to implant fracture.
>
> **Interocclusal Space**
> The restoration consists of the abutment, the abutment screw, and the crown (it may also include a screw to secure the crown to the abutment if it is not cemented). This restorative "stack" is the total of all the components used to attach the crown to the implant. The dimensions of the restorative stack vary slightly depending on the type of abutment and the implant-restorative interface (i.e., internal or external connection). The minimum amount of interocclusal space required for the restorative "stack" on an external hex-type implant is 7 mm.
>
> ---
> [a]All of the minimal space requirements discussed here are generic averages. The actual space limitations for any particular implant system must be determined according to the manufacturer's specifications.

Hard Tissue Evaluation

The amount of available bone is the next criterion to evaluate. Wide variations in jaw anatomy are encountered, and it is therefore important to analyze the anatomy of the dentoalveolar region of interest both clinically and radiographically.

A visual examination can immediately identify deficient areas (Fig. 75.10), whereas other areas that appear to have good ridge width will require further evaluation (Fig. 75.11). Clinical examination of the jawbone consists of palpation to feel for anatomic defects and variations in the jaw anatomy, such as concavities and undercuts. If desired, it is possible with local anesthesia to probe through the soft tissue (intraoral bone mapping) to assess the thickness of the soft tissues and measure the bone dimensions at the proposed surgical site.

The spatial relationship of the bone must be evaluated in a three-dimensional view because the implant must be placed in the appropriate position relative to the prosthesis. It is possible that an adequate

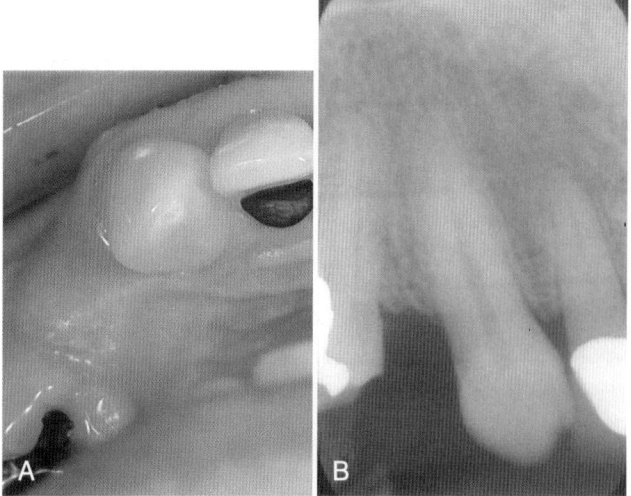

Fig. 75.8 (A) Clinical photograph of maxillary premolar space with apparently adequate space between the remaining teeth for an implant-supported crown. (B) Radiograph clearly shows a lack of space between the roots of the adjacent teeth as a result of convergence into the space (same patient as in part A).

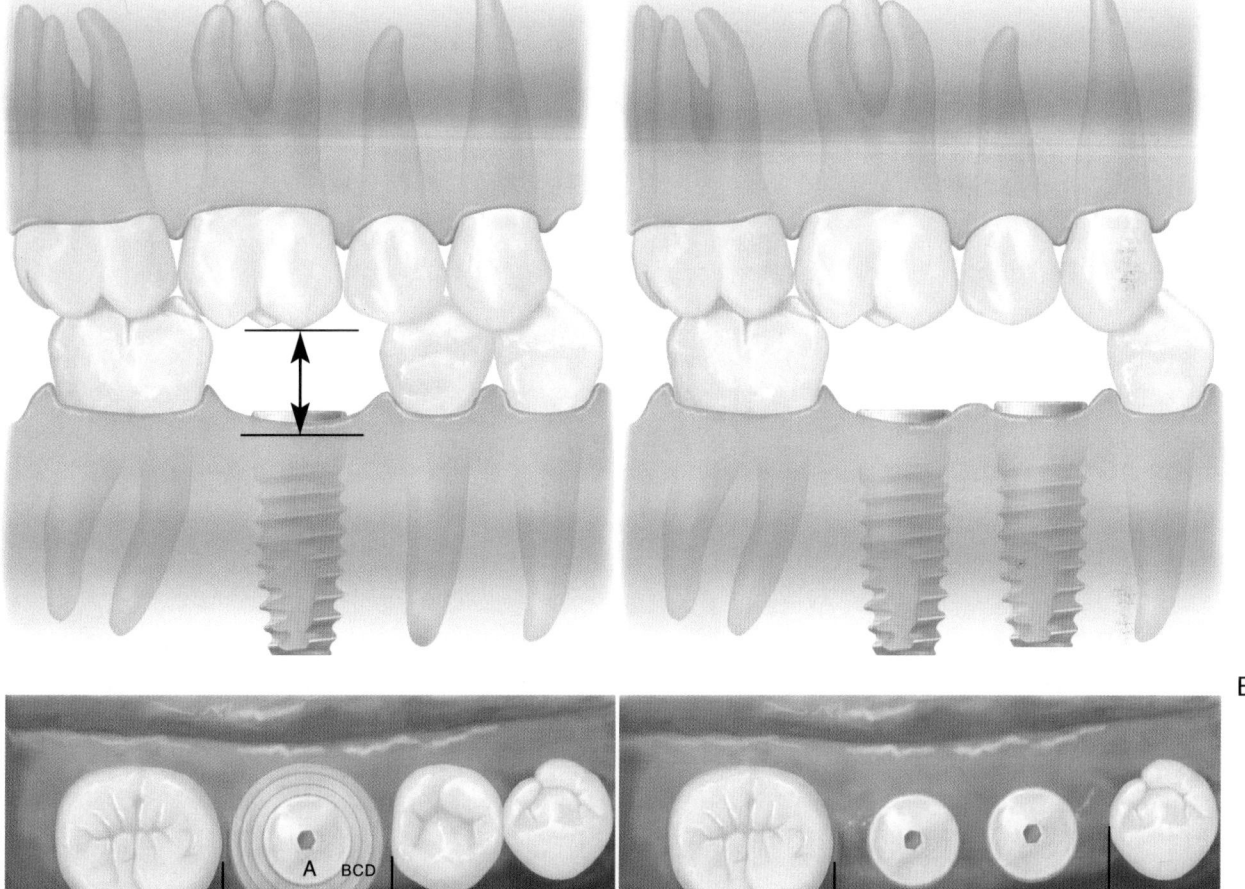

The minimum mesial-distal space (*d*) required for a:
A. Narrow diameter implant (e.g., 3.25 mm) is 6 mm.
B. Standard diameter implant (e.g., 4.1 mm) is 7 mm.
C. Wide diameter implant (e.g., 5.0 mm) is 8 mm.
D. Wide diameter implant (e.g., 6.0 mm) is 9 mm.

The minimum mesial-distal space (*d*) required for two standard diameter implants is 14 mm wide.

Fig. 75.9 (A) Minimum amount of mesial-distal space *(d)* required for placement of single-tooth implant between natural teeth: *A,* 6 mm for narrow-diameter implant (3.25 mm); *B,* 7 mm for standard-diameter implant (4.1 mm); *C* and *D,* 8 mm and 9 mm, respectively, for wide-diameter implants (5 mm and 6 mm). (B) Minimum amount of mesial-distal space *(d)* required for placement of two standard-diameter implants (4.1 mm) between natural teeth is 14 mm. This allows approximately 2 mm between teeth/implants and between implant/implant. Minimum amount of space required between implant/restoration interface and opposing occlusal surfaces for restoration of an implant. This dimension will vary depending on implant design and manufacturer component dimensions. The minimal dimension of 7 mm is based on an externally hexed implant and UCLA abutment.

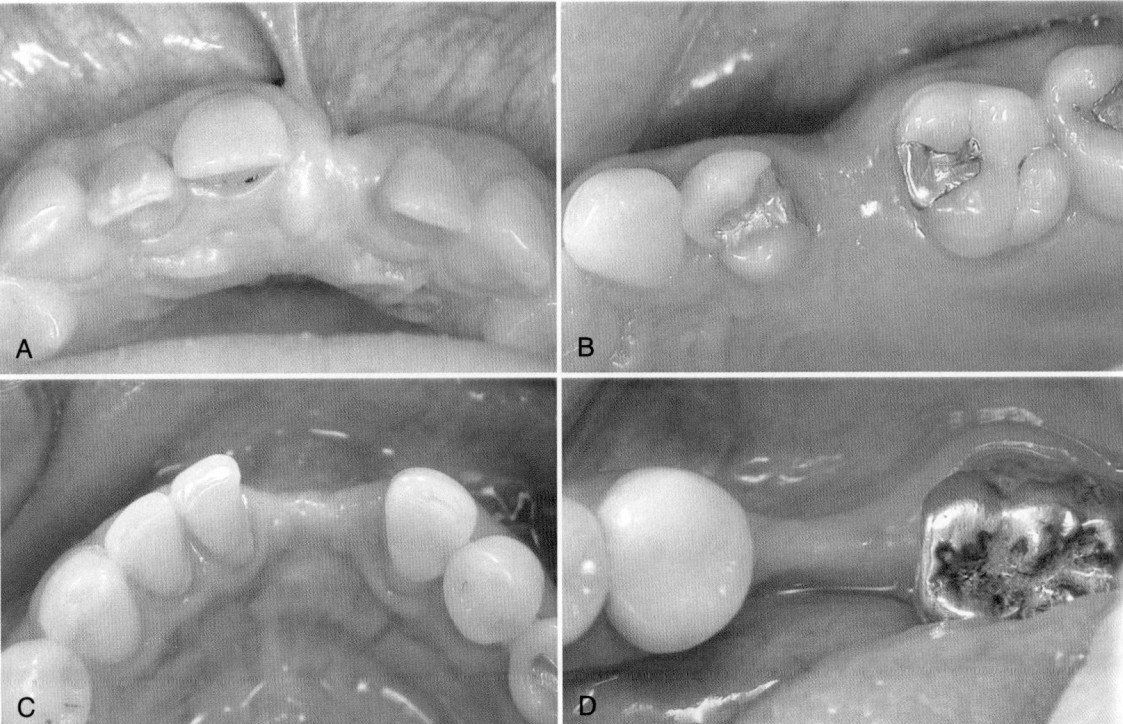

Fig. 75.10 Clinical photographs of edentulous areas with obvious deficient areas of alveolar dimension noted on visual examination: (A) anterior maxilla, (B) posterior maxilla, (C) anterior mandible, and (D) posterior mandible. These clinical images all represent buccal-lingual deficiencies in the alveolar dimensions.

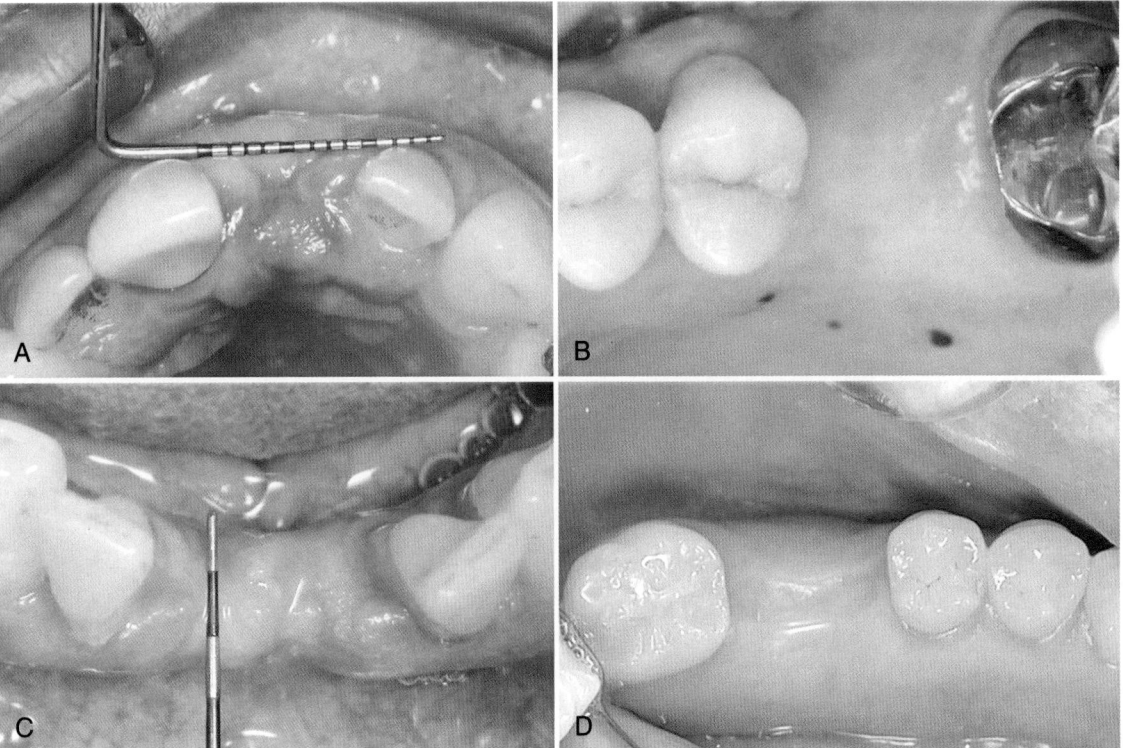

Fig. 75.11 Clinical photographs of edentulous areas with apparent good alveolar dimension noted on visual examination: (A) anterior maxilla, (B) posterior maxilla, (C) anterior mandible, and (D) posterior mandible. It is likely that these sites have adequate bone volume for implant placement. However, it is also possible to find alveolar deficiencies despite the appearance of wide ridges.

dimension of bone is available in the anticipated implant site (see Box 75.1), but that the bone and thus the implant placement might be located too lingual or too buccal for the desired prosthetic tooth replacement.[30] Bone augmentation procedures may be necessary to facilitate the placement of an implant in an acceptable prosthetic position despite the availability of an adequate quantity of bone (i.e., the bone is in the wrong location). Bone augmentation procedures are discussed in Chapters 79 and 80.

Radiographic Examination

Radiographic assessment of the quantity, quality, and location of available alveolar bone in potential implant sites ultimately determines whether a patient is a candidate for implants and if a particular implant site needs bone augmentation. Appropriate radiographic procedures, including periapical radiographs, panoramic projections, and cross-sectional imaging, can help identify vital structures such as the floor of the nasal cavity, maxillary sinus, mandibular canal, and mental foramen (see Chapter 76). In addition to the absolute dimensional measurement of the alveolar bone, it is important to determine whether the volume of bone radiographically (as well as clinically) is located in a position to allow for the proper position of the implant to facilitate restoration of the tooth/teeth in proper aesthetic and functional relationship with the adjacent and opposing dentition. The best way to evaluate the relationship of available bone to the dentition is to image the patient with a diagnostically accurate guide using radiopaque markers that are positioned at the proposed prosthetic locations, ideally with appropriate restorative contours (see Fig. 76.5).

KEY FACT

Implant planning should be "prosthetically driven." This can be achieved with a diagnostic wax-up of the proposed prosthesis and radiographic imaging with radiopaque markers, ideally tooth-shaped, that show the desired tooth position(s) relative to the available bone.

Soft Tissue Evaluation

Evaluation of the quality, quantity, and location of soft tissue present in the anticipated implant site helps to anticipate the type of tissue that will surround the implant(s) after treatment is completed (keratinized vs. nonkeratinized mucosa). For some cases, clinical evaluation may reveal a need for soft tissue augmentation (Box 75.2). Areas with minimal or no keratinized mucosa may be augmented with gingival or connective tissue grafts. Other soft tissue concerns, such as frenum attachments that pull on the gingival margin, should be thoroughly evaluated as well.

Risk Factors and Contraindications

Clearly, there are numerous indications for the use of endosseous dental implants to replace missing teeth. Most patients who are missing one or more teeth can benefit from the application of an implant-retained prosthesis provided they meet the requirements for surgical and prosthetic rehabilitation. Edentulous patients who are unable to function with complete dentures and who have adequate bone for the placement of dental implants can be especially good dental implant candidates. More and more partially edentulous patients are also being treated with dental implant restorations. Many patients, whether they are missing one, several, or all of their teeth, can be predictably restored with implant-retained prostheses.

> **BOX 75.2   How Much Keratinized Tissue Is Required for the Health and Maintenance of Implants?**
>
> Debate continues about whether it is necessary to have a zone of keratinized tissue surrounding implants. Despite strong opinions and beliefs about the need for keratinized mucosa around implants versus this mucosa being unnecessary, neither argument has been proved.
>
> Some studies have concluded that, in the presence of good oral hygiene, a lack of keratinized tissue does not impair the health or function of implants.[54] Others strongly believe that keratinized mucosa has better functional and aesthetic results for implant restorations. Keratinized mucosa is typically thicker and denser than alveolar mucosa (nonkeratinized). It forms a strong seal around the implant with a cuff of circular (parallel) fibers around the implant, abutment, or restoration that is resistant to retracting with mastication forces and oral hygiene procedures. Implants with coated surfaces (i.e., hydroxyapatite [H] or titanium plasma spray [TPS] coating) demonstrate greater peri-implant bone loss and failures in the absence of keratinized mucosa.[13,38]

In this era of high implant success and predictability and thus possible complacency, it is imperative for clinicians to recognize risk factors and contraindications to implant therapy so that problems can be minimized and patients can be accurately informed about risks. As such, the clinician must be knowledgeable in this area and inform patients about risk factors and contraindications before initiating treatment. Contraindications for the use of dental implants, although relatively few and often not well defined, do exist. Some conditions are probably best described as "risk factors" rather than "contraindications" to treatment because implants can be successful in almost all patients; implants may be less *predictable* in some situations, and this distinction should be recognized. Ultimately, it is the clinician's responsibility with the patient to make decisions as to when implant therapy is not indicated.

Table 75.1 lists some conditions and factors that are thought to increase the risk for implant failure or otherwise deem the patient a poor candidate for implant therapy. Some of these conditions are briefly discussed here.

Medical and Systemic Health–Related Issues

Although few absolute medical contraindications to implant therapy exist, some relative contraindications are important to consider. The clinician must consider medical and health-related conditions that affect bone metabolism or any aspect of the patient's capacity to heal normally.[10] This category includes conditions such as diabetes, osteoporosis, and immune compromise; medications; and medical treatments such as chemotherapy and irradiation.

Diabetes Mellitus

Diabetes is a metabolic disease that can have significant effects on the patient's ability to heal normally and resist infections. This is particularly true for patients whose diabetes is not well controlled. Patients with poorly controlled diabetes often have impaired wound healing and a predisposition to infections, whereas patients with well-controlled diabetes experience few, if any, problems (see Chapter 14).

There is concern about the success and predictability of implants in patients with diabetes. Several studies have reported moderate failure rates in patients with diabetes, with implant success ranging from 85.6% to 94.3%.[8,26,36,39] A prospective study demonstrated 2.2% early failures and 7.3% late failures in patients with diabetes.[51] After 5 years, the overall success rate for this group of diabetic patients

TABLE 75.1 Risk Factors and Contraindications for Implant Therapy

	Risk Factor	Contraindication
Medical and Systemic Health–Related Issues		
Diabetes (poorly controlled)	??—Possibly	Relative
Bone metabolic disease (e.g., osteoporosis)	??—Probably	Relative
Radiation therapy (head and neck)	Yes	Relative/absolute
Bisphosphonate therapy (intravenous)	??—Probably	Relative/absolute
Bisphosphonate therapy (oral)	??—Possibly	Relative
Immunosuppressive medication	??—Probably	Relative
Immunocompromising disease (e.g., HIV, AIDS)	??—Possibly	Relative
Psychological and Mental Conditions		
Psychiatric syndromes (e.g., schizophrenia, paranoia)	No	Absolute
Mental instability (e.g., neurotic, hysteric)	No	Absolute
Mentally impaired; uncooperative	No	Absolute
Irrational fears; phobias	No	Absolute
Unrealistic expectations	No	Absolute
Habits and Behavioral Considerations		
Smoking; tobacco use	Yes	Relative
Parafunctional habits	Yes	Relative
Substance abuse (e.g., alcohol, drugs)	??—Possibly	Absolute
Intraoral Examination Findings		
Atrophic maxilla	Yes	Relative
Current infection (e.g., endodontic)	Yes	Relative
Periodontal disease	??—Possibly	Relative

AIDS, Acquired immunodeficiency syndrome; *HIV,* human immunodeficiency virus.

was 90%.[47] None of these studies was able to correlate gender, age, smoking, diabetes type, or level of diabetic control with implant failure. In a meta-analytical review of implant failures in patients who were not diabetics, the early implant failure rate was 3.2% and the late implant failure rate 5.2%.[22] The finding that patients with diabetes experience slightly more late failures may be related to less tissue integrity caused by reduced tissue turnover and impaired tissue perfusion. These results suggest that diabetes may be a risk factor for implants, particularly for late failures. However, the risk does not appear to be particularly high.

Bone Metabolic Disease

Osteoporosis is a skeletal condition characterized by decreased mineral density. The two main classifications are primary (three types) and secondary (multiple types) osteoporosis. *Primary osteoporosis* has been attributed to menopausal changes (type I), age-related changes

(type II), or idiopathic causes (type III). *Secondary osteoporosis* has been attributed to many different diseases and conditions, including diabetes, alcoholism, malnutrition, and smoking.[31]

All the various types of osteoporosis share the same fundamental problem of decreased bone mineral density and the concern that this condition may impair the patient's ability to achieve and maintain implant osseointegration. The premise that implants will not perform as well in a patient with osteoporosis is reasonable given that osseointegration depends on bone formation adjacent to the implant surface and that success rates are highest in dense bone and lowest in poor-quality, loose trabecular bone. However, to date, there is no clear evidence to suggest that implants will not be successful in patients with osteoporosis, so the issue continues to be debated.[9,19] On the positive side, although the evidence is weak, case reports have demonstrated successful implant treatment in patients with osteoporosis.[30] Some investigators advocate the use of longer healing times for osseointegration to occur before loading the implants in patients with osteoporosis.[28] Conversely, in a retrospective analysis of 49 patients who received sinus bone augmentation, individuals (11 patients) with lower bone mass density had significantly lower implant success rates as compared with age- and sex-matched controls.[14] Other parameters evaluated in this study did not demonstrate any significant differences.

Interestingly, there is a trend in aging adults (men older than 50 years and postmenopausal women) for bone mass to decrease progressively through bone demineralization at a rate of 1% to 2% per year and in some individuals as much as 5% to 8% per year throughout their later life.[21,35] If one considers this decline in bone mass with aging along with a continually increasing life expectancy in the population, the number of individuals with osteopenia or osteoporosis will continue to increase, and the concern about this condition's influence on implant success will become increasingly more important for clinicians.

Bisphosphonate Therapy

Some prescribed medications, including steroids and bisphosphonates, may be cause for concern relative to the potential implant patient. A brief statement regarding the risk of bisphosphonate therapy is offered here. Readers are encouraged to review more detailed explanations in Chapters 14 and 39 and to consult online information as well as other resources to get updated information about this important subject as more is learned and recommendations are developed.

Although there is heightened awareness and great concern about risk of bisphosphonate-related osteonecrosis of the jaw (BRONJ), the causal relationship and pathogenesis of the problem has not been defined. A review of available literature offers information that will guide clinicians in their decision making, but it is far from definitive. The prevalence and incidence remains uncertain. In general, the risk of BRONJ is between 1 in 10,000 and 1 in 100,000 but may increase to 1 in 300 after an oral surgical procedure. The great majority of BRONJ cases will likely remain in the population of patients who receive intravenous administration of bisphosphonates. Cofactors, such as smoking, steroid use, anemia, hypoxemia, diabetes, infection, and immune deficiency, have not been firmly established but may be important.[45] Rarely does BRONJ in the oral bisphosphonate patient appear to progress beyond stage 2, and many cases reverse with discontinuation of oral medication. Procedures reported to have contributed to the development of BRONJ include extractions, periodontal surgery, root canal treatment, and dental implant surgery.[46] Dental implant therapy, as well as other surgical procedures, should be avoided in individuals who have been treated with intravenous (IV) bisphosphonate therapy and carefully considered with caution in patients treated with oral bisphosphonate therapy, particularly those with a history of more than 3 years of use.[3]

Immune Compromise and Immune Suppression

Corticosteroid therapy, whether used for hormone replacement, cancer treatment, immune suppression, or another chronic condition, may suppress the immune response, impair wound healing, or compromise the normal adrenal response to stress. See Chapters 14 and 39 for more information on the treatment of patients taking corticosteroids. Individuals undergoing chemotherapy or taking medications that impair healing potential (e.g., steroids) are probably not good candidates for implant therapy because of the effects these agents have on normal healing. This is especially true for cancer chemotherapy. A lowered resistance to infection may also be problematic for these patients. Past history of chemotherapy or immunosuppressive therapy may not be problematic if the patient has recovered from the side effects of treatment.

Patients with an immunocompromising disease, such as human immunodeficiency virus (HIV) infection or acquired immunodeficiency syndrome (AIDS), are not good candidates for implants when their immune system is seriously impaired. Patients with very low or undetectable viral loads and normal (T cell counts) immune function may be candidates for implant therapy (see Chapter 30).

Radiation Therapy

Patients with a history of radiation treatment to the head and neck region may not heal well after surgery. Soft tissue dehiscence may follow surgical manipulation, which may lead to osteoradionecrosis (ORN), a serious condition of nonhealing exposure and infection of bone. This is especially problematic for patients who have received radiation dosages greater than 60 Gy. Surgical procedures, or any procedure that may initiate a wound, are generally avoided in patients with a history of radiation therapy. If deemed necessary, surgical procedures can be done in conjunction with hyperbaric oxygen (HBO) therapy to reduce the risk of ORN.

Several studies have documented poor success rates for implants in patients with a history of radiation therapy.[32,33,44] In a literature review, Sennerby and Roos[50] found irradiation to be associated with high failure rates, as did Esposito and colleagues[24] in their review. Beumer and colleagues[12] reported success rates as low as 60.4% in the irradiated maxilla. Granstrom and colleagues[32] reported a significant improvement in survival rates for implants in patients treated with HBO. However, in a systematic review, Coulthard and colleagues[18] concluded that the evidence is lacking to support the clinical effectiveness of HBO in irradiated patients receiving implants. The application of implants in patients with a history of irradiation, with or without the use of HBO, is not resolved and continues to be debated. Clearly, irradiation is a risk factor for implant success and may be a contraindication.

Psychological and Mental Conditions

In general, any type of psychological abnormality can be considered a contraindication to dental implant treatment because of the patient's uncooperativeness, lack of understanding, or behavioral problems. Physiologically, there is no reason to suspect that implants could not become osseointegrated in these patients. However, the patient's ability to tolerate the number and type of treatment appointments required for implant placement, restoration, and maintenance could be problematic. All psychological conditions have the potential to be absolute contraindications to implant treatment depending on the severity of the condition. The exception might be individuals who demonstrate good cooperative behavior with only mild psychological or mental impairment. The clinician should take great care before accepting a mentally or psychologically impaired individual for treatment with implants.

Habits and Behavioral Considerations

Patients have a variety of habits and behaviors that may increase the risk of failure for dental implants. Smoking, clenching or grinding of teeth, and drug or alcohol abuse are among the most well-known habits that should be identified because of the increased risk for implant failure or complications.

Smoking and Tobacco Use

Moderate to heavy smoking has been documented to result in higher rates of early implant failure and adversely affect the long-term prognosis of dental implant restorations.[6,20,43] This is particularly true for implants placed in poor-quality bone such as the posterior maxilla.[39] The mechanisms of action responsible for higher implant failures associated with smoking are not understood. Plausible explanations include the effect of smoking on white blood cells, vasoconstriction, wound healing, and osteoporosis.[4,37] Smoking is a known risk factor for osteoporosis and thus may adversely affect implant success through its effect on bone metabolism. Smoking cessation may improve the success rate of implants.[5] In a meta-analytical review, Bain and coworkers[7] found that implants with an altered surface microtopography (Biomet 3i, Osseotite; dual acid-etched surface) seemed to significantly lessen the adverse effects of smoking on implant success.

Parafunctional Habits

Parafunctional habits, such as clenching or grinding of teeth (consciously or unconsciously), have been associated with an increased rate of implant failure (e.g., failure to integrate, loss of integration, implant fracture). Repeated lateral forces (i.e., parafunctional habits) applied to implants can be detrimental to the osseointegration process, especially during the early healing period. Patients with known parafunctional habits should be advised of an increased risk of complications or failures as a result of their clenching or grinding. Many consider bruxism to be a contraindication to implant treatment, especially in the case of a short-span, fixed partial denture or a single-tooth implant. If implants are planned for a patient with parafunctional habits, protective measures should be employed, such as creating a narrow occlusal table with flat cusp angles, protected occlusion, and the regular use of occlusal guards.

Substance Abuse

Drug and alcohol abuse should be considered a contraindication for implant therapy for reasons similar to the psychological problems discussed earlier. Patients with drug or alcohol addictions can be irresponsible and noncompliant with treatment recommendations. Depending on the severity and duration of an individual's addiction, some patients may be malnourished or may even have impaired organ function and therefore may not be good surgical candidates because of poor healing capacity. All elective treatments, including implant therapy, should be refused until addictions are treated and controlled.

Posttreatment Evaluation

Periodic posttreatment examination of implants, the retained prosthesis, and the condition of the surrounding peri-implant tissue are important components of successful treatment. Aberrations and complications can often be treated if discovered early, but many problems will go unnoticed by the patient. Thus periodic examination is essential to discovering problems early and to intervening and preventing problems from getting worse. Several parameters are available to evaluate the condition of the prosthesis, the stability of the implants, and the health of surrounding peri-implant tissues after implant integration and prosthetic restoration. Intraoral radiographs should be taken at the time of placement (baseline), at the time of abutment connection (to confirm seating and serve as another baseline), at the time of final restoration delivery (loading), and subsequently to monitor marginal or peri-implant bone changes. Periapical radiographs have excellent resolution and provide adequate details for evaluating bone support around implants if taken at a perpendicular direction.

The long-term success of dental implants is dependent on the health and stability of supporting peri-implant tissues. Good oral hygiene and regular professional care are essential to maintaining peri-implant health, and the importance of good oral hygiene should be stressed as early as possible. Patients should be taught to maintain good oral hygiene. Their performance should be monitored and reinforced at each visit.

See Chapter 86 for a detailed description of important clinical and radiographic monitoring methods as well as oral hygiene and implant maintenance protocols.

Conclusion

Today, clinicians are able to predictably replace missing teeth with endosseous dental implants. Whether missing a single tooth, several teeth, or all teeth, many patients can be candidates for dental implant therapy. It is important for clinicians to recognize factors that influence implant success. In addition to the quantity, quality, and location of available bone, the patient's health, risk factors, and contraindications must be assessed. Patients should be informed about risk factors and provided with treatment options both with and without dental implants. Periodic evaluation, good oral hygiene, and regular maintenance are important aspects of care for the long-term success and the prevention of complications with dental implants.

 A Case Scenario is found on the companion website www.expertconsult.com.

References

 References for this chapter are found on the companion website www.expertconsult.com.

CHAPTER 76

Diagnostic Imaging for the Implant Patient

Sotirios Tetradis | Sanjay M. Mallya | Perry R. Klokkevold

CHAPTER OUTLINE

Standard Projections
Cross-Sectional Imaging
Interactive "Simulation" Software
  Programs

Patient Evaluation
Clinical Selection of Diagnostic
  Imaging

Conclusion

Several radiographic imaging options are available for the diagnosis and treatment planning of patients receiving dental implants.[2,17,18] Options range from standard projections routinely available in the dental office to more complex radiographic techniques typically available only in radiology centers. Standard projections include intraoral (periapical, occlusal) and extraoral (panoramic, lateral cephalometric) radiographs. More complex imaging techniques include cone-beam computed tomography (CBCT) and multislice computed tomography (MSCT). The CBCT and MSCT image data files can be reformatted and viewed on a personal computer using simulation software, making the diagnosis and treatment-planning process interactive and visually more meaningful. Often, combinations of various modalities are used because no single modality can provide all information pertinent to the radiographic evaluation of the implant patient. Familiarity with the benefits and limitations of various techniques and awareness of the specific clinical questions that need to be answered should guide the decision-making process and selection of radiographic examinations for individual patients.

Multiple factors influence the selection of radiographic technique(s) for a particular case, including cost, availability, radiation exposure, and case type. The decision is a balance between these factors and the desire to minimize risk of complications to the patient. Accurately identifying vital anatomic structures and being able to perform implant placement surgery without injury to these structures are critical to treatment success. Diagnostic imaging must always be interpreted in conjunction with a good clinical examination.

This chapter discusses common imaging techniques used for evaluation of the implant patient. Indications for each technique are outlined, along with the advantages and limitations of each technique.

KEY FACT

Accurate identification of vital anatomic structures is critical to treatment success when performing dental implant surgery. Diagnostic imaging must always be interpreted along with a clinical examination.

Standard Projections

Standard diagnostic imaging modalities include periapical, panoramic, lateral cephalometric, and occlusal radiographs. Table 76.1 summarizes the advantages and disadvantages of each modality.

Periapical Radiographs

Periapical radiographs are often the first imaging modality used to evaluate the implant patient.[19,20] These radiographs provide an overall assessment of the quantity and quality of the edentulous alveolar ridge and the adjacent teeth. They are easy to obtain in the dental office, are relatively inexpensive, and deliver low radiation dose to the patient[8] (Table 76.2). Dentists are familiar with the depicted anatomy and possible pathology. Because these direct-exposure projections do not use intensifying screens, intraoral radiographs offer the highest detail and spatial resolution of all radiographic modalities (Fig. 76.1). Thus intraoral radiographs are the projection of choice when subtle, localized pathology, such as a retained root tip, needs to be detected and evaluated.

The most significant disadvantage of periapical radiographs is their susceptibility to unpredictable magnification of anatomic structures, which does not allow reliable measurements.[15] Foreshortening or elongation can be minimized by the use of paralleling technique. However, distortion is particularly accentuated in edentulous areas, where missing teeth and resorption of the alveolus necessitate receptor placement at significant angulation in relation to the long axis of the teeth and alveolar bone. Additionally, periapical radiographs are two-dimensional representations of three-dimensional objects and do not provide any information of the buccal-lingual dimension of the alveolar ridge. Structures that are distinctly separated in the buccal-lingual dimension appear to be overlapping. Also, the periapical image is limited by the size of film or sensor being used. Often, it is not possible to image the entire height of the remaining alveolar ridge, and when extensive mesial-distal areas need to be evaluated, multiple periapical radiographs are required.

Periapical radiographs are useful screening images that offer a detailed view of a small area of the alveolar arch. Limitations that must be considered include the possibility of distortion and the two-dimensional representation of anatomic structures.

Occlusal Radiographs

Occlusal radiographs are intraoral projections that offer easy, economic, low-radiation dose and high-resolution images covering a larger area than periapical projections.[20] Depending on receptor placement and the angulation of the x-ray tube, occlusal radiographs can provide an image of the mandibular width or can depict an extended area of the edentulous ridge. Occlusal radiographs have

TABLE 76.1 Advantages and Disadvantages of the Various Radiographic Projections

Modality	Advantages	Disadvantages
Periapical and occlusal radiography	High resolution and detail, easy acquisition, low radiation exposure, relatively inexpensive	Unpredictable magnification, small imaged area, 2D representation of anatomy
Panoramic radiography	Easy to acquire, images the full dentoalveolar ridge, low radiation dose, relatively inexpensive	Unpredictable magnification, unequal magnification in vertical and horizontal dimensions, 2D representation of anatomy, not detailed
Lateral cephalometric radiography	Easy to acquire, predictable magnification, low radiation dose, relatively inexpensive	Limited use in area of midline, 2D representation of anatomy
Multislice computed tomography	3D representation, no magnification, sufficient detail, digital format, images whole arch	Requires special equipment, expensive, higher radiation dose
Cone-beam computed tomography	3D representation, no magnification, sufficient detail, digital format, images whole arch, low radiation dose	Requires special equipment, relatively expensive

2D, Two-dimensional; *3D,* three-dimensional.

TABLE 76.2 Radiation Dose (Effective Dose in μSv) Received From Common Projections During Evaluation of the Implant Patient Data

Modality	Effective Dose (μSv)
Full-mouth x-ray (FMX) series	177
Panoramic	20
Limited field-of-view CBCT	47
Medium field-of-view CBCT	98
Large field-of-view CBCT	117
MSCT, Maxillofacial	913

CBCT, Cone-beam computed tomography; *CT,* computed tomography; *MSCT,* multislice computed tomography.
Adapted from Mallya SM: Principles of cone beam computed tomography. In Fayad M, Johnson BR, editors: *3D imaging in endodontics: a new era in diagnosis and treatment.* Median effective doses for standard exposure protocols were derived from collation of data from several reports in the literature.

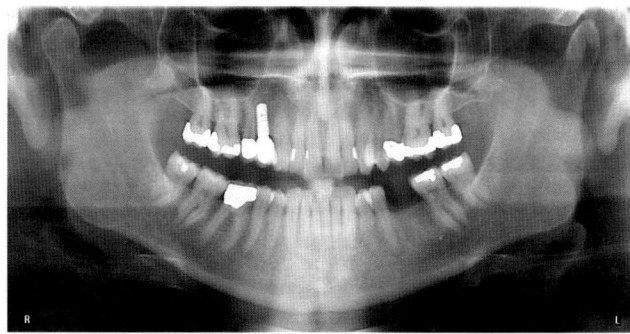

Fig. 76.2 Panoramic radiograph. Both jaws are visualized on the same image. An overall assessment of superoinferior and mesial–distal dimensions of the alveolar ridge can be formulated. Tooth and root positions relative to planned implant sites can be evaluated. Important anatomic structures, such as the maxillary sinus and mandibular canal, can be identified.

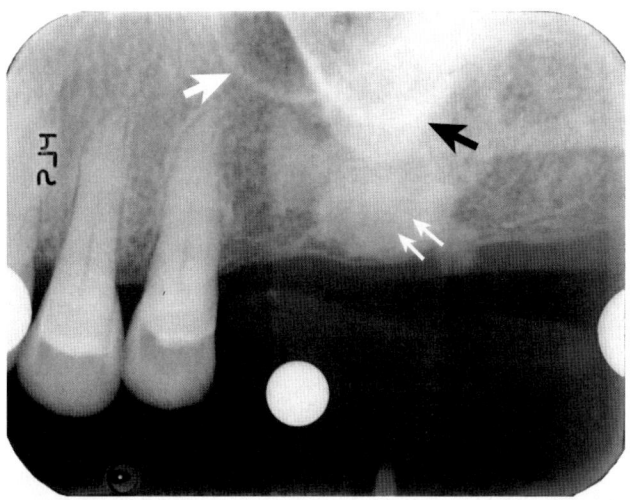

Fig. 76.1 The periapical radiograph offers a high-resolution, detailed image of the edentulous area. Healing of the extraction socket with dense bone (socket sclerosis) can be seen *(small white arrows).* Some anatomic structures, such as the maxillary sinus *(large white arrow)* and the zygomatic process of the maxilla *(black arrow),* can also be visualized.

the same limitations of distortion and overlapping anatomy as periapical radiographs.

Occlusal radiographic projections offer an initial assessment of the implant patient, and they provide an overview of the mandibular width or can visualize larger areas of alveolar ridge compared with periapical radiographic projections.

Panoramic Radiographs

Panoramic radiographs are often used in the evaluation of the implant patient because they offer several advantages over other modalities.[16] Panoramic radiographs deliver low radiation doses (see Table 76.2) to provide a broad picture of both arches and thus allow assessment of longer edentulous spans, angulation of existing teeth and occlusal plane, and important anatomy in implant treatment planning such as the maxillary sinus, nasal cavity, mental foramen, and mandibular canal (Fig. 76.2). Panoramic units are widely available and easy to operate, and dentists are familiar with the anatomy and pathology depicted by the images. Similar to intraoral projections, panoramic images are two-dimensional and thus do not offer diagnostic information for the buccal–lingual width of the alveolar arch.

Panoramic images appear intuitively familiar. However, they combine characteristic physical and radiographic principles that make them distinct from other intraoral and extraoral radiographs. Although outside the scope of this chapter, familiarity with the principles underlying panoramic radiography is central for understanding, and thus compensating for, the limitations and constraints of the images. The reader is referred to other textbooks for detailed discussion of this topic.[7,10] Briefly, the existence of ghost shadows, unpredictable horizontal and vertical magnification, distortion of structures outside the focal trough, projection geometry generated by the negative vertical angulation of the x-ray beam, and the propensity to patient-positioning errors do not allow consistently detailed and accurate measurements to be generated. As a result, panoramic radiographs do not provide the highly detailed images that are generated by intraoral radiographs.

Measurement distortion is more prevalent and varies across the radiographic image. On average, panoramic radiographs are 25% magnifications of actual size. Implant manufacturers often provide transparency sheets with implant size outlines of 25% magnification. However, it is important to appreciate that the 25% magnification is an estimate. The actual magnification may range from 10% to 30% in different areas within the same image and depends greatly on patient positioning during panoramic radiography. For this reason, precise measurements on panoramic projections are not possible. Nonetheless, panoramic radiographs offer an overall view of the maxilla and mandible that can be used to estimate bone measurements and evaluate the approximate relationships between teeth and other anatomic structures. More precise diagnostic imaging should be used to measure the proximity of critical anatomic structures, such as the maxillary sinus or the mandibular canal, to proposed implant positions.

Panoramic projections provide useful information for the initial assessment of the implant patient. However, because of magnification and distortion errors, panoramic radiographs should not be used for detailed measurements of proposed implant sites.

Cross-Sectional Imaging

Cross-sectional diagnostic imaging modalities include MSCT and CBCT. Conventional tomography also provides cross-sectional images with predictable magnification and has been used in the assessment of the implant patient. However, with the introduction and expansion of CBCT imaging, conventional tomography is becoming obsolete and is not described in this chapter.

Cone-Beam Computed Tomography

Cone-beam computed tomography (CBCT) is an imaging modality that offers significant advantages for the evaluation of implant patients.[5,14] CBCT was introduced to dentistry in the late 1990s,[1,12] and several CBCT units are commercially available for imaging of the craniofacial complex. The x-ray source and the detector are diametrically positioned and make a 180- to 360-degree rotation around the patient's head within the gantry. The x-ray beam is collimated and the resultant beam is cone or pyramid shaped. Typically, a single complete rotation, 180 to 500 basis projections of the region of interest, is generated. The computer uses these images to generate a digital, three-dimensional map of the face. Once this map is generated, multiplanar reconstructions—axial, coronal, sagittal, or oblique sections of various thicknesses—can be reconstructed from the data.

> ### KEY FACT
>
> CBCT offers significant advantages for the evaluation of implant patients. The field of view (FOV) is an important feature that describes the extent of the imaged volume from large FOV (greater than 15 cm) to medium FOV (8 to 15 cm) and limited FOV (less than 8 cm). Limited FOV units image a small area, delivering less radiation and producing a higher-resolution image

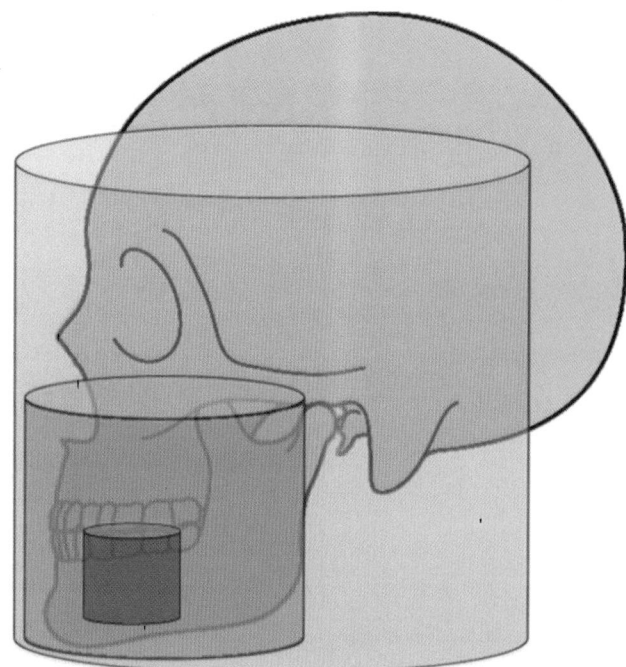

Fig. 76.3 Schematic diagram of the anatomic area imaged with large *(green),* medium *(blue),* and limited *(magenta)* field of view cone-beam computed tomography.

An important feature of the various CBCT units is the field of view (FOV) describing the extent of the imaged volume. CBCT units are typically categorized as large FOV (greater than 15 cm), medium FOV (8 to 15 cm), and limited FOV systems (less than 8 cm). Fig. 76.3 depicts schematically the anatomic area covered by large, medium, and limited FOV scans. In general, large FOV units image a more extensive anatomic area, deliver a higher radiation exposure to the patient, and produce lower-resolution images (Fig. 76.4). Conversely, limited FOV units image a small area of the face, deliver less radiation, and produce a higher-resolution image (Fig. 76.5).

CBCT scans offer several advantages for evaluation of the implant patient, compared with two-dimensional (2D) imaging. True cross sections offer a precise and detailed evaluation of the height and width of the alveolar ridge. The images can be adjusted and printed without magnification, facilitating measurements directly on the prints or films with standard rulers (i.e., not magnified). Vertical and horizontal rulers adjacent to each section allow the clinician to check for magnification and make direct measurements. The digital format allows for image enhancement tools, rapid communication between the radiologist and the surgeon, and generation of multiple copies of the images. Various anatomic structures can be visualized and analyzed at all three coordinate axes, so that their superoinferior, anteroposterior, and buccolingual location can be identified with precision. CBCT images the entire arch, or even both arches, so several edentulous areas can be visualized with a single examination. The bone and soft-tissue contrast and resolution are appropriate for the diagnostic task.

In summary, CBCT scanning is a valuable imaging modality for three-dimensional and cross-sectional evaluation of the implant patient. It has similar advantages and disadvantages as CT scanning. The most significant difference is that CBCT imaging delivers much less radiation exposure to the patient.

Multislice Computed Tomography

Multislice CT (MSCT) was widely used in the evaluation of the implant patient.[3,6] However, with the advent of CBCT, utilization of

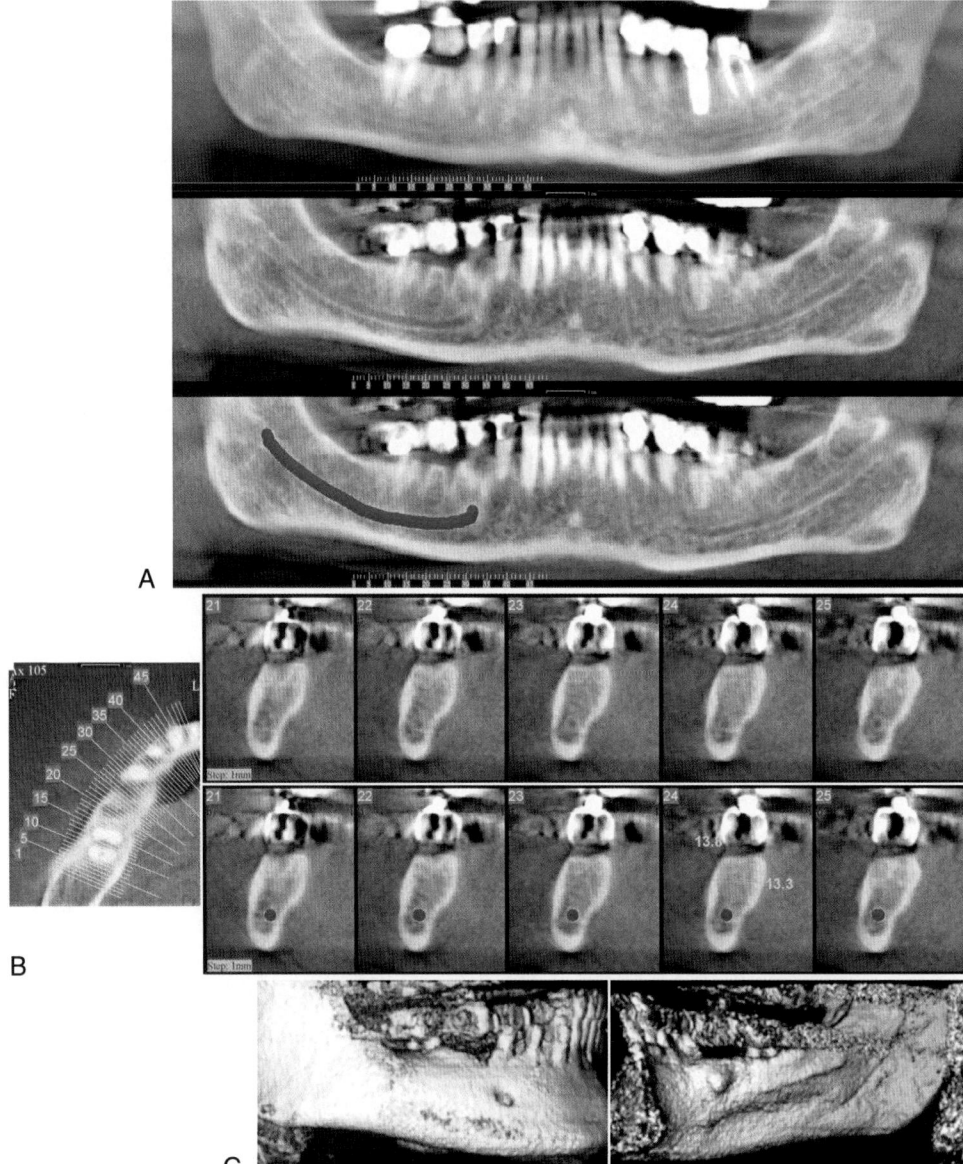

Fig. 76.4 Cone-beam computed tomography images for the evaluation of the edentulous space at the area of missing tooth #30 before implant placement using a large field-of-view unit (NewTom 3G, Verona, Italy, distributed by AFP Imaging, Elmsford, New York). Note the tooth-shaped marker used. (A) A series of "panoramic" reconstructions through the alveolar ridge reveals the relationship of the marker to the adjacent teeth. The top "panoramic" view is 12 mm thick so as to depict most of the extent of the alveolar ridge and adjacent teeth. The middle "panoramic" image is 1 mm thick through the area of the mandibular canal. Note that adjacent teeth are out of the plane of the section and thus not depicted on the image. The bottom "panoramic" view is the same as the middle one, but the position of the mandibular canal has been depicted by the *red line*. (B) Scout axial view and series of cross sections through the area of the marker. The bottom row shows the same axial slices as the top row. However, the position of the *red line* drawn on the panoramic view is also depicted to help localization of the mandibular canal. The height and width of the alveolar ridge have been measured in a selected section. (C) Three-dimensional reconstructions provide an overall impression of the bone contours and shape of the alveolar ridge. Note the small exostosis on the lingual surface of the alveolar ridge.

MSCT has been reduced significantly. However, MSCT is an excellent choice for evaluation of the implant patient if CBCT scanning is not available.[4]

Typical dental views reconstructed from a MSCT scan include a scout view (see Fig. 76.6A) as well as axial (Fig. 76.6B), panoramic (Fig. 76.6C), and cross-sectional (Fig. 76.6D) views of the jaws. Appropriate axial slices through the alveolar ridge of interest are selected as scout views. The curvature of the maxillary or mandibular ridge is then drawn on the axial slices, and panoramic images along the drawn line are created. Finally, cross-sectional slices, typically at every 1 to 2 mm and perpendicular to the drawn curvature, are created. In addition to these flat, two-dimensional views, complex, three-dimensional images with surface rendering can also be generated from the CT data (Fig. 76.6E). These images can provide useful information about the alveolar ridge defects that are easy to comprehend.

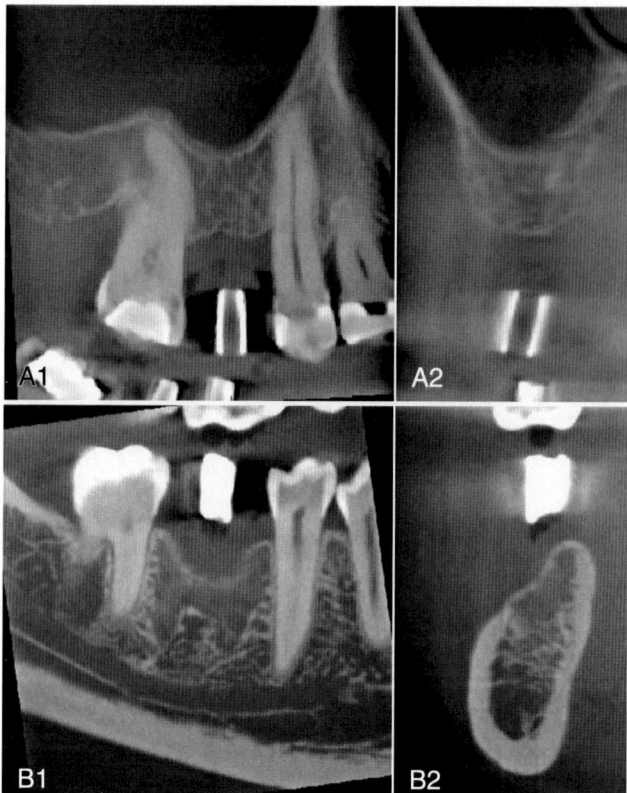

Fig. 76.5 Cone-beam computed tomography images for the evaluation of the edentulous space at the area of missing tooth #4 (A) and missing tooth #30 (B) using a limited field-of-view scan (3D Accuitomo, J. Morita Corporation, Suita City, Osaka, Japan, distributed by J. Morita USA, Inc., Irvine, California). Sagittal and cross-sectional slices are shown. Although the anatomic area imaged is limited, the resolutions of the images are high. (A) Implant site #4 (maxillary right second premolar) in anterior–posterior (A1) and buccolingual (A2) cross-sectional views. (B) Implant site #30 (mandibular right first molar) in anterior–posterior (B1) and buccolingual (B2) cross-sectional views.

MSCT offers the same advantages and disadvantages as MSCT. However, the two modalities have basic differences that result from the different physical principles used during image acquisition. MSCT scans offers a greater *contrast resolution,* or the ability to distinguish two objects with small density differences. In contrast, CBCT scans have a limited capacity to separate muscle from fat or connective tissue compared with MSCT scans. Fortunately, the diagnostic tasks in implant treatment planning do not require high-contrast resolution. Because bone has a much higher radiodensity than surrounding soft tissues, both CBCT and MSCT clearly depict bone morphology and internal trabecular architecture. One of the most significant advantages of CBCT scanning versus MSCT scanning is the significantly lower radiation dose delivered to the patient[9,21,22] (Table 76.2).

MSCT scanning requires specialized equipment and setting. Radiologists and technicians need to be knowledgeable of the anatomy, anatomic variants, and pathology of the jaws, as well as considerations pertinent to implant treatment planning, so that optimal views will be provided. An MSCT scan delivers a much higher radiation dose to the patient than the other modalities used during implant treatment planning[13] (Table 76.2). Because a CT scan images the whole arch, radiation is delivered to the entire imaged area, regardless of how many or how few sites are actually needed. Metallic restorations can cause beam-hardening artifacts that impair the diagnostic quality

of the images. This is particularly challenging in patients with heavily restored dentition. In general, the cost of MSCT is significantly higher than that of CBCT or the other standard intraoral and extraoral projections.

In summary, MSCT scanning offers many advantages during implant treatment planning, including accurate cross-sectional imaging and three-dimensional visualization of anatomic structures. High dose to the patient and artifacts caused by metallic restorations are concerns that should be considered.

Interactive "Simulation" Software Programs

Implant treatment planning can be greatly enhanced by the use of specialized software. In addition to measuring the quantity and quality of bone in potential implant sites, these programs use CT (MSCT or CBCT) scan data to simulate placement of implant and restorations. Using a database of commercially available implant images, the length, width, angulation, and position of implants can be "simulated" in the desired positions and evaluated relative to other structures in three dimensions. In cases of alveolar ridge deficiency or defects, or when sinus bone augmentation is indicated, the additional bone volume needed can be evaluated and quantified. The restoration of the implants can also be simulated and the distribution of mechanical forces onto the implant and adjacent bone predicted.

Software programs specialized in implant treatment planning, such as SIM/Plant (Materialise/Columbia Scientific, Glen Burnie, Maryland), can acquire information directly from CBCT or CT scan data. The clinician can use the reformatted images on a personal computer in an interactive manner to identify anatomic structures, simulate implant placement positions, and better appreciate relationships between planned implant positions and teeth or anatomic structures (Fig. 76.7). InVivo5 planning software (Anatomage, San Jose, California) acquires data directly from CBCT or CT scan DICOM (Digital Imaging and Communications in Medicine) files without the need for reformatting. The clinician can evaluate the case on a personal computer in an interactive manner to identify anatomic structures, simulate implant placement positions, and better appreciate relationships between planned implant positions and teeth or anatomic structures. Once implant positions are confirmed, a computer-generated surgical guide is produced to facilitate the surgical placement of implants in the planned positions (Fig. 76.8).

Patient Evaluation

Evaluation of the implant patient should be disciplined and objective. Specific questions that can affect implant placement and outcome should be considered and examined carefully and explicitly. The advantages and disadvantages of various radiographic projections should be considered and radiographic modalities chosen based on necessary information for the particular patient. The objectives for any radiographic evaluation, regardless of imaging technique used, should include an evaluation to (1) exclude pathology, (2) identify anatomic structures, and (3) measure the quantity, quality, and location of available bone.

> **CLINICAL CORRELATION**
>
> All diagnostic images, regardless of technique, should be evaluated to identify or exclude pathology and to identify normal anatomic structures.

Text continued on p. 762

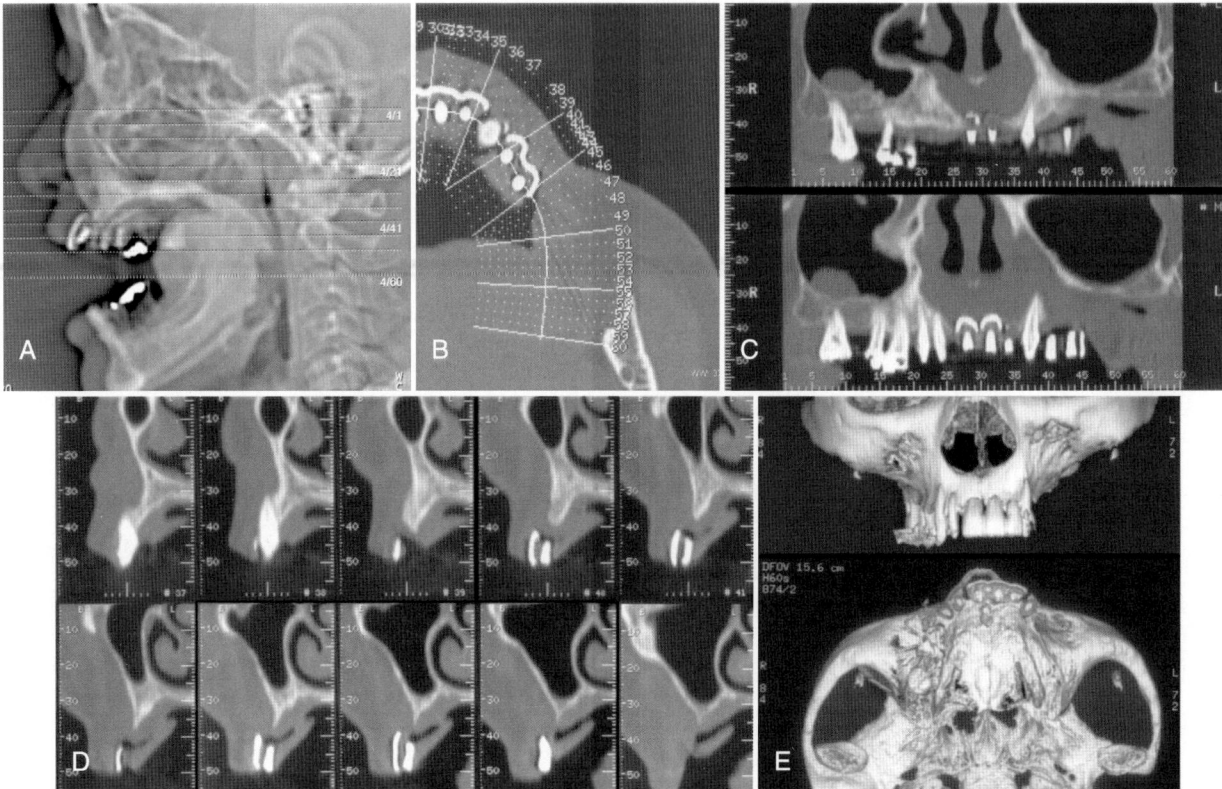

Fig. 76.6 Multislice computed tomography (MSCT) examination for evaluation of edentulous maxilla before implant placement. (A) Scout view of the patient's head; axial sections through the area of interest are indicated. (B) Axial slice through the markers is used to display the orientation of the panoramic and cross-sectional images through the alveolar ridge. (C) Panoramic views through the alveolar ridge demonstrate the relation of the markers to adjacent teeth. (D) Cross-sectional slices through the area of the markers reveal the height and buccolingual dimension of the alveolar ridge, as well as the relation of the markers to the ridge. (E) Three-dimensional reconstructions provide an overall impression of the bone contours and shape of the alveolar ridge.

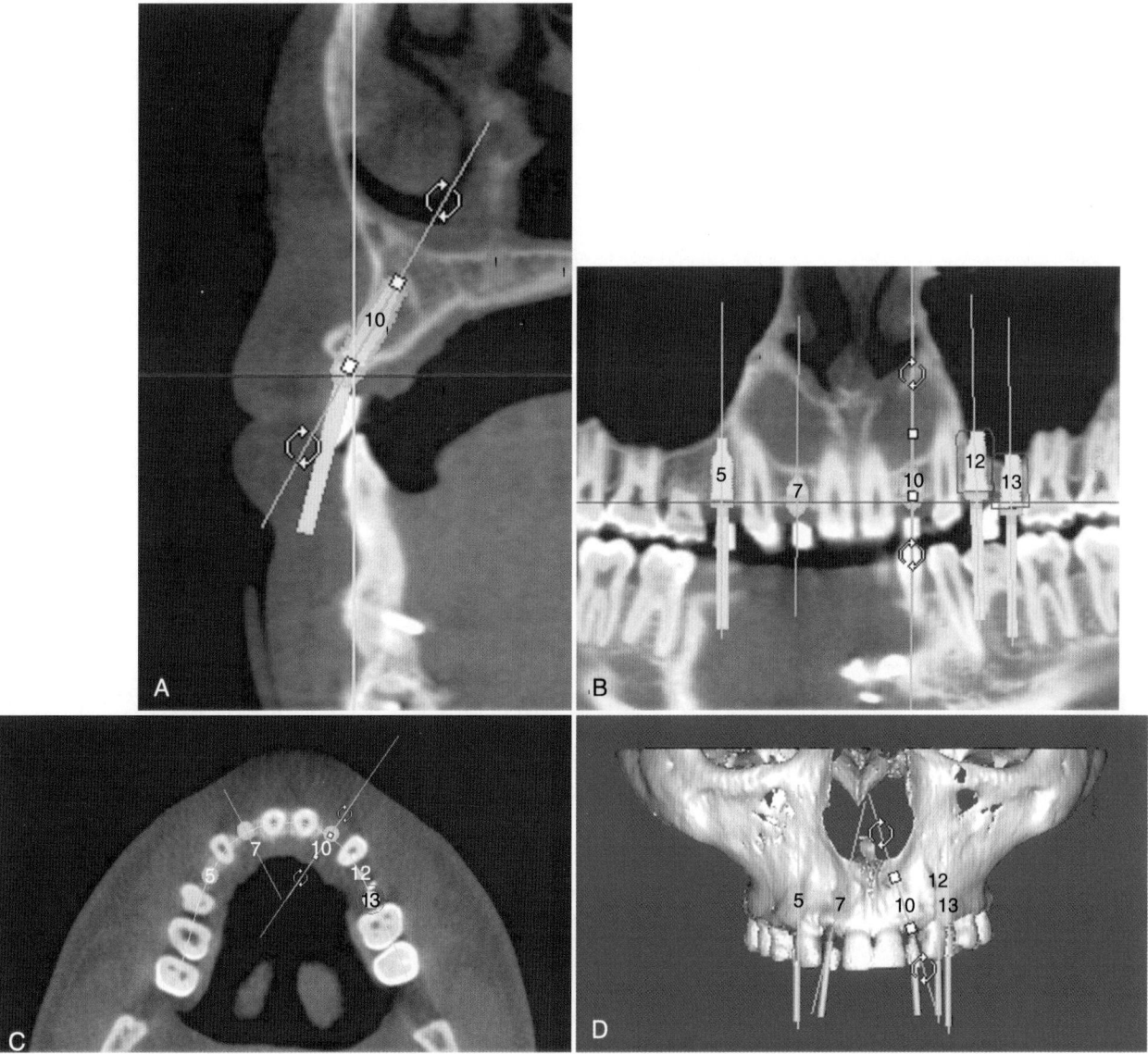

Fig. 76.7 SIM/Plant images. The SIM/Plant software program allows clinicians to measure bone height, width, density, and volume on a personal computer. Scan data are reformatted for interactive evaluation and manipulation. Implant positions can be simulated on the patient's scan data before surgery, allowing the surgeon to anticipate areas of deficiency. (A) Cross-sectional image through simulated implant in anterior maxilla, site #10. (B) Panoramic projection of multiple simulated implant positions, #5, 7, 10, 12, and 13. (C) Axial view of simulated implants. (D) Three-dimensional image of maxilla with simulated implants.

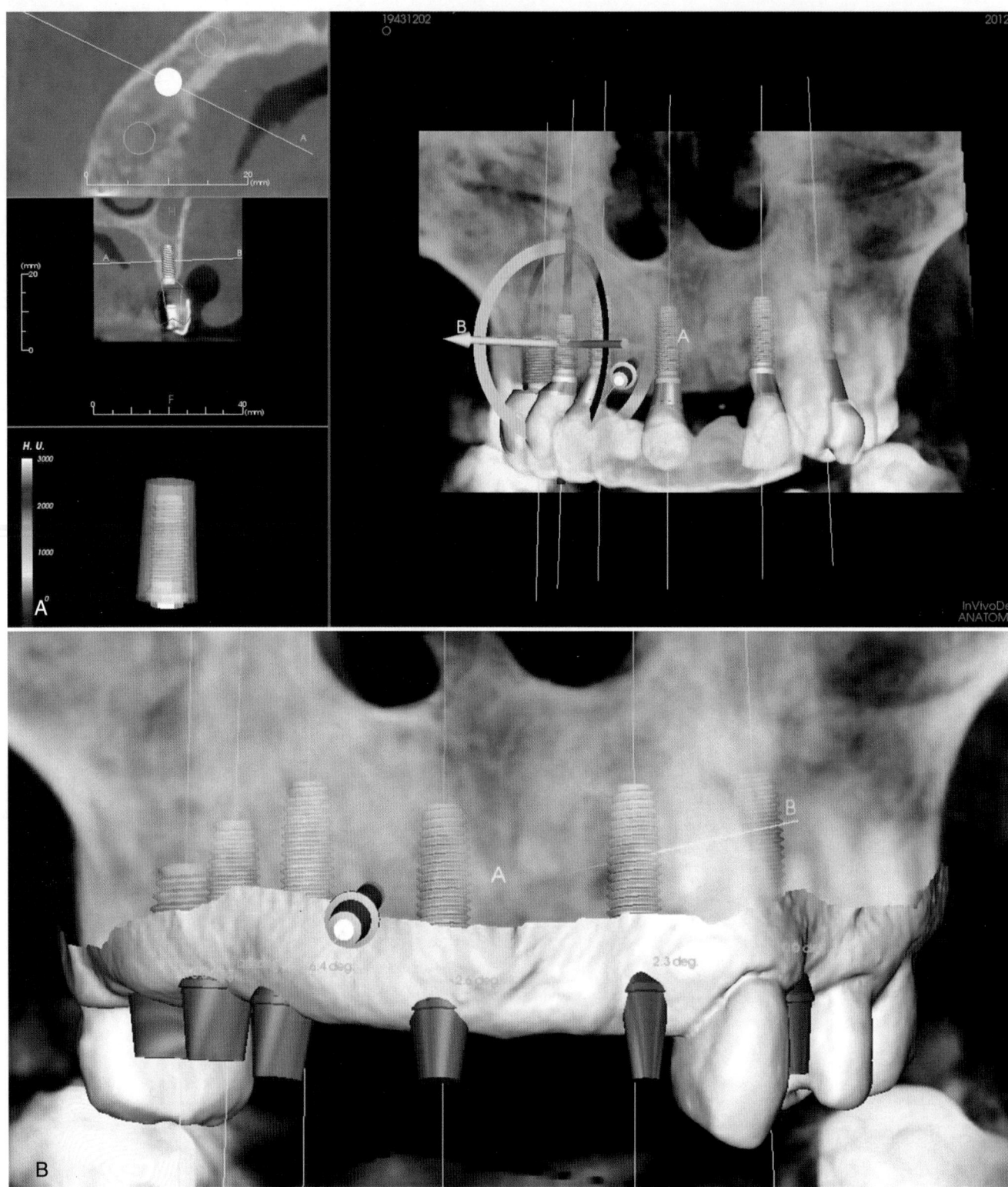

Fig. 76.8 InVivo5 simulation images. The InVivo5 software program allows clinicians to plan implant treatment and simulate virtual implant positions directly from DICOM scan data on a personal computer. (A) Cross section and axial images with three-dimensional simulation of implant positions. (B) Model mockup for computer-generated surgical guide.

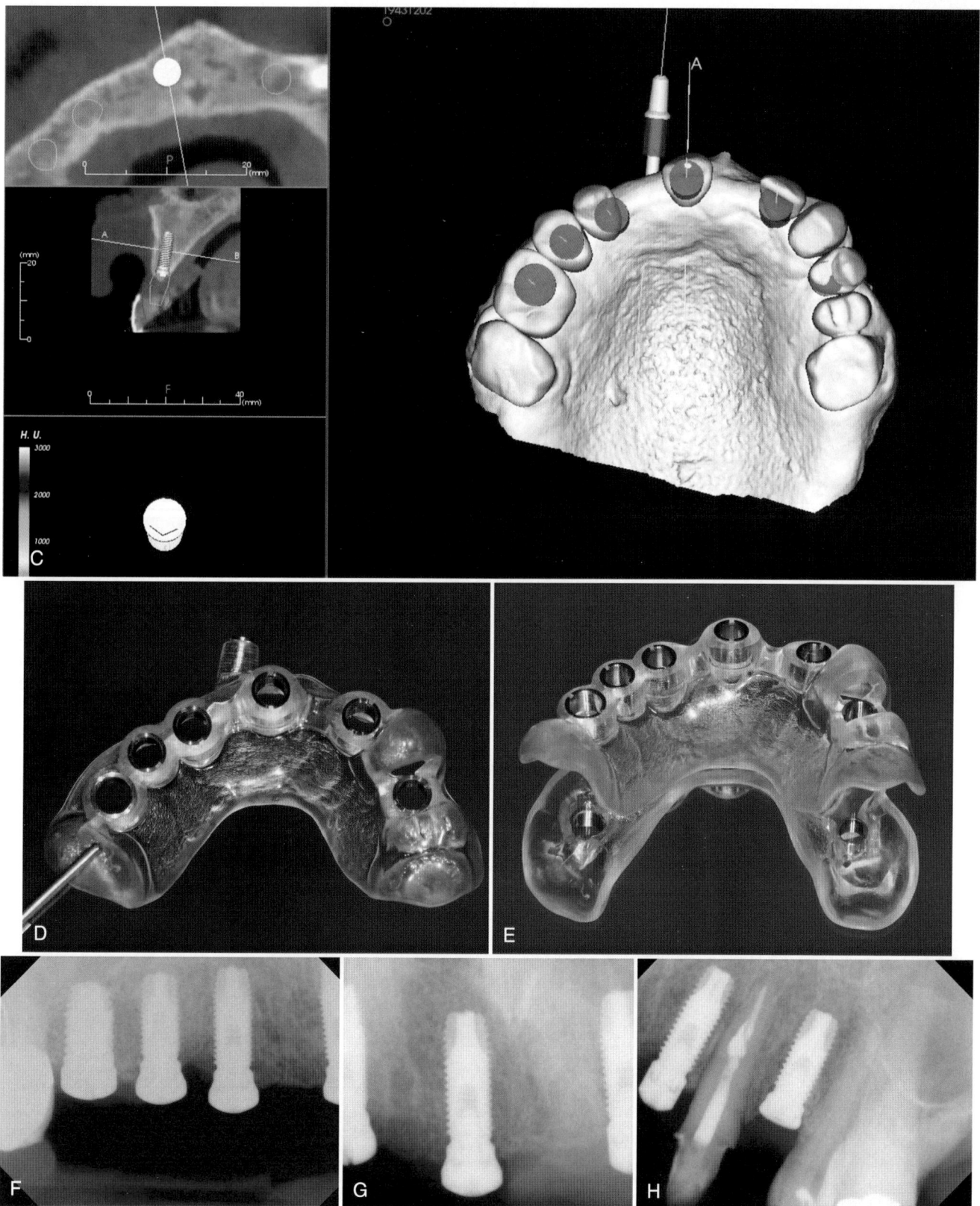

Fig. 76.8, cont'd (D–E) Surgical guide that was created from a simulated plan. (F–H) Periapical radiographs demonstrating the accurate position and alignment of implants that were placed using a computer-generated surgical guide.

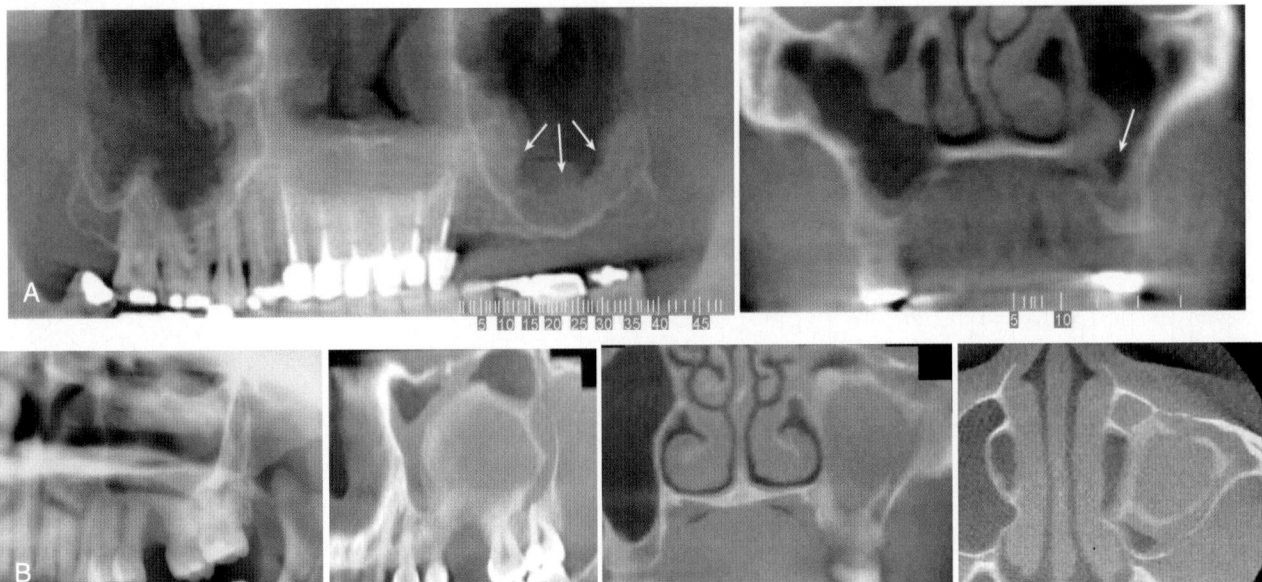

Fig. 76.9 Cone-beam computed tomography examination of the posterior left maxilla. Top row (A) shows reconstructed "panoramic" and coronal sections of the alveolar ridge. Note the thickened mucoperiosteal lining of the floor of the left maxillary sinus *(white arrow)*. The patient has chronic maxillary sinusitis. Bottom row (B) shows conventional panoramic, reconstructed "panoramic," coronal, and axial sections of the alveolar ridge at the area of the missing first maxillary molar. A large radiolucent lesion at the edentulous alveolar ridge elevates the floor of the maxillary sinus and occupies most of the sinus. Biopsy revealed a keratocystic odontogenic tumor that was an incidental finding in this asymptomatic patient.

Exclude Pathology

Healthy bone is a prerequisite for successful osseointegration and long-term implant success. The first step in the radiographic evaluation of the implant site is to establish the health of the alveolar bone and other tissues imaged within a particular projection. Local and systemic diseases that affect bone homeostasis can preclude, modify, or alter the placement of implants. Retained root fragments, residual periodontal disease, cysts, and tumors should be identified and resolved before implant placement. Systemic diseases, such as osteoporosis and hyperparathyroidism, alter bone metabolism and might affect implant osseointegration. Areas of poor bone quality should be identified and, if indicated, adjustments to the treatment plan incorporated. Maxillary sinusitis, polyps, or other sinus pathology should be diagnosed and treated when implants are considered in the posterior maxilla, especially if sinus bone augmentation procedures are planned (Fig. 76.9).

Identify Anatomic Structures

Several important anatomic structures are found close to desired areas of implant placement in the maxilla and mandible (Box 76.1). Familiarity with the radiographic appearance of these structures is important during treatment planning and implant placement. Their exact localization is central to prevent unwanted complications and unnecessary morbidity. Important anatomic structures in the maxilla include the floor and anterior wall of the maxillary sinus, incisive foramen, floor and lateral wall of the nasal cavity, and canine fossa. Important anatomic structures in the mandible that should be recognized include the mandibular canal, anterior loop of the mandibular canal, mental foramen, anterior extension of the canal, and submandibular fossa. The existence of anatomic variants, such as incomplete healing of an extraction site, sinus loculation, division of mandibular canal (Fig. 76.10), or absence of a well-defined corticated canal, should also be recognized. See Chapter 58 for important periodontal and implant surgical anatomy.

BOX 76.1 Anatomic Structures Pertinent to Treatment Planning of the Implant Patient

Maxilla
Maxillary sinus (floor and anterior wall)
Nasal cavity (floor and lateral wall)
Incisive foramen
Canine fossa
Canalis sinuosus

Mandible
Mandibular canal
Anterior loop of the mandibular canal
Anterior extension of the mandibular canal
Mental foramen
Submandibular fossa
Retromolar canal
Lingual inclination of the alveolar ridge

CLINICAL CORRELATION

Several important anatomic structures need to be identified in the jaws prior to implant placement. Violation of structures such as nerves may cause serious complications. Familiarity with the radiographic appearance of vital structures is important, and the existence of anatomic variants should also be recognized.

Assess Bone Quantity, Quality, and Volume

The primary goal of diagnostic imaging for potential implant patients is to evaluate the available bone volume for implant placement in desired anatomic locations. The clinician should estimate and verify exact adequate height, width, and density to the recipient bone while

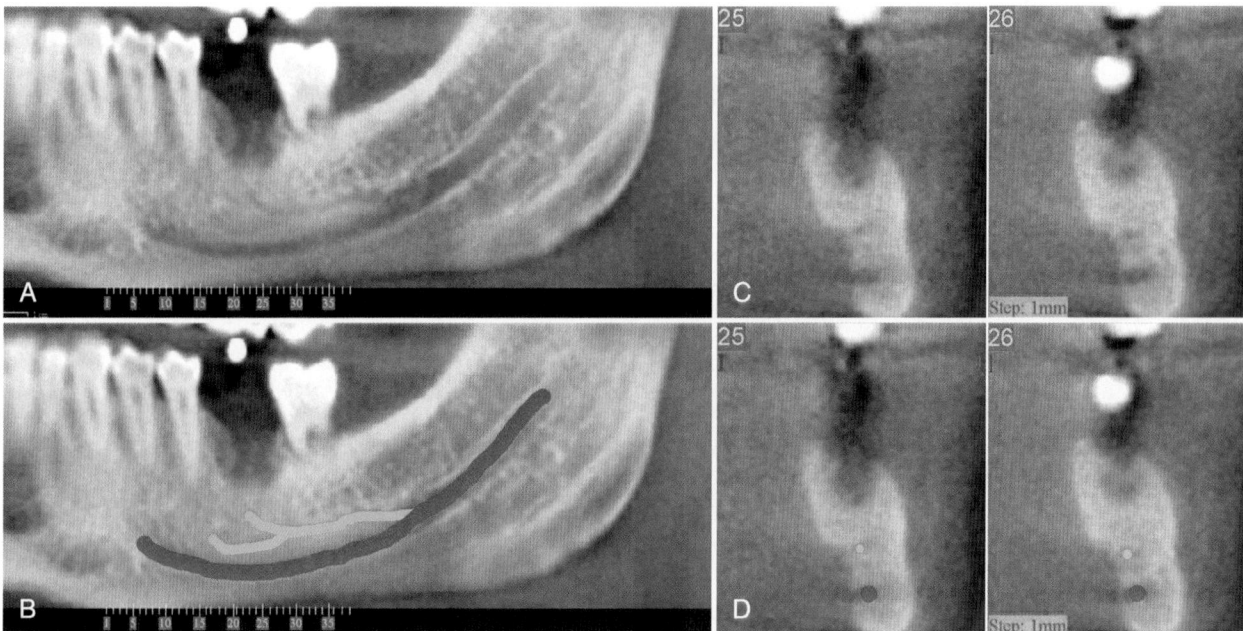

Fig. 76.10 Cone-beam computed tomography examination of the area of missing tooth #19 before implant placement. (A) Panoramic view of the area of interest depicts an accessory mandibular canal. (B) Same panoramic view with the accessory mandibular canal colored blue and the main canal colored red. (C) Cross-sectional views through the area of missing tooth #19. (D) Same cross-sectional images depicting the blue and red markings. Note that the position of the markings coincides with the position of the accessory and main mandibular canals (compare parts C and D).

avoiding damage to critical anatomic structures. Failure to accurately assess the location of important anatomic structures can lead to unnecessary complications. For example, inadvertent penetration and damage to the inferior alveolar nerve can result in serious immediate-term (profuse bleeding), short-term, and long-term (nerve paresthesia/anesthesia) complications. The height and width of the alveolar bone should be accurately detailed. Depending on the technique, diagnostic imaging can estimate or measure the coronal–apical height, the buccal–lingual width, and the mesial–distal spacing available for implants that will be placed in proximity to teeth or relative to other planned implants.

This task can be simple in cases with good bone quality and sufficient bone volume in the desired implant location(s). However, in cases with moderate to severe bone resorption, alveolar defects, or recent extraction sites, obtaining a clear and accurate diagnostic image can be more challenging. The diagnostic imaging may reveal inadequate bone volume for the proposed implant(s) and indicate a need for bone augmentation or, depending on the severity of the deficiency, preclude the patient from the possibility of implant therapy (Fig. 76.11). When ridge augmentation is deemed necessary, radiographic evaluation prior to and after surgery informs treatment planning and ensures grafting integrity and quality (Fig. 76.12).

In addition to the amount, the quality of the available bone should also be evaluated. A uniform, continuous cortical outline and a lacy, well-defined trabecular core reflect the normal bone homeostasis necessary for appropriate bone response around the implant. Thin or discontinuous cortex, sparse trabeculation, large marrow spaces, and altered trabecular architecture should be noted because they might predict poor implant stabilization and less desirable response of the bone. Poor bone quality may necessitate modifications of the treatment planning, such as waiting longer for healing (osseointegration) to maximize bone-to-implant contact before loading.

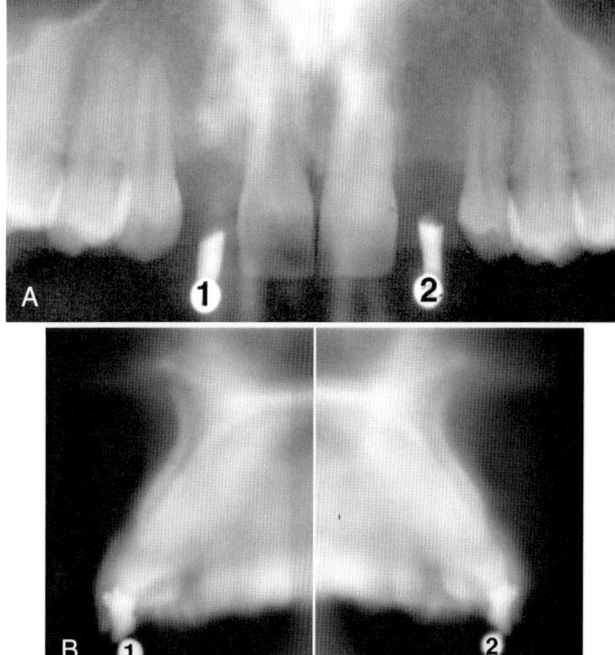

Fig. 76.11 Radiographic evaluation of a patient with congenitally missing maxillary lateral incisors before implant placement. (A) Panoramic radiograph reveals sufficient height and mesial-lateral width of the alveolar ridge. (B) Cross-sectional conventional tomography of the edentulous areas reveals a narrow (<4 mm) buccal-lingual width of the alveolar ridge that needs to be addressed by modifications in the treatment planning, such as bone augmentation.

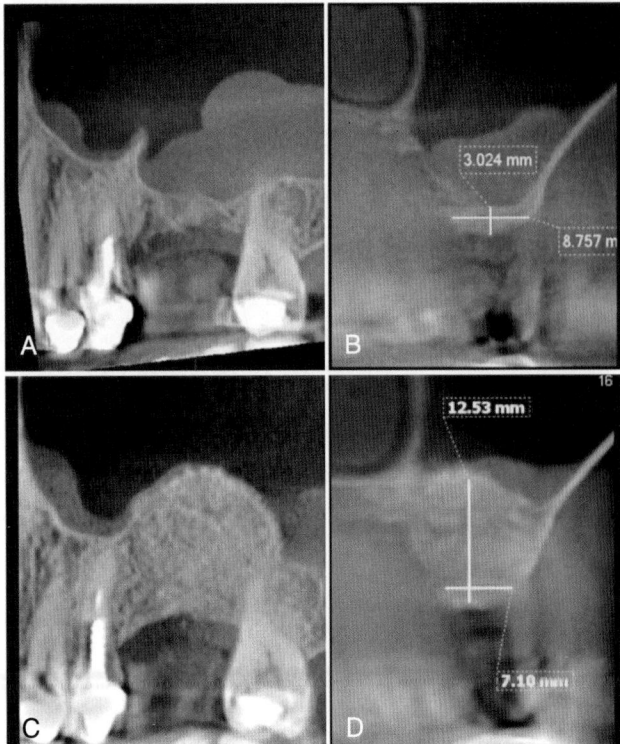

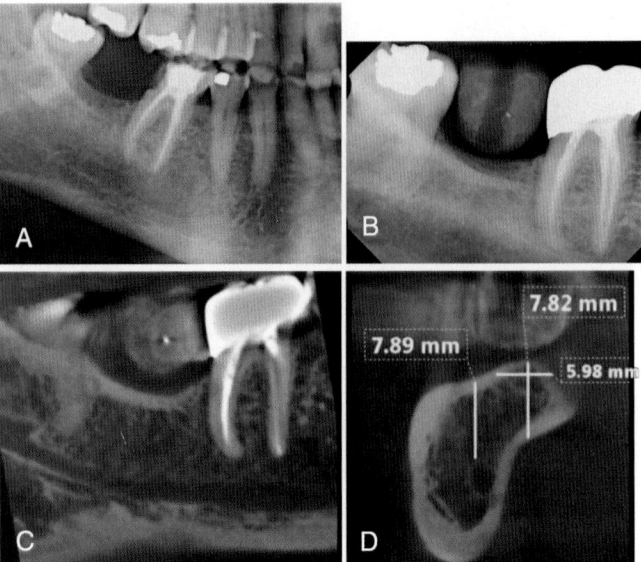

Fig. 76.12 Radiographic evaluation of a patient with missing left maxillary second premolar and first molar. Initial cone-beam computed tomography (CBCT) reveals an atrophic alveolar ridge (A) with inadequate height for implant placement (B). Also note the thickened mucoperiosteum at the floor of the maxillary sinus. CBCT after sinus grafting for ridge augmentation shows the uniformly opaque grafting area blending with alveolar trabeculation and a smooth sinus floor elevation (C), which provides adequate dimensions for implant placement (D).

Fig. 76.13 Radiographic evaluation of a patient with an edentulous posterior left mandible before implant placement. Panoramic (A) and periapical (B) radiographs demonstrate sufficient height of the alveolar ridge with little or no resorption. Cone-beam computed tomography sections (C–D) reveal significant lingual inclination of the alveolar ridge with lingual concavity that is not depicted on conventional radiographs.

Evaluate Relation of Alveolar Ridge With Existing Teeth and Desired Implant Position

Accurate placement (spatial position and angulation relative to adjacent teeth and occlusal plane) will greatly affect the restorative success and long-term prognosis of the implant (see Chapters 75 and 77). A significant variable during the preimplant evaluation is the relation of the desired implant position relative to the existing teeth, alveolar crest, and occlusal plane. Angled or custom abutments can accommodate slight variations in implant position and implant inclination. However, more significant deviations should be avoided.

Prolonged tooth loss is usually associated with atrophy of the alveolar ridge and, in the case of the maxilla, with pneumatization of the sinus floor toward the alveolar crest. Traumatic extractions can compromise the buccal or lingual cortex and alter the shape and buccolingual ridge dimension. Anatomic variants, such as lingual inclination of the alveolus or narrow ridges, should be considered during treatment planning of the implant patient (Fig. 76.13).

An important part of diagnostic imaging must include an evaluation of the available bone relative to the "prosthetically driven" implant position. This aspect of the patient evaluation is best accomplished with diagnostic models, wax-up of planned tooth replacement, and radiographic markers in the desired tooth positions during imaging. Steel balls, brass tubes, and gutta-percha have all been used to establish the proposed tooth positions relative to the existing alveolar bone. The use of these nonanatomic markers is helpful for evaluating bone height and width in specific anatomic locations. However, they do not accurately represent the tooth contours and do not allow the clinician to estimate variations in implant position and angulation relative to the position and emergence of the planned tooth replacement. Therefore it is more desirable and beneficial to use radiopaque tooth-shaped markers so that the existing alveolar bone can be evaluated relative to the entire tooth position/contours (Fig. 76.14; see also Fig. 76.5). This is particularly important for anterior, aesthetic implant cases. Patients should always be imaged with radiographic guides (markers).

Clinical Selection of Diagnostic Imaging

Radiography is an important diagnostic tool for the evaluation of the implant patient. However, radiographic imaging alone is insufficient. It is important to correlate diagnostic information with a good clinical examination. Conversely, a clinical examination is insufficient to provide the information needed to plan implant treatment for a patient without some radiographic imaging.

Clinical Examination

Before taking any radiographs, a complete clinical examination of the implant patient is required. This should include the etiology and duration of tooth loss, any history of traumatic extraction, and a review of records and radiographs, if available. A clinical assessment of the edentulous area, covering mucosa, adjacent and opposing teeth, and occlusal plane, should be performed. Temporomandibular function, mandibular maximal opening, and protrusive and lateral movements should be evaluated.

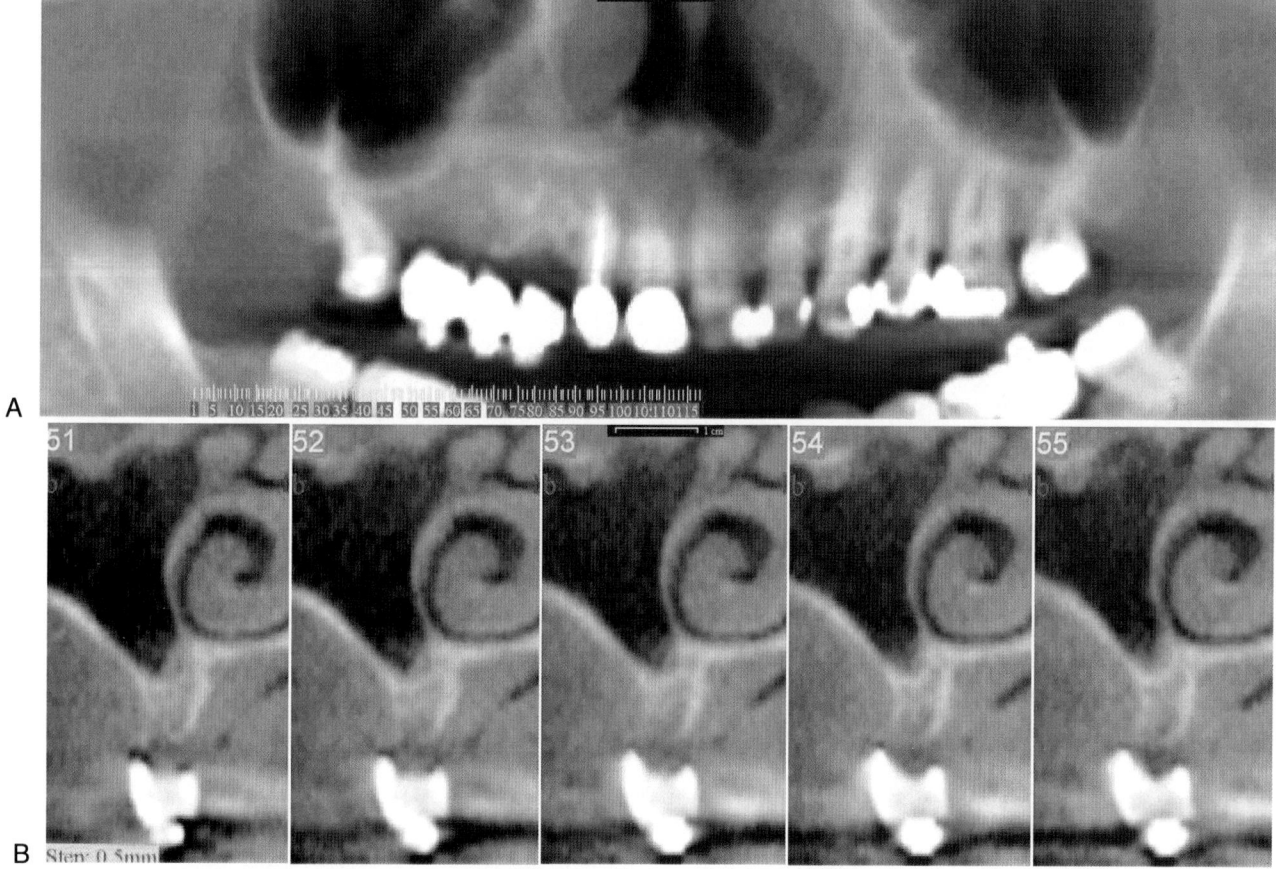

Fig. 76.14 (A) Panoramic view of partially edentulous maxilla with tooth-shaped markers in areas of missing teeth (potential implant sites). (B) Cross-sectional views from a cone-beam computed tomography examination before implant placement in the right maxilla. Appropriately sized and shaped tooth markers placed in the prosthetically desired locations of the planned restorations for the missing teeth help evaluate the existing alveolar ridge relative to the prospective tooth positions and contours.

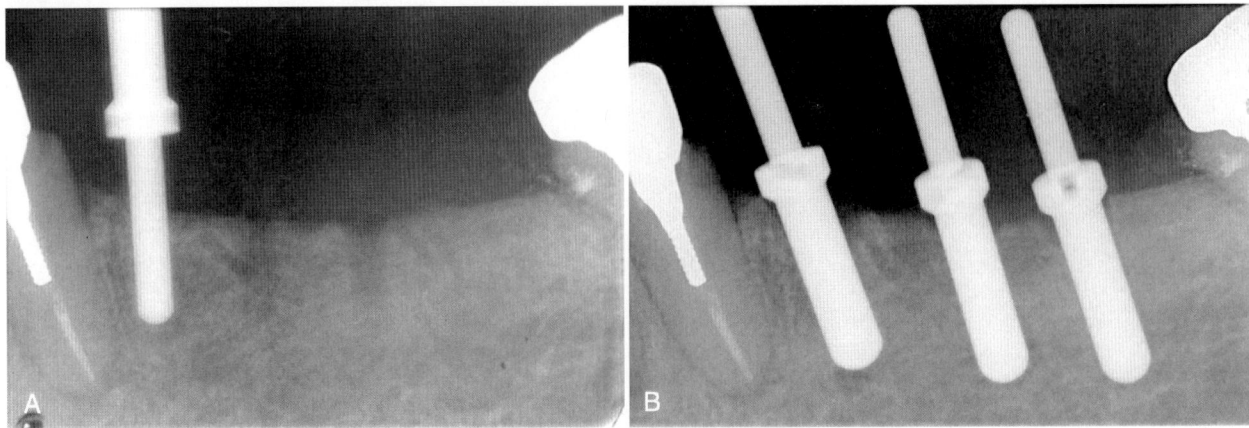

Fig. 76.15 Intraoperative periapical radiographs are valuable in assessing the proximity of adjacent teeth. (A) The 2-mm guide pin is used to determine the direction of the osteotomy site and its proximity to the adjacent root.[17] (B) After angle correction, the osteotomy sites are completed to length with the final drill. Here the 3-mm guide pins confirm the correct angulation and spacing of the final osteotomy site preparation before implant placement.

Screening Radiographs

At this point, an overall assessment of the health of the jaws should be performed. The American Academy of Oral and Maxillofacial Radiology recommends panoramic radiography as the initial evaluation of the dental implant patient, supplemented with periapical radiographs as needed.[17] Periapical radiographs provide a high-resolution image of the alveolus and the surrounding structures, including adjacent teeth. For extended edentulous areas, panoramic, lateral cephalometric, and occlusal radiographs can be used to estimate bone height and width. Any pathology of the bone at the prospective implant site, as well as of the surrounding structures, should be identified and treated as indicated.

KEY FACT

The American Academy of Oral and Maxillofacial Radiology recommends panoramic radiography as the initial evaluation of the dental implant patient, supplemented with periapical radiographs as needed. The organization also recommends that radiographic examination of any potential implant site should include cross-sectional imaging orthogonal to the site of interest.

Fabrication of Radiographic and Surgical Guides

Once the health of the soft and hard tissues is established, casts should be taken and a detailed analysis performed. The clinician should decide on the number of implants and their desired location. Next, a radiographic guide should be fabricated, usually with clear acrylic. The position of the desired implants is indicated by the use of radiopaque objects such as metallic balls, cylinders, or rods; gutta-percha; or composite resin. If CT imaging might be performed, the use of metallic markers should be avoided. The design of such a guide greatly enhances the diagnostic information provided by the radiographs because it correlates the radiographic anatomy with the exact position of the proposed implant location.

Cross-Sectional Imaging

The American Academy of Oral and Maxillofacial Radiology recommends that radiographic examination of any potential implant site should include cross-sectional imaging orthogonal to the site of interest.[17] The potential morbidity of a compromised anatomic structure

and the poor performance and potential failure of a misplaced implant, combined with the wide availability of tomographic facilities, favor the use of cross-sectional imaging in most cases of implant treatment planning. It is crucial that the cross sections are perpendicular to the curvature of the mandible and parallel to the planned implant. Improper patient positioning can lead to an overestimation of the height and width of the available bone. If the surgeon believes that sections were performed at the wrong angulation, new images should be requested. This might necessitate reexposure of the patient.

Intraoperative and Postoperative Radiographic Assessment

Various radiographic modalities can provide valuable information during implant placement. Because of the ease of acquisition and high resolution, periapical radiographs are most commonly used. Intraoperative radiographs can be taken during surgery to evaluate proximity to important anatomic structures. Sequential periapical radiographs guide the clinician to visualize changes in direction and depth of the drilling procedure and parallelism to adjacent teeth and other implants (Fig. 76.15). Digital radiographs are particularly advantageous during an intraoperative assessment of implant placement; images appear on the screen almost instantaneously and can be manipulated to extract the most pertinent diagnostic information (see Chapter 33).

Implant osseointegration, and the level of peri-implant alveolar bone are major determinants of implant prognosis. Panoramic and periapical radiographs offer a fast, easy, and low-radiation depiction of the implant and surrounding tissues and aid in the assessment of implant success. To obtain an accurate assessment of peri-implant bone height, the x-ray beam should be directed perpendicular to the implant. In the case of threaded implants, the implant threads should be distinguishable and not overlapping (Fig. 76.16A).

A 1.2-mm marginal bone loss during the first year after implant placement and 0.1 mm per year afterward are expected; however, further bone loss is considered abnormal.[2] Pathologic bone loss could be localized along the full extend of the implant (peri-implant bone loss) or around the crestal part of the implant ("saucerization"), and it could reflect poor osseointegration, peri-implantitis, or unfavorable stress distribution (Fig. 76.16B–C).

In select cases, when poor implant placement (Fig. 76.17) or compromise of vital anatomic structures (Fig. 76.18) is suspected, advanced imaging (CBCT, CT, or conventional tomography) provides

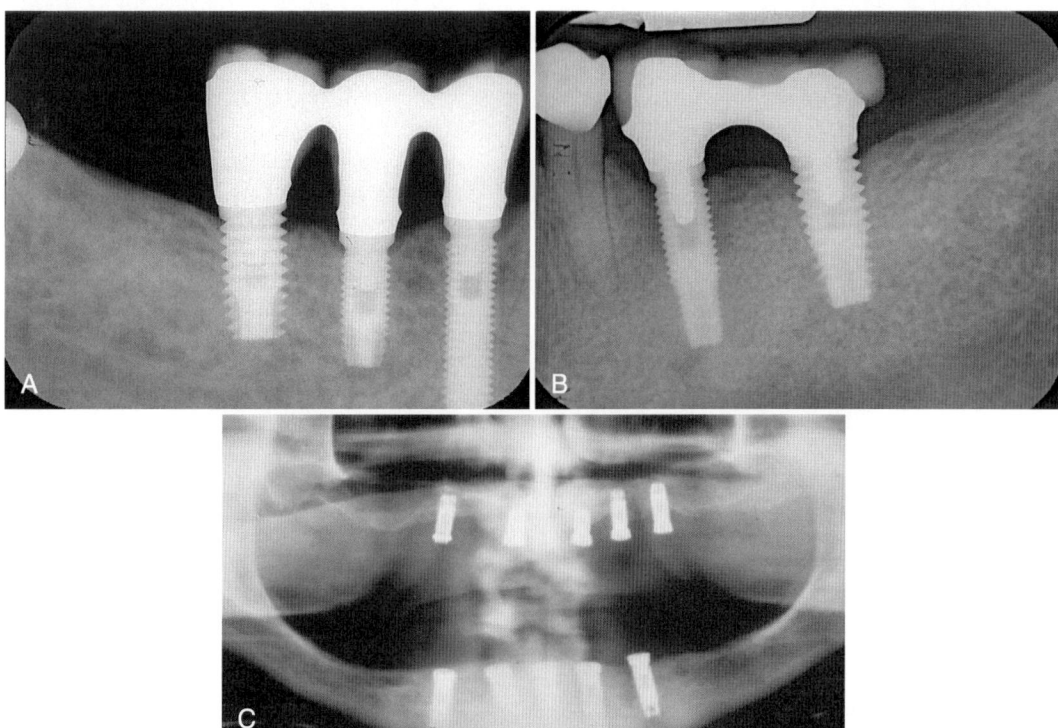

Fig. 76.16 Radiographic follow-up after implant placement in three different patients. (A) Periapical radiograph of three implants in the posterior right mandible. "Normal" bone remodeling around the anterior two implants and slight horizontal bone loss/remodeling around the molar/posterior implant is present. (B) Periapical radiograph of two implants in the left posterior mandible. Severe bone loss (50% of implant length) is seen around the anterior implant, whereas mild bone loss/bone remodeling is observed around the posterior implant. A moderate buccal cantilever in the restoration likely contributed to an adverse occlusal load and the resultant bone loss observed in this case. (C) Panoramic radiograph of maxillary and mandibular implants in an edentulous patient prior to implant loading. The mandibular implants do not show signs of bone loss and appear to be osseointegrated. All maxillary implants show signs of moderate-to-severe peri-implant bone loss, and the success of osseointegration is questionable.

Fig. 76.17 Radiographic follow-up after implant placement. (A) Panoramic radiograph suggests mild-to-moderate bone loss around the neck of all implants. This is especially true for the implants in the left maxilla. These implants appear to be angled, and the distal implant is positioned more apical. The overdenture bar is not completely seated on the left implants. Note that superimposed overlapping anatomic structures in this panoramic radiograph impair the ability to clearly visualize and assess bone loss around implants. (B) Cross-sectional (B1) and sagittal cone-beam computed tomography (B2) images of the anterior implant in the left maxilla. Poor implant placement beyond the buccal cortex of the alveolar ridge (cross section) and peri-implant bone loss (sagittal) are revealed.

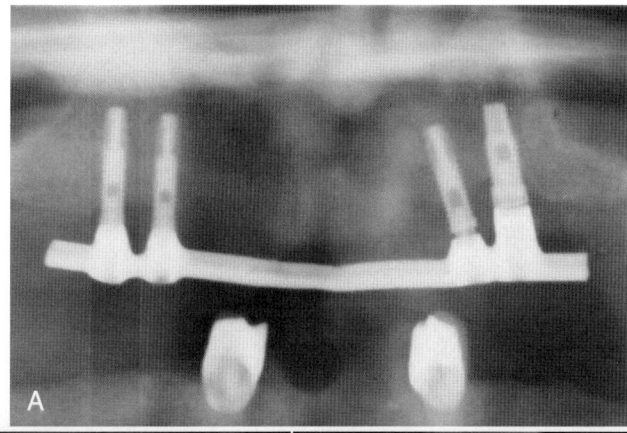

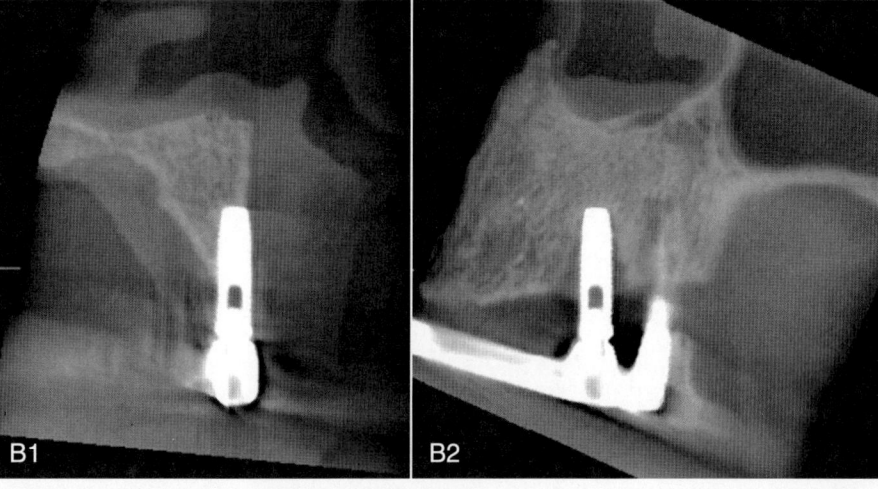

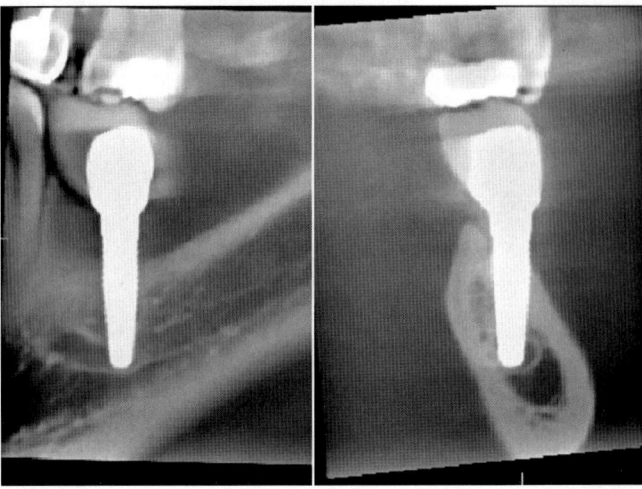

Fig. 76.18 Cone-beam computed tomography sagittal and cross-sectional images clearly demonstrate penetration of the implant into the mandibular canal.

a three-dimensional evaluation of the oral structures in relation to the implants. This information can be very important for proper assessment and treatment planning. The treating dentist should recognize relevant signs and symptoms and order appropriate imaging as soon after implant placement as possible. Implant removal, if necessary, would be less complicated before advanced osseointegration.

Conclusion

Many radiographic projections are available for the evaluation of implant placement, each with advantages and disadvantages. The clinician must follow sequential steps in patient evaluation, and radiography is an essential diagnostic tool for implant design and successful treatment of the implant patient. Selection of appropriate radiographic modalities will provide the maximum diagnostic information, help avoid unwanted complications, and maximize treatment outcomes while delivering an "as low as reasonably achievable" radiation dose to the patient.[11]

Case Scenarios are found on the companion website www.expertconsult.com.

References

References for this chapter are found on the companion website www.expertconsult.com.

CHAPTER 77

Prosthetic Considerations for Implant Treatment

Todd R. Schoenbaum | Evelyn Chung | Ting-Ling Chang | Perry R. Klokkevold

CHAPTER OUTLINE

For online-only content on fully edentulous prosthetic considerations, go to the companion website at www.expertconsult .com.

Ultimately, successful implant treatment requires a team of clinicians dedicated to excellence in surgical and the prosthetic aspects of the process. This chapter reviews the critical aspects of prosthetic implant treatment proven to maximize long-term functional, biologic, and aesthetic success.

Implant Considerations

Understanding the Anticipated Load on the System and Its Relation to Implant Diameter

Selecting the appropriate implants for the partially edentulous patient depends in part on the anticipated loads of that particular tooth location. The larger the anticipated loads, the more robust the implant must be to properly support the prosthesis. Notably, for any given implant design, larger-diameter implants result in stronger prostheses.[14] The implant connection design also plays a significant role and will be discussed later. However, the prosthetic advantages of a larger-diameter implant must be balanced with the surgical needs for sufficient (~1.5 mm) surrounding bone. In some locations, this constraint will present itself in the mesiodistal dimension, whereas in others the constraint will come from the buccolingual dimension of the alveolar ridge.

The anticipated load on the implant is affected by its position in the arch. The more posterior the implant is in the arch, the higher the anticipated load. Estimates have been made relating to the ratio of load from anterior to posterior,[45] but such generalizations oversimplify the complexity of the system. Although a tooth located more posteriorly will receive at least twice the load forces (and therefore require a larger implant diameter), there are several other factors that will influence the result. Anterior–posterior position in the arch is part of this consideration, but so are the number and integrity of the teeth distal to the implant position. A first molar implant with good second molars will receive significantly less force than that same molar with no other molar support.

Often overlooked, the size of the muscles of mastication can provide cursory evidence regarding just how much force a patient is able to produce on his or her dentition. Patients with very large muscles will generate greater forces on their teeth and implants. However, excessive forces do not always show up as attrition. These forces can be delivered in a largely vertical vector with little to no

horizontal component. This information should be checked and recorded at the initial patient examination. Patients with a history of cracked or broken teeth and crowns should be expected to place heavier loads on the implants used to replace them.

In the evaluation of the implant patient, special attention should be given to the arch opposing the location of expected implant treatment. If the opposing dentition is a removable appliance, then the implant will receive significantly lower forces.[48,53] Conversely, if the opposing dentition is implant-supported fixed restorations, the forces are likely to be quite high. This phenomenon is largely due to the lack of a periodontal ligament (PDL) around the implants. If the implant is opposing a removable appliance, it should be determined if there is any likelihood of converting to a fixed implant-supported prosthesis. If this is the case, then the implant in question should be planned with increased loads in mind.

Occlusal guards have long been employed to protect the dentition and prostheses against excessive forces and destructive wear habits. As implants lack the "cushioning effect" that the PDL provides to natural teeth, the occlusal guard can provide the patient with an added layer of protection against overloading of the implant system. The limiting factor with occlusal guards is patient compliance.

Clinicians looking for a more quantified approach to evaluating the loads placed on teeth and implants might consider digital occlusal analysis systems.

CLINICAL CORRELATION

The anticipated load on the implant is affected by its position in the arch. The more posterior the implant, the higher the anticipated load. Estimates have been made relating to the ratio of load from anterior to posterior, but such generalizations oversimplify the complexity of the system. Although a tooth located more posteriorly will receive at least twice the load forces, there are several other factors that will influence the result. Other important factors to consider are the number of implants, the stability of the surrounding dentition, and individual mastication forces.

Larger-diameter implants create stronger prosthetics and are less likely to fracture.[14] The use of larger implants becomes more important under the following circumstances: enlarged masseter/temporalis muscles, a history of broken teeth and crowns, distal-most tooth in the arch, opposing other implants, and patients unwilling to wear an occlusal guard. However, the prosthetic advantages of larger platform implants must be balanced with the realities of the surgical site. In locations with space constraints, other prosthetic modalities may be employed to mitigate the anticipated risks. Innovations in implant connections, manufacturing tolerances, and alloys have created more and more robust systems that will improve the ability to withstand excessive forces.

Narrow-diameter implants have proven to be a reliable and useful approach to compromised spaces (<7 mm).[71] This constraint can be mesiodistal due to adjacent teeth or implants, or it can be buccolingual due to inadequate volume of the alveolar ridge. Use of such implants is best reserved for sites with low expected loads and constrained spaces, namely the incisors of both jaws.

Number of Implants

Partially edentulous patients with multiple adjacent missing teeth can present some unique challenges. If we use 4 mm as the diameter of a "regular" implant, and the guideline of 1.5 mm of circumferential peri-implant bone, we can quickly estimate the amount of space required for implants by multiplying 7 mm times the number of missing teeth.[133] Or more simply, one tooth requires 7 mm of mesiodistal space; two teeth require 14 mm, three teeth require 21 mm, and so on (Fig. 77.1). This is an oversimplification of the planning process, but makes initial estimations of treatment options easier.

Not every missing tooth needs an implant. Two implants with a three-unit fixed dental prosthesis (FDP) have proven to be quite reliable in many situations.[90] Material selection is key; weaker and unproven materials should be used with extreme caution. Gold alloy porcelain-fused-to-metal (PFMs) and zirconia-based FDPs have good (but not perfect) track records. Lithium disilicate materials (and recent derivatives) are not well tested for multiunit FDPs. The use of a pontic between two implants has aesthetic advantages in relation to the volume of the peri-implant tissues. This topic will be covered

more in depth during the discussion on implants in the aesthetic zone.

Cantilevers off one or more implants can be a creative solution to complicated implant treatment planning situations. Such a design is certainly less durable than a noncantilevered approach, but it does have its place. Cantilever FDPs are best reserved to replace multiple missing incisors in patients with nonexcessive occlusal forces.[119] The use of a cantilever pontic should be avoided in most posterior situations, unless multiple implants are splinted and the length of the cantilever is deemed acceptable.

Narrow-diameter implants can be implemented in areas with reduced dimensions, but only to a point. Narrower implants are inherently more fragile and more apt to suffer from catastrophic failure. Their minimal dimensions will make more aesthetic prosthetic materials (i.e., zirconia abutments) a riskier option. Although manufacturers will continue to produce smaller and smaller implants, their use in patients should be considered cautiously until proven to be successful.

When space constraints push the clinician to select smaller and riskier implants, alternative options should be seriously considered: orthodontics, tooth-borne FDPs (Fig. 77.2), bone augmentation, and additional extractions. Though the last option may sound overly aggressive, it can be the best choice in scenarios where adequate space cannot be created. This most commonly presents as a single missing mandibular incisor. The two missing incisors can then be replaced with a single implant. In this scenario the implant can be placed centrally between the two missing teeth or off to one side with a larger cantilever (Fig. 77.3). The centrally located implant will reduce the stress due to the decreased length of the cantilever, but the offset implant may allow for the creation of a more natural gingival architecture around the pontic.

Implant-Abutment Connection

Of all the variations in implant designs, perhaps none is as important to prosthetic success as the connection design. The design of an implant abutment junction (IAJ) will influence everything from incidence of screw loosening, to maintenance of the hard and soft tissues, to leakage *inside* the implant. The implant(s) should be selected for a particular scenario based on a thorough consideration of the connection that best suits the case. There is no "one size fits all" solution. Certain connections are well suited for fully edentulous patients but are poor choices for a single unit, whereas another connection might be well proven in complicated aesthetic treatments but do poorly under heavy loads.

Currently available dental implants are classified into three types (Fig. 77.4) based on their abutment connection design: external connection, internal connection, and solid body (the abutment is contiguous with the implant body).

The external connection implant is commonly referred to as an "external hex" implant due to the presence of a raised hexagon connection on most versions of this design. The external connection is one of the older connection designs still in common use today. It offers the advantages of an extremely extensive array of prosthetic products to address even the most complicated of clinical presentations. It is a robust implant and rarely suffers from fracture of the implant body itself. This is a well-tested and widely accepted implant design.[4,5] It is well suited to the restoration of fully edentulous patients desiring a fixed restoration. The wide platform of the implant creates a stable base, whereas the relatively short connection (0.7 mm tall) allows for easy correction of nonparallel implants.

The primary drawback of the external connection implant is screw loosening.[40,41,61,64] The short connection height does little to share the forces between the abutment and the implant body. Even if the

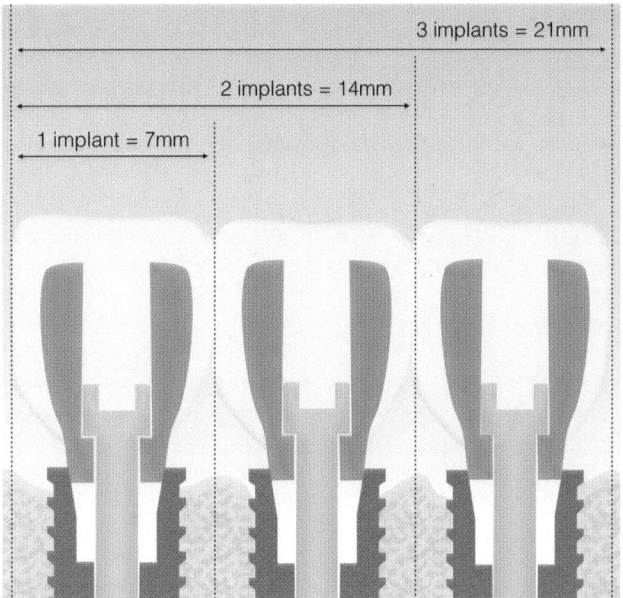

Fig. 77.1 Implants benefit from the presence of 1.5 mm of bone circumferentially. A "normal" diameter implant is ~4 mm. For treatment planning purposes, each implant should have 7 mm of space mesial–distally at the bone crest, two implants would need 14 mm, and so on.

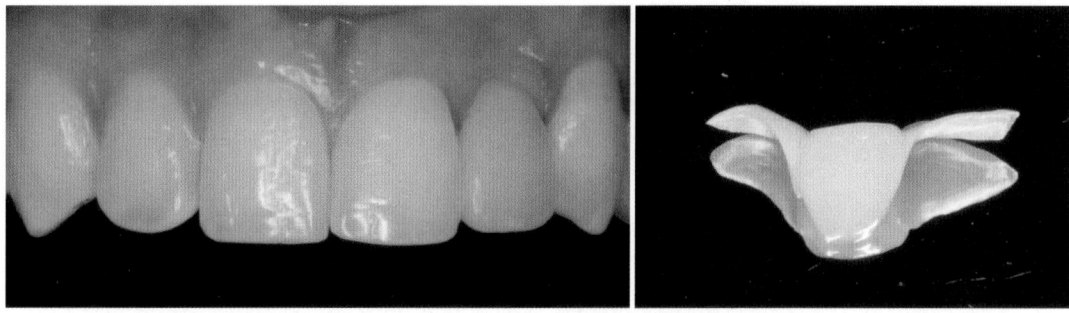

Fig. 77.2 It is important to understand that implants are not the only way to replace missing teeth. In this example a ceramic Maryland bridge is used to replace the upper left lateral incisor.

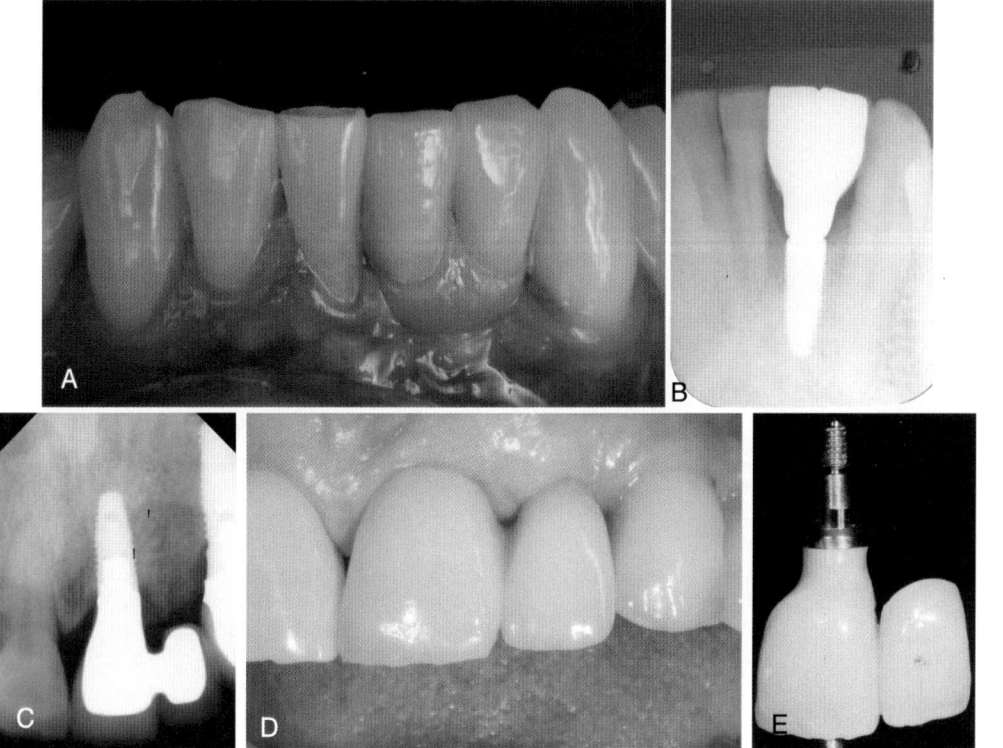

Fig. 77.3 Replacement of two consecutive missing teeth presents a unique challenge. Mesial–distal space requirements often preclude the use of two adjacent implants. The implant can be placed centrally (A–B) or in the position of one of the missing roots (C–E).

hex portion is engaged, there is still very little vertical wall height to transfer the oblique forces of the prosthesis. Inevitably, these forces are transferred largely to the abutment screw, which stretches and deforms under load. Over time this will result in the need to tighten and replace the screws. This problem is significantly reduced with prostheses supported by multiple implants. It is primarily a problem with single tooth replacements on the external connection implant.

KEY FACT

Perhaps the most important implant design factor relative to prosthetic success is the implant-abutment connection design. The design of an implant abutment junction (IAJ) will influence everything from incidence of screw loosening, to maintenance of the hard and soft tissues, to leakage inside the implant.

Compared with more modern implant designs, the external connection loses more crestal bone.[a] This is a multifactorial problem, but it is due in large part to the constant opening and closing of the IAJ under load.[55,95,106] This leads to bacterial infiltrate being pumped into and out of the internal aspects of the implant[5,59] and directly into the peri-implant tissues (Fig. 77.5). A move away from the external connection has mitigated (but not eliminated) both screw loosening and excessive crestal bone loss.

The internal connection (in all its variations) has become the implant of choice for most partially edentulous rehabilitations due to improved reliability compared with the external hex design.[49] For most systems, it is a misnomer to call it an "internal hex." The geometry of the connection itself comes in many variations including hexagons, octagons, 12-pointed stars, trilobes, circles with four flat

---

[a]References 7, 8, 13, 20, 25, 26, 44, 46, 58, 104, 115, 134, 136.

sides, seven-splines, and others. The number of sides to the connection allows the user various positions from which to orient a stock manufacturer abutment. Some manufacturers prescribe which lobe or point of the implant connection should be oriented buccally to address this. Although more sides on the connection allow for more flexibility in positioning a stock abutment, this does increase the difficulty of correctly aligning a custom abutment. There is no overwhelming, independent, peer-reviewed evidence that any one internal connection geometry is superior to all the others.

Many implant systems have begun to incorporate a tapered element into the implant abutment connection. The rationale for incorporating a taper into the connection is to further stabilize the IAJ,[88] thus minimizing leakage, abutment movement, and loosening of screws.

This concept comes from the world of machining tools, like lathes and drill presses. For some unknown reason, the dental profession has taken to referring to any tapered connection implant as a "Morse taper," though few implant designs meet the very specific specifications of any Morse taper variation (~1.5-degree taper).

Regardless, upon fully torquing the abutment screw, implants with a very narrow taper do create a better seal and will have better long-term stability of the abutment and the screw. Both are advantages in terms of maintenance and persevering the peri-implant tissues at a maximum level. Some tapered connection implant systems even require a special tool to remove the abutments, as after screw removal the components can have such a strong friction fit.

When wide diameter external connection implants were introduced, they remained compatible with the abutments from the narrower implants. Some clinicians and scientists began experimenting with using these narrow abutments on wider implants; they referred to these connections as "platform switched."[74] This term has come to encompass any implant that has an abutment that is narrower than the implant neck (Fig. 77.6). The preponderance of evidence suggests that the platform-shifted design maintains bone at a higher level than that of a nonplatform switched design.[b] The reasons for this effect are less leakage at the IAJ (most are tapered connections),[9,38,73,92] less screw loosening,[101,110] less stress on the peri-implant bone,[29,52,85,86] and movement of the nonosseointegrating surface of the abutment away from the bone. The latter concept creates a horizontal space on the implant for supracrestal connective tissue to establish a circumferential peri-implant seal, thereby allowing the bone to maintain its position at a higher level without having to remodel to a lower position.[111,112]

The only potential downside to a platform-switched implant system is that the abutment is narrower and therefore more prone to breakage. Data on this concern are sparse, but it stands to reason that for any material (in particular zirconia), the thinner it is, the more easily it will suffer fracture. Many manufacturers have begun to address this problem by offering their zirconia abutments with a titanium insert that interfaces with the implant body (Fig. 77.7). This has the benefit of placing the more fragile zirconia outside the implant and prevents the possibility of the zirconia wearing the implant connection prematurely.

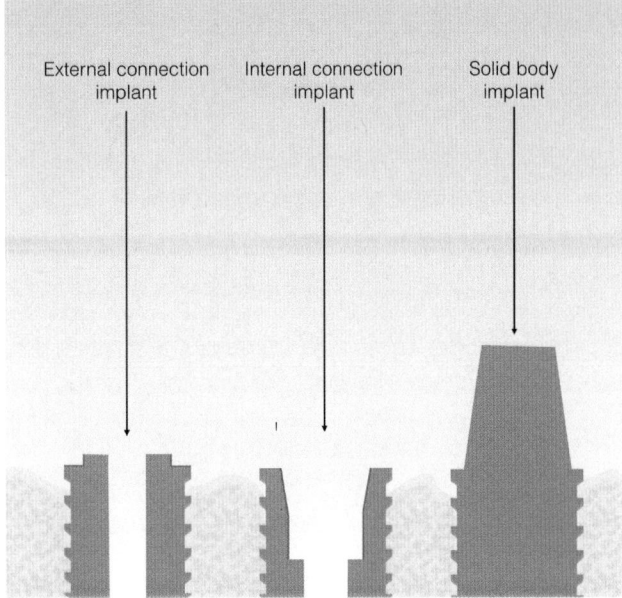

Fig. 77.4 Most currently available implants can be classified as one of three types: external connection, internal connection, or solid body. The external hex connection is primarily indicated for full-arch treatments. The solid body implant must be placed in the ideal position, as there is no way to correct the position with the abutment. The internal connection implant (of which there are many varieties) is indicated for most partially edentulous treatments. Note the abutment engagement areas, as highlighted in *red*.

---

[b]References 7, 8, 13, 20, 25, 26, 44, 46, 58, 104, 115, 134, 136.

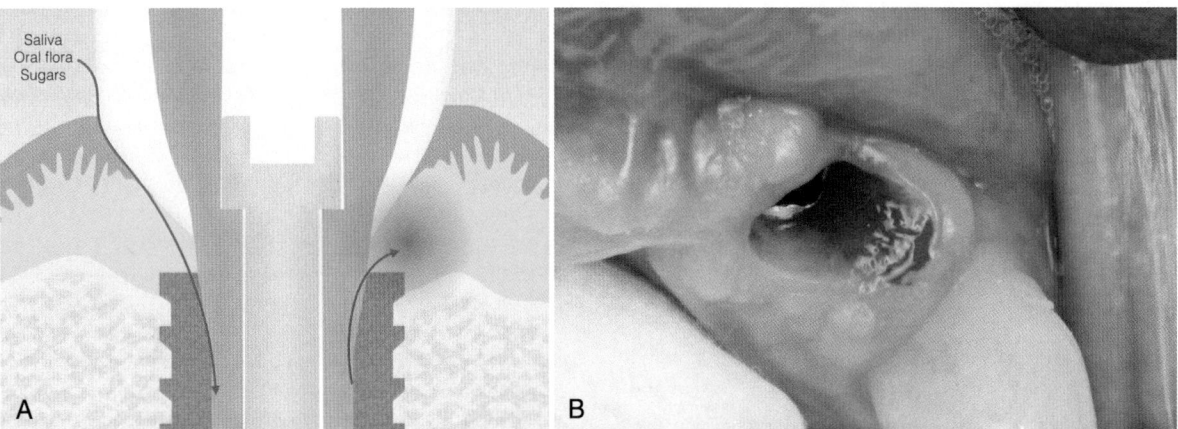

Fig. 77.5 All two-piece implants have hollow internal spaces. Under functional loads, the junction between the implant and the abutment will open slightly and allow saliva, oral flora, and nutrients into the internal aspects of the implant (A). In this oxygen-free environment, anaerobes will proliferate. They will be pumped into the peri-implant tissues and may be partially responsible for typical peri-implant bone loss or inflammation of the peri-implant tissues (B).

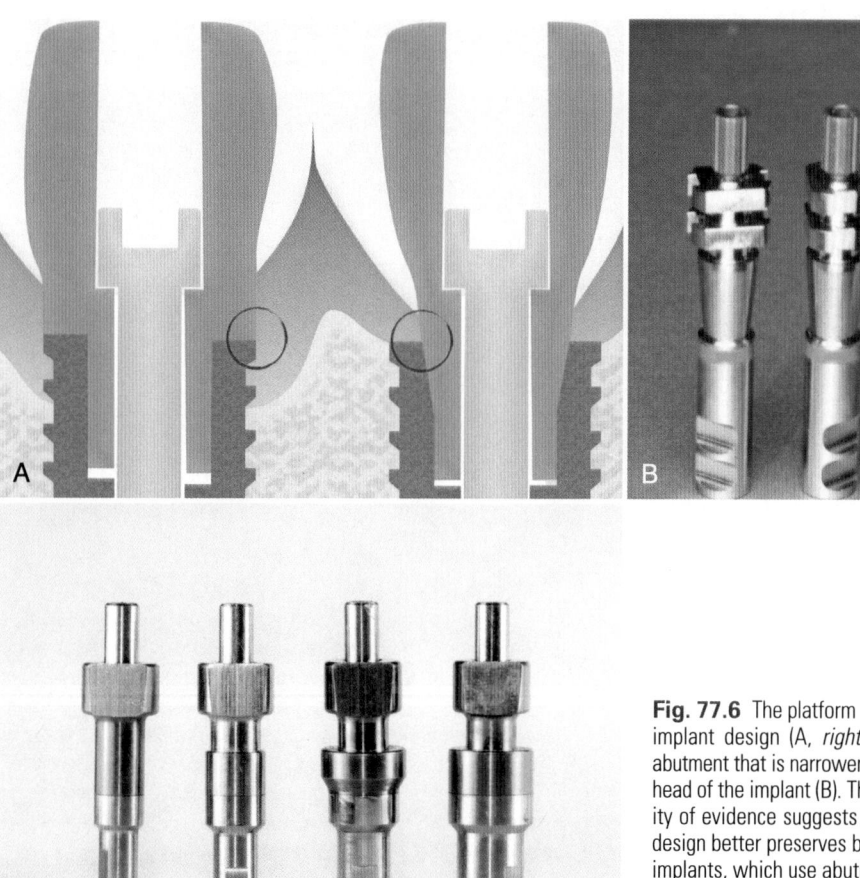

Fig. 77.6 The platform switched implant design (A, *right*) has an abutment that is narrower than the head of the implant (B). The majority of evidence suggests that this design better preserves bone than implants, which use abutments as wide or wider than the head of the implant (C).

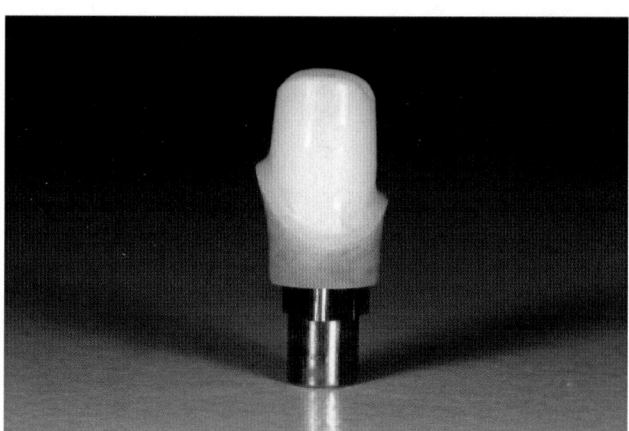

Fig. 77.7 Zirconia abutments are useful to minimize any changes to the color of the peri-implant tissues and allow the use of semitranslucent prosthetic materials. Most manufacturers have developed zirconia abutments, which have a titanium base as shown here. This may make the abutments stronger and will eliminate the failure of the zirconia *inside* the implant body. Such failures are difficult to resolve successfully.

The internal aspect of the implant is hollow to allow for the screw and the abutment connection. However, these spaces inside the implant can serve as a pathogenic reservoir if or when the IAJ leaks.[9,73,92] This internal chamber is anaerobic, body temperature, and when the IAJ leaks it will become filled with oral bacteria, saliva, and nutrients. The chamber is then fertile breeding ground for anaerobic bacteria and their by-products. Continued movement between the abutment and the implant will pump the bacterial exudate into the fragile peri-implant tissues. It appears that this is one of the primary causes of "normal" bone loss around implants. Excessive amounts of pumping may be culpable in idiopathic incidences of peri-implant mucositis and peri-implantitis. Therefore clinicians should opt for implants and abutments that have been shown (over extended periods of time) to reduce the micro-gap and leakage. This is best accomplished with a narrow tapered connection and abutments with titanium interfaces milled by the implant manufacturer. There are additional factors to consider in selecting the appropriate implant for any given scenario, but efforts to minimize the loss of peri-implant tissues is best accomplished with this treatment modality.

The last type of implant connection to address is the "solid body" implant, or an implant in which the abutment and the implant are one contiguous piece. Such implants have been available for some time but have never gained significant popularity. The challenge with solid body implants is not surgical, and they may in fact be better for the peri-implant tissues because there is no microgap and no leakage. The problem is prosthetic. For these implants, there is no screw-retained option for the prosthesis, and the cement margin is determined at the time of placement. The abutment can be prepped to move the margin apically if absolutely necessary, but there is no reasonable way to move the margin coronally. This presents a serious problem when the gingiva has any significant papilla adjacent to the implant, as the cement margin that is placed perhaps 1 mm subgingival on the facial aspect may now be 3 to 7 mm subgingival at the mesial and distal aspect (Fig. 77.8). With no option for a screw-retained restoration, the restoring clinician is now tasked with fully removing cement far too deep subgingival and will inevitably leave cement

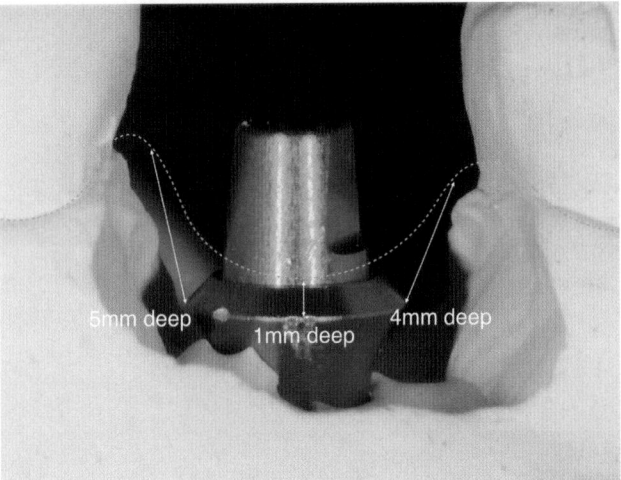

Fig. 77.8 Solid body (and tissue-level) implants present a unique prosthetic challenge due to the margin being on the implant body itself. This often results in mesial and distal margins that are far too deep to reliably remove cement. As such, restorations for tissue-level implants should generally be screw retained. Unfortunately, restorations on solid body implants can only be cemented. Extreme care must be used with solid body implants.

TABLE 77.1	Major Versus Minor Complications in Implant Prosthetics	
Major Complications	**Minor Complications**
Implant failure	Screw loosening
Atypical peri-implant bone loss	Chipped porcelain not requiring prosthesis replacement
Persistent inflammation of the soft tissue	De-cementation of the prosthesis
Infection of the peri-implant tissues	
Failure of the porcelain requiring replacement of the prosthesis	
Loss of the prosthesis	
Fractured screws or abutments	

behind. This residual cement is likely to induce inflammatory reactions and loss of bone, soft tissue, and perhaps the implant itself.[72,145]

The solid body implant offers no recourse should the abutment break. This is of particular concern as the use of solid body zirconia implants becomes more prevalent. Should the abutment on the solid body implant break, the implant must either be extracted or abandoned. Special care should be taken with solid body implants to avoid overprepping the abutment area, leading to weakness and increased risk of fracture.

There are a few esoteric implant-abutment connections on the market as well, including press-fit, cemented abutments (where the abutment is cemented *into* the implant), and others. These will not be discussed here due to space constraints and their relative obscurity at the current time.

 ### Abutment/Prosthesis Considerations for Single Units

Retention Method for Partially Edentulous Treatment: Cemented Prostheses, Screw-Retained Porcelain-Fused-to-Metal Options, Screw-Retained Full Contour Zirconia, and Hybrid Designs

When treatment planning a partially edentulous case for restoration with an implant, one of the major prosthetic decisions to be made is whether to have a crown that is cemented to an abutment or a crown that is contiguous with the abutment and screwed directly to the implant. For the sake of discussion here, the screw-retained option will be defined as a cast gold alloy abutment with appropriate support of feldspathic porcelain that will be layered directly on it (sometimes referred to as UCLA abutments). Variations of the screw-retained crown will be discussed later. Many clinicians have developed personal preferences for screw or cement-retained crowns based on their experiences and failures. Much of an individual clinician's anecdotal experience likely has much to do with the skill of his or her technician when considering screw-retained PFMs. Here we will consider the peer-reviewed evidence to determine the evidence-based advantages and disadvantages of each type of retention.

For *most* single tooth replacements, either screw or cement-retained crowns have proven to have very high levels of long-term

success,[90,113,124,139] provided that the clinician and technician follow critical guidelines. In some clinical scenarios, one type of retention is the overwhelmingly superior choice, but this does not reflect the majority of cases.

It is important to understand the difference between *major* and *minor* complications (Table 77.1). Minor complications are issues that can be resolved with little effort or increased risk, such as loose screws, minor porcelain fracture, and reversible peri-implant mucositis. Major complications are loss of the implant, peri-implantitis, severe bone loss, fractured screws, significant porcelain failure, and loss of the prosthesis.

Screw-retained restorations have a long history of clinical success. Their introduction in 1988[78] allowed clinicians to create more aesthetic restorations than were possible with the available alternatives of the time, and in less vertical space. They can be used in areas with limited interocclusal distances due to their construction design. They can be created with metal occlusal or palatal surfaces for patients with high functional demands. They can have the porcelain carried to within 1 mm of the head of the implant for improved aesthetics. The primary disadvantages of the screw-retained restoration are significantly more prosthetic complications[c]: porcelain fracture (Fig. 77.9),[68,94,113] screw loosening,[d] increased bone loss,[33,54,60,75,94] increased lab costs, and the need for ideal implant angulation. Minor areas of porcelain fracture can be predictably remedied with contouring and polishing. Larger fractures will require replacement of the entire prosthesis, as porcelain cannot be repaired after prolonged exposure to the oral environment. A dedicated technician could strip all the porcelain off the metal framework in an attempt to save the costs of a new abutment and alloy, but it may very well be that the reason for the fracture in the first place was a poorly designed framework. As such, it is advisable to fabricate an entirely new prosthesis should the porcelain fail. Screw loosening has been established repeatedly as significantly more common in screw-retained restorations, in spite of the fact that cemented restorations generally use the same screw and torque specifications. The reason for this phenomenon is not exactly known, though it is likely due to poorly casted abutment interfaces, increased preload due to nonpassive frameworks,[89,125,138] the historic use of weaker gold alloy screws, or damage to the interface during divestment (Fig. 77.10) or finishing. Technicians must exercise care when creating a screw-retained restoration to ensure the integrity of the abutment interface. The UCLA abutment should have a machined interface made by the manufacturer

[c]References 28, 34, 39, 76, 90, 105, 113, 144.
[d]References 16, 34, 39, 76, 90, 99, 113, 143.

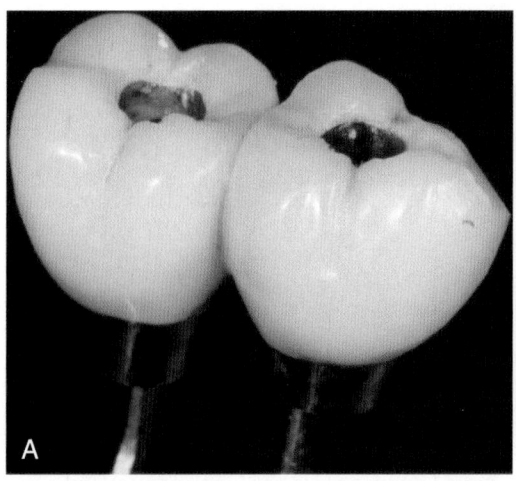
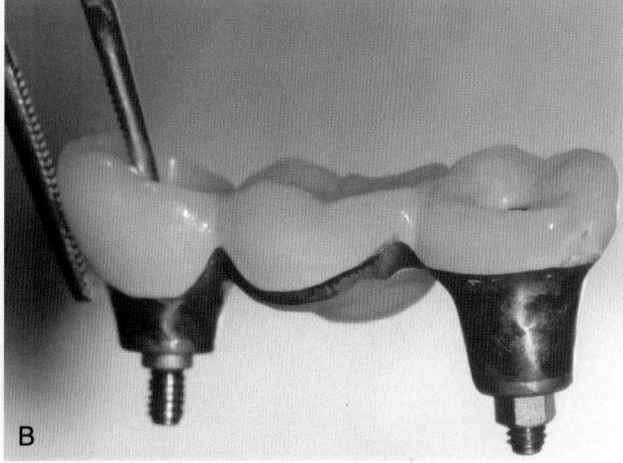

Fig. 77.9 Screw-retained PFM restorations have been shown to have significantly more prosthetic complications, most commonly failure of the porcelain and loose abutment screws. Failure of the porcelain is best addressed by replacement. The new prosthesis will need a more robust framework design or alternative materials. (A) Screw-retained PFM crowns with fractured porcelain. (B) Screw-retained PFM bridge being replaced after screws loosened.

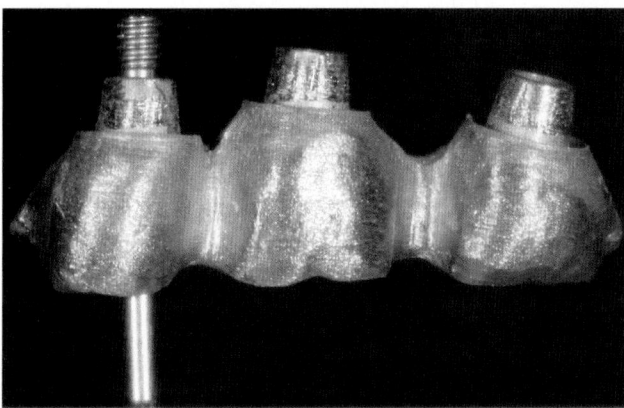

Fig. 77.10 During the fabrication of a screw-retained PFM, the technician must exercise extreme care in creation of the framework so as not to damage the interface area as shown here. The damaged interface will produce a poor-fitting prosthesis leading to increased leakage and screws that loosen more frequently.

to ensure the integrity of the fit between the abutment and the implant. Because the screw access channel must exit the crown, this option is best reserved for when the implant angulation exits directly through the occlusal surface in posterior regions and through the palatal/lingual surface in the anterior regions.

KEY FACT

For most single tooth implant crowns, both screw and cement-retained methods have proven to be highly successful over the long term provided that the clinician and technician follow critical guidelines. In some clinical scenarios, one type of retention is the overwhelmingly superior choice, but this does not reflect the majority of cases.

The common alternative to the screw-retained crown is the cement-retained crown. This system is made up of an abutment (titanium, gold alloy, or zirconia) that is screwed into the implant and a crown that will be cemented to the abutment. The cement-retained crown allows the restoration of implants that are not placed ideally without having to manage a screw access channel exiting

through a crucial aesthetic or functional area. This situation is most common in the aesthetic zone. When implants are placed angled such that and their line of draw exits through the facial surface of the crown, it becomes aesthetically prohibitive to use a "normal" screw-retained crown (Fig. 77.11). There are some workarounds that will be discussed briefly later.

Some clinicians prefer cement-retained restorations because the cementation process is familiar and comfortable. However, the cementation process is not to be taken lightly, as residual cement is one of the major causes (but not the only cause) of peri-implantitis.[1,15,72,145] Cementation details will be discussed later, but note that no attempt should be made to cement an implant crown when margins are more than 1 mm subgingival (Fig. 77.12).[83,84] Cement-retained implant crowns have the main advantage of being far more durable than the screw-retained alternative, a fact confirmed in multiple reviews.[90,113,124,144,146] Porcelain failure of screw-retained crowns has been reported to be as high as 38%, compared with just 4% for cement-retained crowns at an average of 5 years.[94] For this reason cement-retained implant crowns are indicated in scenarios of higher loads (i.e., molars, patients with enlarged masseters). Should the patient break the cemented crown, retrieval of the remaining abutment is greatly simplified. Drilling through even an intact cemented crown to access the screw channel is a relatively simple matter, akin to endodontic access. Lastly, there is the issue of lab cost. The cemented restorations typically lead to far less expensive lab bills compared with the screw-retained PFM options, though the cost of the latter varies significantly with the market price for gold alloy.

One of the reasons cited for selecting a screw-retained restoration is the ease of retrievability. There is a valid concern that should something fail, the cemented crown is more difficult to remove. Although it may seem obvious, removal of the cemented crown is hardly more difficult than for a screw-retained crown (Fig. 77.13).[120] The differences are drilling the access through porcelain or metal instead of composite and the location of access may be difficult to discern. Most clinicians are fairly adept at cutting through porcelain, but locating the access channel can be a slight challenge. Most often, the access is fairly easy to locate based off simple radiographs. More sophisticated approaches to recording the location of the access have been proposed, from stents,[56] to guides,[141] to occlusal markings (Fig. 77.14).[116,122] During the era of weaker abutment screws and external connection implants, screw loosening was a common problem. As

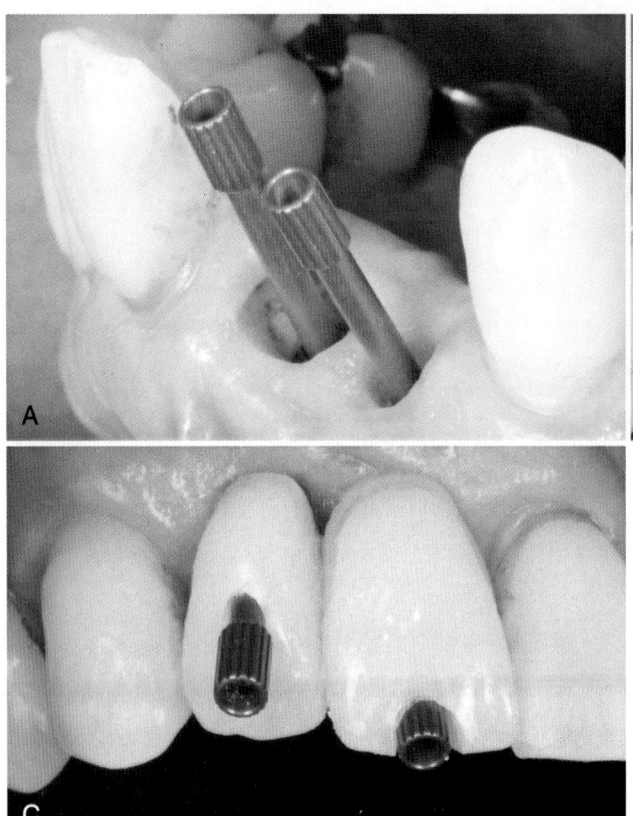

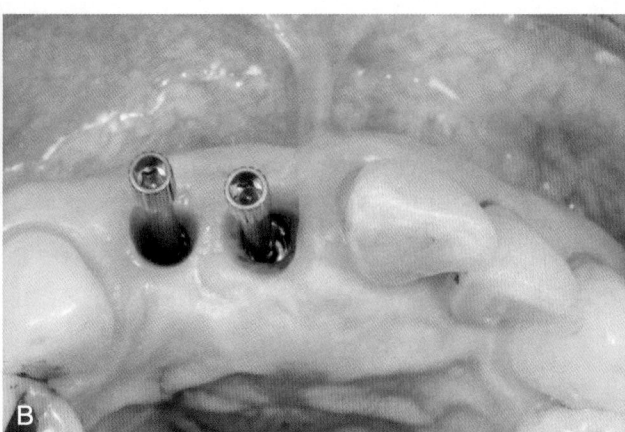

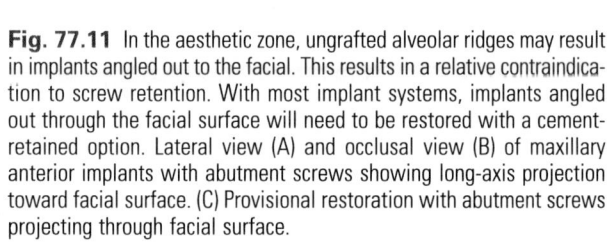

Fig. 77.11 In the aesthetic zone, ungrafted alveolar ridges may result in implants angled out to the facial. This results in a relative contraindication to screw retention. With most implant systems, implants angled out through the facial surface will need to be restored with a cement-retained option. Lateral view (A) and occlusal view (B) of maxillary anterior implants with abutment screws showing long-axis projection toward facial surface. (C) Provisional restoration with abutment screws projecting through facial surface.

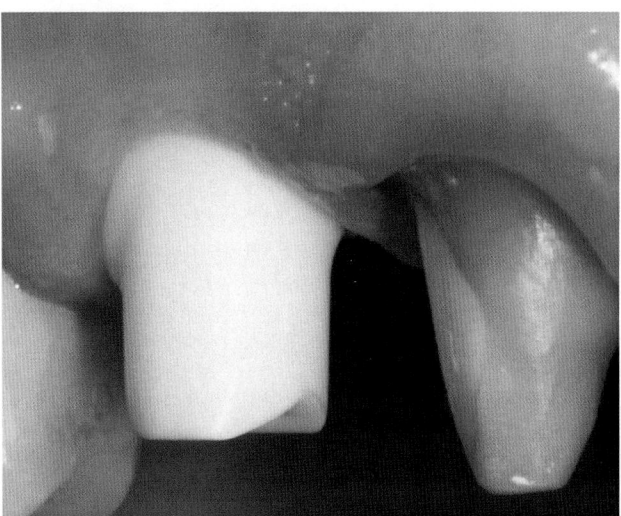

Fig. 77.12 For cemented implant restorations, the abutment must be designed such that the cementation margin is no deeper than 1 mm below the gingival margin. In all but the flattest of ridges, this can only be accomplished with a custom-milled abutment.

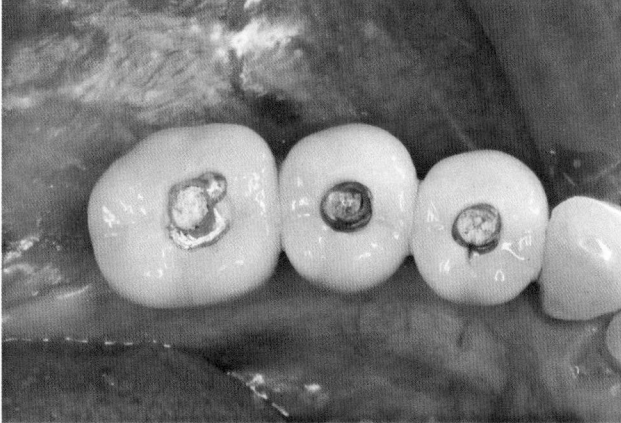

Fig. 77.13 Removal and replacement of failed cement-retained implant crowns are relatively straightforward procedures with most implant designs. The clinician estimates the long access of the implant with radiographs and by palpating the ridge and then simply drills into the screw access through the crown material. The abutments/crowns may still be cemented together and can be removed as one piece.

such, replacement of the screws was a common maintenance requirement and a screw-retained restoration was ideal. Modern implant connections rarely suffer from loose screws, even for single-unit implants.[90,105]

There are a few other crown retention variations that should be mentioned. One is the full-contour zirconia, screw-retained crown This crown is similar in design to the cast gold, screw-retained crown, but it has no feldspathic layering porcelain, and the substructure is zirconia. Though relatively new to market, these restorations may prove to maintain many of the advantages of the screw-retained

system while eliminating its major complication—porcelain fracture. Not all manufacturers offer this restoration, and some variants do not offer a titanium insert to protect the implant from wear and zirconia failure. The titanium insert should be used whenever possible. Some manufacturers offer this restoration with a screw channel that can be angled up to 25 degrees to allow for screw-retained restorations even when the implant is not in the long access of the crown. The screw-retained zirconia option is relatively new and not fully tested in clinical trials. Implement with caution.

Another option is the hybrid crown (sometimes referred to as a screwmentable crown). This system consists of a crown that is cemented to a stock titanium abutment (Fig. 77.15), but the cementation is performed in the laboratory where excess cement can be easily removed. The screw access is predrilled into the crown. This system offers the advantages of minimal risk of retained cement, minimal risk of porcelain fracture when stronger ceramics are used, and a lower lab cost than cast gold alloys. This system is relatively new and not fully tested; in clinical trials implement with caution.

Lastly, there is the option of lingual set screws. This system is most commonly employed in the anterior areas of the mouth when the implants are angled too far toward the facial for a traditional screw-retained restoration and the clinician is uncomfortable with a cemented option. The challenges with lingual set screws are increased lab costs, difficulty in locating technicians competent in the technique, leakage between the crown and the abutment, and challenging screw access.

Abutment Material Selection

In most bone-level implant designs, the junction between the abutment and the implant is near the crestal bone. In this area the connective tissue and the junctional epithelium may be in intimate contact with the abutment. As such, the abutment material and accuracy of the fit play a critical role in preserving the peri-implant bone and soft tissue. Some abutments better preserve the peri-implant tissues than others. The most relevant options for currently available definitive abutment materials are titanium, titanium with a titanium nitride coating, full-contour zirconia, zirconia with a titanium base, and gold alloy (Fig. 77.16). Other less common options include lithium disilicate and chrome-cobalt alloys.

The most rigorous study examining bone and soft tissue reactions to abutment materials found histologic evidence that titanium preserved 1.5 mm more soft tissue and 1 mm more bone compared with the fully cast gold alloy abutment.[2] However, it should be noted that this study was performed in the canine mandible and that when a titanium interface was used in conjunction with a cast gold abutment, there was less bone loss than with the gold alone. It stands to reason that some of the bone and soft tissue loss with gold abutments may have more to do with the less accurate fit of a cast restoration than to the influence of the material itself. More recent clinical studies and reviews have questioned these findings, with gold and titanium showing an equivalent biologic response.[79,137] However, the latter

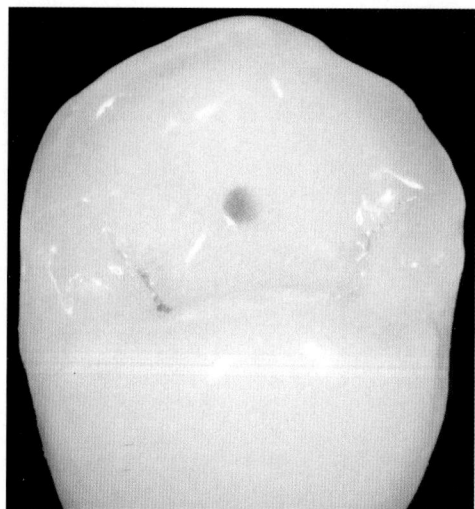

Fig. 77.14 Placement of an occlusal/palatal marker during fabrication of the crown can make finding the screw access more predictable should removal become necessary.

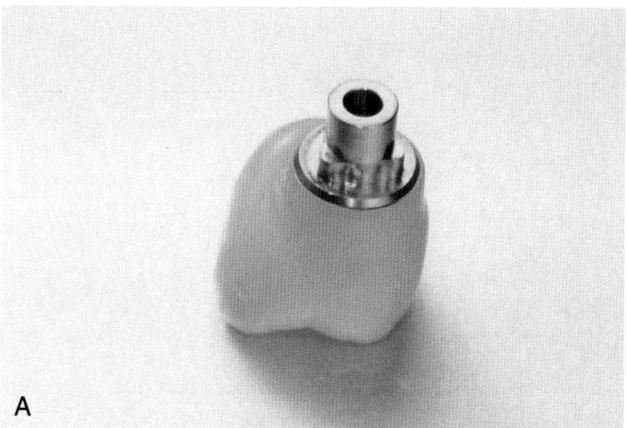

A

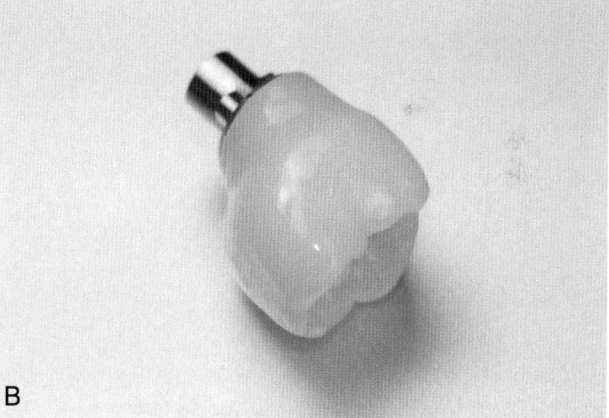

B

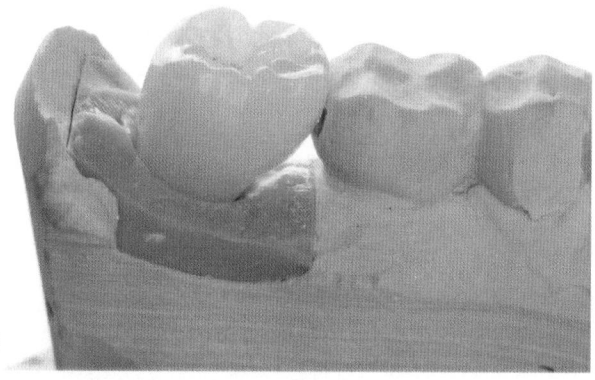

C

Fig. 77.15 The hybrid crown design consists of a titanium base that is connected to a full contour ceramic (generally zirconia) crown. In the laboratory, the technician follows a specific protocol to cement the titanium base to the ceramic crown. This design produces a screw-retained restoration that should be less prone to the problems of a PFM, though few long-term data are yet available. (A) Abutment view of titanium base crown. (B) Crown view of titanium base crown. (C) Titanium base crown in lab model.

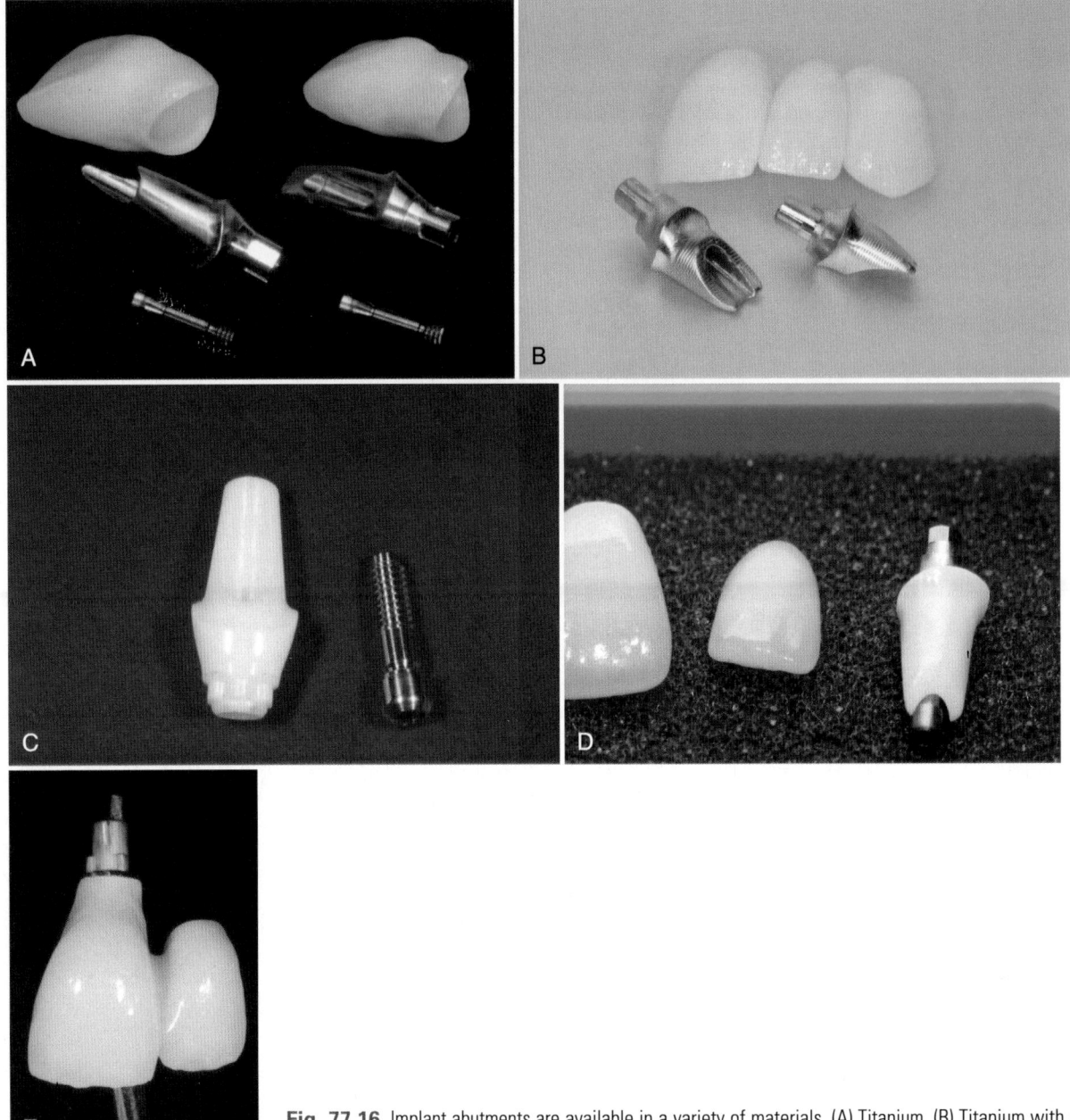

Fig. 77.16 Implant abutments are available in a variety of materials. (A) Titanium. (B) Titanium with a titanium nitride coating. (C) Full contour zirconia. (D) Zirconia with a titanium base. (E) Gold alloy.

were done with radiographic analysis rather than the histologic measurements of the former. As a whole, the data are not yet conclusive on the biocompatibility of the abutment material and its clinical effects on the tissues. Titanium has been repeatedly shown to perform better on a histologic level than gold alloys, but the difference may be of little clinical significance. What is clear is that the interface between the abutment and the implant must be as accurate as possible. This will ensure minimal leakage, minimal screw loosening, and better maintenance of the peri-implant tissues. Abutments that require casting of the implant interface portion cannot match the fit accuracy of the machined interface.[19]

The strength of the abutment is critical in maintaining long-term success with minimal technical complications. Titanium and gold alloy abutments have a long track record of outstanding strength. Some studies have even shown failure of the implant before failure of the titanium abutment.[131] The primary concern regarding strength is related to zirconia abutments.

Zirconia abutments can be used with little risk of fracture in many clinical scenarios,[91] but there are a few caveats. The zirconia abutment should have an implant interface component made of titanium (Fig. 77.17).[131] This minimizes the risk of wear to the implant body, and should the zirconia fracture, it is outside the implant where it is much easier to treat. The zirconia abutment should not be used in cases with extreme loads (i.e., molars, patients with enlarged muscles of mastication, long span FDPs). The zirconia abutments should be made by a reputable manufacturer. Evidence has shown that the manufacturer can have a huge impact on the strength of the material.[69] The abutment walls should be sufficiently thick, no less than 0.7 mm. Every effort should be made to avoid cutting the zirconia after it has been sintered.

Lastly we must consider the effect of the abutment material on the color of the soft tissue. Gray-colored metallic abutments will darken the tissue more than zirconia abutments, but the effect is not as great as might be expected. Zirconia abutments still cause a

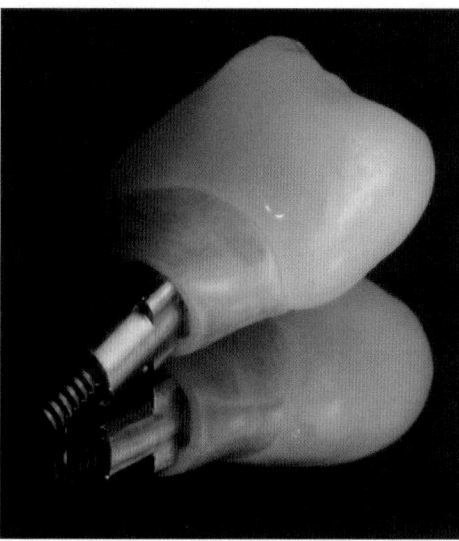

Fig. 77.17 Zirconia implant abutments should be fabricated with a titanium base. This has multiple advantages: increased strength, less complicated failures, and less wear of the internal surface of the implant.

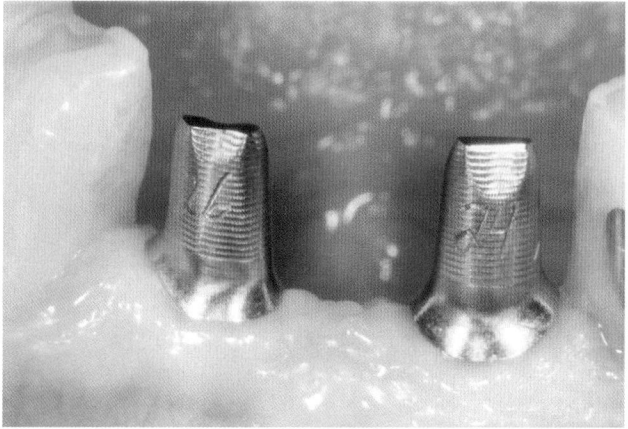

Fig. 77.18 Gold color coating of titanium abutments produces less graying of the soft tissue. This coating is made from titanium nitride or titanium oxide.

significant and perceptible darkening of the soft tissue, confirmed in multiple studies.[17,70,82] Some manufacturers and clinicians have developed techniques to anodize or coat titanium abutments to create gold or pink shades. These may offer some improvement of soft tissue aesthetics. The gold-colored abutments (Fig. 77.18) allow predictable use of semi-translucent ceramics with minimal shade change. The thickness of the overlying tissue has been shown to have a greater influence on the perceived color of the gingiva over an implant than the material used. Thick tissues have an almost nonperceptible color shift, whereas with thin tissues the shift is always perceptible, even with zirconia abutments.[63]

 KEY FACT

It is clear that the interface between the abutment and the implant must be as accurate as possible. An accurate IAJ fit will ensure minimal leakage, minimal screw loosening, and better maintenance of the peri-implant tissues. Clinicians should understand and appreciate that abutments with casting of the implant interface portion cannot match the fit accuracy of the machined interface.

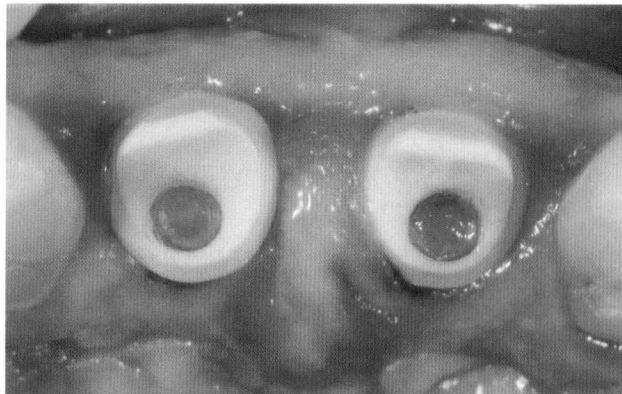

Fig. 77.19 Even in the aesthetic zone, the abutment margins should not be placed deeper than 1 mm subgingivally. The margins should be clearly visible circumferentially. This will minimize the risk of cement-induced peri-implantitis.

Abutment Design and Emergence Profile

The design and contours of the abutment play a key role in the shape and dimensions of the peri-implant tissues. If the abutment is overcontoured it will ultimately lead to a loss of bone and soft tissue. This is a common problem when technicians design and shape the abutment without the soft tissue mask on the model. Such overcontoured abutments may require surgery to deliver because the tissue prevents complete seating of the restoration. Alternatively, the restoration can be reshaped to reduce or eliminate impingement on tissues.

The emergence profile of the abutment is the area of the abutment between the head of the implant and the soft tissue margins. More data are showing that undercontouring the emergence profile helps to protect and maintain the peri-implant bone and soft tissue.[111] The "platform switch" style implant helps to create the narrowed abutment design due to the smaller diameter of the connection interface. In most scenarios, the abutment should be designed to emerge from the implant in a narrowed hourglass shape. The narrowed design may allow for increased blood flow around the implant and provide sufficient room for the soft tissues without bone remodeling.[121,135]

Understanding the effects the emergence profile has on the shape and position of the soft tissue is critical for implant treatment in the aesthetic zone.[117,127] By selectively over- or undercontouring the emergence zone, the soft tissue can be positioned with a high degree of accuracy.[132] More on this technique will be described in the next section with the use of aesthetic zone provisional restoration.

For cement restorations, arguably the most critical aspect of the abutment design is the placement of the margins. The peri-implant soft tissue is never perfectly flat, and as such custom abutments are almost universally indicated to avoid deep subgingival margins with the risk of retained cement and the resulting peri-implantitis. The only way for a stock abutment to be used with minimal risk is to select one with completely supragingival margins, but this can be aesthetically unacceptable. If a common stock abutment is selected to hide the titanium, with a facial margin 1 mm subgingival, in most scenarios the margin at the mesial and distal papilla will be 4 mm or more subgingival. Both in vitro and in vivo studies have shown that for margins beyond 1 mm subgingival, significant amounts of cement will always be left behind.[83,84] No attempt should ever be made to cement restorations on implants with margins more than 1 mm subgingival (Fig. 77.19). A custom abutment can be easily designed to address the natural scalloping of the gingiva. It is fabricated by milling or casting, though casting of custom abutments

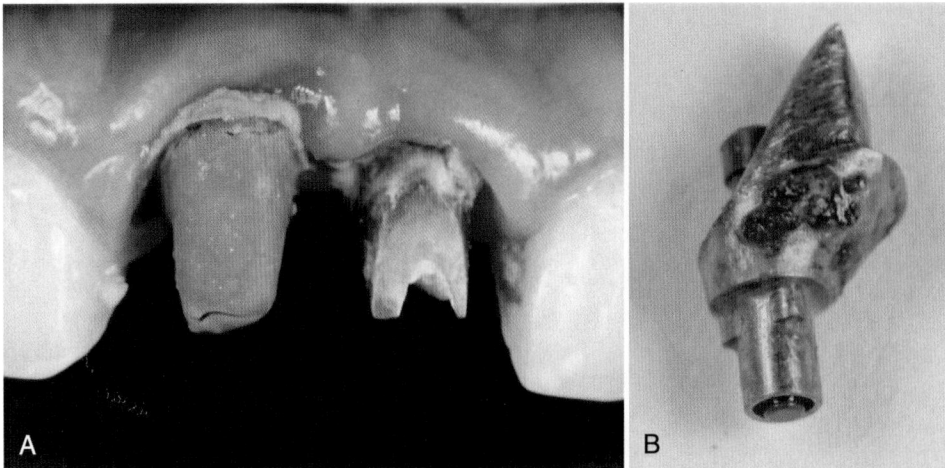

Fig. 77.20 When margins are placed deeper than 1 mm, it is inevitable that cement will be left subgingivally. Regardless of cement type, cement left subgingivally will result in significant loss of bone and soft tissue. Here, a large amount of residual cement has caused catastrophic loss of bone and soft tissue (peri-implantitis). These implants ultimately required extraction and significant reconstruction to treat. (A) Clinical view. (B) Abutment removed.

for cement-retained crowns is no longer the best option due to increased costs, increased screw loosening,[e] and the less accurate fit at the implant.[19]

 CLINICAL CORRELATION

The thickness of the overlying tissue has been shown to have a greater influence on the perceived color of the gingiva over an implant than the abutment/restorative material used. The color shift is almost imperceptible under thick tissues, whereas it is nearly always noticeable when covered by thin tissues, even with zirconia abutments.

Milled custom abutments can be made out of titanium or zirconia. When prescribing these abutments, it is critical to communicate to the technician where the margins should be placed. If left unstated, many technicians will opt to place them deep subgingivally. Several studies[83,84] have clearly shown that cement cannot be predictably removed at depths greater than 1 mm subgingival. If the margins are any deeper than 1 mm, significant amounts of cement will be left behind and will likely start the process of peri-implantitis (Fig. 77.20). It is common for clinicians and technicians to place the margins deeper than 1 mm subgigival in aesthetic cases in an attempt to hide the titanium abutment if recession should occur. This strategy is unwise and will inevitably result in retained cement. The correct approach is to shape the tissue with a provisional, allow it to mature, and place the margin no deeper than 1 mm. The abutment could also be made of zirconia and stained to resemble the root surface. Clinicians should be aware of the significant strength variations in zirconia abutments based on the manufacturer.[69]

CLINICAL CORRELATION

No attempt should ever be made to cement restorations on an implant abutment with margins more than 1 mm below the gingival margin. A custom abutment can be easily designed to address the natural scalloping

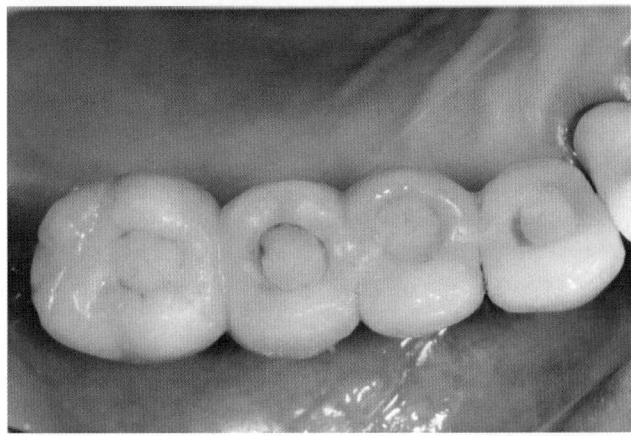

Fig. 77.21 Many in vitro studies have shown that splinting of adjacent implants helps to share occlusal forces between the implants. However, several clinical trials have shown no clinically significant difference in bone levels between splinted and nonsplinted restorations at 3, 5, and 10 years of use.

of the gingiva. The probability of leaving (missing) excess cement trapped below the gingival margin is extremely high and problematic. Studies have clearly shown that cement cannot be removed at depths greater than 1 mm subgingival.

Splinting Adjacent Implants

The rational for splinting adjacent implants (Fig. 77.21) stems from various finite element analysis (FEA)[10,12,142,148] and photo-elastic gel (PEG) experiments.[51] These in vitro studies repeatedly confirm that multiple implants produce less acute forces in the peri-implant bone when splinted compared with multiple individual restorations. However, we do not have a clear notion of how much stress is acceptable for the peri-implant bone and at what threshold we might expect pathologic bone loss. The clinician must consider the length and diameter of the implants as well as the quality and quantity of the bone when determining if multiple implants should be splinted together.

[e]References 16, 34, 39, 76, 90, 99, 113, 143.

Splinted restorations are advisable when the foundation is compromised (i.e., short or narrow implants, compromised bone).[87,147] This will allow the stronger or better supported implants to "assist" the others. The compromise here is that if the weaker implant fails, an entirely new prosthesis may need to be fabricated, usually at a significant expense.

The rationale for splinting adjacent implants involves the intention of "sharing the forces," a concept derived from the in vitro studies of the early 2000s cited earlier. The implication is that clinically we would see fewer implant failures and less bone loss over extended use with splinted restorations. Long-term in vivo randomized controlled trials (RCTs)[30,42,140] have tested this hypothesis in order to quantify the differences in bone loss and implant failure with splinted versus nonsplinted restorations. In the partially edentulous RCT, at 10 years the mean difference in bone loss between splinted and nonsplinted restorations for 132 implants was a mere 0.1 mm.[140] This could hardly be considered clinically significant under most scenarios. In the fully edentulous study with two mandibular implants retaining a full denture, the differences at 3 years were statistically insignificant at most sites and only about 0.5 mm at the most significantly different sites.[42] A prospective split mouth, in vivo trial examining bone levels around splinted and not-splinted restorations showed no significant difference at 36 months.[30] Until better evidence shows otherwise, "sharing forces" in an attempt to reduce bone loss is not a proper consideration for whether or not adjacent implants should be splinted. These data are not necessarily in conflict with the early in vitro experiments, they simply illustrate that higher forces do not necessarily result in more bone loss and that it is difficult to extrapolate data from FEAs and PEGs to clinical realities. Depending on the type of bone and implant, there is likely a threshold below which increased forces will not result in significant bone loss over extended use. Conversely, despite the lack of significance found in these studies, there may be scenarios in which clinical judgment warrants splinting adjacent implants such as multiple implants placed in the posterior maxilla in type IV bone opposing an intact natural dentition or implants.

The downside to splinted restorations is largely related to long-term repair and replacement costs. With patients having implants that must maintain a prosthesis for 30, 40, or 50 years, it is appropriate to consider that the prosthesis will require replacement throughout its life. Most commonly, this is related to porcelain failure on screw-retained PFM FDPs.[94] After a PFM restoration has been in the mouth for any significant period of time, porcelain failure cannot simply be repaired. The restoration must be fully stripped or replaced. Practically speaking, it can be a challenge to find a laboratory willing and able to strip and restack porcelain, and most will opt for complete replacement of the prosthesis. Essentially this has doubled, tripled, or quadrupled the cost of replacement. If an individual unit suffers the same complication, only the unit affected needs to be replaced. Issues related to patient autonomy and desires need to be considered in the replacement of multiple adjacent missing teeth. Some patients may tolerate splinted restorations, whereas others may desire individual units. Oral hygiene techniques and ease of cleansibility will vary between restoration types as well.

KEY FACT

Until evidence shows otherwise, "sharing forces" is not a valid reason to splint adjacent implants. These data are not necessarily in conflict with the early in vitro experiments, they simply illustrate that higher forces do not necessarily result in more bone loss and it is difficult to extrapolate data from finite element analysis and photo-elastic gel studies to clinical realities.

Indications for splinting adjacent implants include significant off-axis forces (i.e., canine replacement), multiple adjacent external hex implants, poor bone, and diminutive implants.[50]

Management of Partially Edentulous Implant Treatment in the Aesthetic Zone

Diagnosis and Treatment Planning

Treatment of the partially edentulous patient in the aesthetic zone is one of the more challenging prosthetic scenarios. The "aesthetic zone" is not simply canine to canine in the maxilla. Each patient must be individually evaluated for lip position and movement (Fig. 77.22) to determine the appropriate level of aesthetic consideration necessary.

The primary challenge in this treatment is the peri-implant soft tissues.[18] If patients show soft tissue during lip movement, then particular attention should be paid to the creation and preservation of natural appearing gingiva. First, there must be sufficient thickness of the gingiva. Thin tissue biotypes are more prone to recession, peri-implant mucositis, papilla loss, and graying.[65,80,81,107,149] The surgical team may need to employ various techniques prior to, or at the time of, implant placement to increase the tissue thickness.

During the treatment planning phase, the clinical team should consider the shape and position of the soft tissue on all teeth or implants in the area. If any of these positions are planning to be modified, the corresponding implant position may change as well.

Management of potential changes to the tissue color can be challenging, as there is a shift in the gingiva around implants to a gray tone.[17] This can be somewhat managed with the use of UCLA or zirconia abutments, though research has clearly shown that there can still be a perceptible color shift with these more aesthetic materials (delta E >3.9).[62] Though zirconia abutments are weaker than titanium, they have shown comparable survival rates for single units in vivo.[150] Some technicians have begun experimenting with the use of fluorescing glazes over the emergence zone of zirconia abutments to decrease the color shift. Some manufacturers and clinicians have coated the titanium abutments with a gold or pink color, again in an attempt to mitigate color changes.

The greatest challenge of implants in the aesthetic zone is papilla management. Implants, even with contemporary designs (i.e., platform switch, conical connections), cannot maintain crestal bone height as much as a healthy tooth. The implant is very different than the natural tooth because it does not have periodontal ligament (and its blood supply) or supracrestal inserting connective tissue fibers. The clinical appearance (i.e., height and fullness) of the papilla between an implant and a tooth ultimately depends on the periodontal attachment level of the adjacent tooth and not the level of bone adjacent to the implant. Should the papilla fail to meet desires and expectations, the open gingival embrasure is generally best managed through additional surgery or closing the space with restorations.[132] Although there have been good attempts to solve the problem of deficient papilla with pink prosthetics, it is all but impossible to resolve it in a manner that is both aesthetically convincing and hygienic in the partially edentulous patient.

Although there will be variations in papilla height adjacent to or between implants, the average papilla height adjacent to a single implant is 4.2 mm.[66] Between adjacent, unrestored natural teeth, the average papilla height is at least 5 mm.[130] Between adjacent (external hex) implants, the average papilla is only 3.4 mm (Table 77.2).[128]

The preceding figures are averages and do not represent the actual value for what is possible for any given patient. The key to predictable,

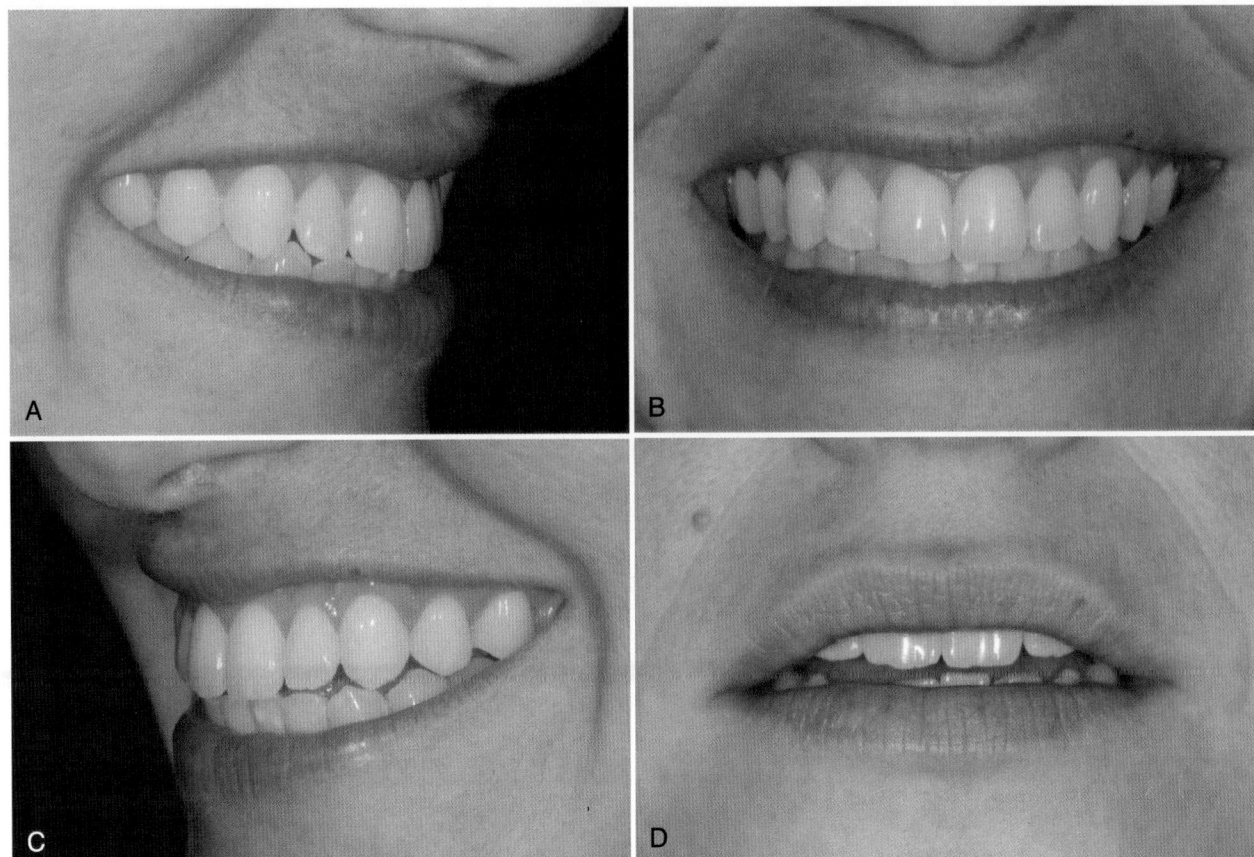

Fig. 77.22 Implant treatment in the aesthetic zone is more challenging than in the functional zone. It is important to keep in mind that the aesthetic zone differs for each patient. It should be evaluated though a series of basic photos: right, center, and left at maximum smile (A–C), and with lips at rest (D). In this patient the aesthetic zone clearly includes the anterior teeth and all premolars.

TABLE 77.2	Anticipated Papilla Height		
	Between Natural Teeth	**Between Tooth and Implant**	**Between Adjacent Implants**
Average expected papilla height (from crest of bone)	≥5 mm (Tarnow, 1992)[130]	4.2 mm (Kan, 2003)[66]	3.4 mm (Tarnow, 2003)[128]

successful treatment in the aesthetic zone is the implant-retained provisional restoration. This will allow the clinical team and the patient to truly test the four key criteria of aesthetics, phonetics, function, and hygiene. Revisions and alterations are much easier to accomplish with provisionals as compared with the definitive prosthesis.

FLASH BACK

The greatest challenge of implants in the aesthetic zone is papilla management. Although there have been good attempts to solve the problem of deficient papilla with pink prosthetics, it is all but impossible to resolve it in a manner that is both aesthetically convincing and hygienic in the partially edentulous patient.

Tissue Shaping and Management

Following integration of the implant and maturation of the soft tissue, there may be the need to correct slight malpositions of the peri-implant tissues. This can be done through modification of the implant abutment, but it should not be done repeatedly to avoid increased tissue changes that lead to bone loss. Significant deficiencies of tissue may be difficult to correct, whereas others may be able to be addressed with additional surgery.

The emergence profile of the provisional restoration can be added to or contoured back to manipulate the soft tissue position. Applying additional contour will move the gingiva apically, whereas undercontouring will allow the tissue to drape more coronally. The abutment can also be modified to apply pressure to the base of the papilla, thus forcing the tip coronally,[132] but this technique should be used with caution around implants due to a diminished blood supply and fragility of the soft tissue.[111] The clinician should minimize the number of reattachments to the head of the implant, as this will weaken the integrity of the tissues and create additional bone loss.[3,112]

Ideally all contours of the soft tissues should be designed in the patient's mouth, and the four keys (aesthetics, phonetics, function, and hygiene) should be tested and approved. If done correctly, the transition from the patient to the technician is seamless with the provisional serving as a blueprint for the definitive prosthesis.

Conclusion

Successful implant treatment requires a team of clinicians and technicians dedicated to excellence in surgical and prosthetic aspects. A thorough understanding of the prosthodontic restoration of implants from implant-abutment connections to hard and soft tissue interfaces and compatibility with the implant/abutment/restoration is essential. This chapter reviewed the critical aspects of prosthetic implant treatment proven to maximize long-term functional, biologic, and aesthetic success.

 A Case Scenario is found on the companion website www.expertconsult.com.

References

 References for this chapter are found on the companion website www.expertconsult.com.

CHAPTER 78

Basic Implant Surgical Procedures

Perry R. Klokkevold

CHAPTER OUTLINE

General Principles of Implant Surgery
Two-Stage "Submerged" Implant Placement
One-Stage "Nonsubmerged" Implant Placement
Conclusion

> Editors' note: An animation (slide show) has been added by the editors as a supplement to the chapter. It was produced by My Dental Hub as a patient education tool and covers the basic elements in a conceptual manner. It is not intended to be a procedural guide for dental professionals.

The surgical procedures for the placement of nearly all endosseous dental implants currently used are based on the original work of Professor Per-Ingvar Brånemark and colleagues in Sweden in the 1960s and 1970s.[4,5] Their landmark research evaluated the biologic, physiologic, and mechanical aspects of the titanium screw-shaped implant, subsequently known commercially as the Nobelpharma "Brånemark" implant system and currently manufactured by Nobel Biocare. The original Brånemark implant was a parallel-walled, cylindrically shaped, threaded implant with an external hex connection and a machined surface. Since their introduction, many designs of root form implants have been developed, modified, and studied. The same fundamental principles of atraumatic, precise implant site preparation applies to all implant systems. Briefly, this includes a gentle surgical technique and progressive, incremental preparation of the bone for a precise fit of the implant at the time of placement.

This chapter outlines the basic surgical procedures for the placement of endosseous dental implants using either one-stage or two-stage protocols. The principles described here are intentionally generic and meant to serve as guidelines that are applicable to most common implant systems (Video 78.1). Each implant system is designed with specific armamentarium and recommendations for use (e.g., drilling speeds), and it is advisable to follow the detailed protocols provided by the manufacturer. For the presentation of a dental implant case, see Video 78.2.

General Principles of Implant Surgery

Patient Preparation

Most implant surgical procedures can be done in the office using local anesthesia. Conscious sedation (oral or intravenous) may be indicated (see Chapter 38) for some patients. The risks and benefits of implant surgery specific to the patient's situation and needs should be thoroughly explained prior to surgery. A written, informed consent should be obtained for the procedure.

Implant Site Preparation

Some basic principles must be followed to achieve osseointegration with a high degree of predictability[3,4,7] (Box 78.1). The surgical site should be kept aseptic, and the patient should be appropriately prepared and draped for an intraoral surgical procedure. Prerinsing with chlorhexidine gluconate for 1 to 2 minutes immediately before the procedure will aid in reducing the bacterial load present around the surgical site. Every effort should be made to maintain a sterile surgical field and to avoid contamination of the implant surface. Implant sites should be prepared using gentle, atraumatic surgical techniques with an effort to avoid overheating the bone.

Successful osseointegration occurs predictably for submerged[4] and nonsubmerged[11] dental implants when proven clinical guidelines are followed. Well-controlled studies of patients with good plaque control and appropriate occlusal forces have demonstrated that root form, endosseous dental implants show little change in bone height around the implant over years of function.[1] After initial bone remodeling in the first year (1 to 1.5 mm of resorption described as "normal remodeling around an externally hexed implant"),[1] the bone level around healthy functioning implants remains stable for many years afterward. The average annual crestal bone loss after the first year in function is expected to be 0.1 mm or less. Hence, implants offer a predictable solution for tooth replacement.

Regardless of the surgical approach, the implant must be placed in healthy bone with good primary stability to achieve osseointegration, and an atraumatic technique must be followed to avoid damage to bone. Drilling of the bone without adequate cooling generates excessive heat, which injures bone and increases the risk of failure.[12] The anatomic features of bone quality (dense compact versus loose trabecular) at the recipient site influences the interface between bone and implant.[9] Compact bone offers a much greater surface area for bone-to-implant contact than cancellous bone. Areas of the jaw exhibiting thin layers of cortical bone and large cancellous spaces, such as the posterior maxilla, have lower success rates than areas of dense bone.[9] The best results are achieved when the bone-to-implant contact is intimate at the time of implant placement.

One-Stage Versus Two-Stage Implant Placement Surgery

Currently, most threaded endosseous implants can be placed using either a one-stage (nonsubmerged) or a two-stage (submerged)

BOX 78.1   Basic Principles of Implant Therapy to Achieve Osseointegration

1. Implants must be sterile and made of a biocompatible material (e.g., titanium).
2. Implant site should be prepared under sterile conditions.
3. Implant site should be prepared with an atraumatic surgical technique that avoids overheating of the bone during preparation of the recipient site.
4. Implants should be placed with good initial stability.
5. Implants should be allowed to heal without loading or micromovement (i.e., undisturbed healing period to allow for osseointegration) for 2 to 4 or 4 to 6 months, depending on the bone density, bone maturation, and implant stability.

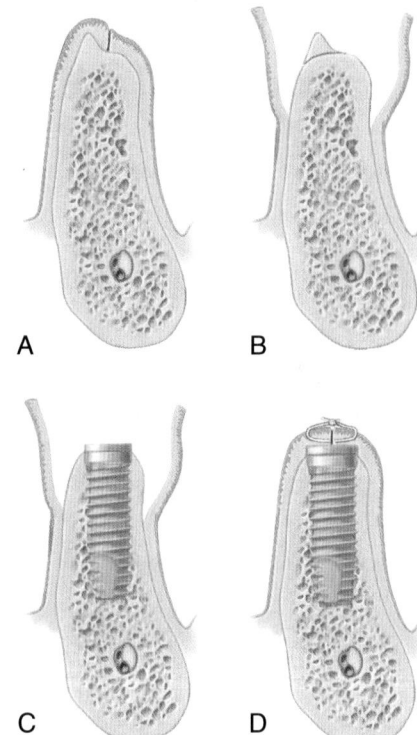

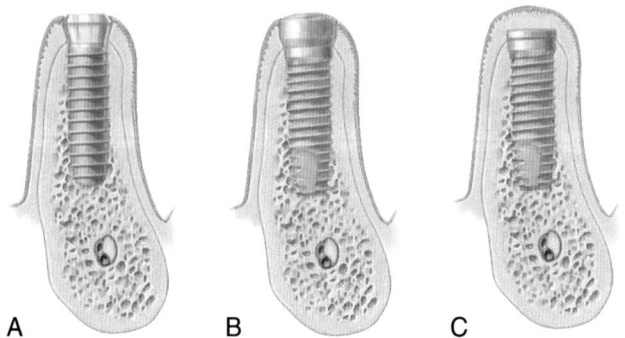

Fig. 78.1 One-stage implant versus two-stage implant surgeries. (A) One-stage surgery with the implant designed so that the coronal portion of the implant extends through the gingiva. (B) One-stage surgery with implant designed to be used for two-stage surgery. A healing abutment is connected to the implant during the first-stage surgery. (C) In the two-stage surgery, the top of the implant is completely submerged under gingiva.

Fig. 78.2 Tissue management for a two-stage implant placement. (A) Crestal incision is made along the crest of the ridge, bisecting the existing zone of keratinized mucosa. (B) Full-thickness flap is raised buccally and lingually to the level of the mucogingival junction. A narrow, sharp ridge can be surgically reduced/contoured to provide a reasonably flat bed for the implant. (C) Implant is placed in the prepared osteotomy site. (D) Tissue approximation achieves primary flap closure without tension.

protocol. In the one-stage approach, the implant or the abutment emerges through the mucoperiosteum/gingival tissue at the time of implant placement, whereas in the two-stage approach, the top of the implant and cover screw are completely covered with the flap closure (Fig. 78.1). Implants are allowed to heal, without loading or micromovement, for a period of time to allow for osseointegration. In two-stage implant surgery, the implant must be surgically exposed following a healing period. Some implants, referred to as "tissue level," are specifically designed with the coronal portion of the implant positioned above the crest of bone and extending through the gingival tissues at the time of placement in a one-stage protocol (Fig. 78.1A). Other implant systems, referred to as "bone level," are designed to be placed at the level of bone and require a healing abutment to be attached to the implant at the time of placement to be used in a one-stage approach[8] (Fig. 78.1B).

A one-stage surgical approach simplifies the procedure because a second-stage exposure surgery is not necessary. The two-stage, submerged approach is advantageous for situations that require simultaneous bone augmentation procedures at the time of implant placement because membranes can be submerged, which will minimize postoperative exposure. Mucogingival tissues can be augmented if desired at the second-stage surgery in a two-stage protocol or as part of the one-stage protocol. Fundamental differences in flap management for these two surgical techniques are described separately.

Two-Stage "Submerged" Implant Placement

In the two-stage implant surgical approach, the first-stage or implant placement surgery ends by suturing the soft tissues together over the implant cover screw so that it remains submerged and isolated from the oral cavity. In areas with dense cortical bone and good initial implant support, the implants are left to heal undisturbed for a period of 2 to 4 months, whereas in areas of loose trabecular bone, grafted sites, and sites with lesser implant stability, implants may be allowed to heal for periods of 4 to 6 months or more. Longer healing periods are indicated for implants in sites with less bone support. During healing, osteoblasts migrate to the surface and form bone adjacent to the implant (osseointegration).[6] Shorter healing periods are indicated for implants placed in good quality (dense) bone and for implants with an altered surface microtopography (e.g., acid etched, blasted, or etched and blasted). Readers are referred to online material and other resources for more information about implant surface microtopography.

In the second-stage (exposure) surgery, the implant is uncovered and a healing abutment is connected to allow emergence of the abutment through the soft tissues. Once healed, the restorative dentist then proceeds with the prosthodontic aspects of the implant therapy (impressions and fabrication of prosthesis).

The following paragraphs describe the steps for osteotomy preparation and the first-stage implant placement surgery of the two-stage protocol. Figs. 78.2 and 78.3 illustrate the procedures via diagrams, and Fig. 78.4 depicts the procedures with clinical photographs.

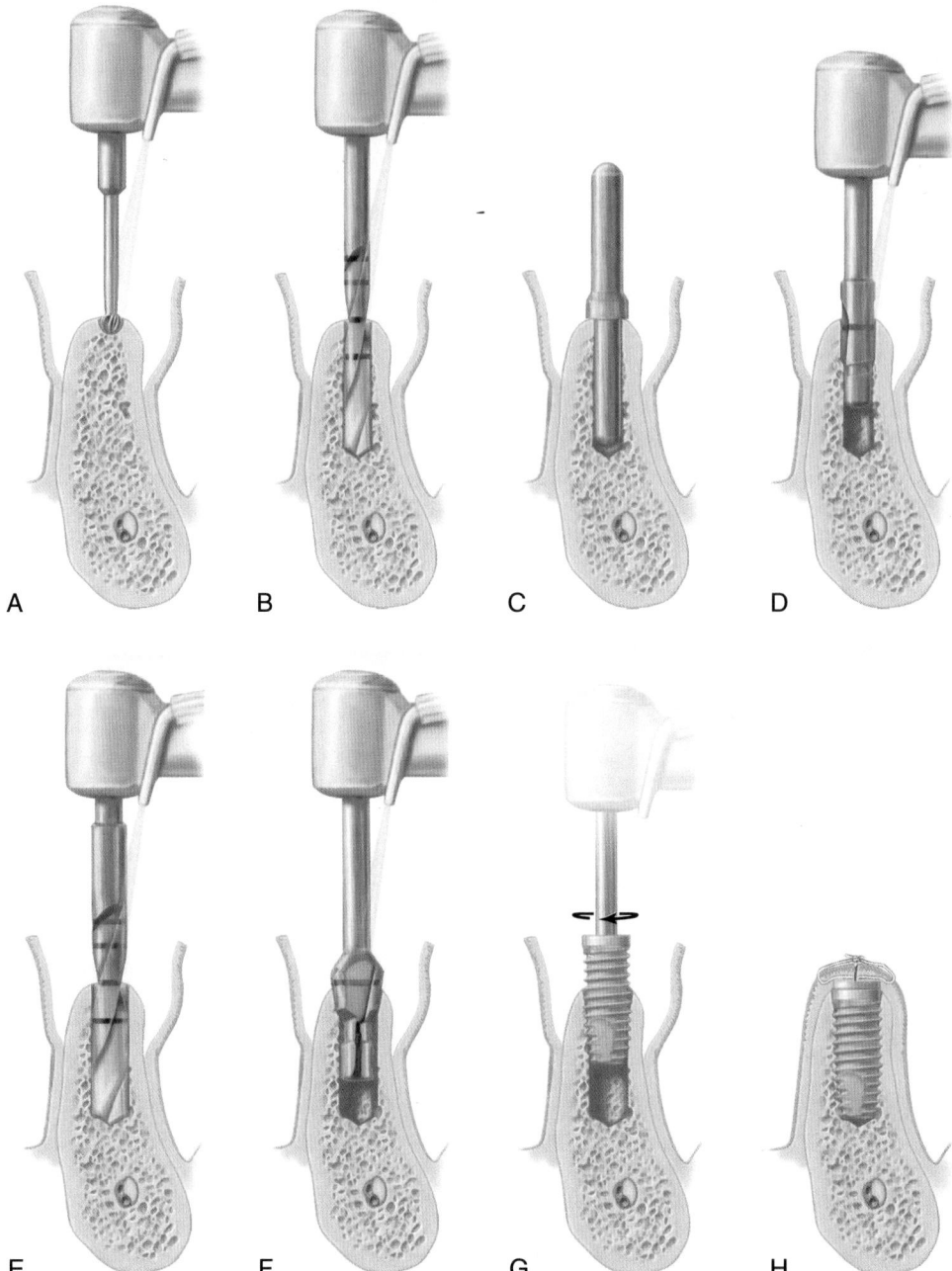

Fig. 78.3 Implant site preparation (osteotomy) for a 4-mm diameter, 10-mm length screw-type, threaded (external hex) implant in a subcrestal position. (A) Initial marking or preparation of the implant site with a round bur. (B) Use of a 2-mm twist drill to establish depth and align the implant. (C) Guide pin is placed in the osteotomy site to confirm position and angulation. (D) Pilot drill is used to increase the diameter of the coronal aspect of the osteotomy site. (E) Final drill used is the 3-mm twist drill to finish preparation of the osteotomy site. (F) Countersink drill is used to widen the entrance of the recipient site and allow for the subcrestal placement of the implant collar and cover screw. Note: An optional tap (not shown) can be used following this step to create screw threads in areas of dense bone. (G) Implant is inserted into the prepared osteotomy site with a handpiece or handheld driver. Note: In systems that use an implant mount, it is removed prior to placement of the cover screw. (H) The cover screw is placed and soft tissues are closed and sutured.

Flap Design, Incisions, and Elevation

Flap management for implant surgery varies slightly, depending on the location and objective of the planned surgery. There are different incision/flap designs, but the most common is the crestal flap design. The incision is made along the crest of the ridge, bisecting the existing zone of keratinized mucosa (see Figs. 78.2A and 78.4B).

A remote incision with a layered suturing technique may be used to minimize the incidence of bone graft exposure when extensive bone augmentation is planned. The crestal incision, however, is preferred in most cases, because closure is easier to manage and typically results in less bleeding, less edema, and faster healing.[10]

A full-thickness flap is raised (buccal and lingual) up to or slightly beyond the level of the mucogingival junction, exposing the alveolar

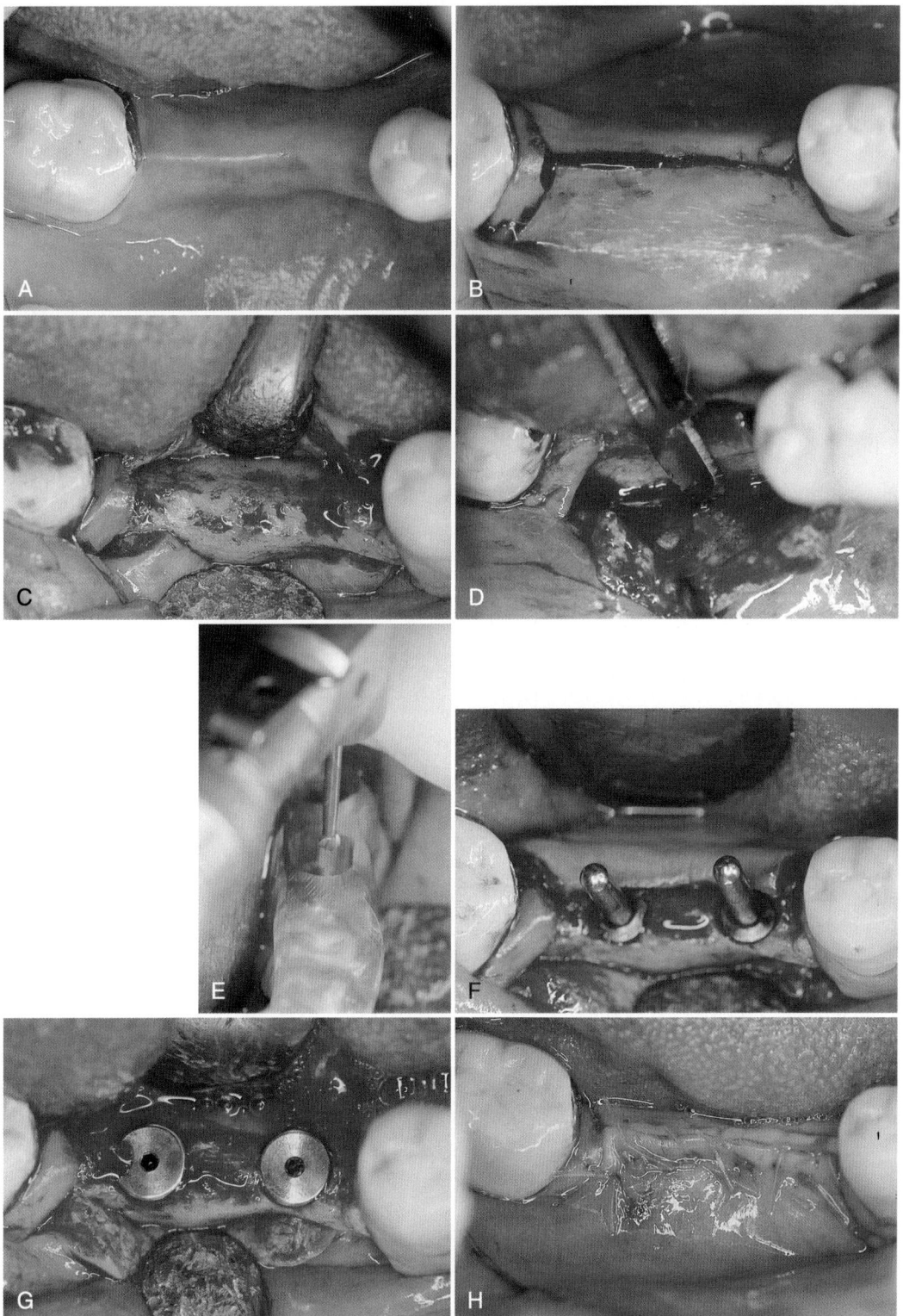

Fig. 78.4 Clinical view of stage-one implant placement surgery. (A) Partial edentulous ridge; presurgical and prosthodontic treatment has been completed. (B) Mesial sulcular and distal vertical incisions are connected by a crestal incision. Notice that bands of gingival collars remain adjacent to the distal molar tooth. (C) Minimal flap reflection is used to expose the alveolar bone. Sometimes a ridge modification is necessary to provide a flap recipient bed. (D) Buccal flap is partially dissected at the apical portion to provide a flap extension. This is a critical step to ensure a tension-free closure of the flap after implant placement. (E) It is important to use the surgical stent to determine the mesial-distal and buccal-lingual dimensions and proper angulation of the implant placement. (F) Frequent use of the guide pins ensures parallelism of the implant placement. (G) After placement of two Nobelpharma implants, the cover screws are placed. The cover screws should be flush with the rest of the ridge to minimize the chance of exposure. This is especially important if the patient will wear a partial denture during the healing phase. (H) Suturing completed. Both regular interrupted and inverted mattress sutures are used intermittently to ensure tension-free, tight closure of the flaps.

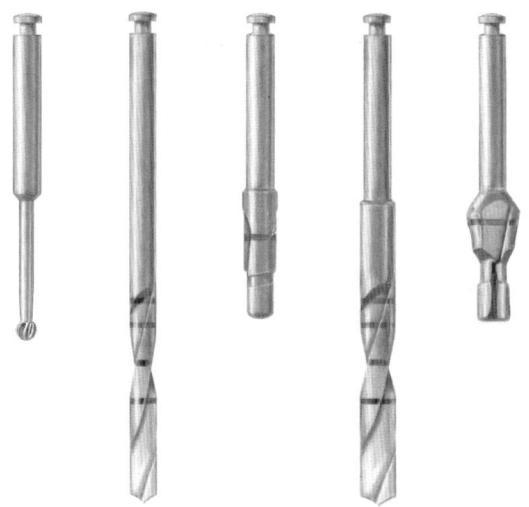

Fig. 78.5 Sequence of drills used for standard-diameter (4-mm) implant site osteotomy preparation: round, 2-mm twist, pilot, 3-mm twist, and countersink. Bone tap (not shown here) is an optional drill that is sometimes used in dense bone before implant placement.

ridge of the implant surgical sites (see Figs. 78.2B and 78.4C). Elevated flaps may be sutured to the buccal mucosa or the opposing teeth to keep the surgical site open during the surgery. The bone at the implant site must be thoroughly debrided of all granulation tissue.

For a "knife-edge" alveolar process with sufficient alveolar bone height and distance from vital structures (e.g., inferior alveolar nerve), a large round bur is used to recontour or flatten the bone to provide a wider, level surface for the implant site preparation (see Fig. 78.2B). However, if the vertical height of the alveolar bone is limited (e.g., <10 mm), the knife-edge alveolar bone height should be preserved. Bone augmentation procedures can be used to increase the ridge width while preserving alveolar bone height (see Chapter 79).

Implant Site Preparation

Once the flaps are reflected and the bone is prepared (i.e., all granulation tissue removed and knife-edge ridges flattened), the implant osteotomy site can be prepared. A series of drills are used to prepare the osteotomy site precisely and incrementally for an implant (Fig. 78.5). A surgical guide or stent is inserted, checked for proper positioning, and used throughout the procedure to direct the proper implant placement (see Fig. 78.4E).

Round Bur

A small round bur (or spiral drill) is used to make the initial penetration into bone for the implant site. The surgical guide is removed, and the initial marks are checked for their appropriate buccal-lingual and mesial-distal location, as well as the positions relative to each other and adjacent teeth (see Fig. 75.9). Slight modifications may be necessary to adjust spatial relationships and to avoid minor ridge defects. Any changes should be compared with the prosthetically driven surgical guide positions. Each marked site is then prepared to a depth of 1 to 2 mm with a round drill, breaking through the cortical bone and creating a starting point for the 2-mm twist drill (see Fig. 78.3A).

The 2-mm Twist Drill

A small twist drill, usually 2 mm in diameter and marked to indicate various lengths (i.e., corresponding to the implant sizes), is used next to establish the depth and align the long axis of the implant recipient site (see Fig. 78.3B). This drill may be externally or internally irrigated. In either case, the twist drill is used at a speed of approximately 800 to 1500 rpm, with copious irrigation to prevent overheating of the bone. Additionally, drills should be intermittently and repeatedly "pumped" or pulled out of the osteotomy site while drilling to expose them to the water coolant and to facilitate clearing bone debris from the cutting surfaces. In other words, clinicians should pump the drill (up and down) intermittently and avoid using a constant "push" of the drill in the apical direction only.

When multiple implants are being placed next to one another, a guide pin should be placed in the prepared sites to check alignment, parallelism, and proper prosthetic spacing throughout the preparation process (see Fig. 78.3C). The relationship to neighboring vital structures (e.g., nerve and tooth roots) can be determined by taking a periapical radiograph with a guide pin or radiographic marker in the osteotomy site (see Fig. 76.15). Implants should be positioned with approximately 3 mm between one another to ensure sufficient space for interimplant bone and soft-tissue health and to facilitate oral hygiene procedures. Therefore the initial marks should be separated by at least 7 mm (center to center) for 4 mm standard-diameter implants. Incrementally more space is needed for wide-diameter implants (see Fig. 75.9).

The 2-mm twist drill is used to establish the final depth of the osteotomy site corresponding to the length of each planned implant. The clinician should also evaluate the bone quality (density) with this drill while preparing the osteotomy to assess the need for modifying subsequent drills used (Box 78.2). If the vertical height of the bone was reduced during the initial ridge preparation, this must be taken into account when preparing the site for a predetermined implant length. For example, if it appears that the implant will be too close to a vital structure, such as the inferior alveolar nerve canal, the depth of the implant osteotomy site and length of the implant may need to be reduced.

The next step is to use a series of drills to incrementally increase the width of the osteotomy site to accommodate the planned implant diameter. The styles, shapes, and final diameter of the drills will differ slightly among different implant systems, but their general purpose is to prepare a recipient site with a precise diameter (and depth) for the selected implant without unduly traumatizing the surrounding bone. It is important to use copious irrigation and a "pumping" action for all drilling.

KEY FACT

A series of drills will be used (speeds determined by manufacturer) sequentially to prepare osteotomy sites. It is essential to prepare sites with copious irrigation to prevent overheating of the bone. Additionally, drills should be intermittently and repeatedly "pumped" or pulled out of the osteotomy site while drilling to expose them to the water coolant and to facilitate clearing bone debris from the cutting surfaces.

Pilot Drill

Following the 2-mm twist drill, a pilot drill with a noncutting 2-mm–diameter "guide" at the apical end and a cutting 3-mm–diameter (wider) midsection is used to enlarge the osteotomy site at the coronal end, thus facilitating the insertion of the subsequent drill in the sequence (see Fig. 78.3D).

The 3-mm Twist Drill

The final drill in the osteotomy site preparation for a standard-diameter (4 mm) implant is the 3-mm twist drill. It is the last drill used to widen the site along the entire depth of the osteotomy from the previous diameter (2 mm) to final diameter (3 mm). This final drill in the

BOX 78.2   Clinical Advice to Enhance Precision of Final Implant Site Preparation

Clinical Situation 1

If the final drill stops advancing in the apical direction before reaching the desired depth, the added hand pressure necessary to achieve the proper depth can cause wobbling and funneling of the recipient site. This is especially true with "cannon" drills (used for cylindrical implants). To minimize this effect, a smaller-diameter drill should be used to prepare the site slightly deeper (e.g., 0.5 mm or less). This narrower drill allows the desired depth to be reached without affecting the side walls and facilitates a more precise osteotomy preparation with the final drill. It is also important to use drills that are sharp, especially for dense bone.

Clinical Situation 2

If the final drill is inserted at an inaccurate angle, the result is funneling of the coronal portion of the implant site. To minimize this potential problem, when drilling multiple implant sites, the operator should always keep a direction indicator in an adjacent site. For single-implant sites, the adjacent teeth and surgical guide should serve as direction indicators. When dealing with dense bone, a precise recipient site can be achieved more predictably if there is minimal diameter change from drill to drill. For example, switching from 3 to 5 mm is much less precise than proceeding from 3 to 3.3 to 4.2 to 5 mm.

Clinical Situation 3

If the bone is "soft" (e.g., loose trabecular bone), it may be advantageous to underprepare the osteotomy site. A slightly underprepared site can be accomplished by using the final drill to a shallower depth than the previous drill (e.g., half the depth of the osteotomy site). This avoids removing too much bone and increases the implant stability or tightness at the time of placement. Another method to achieve an underprepared site is to use a drill with a slightly smaller diameter as the final drill in the preparation (e.g., a 2.75-mm drill as the final drill rather than a 3-mm or a 3.25-mm version as the final drill for a 4-mm implant).

sequence finishes preparing the osteotomy site and consequently is the step that dictates whether the implant will be stable or not (see Fig. 78.3E). It is critically important that the final diameter drilling be accomplished with a steady hand, without wobbling or changing direction so that the site is not overprepared. Finally, depending on bone density, the diameter of this final drill may be slightly increased or decreased to enhance implant support (see Box 78.2).

Countersink Drill (Optional)

When it is desirable to place the cover screw at or slightly below the crestal bone, countersink drilling is used to shape or flare the crestal aspect of the osteotomy site allowing the coronal flare of the implant head and cover screw to fit within the osteotomy site (see Fig. 78.3F). As with all drills in the sequence, copious irrigation and gentle surgical techniques are used.

Bone Tap (Optional)

As the final step in preparing the osteotomy site in dense cortical bone, a tapping procedure may be necessary (not shown on Fig. 78.3). With self-tapping implants being almost universal, there is less need for a tapping procedure in most sites. However, in dense cortical bone or when placing longer implants into moderately dense bone, it is prudent to tap the bone (create threads in the osteotomy site) before implant placement to facilitate implant insertion and to reduce the risk of implant binding (see Fig. 78.3G).

! CLINICAL CORRELATION

When faced with a very soft, poor-quality bone (e.g., loose trabecular bone in the posterior maxilla), tapping is not necessary or recommended (see Box 78.2). It is better to allow the threaded implant to "cut" its own path into the osteotomy site.

Bone tapping and implant insertion are both done at very slow speeds (e.g., 20 to 40 rpm). All other drills in the sequence are used at higher speeds (800 to 1500 rpm).

It is important to create a recipient site that is accurate in size and angulation. In partially edentulous cases, limited jaw opening or proximity to adjacent teeth may prevent appropriate positioning of the drills in posterior edentulous areas. In fact, implant therapy may be contraindicated in some patients because of a lack of interocclusal clearance, lack of interdental space, or a lack of access for the instrumentation. Therefore a combination of longer drills and shorter drills, with or without extensions, may be necessary. Anticipating these needs before surgery facilitates the procedure and improves the results.

! CLINICAL CORRELATION

In areas with loose trabecular bone, such as the posterior maxilla, it may not be necessary to tap the site. If bone is especially loose, it may be beneficial to underprepare the site. For example, the final drill could be omitted to increase the implant stability.

Implant Placement

Implants are inserted with a handpiece rotating at slow speeds (e.g., 25 rpm) or by hand with a wrench. Insertion of the implant must follow the same path or line as the osteotomy site. When multiple implants are being placed, it is helpful to use guide pins in the other sites to have a visual guide for the path of insertion.

Flap Closure and Suturing

Once the implants are inserted and the cover screws secured (see Fig. 78.4G), the surgical sites should be thoroughly irrigated with sterile saline to remove debris and clean the wound. Proper closure of the flap over the implant is essential. One of the most important aspects of flap management is achieving good approximation and primary closure of the tissues in a tension-free manner (see Fig. 78.3H). This is achieved by incising the periosteum (innermost layer of full-thickness flap), which is nonelastic. Once the periosteum is released, the flap becomes very elastic and is able to be stretched over the implant without tension. One suturing technique that consistently provides the desired result is a combination of alternating horizontal mattress and interrupted sutures (see Fig. 78.4H). Horizontal mattress sutures evert the wound edges and approximate the inner, connective tissue surfaces of the flap to facilitate closure and wound healing. Interrupted sutures help to bring the wound edges together, counterbalancing the eversion caused by the horizontal mattress sutures.

The clinician should choose an appropriate suture for the given patient and procedure. For patient management, it is sometimes simpler to use a resorbable suture that does not require removal during the postoperative visit (e.g., 4-0 chromic gut suture). However, when moderate-to-severe postoperative swelling is anticipated, a nonresorbable suture is recommended to maintain a longer closure period (e.g., 4-0 monofilament suture). These sutures require removal at a postoperative visit.

Postoperative Care

Simple implant surgery in a healthy patient usually does not require antibiotic therapy. However, antibiotics (e.g., amoxicillin, 500 mg three times a day [tid]) can be prescribed if the surgery is extensive or if the patient is medically compromised. Postoperative swelling is likely after flap surgery. This is particularly true when the periosteum has been incised (released). As a preventive measure, patients should apply cold packs over the first 24 to 48 hours. Chlorhexidine gluconate oral rinses can be prescribed to facilitate plaque control, especially in the days after surgery when oral hygiene is typically poorer. Adequate pain medication should be prescribed (e.g., ibuprofen, 600 to 800 mg tid).

Patients should be instructed to maintain a relatively soft diet after surgery. Then, as healing progresses, they can gradually return to a normal diet. Patients should also refrain from tobacco and alcohol use after surgery. Provisional restorations, whether fixed or removable, should be checked and adjusted to minimize trauma to the surgical area.

Second-Stage Exposure Surgery

For implants placed using a two-stage "submerged" protocol, a second-stage exposure surgery is necessary. Box 78.3 lists the objectives for second-stage implant exposure surgery. The need for a zone of keratinized tissue surrounding implants is desirable, as one long-term study indicated that the presence of keratinized tissue is strongly correlated with soft- and hard-tissue health.[2]

Simple Circular "Punch" or Crestal Incision

In areas with sufficient zones of keratinized tissue, the gingiva covering the head of the implant can be exposed with a circular or "punch" incision (Fig. 78.6). Alternatively, a crestal incision through the middle of the keratinized tissue and full-thickness flap reflection can be used to expose implants.

Partial-Thickness Repositioned Flap

If a minimal zone of keratinized tissue exists at the implant site, a partial-thickness flap technique can be used to fulfill the objective of the second-stage surgery (exposing the implant) while increasing the width of keratinized tissue. The initial incision is made within the zone of keratinized tissue so that it becomes the outer edge of the reflected split-thickness flap. Vertical releasing incisions are used on both the mesial and the distal end of the flap (Fig. 78.7A–B). A partial-thickness flap is then raised in such a manner that a nonmobile, firm periosteum remains attached to the underlying bone. The flap, containing a narrow band of keratinized tissue, is then repositioned to the facial side of the emerging head of the implant and sutured to the periosteum with a fine needle and resorbable suture such as a 5-0 gut suture (Fig. 78.8). If the initial amount of keratinized tissue is less than 2 mm, the flap may be started at the labial edge of the keratinized tissue allowing that zone to remain on

---

BOX 78.3   Objectives of Second-Stage Implant Surgery

1. To expose the submerged implant without damaging the surrounding bone
2. To control the thickness of the soft tissue surrounding the implant
3. To preserve or create attached keratinized tissue around the implant
4. To facilitate oral hygiene
5. To ensure proper abutment seating
6. To preserve soft-tissue aesthetics

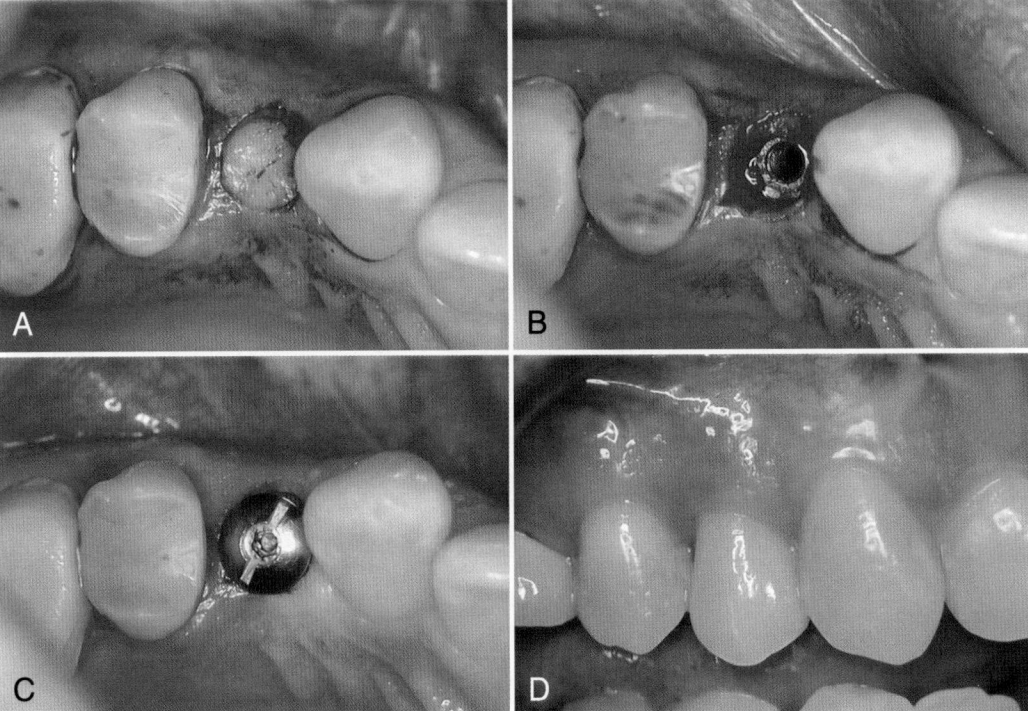

Fig. 78.6 Clinical view of second-stage implant exposure surgery in a case with adequate keratinized tissue. (A) Simple circular "punch" incision used to expose implant when sufficient keratinized tissue is present around the implant. (B) Implant exposed. (C) Healing abutment attached. (D) Final restoration in place, achieving an aesthetic result with a good zone of keratinized tissue.

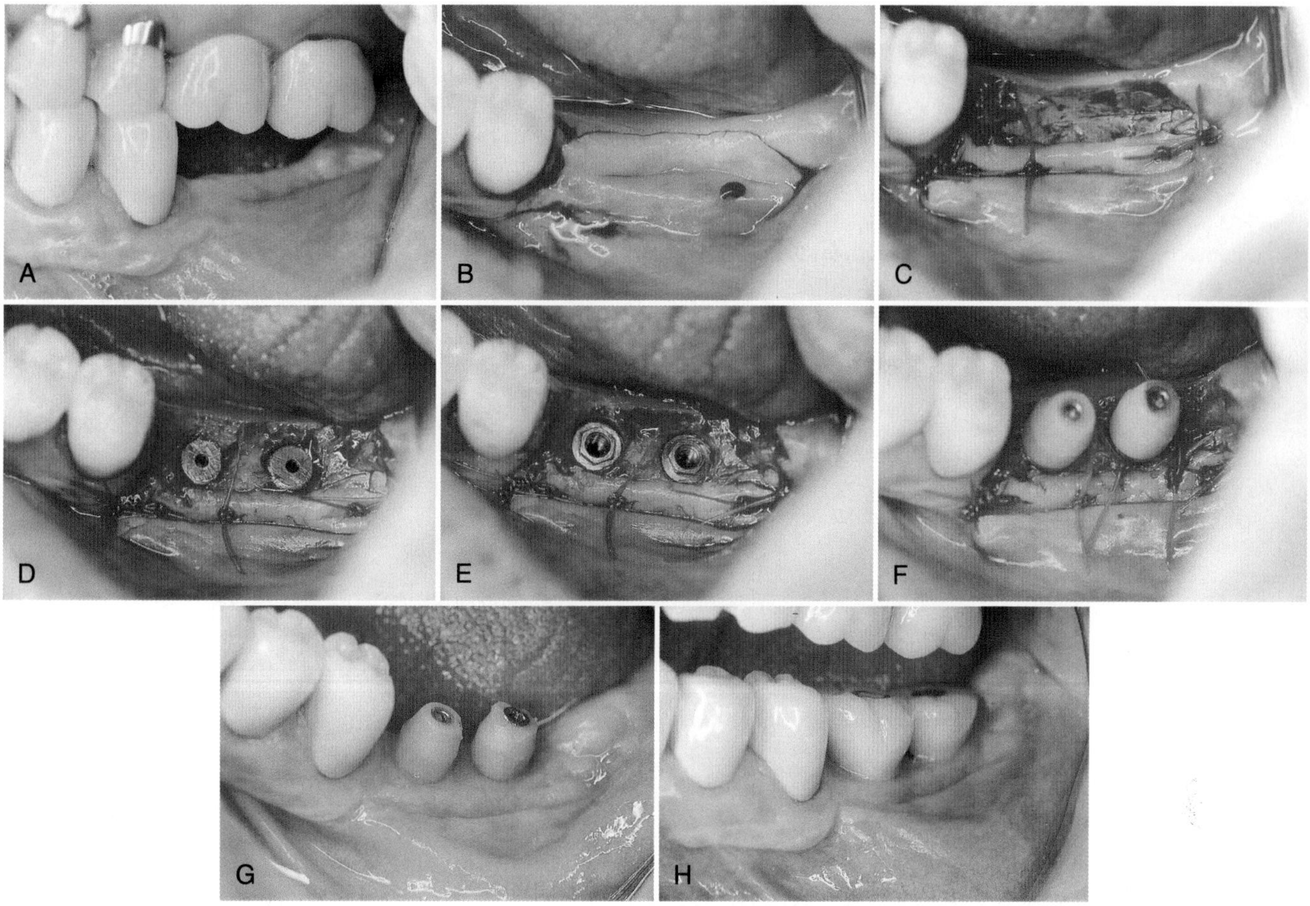

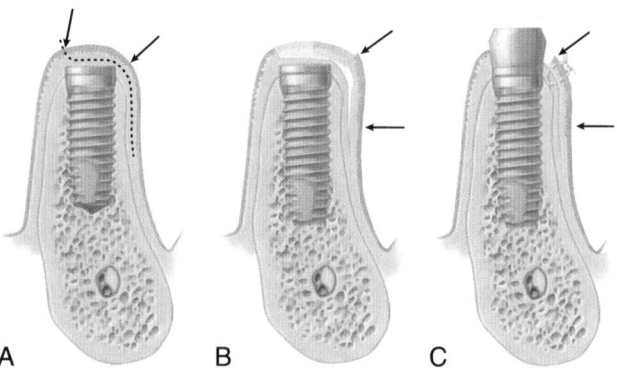

Fig. 78.7 Clinical view of second-stage implant exposure surgery in a case with inadequate keratinized tissue. (A) Two endosseous implants were placed 4 months previously and are ready to be exposed. Note the narrow band of keratinized tissue. (B) Two vertical incisions are connected by crestal incision. If facial keratinized tissue is insufficient, it is necessary to locate the crestal incision more lingually so that there is at least 2 to 3 mm of keratinized band. (C) Buccal partial-thickness flap is sutured to the periosteum apical to the emerging implants. (D) Gingival tissue coronal to the cover screws is excised using the gingivectomy technique. (E) Cover screws are removed, and heads of the implants are cleared. (F) Abutments are placed. Visual inspection ensures intimate contact between the abutments and the implants. (G) Healing at 2 to 3 weeks after second-stage surgery. (H) Four months after the final restoration. Note the healthy band of keratinized attached gingiva around the implants.

Fig. 78.8 Illustration depicting the use of a split-thickness flap that is repositioned to the labial surface to preserve and increase the amount of keratinized tissue. (A) Partial-thickness flap is created from the lingual aspect of the crest toward the labial surface to preserve the keratinized tissue on the crest (over the implant). Note: This tissue might be excised in a simple implant exposure. (B) The split-thickness flap is repositioned to the labial surface. (C) The flap is sutured to the periosteum at a more apical position preserving the amount of keratinized tissue *(arrows)*. Finally, the remaining connective tissue over the cover screw (B) is excised with a sharp blade to expose the implant. Care should be taken to avoid removing keratinized tissue from the lingual aspect of the implant.

the lingual aspect of the implant. A partial-thickness flap is apically displaced and sutured to the periosteum without exposing the alveolar bone (see Fig. 78.7C). A free gingival graft may be harvested from the palate and sutured to the periosteum on the labial surface of the implants to increase the zone of keratinized tissue (not shown).

After the flap is repositioned and secured with periosteal sutures, the excess tissue coronal to the cover screw is excised, usually with a surgical blade (see Fig. 78.8B). However, if removal of this tissue would jeopardize the amount of remaining keratinized tissue around the lingual aspect of the implant, a similar partial-thickness flap can be elevated and repositioned on the lingual side as well. Extra care must be taken when creating a split-thickness flap on the lingual surface of mandibular sites because the tissue is often very thin. Alternatively, a full-thickness lingual flap will be safer and will serve a similar purpose of preserving keratinized tissue on the lingual surface of the implant.

A sharp blade is used to eliminate all tissues coronal to the cover screw (see Fig. 78.7D). The cover screw is then removed, the head of the implant is thoroughly cleaned of any soft- or hard-tissue overgrowth, and the healing abutments or standard abutments are placed on the implant (see Fig. 78.7E–F). The fit of the healing abutments to the implants can often be visually evaluated. However, if it is not possible to visualize clearly the intimate connection between the implant and the abutment, an intraoral periapical x-ray film should be taken to confirm complete seating. Bone may need to be removed around the top of the implant to get the abutment to seat properly. Readers are referred to online material for a discussion of bone profiling.

KEY FACT

In sites with limited keratinized tissue, a partial-thickness flap can be utilized to preserve and reposition the keratinized tissue. A partial-thickness flap is apically displaced and sutured to the periosteum. In cases without keratinized tissue, a free gingival graft may be harvested from the palate and sutured to the periosteum on the labial surface of the implants to increase the zone of keratinized tissue.

Postoperative Care

Once the implant is exposed and soft tissues are sutured, it is important to remind the patient of the need for good oral hygiene around the implant and adjacent teeth. Care should be taken during oral hygiene procedures to avoid dislodging any repositioned or grafted soft tissues. Direct pressure or movement directed toward the soft tissue from a provisional prosthesis can delay healing and should be avoided. Tissues should be monitored regularly, and the provisional prosthesis should be adjusted as needed. Impressions for the final prosthesis fabrication can begin about 2 to 6 weeks after implant exposure surgery, depending on healing and maturation of soft tissues. Fig. 78.7 (parts G and H) shows the postoperative results in a clinical case after 2 to 3 weeks and 4 months, respectively.

One-Stage "Nonsubmerged" Implant Placement

In the one-stage implant surgical approach, a second implant exposure surgery is not needed because the implant is exposed (per gingival) from the time of implant placement (Fig. 78.9). In the standard (classic) implant protocol, the implants are left unloaded and undisturbed for a period similar to that for implants placed in the two-stage approach (i.e., in areas with dense cortical bone and good

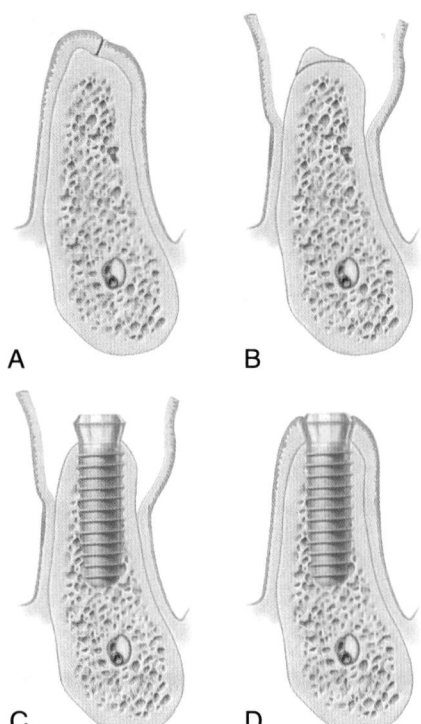

Fig. 78.9 Tissue management for a one-stage implant placement. (A) Crestal incision made along the crest of the ridge, bisecting the existing zone of keratinized mucosa. (B) Full-thickness flap is raised buccally and lingually to the level of the mucogingival junction. A narrow, sharp ridge can be surgically reduced or contoured to provide a reasonably flat bed for the implant. (C) Implant is placed in the prepared osteotomy site. (D) Tissues are adapted around the neck of the implant to achieve flap closure with the implant protruding through the soft tissues.

initial implant support, the implants are left to heal undisturbed for a period of 2 to 4 months, whereas in areas of loose trabecular bone, grafted sites, or minimal implant support, they may be allowed to heal for periods of 4 to 6 months or more).

In the one-stage surgical approach, the implant or the healing abutment protrudes approximately 2 to 3 mm from the bone crest, and the flaps are adapted around the implant/abutment. As with the second-stage surgical procedures described, the soft tissues may be thinned, repositioned, or augmented at the implant placement surgery to increase the zone of keratinized tissue surrounding the implant.

Flap Design, Incisions, and Elevation

The flap design for the one-stage surgical approach is always a crestal incision bisecting the existing keratinized tissue (see Fig. 78.9). Vertical incisions may be needed at one or both ends to facilitate access to the bone or osteotomy site. Tissues can be thinned in posterior areas if desired but are generally not thinned in anterior aesthetic areas. Full-thickness flaps are elevated facially and lingually.

Implant Site Preparation

Implant site preparation for the one-stage approach is identical in principle to the two-stage implant surgical approach. The primary difference is that the coronal aspect of the implant or the healing abutment (two-stage implant) is placed approximately 2 to 3 mm above the bone crest and the soft tissues are approximated around the implant/implant abutment.

Flap Closure and Suturing

The keratinized edges of the flap are sutured with single interrupted sutures around the implant. Depending on the clinician's preference, the wound may be sutured with resorbable or nonresorbable sutures. When keratinized tissue is abundant, scalloping around the implant provides better flap adaptation.

Postoperative Care

The postoperative care for the one-stage surgical approach is similar to that for the two-stage surgical approach except that the cover screw or healing abutment is exposed to the oral cavity. Patients are advised to avoid chewing in the area of the implant. Prosthetic appliances should not be used if direct chewing forces can be transmitted to the implant, particularly in the early healing period (first 4 to 8 weeks). When removable prosthetic appliances are used, they should be adequately relieved and a soft-tissue liner should be applied.

Conclusion

It is essential to understand and follow basic guidelines to predictably achieve osseointegration. Fundamental protocols must be followed for implant placement (stage one) and implant exposure surgery (stage two). These fundamentals apply to all implant systems.

 A Case Scenario is found on the companion website www.expertconsult.com.

References

 References for this chapter are found on the companion website www.expertconsult.com.

CHAPTER 79

Localized Bone Augmentation and Implant Site Development

Perry R. Klokkevold

CHAPTER OUTLINE

Guided Bone Regeneration *(e-only)*
Localized Ridge Augmentation
Alveolar Ridge Preservation/Management of Extractions
Conclusion

 For online-only content on guided bone regeneration, please visit the companion website at www.expertconsult.com.

One of the most critical aspects of creating an aesthetic implant restoration is surgical placement of the implant in a "prosthetically driven" position; doing so will restore the tooth in a natural position and emulate the natural emergence of the tooth from the soft tissues. Implants placed without regard for prosthetic position often leave patients with dental restorations that are functionally and aesthetically compromised. To place implants in an aesthetically and functionally optimal position that is properly surrounded with bone, it is often necessary to reconstruct (or preserve) the alveolar ridge.

Periodontal bone loss, gingival recession, tooth loss, and long-term use of removable appliances typically result in alveolar defects that prevent the placement of implants in an optimal prosthetic position. It also leads to soft-tissue deficiencies that are aesthetically unacceptable. Fortunately, continuous innovations in regenerative materials and advances in surgical techniques have led to advanced implant procedures and an increased predictability in the reconstruction of alveolar ridge defects.[32,43]

Standard implant placement surgery, as described in Chapter 78, is based on adequate bone volume and quality in the desired implant location. The time-tested standard protocol allows for adequate remodeling and maturation of bone, with healing periods of 3 to 6 months. In recent years, the implant procedures have challenged these original conventions by placing implants in areas with inadequate bone volume, simultaneous with bone augmentation, and restoring or loading implants after shorter healing periods. This chapter presents an overview of surgical bone augmentation procedures used to correct or to prevent alveolar ridge deficiencies for the optimal placement of dental implants.

Localized Ridge Augmentation

Patients often present with a request for implants after the tooth or teeth have already been lost, sometimes for years, and the alveolar ridge has resorbed. In these cases, the clinician is obligated to perform augmentation procedures to reconstruct lost alveolar bone dimensions so that implants can be placed in the proper (prosthetically driven) position.

Surgical reconstructive procedures for the preparation and placement of dental implants have become more numerous and complex. Depending on the size and morphology of the defect, various augmentation procedures can be used. These procedures are categorized according to the deficient dimension: horizontal or vertical. The fundamental bone grafting methods used to augment alveolar deficiencies include particulate bone grafts and monocortical block grafts. Barrier membranes can be used with bone grafts to reconstruct all types of alveolar bone defects. See Chapter 80 for a review of procedures used to achieve vertical augmentation. The proven principles of guided bone regeneration (GBR) and flap management must be followed to achieve good results. These include an adequate blood supply; maintaining a stable, protected space for bone growth; and achieving tension-free flap wound closure.

Flap Management

Soft-tissue management is a critical aspect of bone augmentation procedures. Incisions, reflection, and manipulation should be designed to optimize blood supply and wound closure. The design and management of mucoperiosteal flaps must consider the increased dimensions of the ridge after augmentation as well as aesthetics and approximation of the wound margins. The surgical procedure must be executed with the utmost of care to preserve the vascularity of the flap and to minimize tissue injury.[1]

Several flap techniques maintain a "submerged" position of bone grafts and barrier membranes during the entire healing process, including a remote or displaced incision.[11,30] The advantage of a remote incision is that the wound opening is positioned away from the graft. On the other hand, a conventional crestal incision can be used, even in large supracrestal defects, as long as a periosteal releasing incision and coronal advancement of the flap achieve a tension-free closure.[35] Most reports suggest removing sutures approximately 10 to 14 days after surgery. It is also highly advisable to abstain from using removable prosthesis for several weeks (longer is better) after surgery to avoid placing pressure over the wound during the early healing phase.

General concepts for flap management associated with ridge augmentation include the following:

1. It is desirable to make incisions remote relative to the placement of barrier membranes (e.g., vertical releasing incisions at least one tooth away from the site to be grafted). In the anterior maxilla, keeping vertical incisions remote is also an aesthetic advantage.
2. Full mucoperiosteal flap elevation at least 5 mm beyond the edge of the bone defect is desirable.
3. The use of vertical incisions, although often required for surgical access, should be minimized.
4. Use of a periosteal releasing incision to give the flap elasticity and permit tension-free suturing is essential. This permits complete closure without stress on the wound margins.
5. Removable appliances should not be inserted over the wound for 2 to 3 weeks or more to avoid postoperative trauma to the surgical site.
6. Wound closure should incorporate a combination of mattress sutures to approximate connective tissues and interrupted sutures to adapt wound edges.

Horizontal Bone Augmentation

A deficiency in the horizontal dimension of bone may be minimal, such as a dehiscence or fenestration of an implant surface, or it may be more significant, such that the implant would have more than one axial surface exposed while having some bone along the entire vertical length. Dehiscence or fenestration defects can usually be managed during implant placement because most of the implant is covered and stabilized by native bone. If the horizontal deficiency is large and the implant placement would result in significant exposure (i.e., implant body is significantly outside the alveolar bone), it may be better to reconstruct the bone first, in a staged approach, with a subsequent surgery for implant placement.

Although reconstruction of deficient ridges with bone grafts alone (i.e., without barrier membrane) has proved to be effective, variable resorption of the grafted bone has been reported. Preliminary results in a 1- to 3-year study using autografts harvested from the maxillary tuberosity showed an increased ridge width, but resorption of 50% of the graft volume was also noted.[60] Buser and colleagues[11] investigated the lateral ridge augmentation procedure using an autograft from the retromolar or symphysis area covered by a membrane in 40 consecutively treated patients and noted no clinical signs of resorption of the block graft. The researchers emphasized a remote incision technique, perforation of the cortex, stable placement of corticocancellous autografts, precise adaptation and stabilization (with miniscrews) of the polytetrafluoroethylene (ePTFE) membranes, and a tension-free primary soft-tissue closure. After 7 to 13 months, the sites were reopened for membrane removal and implant placement. Of the 40 patients, 38 exhibited excellent ridge augmentation, whereas two sites showed some soft-tissue encapsulation of the grafted bone.

Nevins and Mellonig[47] and Doblin and colleagues[17] reported an increased amount of new bone using freeze-dried bone allografts (FDBAs) with membranes, even in the presence of membrane exposure. The biopsies showed viable bone cells and visible osteocytes in lacunae, and a 9-month specimen showed no remaining allograft material.

On the other hand, there are some contradictory results using demineralized freeze-dried bone allograft (DFDBA) and membrane combinations.[3,8,9] In a human study, seven paired extraction sockets were grafted with either DFDBA or autologous bone. Sites were reentered and biopsied after 3 to 13 months to evaluate bone formation. Histologic specimens revealed dead particles of DFDBA with no evidence of bone formation on the surface and no evidence of osteoclastic resorption. Conversely, the autogenous sites revealed vascular channels with woven and lamellar bone. Some nonvital, cortical bone chips were observed with osteoclastic resorption.

eFig. 79.1 (online) shows an example of the lack of bone formation around DFDBA particles used in a ridge augmentation procedure after more than 20 months of healing under a nonresorbable ePTFE barrier membrane.

KEY FACT

Dehiscence defects can usually be managed with simultaneous bone grafting during implant placement because most of the implant is covered and stabilized by existing native bone. If the horizontal alveolar deficiency is large such that the implant would be positioned with significant exposure (i.e., more than half of the implant diameter placed outside the alveolar bone), it may be better to reconstruct the bone first, in a staged approach, with a subsequent surgery for implant placement.

Particulate Bone Graft

Advantages of particulate bone grafts (or bone chips) are that the smaller pieces of bone demonstrate more rapid ingrowth of blood vessels (revascularization), larger osteoconduction surface, more exposure of osteoinductive growth factors, and easier biologic remodeling compared with a bone block for reconstruction of large defects. However, particulate grafts often lack a rigid, supportive structure and are therefore much more easily displaced as compared with monocortical block grafts.

Autologous particulate bone grafts can be harvested from any edentulous jaw site, either in smaller "particle" or in a larger "block" of bone. If the bone has been harvested in a block, a bone mill is necessary to grind or "particulate" the bone and prepare it for transplantation into the bone defect (eFig. 79.2, online).

Particulate grafts are indicated (1) in defects with multiple osseous walls that will contain the graft, or (2) in dehiscence or fenestration defects when implants are placed during the bone augmentation procedure. If a bone defect does not have sufficient osseous walls to contain the graft, the barrier membrane (placed in contact with the native bone) should be secured along the periphery with tacks, screws, or sutures. This bone graft and secured barrier membrane combination becomes an environment that is stable and supports new bone formation. Fig. 79.1 depicts the use of a barrier membrane in combination with a particulate bone graft to treat a mandibular horizontal defect.

Monocortical Block Graft

Horizontal alveolar deficiencies that might be challenging to reconstruct with particulate grafts can easily be reconstructed with a monocortical block bone graft. The technique uses a cortical block of bone harvested from a remote site and used to increase the width of bone. The block graft taken from an intraoral (e.g., mandibular symphysis or ramus) or extraoral (e.g., iliac crest or tibia) site is fixated to the prepared recipient site with screws. The overlying soft tissues can be separated from the bone graft with a barrier membrane or simply covered with the mucoperiosteal flap. Fixation hardware (screws and plates) should be removed after an adequate period of healing (approximately 6 months). The disadvantage of this technique is the biologic limitation of revascularizing large bone blocks. It

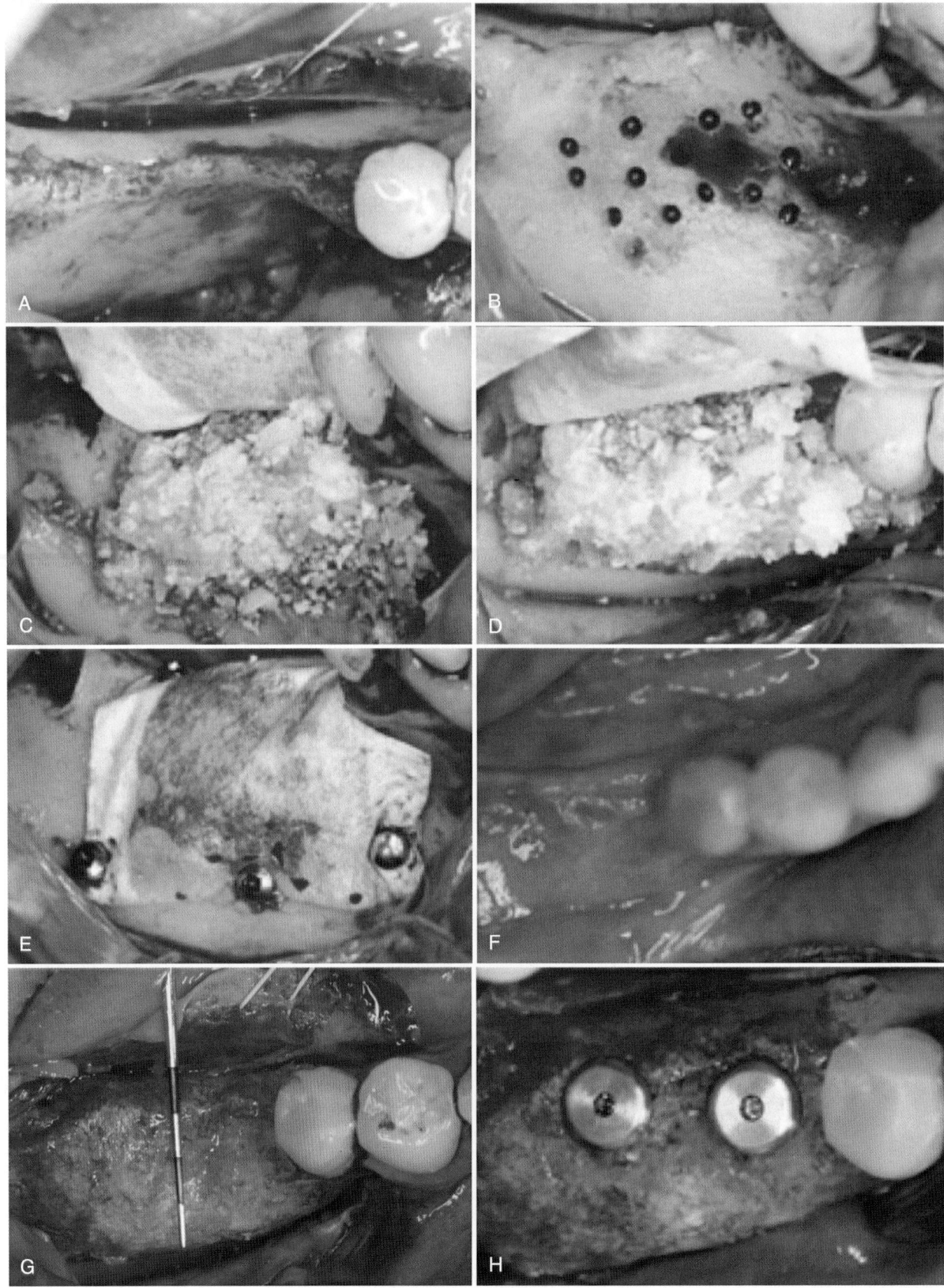

Fig. 79.1 Horizontal bone augmentation with expanded polytetrafluoroethylene (ePTFE) barrier membrane. Bone graft consists of a mixture of autogenous particles harvested from the alveolar ridge and Bio-Oss (Osteohealth Company, Luipold Pharmaceuticals, Inc., Shirley, New York). (A) Partially edentulous posterior mandible with narrow buccolingual dimensions. (B) Cortical perforations made in buccal bone with small round bur to enhance blood supply to the grafted area. (C) Placement of ePTFE barrier membrane and mixture of autogenous and Bio-Oss particulate bone graft. (D) View of part C from occlusal perspective to visualize horizontal augmentation. (E) Barrier membrane secured to native bone with fixation screws. (F) Clinical photograph of healed site prior to membrane removal. Soft-tissue closure maintained throughout healing without membrane exposure. (G) Clinical photograph of healed ridge after membrane removal. Dimensions of alveolar ridge are significantly wider as demonstrated with periodontal probe. (H) Two standard-diameter implants placed in a "prosthetically driven" ideal position. Notice there are no implant exposures. *(Images courtesy Dr. Istvan A. Urban, Budapest, Hungary.)*

therefore is crucial to have sufficient osteogenic cells in the residual surface of the surrounding bone and to limit this technique to horizontal augmentation and only minimal vertical defects.

Fig. 79.2 shows the use of a monocortical block graft to reconstruct a horizontal deficiency in the posterior right mandible. The patient presented with a loss of the buccal cortical plate of bone after a traumatic extraction of endodontically treated tooth #29. The surgical extraction also resulted in an iatrogenic cut into the mesial root of tooth #30, rendering the tooth nonrestorable. The recommended treatment included extraction of tooth #30, monocortical block graft reconstruction of the buccal defect at site #29, and bone augmentation of the extraction socket #30. The procedure for this case follows.

KEY FACT

Large horizontal alveolar deficiencies can be challenging to reconstruct with particulate grafts. In such a situation, it may be more manageable to use a monocortical block bone graft to reconstruct the area. The technique uses a cortical block of bone harvested from a remote site (e.g., mandibular symphysis or ramus) and fixated to the prepared recipient site with screws.

Procedure

Following local anesthesia, an incision was made in keratinized tissue along the crest and around the molar tooth (#30) with a vertical releasing incision mesial to the first bicuspid (#28). A full-thickness flap was elevated to expose the alveolar bone (see Fig. 79.2D). All soft tissues were thoroughly removed from the recipient site before bone grafting. After simple forceps delivery of tooth #30, the defect to be grafted was measured to determine the size of block graft to harvest from the mandibular symphysis. Several bleeding points were created using a small round bur.

The autogenous monocortical block graft was harvested from the mandibular symphysis. It was cut to an appropriate size and mortised to intimately fit the recipient defect site. Once properly positioned, the graft was fixated with two fixation screws (Leibinger, Kalamazoo, Michigan) that passed through the graft and into the existing native alveolar bone. A periosteal releasing incision was used to sever the periosteum from anterior to posterior and facilitate coronal advancement of the mucogingival flap.

After 6 months of healing, a full-thickness mucoperiosteal flap was elevated to expose the alveolar bone sites #29 and 30. Mild resorption of the monocortical block graft is evident. Notice that the position of the head of the fixation screws (especially the posterior screw) is more protruded than the grafted bone as a consequence of bone remodeling and resorption (see Fig. 79.2H–I).

The fixation screws are removed, and the sites are prepared in the usual manner for the placement of two-screw type, wide-diameter implants (Implant Innovations, Palm Beach Gardens, Florida). Care is taken to avoid preparing into the grafted site too wide or too far to the buccal surface because the grafted bone may be vulnerable to fracture or additional resorption (Fig. 79.2J).

Simultaneous Implant Placement

Large alveolar bone defects need to be augmented before implant placement and require a healing period of 6 months or longer. In selected cases, it is possible to perform a bone augmentation procedure simultaneously with the implant placement. It is essential to achieve good implant stability in the existing native bone so that endosseous integration can occur.

A predictable osseous defect to manage with simultaneous implant placement is the implant dehiscence or fenestration defect. *Fenestration* defects are exposures of the implant's axial surface that do not include the coronal aspect of the implant (Fig. 79.3). *Dehiscence* defects expose a part of the axial surface, including the coronal aspect of the implant, while maintaining sufficient bone volume around all remaining implant surfaces (Fig. 79.4). In a dehiscence defect, the implant remains within the confines of the existing bone.

Fenestration and dehiscence defects have been managed with barrier membranes or simply with flap closure. Bone grafts have also been used. The only controlled comparison studies between membrane treatment and periosteal flap coverage of exposed implant surfaces in humans demonstrated that the membrane treatment was far superior with regard to bone fill.[14] Another controlled study in humans showed better results in the membrane groups; four of six sites (67%) treated with a membrane resulted in 95% to 100% elimination of the dehiscence and total coverage of the threads. In the control sites, only two of six sites (33%) showed moderate-to-complete bone fill.[48] All other clinical studies are in the form of case reports.[43] Fig. 79.5M demonstrates coverage of an implant dehiscence using a barrier membrane. Admittedly, without a biopsy it cannot be determined whether the tissue covering the implant is bone or firm connective tissue.[27,31]

A 1-year multicenter study evaluating 55 Brånemark implants (i.e., machined-surface, external hex) with bone dehiscence in 45 patients, treated by ePTFE membrane alone, demonstrated an average bone fill of 82%.[15] The average initial defect height was 4.7 mm. The 1-year follow-up of these implants demonstrated a favorable response to loading. Of the 55 implants, a total of 6 failed, corresponding to a cumulative survival rate of 84.7% in the maxilla and 95% in the mandible, which is similar to previously published results for this implant design.

A clinical report on the use of titanium-reinforced (TR) membranes demonstrated the biologic potential to fill a large protected space in four patients.[29] Bone dehiscence at implant sites ranged from 5 to 12 mm (mean: 8.2 mm). They were covered with a TR membrane alone (no graft). Reentry after 7 to 8 months of submerged healing found complete bone coverage over all implants. Radiographic evaluation demonstrated the implants functioning with normal crestal bone support after 1 year.

No clinical comparisons are available in the literature evaluating the placement of bone grafts with or without barrier membranes on implant dehiscence defects. Most evidence supports the use of graft materials in conjunction with membrane treatment, especially the use of FDBA in conjunction with GBR. In a study with 40 patients, 110 implants were placed in conjunction with barrier membranes and FDBA; a success rate of 96.8% was achieved with complete bone fill (defined as >90% fill of dehiscence).[50] This study reported a membrane exposure rate of 29% but noted little adverse effect on the bone regeneration.

With respect to ridge preservation, Becker and colleagues[7] reported the effect of barrier membranes and autogenous bone grafts on the preservation of ridge width around implants. They evaluated the ridge width around 76 implants in 61 patients from a case series database. Three groups were compared, including 34 implants treated with GBR (barrier membranes), 27 implants treated with autogenous bone grafts, and 15 implants placed without the need for ridge preservation/augmentation procedures (control group). The results revealed that implant sites treated with barrier membranes and autogenous bone grafts lost an average of 0.1 mm and 0.8 mm, respectively, more than the no-augmentation group.

Another study evaluated the possibility of regenerating bone around implants placed in extraction sockets.[35] Bone augmentation was achieved with human DFDBA particles mixed with tetracycline packed around the exposed implant surfaces. Implants and graft material were covered with ePTFE barrier membranes with complete

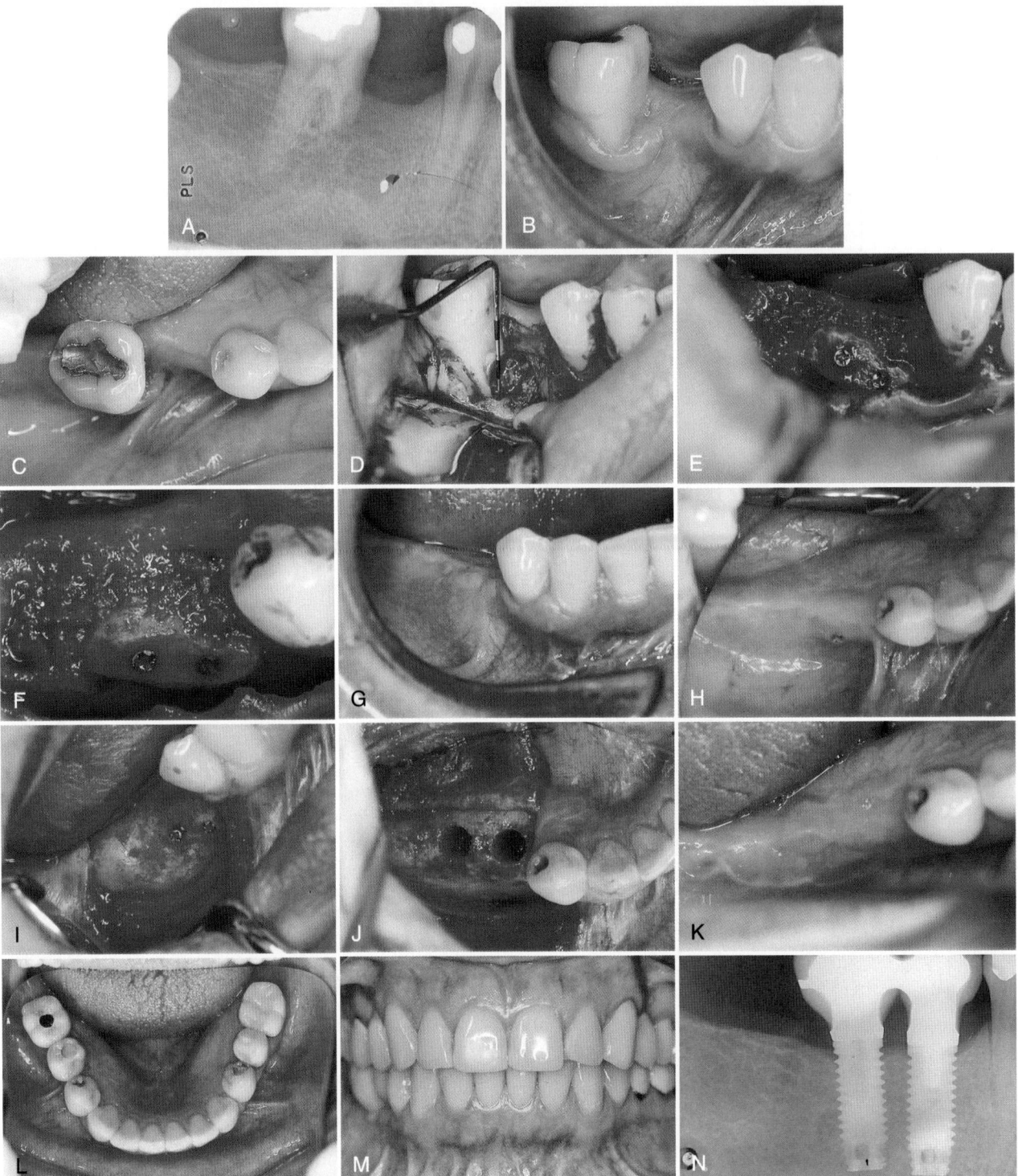

Fig. 79.2 Use of a monocortical block graft to reconstruct a horizontal deficiency in the posterior right mandible. (A) Periapical radiograph shows missing tooth #29 and damaged (i.e., cut) mesial root #30. (B–C) Labial and occlusal views, respectively, of site reveal deficient alveolar ridge on buccal side of #29. (D) Full-thickness flap reflection reveals the extent of missing bone in the buccal aspect of site #29, as well as the periodontal defect and damaged mesial root #30. (E–F) Autogenous monocortical bone block graft secured to native alveolar bone with fixation screws. (G) Good tissue healing after block graft, with evidence of a widened alveolar ridge. (H) After 6 months of healing, posterior fixation screw is observed protruding through the mucosa. (I) Full-thickness flap reveals that bone resorption has resulted in exposure of part of the fixation screw. (J) Osteotomy prepared for wide-diameter implants, taking care to avoid making the labial bone "graft" too thin. (K) Complete closure and good healing of wound after implant placement. (L–M) Clinical photographs of completed restorations. (N) Final radiograph shows good restoration contours on wide-diameter implants.

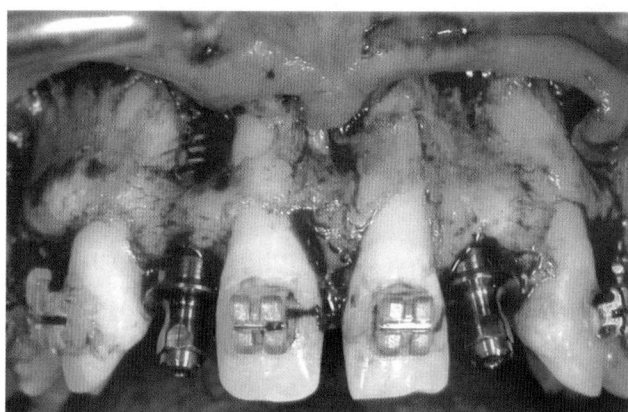

Fig. 79.3 Fenestration defect observed in very thin maxillary anterior sites. Implants placed in the maxillary lateral incisor positions demonstrating fenestration defects caused by the concavities in the apical area. Notice that the natural teeth (centrals and cuspids) also demonstrate fenestrations. Bone will grow across this type of defect in a predictable manner because the implants are stable; the defect is small and surrounded by bone.

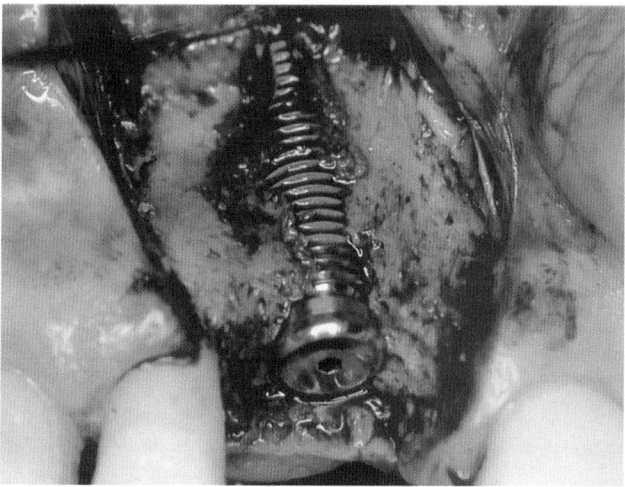

Fig. 79.4 Dehiscence defect observed during placement of an implant in the maxillary central incisor position. Note that the implant is completely surrounded by existing native bone except for the facial surface, which is exposed. Bone will grow across this type of defect in a predictable manner because the implant is stable and the exposed surface is relatively flat with bone on all surfaces.

flap closure for 4 to 6 months. The results demonstrated complete bone regeneration in all cases except when barrier membranes were prematurely exposed and removed. One-year posttreatment histologic evaluation of regenerated bone revealed remnants of the DFDBA graft particles in direct contact with vital bone tissue (woven and lamellar bone). Osteoblasts were observed and appeared to be actively engaged in bone formation adjacent to graft particles. Fig. 79.5 (parts L and M) demonstrates a simultaneous GBR and implant placement in a dehiscence defect.

Complications

Bone augmentation procedures used to increase the bone volume in deficient alveolar ridges have been successful and have enabled the placement of implants into prosthetically driven positions.[56] Unfortunately, these augmentation procedures carry an increased risk of morbidity and can require secondary surgeries to correct problems

resulting from the procedure.[67] The subsequent corrective surgeries required to correct problems add surgical time and complexity to the implant therapy.

Surgical complications are reported for a variety of bone reconstructive techniques.[18] A review assessed the number and types of complications associated with bone reconstructive procedures for endosseous implants.[61] The review of the literature (1976–1994) included 2315 implants in 733 autogenous block, particulate, and various other bone graft materials. Complications reported included bleeding, postoperative infection, bone fracture, nerve dysfunction, perforation of the mucosa, loss of a portion of the bone graft, pain, decubital ulcers, sinusitis, and wound dehiscence. Wound dehiscence seemed to have the most deleterious effect on implant survival. This finding emphasizes the importance of flap management.

Typical findings include less bone fill with early exposure and membrane removal versus retaining the membrane without exposure for 6 to 8 months.[30,58] Buccolingual ridge deficiencies were treated in a prospective study involving 19 patients using ePTFE membranes and miniscrews as fixation and tenting devices.[37] The group of defects, which healed uneventfully, yielded on reentry a 90% to 100% bone regeneration compared with the maximal volume of the space defined by the membrane placement. In the exposed-membrane group, the percentage of regenerated bone ranged from 0% to 62%. When a late membrane removal was performed (3 to 5 months after surgery), the regeneration varied between 42% and 62%. The authors concluded that the length of membrane healing and size of the defect played a significant role in the amount of new bone formation.[37]

CLINICAL CORRELATION

Bone is a unique tissue that has the capacity to regenerate itself completely. Bone augmentation procedures have been shown to be an effective way to increase the bone volume in deficient alveolar ridges, allowing the placement of implants in a proper, "prosthetically driven" position. Clinicians must appreciate that bone augmentation procedures have an increased risk of complications, which may add procedures and complexity to the implant therapy.

A retrospective review of 233 patients treated with a variety of bone augmentation procedures to correct 331 alveolar ridge defects reported the incidence of soft-tissue dehiscence, infection, sensory disturbance, the need for additional augmentation procedures, and early implant failure.[26] Augmentation procedures included GBR, staged horizontal ridge augmentation, staged vertical ridge augmentation, and sinus floor elevation. Soft-tissue dehiscence occurred in 1.7% after GBR and 25.9% after staged horizontal augmentation. Infections were diagnosed in 2% of cases after GBR, 11% after staged horizontal augmentation, and 9% after staged vertical ridge augmentation. The need for additional bone augmentation was identified in 2% following GBR, 37% following staged horizontal ridge augmentation, and 9% after staged vertical ridge augmentation. Early implant failures occurred in 1.6% after GBR and in 12% after staged vertical augmentation. One patient experienced a temporary sensory disturbance following a staged horizontal ridge augmentation procedure.

Other authors have reported successful bone fill in situations in which membranes were removed early due to premature exposure.[47,57] A significantly greater fill of the osseous defect at the grafted sites was noted. The authors concluded that the regeneration of bone around the implants appeared most dependent on the anatomy of the bony defect at the time of implant placement.

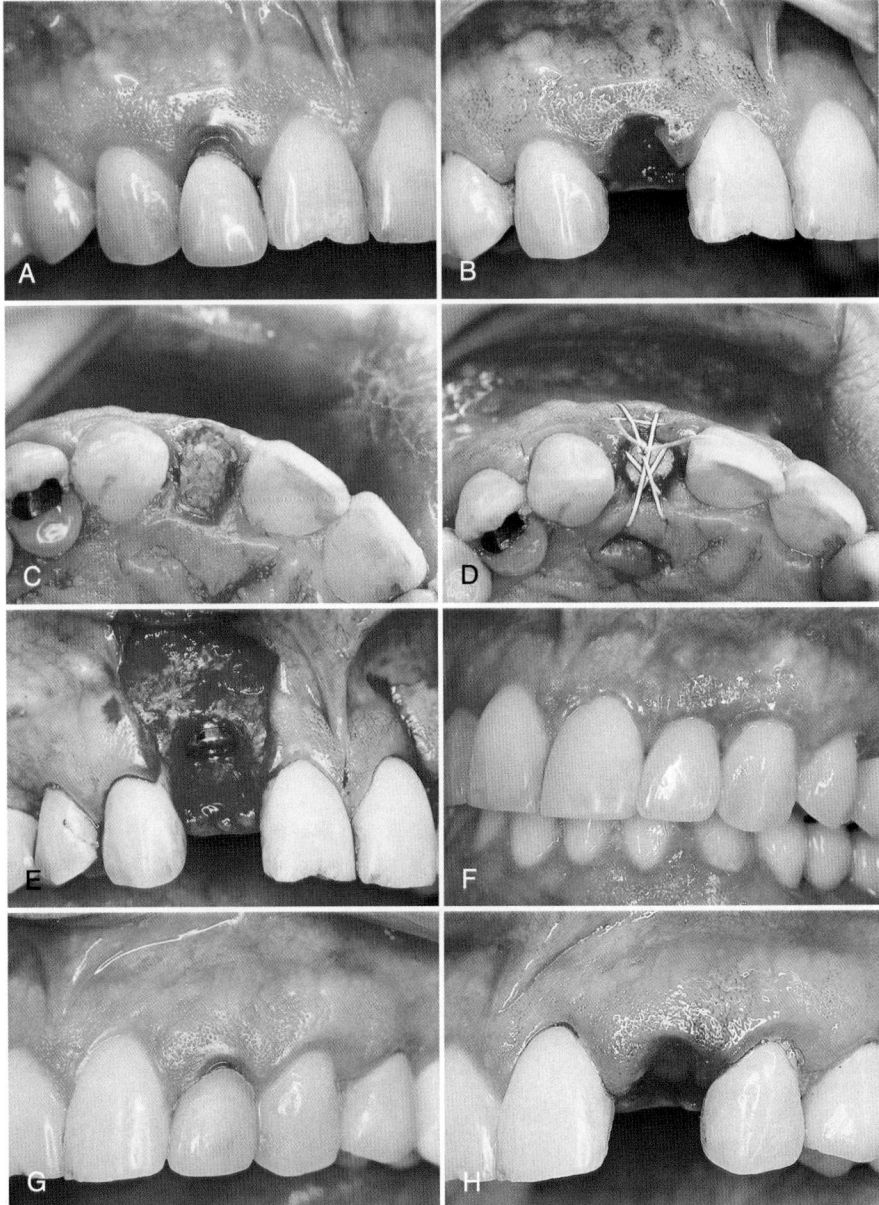

Fig. 79.5 Use of staged (A to H) and delayed (I to O) implant placement after extraction of two maxillary lateral incisors in one individual. (A) Preoperative photograph of tooth #7 with gingival recession and marginal inflammation. (B) Atraumatic extraction or tooth #7 without tissue incision or tissue elevation. Palpation reveals no facial bone present at the time of extraction. (C) Decalcified freeze-dried bone allograft condensed into extraction site. (D) Expanded polytetrafluoroethylene (ePTFE) barrier membrane positioned over graft and held in place with sutures. (E) Six months after the extraction/graft, the implant is placed. Notice the implant is completely covered with bone. (F) Final restoration. (G) Preoperative photograph of tooth #10 with exposed gingival margin. (H) Atraumatic extraction of tooth #10 without tissue incision or tissue elevation. Palpation reveals no facial bone present, and dehiscence is expected.

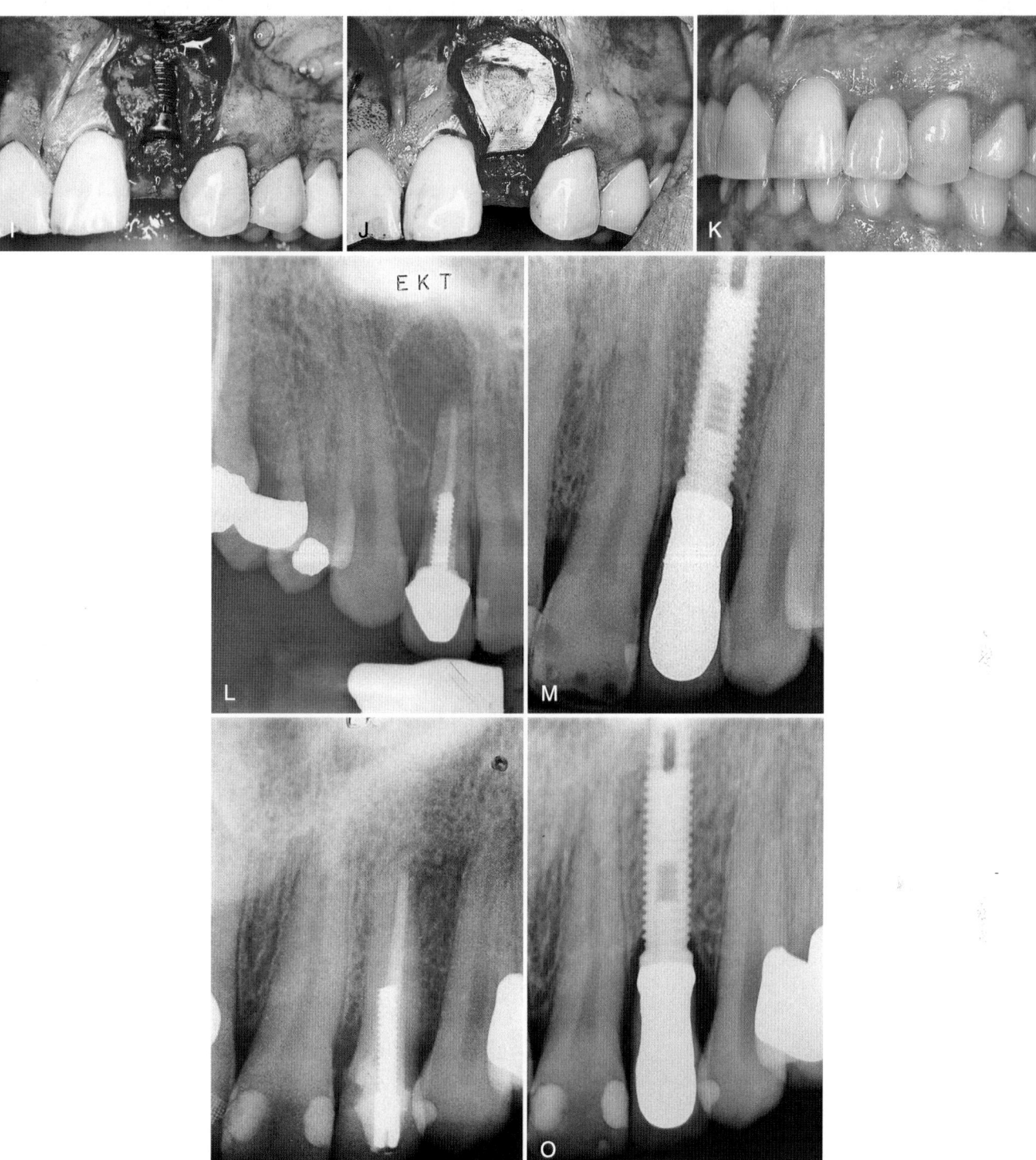

Fig. 79.5, cont'd (I) Two months after extraction, the implant is placed with dehiscence defect. (J) Guided bone regeneration accomplished with ePTFE barrier membrane positioned over the dehiscence. (K) Final restoration. (L) Periapical radiograph of tooth #7 with a large radiolucent lesion around the apex and periodontal bone loss along the distal interproximal area. (M) Final radiograph of delayed implant placement. (N) Periapical radiograph of tooth #10. (O) Final radiograph. *(A, B, C, F, G, J, M, N, and O from Klokkevold PR, Han TJ, Camargo PM: Aesthetic management of extractions for implant site development: delayed versus staged implant placement,* Pract Periodontics Aesthet Dent *11:603, 1999.)*

Although the effect or amount of regenerated bone with regard to membrane exposure is somewhat contradictory, the goal should be to keep the membranes covered during the healing period so that the risk of infection and soft-tissue and aesthetic problems can be minimized or eliminated. Again, the importance of flap management for ridge augmentation procedures should be stressed. See Chapter 85 for more information and details regarding surgical complications and failures.

Alveolar Ridge Preservation/Management of Extractions

Because tooth extraction (or loss) often results in alveolar ridge resorption or collapse, preservation of bone volume at the time of extraction is a desirable goal. Most bone loss after extraction occurs in the first 6 to 24 months.[12] Therefore when clinicians are afforded the opportunity to intervene at the time of extraction, preservation of alveolar bone should be initiated. A conservative approach to the management of extraction sites can eliminate or significantly reduce the necessity of advanced bone augmentation procedures.

When extracting a tooth and preparing for implant placement, alveolar bone resorption should be prevented or at least minimized. Experimental animal studies show that the use of a barrier membrane enhances the predictability of bone fill in the extraction site and therefore maintains original bone volume when compared with mucoperiosteal flap coverage alone.[8] Clinical studies also demonstrate the benefits of a regenerative approach to tooth extraction.[39,40,46] These authors found that a nonresorbable barrier membrane results in minimal resorption of alveolar ridge size and shape.

Although earlier studies have proposed the concept of treating extraction sites without flap closure (i.e., an exposed membrane used to cover the graft), more recent studies conclude that complete wound closure over the physical barrier might be associated with greater bone fill.[6,58] The decision about whether to advance a flap to achieve wound closure must be weighed against the soft-tissue changes that will be created (i.e., mucogingival junction discrepancies and aesthetic problems) and that may require subsequent surgical correction.

The histologic assessment of allograft healing in extraction sockets has been reported.[2,10,13,20,64,66] In a series of clinical studies, the authors evaluated the quality of bone as well as the dimensions of alveolar ridge preservation with various comparison of allograft properties. Extraction sockets were nonmolar sites that were grafted and allowed to heal for a prescribed amount of time. The alveolar dimensions were measured at the time of extraction and again at the time of implant placement. A core biopsy was harvested to assess the percentage of new bone formation, residual bone graft particles, and connective tissue/nonmineralized tissue. In a study[64] evaluating the timing of bone formation in sites grafted with DFDBA, it was determined that more new bone (47.41% vs. 32.63%) was formed in sites allowed to heal for a long term (18–20 weeks) as compared with sites that healed for a short term (8–10 weeks), respectively. Another study[2] evaluating new bone formation with mineralized allograft found no greater new bone formation (45% vs. 45.8%) by waiting longer (27 weeks) as compared with the shorter healing period (14 weeks), respectively. When demineralized allograft was compared with mineralized allograft, there was significantly more new bone formation in sites grafted with DFDBA (38.42%) than in sites grafted with FDBA (24.63%).[66] The DFDBA group also had a significantly lower mean percentage of residual graft particles (8.88% vs. 25.42%). Finally, in another clinical study[20] comparing cortical versus cancellous

FDBA, the authors found no difference in the percentage of new bone formation. There was a significantly greater percentage of residual bone graft particles in the cortical FDBA compared with the cancellous FDBA. Except for a great loss of lingual bone crest in the cancellous group of the latter study, none of the other studies found significant differences in clinical measurements between groups.

The timing of implant placement relative to the time of extraction has been widely debated. Depending on the quantity, quality, and support of existing bone, as well as the preferences of the clinician and patient, the placement of implants after tooth extraction can be immediate, delayed, or staged. By definition, *immediate* implant placement occurs at the time of extraction. Delayed implant placement is performed approximately 2 months after extraction to allow for soft-tissue healing. *Staged* implant placement allows for bone healing within the extraction site, which typically requires 4 to 6 months or longer.

Tooth extraction is managed with an atraumatic surgical technique that uses a narrow, flat instrument (e.g., Periotome, Hu-Friedy, Chicago) directed apically into the sulcus to sever the periodontal ligament and slightly expand the adjacent periodontal tissues. The tooth is elevated and removed with forceps using a gentle, rotational movement. Chapter 83 describes new techniques for atraumatic extraction. Buccolingual forces are avoided to prevent damaging the integrity of the labial bone. No incisions are made, and care is taken to avoid soft-tissue reflection. In this manner, soft tissues maintain their structural anatomy, and the periosteum (blood supply to the bone) remains intact. If the tooth has multiple roots, curved roots, or other anatomic features that make removal difficult, it may be necessary to cut the tooth using a high-speed rotary drill or other cutting device and remove it in smaller pieces. It is important to cut only tooth structure and avoid cutting (overheating) bone when using high-speed rotary drills. The bone within the extraction site is completely debrided of soft tissue with surgical curettes. After debridement, the extraction site is thoroughly irrigated with sterile saline. Finally, the clinician can evaluate the bone level and socket anatomy to determine whether to bone graft the site and when to place the implant (immediate, delayed, or staged placement).

FLASH BACK

The timing of implant placement relative to the time of extraction has been widely debated. Historically, during the early period of osseointegrated implants, immediate or early implant placement was discouraged. Today, these early tenets are being challenged with immediate implant placement and immediate provisionalization.

Delayed Implant Placement

Delayed implant placement shares some advantages of immediate implant placement, including extraction site preservation, and offers additional advantages. Unlike immediate implant placement, which is deficient of soft tissue for coverage, the delayed implant placement technique allows time for soft-tissue healing to close the wound.[28] The delayed placement technique still reduces the length of treatment by a few months because it is not necessary to wait for complete bone healing. Furthermore, because bone formation is active within the first few months after tooth extraction, the delayed technique may facilitate more osteogenesis adjacent to the implant.

The primary advantage of delayed implant placement is that, by allowing for soft-tissue healing and closure of the extraction site, mucogingival flap advancement is not necessary. This alleviates the need for additional surgeries to correct mucogingival discrepancies. Delayed implant placement also allows time for the resolution of infections that may have been present within the extraction site.

As with immediate implant placement, similar limitations of bone support and implant stability exist for delayed placement. The normal osseous healing that occurs within the first 2 months does not significantly affect the anatomy of the alveolar bone. Therefore limitations in bone support after 2 months of healing are similar to those that exist at the time of extraction.

Staged Implant Placement

Staged implant placement allows adequate time for osseous healing. This may be complete osseous healing of an extraction site without a bone graft (if circumferential bone support is good) or with a bone graft. Staged implant placement, by definition, allows for complete hard- and soft-tissue healing and permits the placement of implants into healed bone sites with adequate coverage by hard and soft tissues.[56] This eliminates the necessity of mucogingival flap advancement, allows for the resolution of preexisting infections, and prevents soft-tissue invasion. Furthermore, by using an extended healing period, the grafted bone also has the opportunity to become vascularized. Bone grafts performed simultaneously with implant placement do not share this advantage. The primary disadvantage of staged implant placement is the length of time required for bone healing.

Delayed Versus Staged Technique

Delayed and staged techniques for implant placement are demonstrated here in one individual using two extraction sites with similar bone morphologies in the anterior maxilla (see Fig. 79.5). Both techniques facilitate the aesthetic placement of implants into prosthetically driven positions. Delayed and staged approaches maintain alveolar bone volume, reduce the need for advanced bone augmentation, and eliminate the need for subsequent mucogingival surgery. The timing and management of delayed versus staged implant placement are described in the next section.

To decide which implant placement method to use, the quantity and location of bone surrounding the tooth should be assessed. Once the patient has been anesthetized, a periodontal probe can be used to "sound" for the level of bone support through the soft tissue. Using this method, the bone levels surrounding the tooth can be mapped. Bone support that surrounds the extraction site can also be evaluated and confirmed after tooth removal by palpation, probing, and direct (internal) visualization.

If the tooth to be extracted has sufficient bone support on all surfaces, the extraction site can be expected to fill with bone without additional augmentation procedures, except when the labial bone is very thin. A simple extraction followed by a healing period of 4 to 6 months could be sufficient for complete osseous healing. Subsequently, an implant could be placed in the usual manner without the need for bone augmentation. Conversely, if little or no bone exists on the labial surface, it should be anticipated that the site would require bone augmentation to facilitate placement of the implant. In this case, bone grafting at the time of extraction can be used to maintain the alveolar ridge dimensions occupied by the tooth.

Immediate Implant Placement

The primary advantage of immediate implant placement is the reduction of the healing time, which translates to an earlier restorative time (i.e., shorter time to completion for the patient).[38,44,55,65] Because the implant is placed at the time of extraction, the bone-to-implant healing begins immediately with extraction site healing. Another advantage is that the normal bone healing, which generally occurs within the extraction site, takes effect around the implant. This bone-forming activity may enhance the bone-to-implant contact compared with an implant placed in a site with less osteogenic activity.

Possible disadvantages of immediate implant placement include the need for subsequent mucogingival surgeries to correct tissues moved by repositioned flaps and the need for bone grafting to fill extraction site defects around the implant. If inadequate bone exists to stabilize the implant, immediate implant placement is not recommended.

When a two-stage implant is placed at the time of tooth extraction, the mucogingival flap is advanced, with releasing incisions, to cover the implant completely (an exception would be a one-stage implant). It may also be necessary to graft bone into the extraction site in areas that do not contact the implant to avoid soft-tissue invasion around the implant.[55] A 1-year study of 49 immediate extraction site implants treated by a membrane alone demonstrated a 93.6% bone fill. After 1 year (postloading), the implant success rate was 93.9%.[6]

Although some have advocated submerging implants placed in extraction sockets with flap advancement,[28] others have demonstrated success with a nonsubmerged approach. Implants may be placed in extraction sockets along with bone augmentation without flap advancement using a one-stage implant placement approach. Clinical studies evaluating the outcome of bone augmentation around implants placed in extraction sockets reveal good bone fill.[36] The placement of 21 transmucosal implants in immediate extraction sites treated with a barrier membrane were tested for the implant success rate and the percentage of bone fill. Twenty of the twenty-one transmucosal implants yielded complete bone fill and coverage of the entire plasma-coated implant surface.

A clinical report on the use of resorbable collagen membranes around extraction site implants demonstrated a variable degree of bone fill in nine patients.[49] More clinical review of the use of resorbable membranes for GBR is required because evidence is insufficient to evaluate the predictability.

In a study of 30 patients, the use of autografts alone in 54 extraction sites was highly effective for simultaneously placed implants completely within the envelope of bone.[4] The study showed that extraction sites, including those with a buccal dehiscence, could be treated with autografts alone. However, because nongrafted sites were not included, the absolute need to graft small defects adjacent to implants was not ascertained by this study. In another study, implants placed in extraction sockets were tested for their potential to regenerate bone with allograft alone, a membrane alone, and a combination treatment.[23] Reentry confirmed 100% thread coverage in all but one implant in the "no-wall" group treated with DFDBA alone. A clinical study of five patients evaluated different treatment modalities for extraction site implants together with bone graft combinations.[59] This small study supported the concept that "non–space-making defects" are best treated with a combination of barrier membrane and an autograft or allograft as compared with treatment with a nonreinforced membrane alone (without a graft).

Immediate placement of an implant into the extraction socket in a one-stage approach along with immediate provisionalization is perhaps the best way to manage the hard and soft tissues following extraction (Fig. 79.6). The immediate placement of a provisional restoration is the best way to support the soft tissues (papilla and marginal gingiva) following tooth extraction.

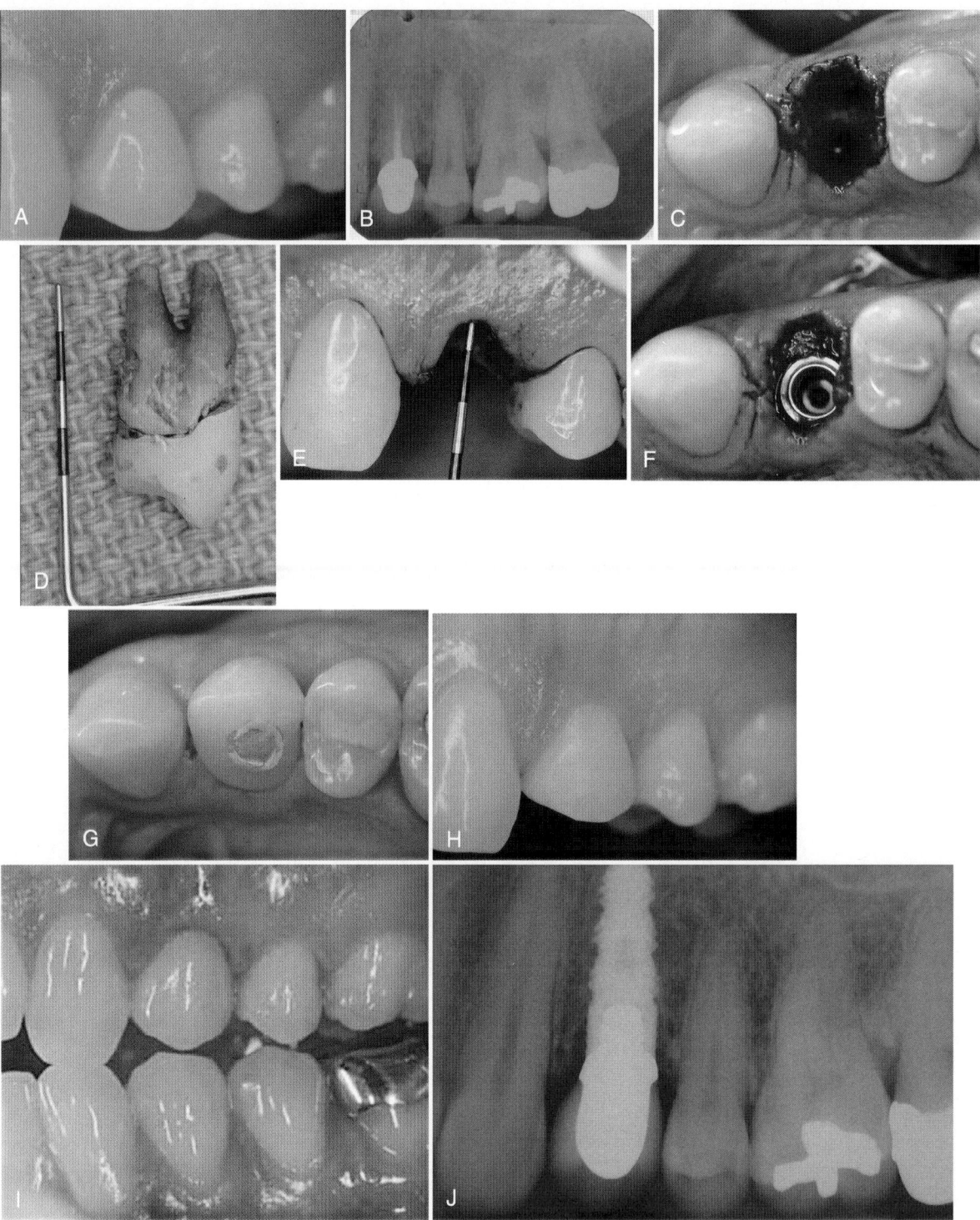

Fig. 79.6 Immediate implant placement after extraction of a maxillary first premolar. (A) Preoperative clinical photograph of tooth #12, which fractured and was deemed nonrestorable. (B) Periapical radiograph of tooth #12. It is root canal–treated and has a full-coverage porcelain-fused-to-metal crown. (C) Atraumatic extraction of tooth #12 without incisions or tissue elevation. (D) Extracted tooth. (E) Palpation and examination with probe reveals intact bony walls around the extraction socket. The facial bone wall is observed to be about 2 mm below the facial gingival margin. (F) The palatal aspect of the extraction socket is prepared, and a tapered implant is placed to emerge through the central fossa. Autogenous bone chips (harvested from the maxillary tuberosity) are condensed into the labial aspect of the extraction socket to support the facial bone and soft-tissue contours. (G) An immediate provisional restoration is fabricated (indirectly in the laboratory) and delivered at the time of implant placement. The palatal cusp is not replaced in this provisional to avoid function and the occlusion is checked for light centric contacts only. (H) Facial view of provisional restoration at the time of delivery. Notice how the interdental papilla and facial gingival margin are well supported by the contours of the provisional restoration. (I) Final restoration at time of delivery (approximately 4 months after implant placement). (J) Final radiograph of definitive restoration.

Conclusion

Localized bone augmentation procedures allow clinicians to reconstruct horizontal alveolar ridge deficiencies and replace missing teeth with dental implants in a prosthetically driven position with natural appearance and function. In many cases, implants can be placed simultaneously with the bone augmentation procedure. In cases of advanced bone resorption, ridge augmentation before implant placement may be a better choice. Bone grafting procedures can also be used to preserve alveolar dimensions following tooth extraction. If adequate bone exists around the extraction socket to stabilize an implant, it may be possible to combine immediate implant placement and bone grafting in a simultaneous procedure. The predictable outcome of these procedures depends on several biologic principles that must be followed. Diagnosis, treatment planning, careful execution of the surgical treatment, postoperative follow-up, and appropriate implant loading are all important factors in achieving success.

 A Case Scenario is found on the companion website www.expertconsult.com.

References

 References for this chapter are found on the companion website www.expertconsult.com.

CHAPTER 80

Advanced Implant Surgical Procedures

Perry R. Klokkevold | *Istvan A. Urban* | *David L. Cochran*

CHAPTER OUTLINE

Maxillary Sinus Elevation and Bone Augmentation
Supracrestal/Vertical Bone Augmentation
Growth Factors in Bone Augmentation *(e-only)*
Conclusion

 For online-only content on growth factors in bone augmentation, go to the companion website at www.expertconsult.com.

The high predictability of endosseous dental implants has led to routine use and an expectation for success. Yet the ultimate success for any individual patient or any particular implant relies on a multitude of factors, the most important of which is the *availability of bone.* The loss of teeth, whether caused by disease or trauma, frequently results in severe deficiency of the alveolar bone. Horizontal bone deficiencies are managed quite predictably with localized bone augmentation procedures (see Chapter 79). However, vertical bone deficiencies can be much more challenging and less predictable. The posterior maxilla is challenging due to a general lack of bone volume and the omnipresent poor bone quality of the area; that is, posterior maxillary bone often consists of a thin cortical shell filled with sparse trabecular bone. Edentulous sites, in any anatomic location, that suffer from significant vertical alveolar bone loss are especially challenging to reconstruct.

This chapter reviews advanced surgical procedures used to treat the most challenging type of bone loss, which is *a deficiency in vertical bone height.* Maxillary sinus elevation and bone augmentation, vertical bone augmentation, and distraction osteogenesis are reviewed. The role of growth factors in bone augmentation procedures is also discussed.

Maxillary Sinus Elevation and Bone Augmentation

Rehabilitation of the edentulous posterior maxilla with dental implants often represents a clinical challenge due to insufficient bone volume resulting from *pneumatization* of the maxillary sinus along with a loss of alveolar crestal bone from disease or remodeling. Prior to the utilization of bone augmentation procedures, patients with missing teeth and deficient bone in the posterior maxilla could only be rehabilitated with removable prostheses, short implants, or cantilevered restorations (i.e., supported by adjacent teeth). Historically, the failure rate for implants in the posterior maxilla has been significantly higher than failure rates for implants in other anatomic locations.[23] Consequently, procedures such as the maxillary sinus elevation and bone augmentation are needed to increase the amount of vertical bone height in the posterior maxilla for the placement of implants.

In 1980, Boyne and James[4] first described a procedure to graft the maxillary sinus floor with autogenous marrow and bone for placing an implant (blade type). Access to the maxillary sinus was gained through a "Caldwell-Luc" procedure (i.e., an opening into the maxillary sinus created at the anterior-superior aspect). Since then, several other techniques have been described, including variations on the lateral window osteotomy and a variety of techniques to lift the sinus floor from a crestal approach.

Various bone graft materials have been used to augment the maxillary sinus. The 1996 Consensus Conference on Maxillary Sinus Bone Grafting reviewed available data and concluded that allografts, alloplasts, and xenografts, alone or in combination with autogenous bone, can be effective as bone substitute graft materials for sinus bone augmentation.[24] More important, it was concluded that the sinus graft procedure with implant placement is a highly predictable and effective therapeutic modality for the rehabilitation of the posterior maxilla. Sinus floor elevation with bone augmentation is now a well-accepted procedure used to increase bone volume in the posterior maxilla. Numerous reports have validated the safety and efficacy of this procedure.[7,13,18,50] Implant success rates are equal to or better than that of implants placed in nongrafted maxillary bone (i.e., areas of the posterior maxilla with adequate height of existing native bone).[50] Thus bone augmentation of the maxillary sinus is a viable option for the vertically deficient posterior maxilla in which the interocclusal dimension is normal or only moderately increased.

CLINICAL CORRELATION

The normal process of pneumatization of the maxillary sinus often results in inadequate bone height to place implants in the posterior maxilla. The lack of bone height is further exacerbated by alveolar bone loss from periodontal disease or tooth loss.

Indications and Contraindications

As with any therapeutic procedure, treatment success depends on appropriate patient selection, careful evaluation of the anatomy, identification and management of any pathology, sound surgical procedures, and appropriate postsurgical management. The primary indication for maxillary sinus elevation and bone augmentation, specific for the placement of endosseous dental implants, is an alveolar bone height in the posterior maxilla that is deficient (e.g., less than 7 mm of existing vertical bone height). Other factors that must be considered include the health of the patient, the condition of the remaining dentition, and the likelihood of a beneficial outcome. A thorough evaluation of the patient and the clinician's assessment will ultimately determine whether the procedure is indicated for any particular individual.

Contraindications to maxillary sinus elevation and bone augmentation are similar to contraindications for other surgical procedures, with the added consideration of contraindications specific to the maxillary sinus (Box 80.1). Patients must be in good general health and free of diseases that affect the maxilla or maxillary sinus. Local factors that are considered contraindications to maxillary sinus elevation and bone augmentation include the presence of tumors, maxillary sinus infection, severe chronic sinusitis, scar or deformity of the sinus cavity from previous surgery, dental infection, severe allergic rhinitis, and chronic use of topical steroids. Systemic contraindications to treatment include radiation therapy, uncontrolled metabolic disease (e.g., diabetes), excessive tobacco use, drug or alcohol abuse, and psychological or mental impairment.

Surgical Procedures for Sinus Elevation

The goal of sinus elevation and bone augmentation is to lift the schneiderian membrane from the floor of the sinus, raising it up into the sinus cavity to create a new, more superiorly located sinus floor with a space between it and the deficient alveolar ridge. The newly created space can then be filled with bone (or a suitable bone substitute material) to increase the total vertical height of bone in the posterior maxilla for implant placement.

The maxillary sinus bone augmentation procedure was first described in the 1960s by Boyne (unpublished oral presentations to United States [US] Navy Dental postgraduates, 1965–1968) and originally used as a preprosthetic surgical procedure for patients with large tuberosities and pneumatized sinuses.[3] To reduce the size of the tuberosity without creating an oral-antral defect, bone was grafted into the sinus cavity to increase the volume of bone within the maxillary tuberosity. After a period of healing, the tuberosity was reduced surgically from the alveolar ridge crest. As stated previously, Boyne and James[4] (1980) were the first to describe the use of the maxillary sinus bone-grafting procedure for placement of an implant (blade type) to retain a dental prosthesis. Greater use and

further development of this procedure evolved along with the success of endosseous dental implants and the desire to replace missing posterior maxillary teeth with implant-retained restorations.

The variety of techniques used for sinus elevation and bone augmentation are defined by the anatomic location of the osteotomy used to gain access to the maxillary sinus. Specifically, four different anatomic locations have been described: (1) the superior lateral wall, or "Caldwell-Luc," opening, which is located high on the lateral wall of the maxilla just anterior to the zygomatic arch; (2) the middle lateral wall opening, which is located midway between the alveolar ridge and the zygomatic arch; (3) the inferior lateral wall opening, which is located at the level of the alveolar ridge; and (4) the crestal osteotomy approach, which is an opening through the alveolar bone crest superiorly toward the floor of the sinus. At present, the most common procedure used for sinus elevation and bone augmentation is the lateral wall antrostomy (middle or inferior approach). The crestal approach osteotomy is also fairly common.

FLASH BACK

Sinus augmentation is the most commonly performed procedure to overcome the problems associated with the pneumatized sinus. Several different approaches have been used to access the maxillary sinus for bone augmentation. Currently, the lateral window approach is the most frequently used technique. The crestal approach is popular as well.

Presurgical Evaluation of Maxillary Sinus

Presurgical evaluation of the maxillary sinus is primarily accomplished using radiographic examination techniques (Fig. 80.1). Several observations about the anatomy can be made with a periapical or panoramic projection, but the internal anatomy is more accurately assessed with a three-dimensional scan, such as computed tomography (CT) or cone beam CT (CBCT) scan. The maxillary sinus should be evaluated for any pathology, masses, or the presence of septa. If three-dimensional scans are available, the lateral wall should also be evaluated for the presence of medium or large intraosseous vascular channels (see Fig. 58.15). Medium- to large-sized vessels occasionally traverse the lateral wall of the maxillary sinus, and identifying them prior to surgery helps to avoid a bleeding problem during surgery (see Chapter 58).[31]

Simultaneous Implant Placement

Simultaneous implant placement is possible with sinus elevation and bone augmentation procedures as long as the implant can be stabilized in the desired location with the existing native bone (eFig. 80.1).

It has been suggested that a minimum of 5 mm of existing native bone in the alveolar crest is required for simultaneous implant placement. However, some clinicians claim that it is possible to place implants simultaneously with as little as 1 mm of remaining bone.[29,58] The most important factor in determining whether implants can be placed at the time of sinus bone augmentation is the ability to achieve implant stability in the existing bone rather than any predetermined measure of bone height. Factors that influence implant stability include bone height, bone quality, precision of osteotomy preparation, and the surgeon's skill. If the amount and quality of existing native bone is not sufficient to place and stabilize implants at the time of bone augmentation, then implants should be placed at a subsequent surgery after an appropriate healing period (Fig. 80.2).

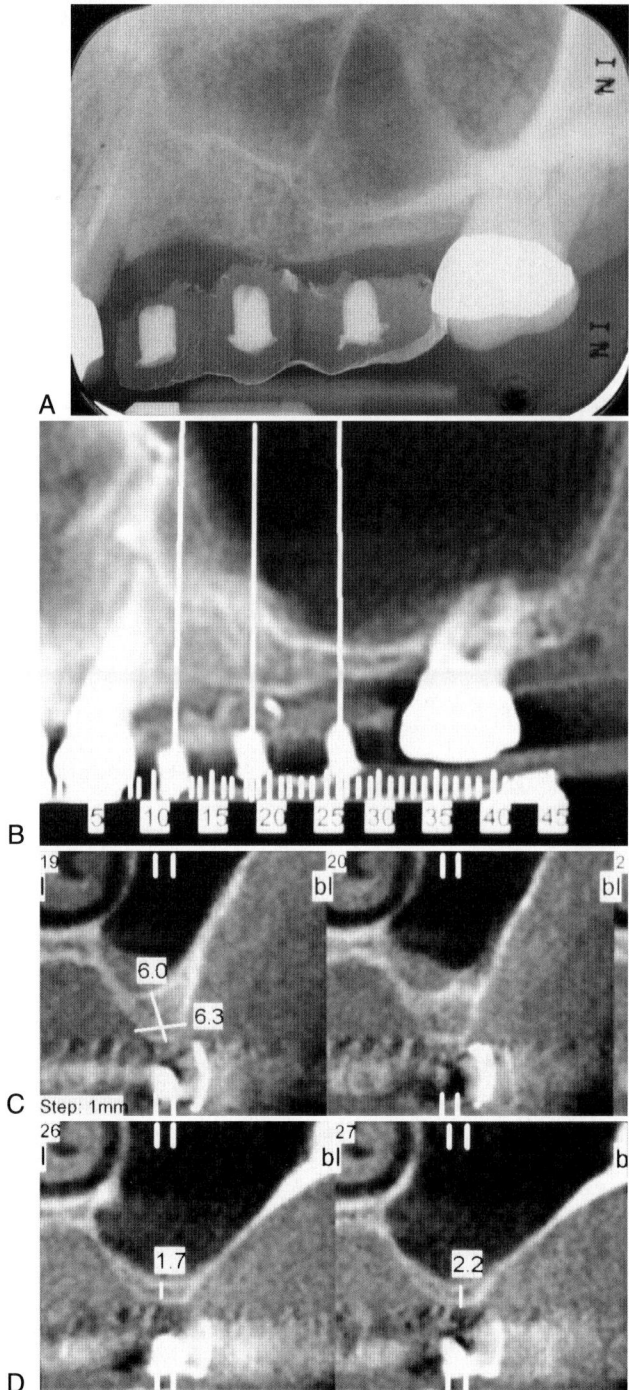

Fig. 80.1 Presurgical evaluation of the maxillary sinus. (A) Periapical radiograph. (B) Panoramic projection from cone beam scan. Note the presence of maxillary septa in the premolar region. (C) Cross-sectional image in premolar region showing about 6 mm of bone height and the presence of maxillary septa. (D) Cross-sectional image in molar region showing about 2 mm of bone height.

Bone Graft Materials

Autogenous bone is often referred to as the gold standard for bone augmentation because of its osteoconductive, osteoinductive, and osteogenic properties.[4] However, harvesting autogenous bone from intraoral or extraoral locations creates a second surgical site with additional morbidity. Numerous studies have demonstrated clinical success using many variations of bone graft materials and combinations.[24,50]

Several clinical studies and reports have attempted to evaluate the maxillary sinus augmentation procedures using a variety of bone-grafting materials, including autogenous bone from the iliac crest or oral cavity and bone substitutes such as freeze-dried demineralized bone, resorbable and nonresorbable hydroxyapatite, and xenografts. However, only a few studies have critically evaluated the long-term clinical outcome of this procedure, and most have used a small study population. Short- to long-term clinical studies of dental implants placed into grafted sinuses demonstrate an equivalent or higher survival rate as compared with implants placed in native maxillary bone (i.e., without the need of sinus augmentation).[24,50] The results of these studies support the clinical predictability of maxillary sinus augmentation procedures for the rehabilitation of the edentulous posterior maxilla with implant-supported prostheses (Fig. 80.3).

The use of bone-substitute graft materials can reduce the morbidity introduced by a second surgical site while maintaining equally good implant success rates.[24] Anorganic bovine bone-derived mineral (ABBM) (Bio-Oss, Geistlich Pharma AG, Wolhusen, Switzerland) has also been utilized successfully for sinus augmentation.[55] (ABBM has also been referred to in the literature as *deproteinized bovine bone mineral, deproteinized anorganic bovine bone,* and *anorganic bovine bone.*) This graft material has demonstrated good dimensional stability and high implant survival rates.[13] These bone-substitute graft materials form an osteoconductive scaffold for bone growth but do not have any osteoinductive properties. A possible exception is demineralized freeze-dried bone allograft (DFDBA). This material has demonstrated osteoinductive potential but has not proved to be particularly advantageous in the maxillary sinus bone augmentation.[24,54] In fact, the bone volume gained with the use of DFDBA is less than that achieved with mineralized graft materials. Presumably the lesser bone volume achieved with DFDBA is a result of moderate postoperative shrinkage of this material.

Crestal Osteotomy Technique

In cases with moderate bone height (e.g., 7–9 mm) that require limited sinus bone augmentation, a crestal approach to elevation may be desirable. The osteotome technique is a procedure that uses osteotomes (eFig. 80.2) to compress bone (internally from the alveolar crest upward) against the floor of the sinus, ultimately leading to a controlled "inward fracture" of the sinus floor bone along with the schneiderian membrane, creating a "tented" space for grafting.

The osteotome sinus floor elevation (OSFE) technique was described by Summers.[42,43] It is considered to be a conservative approach to sinus elevation, but it is also a "blind" technique because it does not allow the operator to visualize the schneiderian membrane during the osteotomy. For this reason, it is a technique-sensitive procedure as well (i.e., the operator must "feel" the bone fracture and the membrane elevation). The increased vertical bone height can only be observed with radiographs that, if successful, will show a raised radio-opaque dome at the treatment site within the sinus cavity. Radiolucent graft materials such as DFDBA will not be apparent in the immediate postoperative radiograph.

Procedure

An osteotomy site is prepared with a series of drills (e.g., initial drills used for implant site preparation) to a depth that is approximately 1 to 2 mm from the floor of the maxillary sinus. Osteotomes are used to increase compressive forces gradually against the floor of the sinus by adding incremental quantities of graft material until the floor of the sinus fractures inward (Fig. 80.4). The impact force needed to fracture the sinus floor is typically achieved with careful tapping of the osteotome with a mallet. Care must be taken to prevent

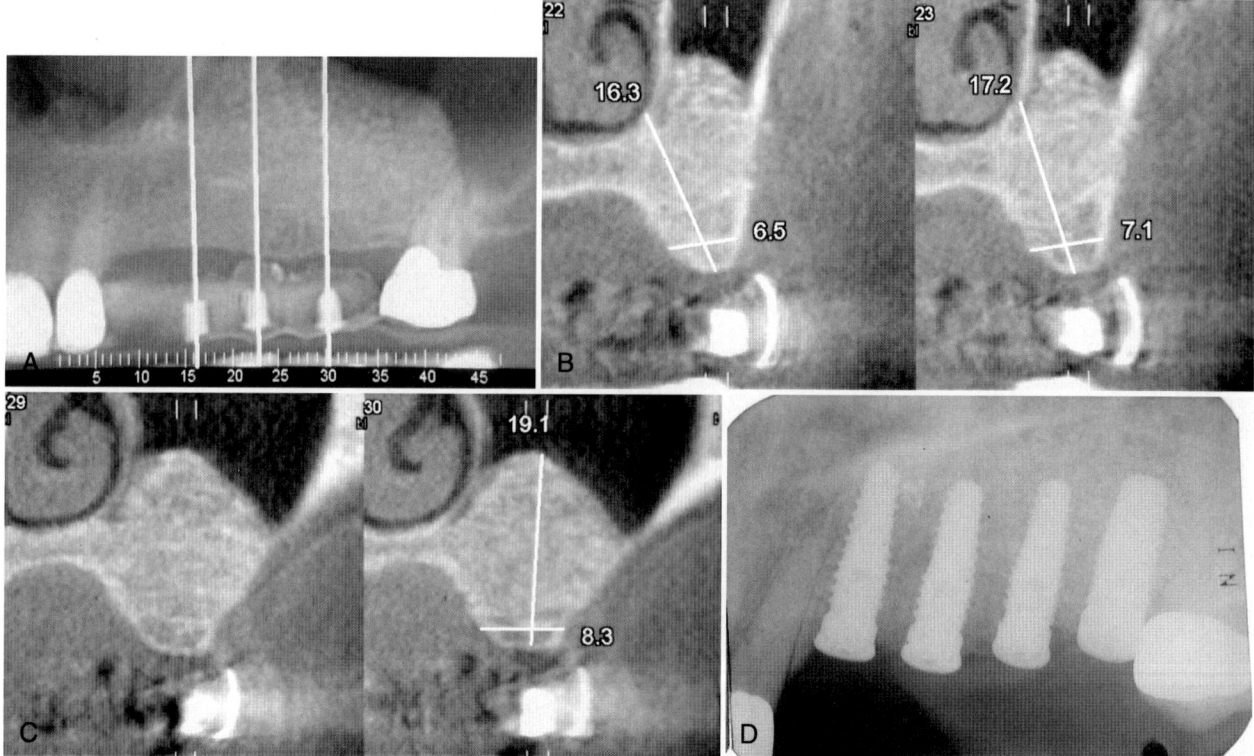

Fig. 80.2 Staged implant placement after sinus elevation and bone augmentation procedure. Same patient as in Fig. 80.1. See preoperative radiograph and preoperative cross-sectional images. (A) Postsurgical panoramic view of bone-augmented maxillary sinus. The maxillary left cuspid has been extracted because of a vertical fracture. (B) Postsurgical cross-sectional image in premolar region demonstrating more than 17-mm vertical bone height. (C) Postsurgical cross-sectional image in molar region demonstrating 19.1-mm vertical bone height. (D) Postsurgical radiograph of implants placed in the previously grafted maxillary sinus (and cuspid site).

over-insertion of osteotomes beyond the level of existing sinus floor bone to avoid instrument perforation through the schneiderian membrane. After the controlled inward fracture of the maxillary sinus floor, bone graft materials continue to be slowly introduced, through the osteotomy site and into the maxillary sinus, which continues to elevate the membrane and thus allows a vertical expansion of the bone height in a localized area of the maxillary sinus. This latter elevation of the membrane is achieved by simply pushing graft material into the site with the osteotome alone (i.e. without using the mallet). Once the sinus membrane is elevated with bone graft material to the desired height, the implant osteotomy can be completed. The final implant osteotomy drill is used to finish preparing the lateral walls to a depth of the native bone only (i.e., full depth drilling is not necessary) and the implant is inserted. Multiple individual sites can be elevated and prepared simultaneously through separate osteotomy sites.

Published reports of this technique have demonstrated increased bone height from 2 to 7 mm (average, 3.8 mm).[47] Thus the crestal approach is a useful technique for increasing the vertical height of bone up to approximately 4 mm. If more vertical bone height is needed, the lateral wall osteotomy approach may be more advantageous. In addition to the usual precautions and contraindications for sinus elevation and bone augmentation procedures, the osteotome technique may be contraindicated for sinuses that have an acutely sloped floor or septa in the location of the planned osteotomy. An acutely sloped sinus floor will tend to deflect the osteotome in an undesirable direction rather than allowing the osteotome to penetrate into the sinus space, and the presence of septa makes it virtually impossible to fracture the sinus floor inward. Box 80.2 provides

additional precautions and clinician comments on using the osteotome technique. Several new instruments and techniques have emerged that improve the ability to create a crestal approach osteotomy while avoiding trauma or injury to the schneiderian membrane. These instruments/techniques vary from selective rotary drill systems to piezoelectric bone surgery. See Chapter 83 for a description of piezoelectric bone surgery.

KEY FACT

Published reports of the crestal osteotomy technique have demonstrated increased bone height from 2 to 7 mm (average, 3.8 mm). Significantly more bone height increase is typically possible with the lateral window approach. When more than 4 mm of bone height increase is desired, the lateral window approach may be advantageous.

Lateral Window Technique

The lateral window technique is probably the most effective and efficient way to access the maxillary sinus for bone augmentation. In this procedure, an opening into the maxillary sinus is created in the lateral wall to elevate the schneiderian membrane and to place bone graft in the space immediately superior to the existing alveolar bone. The lateral wall osteotomy can be prepared with a high-speed drill (carbide or diamond) or a piezoelectric bone surgery device (see Chapter 83). It is also possible to prepare the lateral wall osteotomy with rotary instruments that are designed to selectively cut bone. Some clinicians will prepare the lateral window outline

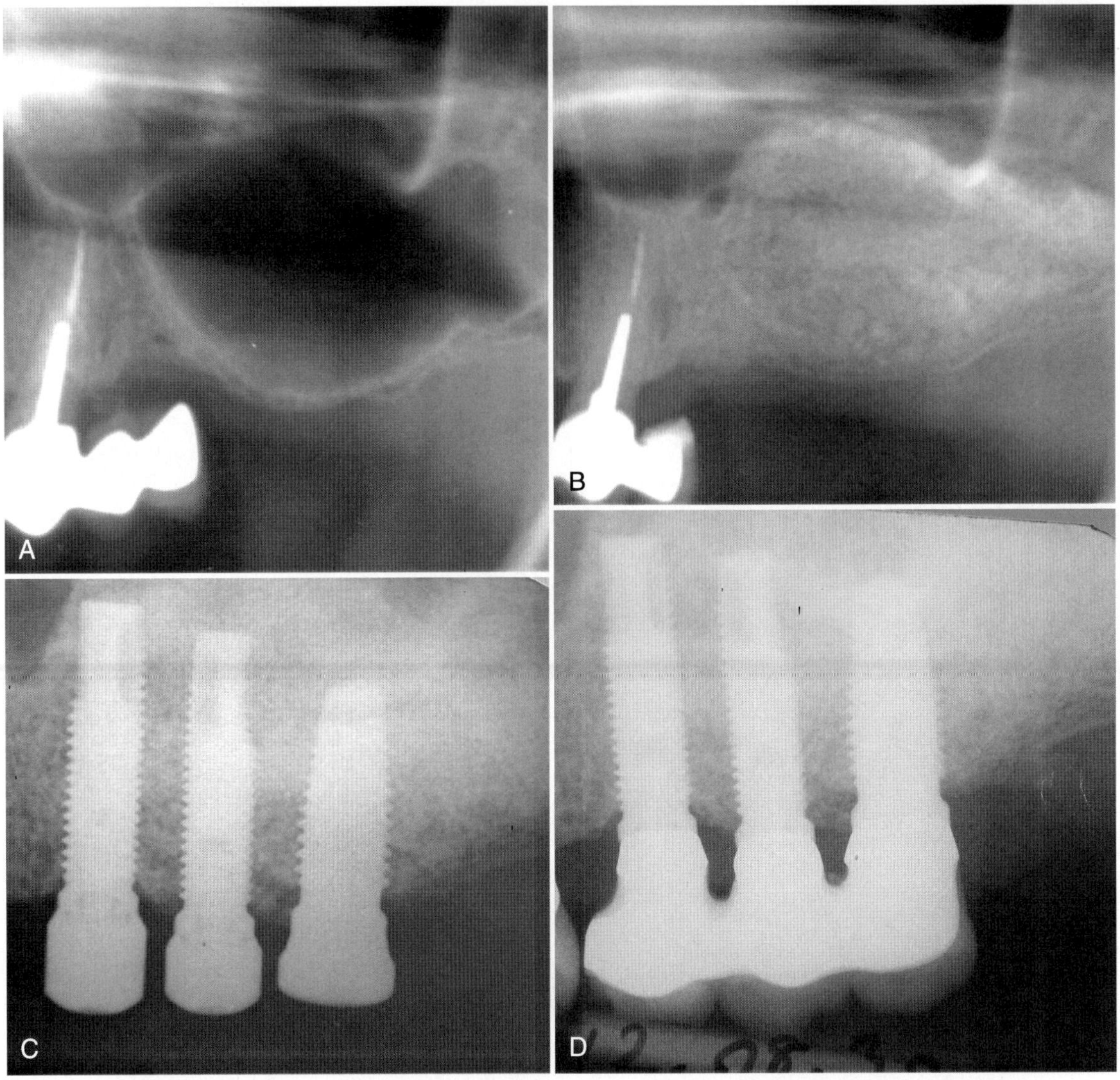

Fig. 80.3 Long-term follow-up of patient presenting with minimal residual crestal bone height. (A) Preoperative radiograph demonstrates minimal residual crestal bone height. (B) Postoperative radiograph demonstrates sinus graft healing after 6 months. (C) Abutment connection of implants after 6 months of submerged healing. The three distal implants were placed into augmented bone. (D) Periapical radiograph demonstrates stability of crestal bone around implants at 10 years loading. *(From Urban IA, Lozada JL: A prospective study of implants placed in augmented sinuses with minimal and moderate residual crestal bone: results after 1 to 5 years, Int J Oral Maxillofac Implants 25:1203–1212, 2010.)*

BOX 80.2   Clinician Comments on Use of the Osteotome Technique

Clinical Perspective 1

The osteotome procedure involves repeated tapping of osteotomes with a mallet to create the necessary pressure to fracture the floor of the maxillary sinus. This tapping can be bothersome to some individuals, especially patients who are not sedated for the procedure. The tapping procedure tends to be more bothersome for patients with dense cortical bone and for those with loose trabecular bone. In fact, a specific postoperative complication, called *benign paroxysmal positional vertigo* (BPPV), has been associated with the osteotome sinus elevation technique. During the osteotomy preparation and sinus floor elevation, the trauma induced by percussion of the osteotome

with the surgical hammer, along with hyperextension of the neck during the operation, can displace otoliths in the inner ear and induce BPPV.

Clinical Perspective 2

The osteotome technique requires that the osteotome be properly aligned in the direction of the long axis of the planned implant. Thus patients must be able to open wide enough to allow a direct insertion of the osteotome into the osteotomy site. Offset osteotomes are available that can facilitate the correct angulation (see eFig. 80.2B, online).

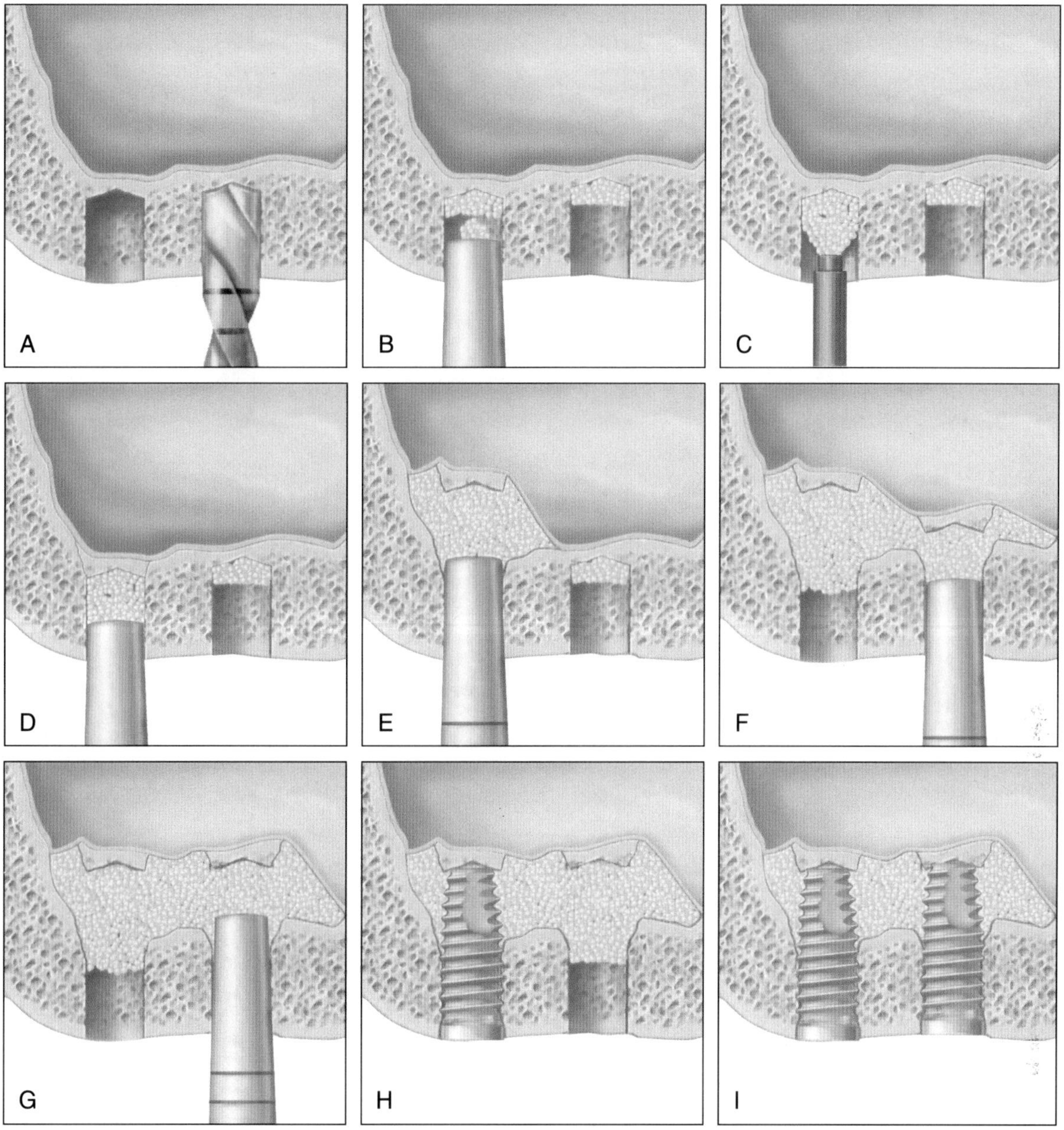

Fig. 80.4 Illustration of the osteotome sinus floor elevation (OSFE) technique. (A) Osteotomy prepared with drills to a depth that is near the maxillary sinus floor. (B) Graft material introduced into osteotomy and condensed with osteotome. (C) Additional bone graft material is added to the osteotomy. (D) Bone graft continues to be condensed by osteotomes. (E) This process is continued until floor of sinus is "fractured" up internally and the floor is lifted with the bone graft material. (F) Continuation of process shown in E for second site. (G) Bone graft material continues to be added gradually to both sites with osteotome condensation to elevate the schneiderian membrane away from the bone (maxillary sinus walls) until sufficient height and volume are created for the placement of implants. (H) The coronal aspect of the osteotomy is carefully prepared for the placement of implants (instrumentation not shown), and the implant is placed. (I) Final view of two implants placed in the grafted maxillary sinus using the OSFE technique.

only, leaving the center bone attached to the membrane as it is elevated and rotated into the sinus, thus becoming the superior wall of the space created for bone grafting (Fig. 80.5A–C). Other clinicians prefer to eliminate the bony window entirely by reducing or removing it completely (Fig. 80.5D–F). With the former technique, it is important to create a window that is small enough, relative to the mediolateral width of the maxillary sinus, to allow the "window" to be pushed completely into the sinus cavity without prematurely hitting the medial wall. If the window cannot be inserted completely, it must be carefully separated from the membrane and removed. The bone

removed from the lateral window osteotomy can be harvested and incorporated into the bone graft.

Once the lateral window osteotomy is created, elevation of the schneiderian membrane is accomplished with hand instruments that are inserted along the internal aspect of the bony walls of the sinus (eFig. 80.3). Great care is taken to avoid perforation of the membrane. Small instruments (e.g., De Marco curette) are introduced along the inferior, anterior, posterior, and superior aspects of the prepared window, gradually inserting further along the bone until the membrane begins to separate and lift away from the bone. Subsequently, larger

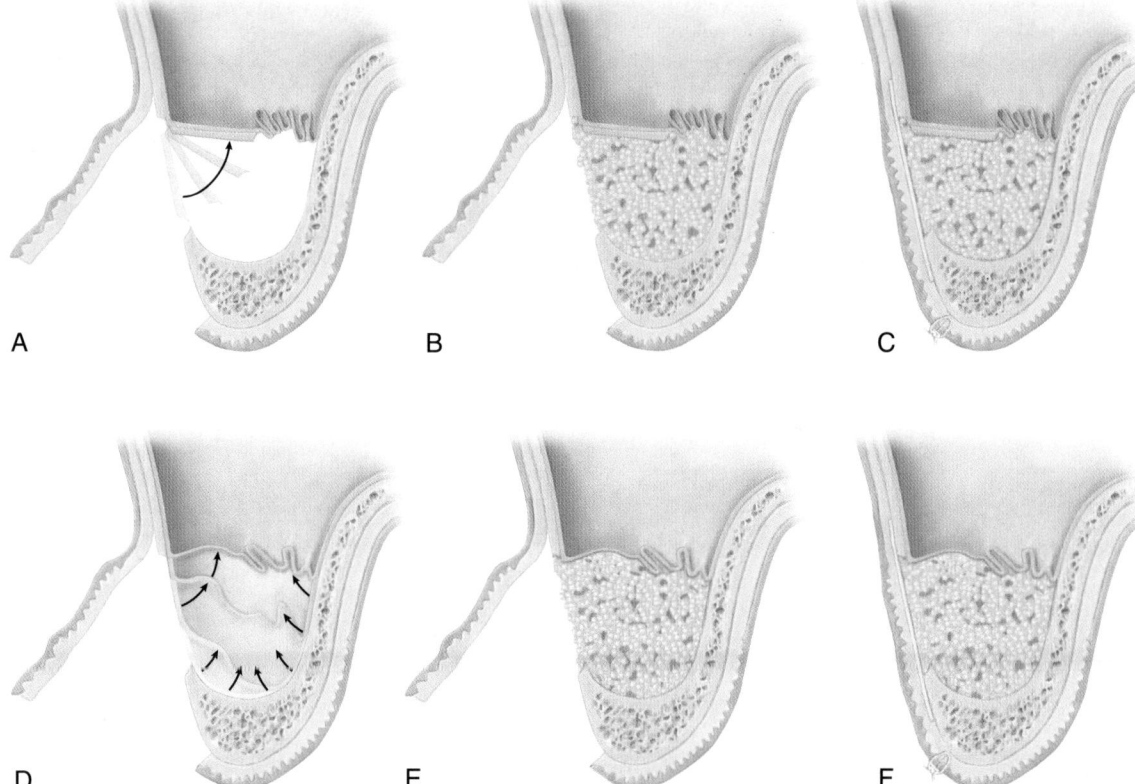

Fig. 80.5 Illustrations showing two techniques for the lateral window procedure to access the maxillary sinus for bone augmentation. The first technique (A–C) preserves the bone of the lateral window, elevating it up into the sinus cavity to create a new sinus floor. The second technique (D–F) completely removes the lateral window as part of the preparation. (A) Lateral window is cut at the periphery of the access window, leaving the lateral bony wall in the center of the window intact. The bony window is then pushed inward to become the new, elevated sinus floor/superior wall of the grafted maxillary sinus space. (B) Bone graft material is packed into the newly created space. (C) A barrier membrane is placed over the lateral window and bone graft material. The full-thickness flap is sutured over the barrier membrane. (D) Lateral window is removed entirely during the preparation of the osteotomy. The schneiderian membrane is elevated inward and upward to become the superior containment of the grafted maxillary sinus space without a superior bony wall. (E) Bone graft material is packed into the newly created space. (F) A barrier membrane is placed over the lateral window and bone graft material. The full-thickness flap is sutured over the barrier membrane.

instruments (e.g., Gracey curette) are gently introduced along the bone to continue lifting the membrane to the desired levels (height, width, and depth). Instruments must always be kept in contact with the bone surface while elevating the schneiderian membrane to avoid perforation. An implant surgical guide should be used to estimate the planned anterior-posterior implant positions and to assess the dimensions of needed sinus augmentation. Once elevated, the space can be grafted with bone (autogenous, bone substitute, or a combination). If implants will be simultaneously placed, the implant osteotomy sites should be prepared, and implants placed after the medial, anterior, and posterior aspects of the sinus are filled with bone graft, thereby supporting the schneiderian membrane up and away from the drills and implants. After implant placement, the remaining lateral aspect is packed with bone graft. Finally, the lateral window and bone graft are covered with a barrier membrane (e.g., resorbable membrane) and the flap is sutured. Covering the lateral window osteotomy with a barrier membrane has been shown to increase the amount of vital bone and has a positive effect on implant survival.[45,56]

Risks and Complications

The maxillary sinus elevation and bone augmentation procedure is technique sensitive, requiring meticulous surgical skills. Risks and

complications of the procedure include tearing or perforation of the schneiderian membrane, intraoperative/postoperative bleeding, postoperative infection, and loss of bone graft or implants (see Chapter 85).

The reported incidence of perforation or tearing of the schneiderian membrane varies greatly (up to 60%) and depends largely on the anatomy of the sinus as well as the skill and experience of the operator.[9,26,30,36] The presence of septa in the maxillary sinus increases the likelihood of membrane perforation.

Positioning of the sinus window within 2 to 4 mm from the anterior and inferior borders of the sinus makes it easier to get direct access to the bony walls. This may lessen the amount of membrane perforation during the elevation of the sinus membrane.

If the perforation is small, it can often be managed with a resorbable barrier membrane placed over the opening, followed by careful packing of the bone augmentation material. If a perforation or tear is extensive (see Fig. 85.18), it may be necessary to abort the procedure, close the wound, and attempt it again at a later date.

Infections have been reported in a small but significant number of cases (up to 10%) after maxillary sinus elevation and bone augmentation procedures.[36,53] Prevention of infection is crucial for bone augmentation procedures. Surgery should always be performed using sterile techniques. Patients should use a presurgical antimicrobial mouth rinse (e.g., chlorhexidine), and postoperative antibiotics should be prescribed. The signs and symptoms of sinus graft infection as well as a detailed protocol for its treatment was described in a clinical study.[53]

Opening a window through the lateral wall is accomplished by completely cutting through the bone of the lateral wall up to the schneiderian membrane. The membrane is highly vascularized and may bleed significantly.[1,31] However, a more serious bleeding problem can arise if an intraosseous artery is severed in the process. Bone wax and topical hemostatic agents must be available to manage such an urgent surgical complication. If a medium-to-large intraosseous vascular channel is identified presurgically via three-dimensional imaging such as a cone beam scan (CBCT), the surgical approach can be modified to minimize the risk of a bleeding complication.

KEY FACT

Maxillary sinus augmentation is a predictable technique to gain vertical bone height in the posterior maxilla. However, despite the high success rates, various intraoperative and postoperative complications have been reported. Patient selection, patient preparation, and precise surgical techniques are the key factors for reducing the incidence of sinus complications.

 ## Supracrestal/Vertical Bone Augmentation

Supracrestal or vertical bone augmentation presents one of the greatest challenges of bone regeneration in implant dentistry. This is primarily due to difficulty of the surgical procedure and the potential for postoperative complications. Because vertical augmentation can be a challenging procedure with a relatively high rate of complications, it is necessary to justify this particular treatment for each patient. The rate of complications associated with vertical bone augmentation procedures, including membrane exposure or postoperative infection, is reported to range from 2.87% to 17%.[40,41,46,49] Alternative treatment options, albeit with limited outcomes, need to be considered. For example, regenerating a vertically deficient ridge may not be necessary if (1) implants can be placed in adjacent sites, (2) short implants can be used, (3) cantilevers or conventional bridges can be used, or (4) in the case of vertical deficiencies in aesthetic areas, pink ceramic can be used to create an illusion of "normal" soft tissue anatomy.

Historical attempts to vertically increase alveolar bone height using modalities such as onlay bone grafting have failed. More recent treatment modalities developed for vertical bone growth include vertical guided bone regeneration (GBR) and distraction osteogenesis. The techniques and evidence of success are presented.

Guided Bone Regeneration

The surgical technique of GBR for supracrestal regeneration was described in the 1990s.[43] Although available evidence is limited, both animal and human studies demonstrate successful vertical bone augmentation with histologic evidence.[25,41] Some studies have evaluated the effect of space creation by a membrane alone, whereas others have used an autogenous bone graft to maintain space under the membrane. Using titanium-reinforced (TR) membranes without bone graft (space filled with blood clot only) in a canine model, Jovanovic and colleagues[25] demonstrated a gain of 1.82 mm of vertical bone height around simultaneously placed implants. In

a clinical study, Simion and coworkers[41] treated five patients with GBR to gain vertical bone height around 15 implants placed in a supracrestal position with 4 to 7 mm of the implant exposed. Titanium miniscrews were placed distal to the implants in a supracrestal position with 3 to 4 mm exposed. The implants and miniscrews were covered with a titanium-reinforced expanded polytetrafluoroethylene (e-PTFE) barrier membrane. Clinical evaluation at implant exposure surgery revealed an average of 3 mm (range from 1 to 4 mm) of vertical bone gain after 9 months. Histomorphometric evaluation of harvested miniscrews showed good bone-to-implant contact (42.5% ± 3.6%) with the regenerated bone. These studies suggest that supracrestal bone formation up to 3 mm is predictable using the GBR technique with a titanium-reinforced barrier membrane–blood clot combination.

Studies showed that supracrestal bone formation is more predictable using a bone graft filler material placed under the TR membrane.[39] Therefore at present, advanced surgical GBR augmentation for vertical bone gain should be achieved with a nonresorbable TR membrane that is supported by a bone graft (Fig. 80.6). The long-term results of vertical GBR after 1 to 5 years of prosthetic loading were examined in a retrospective multicenter study evaluating 123 implants.[39] Three treatment modalities (nonresorbable regenerative membranes in combination with blood clot only, DFDBA, and autogenous bone chips) were studied, and the results from this investigation revealed that vertical bone regeneration greater than 4 mm could only be achieved with the use of autogenous bone chips. These authors reported an overall success rate of 97.5%, leading them to conclude that vertically augmented bone using GBR techniques supports implant placement in a fashion similar to native, nonregenerated bone.

Urban and colleagues[49] used TR membranes with autogenous particulated bone for vertical bone augmentation before implant placement. The study included 35 patients with 36 vertical bone defects. Eighty-two implants were placed in a staged approach, and a resorbable collagen membrane (Bio-Gide Resorbable Bilayer Membrane, Osteohealth, Shirley, New York) was placed over the newly formed crestal bone during the implant placement surgery to protect the graft from early resorption after removal of the ePTFE membrane. Implants were followed from 1 to 6 years after prosthetic loading. Treatment groups included single and multiple tooth sites, as well as vertical defects in the posterior maxilla. Vertical bone augmentation of the posterior maxillary ridge was done simultaneously with sinus bone augmentation (eFig. 80.4). At membrane removal, the mean vertical bone augmentation was 5.5 mm (±2.29 mm). The mean combined crestal remodeling was 1.01 mm (±0.57 mm) at 12 months, which remained stable through the 6-year follow-up period. There were no statistically significant differences between the treatment groups in mean marginal bone remodeling. The overall implant survival rate was 100% with a cumulative success rate of 94.7%.

The efficacy of a 1:1 mixture of ABBM and autogenous particulated bone graft using ePTFE membranes was evaluated histologically and histomorphometrically in 8 patients (10 ridge defects).[38] After a healing period of 6 to 9 months, a mean vertical gain of 3.15 mm (SD ±1.12 mm) was achieved. A clinical and histologic study evaluating the same graft material and using dense-PTFE membranes in 19 patients achieved an average bone gain of 5.45 mm (SD 1.93).[51] In both studies histologic evaluation showed that ABBM was surrounded by a dense network of newly formed bone at varying degrees of maturation.

Simion and coworkers reported the long-term results of machined surface implants placed in vertically augmented bone achieved with GBR. Patients were followed from 13 to 21 years with a mean

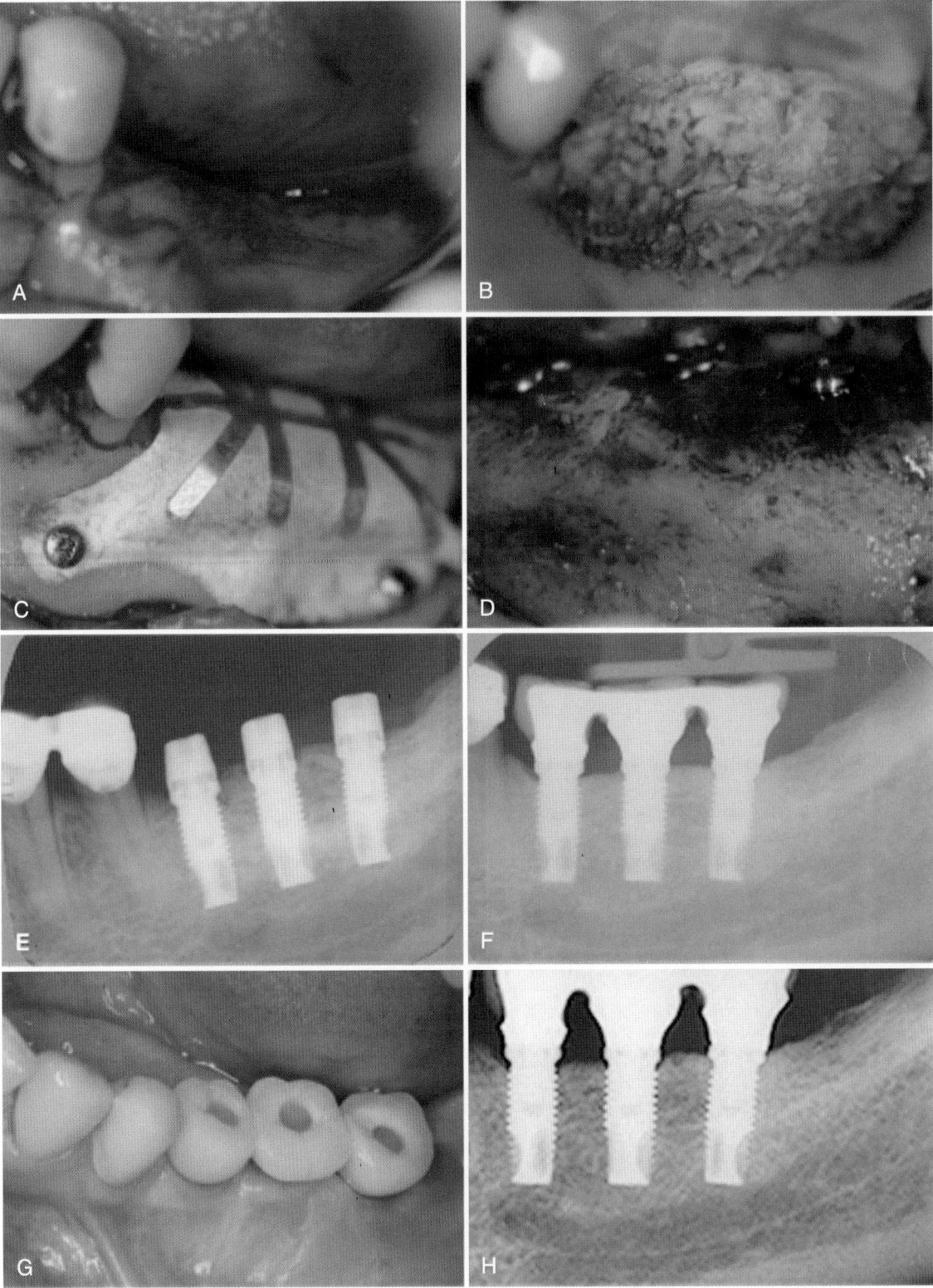

Fig. 80.6 Representative case of a posterior mandibular vertical ridge augmentation. (A) Atrophic posterior mandibular area. (B) Particulated chin bone graft is placed on the ridge. Cortical bone was perforated, and guided tissue regeneration membrane/titanium-reinforced (GTRM-TR) membrane was secured on the lingual side before applying bone graft. (C) GTRM-TR membrane is secured over the graft with titanium pins. (D) Three implants are in place in the newly formed posterior mandibular ridge. Note the well-integrated bone graft. (E) Periapical radiograph at abutment connection. (F) Periapical radiograph at 8-year follow-up with implants in function. (G) Clinical picture demonstrates healthy peri-implant mucosa. (H) Periapical radiograph at 13-year follow-up with implants in function. *(A–G from Urban IA, Jovanovic SA, Lozada JL: Vertical ridge augmentation using guided bone regeneration (GBR) in three clinical scenarios prior to implant placement: a retrospective study of 35 patients 12 to 72 months after loading,* Int J Oral Maxillofac Implants *24:502–510, 2009.)*

follow-up of 16 years. The average marginal bone loss between baseline (1-year postloading) and the final evaluation was 1.06 mm.[37]

There are limited clinical data on the outcomes of simultaneous GBR for horizontal or vertical bone gain for the reconstruction of severely atrophic edentulous maxilla. Urban and colleagues[52] evaluated 16 consecutively treated patients (mean age: 64 years) for vertical and/or horizontal bone augmentation with GBR in combination with bilateral sinus augmentation utilizing a mixture of autologous and anorganic bovine bone. Implant survival, bone gain, intraoperative/postoperative complications, and peri-implant bone loss were calculated up to the last follow-up exam. One hundred and twenty-two dental implants were placed into augmented sites and have been followed for up to 15 years (average follow-up of 6.5 years). The vertical bone gain was 5.1 mm; horizontal bone gain was 7 mm. The mean peri-implant bone loss values were consistent within the standards for implant success (1.4 ± 1 mm). At the patient level,

only one patient who had three implants presented with severe peri-implant bone loss (Fig. 80.7).

KEY FACT

Vertical ridge augmentation is one of the most challenging clinical procedures in reconstructing alveolar ridges. Despite the potential for complications with this treatment approach, high success and good long-term implant survival rates have been documented.

Conclusion

Bone augmentation and advanced implant surgery procedures allow clinicians to reconstruct vertical alveolar bone deficiencies and replace missing teeth with endosseous dental implants. Diagnosis, treatment

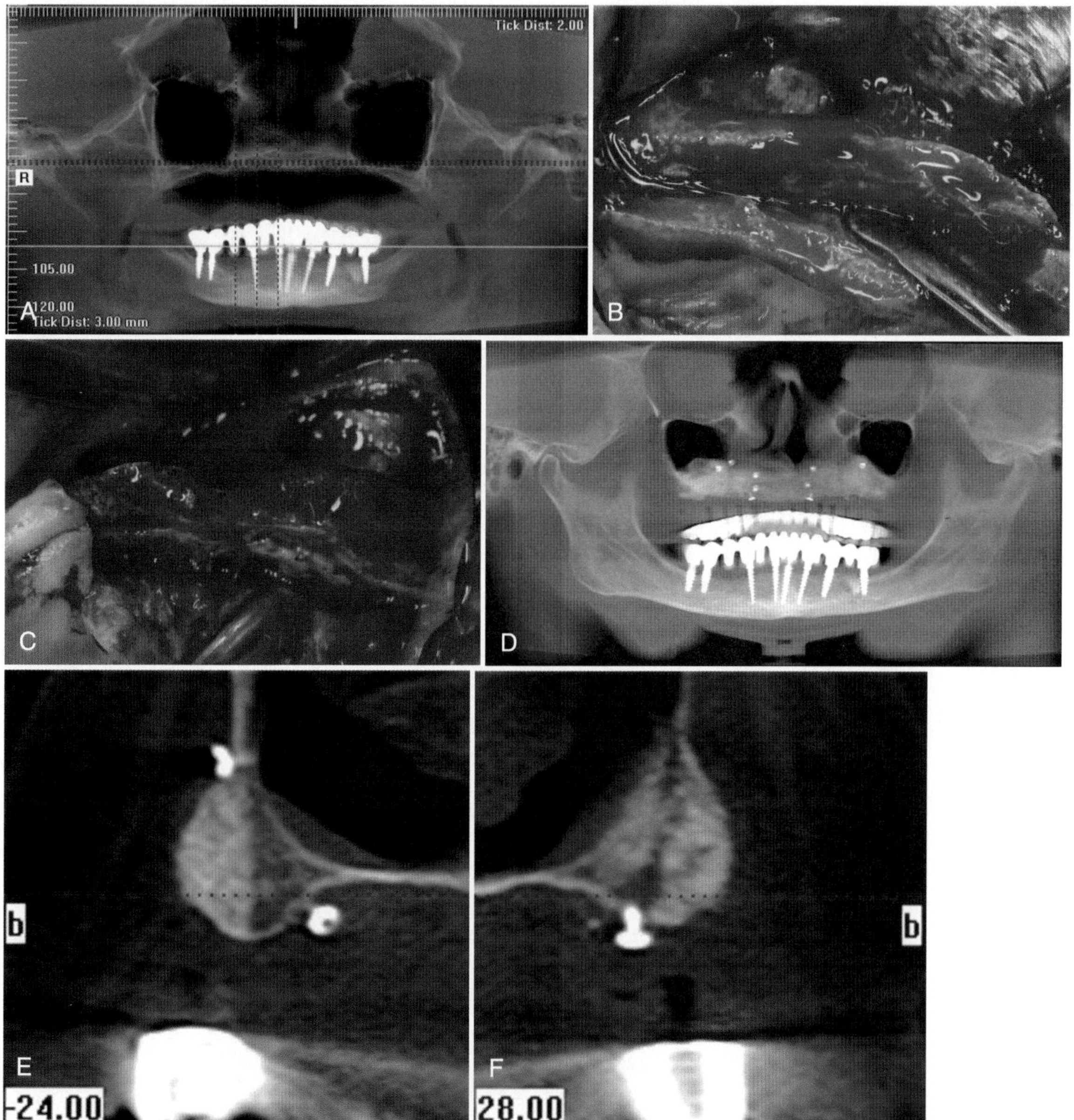

Fig. 80.7 Five-year follow-up of a 60-year-old female after reconstruction of an edentulous and severely resorbed maxilla. (A) Panoramic view of a severely resorbed maxillary case. (B–C) Occlusal views of the ridge atrophies. (D–F) Panoramic and cross-sectional views of the reconstructed ridge.   *Continued*

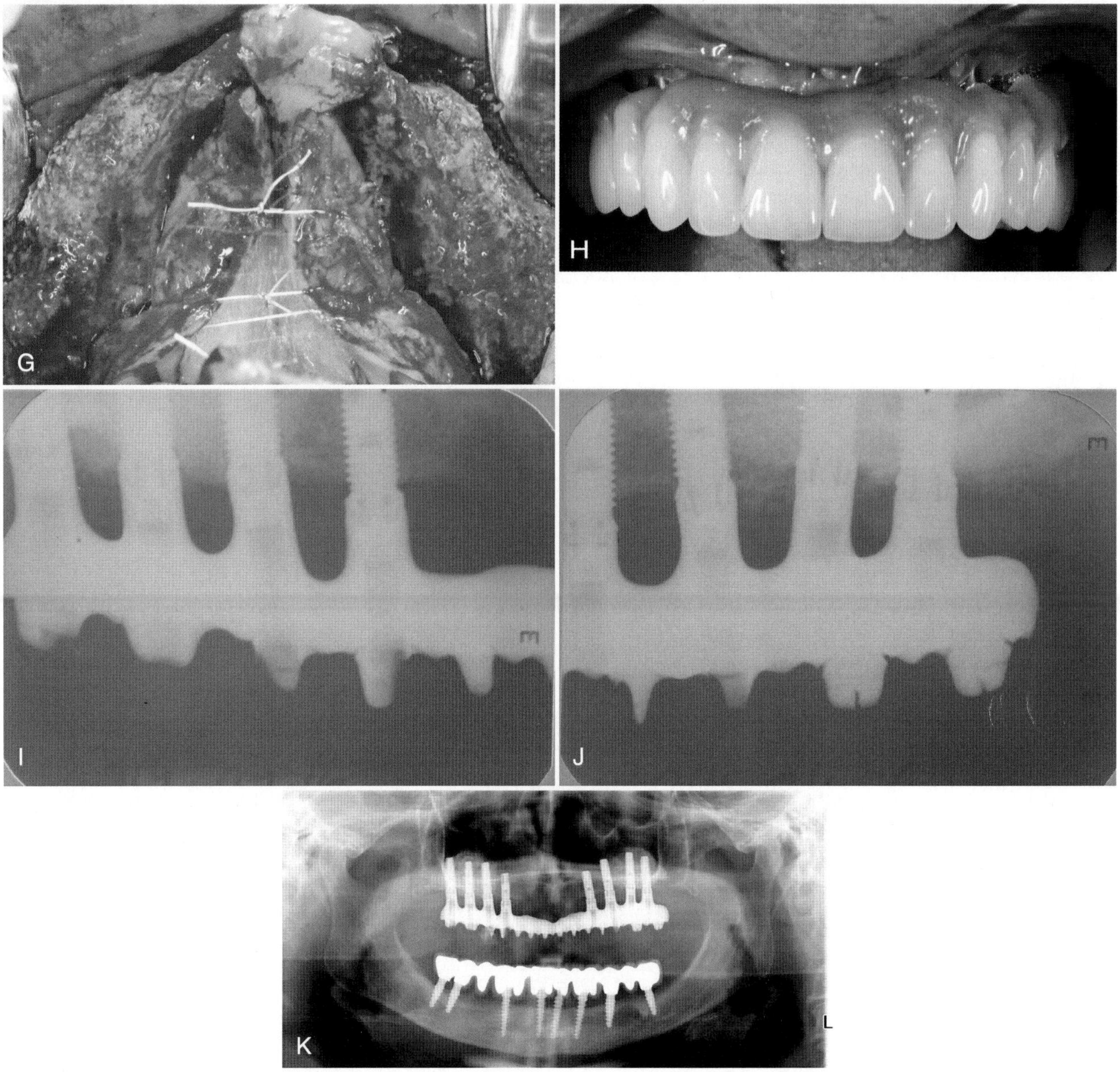

Fig. 80.7, cont'd (G) Occlusal view of the regenerated maxilla. (H) Labial view of the final fixed implant–supported maxillary complete denture (bridge). (I–J) Periapical radiographs after 5 years of loading. (K) Panoramic radiograph of the reconstruction. Note that the lower jaw was reconstructed before the patient sought treatment from the author.

planning, careful execution of the surgical treatment, postoperative follow-up, and appropriate implant loading are all important factors in achieving a predictable outcome and success with these procedures. Sinus elevation and bone augmentation has become a widely used and predictable procedure to augment the deficient posterior maxilla (i.e., pneumatized maxillary sinus). Reconstruction of vertically deficient ridges remains a significant challenge despite the reported progress and success of new techniques.

 A Case Scenario is found on the companion website www.expertconsult.com.

References

 References for this chapter are found on the companion website www.expertconsult.com.

CHAPTER 81

Aesthetic Management of Difficult Cases (Minimally Invasive Approach)

Thomas J. Han | Kwang-Bum Park | Perry R. Klokkevold

CHAPTER OUTLINE

Surgical Strategy for Predictable Aesthetics
Immediate Implant Placement for Predictability and Aesthetics
Surgical Management of Difficult Cases (Minimally Invasive Approach)
Conclusion

 For online-only content on surgical strategy for predictable aesthetics, as well as two additional case presentations for the surgical management of difficult cases, please visit the companion website at www.expertconsult.com.

In recent years, implant dentistry has been increasingly influenced by aesthetic considerations. In addition to successful osseointegration, harmonious soft and hard tissues must surround the implant restorations so that they look natural and healthy. A major challenge in implant dentistry is that, in many instances, dental implants need to be placed in an aesthetic zone with extensive alveolar bone deficiency from tooth loss, dentoalveolar infection, or other disorders (Fig. 81.1). Gingival morphology follows the shape of the underlying bone, and it is difficult to build aesthetically acceptable gingiva in areas with deficient supporting bone. Furthermore, using conventional surgical approaches to accomplish the goal in a patient-friendly manner with minimal trauma and clinical predictability is an extremely demanding task.

Treatment planning in a complex implant case today is often confusing because of the many different surgical and restorative approaches to solve the same problem. Many times these procedures seem to conflict. When considering the surgical placement of implants, clinicians must consider the approach (conventional two-stage approach versus a one-stage approach) and the timing of implant placement (immediate versus delayed or staged placement). For bone augmentation procedures, the clinician may choose the more conventional approach of augmenting the ridge first and placing the implant or implants after healing, or the simultaneous implant placement technique with bone augmentation approach in which bone grafting is done at same time as implant placement. All of these approaches can provide a successful outcome if patient selection is appropriate and techniques are performed properly.[9,22,24,32] However, depending on the situation, some of these techniques are more advantageous than others in achieving aesthetic results with better predictably and less patient discomfort.

It is easy for a clinician "dogmatically" to choose one approach, usually the one that the clinician feels most comfortable with, and to treat all patients with the same approach. However, with heightened expectations of aesthetics pushing the art and science of dentistry, it is necessary more than ever for clinicians to understand fully all the available options of treatment and decide appropriately which, where, when, and how to use these options for each patient.

An important clinical development in dental implant surgery is the concept of a "minimally invasive" approach to treatment. Specifically, the drive is toward minimally invasive implant placement. With advances in technologies, materials, and biologic sciences in dentistry, this approach to implant surgery is becoming more popular among clinicians and will most likely dominate the way dental implants will be placed in the near future.

Minimally invasive surgery in implant dentistry implies a surgical approach that minimizes the extent and number of surgical procedures while providing aesthetics, predictability, and longevity with minimal surgical morbidity and discomfort to patients. The surgical approach most often required to achieve these goals for anterior implant therapy involves immediate implant placement, a one-stage surgical approach, with or without flap, and simultaneous bone grafting. Furthermore, these surgical techniques need to be guided by a consistent surgical strategy that provides predictable aesthetic results in implant dentistry. A minimally invasive approach to implant therapy in posterior sextants in which aesthetics is not a major concern can be predictably achieved with the use of short, wide implants.[2,15,16,27]

This chapter introduces surgical strategies that enhance the aesthetic predictability in implant dentistry. The minimally invasive surgical approach to manage difficult aesthetic and anatomically deficient cases is discussed with examples. The one-stage, immediate implant placement technique, which is the foundation of a patient-friendly approach to aesthetic implant dentistry, is presented in detail. The thought processes involved in case selection, their scientific rationale, and proper techniques of soft and hard tissue management are described with cases.

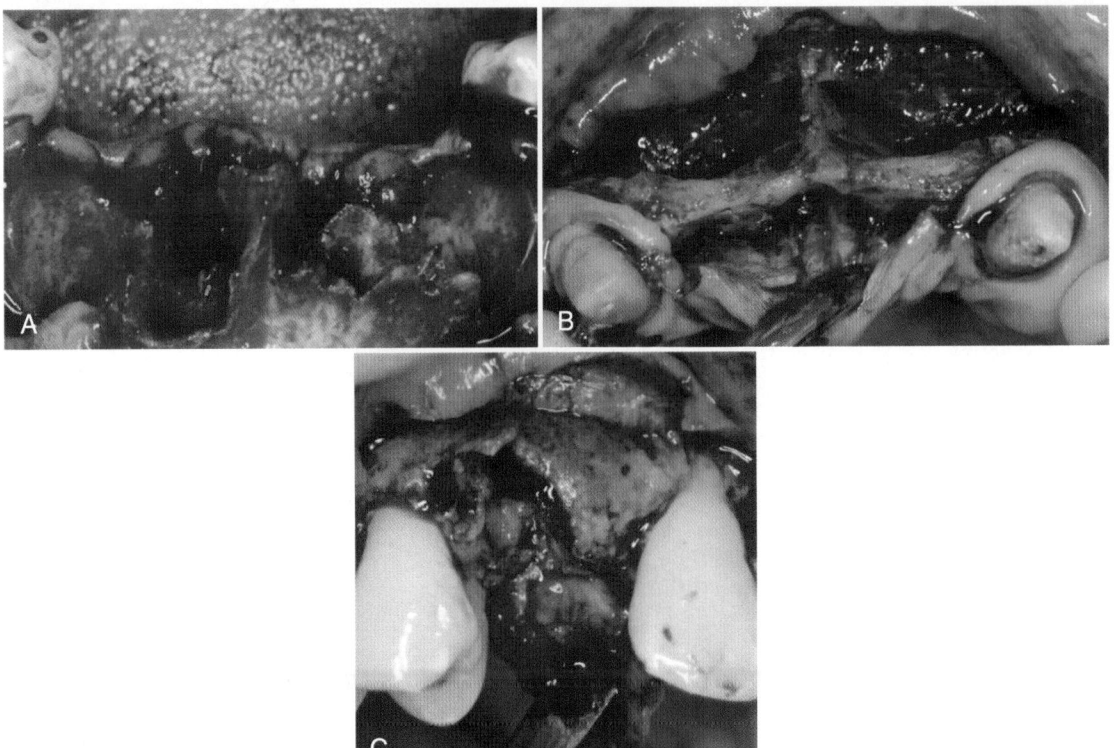

Fig. 81.1 Implant sites in the anterior, aesthetic zone with extensive bone loss. (A) Anterior mandibular site showing extensive bone loss following extraction of hopelessly infected mandibular incisors. (B) Extremely narrow (labial-palatal) ridge width in the anterior maxilla that was missing central and lateral incisors for many years. (C) Moderate bone loss associated with the extraction socket of a maxillary cuspid.

KEY FACT

Minimally invasive surgery is an approach that minimizes the extent of surgical invasiveness, as well as the number of surgical procedures, while providing aesthetics and predictability with minimal surgical morbidity and discomfort to patients. The surgical approach most often required to achieve these goals for anterior implant therapy involves immediate implant placement, a one-stage surgical approach, with or without flap, and simultaneous bone grafting.

 ## Surgical Strategy for Predictable Aesthetics

Adherence to the following surgical strategies enhances predictability and outcomes for aesthetic dental implant surgical procedures with minimal discomfort to patients (see the online description of the following key points):

1. Determine the level of surgical aesthetic goal to be achieved.
2. Visualize the final outcome.
3. Preserve existing tissues important for aesthetics.
4. Always overbuild bone and soft tissue in augmentation surgical procedures.

Immediate Implant Placement for Predictability and Aesthetics

Immediate implant placement in a one-stage approach, in which a healing abutment or provisional restoration is attached to the implant and remains exposed, provides more predictable preservation of the interproximal peri-implant gingival tissue with less patient discomfort

and treatment time.[21,22] This approach to implant placement is the foundation of a minimally invasive approach to aesthetic implant dentistry. However, as with any surgical technique, it takes learning and practice to perform it properly. The criteria and techniques for proper immediate implant placement have previously been established and reported with successful long-term outcomes.[18,32]

One of the more difficult aspects of immediate implant placement is positioning the implant with sufficient primary stability in an extraction socket, often without elevating a flap. The alveolar architecture in relation to the angle of the implant to be inserted, the presence or absence of a bone concavity apical to the extracted tooth, the amount of existing bone apical and palatal to the extraction socket that can provide primary stability for the immediate implant, and the quality of the bone and soft tissues of the ridge should all be thoroughly evaluated clinically and radiographically before surgery.[18,32] Many clinicians perform successful immediate implant placement without the aid of three-dimensional scans (e.g., computed tomography [CT] or cone beam CT [CBCT]). However, if the tooth involved is long and large or if the patient has an alveolar concavity or other anatomic variations, the use of a CT or CBCT scan is advised.

A major disadvantage of placing implants immediately in the changing alveolar bone of an extraction socket is that it may result in progressive recession of the gingival labial margin over the implant restoration.[4,17] Therefore, when placing an immediate implant with a one-stage surgical approach in an aesthetic zone, a prudent strategy would be to improve the quality and quantity of labial gingival tissue, which seems to be vital for the stability of the labial gingival margin involving immediate implants.[19,31] One of the most effective ways to keep the implanted socket from collapsing and improve the labial gingival biotype is simultaneously to fill the labial socket void with particulate bone and augment the labial gingival tissue with soft tissue.[3,23,26,30,32]

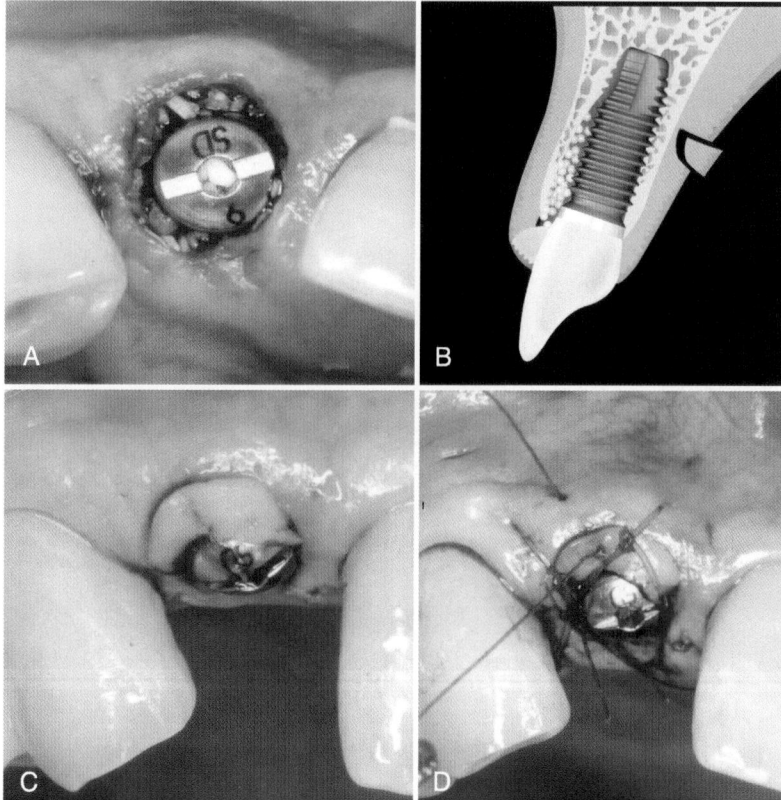

Fig. 81.2 (A) Bone graft material is lightly packed into the extraction socket gap between the labial wall and the implant surface. (B) Diagram of crescent-shaped, free gingival graft tissue being harvested from the palate. (C) Clinical photograph of crescent-shaped, free gingival graft tissue positioned over the bone graft to fit snugly in the gap between the gingival wall and the implant surface. (D) Crescent-shaped, free gingival graft is sutured in place using 5-0 gut sutures. The sutures pass through the gingival graft toward the labial gingival margin and are tied. Then, without cutting the ends, the suture is passed over the graft and tied to the palatal gingival tissue. Three sutures are needed to keep the graft in position.

An effective bone and gingival tissue augmentation technique used with flapless immediate implant placement in a one-stage approach is the bone and crescent-shaped free gingival grafting technique.[18] In this technique, the space between the inner surface of the labial bony wall and the labial surface of the implant is filled with slow-resorbing mineralized, freeze-dried particulate bone allograft or particulate xenograft to help preserve the horizontal dimension of the ridge (Fig. 81.2A). Then, a crescent-shaped soft tissue graft is harvested from the ipsilateral palate (Fig. 81.2B) and is transplanted into the labial recipient site coronal to the particulate bone graft (Fig. 81.2C). To provide or maintain the blood supply to the donor tissue, it is important that the outer surface of the crescent graft fits in intimate contact with the bleeding lamina propria of the labial gingiva. Proper suturing ensures good proximity and prevents the graft from being displaced coronally out of the recipient site (Fig. 81.2D).

The advantages of this approach to gingival augmentation are simplicity and minimal surgical morbidity. In addition to providing a sealed protection for the bone graft, it prevents resorption of the sensitive labial crestal bone. Preparation of the recipient site involves no surgical manipulation other than de-epithelialization, as described. Gingival walls are completely intact with a full blood supply. The donor site wound is small (approximately 3 mm depth × 3 mm height at the widest point) with intact epithelium around the wound, which epithelializes within a week and causes minimal discomfort for the patient. Because each donor tissue graft is small, multiple grafts can be harvested from a single palate, so that multiple immediate implants can be augmented at same time. Furthermore, this gingival augmentation technique frequently improves an unfavorable initial gingival margin because the grafted gingival margin is always coronal to the existing gingival margin. This minimizes a need for other time-consuming techniques, such as orthodontic extrusion, or a delayed approach to implant placement when the initial gingival margin is not aesthetic or ideal, as recommended by many investigators.[5,33]

The risk-to-benefit ratio of the crescent grafting technique is favorable enough that if the graft does not survive, or if more than expected horizontal resorption of the ridge occurs, traditional techniques (e.g., subepithelial connective tissue graft) can be performed to augment the results. This is usually possible without refabrication of the implant restoration because the vertical height of the interdental papilla is sufficiently preserved with immediate implant placement in a one-stage approach.

KEY FACT

An effective bone and gingival tissue augmentation technique used with flapless immediate implant placement in a one-stage approach is the bone and crescent-shaped free gingival grafting technique. To provide and maintain the blood supply to the donor tissue, it is important that the outer surface of the crescent graft fits in intimate contact with the bleeding lamina propria of the labial gingiva. Proper suturing ensures good proximity and prevents the graft from being displaced coronally. The crescent graft technique enhances gingival thickness following extraction and immediate implant placement.

Surgical Management of Difficult Cases (Minimally Invasive Approach)

The failure to satisfy the aesthetic needs of a patient frequently starts with an inadequate examination of the soft and hard tissues surrounding the surgical site and the natural dentition. This can result in an incorrect diagnosis, which leads to an incorrect treatment plan. The wrong treatment plan combined with selection of inappropriate surgical approaches or techniques can result in a disastrous aesthetic outcome and unnecessary patient suffering. The first two case presentations describe the examination and thought processes involved in determining the diagnosis and treatment planning of complex anterior cases with extensive alveolar bone loss. The proper application of the surgical strategies and the minimally invasive techniques, previously described, are illustrated. The final case presentation illustrates the minimally invasive approach to posterior implant therapy with the use of short, wide implants, in which aesthetics is not the major concern.[2,15,16,27]

Components of Aesthetic Examination

The patient's chief complaint, aesthetic zone, tooth positions, gingival form, osseous crest position, biotype, tooth shape, horizontal and vertical ridge deficiency, and occlusal status all play important roles in deriving an accurate aesthetic treatment plan for the patient. Therefore developing the necessary skill and knowledge to examine and recognize problems of these components is an essential first step to clinical success.

Case Presentation 1

The first case presented is in a patient with a simultaneous bone and soft tissue augmentation with multiple maxillary anterior immediate implants placed in a one-stage, flapless approach.

Patient Dental History and Chief Complaint

The patient is a 70-year-old woman with severe mobility and discomfort of the maxillary four incisors. Except for a generalized feeling of weakness, she is healthy and does not have any medical contraindications to dental treatment. She presented with a desire to replace her maxillary incisors with dental implants, but she is very concerned about the physical discomfort she may experience from the implant surgery. She does not want to wear a removable prosthesis at all, not even for a short time. She is content with her present dental aesthetics.

Examination and Diagnosis

The maxillary incisors exhibit moderate to severe periodontitis with 4- to 7-mm periodontal probing depths. They exhibit severe (2+) mobility with fremitus. The periodontal and restorative prognosis of these teeth is poor. She has an excessive overbite with evidence of moderate mandibular incisor wear, indicating possible parafunctional habits. Her incisors are slightly elongated, but the dentogingival symmetry is acceptable (Fig. 81.3A). The shape of the incisors is slightly triangular with sufficient interdental papilla volume and height. Interproximal gingival tissue is not swollen or edematous. Her gingival biotype appears to be on the thin side with slight marginal inflammation, and the position of the labial gingival margins is already high (i.e., maximal apical position). Any further recession will be unaesthetic.

Radiographic evaluation demonstrates moderate to severe vertical and horizontal periodontal bone loss. The osseous crest position, in relation to the gingival margins, appears too apical to provide adequate gingival support (see Fig. 81.3B). The restorative and periodontal status of the canines is healthy.

Treatment Objectives

Considering her age, reasonable aesthetic expectation, concern for surgical morbidity, and a lack of willingness to wear a removable provisional prosthesis, the treatment objective for this patient would be to use a surgical approach that minimizes the extent and number of surgical procedures while providing predictability, longevity, and acceptable aesthetics. Recommending orthodontic extrusion or multiple surgical procedures to achieve ideal aesthetics on this patient would be considered an excessive treatment plan and would not provide any additional value or benefits for her.

Treatment Options

Considerations for extracting four maxillary incisors include the need to remove sound porcelain-fused-to-metal crowns from the canines to replace them as part of a six-unit fixed prosthesis. This option has a questionable long-term functional and aesthetic prognosis. Her dentition exhibits evidence of excessive overbite and parafunctional habit, which may have contributed to the alveolar bone loss of the incisors in the first place. The convex shape of the ridge and the lack of osseous support will most likely result in substantial horizontal and vertical resorption of the edentulous ridge under the pontics of the fixed bridge, even with extraction socket grafting and ovate provisionalization. This will compromise the long-term aesthetics.

Even if this patient can tolerate the temporary removable partial denture, which she said she cannot, this option poses a considerable aesthetic challenge. The ridge surrounding the extraction sockets will rapidly lose vertical and horizontal dimensional soon after the extractions.[3] The loss of vertical height in the interproximal gingival areas creates an aesthetic problem that is very difficult to correct. It often requires multiple surgical procedures that have a high incidence of surgical morbidity and rarely achieve the desired ideal aesthetic result. This is especially true in a case such as this in which the patient has extensive periodontal vertical and horizontal bone loss. The anticipated vertical ridge collapse after the extraction is substantial, even with bone grafting of the extraction sockets. More important, the need for multiple surgical procedures to achieve "acceptable" aesthetic results for this patient may be too traumatic for her.

Extracting four maxillary incisors, immediately placing two implants, and replacing the teeth with a 4-unit provisional fixed partial denture supported by two implants is an acceptable but risky treatment option. Immediate provisionalization of the two immediately placed implants, with her occlusion and suspected parafunctional habit, carries the risk of early excessive loading and implant failure. Additionally, it will be challenging to maintain the vertical and horizontal ridge dimensions in the edentulous area under the pontics. Most likely it will require additional soft tissue augmentation procedures to achieve "acceptable" aesthetics in the pontic area (i.e., missing central incisor area).

> ⚠ **CLINICAL CORRELATION**
>
> A common cause of aesthetic failure is inadequate examination of the soft and hard tissues surrounding the surgical site and the natural dentition. If the examination is incomplete or findings are misinterpreted, an incorrect diagnosis will be made, which in turn will lead to an incorrect treatment plan. The judgment to formulate an appropriate treatment plan depends on making an accurate diagnosis!

Extracting four maxillary incisors, immediately placing four implants in the sockets, and replacing the missing teeth with a four-unit

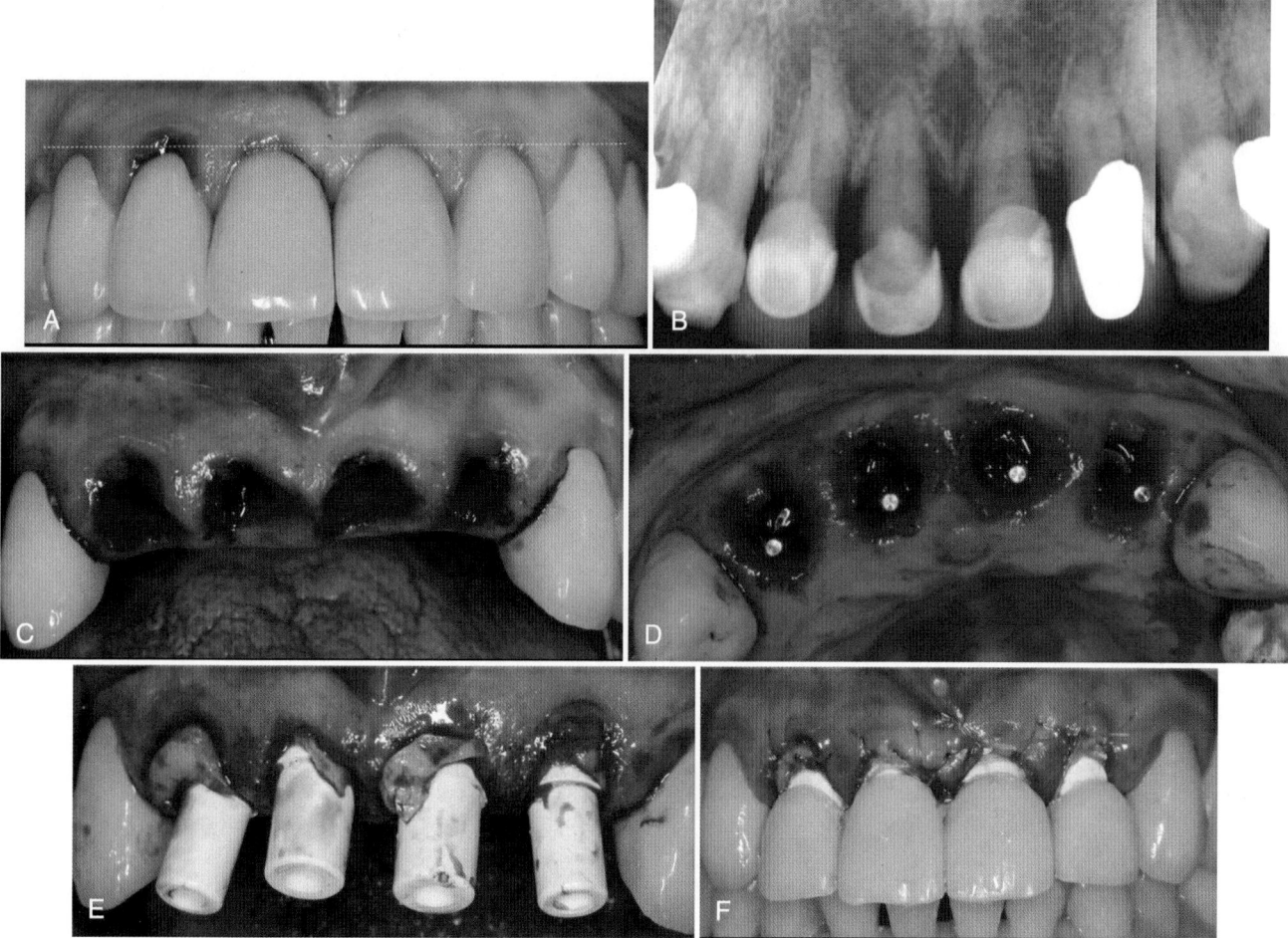

Fig. 81.3 (A) Clinical photograph of periodontally compromised maxillary anterior teeth with long clinical crowns. The presenting aesthetic status is not ideal. However, the dentogingival symmetry is fair because the gingival margin is approximately the same for all incisors (cuspid, lateral, and central). (B) Periapical radiographs of the maxillary anterior teeth reveal moderate to severe horizontal periodontal bone loss with vertical intrabony defects. (C) Simple, atraumatic extraction of the maxillary incisors reveals sockets with unsupported interdental tissues. Note the absence of incisions or flap reflection, which has preserved the blood supply and integrity of the interdental soft tissues. (D) Guide pins placed in prepared implant sites reveal good position within the extraction sockets achieving good primary stability from the palatal aspect of the socket. (E) Implants with temporary abutments and crescent-shaped, free gingival grafts (not yet sutured). (F) Implant provisional abutments are prepared, and provisional restorations are fabricated using conventional methods.

Continued

provisional fixed partial denture supported by four implants is another acceptable option. Splinting four provisionals together should provide sufficient resistance and protection to the implants from early excessive loading. Some clinicians do not recommend placing implants next to each other in the lateral and central incisor positions because they are often positioned too close and it is very difficult to create or maintain an interdental papilla that emulates an interdental papilla between an implant and a tooth or between two natural teeth.[39] However, the more recent use of implants with a platform-switching design may change the spatial requirements for achieving an interdental papilla between implants. The bone between implants appears to be better protected, and as a result the vertical height of the interproximal tissue may be better preserved.[8,25] If procedures are carried out properly, this option can provide a long-term functional and aesthetic result, with minimal discomfort to the patient.

1. Extract four maxillary incisors and replace them with a conventional (six-unit) fixed prosthesis supported by the canines.
2. Extract four maxillary incisors and wait for healing of the sockets and ridge while temporarily replacing the missing teeth with a removable partial denture. Plan to place two or four implants after 3 to 6 months of healing by using either a one- or two-stage approach.
3. Extract four maxillary incisors, immediately place two implants in the lateral positions, and replace the missing teeth with a four-unit provisional fixed partial denture supported by two implants.
4. Extract four maxillary incisors, immediately place four implants in the sockets, and replace the missing teeth with a four-unit provisional fixed partial denture supported by four implants.

Surgical Strategy for Predictable Aesthetics

Because of the patient's age and reasonable expectation, the level of the aesthetic goal determined for this patient is not ideal but is acceptable. This level of aesthetics can be predictably achieved in a minimally invasive, patient-friendly manner. By mentally visualizing the surgical and prosthetic goal, an acceptable aesthetic outcome can be achieved for this patient if the existing heights of the interproximal gingival tissues can be maintained. Additionally, if the existing biotype and

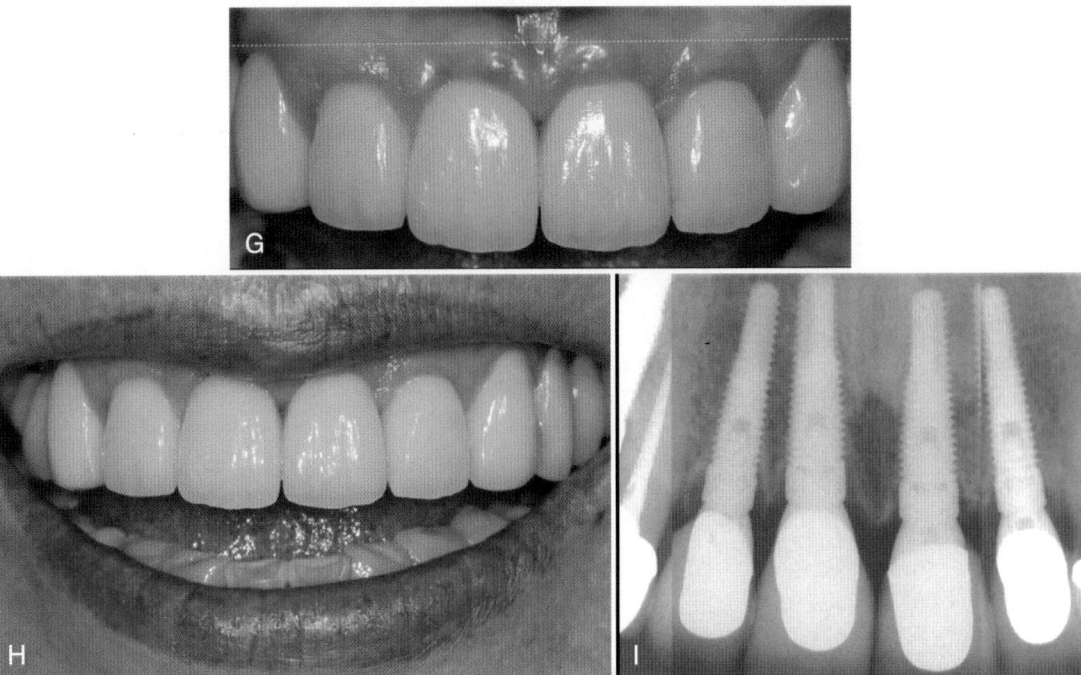

Fig. 81.3, cont'd (G) One-year postloading results show nearly complete preservation of the interproximal papilla height and improved labial gingival biotype. Labial gingival margins are substantially coronal in position as compared with the initial levels. (H) The final restorations have a more normal length, offering the patient a much more youthful smile. Preexisting moderate to severe attrition is noted on the incisal edges of the mandibular anterior teeth. (I) Periapical radiographs at 1 year of the implants with final restorations reveal good preservation of interproximal bone height with minimal saucerization. The platform-switched implant restorations likely contribute to the preservation of bone.

the level of the labial gingival margin can be overbuilt with hard and soft tissue augmentation, the final aesthetic outcome will be enhanced. If this can be accomplished with simultaneous implant placement, it will minimize the number of surgical procedures required. In this case, especially because the patient appears to have parafunctional habits, it is desirable to place more implants and use them to support the immediate provisionalization.

Considering all of these treatment options, the treatment that is most compatible with this patient's surgical strategy for predictability, acceptable aesthetics, and long-term results is treatment option 4, extraction of the incisors followed by immediate placement of four implants with an immediate provisional restoration supported by the implants.

Treatment Plan and Rationale

Four maxillary incisors are to be extracted and four implants placed immediately in a one-stage approach with simultaneous bone and soft tissue grafting. The bone and crescent-shaped free-gingival grafting technique will be used to overbuild labial gingival biotype.[18] A tapered implant with platform-switching design is to be used. The tapered design has been shown to promote primary stability in sockets, and the platform-switching design better maintains the interimplant bone.[8,25] An immediate provisional restoration without centric contacts will be attached to the implants.

Treatment Sequence

In complex treatment involving dental implants, the treatment plan must be sequenced and coordinated between the restorative dentist and the surgeon before starting the treatment. This is especially true when immediate provisionalization is planned. This will enhance success and help make the treatment more patient friendly.

Surgical Procedure

Once the patient is anesthetized, the incisors are extracted atraumatically, thus ensuring that gingival tissues, especially the interdental papilla, are not damaged (see Fig. 81.3C). The sockets are prepared to receive implants by removing the sulcular epithelium and by completely and thoroughly removing all granulation tissue. Immediately placed implants must have complete primary stability at the time of placement. Proper vertical position, buccolingual position, and mesiodistal position, as well as buccolingual angulation, are all critical factors for a successful outcome. Implants in anterior sockets are prepared and placed toward the palate (see Fig. 81.3D) to ensure sufficient labial bone thickness for labial margin stability.[9] Once the provisional healing abutments are accurately seated (may require bone profiler), the labial void of the sockets is grafted with particulate bone, and a crescent-shaped free gingival tissue graft is harvested and placed over the graft (see Fig. 81.3E), as described previously and in the literature.[18] By using this technique, all four teeth can be augmented in one surgical procedure with minimal discomfort to the patient. Once the soft tissue crescent grafts are secured with sutures, the provisional abutments are prepared for provisional crowns. The provisional crowns (splinted) are fabricated using conventional methods (see Fig. 81.3F). Contours of the provisional crowns may need to be modified as healing and remodeling occurs. Impression taking for the final restoration is relatively easy because the provisional abutments placed at the time of surgery and modified during healing nicely shape the tissues for an optimal prosthetic emergence profile.

Results

The 1-year result shows nearly complete preservation of the interproximal papilla height and an improved labial biotype with labial gingival margins that are substantially coronal to the original gingival margin level (see Fig. 81.3G). The final result consists of crowns with a more normal incisor length and a more youthful smile (see Fig. 81.3H). Some gingival irregularity is noted, and it appears to be a result of the soft tissue grafting. These areas could easily be smoothed with gingivoplasty, but the patient refused. Radiographs reveal preservation of interproximal bone with minimal saucerization around the implants with a platform-switch design (see Fig. 81.3I).

After the surgical strategies described and with the use of minimally invasive surgical techniques, this 70-year-old patient received immediate implant-supported replacement of severely compromised maxillary incisors with an acceptable (or better) aesthetic result and minimal treatment discomfort. With one surgery, including the extractions, she was provided with a fixed implant restoration on four implants. In the same surgery, the bone and soft tissue were augmented while preserving the interdental papilla. She experienced very little postoperative pain and was pleased with her new, more youthful-looking smile. The treatment time was only 6 months from extraction to final restoration. She was never without teeth and never wore a removable prosthesis. The improvement of the labial gingival margin was achieved without orthodontic extrusion or multiple surgical procedures.

Conclusion

The clinical science in dentistry has evolved to where placement of dental implants and restoring them require sufficient knowledge in several disciplines of dentistry. In addition to mastering surgical objectives and techniques, periodontists must be able to evaluate and accurately diagnose (and treat or refer) a wide range of related "restorative" issues including but not limited to aesthetics, occlusion, temporomandibular joint function, vertical dimension, and dental–skeletal relationships. These "other" aspects of diagnosis are essential for the development of an appropriate treatment plan, which is necessary for a successful outcome in aesthetic implant dentistry.

In addition, with heightened expectations of aesthetics pushing the art and science of dentistry, it is necessary more than ever for clinicians to understand fully all the available treatment options and to be able to determine appropriately which option to choose, when to use certain techniques, and how to apply them for each patient's scenario.

The minimally invasive approach and techniques presented in this chapter are not the only ways to manage difficult aesthetic cases, and some clinicians may consider them controversial. Certainly, these techniques require learning and practice to make them effective in each clinician's hands. However, they present a sound approach to what is possible in hard and soft tissue management for aesthetic implant surgery and provide effective strategies and techniques for solving many difficult aesthetic cases in a patient-friendly manner.

 A Case Scenario is found on the companion website www.expertconsult.com.

References

 References for this chapter are found on the companion website www.expertconsult.com.

CHAPTER 82

Dental Implant Microsurgery: Immediate Placement

Dennis A. Shanelec | *Leonard S. Tibbetts*

The success of dental implants in extraction sites combined with immediate provisionals for newly placed dental implants has brought a convergence in restorative and surgical practice for treatment planning of dental implants. This convergence reaches its summit in the approach to failing teeth in the maxillary aesthetic zone. For anatomic reasons, maxillary anterior teeth are at high risk for traumatic injury[13,14] (Fig. 82.1). Traumatized teeth frequently receive endodontic treatment that may be followed by horizontal or vertical root fracture.[1,2,15] Dentistry's historic answer to tooth loss has been the fixed bridge. Tooth preparation necessary for a fixed bridge often results in significant reduction of tooth structure.[22] Inherent aesthetic limitations of fixed bridges include loss of gingival papillae and resorption of the buccal alveolar plate. For these reasons, dental implants are a preferred choice for tooth replacement in the maxillary aesthetic zone.

Implant Microsurgery

Microsurgery is associated with enhanced soft tissue procedures and fine suturing. This is part of the scope of implant microsurgery, but additional benefits include dental implant drilling precision. The ability to discern minute dimensional differences permits implant osteotomy preparations centered exactly between reference points such as adjacent teeth, adjacent implants, or buccal and lingual ridge anatomy. More profoundly, the microscope allows immediate detection of subtle changes in drill position so appropriate feedback corrections can be applied to the handpiece. Enhanced angular perception is also important. The drill's angular position can be oriented relative to small landmarks such as the implant platform surface level or the angle of adjacent implant healing caps. This permits optimal parallel positioning and depth of adjacent implants. The implant drill angle can also be accurately oriented to root surface angulation using just 3 to 4 mm of root anatomy exposed between the cementoenamel junction and the osseous crest. These reference points are simply not visible without a microscope. The detection of subtle angulation reference points and changes in drill position permit feedback correction, which is important for osteotomy preparation in extraction sockets. The microscope-enhanced accuracy of osteotomy microsurgery permits socket implant placement in an ideal position followed by an aesthetic implant-supported provisional (Fig. 82.2). As a flapless procedure, this is accomplished with minimal patient morbidity.[22]

KEY FACT

The microscope facilitates detection of subtle changes in drill position. Enhanced angular perception is possible by focusing on small landmarks such as the implant platform or healing abutment surface of an adjacent implant. This permits optimal parallel positioning of the drill angle. These reference points are not visible without a microscope. Detection of subtle angulation reference points and changes in drill position permit feedback correction, which is important for osteotomy preparation in extraction sockets.

Microsurgical Tooth Extraction

Tooth extraction has been traumatic for centuries. Conventional tooth extraction may require mucogingival flaps and bone removal, resulting in compromised aesthetics. Using a microscope with minimally invasive principles reduces trauma and results in predictable aesthetic outcomes.[6] Instrument selection influences the trauma of tooth removal. Periotome luxation or leveraged mechanical extraction using tapped root anchorage systems can carefully separate a tooth from its surrounding ligament and lift it vertically from the socket. This limits injury to papillae and preserves natural gingival anatomy (Fig. 82.3). Subtle nuances in luxation direction can be microscopically detected for root removal in a proper anatomic path of extraction. Increased visibility under the microscope permits most extractions without mucogingival flaps. Greater visibility also permits atraumatic sectioning of ankylosed roots to leave alveolar bone and soft tissue uninjured. Apical granulomatous lesions can be completely debrided with full visibility. Such minimally invasive microsurgical techniques translate into reduced patient morbidity with enhanced healing.

Implant Drilling in the Extraction Site

Microsurgical implant drilling in the extraction socket is unique. Under the microscope, a socket appears as large as a room, with its apex and walls clearly visible. A different set of skills is required for socket drilling. For placement of maxillary anterior implants, the most favorable bone lies to the palatal (Fig. 82.4). Drilling therefore must be done at an angle to the palatal socket wall. Twist drills innately track toward the direction of less dense bone and into the open socket. Drilling of sockets under a microscope utilizes visual feedback to constantly redirect the drill to the correct position and

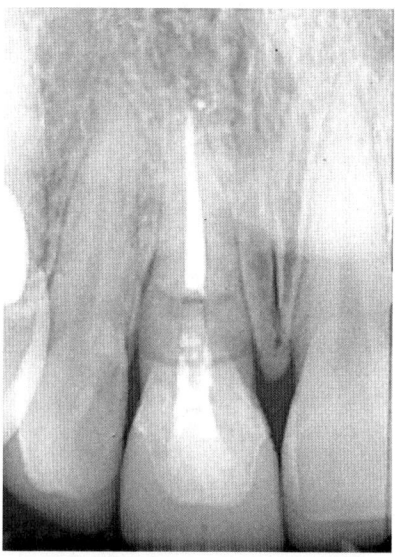

Fig. 82.1 **Periapical radiograph of typical fractured central incisor.**

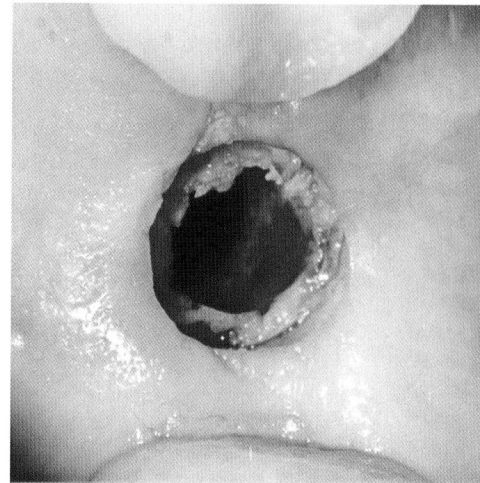

Fig. 82.2 **Flapless dental implant microsurgery.**

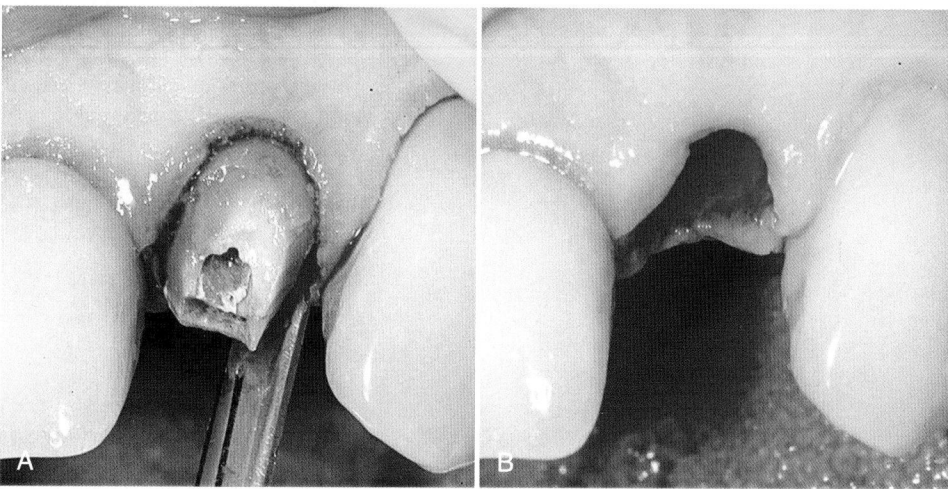

Fig. 82.3 (A) Periotome extraction of lateral incisor. (B) Noninvasive extraction of lateral incisor. Tissue contours are preserved.

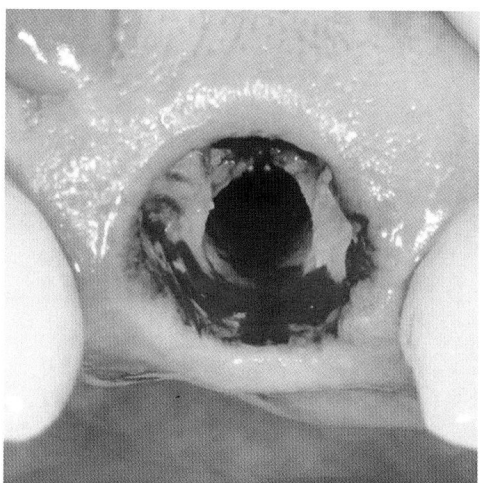

Fig. 82.4 **Palatal wall socket osteotomy.**

angulation. This avoids the common mistake of placing an implant too far toward the buccal. With the magnification and lighting a microscope provides, implants can be placed in the palatal socket wall with good initial stability and ideal aesthetic position. Microscope-enhanced dimensional and angular perceptions allow adjustments to correct drilling speed. Too little or too much drill pressure or excessive drill speed causes frictional heat. This adversely affects implant osteointegration. Detecting micromovement of the advancing drill ensures that proper pressure and rotational speed are applied to varying bone densities encountered in the socket. The angular velocity at the cutting edge of a 4-mm drill is several times faster than the velocity at the cutting edge of a 2-mm drill. For this reason, pressure and rotation of larger diameter drills must be decreased to compensate for their faster cutting speed. Enhanced visual feedback for speed and pressure correction is accomplished through directly viewing the advancing drill under the microscope.

Bone Grafting

The osteotomy in an extraction socket is prepared in the palatal wall. This placement results in a gap between the implant and the buccal socket wall. To avoid displacing a particulate graft, the provisional is finished before a socket bone graft is placed. The socket is filled with xenograft to within a millimeter of its crest. Xenograft is selected to reduce remodeling resorption of the buccal bone. Filtered bone from the osteotomy preparation is rinsed with 3% tetracycline solution and then condensed on the top of the xenograft. Finally, it is covered with a layer of microfibrillar collagen to contain the graft.

Buccal Gingival Grafting

Recession on the buccal gingival margin around anterior implants placed in extraction sockets has been well documented.[11,17] Multiple factors, such as the periodontal biotype, presence or absence of the buccal cortical plate, surgical trauma, implant position, and the emergence profile of both the provisional and final restorations, are associated with such recession.[9,12,16,18–20] A subepithelial connective tissue graft is therefore harvested from the palate and transferred into a split-thickness envelope incision on the buccal of the implant. A connective tissue graft is done to maintain or augment gingival height and thickness that may have been lost as the result of injury (Fig. 82.5). Even gingival tissue at a normal height can be expected to recede as much as 1.5 mm unless gingival grafting is performed. Placing a subepithelial connective tissue graft concurrent with implant placement ensures stability of the postoperative gingival level.[7,21]

Immediate Provisional Fabrication

To preserve natural aesthetics and provide support for gingival anatomy, an implant provisional must emerge from the surrounding gingival tissue in exactly the same way as the extracted tooth.[4,23] The surgical microscope gives dentists the visibility necessary to fabricate ideal anatomy for implant provisional crowns The provisional crown on the implant serves a number of functions, as follows:

1. It provides optimal aesthetics and function.
2. It minimizes tissue collapse by supporting the gingival tissue.
3. It obturates the surgical extraction socket to contain particulate and soft tissue grafts.

Creating an implant provisional crown begins before the tooth is removed.[8] A clear silicone impression captures the dentogingival junction and its proximal tooth contours (Fig. 82.6). Tooth color matching is done, and a light-cured flowable composite resin duplicate of the tooth is created using the impression (Fig. 82.7). The duplicate crown is trimmed to the exact location of the dentogingival junction and then hollowed to create a shell crown. It is fitted to a screw-retained titanium provisional abutment that is opaque for a color match (Fig. 82.8). Great attention is paid to the incisal edge position of the shell crown before luting it to the abutment with flowable composite resin. Screw access for removal of the provisional is accomplished by drilling through the incisal one-third of the provisional crown.

The luted abutment and crown are removed and placed on a laboratory handle to facilitate shaping and polishing (Fig. 82.9). Subgingival provisional contours created under the microscope provide tissue support and well-finished margins. Each provisional crown has a uniquely shaped subgingival emergence profile that duplicates the original tooth. Voids and rough edges are eliminated, and the provisional is carefully shaped under the microscope to provide gingival support (Fig. 82.10). Shaping the provisional is accomplished with a 12-fluted finishing bur, glass nail file, and a prophylaxis cup

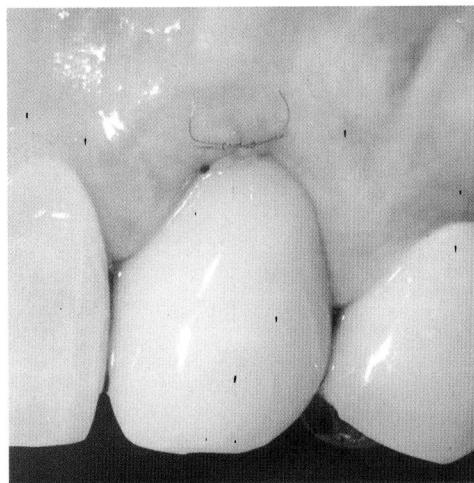

Fig. 82.5 Facial connective tissue graft placed under gingival margin and secured with a fine suture.

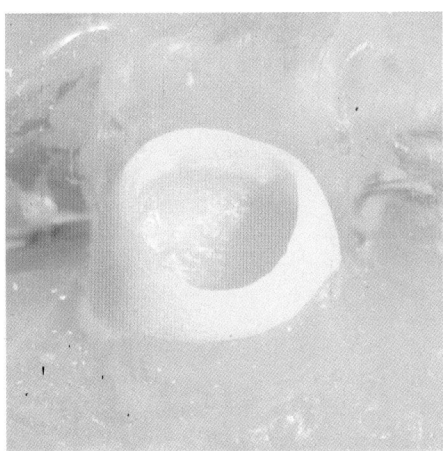

Fig. 82.7 Shell composite crown created from impression.

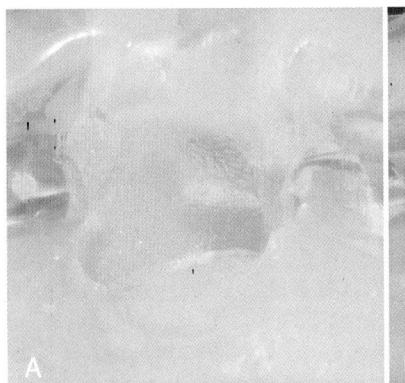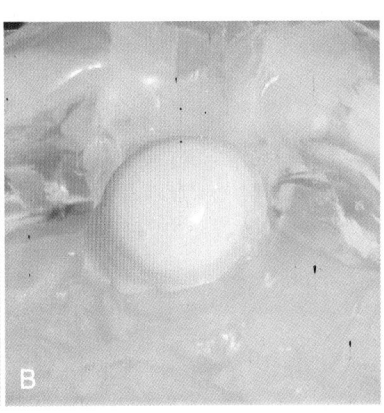

Fig. 82.6 (A) Clear silicone impression of failing tooth crown. (B) Clear silicone impression filled with composite.

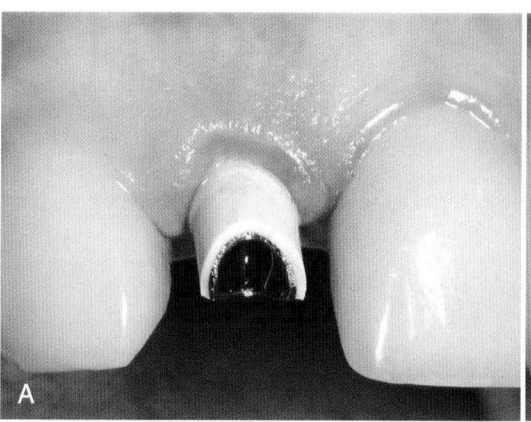
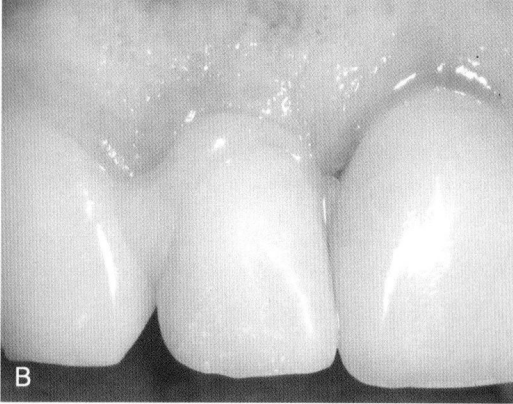

Fig. 82.8 (A) Opaque titanium temporary abutment. (B) Composite crown luted to opaque titanium temporary abutment.

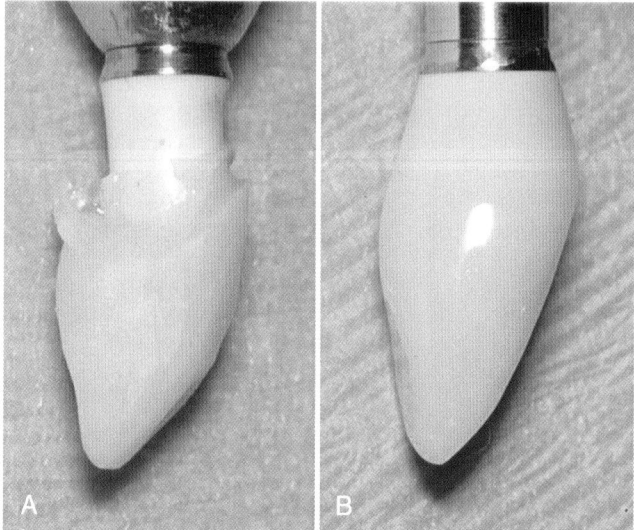

Fig. 82.9 (A) Screw-retained provisional before finishing. (B) Screw-retained provisional after finishing.

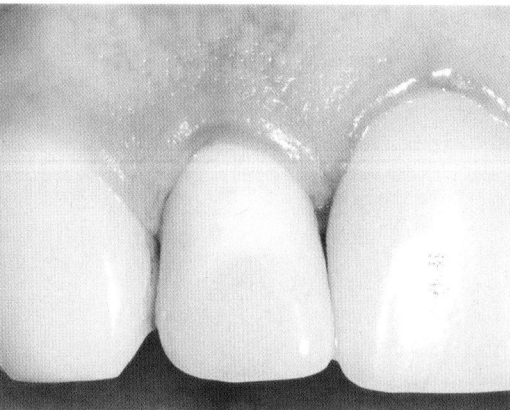

Fig. 82.10 Provisional restoration supporting gingival tissue.

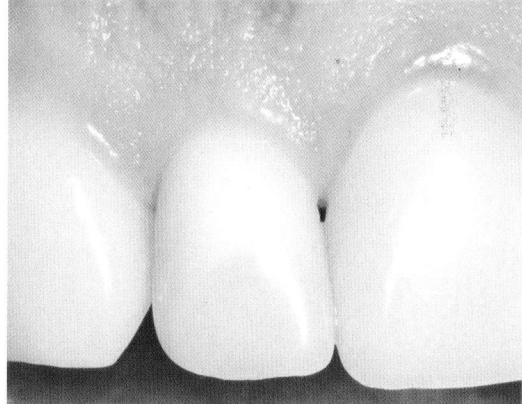

Fig. 82.11 Provisional 1 week after implant microsurgery.

with pumice. Attention to detail is critical. As a final step, the provisional crown is glazed and thoroughly cured. Light curing the composite ensures that no free monomer is present to irritate soft tissue or bone. The machined titanium provisional abutment ensures good marginal fit and reduces the possibility of loosening.

 CLINICAL CORRELATION

An immediate provisional restoration delivered with the immediately placed implant provides optimal aesthetics and function, minimizes tissue collapse by supporting the gingival tissue, and helps to obturate the surgical extraction socket to contain particulate and soft tissue grafts.

Immediate Implant Occlusion

Early loading bone trauma is minimized in multiple immediate implant provisional cases by splinting. Early loading bone trauma in single implant cases is reduced by lessening occlusal forces. Symmetric and light mesial and distal proximal contacts are established, and the provisional is taken out of centric and lateral occlusal contact by using 1-mm green occlusal indicator wax. This technique allows patients to leave the dental office with a nonloaded aesthetic provisional tooth securely anchored to the implant (Fig. 82.11).

Custom Impression Transfer Coping

A custom impression transfer coping is necessary to preserve and communicate gingival supporting contours to the ceramicist. The chairside-created provisional anatomy must be precisely reproduced for the dental laboratory via the custom impression transfer coping.[5,10] To make the custom transfer coping, an impression of the gingival third of the provisional crown is made with an implant analog attached (Fig. 82.12). This registers the implant platform orientation and preserves the provisional anatomy. The crown is removed, and a standard impression coping is attached to the implant analog. Acrylic powder fills the gap between the impression coping and the clear silicone impression. Monomer liquid is then infused into the powder to create a hard acrylic copy of provisional anatomy (Fig. 82.13).[3,5] Using a 25-gauge needle to apply monomer to the powder from the base upward minimizes inclusion of air bubbles in the custom transfer coping. For orientation, a mark is initially applied to the labial surface of the provisional impression. It is transferred to the custom transfer coping to provide orientation for the restorative dentist during final impressions. This technique allows precise communication from the surgeon to the restorative dentist to the ceramicist of the anatomy

required for a final restoration that aesthetically supports gingival tissue.

Final Implant Restoration

Final impressions are taken using the custom impression transfer coping. Computer-assisted scanning and machining create a zirconia abutment and zirconia coping for an all-ceramic crown (Fig. 82.14).

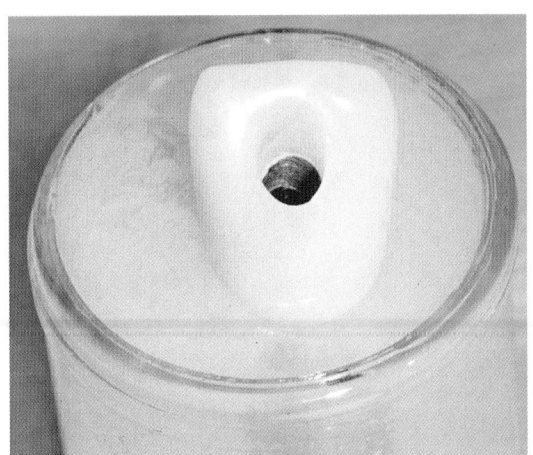

Fig. 82.12 Clear silicon impression of provisional.

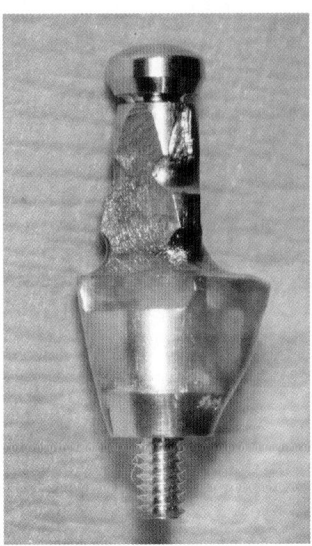

Fig. 82.13 Custom impression transfer coping reproducing emergence profile.

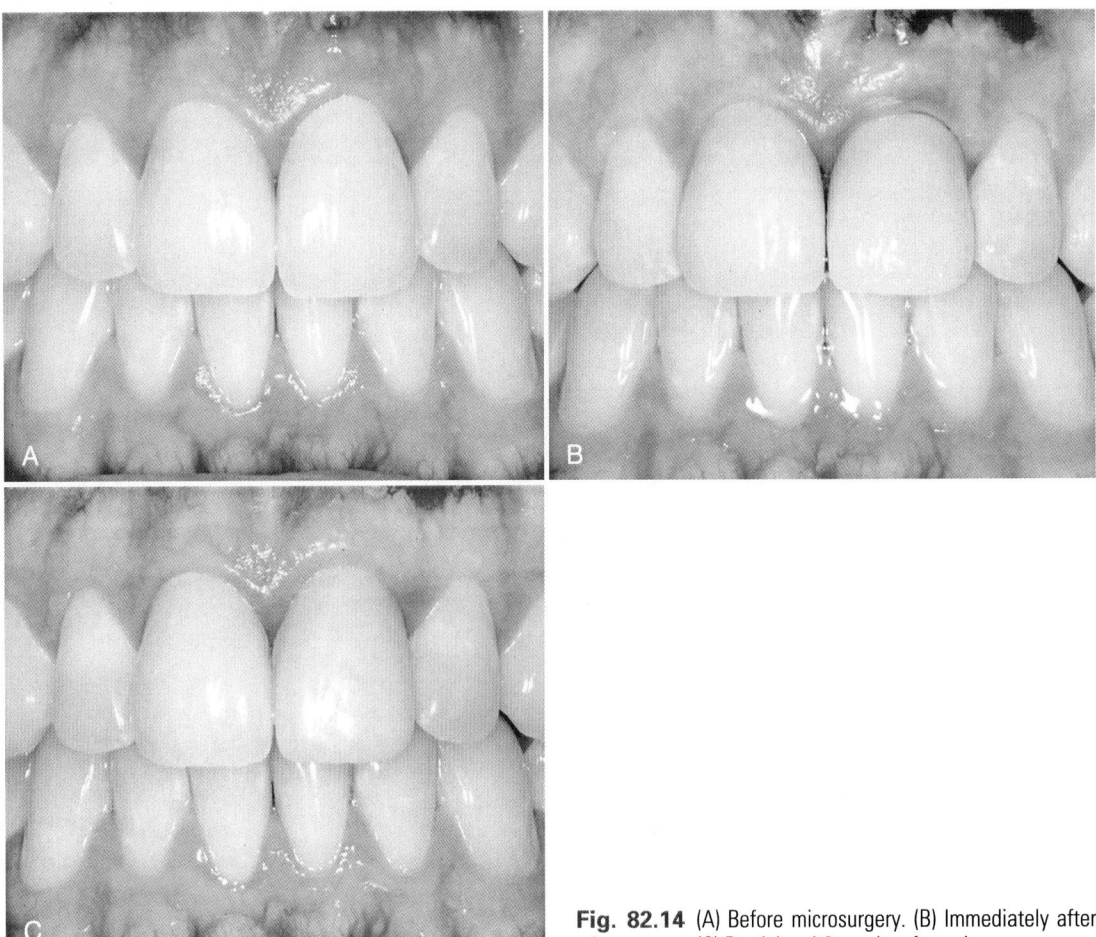

Fig. 82.14 (A) Before microsurgery. (B) Immediately after microsurgery. (C) Provisional 8 weeks after microsurgery.

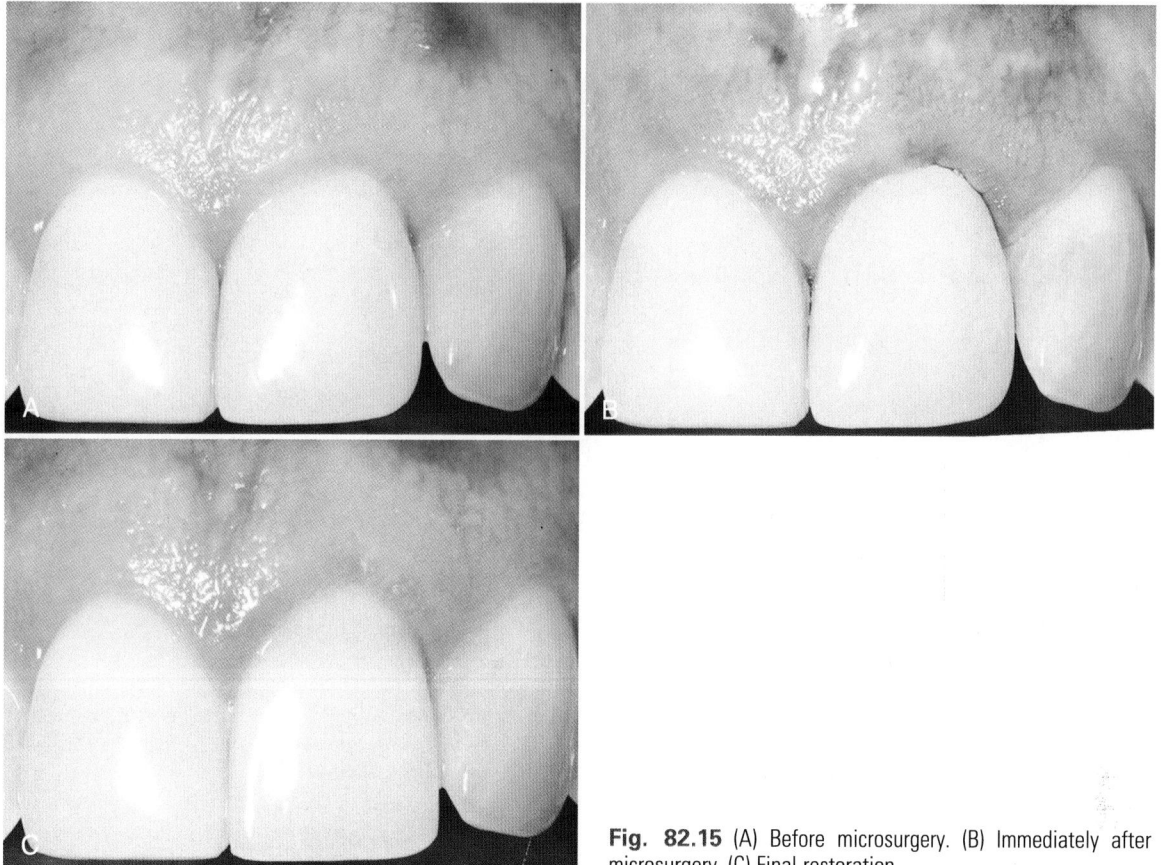

Fig. 82.15 (A) Before microsurgery. (B) Immediately after microsurgery. (C) Final restoration.

Zirconia has the benefit of tissue biocompatibility and light translucency. The sequence described ensures a final implant abutment and crown that exactly matches both the provisional emergence profile and the original tooth shape. Working as a team, the surgeon, restorative dentist, and laboratory technician can create a final restoration in harmony with preserved gingival architecture (Fig. 82.15).

Conclusion

Some of the advantages of microsurgery for extraction and implant placement have been described with an emphasis on tissue management and the ability to enhance visualization of details, which translate into better results. This microsurgery protocol advances dentistry from an era of traumatic tooth extraction to one of seamless immediate tooth replacement using implant microsurgery.

References

🌐 References for this chapter are found on the companion website www.expertconsult.com.

CHAPTER 83

Piezoelectric Bone Surgery

Tomaso Vercellotti | Perry R. Klokkevold | Giuseppe Vercellotti

CHAPTER OUTLINE

Clinical Characteristics of Ultrasonic Cutting
Clinical Applications
Advanced Clinical Applications *(e-only)*
Conclusion

 For online-only content on advanced clinical applications including sinus lift, ridge expansion, and bone harvesting, please visit the companion website at www.expertconsult.com.

Ultrasound has been used for many years in periodontics to remove tartar, debride root surfaces, and degranulate periodontal defects. In recent decades a novel family of ultrasonic-powered devices has been developed that is revolutionizing oral and maxillofacial bone surgery.

This surgical technique, known as piezoelectric bone surgery, was invented by Vercellotti and developed by Mectron Medical Technology (Carasco, Italy). The Piezosurgery device (Fig. 83.1) consists of a piezoelectric ultrasonic transducer powered by an ultrasonic generator, capable of driving a range of specially designed cutting inserts.[25,30] The Piezosurgery device employs ultrasonic vibrations to cut mineralized tissues. To this end, a primary frequency at 30 kHz is overmodulated by the superimposition of a sound wave (30 to 60 Hz) to generate a hammering action that effectively cuts bone without harming soft tissues and with minimal heat production. Box 83.1 describes the main cutting properties of Piezosurgery by Mectron, and Box 83.2 describes Piezosurgery inserts. Piezoelectric bone surgery techniques have been developed for clinical applications in dentistry and are becoming state of the art for a variety of procedures.[26–28,30,37,38] Piezosurgery Medical has expanded development of clinical applications to other fields of medicine. The extraordinary cutting properties of piezoelectric bone surgery have been introduced and applied in maxillofacial surgery, facial plastic surgery, otolaryngologic surgery, cranial and spinal neurosurgery, and minute orthopedic surgery.[7–17]

 KEY FACT

Ultrasonic scalers use only one frequency and have insufficient power to cut mineralized tissues. In comparison, Mectron surgical devices rely on the juxtaposition of a sound wave (30 to 60 Hz) to the primary ultrasonic wave (24 to 36 kHz) to cut bone without overheating. This phenomenon is known as frequency overmodulation.

The most compelling characteristics of piezoelectric bone surgery are low surgical trauma, exceptional control during surgery, and a fast healing response of tissues. Clinical studies demonstrate that the specificity of operation and the techniques employed with piezoelectric bone surgery make it possible to exploit differences in hard and soft tissue anatomy advantageously.[7,32,34,36] This not only increases treatment effectiveness but also improves postoperative recovery and healing. Experimental studies on animals have shown faster tissue healing when compared with traditional cutting instruments.[7]

 KEY FACT

Piezosurgery's cutting action is selective, that is, cuts only mineralized tissues while sparing soft tissues. Selective cutting is made possible by the application of ultrasonic frequencies between 24 and 36 kHz.

Ideally, surgical trauma should be minimized to obtain optimal healing, which depends on gentle management. Surgery, by definition, alters normal physiology by interrupting the vascular supply of tissues. The degree of surgical invasiveness is extremely important for the quality of tissue healing and may affect whether wounds heal by repair or regeneration. Indeed, when surgical trauma is kept to a minimum, it generates enough stimulation to favor healing mechanisms that lead to regeneration, which is actually promoted by ultrasonic frequencies. Conversely, surgical techniques that are more traumatic often lead to greater inflammatory responses with slow healing that may lead to repair and scarring rather than regeneration. For this reason, it is desirable to choose the least traumatic surgical instruments and techniques for any surgical procedure. Piezoelectric bone surgery was conceived and developed precisely to overcome the limits of traditional bone-cutting instruments and to achieve the most effective treatment with the least morbidity.

From a mechanical standpoint, the effect of burs or twist drills on bone is characterized by lamellar fracturing in areas adjacent to the cut surface and the deposition of large bone fragments and debris in the endosteal spaces. This finding is thought to be, at least in part, responsible for the inflammatory process that takes place in immediate postsurgical wound healing and for the delay of osteogenesis observed in these wounds. In contrast, the micromechanical cutting action of piezoelectric bone surgery results in micronization of the cut bone and does not cause lamellar fracturing in adjacent bone; this feature

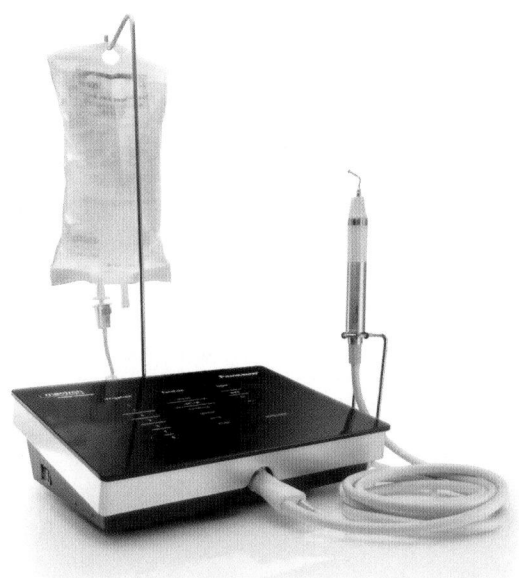

Fig. 83.1 Piezosurgery device by Mectron Medical Technology. *(Courtesy Mectron Medical Technology, Carasco, Italy.)*

may favor exposure and release of bone morphogenetic proteins (BMPs) and be responsible for the early onset of osteogenesis at these sites (see later). Furthermore, the inflammatory response may be diminished because little or no need exists to remove damaged bone and surgical debris as compared with conventional rotary-drilled sites (Fig. 83.2).

KEY FACT

The most compelling characteristics of piezoelectric bone surgery are low surgical trauma, exceptional precision and control, and fast healing. Clinical studies demonstrate that the specificity of operation and the techniques used with piezoelectric bone surgery make it possible to exploit differences in hard and soft tissue anatomy advantageously.

Clinical Characteristics of Ultrasonic Cutting

The primary clinical characteristics of the Piezosurgery cutting action include microprecision, selective cutting, maximum visibility, and excellent healing.

Microprecision

Piezosurgery cuts mineralized tissues with microprecision and extraordinary surgical control. Piezoelectric osteotomies are easy to create, but it is important to recognize that the technique and instrument handling are different from the technique using a traditional handpiece with rotary instruments. The Piezosurgery insert is applied to the bone with a relatively light stroke similar to the smooth precision used to draw a picture. Heavy pressure or force is not required and can, in fact, antagonize the ultrasonic frequency, thus reducing efficiency and transforming mechanical energy into thermal energy (Fig. 83.3). The microprecision of this instrument is made possible by the ultrasonic frequency, which produces mechanical microshock waves at a linear range of approximately 80 µm. The extraordinary surgical control that characterizes Piezosurgery is due to the fact that its microvibrations require only light pressure (approximately 300 g) to be applied to the handpiece. Indeed, the pressure applied

by the surgeon to the Piezosurgery handpiece is much lower than the pressure typically applied to a rotary or oscillating type handpiece (approximately 5000 g), which uses mechanical macrovibrations for cutting. This characteristic provides maximum control during surgery and makes this technique unique, especially in areas with delicate anatomy.

KEY FACT

Heavy pressure or force is not required to operate the piezoelectric bone surgical handpiece. In fact, forceful handling antagonizes the ultrasonic frequency, thus causing a reduction in the cutting efficiency and transforming mechanical energy into thermal energy.

Selective Cutting

Piezosurgery's cutting action is selective because it cuts only mineralized tissues, which are characterized by greater mechanical resistance to the action of the ultrasonic microvibrations. Indeed, the linear motion of the vibrations, which is in the order of approximately 80 µm, is absorbed and dispersed by the elastic nature of soft tissues. These microvibrations are physically unable to cut soft tissue, where

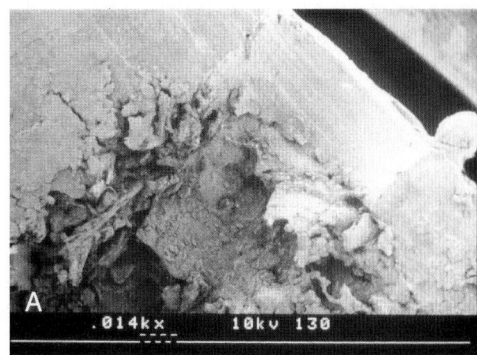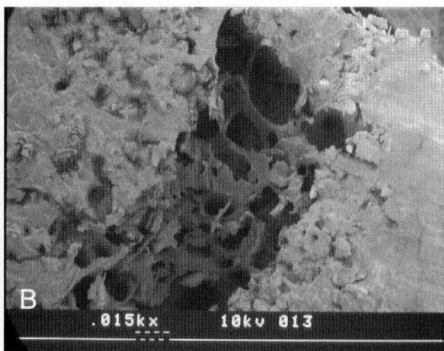

Fig. 83.2 Comparison of bone surfaces prepared with rotary instrumentation and Piezosurgery (Mectron Medical Technology, Carasco, Italy). (A) Rotary technique: in vitro photograph of the implant site following preparation with twist drill of 3.15 mm. The site is ready to receive the implant. Note the compact surface of the cortical bone where no vascular canals are visible. The underlying spongiosa is irregular due to the presence of bone debris in the endosteal spaces. (B) Piezoelectric technique: in vitro image of implant site preparation with 3-mm ultrasonic inserts. The site is ready to receive the implant. Note the cortical bone microporosity where open vascular canals are clearly visible. The underlying spongiosa is intact and free from bone debris. *(Courtesy of Dr. Alberto Rebaudi, Genoa, Italy.)*

BOX 83.2   Description of Piezosurgery Inserts

The mechanical action of bone cutting takes place thanks to the linear microvibrations of inserts with a variable range from 20 to 80 μm, depending on the setting selected. Piezosurgery inserts are classified based on their functional and clinical characteristics.

Functional Classification

Sharp: These inserts have sharp ends for osteotomy and osteoplasty. They are made of nitride titanium steel and are gold in color.

Smoothing: These nitride titanium inserts are diamond coated and gold in color. Their different granulometry produces a smoothing action that is generally used to complete the cut near soft tissue.

Blunt: These steel-colored inserts are characterized by rounded ends and are generally used to refine the cut in contact with soft tissue.

The inserts described in the functional classification as sharp, smoothing, and blunt have clinical classification codes that relate to their specific use.

Clinical Classification

OT: The identification code for inserts used to perform osteotomy is *OT* followed by a number.

OP: The identification code for inserts used to perform osteoplasty is *OP* followed by a number.

EX: The identification code for inserts used to perform extraction is *EX* followed by a number.

IM: The identification code for inserts used to perform implant site preparation is *IM* followed by a number.

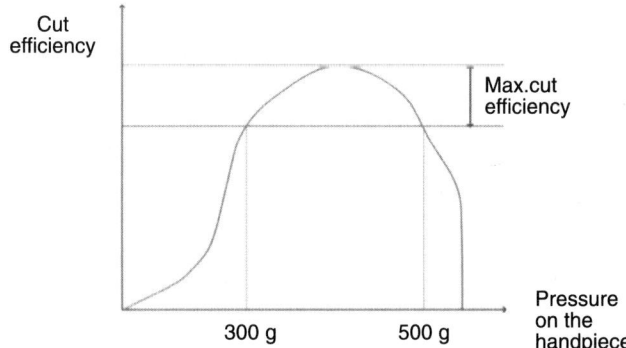

Fig. 83.3 Graph illustrating the relationship between Piezosurgery (Mectron Medical Technology, Carasco, Italy) cutting efficiency and pressure applied on the handpiece. Note that optimal cutting efficiency is found between 300 and 500 g; pressure in excess of 500 g leads to a sudden and complete loss of cutting efficiency. *Max.,* Maximum.

---

cutting dramatically reduces the risk of accidental damage to delicate anatomic structures.

Maximum Visibility

Piezosurgery allows maximum visibility by creating a surgical field that is blood free during cutting because of the cavitation of the cooling irrigation solution. Cavitation is a physical phenomenon that, from a clinical standpoint, happens with the nebulization of the saline solution when it contacts the insert vibrating at ultrasonic frequency. The slight hydropneumatic pressure applied by the nebulized irrigation fluid induces hemostasis in both hard and soft tissues. An important advantage of the cavitation effect is the thorough debridement of the surgical site at the time of the mechanical removal of inflammatory tissue by means of dedicated Piezosurgery inserts. This effect is only temporary, and bleeding resumes shortly after the cutting (and cavitation) action is stopped. Clinically, it is important to ensure proper irrigation and intermittent cutting action to maintain optimal surface microcirculation, especially for long surgical procedures. An added benefit of the temporary hemostasis induced by the cavitation effect is the notably reduced blood loss, especially during longer procedures, which leads to decreased postoperative edema.

kinetic energy is easily dissipated and—when in low dosage—stimulates tissue healing by promoting mitotic divisions (see later). Clearly, the most significant demonstrated benefit of Piezosurgery selective cutting is the ability to preserve the integrity of soft tissues, such as the alveolar nerve, the infraorbital nerve, the maxillary sinus membrane, blood vessels, and the dura mater, while effectively cutting the mineralized tissue (bone) in close proximity to these tissues. A study conducted by Schaeren and colleagues[17] revealed that even prolonged contact for up to 5 seconds between Piezosurgery inserts and a peripheral nerve did not dissect the nerve. Combined with maximum operator control, the safety of Piezosurgery's selective

Excellent Healing

Clinical studies comparing use of piezoelectric bone surgery with traditional rotary instruments for third molar extractions[3,6,18] and periodontal surgery[34] have reported better recovery and fewer postoperative symptoms in patients treated with Piezosurgery. Postoperative healing after piezoelectric bone surgery is characterized by minimal swelling and little bleeding, and the rate of postoperative morbidity is lower compared with traditional techniques.[33]

Improved Hard Tissue Healing

The improved healing response observed at Piezosurgery-treated sites may be explained by the stimulation of healing mechanisms promoted by the device's secondary wave, which operates in the range of 30 to 60 Hz. Indeed, research has shown that the application of low-intensity, high-frequency vibrations in the range of 10 to 50 Hz (i.e., the frequency of postural muscle contractions) to bone tissues mimics mechanical loading and induces the release of several growth factors, including BMPs responsible for osteoblast differentiation and new bone formation.[4,5,23] In an animal study comparing the biomolecular profile of sites prepared with piezoelectric bone surgery or rotary drills, BMP-4 increased earlier at implant sites prepared with piezoelectric bone surgery.[7] As compared with drilled sites, the levels of BMP-4 at Piezosurgery-treated sites were 18.5 times higher at 7 days, 15 times higher at 14 days, and 2 times lower at 56 days. The peak levels of BMP-4 were observed at 14 days for Piezosurgery-treated sites. The level of BMP-4 at drilled sites did not reach the same level of BMP-4 achieved at Piezosurgery-treated sites until day 56. A greater increase in the level of transforming growth factor beta 2 (TGF-β2) was also noted at implant sites prepared with piezoelectric bone surgery techniques. As compared with drilled sites, the levels of TGF-β2 at Piezosurgery-treated sites were 3.5 times higher at 7 days, 19 times higher at 14 days, and diminished below baseline at 56 days. The level of TGF-β2 at drilled sites never exceeded baseline levels.

Proinflammatory cytokine tumor necrosis factor alpha, proinflammatory and bone-resorbing cytokine interleukin-1β (IL-1β), and antiinflammatory cytokine IL-10 were also measured. In general, the expression of these proinflammatory cytokines was higher in the early experimental phases of drilled sites only, which also showed more inflammatory cells. The piezoelectric bone surgery–treated sites showed a higher expression of the proinflammatory and bone-resorbing cytokine IL-1β at 56 days. This last finding may be indicative of bone remodeling at day 56 in piezoelectric bone surgery–treated sites (IL-1β is involved in osteoclast differentiation). The lower expression of inflammatory factors following the application of Piezosurgery may be explained in terms of reduced trauma to the cut tissues compared with the use of rotatory instruments; this reduced trauma is made possible by the technology's microvibrations and lack of friction overheating.

Improved Soft Tissue Healing

Research on a novel application of Piezosurgery to detach the periosteum from underlying bone tissue investigated the effect of this technology on the integrity and healing of mucoperiosteal flaps.[21] Periosteal activation following surgical intervention is responsible for chondrogenesis, osteogenesis, and angiogenesis, which ultimately promote vascularization and bone remodeling. Periosteal healing response following trauma is directly related to the integrity of the periosteum, which provides nourishment to the underlying bone and is essential in osteoinduction and osteoconduction. To ensure proper healing and clinical success, periosteal integrity should therefore be preserved to the maximum extent possible, especially in patients with compromised health. However, the use of manual instrumentation for periosteal elevation has been shown to damage the cells of the osteogenic layer mechanically. Histologically, the periosteum detached with manual elevators shows visible tears, and individual tissue layers are not clearly visible. In contrast, the use of dedicated Piezosurgery inserts specifically designed for periosteal separation from bone was found to be associated with a clean separation of the tissues, with preservation of the outer fibrous layer and the inner cambium layer. Additionally, fat vacuoles and collagenous connective tissue can also be discerned (Fig. 83.4).[21] At the biomolecular level, expression of collagen (II and IV) and osteocalcin in the 8 days following surgery was significantly greater at Piezosurgery-treated sites, thus indicating a more robust healing response. These findings complement the clinical observation that, following piezoelectric bone surgery procedures, gingival tissues show optimal healing and typically appear light in color when compared with the appearance of autogenous gel of platelet-rich plasma.

Clinical Applications

The clinical use of Piezosurgery in osseous surgery advantageously promotes all the benefits of microsurgery, especially when working under optical magnification. Piezosurgery has become an essential instrument in dentistry and in periodontal daily practice to minimize patients' morbidity and increase overall clinical predictability. Piezoelectric bone surgery has many important clinical applications in dentistry. In fact, nearly all techniques previously performed with burs, twist drills, chisels, or oscillating saws have the potential to be performed with Piezosurgery. For 18 consecutive years, one of the authors (T.V.) has used Piezosurgery on a daily basis for oral, periodontal, and implant surgical procedures, thus enabling him to develop techniques and protocols for each. Readers are referred to online materials and other publications for detailed descriptions and step-by-step instructions on these Piezosurgery protocols.[31] A brief overview of basic clinical applications using piezoelectric surgery is described here.

Periodontal Surgery

The use of Piezosurgery in periodontal surgery simplifies and improves both soft and hard tissue management (Table 83.1).[39] In osseous

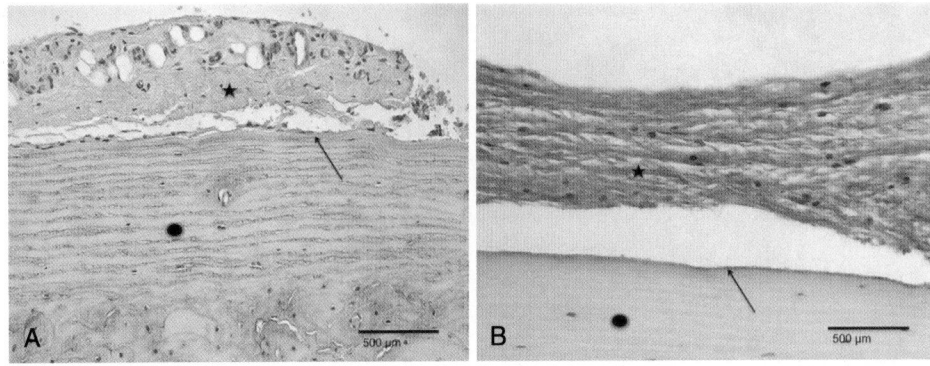

Fig. 83.4 Comparison between periosteal surface elevated with manual instruments and Piezosurgery PR (Mectron Medical Technology, Carasco, Italy) insert tips. (A) Histologic section depicting subperiosteal preparation using manual instrumentation. Note the irregular separation between periosteum *(star)* and bone *(closed circle)* at the boundary between the two layers *(arrow)*. The periosteum shows evidence of mechanical tears. (B) Histologic section showing clear separation between periosteum *(star)* and bone *(closed circle)* at the boundary between the two layers *(arrow)* following preparation with novel piezoelectric inserts. The periosteum is intact and shows no signs of mechanical damage. *(Adapted from Stoetzer M, Magel A, Kampmann A, Lemound J, Gellrich NC, von See C. Subperiosteal preparation using a new piezoelectric device: a histological examination. GMS Interdiscip Plast Reconstr Surg DGPW 3:Doc18, 2014.)*

TABLE 83.1   Piezoelectric Periodontal Surgery Protocol

Management by Tissue Type	Procedure	Inserts Used[a]
Soft Tissue	Soft tissue removal	OP3, PS2, SLC
Hard Tissue		
Bone	Alveolar bone ostectomy	OT13, OT14, OP3, SLC
	Crestal bone osteoplasty	OP3, SLC
	Interproximal osteoplasty	OP4, OP8, OP9
Root	Scaling	PS2
	Debridement	OP5, OP5A
	Planing	PP1

[a]Piezosurgery, Mectron Medical Technology, Carasco, Italy.

resective periodontal surgery, piezoelectric bone surgery represents a notable evolution from the past because it allows the application of concepts of bone microsurgery. In periodontal soft tissue management, after raising the primary flap with a traditional technique, it is easier to detach the secondary flap and remove inflammatory granulation tissue by using a scaler-shaped insert (Piezosurgery insert PS2) (Fig. 83.5A) or an insert in the shape of a rounded scalpel (Piezosurgery insert OP3). Contrary to traditional manual techniques, this phase has little bleeding and better visibility as the result of the cavitation of the saline solution (coolant). Hard tissue management is also improved: with the proper inserts and power mode, the ultrasound device facilitates effective scaling, debridement, and root planing (see Fig. 83.5B and C). In particular, debridement with special diamond-coated inserts enables thorough cleaning even for interproximal bone defects, which can therefore be remodeled into even surfaces (see Fig. 83.5D). The mechanical action of ultrasonic microvibrations, together with cavitation of the irrigation fluid (pH neutral; isotonic saline solution) eliminates bacteria, toxins, dead cells, and debris, thus creating clean physiology for healing of the wound. Healing is improved by applying ultrasound to produce micropits at the base of the defect to activate cellular response of healing mechanisms. In hard tissue management, the ostectomy maneuver with Piezosurgery is extremely precise and does not pose any risk of damaging the root surface. Typically, to avoid damaging

the radicular cementum, conventional ostectomy techniques are incomplete and leave residual "widow's peaks" that require manual removal using hand chisels. When using Piezosurgery for resective procedures, because it is possible to work on the root surface without damaging it, it is possible to perform thorough ostectomies that do not leave behind more than "micro" widow's peaks. These minimal formations are easily removed when using the final insert for root planing procedures (Piezosurgery insert PP1). When working on reshaping the crestal bone surface, the osteoplasty maneuver at low irrigation allows collecting autogenous particulate bone that can be immediately grafted into small bony defects (see Fig. 83.5E). The use of this technology not only reduces the invasiveness of traditional surgery by making it faster and by ensuring thorough cleaning of the periodontium, but it also favors tissue healing by using bone removed in the osteoplasty procedure to graft small osseous defects, thus preserving bone architecture.

CLINICAL CORRELATION

The clinical use of Piezosurgery in osseous surgery advantageously promotes all the benefits of microsurgery, especially when working under optical magnification. It simplifies and improves both soft and hard tissue management.

It is our opinion that Piezosurgery in periodontal surgery can redefine the guidelines that mark the border between resective treatment and regenerative treatment. Indeed, the choice between a resective technique and a regenerative technique generally depends on the depth of the bone defect, whether it is more or less than 3.5 mm. Thanks to piezoelectric bone surgery, defects greater than 3.5 mm can now be grafted with particulate bone and covered with resorbable membranes.

The ability to work on the bone defect under magnification (e.g., surgical microscope) makes it possible to exploit the benefits of Piezosurgery microprecision in preparing the recipient site and stabilizing micrografts (see Fig. 83.5F to H).

Crown Lengthening

Clinical crown lengthening is the most common periodontal surgical (ostectomy) operation performed in otherwise healthy periodontal

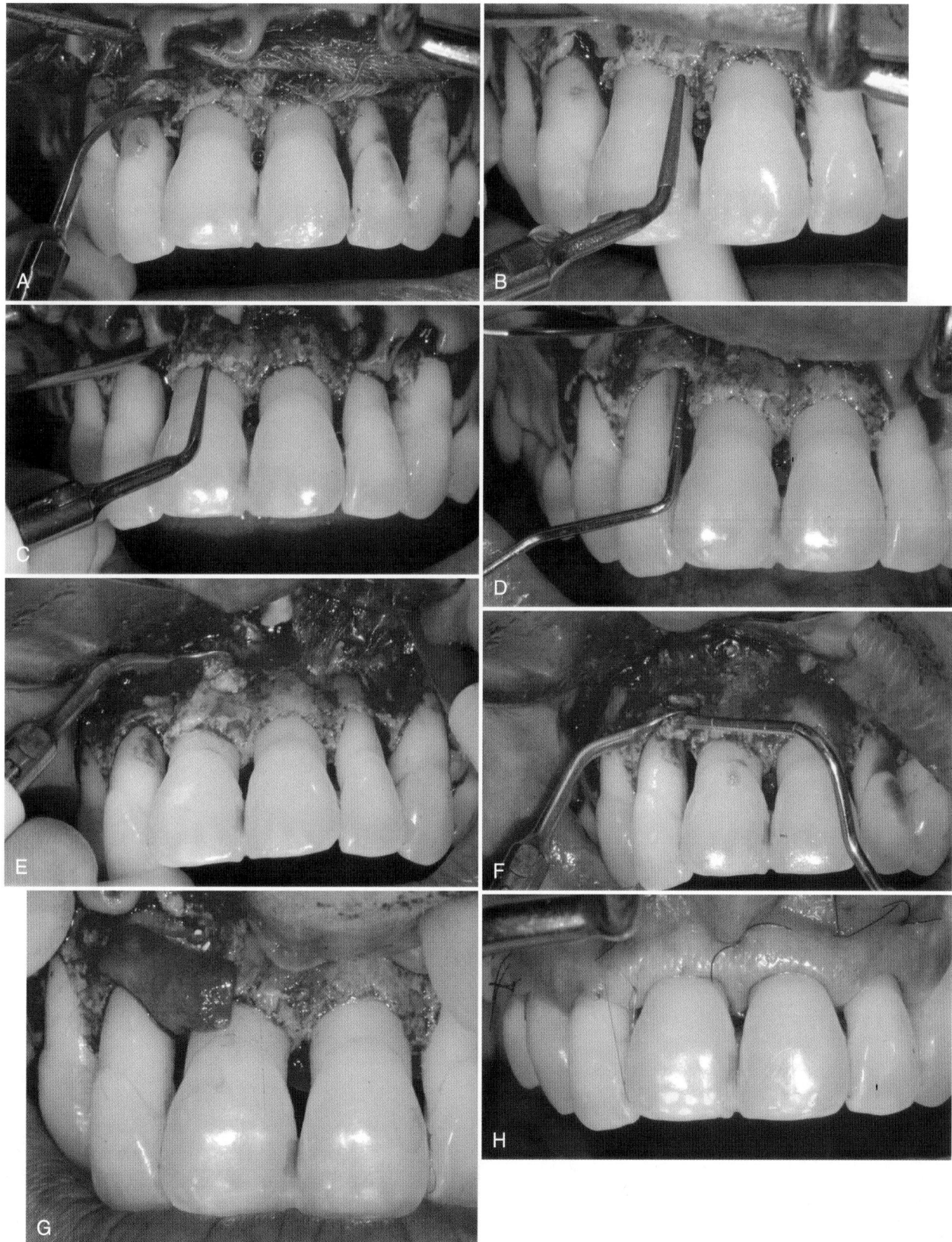

Fig. 83.5 Clinical case demonstrating the use of piezoelectric bone surgery for periodontal surgery. (A) Ultrasonic scaling using Piezosurgery PS2 insert (Mectron Medical Technology, Carasco, Italy). (B) Root surface debridement using Piezosurgery diamond-coated OP5 insert. (C) Ultrasonic root planing using Piezosurgery blunt insert PP1. (D) Interproximal infrabony defect with probe. (E) Autogenous bone chip–harvesting technique using Piezosurgery osteoplasty insert OP3. (F) Autogenous bone-grafting technique. (G) Collagen membrane stabilizing microbone grafting. (H) Flap repositioned and sutured.

conditions. The indication for this procedure is usually associated with a need or desire to expose more tooth structure because of short clinical crowns and/or loss of clinical tooth structure. In general, the goal is to reposition the periodontal bone and soft tissues to a more apical position with appropriate biologic dimensions to avoid periodontal inflammation after tooth restoration.

The clinical crown lengthening technique entails performing a periradicular ostectomy of a few millimeters (1 to 2 mm) combined with an osteoplasty technique to allow for repositioning of the periodontal flap in a more apical position with favorable periodontal tissue architecture. The positive result obtained is that the health of the treated part is preserved even though the normal gingival morphology is altered. Clinical application must include aesthetic assessment, as well as an assessment of the position and health of the adjacent periodontium.

The traditional surgical technique entails raising of a full-thickness flap, ostectomy with manual instruments, osteoplasty with a bur for crest bone architecture recontouring, periradicular bone removal, root planing, and, finally, replacing the flap in an apical position.

The ostectomy is simple to perform using Piezosurgery in direct contact with the root surface because control of the instrument during surgery is precise, even in very difficult proximity cases (Piezosurgery OP3 insert). The root planing phase can be performed very effectively using blunt ultrasonic inserts (Piezosurgery PP1 insert).

Saline solution cavitation reduces bleeding during surgery and facilitates debridement of the surgical area. This effect is likely responsible for the excellent soft tissue healing result, which is always characterized by a light color and the absence of edema.

A histologic animal study conducted at Harvard University in Cambridge, Massachusetts, showed a better healing response for bone and root cementum in teeth that were crown lengthened using Piezosurgery as compared with teeth that were crown lengthened with traditional rotary instruments.[36] Concerning the latter, the tungsten carbide bur was found to be more favorable than the diamond-coated bur for the bone-healing process.

The crown lengthening technique performed with Piezosurgery using appropriate inserts makes it possible to reduce bone effectively while preserving root surface integrity.

Tooth Extraction

Today, tooth extraction is considered the first step in the preparation for implant placement. Maintaining the integrity of the alveolar bone walls is an essential part of this process. Consequently, whether an implant is being placed at the time of extraction or not, the selection of instruments and techniques that minimize trauma to socket walls is critical.

Anatomic differences greatly influence the difficulty of extraction and the challenge of maintaining alveolar bone walls. A newer periodontal classification for dental extractions has been developed (Table 83.2) that makes it easier to choose the best surgical tooth extraction technique for different anatomic situations (Table 83.3).[37] The aim is always to preserve the integrity of the alveolar walls and the morphology of soft tissue. This classification divides anatomy into four types depending on the anatomic characteristics of periodontal biotype and anatomy or pathology of the periodontal ligament. Classifying anatomy into type 1, 2, 3, or 4 simplifies the diagnostic process and the subsequent surgical decision. Each type corresponds to a different anatomic issue, which requires a specific extraction technique and determines the most effective surgical instruments.

Type 1 anatomy describes a normal periodontal biotype and a normal periodontal ligament (i.e., no pathologic features). This anatomic condition poses little surgical difficulty. A traditional extraction technique using manual instruments is sufficient.

TABLE 83.2　Periodontal Classification for Dental Extraction

Periodontal Biotype Thickness	Periodontal Ligament	Diagnosis	Anatomic Classification
Normal	Normal	Normal	Type 1
Thin	Normal	Thin	Type 2
Normal	Ankylotic	Ankylotic	Type 3
Thin	Ankylotic	Thin and ankylotic	Type 4

TABLE 83.3　Root Extraction Surgical Classification by Tomaso Vercellotti

Anatomic Classification	Periodontal Diagnosis	Tissue Damage Risk	Surgery Difficulty	Technique	Maneuver	Surgical Instrument	Piezosurgery[a] Insert
Type 1	Normal	Low	Easy	Standard	Periotomy External Luxation Removal	Periotome Elevator Forceps	
Type 2	Thin	High	Medium	Advanced	Periotomy Root sectioning Internal luxation Removal	Periotome Piezosurgery Elevator Forceps	OT7S-3, EX1-3, OP5
Type 3	Ankylotic	Low	Complex	Advanced	Periotomy Rootplasty External luxation Removal	Periotome Piezosurgery Elevator Forceps	OT7S-3, EX1-3, OP5
Type 4	Thin and ankylotic	Very high	Severe	Advanced	Periotomy Root resection and rootplasty Internal luxation Removal	Periotome Piezosurgery Elevator Forceps	OT7S-3, EX1-3, OP5

[a]Mectron Medical Technology, Carasco, Italy.

Type 2 anatomy describes a thin periodontal biotype with a normal periodontal ligament. The surgical difficulty for tooth removal is minimal. However, preserving the integrity of the thin alveolar buccal walls makes the extraction more complex. In this situation, the normal displacement operation runs the risk of creating a dehiscence from fracturing the thin buccal cortical plate. To avoid this risk, it is recommended that the surgeon use a root fractioning technique that makes it possible to obtain root mobility inside the alveolus to eliminate the risk of damaging the thin labial and crestal bone is recommended.

Type 3 anatomy describes a normal periodontal biotype with an ankylotic periodontal ligament. The surgical difficulty for tooth removal is high because it is not possible to obtain the mobility necessary for displacement. The traditional technique uses a periradicular osteotomy with burs. This is possible without much consequence for mandibular third molars but often results in serious damage to the buccal alveolar walls. The recommended technique creates the space necessary for extraction by operating only on the root surface through a rootplasty maneuver. The tooth is removed from the socket by consuming the root surface without touching the alveolar bone. This technique is easy to perform with excellent control using specific Piezosurgery inserts (OP5), used like a bur around the root (eFig. 83.1).

Type 4 anatomy describes a thin periodontal biotype and an ankylotic periodontal ligament, which is a combination of the challenging aspects of type 2 and type 3 anatomy. The surgical difficulty for tooth removal is the highest. In all cases where aesthetics is important, a root-sectioning technique that divides the root into segments with a mesiodistal cut is recommended. This allows the separate pieces (e.g., buccal and palatal) to be removed internal to the socket with minimal force applied just to the mesiodistal socket walls.

To ensure success of the procedure, it is important for the clinician to master the proper technique to perform extractions with Piezosurgery. As in all other procedures, inserts must never be allowed to rest in one single place when the ultrasonic vibration is active. This is particularly important when working in the periodontal ligament space. To avoid pinching of the insert and consequently having the ultrasonic vibration converted into thermal energy, it is important to keep the insert constantly moving.

Implant Site Preparation

Special Piezosurgery inserts developed for bone perforation have enabled the development of a newer technique for ultrasonic implant site preparation (UISP). Extensive clinical experience has culminated in the development of a protocol with significant clinical advantages. One article described the protocol in detail and reported the results of a multicenter case series study analyzing 3579 implants with a 1- to 3-year follow-up.[41] The preliminary results indicated that implant site preparation with Piezosurgery is a valid alternative to preparation with conventional rotary instrumentation, with an overall osseointegration percentage of 97.82% (97.14% maxilla, 98.75% mandible) and an overall implant survival rate of 97.74% (96.99% maxilla, 98.75% mandible). These results are extremely encouraging, especially considering that implant placement was often combined with bone regenerative techniques. Given certain specific advantages of UISP, it is preferable to conventional techniques in the presence of soft bone and limited residual volume, as well as in proximity to delicate anatomic structures such as the inferior alveolar nerve or the schneiderian membrane.

The first advantage of UISP is related to the cutting characteristics of Piezosurgery, which facilitate differential preparation of the cortical and cancellous bone. A surgical classification system of bone quality at the implant site was developed that simplifies the diagnosis and

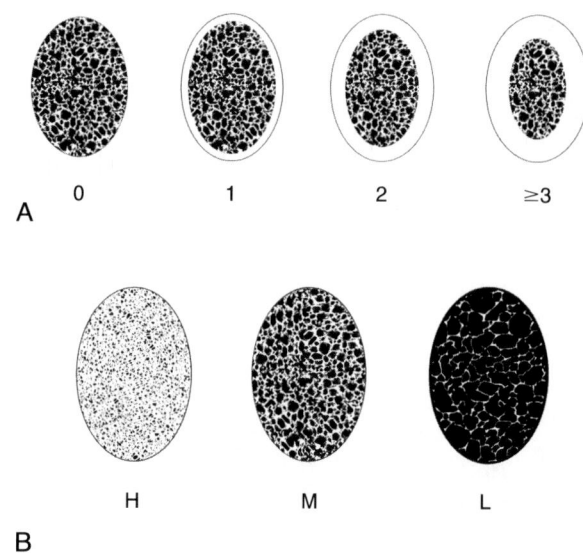

Fig. 83.6 Surgical bone classification by Tomaso and Giuseppe Vercellotti. (A) Cortical crestal thickness in millimeters. (B) Radiographic cancellous bone classification *H,* High; *L,* low; *M,* medium.

surgical decision-making process by exploiting differences in bone anatomy (Fig. 83.6). The differential implant site preparation (DISP) technique can be used within the initial osteotomy site to correct the implant axis by selectively directing the cutting action in the desired direction.[30] DISP can also be used in combination with twist drills to facilitate preservation of alveolar crestal bone while achieving maximum primary stability.[42]

The second advantage of UISP is the fast clinical healing of both soft and hard tissue. Animal research demonstrates that new bone formation (neo-osteogenesis) is active at implant sites prepared with piezoelectric bone surgery earlier than at sites prepared with traditional techniques.[7] A histomorphometric study on mini-pigs showed more bone formation and a greater density of periimplant osteoblasts at implant sites prepared with Piezosurgery as compared with sites prepared with twist drills.[7] Clinically, the minimally invasive nature of the surgery and the stimulation of bone healing translate into better primary stability and likely faster osseointegration compared with conventional instrumentation. In a randomized controlled clinical trial, patients received two identical adjacent implants in the upper premolar area: the test site was prepared with Piezosurgery, and the control site was prepared using twist drills.[19] Resonance frequency analysis (RFA) measurements were taken by a blinded operator on the day of surgery and at scheduled intervals throughout the first 90 days postoperatively. At the end of this time period, following failure of one implant in the control group, 97.5% of implants were osseointegrated. An initial decrease in mean implant stability quotient (ISQ) values was observed in both groups; however, the decrease in the Piezosurgery group was significantly less than in the control group. The Piezosurgery group also exhibited an earlier stability level reversal, indicating that an overall achievement of better primary stability compared with implants placed with twist drills. The surgical technique entails an osteotomy preparation using a series of Piezosurgery inserts. The preparation is initiated with the narrow, pointed IM1 insert (Fig. 83.7A). Parallel pins are used throughout the procedure to check alignment (see Fig. 83.7B). The 2-mm–diameter IM2 insert is used to prepare the osteotomy further (see Fig. 83.7C). The coronal aspect of the preparation is widened with the pilot 2/3 insert (see Fig. 83.7D), and the osteotomy is finished with the IM3 insert (see Fig. 83.7E). Final cortical preparation is accomplished

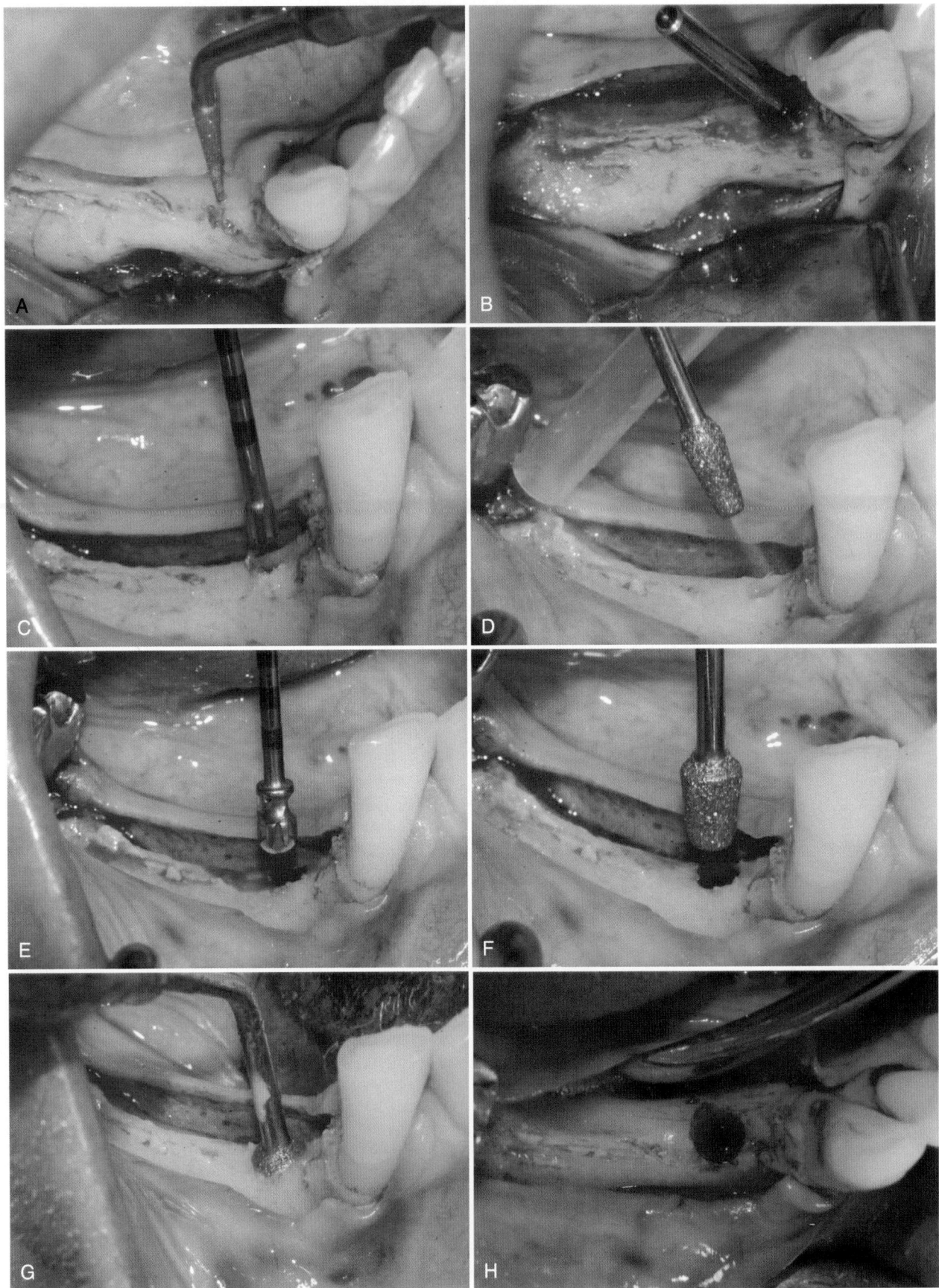

Fig. 83.7 Implant site preparation and placement. (A) Piezosurgery insert (IM1) used to start the implant site preparation (Mectron Medical Technology, Carasco, Italy). (B) Parallel pin in place to check the direction of osteotomy. (C) Piezosurgery 2-mm–diameter insert (IM2) for pilot osteotomy. (D) Piezosurgery insert for cortical preparation (pilot 2/3). (E) Cancellous bone preparation with Piezosurgery insert IM3. (F) Piezosurgery diamond-coated insert (IM4) for final cortical bone preparation. (G) Piezosurgery pilot insert 3/4 in action. (H) Occlusal view of completed implant site preparation.

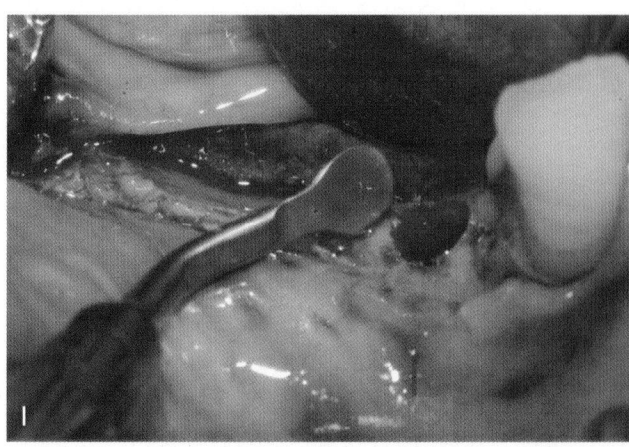
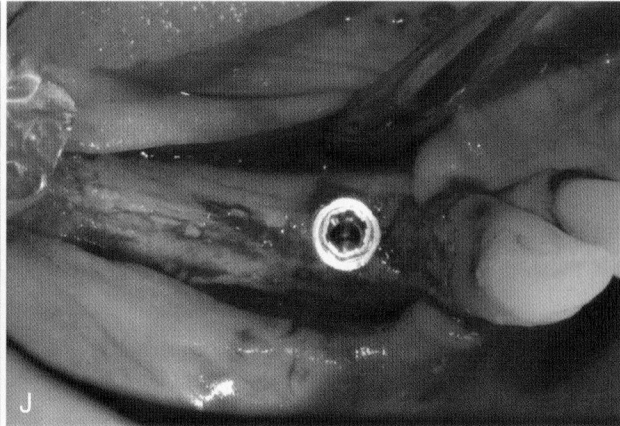

Fig. 83.7, cont'd (I) Osteoplasty of crestal bone in the peri-implant area using Piezosurgery insert OP3. (J) Occlusal view of well-placed implant despite the narrow ridge.

with the IM4 insert (see Fig. 83.7F). After use of the pilot 3/4 insert (Fig. 83.7G), the implant osteotomy is completed (see Fig. 83.7H). If desired, before implant placement, osteoplasty of the crestal bone is possible with the OP3 insert (see Fig. 83.7I). Fig. 83.7J shows a final occlusal view of an implant placed in a narrow ridge.

Conclusion

Piezoelectric bone surgery is a well-known surgical technique for bone surgery with many clinical applications in dentistry. The extraordinary cutting properties and applications of piezoelectric bone surgery are described in this chapter. The most compelling characteristics of piezoelectric bone surgery are low surgical trauma, exceptional precision, and fast healing response. As a result, Piezosurgery has the ability to increase treatment effectiveness while improving postoperative recovery and healing.

Although a great deal of scientific research focuses on new products for tissue engineering and bone regeneration, the importance of minimal surgical trauma for optimal bone healing and regeneration should not be overlooked. A new appreciation for the effectiveness of Piezosurgery has the potential to redefine the concept of minimally invasive surgery in osteotomy and osteoplasty procedures.

 Case Scenarios are found on the companion website www.expertconsult.com.

References

 References for this chapter are found on the companion website www.expertconsult.com.

CHAPTER 84

Digitally Assisted Implant Surgery

Daniel H. Etienne | *Raymond R. Derycke* | *Perry R. Klokkevold*

CHAPTER OUTLINE

Digitally Assisted Implant Surgery
Conclusion

 For online-only content on technical principles and limitations and on system risk analysis, please visit the companion website at www.expertconsult.com.

The surgical procedures for the placement of implants have more or less remained the same since the introduction of osseointegrated dental implants. Briefly, implant placement surgery involves the elevation of a full-thickness flap to expose bone; a sequential series of drills with increasing diameters is used with profuse irrigation to prepare a precise implant site osteotomy in the bone (see Chapter 78). The site is prepared, and the implant is positioned in a manner that avoids important anatomic structures, such as the inferior alveolar nerve, sinus cavities, and teeth. The ultimate goal is to position the implant for optimal functional support of the planned prosthetic tooth replacement(s) with proper emergence and natural aesthetics.

Clinicians determine implant positions based on presurgical diagnostic imaging, study models, and the use of a diagnostic wax-up of the planned tooth replacement(s). The final position of the implant(s) results from the surgeon's interpretation of diagnostic information and his or her ability to translate that information to the patient at the time of surgery. A conventional surgical "guide" is typically an acrylic stent, fabricated by a laboratory technician, that is positioned in the mouth and used to direct drills through openings in proposed tooth sites. It may or may not have precise guide channels for implant positioning. The clinician uses the guide along with his or her interpretation of diagnostic information, clinical experience, and surgical skills to place the implant(s). The use of a conventional surgical guide has several limitations and potential sources of error, including inaccuracies in the stent during fabrication, movement of the stent during surgery, and variations in the clinician's use of the stent, which can lead to imprecise implant positioning.

Advances in implant surgical technology include simulation software, computer-generated surgical guides, and real-time digital tracking or guidance.

- Implant planning or simulation software is used preoperatively with the patient's scan data to "simulate" implant placement into a virtual patient. The software allows the clinician to view a three-dimensional (3D) computer image of the patient's jaw created from the computed tomography (CT) or cone beam CT (CBCT) scan data.[46]
- Computer-generated surgical guides with drill sleeves are produced using various techniques from the presurgical "virtual" implant placement data. These guides are used to place implants more accurately based on the "planned" locations.[18,28,38]

- Digitally assisted implant surgery or real-time micro positioning implant surgery (RTMIS) uses simultaneous tracking and "guidance" of the implant instrumentation to follow the planned treatment accurately during surgery.[10] Computer imaging from scan data is observed interactively with implant placement instrumentation during the surgical procedure.

This chapter provides an overview of the terminology, technical requirements, and limitations of digitally assisted implant surgery.

Digitally Assisted Implant Surgery

Real-Time Micro Positioning Implant Surgery: Overview

RTMIS is the most sophisticated and perhaps the most promising of these technologies because it has the greatest potential to reduce surgical time, minimize surgical invasiveness, and result in a more precise translation of implant planning to the actual surgical procedure.[6,22,45] However, as with many newer technologies, conflicting reports regarding its accuracy exist.[24,42] The computerized surgical and prosthetic chain of treatment requires precision at many levels.[33]

Uses and Requirements

Computerized navigation surgery evolved from early applications in neurosurgical procedures and continues to evolve today with applications in many surgical specialties.[36,39] Clearly, the principal advantage of using a computer to assist surgery is the precision it offers. Moreover, real-time safety control is obtained with multiple imaging sources facilitating a minimally invasive approach to surgical procedures. As in medicine, 3D imaging is used in dentistry to facilitate presurgical planning and to guide the surgical procedure. In the case of implant surgery, this allows precise implant positioning while avoiding injury to nearby important anatomic structures. Computers have been used to enhance dental implant surgery in a variety of ways, from simple imaging software used to visualize implant positions in a 3D virtual patient to more complex, simultaneous image monitoring and instrument navigation used to perform the surgery.[10,19]

As an example, the aerospace industry uses computer assembling software with augmented reality and real-time stock management to reduce complete assembly time of an Airbus A350 aircraft by

30%.[20,21] Similarly, in dentistry, the goals of computer-assisted implant placement are to reduce surgical time, enhance precision, and facilitate prosthetic treatment by combining real-time surgical navigation with computer-aided design (CAD) and computer-aided manufacturing (CAM).

The European Commission (EC) has established a Global Medical Device Nomenclature and an internationally agreed-on classification system for medical devices with four classes from low risk to high risk. The Food and Drug Administration (FDA) in the United States has a Unique Device Identification for the registration of medical devices with three classes from low to middle and high risks.

- Class 1 medical devices are deemed low risk and are therefore subject to the least regulatory control. They do not need to be evaluated by a certified body. In dentistry, a computer-generated surgical guide is considered a class 1 medical device. Regulation committees do not categorize it as an assisting device.
- Class 2 medical devices are a higher risk than class 1. The EC class 2 is subdivided into class 2A and class 2B, where 2A is an assisting device without automation and 2B is a device with automatic assisting. Real-time micro positioning (RTM) device is a class 2 FDA or class 2A EC. In contrast to a class 1 medical device, a class 2 or 2A medical device must show innovation and improvement of a clinician's decision making and offer new evidence of benefit to the patient.

The use of RTMIS requires an accurate alignment (identification and registration) of the patient anatomy with the patient's volumetric data obtained from radiographic imaging (CT scan, CBCT data) and through a tracking system with a 3D contact probe or ultrasound 3D mapping (Fig. 84.1). The system allows matching between imaging and real patient positions, and it permits tracking of the precise movements of the surgical instrumentation (e.g., handpiece, drills) in relation to the actual patient. Various modalities have been developed to acquire and register image data and to coordinate and track movements.[6]

Sequence of Steps

The clinical sequence of steps (Fig. 84.2) required for conventional RTMIS is as follows:

1. *Data acquisition.* The patient is scanned for image data acquisition with fiducial (artificial) radiographic markers (e.g., stent with markers or intentionally placed pins or screws into jaw) or anatomic (natural) markers such as teeth or bony landmarks. If fiducial markers are placed in a stent, the patient must have the stent in place when scanned.
2. *Identification.* The anatomic or fiducial markers are identified with a probe tracked by the system. If markers were incorporated into a radiographic stent, the stent will again be placed in the mouth, and the markers will be identified by hand with a probe tracked by the stereovision system.
3. *Registration.* After identification of the predetermined markers, the software indicates the best localization or "match" on the arch between the image data and the patient. An invalidated registration may be caused by an improper initialization or CT scan data.
4. *Navigation.* Ultimately, the operator is able to visualize surgical instrument navigation (movement). The drilling instruments are guided to a target point of impact with a 3D spatial orientation.
5. *Accuracy.* Sustained accuracy procedures are critical during surgery and should prove the reliability of the system's overall accuracy. This sustained accuracy procedure is completed by contacting the handpiece or drill on selected teeth while visualizing markers, which can be viewed by the stereovision system.

ASSISTING DATA CHAIN

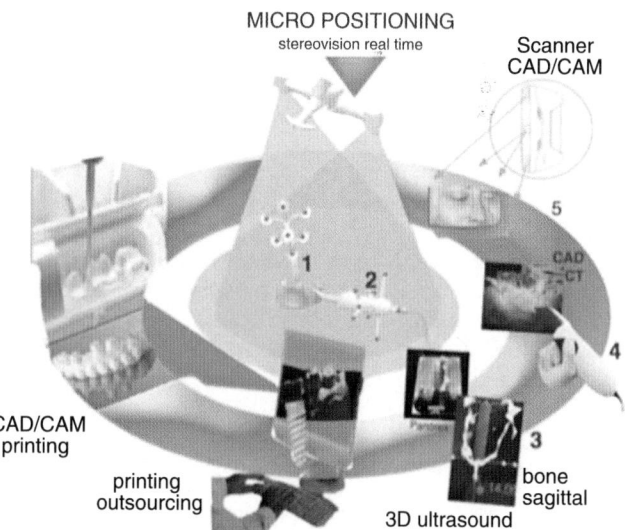

Fig. 84.2 Assisting data chain with real-time micro positioning implant surgery. The basic setup for a navigation system consists of stereovision cameras with several tools: *(1)* infrared receptor allows real-time patient tracking; *(2)* the contra-angle probe and the ultrasound probe have markers that are tracked in real time by the cameras; *(3)* ultrasound three-dimensional *(3D)* mapping shows bone surface and adjacent root morphology; *(4)* computer-aided design and computer-aided manufacturing *(CAD/CAM)* registered with ultrasound and computed tomography *(CT)* scan; and *(5)* extraoral scanning for matching other 3D imaging.

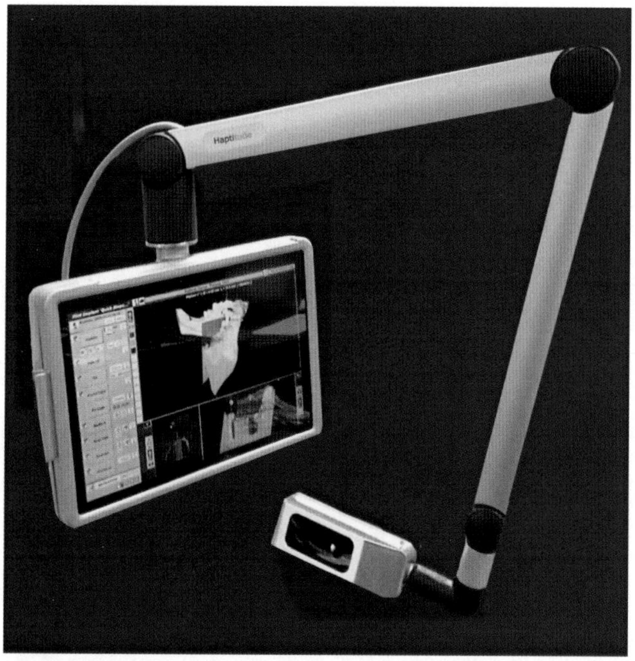

Fig. 84.1 Dental implant real-time navigation system (Open Pilot System, Stereovision Haptitude) with infrared stereovision cameras and a monitor display showing the three-dimensional ultrasonic reconstruction of a mandible with the planed implant position in a coronal and a panoramic view. On the panoramic view, a two-dimensional x-ray film is overlaid on the ultrasonic image. *(Courtesy Haptitude.)*

6. *Feedback.* Variations from the ideal position can be restricted by the software through inactivation of the drill (stop-and-go action) or by an audible or visual cue.

KEY FACT

Real-time micro positioning implant surgery requires an accurate alignment of the patient's anatomy with the patient's volumetric data from radiographic imaging (computed tomography scan, cone beam computed tomography data). A tracking system with a three-dimensional contact probe or ultrasound three-dimensional mapping is used for identification and registration.

Data Acquisition and Registration

CT scans and CBCT scans are widely used for 3D imaging of patients (see Chapter 76). Factors that must be considered when deciding to use a CT scan include radiation exposure, limitations in accuracy, and the possibility of diffracted images as a result of metallic restorations. The evolution of scanner technology (spiral CT scan, CBCT scan) has made it possible to reduce the radiation dose to the level of a conventional panoramic radiograph while maintaining adequate diagnostic quality for preoperative implant planning.[11,15]

Radiographically identifiable markers are important for RTMIS just as they are for implant planning with conventional diagnostic methods. However, unlike conventional planning, in which orientation and simulation of implant positions are related to the planned prosthetic crown positions, RTM markers must relate the image data to the actual patient's anatomy. In other words, the position of the surgical instrumentation (and ultimately the drills and the implant) must be related to the scan image data of the patient's jaw morphology and the image data must be precisely aligned with the actual patient's anatomy. Thus, it is critically important to scan the patient with markers that are identified in the scan and correlated with the patient. Correlation between the scan and the patient's markers is called *registration*. This process is a statistical matching from point to point, point to surface, or surface to surface. CBCT scans present less diffraction with metal, and registration is easier than with CT scans.

A 3D localization of the template is made with different methods of registration. The operator contacts the marker on the template with an instrument that is seen by the system camera. RTM data are obtained when these markers are attached to the patient.

The operator needs to validate whether the template and the patient are correlated in a true position because deviations may result due to mathematic formulations of the data in the registration process. This critical step is used to control the accuracy of the patient's position. In the absence of a template, anatomic markers such as teeth or specific bony landmarks and/or artificial markers (fiducial) such as small tacks or screws that are secured in the bone can be used. The operator checks the accuracy with a pointer instrument that has its own markers used to touch different sites of the mouth. The precision is visualized by localization of the images on the screen and the real position of the instrument in the patient's mouth.

KEY FACT

The orientation of surgical instrumentation (i.e., drills) must be related to the scan image data of the patient's jaw morphology, and the image data must be precisely aligned with the actual patient's anatomy. The critically important correlation between scan data and the actual patient is called *registration*. Markers in the scan are matched with markers in the patient by using a point-to-point, point-to-surface, or surface-to-surface method.

Navigation and Positional Tracking

Numerous commercial products exist for navigation or positional tracking, but few meet the *computer-aided surgery* (CAS) requirements in terms of accuracy[8,48] (approximately 0.1 mm at a distance of 1 m[4]), reliability, and clinical usability. The "real-time" navigational technology is based on global positioning system technology.[41] Some of the technologies used in medical CAS to track movement include mechanical, magnetic, and optical tracking systems.

Mechanical tracking systems use a six-axis coding robot with a passive arm. The system is very reliable and highly accurate but has limitations when more than one instrument or patient marker needs to be located. Thus mechanical tracking is less desirable for implant CAS, which requires the use of several different instruments and multiple markers.

Magnetic tracking systems use a magnetic source and a field receiver. The system loses accuracy in the presence of magnetic field interference. Relative inaccuracies result from changes in the magnetic field, which may be caused by any metallic mass that may be present, such as a drill motor (with or without activation).[3,4] Thus the obligatory presence of drill motors in the operating room during implant surgery makes magnetic trackers impractical for implant CAS.

Optical tracking systems are recognized for their dependability and accuracy. Positioning is made by intersecting the vision plane between two or three cameras to locate markers with stereovision. A passive system absorbs and processes ambient light, whereas an active system interprets reflected light.

Active markers with infrared light–emitting diodes (IREDs) have been widely used with superb accuracy but are sensitive to reflections and interference with the line of sight between the IRED markers and the cameras.[25,31] Although variations in optical localizers are adequate for medical applications,[1,12] they need to be improved for use in dental implant surgery. This is particularly problematic with the typical seating arrangement of surgeon and assistant (i.e., the direct line of sight to the cameras may be interrupted by the operators). A stereovision with natural-light cameras is a less expensive alternative compared with IREDs. However, natural-light systems are more sensitive to surrounding light, background, and the shape of markers. In comparison, infrared cameras are less sensitive to these light variations.

With optical tracking devices, the surrounding light in the operating room is important, and the choice of an infrared tracking device is more relevant. Patients' motion will be tracked efficiently if the marker is stable during surgery. In case of loose teeth or unstable markers, cortical bone screws should be used.

External Viewer, Augmented Reality, and Three-Dimensional Projection Screens

Once registration between the data and the actual patient has been established, the instrumentation can be coordinated with the system and observed by the surgeon or operator (Figs. 84.3 and 84.4). Instrument movement relative to the image data (and through registration to the patient) may be viewed on an external monitor, visually projected in the surgeon's field of vision (resulting in a superimposed visual image seen over the surgical field) by using a head-mounted projection system or projected on a 3D projection screen (Fig. 84.5).[47] In this manner, the image on the external monitor (see Fig. 84.4), the surgical field, or the 3D projection screen (Fig. 84.6) guides the surgeon to perform the planned procedure.

Side viewers display target data in two dimensions and require the surgeon to look away from the surgical field. However, see-through viewers display target data transparently in the surgeon's field of

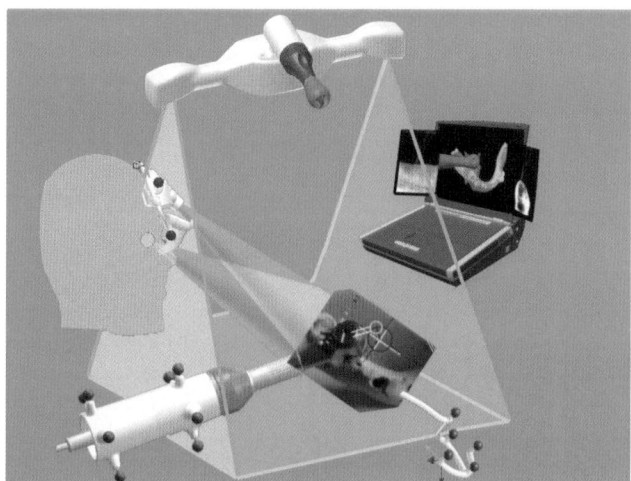

Fig. 84.3 Global setup for surgical navigation. The basic setup for a navigation system consists of stereovision cameras with several tools. The contra-angle probe, the ultrasound probe, and the patient jig need to have markers, which are tracked by the cameras. The occlusal stent, with markers in the standard process and without markers in ultrasound registration, used during computed tomography scan acquisition will be recognized in its three dimensions for prosthetic planning.

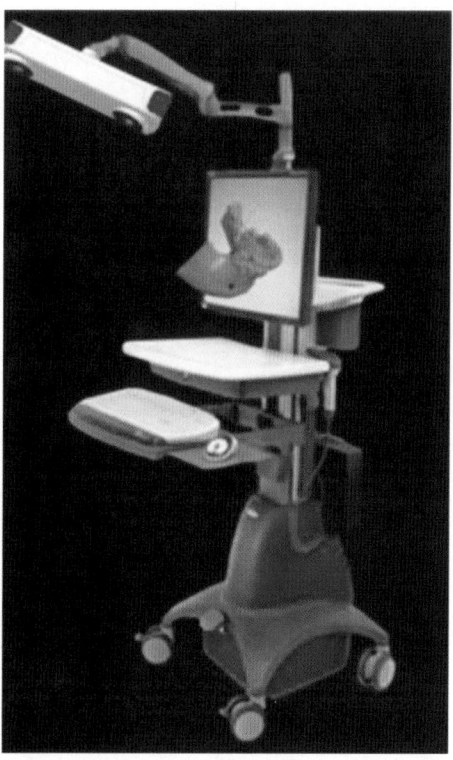

Fig. 84.5 Dental implant real-time navigation system with infrared stereovision cameras and a three-dimensional monitor display showing the reconstruction of a computed tomography–scanned mandible.

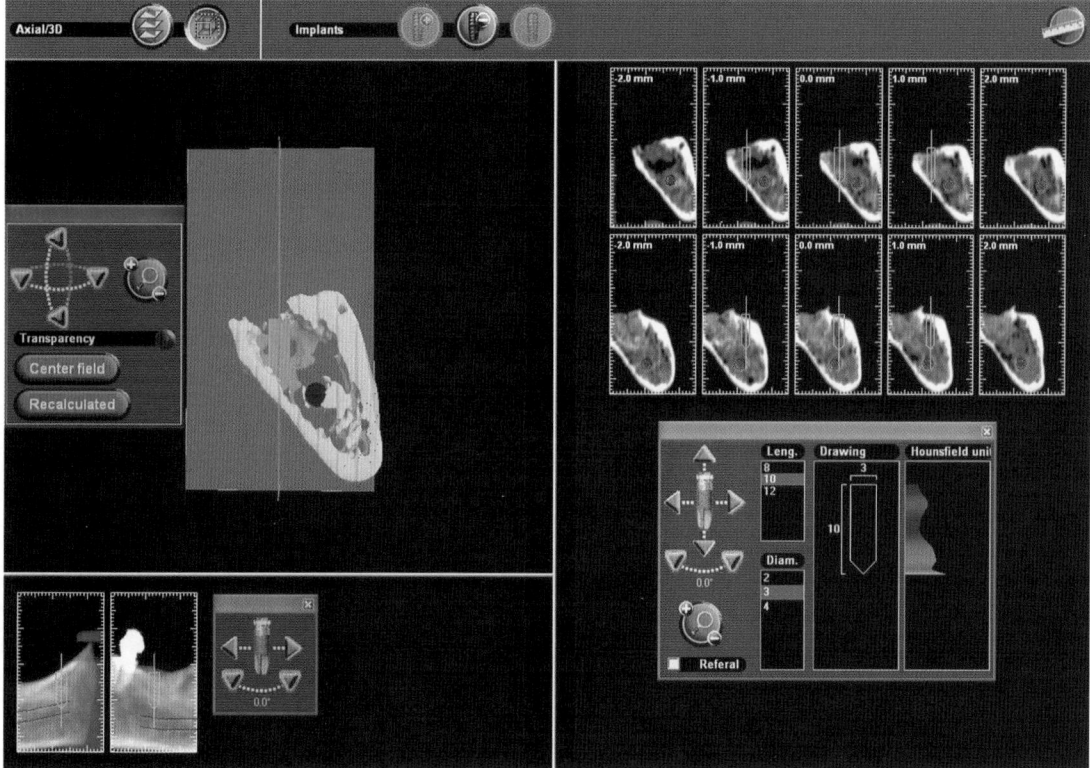

Fig. 84.4 Images of a computer screen and the surgeon's view of computer-aided implant surgery navigation simulated with a dry mandible. During navigation, the surgeon concentrates on visual cues seen on the eye viewer. *(Courtesy Haptitude.)*

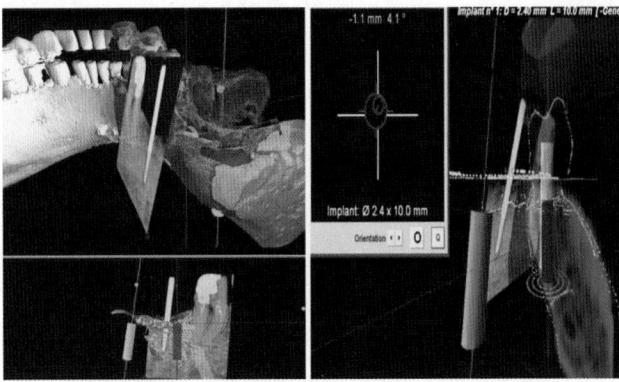

Fig. 84.6 Screen views available during surgery. *Upper left,* The computed tomography (CT) scan reconstruction of the mandible and teeth is observed in *yellow.* Surface mapping of bone and crown morphology *(dark green/blue)* obtained from ultrasound or optical scanner. The computer compares the data from the three-dimensional (3D) topography to the two-dimensional (2D) x-ray film. *Lower left,* The 2D x-ray film is matched to a 3D topography of the patient's "matrix" with the simulated implant positions in *green* and *red. Upper right,* The target and position of the drill and implant are observed. *Lower right,* Real-time navigation with a combination of superimposed images from a 2D x-ray film, optical scanner, CT scan, and 3D ultrasound scan. *(Courtesy Haptitude.)*

view and allow the operator to observe the surgical field continuously. An augmented-reality viewer[26] allows the surgeon to see target data in three dimensions, superimposed over the surgical site through projected images in both eyes.[49] The augmented-reality method allows the operator to adapt to the system more naturally and therefore more rapidly, but it does not appear to have advantages over the use of two-dimensional (2D) side-viewer devices in terms of accuracy.[43] Both systems allow simultaneous viewing of virtual information of the implant (axis and target) and a real vision of the surgical site. Augmented-reality devices are very sensitive to calibration before surgery and require care and monitoring intraoperatively to prevent misalignment during surgery. The relative stability of a headset is critical to maintaining accuracy.

Alternatively, 3D projection screens provide a "real 3D vision" viewed on a specialized monitor (see Fig. 84.5) without the need for viewers (i.e., operator glasses).

Two types of 3D projection screens are available, as follows:

1. The multiplane device has a screen that provides three simulated real-time planes. The object is projected in the screen with a back-field simulated projection. A plane within the screen surface and the forward plane are at a maximum focus of 10 to 20 cm. This device provides a 3D view that is extremely dependent on the shape.
2. A newer-generation device uses nanolenses on each pixel of screen resolution. It provides a natural light-splitting effect similar to the effect of a natural eye separating the three basic colors. Consequently, it is perceived as a natural view. A lateral displacement of the operator's head provides 8 to 12 simulated views, which together create a natural "volume" effect. No adaptation time is required, and viewing is intuitive.

This 3D projection screen technology cannot provide a true holographic 3D view because of the eye's plane of focus on a flat screen, but it does provide a 3D "real volumetric view." The actual 3D projected screen technology does not provide enough high-quality texture, but it is overviewed with simple shape symbols (e.g., cross, circle). Another difficulty is introduced by the nonlinear depth scale of the screen, which is perceived by the operator's brain as nonlogical

and induces a decrease in intuitive hand localization. In addition to this improvement in 3D vision, a 3D sequence of images can be modified for specific applications such as navigation. For example, a 3D sequence of eight views can be modified to facilitate the observation of a projected view of the object at 90 degrees with a minimal head side shift of only 5 degrees. These real-time, 3D front and side views provide intuitive 3D data views in spite of the 2D parameters used to visualize them.

Registration: A Mathematical Complexity

After scan acquisition, the 3D image data of markers or ultrasound bone surface are identified by software as anatomic geometric elements. Then correlation (registration) between marker and surface should be done with the tracking device and the tracked tool. The tracking device gives real-time patient and tool position with its axis. The patient's and localized marker or surface positions could be placed into the patient's referral (fiducial). Several devices have been used to capture the actual patient's anatomy or fiducial marker at surgery, including a touch pointer and an ultrasound probe. The touch pointer allows the operator to touch specific anatomic points (or fiducial markers), whereas an ultrasound tracking device records multiple points of reference on a surface. A hand pointer device is fairly accurate, but if the clinician is not careful, the tendency is to define points that are not in contact with a real surface, thus creating false mapping. The ultrasound probe has a lower accuracy[32] than the touch pointer presenting a maximal (Mx) deviation of 5% of the thickness tissue in the 5 MHz range (i.e., 0.05 mm inaccuracy with 10-mm soft palate tissue), but it has the advantage of capturing continuous data of bone morphology through the mucosa or gingiva.[29,40]

Three registration methods are used to match anatomic points of the preoperative image data and the intraoperative patient's anatomy: (1) point imaging to patient's point, (2) surface to point, and (3) surface to surface. Point-based and line-based methods are described here to illustrate the requirements for adequate registration.

In the point-based method, a few particular points are identified in the preoperative image data (anatomic points) or artificial (fiducial) markers and the patient's anatomy. Points must be well defined and stable so that they can be precisely matched, and the computer calculates a transformation equation that minimizes the mean distance between matched points to complete the registration. The registration accuracy can be predicted, depending on the distribution of points (e.g., an equilateral tripod gives more accurate results than three colinear points).[16,35]

With specific algorithms, a triangle in the preoperative set of points and a triangle in the intraoperative set of points are computed, compared, and then registered. An average accuracy is around 0.5 to 1 mm with an Mx deviation >2 mm with algorithm type iterative closest point (ICP) modified (most common).

Surface-to-surface methods are derived from point-based methods. All lines and surfaces measured on image planning (after segmentation of anatomic structure of the jawbone in the CT scan) and the points taken on the patient's anatomy by the tracking device are known as a *set of points.* These sets may be dense or sparse; a segmented bone surface may have hundreds or thousands of points. When the segmented surface is dense, one can assume that almost all points measured with the tracking device will be identified as points of the segmented surface. Algorithms have been developed to match preoperative and intraoperative data, but the number of possible errors in the identification process increases dramatically with line-based or curve-based methods.[34] Surface to surface is the most accurate method by far, but it is still a very operative- and experience-dependent process.

Tracking Device

Ideally, a practitioner would like <0.3-mm accuracy due to prosthetic requirements. Without guidance, an operator may attain 0.5-mm accuracy. RTM with magnetic trackers, ultrasound space tracking, and an inertial system shows a mean deviation >0.3 mm. The combination computer-guided template and RTM has 0.3-mm accuracy. Actual stereovision tracking or, in the future, a laser ultrafast scanner will show a mean 0.1 mm accuracy on the contra-angle working tip. Nevertheless, laser scanning real-time systems based on shape recognition will need at least a frame rate of 15 to 20/sec to be compatible with a real-time mode.

In dentistry, cameras sensitive to an infrared range of 800 to 900 nm are used to cope with the surgical light artifacts or the strong contrast in light spots. Two cameras are used, and they have to be synchronized. More have around 4.5 µm of pixel size, with an average dimension of 1600×1200. Importantly, camera specifications have to be adapted for a particular tracking device and the environment where the cameras will be used. A deviation of 0.1 to 2 mm may result from improper use.

To illustrate these considerations, a distance range of 40 to 90 cm from the cameras to the patient's head is required, with the greatest accuracy in the center field. The field of view must be sufficiently large to see most of the markers; if the number of markers is insufficient, a deviation >2 mm may occur. In addition is the issue of dynamics; for example, rapid capture of a point of reference for registration with a CT scan or a poor axis of view for cameras will produce 0.3- to 2-mm inaccuracy. This is due to the speed of frames/second (f/sec). A speed acquisition imaging >40 f/sec appears mathematically favorable (the normal speed of the human eye is 15 f/sec), and algorithms matching CAD frames with other captured images perform more favorably in detecting tool position in a relatively static position.

One difficulty with cameras and real-time monitoring is that the patient and instrument markers have to be seen at the same time without being covered by the contra-angle body, depending on the head position and the surgical site. This situation is avoided when the cameras are placed in front of the patient, above the operator's head, and with the use of a larger camera field.

Cameras are accurate in height and width but less in depth, which is limited by the pixel size of the sensors.

Clinical Advantages of RTMIS

- Improved precision
- Noninvasive implant surgery (without or with limited flap reflection)
- Reduced postoperative complications
- Perspectives for improved prosthetic treatment

Challenges With RTMIS

- Learning curve
- Time spent for preparing simulation (if done by the surgeon)
- Time spent for installation (but overall, surgery is shorter)
- Cost

Benefit of Ultrasound Mapping

- Immediate chairside real-time 3D imaging
- Data obtained at the same time as the patient's position
- Absence of registration
- Bone surface visualization, sinus floor, root morphology
- Same accuracy as CBCT <0.3 mm

Conclusion

Patient and clinician demand exists for a minimally invasive approach to implant surgery. RTM implant placement secures implant placement for all operators, but experience is still important for an evaluation of the clinical indication, risk in tissue management, and prosthetic case requirements. The ideal training to obtain a required competence with a digital system needs to be defined, with simplification of all procedures, and it may be an evolution toward a surgical team. With an integration of CAD and CAM prosthetic procedures, laboratory technicians will affect the overall treatment of patients receiving implants by reducing the treatment time and eventually the cost as well.

 A Case Scenario is found on the companion website www.expertconsult.com.

References

 References for this chapter are found on the companion website www.expertconsult.com.

CHAPTER 85

Implant-Related Complications and Failures

Stuart J. Froum | Perry R. Klokkevold | Sang Choon Cho | Scott H. Froum

CHAPTER OUTLINE

Definitions of Implant Survival and
 Success
Types and Prevalence of Implant
 Complications
Types of Dental Implants
Surgical Complications

Biologic Complications
Complications Related to
 Augmentation Procedures *(e-only)*
Complications Related to
 Placement and Loading Protocols
 (e-only)

Prosthetic or Mechanical
 Complications
Aesthetic and Phonetic
 Complications
Conclusions

 Content on complications related to augmentation procedures and to placement and loading protocols can be accessed on the companion website at www.expertconsult.com.

The successful use of osseointegrated dental implants has dramatically changed dentistry and significantly improved dentists' ability to provide tooth replacement options for patients.[3,115] Despite implants' long-term predictability and success, implant-related complications and failures happen in some cases.[4,29] Complications can be surgical, biologic, mechanical, or aesthetic. Some complications are relatively minor and easy to manage, but others are more significant and challenging to resolve. The most serious complications can result in failure of prostheses, loss of implants, and severe loss of supporting bone.

Surgical complications are those problems or adverse outcomes that result from surgery, including procedures used for implant site development, implant placement, implant exposure, and tissue augmentation. Implant complications commonly arise from placement of an implant in a nonideal position. Malpositioned implants, which usually result from poor preoperative treatment planning or errors in surgical technique, can lead to an array of implant problems ranging in severity from minor to major. Surgical complications include compromised aesthetic and prosthetic results, soft tissue and bone dehiscences, impingement on and damage to anatomic structures, and implant failure. Unfortunately, the problems that arise from implant malposition are often not recognized until after osseointegration, when the prosthesis is being fabricated.

Biologic complications involve the hard and soft tissues that support the implant. Peri-implant tissue changes can be limited to inflammation of surrounding soft tissues or be more significant, such as progressive loss of supporting bone. The ultimate biologic complication is implant loss or failure, which can produce soft and hard tissue defects. Loss of implants can be caused by failure to achieve osseointegration in the early stages before restoration or by loss of osseointegration as a result of destruction of supporting bone after the restoration is installed and functioning.

Prosthetic or *mechanical complications* and failures typically occur in the form of material failure, such as abutment and prosthetic screw loosening or fractures. The prosthesis can be rescued from many mechanical problems if they are minor and recognized early.

However, some complications, such as implant fractures, are devastating and not salvageable.

Aesthetic complications arise when the patient's expectations are not met. Satisfaction with the aesthetic outcome of the implant prosthesis varies from patient to patient. The risk of aesthetic complications is increased among patients with high aesthetic expectations and suboptimal patient-related factors, such as a high smile line, thin gingival tissues, or inadequate bone quantity and quality.

This chapter reviews common implant-related complications. A summary of the literature offers some insight into the prevalence of implant-related complications. Implant failure and surgical complications related to site development and variations in implant placement protocols are discussed.

Definitions of Implant Survival and Success

The criteria used to define and report implant success or failure can vary substantially among publications. Selection of success criteria can be based on the author's preference, study population, or some other study objective. Because the level of success reported in an article is based on the criteria used to define success, recognizing the tremendous variation in the way investigators measure and interpret success is crucial. Sometimes, outcomes are measured by the presence or absence of implants at the time of the last examination, which is a measure only of implant survival and should not be confused with implant success. In contrast to this simplified reporting, some investigators use detailed criteria to measure implant success and failure, with variations of successful outcomes separated and defined by additional criteria.

Implant survival is defined as an implant that remains in place at the time of evaluation, regardless of any untoward signs, symptoms, or history of problems. There is a difference between implants that are functioning under an implant-retained restoration and those that are not connected to a restoration and not providing support or function. These implants are sometimes referred to as *sleepers*, and they should not be considered successful merely because they remain osseointegrated. Sleeper implants instead should be included in the discussion as surviving but counted as *failures* because they did not fulfill the originally intended treatment objective.

Implant success is defined by the presence of the implant and the criteria evaluating its condition and function at the time of examination. Various criteria for implant success and failure have been published, but not all investigators agree with or use them. In the classic definition, Albrektsson and colleagues[6] defined success as an implant with no pain, no mobility, no radiolucent peri-implant areas, and no more than 0.2 mm of bone loss annually after the first year of loading. Roos-Jansaker and associates[157] added to this by defining a successful implant as one that loses no more than 1 mm of bone during the first year of function.

Sometimes, the criteria are used as proposed, but in other cases, they are used by investigators with modifications and additional criteria. This makes it difficult to compare studies and draw conclusions about any aspect of implant success or failure based on one or a few studies.

Strictly defined, implant success is any implant-retained restoration in which (1) the original treatment plan is performed as intended without complications, (2) all implants that were placed remain stable and functioning without problems, (3) the peri-implant hard and soft tissues are healthy, and (4) the patient and treating clinicians are pleased with the results. When these strict criteria are used, the rate of implant success (i.e., absence of complications) is only about 61% after 5 years for implant-supported fixed partial dentures (FPDs) and 50% after 10 years for combined tooth–implant FPDs.[113]

An additional criterion of implant success that is not typically reported but should be considered is the aesthetic success or patient satisfaction with the outcome. Several methods have been proposed to evaluate aesthetic results. A restorative index was proposed by Jensen and coworkers[95] to appraise the aesthetics of the final restoration. The index uses a scale of 1 to 10, with 1 being an extremely poor result and 10 being a superlative aesthetic result. Based on subjective and objective criteria, the index evaluates the size and shape of the implant restoration compared with the equivalent contralateral tooth, how well it blends into the arch, and the papillae, gingival form, color, and other factors considered essential in determining an aesthetic result. The pink aesthetic score is an index proposed by Furhauser and colleagues[72] that considers seven soft tissue parameters, including evaluation of the color, contour, and texture of the surrounding soft tissues (i.e., papilla and facial mucosa). Each parameter is given a score of 0, 1, or 2, which allows the best score of 14 to determine the highest level of aesthetics.

Other indices were proposed for single-tooth implant restorations in the aesthetic zone.[23,122] Proposed by Belser and colleagues,[23] one index combines a modified pink aesthetic score with a white aesthetic score that focuses on the visible part of the implant restoration. Scoring includes five parameters: general tooth form, hue, value, surface texture, and translucency. The maximum white aesthetic score is 10. These indices are aimed at quantifying the aesthetic result, which can provide an objective method of judging implant aesthetic success.

KEY FACT

Implant survival indicates that the implant has become osseointegrated but does not consider associated problems. An implant that is not restored can be included in survival percentages while failing to fulfill its intended purpose. *Implant success* is defined by criteria evaluating the condition and function of the implant. Because different criteria have been used to define implant success, it is difficult to make comparisons between studies and often impossible to make conclusions about implant success or failure based on only one or a few studies.

Types and Prevalence of Implant Complications

The prevalence of implant-related complications has been reported in several reviews. However, a systematic review of the incidence of complications in studies of at least 5 years' duration revealed that biologic complications were considered in only 40% to 60% and technical complications in only 60% to 80% of the studies. The review found that the incidence of technical complications related to implant components and suprastructures was higher for overdentures than for fixed restorations.[24]

In a systematic review of reports on the survival and complication rates of implant-supported FPDs, Lang and associates[113] found that the most common technical complication was fracture of veneers (13.2% after 5 years), followed by loss of the screw access hole restoration (8.2% after 5 years), abutment or occlusal screw loosening (5.8% after 5 years), and abutment or occlusal screw fracture (1.5% after 5 years and 2.5% after 10 years). Fracture of implants occurred infrequently (0.4% after 5 years and 1.8% after 10 years).

A retrospective evaluation of 4937 implants by Eckert and colleagues[54] found that implant fractures occurred more frequently in partially edentulous restorations (1.5%) than in restorations of completely edentulous arches (0.2%), and all observed implant fractures occurred with commercially pure, 3.75-mm diameter threaded implants.

In a literature review that included all types of implant-retained prostheses, Goodacre and colleagues[77] found that the most common technical complications were loosening of the overdenture retentive mechanism (33%), resin veneer fractures with FPDs (22%), overdentures needing to be relined (19%), and overdenture clip or attachment fracture (16%). With the inclusion of edentulous patients having overdentures, their review seemed to indicate a significantly higher percentage of complications than Pjetursson's systematic review[145] of patients with implant-supported FPDs. Goodacre and associates[76] found it impossible to calculate an overall prosthesis complication rate because most studies included in their review did not report several of the complication categories.

The most common complication reported for single crowns was abutment or prosthesis screw loosening. The rate of abutment screw loosening varied dramatically from one study to another, ranging from 2% to 45%.[77] The highest rate of abutment screw loosening was associated with single crowns, followed by overdentures. The rate of prosthesis screw loosening was similar, ranging from 1% to 38% in various studies. A higher frequency was reported for single crowns in the posterior areas (i.e., premolar and molar) than in the anterior region.

Implant fracture is an uncommon but significant complication. Goodacre and colleagues[76] reported a 1.5% incidence in their literature review. The incidence of implant fracture was higher in FPDs supported by only two implants. Consistent with this finding, Rangert and coworkers[149] reported that most implant fractures occurred in single- and double-implant–supported restorations. They also found that most of these fractures were in posterior partially edentulous segments, in which the generated occlusal forces can be greater than in anterior segments (Fig. 85.1).

In a systematic review of prospective longitudinal studies (i.e., minimum of 5 years' duration) reporting biologic and technical complications associated with implant therapy (i.e., all restoration types included), Berglundh and colleagues[24] found that the incidence of technical complications was consistent with Pjetursson's findings, with implant fracture occurring in less than 1% (0.08% to 0.74%) of cases. Consistent with the findings in Goodacre's review, technical complications were higher for implants used in overdenture therapy than implants supporting fixed prostheses.

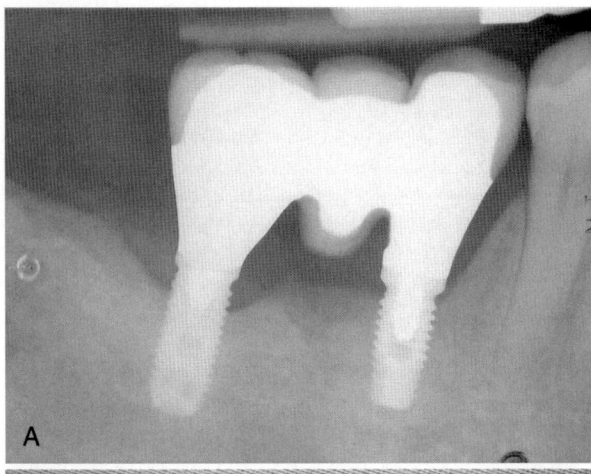

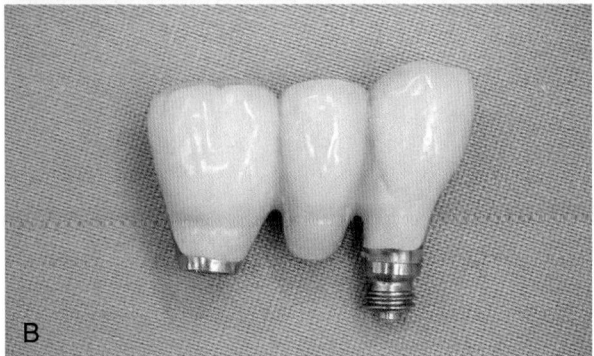

Fig. 85.1 (A) Radiograph of a three-unit, posterior, fixed partial denture supported by two standard-diameter, screw-shaped threaded implants. Notice the long crown height, relatively short implant length, and bone loss around the posterior implant. (B) Photograph of the ultimate implant-supported restoration failure. The anterior implant fractured between the second and third threads, which resulted in loss of the restoration.

In Lang and associates' systematic review[113] of survival and complication rates for implant-supported FPDs, biologic complications such as peri-implantitis and soft tissue lesions occurred in 8.6% of patients after 5 years. In a later literature review of the prevalence of peri-implant diseases, Zitzmann and Berglundh[191] reported that although cross-sectional studies were rare, data from the only two studies available showed that peri-implant mucositis occurred in 80% of patients and 50% of implant sites. Peri-implantitis was identified in 28% and 56% or more of patients and in 12% and 43% of implant sites in the two studies that followed patients with functional implants for at least 5 years.

A critical review of the literature by Esposito and associates[64] included 73 publications reporting early and late failures of Brånemark implants; biologically related implant failures were relatively low at 7.7%. Treatments involved all anatomic areas and all types of prosthetic design. The study authors concluded that the predictability of implant treatment was especially good for partially edentulous patients compared with totally edentulous patients; failures in the latter population were twice as high as those in the other group. The incidence of implant failure was three times higher for the edentulous maxilla than for the edentulous mandible, whereas failure rates for the partially edentulous maxilla were similar to those for the partially edentulous mandible.

Risk factors such as smoking, diabetes, and periodontal disease can contribute to implant failure and complications. Several studies with numerous implants and years of follow-up have concluded that smoking is a definite risk factor for implant survival.[13,50,51,56,134] A

systematic review of the effect of risk factors on implant outcomes concluded that smoking had an adverse effect on implant survival and success; the effects were more pronounced in areas of loose trabecular bone (i.e., posterior maxilla).[107] The review suggested that type 2 diabetes could have an adverse effect on implant survival rates but did not have enough studies to permit a definitive conclusion.[107] The same review concluded that although patients with a history of treated periodontitis did not show a decrease in implant survival, they did experience more biologic implant complications and lower success rates, especially with longer-term follow-up.[107]

Types of Dental Implants

Analysis of the data on the prevalence of implant complications (i.e., failure, fracture, and peri-implantitis) in published systematic reviews should consider the fact that many of these studies reported on implants with earlier designs (i.e., machined surfaces and external connections). Most current implant systems feature surfaces with an altered microtopography (i.e., rough), and many have internal connections. The prevalence and type of complications associated with the newer implant designs may be different.

Many modifications have been developed to try to improve the long-term success rates of implants. More than 1300 types of dental implants are available with different materials, shapes, sizes, lengths, and surface characteristics or coatings. Although it has been suggested that machined surfaces are more resistant to plaque accumulation and peri-implantitis, there is limited evidence to show that implants with relatively smooth surfaces (i.e., machined) are less prone to bone loss from chronic infection than implants with rough surfaces. To date, there is no evidence showing that any particular type of dental implant has superior long-term success.[59]

Different implant designs and surfaces must be studied in prospective human trials over long periods. Until those data become available, clinicians should be aware that historical data reporting success rates for earlier implant designs may not reflect the outcomes for current implants. Moreover, new implant surfaces and designs are commonly introduced with limited or no data available on potential complications.[a]

Surgical Complications

As with any surgical procedure, implant surgery has risks. Proper precautions must be taken to prevent injuries, including (1) a thorough review of the patient's medical history, (2) a comprehensive clinical and radiographic examination, (3) establishment of a comprehensive interdisciplinary treatment plan, and (4) good surgical techniques.

Surgical complications include perilous bleeding, damage to adjacent structures such as teeth, injury to nerves, and iatrogenic jaw fracture. Postoperative complications include bleeding, hematoma, and infection. They may be minor, transient, and easily managed or more serious and require postoperative treatment.

Hemorrhage and Hematoma

Bleeding during surgery is expected and usually easily controlled. However, if a sizable vessel is incised or otherwise injured during surgery, the hemorrhage can be difficult to control. Smaller vessels naturally constrict or retract to slow the hemorrhage. If bleeding continues, it may be necessary to apply pressure or suture the hemorrhaging vessel. Cauterizing the hemorrhaging vessel also may be warranted. This can be especially difficult if there is a vascular injury to an artery that is inaccessible, such as in the floor of the mouth or

[a]References 8, 10, 41, 52, 141, 142, 173, 178, 192.

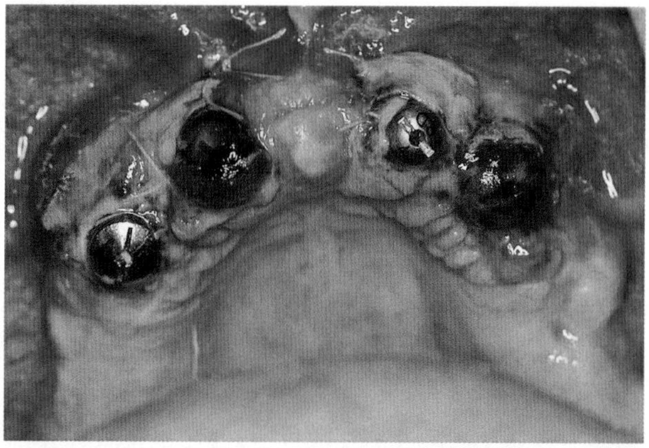

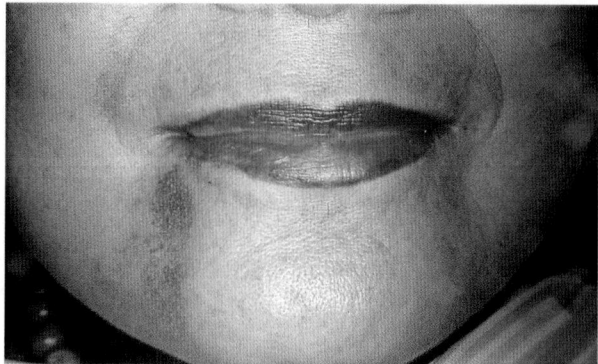

Fig. 85.2 Clinical photograph of postoperative bleeding around healing abutments after second-stage implant exposure surgery.

Fig. 85.3 Clinical photograph of postoperative (extraoral) bruising indicative of subdermal bleeding into connective tissue spaces. This is a normal expectation that resolves in 7 to 14 days.

posterior maxilla. Serious bleeding from an inaccessible vessel can be life-threatening, not by exsanguination but rather as a result of airway obstruction. This is most problematic when the point of bleeding is inaccessible and internal (i.e., in connective tissues and soft tissue spaces).

Postoperative bleeding is an equally important problem to manage (Fig. 85.2). Patients should be given postoperative instructions on normal expectations for bleeding and how to prevent and manage minor bleeding. Historically, standard practice is that they should be advised, with their physician's approval, to discontinue or reduce medications that increase bleeding tendency 3 to 10 days before surgery. However, recent evidence suggests that this may not be necessary and may increase the risk of hematologic or cardiovascular problems[96,97,134,159] (see Chapter 39).

Dental health care providers should consult with medical health care providers regarding the best management for each patient. Dental health care providers and patients should always include the treating medical practitioner in management decisions if postoperative bleeding is excessive or persistent.

Submucosal or subdermal hemorrhage into the connective tissues and soft tissue spaces can result in hematoma formation. Postoperative bruising is a typical example of minor submucosal or subdermal bleeding into the connective tissues (Fig. 85.3). Bruising and small hematomas typically resolve without special treatment or consequence. However, larger hematomas or those that occur in medically compromised individuals are susceptible to infection as a result of the noncirculating blood that sits in the space. It is prudent to prescribe antibiotics for patients who develop a noticeably large hematoma.

Referral to the appropriate medical physician may be warranted for nonresolving hematomas.[88]

Although the incidence of a life-threatening hemorrhage from implant surgery is extremely low, the seriousness of the problem warrants the attention of everyone who participates in this type of surgery. Potentially fatal complications have been reported for implant surgical procedures in the mandible, especially the anterior region.[b] Massive internal bleeding in the highly vascular region of the floor of the mouth can result from instrumentation or implants that perforate the lingual cortical plate and sever or injure the arteries running along the lingual surface. Depending on the severity and location of the injury, bleeding may become apparent immediately or only after some delay. In either case, the progressively increasing hematoma dissects and expands to displace the tongue and soft tissues of the floor of the mouth, ultimately leading to upper airway obstruction.

Emergency treatment includes airway management (primary importance) and surgical intervention to isolate and stop the bleeding. Clinicians must be aware of this risk and be prepared to act quickly. It is important to recognize that bleeding, although considered a complication at the time of surgery, can become a serious complication in the hours and days after surgery.[47]

> ## CLINICAL CORRELATION
>
> Although the incidence of a life-threatening hemorrhage from implant surgery is extremely low, it is a serious problem that can occur. Implant surgical procedures in the anterior mandible have been associated with potentially fatal complications. Massive internal bleeding in the floor of the mouth from inadvertent injury to lingual arteries can cause an expanding hematoma that displaces the tongue and soft tissues, obstructing the upper airway. Emergency treatment includes airway management and surgical intervention to isolate and stop the bleeding. Clinicians must be aware of this risk and be prepared to act quickly.

Neurosensory Disturbances

One of the more problematic surgical complications is an injury to nerves. Neurosensory alterations caused by damage to a nerve can be temporary or permanent. Neuropathy can be caused by a drilling injury (i.e., cut, tear, or puncture of the nerve) or by implant compression or damage to the nerve (Fig. 85.4; see Fig. 76.18). In either case, the injury causes neuroma formation, and two patterns of clinical neuropathy may follow. *Hypoesthesia* is a neuropathy defined by impaired sensory function that is sometimes associated with phantom pain. *Hyperesthesia* is a neuropathy defined by pain with minimal or no sensory impairment.[79] Some neuropathies resolve, whereas others persist. The type of neuropathy does not indicate the potential for recovery.

For several reasons, it is likely that neurosensory disturbances occur more frequently after implant surgery than is reported in the literature. First, many of the changes are transient in nature, and most patients recover completely or at least recover to a level that is below a threshold of annoyance or daily perception. Second, wide variation exists in the postoperative evaluation of patients by clinicians. Some clinicians do not assess or inquire about postsurgical neurosensory disturbances, allowing this complication to go unnoticed. Likewise, some patients expect altered sensation as part of surgery and may never acknowledge or comment on its presence, especially if the disturbance is minor. It is therefore likely that minor neuropathies exist but go unrecognized and unreported.

According to a systematic review of inferior alveolar nerve injuries after implant placement, the importance of early diagnosis and

---

[b]References 19, 45, 47, 67, 89, 137, 139, 176.

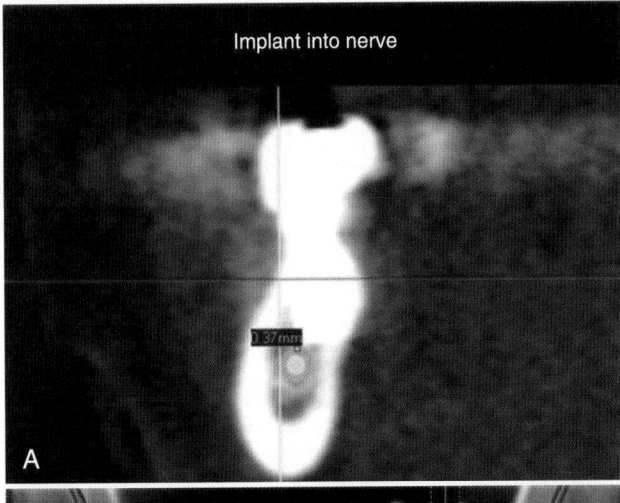

Implant into nerve

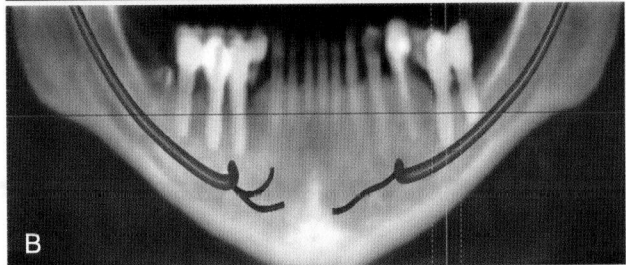

Fig. 85.4 (A) Cross-sectional computed tomography (CT) image shows the implant impinging on the inferior alveolar nerve canal. (B) Panoramic CT scan shows the implant in the lower left first molar area impinging on the inferior alveolar nerve canal. The nerve is marked by tracing with software.

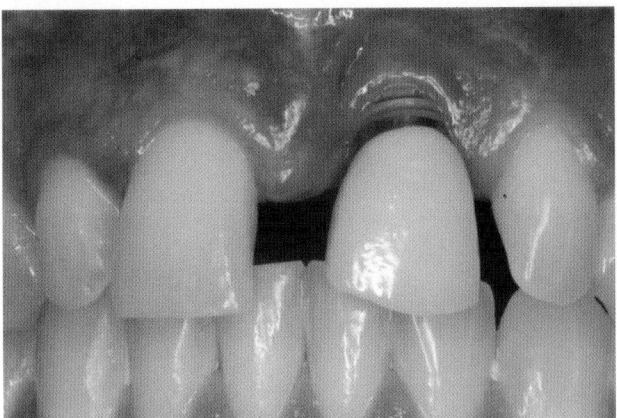

Fig. 85.5 Clinical photograph of gingival recession around a maxillary anterior implant (left central incisor) resulting in exposure of the crown margin, the implant collar, and several threads of the implant.

treatment is considered essential for preventing long-term, permanent neurologic problems. If a diagnosis is established and treatment is rendered within the first 36 hours, a high percentage of successful outcomes can be achieved. An estimated 25% of patients with iatrogenic paresthesia suffer permanent effects.[104] Several researchers and clinicians proposed that early implant removal (i.e., within the first 24 to 36 hours after implant placement) may lead to better healing with the return of sensation.[104,105]

Neurosensory disturbances reported in the literature are most prevalent and significant when they are more serious and occur more frequently, such as those associated with lateral transposition of the mandibular nerve.[93,101] This relatively uncommon procedure is used to reposition the nerve and allow longer implants to be placed in the atrophic posterior mandible. Lateral nerve transposition procedures are associated with an almost 100% incidence of neurosensory dysfunction immediately after surgery. More than 50% (range, 30% to 80%) of these neurosensory changes are permanent.[101] Several articles have been written on the treatment of neurosensory disturbances.[7,128,151]

Implant Malposition

Many of the complications that arise during implant surgery can be attributed to the dental implant being placed in an undesired or unintended position. Malpositioning of dental implants is usually the result of poor treatment planning before surgery, lack of surgical skill, or poor communication between the implant surgeon and the restorative dentist. Optimal implant aesthetics and the avoidance of positional complications can be achieved by placing the implant in a prosthetically driven manner.[123,140] The implant should be placed with reference to the three dimensions dictated by the position of the final restoration and not by the availability of bone.

Angulation is another important determinant of implant position that affects outcome aesthetics. The ideal implant position entails an accurate preparation, insertion, and placement into the alveolus in a proper three-dimensional geometry according to apicocoronal, mesiodistal, and buccolingual parameters and implant angulation relative to the final prosthetic restoration and gingival margins[108,160] (see Chapter 78).

Apicocoronally, the implant should be placed so the platform is about 3 mm apical to the gingival margin of the anticipated restoration.[28] The implant position varies slightly from one implant system to another, depending on abutment design and space requirements. If the implant platform is placed too far coronally, there will not be sufficient room to develop a natural-looking emergence profile, and the tooth may have a boxy, unaesthetic appearance. If the platform is placed at or above the level of the gingival margin, metal collar or implant exposure can occur, yielding an unaesthetic result (Fig. 85.5). If the implant platform is placed too far apically, a long transmucosal abutment will be necessary to restore the implant. This can lead to a deep pocket and difficult hygiene access for the patient and clinician.

The implant should be placed at a distance of 1.5 to 2 mm from an adjacent natural tooth and 2 to 3 mm from an adjacent implant to maintain an adequate biologic dimension.[81] Similar to natural teeth, violation of biologic width around an implant can lead to bone loss.[87] Implants that are placed too close to each other (Fig. 85.6) or to natural teeth can be difficult to restore. Impression copings and impression-taking techniques must be modified. Improperly spaced implants invariably lead to chronic inflammation and peri-implantitis.[57,181] Conversely, an implant placed at an excessive distance from an adjacent tooth or implant may require prosthetic compensation in the form of mesial or distal cantilevers, which can predispose the implant to biologic (i.e., bone loss) and mechanical (i.e., screw loosening,[77] screw fracture,[179] and implant fracture[149]) complications and difficulties with hygiene.[181]

Ideally, an implant should be placed buccolingually so there is at least 2 mm of bone circumferentially around it.[172] Implant exposure through the lingual or buccal cortex can predispose an individual to abscess and suppuration.[38] Implants that are placed too palatally or lingually require prosthetic compensation in the form of a buccal ridge lap, which may be difficult for the patient to clean and can lead to tissue inflammation.[22]

To obtain ideal aesthetics, to avoid potential aesthetic complications, and to correct bodily placement of the dental implant, it must be correctly angulated on insertion. In most anterior cases, it is desirable to have the long axis of the implant directed so it is emerging toward the cingulum. In the posterior region, the implant axis should be directed toward the central fossa or the stamp cusp of the opposing tooth. Implants that are placed with mild to moderate misangulations

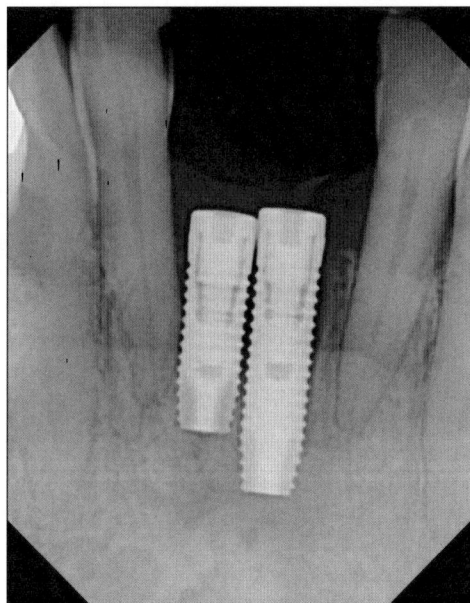

Fig. 85.6 Radiograph of two mandibular anterior implants placed too close together (i.e., no proximal space), resulting in implants that are impossible to restore.

can often be corrected prosthetically with implant abutments. Minor misangulations (i.e., 15 to 20 degrees) can be corrected with pre-fabricated or customized angled abutments; moderate misangulations (i.e., 20 to 35 degrees) can usually be managed with customized UCLA-type abutments; and extreme errors in implant angulations (>35 degrees) may make an implant unrestorable and require it to be left submerged (i.e., a sleeper) or be removed (Fig. 85.7).

The ultimate complication of malpositioning is implant or instrument invasion into vital structures. The most common violation of neighboring anatomy is placement of the dental implant into the adjacent tooth root. Surgical procedures used to prepare osteotomy sites and place implants adjacent to teeth can injure them by directly cutting into the tooth structure or by damaging nearby supporting tissues and nerves. Instrumentation (e.g., drills) directed at or near the adjacent tooth can injure the periodontal ligament, tooth structure, and nerve of the tooth. Depending on the extent of the injury, the tooth can require endodontic therapy or extraction.

On insertion, dental implants follow the trajectory of the osteotomy prepared by the drill. Care must be taken when preparing the osteotomy to stay true to the planned path of insertion. Radiographs taken periodically during implant surgery with a guide pin in the osteotomy site can greatly reduce the potential for damaging adjacent teeth (see Fig. 76.15). Radiographic analysis before implant surgery should include detection of curved, convergent, or dilacerated root structures of adjacent teeth that can limit implant placement.

Particular care must be taken when placing implants in the mandible so as to not encroach on the inferior alveolar canal or the mental foramen (see Chapter 58 for a description of the anatomy). Encroachment on the mandibular canal or mental foramen during osteotomy or implant placement by direct contact or mechanical compression of bone can injure nerves and blood vessels. Paresthesia,

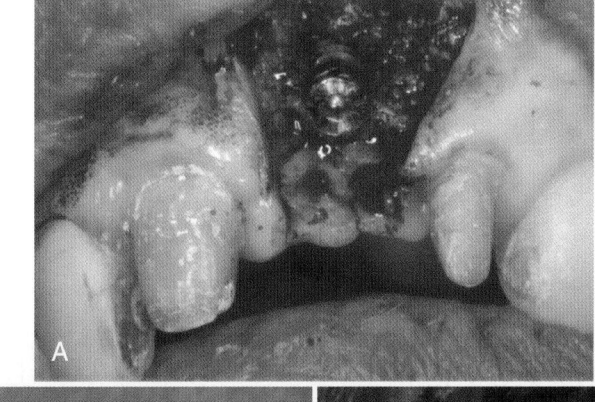

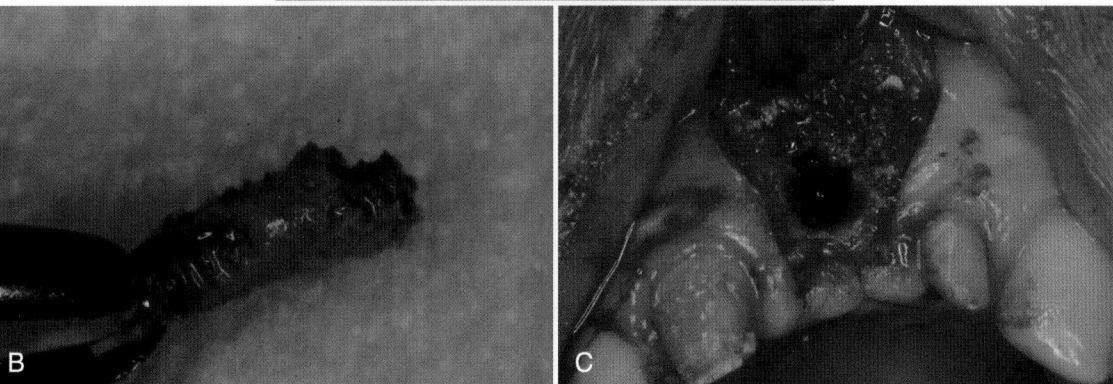

Fig. 85.7 Clinical photograph of a maxillary anterior implant (i.e., left central incisor) placed with an extreme facial angulation, resulting in an implant that emerges through the gingiva at a level that is more apical than the adjacent natural tooth gingival margins. (A) Surgical exposure of the malpositioned implant. (B) Surgically removed implant. (C) Alveolar defect resulting from surgical removal of the malpositioned implant.

hypoesthesia, hyperesthesia, dysesthesia, or anesthesia of the lower lip, skin, mucosa, and teeth can result, as can arterial or venous bleeding.[78] The reported incidence of sensory disturbances after mandibular implant placement is 0% to 40%.[18,104]

In the maxilla, care must be taken to avoid dental implant perforation into the maxillary sinus or nasal cavity. Displacement of the entire dental implant into the maxillary sinus cavity may require a Caldwell-Luc procedure for retrieval. The online section on Sinus Bone Augmentation provides further information about complications related to the maxillary sinus.

The risks of surgery always exist, but the complications can be minimized by an understanding of the causes and with proper diagnosis and treatment planning. Three-dimensional imaging (i.e., computed tomography [CT] and cone beam CT [CBCT]) provides the surgeon with useful preoperative information for diagnosis and treatment planning (see Chapter 76). Careful surgical exposure for direct visualization and identification of the mental nerve are indicated. The surgeon should establish a *zone of safety* and keep instrumentation and implants a safe margin (≥2 mm) away from the nerve.[78]

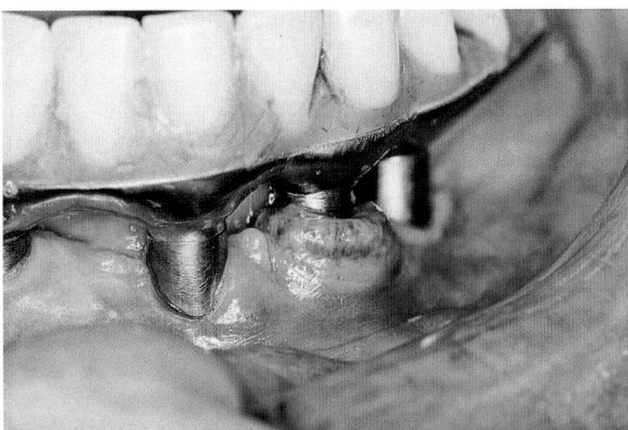

Fig. 85.8 Inflammatory proliferation caused by a loose-fitting connection between the abutment and the implant. *(Courtesy Dr. John Beumer, UCLA Maxillofacial Prosthetics, Los Angeles, CA.)*

 KEY FACT

Malpositioned implants can be avoided by proper planning, good communication, and meticulous surgical skills. Radiographs taken periodically during implant surgery with guide pins in the osteotomy site can greatly reduce damage to adjacent teeth. Radiographic analysis before implant surgery should include detection of curved, convergent, or dilacerated root structures of adjacent teeth that can limit implant placement.

Biologic Complications

Biologic complications involve pathology of the surrounding peri-implant hard and soft tissues. Frequently, soft tissue problems are an inflammatory response to bacterial accumulation around implants. Bacteria can accumulate at the junction of an ill-fitting implant–abutment or abutment–crown connection. Some of the highly textured, macroscopically rough implant surfaces (e.g., titanium plasma–sprayed [TPS] or hydroxyapatite [HA] coating) may also perpetuate the accumulation of bacteria on the implant surface.

Inflammation and Proliferation

Because inflammation of the peri-implant soft tissues is similar to the inflammatory response in gingival and other periodontal tissues, the clinical appearance also is similar. Inflamed peri-implant tissues demonstrate the same erythema, edema, and swelling around teeth. Occasionally, the reaction of peri-implant soft tissues to bacterial accumulation is profound and unusual, with dramatic inflammatory proliferation (Fig. 85.8). This type of lesion is somewhat characteristic around implants and indicates a loose-fitting implant-to-abutment connection or trapped excess cement that remains buried within the soft tissue space (i.e., pocket).

The precipitating local factor ultimately becomes infected with bacterial pathogens, leading to mucosal hypertrophy or proliferation and possible abscess formation (Fig. 85.9). Correction of the precipitating factors (e.g., loose connection, retained cement) can effectively resolve the lesion. Another type of lesion resulting from a loose abutment connection is a fistula (Fig. 85.10), and correcting the etiologic factor can quickly resolve it.

Dehiscence and Recession

Dehiscence or recession of the peri-implant soft tissues occurs when support for the tissues is lacking or has been lost. Recession is a common finding after implant restoration and should be anticipated, especially when soft tissues are thin and not well supported (Fig. 85.11). Improper implant positioning also predisposes peri-implant tissues to recession. Placement or angulation of the implant too far buccally causes the buccal plate to resorb, resulting in greater recession.[171]

Another factor is the thickness of the buccal plate of bone. Spray and colleagues[172] recommended a buccal bone thickness of 2 mm or greater to support the buccal soft tissue. If it is insufficient, preoperative or simultaneous site development using guided bone regeneration is indicated. Recession is a problem that is particularly disconcerting in anterior aesthetic areas. Patients with a high smile line or high aesthetic demands consider recession a failure (Fig. 85.12).

The anatomy and soft tissue support around implants are different from those around teeth. Periodontal tissues have the advantage of soft tissue support supplied by circumferential and transseptal connective tissue fibers that insert into the cementum at a level that is more coronal than the supporting bone. In the absence of inflammation, these fibers support periodontal soft tissues far above the level of crestal bone. As a result, gingival margins and interdental papillae are supported and maintained higher around teeth than around implants, even when the periodontal tissues are very thin.

Peri-implant soft tissues, however, depend entirely on the surrounding bone for support. Soft tissue thickness accounts for some soft tissue height, but there are no supracrestal inserting connective tissue fibers to aid the soft tissue support around an implant. The soft tissue height around implants is typically limited to about 3 or 4 mm, and bone loss around implants often leads to recession.

 FLASH BACK

The peri-implant soft tissue seal is weaker than the periodontal soft tissue seal. The soft tissue seal around implants depends on tissue thickness and a long junctional epithelial attachment with hemidesmosomes. It is inferior to the periodontal attachment around natural teeth because it lacks the inserting connective tissue fibers (i.e., Sharpey fibers) of the periodontium. Periodontal papillae and gingival margins are also supported at a higher supracrestal level compared with peri-implant soft tissues. Periodontal soft tissues are supported by circumferential and transseptal connective tissue fibers that insert into the cementum at a level that is more coronal than the supporting bone.

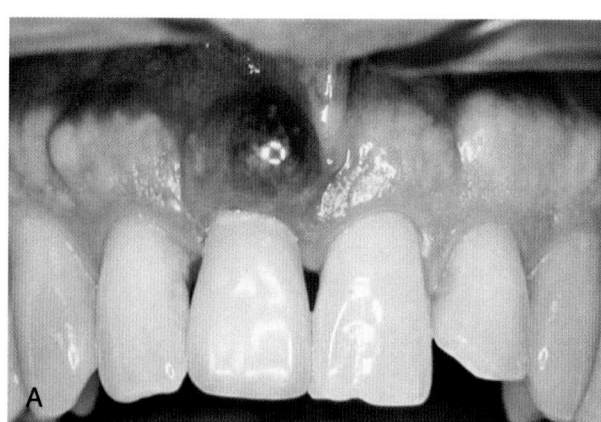
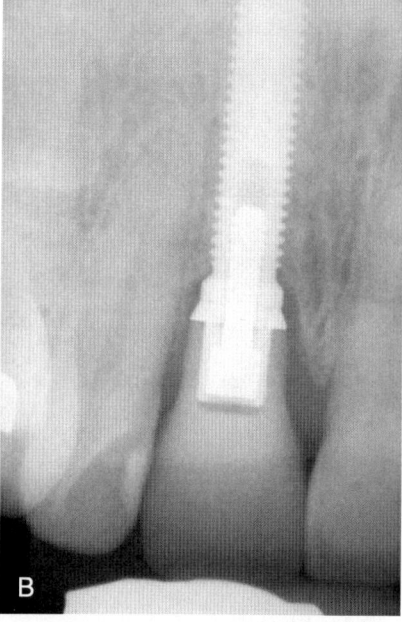

Fig. 85.9 (A) Clinical photograph of an abscess caused by excess cement trapped within the soft tissues. (B) Radiograph of an implant with a cemented crown (same patient as in A). Notice the subgingival depth of the crown–abutment (cement line) junction, which is below the level of the adjacent interproximal bone and therefore impossible to adequately access with an explorer to remove the excess cement. *(Courtesy Dr. John Beumer, UCLA Maxillofacial Prosthetics, Los Angeles, CA.)*

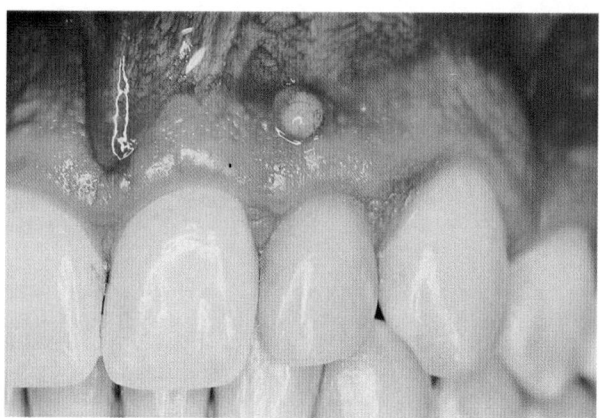

Fig. 85.10 Fistula caused by a loose implant–abutment connection (i.e., maxillary left lateral incisor).

Peri-Implantitis and Bone Loss

Peri-implantitis is an inflammatory process that affects the tissues around an osseointegrated implant and results in the loss of supporting bone.[129] The reported prevalence of peri-implantitis varies from less than 7% to 37% of implants.[106] The variation can be attributed to differences in studied populations, length of follow-up time, implant variables, and the criteria used to define peri-implantitis.[109,158] Two systematic reviews concluded that peri-implantitis affected 10% of implants and 20% of patients during the 5 to 10 years after placement.[11,131]

A classification for early, moderate, and advanced peri-implantitis based on the degree of bone loss was proposed to improve communication when describing prevalence and treatment.[71] Soft tissue measurements using manual or automated probes have been suggested to diagnose a compromised implant site.[71a] Although some reports state that probing is contraindicated, careful monitoring of probing depth over time seems useful in detecting changes of the peri-implant

tissue.[44,148,174,175] Standardized radiographic techniques, with or without computerized analysis, have been useful in evaluating peri-implant bone levels.[4,25,29,99,148] Periodic evaluation of tissue appearance, probing depth changes, and radiographic assessment are the best means of detecting changes in bone support.

Clinicians should monitor the surrounding tissues for signs of peri-implant disease by observing changes in probing depth and radiographic evidence of bone destruction, suppuration, calculus buildup, swelling, color changes, and bleeding.[130,136] Peri-implantitis can be perpetuated by bacterial infection that has contaminated a rough (e.g., TPS- or HA-coated) implant surface and by excessive biomechanical forces.[188,189] The classic trough-type defect is typically associated with peri-implantitis (Fig. 85.13). In cases with severely reduced bone support extending into the apical half of the implant (Fig. 85.14) or in cases demonstrating mobility, implant removal should be considered.[6,135]

The number and distribution of implants and the occlusal relationships influence the biomechanical forces applied to implants.[147,153] A review by Lindhe and Meyle from the Consensus Report of the Sixth European Workshop on Periodontology concluded that risk indicators for peri-implantitis included (1) poor oral hygiene, (2) a history of periodontitis, (3) diabetes, (4) cigarette smoking, (5) alcohol consumption, and (6) implant surface.[117] Risk factors 1 to 4 have been recognized and reported in the literature.[107] The report suggests that although data for risk factors 5 and 6 are limited, they appear to be relevant to peri-implantitis.[117] One study found little evidence to support smoking as a risk factor for peri-implantitis.[167] Another proposed risk factor involves individual genetic polymorphisms.[33,112] More research is needed to study the relation of this risk factor to the development of peri-implantitis.

Other risk factors, including excess and retained cement, have been implicated in peri-implantitis. One article said that excess dental cement was associated with signs of peri-implant disease in 81% of cases evaluated using a dental endoscope.[187] The radiopacity of some commonly used cements affects their detectability.[183] This emphasizes

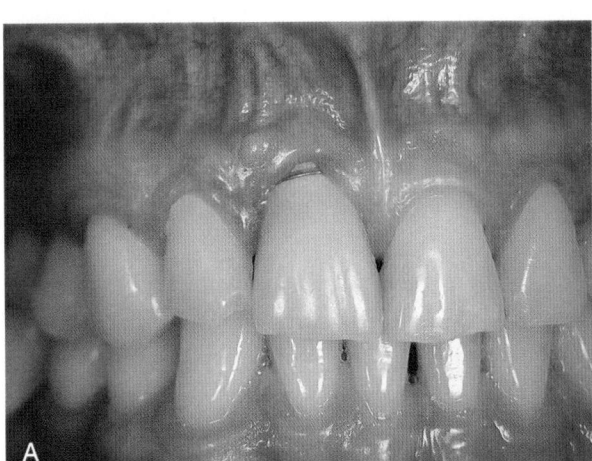
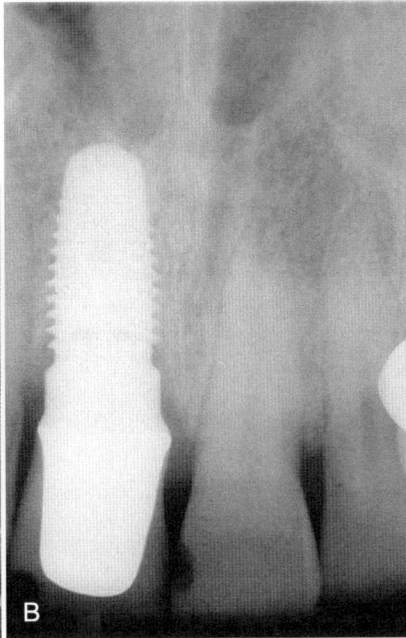

Fig. 85.11 (A) Clinical photograph of a single-tooth implant crown (maxillary right central) with moderate recession that occurred 1 year after the final restoration. In this case, recession most likely occurred because the labial bone around this wide-diameter implant was very thin or nonexistent. (B) Radiograph of a wide-diameter (6-mm) implant supporting a maxillary central incisor crown (same patient as in A).

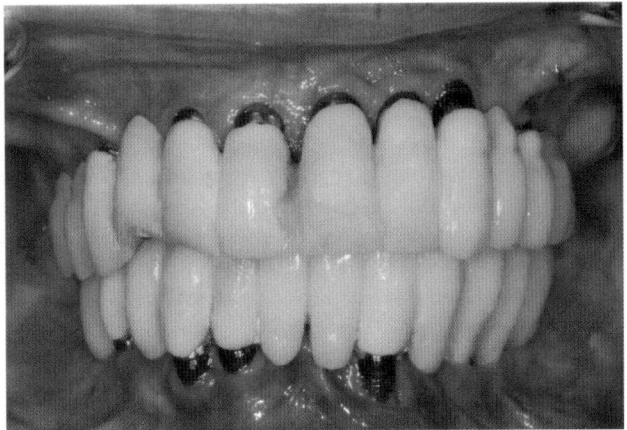

Fig. 85.12 Poor aesthetics resulting from gingival recession and exposure of the crown margins, implant collars, and threads of several maxillary and mandibular implants supporting full-arch, fixed partial dentures. Notice the thin labial tissues and erythema, especially around the mandibular implant sites.

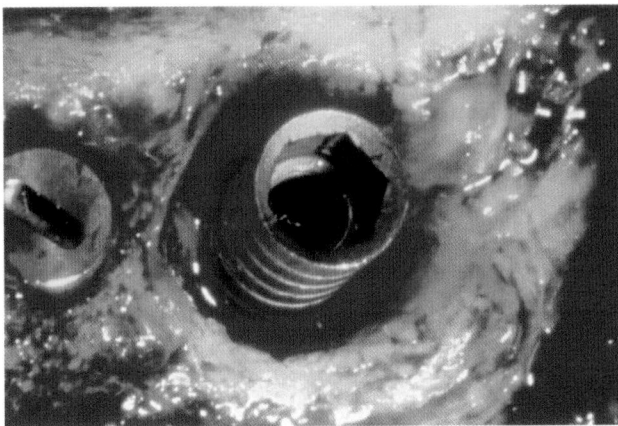

Fig. 85.13 Moderately advanced bone loss around an implant with the typical circumferential trough type of bony defect. *(From Garg AK:* Implant dentistry: a practical approach, *ed 2, Mosby, St. Louis, 2010.)*

the importance of proper cementation, use of screw-retained rather than cemented restorations when possible, and careful clinical examination after final crown cementation on implants.

Other proposed peri-implantitis predisposing factors include the presence of aggressive bacteria, excessive mechanical stress, and corrosion. Each was documented as a factor that could act synergistically with biofilm or existing peri-implantitis to worsen the condition.[133]

Nine systematic reviews[c] concluded that no predicable method of treatment for peri-implantitis could be recommended. However, a clinical study of 170 consecutively treated implants with peri-implantitis using a regenerative protocol reported a more than 98% success rate.[70]

---

[c]References 34, 40, 58, 62, 86, 110, 138, 152, 155, 158.

Implant Loss or Failure

Implant loss or failure is considered relative to the time of placement or restoration. Early implant failures occur before implant restoration. Late implant failures occur after the implant has been restored. When an implant fails before restoration, it probably did not achieve osseointegration, or the integration was weak or jeopardized by infection, movement, or impaired wound healing (Fig. 85.15). Late implant failures occur after prosthesis installation for a variety of reasons, including infection and implant overload (Fig. 85.16). In a review of the literature to evaluate biologic causes for implant failure, Esposito and colleagues[63] found that infections, impaired healing, and overload were the most important contributing factors. Two systematic reviews of the literature concluded that a single dose of preoperative antibiotic therapy could decrease the failure rate of dental implants.[60,168]

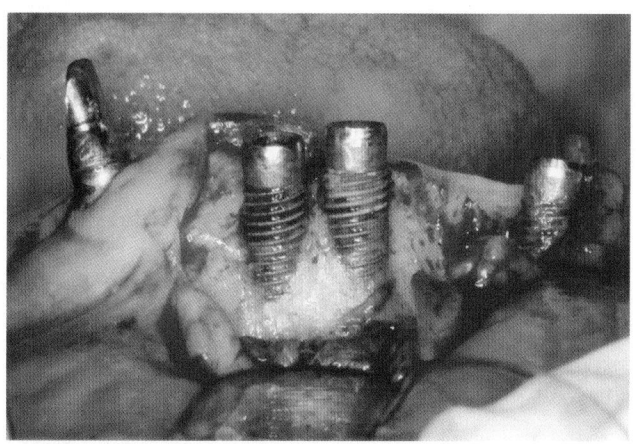

Fig. 85.14 Severe horizontal and vertical bone loss around several mandibular implants.

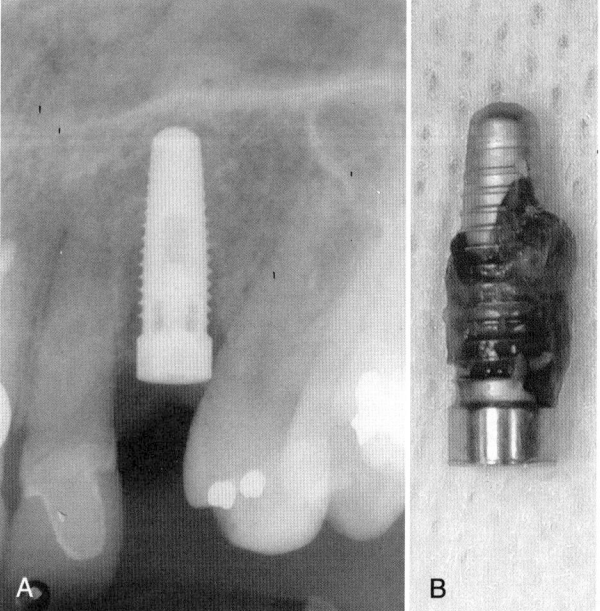

Fig. 85.15 (A) Radiograph of an early failed implant caused by lack of osseointegration. In addition to the crestal bone loss, notice the radiolucency along the sides of the implant. (B) Photograph of the failed (nonintegrated) implant (shown in A) that was easily removed along with surrounding connective tissue.

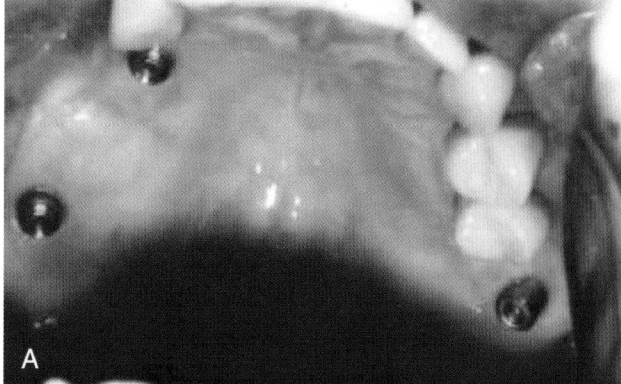

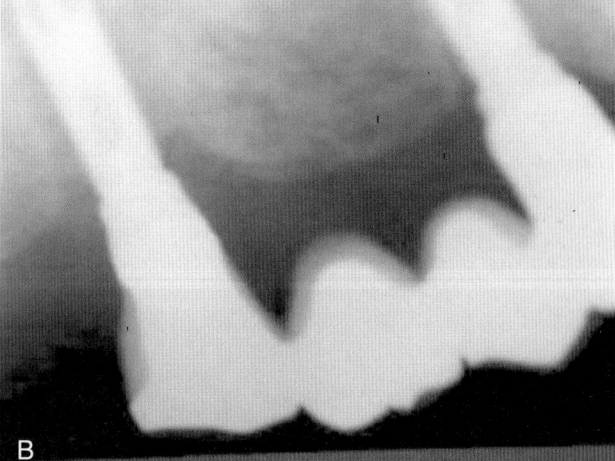

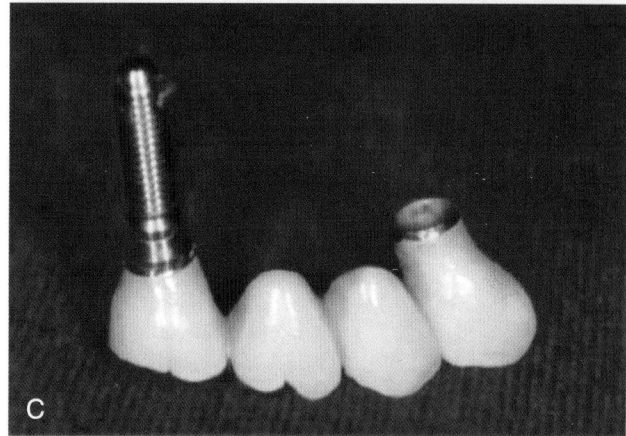

Fig. 85.16 A four-unit fixed partial denture in the posterior maxilla was supported by only two implants. (A) Clinical photograph of implant abutments in the posterior maxilla. (B) Radiograph taken 30 months after restoration. Notice the bone loss around the distal implant. (C) Failed distal implant attached to a failed prosthesis. The biologic failure of one (posterior) implant resulted in a long-span cantilever extension from the other (anterior) implant that ultimately led to its mechanical failure (i.e., abutment screw fracture). *(Courtesy Dr. John Beumer, UCLA Maxillofacial Prosthetics, Los Angeles, CA.)*

A review of the reasons for failure of oral implants concluded that several situations increased the failure rate: a low insertion torque on immediately placed or early loaded implants, inexperienced surgeons, implants inserted in the maxilla and posterior regions of the jaws, implants placed in heavy smokers, implant insertion in poor-quality (i.e., type III and IV) bone, lack of initial stability, and prosthetic rehabilitation with implant-supported overdentures.[39]

The risk of implant failure varies among patients, but patterns of loss tend to cluster. A second attempt at dental implant placement should be approached cautiously if placing the implant in the same site as the one that previously failed. It is often challenging to achieve adequate diameter, length, and stability of replacement implants due to the residual defect created by removal of the failed implant. In 2007, Grossmann and Levin reported an overall survival rate of 71% for dental implants that were placed in sites of previously failed single implants. In that study, all of the original implants failed during the early healing phase (mean of 2.3 to 3.2 months after

placement).[80] In a 2008 study, Machtei and colleagues[119] reported an overall survival rate of 83.5% for the second attempt at dental implants. They concluded that replacing failed implants resulted in a lower survival rate compared with that for implants placed in pristine sites. This could not be associated with conventional implant- or patient-related factors. They suggested that a site-specific negative effect might be associated with this phenomenon.[119]

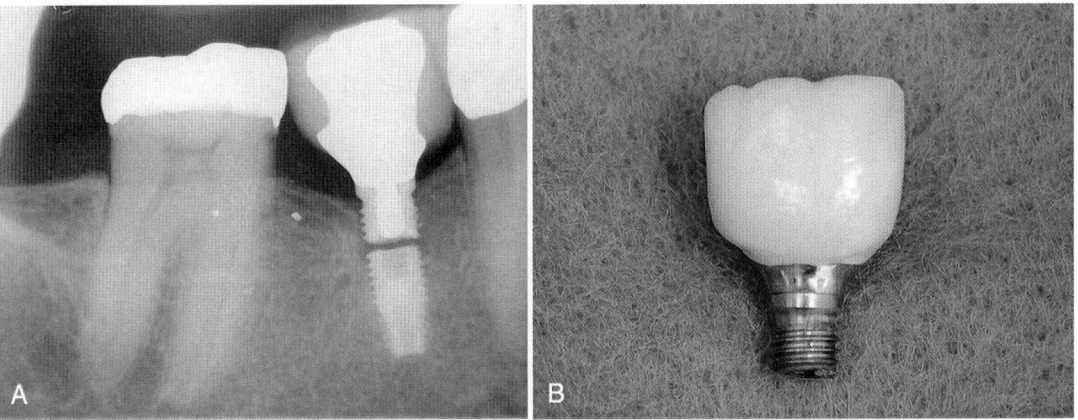

Fig. 85.17 (A) Radiograph of a fractured standard-diameter implant used to support a molar-sized single crown in the posterior mandible. (B) Crown and coronal portion of the implant (same as shown in A) that fractured between the third and fourth threads.

In 2011, Machtei and coworkers reported a lower survival rate (60%) for third reimplanted sites.[118] This outcome represents a further diminished prognosis compared with implants in original sites or after a second attempt.[43] Replacement of a failed implant poses a challenge in achieving osseointegration in a healed bone site and can reduce the implant survival rate.[118]

Prosthetic or Mechanical Complications

Prosthetic or mechanical complications occur when the strength of materials is no longer able to resist the forces that are being applied. As materials fatigue, they begin to stretch and bend. Ultimately, depending on the applied forces, they will fracture. Material failures lead to prosthetic complications such as loose, broken, and failed restorations.

Screw Loosening and Fracture

Screw loosening has occurred frequently in screw-retained FPDs. Screw-retained single crowns attached to externally hexed implants (i.e., those with narrow- or standard-diameter restorative interface connection surfaces) are particularly prone to this type of mechanical complication. Screw loosening has been reported for 6% to 49% of cases at the first annual checkup.[91,132] Screw loosening was a more prevalent problem with earlier designs. For example, abutment screws were previously made with titanium, which did not offer the clamping forces of current materials. Newer abutment designs and improved abutment screws enable an increased clamping force to be achieved without excessive torque, which has helped to reduce the rate of screw loosening.

Abutment or prosthesis screw loosening is often corrected by retightening the screws, but if screws continue to be stretched over time, they become fatigued and eventually fracture. This problem is evident in the patient with a loose single crown. In the patient with a prosthesis retained by multiple implants, the ability to detect a loose screw is greatly diminished, and the problem may go unnoticed until additional screws stretch, fatigue, and fracture. In either case, the biomechanical support (and resistance) for the restoration must be evaluated and, if possible, changed to prevent recurrence of the problem.

Implant Fracture

The ultimate mechanical failure is implant fracture because it results in loss of the implant and possibly of the prosthesis (Fig. 85.17). Removal of a fractured implant creates a large osseous defect. Factors such as fatigue of implant materials (Fig. 85.18) and weakness in

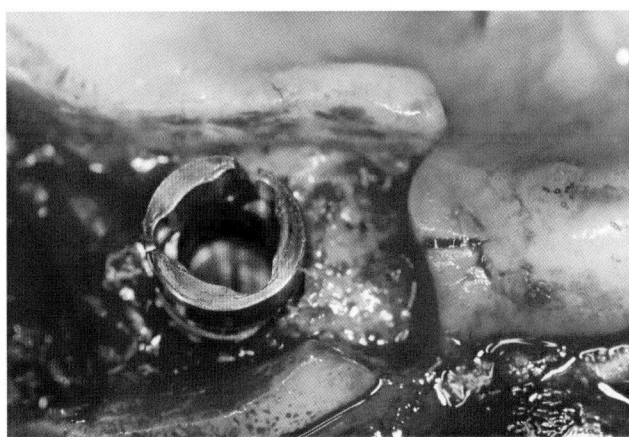

Fig. 85.18 The implant fractured at the internal connection collar. Fracture was caused by rotational forces applied to the implant at the time of placement into dense bone and was likely the result of combined material weakness and density of the prepared site.

prosthetic design or dimension are the usual causes of implant fractures.[4,16] Balshi[16] listed three categories of causes that may explain implant fractures: (1) design and material, (2) nonpassive fit of the prosthetic framework, and (3) physiologic or biomechanical overload. Patients with bruxism seem to be at higher risk for these events and therefore need to be screened, informed, and treated accordingly.[15,16] These patients should be fitted with occlusal guards in conjunction with placement of the final prostheses.

Fracture of Restorative Materials

Fracture or failure of materials used for implant-retained restorations can be a significant problem. This is particularly true for veneers (i.e., acrylic, composite, or ceramic) that are attached to superstructures (Fig. 85.19).

Aesthetic and Phonetic Complications
Aesthetic Complications

The challenge of modern implant dentistry is achieving an aesthetic and functional implant restoration. Harmonious tooth shape and size and ideal soft tissue contours are key factors for successful aesthetic outcomes.[108]

Aesthetic complications arise when patient expectations are not met. Patients' degree of satisfaction with the aesthetic outcome of

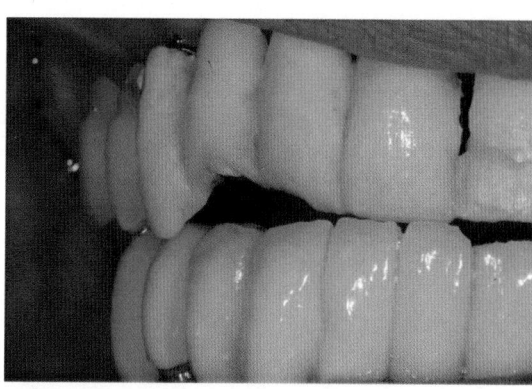

Fig. 85.19 Fractured porcelain from incisal edges of an implant-supported fixed partial denture.

implant prostheses varies. The risk of aesthetic complications is increased for patients with high aesthetic expectations and suboptimal patient-related factors such as a high smile line, thin periodontal soft tissues, or inadequate bone quantity and quality. In addition to the appearance of the final restoration, factors such as a patient's perception and desires determine the acceptance of the results. Aesthetic complications can result from poor implant position, deficiencies in the existing anatomy of edentulous sites that were reconstructed with implants, and prosthetic-related factors such as color mismatch.[14]

Important prerequisites for achieving optimal gingival tissue contour are sufficient peri-implant bone to support the soft tissues and a sufficient zone of keratinized tissue. Soft and hard tissue defects can be treated by a variety of augmentation procedures.

Implant placement in the aesthetic zone requires precise three-dimensional tissue reconstruction and ideal implant placement.[81,160] This reconstructive procedure enables the restorative dentist to develop a natural emergence profile of the implant crown. If the amount of available bone does not allow for ideal implant placement and the implant is positioned too far apically or buccally or in the proximal space, an unaesthetic emergence profile can result (Fig. 85.20).

If crown contours and dimensions are not ideal or gingival harmony around the implant restoration is unaesthetic, the patient may consider the implants or restorations to be failures because the outcome does not represent a natural appearance (Fig. 85.21). Gingiva-colored materials used to replace lost gingival anatomy offer an alternative to surgical augmentation in patients undergoing implant therapy (Fig. 85.22). These restorations provide numerous advantages over conventional restorations, including improved lip support, masking of interproximal spaces, and restoration of gingival symmetry in selected cases.[85]

If the patient is truly dissatisfied with the aesthetic result and there is a problem with the position of the implants that can be corrected (i.e., the patient's expectations are reasonable), the implants can be removed. The case can be reevaluated and possibly retreated. However, the clinician should consider prosthetic solutions before implant removal. Using angulated abutments, superstructures, or gingiva-colored materials, or submerging the implant with a conventional fixed partial denture may result in an acceptable aesthetic result, avoiding multiple operations to rebuild hard and soft tissues if an integrated implant is removed.

Careful patient evaluation and treatment planning with a solid understanding of and appreciation for the predictability and limitations of implant procedures can minimize aesthetic complications. Patients with a high smile line, high aesthetic demands, thin periodontium, or lack of hard and soft tissue support in the anterior aesthetic region should be treated only after extensive interdisciplinary treatment planning by experienced clinicians.

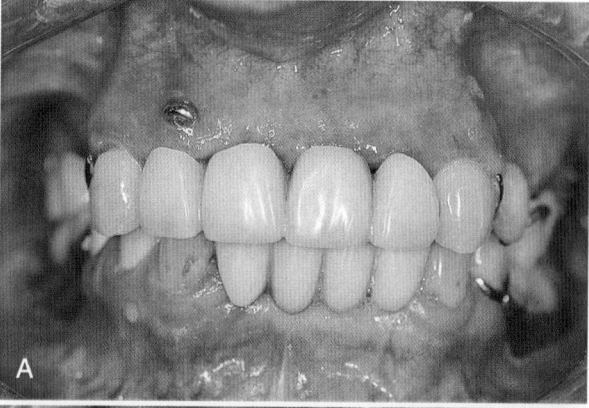

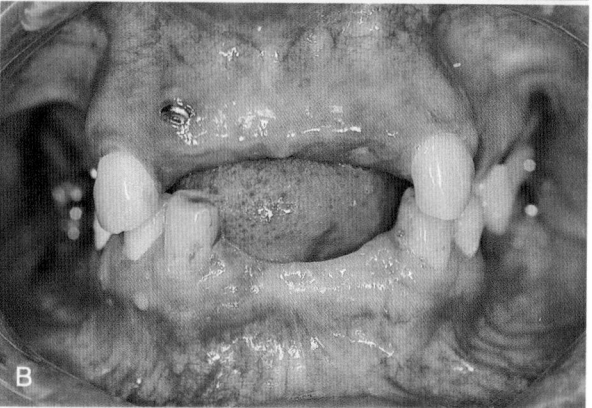

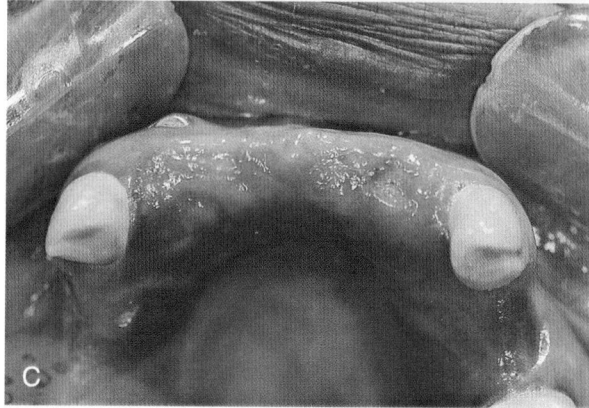

Fig. 85.20 Poor implant position makes it impossible to correct the problem with an aesthetic, natural-appearing restoration. (A) Anterior view with the removable partial dentures inserted. (B) Anterior view without the removable partial dentures. Notice the high level of implant cover screw/head exposure (maxillary right lateral incisor) that is significantly apical to the level of the adjacent natural tooth (cuspid) gingival margin. (C) Occlusal view of the same patient. Notice the labial projection of the same implant (maxillary right lateral incisor) and the palatal position of the implant in the premolar area. Any attempt to restore the anterior implants would not be aesthetically acceptable.

KEY FACT

Aesthetic complications arise when a patient's expectations are not met. Satisfaction with the aesthetic outcome varies tremendously among patients, and the increased risk of aesthetic complications correlates with high aesthetic expectations and less than optimal patient-related factors, such as a high smile line, thin periodontal soft tissues, or inadequate bone quantity and quality. Risk factors should be carefully evaluated and discussed with the patient before initiating therapy, and the ability to meet the patient's expectations should be carefully considered.

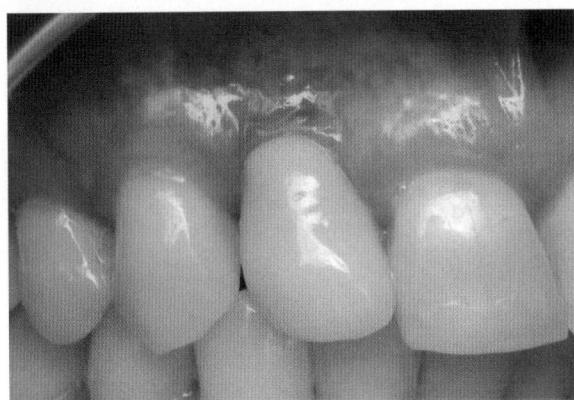

Fig. 85.21 High gingival margin on single-tooth implant crown in the maxillary lateral incisor position, showing the discrepancy between gingival margin levels of the implant and the adjacent natural teeth.

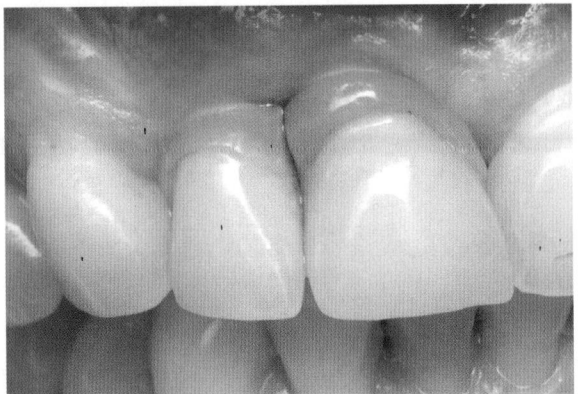

Fig. 85.22 Pink porcelain was used on an implant-supported fixed restoration to mask the high gingival margin and long implant crowns resulting from an uncorrected alveolar ridge defect.

Phonetic Problems

Implant prostheses that are fabricated with unusual palatal contours (i.e., restricted or narrow palatal space) or that have spaces under and around the superstructure can create phonetic problems for the patient. This is particularly problematic when full-arch, implant-supported, fixed restorations are fabricated for patients who have a severely atrophied maxilla. Horizontal bone loss in the premaxilla often causes palatal positioning of the dental implants, resulting in the prosthesis covering the incisive papilla region. Because some sounds are formed when the tip of the tongue lightly touches the palate at the incisive papilla region, covering this area can interfere with proper enunciation. Titanium-framed full restorations allow a thinner bulk of material in this region and can minimize phonetic complications.

These complications are exacerbated when using an immediate fixed provisional restoration. Phonetic problems can be common in full-denture cases. However, with dentures, the clinician can figure out many of the speech issues in wax before the final restoration, making it easier to focus on the specific problem area. Ideal tooth setup and multiple adjustments are needed to minimize phonetic problems. These patients are probably best served with an implant-assisted maxillary overdenture because the design facilitates replacement of missing alveolar structure and avoids creating spaces that allow air to escape during speech.

Conclusions

Although implants offer a highly predictable treatment option for the replacement of single and multiple missing teeth, surgical, biologic, mechanical, prosthetic, and aesthetic complications can occur. Careful diagnosis and treatment planning with the use of diagnostic imaging, surgical guides, meticulous techniques, and adherence to proven principles can prevent many of the problems discussed in this chapter.

A thorough understanding of anatomy, biology, and wound healing can reduce the incidence of complications. There is no substitute for good training, knowledge, and clinical experience. The clinician who places or restores implants must be well prepared to diagnose, prevent, and manage complications.

 A Case Scenario is found on the companion website www.expertconsult.com.

References

 References for this chapter are found on the companion website www.expertconsult.com.

Supportive Implant Treatment

Jonathan H. Do | Perry R. Klokkevold

Dental implant therapy does not end with the final prosthetic restoration of the implant. Predictability and long-term success of a dental implant and its restoration require sound treatment planning, precise surgical and restorative execution, and impeccable long-term maintenance, which depend on patient compliance with home care and professional supportive implant treatment.

Peri-implant maintenance begins as the implant becomes exposed to the oral cavity and continues at regular intervals during the life of the implant. The recall interval is determined by the patient's oral hygiene and susceptibility to biofilm-induced inflammatory diseases. For the first year after treatment, recall maintenance visits should be scheduled at 3-month intervals and then adjusted to suit the patient's needs. Patients who have good oral hygiene, minimal deposits, and disease resistance require infrequent professional hygiene maintenance, whereas those who have poor oral hygiene, heavy deposits, and disease susceptibility require more frequent follow-up care.

Rationale for Supportive Implant Treatment

Although dental implants are not vulnerable to dental caries, they are susceptible to mechanical complications and peri-implant, biofilm-induced inflammatory tissue changes. A 10-year retrospective study[48] of 397 fixed-implant reconstructions in 300 patients observed a mechanical complication rate of 24.7%. The most frequent complication was ceramic chipping (20.31%), followed by occlusal screw loosening (2.57%) and loss of retention (2.06%). Although relatively infrequent, occlusal screw loosening can result in a subgingival gap at the implant–abutment junction that retains plaque and stimulates an inflammatory reaction in soft and hard tissues.

Biologically, biofilm accumulation due to inadequate or no access for oral hygiene can result in peri-implant mucositis and peri-implantitis. Peri-implant mucositis is characterized by inflammation confined to the soft tissue and is reported to affect up to 80% of patients with dental implants.[25] Peri-implantitis is characterized by peri-implant inflammation with progressive crestal bone loss beyond the initial remodeling. The prevalence of peri-implantitis among patients is 11.2% to 53%.[27,37,38-40] Poor oral hygiene, residual cement, current or history of periodontitis, cigarette smoking, and diabetes mellitus are risk factors for peri-implant diseases.[1,9]

The relationship between peri-implant mucositis and peri-implantitis is similar to that between gingivitis and periodontitis. Although peri-implant mucositis does not necessarily progress to peri-implantitis,

it is likely the precursor to peri-implantitis.[1] The inflammatory response in peri-implant disease appears to be similar to that in periodontal disease.[41] However, the severity and rate of disease progression appear to be more pronounced around implants. This may be caused by the absence of a self-limiting process, which is observed in periodontitis, around implants that separates the inflammatory cell infiltrate from the bone.[6] Experimental models demonstrated that peri-implant mucositis was reversible at the biomarker level (i.e., matrix metalloproteinase 8 [MMP-8] and interleukin-1β [IL-1β]).[41]

A review of the literature[36] reported that peri-implant mucositis could be effectively treated with nonsurgical mechanical therapies, but these modalities tended to be ineffective against peri-implantitis. Results of surgical treatment for peri-implantitis are not predictable. Prevention, early detection, and early treatment of peri-implant diseases are therefore crucial. Periodic and well-regimented supportive implant treatment is essential to the long-term success of dental implant therapy.

KEY FACT

Implants are susceptible to mechanical complications and biofilm-induced inflammatory diseases, such as peri-implant mucositis and peri-implantitis.

Examination of Implants

The supportive implant treatment appointment should include: an inquiry about new concerns, problems, or pain; review of changes in the patient's medical and oral status; evaluation and reinforcement of oral hygiene; examination and evaluation of soft and hard tissue health; evaluation of implants and the associated implant restorations' stability and integrity; and professional supportive treatment. Assessment should determine the appropriate recall interval and plan for the next visit.

Examination begins with visual inspection for biofilm and calculus accumulation; signs of inflammation and swelling; peri-implant soft tissue quality, color, consistency, and contour; and aberrations in the implant prosthesis. Peri-implant soft tissue can be digitally palpated to detect edema, tenderness, exudation, or suppuration. Peri-implant probing can be done to assess the condition and level of soft and hard tissues surrounding implants. When indicated, radiographic images can be obtained to help verify the level of the peri-implant crestal bone. Determination of implant stability or mobility

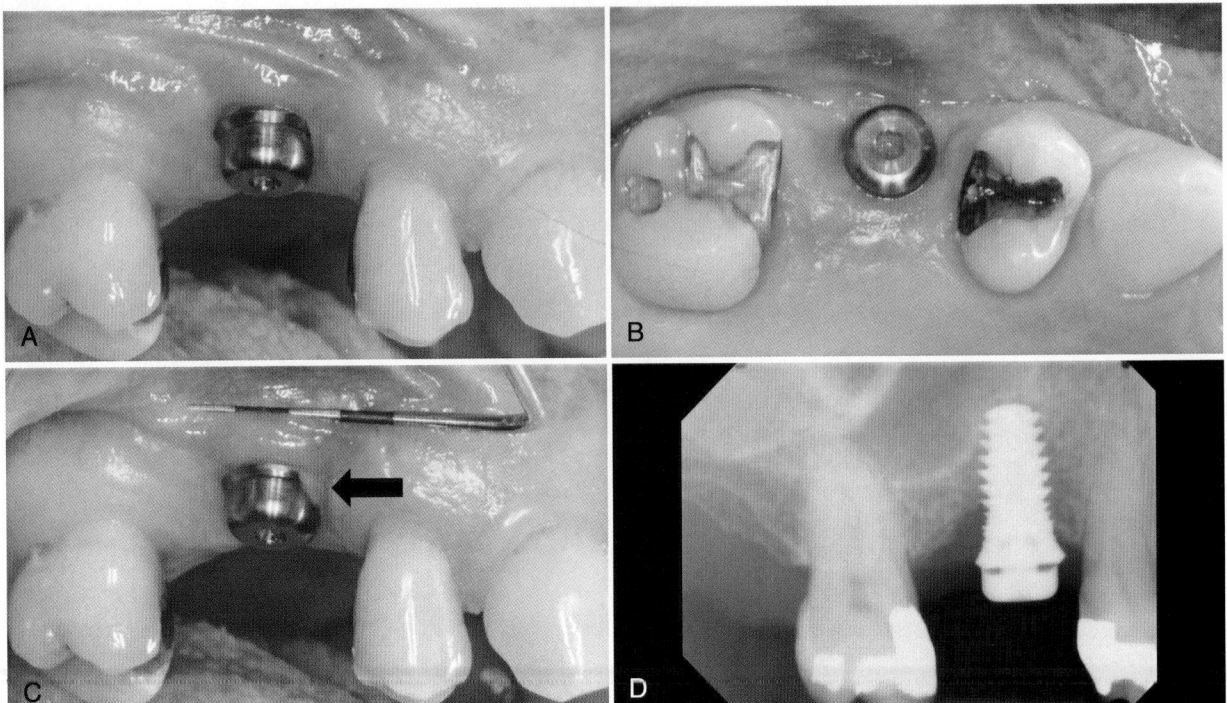

Fig. 86.1 Peri-implantitis. (A and B) Minimal biofilm accumulation is seen. The peri-implant mucosa exhibits minimal erythema and edema. Notice the buccal placement of the implant in B. (C) Manipulation of tissue indicates a lack of buccal keratinized attached gingiva and exudation from the peri-implant sulcus *(arrow)*. (D) The periapical radiograph shows peri-implant bone loss to the apex of the implant.

and percussion testing can help verify implant osseointegration (Fig. 86.1).

Peri-implant Probing

Probing of implants can be done with light force (i.e., 0.25 N) using a traditional steel probe without adverse effects to the peri-implant mucosa.[15] Implant probing should be recorded at the time of final restoration as the baseline measurement and done at least annually thereafter.[25]

Clinicians should use caution when evaluating peri-implant probing because these measures cannot be interpreted the same as probing depths around teeth. Although periodontal probing around natural teeth is useful for assessing the health of periodontal tissues, the sulcus or pocket depth, and the level of attachment, probing around implants may not provide comparable results.[7] Due to distinct differences in the tissues that surround and support teeth compared with those that surround and support implants, the probe inserts and penetrates differently. Around teeth, the periodontal probe is resisted by the health of the periodontal tissues and importantly by the insertion of supracrestal connective tissue fibers into the cementum of the root surface. These fibers, which are unique to teeth, are the primary source of resistance to the probe.[3] There is no equivalent fiber attachment around implants. Connective tissue fibers around implants usually run parallel to the implant or restorative surface and do not have perpendicular or inserting fibers (see Chapter 74). The primary

source of resistance to the probe depends on the conditions around the implant.[12,24] At noninflamed sites, the most coronal aspect of connective tissue adhesion to the implant resists the probe. At inflamed sites, the probe tip consistently penetrates farther into the connective tissue until less inflamed connective tissue is encountered, which is often close to or at the level of bone.

The value of peri-implant probing is different from periodontal probing and offers comparatively limited information. Probing around implants can measure the level of the mucosal margin relative to a fixed position on the implant or restoration and can also measure the depth of tissue around the implant. The peri-implant probing depth is often a measure of the thickness of the surrounding connective tissues and correlates most consistently with the level of surrounding bone. However, peri-implant probing is affected by several conditions, including the size of the probe, the force and direction of insertion, the health and resistance of peri-implant tissues, the level of bone support, and the features of the implant, abutment, and prosthesis design (Fig. 86.2).

A comparison[45] of probing pocket depth of implants with peri-implantitis before and after the removal of the prosthetic restorations reported similar probing depths in only 37% of sites. In 39% of sites, the difference was ±1 mm; in 15% of sites, it was ±2 mm; and in 9% of sites, it was ±3 mm. Probing measurements can be an accurate measure of soft tissue thickness around an implant (i.e., peri-implant soft tissue above the bone level), but in many cases or sites, the inability to properly angle and direct the probe along the implant can lead to inaccurate assessment of soft tissue thickness. In these situations, the clinician must appreciate the limitations and know that other clinical parameters and radiographs are required to help evaluate the peri-implant's condition.

Probing around implants is likely to vary more than around teeth. Studies have shown that a change in probing force around implants results in more dramatic changes than a similar change in probing

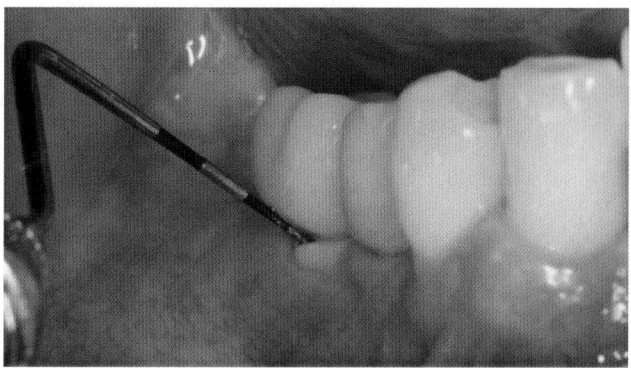

Fig. 86.2 Buccal probing of the implant is impeded by the implant restoration.

force around teeth.[29] The probing depth around implants presumed to be healthy (and without bleeding) has been documented as about 3 mm around all surfaces.[2,8] The absence of bleeding on probing around teeth has been established as an indicator of health and a predictor of periodontal stability.[21] Studies comparing bleeding on probing around teeth and implants in the same patient have reported that bleeding around implants occurs more frequently.

Bleeding on probing at implant sites can indicate inflammation in the peri-implant mucosa. However, the ability to use bleeding on probing as an indicator for assessing diseased or healthy sites around implants has not been established. Due to the potential for false-positive bleeding (i.e., provoked bleeding) with probing, the use of marginal bleeding, which is a more sensitive indicator of inflammation and is less likely to elicit false-positive bleeding, has been proposed to assess peri-implant inflammation.[50] Marginal bleeding can be evaluated by running a probe circumferentially along the coronal portion in the implant sulcus. Overall, the value of peri-implant probing is in monitoring changes in the probing pocket depth over time rather than the initial value because some implants are placed apically for aesthetics.[1]

> ### CLINICAL CORRELATION
>
> Probing of implants can be accomplished with a traditional steel probe. It is valuable for detecting tactilely inflammatory changes in the tissue, such as loss of tissue to resistance to probe penetration, sponginess of peri-implant mucosa, and bleeding on probing, and for monitoring changes in probing depth over time.

Microbial Testing

Studies in animals and humans have demonstrated the development of peri-implant mucosal inflammation in response to the accumulation of bacterial plaque.[5,33,41,51] Microbiologic studies suggest that greater probing depths (i.e., pockets) around implants harbor higher levels of pathogenic microorganisms.[30,35,43] Studies have also documented similarities in the microbial composition of plaque in healthy periodontal sites compared with healthy peri-implant sites.[31] Evidence indicates that the microbiota of diseased periodontal pockets harbor the same pathogenic microorganisms as those observed in inflamed peri-implant sites (i.e., peri-implantitis).[31,43] However, there is no evidence to prove that periodontal pathogens cause peri-implant disease, and the pathogenesis of inflammatory disease around implants has not been defined.[10]

One report[1] accepted the idea that peri-implant disease, like periodontal disease, occurs primarily as a result of an overwhelming bacterial insult and subsequent host response. Human biopsies indicate that peri-implantitis and periodontitis exhibit similar histologic features, including an inflammatory cell infiltrate in the connective tissue dominated by B lymphocytes and plasma cells and by up-regulation of inflammatory biomarkers. No evidence indicates that laboratory tests for the identification of suspected periodontal pathogens are of use in the evaluation of implants.[14] The usefulness of microbial testing may be limited to the evaluation of peri-implant sites that are showing signs of infection and bone loss, allowing the clinician to prescribe appropriate antibiotics.

Stability Measures

The assessment of implant stability or mobility is an important measure for determining whether osseointegration is being maintained. Important as it is, however, this measure has extremely low sensitivity but high specificity. An implant can exhibit significant bone loss and remain stable; the stability measure in this case has a low sensitivity for the detection of bone loss. Conversely, if implant mobility is detected, it is likely that the implant is not surrounded by bone; mobility is highly specific for the detection of implant failure or lack of osseointegration. Mobility demands differentiation of loss of implant osseointegration from a loose implant restoration.

There is great interest in evaluating the stability of bone-to-implant contact in a noninvasive manner. Two noninvasive techniques for evaluating implant stability are impact resistance (e.g., Periotest) and resonance frequency analysis (RFA). Originally designed to evaluate tooth mobility quantitatively, the Periotest (Gulden, Bensheim, Germany) is a noninvasive electronic device that provides an objective measurement of the reaction of the periodontium to a defined impact load applied to the tooth crown. The Periotest value depends to some extent on tooth mobility but mainly on the dampening characteristics of the periodontium. Despite dependence on the periodontium, the Periotest has been used to evaluate implant stability. However, unlike teeth, the movement of implants and surrounding bone is minuscule, and Periotest values therefore fall within a much smaller range compared with those for teeth. Detection of horizontal mobility may be a significant advantage of the Periotest because it is much more sensitive to horizontal movement than similar detection by other means, such as manual assessment.[14]

Another noninvasive method used to measure the stability of implants is RFA,[28] which uses a transducer that is attached to the implant or abutment. A steady-state signal is applied to the implant through the transducer, and the response is measured. The RFA value is a function of the stiffness of the implant in the surrounding tissues. The stiffness is influenced by the implant, the interface between the implant and the bone and soft tissues, and the surrounding bone itself. The height of the implant or abutment above the bone influences the RFA value. Unlike the Periotest, the RFA does not depend on movement in only one direction. The absolute RFA values vary from one implant design to another and from one site to another, but there is high consistency for any one implant or location.

The value of RFA is most appreciated with repeated measures of the same implant over time because it is very sensitive to changes in the bone–implant interface. Small changes in tissue support can be detected using this method. An increase in RFA value indicates increased implant stability, whereas a decrease indicates loss of stability. However, this is a relative measure, and it has not been determined whether RFA is capable of detecting impending failure before the implant fails.

Much interest and research have focused on the use of noninvasive methods to evaluate implant stability. Mobility remains the cardinal sign of implant failure, and detecting mobility is therefore an important parameter.

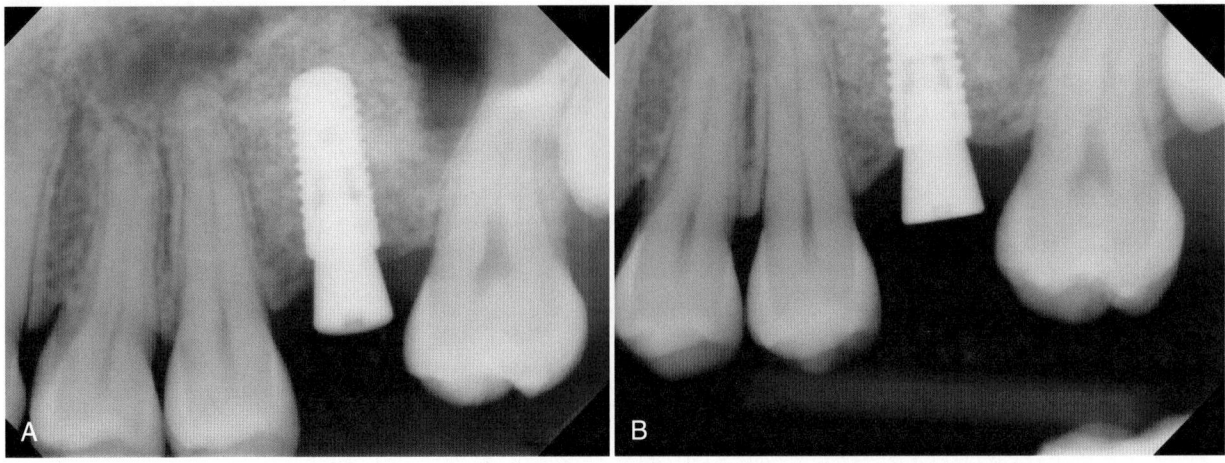

Fig. 86.3 (A) A periapical radiograph captures the whole implant. (B) A second perpendicular periapical radiograph is necessary to assess the crestal bone level. Platform switching is seen at the implant–abutment junction.

Implant Percussion

Tapping an implant's healing abutment or restoration with an instrument produces a sound that can help determine its osseointegration. A solid resonating sound and the absence of pain usually indicate osseointegration. A dull sound can indicate that the implant is fibrous encapsulated; radiographic and other clinical findings are needed for diagnosis. Video 86.1 demonstrates percussion testing, which distinguishes between an osseointegrated implant and a failed implant.

Radiographic Examination

Perpendicular intraoral periapical radiographs should be taken at implant placement, at abutment connection, and at final restoration for baseline documentation of bone levels and annually[11] thereafter to monitor marginal or peri-implant bone changes. In the setting of peri-implant inflammation, a periapical radiograph is indicated for peri-implant bone evaluation and disease diagnosis. Periapical radiographs have excellent resolution and, when taken perpendicular to an implant, can provide valuable details of the implant-abutment junction, mesial and distal crestal bone level relative to the implant platform, and bone-to-implant interface along the length of the implant (Fig. 86.3). Periapical radiographs are difficult to standardize and great variation is inherent in the acquisition process, but they are relatively simple, inexpensive, and readily available in the dental office. It is diagnostically important to obtain images that clearly show implant threads (i.e., not blurred by nonperpendicular angulation) and the restorative implant–abutment connection.

The objective of the radiographic examination is to measure the height of bone adjacent to the implant, evaluate the quality of bone along the length of the implant, and detect peri-implant radiolucencies. Although the predictive value of assessing implant stability with radiographs is low, films do offer a reasonable method to measure changes in bone levels.[46] The predictive value of detecting implant failure or loss of stability is good when radiolucent lesions are discovered with periapical radiographs. Identification of unstable implants is reliable when radiographs are obtained as part of an annual examination and when examining patients on a routine long-term basis.[19]

The radiographic examination remains one of the primary tools for detection of failed or failing implants in routine clinical evaluations, although it is not as accurate as mobility tests. In one study designed to evaluate the accuracy and precision of radiographic diagnosis of mobility, the probability of predicting implant mobility in a population

with a low prevalence of implant failures was low.[46] Other studies, however, have demonstrated a much higher predictive value for radiographic diagnosis of implant mobility.[18,19] Investigators concluded that the most important factors for making an accurate radiographic diagnosis are the quality of the radiograph and the experience of the clinician.[19,46]

◄◄   FLASH BACK

Intraoral periapical radiographs of implants must be taken with the x-ray beam perpendicular to the implant fixture to enable clear visualization of implant threads and the mesial and distal crestal bone levels.

Assessment of Peri-Implant Health
Evaluation of Biofilm Control

Impeccable biofilm control is crucial to peri-implant tissue health. Poor biofilm control is associated with peri-implant disease (odds ratio =14.3).[25] It is advantageous to evaluate biofilm control before tissue manipulation. The amount and location of biofilm and calculus accumulation should be assessed visually. Poor control is typically associated with biofilm and calculus retention and with erythematous and edematous gingival tissue. When biofilm control is inadequate, the patient should be asked to demonstrate his or her oral hygiene routine in front of a mirror so that the clinician can evaluate the patient's technique. If the patient fails to remove biofilm in any areas, the patient's attention should be directed to the location of the biofilm. An instrument can be used to remove the biofilm, with the patient paying attention so that he or she can see its color and consistency. At this time, oral hygiene instruction should be demonstrated and reinforced.

Evaluation of Peri-Implant Health and Disease

Peri-implant mucosal health is characterized by pink, firm, and well-adapted gingival tissue. Peri-implant disease is associated with clinical erythema, edema, and loss of tissue tightness around the implant. Peri-implant mucosa can be nonkeratinized and unattached (see Fig. 86.1C) or keratinized and attached (Fig. 86.4C). In the setting of keratinized, attached mucosa, a gingival seal or gingival cuff is established around the implant.[4] The gingival cuff can protect the underlying bone and reduce subgingival plaque formation. Due to the mobile nature of oral mucosa, the protective

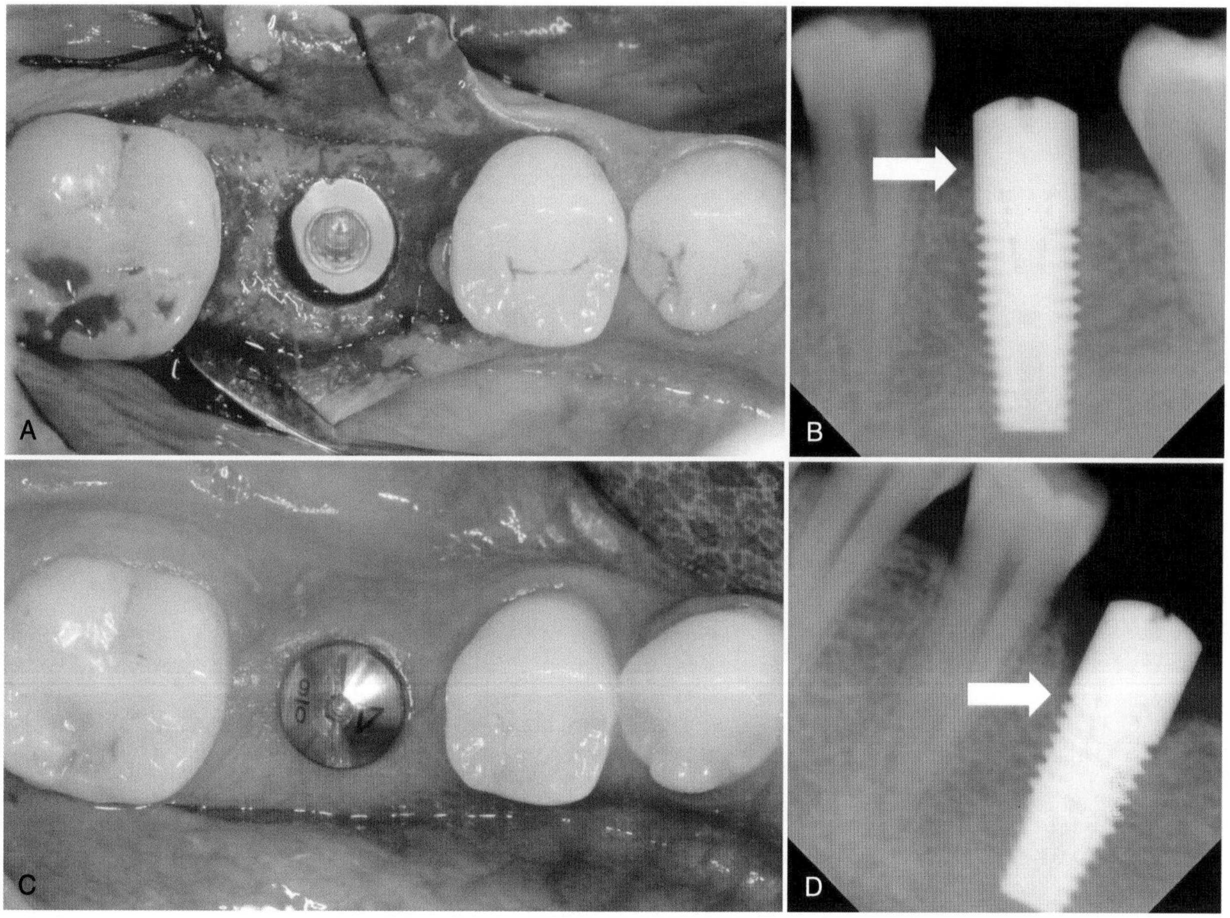

Fig. 86.4 (A) Subcrestal placement of an implant with adequate buccal and lingual bone thickness. (B) Periapical radiograph at the time of implant placement. (C) Implant at the 5-month osseointegration check exhibits adequate peri-implant keratinized attached tissue. (D) It also shows crestal bone remodeling to the first thread. *Arrows* indicate the mesial crestal bone level.

function of nonkeratinized, unattached peri-implant mucosa may not be as effective. However, the presence of keratinized, attached gingiva, which can facilitate oral hygiene, is not a requisite for peri-implant health if biofilm is well controlled.[44,49] Nonetheless, sites deficient in keratinized, attached tissue typically exhibit vertical or horizontal ridge deficiencies, shallow vestibular depths, and long or bulky restorations. All of these factors can impede oral hygiene access and contribute to biofilm accumulation and peri-implant inflammation.

 KEY FACT

Peri-implant health is characterized by pink, firm, and well-adapted peri-implant mucosa. Peri-implant disease is associated with erythema, edema, and loss of tissue tightness around the implant.

In cases of inflammation, the peri-implant tissue must be palpated for tenderness and suppuration, the implant must be probed, and periapical radiographs must be obtained and compared with baseline images to determine peri-implant bone loss. Suppuration often indicates peri-implantitis.[25] Radiographic crestal bone loss beyond the implant baseline level at the time of final prosthesis delivery in conjunction with bleeding on probing is characteristic of peri-implantitis.[22] Due to potential measurement errors, a threshold of

detectable bone loss of 1.0 to 1.5 mm is recommended for the diagnosis of peri-implantitis.[42] In the absence of a baseline radiograph, a vertical distance of 2 mm from the expected marginal bone level after the initial crestal bone remodeling is recommended as the threshold for diagnosing peri-implantitis.[42]

The amount of initial marginal bone remodeling depends on the design of the implant–abutment junction. Platform-switched implants (Fig. 86.5C; see Fig. 86.3), in which the abutment is internally offset relative to the implant fixture at the implant–abutment junction, may exhibit less crestal bone remodeling than non–platform-switched implants (see Fig. 86.4), in which the abutment is flush or even with the implant fixture at the implant–abutment junction.

Evaluation of Implant Osseointegration

Implant osseointegration must be determined before fabrication and delivery of the final implant prosthesis. Implant osseointegration can be definitively determined only histologically, which requires the implant and the surrounding bone to be removed. A combination of radiographic and clinical parameters are used to assess implant osseointegration or to rule out lack of osseointegration. They include absence of peri-implant inflammation and pain in response to palpation and percussion, a solid resonating sound in reaction to percussion, complete radiographic bone-to-implant contact along the implant surface (i.e., absence of radiolucencies along the bone–implant interface), and implant stability.

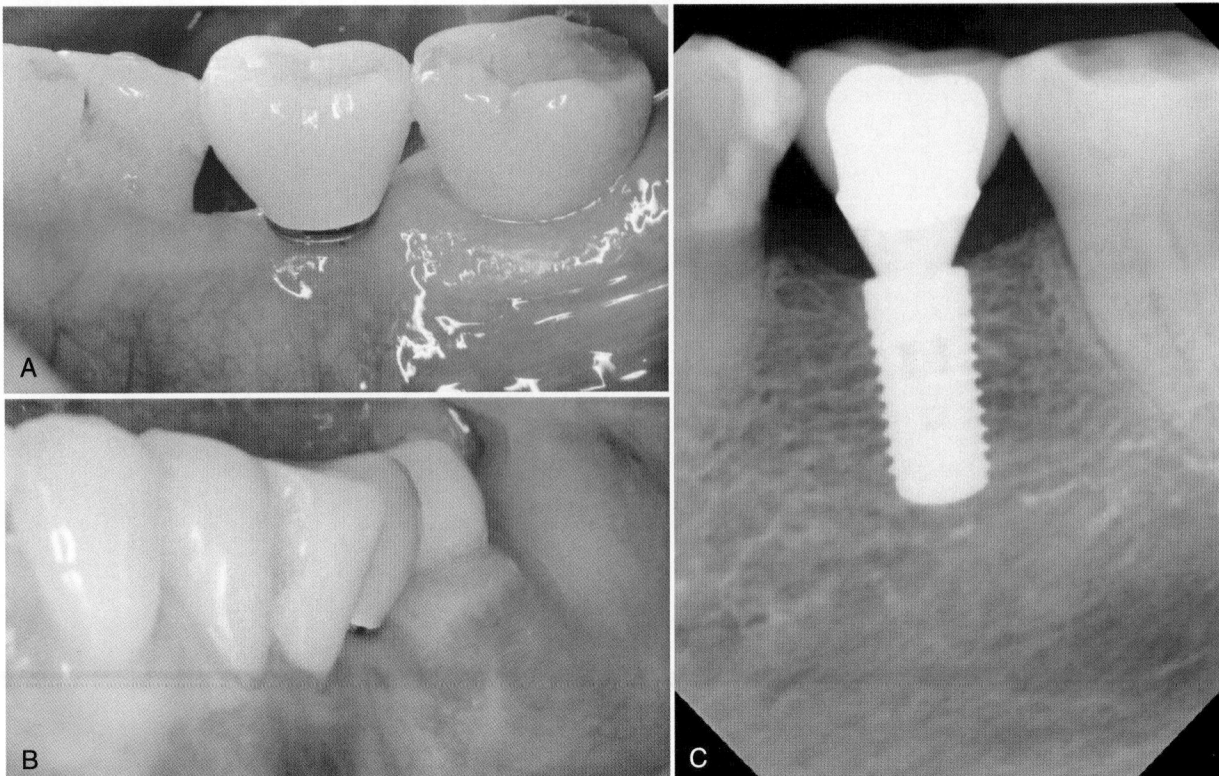

Fig. 86.5 Restoration is designed with adequate hygiene access. (A) Lingual view. (B) Mesial view of the buccal contour. (C) The periapical radiograph shows a gradual transition from the implant fixture to the restoration. Platform switching is seen at the implant–abutment junction.

Evaluation of Implant Restorations

Implant superstructures, frameworks, and restorations should be fabricated to accommodate and facilitate oral hygiene (e.g., embrasure spaces made to allow passage of a proxy brush) (see Fig. 86.4). Occlusal schemes of implant restorations should provide adequate posterior support, maximize axial loading, and minimize incline contacts, nonaxial loading, and interferences in excursive movements.

During delivery, radiographs perpendicular to the implant should be obtained for baseline documentation and to verify complete seating of the restorations. After delivery, cement-retained implant restorations should be thoroughly evaluated for residual excess cement, which must be removed. During follow-up visits, implant restorations should be carefully examined for heavy contacts, fractures, loose screws, and in removable prostheses, worn-out retentive components (i.e., Hader clips and locator attachment inserts). Occlusion should be adjusted accordingly to prevent implant overload and fractures of implant parts. Loose abutment and set screws must be evaluated, possibly replaced, and properly torqued down. Worn-out retentive components must be replaced periodically to ensure proper retention, stability, and function of the removable prosthesis. Occlusal wear of teeth and fit of tissue-borne surfaces of an implant prosthesis should be assessed and corrected as indicated. In patients with oral parafunctions and heavy occlusal forces, occlusal guards are recommended to protect implants and restorations.

Implant Maintenance

Methods for Patient Oral Hygiene

The importance of good oral hygiene should be stressed even before implants are placed, and peri-implant oral hygiene for biofilm control should begin as early as possible after the implant is exposed to the oral cavity. A cotton tip, cotton gauze, or soft toothbrush can be used to gently remove biofilm from healing abutments or provisional restorations during the early postoperative phase of healing. Before implant osseointegration, the use of powered toothbrushes should be avoided.

After implant osseointegration has been achieved and verified, brushing with dentifrice can help remove deposits and increase smoothness of exposed implant and restoration surfaces.[32] Other dental hygiene aids, such as dental floss, rubber tips, and interdental brushes, can be employed (Fig. 86.6). Oral hygiene should emphasize removal of biofilm and deposits along the gingival margin. Evidence for the use of a powered oral irrigator around implants is limited. One study reported that subgingival irrigation of 0.06% chlorhexidine gluconate with a Waterpik device (Water Pik, Inc., Fort Collins, CO) was more effective at reducing biofilm and gingival inflammation and produced fewer stains than rinsing with 0.12% chlorhexidine gluconate once daily.[16]

Methods for Professional Recall Maintenance

Professional maintenance consists of the removal of dental biofilm and calculus from implant components exposed to the oral environment.[26] Like root surfaces, the transmucosal surfaces of implants should be smooth to minimize plaque accumulation and to facilitate oral hygiene practices.[23] At sites with excellent biofilm control and peri-implant health, the need for professional instrumentation is minimal, and instrumentation should be limited to prevent iatrogenic damage to implant components that can contribute to plaque and calculus accumulation. In the setting of biofilm, calculus, and tenacious deposits, care should be taken to minimize damage to transmucosal implant surfaces. However, priority should be placed on the complete removal of implant surface deposits.

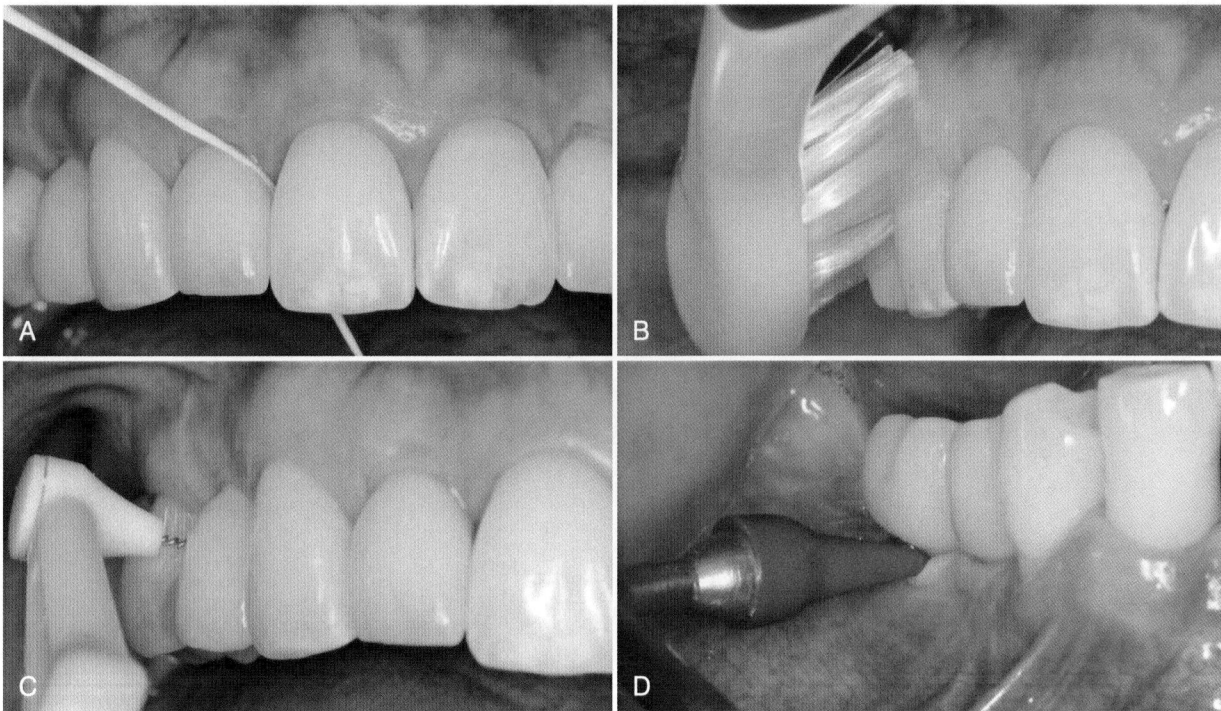

Fig. 86.6 Methods for patient oral hygiene are shown. (A) Flossing. (B) Bass method of brushing with an extra-soft toothbrush. (C) Interproximal brushing. (D) Removal of biofilm with a rubber tip. Hygiene methods remove biofilm along the gingival margin.

All metal instruments, including metal curettes and scalers, and ultrasonic scalers increase the surface roughness of polished titanium.[26] The use of plastic, Teflon-coated, and carbon and gold-coated curettes and nonmetal ultrasonic tips have been advocated to protect the titanium implant surface and the titanium abutment from contamination by other metals and to reduce the likelihood of scratching the surface. Unfortunately, the large size and flexibility of nonmetal curettes may not allow effective biofilm and calculus removal,[34] and Teflon- and gold-coated curettes cannot be sharpened.

Most implant prostheses are made with gold alloys or ceramic materials, which are usually identical to the materials used in restorations for the natural dentition. The location of the connection between the restorative material and the implant is typically below the mucosa and often near the crest of bone; most calculus removal is done above this level. The fear of contaminating the titanium implant is therefore unwarranted. Gold alloy or ceramic surfaces can be debrided with most scalers and curettes (e.g., plastic, gold-coated, stainless steel) without damaging the surface. Rubber cups and polishing paste can be used to remove biofilm and to enhance the smoothness of machined and polished surfaces. Magnetostrictive and piezoelectric ultrasonic instruments with metal tips (e.g., Cavitron) should be used with caution because of irregularities that can easily be created in the surface.

Treatment of Peri-Implant Diseases

The goals of treatment are elimination of all peri-implant infectious and inflammatory processes, prevention of disease progression, and preservation and restoration of function and aesthetics. Treatment begins with patient education about the causes, pathogenesis, and prevention of peri-implant diseases, along with oral hygiene instruction. Although bacteria are the main etiologic factor, systemic (e.g., smoking, poorly controlled diabetes) and local factors (e.g., residual

excess cement, poorly designed restorations that inhibit hygiene access) should be identified and modified.

Peri-Implant Mucositis

Peri-implant mucositis can be effectively treated with nonsurgical mechanical therapy.[36] Treatment requires complete removal of supramucosal and submucosal biofilm, calculus, and deposits using curettes, ultrasonic scalers, and polishing cups with prophy paste. Antimicrobials (e.g., chlorhexidine irrigation, mouthrinse) can be used with mechanical debridement to enhance treatment outcome.[36]

Peri-Implantitis

The treatment of peri-implantitis includes nonsurgical and surgical interventions, which can be combined with the adjunctive use of antimicrobials. Nonsurgical interventions consist of antimicrobial rinse and irrigation, local antibiotics, ultrasonic debridement, mechanical debridement with air-abrasive devices, and laser therapy. Surgical treatment includes full-thickness flap elevation for access, followed by degranulation, surface debridement by laser or mechanical instruments, surface decontamination with laser or antimicrobials, and bone augmentation. The data from two systematic reviews[13,47] are insufficient to suggest which intervention for peri-implantitis is most effective or to allow specific recommendations for the use of locally or systematically administered antibiotics.

Implant surface decontamination or disinfection remains challenging, especially for implants with roughened surfaces. For some treatment modalities, recurrence of peri-implantitis appears to be high (up to 100%) after 1 or more years of treatment, and retreatment may be necessary. Surgical access appears to be necessary to arrest peri-implant bone loss. Surgical treatment can result in gingival recession and compromised aesthetics. At sites with high aesthetic demands, definitive treatment of peri-implantitis can include the removal of the implant, grafting of the site, and placement of another implant.

KEY FACT

Treatment of peri-implant mucositis is effective, whereas treatment of peri-implantitis is unpredictable. Prevention, early detection, and treatment of peri-implant inflammatory diseases are essential for successful outcomes.

Referral of Patients to the Periodontist

The previously described guidelines allow many implants to be maintained quite well by primary dental care providers (i.e., general dentists). Referral to a periodontist should be considered if peri-implantitis or peri-implant mucositis is diagnosed and cannot be resolved with improved oral hygiene and professional maintenance care. Early referral is advantageous to stop progression and limit the extent of bone loss.

 A Case Scenario is found on the companion website www.expertconsult.com.

References

 References for this chapter are found on the companion website www.expertconsult.com.

CHAPTER 87

Results of Implant Treatment

Perry R. Klokkevold

CHAPTER OUTLINE

Defining Implant Outcomes
Factors That Influence Implant Outcomes
Aesthetic Results and Patient Satisfaction
Conclusions

The landmark Göteborg study and the replica study at the University of Toronto supported expectations for the success and predictability of root-form dental implants. The study, conducted over a 15-year period at the University of Göteborg, Sweden, by P.I. Bränemark and coworkers, began in 1965 and concluded in 1980. The results, which were reported in several articles, defined the concept of osseointegration, described protocols for success, and shared clinical experiences.

The most significant article from the study, published in 1981, was on osseointegrated implants in the treatment of the edentulous jaw.[2] The Göteborg study included 2768 root-form implants placed into 410 edentulous jaws in 371 consecutive patients. The data were most often reported in subsets according to the three study phases (i.e., initial, developmental, and routine). Cases treated in the routine period with standardized procedures and an observation time of 5 to 9 years were thought to reflect the potential of the method and were the basis of data reported in that historic publication. The subset consisted of 895 implants placed in 130 jaws. The implant survival rate was 81% in the maxilla and 91% in mandible. The prosthesis survival (i.e., continuous stability) rate was 89% in the maxilla and 100% in the mandible.

The replica study, which was conducted at the University of Toronto, demonstrated that comparable results could be predictably achieved using the same implant design and treatment protocols.[5,78–80] Together, these studies demonstrated that implant survival of 81% or more and prosthesis survival of 89% or more could be expected in the edentulous patient.

In the decades since the landmark discovery of osseointegration and the documentation of its clinical effectiveness, clinicians have had tremendous success in replacing missing teeth with endosseous root-form dental implants in both partially edentulous and edentulous patients.[1,48] Despite the high level of success and long-term predictability, a 100% success rate cannot be achieved. Complications and implant failures do occur.[2,12] Some implants fail to achieve osseointegration; some achieve osseointegration but lose bone progressively over time, leading to failure; and other implants rapidly lose bone and fail in a short time. Some implants achieve and maintain osseointegration but fail because they do not meet the aesthetic expectations of the patient or clinician.

The reporting of implant success varies widely in the literature, which makes defining an absolute implant success rate impractical. This chapter considers implant treatment results in light of the factors that influence implant survival and success. The intent is to outline important aspects that need to be considered in evaluating implant outcomes and offer guidelines for understanding published results.

Defining Implant Outcomes

Implant outcomes are reported in a variety of ways in the literature. Various levels of implant success and failure are described in case reports, case series, retrospective studies, controlled studies, and prospective studies. The type of study and method of reporting are decided by the authors and often influenced by the data collected and the study objectives. Each type of study or report has recognized limitations, but because of tremendous variation that exists in the ways individual investigators measure, interpret, and report implant outcomes, differences in the results from one study to another may not be obvious.

Some implant outcomes are reported as the presence or absence of the implant at the time of the last examination, regardless of whether the implant was functional, suffered from bone loss, or had other problems. This type of assessment is a measure of implant *survival* and should not be confused with implant *success*. In contrast to such an overly simplified assessment, some investigators report implant outcomes using specific criteria to determine implant success.

Implant success is defined by specific criteria used to evaluate the condition and function of the implant. Criteria for implant success have been proposed in the literature but have not been used consistently. The problem is that a universally accepted definition of implant success has not been established. In the classic definition, Albrektsson and colleagues[3] defined success as an implant with no pain, no mobility, no radiolucent peri-implant areas, and less than 0.2 mm of bone loss annually after the first year of loading.[3] Bone loss in the first year was recognized, but it was not defined or quantified as part of the success criteria until later in a separate definition by Roos and associates.[61]

The challenge in comparing reported data between studies is that investigators use different criteria for success in their work. As a result, it is difficult or impossible to make comparisons between studies, and drawing conclusions about implant success or failure from data reported in different studies is tenuous.

Success rates are dramatically affected by variations in the criteria used to define them. In strict terms, if implant success is considered to be an outcome without adverse effects or problems, the treatment would be performed as planned, implants would remain stable and functioning without problems, peri-implant tissues would be stable

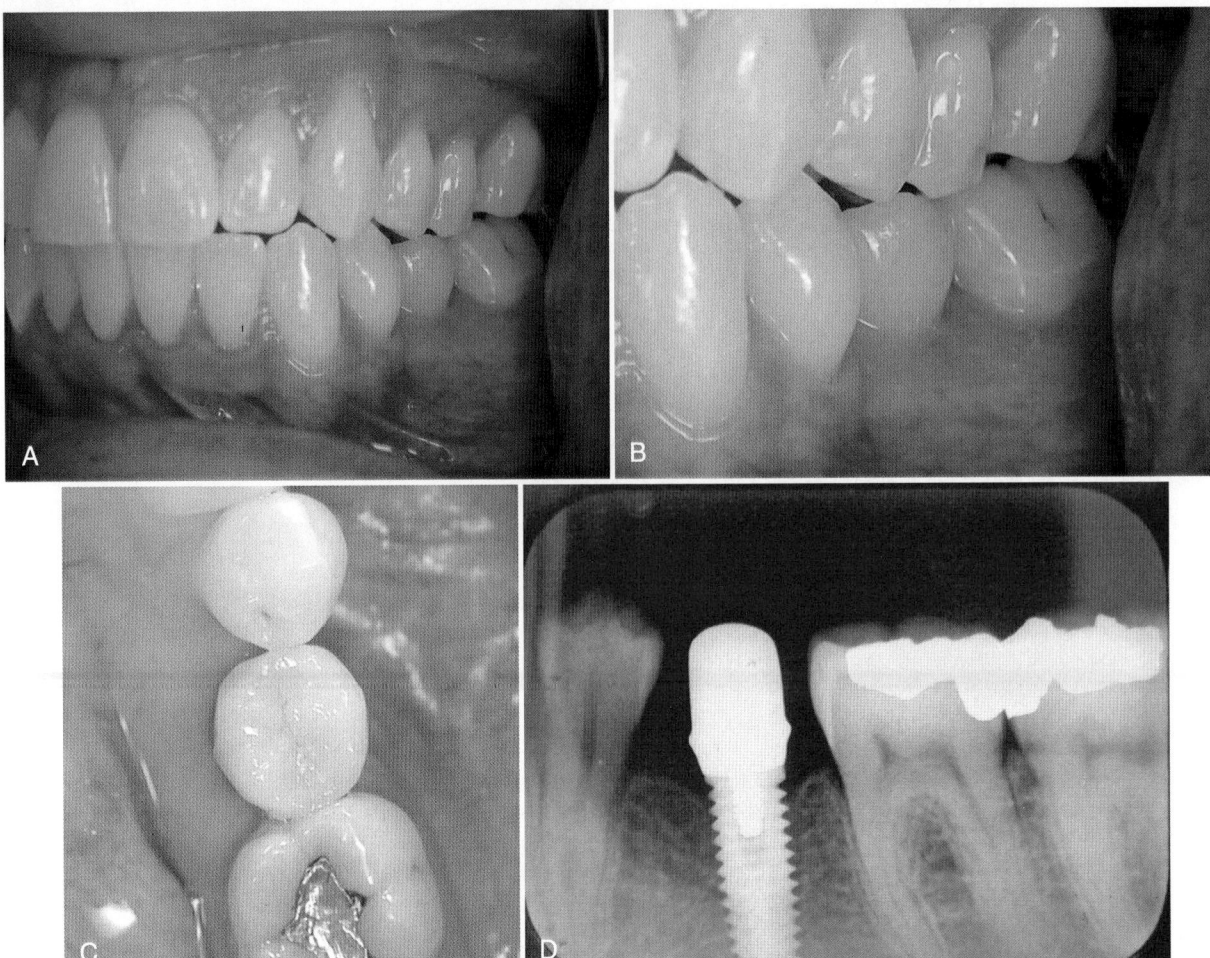

Fig. 87.1 Clinical implant success was demonstrated when a single implant was placed in the mandible to replace the lower second premolar (as planned). The implant osseointegrated, and function was successfully restored. The patient and clinicians were pleased with the outcome. (A) Photograph of the dentition in occlusion (from the left side). (B) Close-up photograph of the dentition in occlusion. The mandibular second premolar is an implant-supported crown. (C) Occlusal view of an implant-supported crown in the second premolar position. Replacement of the mandibular second premolar with an implant is a conservative treatment, obviating the need to prepare adjacent teeth. (D) Periapical radiograph of the posterior mandibular teeth and implant in the second premolar position. Bone support is good, and bone loss is minimal and consistent with expectations for this implant design.

and healthy, and the patient and treating clinician would be pleased with the outcome (Fig. 87.1). Use of strict criteria would produce implant success rates lower than those determined using less stringent criteria.

Table 87.1 illustrates the powerful effect that small changes in success criteria have on reported success rates. The data demonstrate that changing the criteria of success to include a probing pocket depth (PPD) of 5 mm or less to 6 mm or less changed the implant success rates from 52.4% to 62% and from 79.1% to 81.3% for patients with and without a history of periodontitis, respectively.[42] This also shows that implant survival is quite different from implant success.

KEY FACT

Implant success is defined by specific criteria used to evaluate the condition and function of the implant. Criteria for implant success have been proposed in the literature but not used consistently. Depending on the criteria used, the rates of implant success reported in studies can vary substantially.

Implant survival is defined as an implant that remains in place at the time of evaluation, regardless of untoward signs and symptoms or a history of problems. Extant implants that are healthy and functioning under an implant-retained restoration are different from those that are suffering from peri-implant bone loss or those that are not connected to a restoration and not functioning (Fig. 87.2), but these operational differences do not affect calculations of implant survival. Implants that are osseointegrated but not functional are referred to as *sleepers* and should not be considered successful merely because they are present and osseointegrated.

Implant survival and implant success are different outcome measures. Consider the dramatic difference between survival and success rates for implants reported in a systematic review (21 studies included) of implants supporting fixed partial dentures.[59] The 5-year implant survival rate was 95.4%, whereas the overall 5-year success rate (individual implant success rates were not calculated), defined as free of complications, was only 61.3%.[59]

In a 10-year retrospective study of 397 fixed implant reconstructions in 300 patients, the observed mechanical complication rate

TABLE 87.1 Effect of Slight Modifications of Implant Success Criteria on Successful Outcomes[a]

Group	PPD ≤5 mm, No BOP, BL <0.2 mm/ yr (%)	PPD ≤6 mm, No BOP, BL <0.2 mm/ yr (%)	PPD ≤5 mm, No BOP (%)	PPD ≤6 mm, No BOP (%)	Implant Survival (%)
Group A	52.4	62	71.4	81	90.5
Group B	79.1	81.3	94.5	96.7	96.5

[a]The initial success criteria at 10 years were set as a PPD ≤5 mm, no BOP, and BL <0.2 mm annually. The implant success rates for group A (i.e., patients with a history of periodontitis) and group B (i.e., patients with periodontal health) using these initial criteria are listed in the first column. Notice how dramatically the success rates change when the criteria used to define success are modified to include PPD ≤6 mm (i.e., second column). The next two columns show the success rates for each group using PPD ≤5 mm and ≤6 mm when the criteria are modified to omit bone loss as a determinant. The last column shows the implant survival rate for each group, which demonstrates that the survival rate is different than the success rate.

PPD, Probing pocket depth; *BOP*, bleeding on probing; *BL*, bone loss.
Data from Karoussis IK, Salvi GE, Heitz-Mayfield LJ, et al: Long-term implant prognosis in patients with and without a history of chronic periodontitis: a 10-year prospective cohort study of the ITI Dental Implant System. *Clin Oral Implant Res* 14:329–339, 2003.

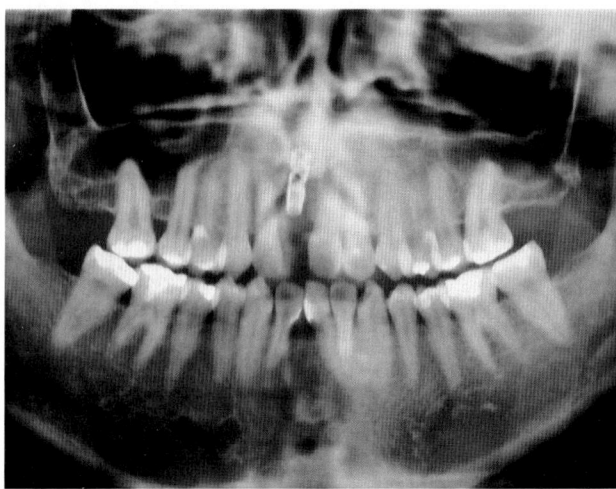

Fig. 87.2 Panoramic radiograph shows an implant placed in the position of a missing maxillary right central incisor. The implant appears to be placed in a nonrestorable position. It is osseointegrated and could technically be counted as a surviving implant, but it must be considered a failure because it does not meet the intended goal and function has not been restored.

was 24.7%.[77] The most frequent complication was ceramic chipping (20.31%), followed by occlusal screw loosening (2.57%) and loss of retention (2.06%).[77] Although relatively uncommon, occlusal screw loosening can result in a subgingival gap at the implant–abutment junction that retains plaque and stimulates an inflammatory reaction in the soft and hard tissues, leading to bone loss around the implant. Although surviving, these implants would fail to meet optimal success criteria.

Defining implant results in absolute terms is difficult and confusing. Implant survival, which typically is reported in studies, can overestimate good implant outcomes. Implant success, which is less often reported, could offer a better measure if specific success criteria were universally defined, accepted, and used. Implant success is difficult or impossible to compare across studies because of differences in evaluation criteria used by investigators. Implant success in a single study or series of studies using the same success criteria is meaningful only in the context of that study or series.

Currently, the usefulness of implant success rates from different studies is limited. Implant survival is important but is only an indicator of surviving implants and does not reveal whether they are functioning or had problems associated with them over time. The incidence of peri-implant problems is more significant than once thought. A systematic review of the literature evaluating the prevalence of peri-implant disease reported that peri-implant mucositis and peri-implantitis occurred in 19% to 65% and 1% to 47% of cases, respectively.[22]

Factors That Influence Implant Outcomes

Many issues influence implant outcomes, including available bone, implant design, placement and loading protocols, and host-related factors.

Anatomic Location

Osseointegration depends on the availability of an adequate quantity and quality of bone at the implant site. Areas with abundant bone volume in the desired location are better than those with deficient bone volume. Areas with good bone density provide more predictable outcomes than those with poor bone density.

The bone classification system described by Lekholm and Zarb[49] defines bone with different levels of support for implants and the likely impact on survival and success. The quality of bone support is greatly influenced by the anatomic location, and implant outcomes are sometimes categorized according to location. Extreme examples are the anterior mandible and the posterior maxilla. The anterior mandible typically consists of dense cortical bone, which offers great support and high bone-to-implant contact, whereas the posterior maxilla is often limited in volume because of alveolar resorption and sinus pneumatization and typically consists of a loose, trabecular structure and a thin cortical bone shell.

Implants placed in the posterior maxilla are less well supported compared with implants placed in the anterior mandible. Jaffin and Berman[36] demonstrated the significance of bone quality on implant survival in a report of 1054 Brånemark implants. Ninety percent of the implants were placed in type I, II, or III bone, with a failure rate of only 3%. Of the 10% that were placed in type IV bone, 35% failed.[36] Excluding those placed in the mandible, 23 (44%) of 52 implants placed in type IV bone in the maxilla failed, for a dismal survival rate of 56%. The study authors concluded that bone quality was the single greatest determinant of implant loss.

Anatomic location has a significant effect on implant outcome, particularly for the posterior maxilla. The implants used in the study by Jaffin and Berman[36] had machined surfaces, and current implants with altered microtopography are thought to perform better in the posterior maxilla due to increased bone-to-implant contact. When all 1054 implants (placed in all types of bone) are considered together, the combined implant survival rate (93.9%) in the study is within or slightly higher than the reported range in the Göteborg study (done with similar implants).

Implant Design

Implant design influences outcome. Hundreds of companies manufacture and market dental implants worldwide, and the number continues to grow. Implant dimensions, geometries, and surface characteristics vary tremendously and continue to evolve as innovation and research findings pave the way for changes that are thought to improve outcomes. Very few implant designs have been studied.

They instead rely on being clinically similar to researched and approved designs without additional studies or documentation to support their effectiveness. In most cases, it is impossible to appreciate the effect of a particular implant design features on outcomes. Nonetheless, novel implant designs are being used, and outcomes are being reported in studies that evaluate other aspects of treatment that are not specific to the design, which makes comparisons and assessments more confusing and unreliable.

The studies that have documented the success of dental implants based on design characteristics have shaped current standards for selection and use. For example, many clinicians adhere to the premise that longer implants, threaded implants, and rough-surfaced implants are better than shorter, unthreaded, and smooth designs. As changes in design and use have evolved over time, some beliefs have been disproved, and continued advances and research will undoubtedly refute other firmly held beliefs.

Clinicians would like to know whether one implant design performs better than the rest, but it is almost impossible to determine which design characteristics are important, because there are many variables to consider and implants are successful most of the time. Given the generally high rate of success, it appears that subtle differences in implant design are probably not significant for most patients and situations.[24,28] However, in patients with inadequate sites or challenging circumstances, certain implant designs may perform better than others. An example is the effect of implant surface characteristics. Implants with altered surface microtopography (i.e., acid-etched or blasted) enhance the bone-to-implant interface[44,45] and can improve outcomes, especially in compromised sites.[71,72] Lower success rates have been associated with smooth-surface (i.e., machined) implants.[37,60,64]

Implant length is another consideration. Many studies have supported the dogma that longer is better for implant success,[65,66] but later studies have challenged it.[31] Another important feature is the macro-thread design of implants. Clinical research[52] evaluating the stability (assessed by resonance frequency analysis) of a novel implant designed with a wide thread depth and increased pitch found that it did not cause the typical decrease in stability in the early postoperative healing period. This finding may have an impact on early and immediate loading protocols.

KEY FACT

Many features influence outcomes, including available bone, implant design, placement and loading protocols, and host-related factors. Defining implant results in absolute terms can be difficult and confusing.

Placement and Loading Protocols

The traditional placement protocol required a healed edentulous ridge into which implants were placed and allowed to osseointegrate for a period without occlusal loading (see Chapter 78). The nonloading period after implant placement was empirically determined to be 3 to 4 months in the mandible and 6 months in the maxilla.[10] A strongly held belief was that early loading would lead to higher failure rates.[11]

In contrast to the early standards, some current protocols advocate dramatically different approaches, including implant placement immediately after tooth extraction and implant occlusal loading immediately or shortly after placement. Each of these approaches has distinct advantages, but they are accompanied by challenges that have the potential to adversely affect outcomes.

Immediate Implant Placement

The immediate implant placement protocol describes the procedure in which an implant is placed in an extraction socket after tooth removal and socket debridement. This procedure, described by Schulte and colleagues[68] in 1978 and by Lazzara in 1989,[47] has been reported with survival rates equivalent to those of implants placed into healed ridges.[14,51] The advantages of immediate placement include decreased surgery, cost, and healing time.[69] Immediate implant placement introduces an additional risk of complications, including poor implant position, compromised aesthetic outcome, and implant failure (see Chapter 85). Despite the increased risk, a high long-term (1- to 16-year) survival rate of 96% has been reported for implants immediately placed into extraction sockets.[74]

Immediate Occlusal Loading

Brånemark established the concept of the osseointegrated dental implant as a predictable treatment modality for the edentulous patient on the empirically based requirement that the implant remain submerged and unloaded for a healing period of 3 to 6 months.[10] This original protocol, requiring the implant to remain stress free, was based on the concern that premature loading would cause micromotion of the dental implant, leading to fibrous encapsulation and implant failure. However, studies have shown this assumption to be incorrect, demonstrating that immediately loaded implants can achieve success rates (>90%) similar to those for conventionally loaded dental implants.[15,19,29,33,40] The long-term predictability of immediately loaded implants requires strict surgical and prosthodontic protocols.[7]

Bone Augmentation

A common problem encountered in implant dentistry is insufficient bone quantity to allow implant placement. Deficiencies in alveolar bone result from developmental defects, periodontal disease, tooth loss, or trauma.[6,13,67] For most cases with alveolar ridge resorption, bone regenerative procedures are required to correct the defects before or simultaneously with implant placement (see Chapters 79 and 80). The question is whether implants placed in sites that are reconstructed with bone augmentation procedures can achieve the same survival and success rates as implants placed in native bone sites.

The results of implants and bone augmentation procedures reported in the literature have been assessed by expert clinicians in several workshops.[16,30,34,35] One systematic review of the literature (2003 Workshop on Contemporary Science in Clinical Periodontics), including 13 studies (i.e., guided bone regeneration) with 1741 patients and 5 studies (i.e., distraction osteogenesis) with 92 patients, found that survival rates of dental implants in augmented bone achieved a high level of predictability that was similar to that for implants placed in natural (nongrafted) bone.[30]

Another systematic review of the literature (2008 Consensus Report of the Sixth European Workshop on Periodontology[73]) pointed out that bone augmentation procedures can fail and that implants placed in these areas do not enjoy the high long-term survival rates of dental implants placed in pristine sites.[73] The 2003 systematic review did not include an assessment of whether bone augmentation procedures failed; it intentionally focused on implants placed in sites that were successfully treated with bone augmentation. More research is needed to determine the long-term performance of dental implants placed in augmented bone and the clinical benefits of bone augmentation with respect to alternative treatments (e.g., use of short implants).

Risk Factors

Most patients enjoy similar rates of survival and success with dental implants. Only a few patients experience implant failure.

In addition to the factors previously discussed, host-related factors can adversely affect healing, osseointegration, and maintenance of dental implants. Smoking, diabetes, and periodontitis have been identified as risk factors that can adversely affect implant outcomes. In a systematic review of the literature, Klokkevold and Han[43] evaluated the influence of smoking, diabetes, and periodontal disease on outcomes and found that smoking has an adverse effect on implant survival and success, with the effects being more pronounced in areas of loose trabecular bone (e.g., posterior maxilla).

The review also suggested that type 2 diabetes had an adverse effect on implant survival rates, but the limited number of included studies did not permit a definitive conclusion.[43] The review did conclude that although patients with a history of treated periodontitis did not show a decrease in implant survival, they did experience more complications and lower success rates, especially when the implants were followed over longer periods (10+ years).[43]

Smoking

Above all other risk factors, smoking has a significant negative impact on implant survival and success. In a study of 2194 implants, Bain and Moy reported a significantly greater rate of failure among smokers (11.28%) than nonsmokers (4.76%).[8] De Bruyn and Colleart reported an early failure rate of 9% among smokers compared with 1% among nonsmokers.[18] Two other studies, one of 10 years[25] and the other with follow-up assessment of 6 months to 21 years,[56] concluded that smoking was a definite risk factor for implant survival.[20,21]

Diabetes

The role of diabetes mellitus as a risk factor for implant outcomes is less clear. Although a metabolic disease such as diabetes was expected to have an adverse effect on bone healing[75] and tissue support for implants, the research has not definitively determined that diabetes has a negative impact on implant survival or success.[4]

Moy and coworkers[56] reported a significantly lower success rate (68.7%) for patients with diabetes compared with the success rate (85.1%) for the entire study population (1140 patients with 4680 implants); individual implant survival and success rates were not reported. However, the low success rate (i.e., high failure rate) may be an overestimate of the actual implant failure rate for patients with diabetes, because it counts the number of patients with failures regardless of how many implants they had (i.e., implants successfully inserted and maintained in these patients are not counted). There were 48 patients with diabetes in the study, 4.2% of the 1140 total. Of these, 15 patients experienced implant failures.

Conversely, in a systematic review of the literature (33 studies), Javed and Romanos found that patients with good metabolic control (i.e., glycated hemoglobin [HbA1c] levels in the normal range) achieve success rates with osseointegrated implants that are similar to those for patients without diabetes.[38] Dowell and coworkers[23] also found similar success for implants placed in patients with controlled diabetes.

Periodontitis

A limited number of studies have assessed the prognosis of implant treatment in patients with a history of periodontitis.[41] Most of these studies suggest that implants are equally successful in patients with a history of chronic periodontitis. Short-term studies demonstrate 90% to 100% implant survival in patients with a history of chronic periodontitis.[53,55] Long-term studies report 90% to 97% implant survival rates for patients with a history of chronic periodontitis.[42,50,62,76] Short-term implant survival rates for patients treated for aggressive periodontitis are 95% to 100%.[53,54] One long-term study reported an 88.8% implant survival rate over 5 years for patients treated for aggressive periodontitis.[55]

Implant survival in patients with a history of periodontitis appears to be highly predictable. However, the lack of long-term studies to support implant survival in patients treated for aggressive periodontitis leaves the prognosis for these patients open to question.[41]

Long-term studies evaluating implant treatment in periodontally compromised patients suggest that they may experience more peri-implant problems.[42] When these patients are followed for extended periods, there appear to be more complications (i.e., peri-implantitis) associated with implants than in periodontally healthy patients. In a 10-year prospective study of patients with and without a history of chronic periodontitis, the rate of biologic complications (i.e., peri-implantitis) was higher for those with a history of chronic periodontitis (28.6%) than those with periodontal health (5.8%).[42] This controlled study by Karoussis and coworkers[42] found a statistically significant difference in mean peri-implant bone loss between patients with a history of chronic periodontitis and patients who were periodontally healthy.

Peri-implant problems may be attributed to a continuous increase in the percentage of implants exhibiting probing pocket depths of 4 mm or deeper over time.[26] A systematic review of implant outcomes in patients treated for periodontitis concluded that these individuals had a greater incidence of biologic complications and lower success and survival rates compared with periodontally healthy subjects.[70]

KEY FACT

Smoking, diabetes, and periodontitis are risk factors that can adversely affect implant outcomes.

Aesthetic Results and Patient Satisfaction

The ultimate goal of treatment is to achieve natural-appearing, optimally functioning, implant-supported tooth replacements. Proper tooth dimensions and contours, and ideal soft tissue support are key factors for successful aesthetic outcomes.[46] If crown form, dimension, and shape and gingival harmony around the implants are not ideal, the patient may consider the implant restoration unacceptable, because the result does not represent a natural dental profile (Fig. 87.3). For some patients, such as those with severe alveolar deficiency, an ideal

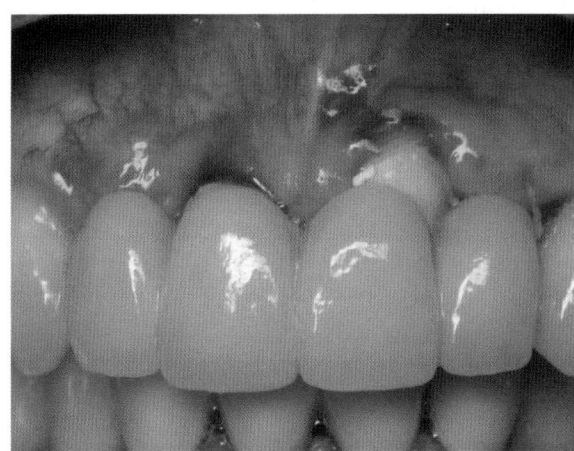

Fig. 87.3 Clinical photograph shows a maxillary anterior fixed restoration supported by two malpositioned implants in the central incisor positions. The patient was dissatisfied with the aesthetic outcome. The left implant was positioned between the central and lateral incisor and angled toward the facial surface at a level above the gingival margin. A tooth-colored material was used to mask the exposed framework in the gingival area.

aesthetic outcome may be impossible because reconstructive surgical procedures are complex, require extensive time, and remain unpredictable. For others, a less-than-ideal aesthetic outcome may be acceptable (see Chapter 81).

Aesthetic problems and patient dissatisfaction happen when results are inferior to what was expected. Satisfaction with the aesthetic outcome of the implant prosthesis varies from patient to patient, depending on a number of factors. The risk for aesthetic failure is increased for patients with high aesthetic expectations. The risk is also higher when patients present with patient-related risk factors such as a high smile line, thin periodontal soft tissues, and compromised bone support. Two recent systematic reviews reported that the patient's perceptions and desires greatly influence and determine how well he or she accepts the implant outcome.[17,57]

Although infrequently reported, aesthetic success and patient satisfaction need to be included when considering the results of implant therapy. Despite several proposed methods for evaluating aesthetic results, reports of aesthetic parameters in the scientific literature are scarce.[9] A restorative index appraises the white aesthetics of the final restoration,[39] a soft tissue or pink aesthetic score considers soft-tissue parameters,[32] and an aesthetic index uses a combination of pink and white aesthetic scores, focusing on the visible part of the implant restoration.[8] These indices quantify the aesthetic result, providing an objective method of judging aesthetic success.

In a survey of patient satisfaction, more than 90% of patients were completely satisfied in terms of function and aesthetics.[58] A questionnaire was given to 104 patients 5 to 15 years (mean, 10.2 years) after implant placement to assess subjective perceptions of treatment. Of these patients, 48% were treated with single implant crowns and 52% were treated with fixed partial dentures. The survival rate for all implants was 93%. Most patients had favorable responses to the questions regarding function, aesthetics, hygiene, and cost. Table 87.2 lists the percentage of patients responding as highly satisfied or satisfied for each category. Comparing chewing comfort for teeth or implants, 72.1% perceived no difference, 17.3% felt more secure chewing on teeth, and 7.7% felt more secure chewing on implants.

In another survey, patient satisfaction with implant-supported prostheses in totally edentulous jaws was evaluated.[63] Experience with an implant-supported prosthesis was assessed over a period of 10 years, and 97% of the 135 patients reported overall satisfaction with treatment. Chewing satisfaction was reported as good or very good by all but one patient (99.3% positive response rate). Improved lifestyle and greater self-confidence in public were reported by 75% and 82% of patients, respectively.

A systematic review of the literature, which included all randomized controlled trials published in English or French up to April 2007 comparing conventional mandibular dentures and implant overdentures in adult edentulous patients, identified eight publications for meta-analysis.[27] The study reported that patients were more satisfied with implant overdentures than with conventional mandibular dentures. However, there was a lack of evidence to show a patient's perception of the impact of mandibular implant overdentures on general health.

TABLE 87.2   Patient Satisfaction With Implant Treatment

Implant Experience	Highly Satisfied or Satisfied (%)[a]
Function or chewing	97
Phonetics	96
Aesthetics	97
Oral hygiene ease	93
Complete fulfillment	92
Would do treatment again	94
Would recommend to friend or relative	89
Reasonable or justified cost	87

[a]Percentage of patients subjectively responding with *highly satisfied* or *satisfied* to survey questions about their implant experience. More than 90% responded favorably and thought implant treatment was a positive experience.
Data from Pjetursson BE, Karoussis I, Burgin W, et al: Patients' satisfaction following implant therapy. A 10-year prospective cohort study. *Clin Oral Implants Res* 16:185–193, 2005.

CLINICAL CORRELATION

Aesthetic problems and dissatisfaction happen when results do not match a patient's expectations. Satisfaction with the aesthetic outcome of an implant prosthesis varies among patients. The risk of failure is greater among those with high aesthetic demands and risk factors such as a high smile line, thin periodontal soft tissues, or compromised bone support.

Conclusions

The use of dental implants to replace missing teeth is highly predictable, advantageous, and beneficial for patients. Because of variations in implant designs, study protocols, and populations studied, results are difficult to compare and an absolute definition of implant success remains elusive. The results of implant treatment are reported using a wide range of criteria from being present (i.e., survival) to being functional without complications (i.e., success).

It is challenging to compare the results of studies because the number of variables continues to change. Clinical research suggests that certain risk factors can decrease success rates for some patients. Understanding what is being reported in the literature helps patients and clinicians appreciate implant treatment results.

 A Case Scenario is found on the companion website www.expertconsult.com.

References

 References for this chapter are found on the companion website www.expertconsult.com.

INDEX

Page number followed by *f* indicates figure, by *t* table, and by *b* box.

For entries that have an *e* included in the page number (e.g., 179.*e*2 or *e*60*f*), go to the companion website at www.expertconsult.com, and after registering, search for the term on the book website.

873

For entries that have an *e* included in the page number (e.g., 179.*e2* or *e60f*), go to the companion website at www.expertconsult.com, and after registering, search for the term on the book website.

For entries that have an e included in the page number (e.g., 179.e2 or e60f), go to the companion website at www.expertconsult.com, and after registering, search for the term on the book website.

For entries that have an *e* included in the page number (e.g., 179.*e2* or *e*60*f*), go to the companion website at www.expertconsult.com, and after registering, search for the term on the book website.

For entries that have an *e* included in the page number (e.g., 179.*e2* or *e60f*), go to the companion website at www.expertconsult.com, and after registering, search for the term on the book website.

For entries that have an *e* included in the page number (e.g., 179.*e2* or *e60f*), go to the companion website at www.expertconsult.com, and after registering, search for the term on the book website.

For entries that have an *e* included in the page number (e.g., 179.*e2* or *e60f*), go to the companion website at www.expertconsult.com, and after registering, search for the term on the book website.

For entries that have an *e* included in the page number (e.g., 179.*e*2 or *e*60*f*), go to the companion website at www.expertconsult.com, and after registering, search for the term on the book website.